cpt® CODING ESSENTIALS

Anesthesia and Pain Management | 2019

CPT® Coding Essentials Anesthesia and Pain Management 2019

Copyright © 2018 American Medical Association

All rights reserved

Current Procedural Terminology (CPT®), the Introduction, CPT code descriptions, parentheticals, CPT Coding Guidelines, AMA Coding Notes, and *CPT Assistant* citations are copyright 2018 American Medical Association. All rights reserved.

All other content herein, including chapters, appendices, illustrations, definitions, and crosswalks are copyright DecisionHealth. All rights reserved.

Fee schedules, relative value units, conversion factors and/or related components are not assigned by the AMA, are not part of CPT, and the AMA is not recommending their use. Neither DecisionHealth nor the AMA directly or indirectly practices medicine or dispenses medical services. The AMA and DecisionHealth assume no liability for data contained or not contained herein. The AMA and DecisionHealth disclaim responsibility for any consequences or liability attributable to or related to any use, nonuse or interpretation of information contained in this product.

This publication does not replace the AMA's Current Procedural Terminology codebook or other appropriate coding authority. The coding information in this publication should be used only as a guide.

Disclaimer

No part of this publication may be reproduced, stored in a retrieval system, or transmitted in any form or by any means, electronic, mechanical, photocopy, or otherwise without prior written permission of DecisionHealth and the American Medical Association.

This publication is sold with the understanding that neither DecisionHealth nor the American Medical Association is engaged in rendering legal, medical, accounting, or other professional services in specific situations. Although prepared for professionals, this publication should not be used as a substitute for professional services in specific situations. If legal or medical advice is required, the services of a professional should be sought.

Printed in the United States of America

ISBN: 978-1-62202-757-6
OP259819

Additional copies of this book or other AMA products may be ordered by calling 800-621-8335 or visiting the AMA Store at amastore.com. Refer to product number OP259819.

AMA publication and product updates, errata, and addendum can be found at **amaproductupdates.org.**

Published by DecisionHealth, a division of Simplify Compliance
100 Winners Circle, Suite 300
Brentwood, TN 37027
www.codingbooks.com

Contents

Codes List

The CPT surgery and ancillary codes and code ranges that appear in this book are listed below.

Surgery Codes

00100
00102
00103
00104
00120
00124
00126
00140
00142
00144
00145
00147
00148
00160
00162
00164
00170
00172
00174
00176
00190
00192
00210
00211
00212
00214
00215
00216
00218
00220
00222
00300
00320
00322
00326
00350
00352
00400
00402
00404
00406
00410
00450
00454
00470
00472
00474
00500
00520
00522
00524
00528
00529
00530
00532
00534
00537
00539
00540
00541
00542
00546
00548
00550
00560
00561
00562
00563
00566
00567
00580
00600
00604
00625
00626
00630
00632
00635
00640
00670
00700
00702
00730
00731-00732
00750
00752
00754
00756
00770
00790
00792
00794
00796
00797
00800
00802
00811-00812
00813
00820
00830
00832
00834
00836
00840
00842
00844
00846
00848
00851
00860
00862
00864
00865
00866
00868
00870
00872
00873
00880
00882
00902
00904
00906
00908
00910
00912
00914
00916
00918
00920
00921
00922
00924
00926
00928
00930
00932
00934
00936
00938
00940
00942
00944
00948
00950
00952
01112
01120
01130
01140
01150
01160
01170
01173
01200
01202
01210
01212
01214
01215
01220
01230
01232
01234
01250
01260
01270
01272
01274
01320
01340

01360
01380
01382
01390
01392
01400
01402
01404
01420
01430
01432
01440
01442
01444
01462
01464
01470
01472
01474
01480
01482
01484
01486
01490
01500
01502
01520
01522
01610
01620
01622
01630
01634
01636
01638
01650
01652
01654
01656
01670
01680
01710
01712
01714
01716
01730
01732
01740
01742
01744
01756
01758
01760
01770
01772
01780
01782
01810
01820
01829
01830
01832
01840
01842
01844
01850
01852
01860
01916
01920
01922
01924
01925
01926
01930
01931
01932
01933
01935
01936
01951
01952
01953
01958
01960
01961
01962
01963
01965
01966
01967
01968
01969
01990
01991
01992
01996
20526
20550-20551
20552-20553
20600-20604
20605-20606
20610-20611
27096
28890
36000
36010
36011-36012
36013-36015
36100
36140
36400-36406
36410
36415
36420-36425
36430
36440
36555-36556
36557-36558
36560-36561
36563
36565-36566
36568-36569
36570-36571
36572-36573
36575-36576
36578
36580-36581
36582-36583
36584-36585
36589-36590
36591
36592
36593
36595
36596
36597
36598
36600
36620-36625
61050-61055
62270-62272
62273
62280-62282
62284
62290-62291
62302-62305
62320-62321
62322-62323
62324-62325
62326-62327
62350-62351
62355
62360-62362
62367-62368
62369-62370
62380
63650-63655
63661-63662
63663-63664
63685-63688
64400-64405
64408
64410
64413
64415-64416
64417-64418
64420-64421
64425
64430
64435
64445
64446
64447
64448
64449
64450
64455
64461-64463
64479-64480
64483-64484
64486-64489
64490-64492
64493-64495
64505
64510
64517
64520
64530
64555
64561
64575
64580
64581
64585
64590
64595
64600-64610
64612
64615
64616
64620
64630
64632
64633-64636
64640
64642-64643
64644-64645
64646-64647
64680
64681

Ancillary Codes

71045-71048
72020
72040-72052
72070-72074
72080
72081-72084
72100-72114
72120
72125-72127
72128-72130
72131-72133
72141-72142
72146-72147
72148-72149
72156-72158
72200-72202
72240-72270
72275
72285
72295
75901
75902
76800
76942
77001
77002
77003
77021
80047-80048
80050
80051
80053
80171
80175
80177
80199
80203
80305-80307
80323
80329-80331
80332-80334
80335-80337
80338
80345
80346-80347
80348
80349
80353
80354
80355
80357
80358
80361
80362-80364
80365
80366
80368
80369-80370
80372
80373
82286
82310
82330
82374
82435
82947-82948
83873
84132
84260
84295
85002
85004
85013-85014
85018
85025-85027
85041
85045-85046
85048
85049
85345
85610-85611
85651-85652
90791-90792
90832-90838
90863
90865
90867-90869
90870
90875-90876
90880
90882
90885
90887
90889
90901
92960-92961
93000-93010
93040-93042
93318
94002-94004
94760-94762
95812-95813
95831-95834
95851-95852
95857
95860-95864
95866
95867-95868
95869
95870
95872
95873
95874
95905
95907-95913
95921-95922
95923
95925-95927
95928-95929
95970-95972
95990-95991
96150-96151
96152-96155
96360-96361
96365-96368
96369-96371
96372
96373
96374-96376
97810-97814
99000-99001
99024
99026-99027
99050
99051
99053
99056
99058-99060
99070
99071
99100
99116
99135
99140
99151-99153
99155-99157
99605-99607
0106T-0110T
0213T-0215T
0216T-0218T
0228T-0229T
0230T-0231T
0278T
0440T-0442T

Introduction

Unlike other specialty coding books on the market, *CPT® Coding Essentials for Anesthesia and Pain Management 2019* combines anesthesia and pain management-specific procedural coding and reimbursement information with verbatim guidelines and parenthetical information from the Current Procedural Terminology (CPT®) codebook. Additionally, *CPT® Coding Essentials for Anesthesia and Pain Management 2019* enhances that CPT-specific information by displaying pertinent diagnostic codes, procedural descriptions, illustrations, relative value units (RVUs), and more on the same page as the CPT code being explained. This one book provides anesthesia and pain management coding and billing knowledge that otherwise might take years of experience or multiple resources to accumulate. It sets a foundation for anesthesia and pain management coders and subspecialty coding experts that facilitates correct code assignment.

This book includes reporting rules for CPT code submission as written and enforced by the Centers for Medicare and Medicaid Services (CMS). *CPT® Coding Essentials for Anesthesia and Pain Management 2019* is not intended to equip coders with information to make medical decisions or to determine diagnoses or treatments; rather, it is intended to aid correct code selection that is supported by physician or other qualified health care professional (QHCP) documentation. This reference work does not replace the need for a CPT codebook.

About the *CPT® Coding Essentials* Editorial Team and Content Selection

The *CPT® Coding Essentials* series is developed by a team of veteran clinical technical editors and certified medical coders. When developing the content of this book, the team members consider all annual new, revised, and deleted medical codes. They adhere to authoritative medical research; medical policies; and official guidelines, conventions; and rules to determine the final content presented within this book. Additionally, the team monitors utilization and denial trends when selecting the codes highlighted in *CPT® Coding Essentials for Anesthesia and Pain Management 2019.*

The main section of *CPT® Essentials for Anesthesia and Pain Management 2019* is titled "CPT® Procedural Coding." This section is organized for ease of use and simple lookup by displaying CPT codes in numeric order. Each code-detail page of this section presents a single code or multiple codes representing a code family concept.

The procedures featured in the *CPT® Coding Essentials for Anesthesia and Pain Management 2019* are those commonly performed by an anesthesiologist or pain management specialist, but more difficult to understand or miscoded in claims reporting. This book does not provide a comprehensive list of all services performed in the specialty, nor all sites within impacted body systems. Similarly, the CPT to ICD-10-CM crosswalks are intended to illustrate those conditions that would most commonly present relative to the procedure and the specialist. The crosswalks are not designed to be an exhaustive list of all possible conditions for each procedure, nor medical necessity reasons for coverage.

The "CPT Procedural Coding" section is complemented by other sections that review anesthesia and pain management terminology and anatomy, ICD-10-CM conventions and coding, ICD-10-CM documentation tips, and ICD-10 procedure coding system (ICD-10-PCS) coding and format. The appendices contain data from the CMS National Correct Coding Initiative, multiple ICD-10-CM compliant anesthesia and pain management condition documentation checklists, and evaluation and management (E/M) documentation guidelines.

Sections Contained Within This Book

What follows is a section-by-section explanation of *CPT® Coding Essentials for Anesthesia and Pain Management 2019.*

Terminology, Abbreviations, and Basic Anatomy

This section provides a quick reference tool for coders who may come across unfamiliar terminology in medical record documentation. This review of basic terminology displays lists of alphabetized Greek and Latin root words, prefixes, and suffixes associated with anesthesia and pain management.

The combination of root words with prefixes and suffixes is the basis of medical terminology and enables readers to deduce the meaning of new words by understanding the components. For example, *neuro* is a root word for *nerve,* and *–algia* is a suffix for *pain*; thus, *neuralgia* describes nerve pain.

Also included in this section are a glossary of anesthesia and pain management-specific terms and a list of anesthesia and pain management acronyms and abbreviations. Keep in mind that these glossary definitions are anesthesia and pain management-specific. The same word may have a different meaning in a different specialty. In some cases, a parenthetical phrase after the anesthesia and pain management term may provide the reader with a common acronym or synonym for that term. Pay particular attention to the use of capitalization in the abbreviation and acronym list, as the same letters sometimes have varied meaning in clinical nomenclature, depending on capitalization.

Introduction to ICD-10-CM and ICD-10-PCS

For coders who want a review, *CPT® Coding Essentials for Anesthesia and Pain Management 2019* recaps the development of the ICD-10-CM and ICD-10-PCS code sets and outlines important concepts pertaining to the ICD-10-CM code set.

Lists of common diagnoses and conditions from the ICD-10-CM code sets for each selected CPT code or code range may be found within the "CPT Procedural Coding" section.

The ICD-10-CM content provided within this book complements your use of the *ICD-10-CM 2019* codebook. This section provides a chapter-by-chapter overview of ICD-10-CM that includes common new diagnoses and their codes, as well as identification of new or substantially changed chapter-specific guidelines for 2019.

ICD-10-PCS was commissioned by CMS and developed by 3M Health Information Systems for inpatient reporting of procedures to replace ICD-9-CM Volume 3. ICD-10-PCS is not used for reporting physician services; however, an understanding of ICD-10-PCS is essential to physician practices because physician inpatient surgical documentation is used by hospitals for the abstraction of ICD-10-PCS codes for hospital billing. The nomenclature and structure of ICD-10-PCS diverges significantly from ICD-9-CM Volume 3 and from CPT codes. An overview of this structure is reviewed in this section.

ICD-10-CM Anatomy and Physiology

Advanced understanding of the nervous system, anatomy and pathophysiology is essential to accurate coding for anesthesia and pain management. A detailed study of the anatomy and physiology of anesthesia and pain management gives beginner or intermediate anesthesia and pain management coders the information boost they may need to accurately abstract the medical record.

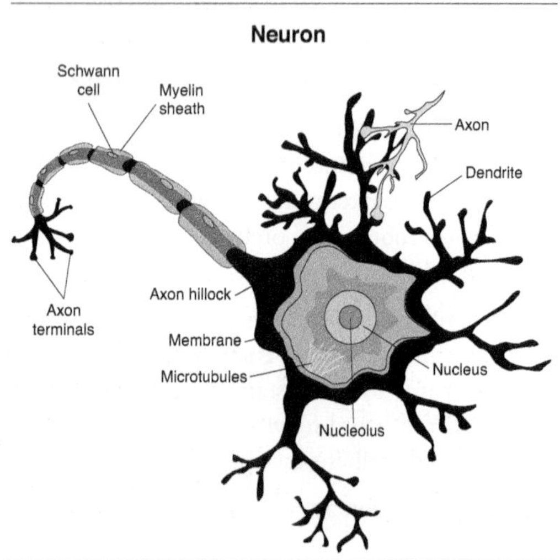

The anatomy and physiology explanations are accompanied by labeled and detailed illustrations for anesthesia and pain management, beginning at the cellular level and extending to the functions and interactions of the various body parts. This section also includes discussion of common disorders of the nervous system and other anatomical systems affected by anesthesia, their pathophysiology, as well as coding exercises to assess mastery of the anesthesia and pain management coding topic.

ICD-10-CM Documentation

Accurate, complete coding of diseases, disorders, injuries, conditions, and even signs and symptoms using ICD-10-CM codes requires extensive patient encounter documentation. This section highlights commonly encountered anesthesia and pain management conditions that require a high level of specificity for documentation and reporting.

The documentation information is presented in an easy-to-understand bulleted format that enables the physician, QHCP, and/or coder to quickly identify the specificity of documentation required for accurate ICD-10-CM code abstraction. This section also includes coding exercises to assess mastery of the anesthesia and pain management documentation topic.

CPT® Procedural Coding

"CPT Procedural Coding" is the main section of this book and displays pertinent coding and reimbursement data for each targeted CPT code or code family on code-detail pages. The following is presented within each surgical code detail page:

- CPT code and verbatim description with icons (when required)
- Parentheticals (when they exist)
- Official AMA Coding Guidelines
- Plain English descriptions
- Illustrations
- ICD-10-CM diagnostic codes
- AMA *CPT® Assistant* newsletter references
- CMS Pub 100 references
- CMS base units or relative value units
- CMS global periods
- CMS modifier edits

Category III codes and codes from diagnostic chapters will contain a truncated version of the code-detail page content, as diagnostic tests are too broad for all data elements contained in the code-detail pages.

AMA Coding Guidelines

The guidelines and parenthetical instructions included in the CPT codebook provide coders with insight into how the AMA CPT Editorial Panel and CPT Advisory Committee intend the codes to be used. This information is critical to correct code selection, and until now, has been unavailable in books other than the official AMA CPT codebook.

Section guidelines for the pertinent sections of the CPT codebook (Anesthesia, Surgery, Radiology, Pathology, and Medicine) appear before the code-detail pages associated with the respective CPT section. Guidelines that appear elsewhere within a CPT codebook section are displayed on the code-detail page, whenever appropriate. The reproduction of anesthesia and pain management coding guidelines and parenthetical information in *CPT® Coding Essentials for Anesthesia and Pain Management 2019* is verbatim from the AMA CPT codebook.

CPT Codes and Descriptions

CPT codes are listed in numerical order and include anesthesia, surgery, radiology, laboratory, and medicine codes pertinent to anesthesia and pain management.

The CPT code set has been developed as stand-alone descriptions of medical services. However, not all descriptions of CPT codes are presented in their complete form within the code set. In some cases, one or more abbreviated code descriptions (known as *child codes*) appear indented and without an initial capital letter. Such codes refer back to a common portion of the preceding code description (known as a *parent code*) that includes a semi-colon (;) and includes all of the text prior to the semi-colon. An example of this parent–child code system follows:

00120 Anesthesia for procedures on external, middle, and inner ear including biopsy; not otherwise specified

00124 otoscopy

00126 tympanotomy

The full descriptions for indented codes 00124 and 00126 are:

00124 Anesthesia for procedures on external, middle, and inner ear including biopsy; otoscopy

00126 Anesthesia for procedures on external, middle, and inner ear including biopsy; tympanotomy

When a group of similar codes is found on a code-detailed page in *CPT® Essentials*, a full description of each code will be displayed.

Icons

Icons on the code-detail page may affect ICD or CPT codes. The male (♂) and female (♀) edit icons are applied to ICD codes. New or revised CPT codes are identified with a bullet (●) or triangle (▲), respectively. The plus sign (+) identifies add-on codes. Add-on codes may never be reported alone, but are always reported secondarily to the main procedure, and should never be reported with modifier 51, *Multiple Procedures*.

A bullet with the numeral 7 within it (❼) is displayed next to ICD-10-CM codes that require a seventh character. Consult the ICD-10-CM codebook for appropriate seventh characters.

The bolt symbol (⚡) identifies CPT codes for vaccines pending FDA approval.

The star symbol (★) identifies CPT codes that may be used to report telemedicine services when appended by modifier 95.

The right/left arrows symbol (⇄) identifies where the full range of lateral codes would be appropriate. In an effort to conserve space in the *CPT® Coding Essentials* series, we have chosen to use this icon to denote laterality.

New to this 2019 edition of the *CPT® Coding Essentials* series is an icon (▯) to denote the *CPT® QuickRef*, a mobile app created by the AMA and available from the App Store and Google Play. The icon indicates that additional dynamic information can be accessed within the app (in-app purchases required).

Parenthetical Information

The CPT code set sometimes provides guidance in the form of a parenthetical instruction. For example:

(For donor nephrectomy, use 00862)

Code-detail pages include parenthetical instructions specific to both the code and the section within which the code is placed within the CPT code set. Not all codes and/or sections have associated parenthetical statements.

CPT® Assistant References

CPT® Assistant is a monthly newsletter published by the AMA that provides supplemental guidance to the CPT codebook. If a CPT code is the subject of discussion in a past issue of *CPT® Assistant*, the volume and page numbers are noted beneath the code to direct readers to the relevant newsletter archives to keep abreast of compliant coding rules.

Plain English Description

A simple description of what is included in the service represented by each CPT code is provided as a guide for coders to select the correct CPT code while reading the medical record. Not all approaches or methodologies are described in the Plain English Description; rather, the most common approaches or methodologies are provided. In some cases, the description provides an overview to more than one code, as some code-detail pages have multiple codes listed.

Illustrations

Streamlined line drawings demonstrate the anatomical site of the procedure, illustrating the basics of the procedure to assist in code selection. In some cases, not all codes on the code-detail page and not all approaches or methodologies are captured in the single illustration.

Diagnostic Code Crosswalk

ICD-10-CM codes commonly associated with the service represented on the code-detail page are listed with their official code descriptions. Keep in mind that in some cases, only the most common diagnoses for a procedure are listed due to space constraints.

While most codes support the medical necessity of the procedure performed, medical necessity rules vary by payer, and the acceptability of these diagnoses for medical necessity purposes cannot be guaranteed.

The mappings from CPT to ICD-10-CM in *CPT® Coding Essentials for Anesthesia and Pain Management 2019* were prepared by clinical coding experts.

The most common ICD-10-CM codes appropriate to the procedure or services represented on the code-detail page are provided. When a seventh character is required for a code, a bullet with the numeral 7 within it (❼) alerts the coder. Sometimes, a seventh character is appended to a code with only three, four, or five characters. In those cases, place holding Xs are to be appended to the codes so that only the seventh character must be added. For example, the following ICD-10-CM diagnosis code:

T88.4 Failed or difficult intubation

requires a seventh character; therefore, it is displayed with six characters in this manner:

(❼) T88.4XX Failed or difficult intubation

Within ICD-10-CM, many diagnoses have different codes based on laterality (for example, right plantar nerve, left plantar nerve, unspecified plantar nerve). Due to space constraints, not every laterality code is listed. Rather, a representative code is listed along with an icon indicating that other laterality code versions are available.

The provided crosswalks are not meant to replace your ICD-10-CM codebook. Please consult your manual for all seventh characters needed to complete listed codes and additional laterality choices, as well as ICD-10-CM coding conventions essential to proper use.

Pub 100

CMS Pub 100 (Publication 100-04, "Medicare Claims Processing Manual") is an online resource of federal coding regulations that often relate to CPT coding. If a CPT code or its associated procedure is the topic of discussion in a CMS Pub 100 entry, the Pub 100 reference is noted so that coders may access it online at www.cms.gov/regulations-and-guidance/guidance/manuals/internet-only-manuals-IOMs.html.

Payment Grids

Information in the payment grids that appear on the code-detail pages comes from CMS. These grids identify the base units used to compute allowable amounts for anesthesia services or the relative value of providing a specific professional service in relation to the value of other services, the number of postoperative follow-up days associated with each CPT code, and other reimbursement edits. All data displayed in the payment grids are relevant to physicians participating in Medicare.

Global Period

During the follow-up, or global surgery period, any routine care associated with the original service is bundled into the original service. This means that, for example, an evaluation and management (E/M) visit to check the surgical wound would not be billable if occurring during the global surgery period.

Possible global periods under Medicare are 0, 10, and 90 days. XXX indicates that the global period concept does not apply to the service.

Base Units

All Anesthesia charges are based on units. Base unit amounts are published yearly and are based on the complexity of the case and the expected workload of the anesthesia provider required to perform the work. Base units are then added to time units and then any modifiers to derive payment.

Relative Value Units (RVUs)

Relative value unit (RVU) data shows the breakout of work, practice expense (PE), and malpractice expense (MP) associated with a code, and provides a breakout for the service depending on whether it was performed in the physician's office or in a facility not belonging to the physician. Understandably, the physician payment for a surgical procedure is reduced if a procedure is hosted by a facility, as the facility would expect payment to cover its share of costs. A physician who performs the surgery in his or her own office is not subject to the same cost-sharing. This cost difference shows up in the PE column.

The payment information provided is sometimes used to set rates or anticipate payments. Payment information may be affected by modifiers appended to the CPT code.

Modifiers

Sometimes, modifiers developed by the AMA and by CMS may be appended to CPT codes to indicate that the services represented by the codes have been altered in some way. For example, modifier 26 reports the professional component of a service that has both a professional and a technical component. A patient who undergoes an ultrasound might have a technician perform the ultrasound itself, while the physician interprets the ultrasound results to determine a diagnosis. The technician's service would be reported with the same ultrasound CPT code as the physician, but the physician would use modifier 26 to indicate the professional component only, and the technician would report modifier TC, which is a Healthcare Common Procedure Coding System (HCPCS) Level II modifier identifying the service as the technical portion only. If the physician performs the ultrasound and interprets the results, no modifier is required.

When such circumstances affect the code, users may find the payment information provided for the full code, the professional services–only code, and the technical component–only code.

Many modifiers affect payment for services or with whom payment is shared when multiple providers or procedures are involved in a single surgical encounter. CMS provides definitions for the payments, based on the number listed in the modifier's field.

Modifier 50 (bilateral procedure)

0 150% payment adjustment for bilateral procedures does not apply. If a procedure is reported with modifier 50 or with modifiers RT and LT, Medicare bases payment for the two sides on the lower of (a) the total actual charge for both sides or (b) 100% of the fee schedule amount for a single code. For example, the fee schedule amount for code XXXXX is $125. The physician reports code XXXXXLT with an actual charge of $100 and XXXXXRT with an actual charge of $100.

Payment would be based on the fee schedule amount ($125) because it is lower than the total actual charges for the left and right sides ($200). The bilateral adjustment is inappropriate for codes in this category (a) due to physiology or anatomy or (b) because the code descriptor specifically states that it is a unilateral procedure and there is an existing code for the bilateral procedure.

1 150% payment adjustment for bilateral procedures applies. If a code is billed with the bilateral modifier or is reported twice on the same day by any other means (such as with RT and LT modifiers or with a 2 in the units field), payment is based for these codes when reported as bilateral procedures on the lower of (a) the total actual charge for both sides or (b) 150% of the fee schedule amount for a single code. If a code is reported as a bilateral procedure and is reported with other procedure codes on the same day, the bilateral adjustment is applied before any applicable multiple procedure rules are applied.

2 150% payment adjustment for bilateral procedure does not apply. RVUs are already based on the procedure being performed as a bilateral procedure. If a procedure is reported with modifier 50, or is reported twice on the same day by any other means (such as with RT and LT modifiers with a 2 in the units field), payment is based for both sides on the lower of (a) the total actual charges by the physician for both sides, or (b) 100% of the fee schedule amount for a single code. For example, the fee schedule amount for code YYYYY is $125. The physician reports code YYYYYLT with an actual charge of $100 and YYYYYRT with an actual charge of $100.

Payment would be based on the fee schedule amount ($125) because it is lower than the total actual charges for the left and right sides ($200). The RVUs are based on a bilateral procedure because (a) the code descriptor specifically states that the procedure is bilateral, (b) the code descriptor states that the procedure may be performed either unilaterally or bilaterally, or (c) the procedure is usually performed as a bilateral procedure.

3 The usual payment adjustment for bilateral procedures does not apply. If a procedure is reported with modifier 50, or is reported for both sides on the same day by any other means (such as with RT and LT modifiers or with a 2 in the units field), Medicare bases payment for each side or organ or site of a paired organ on the lower of (a) the actual charge for each side or (b) 100% of the fee schedule amount for each side. If a procedure is reported as a bilateral procedure and with other procedure codes on the same day, the fee schedule amount for a bilateral procedure is determined before any applicable multiple procedure rules are applied. Services in this category are generally radiology procedures or other diagnostic tests that are not subject to the special payment rules for other bilateral procedures.

9 Concept does not apply.

Modifier 51 (multiple procedures)

This modifier indicates which payment adjustment rule for multiple procedures applies to the service.

0 No payment adjustment rules for multiple procedures apply. If the procedure is reported on the same day as another procedure, payment is based on the lower of (a) the actual charge or (b) the fee schedule amount for the procedure.

1 This indicator is only applied to codes with a procedure status of "D." If a procedure is reported on the same day as another procedure with an indicator of 1, 2, or 3, Medicare ranks the procedures by the fee schedule amount, and the appropriate reduction to this code is applied (100%, 50%, 25%, 25%, 25%, and by report). Carriers and Medicare Administrative Contractors (MACs) base payment on the lower of (a) the actual charge or (b) the fee schedule amount reduced by the appropriate percentage.

2 Standard payment adjustment rules for multiple procedures apply. If the procedure is reported on the same day as another procedure with an indicator of 1, 2, or 3, carriers and MACs rank the procedures by the fee schedule amount and apply the appropriate reduction to this code (100%, 50%, 50%, 50%, 50%, and by report). MACs base payment on the lower of (a) the actual charge or (b) the fee schedule amount reduced by the appropriate percentage.

3 Special rules for multiple endoscopic procedures apply if a procedure is billed with another endoscopy in the same family (that is, another endoscopy that has the same base procedure). The base procedure for each code with this indicator is identified in field 31G of Form CMS-1500 or its electronic equivalent claim. The multiple endoscopy rules apply to a family before ranking the family with other procedures performed on the same day (for example, if multiple endoscopies in the same family are reported on the same day as endoscopies in another family or on the same day as a non-endoscopic procedure). If an endoscopic procedure is reported with only its base procedure, the base procedure is not separately paid. Payment for the base procedure is included in the payment for the other endoscopy.

4 Diagnostic imaging services are subject to Multiple Procedure Payment Reduction (MPPR) methodology. Technical Component (TC) of diagnostic imaging services are subject to a 50% reduction of the second and subsequent imaging services furnished by the same physician (or by multiple physicians in the same group practice using the same group National Provider Identifier [NPI]) to the same beneficiary on the same day, effective for services July 1, 2010, and after. Physician Component (PC) of diagnostic imaging services are subject to a 25% payment reduction of the second and subsequent imaging services effective Jan. 1, 2012.

5 Selected therapy services are subject to MPPR methodology. Therapy services are subject to 20% of the Practice Expense (PE) component for certain therapy services furnished in office or other non-institutional settings, and a 25% reduction of the PE component for certain therapy services furnished in institutional settings. Therapy services are subject to 50% reduction of the PE component for certain therapy services furnished in both institutional and non-institutional settings.

6 Diagnostic services are subject to the MPPR methodology. Full payment is made for the TC service with the highest payment under the Medicare Physician Fee Schedule (MPFS). Payment is made at 75% for subsequent TC services furnished by the same physician (or by multiple physicians in the same group practice using the same group NPI) to the same beneficiary on the same day.

7 Diagnostic ophthalmology services are subject to the MPPR methodology. Full payment is made for the TC service with the highest payment under the MPFS. Payment is made at 80% for subsequent TC services furnished by the same physician (or by multiple physicians in the same group practice using the same group NPI) to the same beneficiary on the same day.

9 Concept does not apply.

Modifier 62 (two surgeons)

This field provides an indicator for services for which two surgeons, each in a different specialty, may be paid.

0 Co-surgeons not permitted for this procedure.

1 Co-surgeons could be paid. Supporting documentation is required to establish medical necessity of two surgeons for the procedure.

2 Co-surgeons permitted. No documentation is required if two specialty requirements are met.

9 Concept does not apply.

Modifier 66 (surgical team)

This field provides an indicator for services for which team surgeons may be paid.

0 Team surgeons not permitted for this procedure.

1 Team surgeons could be paid. Supporting documentation is required to establish medical necessity of a team; paid by report.

2 Team surgeons permitted; paid by report.

9 Concept does not apply.

Modifier 80 (assistant surgeon)

This field provides an indicator for services for which an assistant at surgery is never paid.

0 Payment restriction for assistants at surgery applies to this procedure unless supporting documentation is submitted to establish medical necessity.

1 Statutory payment restriction for assistants at surgery applies to this procedure. Assistants at surgery may not be paid.

2 Payment restriction for assistants at surgery does not apply to this procedure. Assistants at surgery may be paid.

9 Concept does not apply.

Because many of the services represented by CPT codes in the Radiology, Pathology, and Medicine chapters of the CPT codebook are diagnostic in nature, crosswalks to the ICD-10-CM code set are too numerous to list. Instead, a narrative description of the service is followed by RVU, modifier, and global information. The official CPT parenthetical information associated with the CPT code is included as well.

The following page presents a guide to the information contained within a code-detail page.

HCPCS Level II Codes

The Healthcare Common Procedure Coding System (HCPCS, pronounced "hick-picks") is a collection of code sets that are used to report health care procedures, supplies, and services. HCPCS Level I codes are CPT codes, developed and copyrighted by the American Medical Association. HCPCS Level II codes include alphanumeric codes developed by CMS to report services, procedures, and supplies not reported with CPT codes. These codes include; ambulance services; durable medical equipment, prosthetics, orthotics, and supplies (DMEPOS); drugs; and quality measure reporting. HCPCS Level II codes also include American Dental Association codes for current dental terminology, or CDT codes, and hundreds of two-character modifiers. These modifiers are used to identify anatomic sites, describe the provider of care or supplies, or describe specific clinical findings.

Modifiers

HCPCS Level II and CPT modifiers appropriate to anesthesia and pain management coding are included in this chapter. A modifier provides the means to report or indicate that a service reported with a CPT or HCPCS Level II code has been altered by some specific circumstance but not changed in its definition or code. The service may have been greater, or lesser, or may have been performed by multiple physicians who will share in reimbursement for the service. Modifiers also enable health care professionals to effectively respond to payment policy requirements established by other entities, and often affect reimbursement.

Modifiers may be part of the CPT code set or part of the HCPCS Level II code set. Both types are included in this chapter. CMS rules specific to the assignment of modifiers are presented in numeric (CPT modifiers) or alphanumeric order (HCPCS Level II modifiers).

In addition to modifiers developed by the AMA and by CMS, a set of modifiers has been developed by the American Society of Anesthesiologists (ASA) to describe the well-being of the patient undergoing anesthesia. The modifier section of this book also describes the ASA physical status modifiers P1 through P6.

Appendices

What follows is an explanation the appendices contained within *CPT® Coding Essentials for Anesthesia and Pain Management 2019.*

Appendix A: National Correct Coding Initiative Edits

The National Correct Coding Initiative (CCI) was developed by CMS to restrict the reporting of inappropriate code combinations and reduce inappropriate payments to providers. The CCI edits essentially identify when a lesser code should be bundled into the parent code and not separately reported, and when two codes are mutually exclusive. In either case, only one of the codes is eligible for reimbursement. In other cases, it is only appropriate to report both codes concurrently if modifier 59 is appended to identify that one of the codes reported is a distinct procedural service.

Each of the CCI edits presented in this appendix includes a superscript that identifies how the edit should be applied. With a superscript of 0 (12001^{0}), the two codes may never be reported together. With a superscript of 1 (12001^{1}), a modifier may be applied and both codes reported, if appropriate. A superscript of 9 (12001^{9}) indicates that the modifier issue is not applicable to this code pairing, and the two codes should not be reported together. Remember, the modifier can only be used when the paired codes represent distinct procedural services. The modifier would be appended to the lesser of the two codes, as defined by their RVUs.

The CCI edits for each of the anesthesia and pain management CPT codes found in this guide are included in this appendix, listed in numeric order for simple lookup. CCI edits are updated quarterly. Those listed in this guide are effective Jan. 1, 2019, through March 31, 2019. Future quarterly CCI edits can be found online at https://www.cms.gov/Medicare/Coding/NationalCorrectCodInitEd/Version_Update_Changes.html.

Appendix B: Clinical Documentation Checklist

One of the biggest challenges of ICD-10-CM is ensuring that the clinical documentation from providers is sufficient. There are two main problems in documentation associated with ICD-10-CM:

- The terminology has in some cases changed from the old system, and providers may need to adjust their documentation for clarity
- The level of detail required in ICD-10-CM is much greater than previously required for code abstraction

The Clinical Documentation Checklist for Anesthesia and Pain Management was developed to be used as a communication tool between coder and physician, or as a document that can be reproduced as a template for documentation by the physician. Essentially, the checklist identifies those documentation details required for complete and accurate code selection. For example, in ICD-10-CM, secondary diabetes is divided into diabetes due to underlying condition (E08) and diabetes induced by drugs or chemicals (E09). Furthermore, another category, other specified diabetes mellitus (E13), has been added. This category is selected for patients who have monogenic diabetes, which includes maturity onset diabetes of the young (MODY), postpancreatectomy diabetes, or when the cause of secondary diabetes is not documented. Type 1 is reported with E10 codes, and type 2 with E11 codes.

Official CPT code description(s) for the master code(s) enable coders to double-check their code selections.

Master code or code family for this code-detail page. All information on this page links to or crosswalks to this code(s).

Citations for *CPT® Assistant* are provided so coders know when to seek further information from this authoritative reference.

RVUs are national Medicare relative value units, or a breakdown of the costs of medical care based on CPT code. Physician work, practice expense, malpractice expense, and total expense differ for facility and nonfacility, so both are listed. RVUs may be used to predict or set fees for physician payment. RVUs shown are for physicians participating in the Medicare program. For anesthesia based codes, base units are displayed.

36430

36430 Transfusion, blood or blood components

(When a partial exchange transfusion is performed in a newborn, use 36456)

AMA Coding Guideline

Venous Procedures

...cture, needle or catheter for diagnostic ...r intravenous therapy, percutaneous. ...codes are also used to report the therapy ...ified. For collection of a specimen from an ...hed catheter, use 36592. For collection of ...men from a completely implantable venous ...device, use 36591.

Parenthetical instructions that are part of the official CPT codebook give crucial direction to prevent coding errors.

...lar Introduction and Injection ...dures

Listed services for injection procedures include necessary local anesthesia, introduction of needles or catheter, injection of contrast media with or without automatic power injection, and/or ... pre- and postinjection care specifically ...the injection procedure.

...vascular catheterization should be coded ...introduction and all lesser order selective ...tion used in the approach (eg, the ...for a selective right middle cerebral ...eterization includes the introduction and ...catheterization of the right common and ...rotid arteries).

...second and/or third order arterial ...tion within the same family of arteries or ...lied by a single first order vessel should be expressed by 36012, 36218, or 36248. Additional first order or higher catheterization in vascular families supplied by a first order vessel different from a previously selected and coded family should be separately coded using the conventions described above.

Plain English Descriptions of the procedure or service explain what the master code represents, enabling the coder to verify code selections against the medical record.

Surgical Procedures on Arteries and Veins

Primary vascular procedure listings include establishing both inflow and outflow by whatever procedures necessary. Also included is that portion of the operative arteriogram performed by the surgeon, as indicated. Sympathectomy, when done, is included in the listed aortic procedures. For unlisted vascular procedure, use 37799.

Please see the Surgery Guidelines section for the following guidelines:

- *Surgical Procedures on the Cardiovascular System*

AMA Coding Notes

Vascular Introduction and Injection Procedures

(For radiological supervision and interpretation, see Radiology)

(For injection procedures in conjunction with cardiac catheterization, see 93452-93461, 93563-93568)

(For chemotherapy of malignant disease, see 96401-96549)

AMA *CPT Assistant* □

36430: Aug 97: 18, Nov 99: 32-33, Aug 00: 2, Mar 01: 10, Oct 03: 2, Jul 06: 4, Jul 07: 1, Jul 17: 4

Plain English Description

Blood and blood components include whole blood, platelets, packed red blood cells, and plasma products. Transfusions are performed to replace blood that is lost or depleted due to an injury, surgery, sickle cell disease, or treatment for a malignant neoplasm. Red blood cells are given to increase the number of blood cells that transport oxygen and nutrients throughout the body, platelets to control bleeding and improve blood clotting, and plasma to replace total blood volume and provide blood factors that improve blood clotting. The skin is prepped over the planned transfusion site and an intravenous line inserted. Any medication ordered by the physician is administered prior to the transfusion. The blood and/or blood components are administered. The patient is monitored during the transfusion for any signs of adverse reaction.

Transfusion, blood or blood components

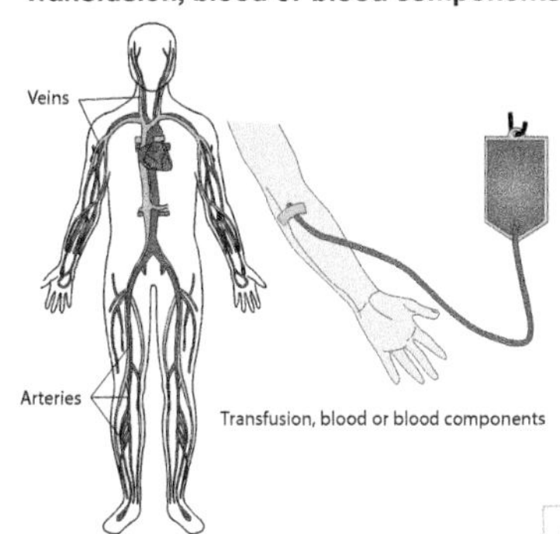

Simple line illustrations bring clarity and understanding to complex procedures.

ICD-10-CM Diagnostic Codes

There are too many ICD-10-CM codes to list. Refer to ICD-10-CM code book for associated diagnostic codes.

Common diagnoses associated with the procedure are linked to the ICD-10-CM code set. Icons identify when a seventh character is required, and Xs have been added to codes as placeholders to prevent errors when assigning the seventh character. Diagnoses that are limited to one sex are noted with an icon. Diagnoses that apply to multiple sides/regions of the body are noted with an icon.

CCI Edits

Refer to Appendix A for CCI edits.

Pub 100

36430: Pub 100-03, 1, 110.16, Pub 100-03, 1, 110.7, Pub 100-04, 4, 231.8

Facility RVUs □

Code	Work	PE Facility
36430	0.00	0.98

Non-facility RVUs □

Code	Work	PE Non-Facility		
36430	0.00	0.98	0.02	1.00

Modifiers (PAR) □

Code	Mod 50	Mod 51
36430	0	0

From the CMS database, key CPT code modifiers affecting relative values when they indicate multiple procedures or multiple providers, as in co-surgery, team surgery, or assistant surgery are listed here.

Global Period

Code	Days
36430	XXX

The Medicare global period indicates the number of postoperative days during which any routine care associated with the original service is bundled into the original service. Possible global periods are 0, 10, and 90 days.

● New ▲ Revised ✚ Add On ⊘Modifier 51 Exempt ★Telemedicine □CPT QuickRef ⁄FDA Pending ⇄ Laterality ❼Seventh Character ♂Male ♀Female

CPT © 2018 American Medical Association. All Rights Reserved.

Appendix C: Documentation Guidelines for Evaluation and Management (E/M) Services

As the author and owner of E/M codes found in the CPT codebook, the AMA has developed detailed guidelines on how to determine which code is appropriate to report, based on the medical record for the encounter. These guidelines look at the quality and quantity of the data in the record:

- History
- Examination
- Medical decision making
- Counseling
- Coordination of care
- Nature of the presenting problem
- Length of the visit

In 1995, CMS published its own Documentation Guidelines (DGs). Recognizing that the 1995 DGs did not appropriately reflect the work performed in some specialties, CMS published a second set of DGs in 1997. Both sets are still in use. The 1995 DGs are appropriate for multi-system examinations; for example, an internal medicine physician. The 1997 DGs are appropriate for in-depth, single-system examinations, for example, from a retinal specialist.

For Medicare and Medicaid, either the 1995 or 1997 DGs are to be followed, depending on the preference of the provider or coder. The CPT guidelines, while largely incorporated into the 1995 and 1997 DGs, still have unique features accepted by some private payers. Unabridged copies of all three sets of DGs are presented in Appendix C.

Terminology, Abbreviations, and Basic Anatomy

The Terminology, Abbreviations, and Basic Anatomy chapter can be used as a reference tool if there is confusion when reading medical record documentation and when a more extensive understanding of medical terminology is needed. The following includes terms, abbreviations, symbols, prefixes, suffixes, and anatomical illustrations that will help clarify some of the more difficult issues, and give a firmer understanding of information, that is in medical record documentation.

Medical Terminology

A majority of medical terms are composed of Greek and Latin word parts and are broken down into different elements. One element is the root word. The root word is the foundation of the medical term and contains the fundamental meaning of the word. All medical terms have one or more roots.

Examples:

hydr = water

lith = stone

path = disease

Combining forms (or vowel, usually "o") links the root word to the suffix or to another root word. This combining vowel does not have a meaning on its own; it only joins one part of a word to another.

Prefixes and suffixes are two of the other elements used in medical terminology and consist of one or more syllables (prepositions or adverbs) placed before or after root words to show various kinds of relationships. Prefixes are before the root word and suffixes are after the root word and consist of one or more letters grouped together. They are never used independently; however, they can modify the meaning of the other word parts. Many prefixes and suffixes are added to other words with a hyphen, but medical dictionary publishers are opting to drop the hyphen on many of the more common prefixed medical words.

Examples:

Prefixes:

micro = small

peri = surrounding

Suffixes:

algia = pain

an = pertaining to

The following are lists of prefixes and suffixes typically seen in Anesthesia/Pain Management:

Root Words/Combining Forms

abdomin/o	abdomen
acous/o	hearing
acr/o	extremities, top, extreme point
aden/o	gland
adip/o	fat
andr/o	male
ankyl/o	stiff, bent, crooked
anter/o	front
arthr/o	joint
ather/o	yellowish, fatty plaque
audi/o	hearing
aur/o	ear
aut/o	self
axill/o	armpit
balan/o	glans penis
bi/o	life
blast/o	developing cell
blephar/o	eyelid
brach/o	arm
bronch/o	bronchial tubes
carcin/o	cancer
card/o	heart
cheil/o	lip
chol/o	gall, bile
cholangi/o	bile duct
chondr/o	cartilage
cis/o	to cut
colp/o	vagina
coron/o	heart
cost/o	ribs
crani/o	skull
cry/o	cold
cutane/o	skin
cyan/o	blue
cyt/o	cell
cyst/o	urinary bladder
dacry/o	tear duct, tear
derm/o	skin
dermat/o	skin
dipl/o	double, two
dips/o	thirst
dist/o	distant, far

ech/o	sound
encephal/o	brain
enter/o	intestine
erythr/o	red
erythem/o	red
eti/o	cause of disease
galact/o	milk
gastr/o	stomach
gloss/o	tongue
gluc/o	sugar
glyc/o	sugar
gon/o	seed
gravid/o	pregnancy
gynec/o	female, woman
hemat/o	blood
hepat/o	liver
hidr/o	sweat
hist/o	tissue
home/o	sameness
inguin/o	groin
isch/o	to hold back
kal/o	potassium
kerat/o	horny tissue, hard
labi/o	lip
lapar/o	abdomen, abdominal
laryng/o	larynx
lei/o	smooth
leuk/o	white
lingu/o	tongue
lith/o	stone
lord/o	swayback, curvature in lumbar region
mamm/o	breast
mast/o	breast
melan/o	black
ment/o	mind
metr/o	uterus
morph/o	shape, form
my/o	muscle
myc/o	fungus
myel/o	spinal cord
myring/o	eardrum
natr/o	sodium
necr/o	death (of cells or all of the body)
nephr/o	kidney
neur/o	nerve
noct/o	night
odont/o	tooth
olig/o	few, scanty
omphal/o	naval, umbilicus
onc/o	tumor
onych/o	nail
oophor/o	ovary
opt/o	eye
ophthalm/o	eye
or/o	mouth
orch/o	testis
orchi/o	testis
orchid/o	testis
orth/o	straight
oste/o	bone
ot/o	ear
ov/o	egg
ovul/o	egg
pachy/o	thick
path/o	disease
phag/o	to eat, swallow
phleb/o	vein
phon/o	voice
phot/o	light
phren/o	diaphragm
plas/o	formation, development
pneumon/o	lungs
poli/o	gray matter
proct/o	rectum and anus
pulmon/o	lungs
psych/o	mind
py/o	pus
quadr/o	four
ren/o	kidney
rhin/o	nose
rhytid/o	wrinkle
rhiz/o	nerve root
salping/o	fallopian tubes
sial/o	salivary gland
sarc/o	flesh
sect/o	to cut
spir/o	breathing
spondyl/o	vertebra
squam/o	scale-like
staphyl/o	clusters
steat/o	fat
strept/o	twisted chains
terat/o	monster
thec/o	sheath
thorac/o	chest
thromb/o	clot
trich/o	hair
tympan/o	eardrum
ung/o	nail
vas/o	vessel
ven/o	vein
viscer/o	internal organs

xanth/o	yellow
xer/o	dry

Prefixes

a(d)-	towards
a(n)-	without
ab-	from
ab(s)-	away from
ad-	towards
allo-	other, another
ambi-	both
amphi-	on both sides, around
ana-	up to, back, again, movement from
aniso-	different, unequal
ante-	before, forwards
anti-	against, opposite
ap-, apo-	from, back, again
bi(s)-	twice, double
bio-	life
brachy-	short
cata-	down
circum-	around
con-	together
contra-	against
cyte-	cell
de-	from, away from, down from
deca-	ten
di(s)-	two
dia-	through, complete
di(a)s	separation
diplo-	double
dolicho-	long
dur-	hard, firm
dys-	bad, abnormal
e-, ec-	out, from out of
ecto-	outside, external
ek-	out
em-	in
en-	into
endo-	into
ent-	within
epi-	on, up, against, high
eso-	will carry
eu-	well, abundant, prosperous
eury-	broad, wide
ex-, exo-	out, from out of
extra-	outside, beyond, in addition
haplo-	single
hapto-	bind to
hemi-	half
hept-	seven
hetero-	different
hex-	six
homo-	same
hyper-	above, excessive
hypo-	below, deficient
im-, in-	not
in-	into, to
infra-	below, underneath
inter-	among, between
intra-	within, inside, during
intro-	inward, during
iso-	equal, same
juxta-	adjacent to
kata-	down, down from
macro-	large
magno-	large
medi-	middle
mega-	large
megalo-	very large
meso-	middle
meta-	beyond, between
micro-	small
neo-	new
non-	not
ob-	before, against
octa-	eight
octo-	eight
oligo-	few
pachy-	thick
pan-	all
para-	beside, to the side of, wrong
pent-	five
per-	by, through, throughout
peri-	around, round-about
pleo-	more than usual
poly	many
post-	behind, after
pre-	before, in front, very
pros-	besides
prox-	besides
pseudo-	false, fake
quar(r)-	four
re, red-	back, again
retro-	backwards, behind
semi-	half
sex-	six
sept-	seven
sub-	under, beneath
super-	above, in addition, over
supra-	above, on the upper side
syn-	together, with
sys-	together, with

tetra-	four
thio-	sulfur
trans-	across, beyond
tri-	three
uni-	one
ultra-	beyond, besides, over

Suffixes

-ase	fermenter
-ate	do
-cide	killer
-c(o)ele	cavity, hollow
-ectomy	removal of, cut out
-form	shaped like
-ia	got
-iasis	full of
-ile	little version
-illa	little version
-illus	little version
-in	a substance, chemical, chemical compound
-ism	theory, characteristic of
-itis	inflammation
-ity	makes a noun of quality
-ium	thing
-ize	do
-logy	study of, reasoning about
-megaly	large
-noid	mind, spirit
-oid	resembling, image of
-ogen	precursor
-ol(e)	alcohol
-ole	little version
-oma	tumor (usually)
-osis	full of
-ostomy	"mouth-cut"
-pathy	disease of, suffering
-penia	lack
-pexy	fix in place
-plasty	re-shaping
-philia	affection for
-rhage	burst out
-rhea	discharge, flowing out
-rhexis	shredding
-pagus	Siamese twins
-sis	idea (makes a noun, typically abstract)
-thrix	hair
-tomy	cut
-ule	little version
-um	thing (makes a noun, typically concrete)

Anesthesia/Pain Management Terms

The following definitions are medical terms commonly seen while coding/billing for Anesthesia/Pain Management:

Acupressure – A therapy developed by the ancient Chinese and used in eastern cultures for thousands of years. Practitioners apply varying physical pressure, through touch, to specific body sites in order to channel and stimulate energy flow.

Acupuncture – An ancient Chinese practice, using needles inserted into specific sites in the body, along "meridians," to stimulate body systems. This therapy is used for a wide variety of purposes including relaxation, pain relief, and treating illness and disease.

Acute Pain – The physiological response to trauma, injury, surgery or illness. It is generally time limited from days to weeks.

Adjuvant – Generally used to describe an "add-on" or additional therapy.

Adjuvant Analgesic – Generally used to describe drugs that have a primary use other than pain control but have secondary pain-relieving qualities.

Algology – The science and study of pain.

Allodynia – Pain due to a stimulus that does not normally provoke pain. The original definition adopted by the IASP committee was pain due to non-noxious stimulus to the normal skin. Allodynia involves a change in the quality of a sensation, tactile, thermal, or of any other kind. The usual response to a stimulus was not painful, but the present response is.

Analgesia – Absence of pain in response to stimulation that would normally be painful.

Analgesic – Generally refers to a pain relief medication; also a pain-relieving effect, such as "the acupuncture was analgesic."

Anesthesia – The absence of sensation, either in a region of skin, a region of the body, or as a total loss of consciousness. "Local" anesthesia affects (numbs) a specific area of the body and "general" anesthesia results in unconsciousness; anesthesiologist induces sleep and maintains unconsciousness to avoid sensation.

Anesthesia Dolorosa – Where pain is present in an area that is anesthetic.

Anesthesia – A medical specialty devoted to the science of anesthesia; a subspecialty of Anesthesia is the study of pain control drugs and procedures.

Anesthetic – An agent or agents that produce regional anesthesia (certain part of the body) or general anesthesia (loss of consciousness).

Angina – Usually pain syndromes associated with cardiac disease. May indicate a feeling of oppression or tightness of the chest or throat.

Anterior – A term used by medical professionals meaning at the front of, or close to the front of the body. (*See* Posterior)

Anticonvulsants – Group of drugs used to prevent seizures, also used as adjuvant analgesics in chronic pain treatment to alter transmission of the pain signal.

Arthralgia – Pain in a joint, usually due to arthritis.

Arthritis – Basically, chronic or ongoing inflammation of a joint. There are many different arthritic conditions because it lacks the negative stigma associated with the term "narcotics."

Biofeedback – A non-drug technique used to treat a wide variety of pain conditions. A non-invasive electronic device is used to monitor various biologic responses (such as heart rate). Information is gathered, and then used to teach the patient various control techniques.

Causalgia – A syndrome of sustained burning pain, allodynia, and hyperpathia after a nerve injury, often combined with vasomotor and sudomotor dysfunction and later trophic changes.

Central Pain – Pain associated with a lesion of the central nervous system.

Chronic – Long term or ongoing.

Chronic Pain – An ongoing or persistent pain syndrome; generally lasting more than six months.

Complex Regional Pain Syndrome – Chronic pain condition that can affect any area of the body. It is subdivided into two types. Type 1 is typically triggered by an injury, often minor, that does not directly involve the nerves. It may also be triggered by an illness or have no known cause. Type 2, more commonly referred to as causalgia, is the result of an injury to a nerve. Both types are characterized by neuropathic pain that can be severe or even disabling. In addition, the affected body site, which is usually an extremity, may show evidence of sympathetic nervous system changes such as abnormal circulation, temperature, and sweating. Loss of function of the extremity, muscle atrophy, and hair and skin changes may also eventually occur.

Contraindicated – A term frequently used in pain management to mean that a medication or treatment is not to be used in a specific patient because it may cause serious side effects or reactions.

Cutaneous – Generally referring to the skin and/or the tissues directly underneath the skin.

Cutaneous Intervention – A variety of treatments through the skin used to promote healing or pain relief, including heat, cold, massage, acupressure, ultrasound, hydrotherapy, TENS, and vibration.

Deafferentation Pain – Pain due to loss of sensory input into the central nervous system (as can occur with avulsion of the brachial plexus), or other types of peripheral nerve lesions. Can also be due to pathologic lesions of the central nervous system.

Dermatome – A term related to very specific sections of the body that are associated with the distribution of the large nerves coming from the spine. Dermatomes are helpful in locating which area in the spine is malfunctioning.

Dysesthesia – An abnormal unpleasant sensation, can be spontaneous or evoked. A dysesthesia is always unpleasant. The patient must decide whether a sensation is pleasant or unpleasant.

Edema – Swelling; generally, an abnormal accumulation of body fluids, often accompanying inflammation.

Endorphin – A substance the body manufactures that acts like morphine in the brain and central nervous system. This natural pain-relieving agent can be stimulated by exercise.

Epidural Space – A space located between the spinal cord and the vertebral column in the spine.

Epidural Steroid Injection – An injection of steroid medication into the epidural space of the spine; used in some forms of back pain.

Epidurogram – An x-ray test using contrast dye to confirm epidural catheter placement and obtain information about a patient's epidural space.

Fibromyalgia – A muscle and connective tissue disorder characterized by symptoms of pain, tenderness, and stiffness of tendons, muscles, and surrounding soft tissue.

Fibrosis – Scarring of tissue; abnormal formation of fibrous tissue.

General Anesthesia – During surgery, using a mixture of medications and gas, a gradual titration of the medication under the direction of the physician.

Hyperalgesia – An increased response to a stimulus that is normally painful.

Hyperesthesia – Increased sensitivity to any stimulation.

Hyperpathia – Abnormally exaggerated subjective response to painful stimuli. May occur with hyperesthesia, hyperalgesia, or dysesthesia. The pain is often explosive in character.

Hypoalgesia – Diminished sensation to noxious stimulation.

Hypoesthesia – Abnormally decreased sensitivity, particularly to touch in its absence.

Intramuscular (IM) – An injection of medication or fluids into a muscle.

Intravenous (IV) – An injection of medication or fluids into a vein.

Migraine Aura, Persistent, without Cerebral Infarction – This is a rare complication of a migraine and is characterized by the presence of a migraine aura lasting for more than one week without radiographic evidence of a cerebral infarction.

Migraine, Chronic – A diagnosis of chronic migraine is made when a patient has 15 or more headache days per month.

Migraine, Episodic – The term episodic migraine may be used to differentiate a patient who does not have chronic migraines from one who does. This term is not used in ICD-10-CM codes.

Migraine, Hemiplegic – Symptoms are the same as a migraine with aura. In addition, the migraine is accompanied by muscle/motor weakness. Hemiplegic migraines are further differentiated as familial or sporadic. A familial hemiplegic migraine is one in which the patient has at least one first- or second-degree family member who has also been diagnosed with hemiplegic type migraines. Sporadic hemiplegic migraine is one in which the patient does not have any first or second degree family members who have also been diagnosed with hemiplegic type migraines.

Migraine with Aura – Symptoms are the same as a migraine without aura. In addition, the migraine is accompanied by visual, sensory, or speech disorders.

Migraine without Aura – The most common type of migraine. Symptoms typically include: unilateral headache, pulsating pain, moderate to severe in intensity, aggravated by physical activity, associated with nausea/vomiting, sensitivity to light (photophobia) and/or sound (phonophobia), duration typically 4-72 hours.

Myopathy – Any abnormal disease or condition of muscle tissue, often involving pain.

Myotome – A term related to sections of the body that are associated with a muscle or muscle group including the insertions sites at either end of the muscle fibers.

Nervous System – The organs and tissues of the body that provide for communication with other body systems and including the higher centers of reasoning; the brain and spinal cord are components of the central nervous system, and the nerves outside those structures make up the peripheral nervous system.

Neuralgia – Pain in the distribution of a specific nerve or nerves.

Neuritis – Acute and/or chronic inflammation of nerves.

Neuropathic Pain – Pain syndrome in which the predominant mechanism is aberrant somatosensory processing. May be restricted to pain originating in peripheral nerves and nerve roots.

Neuropathy – A functional disturbance or pathological change in the peripheral nervous system, sometimes limited to non-inflammatory lesions as opposed to neuritis.

Nociceptor – A receptor for pain, preferentially sensitive to a noxious stimulus or to a stimulus that would become noxious if continued. Pain is a perception that takes place at higher levels of the central nervous system.

Non-Steroidal Anti-inflammatory Drug (NSAID) – This is a specific class of drugs that reduces inflammation and swelling in and around the site of injury or irritation. These drugs (such as ibuprofen) are widely used in acute pain management and in chronic inflammatory conditions such as arthritis.

Noxious Stimulus – Stimulus that is potentially or actually damaging to body tissue.

Opioid – A narcotic used to help treat pain.

Osteoarthritis – The most common form of arthritis often associated with aging. It may occur in one joint or in many and is often degenerative in nature.

Pain – Sensation of discomfort, distress, or agony, resulting from the stimulation of specialized nerve endings. It serves as a protective mechanism (induces the sufferer to remove or withdraw).

Pain Threshold – Pain threshold is the least experience of pain that a subject can recognize.

Pain Tolerance Level – The greatest level of pain that a patient is able to tolerate.

Paresthesia – An abnormal sensation, such as burning, or prickling, that may be spontaneous or in response to stimulus. It has the same clinical limitations as the pain tolerance level.

Patient-Controlled Analgesia (PCA) – An intravenous drug delivery system, generally used after surgery, that allows patients to control the amount of pain medicine they receive, by pushing a button that causes the system to administer a dose of medicine. Patients are taught to administer pain medication depending on the level of pain. This method has been shown to provide effective pain relief using less medication.

Physiological Dependence – A condition that occurs with opioids and other drugs whereby the body becomes accustomed to a chemical. Often confused with addiction or psychological dependence, this condition is common and not associated with drug abuse. The hallmark of physiological dependence is the need to avoid abrupt discontinuation of the drug, which will cause a predictable withdrawal syndrome. Discontinuation of the drug can be easily accomplished by tapering the dose of the medication slowly under the direction of the physician.

Posterior – Close to, or at the back of the body. Also called "dorsal."

Pruritus – Itching.

Pseudoaddiction – A drug seeking behavior pattern of pain patients who are not getting adequate pain relief. For example, a patient is given a pain pill that only last for four hours, but only allowed to take it every six hours. This behavior can be mistaken for addiction and other psychological and behavioral factors, including overwhelming obsession with obtaining and using drugs, despite harm to self or others. Addiction is feared, but very rare in chronic pain analgesic users. Also known as "psychological dependence."

Psychosomatic – A term used to describe a physical disorder thought to be caused partly or entirely by psychological problems.

Radiculalgia – Pain along the distribution of one or more sensory nerve roots.

Radiculitis – Inflammation of one or more nerve roots.

Radiculopathy – A usually painful disturbance of function or pathologic change in one or more spinal nerve roots.

Referred Pain – Pain that is felt in a place different from the place of origin. For example, pain from pressure in the liver is often felt in the right upper chest or shoulder.

Somatosensory – Pertaining to sensations received from all tissues of the body (skin, muscles).

Sonogram – Using high frequency sound waves. Also a technique to apply heat during physical therapy.

Titration – Increasing or decreasing a medication in an incremental manner, to reach a desired level. This method is used to allow the body to adjust, or to find an effective dose. Titration is used with anti-depressants, steroids, opioids and other drugs.

Tolerance – A physiological phenomenon that develops in some patients with long term opioid use where the body requires increasing amounts of drug to achieve the same level of effect. There are several theories that may explain tolerance including the body becoming a more effective metabolizer of the medication, and the body making less receptor sites for a drug after long exposure. Often confused with addiction.

Transcutaneous Electrical Nerve Stimulation (TENS) – A cutaneous intervention that relieves pain by sending electrical stimulation to nerve fibers and interfering with pain signal transmission. This method employs electrodes placed on the skin in various locations, using various degrees of intensity to achieve pain relief.

Transdermal – Referring to delivery through the skin. Patches that deliver medication are transdermal.

Trigger Point – A hypersensitive area in muscle or connective tissue with pain locally as well as referred pain and tenderness.

Withdrawal – A syndrome that occurs when opioids and some other drugs are abruptly discontinued, or a condition marked by a pattern of behavior observed in schizophrenia and depression, characterized by a pathological retreat from interpersonal content and social involvement and leading to pre-occupation.

Abbreviations/Acronyms

The following abbreviations and acronyms are commonly seen in documentation for Anesthesia/Pain Management:

A	without, lack of, Apathy (lack of feeling); apnea (without breath); aphasia (without speech); anemia (lack of blood)
A & P	anterior and posterior; auscultation and percussion
Ab	antibody
ab	away from, Abductor, (leading away from); aboral (away from mouth)
Abd	abdomen
ABG	arterial blood gases
ABP	arterial blood pressure
Ac	before meals
ACBG	aortocoronary bypass graft
ACE	angiotensin converting enzyme
ACL	anterior cruciate ligament
ACT	anticoagulant therapy; active motion
ACTH	adrenocorticotropic hormone
Ad	to, toward, near to, Adductor, (leading toward); adhesion, (sticking to); adnexa (structures joined to); adrenal (near the kidney)
ADH	antidiuretic hormone
ADL	activities of daily living
Ad lib	as desired
AFB	acid-fast bacilli
AFIB	atrial fibrillation
AFP	alpha-fetoprotein
AGA	appropriate for gestational age
AI	aortic insufficiency
AICD	automated implantable cardio-defibrillator
AIDS	acquired immune deficiency syndrome
AKA	above knee amputation
Allo	other, another
ALP	alkaline phosphatase
AMA	against medical advice
AMB	ambulatory
Ambi	both, Ambidextrous, (ability to use hands equally); ambilateral (both sides)
AMI	acute myocardial infarction
Amphi	about, on both sides, both, Amphibious, (living on both land and water)
Ampho	both, Amphogenic, (producing offspring of both sexes)
a(n)	without
Ana	up, back, again, excessive, Anatomy, (a cutting up); anagenes (reproduction of tissue); anasarca (excessive serum in cellular tissues of body)
Ante	before, forward, Antecubital, (before elbow); anteflexion, (forward bending)
Anti	against, opposed to, reversed Antiperistalsis (reversed peristalsis); antisepsis (against infection)
AP	apical pulse
Apo	from, away from Aponeurosis (away from tendon); apochromatic (abnormal color)
APSGN	acute poststreptococcal glomerulonephritis
ARF	acute renal failure
AS	aortic stenosis
ASCVD	arteriosclerotic cardiovascular, disease
ATN	acute tubular necrosis
AU	both ears
AV	aortic valve
AVB	atrio-ventricular block
AVR	aortic valve replacement
BE	barium enema
BBS	bilateral breath sounds
BG	blood glucose
BI	brain injury
bi	twice, double Biarticulate (double joint); bifocal (two foci); bifurcation (two branches)
BID	twice a day
bilat	bilateral
B/K	below knee
BM	bowel movement or breast milk
BMR	basal metabolic rate
BP	blood pressure
BPH	benign prostatic hypertrophy
Brachy	short
BRP	bathroom privileges
BS	bowel sounds
BSA	body surface area
BSE	breast self-examination
BT	bowel tones
BUN	blood urea nitrogen
bx	biopsy
C	Celsius(centigrade)
c (C)	with
C&S	culture and sensitivity
c/o	complaint of
Ca	calcium, cancer, carcinoma
CA	cardiac arrest
CABG	coronary artery bypass graft
CAD	coronary artery disease

CAPD	continuous ambulatory peritoneal dialysis
CAT	computerized tomography scan
Cata	down, according to, complete Catabolism (breaking down); catalepsia (complete seizure); catarrh (flowing down)
CATH LAB	cardiac catheterization lab
CBC	complete blood count
CBD	common bile duct
CBE	clinical breast examination
CBI	continuous bladder irrigation
CBR	complete bed rest
CC	chief complaint
CCK	cholecystokinin
CCPD	continuous cyclic peritoneal dialysis
CCU	cardiac care unit
CD	cardiovascular disease
CEA	cultured epithelial autograft
CFT	complement-fixation test
CHD	coronary heart disease
CHF	congestive heart failure
CI	cardiac insufficiency
CICU	cardiac intensive care unit
CIHD	chronic ischemic heart disease
Circum	Around, about Circumflex (winding about); circumference (surrounding); circumarticular (around joint)
CMS	circulation, motion, sensation
CO	cardiac output
Com	With, together, Commissure (sending or coming together)
Con	With, together, Conductor (leading together); concrescence (growing together); concentric (having a common center)
Contra	Against, opposite Contralateral (opposite side); Contraception (prevention of conception); contraindicated (not indicated)
CO2	carbon dioxide
COPD	chronic obstructive pulmonary disease
CP	chest pain, cleft palate
CPAP	continuous positive airway pressure
CPR	cardiopulmonary resuscitation
CPPD	chest percussion and post drainage
CRF	chronic renal failure
CRPS	complex regional pain syndrome
CRRT	continuous renal replacement therapy
CRT	capillary refill time
CSF	cerebrospinal fluid, colony stimulating factors
CT	chest tube, computed tomography
CVA	cerebral vascular accident, costovertebral angle
CVP	central venous pressure
CX	circumflex
Cx'd	cancelled
CXR	chest x-ray

D5W	Dextrose 5% in water
D5LR	Dextrose 5% with lactated ringers
DAT	diet as tolerated
DBP	diastolic blood pressure
DC (dc)	discontinue
DEX (DXT)	blood sugar
De	Away from, Dehydrate (remove water from); dedentition (removal of teeth); decompensation (failure of compensation)
deca	ten
Di	Twice, double, Diplopia (double vision); dichromatic (two colors); digastric (double stomach)
Dia	Through, apart, across, completely Diaphragm (wall across); diapedesis (ooze through); diagnosis (complete knowledge)
DIC	disseminated intravascular coagulation
Diplo	double
Dis	Reversal, apart from, separation disinfection (apart from infection); disparity (apart from equality); dissect (cut apart)
DKA	diabetic ketoacidosis
DM	diabetes mellitus
DNA	deoxyribonucleic acid
DNR	do not resuscitate
DTR	deep tendon reflex
DVT	deep vein thrombosis
Dx	diagnosis
Dys	Bad, difficult, disordered, Dyspepsia (bad digestion); dyspnea (difficult breathing); dystopia (disordered position)
E, ex	Out, away from, Enucleate (remove from); eviscerate (take out viscera or bowels); exostosis (outgrowth of bone)
EBV	Epstein-Barr Virus
Ec	Out from, Ectopic (out of place); eccentric (away from center); ectasia (stretching out or dilation)
ECF	extracellular fluid, extended care facility
ECG (EKG)	electrocardiogram/electrocardiograph
Ecto	On outer side, situated on Ectoderm (outer skin); ectoretina (outer layer of retina)
EENT	eye, ear, nose and throat
Em, en.	Empyema (pus in); encephalon (in the head)
EMG	electromyogram
Endo	Within, Endocardium (within heart); endometrium (within uterus)
Ent	within
Epi	Upon, on, Epidural (upon dura); epidermis (on skin)
ERCP	endoscopic retrograde cholangiopancreatography
ESRD	end stage renal disease
ET	endotracheal tube
Exo	Outside, on outer side, outer layer, Exogenous (produce outside); exocolitis (inflammation of outer coat of colon)
Extra	Outside, Extracellular (outside cell); extrapleural (outside pleura)
F & R	force and rhythm
FA	fatty acid
FBS	fasting blood sugar

FD	fatal dose, focal distance
FDA	Food & Drug Administration
Fx	fracture
FUO	fever of unknown origin
FVD	fluid volume deficit
GB	gallbladder
GFR	glomerular filtration rate
GI	gastrointestinal
GU	genitourinary
HA	headache
Haplo	single
Hapto	bind to
Hb	hemoglobin
HCG	human chorionic gonadotropin
HCVD	hypertensive cardiovascular disease
HCO3	bicarbonate
HCT	hematocrit
HD	heart disease, hemodialysis
HDL	high density lipoprotein
HEENT	head, eye, ear, nose and throat
Hemi	Half, Hemiplegia (partial paralysis); hemianesthesia (loss of feeling on one side of body)
hept	seven
hetero	different
hex	six
Hgb	hemoglobin
HIV	human immunodeficiency virus
HM	heart murmur
h/o	history of
homo	same
HPI	history of present illness
HRT	hormone replacement therapy
HS	hour of sleep
HTN (BP)	hypertension
Hx	history
Hyper	Over, above, excessive Hyperemia (excessive blood); hypertrophy (overgrowth); hyperplasia (excessive formation)
Hypo	Under, below, deficient Hypotension (low blood pressure); (deficiency or underfunction of thyroid)
I & O	intake and output
IBC	iron binding capacity
IBD	inflammatory bowel disease
IBS	irritable bowel syndrome
IBW	ideal body weight
ICCE	intracapsular cataract extraction
ICF	intermediate care facility
ICP	intracranial pressure
ICS	intercostal space

ICT	inflammation of connective tissue
ICU	intensive care unit
IDDM	insulin dependent diabetes mellitus
IE	inspiratory exerciser
IH	infectious hepatitis
IHD	ischemic heart disease
IHR	intrinsic heart rate
IIP	implantable insulin pump
IM	intramuscular
Im, in	In, Into, Immersion (act of dipping in); infiltration (act of filtering in); injection (act of forcing liquid into)
Imp	impression
IMV	intermittent mandatory ventilation
Infra	Below, Infraorbital (below eye); infraclavicular (below clavicle or collarbone)
Inter	Between, Intercostal (between ribs); intervene (come between)
Intra	Within, Intracerebral (within cerebrum); intraocular (within eyes); intraventricular (within ventricles)
Intro	Into, within, Introversion (turning inward); introduce (lead into)
IPD	intermittent peritoneal dialysis
IPPB	intermittent positive pressure breathing
Iso	equal, same
ITP	immune thrombocytopenic purpura
IV	intravenous
IVF	in vitro fertilization
IVP	intravenous pyelography
JAMA	Journal of the American Medical Association
Juxta	adjacent to
JVP	jugular venous pressure
K	potassium
Kata	down, down from
KCl	potassium chloride
KI	potassium iodide
KUB	kidney, ureter, bladder
KVO	keep vein open
L & A	light and accommodation
LB	large bowel
LDL	low density lipoprotein
LE	lupus erythematosus
LFTs	liver function tests
LLQ	left lower quadrant
LMP	last menstrual period
LP	lumbar puncture
LUQ	left upper quadrant
Lytes	electrolytes
Macro	large
Magno	large
MAP	mean arterial pressure

MAR	medication administration record
MDI	multiple daily vitamin
Medi	middle
Mega	large
Megalo	very large
Meso	middle
Meta	Beyond, after, change Metamorphosis (change of form); metastasis change (beyond original position); metacarpal (beyond wrist)
MI	myocardial infarction
Micro	small
MLC	midline catheter
MM	mucous membrane
MoAbs	monoclonal antibodies
MOM	Milk of Magnesia
MRDD	mental retarded/developmentally disabled
MRI	magnetic resonance imaging
MRM	modified radical mastectomy
MS	multiple sclerosis, morphine sulfate
MV	Mitral Valve
MVP	mitral valve prolapse
Na	sodium
NaCl	sodium chloride
NAD	no apparent distress
NED	no evidence of disease
Neg	negative
Neo	new
NICU	neonatal intensive care unit
NIDDM	noninsulin dependent diabetes mellitus
NKA	no known allergies
NKDA	no known drug allergies, non-ketotic diabetic acidosis
NKMA	no known medication allergies
noc	night
non	not
NPD	nightly peritoneal dialysis
NPO	nothing by mouth
NS (NIS)	normal saline
NSAID	nonsteroidal anti-inflammatory drug
NS	normal saline
NSR	normal sinus rhythm
NTD	neural tube defect
NV	nausea & vomiting
NYD	not yet diagnosed
O2	oxygen
Ob	before, against
Octa	eight
Octo	eight
Oligo	few
OOB	out of bed
Opistho	Behind, backward, Opisthotic (behind ears); opisthognathous (beyond jaws)
ORIF	open reduction internal fixation
OS	left eye
OT	occupational therapy
OU	both eyes
P	after
P	pulse
PABA	para-aminobenzoic acid
Pachy	thick
Pan	all
Para	Beside, beyond, near to Paracardiac (beside the heart); paraurethral (near the urethra)
PCA	patient controlled analgesia, posterior communicating artery
PCN	penicillin, primary care nurse
PCV	packed cell volume
PD	peritoneal dialysis
PDA	patent ductus arteriosus
PDD	pervasive development disorder
PDR	physician's desk reference
PE	physical examination
PEG	percutaneous endoscopic gastrostomy
PEJ	percutaneous endoscopic jejunostomy
Peri	around, Periosteum (around bone); periatrial. (around atrium); peribronchial (around bronchus)
PERL	pupils equal, react to light
Permeate	(pass through); perforate (bore through); peracute (excessively acute)
PERRLA	pupils equal, round, react to light, accommodation
PET	positron emission tomography
PFT	pulmonary function test
PG	prostaglandin
PH	past history
PI	present illness
PICC	peripherally inserted central venous catheter
PID	pelvic inflammatory disease
Pleo	more than usual
PMI	point of maximal impulse
PMH	past medical history
PNH	paroxysmal nocturnal hemoglobinuria
PO	by mouth
Poly	many
Post	after, behind, Postoperative (after operation); postpartum (after childbirth); postocular (behind eye)
post op	post-operative
PRBC	packed red blood cells
Pre	before, in front of, Premaxillary (in front of maxilla); preoral (in front of mouth)

pre op	pre-operative
prep	preparation
PRN	as needed
Pro	before, in front of, Prognosis (foreknowledge); prophase (appear before)
pros	besides
prox	besides
PS	pyloric stenosis
PSA	prostate specific antigen
Pseudo	false, fake
PT	prothrombin time
P.T.	physical therapy
PTT	partial thromboplastin time
PUD	peptic ulcer disease
PVD	peripheral vascular disease
Px	pneumothorax
Q	every
QD	everyday
QH	every hour
Q2H	every 2 hours
QID	four times a day
qns	quantity not sufficient
QOD	every other day
Qs	quantity sufficient, quantity required
quar(r)	four
R	respirations
RAD	reactive airway disease
RAI	radioactive iodine
RAIU	radioactive iodine uptake
RBC	red blood cells
RDW	red cell distribution width
Re	back, again, contrary, Reflex (bend back); revert (turn again to); regurgitation (backward flowing, contrary to normal)
REEDA	redness, edema, ecchymosis, drainage, approximation
Retro	backward, located behind Retrocervical (located behind cervix); retrograde (going backward); retrolingual. (behind tongue)
RHD	rheumatic heart disease, relative hepatic dullness
RLQ	right lower quadrant
RM	respiratory movement
RO	rule out
ROM	range of motion
ROS	review of systems
RT or R	right
RUQ	right upper quadrant
Rx	prescription, pharmacy
S(s)	without
S/S	signs & symptoms
SAB	spontaneous abortion

SAST	serum aspartate aminotransferase
SB	spina bifida
SBO	small bowel obstruction
Semi	half, Semi cartilaginous (half cartilage); semi lunar(half-moon); semiconscious (half conscious)
SGPT	serum glutamic-pyruvic transaminase
SLE	systemic lupus erythematosus
SNF	skilled nursing facility
SOB	shortness of breath
SOBOE	shortness of breath on exertion
SOP	standard operating procedure
SR	sinus rhythm
SS	social services
STAT	immediately
STD	sexually transmitted disease
STH	somatotropic hormone
STM	short term memory
Sub	under, Subcutaneous (under skin); subarachnoid (under arachnoid); (under nail)
SUI	stress urinary incontinence
super	above, upper, excessive, Supercilia (upper brows); supernumerary (excessive number); supermedial (above middle)
supra	above, upper, excessive Suprarenal (above kidney); suprasternal (above sternum); suprascapular (on upper part of scapula)
SVR	systemic vascular resistance
sym	together, with, Symphysis (growing together); synapsis (joining together); synarthrosis (articulation of joints together)
syn	together, with
sys	together, with
Sx	symptoms
T	temperature
T3	triiodothyronine
T4	thyroxine
TBSA	total body surface area
TCDB	turn, cough, deep breathe
TDM	treadmill
TED (hose)	thrombo-embolism deterrent
TEP	transesophageal puncture
Tetra	four
Thio	sulfur
THR	total hip replacement
THTM	thallium treadmill
TIA	transient ischemic attack
TIBC	total iron binding capacity
TID	three times a day
TIL	tumor infiltrating lymphocytes
TKR	total knee replacement
TNF	tumor necrosis factor

TNM	tumor, node, metastases
TNTC	too numerous to mention
TP	tuberculin precipitation
TPN	total parenteral nutrition
TPR	temperature, pulse, respiration
Trans	across, through, beyond, Transection (cut across); transduodenal (through duodenum); transmit (send beyond)
TTN	transient tachypnea of the newborn
TTP	thrombotic thrombocytopenia purpura
Tri	three
TUPR	transurethral prostatic resection
TURP	transurethral resection of the prostate
TWB	touch weight bear
TWE	tap water enema
Tx	treatment, traction
UA	urinalysis
UAO	upper airway obstruction
UBW	usual body weight
UGA	under general anesthesia
UGI	upper gastrointestinal
Ultra	beyond, in excess, Ultraviolet (beyond violet end of spectrum); ultrasonic (sound waves beyond the upper frequency of hearing by human ear)
Uni	one
up ad lib	up as desired
UPJ	ureteropelvic junction
URI	upper respiratory infection
US	ultrasonic, ultrasound
USA	unstable angina
UTI	urinary tract infection
UVJ	ureterovesical junction
VA	visual acuity
VBP	venous blood pressure
VBAC	vaginal birth after caesarean
VC	ventricular contraction
VENT	ventral
VF/Vfib	ventricular fibrillation
VLDL	very low density lipoprotein
VP	venous pressure, venipuncture
VPB	ventricular premature beats
VPC	ventricular premature contractions
VS	vital signs
VSD	ventricular septal defect
VT/Vtach	ventricular tachycardia
W	vessel wall
W/C	wheelchair
WBC	white blood cell
WD	well developed
WHO	World Health Organization
WN	well nourished
WNL	within normal limits
X	times

Anatomy

Anatomy is the science of the structure of the body. This section will address systemic, regional, and clinical anatomy as it applies to coding in the Anesthesia setting. Anatomical terms have distinct meanings and are a major part of medical terminology.

Anatomical Positions

Often in medical records, anatomical positional terms are used to identify specific areas of body parts and body positions. The following list is commonly used terms that may be found in medical documentation:

- Superior = Nearer to head
- Inferior (caudal) = Nearer to feet
- Anterior (ventral) = Nearer to front
- Proximal = Nearer to trunk or point of origin (e.g., of a limb)
- Distal = Farther from trunk or point of origin (e.g., of a limb)
- Superficial = Nearer to or on surface
- Deep = Farther from surface
- Posterior (dorsal) = Nearer to back
- Medial = Nearer to median plane
- Lateral = Farther from median plane

Anatomical Planes

Anatomical descriptions are based on four anatomical planes that pass through the body in the anatomical position:

- Median plane (midsagittal plane) is the vertical plane passing longitudinally through the body, dividing it into right and left halves
- Paramedian (parasagittal) plane is a sagittal plane that divides the body into unequal right and left regions.
- Coronal (frontal) planes are vertical planes passing through the body at right angles to the median plane, dividing it into anterior (front) and posterior (back) portions
- Horizontal planes are transverse planes passing through the body at right angles to the median and coronal planes; a horizontal plane divides the body into superior (upper) and inferior (lower) parts (it is helpful to give a reference point such as a horizontal plane through the umbilicus).

Anatomical Movement Terms

Various terms are used to describe movements of the body. Movements take place at joints where two or more bones or cartilages articulate with one another. They are described as pairs of opposites.

Flexion	Bending of a part or decreasing the angle between body parts.
Extension	Straightening a part or increasing the angle between body parts.
Abduction	Moving away from the median plane of the body in the coronal plane.
Adduction	Moving toward the median plane of the body in the coronal plane. In the digits (fingers and toes), abduction means spreading them, and adduction refers to drawing them together.
Rotation	Moving a part of the body around its long axis. Medial rotation turns the anterior surface medially and lateral rotation turns this surface laterally.
Circumduction	The circular movement of the limbs, or parts of them, combining in sequence the movements of flexion, extension, abduction, and adduction.
Pronation	A medial rotation of the forearm and hand so that the palm faces posteriorly.
Supination	A lateral rotation of the forearm and hand so that the palm faces anteriorly, as in the anatomical position.
Eversion	Turning sole of foot outward.
Inversion	Turning sole of foot inward.
Protrusion (protraction)	To move the jaw anteriorly.
Retrusion (retraction)	To move the jaw posteriorly.

Anatomical Planes

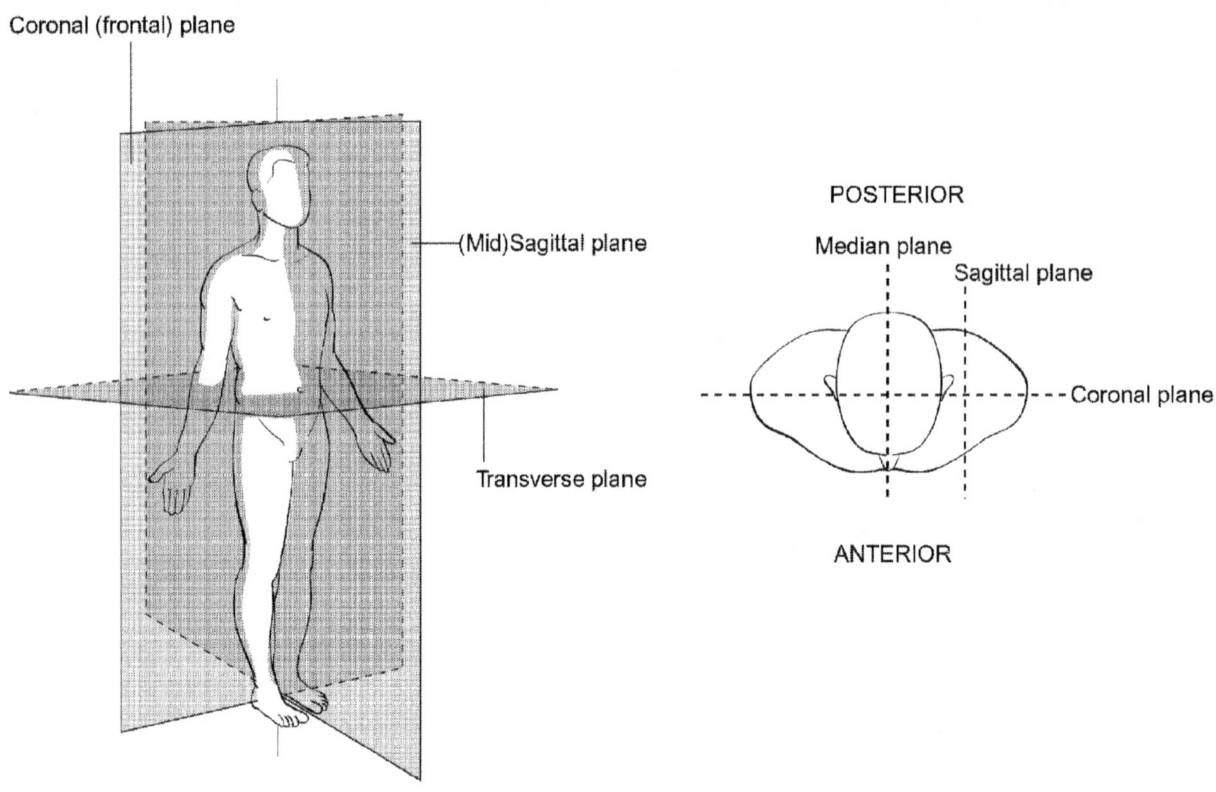

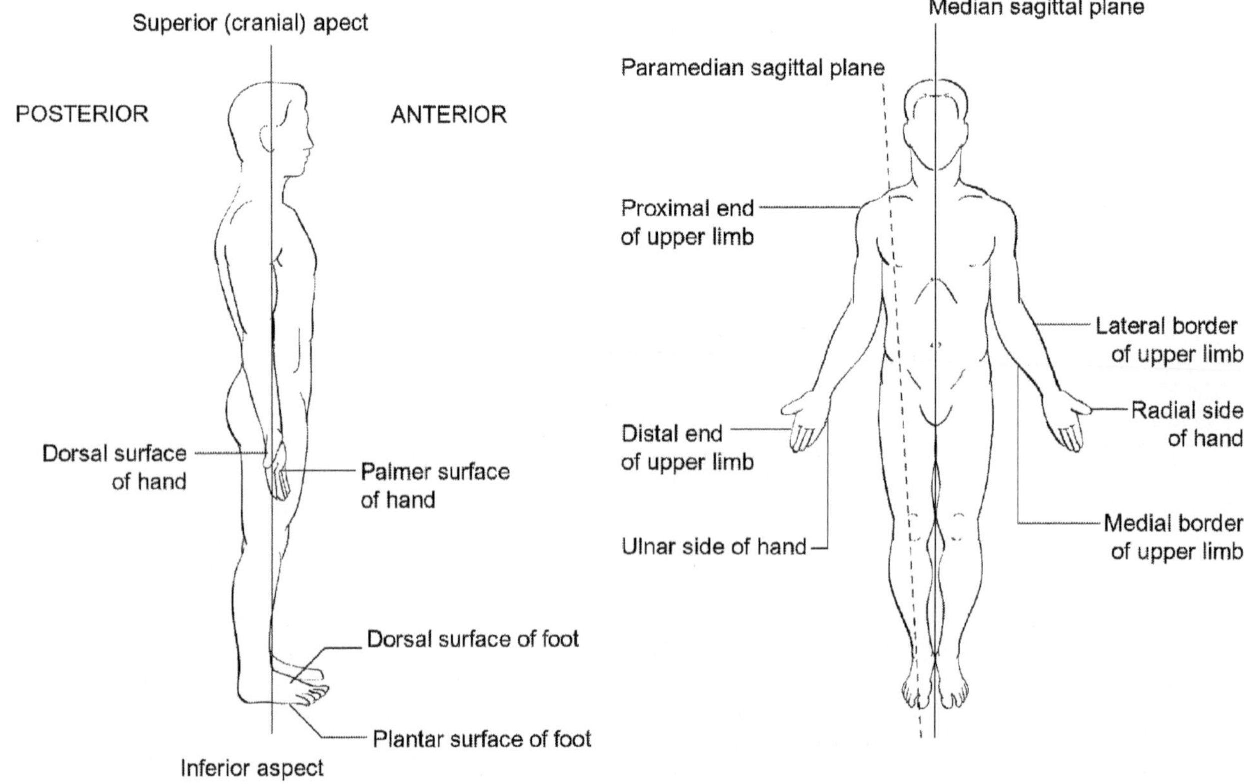

© Fairman Studios, LLC, 2002. All Rights Reserved.

Anesthesia/Pain Management Anatomy

The illustrations on the following pages detail anatomical images which relate to Anesthesia/Pain Management:

Male Figure
(Anterior View)

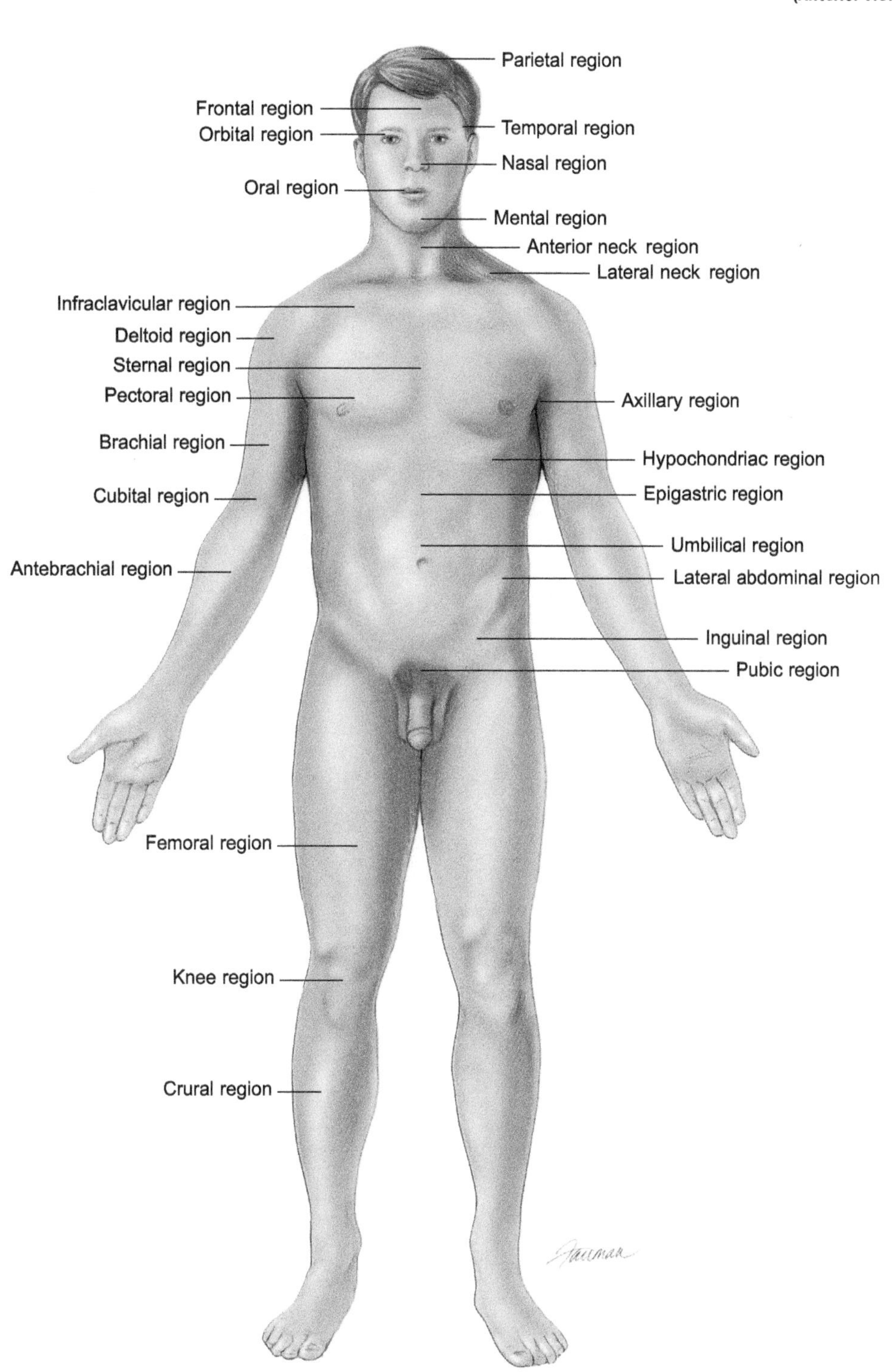

© Fairman Studios, LLC, 2002. All Rights Reserved.

Female Figure
(Anterior View)

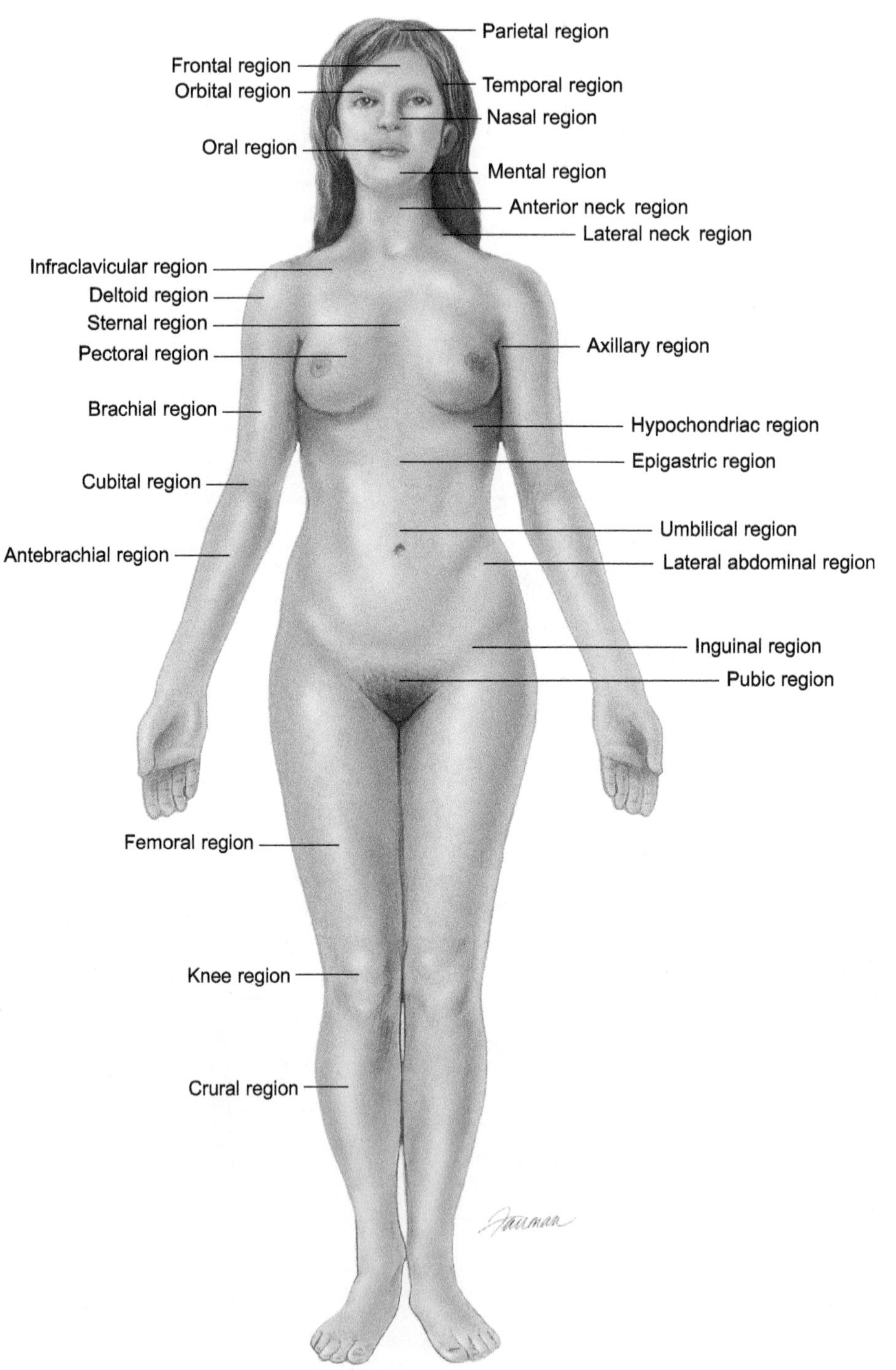

© Fairman Studios, LLC, 2002. All Rights Reserved.

Muscular System
(Anterior View)

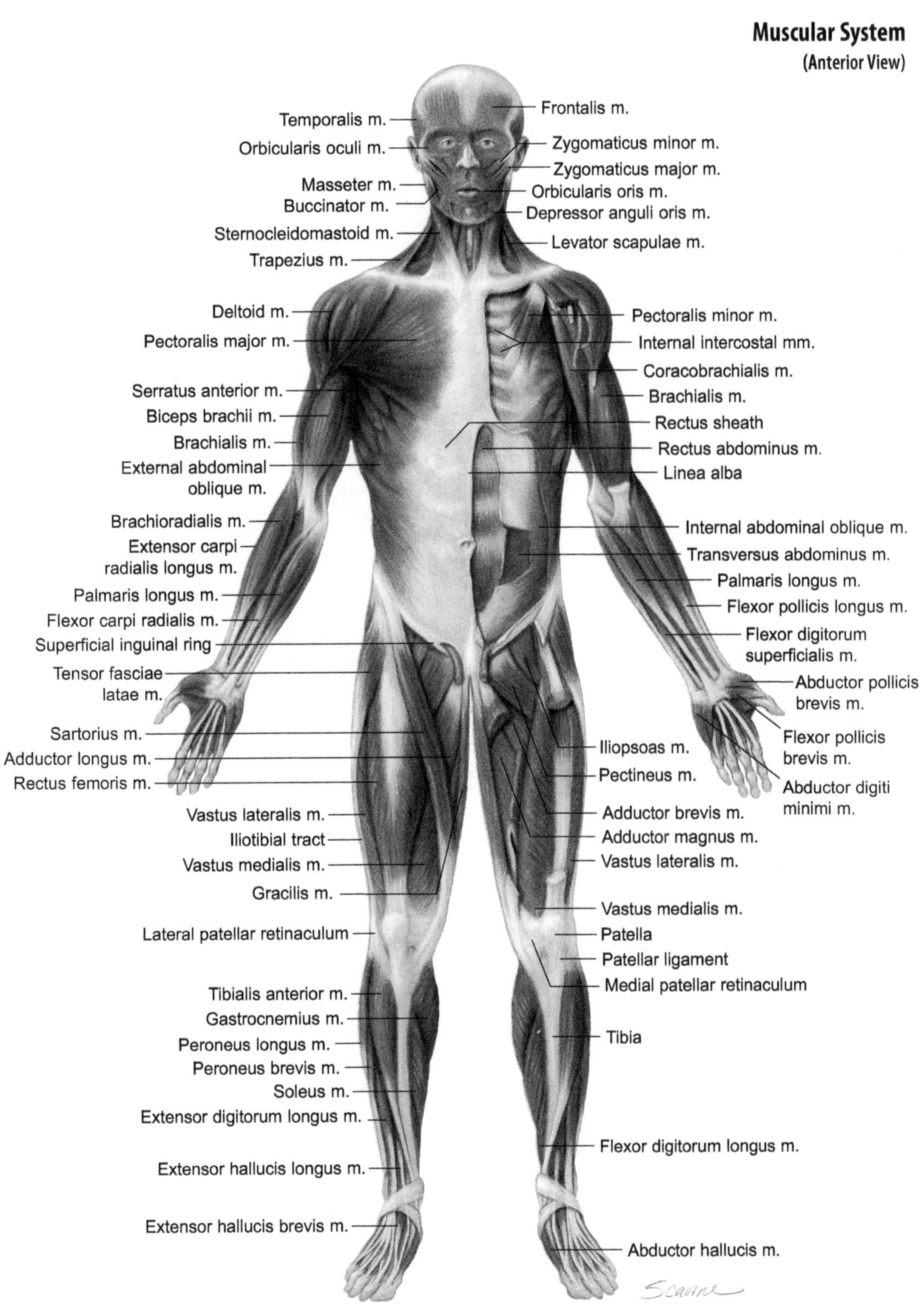
Temporalis m.
Orbicularis oculi m.
Masseter m.
Buccinator m.
Sternocleidomastoid m.
Trapezius m.
Frontalis m.
Zygomaticus minor m.
Zygomaticus major m.
Orbicularis oris m.
Depressor anguli oris m.
Levator scapulae m.
Deltoid m.
Pectoralis major m.
Serratus anterior m.
Biceps brachii m.
Brachialis m.
External abdominal oblique m.
Brachioradialis m.
Extensor carpi radialis longus m.
Palmaris longus m.
Flexor carpi radialis m.
Superficial inguinal ring
Tensor fasciae latae m.
Sartorius m.
Adductor longus m.
Rectus femoris m.
Vastus lateralis m.
Iliotibial tract
Vastus medialis m.
Gracilis m.
Lateral patellar retinaculum
Tibialis anterior m.
Gastrocnemius m.
Peroneus longus m.
Peroneus brevis m.
Soleus m.
Extensor digitorum longus m.
Extensor hallucis longus m.
Extensor hallucis brevis m.
Pectoralis minor m.
Internal intercostal mm.
Coracobrachialis m.
Brachialis m.
Rectus sheath
Rectus abdominus m.
Linea alba
Internal abdominal oblique m.
Transversus abdominus m.
Palmaris longus m.
Flexor pollicis longus m.
Flexor digitorum superficialis m.
Abductor pollicis brevis m.
Flexor pollicis brevis m.
Abductor digiti minimi m.
Iliopsoas m.
Pectineus m.
Adductor brevis m.
Adductor magnus m.
Vastus lateralis m.
Vastus medialis m.
Patella
Patellar ligament
Medial patellar retinaculum
Tibia
Flexor digitorum longus m.
Abductor hallucis m.

© Fairman Studios, LLC, 2002. All Rights Reserved.

Skeletal System

(Vertebral Column – Left Lateral View)

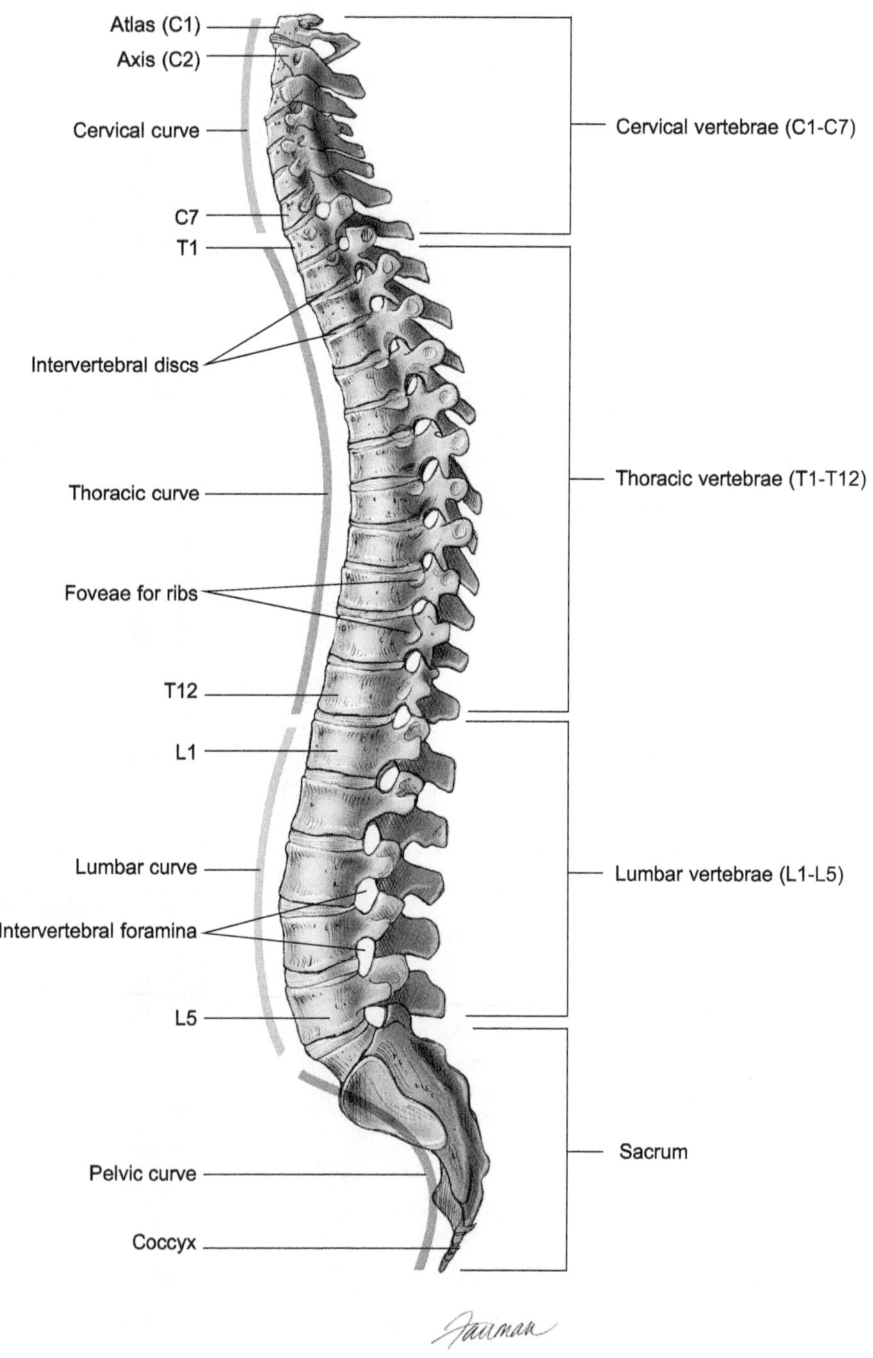

© Fairman Studios, LLC, 2002. All Rights Reserved.

Brain

(Inferior View)

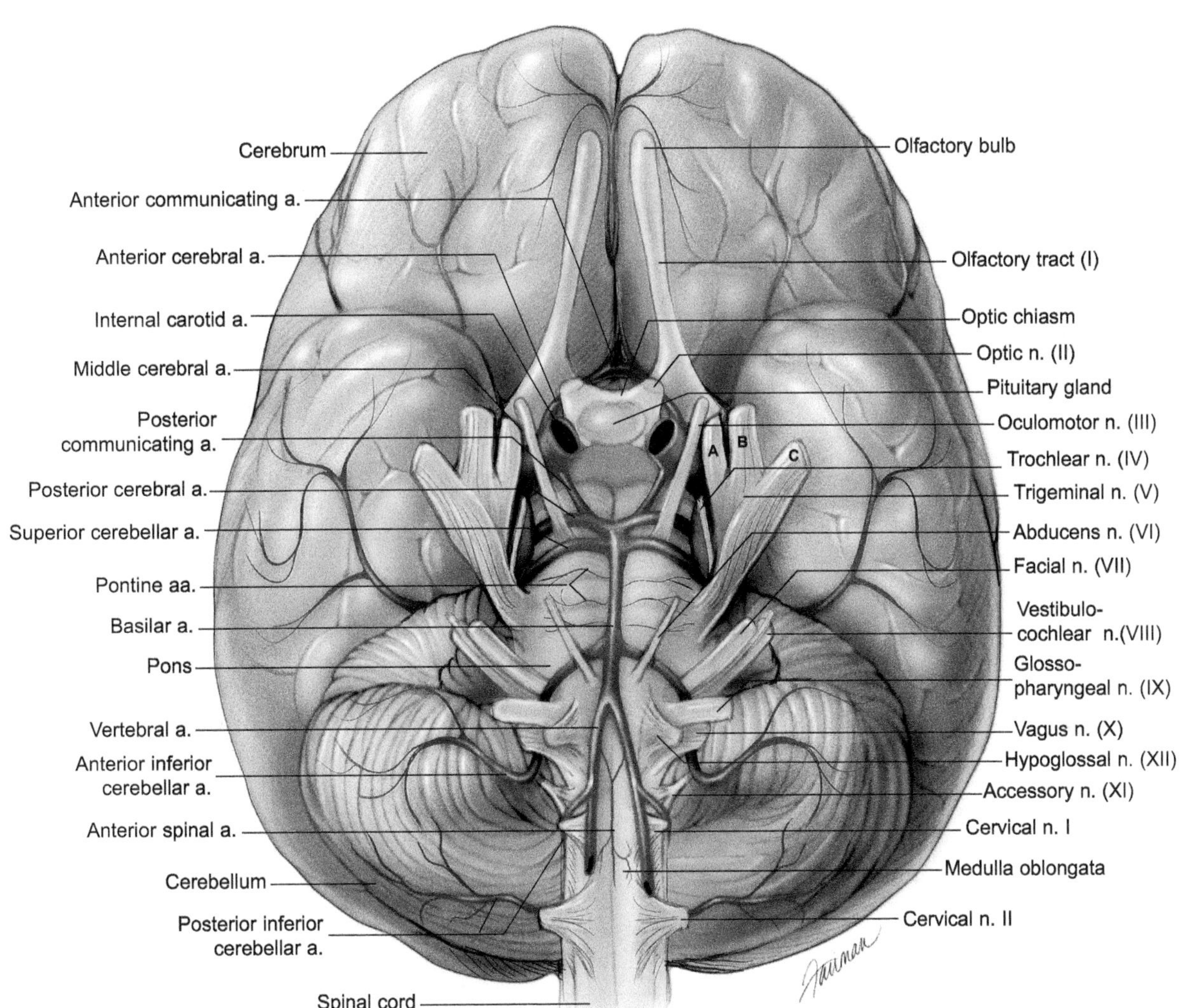

Trigeminal Nerve (V) branches:

A	Ophthalmic branch
B	Maxillary branch
C	Mandibular branch

© Fairman Studios, LLC, 2002. All Rights Reserved.

Nervous System

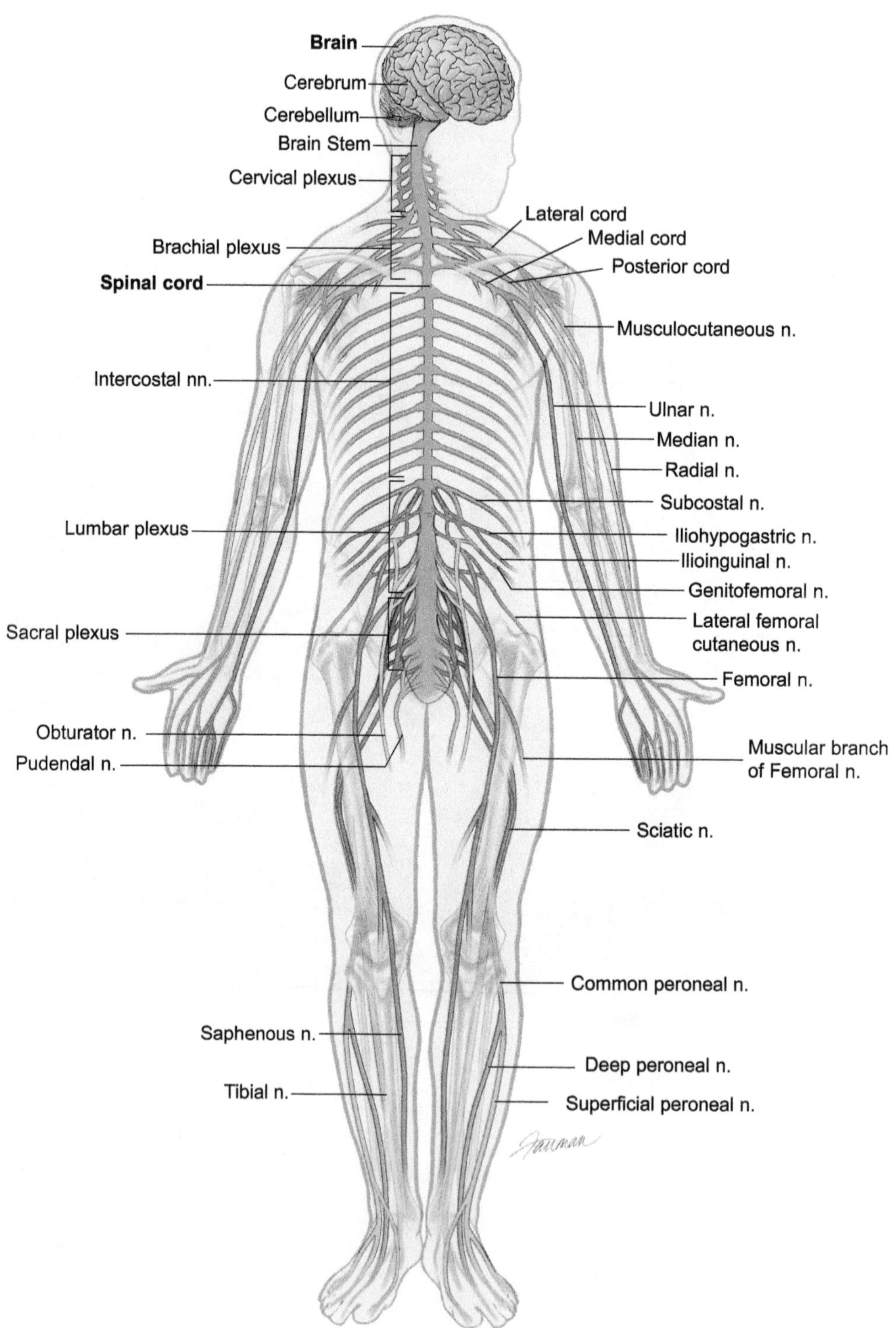

© Fairman Studios, LLC, 2002. All Rights Reserved.

Cranial Nerves (12)

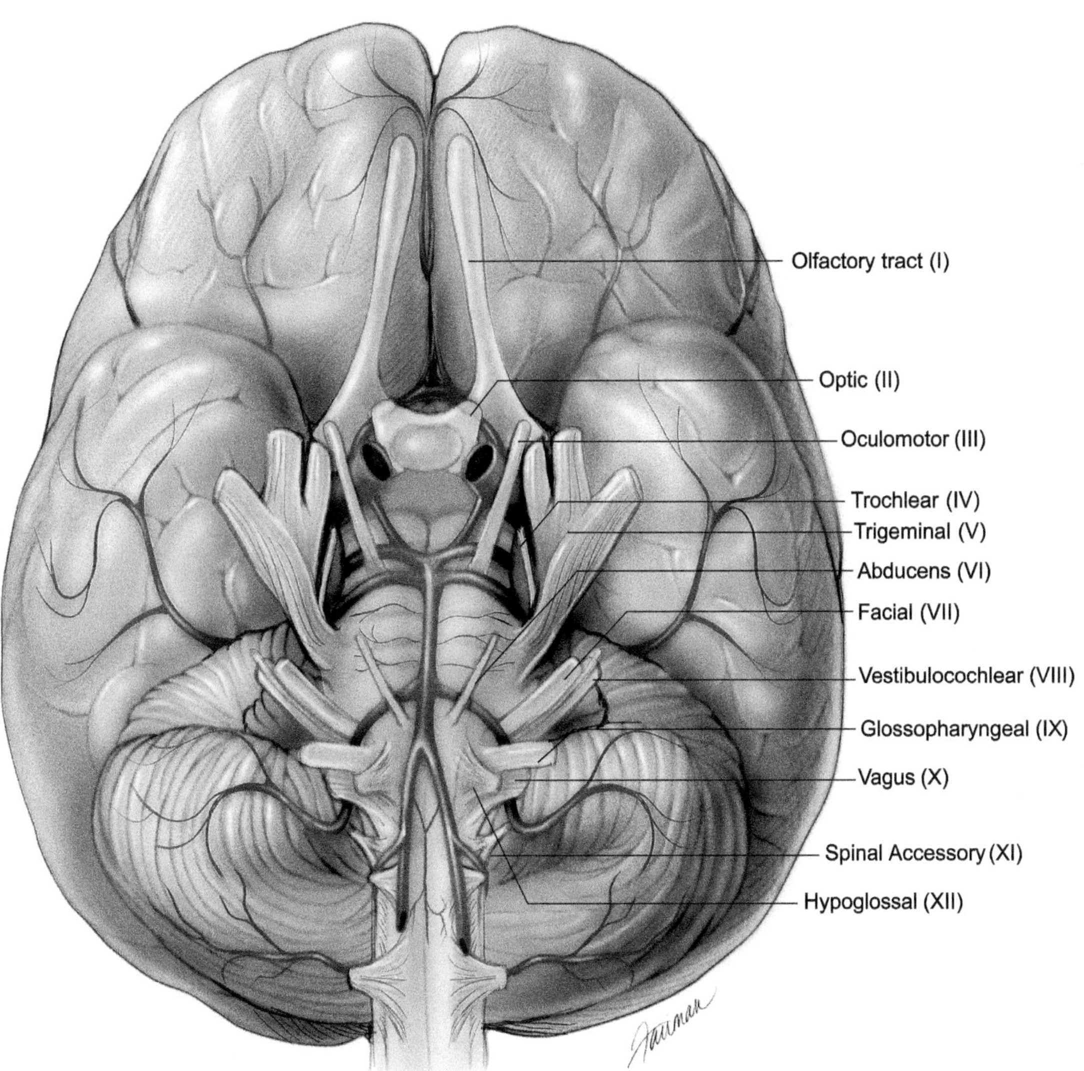

© Fairman Studios, LLC, 2002. All Rights Reserved.

Cerebral Vasculature

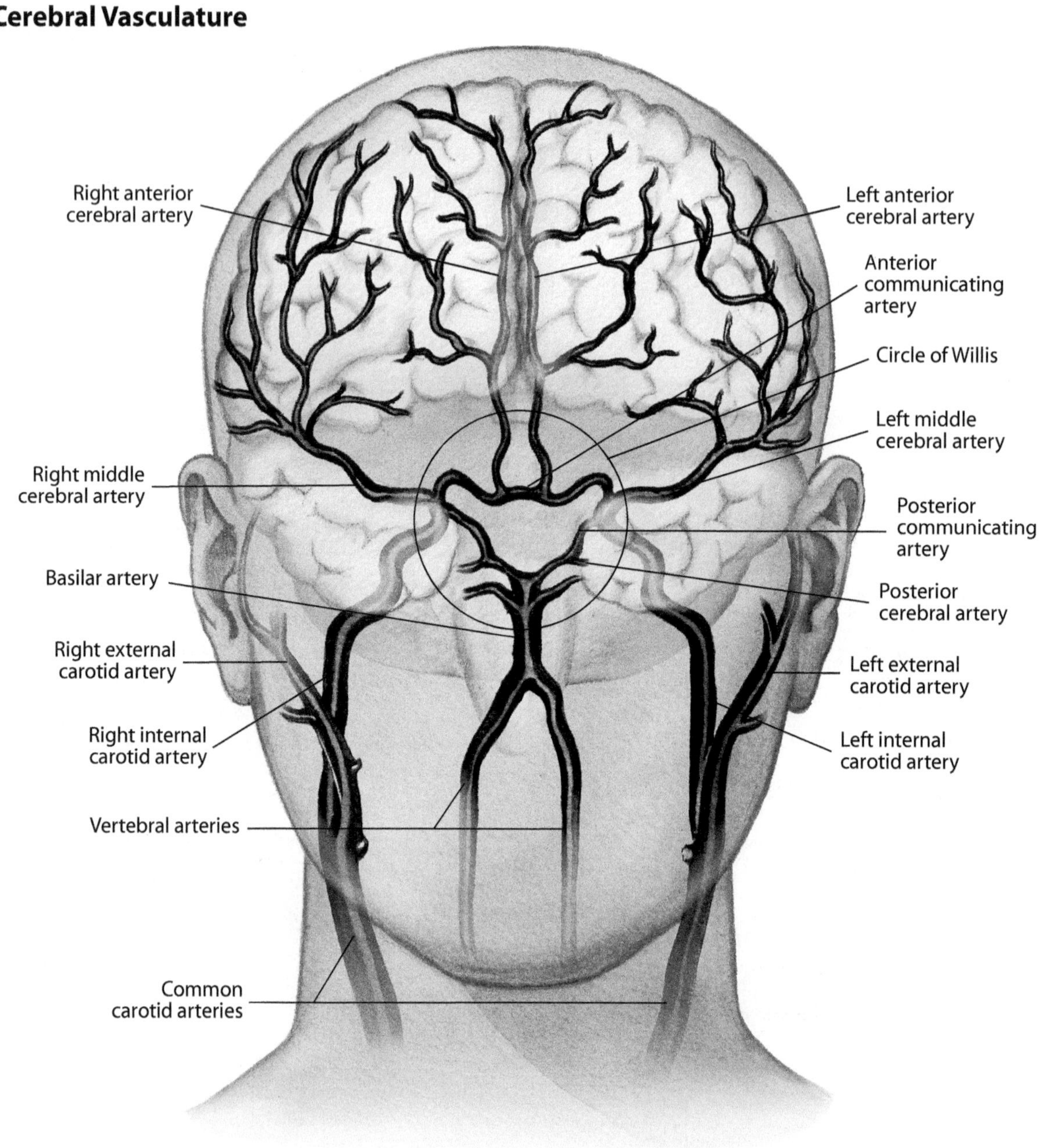

© BradleyClarkArt.com. All Rights Reserved.

Vascular System

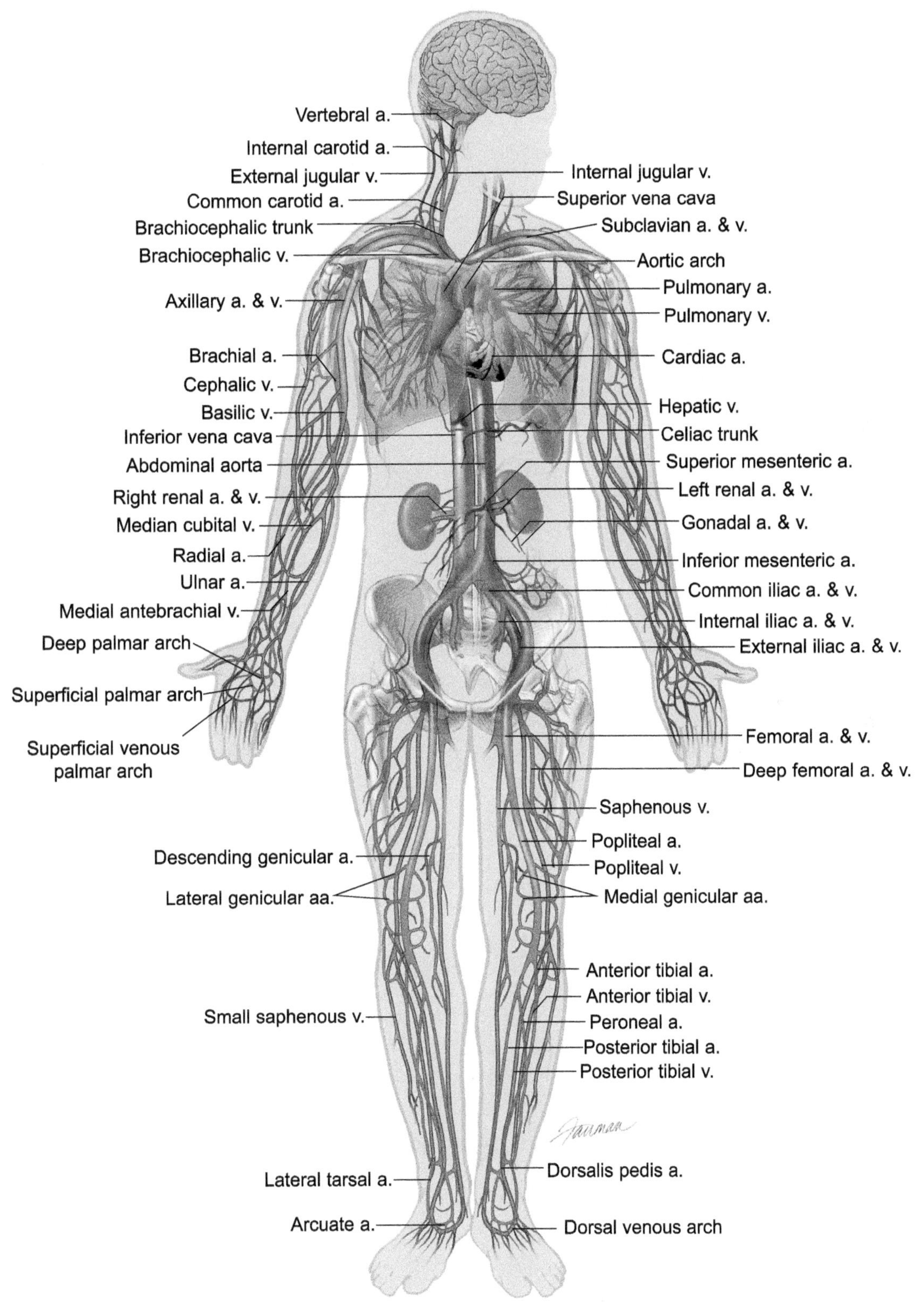
Vertebral a.
Internal carotid a.
External jugular v.
Common carotid a.
Brachiocephalic trunk
Brachiocephalic v.
Axillary a. & v.
Brachial a.
Cephalic v.
Basilic v.
Inferior vena cava
Abdominal aorta
Right renal a. & v.
Median cubital v.
Radial a.
Ulnar a.
Medial antebrachial v.
Deep palmar arch
Superficial palmar arch
Superficial venous palmar arch
Internal jugular v.
Superior vena cava
Subclavian a. & v.
Aortic arch
Pulmonary a.
Pulmonary v.
Cardiac a.
Hepatic v.
Celiac trunk
Superior mesenteric a.
Left renal a. & v.
Gonadal a. & v.
Inferior mesenteric a.
Common iliac a. & v.
Internal iliac a. & v.
External iliac a. & v.
Femoral a. & v.
Deep femoral a. & v.
Saphenous v.
Popliteal a.
Popliteal v.
Medial genicular aa.
Descending genicular a.
Lateral genicular aa.
Anterior tibial a.
Anterior tibial v.
Peroneal a.
Posterior tibial a.
Posterior tibial v.
Small saphenous v.
Lateral tarsal a.
Arcuate a.
Dorsalis pedis a.
Dorsal venous arch

© Fairman Studios, LLC, 2002. All Rights Reserved.

Introduction to ICD-10-CM and ICD-10-PCS Coding

ICD-10-CM

The International Classification of Diseases (ICD) is designed to promote international comparability in the collection, processing, classification, and presentation of mortality statistics. This includes providing a format for reporting causes of death on the death certificate. The reported conditions are translated into medical codes through use of the classification structure and the selection and modification rules contained in the applicable revision of the ICD, published by the World Health Organization (WHO). These coding rules improve the usefulness of mortality statistics by giving preference to certain categories, consolidating conditions, and systematically selecting a single cause of death from a reported sequence of conditions.

ICD-10 is used to code and classify mortality data from death certificates, having replaced ICD-9 for this purpose as of January 1, 1999. The ICD-10 is copyrighted by the WHO, which owns and publishes the classification. WHO has authorized the development of an adaptation of ICD-10 for use in the United States for U.S. government purposes.

Development of ICD-10-CM

The National Center for Health Statistics (NCHS) is the Federal agency responsible for use of the *International Statistical Classification of Diseases and Related Health Problems,* 10th revision (ICD-10) in the United States. The NCHS has developed ICD-10-CM, a clinical modification of the classification for morbidity purposes. As agreed, all modifications must conform to WHO conventions for the ICD. ICD-10-CM was developed following a thorough evaluation by a Technical Advisory Panel and extensive additional consultation with physicians, clinical coders, and others to assure clinical accuracy and utility.

The entire draft of the Tabular List of ICD-10-CM, and the preliminary crosswalk between ICD-9-CM and ICD-10-CM were made available on the NCHS website for public comment. The public comment period ran from December 1997 through February 1998. The American Hospital Association (AHA) and the American Health Information Management Association (AHIMA) conducted a field test in the summer of 2003, with a subsequent report. All comments and suggestions from the open comment period and the field test were reviewed, and additional modifications were made based on these comments and suggestions.

On August 22, 2008, Health and Human Services (HHS) published a proposed rule to adopt ICD-10-CM (and ICD-10-PCS) to replace ICD-9-CM in HIPAA transactions. The comment period for this proposed rule closed October 21, 2008. On January 16, 2009, the final rule on adoption of ICD-10-CM and ICD-10-PCS was published, specifying an anticipated implementation date of October 1, 2013. On August 24, 2012, the HHS announced a rule delaying the implementation date. The final initial implementation date was October 1, 2015. The 2019 ICD-10-CM updates went into effect on October 1, 2018.

The ICD-10-CM Coordination and Maintenance Committee

Annual modifications are made through the ICD-10-CM Coordination and Maintenance Committee. The Committee is made up of representatives from two Federal Government agencies, the National Center for Health Statistics (NCHS) and the Centers for Medicare and Medicaid Services (CMS). The Committee holds meetings twice a year which are open to the public. Modification proposals submitted to the Committee for consideration are presented at the meetings for public discussion. Approved modification proposals are incorporated into the official government version and become effective for use October 1 of the following year.

Official Coding Guidelines

In order to code effectively, the Official Guidelines for Coding and Reporting must be reviewed. Some of the current Guidelines are listed in the table below to illustrate important features.

ICD-10-CM General Coding Guidelines
Locating a Code in ICD-10-CM
To select a code in the classification that corresponds to a diagnosis or reason for visit documented in a medical record, first locate the term in the Alphabetic Index, and then verify the code in the Tabular List. Read and be guided by instructional notations that appear in both the Alphabetic Index and the Tabular List. It is essential to use both the Alphabetic Index and Tabular List when locating and assigning a code. The Alphabetic Index does not always provide the full code. Selection of the full code, including laterality and any applicable 7th character can only be done in the Tabular List. A dash (-) at the end of an Alphabetic Index entry indicates that additional characters are required. Even if a dash is not included at the Alphabetic Index entry, it is necessary to refer to the Tabular List to verify that no 7th character is required.
Level of Detail in Coding
Diagnosis codes are to be used and reported at their highest number of characters available. ICD-10-CM diagnosis codes are composed of codes with 3, 4, 5, 6 or 7 characters. Codes with three characters are included in ICD-10-CM as the heading of a category of codes that may be further subdivided by the use of fourth and/or fifth characters and/or sixth characters, which provide greater detail. A three-character code is to be used only if it is not further subdivided. A code is invalid if it has not been coded to the full number of characters required for that code, including the 7th character, if applicable.
Codes from A00.0 through T88.9, Z00-Z99.89
The appropriate code or codes from A00.0 through T88.9, Z00-Z99.89 must be used to identify diagnoses, symptoms, conditions, problems, complaints or other reason(s) for the encounter/visit.
Signs and Symptoms
Codes that describe symptoms and signs, as opposed to diagnoses, are acceptable for reporting purposes when a related definitive diagnosis has not been established (confirmed) by the provider. Chapter 18 of ICD-10-CM, Symptoms, Signs, and Abnormal Clinical and Laboratory Findings, Not Elsewhere Classified (codes R00.0 - R99) contains many, but not all, codes for symptoms. **See Section I.B.18 Use of Signs/Symptom/Unspecified Codes.**

ICD-10-CM Coding for Anesthesia/ Pain Management

Anesthesia

Because anesthesia services are provided for surgical procedures on all body systems, anesthesiologists need to be familiar with all chapters of ICD-1Ø-CM. For this reason, an overview of all chapters is provided. Examples of specific conventions that anesthesiologists should be aware of include:

- Laterality is a component of many codes
- Codes for complications of pregnancy are specific to the trimester during which the complication occurred
- For multiple gestation, some codes require identification of the fetus affected by the complication

Codes that are specifically related to complications and adverse effects of anesthesia or anesthetics are found mainly in four sections: complications of anesthesia related to pregnancy, labor and delivery, or the puerperium (O29, O74, O89); poisoning, adverse effect, or underdosing of anesthetics (T41); external causes such as endotracheal tube wrongly placed during anesthetic procedure (Y65.3), Anesthesia devices associated with adverse incidents (category Y7Ø), and other complications of surgical and medical care, such as hypothermia due to anesthesia (T88, 51).

Pain Medicine

Those specializing in pain management services need to understand ICD-1Ø-CM codes for pain and pain related conditions such as neoplasms, musculoskeletal system disorders, and nervous system disorders. The most frequently reported codes for pain and pain syndromes are found in three chapters which are:

- Chapter 6 – Diseases of the Nervous System
- Chapter 13 – Diseases of the Musculoskeletal System and Connective Tissue
- Chapter 18 – Symptoms, Signs, and Abnormal Clinical/ Laboratory Findings, NOS

In Chapters 4 and 5, anatomy and physiology, documentation, and coding for pain and pain syndromes will be discussed in detail. However, before the information in those chapters can be fully understood, an introduction to ICD-1Ø-CM coding is needed.

Overview of ICD-10-CM

ICD-1Ø-CM makes use of a two volume format. Volume I is the Tabular List and Volume 2 is the Alphabetic Index. The Alphabetic Index contains the Neoplasm Table, Table of Drugs and Chemicals, and an Alphabetic Index to External Causes. The code set also contains Official Guidelines for Coding and Reporting. While the following overview will help coders begin to understand ICD-1Ø-CM, it should not be used as the only source of information. Coders should obtain the most recent copy of the Official Guidelines for Coding and Reporting to begin a more comprehensive review. A copy of the current ICD-1Ø-CM Code Set is also recommended.

ICD-10-CM Official Guidelines for Coding and Reporting

The structure and format of the Guidelines for Coding and Reporting are as follows:

- Section I. Conventions, general coding guidelines and chapter-specific guidelines
- Section II. Selection of principal diagnosis
- Section III. Reporting additional diagnoses
- Section IV. Diagnostic coding and reporting guidelines for outpatient services
- Appendix I. Present on admission reporting guidelines

Section I – Conventions, General Coding Guidelines and Chapter-Specific Guidelines

Section I of the Guidelines is divided into three general areas:

A. Conventions of the ICD-10-CM
B. General Coding Guidelines
C. Chapter-Specific Coding Guidelines

Conventions

ICD-10-CM uses placeholders for codes with 7th character extensions and two types of excludes notes.

7th Characters

Certain categories have applicable 7th characters. The meanings of the 7th character are dependent on the chapters, and in some cases the categories, in which they are used. The applicable 7th characters and their definitions are found under each category or subcategory to which they apply in the Tabular List. When 7th character designations are listed under a category or subcategory, the 7th character is required for all codes in that category or subcategory. Failing to assign a 7th character results in an invalid diagnosis code that will not be recognized by payers. Because the 7th character must always be in the 7th place in the data field, codes that are not 6 characters in length require the use of the placeholder 'X' to fill the empty characters. There are a number of chapters that make use of 7th characters including:

- Chapter 7 – Diseases of the Eye and Adnexa (H00-H59). The 7th character is used for glaucoma codes to designate the stage of the glaucoma.
- Chapter 13 – Diseases of the Musculoskeletal System and Connective Tissue (M00-M99). A 7th character is required for chronic gout codes to identify the condition as with or without tophus. The 7th character is also used for stress fractures and pathological fractures due to osteoporosis, neoplastic or other disease to identify the episode of care (initial, subsequent, sequela). For subsequent encounters the 7th character also provides information on healing (routine, delayed, with nonunion, with malunion).
- Chapter 15 – Pregnancy, Childbirth, and the Puerperium (O00-O9A). The 7th character identifies the fetus for those conditions that may affect one or more fetuses in a multiple gestation pregnancy. The 7th character identifies the specific fetus as fetus 1, fetus 2, fetus 3, and so on – NOT the number of fetuses.
- Chapter 18 – Symptoms, Signs and Abnormal Clinical/Laboratory Findings, NOS (R00-R99). There are subcategories for coma that identify elements from the coma scale and the 7th character provides information on when the coma scale assessment was performed.
- Chapter 19 – Injury, Poisoning and Certain Other Consequences of External Causes (S00-T88). The 7th character is used to identify the episode of care (initial, subsequent, sequela). For fractures it identifies the episode of care, the status of the fracture as open or closed, and fracture healing for subsequent encounters as routine, delayed, nonunion, or malunion.
- Chapter 20 – External Causes of Morbidity (V01-Y99). The 7th character is used to identify the episode of care (initial, subsequent, sequela).

Examples of codes with applicable 7th characters:

- M48.46XA Fatigue fracture of vertebra, lumbar region, initial encounter for fracture
- M80.051D Age-related osteoporosis with current pathological fracture, right femur, subsequent encounter for fracture with routine healing
- O33.4XX0 Maternal care for disproportion of mixed maternal and fetal origin, fetus not applicable or unspecified. Note: 7th character 0 is used for single gestation
- O36.5932 Maternal care for other known or suspected poor fetal growth, third trimester, fetus 2
- S52.121A Displaced fracture of head of right radius, initial encounter for closed fracture
- T88.2XXS Shock due to anesthesia, sequela
- W11.XXXA Fall on and from ladder, initial encounter

Note the use of the placeholder 'X' for those codes that are less than 6 characters in the examples above.

Excludes Notes

There are two types of excludes notes in ICD-10-CM which are designated as Excludes1 and Excludes2. The definitions of the two types differ, but both types indicate that the excluded codes are independent of each other. A type 1 Excludes note, identified in the Tabular as ***Excludes1***, is a pure excludes. It means that the condition referenced is "NOT CODED HERE." For an Excludes1 the two codes are never reported together because the two conditions cannot occur together, such as a congenital and acquired form of the same condition. An exception to the Excludes1 definition is the circumstance when the two conditions are unrelated to each other. If it is not clear whether the two conditions involving an Excludes1 note are related or not, query the provider. For example, code F45.8, Other somatoform disorders, has an Excludes1 note for "sleep related teeth grinding (G47.63)," because "teeth grinding" is an inclusion term under F45.8. Only one of these two codes should be assigned for teeth grinding. However, psychogenic dysmenorrhea is also an inclusion term under F45.8, and a patient could have both this condition and sleep related teeth grinding. In this case, the two conditions are clearly unrelated to each other, and so it would be appropriate to report F45.8 and G47.63 together.

A type 2 Excludes note, identified in the Tabular as ***Excludes2***, indicates that the excluded condition is "NOT INCLUDED HERE." This means that the excluded condition is not part of the condition represented by the code, but the patient may have both conditions at the same time and the two codes may be reported together when the patient has both conditions.

General Coding Guidelines

When locating a code in ICD-10-CM, it is important to note that the 7th characters do not appear in the Alphabetic Index. The Tabular List must be checked to determine whether a 7th character should be assigned, and if so, which one to select.

Also, notice that the guideline for borderline diagnoses provides three scenarios. First, if the diagnosis provided at the time of discharge is documented as "borderline," the condition is coded as if it were confirmed. This guideline applies to both inpatient and outpatient encounters. Second, if there is a specific code listed in the Alphabetic Index for conditions documented as borderline, such as borderline diabetes, the code identified in the alphabetic index should be assigned. Third, if the documentation is unclear regarding a borderline condition, the provider/attending physician should be queried.

Finally, the assignment of a diagnosis code is based on the provider's diagnostic statement that the condition exists. The provider's statement that the patient has a particular condition is sufficient. Code assignment is not based on clinical criteria used by the provider to establish the diagnosis.

Chapter-Specific Coding Guidelines

The information that follows provides an overview of each chapter and highlights some of the more significant aspects of the guidelines. Using this overview is a good starting point for learning about ICD-1Ø-CM; however, this resource must be combined with more intensive training using the Official Guidelines for Coding and Reporting and the current code set in order to attain the proficiency needed to assign ICD-1Ø-CM codes to the highest level of specificity accurately.

Chapter 1 – Certain Infectious and Parasitic Diseases (A00-B99)

Infectious and parasitic diseases are those that are generally recognized as communicable or transmissible. Examples of diseases in Chapter 1 include: scarlet fever, sepsis due to infectious organisms, meningococcal infection, and genitourinary tract infections. It should be noted that not all infectious and parasitic diseases are found in Chapter 1. Localized infections are found in the body system chapters. Examples of localized infections found in other chapters include strep throat, pneumonia, influenza, and otitis media.

Chapter Guidelines

Guidelines in Chapter 1 relate to coding of infections that are classified in chapters other than Chapter 1 and for infections resistant to antibiotics. Note that only severe sepsis and septic shock require additional codes from Chapter 18 – Symptoms, Signs, and Abnormal Clinical Findings NOS. Exceptions include sepsis complicating pregnancy, childbirth and the puerperium and congenital/newborn sepsis which are found in Chapters 15 and 16 respectively. In order to report sepsis, severe sepsis, and septic shock accurately, both the guidelines and coding instructions in the Tabular List must be followed.

Some infections are classified in chapters based on the body system that is affected rather than in Chapter 1. For infections that are classified in other chapters that do not identify the infectious organism, it is necessary to assign an additional code from the following categories in Chapter 1:

- B95 Streptococcus, Staphylococcus, and Enterococcus as the cause of diseases classified elsewhere
- B96 Other bacterial agents as the cause of diseases classified elsewhere
- B97 Viral agents as the cause of diseases classified elsewhere

Codes for infections classified to other chapters that require an additional code from Chapter 1 are easily identified by the instructional note, "Use additional code (B95-B97) to identify infectious agent."

In addition to the extensive guidelines related to MRSA infections, there are also guidelines for reporting bacterial infections that are resistant to current antibiotics. An additional code from category Z16 is required for all bacterial infections documented as antibiotic resistant for which the infection code does not also capture the drug resistance.

Chapter 2 – Neoplasms (C00-D49)

Codes for all neoplasms are located in Chapter 2. Neoplasms are classified primarily by site and then by behavior (benign, carcinoma in-situ, malignant, uncertain behavior, and unspecified). In some cases, the morphology (histologic type) is also included in the code descriptor. Many neoplasm codes have more specific site designations and laterality (right, left, bilateral) is a component of codes for paired organs and the extremities. In addition, there are more malignant neoplasm codes that capture morphology.

Chapter Guidelines

Careful review of the guidelines related to neoplasms, conditions associated with malignancy, and adverse effects of treatment for malignancies is required. The guidelines provide instructions for coding primary malignancies that are contiguous sites versus primary malignancies of two sites where two codes are required. Another coding challenge related to neoplasms is determining when the code for personal history should be used rather than the malignant neoplasm code. For blood cancers this is further complicated because it is necessary to determine whether the code for "in remission" or "personal history" should be assigned.

Primary malignancies that overlap two or more sites that are next to each other (contiguous) are classified to subcategory/code .8 except in instances where there is a combination code that is specifically indexed elsewhere. When there are two primary sites that are not contiguous, a code is assigned for each specific site. For example, a large (primary) malignant mass in the right breast (female) that extends from the upper outer quadrant to the lower outer quadrant would be reported with code C5Ø.811 Malignant neoplasm of overlapping sites of right female breast. However, if there are two distinct lesions in the right breast (female), a Ø.5 cm lesion in the upper outer quadrant and a noncontiguous 1 cm lesion in the lower outer quadrant, two codes would be required, C5Ø.411 for the Ø.5 cm lesion in the upper outer quadrant and C5Ø.511 for the 1 cm lesion in the lower outer quadrant.

Malignant neoplasms of ectopic tissue are coded to the site of origin. For example, ectopic pancreatic malignancy involving the stomach is assigned code C25.9 Malignant neoplasm of pancreas, unspecified.

There are guidelines for anemia associated with malignancy and for anemia associated with treatment. When an admission or encounter is for the management of anemia associated with a malignant neoplasm, the code for the malignancy is sequenced first followed by the appropriate anemia code, such as D63.Ø Anemia in neoplastic disease. For anemia associated with chemotherapy or immunotherapy, when the treatment is for the anemia only, the anemia code is sequenced first followed by the appropriate code for the neoplasm and code T45.1X5- Adverse effect of antineoplastic and immunosuppressive drugs. For anemia associated with an adverse effect of radiotherapy, the anemia should be sequenced first, followed by the code for the neoplasm and code Y84.2 Radiological procedure and radiotherapy as the cause of abnormal reaction in the patient.

Code C8Ø.Ø Disseminated malignant neoplasm, unspecified is reported only when the patient has advanced metastatic disease with no known primary or secondary sites specified. It should not be used in place of assigning codes for the primary site and all known secondary sites. Cancer unspecified is reported with code C8Ø.1 Malignant (primary) neoplasm, unspecified. This code should be used only when no determination can be made as to the primary site of the malignancy. This code would rarely be used in the inpatient setting.

The guidelines provide detailed information on sequencing of neoplasm codes for various scenarios, such as sequencing for an encounter for a malignant neoplasm during pregnancy. Be sure to review the Official Guidelines for Coding and Reporting for this chapter before assigning a code.

Coding for a current malignancy versus a personal history of malignancy is dependent on two factors. First, it must be determined whether the malignancy has been excised or eradicated. Next, it must be determined whether any additional treatment is being directed to the site of the primary malignancy.

Primary malignancy excised/or eradicated?	Still receiving treatment directed at primary site?	Code Assignment
No	Yes	Use the malignant neoplasm code
Yes	Yes	Use the malignant neoplasm code
Yes	No	Use a code from category Z85 Personal history of primary or secondary malignant neoplasm

There are also guidelines related to coding for leukemia in remission versus coding for personal history of leukemia. These guidelines also apply to multiple myeloma and malignant plasma cell neoplasms. Categories with codes for "in remission" include:

- C90 Multiple myeloma and malignant plasma cell neoplasms
- C91 Lymphoid leukemia
- C92 Myeloid leukemia
- C93 Monocytic leukemia
- C94 Other leukemias of specified cell type

Coding for these neoplasms requires first determining, based on the documentation, whether or not the patient is in remission. If the documentation is unclear as to whether the patient has achieved remission, the physician should be queried.

Coding is further complicated because it must also be determined whether a patient who has achieved and maintained remission is now "cured," in which case the applicable code for personal history of leukemia or personal history of other malignant neoplasms of lymphoid, hematopoietic and related tissues should be assigned. If the documentation is not clear, the physician should be queried. Categories that report a history of these neoplasms include:

- Z85.6 Personal history of leukemia
- Z85.79 Personal history of other malignant neoplasms of lymphoid, hematopoietic and related tissues

Multiple myeloma, malignant plasma cell neoplasm, leukemia eradicated?	Still receiving treatment for the neoplasm?	Documentation that patient is currently in remission or has maintained remission and is now "cured"?	Code Assignment
No	Yes	No	Use the malignant neoplasm code with fifth character '0' for not having achieved remission or fifth character '2' for in relapse
Yes	No	In remission	Use the malignant neoplasm code with fifth character '1' for in remission
Yes	No	Maintained remission/cured	Use a code from category Z85 Personal history of primary or secondary malignant neoplasm

Chapter 3 – Diseases of the Blood and Blood-Forming Organs and Certain Disorders Involving the Immune Mechanism (D50-D89)

Diseases of the blood and blood-forming organs include disorders involving the bone marrow, lymphatic tissue, platelets and coagulation factors. Certain disorders involving the immune mechanism such as immunodeficiency disorders (except HIV/AIDS) are also classified to Chapter 3.

Chapter Guidelines

There are no chapter-specific guidelines for Chapter 3. However, Chapter 2 guidelines should be reviewed for anemia associated with a malignancy or with treatment of a malignancy.

Chapter 4 – Endocrine, Nutritional, and Metabolic Diseases (E00-E89)

Chapter 4 covers diseases and conditions of the endocrine glands which include the pituitary, thyroid, parathyroids, adrenals, pancreas, ovaries/testes, pineal gland and thymus; malnutrition and other nutritional deficiencies; overweight and obesity; and metabolic disorders such as lactose intolerance, hyperlipidemia, dehydration, and electrolyte imbalances. One of the most frequently treated conditions, diabetes mellitus, is found in this chapter.

Diabetes Mellitus

Diabetes mellitus, one of the most common diseases treated by physicians, is classified in Chapter 4 and since complications of diabetes can affect one or more body systems all physician specialties must be familiar with diabetes coding. Two significant concepts to note in diabetes coding include 1) the code categories, and 2) that single codes capture the type of diabetes, the body system affected, and specific manifestations/complications affecting that body system. Diabetes mellitus code categories include:

- E08 Diabetes mellitus due to an underlying condition. Examples of underlying conditions include:
  - Congenital rubella
  - Cushing's syndrome
  - Cystic fibrosis
  - Malignant neoplasm
  - Malnutrition
  - Pancreatitis and other diseases of the pancreas
- E09 Drug or chemical induced diabetes mellitus
- E10 Type 1 diabetes mellitus
- E11 Type 2 diabetes mellitus
- E13 Other specified diabetes mellitus. This category includes diabetes mellitus:
  - Due to genetic defects of beta-cell function
  - Due to genetic defects in insulin action
  - Postpancreatectomy
  - Postprocedural
  - Secondary diabetes not elsewhere classified

Combination codes capture information about the body system affected and specific complications/manifestations affecting that body system. Specific information regarding the following complications is captured in a single code:

- No complications
- Ketoacidosis which is further differentiated as with or without coma
- Kidney complications with specific codes for diabetic nephropathy, chronic kidney disease, and other diabetic kidney complications
- Ophthalmic complications with specific codes for diabetic retinopathy including severity (nonproliferative - mild, moderate, severe; proliferative; unspecified) and whether there is any associated macular edema; diabetic cataract; and other ophthalmic complications
- Diabetic neurological complications with specific codes for amyotrophy, autonomic (poly)neuropathy, mononeuropathy, polyneuropathy, other specified neurological complication
- Diabetic circulatory complications with specific codes for peripheral angiopathy differentiated as with gangrene or without gangrene
- Diabetic arthropathy with specific codes for neuropathic arthropathy and other arthropathy
- Diabetic skin complication with specific codes for dermatitis, foot ulcer, other skin ulcer, and other skin complication
- Diabetic oral complications with specific codes for periodontal disease and other oral complications
- Hypoglycemia which is further differentiated as with or without coma
- Hyperglycemia
- Other specified complication
- Unspecified complication

"Uncontrolled" and "not stated as uncontrolled" are not components of the diabetes codes. This does not mean that diabetes documented as uncontrolled or poorly controlled cannot be captured. Uncontrolled or poorly controlled diabetes is captured with the code for the specified type diabetes mellitus with hyperglycemia (EØ8.65, EØ9.65, E1Ø.65, E11.65, or E13.65).

Chapter Guidelines

All chapter-specific guidelines for Chapter 4 relate to coding diabetes mellitus. Some of the guidelines are discussed below.

Diabetics may have no complications, a single complication or multiple complications related to their diabetes. For diabetics with multiple complications it is necessary to report as many codes within a particular category (EØ8-E13) as are necessary to describe all the complications of the diabetes mellitus. Sequencing is based on the reason for the encounter. In addition, as many codes from each subcategory as are necessary to completely identify all of the associated conditions that the patient has should be assigned. For example, if an ophthalmologist is evaluating a patient with type 1 diabetes who has mild nonproliferative diabetic retinopathy without macular edema and diabetic cataracts, two codes from the subcategory for type 1 diabetes with ophthalmic complications must be assigned, code E1Ø.329 for mild nonproliferative retinopathy without macular edema and code E1Ø.36 to capture the diabetic cataracts.

The physician should always be queried when the type of diabetes is not documented. However, the guidelines do provide instructions for reporting diabetes when the type is not documented. Guidelines state that when the type of diabetes mellitus is not documented in the medical record the default is E11 Type 2 diabetes mellitus. In addition, when the type of diabetes is not documented but there is documentation of long-term insulin or hypoglycemic drug use, a code from category E11 Type 2 diabetes mellitus is assigned along with code Z79.4 Long-term (current) use of insulin or Z79.84, Long term (current) use of oral hypoglycemic drugs.

Diabetes mellitus in pregnancy and gestational diabetes are reported with codes from Chapter 15 Pregnancy, Childbirth, and the Puerperium as the first listed diagnosis. For pre-existing diabetes mellitus, an additional code from Chapter 4 is reported to identify the specific type and any systemic complications or manifestations.

Complications of insulin pump malfunction may involve either overdosing or underdosing of insulin. Underdosing of insulin or other medications is captured by the addition of a column and codes in the Table of Drugs and Chemicals specifically for underdosing. Underdosing of insulin due to insulin pump failure requires a minimum of three codes. The principal or first-listed diagnosis code is the code for the mechanical complication which is found in subcategory T85.6-. Fifth, sixth and seventh characters are required to capture the specific type of mechanical breakdown or failure (fifth character), the type of device which in this case is an insulin pump (sixth character '4'), and the episode of care (seventh character). The second code T38.3X6- captures underdosing of insulin and oral hypoglycemic [antidiabetic] drugs. A seventh character is required to capture the episode of care. Then additional codes are assigned to identify the type of diabetes mellitus and any associated complications due to the underdosing.

Secondary diabetes mellitus is always caused by another condition or event. Categories for secondary diabetes mellitus include: E08 Diabetes mellitus due to underlying condition, E09 Drug and chemical induced diabetes mellitus, and E13 Other specified diabetes mellitus. For patients with secondary diabetes who routinely use insulin or hypoglycemic drugs, code Z79.4 Long-term (current) use of insulin or Z79.84, Long term (current) use of oral hypoglycemic drugs should be reported. Code Z79.4 is not reported for temporary use of insulin to bring a patient's blood sugar under control during an encounter. Coding and sequencing for secondary diabetes requires review of the guidelines as well as the instructions found in the tabular. For example, a diagnosis of diabetes due to partial pancreatectomy with postpancreatectomy hypoinsulinemia requires three codes. Code E89.1 Postprocedural hypoinsulinemia is the principal or first-listed diagnosis followed by a code or codes from category E13 that identifies the type of diabetes as "other specified" and the complications or manifestations, and lastly code Z90.411 is reported for the acquired partial absence of the pancreas.

Chapter 5 – Mental and Behavioral Disorders (F01-F99)

Mental disorders are alterations in thinking, mood, or behavior associated with distress and impaired functioning. Many mental disorders are organic in origin, where disease or injury causes the mental or behavioral condition. Examples of conditions classified in Chapter 5 include: schizophrenia, mood (affective) disorders such as major depression, anxiety and other nonpsychotic mental disorders, personality disorders, and intellectual disabilities.

Chapter Guidelines

Detailed guidelines are provided for coding certain conditions classified in Chapter 5, including pain disorders with related psychological factors, and mental and behavioral disorders due to psychoactive substance use, abuse, and dependence.

Pain related to psychological disorders may be due exclusively to the psychological disorder, or may be due to another cause that is exacerbated by the psychological factors. Documentation of any psychological component associated with acute or chronic pain is essential for correct code assignment. Pain exclusively related to psychological factors is reported with code F45.41, which is the only code that is assigned. Acute or chronic pain disorders with related psychological factors are reported with code F45.42 Pain disorder with related psychological factors and a second code from category G89 Pain not elsewhere classified for documented acute or chronic pain disorder.

Mental and behavioral disorders due to psychoactive substance use are reported with codes in categories F10-F19. Both the guidelines and tabular instructions must be followed to code mental and behavioral disorders due to psychoactive substance use correctly. As with all other diagnoses, the codes for psychoactive substance use, abuse, and dependence may only be assigned based on provider documentation and only if the condition meets the definition of a reportable diagnosis. In addition, psychoactive substance use codes are reported only when the condition is associated with a mental or behavioral disorder and a relationship between the substance use and the mental or behavioral disorder is documented by the physician.

The codes for mental and behavioral disorders caused by psychoactive substance use are specific as to substance; selecting the correct code requires an understanding of the differences between use, abuse, and dependence. Physicians may use the terms use, abuse and/or dependence interchangeably; however, only one code should be reported for each behavioral disorder documented when the documentation refers to use, abuse and dependence of a specific substance. When these terms are used together or interchangeably in the documentation the guidelines are as follows:

- If both use and abuse are documented, assign only the code for abuse
- If both use and dependence are documented, assign only the code for dependence
- If use, abuse and dependence are all documented, assign only the code for dependence
- If both abuse and dependence are documented, assign only the code for dependence

Coding guidelines also provide instruction on correct reporting of psychoactive substance dependence described as "in remission." Selection of "in remission" codes in categories F10-F19 requires the physician's clinical judgment. Codes for "in remission" are assigned only with supporting provider documentation. If the documentation is not clear, the physician should be queried.

Chapter 6 – Diseases of Nervous System and Sense Organs (G00-G99)

Diseases of the Nervous System include disorders of the brain and spinal cord (the central nervous system) such as cerebral degeneration or Parkinson's disease, and diseases of the peripheral nervous system, such as polyneuropathy, myasthenia gravis, and muscular dystrophy. Codes for some of the more commonly treated pain diagnoses are also found in Chapter 6 including: migraine and other headache syndromes (categories G43-G44); causalgia (complex regional pain syndrome II) (CRPS II) (G56.4-, G57.7-); complex regional pain syndrome I (CRPS I) (G90.5-); neuralgia and other nerve, nerve root and plexus disorders (categories G50-G59); and pain, not elsewhere classified (category G89). Excluded from Chapter 6 are codes related to diseases of the eye and adnexa and ear and mastoid processes that are covered in Chapters 7 and 8 respectively.

Chapter Guidelines

Chapter-specific coding guidelines for the nervous system and sense organs cover dominant/nondominant side for hemiplegia and monoplegia, and pain conditions reported with code G89 Pain not elsewhere classified.

Codes for hemiplegia and hemiparesis (category G81) and monoplegia of the lower limb (G83.1-), upper limb (G83.2-), and unspecified limb (G83.3-) are specific to the side affected and whether that side is dominant or non-dominant. Conditions in these categories/subcategories are classified as:

- Unspecified side
- Right dominant side
- Left dominant side
- Right non-dominant side
- Left non-dominant side

When documentation does not specify the condition as affecting the dominant or non-dominant side the guidelines provide specific instructions on how dominant and non-dominant should be determined. For ambidextrous patients, the default is dominant. If the left side is affected, the default is non-dominant. If the right side is affected, the default is dominant.

There are extensive guidelines for reporting pain codes in category G89, including sequencing rules and when to report a code from category G89 as an additional code. It should be noted that pain not specified as acute or chronic, post-thoracotomy, postprocedural, or neoplasm-related is not reported with a code from category G89. Codes from category G89 are also not assigned when the underlying or definitive diagnosis is known, unless the reason for the encounter is pain management rather than management of the underlying condition. For example, when a patient experiencing acute pain due to vertebral fracture is admitted for spinal fusion to treat the vertebral fracture, the code for the vertebral fracture is assigned as the principal diagnosis, but no pain code is assigned. When pain control or pain management is the reason for the admission/encounter, a code from category G89 is assigned and in this case the G89 code is listed as the principal or first-listed diagnosis. For example, when a patient with nerve impingement and severe back pain is seen for a spinal canal steroid injection, the appropriate pain code is assigned as the principal or first-listed diagnosis. However, when an admission or encounter is for treatment of the underlying condition and a neurostimulator is also inserted for pain control during the same episode of care, the underlying condition is reported as the principal diagnosis and a code from category G89 is reported as a secondary diagnosis. Pain codes from category G89 may be used in conjunction with site-specific pain codes that identify the site of pain (including codes from chapter 18) when the code provides additional diagnostic information such as describing whether the pain is acute or chronic. In addition to the general guidelines for assignment of codes in category G89, there are also specific guidelines for postoperative pain, chronic pain, neoplasm related pain and chronic pain syndrome.

Postoperative pain may be acute or chronic. There are four codes for postoperative pain: G89.12 Acute post-thoracotomy pain, G89.18 Other acute post-procedural pain, G89.22 Chronic post-thoracotomy pain, and G89.28 Other chronic post-procedural pain. Coding of postoperative pain is driven by the provider's documentation. One important thing to remember is that routine or expected postoperative pain occurring immediately after surgery is not coded. When the provider's documentation does support reporting a code for post-thoracotomy or other postoperative pain, but the pain is not specified as acute or chronic, the code for the acute form is the default. Only postoperative pain that is not associated with a specific postoperative complication is assigned a postoperative pain code in category G89. Postoperative pain associated with a specific postoperative complication such as painful wire sutures is coded to Chapter 19, Injury, Poisoning, and Certain Other Consequences of External Causes with an additional code from category G89 to identify acute or chronic pain.

Chronic pain is reported with codes in subcategory G89.2- and includes: G89.21 Chronic pain due to trauma, G89.22 Chronic post-thoracotomy pain, G89.28 Other chronic post-procedural pain, and G89.29 Other chronic pain. There is no time frame defining when pain becomes chronic pain. The provider's documentation directs the use of these codes. It is important to note that central pain syndrome (G89.Ø) and chronic pain syndrome (G89.4) are not the same as "chronic pain," so these codes should only be used when the provider has specifically documented these conditions.

Code G89.3 is assigned when the patient's pain is documented as being related to, associated with, or due to cancer, primary or secondary malignancy, or tumor. Code G89.3 is assigned regardless of whether the pain is documented as acute or chronic. Sequencing of code G89.3 is dependent on the reason for the admission/encounter. When the reason for the admission/encounter is documented as pain control/pain management, code G89.3 is assigned as the principal or first-listed code with the underlying neoplasm reported as an additional diagnosis. When the admission/encounter is for management of the neoplasm and the pain associated with the neoplasm is also documented, the neoplasm code is assigned as the principal or first-listed diagnosis and code G89.3 may be assigned as an additional diagnosis. It is not necessary to assign an additional code for the site of the pain.

Chapter 7 – Diseases of Eye and Adnexa (H00-H59)

Chapter 7 classifies diseases of the eye and the adnexa. The adnexa includes structures surrounding the eye, such as the tear (lacrimal) ducts and glands, the extraocular muscles, and the eyelids. Coding diseases of the eye and adnexa can be difficult due to the complex anatomic structures of the ocular system. Laterality is required for most eye conditions. For conditions affecting the eyelid, there are also specific codes for the upper and lower eyelids.

Not all eye conditions are found in Chapter 7. For example, some diseases that are coded to other chapters have associated eye manifestations, such as eye disorders associated with infectious diseases (Chapter 1) and diabetes (Chapter 4). There are also combination codes for conditions and common symptoms or manifestations. Most notable are combination codes for diabetes mellitus with eye conditions (EØ8.3-, EØ9.3-, E1Ø.3-, E11.3-, E13.3-). Because the diabetes code captures the manifestation, these conditions do not require additional manifestation codes from Chapter 7.

Chapter Guidelines

All guidelines for Chapter 7 relate to assignment of codes for glaucoma. Glaucoma codes (category H4Ø) are specific to type and in most cases laterality (right, left, bilateral) is a component of the code. For some types of glaucoma, the glaucoma stage is also a component of the code. Glaucoma stage is reported using a 7th character extension as follows:

- 0 – Stage unspecified
- 1 – Mild stage
- 2 – Moderate stage
- 3 – Severe stage
- 4 – Indeterminate stage

Indeterminate stage glaucoma identified by the 7th character 4 is assigned only when the stage of the glaucoma cannot be clinically determined. If the glaucoma stage is not documented, 7th character Ø, stage unspecified, must be assigned.

Because laterality is a component of most glaucoma codes, it is possible to identify the specific stage for each eye when the type of glaucoma is the same, but the stages are different. When the patient has bilateral glaucoma that is the same type and same stage in both eyes, and there is a bilateral code, a single code is reported with the seventh character for the stage. When laterality is not a component of the code (H4Ø.1Ø-, H4Ø.11-, H4Ø.2Ø-) and the patient has the same stage of glaucoma bilaterally, only one code for the type of glaucoma with the appropriate 7th character for stage is assigned. When the patient has bilateral glaucoma but different types or different stages in each eye and the classification distinguishes laterality, two codes are assigned to identify appropriate type and stage for each eye rather than the code for bilateral glaucoma. When there is not a code that distinguishes laterality (H4Ø.1Ø-, H4Ø.11-, H4Ø.2Ø-) two codes are also reported, one for each type of glaucoma with the appropriate seventh character for stage. Should the glaucoma stage evolve during an admission, the code for the highest stage documented is assigned.

Chapter 8 – Diseases of the Ear and Mastoid Process (H60-H95)

Chapter 8 classifies diseases and conditions of the ear and mastoid process by site, starting with diseases of the external ear, followed by diseases of the middle ear and mastoid, then diseases of the inner ear. Several diseases with associated ear manifestations are classified in other chapters, such as otitis media in influenza (JØ9. X9, J1Ø.83, J11.83), measles (BØ5.3), scarlet fever (A38.Ø), and tuberculosis (A18.6).

Chapter Guidelines

Currently, there are no chapter-specific guidelines for diseases of the ear and mastoid process.

Chapter 9 – Diseases of the Circulatory System (I00-I99)

This chapter conditions affecting the heart muscle and coronary arteries, diseases of the pulmonary artery and conditions affecting the pulmonary circulation, inflammatory disease processes such as pericarditis, valve disorders, arrhythmias and other conditions affecting the conductive system of the heart, heart failure, cerebrovascular diseases, and diseases of the peripheral vascular system.

Hypertension

Essential hypertension is reported with code I1Ø Essential hypertension and is not designated as benign, malignant and unspecified. The classification presumes a causal relationship between hypertension and heart involvement and between hypertension and kidney involvement, as the two conditions are linked by the term "with" in the Alphabetic Index.

For hypertension and conditions not specifically linked by relational terms such as "with," "associated with" or "due to" in the classification, provider documentation must link the conditions in order to code them as related.

These conditions should be coded as related even in the absence of provider documentation explicitly linking them, unless the documentation clearly states the conditions are unrelated.

There are categories for hypertensive heart disease (I11), hypertensive chronic kidney disease (I12), hypertensive heart and chronic kidney disease (I13), and secondary hypertension (I15).

Myocardial Infarction

The period of time for initial treatment of acute myocardial infarction (AMI) is 4 weeks. Codes for the initial treatment should be used only for an AMI that is equal to or less than 4 weeks old (category I21). If care related to the AMI is required beyond 4 weeks, an aftercare code is reported. Codes for subsequent episode of care for AMI (category I22) are used only when the patient suffers a new AMI during the initial 4-week treatment period of a previous AMI. In addition, codes for initial treatment of acute type 1 ST elevation myocardial infarction (STEMI) are more specific to site requiring identification of the affected coronary artery. Type 1 anterior wall AMI is classified as involving the left main coronary artery (I21.Ø1), left anterior descending artery (I21.Ø2), and other coronary artery of anterior wall (I21.Ø9). A type 1 AMI of the inferior wall is classified as involving the right coronary artery (I21.11) or other coronary artery of the inferior wall (I21.19). Codes for other specified sites for type 1 STEMI include an AMI involving the left circumflex coronary artery (I21.21) or other specified site (I21.29). There is also a code for an initial type 1 STEMI of an unspecified site (I21.3). Type 1 NSTEMI (I21.4) is not specific to site. A subsequent type 1 STEMI within 4 weeks of the first AMI is classified as involving the anterior wall (I22.Ø), inferior wall (I22.1), or other sites (I22.8). There is also a code for a subsequent STEMI of an unspecified site (I22.9). No site designation is required for a subsequent type 1 NSTEMI (I22.2).

ICD-1Ø-CM provides codes for different types of myocardial infarction. Type 1 myocardial infarctions are assigned to codes I21.1-I21.4. Type 2 myocardial infarction, and myocardial infarction due to demand ischemia or secondary to ischemic balance, is assigned to code I21.A1, Myocardial infarction type 2 with a code for the underlying cause. Assign code I21.A1 when a type 2 AMI code is described as NSTEMI or STEMI. Acute myocardial infarctions type 3, 4a, 4b, 4c, and 5 are assigned to code I21.A9, Other myocardial infarction type.

Coronary Atherosclerosis

Codes for coronary atherosclerosis (I25.1-, I25.7-, I25.81-) continue to be classified by vessel type, but codes also capture the presence or absence of angina pectoris. When angina is present the codes capture the type of angina (unstable, with documented spasm, other forms of angina, unspecified angina).

Nontraumatic Subarachnoid/Intracerebral Hemorrhage

These codes are specific to site. For nontraumatic subarachnoid hemorrhage (category I6Ø), the specific artery must be identified, and laterality is also a component of the code. For example, code I6Ø.11 reports nontraumatic subarachnoid hemorrhage from right middle cerebral hemorrhage. Nontraumatic intracerebral hemorrhage (category I61) is specific to site as well with the following site designations: subcortical hemisphere, cortical hemisphere, brain stem, cerebellum, intraventricular, multiple localized, other specified, and unspecified site.

Cerebral Infarction

Codes for cerebral infarction (category I63) are specific to type (thrombotic, embolic, unspecified occlusion or stenosis), site, and laterality. The site designations require identification of the specific precerebral or cerebral artery.

Chapter Guidelines

Guidelines for coding diseases of the circulatory system cover five conditions which include hypertension, acute myocardial infarction, atherosclerotic coronary artery disease and angina, intraoperative and postprocedural cerebrovascular accident, and sequelae of cerebrovascular disease.

As was stated earlier, hypertension is not classified as benign, malignant, or unspecified. Hypertension without associated heart or kidney disease is reported with the code I1Ø Essential hypertension.

There are combination codes for atherosclerotic coronary artery disease with angina pectoris. Documentation of the two conditions are reported with codes from subcategories I25.11- Atherosclerotic heart disease of native coronary artery with angina pectoris, and I25.7- Atherosclerosis of coronary artery bypass grafts and coronary artery of transplanted heart with angina pectoris. It is not necessary to assign a separate code for angina pectoris when both conditions are documented because the combination code captures both conditions. A causal relationship between the atherosclerosis and angina is assumed unless documentation specifically indicates that the angina is due to a condition other than atherosclerosis.

Intraoperative and postprocedural complications and disorders of the circulatory system are found in category I97. Codes from category I97 for intraoperative or postprocedural cerebrovascular accident are found in subcategory I97.8-. Guidelines state that a cause and effect relationship between a cerebrovascular accident (CVA) and a procedure cannot be assumed. The physician must document that a cause and effect relationship exists. Documentation must clearly identify the condition as an intraoperative or postoperative event. The condition must also be clearly documented as an infarction or hemorrhage. Intraoperative and postoperative cerebrovascular infarction (I97.81-, I97.82-) are classified in the circulatory system chapter while intraoperative and postoperative cerebrovascular hemorrhage (G97.3-, G97.5-) are classified in the nervous system chapter.

Category I69 Sequelae of cerebrovascular disease is used to report conditions classifiable to categories I6Ø-I67 as the causes of late effects, specifically neurological deficits, which are classified elsewhere. Sequelae/late effects are conditions that persist after the initial onset of the conditions classifiable to categories I6Ø-I67. The neurologic deficits may be present at the onset of the cerebrovascular disease or may arise at any time after the onset. If the patient has a current CVA and deficits from an old CVA, codes from category I69 and categories I6Ø-I67 may be reported together. For a cerebral infarction without residual neurological deficits, code Z86.73 Personal history of transient ischemic attack (TIA) is reported instead of a code from category I69 to identify the history of the cerebrovascular disease

Acute myocardial infarction (AMI) is reported with codes that identify type I AMI as ST elevation myocardial infarction (STEMI) and non ST elevation myocardial infarction (NSTEMI). Initial acute type I myocardial infarction is assigned a code from category I21 for STEMI/NSTEMI not documented as subsequent or not occurring within 28 days of a previous myocardial infarction. All encounters for care of the AMI during the first four weeks (equal to or less than 4 full weeks/28 days), are assigned a code from category I21. Encounters related to the myocardial infarction after 4 full weeks of care are reported with the appropriate aftercare code. Old or healed myocardial infarctions are assigned code I25.2 Old myocardial infarction.

Code I21.9 Acute myocardial infarction, unspecified is the default for unspecified acute myocardial infarction or unspecified type. If only type 1 STEMI or transmural MI without the site is documented, assign code I21.3 ST elevation (STEMI) myocardial infarction of unspecified site.

Subsequent type 1 or unspecified AMI occurring within 28 days of a previous AMI is assigned a code from category I22 for a new STEMI/NSTEMI documented as occurring within 4 weeks (28 days) of a previous myocardial infarction. The subsequent AMI may involve the same site as the initial AMI or a different site. Codes in category I22 are never reported alone. A code from category I21 must be reported in conjunction with the code from I22. Codes from categories I21 and I22 are sequenced based on the circumstances of the encounter.

Do not assign code I22 for subsequent myocardial infarctions other than type 1 or unspecified. For subsequent type 2 AMI assign only code I21.A1. For subsequent type 4 or type 5 AMI, assign only code I21.A9.

Chapter 10 – Diseases of the Respiratory System (J00-J99)

Diseases of the respiratory system include conditions affecting the nose and sinuses, throat, tonsils, larynx and trachea, bronchi, and lungs. Chapter 1Ø is organized by the general type of disease or condition and by site with diseases affecting primarily the upper respiratory system or the lower respiratory system in separate sections.

Chapter Guidelines

The respiratory system guidelines cover chronic obstructive pulmonary disease (COPD) and asthma, acute respiratory failure, influenza due to avian influenza virus, and ventilator associated pneumonia.

Codes for COPD in category J44 differentiate between uncomplicated cases and those with an acute exacerbation. For coding purposes an acute exacerbation is defined as a worsening or decompensation of a chronic condition. An acute exacerbation is not the same as an infection superimposed on a chronic condition, though an exacerbation may be triggered by an infection.

Guidelines for reporting acute respiratory failure (J96.Ø-) and acute and chronic respiratory failure (J96.2-) relate to sequencing of these codes. Depending on the documentation these codes may be either the principal or first-listed diagnosis or a secondary diagnosis. Careful review of the provider documentation and a clear understanding of the guidelines including the definition of principal diagnosis are required to sequence these codes correctly.

There are three code categories for reporting influenza which are as follows: JØ9 Influenza due to certain identified influenza viruses, J1Ø Influenza due to other identified influenza virus, and J11 Influenza due to unidentified influenza virus. All codes in category JØ9 report influenza due to identified novel influenza A virus with various complications or manifestations such as pneumonia, other respiratory conditions, gastrointestinal manifestations or other manifestations. Identified novel influenza A viruses include avian (bird) influenza, influenza A/H5N1, influenza of other animal origin (not bird or swine), swine influenza. Codes from category JØ9 are reported only for confirmed cases of avian influenza and the other specific types of influenza identified in the code description. This is an exception to the inpatient guideline related to uncertain diagnoses. Confirmation does not require a positive laboratory finding. Documentation by the provider that the patient has avian influenza or influenza due other identified novel influenza A virus is sufficient to report a code from category JØ9. Documentation of "suspected," "possible," or "probable" avian influenza or other novel influenza A virus is reported with a code from category J1Ø.

Ventilator associated pneumonia (VAP) is listed in category J95 Intraoperative and postprocedural complications and disorders of respiratory system not elsewhere classified, and is reported with code J95.851. As with all procedural and postprocedural complications, the provider must document the relationship between the conditions, in this case VAP, and the procedure. An additional code should be assigned to identify the organism. Codes for pneumonia classified in categories J12-J18 are not assigned additionally for VAP. However, when a patient is admitted with a different type of pneumonia and subsequently develops VAP, the appropriate code from J12-J18 is reported as the principal diagnosis and code J95.851 is reported as an additional diagnosis

Chapter 11 – Diseases of the Digestive System (K00-K95)

Diseases of the digestive system include conditions affecting the esophagus, stomach, small and large intestines, liver, and gallbladder. Some of the most frequently diagnosed digestive system diseases and conditions, such as cholecystitis and cholelithiasis, have specific elements incorporated into the codes. For example, cholecystitis is classified as acute, chronic, or acute and chronic regardless of whether the cholecystitis occurs alone or with cholelithiasis. Combination codes for cholelithiasis with cholecystitis identify the site of the calculus as being in the gallbladder and/or bile duct and the specific type of cholecystitis. Combination codes also report cholelithiasis of the bile duct with cholangitis. There are other digestive system conditions that require an acute or chronic designation as well as more combination codes that capture diseases of the gallbladder and associated complications.

Chapter Guidelines

Currently there are no guidelines for the digestive system.

Chapter 12 – Diseases of the Skin and Subcutaneous Tissue (L00-L99)

Diseases of the skin and subcutaneous tissue include diseases affecting the epidermis, dermis and hypodermis, subcutaneous tissue, nails, sebaceous glands, sweat glands, and hair and hair follicles. Common conditions of the skin and subcutaneous tissue include boils, cellulitis, abscess, pressure ulcers, lymphadenitis, and pilonidal cysts.

Chapter Guidelines

All guidelines related to coding of diseases of the skin and subcutaneous tissue relate to pressure ulcers and non-pressure chronic ulcers. Codes from category L89 Pressure ulcer are combination codes that identify the site of the pressure ulcer as well as the stage of the ulcer. For patients with multiple pressure ulcers, multiple codes should be assigned to capture all pressure ulcer sites.

Pressure ulcer stages are based on severity. Severity is designated as:

- Stage 1 – Pressure ulcer skin changes limited to persistent focal edema
- Stage 2 – Pressure ulcer with abrasion, blister, partial thickness skin loss involving epidermis and/or dermis
- Stage 3 – Pressure ulcer with full thickness skin loss involving damage or necrosis of subcutaneous tissue
- Stage 4 – Pressure ulcer with necrosis of soft tissues through to underlying muscle, tendon, or bone
- Unstageable – Pressure ulcer stage cannot be clinically determined
- Unspecified – Pressure ulcer stage is not documented

Assignment of the pressure ulcer stage code should be guided by clinical documentation of the stage or documentation of the terms found in the Alphabetic Index. For clinical terms describing the stage that are not found in the Alphabetic Index and when there is no documentation of the stage, the provider should be queried. Assignment of the code for unstageable pressure ulcer (L89.--Ø) should be based on the clinical documentation. These codes are used for pressure ulcers whose stage cannot be clinically determined (e.g., the ulcer is covered by eschar or has been treated with a skin or muscle graft) and pressure ulcers that are documented as deep tissue injury, but not documented as due to trauma. Unstageable pressure ulcers should not be confused with the codes for unspecified stage (L89.--9). When there is no documentation regarding the stage of the pressure ulcer, the appropriate code for unspecified stage (L89.--9) is assigned.

Patients admitted with pressure ulcers documented as healing should be assigned the appropriate pressure ulcer stage code based on the documentation in the medical record. If the documentation does not provide information about the stage of the healing pressure ulcer, a code for unspecified stage is assigned. If the documentation is unclear as to whether the patient has a current (new) pressure ulcer or if the patient is being treated for a healing pressure ulcer, query the provider. No code is assigned if the documentation states that the pressure ulcer is completely healed.

If a patient is admitted with a pressure ulcer at one stage and it progresses to a higher stage, two separate codes should be assigned: one code for the site and stage of the ulcer on admission and a second code for the same ulcer site and the highest stage reported during the stay. For ulcers that were present on admission but healed at the time of discharge, assign the code for the site and stage of the pressure ulcer at the time of admission.

Non-pressure ulcers described as healing should be assigned the appropriate non-pressure ulcer code based on the documentation in the medical record. If the documentation does not provide information about the severity of the healing non-pressure ulcer, assign the appropriate code for unspecified severity. For ulcers that were present on admission but healed at the time of discharge, assign the code for the site and severity of the non-pressure ulcer at the time of admission.

If the patient is admitted with a non-pressure ulcer at one severity level and it progresses to a higher severity level, two separate codes should be assigned: one code for the site and severity level of the ulcer on admission and a second code for the same ulcer site and the highest severity level reported during the stay.

Chapter 13 – Diseases of the Musculoskeletal System and Connective Tissue (M00-M99)

Coding of musculoskeletal system and connective tissue conditions requires both precise site specificity and laterality. For example, conditions affecting the cervical spine require identification of the site as occipito-atlanto-axial, mid-cervical or cervicothoracic. Laterality is also included for most musculoskeletal and connective tissue conditions affecting the extremities. For some conditions only right and left are provided, but for other conditions that frequently affect both sides, codes for bilateral are also listed. For example, osteoarthritis of the hips has designations for bilateral primary osteoarthritis (M16.Ø), bilateral osteoarthritis resulting from hip dysplasia (M16.2), bilateral post-traumatic osteoarthritis (M16.4), and other bilateral secondary osteoarthritis of the hip (M16.6). In addition, there are 7th characters for some code categories.

7th Characters

In Chapter 13, 7th characters are required for chronic gout to identify the presence or absence of tophus (tophi). Tophi are solid deposits of monosodium urate (MSU) crystals that form in the joints, cartilage, bones, and elsewhere in the body. Chronic gout is reported with codes in category M1A. The required 7th characters identify chronic gout as without tophus (Ø) or with tophus (1).

Fatigue and compression fractures of the vertebra, stress fractures, and pathological fractures due to osteoporosis, neoplastic or other disease also require 7th characters to identify the episode of care. For fatigue fractures of the vertebra (M48.4-) and collapsed vertebra (M48.5-) the 7th character designates episode of care as: initial encounter for fracture (A), subsequent encounter for fracture with routine healing (D), subsequent encounter for fracture with delayed healing (G), and sequela (S). For age-related osteoporosis with current pathological fracture (M8Ø.Ø-), other osteoporosis with current pathological fracture (M8Ø.1-), stress fracture (M84.3-), pathological fracture not elsewhere classified (M84.4-), pathological fracture in neoplastic disease (M84.5-), and pathological fracture in other disease (M84.6-), 7th character designations include those listed for fatigue and compression fractures of the vertebra, and also include two additional 7th characters for subsequent encounter with nonunion (K) or malunion (P). The table below explains and defines the 7th characters used for fractures classified in Chapter 13.

Character	Definition	Explanation
A	Initial encounter for fracture	Use 'A' for as long as the patient is receiving active treatment for the pathologic fracture. Examples of active treatment are: surgical treatment, emergency department encounter, evaluation and treatment by a new physician
D	Subsequent encounter with routine fracture healing	For encounters after the patient has completed active treatment and when the fracture is healing normally
G	Subsequent encounter for fracture with delayed healing	For encounters when the physician has documented that healing is delayed or is not occurring as rapidly as normally expected
K	Subsequent encounter for fracture with nonunion	For encounters when the physician has documented that there is nonunion of the fracture or that the fracture has failed to heal. This is a serious fracture complication that requires additional intervention and treatment by the physician
P	Subsequent encounter for fracture with malunion	For encounters when the physician has documented that the fracture has healed in an abnormal or nonanatomic position. This is a serious fracture complication that requires additional intervention and treatment by the physician

S	Sequela	Use for complications or conditions that arise as a direct result of the pathological fracture, such as a leg length discrepancy following pathological fracture of the femur. The specific type of sequela is sequenced first followed by the pathological fracture code.

Chapter Guidelines

Chapter specific guidelines are provided for musculoskeletal system and connective tissue coding related to the following: site and laterality, acute traumatic versus chronic or recurrent musculoskeletal conditions, osteoporosis, and pathological fractures. Guidelines related to coding of pathological fractures relate to the use of 7th characters which are discussed above.

Most codes in Chapter 13 have site and laterality designations. Site represents either the bone, joint or muscle involved. For some conditions where more than one bone, joint, or muscle is commonly involved, such as osteoarthritis, there is a "multiple sites" code available. For categories where no multiple site code is provided and more than one bone, joint or muscle is involved, it is necessary to report multiple codes to indicate the different sites involved. Because some conditions involving the bones occur at the upper and/or lower ends at the joint, it is sometimes difficult to determine whether the code for the bone or joint should be reported. The guidelines indicate that when a condition involves the upper or lower ends of the bones, the site code assigned should be designated as the bone, not the joint.

Many musculoskeletal conditions are a result of a previous injury or trauma to a site, or are recurrent conditions. Musculoskeletal conditions are classified either in Chapter 13, Diseases of the Musculoskeletal System and Connective tissue or in Chapter 19, Injury, Poisoning, and Certain Other Consequences of External Causes. The table below identifies where various conditions/injuries are classified.

Condition	Chapter
Healed injury	Chapter 13
Recurrent bone, joint, or muscle condition	Chapter 13
Chronic or other recurrent conditions	Chapter 13
Current acute injury	Chapter 19

Osteoporosis is a systemic condition, meaning that all bones of the musculoskeletal system are affected. Therefore, site is not a component of the codes under category M81 Osteoporosis without current pathological fracture. The site codes under M8Ø Osteoporosis with current pathological fracture identify the site of the fracture not the osteoporosis. A code from category M8Ø, not a traumatic fracture code, should be used for any patient with known osteoporosis who suffers a fracture, even if the patient had a minor fall or trauma, if that fall or trauma would not usually break a normal, healthy bone. For a patient with a history of osteoporosis fractures, status code Z87.31, Personal history of osteoporosis fracture should follow the code from category M81.

Chapter 14 – Diseases of the Genitourinary System (N00-N99)

The Genitourinary System (or the Urogenital System) includes the organs and anatomical structures involved with reproduction and urinary excretion in both males and females. Female genitourinary disorders include pelvic inflammatory diseases, vaginitis, salpingitis and oophoritis. Common male genitourinary disorders include prostatitis, benign prostatic hyperplasia, premature ejaculation and erectile dysfunction.

Chapter Guidelines

All coding guidelines relate to coding of chronic kidney disease. The guidelines cover stages of chronic kidney disease (CKD), CKD and kidney transplant status, and CKD with other conditions.

Chapter 15 – Pregnancy, Childbirth and the Puerperium (O00-O9A)

The majority of codes for complications that occur during pregnancy require identification of the trimester.

Trimester

The trimester is captured by the fourth, fifth or sixth character. The fourth, fifth or sixth character also captures the episode of care for complications that can occur at any point in the pregnancy, during childbirth or postpartum, such as eclampsia (O15). Some complications of pregnancy that typically occur or are treated only in a single trimester such as ectopic pregnancy (OØØ) do not identify the trimester. In addition, complications that occur only during childbirth or the puerperium contain that information in the code description, such as obstructed labor due to generally contracted pelvis (O65.1) or puerperal sepsis (O85).

7th Character

A 7th character identifying the fetus is required for certain categories. Some complications of pregnancy and childbirth occur more frequently in multiple gestation pregnancies. These complications may affect one or more fetuses and require a 7th character to identify the fetus or fetuses affected by the complication. The following categories/subcategories require identification of the fetus:

- O31 Complications specific to multiple gestation
- O32 Maternal care for malpresentation of fetus
- O33.3 Maternal care for disproportion due to outlet contraction of pelvis
- O33.4 Maternal care for disproportion of mixed maternal and fetal origin
- O33.5 Maternal care for disproportion due to unusually large fetus
- O33.6 Maternal care for disproportion due to hydrocephalic fetus
- O35 Maternal care for known or suspected fetal abnormality and damage
- O36 Maternal care for other fetal problems
- O40 Polyhydramnios
- O41 Other disorders of amniotic fluid and membranes

- O60.1 Preterm labor with preterm delivery
- O60.2 Term delivery with preterm labor
- O64 Obstructed labor due to malposition and malpresentation of fetus
- O69 Labor and delivery complicated by umbilical cord complications

The 7th character identifies the fetus to which the complication code applies. For a single gestation, when the documentation is insufficient, or when it is clinically impossible to identify the fetus, the 7th character 'Ø' for not applicable/unspecified is assigned. For multiple gestations, each fetus should be identified with a number as fetus 1, fetus 2, fetus 3, etc. The fetus or fetuses affected by the condition should then be clearly identified using the number assigned to the fetus. For example, a triplet gestation in the third trimester with fetus 1 having no complications, fetus 2 in a separate amniotic sac having polyhydramnios, and fetus 3 having hydrocephalus with maternal pelvic disproportion would require reporting of the complications as follows: Fetus 1 – No codes; Fetus 2 – O4Ø.3XX2, Polyhydramnios, third trimester, fetus 2; Fetus 3 – O33.6XX3, Maternal care for disproportion due to hydrocephalic fetus, fetus 3. An additional code identifying the triplet pregnancy would also be reported. Applicable 7th characters are:

- 0 – not applicable or unspecified
- 1 – fetus 1
- 2 – fetus 2
- 3 – fetus 3
- 4 – fetus 4
- 5 – fetus 5
- 9 – other fetus

Chapter Guidelines

Chapter 15 guidelines include information covering general rules and sequencing of codes and coding rules for specific conditions. Only guidelines related to trimester, pre-existing conditions versus conditions due to pregnancy, and gestational diabetes are discussed here. Consult the Official Guidelines for Coding and Reporting for the complete Chapter 15 guidelines.

Most codes for conditions and complications of pregnancy have a final character indicating the trimester. Assignment of the final character for trimester is based on the provider's documentation which may identify the trimester or the number of weeks gestation for the current encounter. Trimesters are calculated using the first day of the last menstrual period and are as follows:

- First trimester – less than 14 weeks 0 days
- Second trimester – 14 weeks 0 days to less than 28 weeks 0 days
- Third trimester – 28 weeks 0 days to delivery

There are codes for unspecified trimester; however, these codes should be used only when the documentation is insufficient to determine the trimester and it is not possible to obtain clarification from the provider. If a delivery occurs during the admission and there is an "in childbirth" option for the complication, the code for "in childbirth" is assigned.

When an obstetric patient is admitted and delivers during that admission, the condition that prompted the admission should be sequenced as the principal diagnosis. If multiple conditions prompted the admission, sequence the one most related to the delivery as the principal diagnosis. A code for any complication of the delivery should be assigned as an additional diagnosis.

For inpatient services, when an inpatient admission encompasses more than one trimester, the code is assigned based on when the condition developed not when the discharge occurred. For example, if the condition developed during the second trimester and the patient was discharged during the third trimester, the code for the second trimester is assigned. If the condition being treated developed prior to the current admission/encounter or was a pre-existing condition, the trimester character at the time of the admission/encounter is used.

Certain categories in Chapter 15 distinguish between conditions that existed prior to pregnancy (pre-existing) and those that are a direct result of the pregnancy. Two examples are hypertension (O1Ø, O11, O13) and diabetes mellitus (O24). The physician must provide clear documentation as to whether the condition existed prior to pregnancy or whether it developed during the pregnancy or as a result of the pregnancy. Categories that do not distinguish between pre-existing conditions and pregnancy related conditions may be used for either. If a puerperal complication develops during the delivery encounter and a specific code for the puerperal complication exists, the code for the puerperal complication may be reported with codes related to complications of pregnancy and childbirth.

Gestational diabetes can occur during the second and third trimesters in women without a pre-pregnancy diagnosis of diabetes mellitus. Gestational diabetes may cause complications similar to those in patients with pre-existing diabetes mellitus. Gestational diabetes is classified in category O24 along with pre-existing diabetes mellitus. Subcategory O24.4- Gestational diabetes mellitus, cannot be used with any other codes in category O24. Codes in subcategory O24.4- are combination codes that identify the condition as well as how it is being controlled. In order to assign the most specific code, the provider must document whether the gestational diabetes is being controlled by diet or insulin. If documentation indicates the gestational diabetes is being controlled with both diet and insulin, only the code for insulin-controlled is assigned. Code Z79.4 for long-term insulin use is not reported with codes in subcategory O24.4-. Codes for gestational diabetes are not used to report an abnormal glucose tolerance test which is reported with code O99.81 Abnormal glucose complicating pregnancy, childbirth, and the puerperium.

Chapter 16 – Newborn (Perinatal) Guidelines (P00-P96)

Perinatal conditions have their origin in the period beginning before birth and extending through the first 28 days after birth. Codes from this chapter are used only on the newborn medical record, never on the maternal medical record. These conditions must originate during this period but for some conditions morbidity may not be manifested or diagnosed until later. As long as the documentation supports the origin of the condition during the perinatal period, codes for perinatal conditions may be reported. Examples of conditions included in this chapter are maternal conditions that have affected or are suspected to have affected the fetus or newborn, prematurity, light for dates, birth injuries, and other conditions originating in the perinatal period and affecting specific body systems.

Chapter Guidelines

The principal diagnosis for the birth record is always a code from Chapter 21, category Z38 Liveborn according to place of birth and type of delivery. Additional diagnoses are assigned for all clinically significant conditions identified on the newborn examination. Other guidelines relate to prematurity, fetal growth retardation, low birth weight and immaturity status.

In determining prematurity, different providers may utilize different criteria. A code for prematurity should not be assigned unless specifically documented by the physician. Two code categories are provided for reporting prematurity and fetal growth retardation, PØ5 Disorders of newborn related to slow fetal growth and fetal malnutrition and PØ7 Disorders of newborn related to short gestation and low birth weight, not elsewhere classified. Assignment of codes in categories PØ5 and PØ7 should be based on the recorded birth weight and estimated gestational age.

To identify those instances when a healthy newborn is evaluated for a suspected condition that is determined after study not to be present, assign a code from category ZØ5, Observation and evaluation of newborns and infants for suspected conditions ruled out. Do not use a code from category ZØ5 when the patient has identified signs or symptoms of a suspected problem; in such cases code the sign or symptom. A code from category ZØ5 may also be assigned as a principal or first-listed code for readmissions or encounters when the code from category Z38 code no longer applies. Codes from category ZØ5 are for use only for healthy newborns and infants for which no condition after study is found to be present. On a birth record, a code from category ZØ5 is to be used as a secondary code after the code from category Z38, Liveborn infants according to place of birth and type of delivery.

Chapter 17 – Congenital Malformations, Deformations, and Chromosomal Abnormalities (Q00-Q99)

Congenital anomalies are conditions that are present at birth. Congenital anomalies include both congenital malformations, such as spina bifida, atrial and ventricular septal heart defects, undescended testes, and chromosomal abnormalities such as trisomy 21 also known as Down's syndrome. Chapter 17 is organized with congenital anomalies, malformations, or deformations grouped together by body system followed by other congenital conditions such as syndromes that affect multiple systems with the last block of codes being chromosomal abnormalities.

Codes for congenital malformations, deformations and chromosomal abnormalities require specificity. For example, codes for encephalocele (category QØ1) are specific to site and must be documented as frontal, nasofrontal, occipital, or of other specific sites. Cleft lip and cleft palate (categories Q35-Q37) require documentation of the condition as complete or incomplete but do require more specific documentation of the site of the opening in the palate as the hard or soft palate and the location of the cleft lip as unilateral, in the median, or bilateral.

Chapter Guidelines

When a malformation, deformation, or chromosomal abnormality is documented, the appropriate code from categories QØØ-Q99 is assigned. A malformation, deformation, or chromosomal abnormality may be the principal or first-listed diagnosis or it may be a secondary diagnosis. For the birth admission the principal diagnosis is always a code from category Z38 and any congenital anomalies documented in the birth record are reported additionally. In some instances, there may not be a specific diagnosis code for the malformation, deformation, or chromosomal abnormality. In this case the code for other specified is used and additional codes are assigned for any manifestations that are present. However, when there is a specific code available to report the congenital anomaly, manifestations that are an inherent component of the anomaly should not be coded separately. Additional codes may be reported for manifestations that are not an inherent component of the anomaly. Although present at birth the congenital malformation, deformation, or chromosomal abnormality may not be diagnosed until later in life and it is appropriate to assign a code from Chapter 17 when the physician documentation supports a diagnosis of a congenital anomaly. If the congenital malformation or deformity has been corrected a personal history code should be used to identify the history of the malformation or deformity.

Chapter 18 – Symptoms, Signs, and Abnormal Clinical and Laboratory Findings, Not Elsewhere Classified (R00-R99)

Codes for symptoms, signs, abnormal results of laboratory or other investigative procedures, and ill-defined conditions without a diagnosis classified elsewhere are classified in Chapter 18. There are 7 code blocks that identify symptoms and signs for specific body systems followed by a code block for general symptoms and signs. The last 5 code blocks report abnormal findings for laboratory tests, imaging and function studies, and tumor markers. Examples of signs and symptoms related to specific body systems include: shortness of breath (RØ6.Ø2), epigastric pain (R1Ø.13), cyanosis (R23.Ø), ataxia (R27.Ø), and dysuria (R3Ø.Ø). Examples of general signs and symptoms include: fever (R5Ø.9), chronic fatigue (R53.82), abnormal weight loss (R63.4), systemic inflammatory response syndrome (SIRS) of non-infectious origin (R65.1-), and severe sepsis (R65.2-). Examples of abnormal findings include: red blood cell abnormalities (R71.-), proteinuria (R8Ø-), abnormal cytological findings in specimens from cervix uteri (R87.61-), and inconclusive mammogram (R92.2).

Combination Codes

A number of codes identify both the definitive diagnosis and common symptoms of that diagnosis. When using these combination codes, an additional code should not be assigned for the symptom. For example, R18.8 Other ascites is not reported with the combination code K7Ø.31 Alcoholic cirrhosis of the liver with ascites because code K7Ø.31 identifies both the definitive diagnosis (alcoholic cirrhosis) and a common symptom of the condition (ascites).

Coma Scale

One significant ICD-10-CM coding concept relates the coma scale codes (R40.2-). Coma scale codes can be used by trauma registries in conjunction with traumatic brain injury codes, acute cerebrovascular disease, and sequela of cerebrovascular disease codes or to assess the status of the central nervous system. These codes can also be used for other non-trauma conditions, such as monitoring patients in the intensive care unit regardless of medical condition. The coma scale codes are sequenced after the diagnosis code(s).

The coma scale consists of three elements, eye opening (R40.21-), verbal response (R40.22-), and motor response (R40.23-) and a code from each subcategory must be assigned to complete the coma scale. If all three elements are documented, codes for the individual scores should be assigned. In addition, a 7th character indicates when the scale was recorded. The 7th characters identify the time/place as follows:

- 0 – Unspecified time
- 1 – In the field (EMT/ambulance)
- 2 – At arrival in emergency department
- 3 – At hospital admission
- 4 – 24 hours or more after hospital admission

If all three elements are not known but the total Glasgow coma scale is documented, the code for the total Glasgow coma score is assigned. The Glasgow score is classified as follows:

- Glasgow score 13-15
- Glasgow score 9-12
- Glasgow score 3-8
- Other coma without documented Glasgow coma scale score or with partial score reported

Chapter Guidelines

There are a number of general guidelines for the use of symptom codes and combination codes that include symptoms as well as some specific guidelines related to repeated falls, the coma scale (discussed above), functional quadriplegia, and systemic inflammatory response syndrome (SIRS) due to non-infectious process. There are also some guidelines referencing signs and symptoms in Section II Selection of Principle Diagnosis. For example, the first guideline related to the use of symptom codes indicates that these codes are acceptable for reporting purposes when a related definitive diagnosis has not been established (confirmed) by the provider. It may also be appropriate to report a sign or symptom code with a definitive diagnosis. However, this is dependent upon whether or not the symptom is routinely associated with the definitive diagnosis/disease process. When the sign or symptom is not routinely associated with the definitive diagnosis, the codes for signs and symptoms may be reported additionally. The definitive diagnosis should be sequenced before the symptom code. When the sign or symptom is routinely associated with the disease process, the sign or symptom code is not reported additionally unless instructions in the Tabular indicate otherwise.

There is a code for repeated falls (R29.6) and another code for history of falling (Z91.81). The code for repeated falls is assigned when a patient has recently fallen and the reason for the fall is being investigated. The code for history of falling is assigned when a patient has fallen in the past and is at risk for future falls. Both codes may be assigned when the patient has had a recent fall that is being investigated and also has a history of falling.

Functional quadriplegia (R53.2) is the lack of ability to use one's limbs or to ambulate due to extreme debility, which includes severe physical disability or frailty. Functional quadriplegia is not associated with a neurologic deficit or injury and code R53.2 should not be used for cases of neurologic quadriplegia. It should only be assigned if functional quadriplegia is specifically documented in the medical record.

Guidelines related to SIRS due to a non-infectious process (R65.1-) relate to sequencing of codes. Also discussed is the need to verify whether any documented acute organ dysfunction is associated with the SIRS or due to the underlying condition that caused the SIRS or another related condition as this affects code assignment.

Chapter 19 – Injury, Poisoning, and Certain Other Consequences of External Causes (S00-T88)

Codes for injury, poisoning and certain other consequences of external causes are found in Chapter 19. One of the important characteristics to note is that injuries are organized first by body site and then by type of injury. Another is that laterality is included in the code descriptor. The vast majority of injuries to paired organs and the extremities identify the injury as the right or left. In addition, most injuries are specific to site. For example, codes for an open wound of the thorax (category S21), are specific to the right back wall, left back wall, right front wall or left front wall. For open wounds of the abdominal wall (S31.1-, S31.6-), the site must be identified as right upper quadrant, left upper quadrant, epigastric region, right lower quadrant, or left lower quadrant. Also, the vast majority of codes require a 7th character to identify episode of care. Episode of care designations have been discussed previously and many of the same designations are used in Chapter 13. However, there are some additional 7th characters for episode of care that are used only in this chapter for fractures of the long bones. Additionally, the codes for poisoning, adverse effects and toxic effects are combination codes that capture both the drug and the external cause. The Table of Drugs and Chemicals includes an underdosing column.

Application of 7th Characters

Most categories in the injury and poisoning chapter require assignment of a 7th character to identify the episode of care. For most categories there are three (3) 7th character values to select from: 'A' for initial encounter; 'B' for subsequent encounter and 'S' for sequela. Categories for fractures are an exception with fractures having 6 to 16 7th character values in order to capture additional information about the fracture including, whether the fracture is open or closed and whether the healing phase is routine or complicated by delayed healing, nonunion, or malunion. Detailed guidelines are provided related to selection of the 7th character value. Related guidelines and some examples of encounters representative of the three episodes of care 7th character values found in the majority of categories are as follows:

A Initial encounter. Initial encounter is defined as the period when the patient is receiving active treatment for the injury, poisoning, or other consequences of an external cause. An 'A' may be assigned on more than one claim. For example, if a patient is seen in the emergency department (ED) for a head injury that is first evaluated by the ED physician who requests a CT scan that is read by a radiologist and a consultation by a neurologist, the 7th character 'A' is used by all three physicians and also reported on the ED claim. If the patient required admission to an acute care hospital, the 7th character 'A' would be reported for the entire acute care hospital stay because the 7th character extension 'A' is used for the entire period that the patient receives active treatment for the injury.

D Subsequent encounter. This is an encounter after the patient has completed the active phase of treatment and is receiving routine care for the injury or poisoning during the period of healing or recovery. Unlike aftercare following medical or surgical services for other conditions which are reported with codes from Chapter 21, Factors Influencing Health Status and Contact with Health Services (Z00-Z99), aftercare for injuries and poisonings is captured by the 7th character D. For example, a patient with an ankle sprain may return to the office to have joint stability re-evaluated to ensure that the injury is healing properly. In this case, the 7th character 'D' would be assigned.

S Sequela. The 7th character extension 'S' is assigned for complications or conditions that arise as a direct result of an injury. An example of a sequela is a scar resulting from a burn.

Fracture Coding

Two things of note related to fracture coding include the 7th character extensions which differ from the 7th character extensions for other injuries, and the incorporation of information from certain fracture classification systems in the code descriptors. In fact, for open fractures of the long bones, correct assignment of the 7th character requires an understanding of the Gustilo classification system. For most fractures the 7th character extensions are the same as those detailed in Chapter 13 for pathological fractures. The designations are again summarized here and are as follows:

7th Character	Description
A	Initial encounter for closed fracture
B	Initial encounter for open fracture type
D	Subsequent encounter for fracture with routine healing
G	Subsequent encounter for fracture with delayed healing
K	Subsequent encounter for fracture with nonunion
P	Subsequent encounter for fracture with malunion
S	Sequela

For fractures of the shafts of the long bones, the 7th characters further describe the fracture as open or closed. When documentation does not indicate whether the fracture is open or closed, the default is closed. For open fractures, the 7th character also captures the severity of the injury using the Gustilo classification. The Gustilo classification applies to open fractures of the long bones including the humerus, radius, ulna, femur, tibia, and fibula. The Gustilo open fracture classification groups open fractures into three main categories designated as Type I, Type II and Type III with Type III injuries being further divided into Type IIIA, Type IIIB, and Type IIIC subcategories. The categories are defined by characteristics that include the mechanism of injury, extent of soft tissue damage, and degree of bone injury or involvement. The table below identifies key features of Gustilo fracture types. When the Gustilo classification type is not specified for an open fracture, the 7th character for open fracture type I or II should be assigned.

Type	Wound/ Contamination	Soft Tissue Damage	Type of Injury	Most Common Fracture Type(s)
Gustilo Type I	< 1 cm/Wound bed clean	Minimal	Low-energy	Simple transverse, short oblique, minimally comminuted
Gustilo Type II	> 1 cm/ Minimal or no contamination	Moderate	Low-energy	Simple transverse, short oblique, minimally comminuted
Gustilo Type III	> 1 cm/ Contaminated wound	Extensive Type IIIA – • Adequate soft tissue coverage open wound • No flap coverage required Type IIIB • Extensive soft tissue loss • Flap coverage required Type IIIC • Major arterial injury • Extensive repair • May require vascular surgeon for limb salvage	High-energy	Unstable fracture with multiple bone fragments including the following: • Open segmental fracture regardless of wound size • Gun-shot wounds with bone involvement • Open fractures with any type of neurovascular involvement • Severely contaminated open fractures • Traumatic amputations • Open fractures with delayed treatment (over 8 hours)

The applicable 7th character extensions for fractures of the shafts of the long bones are as follows:

7th Character	Description
A	Initial encounter for closed fracture
B	Initial encounter for open fracture type I or II
C	Initial encounter for open fracture type IIIA, IIIB, or IIIC
D	Subsequent encounter for closed fracture with routine healing
E	Subsequent encounter for open fracture type I or II with routine healing
F	Subsequent encounter for open fracture type IIIA, IIIB, or IIIC with routine healing
G	Subsequent encounter for closed fracture with delayed healing
H	Subsequent encounter for open fracture type I or II with delayed healing
J	Subsequent encounter for open fracture type IIIA, IIIB, or IIIC with delayed healing
K	Subsequent encounter for closed fracture with nonunion
M	Subsequent encounter for open fracture type I or II with nonunion

7th Character	Description
N	Subsequent encounter for open fracture type IIIA, IIIB, or IIIC with nonunion
P	Subsequent encounter for closed fracture with malunion
Q	Subsequent encounter for open fracture type I or II with malunion
R	Subsequent encounter for open fracture type IIIA, IIIB, or IIIC with malunion
S	Sequela

Chapter Guidelines

There are detailed guidelines for reporting of injury, poisoning and certain other consequences of external causes. The following topics are covered in the chapter-specific guidelines: application of 7th characters; coding of injuries, traumatic fractures, burns and corrosions; adverse effects, poisoning, underdosing and toxic effects; adult and child abuse, neglect and other maltreatment; and complications of care.

The principles for coding traumatic fractures are the same as coding of other injuries. Applicable 7th characters for fractures have already been discussed. Two additional guidelines of note provide default codes when certain information is not provided. A fracture not indicated as open or closed is coded as closed. A fracture not indicated as displaced or nondisplaced is coded as displaced.

Burns are classified first as corrosion or thermal burns and then by depth and extent. Corrosions are burns due to chemicals. Thermal burns are burns that come from a heat source but exclude sunburns. Examples of heat sources include: fire, hot appliance, electricity, and radiation.

The guidelines are the same for both corrosions and thermal burns with one exception: corrosions require identification of the chemical substance. The chemical substance that caused the corrosion is the first-listed diagnosis and is found in the Table of Drugs and Chemicals. Codes for drugs and chemicals are combination codes that identify the substance and the external cause or intent, so an external cause of injury code is not required. However, external cause codes should be assigned for the place of occurrence, activity, and external cause status when this information is available. The correct code for an accidental corrosion is found in the column for poisoning, accidental (unintentional).

Codes for adverse effects, poisoning, underdosing and toxic effects are combination codes that include both the substance taken and the intent. If the intent of the poisoning is unknown or unspecified, code the intent as accidental intent. The undetermined intent is only for use if the documentation in the record specifies that the intent cannot be determined. No additional external cause code is reported with these codes. Underdosing is defined as taking less of a medication than is prescribed by the provider or the manufacturer's instructions. Underdosing codes are never assigned as the principal or first-listed code. The code for the relapse or exacerbation of the medical condition for which the drug was prescribed is listed as the principal or first-listed code and the underdosing code is listed secondarily. An additional code from subcategories Z91.12- or Z91.13- should also be assigned to identify the intent of the noncompliance if known. For example, code Z91.120 would be assigned for intentional underdosing due to financial hardship.

Complications of surgical and medical care not elsewhere classified are reported with codes from categories T80-T88. However, intraoperative and post-procedural complications are reported with codes from the body system chapters. For example, ventilator associated pneumonia is considered a procedural or post-procedural complication and is reported with code J95.851 Ventilator associated pneumonia from Chapter 10 – Diseases of the Respiratory System. Complication of care code assignment is based on the provider's documentation of the relationship between the condition and the care or procedure. Not all conditions that occur following medical or surgical treatment are classified as complications. Only conditions for which the provider has documented a cause-and-effect relationship between the care and the complication should be classified as complications of care. If the documentation is unclear, query the provider. Some complications of care codes include the external cause in the code. These codes include the nature of the complication as well as the type of procedure that caused the complication. An additional external cause code indicating the type of procedure is not necessary for these codes.

Pain due to medical devices, implants, or grafts require two codes, one from the T-codes to identify the device causing the pain, such as T84.84- Pain due to internal orthopedic prosthetic devices, implants, and grafts and one from category G89 to identify acute or chronic pain due to presence of the device, implant, or graft.

Transplant complications are reported with codes from category T86. These codes should be used for both complications and rejection of transplanted organs. A transplant complication code is assigned only when the complication affects the function of the transplanted organ. Two codes are required to describe a transplant complication, one from category T86 and a secondary code that identifies the specific complication. Patients who have undergone a kidney transplant may have some form of chronic kidney disease (CKD) because the transplant may not fully restore kidney function. CKD is not considered to be a transplant complication unless the provider documents a transplant complication such as transplant failure or rejection. If the documentation is unclear, the provider should be queried. Other complications (other than CKD) that affect function of the kidney are assigned a code from subcategory T86.1- Complications of transplanted kidney and a secondary code that identifies the complication.

Chapter 20 – External Causes of Morbidity (V00-Y99)

Codes for external causes of morbidity are found in Chapter 20. External cause codes classify environmental events and other circumstances as the cause of injury and other adverse effects.

Codes in this chapter are always reported as a secondary code with the nature of the condition or injury reported as the first-listed diagnosis. Codes for external causes of morbidity relate to all aspects of external cause coding including cause, intent, place of occurrence, and activity at the time of the injury or other health condition.

External cause codes are most frequently reported with codes in Chapter 19, Injury, Poisoning and Certain Other Consequences of External Causes (S00-T88). There are conditions in other chapters that may also be due to an external cause. For example, when a condition, such as a myocardial infarction, is specifically stated as due to or precipitated by strenuous activity, such as shoveling snow, then external cause codes should be reported to identify the activity, place and external cause status. As was discussed previously, separate reporting of external cause codes is not necessary for poisoning, adverse effects, or underdosing of drugs and other substances (T36-T50), or for toxic effect of nonmedicinal substances (T51-T65), since the external cause is captured in a combination code from Chapter 19.

External Cause Coding and Third Party Payer Requirements

While not all third party payers require reporting of external cause codes, they are a valuable source of information to public health departments and other state agencies regarding the causes of death, injury, poisoning and adverse effects. In fact, more than half of all states have mandated that hospitals collect external cause data using statewide hospital discharge data systems. Another third of all states routinely collect external cause data even though it is not mandated. There are also 15 states that have mandated statewide hospital emergency department data systems requiring collection of external cause data.

These codes provide a framework for systematically collecting patient health-related information on the external cause of death, injury, poisoning and adverse effects. These codes define the manner of the death or injury, the mechanism, the place of occurrence of the event, the activity, and the status of the person at the time death or injury occurred. Manner refers to whether the cause of death or injury was unintentional/accidental, self-inflicted, assault, or undetermined. Mechanism describes how the injury occurred such as a motor vehicle accident, fall, contact with a sharp object or power tool, or being caught between moving objects. Place identifies where the injury occurred, such as a personal residence, playground, street, or place of employment. Activity indicates the activity of the person at the time the injury occurred such as swimming, running, bathing, or cooking. External cause status is used to indicate the status of the person at the time death or injury occurred such as work done for pay, military activity, or volunteer activity.

7th Characters

Most external cause codes require a 7th character to identify the episode of care. The 7th characters used in Chapter 20 are A, D and S. These external cause codes have the same definitions as they do for most injury codes found in Chapter 19. Initial encounter is defined as the period when the patient is receiving active treatment for the injury, poisoning, or other consequences of an external cause and is reported with 7th character 'A'. Subsequent encounters are identified with 7th character 'D'. This is an encounter after the active phase of treatment and when the patient is receiving routine care for the injury or poisoning during the period of healing or recovery. Sequela is identified by 7th character 'S' which is assigned for complications or conditions that arise as a direct result of an injury.

Chapter Guidelines

As with other chapter guidelines, the guidelines for Chapter 20 External Causes of Morbidity are provided so that there is standardization in the assignment of these codes. External cause codes are always secondary codes, and these codes can be used in any health care setting. An overview of the guidelines is provided here. For the complete guidelines related to external causes, the Official Guidelines for the Code Set should be consulted.

The general external cause coding guidelines relate to all external cause codes including those that describe the cause, the intent, the place of occurrence, the activity of the patient, and the patient's status at the time of the injury. External cause codes may be used with any code in ranges A00.0-T88.9 or Z00-Z99 when the health condition is due to an external cause. The most common health conditions related to external causes are those for injuries in categories S00-T88. It is appropriate to assign external cause codes to infections and diseases in categories A00-R99 and Z00-Z99 that are the result of an external cause, such as a heart attack resulting from strenuous activity.

External cause codes are assigned for the entire length of treatment for the condition resulting from the external cause. The appropriate 7th character must be assigned to identify the encounter as the initial encounter, subsequent encounter, or sequela. For conditions due to an external cause, the full range of external cause codes are used to completely describe the cause, intent, place of occurrence, activity of patient at time of event, and patient's status. No external cause code is required if the external cause and intent are captured by a code from another chapter. For example, codes for poisoning, adverse effect and underdosing of drugs, medicaments, and biological substances in categories T36-T50 and toxic effects of substances chiefly nonmedicinal as to source in categories T51-T65 capture both the external cause and the intent.

When applicable, place of occurrence (Y92), activity (Y93), and external cause status (Y99) codes are sequenced after the main external cause codes. Regardless of the number of external cause codes assigned, there is generally only one place of occurrence code, one activity code, and one external cause status code assigned. However, if a new injury should occur during hospitalization, it is allowable in such rare instances to assign an additional place of occurrence code. Codes from these categories are only assigned at the initial encounter for treatment so these codes do not make use of 7th characters. If the place, activity, or external cause status is not documented, no code is assigned. These codes do not apply to poisonings, adverse effects, misadventures, or sequela.

If the intent (accident, self-harm, assault) of the cause of an injury or other condition is unknown or unspecified, code the intent as accidental. All transport accident categories assume accidental intent. A code for undetermined intent is assigned only when the documentation in the medical record specifies that the intent cannot be determined.

The external cause of sequelae are reported using the code for the external cause with the 7th character extension 'S' for sequela. An external cause code is assigned for any condition described as a late effect or sequela resulting from a previous injury.

Chapter 21 – Factors Influencing Health Status and Contact with Health Services (Z00-Z99)

The codes for factors influencing health and contact with health services represent reasons for encounters. These codes are located in Chapter 21 and the initial alpha character is Z so they are referred to as Z-codes. While code descriptions in Chapter 21, such as Z00.110 Health examination of newborn under 8 days old may appear to be a description of a service or procedure, codes in this chapter are not procedure codes. These codes represent the reason for the encounter, service, or visit. The procedure must be reported with the appropriate procedure code.

Chapter Guidelines

There are extensive chapter-specific coding guidelines for factors influencing health status and contact with health services. The guidelines identify broad categories of Z-codes, such as status Z-codes and history Z-codes. Each of these broad categories contains categories and subcategories of Z-codes for similar types of patient visits/encounters with similar reporting rules. Z-codes may be used in any health care setting and most Z-codes may be either a principal/first-listed or secondary code depending on the circumstances of the encounter. However, certain Z-codes, such as Z02 Encounter for administrative examination, may only be used as a first-listed or principal diagnosis. An overview of the guidelines for the broad categories of Z-codes is provided here. Consult the Official Guidelines for the complete guidelines for Chapter 21.

Contact/Exposure – There are two categories of contact/exposure codes which may be reported as either a first-listed or secondary diagnosis although they are more commonly reported as a secondary diagnosis. Category Z20 indicates contact with, and suspected exposure to communicable diseases. These codes are reported for patients who do not show signs or symptoms of a disease but are suspected to have been exposed to it either by a close personal contact with an infected individual or by currently being in or having been in an area where the disease is epidemic. Category Z77 indicates contact with or suspected exposure to substances that are known to be hazardous to health. Code Z77.22 Exposure to tobacco smoke (second hand smoke) is included in this category.

Inoculations and Vaccinations – Inoculations and vaccinations may also be either the first-listed or a secondary diagnosis. There is a single code Z23 Encounter for immunization for reporting inoculations and vaccinations. A procedure code is required to capture the administration of the immunization of vaccination and to identify the specific immunization/vaccination provided.

Status – Status codes indicate that a patient is either a carrier of a disease or has the sequelae or residual of a past disease or condition. Codes for the presence of prosthetic or mechanical devices resulting from past treatment are categorized as status codes. Status codes should not be confused with history codes which indicate that a patient no longer has the condition. Status codes are not used with diagnosis codes that provide the same information as the status code. For example, code Z94.1 Heart transplant status should not be used with a code from subcategory T86.2- Complications of heart transplant because codes in subcategory T86.2- already identify the patient as a heart transplant recipient.

History (of) – There are two types of history Z-codes, personal and family. Personal history codes explain a patient's past medical condition that no longer exists and is not receiving any treatment, but that has the potential for recurrence, and therefore may require continued monitoring. Family history codes are for use when a patient has a family member who has had a particular disease that causes the patient to be at higher risk of also contracting the disease.

Screening – Screening is testing for disease or disease precursors in seemingly well individuals so that early detection and treatment can be provided for those who test positive for the disease (e.g. screening mammogram). The testing of a person to rule out or confirm a suspected diagnosis because the patient has some sign or symptom is a diagnostic examination not a screening and a sign or symptoms code is used to explain the reason for the visit.

Observation – There are three observation categories (Z03-Z05) for use in very limited circumstances when a person is being observed for a suspected condition that has been ruled out. The observation codes are to be used as principal diagnosis only. The only exception to this is when the principal diagnosis is required to be a code from category Z38, Liveborn infants according to place of birth and type of delivery. Then a code from category Z05, Encounter for observation and evaluation of newborn for suspected diseases and conditions ruled out, is sequenced after the Z38 code. Additional codes may be used in addition to the observation code, but only if they are unrelated to the suspected condition being observed.

Aftercare – Aftercare visit codes cover situations when the initial treatment of a disease has been performed and the patient requires continued care during the healing or recovery phase, or for the long-term consequences of the disease. Aftercare for injuries is not reported with Z-codes. The injury code is reported with the appropriate 7th character for subsequent care. Aftercare Z-codes/categories include Z42-Z49 and Z51. Z51 includes other aftercare and medical care.

Follow-up – The follow-up Z-codes are used to explain continuing surveillance following completed treatment of a disease, condition, or injury. They imply that the condition has been fully treated and no longer exists. Do not confuse follow-up codes with aftercare codes or injury codes with 7th character 'S'. Follow-up Z-codes/categories include: Z08-Z09 and Z39.

Donor – Codes in category Z52 Donors of organs and tissues are used for living individuals who are donating blood or other body tissue. These codes are only for individuals donating for other individuals, not for self-donations. The only exception to this rule is blood donation. There are codes for autologous blood donation in subcategory Z52.01-. Codes in category Z52 are not used to identify cadaveric donations.

Counseling – Counseling Z-codes are used when a patient or family member receives assistance in the aftermath of an illness or injury or when support is required in coping with family or social problems. They are not used in conjunction with a diagnosis code when the counseling component of care is considered integral to standard treatment. Counseling Z-codes/categories include: Z30.Ø-, Z31.5, Z31.6-, Z32.2-Z32.3, Z69-Z71, and Z76.81.

Encounters for Obstetrical and Reproductive Services – Routine prenatal visits and postpartum care are reported with Z-codes. Codes in category Z34 Encounter for supervision of normal pregnancy are always the first-listed diagnosis and are not to be used with any other code from the OB chapter. Codes in category Z3A Weeks of gestation may be assigned to provide additional information about the pregnancy. Codes in category Z37 Outcome of delivery should be included on all maternal delivery records. Outcome of delivery codes are always secondary codes and are never used on the newborn record. Examples of other conditions reported with Z-codes include family planning, and procreative management and counseling. Codes in category Z3A, Weeks of gestation, may be assigned to provide additional information about the pregnancy. Category Z3A codes should not be assigned for pregnancies with abortive outcomes (categories OØØ-OØ8), elective termination of pregnancy (code Z33.32), nor for postpartum conditions, as category Z3A is not applicable to these conditions. The date of the admission should be used to determine weeks of gestation for inpatient admissions that encompass more than one gestational week.

Newborns and Infants – There are a limited number of Z-codes for newborns and infants. Category Z38 Liveborn infants according to place of birth and type of delivery is always the principle diagnosis on the birth record. Subcategory ZØØ.11- Newborn health examination reports routine examination of the newborn. A 6th character is required that identifies the age of the newborn as under 8 days old (Ø) or 8-28 days old (1).

Routine and Administrative Examinations – An example of a routine examination is a general check-up. An example of an examination for administrative purposes is a pre-employment physical. These Z-codes are not to be used if the examination is for diagnosis of a suspected condition or for treatment purposes. In such cases the diagnosis code is used. During a routine exam, should a diagnosis or condition be discovered, it should be coded as an additional code. Some of the codes for routine health examinations distinguish between "with" and "without" abnormal findings. An examination with abnormal findings refers to a condition/diagnosis that is newly identified or a change in severity of a chronic condition (such as uncontrolled hypertension, or an acute exacerbation of chronic obstructive pulmonary disease) during a routine physical examination. Code assignment depends on the information that is known at the time the encounter is being coded. For example, if no abnormal findings were found during the examination, but the encounter is being coded before the test results are back, it is acceptable to assign the code for "without abnormal findings" diagnosis. When assigning a code for "with abnormal findings," additional codes should be assigned to identify the specific abnormal findings. Z-codes/categories for routine and administrative examinations include ZØØ-ZØ2 (except ZØ2.9) and Z32.Ø-.

Miscellaneous Z-Codes – The miscellaneous Z-codes capture a number of other health care encounters that do not fall into one of the other categories. Certain of these codes identify the reason for the encounter; others are for use as additional codes that provide useful information on circumstances that may affect a patient's care and treatment. Miscellaneous Z-codes/categories are as follows: Z28 (except Z28.3), Z29, Z4Ø-Z41 (except Z41.9) Z53, Z55-Z6Ø, Z62-Z65, Z72-Z75 (except Z74.Ø1 and only when the documentation specifies that the patient has an associated problem), Z76.Ø, Z76.3, Z76.5, Z91.1-, Z91.83, Z91.84-, and Z91.89.

Introduction to ICD-10-PCS

ICD-1Ø-PCS is a procedure coding system used to report inpatient procedures beginning October 1, 2Ø15. As inpatient procedures associated with changing technology and medical advances are developed, the structure of ICD-1Ø-PCS allows them to be easily incorporated as unique codes. This is possible because during the development phase, four attributes were identified as key components for the structure of the coding system – completeness, expandability, multiaxial, and standardized terminology. These components are defined as follows:

Completeness

Completeness refers to the ability to assign a unique code for all substantially different procedures, including unique codes for procedures that can be performed using different approaches.

Expandability

Expandability means the ability to add new unique codes to the coding system in the section and body system where they should reside.

Multiaxial

Multiaxial signifies the ability to assign codes using independent characters around each individual axis or component of the procedure. For example, if a new surgical approach is used for one of the root operations on a specific body part, a value for the new surgical approach can be added to the approach character without a need to add or change other code characters.

Standardized Terminology

ICD-1Ø-PCS includes definitions of the terminology used. While the meaning of specific words varies in common usage, ICD-1Ø-PCS does not include multiple meanings for the same term, and each term is assigned a specific meaning. For example, the term "excision" is defined in most medical dictionaries as surgical removal of part or all of a structure or organ. However, in ICD-1Ø-PCS excision is defined as "cutting out or off, without replacement, a portion of a body part." If all of a body part is surgically removed without replacement, the procedure is defined as 'resection' in ICD-1Ø-PCS.

General Development Principles

In the development of ICD-10-PCS, several general principles were followed:

Diagnostic Information is Not Included in Procedure Description

When procedures are performed for specific diseases or disorders, the disease or disorder is not contained in the procedure code. There are no codes for procedures exclusive to aneurysms, cleft lip, strictures, neoplasms, hernias, etc. The diagnosis codes, not the procedure codes, specify the disease or disorder.

Not Otherwise Specified (NOS) Options are Restricted

Certain NOS options made available in ICD-10-PCS are restricted to the uses laid out in the ICD-10-PCS draft guidelines. A minimal level of specificity is required for each component of the procedure.

Limited Use of Not Elsewhere Classified (NEC) Option

Because all significant components of a procedure are specified, there is generally no need for an NEC code option. However, limited NEC options are incorporated into ICD-10-PCS where necessary. For example, new devices are frequently developed, and therefore it is necessary to provide an "Other Device" option for use until the new device can be explicitly added to the coding system.

Level of Specificity

All procedures currently performed can be specified in ICD-10-PCS. The frequency with which a procedure is performed was not a consideration in the development of the system. Rather, a unique code is available for variations of a procedure that can be performed.

ICD-10-PCS Structure

ICD-10-PCS has a seven character alphanumeric code structure. Each character contains up to 34 possible values. Each value represents a specific option for the general character definition (e.g., stomach is one of the values for the body part character). The ten digits 0-9 and the 24 letters A-H, J-N and P-Z may be used in each character. The letters O and I are not used in order to avoid confusion with the digits 0 and 1.

Procedures are divided into sections that identify the general type of procedure (e.g., medical and surgical, obstetrics, imaging). The first character of the procedure code always specifies the section. The sections are shown in Table 1.

Table 1: ICD-10-PCS Sections

0	Medical and Surgical
1	Obstetrics
2	Placement
3	Administration
4	Measurement and Monitoring
5	Extracorporeal or Systemic Assistance and Performance
6	Extracorporeal or Systemic Therapies
7	Osteopathic
8	Other Procedures
9	Chiropractic
B	Imaging
C	Nuclear Medicine
D	Radiation Therapy
F	Physical Rehabilitation and Diagnostic Audiology
G	Mental Health
H	Substance Abuse Treatment
X	New Technology

The second through seventh characters mean the same thing within each section, but may mean different things in other sections. In all sections, the third character specifies the general type of procedure performed (e.g., resection, transfusion, fluoroscopy), while the other characters give additional information such as the body part and approach. In ICD-10-PCS, the term "procedure" refers to the complete specification of the seven characters.

ICD-10-PCS Format

The ICD-10-PCS is made up of three separate parts:

- Tables
- Index
- List of codes

The Index allows codes to be located by an alphabetic lookup. The index entry refers to a specific location in the Tables. The Tables must be used in order to construct a complete and valid code. The List of Codes provides a comprehensive listing of all valid codes, with a complete text description accompanying each code.

Tables in ICD-10-PCS

Each page in the Tables is composed of rows that specify the valid combinations of code values. ***Table 2*** is an excerpt from the ICD-10-PCS tables. In the system, the upper portion of each table specifies the values for the first three characters of the codes in that table. In the administration section, the first three characters are the section, the body system and the root operation.

In ICD-10-PCS, the values 3E0 specify the section Administration (3), the body system Physiological Systems/Anatomical Region (E), and the root operation Introduction (0). As shown in Table 2, the root operation (i.e., introduction) is accompanied by its definition. The lower portion of the table specifies all the valid combinations of the remaining characters four through seven. The four columns in the table specify the last four characters. In the administration section they are labeled Body System, Approach, Substance and Qualifier, respectively. Each row in the table specifies the valid combination of values for characters four through seven. The Tables contain only those combinations of values that result in a valid procedure code.

Table 2: Excerpt from the ICD-10-PCS tables

3 Administration **E Physiological Systems/Anatomical Regions** **0 Introduction: Putting in or on a therapeutic, diagnostic, nutritional, physiological, or prophylactic substance except blood or blood products**			
Character 4	**Character 5**	**Character 6**	**Character 7**
T Peripheral Nerves and Plexi X Cranial Nerves	3 Percutaneous	3 Anti-inflammatory B Anesthetic Agent T Destructive Agent	Z No Qualifier

There are 6 code options for the table above:

3E0T33Z	Introduction (injection) anti-inflammatory peripheral nerves and plexi
3E0T3BZ	Introduction (injection) anesthetic agent peripheral nerves and plexi
3E0T3TZ	Introduction (injection) destructive agent peripheral nerves and plexi
3E0X33Z	Introduction (injection) anti-inflammatory peripheral cranial nerves
3E0X3BZ	Introduction (injection) anesthetic agent cranial nerves
3E0X3TZ	Introduction (injection) destructive agent cranial nerves

ICD-10-CM Anatomy and Physiology

Section 1. Nervous System

Chapter Objectives

After studying this chapter, you should be able to:

- Describe the function of the nervous system
- Classify nervous system organs into central and peripheral divisions
- Explain the functions of neuroglia and neurons
- Describe the different types of neuroglial cells
- Identify the two principle tissues types in the nervous system
- Identify the two principle divisions of the nervous system
- Identify central nervous system organs
- Identify three principle areas of the brain
- Identify the protective coverings of the brain and spinal cord
- Identify the two principle divisions of the peripheral nervous system
- Identify peripheral nervous system organs
- Describe nervous system functions
- Explain how nerve impulses are initiated and transmitted
- Describe a reflex arc
- Define the terms irritability and conductivity as they pertain to transmission of nerve impulses
- Describe a variety of diseases and disease processes affecting the nervous system
- Identify how these diseases and disease processes affect and alter nervous system function
- Assign ICD-10-CM codes to diseases, injuries, and other conditions affecting the nervous system
- Define the following terms: central nervous system, peripheral nervous system, neuron, neuroglia, nerve root, nerve, ganglion, nerve reflex, meninges, dura mater, pia mater, arachnoid, encephalon, intracranial, extracranial, extradural, subdural, intraspinal

Overview

The nervous system is the control, regulatory, and communication center of the body. Important functions that the nervous system performs are the maintenance of homeostasis, the stimulation of movement, and the ability to analyze and respond to the world around each person. The nervous system senses both changes within the body, also referred to as the internal environment, and changes around the body, also referred to as the external environment. It then interprets these changes, integrates them, decides on a course of action, and then elicits a response by sending impulses through the body.

The nervous system is divided into two portions – the central nervous system or CNS, and the peripheral nervous system or PNS. The nervous system is composed of four principle organs. These include the brain, spinal cord, nerves, and ganglia. The brain and spinal cord are part of the central nervous system and the nerves and ganglia are part of the peripheral nervous system. The peripheral nervous system has two divisions – the somatic nervous system and the autonomic nervous system.

The somatic nervous system contains nerve fibers that connect the central nervous system with skeletal muscles and skin. The autonomic nervous system contains nerve fibers that connect the central nervous system with cardiac muscle, smooth muscle, and glands.

Cells

The nervous system is composed of two cell types, neurons and neuroglia.

Neurons

Neurons, also called nerve cells, are the cells that conduct impulses from one part of the body to another. These cells have three distinct portions: a cell body, dendrites, and an axon. The dendrites pick up a stimulus and transmit that stimulus to the cell body. The axon picks up the stimulus from the cell body and conducts it away from the cell body to another neuron or another organ of the body.

Neurons are subdivided based on their function into sensory neurons and motor neurons. Sensory neurons carry impulses from receptors in the skin and sense organs to the spinal cord and brain. Motor neurons, also called efferent neurons, carry impulses from the brain and spinal cord to muscles or glands.

Neuron

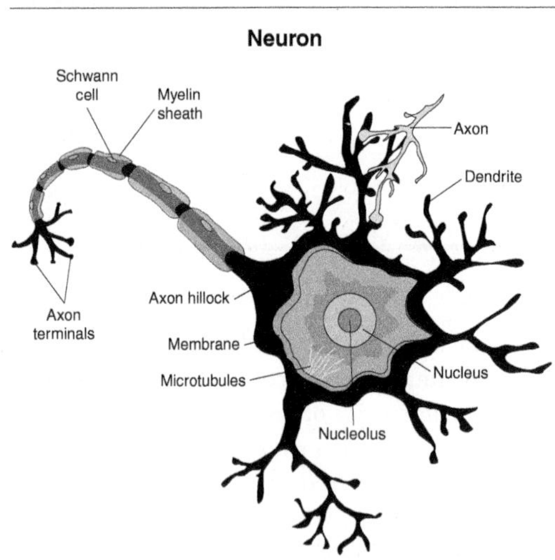

Neuroglia

Neuroglia, also called glial cells, form the connective tissue of the nervous system. These cells combine to form a thick tissue that supports the nerve cells and nerve tissue. In the central nervous system there are four primary types of glial cells, including oligodendrocytes, astrocytes, microglia, and ependymal cells. In the peripheral nervous system, connective tissue cells that serve the same function as oligodendrocytes are called Schwann cells.

Neuroglia are of special interest to the medical coder because they are a common source of tumors of the nervous system. Two common types of central nervous system connective tissue tumors are astrocytomas and gliomas. Schwannomas or neurilemomas are connective tissue tumors found in the peripheral nervous system.

Oligodendrocytes

Oligodendrocytes in the central nervous system are connective tissue cells that form rows of semirigid tissue between neurons in the brain and spinal cord. The oligodendrocytes produce a thick, fatty sheath called the myelin sheath that covers the neurons of the central nervous system. These myelinated nerve fibers in the brain and spinal column make up the white matter in the central nervous system.

Astrocytes

Astrocytes are star-shaped cells that wrap around nerve cells to form a supporting network around the neurons in the brain and spinal cord. They also attach neurons to blood vessels.

Microglia

Microglia are specialized neuroglia that protect the nervous system from disease by engulfing pathogens and clearing away debris. This process is known as phagocytosis.

Schwann cells

The axons of some neurons in the peripheral nervous system are also covered with a myelin sheath formed by flattened Schwann cells. Each Schwann cell produces a portion of the myelin sheath by wrapping itself around the axon and encircling a portion of axon multiple times. The cytoplasm is forced into the inside layer of the Schwann cell forming the myelin sheath. The cell membrane of the Schwann cell wraps itself around the neuron forming a delicate, continuous sheath called the neurilemma that encloses the myelin and assists in the regeneration of injured axons. Other axons are not covered by Schwann cells and these are called unmyelinated axons.

Schwann cell wrapped around axon of neuron

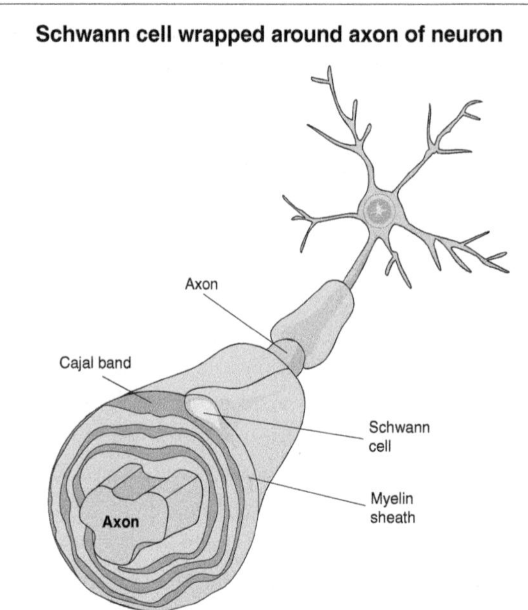

Tissues

Nervous system organs are composed of two principle tissues, nervous and connective tissue. The brain, spinal cord, and nerves are composed of nervous tissue. Nervous tissue is composed of neurons that generate and conduct impulses. The connective tissue is composed of neuroglia. Nervous system connective tissue is a nonconductive tissue that supports and insulates the nervous tissue.

Neural tissue is generally neatly arranged together with the axons of a group of neurons all pointed in the same direction. Myelinated axons which are white in color form the white matter of the brain. Nerve cell bodies and dendrites or unmyelinated axons form the gray matter.

Organs

The nervous system is divided into two parts, the central nervous system (CNS) and the peripheral nervous system (PNS). The CNS is comprised of the brain and spinal cord. The PNS consists of nerves, nerve plexuses, and ganglia.

Brain

The brain is the control center of the body, and along with the endocrine system, it is responsible for maintaining homeostasis. Studying the regions of the brain can be quite confusing as there are a number of ways of dividing brain structures. Some references divide the brain into three principle regions, the forebrain (containing the cerebrum, thalamus, hypothalamus, and pituitary gland), midbrain, and hindbrain (containing the cerebellum, medulla oblongata, and pons). Other references discuss the major structures which include the cerebrum, cerebellum and brainstem (which contains the medulla oblongata, pons, and midbrain). Still others refer to the prosencephalon (forebrain), mesencephalon (midbrain) and rhombencephalon (hindbrain). The prosencephalon is then further subdivided into the telencephalon (region containing the cerebrum) and diencephalon (region containing the thalamus, hypothalamus, and pituitary gland). In this section, the following structures will be described: cerebrum, thalamus, hypothalamus, cerebellum, and brainstem.

Brain

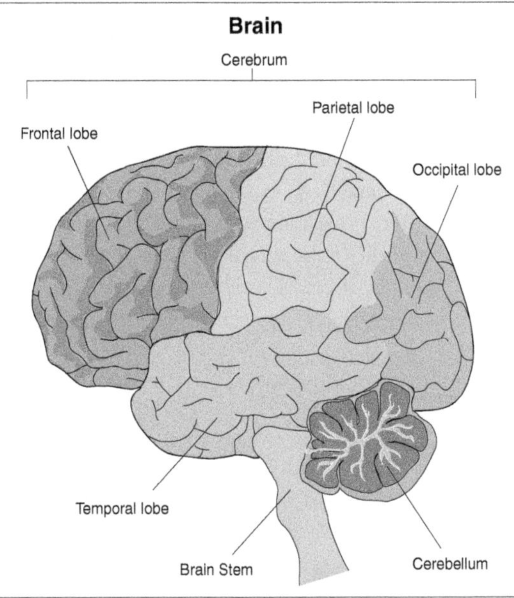

Cerebrum

The cerebrum is the largest portion of the brain. The surface is composed of gray matter which is referred to as the cerebral cortex. The cortex consists of six layers of nerve cell bodies and contains millions of cells. Under the cortex is the cerebral white matter which is composed of the myelinated axons of millions of nerve cells.

As the brain forms during embryonic development, the cortex is much larger than the white matter. As the brain grows, the cortex rolls and folds upon itself creating upfolds called gyri or convolutions, deep downfolds called fissures, and shallow downfolds called sulci. The most prominent fissure is called the longitudinal fissure because it almost completely separates the brain into two halves called the right and left hemispheres. They are connected by a large bundle of transverse nerve cell fibers called the corpus callosum. The right and left cerebral hemispheres are each divided into four lobes which include the frontal lobe, parietal lobe, temporal lobe, and occipital lobe.

The myelinated nerve fibers of the white matter are arranged to transmit impulses in three directions. They are named based on the direction of the nerve impulses they transmit. Association fibers transmit impulses from one part of the cerebral cortex to another within the same hemisphere. Commissural fibers transmit impulses from one hemisphere to another. Projection fibers transmit impulses from the cerebrum to other parts of the brain and spinal cord.

The functions of the cerebrum are numerous and complex but they can be divided into three general functions that include motor functions, which govern muscle movement; sensory functions, which interpret sensory input; and association functions, which are concerned with emotional and intellectual processes.

Brain cells within the cerebrum generate electrical potentials called brain waves. These brain waves pass through the skull and can be detected with sensors called electrodes. Brain waves can be recorded and graphed using an electroencephalograph. The recording is called an electroencephalogram or EEG.

An EEG is used in a clinical setting for many different purposes:

- to diagnose conditions such as epilepsy or narcolepsy
- to determine the cause of nontraumatic loss of consciousness or dementia
- to determine the extent of brain injury following trauma
- to help determine whether a behavior or condition is the result of a physiological condition of the brain, spinal cord, or nerves or whether it is a mental health condition

Thalamus

The thalamus is a large oval structure that lies above the midbrain. One function of the thalamus is to relay all sensory impulses excluding those for smell to the cerebral cortex. A second function is to interpret and produce conscious recognition of pain. It also controls sleep and awake states.

Hypothalamus

The hypothalamus is located below the thalamus. Even though it is relatively small in size, it controls many body activities related to homeostasis. Key functions of the hypothalamus include:

- Controlling and integrating functions of the autonomic nervous system, such as:
  - Heartbeat
  - Movement of food through the digestive tract
  - Contraction of the urinary bladder
- Receiving and interpreting sensory impulses from the viscera
- Monitoring and working with the endocrine system to maintain homeostasis
- Controlling body temperature
- Responding to changes in mental states such as fear by initiating changes in heart rate, respiratory rate, etc.
- Regulating food intake by stimulating the hunger and satiety sensations
- Regulating fluid intake by stimulating the thirst sensation
- Regulating biorhythms that control wake and sleep patterns

Cerebellum

The cerebellum is located below the posterior aspect of the cerebrum and is separated from it by the transverse fissure. Like the cerebrum, the cerebellum has two hemispheres that are separated by a structure called the vermis. The cerebellum is composed of both gray matter and white matter and attached to the brain stem by paired bundles of fibers called the cerebellar peduncles. The cerebellum is the motor area of the brain and controls unconscious movements in the skeletal muscles that are required for coordination, posture, and balance.

Injury to the cerebellum caused by trauma or disease is characterized by certain symptoms such as lack of muscle coordination, also referred to as ataxia. To examine a patient for ataxia, the physician may ask the patient to hold the arms out to the side and then touch the index finger to the nose. Ataxia involving the speech muscles may be indicated by a change in speech pattern. Cerebellar damage may also affect gait causing the patient to stagger or exhibit other abnormal walking movements.

Thalamus and Brainstem

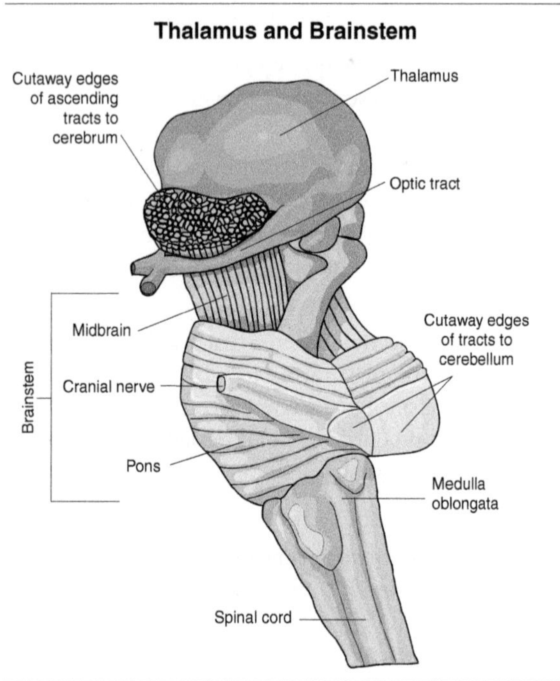

Brain Stem

The brain stem consists of the following structures:

- Medulla oblongata
- Pons
- Midbrain

Medulla oblongata

The medulla oblongata is the most inferior portion of the brain and also forms the upper portion of the spinal cord. One primary function of the medulla is the conduction of nerve impulses between the spinal cord and brain. Two sets of structures in the medulla form the principle conduction pathways. These include the two pyramids on the ventral aspect of the medulla and two nuclei on the dorsal aspect. The two pyramids are composed of motor tracts running from the cortex to the spinal cord. At the junction of the two pyramids are nerve fibers. Some nerve fibers that originate in one side cross to the opposite side, which is why motor areas in the right cerebral cortex control voluntary movement on the left side of the body and those in the left cerebral cortex control voluntary movement on the right side of the body. The two nuclei, called the nucleus gracilis and nucleus cuneatus, receive sensory impulses from the ascending tracts of the spinal cord. The nuclei then relay these impulses to the opposite side of the medulla. Impulses received on one side of the body are processed on the opposite side of the brain.

Four pairs of cranial nerves also originate in the medulla oblongata. These include the glossopharyngeal (cranial nerve IX), the vagus nerve (X), the accessory nerve (XI), and the hypoglossal nerve (XII).

Three vital reflex centers are also located in the medulla. The cardiac center regulates heartbeat; the respiratory center adjusts the rate and depth of breathing; and the vasoconstrictor center regulates the diameter of the blood vessels.

Given the vital activities performed by the medulla, it is not surprising that trauma to this area can be fatal. Non-fatal injuries may cause cranial nerve malfunctions, paralysis or loss of sensation, or respiratory irregularities.

Pons

The pons lies above the medulla and anterior to the cerebellum. Pons means bridge and just as its name implies it serves as a bridge between the spinal cord and the brain. It also connects the various parts of the brain with each other. Four cranial nerves originate in the pons. These include the trigeminal nerve (cranial nerve V), abducens (VI), facial nerve (VII), and vestibulocochlear nerve (VIII).

Midbrain

The midbrain is a short, constricted structure that connects the pons and the cerebellum. Two cranial nerves originate in the midbrain, the oculomotor nerve (III) and the trochlear nerve (IV).

Spinal Cord

The spinal cord begins as a continuation of the medulla extending from the foramen magnum to the level of the second lumbar vertebra. The diameter of the spinal cord is enlarged in two regions where spinal nerves that supply the extremities are contained. The first enlarged area is in the cervical region and contains nerves that supply the upper extremities. It extends from the fourth cervical vertebra to the first thoracic vertebra. The second enlarged area is in the lumbar region and contains nerves that supply the lower extremities. This enlarged area is widest at the T12-L1 interspace. The spinal cord then tapers, ending in the conus medullaris at the second lumbar vertebra. Spinal nerves arise from the conus medullaris. These spinal nerves which look like coarse strands of hair do not leave the vertebral canal immediately. They run through the subarachnoid space and exit at the interspaces between the lumbar vertebrae. This bundle of nerve roots in the lumbosacral region is also referred to as the cauda equina, which is Latin for horse's tail.

Spinal column with spinal nerves

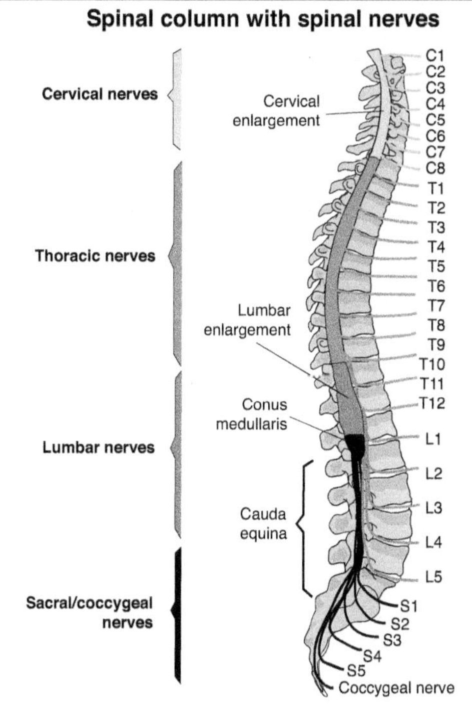

The term cauda or tail is one that medical coders should recognize as the directional term caudad is frequently seen in operative, radiology, and other medical reports. Caudad means toward the tail or situated in relation to a specific reference point. In contrast, the term cephalad is a directional term meaning toward the head.

Meninges

The brain and spinal cord are delicate vital structures that are protected by three membranes called the meninges. The outer membrane is composed of a tough fibrous tissue called the dura mater. The middle membrane is a delicate fibrous tissue called the arachnoid. The inner membrane, called the pia mater, is a transparent layer containing blood vessels and is adherent to the surfaces of the brain and spinal cord.

The medical coder should be familiar with the meninges because they are referenced when coding certain types of injuries, such as a subdural or subarachnoid hemorrhage, and infection or inflammation, such as viral or bacterial meningitis.

Cerebrospinal Fluid

The central nervous system is further protected by cerebrospinal fluid contained in the space between the arachnoid membrane and pia mater. This space is also called the subarachnoid space. The cerebrospinal fluid circulates around the brain and spinal cord and through the ventricles of the brain. The ventricles are cavities within the brain that communicate with each other and with the central canal of the spinal cord. Cerebrospinal fluid is continuously formed within the ventricles and then drains into the subarachnoid spaces.

Obstruction of the flow of cerebrospinal fluid can cause hydrocephalus which may be congenital or acquired.

Brain ventricles and CSF flow

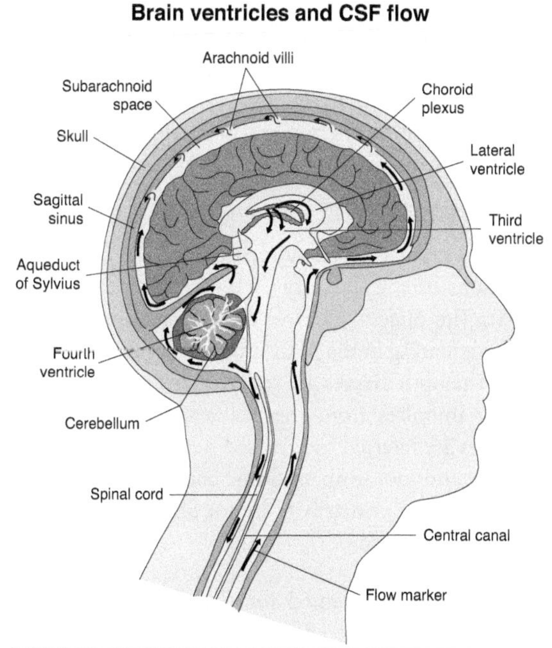

Peripheral Nervous System

The peripheral nervous system (PNS) is essentially all neural tissue that lies outside of the brain and spinal cord. The PNS is subdivided into somatic and autonomic systems.

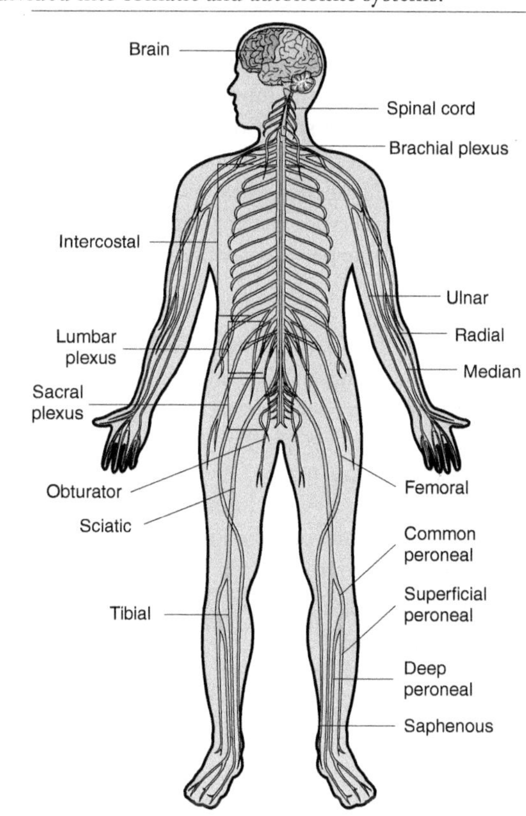

Somatic Nervous System

The somatic nervous system is composed of motor fibers that run from the CNS to the skeletal muscles and sensory fibers that run from the skeletal muscles, skin, and viscera to the CNS.

The somatic nervous system consists of 12 pairs of cranial nerves that originate from the brain and 31 pairs of spinal nerves that originate from the spinal cord. Cranial nerves are distributed primarily to the head, neck, and viscera of the thorax and abdomen, while spinal nerves are primarily distributed to the arms, legs, and trunk.

Cranial Nerves

Ten of the 12 cranial nerves originate from the brain stem. The two exceptions are the olfactory nerves (cranial nerve I) and optic nerves (II). The olfactory nerves consist of numerous olfactory filaments originating in the nasal mucosa that convey impulses to the brain. The optic nerves are really extensions of the forebrain and convey impulses from the retina to the forebrain. Some cranial nerves are referred to as mixed nerves in that they contain both sensory and motor fibers. Some contain only sensory fibers while others consist primarily of motor fibers.

Spinal Nerves

The spinal nerves are named for the region of the vertebral column from which they emerge. There are 8 pairs of cervical nerves, 12 pairs of thoracic nerves, 5 pairs of lumbar nerves, 5 pairs of sacral nerves, and 1 pair of coccygeal nerves. Each spinal nerve is a mixed nerve that is indirectly attached to the spinal cord by two short roots. The dorsal root, also referred to as the posterior or sensory root, contains afferent nerve fibers that conduct impulses into the spinal cord. The ventral root, also referred to as the anterior or motor root, contains axons of motor neurons that conduct impulses away from the spinal cord. Before leaving the spinal canal via the intervertebral foramen, the two roots combine to form the spinal nerve. After the spinal nerve leaves the spinal canal it divides into dorsal (posterior), ventral (anterior), and visceral branches. The dorsal and ventral branches are part of the somatic nervous system while the visceral branches are part of the autonomic nervous system.

Nerve Plexus

Only the ventral branches of spinal nerves T2-T12 are distributed directly to the skin and muscle. The other spinal nerves combine to form plexuses which are complex networks of nerve fibers. The cervical plexus is formed by spinal nerves C1-C4; the brachial plexus is formed by spinal nerves C5-T1; the lumbar plexus is formed by spinal nerves L1-L4; the sacral plexus is formed by spinal nerves L5-S3; and the coccygeal plexus by spinal nerves S4-C1. Nerves that emerge from these plexuses are generally named for the regions they supply. Each of these nerves is subdivided into branches that are usually named for the specific structures they supply.

Spinal nerves/nerve plexus

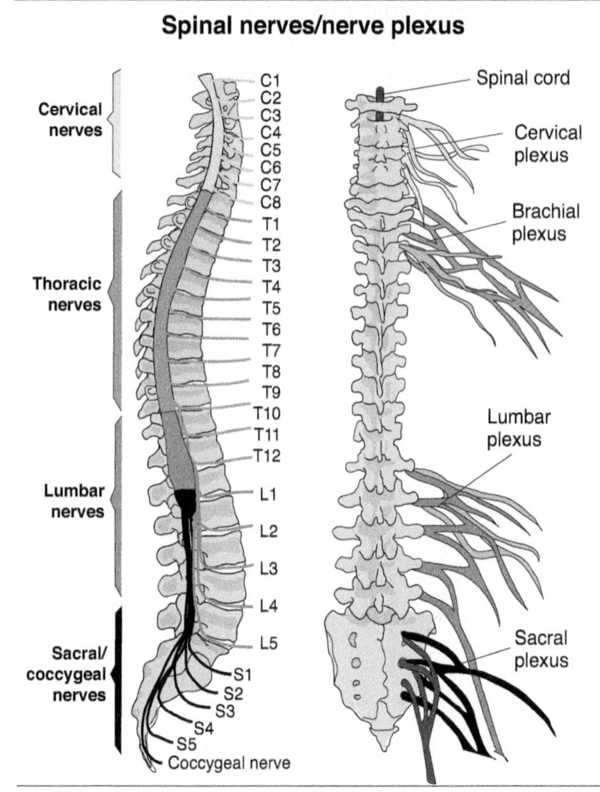

Autonomic Nervous System

The autonomic nervous system controls the smooth muscle, cardiac muscle, and glands. It functions automatically and involuntarily and is regulated by centers in the brain, including the cerebral cortex, hypothalamus, and the medulla oblongata. The autonomic nervous system affects visceral functions and consists entirely of motor fibers that transmit impulses from the CNS to smooth muscle, cardiac muscle, and glandular epithelium.

Examples of visceral functions affected by the autonomic nervous system include:

- Dilation and constriction of blood vessels
- Control of the force and rate of heartbeats
- Relaxation of bladder to allow urination
- Regulation of gastric peristalsis
- Regulation of glandular secretions

The autonomic nervous system is subdivided into parasympathetic and sympathetic functions. Generally, the parasympathetic division works to restore and conserve energy while the sympathetic division expends just enough energy to maintain homeostasis. However, in a situation of extreme threat, the sympathetic division dominates the parasympathetic producing the "fight or flight" response.

Autonomic Nerve Pathways

The autonomic nerve pathways always consist of two neurons. The cell body of the first neuron, also called the preganglionic neuron, is contained in the brain or spinal cord. The axon of the first neuron, also called preganglionic fiber, passes out of the CNS as part of a cranial or spinal nerve. It then separates from the somatic nerve and runs to an autonomic ganglion. There it synapses with the second neuron, also called the postganglionic neuron. The postganglionic axon or fiber then transmits the impulse to the smooth muscle, cardiac muscle, or glandular epithelium.

Function

As was stated earlier, the nervous system is the control, regulatory, and communication center of the body. Nervous system tissue is defined by two distinctive characteristics. The first is its ability to carry electrical messages called nerve impulses to and from the CNS. The second is the very limited ability of nervous tissue to regenerate.

The nervous system has three general overlapping functions: sensory, integrative, and motor.

Sensory

Sensory input is gathered by millions of sensory receptors that detect changes occurring inside and outside the body. These sensory receptors monitor external stimuli such as temperature, light, and sound, as well as internal stimuli such as blood pressure, pH, and carbon dioxide concentration.

Integration

The sensory input is then converted into nerve impulses which are electrical signals that are transmitted to the central nervous system. These nerve impulses create sensations, produce thoughts, or add to memory. Conscious and unconscious decisions are then made in the central nervous system, which is the integrative function of the nervous system.

Motor

Once the central nervous system has integrated the sensory input, the nervous system initiates a response by sending signals to tissues, organs, or glands which elicit a response such as muscle contraction or gland secretion. Tissues, organs, and glands are called effectors because they cause an effect in response to directions received from the central nervous system. This response is referred to as motor output or motor function.

Nerve Impulses

Nerve cells respond to stimuli and convert them into nerve impulses. This is called irritability. Once the stimuli are converted into a nerve impulse, the nerve cells have the ability to transmit that impulse to another nerve cell or to another tissue. This is called conductivity.

Irritability

Any stimulus that is strong enough to initiate transmission of a nerve impulse is referred to as a threshold impulse. A stimulus that is too weak to initiate a response is called a subthreshold stimulus. However, a series of subthreshold stimuli that are applied quickly to a neuron can have a cumulative effect that may initiate a nerve impulse. This is called summation of inadequate stimuli.

The speed with which an impulse is transmitted depends on the size, type, and condition of the nerve fiber. Myelinated fibers with larger diameters transmit nerve impulses faster than mid-sized and small fibers or unmyelinated fibers. Sensory and motor fibers that detect and respond to potentially dangerous situations in the outside environment are generally larger in diameter than those that control or respond to less critical stimuli.

Conductivity

Conductivity is the ability of the nerve cell to transmit an impulse to another nerve cell or another tissue via a conduction pathway. The reflex arc is the most basic type of conduction pathway. There are five basic components to a reflex arc that are required to transmit an impulse.

1. A receptor consisting of the distal end of a dendrite of a sensory neuron responds to a stimulus in the internal or external environment and produces a nerve impulse.
2. The impulse is passed by the receptor to the CNS.
3. The incoming impulse is directed to a center usually within the CNS where it is blocked, transmitted, or rerouted. This is usually accomplished with an association neuron that lies between the sensory neuron and the motor neuron.
4. The motor neuron transmits the impulse to the tissue, organ, or gland that must respond to the stimulus.
5. The tissue, organ, or gland, called an effector, responds to the stimulus.

The axons of neurons in a reflex arc do not ever touch the dendrites of the adjacent neuron in the nerve conduction pathway. The impulse must travel across a minute gap called a synapse. In addition, impulses can travel in only one direction from axon to synapse to dendrite.

Axon/synapse/dendrite

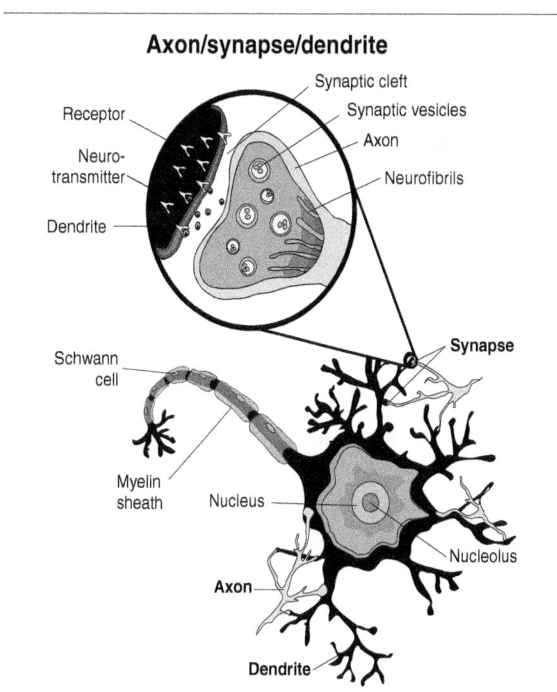

Nervous Tissue Injury

Unlike other tissues, nervous tissue has a very limited ability to regenerate. Specifically, if the cell body of a neuron is destroyed, the neuron cannot regenerate nor can other neurons reproduce and replace the damaged neuron. However, the human body is able to repair damaged nerve cells in which the cell body is intact and the axon has a neurilemma. Nerve cells in the peripheral nervous system generally have axons with a neurilemma while those in the brain and spinal cord do not. This means that a nerve injury of the hand has a good chance of healing while an injury of the brain or spinal cord is more often permanent.

ICD-10-CM Nervous System Coding Guidelines

See the table below for guidelines for *Chapter 5, Mental and Behavioral Disorders and Chapter 6, Diseases of the Nervous System.*

Chapter 5: Mental, Behavioral and Neurodevelopmental Disorders (F01 – F99)

1. Pain disorders related to psychological factors

Assign code F45.41, for pain that is exclusively related to psychological disorders. As indicated by the Excludes 1 note under category G89, a code from category G89 should not be assigned with code F45.41.

Code F45.42, Pain disorders with related psychological factors, should be used with a code from category G89, Pain, not elsewhere classified, if there is documentation of a psychological component for a patient with acute or chronic pain.

See Section I.C.6. Pain.

2. Mental and behavioral disorders due to psychoactive substance use

a. In Remission

Selection of codes for "in remission" for categories F10-F19, Mental and behavioral disorders due to psychoactive substance use (categories F10-F19 with -.21) requires the provider's clinical judgment. The appropriate codes for "in remission" are assigned only on the basis of provider documentation (as defined in the Official Guidelines for Coding and Reporting).

b. Psychoactive Substance Use, Abuse And Dependence

When the provider documentation refers to use, abuse and dependence of the same substance (e.g. alcohol, opioid, cannabis, etc.), only one code should be assigned to identify the pattern of use based on the following hierarchy:

i. If both use and abuse are documented, assign only the code for abuse

ii. If both abuse and dependence are documented, assign only the code for dependence

iii. If use, abuse and dependence are all documented, assign only the code for dependence

iv. If both use and dependence are documented, assign only the code for dependence.

c. Psychoactive Substance Use

As with all other diagnoses, the codes for psychoactive substance use (F10.9-, F11.9-, F12.9-, F13.9-, F14.9-, F15.9-, F16.9-) should only be assigned based on provider documentation and when they meet the definition of a reportable diagnosis (see Section III, Reporting Additional Diagnoses). The codes are to be used only when the psychoactive substance use is associated with a mental or behavioral disorder, and such a relationship is documented by the provider.

Chapter 6: Diseases of the Nervous System G00-G99)

1. Dominant/nondominant side

Codes from category G81, Hemiplegia and hemiparesis, and subcategories, G83.1, Monoplegia of lower limb, G83.2, Monoplegia of upper limb, and G83.3, Monoplegia, unspecified, identify whether the dominant or nondominant side is affected. Should the affected side be documented, but not specified as dominant or nondominant, and the classification system does not indicate a default, code selection is as follows:

- For ambidextrous patients, the default should be dominant.
- If the left side is affected, the default is non-dominant.
- If the right side is affected, the default is dominant.

2. Pain – Category G89

a. General coding information

Codes in category G89, Pain, not elsewhere classified, may be used in conjunction with codes from other categories and chapters to provide more detail about acute or chronic pain and neoplasm-related pain, unless otherwise indicated below.

If the pain is not specified as acute or chronic, post-thoracotomy, postprocedural, or neoplasm-related, do not assign codes from category G89.

A code from category G89 should not be assigned if the underlying (definitive) diagnosis is known, unless the reason for the encounter is pain control/ management and not management of the underlying condition.

When an admission or encounter is for a procedure aimed at treating the underlying condition (e.g., spinal fusion, kyphoplasty), a code for the underlying condition (e.g., vertebral fracture, spinal stenosis) should be assigned as the principal diagnosis. No code from category G89 should be assigned.

Category G89 codes as principal diagnosis or the first-listed code

Category G89 codes are acceptable as principal diagnosis or the first-listed code:

- When pain control or pain management is the reason for the admission/encounter (e.g., a patient with displaced intervertebral disc, nerve impingement and severe back pain presents for injection of steroid into the spinal canal). The underlying cause of the pain should be reported as an additional diagnosis, if known.
- When a patient is admitted for the insertion of a neurostimulator for pain control, assign the appropriate pain code as the principal or first-listed diagnosis. When an admission or encounter is for a procedure aimed at treating the underlying condition and a neurostimulator is inserted for pain control during the same admission/ encounter, a code for the underlying condition should be assigned as the principal diagnosis and the appropriate pain code should be assigned as a secondary diagnosis.

Use of Category G89 Codes in Conjunction with Site Specific Pain Codes

a. Assigning Category G89 and Site-Specific Pain Codes

Codes from category G89 may be used in conjunction with codes that identify the site of pain (including codes from chapter 18) if the category G89 code provides additional information. For example, if the code describes the site of the pain, but does not fully describe whether the pain is acute or chronic, then both codes should be assigned.

b. Sequencing of Category G89 Codes with Site-Specific Pain Codes

The sequencing of category G89 codes with site-specific pain codes (including chapter 18 codes), is dependent on the circumstances of the encounter/admission as follows:

- If the encounter is for pain control or pain management, assign the code from category G89 followed by the code identifying the specific site of pain (e.g., encounter for pain management for acute neck pain from trauma is assigned code G89.11, Acute pain due to trauma, followed by code M54.2, Cervicalgia, to identify the site of pain).
- If the encounter is for any other reason except pain control or pain management and a related definitive diagnosis has not been established (confirmed) by the provider, assign the code for the specific site of pain first, followed by the appropriate code from category G89.

Pain due to devices, implants and grafts

See Section I.C.19. Pain due to medical devices

Postoperative Pain

The provider's documentation should be used to guide the coding of postoperative pain, as well as Section III Reporting Additional Diagnoses and Section IV Diagnostic Coding and Reporting in the Outpatient Setting.

The default for post-thoracotomy and other postoperative pain not specified as acute or chronic is the code for the acute form.

Routine or expected postoperative pain immediately after surgery should not be coded.

a. Postoperative pain not associated with specific postoperative complication

Postoperative pain not associated with a specific postoperative complication is assigned to the appropriate postoperative pain code in category G89.

b. Postoperative pain associated with specific postoperative complication

Postoperative pain associated with a specific postoperative complication (such as painful wire sutures) is assigned to the appropriate code(s) found in Chapter 19, Injury, poisoning, and certain other consequences of external causes. If appropriate, use additional code(s) from category G89 to identify acute or chronic pain (G89.18 or G89.28).

Chronic pain

Chronic pain is classified to subcategory G89.2. There is no time frame defining when pain becomes chronic pain. The provider's documentation should be used to guide use of these codes.

Neoplasm Related Pain

Code G89.3 is assigned to pain documented as being related, associated or due to cancer, primary or secondary malignancy, or tumor. This code is assigned regardless of whether the pain is acute or chronic.

This code may be assigned as the principal or first-listed code when the stated reason for the admission/encounter is documented as pain control/pain management. The underlying neoplasm should be reported as an additional diagnosis.

When the reason for the admission/encounter is management of the neoplasm and the pain associated with the neoplasm is also documented, code G89.3 may be assigned as an additional diagnosis. It is not necessary to assign an additional code for the site of the pain.

See Section I.C.2 for instructions on the sequencing of neoplasms for all other stated reasons for the admission/encounter (except for pain control/pain management).

Chronic pain syndrome

Central pain syndrome (G89.0) and chronic pain syndrome (G89.4) are different than the term "chronic pain," and therefore these codes should only be used when the provider has specifically documented this condition.

See Section I.C.5. Pain disorders related to psychological factors

Documentation Elements of Nervous System

Key documentation elements for nervous system coding include the following:

- Dominant versus nondominant side
- Laterality
  - right
  - left
  - bilateral
- Episode of care for injuries and other external causes of mortality or morbidity
  - Initial encounter
  - Subsequent encounter
  - Sequela
- Loss of consciousness time duration

Diseases, Disorders, Injuries, and Other Conditions of the Nervous System

This section of the chapter looks at a variety of diseases, disorders, injuries, and other conditions involving the nervous system. The information presented in the anatomy and physiology section is expanded here to provide a better understanding regarding the part of the nervous system that is affected and how these conditions affect nervous system function. Specific information is provided for more commonly encountered conditions involving the nervous system.

Following the discussion of the various diseases, disease processes, disorders, injuries, and conditions, some diagnostic statements are provided with examples for coding in ICD-10-CM. The coding practice is followed by questions to help reinforce the student's knowledge of anatomy, physiology, and coding concepts. Answers to the coding questions can be found by reviewing the text or referring to the ICD-10-CM coding books.

Section 1.1 – Infectious/Parasitic Diseases

There are a number of infectious and parasitic diseases that affect the nervous system. Coding infectious and parasitic diseases can be problematic because some of these conditions are found in *Chapter 6 – Diseases of the Nervous System* while others are found in *Chapter 1 – Infectious and Parasitic Diseases.* In addition, some infections are captured by a single code while others have instructions to code the underlying disease first and still others have instructions to use a second code to identify the organism. Some of the more common infectious and parasitic diseases affecting the nervous system are described here.

Section 1.1a – Encephalitis and encephalomyelitis

Encephalitis is an inflammation of the encephalon. The encephalon is the portion of the nervous system enclosed within the cranium, which is more commonly referred to as the brain. The term encephalitis most commonly refers to an inflammation of the brain resulting from a viral infection. Encephalomyelitis refers to an inflammation of the brain and spinal cord.

West Nile encephalitis is a severe form of West Nile virus infection that becomes neuroinvasive and affects the brain. Although 4 out of 5 people infected with the West Nile virus do not develop any disease, about 20% will develop mild or moderate disease symptoms of fever, headache, body aches, fatigue, swollen glands, and a skin rash that can last a few days or several weeks. In less than 1% of infected persons, the disease affects the central nervous system, causing encephalitis, meningitis, or poliomyelitis. Symptoms manifest as headache, high fever, stiff neck, disorientation, stupor, muscle weakness, tremors or convulsions, even coma and paralysis.

Section 1.1a Coding Practice

Condition	ICD-10-CM
West Nile infection complicated by encephalitis	A92.31
Admission for treatment of acute disseminated encephalitis due to adverse effect of H. influenzae vaccine	G04.02, T50.B95A
Rasmussen encephalitis	G04.81
Idiopathic encephalitis	G04.90

Section 1.1a Questions

Can the code for West Nile encephalitis be found under the term 'Infection' or 'Encephalitis'? If not, what term in the Alphabetic Index is used to locate the correct code for West Nile encephalitis?

Why is the vaccine coded in addition to the encephalitis when the vaccine is determined to be the cause of the encephalitis?

Which diagnosis listed above is reported with an unspecified or NOS code?

Which diagnosis listed above is reported using an NEC code?

What additional information is provided in the ICD-10-CM code when coding an adverse effect of vaccine?

See end of chapter for Coding Practice answers.

Section 1.1b – Herpes Zoster

Herpes zoster is caused by the varicella virus, more commonly referred to as chicken pox. Anyone who has had chicken pox can develop herpes zoster, also called shingles. After the initial varicella infection resolves, the varicella virus remains in a dormant state in some nerve cells. If the virus reactivates, it results in herpes zoster characterized initially by burning, itching, tingling or extreme sensitivity of the skin usually limited to one location on one side of the body. Next, a red rash develops followed by groups of blisters at the site of the rash. The outbreak lasts for 2-3 weeks. Following the outbreak, an individual can develop another condition called post-herpetic neuralgia.

Section 1.1b Coding Practice

Condition	ICD-10-CM
Herpes zoster encephalitis	B02.0
Herpes zoster meningitis	B02.1
Herpes zoster myelitis	B02.24
Herpes zoster trigeminal neuralgia	B02.22
Herpes zoster	B02.9

Section 1.1b Questions

What part of the nervous system is affected in herpes zoster encephalitis? In herpes zoster meningitis?

Which codes report an uncomplicated herpes zoster infection?

Which diagnoses report complications of herpes zoster?

Which codes report post-herpetic outbreak conditions?

How is post-herpetic radiculopathy reported?

See end of chapter for Coding Practice answers.

Section 1.1c – Meningitis

Meningitis is an inflammation of the meninges, which are the membranous coverings of the brain and spinal cord. They consist of three layers. The outer membrane is a tough fibrous tissue called the dura mater. The middle membrane is a delicate fibrous tissue called the arachnoid. The inner membrane, called the pia mater, is a transparent membrane that adheres to the brain and spinal cord. Meningitis usually involves the dura mater and/or the arachnoid. When the arachnoid is affected, the condition may be referred to as arachnoiditis. Meningitis may be the result of a bacterial or viral infection or due to another noninfectious cause. The condition may be acute or chronic.

Section 1.1c Coding Practice

Condition	ICD-10-CM
Meningitis due to Lyme disease	A69.21
Meningitis due to coccidioidomycosis	B38.4
Bacterial meningitis due to H. influenzae	G00.0
Spinal meningitis	G03.9
Meningitis due to Streptococcus pneumoniae infection	G00.2, B95.3
Viral meningitis	A87.9

Section 1.1c Questions

Why is only one code required for reporting meningitis due to Lyme disease?

____

____

Which conditions listed above are reported using ICD-10-CM unspecified or NOS codes?

____

____

Why are two codes reported for meningitis due to Streptococcus pneumoniae infection?

____

____

See end of chapter for Coding Practice answers.

Section 1.2 – Neoplasms

Neoplasms of the nervous system, like all neoplasms, are abnormal tissues in which the cells grow and divide more rapidly than that of normal tissue. Primary CNS neoplasms can occur in tissues of the brain or spinal cord but brain tumors are more common than spinal cord tumors. Brain tumors may be benign or malignant with statistics showing that almost half of all brain tumors are benign. However, even benign brain tumors can recur and can be fatal. The CNS, particularly the brain, is also a common site of secondary malignant or metastatic brain tumors. The PNS may also be the site of either benign or malignant neoplastic disease.

Gliomas

The most common types of nervous system tumors are connective tissue tumors called gliomas. Gliomas are differentiated by the type of connective tissue from which they arise and include:

Astrocytoma – A malignant neoplasm arising from astrocytes, the star-shaped glial cells that wrap around nerve cells to form a supporting network around the neurons in the brain and spinal cord. Astrocytomas may be subclassified by tumor grade as follows:

- Grade I, also called pilocytic astrocytomas
- Grade II, also called fibrillary astrocytomas
- Grade III, also called anaplastic astrocytomas
- Grade IV, also called glioblastoma multiforme

Brain stem glioma – A malignant tumor located in the lower part of the brain.

Ependymoma – A tumor that arises from the cells that line the ventricles and the subarachnoid space surrounding the brain and spinal cord through which cerebrospinal fluid flows. These tumors may be benign, malignant, or of uncertain behavior.

Oligodendroglioma – A tumor that arises from oligodendrocytes – cells that produce a thick, fatty sheath that covers and protects the nerve cells. These slow-growing malignant tumors are most common in the cerebrum.

Schwannoma – A tumor of the myelin sheath arising from Schwann cells. These tumors are peripheral nervous system tumors that can be benign or malignant. The most common type of benign schwannoma is an acoustic neuroma, which is a tumor of the vestibulocochlear cranial nerve (CN VIII). The most common sites for malignant schwannomas are the sciatic nerve, brachial plexus, and sacral plexus.

Other Nervous System Neoplasms

Medulloblastoma – A tumor of the cerebellum usually in the region of the fourth ventricle or central part of the cerebellum, or less frequently in the cerebellar hemispheres.

Meningioma – A tumor that develops in the membrane covering the brain and spinal cord. The majority of meningiomas are benign, although approximately 10% are classified as atypical or malignant.

Neuroma – A neuroma is a benign lesion of a nerve or a thickening of nervous tissue. Some specific types of neuromas, such as acoustic neuromas, are classified as neoplasms and reported with codes from the neoplasm chapter whereas other neuromas, such as Morton's neuromas, are classified as mononeuropathies and are coded in the nervous system chapter.

Neurofibromatosis – The term neurofibromatosis is most commonly associated with a genetic condition that causes benign tumors to grow on nervous tissue causing skin and bone abnormalities. This condition is known as neurofibromatosis type 1 (NF1) and is reported with a code from the chapter on congenital malformations, deformations, and chromosomal abnormalities. A less common type, neurofibromatosis type 2 (NF2), causes bilateral neurofibroma-like tumors of the acoustic nerve. NF2 is reported as a benign tumor of the acoustic nerve with a code from the neoplasm chapter. There is also a malignant form of neurofibromatosis, which is reported with a code from the neoplasm chapter.

Secondary Nervous System Neoplasms

Secondary neoplasms of the nervous system are neoplasms that have metastasized from another site to the nervous system. A common site of metastatic lesions is the brain. For example, primary malignant neoplasms of the breast or lung often metastasize to the brain.

Section 1.2 Coding Practice

Condition	ICD-10-CM
Low grade, pilocytic astrocytoma of the cerebellum	C71.6
Benign ependymoma at the base of the spinal cord	D33.4
Von Recklinghausen's disease	Q85.01
Malignant schwannoma, left sciatic nerve	C47.22
Meningothelial meningioma of the right frontal parasagittal region of the brain	D32.0
Subependymal glioma of the brain	D43.2
Spinal cord tumor, lumbosacral region	D49.7
Right upper outer quadrant breast cancer previously excised with admission for surgical treatment of metastasis to brain.	C79.31, Z85.3

Section 1.2 Questions

Why is neurofibromatosis type 1 reported with a code from Chapter 17, Congenital Malformations, Deformations, and Chromosomal Abnormalities?

What information is provided in the ICD-10-CM code for malignant schwannoma of the left sciatic nerve?

How are malignant neoplasms of peripheral nerves classified?

Even though meningothelial meningioma is not specifically described as a benign tumor, it is reported with a code for a benign neoplasm. Why?

See end of chapter for Coding Practice answers.

Section 1.3 – Systemic Atrophies Affecting the CNS

Systemic atrophies affecting the CNS are a group of motor neuron diseases that affect muscle control and strength. Many of these conditions have a hereditary component, meaning that they are caused by inherited genetic disorders. Terms used to describe these systemic atrophies include atrophy, ataxia, palsy, and sclerosis.

Huntington's disease is an autosomal dominant inherited disorder that manifests in adulthood and causes degeneration and death of certain nerve cells in the brain, accompanied by brain atrophy primarily in the basal ganglia and cerebral cortex. Symptoms of Huntington's disease include involuntary muscle movement, dementia, and behavioral changes.

Hereditary spastic paraplegia (HSP), also called familial spastic paraplegia (FSP), is a group of disorders, all of which are characterized by progressive weakness and spasticity or stiffness in the legs. Symptoms begin with mild stiffness of the legs and minor gait impairment. The condition usually progresses slowly with individuals eventually requiring the assistance of a cane, crutches, or wheelchair. Some forms of HSP are accompanied by other symptoms including optic nerve and retinal diseases, cataracts, generalized lack of muscle coordination (ataxia), epilepsy, cognitive impairment, peripheral neuropathy, and deafness. Several genetic disorders have been identified in individuals with HSP. Genetic testing can help identify the specific form of the disease.

Amyotrophic lateral sclerosis (ALS), also called Lou Gehrig's disease, is a progressive, fatal neurological disease. ALS belongs to a group of motor neuron diseases which are characterized by gradual degeneration and death of motor neurons. Motor neurons located in the brain, brain stem, and spinal cord are the control and communication pathways between the nervous system and voluntary muscles. Messages from upper motor neurons in the brain and brainstem are transmitted to lower motor neurons in the spinal cord and then along nerve fibers to specific voluntary muscles. In ALS, both upper and lower motor neurons degenerate and die. Because muscles no longer receive messages to move, the muscles weaken and atrophy. Eventually, the motor neurons in the brain lose the ability to control voluntary movement and all muscle control is lost. When control of the diaphragm and chest wall is lost, the individuals lose the ability to breathe on their own and ventilator support is necessary. Most people with ALS die from respiratory failure within 3-5 years of disease onset.

Amyotrophic lateral sclerosis (ALS)

Also known as Lou Gehrig's Disease, ALS is caused by the degeneration and death of motor neurons in the spinal cord and brain

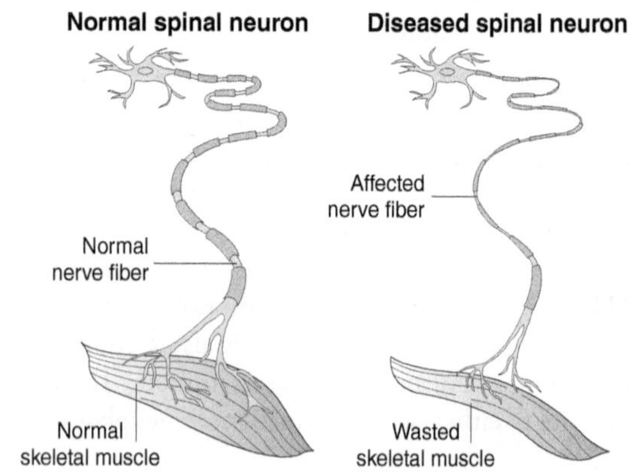

Section 1.3 Coding Practice

Condition	ICD-10-CM
Familial spastic paraplegia	G11.4
Late stage amyotrophic lateral sclerosis requiring ventilator support	G12.21, Z99.11
Huntington's dementia	G10
Spinal muscle atrophy, juvenile, type III	G12.1

Section 1.3 Questions

What terms in the ICD-10-CM Alphabetic Index are used to identify the code for continuous ventilator support?

What is another term for juvenile spinal muscle atrophy III?

See end of chapter for Coding Practice answers.

Section 1.4 – Parkinson's Disease

Parkinson's disease is a brain disorder in which nerve cells in an area of the brain known as the substantia negra become impaired or die. These nerve cells produce the chemical dopamine which is necessary for muscle coordination. Symptoms of Parkinson's disease include tremor, slow movement, rigidity, and problems with balance. Parkinson's disease can be primary or secondary. Primary Parkinson's disease is defined as disease that cannot be linked to another condition as the cause. Secondary Parkinson's disease is disease that can be linked to chemical or environmental toxins such as certain drugs, to a brain inflammation such as encephalitis, to cerebrovascular disease, or to another physiological condition.

Section 1.4 Coding Practice

Condition	ICD-10-CM
Parkinson's disease without dementia	G20
Parkinson's disease secondary to long-term haloperidol use, taken as prescribed	T43.4X5S, G21.11
Admission for malignant neuroleptic syndrome due to olanzapine (antipsychotic NEC), used as prescribed	T43.505A, G21.0
Atypical parkinsonism due to vascular compromise caused by cerebrovascular arteriosclerosis	I67.2, G21.4

Section 1.4 Questions

Why is the adverse effect code reported first?

How is Parkinson's disease with related dementia coded?

See end of chapter for Coding Practice answers.

Section 1.5 – Alzheimer's Disease and Other Degenerative Diseases of the Nervous System

Alzheimer's disease is a progressive fatal brain disease. The disease destroys brain cells, which leads to memory loss, confusion, disruption of thought processes, and behavioral disorders. In individuals with Alzheimer's disease, nerve impulses that form memory and influence thinking are disrupted both within the damaged nerve cells and at nerve synapses. This means that nerve impulses are not transmitted along nerve fibers or from one nerve cell to the next in the brain. Eventually, the nerve cells die and brain tissue atrophies. Damage occurs in the cortex which is responsible for thinking, planning, and remembering and is especially severe in the hippocampus which is responsible for the formation of new memories. As the brain atrophies, the fluid-filled ventricles enlarge.

Other degenerative diseases of the brain include frontotemporal dementia, senile degeneration of the brain not elsewhere classified, and degeneration due to alcohol abuse.

Section 1.5 Coding Practice

Condition	ICD-10-CM
Alzheimer's disease without behavioral disturbance	G30.9, F02.80
Alcoholic encephalopathy due to chronic alcoholism	G31.2, F10.20
Frontal lobe degeneration with dementia including agitated and aggressive behavior	G31.09, F02.81
Sub-acute necrotizing encephalopathy	G31.82

Section 1.5 Questions

What instruction for coding alcoholic encephalopathy is present in ICD-10-CM?

Under what term is the code for Alzheimer's disease found in the Alphabetic Index?

How is Alzheimer's disease classified in ICD-10-CM?

See end of chapter for Coding Practice answers.

Section 1.6 – Multiple Sclerosis and Other Demyelinating Diseases of the Nervous System

Multiple sclerosis is a chronic demyelinating disease of the central nervous system that may be disabling. While the cause is not known, it is believed to be an autoimmune disorder in which the body's defense system attacks myelin that surrounds and protects nerve fibers in the brain, spinal cord, and optic nerves. The nerve fibers may also be damaged. The damaged myelin then forms patches of scar tissue, also referred to as sclerosis or plaque. Symptoms include fatigue; weakness; numbness (paresthesia); dizziness (vertigo); disturbances in gait, balance, and coordination; bladder and bowel dysfunction; vision problems; and mood changes.

While multiple sclerosis is the most common type of demyelinating disease, there are a number of other types such as optic neuritis with demyelination, diffuse sclerosis of the central nervous system, and necrotizing myelitis of the central nervous system.

Another common condition acute transverse myelitis is a spinal cord disorder which is an acute inflammation of the white and gray matter of one or more spinal cord segments, usually in the thoracic spine. Symptoms include bilateral motor, sensory and sphincter deficits below the level of the lesion that can progress over a short period to paraplegia, loss of sensation below the lesion, urinary retention and bowel incontinence. Acute transverse myelitis is most commonly caused by multiple sclerosis however it has also been linked to neuromyelitis optica, infections, immunizations, autoimmune inflammation, vasculitis and certain drugs.

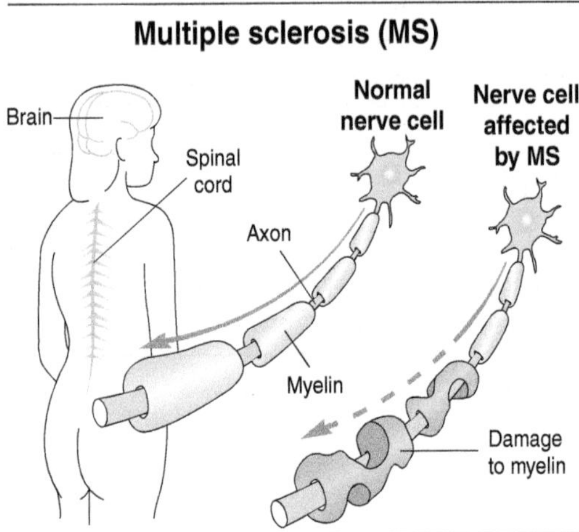

Section 1.6 Coding Practice

Condition	ICD-10-CM
Multiple sclerosis	G35
Demyelinating callosal encephalopathy	G37.1
Patient with multiple sclerosis is now diagnosed with neuromyelitis optica	G36.0 G35
Periaxial encephalitis	G37.0
Sub-acute necrotizing myelitis of the central nervous system (CNS)	G37.4

Section 1.6 Questions

In addition to Multiple Sclerosis, what other code categories are available for demyelinating diseases of the central nervous system?

How is Schilder's disease coded?

How is multiple sclerosis with acute transverse myelitis coded?

See end of chapter for Coding Practice answers.

Section 1.7 – Epilepsy, Seizure Disorders, and Seizures

Epilepsy, also referred to as a seizure disorder, is caused by a surge of electrical signals in all or a part of the brain. Seizure manifestations as well as the length of the seizure may vary considerably. A seizure may be exhibited by convulsions, loss of consciousness, blank staring, or jerky movements of the arms or legs. The seizure may last for a few seconds to several minutes. Only when an individual has two or more incidents of unprovoked seizure activity is a diagnosis of epilepsy made. There are many different types of epileptic seizures but these are generally divided into two broad categories, localization-related seizures, also referred to as focal or partial seizures, and generalized seizures. These two broad categories are then further defined by whether the seizures are intractable or not and whether they present with status epilepticus or without status epilepticus. Intractable epilepsy is epilepsy that is not well controlled. Status epilepticus refers to recurrent or continuous seizure activity lasting more than 30 minutes.

A nonspecific diagnosis of seizure or convulsion disorder is reported with codes from the signs and symptoms chapter.

Section 1.7 Coding Practice

Condition	ICD-10-CM
Epilepsy with myoclonic seizures, intractable without status epilepticus	G40.319
Somatomotor epilepsy	G40.109
Petit mal seizures with status epilepticus	G40.A01
Seizure NOS	R56.9

Section 1.7 Questions

How is epilepsy with intractable seizures and status epilepticus coded?

Why is seizure NOS coded as a sign or symptom and not as epilepsy?

See end of chapter for Coding Practice answers.

Section 1.8 – Migraine

A migraine is a headache that can be extremely painful and can last for several hours or days. Some migraines are preceded by an aura or sensory warning that a migraine is imminent. The aura may consist of flashes of light, blind spots, and/or tingling in the arms or legs. The cause of migraines is not entirely understood, but they may be caused by changes in the trigeminal nerve and/or changes in serotonin levels in the brain. The trigeminal nerve is a major pain pathway. It is also known that serotonin levels drop during a migraine, which may cause the release of neuropeptides that then travel to the meninges causing the headache pain. It is also known that both internal and external environmental factors can trigger migraines. Known triggers include: hormone changes, some foods, stress, sensory stimuli, changes in wake-sleep patterns, physical exertion including sexual activity, changes in the weather or barometric pressure, and some medications.

Status migrainosus refers to a debilitating migraine lasting more than 72 hours. When coding status migrainosus, both the length of time and the debilitating nature of the attack must be documented.

Section 1.8 Coding Practice

Condition	ICD-10-CM
Migraine with aura, controlled with verapamil	G43.109
Persistent migraine aura, without cerebral infarction not intractable	G43.509
Migraine related to menstrual cycle, responsive to Imitrex	G43.829
Debilitating classic migraine for the past 4 days, unresponsive to medication	G43.111
Migraine with cyclical vomiting, not intractable, without status migrainosus	G43.A0

Section 1.8 Questions

When coding for migraine what types of information need to be documented?

How are migraine variants coded in ICD-10-CM?

See end of chapter for Coding Practice answers.

Section 1.9 – Transient Ischemic Attacks

A transient ischemic attack (TIA) is a mini-stroke that typically lasts only a few minutes. A TIA is caused by an interruption of blood supply to a part of the brain. Symptoms may be similar to those of a stroke but typically resolve within 24 hours. Symptoms include: numbness or weakness in the face, arm, or leg usually only on one side; confusion; difficulty speaking or understanding speech; vision changes in one or both eyes; difficulty walking; dizziness; or loss of balance or coordination.

Section 1.9 Coding Practice

Condition	ICD-10-CM
TIA	G45.9
Recurrent focal cerebral ischemia	G45.8
Vertebrobasilar artery insufficiency	G45.0
Internal carotid artery syndrome	G45.1

Section 1.9 Questions

Why are transient ischemic attacks and related artery syndromes coded in the nervous system chapter instead of the circulatory system chapter?

How is cerebral artery spasm coded?

See end of chapter for Coding Practice answers.

Section 1.10 – Trigeminal Neuralgia and Other Nerve Disorders

Neuralgia refers to pain along the path of a nerve. Neuralgia may be caused by infection or inflammation, trauma, compression, or chemical irritation. The most common site of neuralgia is along the trigeminal nerve, also referred to as cranial nerve V (CN V). The trigeminal nerve is the main sensory nerve that innervates the side of the face and eye area. Symptoms include very painful, sharp spasms that typically last only a few seconds or minutes. Pain usually occurs on only one side of the face around the eye, cheek, and/or lower aspect of the face.

Other nerve disorders covered in this section include disorders of the facial nerve such as paralysis, twitching, and weakness. These types of disorders may be caused by an infection, injury, or tumor, but are more commonly idiopathic which means they are of unknown origin. If the nerve disorder is due to an infection, injury, or tumor, a code from one of those chapters would be used instead of a nervous system chapter code. Also, many disorders of optic or acoustic nerves are covered in the chapters on the eye or ear.

Nonspecific diagnoses of neuralgia and neuritis are not reported with codes from the nervous system chapter. Instead, these nonspecific diagnoses are found in the musculoskeletal chapter.

Use caution when coding nerve disorders with the terminology of neuralgia, neuritis and neuropathy. Neuritis is an inflammation of the nerve and should not be coded in this section of ICD-10-CM.

Section 1.10 Coding Practice

Condition	ICD-10-CM
Trigeminal neuralgia	G50.0
Bell's palsy	G51.0
Glossopharyngeal neuralgia	G52.1
Neuralgia NOS	M79.2

Section 1.10 Questions

Neuralgia NOS is reported with a code from the musculoskeletal system chapter. Why is it listed in the musculoskeletal system chapter and not in the nervous system chapter?

How is clonic hemifacial spasm coded?

See end of chapter for Coding Practice answers.

Section 1.11 – Thoracic Outlet Syndrome and Other Nerve Root and Plexus Disorders

Nerve root and plexus disorders are typically caused by compression of these structures. Compression causes symptoms of pain and numbness. Compression caused by intervertebral disc disorders is considered to be a musculoskeletal condition and is reported with codes from the musculoskeletal system chapter.

The term 'thoracic outlet syndrome' refers to a condition in which the neurovascular structures just above the first rib and below the clavicle are compressed resulting in a number of symptoms. The brachial plexus is most commonly affected, although the subclavian artery or vein may also be compressed. The brachial plexus is formed by spinal nerves C5-T1. In thoracic outlet syndrome involving nervous system structures, usually the lower spinal nerve roots of C8-T1 are compressed causing pain and numbness along the ulnar nerve distribution. Sometimes the upper three spinal nerve roots C5-C7 are compressed causing pain and numbness in the neck, upper chest, upper back, and outer arm along the radial nerve distribution.

Section 1.11 Coding Practice

Condition	ICD-10-CM
Thoracic outlet syndrome	G54.0
Sacral plexus compression caused by metastatic lesions to the presacral soft tissues. Patient previously had a prostatectomy for prostate cancer	C79.89, G55, Z85.46
Supraclavicular lymphadenopathy due to non-Hodgkin's non-follicular lymphoma with compression of right brachial plexus	C83.91, G55
One year status post below-elbow amputation of right arm with painful phantom limb syndrome	G54.6, Z89.211

Section 1.11 Questions

What information is necessary to code amputation status accurately in ICD-10-CM?

What terminology is used in ICD-10-CM for diagnoses of brachial or lumbosacral plexus lesions and nerve root lesions?

____

____

How is compression of a nerve plexus coded when it is caused by another condition?

____

____

See end of chapter for Coding Practice answers.

Section 1.12 – Myasthenia Gravis, Muscular Dystrophy, and Other Diseases of the Myoneural Junction

Myoneural junction disorders, also called neuromuscular disorders, are caused by a defect in the transmission of nerve impulses from nerves to muscles. Transmission is interrupted at the (myoneural) junction where nerve cells connect to muscle tissue. Normally, when nerve impulses travel down a motor nerve, acetylcholine, a neurotransmitter, is released at the nerve ending. The acetylcholine travels across the neuromuscular junction and binds to receptors in the muscle, which activate causing the muscle to contract.

Myasthenia gravis is a chronic autoimmune neuromuscular disease caused by a defect in the transmission of nerve impulses from the nerve to the muscle it innervates. In myasthenia gravis, the body produces antibodies that block, alter, or destroy the acetylcholine receptors in the muscle tissue which prevents normal muscle contraction from occurring. Often the condition is more pronounced in muscles that control eye and eyelid movement, facial expression, chewing, talking, and swallowing; however, muscles that control breathing and movement in the neck and extremities may also be affected.

Muscular dystrophy is a group of more than 30 distinct genetic diseases that are characterized by progressive degeneration and weakness of the skeletal muscles that control movement. Some forms occur in infancy and childhood while others are not symptomatic until adolescence or adulthood. The different types also differ in respect to extent of muscle weakness, rate of progression, and pattern of inheritance. Duchenne's muscular dystrophy is the most common type and primarily affects boys. It is caused by the absence of dystrophin, a protein required to maintain the integrity of muscle tissue. Fascioscapulohumeral muscular dystrophy is the most common type manifesting in adolescence and affects muscles of the face, chest, shoulders, arms, and legs. Myotonic muscular dystrophy is the most common type manifesting in adulthood and is characterized by prolonged muscle spasms, cataracts, cardiac abnormalities, and endocrine disturbances.

Section 1.12 Coding Practice

Condition	ICD-10-CM
Myasthenia gravis	G70.00
Duchenne's muscular dystrophy	G71.0
Fascioscapulohumeral muscular dystrophy	G71.0
Myotonic muscular dystrophy	G71.11
Myasthenic syndrome due to uninodular goiter with thyrotoxicosis	E05.10, G73.3

Section 1.12 Questions

How is myasthenia gravis without documentation of exacerbation coded?

____

____

Is thyrotoxicosis the same thing as a thyrotoxic storm? If not, what is the difference?

____

____

How is initial encounter for accidental mercury induced myoneural disorder coded?

____

____

See end of chapter for Coding Practice answers.

Section 1.13 – Cerebral Palsy and Other Paralytic Syndromes

Cerebral palsy is a general term that can refer to a number of neurological disorders that manifest in infancy or early childhood. Cerebral palsy is caused by abnormalities in the brain in the areas that affect muscle control and movement. Most children are born with cerebral palsy but some develop it in infancy or early childhood following a brain infection or head injury. Cerebral palsy can cause a lack of muscle coordination when performing voluntary movements (ataxia); stiff or tight muscles and exaggerated reflexes (spasticity); muscle tone that is either too tight and stiff or too floppy; and gait abnormalities like dragging one foot or leg while walking, walking on toes, or moving with a crouched or scissored gait.

Also included in this section are hemiplegia, paraplegia, diplegia of upper limbs, and monoplegia, as well as other paralytic syndromes. These codes are used for a diagnosis of one of these conditions without further specification, when the condition is stated as old or longstanding, or in multiple coding scenarios.

Section 1.13 Coding Practice

Condition	ICD-10-CM
Congenital spastic diplegic cerebral palsy	G80.1
Long-term left-sided spastic hemiplegia (right side dominant)	G81.14
Long-standing locked-in state following brain stem stroke	I69.398, G83.5
Old cerebral infarction with right side dominant hemiplegia	I69.351

Section 1.13 Questions

Hereditary spastic paraplegia is not included in this code category. Where is it found and why is it listed in another category?

____

____

What does the term diplegic mean?

____

____

When hemiplegia is the result of a cerebral infarction, is a separate code required to describe the hemiplegia?

____

____

See end of chapter for Coding Practice answers.

Section 1.14 – Other Disorders of the Nervous System

The last section in the nervous system chapter includes pain and other disorders of the nervous system, including those of the autonomic nervous system, acquired hydrocephalus, complications of surgical procedures, and other conditions.

Pain

Pain codes in this section are for central pain syndrome, acute or chronic pain that is not classified elsewhere, neoplasm related pain, and chronic pain syndromes. More specific codes for pain are found in other chapters and in the chapter for signs, symptoms, and abnormal clinical and laboratory findings.

Disorders of the Autonomic Nervous System

The autonomic nervous system acts automatically and involuntarily to control smooth muscle, cardiac muscle, and glands. Disorders of the autonomic nervous system can affect heart rhythm, blood pressure, muscle tone, and facial sweating. Complex regional pain syndrome, a condition usually affecting a single extremity and characterized by burning or aching pain in the affected limb, swelling, skin discoloration, altered temperature, abnormal sweating, and hypersensitivity, is also found in this section.

Acquired Hydrocephalus

Acquired hydrocephalus occurs any time after birth and can occur at any age. It can be caused by injury or disease such as hemorrhage, neoplasm, cystic lesion, or infection. Hydrocephalus is broadly categorized as communicating or non-communicating. In communicating hydrocephalus, the flow of CSF is blocked after it exits the ventricles, but can still flow between ventricles. In non-communicating hydrocephalus, the flow of CSF is blocked along one of the narrow passageways connecting the ventricles which prevents flow between them. A common site of blockage is the aqueduct of Sylvius, which is a small passage between the third and fourth ventricles in the middle of the brain.

Complications of Procedures

Complications of surgical procedures and other procedural interventions covers a wide variety of conditions including cerebrospinal fluid leak or spinal headache following spinal puncture, intracranial hypotension following shunting procedure, intraoperative or post-procedural hemorrhage or hematoma of a nervous system structure, as well as other complications.

Section 1.14 Coding Practice

Condition	ICD-10-CM
Post-traumatic hydrocephalus	G91.3
Admission for pain management of acute tumor-related pain from primary malignancy of pancreas	G89.3, C25.9
Arnold-Chiari malformation type 1	G93.5
Carotid sinus syndrome	G90.01
Prolonged post-procedural encephalopathy following coronary artery bypass procedure	G97.82, G93.49, Z95.1

Section 1.14 Questions

What type of nervous system disorder is carotid sinus syndrome?

What term is used to find the correct code for Arnold-Chiari malformation type 1?

Why is a complication code from the nervous system chapter used to report encephalopathy following CABG?

Where are intraoperative and post-procedural complications affecting the nervous system found?

See end of chapter for Coding Practice answers.

Section 1.15 – Nervous System Conditions Originating in the Perinatal Period

These nervous system conditions originate in the perinatal period which is defined as the period before birth through the first 28 days after birth. Conditions that originate in the perinatal period and persist or cause morbidity later in life are also reported with codes from the chapter for certain conditions originating in the perinatal period. Examples of nervous system conditions listed in this chapter include newborn convulsions, disturbances of cerebral status, and disorders of muscle tone.

Cerebral or periventricular leukomalacia is an injury to the white matter of the cerebrum often associated with premature birth. It is considered to be a precursor for neurological impairment and cerebral palsy.

Transient neonatal myasthenia gravis is a neuromuscular postsynaptic transmission defect that sometimes occurs in infants born to mothers with myasthenia gravis. Sucking, swallowing, and respiratory difficulties are the most common symptoms. The condition generally resolves spontaneously, but supportive management and administration of medication prior to feedings is sometimes necessary until the condition resolves.

Section 1.15 Coding Practice

Condition	ICD-10-CM
Floppy baby syndrome	P94.2
Convulsions NOS in newborn	P90
Neonatal periventricular leukomalacia	P91.2
Transient neonatal myasthenia gravis	P94.0

Section 1.15 Questions

Myasthenia gravis in adults is classified as a myoneural disorder. How is transient neonatal myasthenia gravis classified?

See end of chapter for Coding Practice answers.

Section 1.16 – Congenital Malformations of the Nervous System

Many anomalies of the nervous system can be either congenital or acquired. Acquired anomalies are reported with codes from the nervous system chapter (G codes) while most congenital anomalies are reported with codes from the chapter on congenital malformations, deformation, and chromosomal abnormalities (Q codes). Types of conditions included in this section are congenital malformations of the brain, malformations of the spinal cord and meninges, and agenesis or displacement of a nerve or nerve plexus.

Anencephaly is a neural tube defect that results when the portion of neural tube that will form the brain fails to close during the third or fourth week of fetal development. This results in absence of a major portion of the brain including the forebrain and cerebrum. In many cases, the skull, soft tissues of the scalp and skin also fail to form leaving the brain stem and other brain tissue exposed. Anencephalic newborns are unable to see, hear, and feel pain. The absence of the cerebrum leaves the newborn in an unconscious state with only reflex actions such as breathing intact. Most live-born newborns with anencephaly die within hours or days of birth.

An **encephalocele** is also a neural tube defect that causes sac-like protrusions of the brain and cerebral meninges through openings in the skull. This condition results from failure of the neural tube to close properly during fetal development and can result in deformities in the midline of the upper part of the skull, the area between the forehead and nose, or in the back of the skull. Newborns with encephaloceles usually have dramatic deformities evident at birth. Encephaloceles may present with craniofacial deformities or other brain malformations. Newborns with encephaloceles may have other medical conditions including hydrocephalus, spastic quadriplegia, microcephaly, ataxia, developmental delay, vision problems, mental and growth retardation, and seizures.

Spina bifida is another neural tube defect caused by failure of the spinal portion of the neural tube to close properly during the first month of fetal development. The extent of the defect can vary from an open defect with significant damage to the spinal cord and nerves to a closed defect with only failure of the vertebrae to form properly in that region. The three most common types are myelomeningocele, meningocele, and spina bifida occulta. Myelomeningocele is the most severe form and is characterized by protrusion of the spinal cord and meninges from a defect in the spine. Meningocele is characterized by normal development of the spinal cord but with protrusion of meninges through a defect in the spine. Spina bifida occulta is the least severe form characterized by failure of the vertebrae to form properly over the spinal cord and meninges which are covered only by a layer of skin. Spina bifida may occur with or without hydrocephalus.

Section 1.16 Coding Practice

Condition	ICD-10-CM
Spina bifida occulta	Q76.0
Myelomeningocele, thoracolumbar region, with hydrocephalus	Q05.1
Hemianencephaly	Q00.0
Meningoencephalocele frontal region	Q01.0
Congenital phrenic nerve agenesis with resulting pulmonary hypoplasia	Q07.8, Q33.6

Section 1.16 Questions

Why is spina bifida occulta listed under congenital malformation of the spine instead of under congenital malformations of the nervous system?

See end of chapter for Coding Practice answers.

Section 1.17 – Signs, Symptoms, and Abnormal Findings

There are a number of signs, symptoms, and abnormal clinical and laboratory findings that are indicators of nervous system diseases and disorders.

Signs and symptoms specific to the nervous system include:

- Abnormal involuntary movement
- Abnormalities of gait and mobility
- Lack of coordination
- Abnormal reflexes
- Transient paralysis
- Repeated falls
- Facial droop

More general signs and symptoms that could be an indicator of nervous system disease include:

- Drowsiness
- Stupor
- Coma
- Disorientation
- Amnesia
- Other altered mental status
- Vertigo
- Speech disturbances
- Malaise
- Fatigue
- Convulsions

Abnormal laboratory findings include:

- Abnormal blood work
- Abnormal urine tests
- Abnormal cerebrospinal fluid findings
- Elevated tumor associated antigens (TAA) or tumor specific antigens (TSA)

Abnormal findings on diagnostic imaging include:

- Space occupying lesion of CNS
- Abnormal echoencephalogram
- Unspecified white matter disease

Abnormal results of function studies include those identified by:

- Electroencephalogram (EEG)
- Brain scan
- Nerve stimulation studies
- Electromyogram (EMG)

Section 1.17 Coding Practice

Condition	ICD-10-CM
Generalized weakness	R53.1
Lethargy	R53.83
Transient alteration of awareness	R40.4
Abnormal cell counts in CSF	R83.6
Abnormal PET scan, brain	R94.02

Section 1.17 Question

What types of malaise and fatigue are identified in ICD-10-CM?

See end of chapter for Coding Practice answers.

Section 1.18 – Nervous System Injuries, Poisonings, and Other External Causes

Injuries to the nervous system are defined as those conditions that are due to some type of trauma. Some nervous system conditions, such as a subarachnoid hemorrhage, may be of traumatic or nontraumatic origin. Documentation is of paramount importance in determining whether to select a code from the chapter for nervous system diseases or from the chapter for injuries, poisoning, and certain other consequences of external causes.

Injuries, poisonings, and other external causes require a seventh character extender to define the episode of care. Episode of care for injuries to the nervous system must be specified as:

A Initial encounter

D Subsequent encounter

S Sequela

Poisonings from drugs, chemicals, or other substances include toxic and adverse effects of drugs as well as a new underdosing category. The correct poisoning code is initially identified in the Table of Drugs and Chemicals and then verified in the Tabular list. Poisonings, toxic and adverse effects, and underdosing usually require the use of multiple codes to identify the drug or chemical as well as the specific manifestations or other conditions associated with the poisoning.

Other consequences of external causes cover a wide variety of conditions. Examples of conditions related to the nervous system and to mental and behavioral disorders include:

- Abuse or neglect

- Traumatic shock
- Complications related to medical or surgical procedures
- Complications related to nervous system devices

Codes in this chapter may also require the use of external cause codes to provide data for how the injury occurred, the intent (unintentional/accidental versus intentional/suicide/assault), the place of occurrence, and the activity being performed.

Section 1.18 Coding Practice

Condition	ICD-10-CM
Admitted for subdural hemorrhage sustained in a fall when the patient slipped on ice while walking in the driveway of his home. Loss of consciousness less than 30 minutes	S06.5X1A, W00.0XXA, Y93.01, Y92.014
Initial visit for displacement of electrode used for deep brain stimulation in patient with essential tremor	T85.120A, G25.0
Follow-up visit for re-evaluation of injury of lumbosacral sympathetic nerve	S34.5XXD
Healed displaced fracture of the right anterior acetabular wall with concomitant femoral nerve injury. Two years status post injury, motor function has returned but the patient continues to have symptoms consistent with meralgia paresthetica.	G57.11, S32.411S, S74.11XS

Section 1.18 Questions

What are the time frames regarding the loss of consciousness related to head trauma?

Which codes listed in the coding practice examples above are external cause codes?

Which types of external cause codes require a 7th character extension to identify the episode of care?

What does the 7th character extension for the external cause codes specify?

See end of chapter for Coding Practice answers.

Section 1.19 – Mental and Behavioral Disorders

Mental and behavioral disorders have a dedicated chapter in ICD-10-CM. However, because mental and behavioral disorders are clearly related to, or are an integral part of nervous system function, mental and behavioral disorders are discussed here in the nervous system section of this course. There are several broad classifications of mental and behavioral disorders including:

Disorders Due to Physiological Condition – Mental disorders in this section are all caused by some type of physiological condition such as cerebral disease, brain injury, or some other type of cerebral dysfunction. Many codes in this section require that the underlying physiological condition be coded first.

Disorders Due to Psychoactive Substance Use and Dependence – Codes in this section include alcohol, drug, and inhalant use, abuse, and dependence; nicotine dependence; and other psychoactive substance related disorders. Note that nicotine use is not coded from this section but is instead reported with a code from Chapter 21 as a factor influencing health status.

Psychotic Disorders – Some of the more common types of psychotic disorders include schizophrenia, bipolar disorder, and major depressive disorders.

Non-Psychotic Disorders – Anxiety and dissociative and stress-related mental disorders are types of non-psychotic disorders.

Other Disorders – Other disorders and conditions reported with codes from Chapter 5 include: eating disorders, sleep disorders, sexual dysfunction not due to a substance or physiological condition, personality disorders, mental retardation, some developmental disorders, and behavioral and emotional disorders of childhood and adolescence.

Section 1.19 Coding Practice

Condition	ICD-10-CM
Late onset Alzheimer's disease with dementia and combative behavior	G30.1, F02.81
Parkinson's disease with dementia	G31.83, F02.80
Post-concussion syndrome following concussion three weeks ago with loss of consciousness less than 30 minutes.	S06.0X1S, F07.81
Acute alcohol intoxication with blood alcohol level 22 mg/100 ml	F10.920, Y90.1
Recurrent major depression of moderate severity	F33.1
Chronic posttraumatic stress syndrome	F43.12
Developmental dyslexia	F81.0

Section 1.19 Questions

Is FØ2.8Ø ever reported as the primary (first listed) diagnosis code?

Why are two codes required to report post-concussion syndrome?

Why is code Y9Ø.1 used in conjunction with F1Ø.92Ø in the example above?

See end of chapter for Coding Practice answers.

Terminology

Arachnoid – One of the three membranes that protect the brain and spinal cord. The arachnoid is the middle membrane and is composed of delicate fibrous tissue.

Autonomic nervous system – The part of the nervous system that controls the smooth muscle, cardiac muscle, and glands. It functions automatically and involuntarily being regulated by several centers in the brain, including the cerebral cortex, hypothalamus, and the medulla oblongata. The autonomic system consists entirely of motor fibers that transmit impulses from the CNS to smooth muscle, cardiac muscle, and glandular epithelium and affects visceral functions.

Central nervous system (CNS) – One of two primary divisions of the nervous system, the CNS is composed of two organs, the brain and spinal cord.

Dura mater – One of three membranes that protect the brain and spinal cord. The dura mater is the outer membrane and is composed of a tough fibrous tissue.

Encephalon – The brain.

Extradural – Lying outside of the dura mater.

Extracranial – Lying outside the cranial cavity or skull.

Ganglion – A group of nerve cell bodies; a term usually used to refer to a group of nerve cell bodies located in the peripheral nervous system.

Intracranial – Lying within the cranial cavity or skull.

Intraspinal – Lying within the vertebral canal.

Meninges – The three membranes that cover the brain and spinal cord which include an outer membrane called the dura mater, a middle membrane called the arachnoid, and an inner membrane called the pia mater.

Nerve – A cordlike structure composed of one or more myelinated and/or unmyelinated nerve fibers that lie outside the central nervous system protected by connective tissue and nourished with blood vessels. Nerves transmit nerve impulses to and from the central nervous system.

Nerve reflex – An automatic response to a nerve stimulus.

Neuroglia – Connective tissue cells of the central nervous system.

Neuron – Nerve cell; the functional unit of the nervous system consisting of a cell body, dendrites, and an axon.

Peripheral nervous system – All neural tissue that lies outside the skull and vertebral column which includes nerve roots, nerves, nerve plexuses, and ganglions.

Pia mater – One of three membranes that protect the brain and spinal cord. The pia mater is the inner transparent layer containing blood vessels and is adherent to the surfaces of the brain and spinal cord.

Spinal nerve root – One of two bundles of nerve fibers, a sensory bundle and a motor bundle, that emerge from the spinal cord and then combine to form the mixed spinal nerve.

Subdural – Lying under the outermost membrane that covers the brain and spinal cord.

Quiz—Section 1. Nervous System

1. Gliomas are:
   a. Malignant tumors of connective tissue cells in the CNS
   b. Malignant tumors of connective tissue cells in the PNS
   c. Malignant, benign, or uncertain behavior tumors of the connective tissue cells in the CNS
   d. Malignant, benign, or uncertain behavior tumors of the nerve cells (neurons) in the CNS

2. The white matter of the brain is composed of:
   a. Myelinated nerve fibers
   b. Unmyelinated axons
   c. Neurons
   d. Schwann cells

3. The cerebellum is the ______________ area of the brain.
   a. Sensory
   b. Motor
   c. Pain sensor
   d. Autonomic

4. Cauda equina refers to:
   a. A portion of the brain stem
   b. The mid-portion of the spinal cord
   c. The spinal nerve roots in the lumbosacral region
   d. The paired coccygeal nerves

5. Irritability is defined as:
   a. The ability of nerve cells to respond to stimuli and convert them into nerve impulses
   b. Any stimulus that is strong enough to initiate transmission of a nerve impulse
   c. A series of subthreshold stimuli
   d. The ability of the nerve cell to transmit an impulse to another nerve cell or another tissue

6. The code for a neuroma at an amputation site is reported with a code from:
   a. Chapter 2 Neoplasms
   b. Chapter 6 Diseases of the Nervous System
   c. Chapter 19 Injury, poisoning, and certain other consequences of external causes
   d. Multiple codes are required from different chapters

7. Infections of the nervous system:
   a. Are always reported with a code from Chapter 1 Infections
   b. Are always reported with a code from Chapter 6 Diseases of the Nervous System
   c. May be reported with a code from either chapter
   d. May require a single code from Chapter 1 Infections, a single code from Chapter 6 Diseases of the Nervous System, or one or more codes from both chapters

8. The human body is able to repair damaged nerve cells when the cell body is intact and the axon has a neurilemma. True or False?
   a. True
   b. False

9. Which disease listed below is NOT categorized as a demyelinating disease?
   a. Acute hemorrhagic leukoencephalitis
   b. Myasthenia gravis
   c. Multiple sclerosis
   d. Periaxial encephalitis

10. When reporting conditions such as hemiplegia and nerve injuries, documentation required to assign the most specific code includes information regarding which side(s) of the body that is (are) affected. This coding concept is known as:
    a. Dominant side identification
    b. Seventh character extension
    c. Sequencing
    d. Laterality

See next page for answers.

Quiz Answers—Section 1. Nervous System

1. Gliomas are:

   c. Malignant, benign, or uncertain behavior tumors of the connective tissue cells in the CNS

2. The white matter of the brain is composed of:

   a. Myelinated nerve fibers

3. The cerebellum is the _______________ area of the brain.

   b. Motor

4. Cauda equina refers to:

   c. The spinal nerve roots in the lumbosacral region

5. Irritability is defined as:

   a. The ability of nerve cells to respond to stimuli and convert them into nerve impulse

6. The code for a neuroma at an amputation site is reported with a code from:

   c. Chapter 19, Injury, Poisoning, and Certain Other Consequences of External Causes

7. Infections of the nervous system:

   d. May require a single code from Chapter 1 Infections, a single code from Chapter 6 Diseases of the Nervous System, or one or more codes from both chapters

8. The human body is able to repair damaged nerve cells when the cell body is intact and the axon has a neurilemma: True or False?

   a. True

9. Which disease listed below is NOT categorized as a demyelinating disease:

   b. Myasthenia gravis

10. When reporting conditions such as hemiplegia and nerve injuries documentation required to assign the most specific code includes information on which side(s) of the body is affected. This coding concept is known as:

    d. Laterality

Section 2. Musculoskeletal System

Chapter Objectives

After studying this chapter, you should be able to:

- Describe the functions of the musculoskeletal system
- Describe the different types of bone, cartilage, and muscle cells
- Identify the two principle tissues types in the skeletal system
- Describe the characteristics of compact and cancellous bone
- Identify the five principle bone types
- Identify the basic structural elements of a typical long bone
- Explain how bones are formed and the growth process of developing bone (i.e. immature bone)
- Define the terms axial and appendicular skeleton
- Describe the three types of cartilage
- Describe the characteristics of the three types of joints
- Identify the six types of synovial joints
- Describe the three different types of muscle tissue and where these three tissue types are found
- Explain how the nearly 700 muscles in the human body are named
- Identify musculoskeletal system organs
- Understand ICD-10-CM coding guidelines for the musculoskeletal system
- Understand documentation elements required to assign the diagnosis code to the highest level of specificity
- Describe a variety of diseases and disease processes affecting the musculoskeletal system
- Identify how these diseases and disease processes affect and alter musculoskeletal system function
- Define the characteristics of different types of bone fractures
- Assign ICD-10-CM codes to diseases, injuries, and other conditions affecting the musculoskeletal system
- Use the Gustilo open fracture classification system to assign the correct seventh digit extension for open fractures
- Define the following terms: osteoblasts, osteocytes, osteoclasts, chondroblasts, chondrocytes, chondroclasts

Overview

The musculoskeletal system is actually two body systems, the muscular system and the skeletal system. However, because of the interrelated nature of the two systems, they are often discussed together.

The skeletal system provides the structural framework needed to support the body and protect internal organs. Bones and joints also provide leverage needed for movement. The muscular system, specifically skeletal muscle, provides the body with the ability to move and also protects underlying body structures.

Skeletal System

The skeletal system performs a number of important functions. These include:

- Support – The skeletal system supports the soft tissues of the body. The support provided gives the body its shape and allows the body to maintain an erect posture.
- Protection – The skeletal system protects the brain, spinal cord, and thoracic structures including the lungs, heart, and major blood vessels.
- Leverage – Some bones of the skeletal system serve as levers. Muscles attach to these bones and when the muscles contract, the bones function as levers that produce movement.
- Storage – The bones provide storage of mineral salts. Two mineral salts stored in the bones are calcium and phosphorous.
- Blood cell production – The medullary cavities and epiphyses of long bones contain myeloid tissue, more commonly referred to as bone marrow, where blood-forming (hematopoietic) cells are found.

Cells

Cells unique to the skeletal system include osteoblasts, osteocytes, and osteoclasts found in bone and chondroblasts, chondrocytes, and chondroclasts found in cartilage.

Bone is continually reshaping itself. The osteoblasts, osteocytes, and osteoclasts work together to build up, maintain, and break down osseous tissue.

Osteoblasts are bone forming cells that cover new bone. These cells make collagen and hydroxyapatite which are part of the intercellular tissue needed for new bone formation. Collagen is a protein that is a primary component of the white fibers in bone and cartilage. Hydroxyapatite is a mineral that is part of the lattice structure of bone. Some osteoblasts become buried in this intercellular tissue, also called matrix, at which point they become osteocytes. The bone building process occurs in waves as a layer of osteoblasts become buried in matrix and form new layers of bone.

Osteocytes are mature osteoblasts that are incorporated into the bone matrix. Osteocytes maintain bone structure and occupy small cavities present in osseous tissue which are called lacunae. The cytoplasmic processes of osteocytes extend into small canals or channels in osseous tissue called canaliculi. This allows osteocytes to make contact with other osteocytes by means of gap junctions. Osteocytes are highly differentiated and function as mechanosensory cells. This means that mechanical stimuli, such as mechanical stress, can activate osteocytes which respond by sending signals to osteoblasts and osteoclasts which then build up or break down the bone.

Osteoclasts are large, multinucleated cells that function in the absorption and removal of osseous tissue. Osteoclasts make collagenase, an enzyme that breaks down collagen, and also secrete acids that dissolve hydroxyapatite so that the bone matrix can be resorbed and removed.

Like bone, cartilage is also continually reshaping itself. Chondroblasts, chondrocytes, and chondroclasts function in much the same way as bone cells to build, maintain, and break down cartilage. Chondroblasts are dividing cells that build cartilage. Chondrocytes are mature cartilage cells that occupy the cartilage lacunae and maintain cartilage structure. Chondroclasts break down and resorb calcified cartilage.

Tissue

The skeletal system is composed of two types of connective tissue—bone, also called osseous tissue, and cartilage. Connective tissue is the binding and supporting tissue of the body and has widely scattered cells and an abundance of intercellular material called matrix.

Bone

Bone like other connective tissues contains a great deal of intercellular substance surrounding widely scattered cells. Bone is differentiated by the presence of mineral salts, primarily calcium phosphate and calcium carbonate, which form part of the intercellular substance. These mineral salts give bone its hardness. Collagenous fibers are embedded in the intercellular substance providing further reinforcement and strength to bones.

Bones appear to be solid structures. However, bone tissue is actually porous, which means it contains pores or small holes. The pores are filled with living bone cells and blood vessels that supply the cells with nutrients. Bone tissue is classified as cancellous or compact. Cancellous bone, also called spongy bone contains large spaces filled with bone marrow. Compact bone, also called dense bone, contains spaces that are fewer in number and smaller than those found in cancellous bone.

Other characteristics of compact bone include:

- Concentric rings, called lamellae, formed by hard, calcified, intercellular substance
- Blood vessels and nerves penetrating compact bone through structures called Volkmann's canals where they connect with blood vessels and nerves in the medullary cavity
- Longitudinal canals called Haversian canals that are circular cavities formed by the lamellae
- Small spaces between the lamellae called lacunae

Other characteristics of cancellous bone include:

- Thin, irregular latticework bone plates called trabeculae
- Spaces between the trabeculae filled with bone marrow
- Lacunae, which contain osteocytes, within the trabeculae
- Blood vessels from the periosteum penetrating the spongy bone
- Blood circulating through the bone marrow cavities providing nourishment to the osteocytes in the trabeculae

Types of Bone

Bones are classified into five principle types based on their shape and the following characteristics:

- Long bones
  - Greater length than width
  - Divided into a diaphysis in the middle and two epiphyses at the ends
  - Slightly curved to help distribute weight and stress along the length of the bone
  - Contain significantly more compact bone than spongy bone
- Short bones
  - Cube-shaped
  - Consist primarily of spongy bone covered by a thin layer of compact bone
- Flat bones
  - Thin and flat in shape
  - Consist of two thin plates of compact bone with a thin layer of spongy bone between the two plates
- Irregular bones
  - Complex shapes
  - Vary in the amount of compact and spongy bone
- Sesamoid bones
  - Usually small bones with the exception of the patellae in the knee joints which are larger than other sesamoid bones
  - Found in tendons where pressure develops

Types of bones

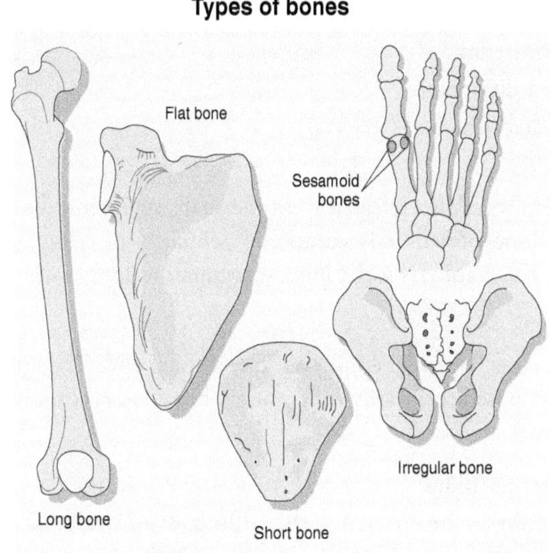

Cartilage

Cartilage is composed of a dense network of collagenous fibers combined with some elastic fibers. The collagenous and elastic fibers are embedded in a gel-like substance. Mature cartilage cells called chondrocytes are distributed singly or in groups in lacunae throughout the matrix. Cartilage is covered by perichondrium which is a dense irregular connective tissue membrane.

There are three types of cartilage which include:

- Hyaline cartilage
- Fibrocartilage
- Elastic cartilage

Hyaline cartilage is the most abundant type of cartilage in the body. This type of cartilage provides both flexibility and support. It covers the ends of bones that form joints where it is called articular cartilage. It is found at the ends of the ribs where it is called costal cartilage. It also forms part of the nose, larynx, trachea, bronchi, and bronchial tubes. Hyaline cartilage is bluish-white in color and has a glossy appearance. Microscopically, the collagenous fibers appear transparent and the lacunae are filled with an abundance of chondrocytes.

Fibrocartilage is strong and rigid. It joins the anterior pelvic bones at the symphysis pubis and also forms the discs that lie between the vertebrae. Microscopically, fibrocartilage has bundles of visible collagenous fibers with chondrocytes scattered throughout.

Elastic cartilage provides strength and maintains shape in the structures it forms. It is found in the larynx, external ear, and Eustachian tubes. Microscopically, elastic cartilage has threadlike elastic fibers that contain chondrocytes scattered throughout the lacunae.

Bone Anatomy

Bones vary somewhat in structure based on their type. A typical long bone is composed of the following parts:

- Diaphysis
- Epiphyses
- Articular cartilage
- Periosteum
- Medullary cavity
- Endosteum

Diaphysis

The diaphysis, also referred to as the shaft, is the middle section of the long bones. It is composed primarily of compact bone tissue. The diaphysis is the longest segment of long bones.

Epiphysis

Long bones have two epiphyses, one at each end. The epiphyses are composed primarily of spongy bone and contain bone marrow.

Articular Cartilage

The epiphyses are covered with a thin layer of hyaline cartilage, which is called articular cartilage when it is present in a joint that forms an articulation with another bone.

Long bone cross section

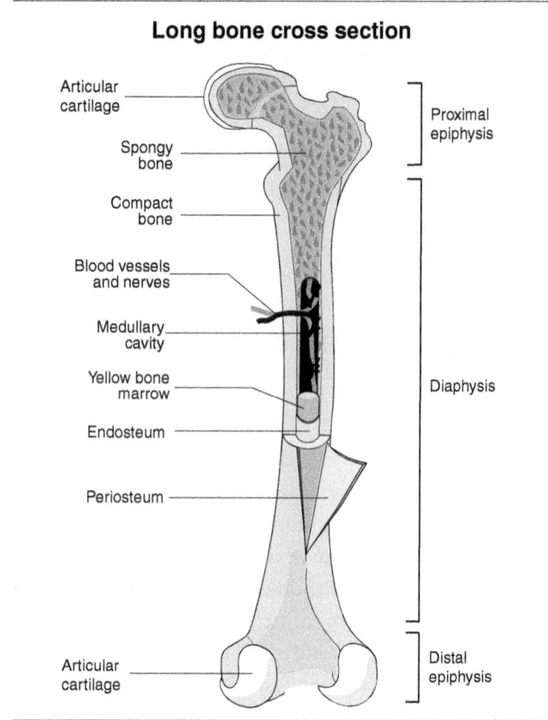

Periosteum

Periosteum is the dense, white, fibrous membrane that covers the external surface of the bone. It is composed of two layers. The outer fibrous connective tissue layer contains blood vessels, lymphatic vessels, and nerves that penetrate the deeper bone tissues. The inner layer contains elastic fibers, blood vessels, and osteoblasts from which new bone arises. The primary functions of the periosteum include:

- Bone growth
- Bone repair
- Supply of nutrients
- Points of attachments for ligaments and tendons

Medullary Cavity

The medullary cavity is the space within the diaphysis that contains bone marrow also called myeloid tissue. Bone marrow gives rise to blood cells and is discussed in Chapter 1.

Endosteum

The endosteum is a thin membrane that lines the medullary cavity and contains osteoblasts.

Bone Formation and Growth

Bone forms by a process called ossification. During embryonic development, the skeleton is composed of fibrous membranes and hyaline cartilage. These tissues are shaped like the bones they will become, providing the framework for the ossification process. There are two general types of bone formation, intramembranous ossification and endochondral ossification. Intramembranous ossification occurs in the fibrous membranes where bone forms directly on or within the membranous framework. Only a few flat bones such as the bones of the roof of the skull and the jaw begin as fibrous membranes and become bone by intramembranous ossification. Most bones begin as hyaline cartilage and become bone by endochondral ossification.

The process by which hyaline cartilage ossifies and grows is as follows in long bones:

1. The embryonic cartilage model develops.
2. A collar of spongy bone begins to form near the middle in what will become the diaphysis.
3. Once a collar of spongy bone has been laid down along the length of the diaphysis, a primary ossification center develops in the middle of the diaphysis and ossification continues along the entire length of the diaphysis and extends into the epiphyses.
4. Blood vessels begin to penetrate the bone.
5. The medullary cavity forms.
6. The periosteum covering the collar thickens and lengthens laying down successive layers of bone that become thickest at the ends of the bone (epiphyses).
7. Secondary ossification centers form in the epiphyses. In the long bones this occurs shortly after birth and in early childhood.
8. At the time that the secondary ossification centers form, almost all of the cartilage has been replaced by bone with the exception of the cartilage on the ends which becomes the articular cartilage and the cartilage between the diaphysis and the epiphysis which becomes the epiphyseal plate, also called the growth plate. The epiphyseal plate allows the bone to increase in length until full growth is attained at which time the cartilage in the epiphyseal plate is replaced with bone.

Axial and Appendicular Skeleton

The 206 bones of the adult human skeleton are divided into two groups, the axial skeleton and the appendicular skeleton.

The axial skeleton contains those bones that form the axis or center of the human body. These are the bones that form the head and trunk of the human body. The axial skeleton is comprised of eighty bones:

- Cranial bones – 8
- Facial bones – 14

Skull
Lateral view

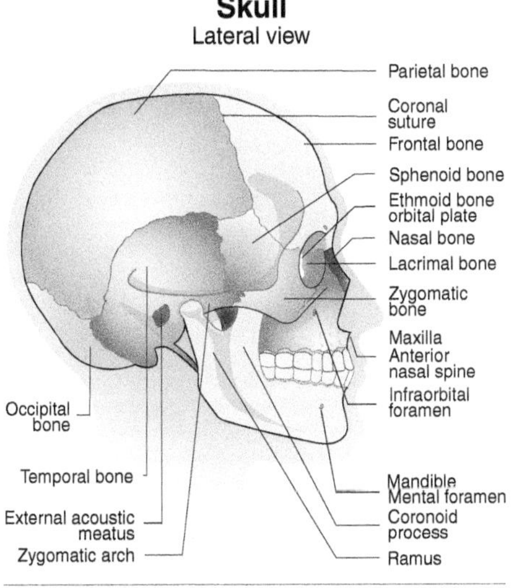

- Hyoid – 1
- Ossicles (bones of the ear) – 6 (3 on each side)
- Vertebral column – 26

Vertebral disc anatomy

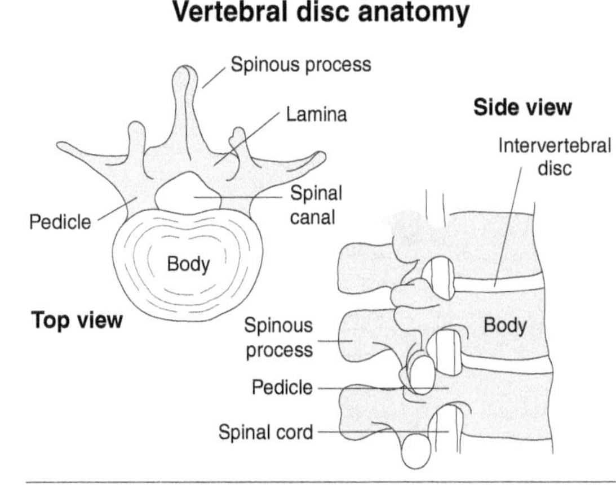

Vertebral column

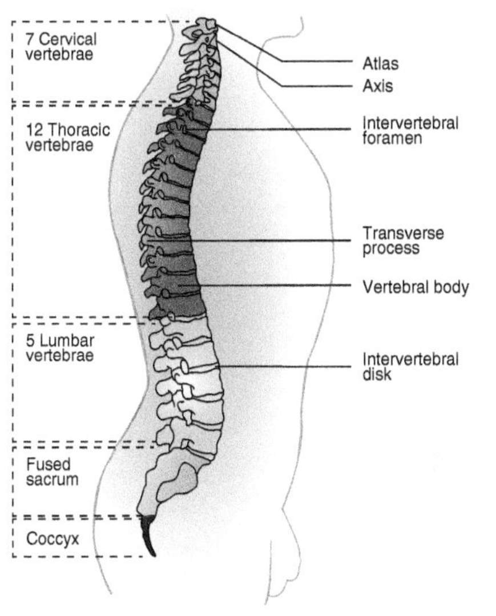

- Sternum – 1
- Ribs – 24

Ribs and sternum

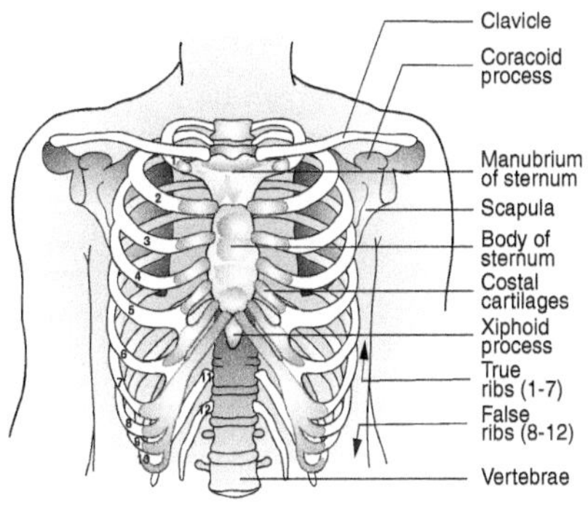

The appendicular skeleton contains the bones that form the appendages, more commonly known as the upper and lower extremities or arms and legs, shoulder and pelvic girdle. There are 126 bones that make up the appendicular skeleton:

- Shoulder girdle
  - Clavicle – 2
  - Scapula – 2

Shoulder girdle

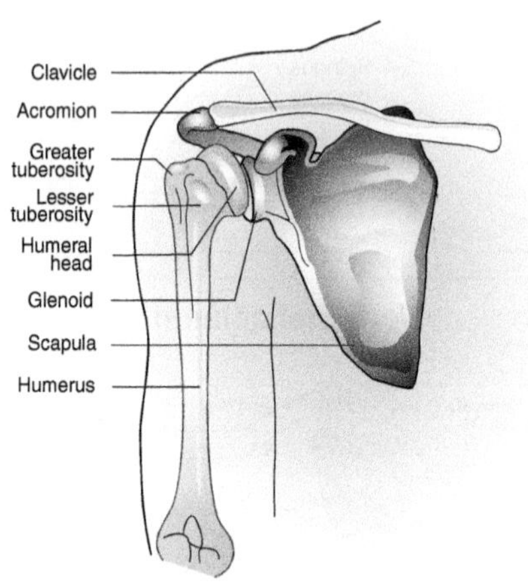

- Upper extremities
  - Humerus – 2
  - Ulna – 2
  - Radius – 2
  - Carpals – 16
  - Metacarpals – 10
  - Phalanges – 28
- Pelvic Girdle
  - Coxal or pelvic bone – 2

Pelvic Girdle

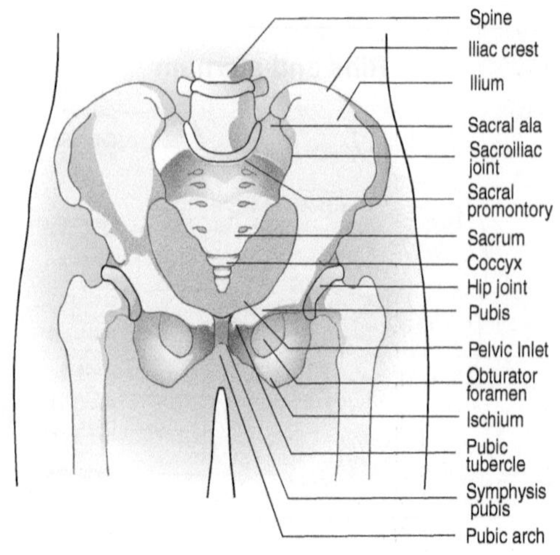

- Lower extremities
  - Femur – 2
  - Fibula – 2
  - Tibia – 2
  - Patella – 2
  - Tarsus – 2
  - Metatarsus – 10
  - Phalanges – 28

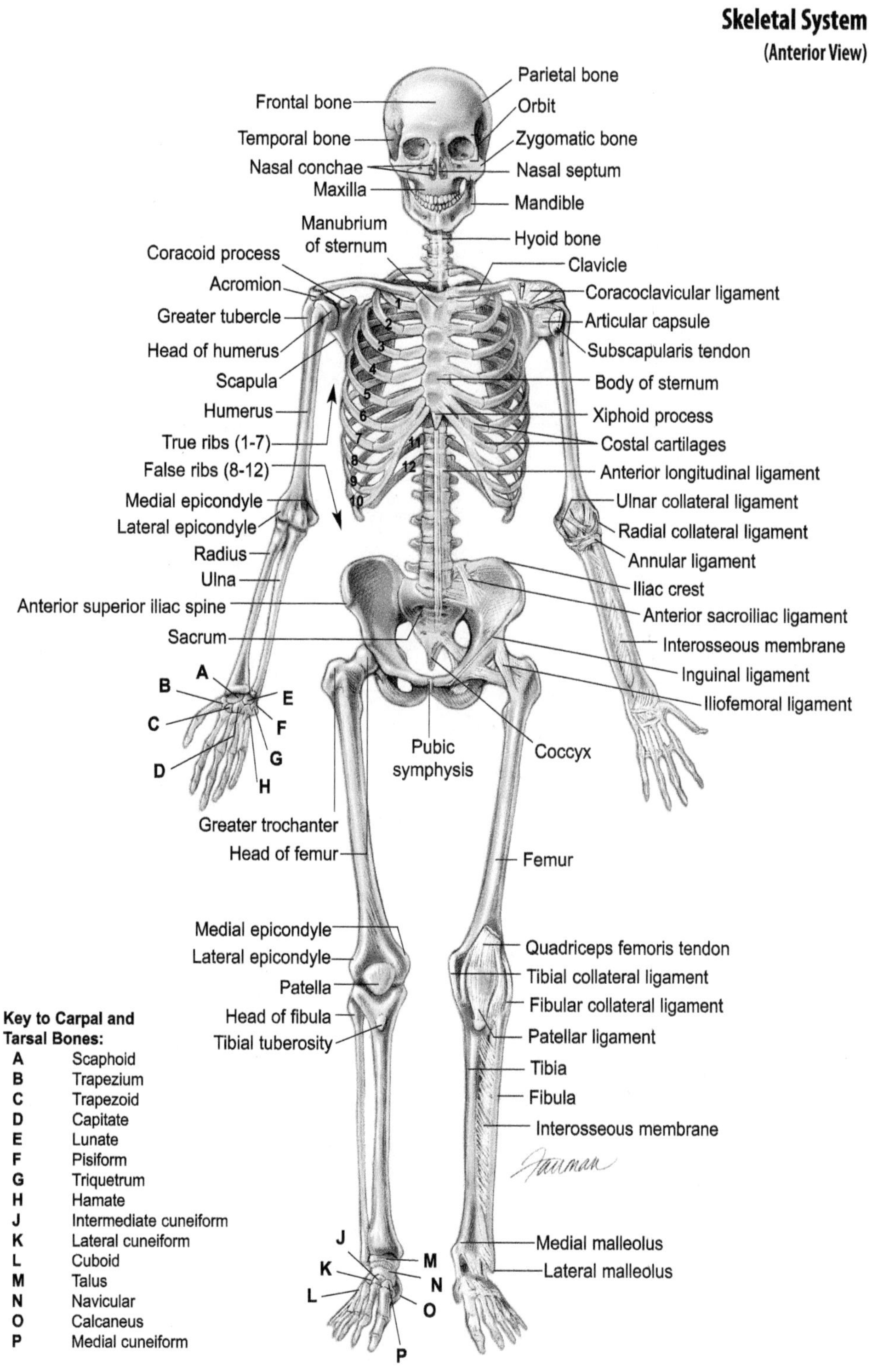

Key to Carpal and Tarsal Bones:

A	Scaphoid
B	Trapezium
C	Trapezoid
D	Capitate
E	Lunate
F	Pisiform
G	Triquetrum
H	Hamate
J	Intermediate cuneiform
K	Lateral cuneiform
L	Cuboid
M	Talus
N	Navicular
O	Calcaneus
P	Medial cuneiform

© Fairman Studios, LLC, 2002. All Rights Reserved.

ICD-10-CM Anatomy & Physiology

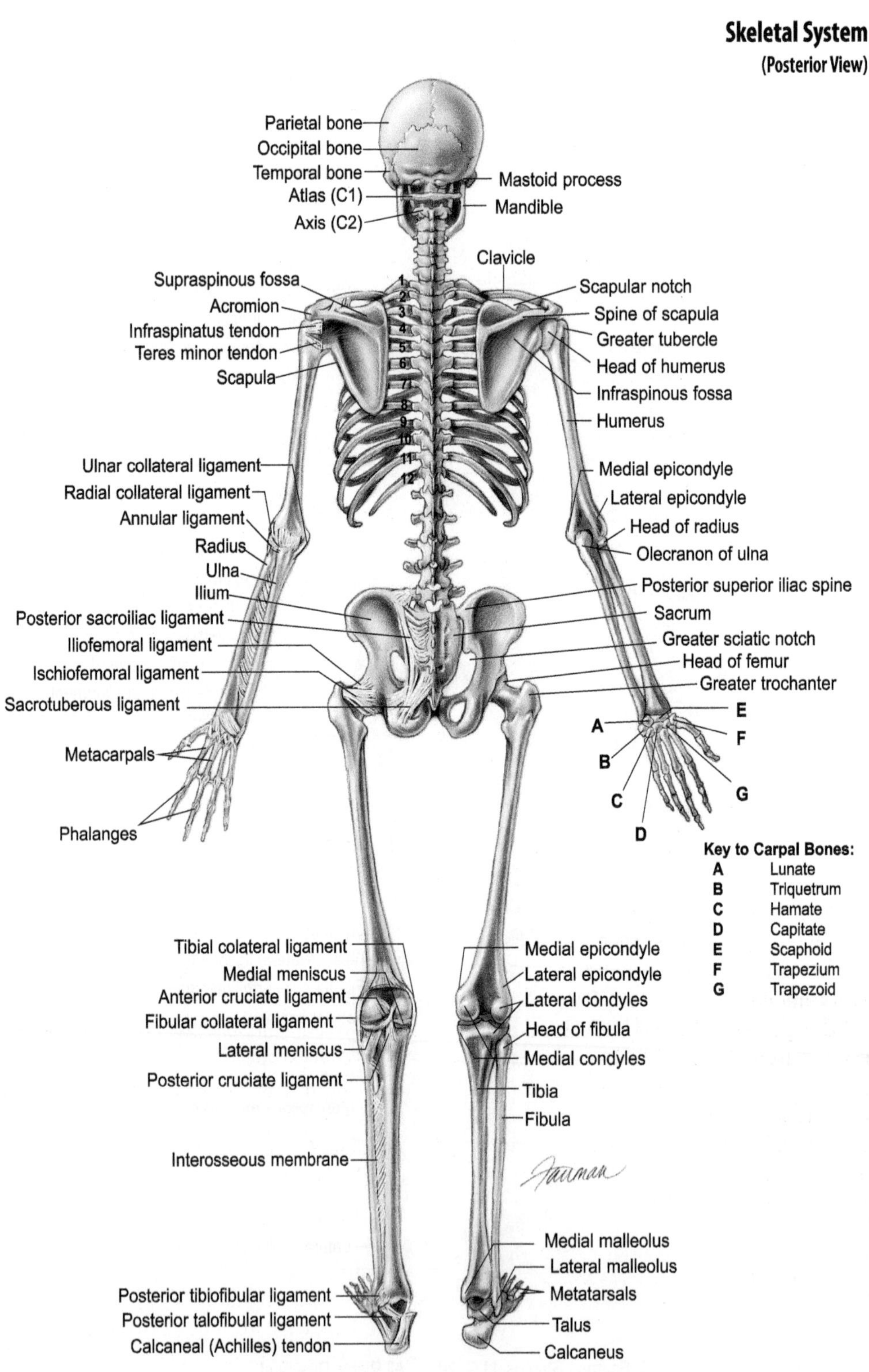
Skeletal System
(Posterior View)
Parietal bone
Occipital bone
Temporal bone
Atlas (C1)
Axis (C2)
Mastoid process
Mandible
Clavicle
Supraspinous fossa
Acromion
Infraspinatus tendon
Teres minor tendon
Scapula
Scapular notch
Spine of scapula
Greater tubercle
Head of humerus
Infraspinous fossa
Humerus
Ulnar collateral ligament
Radial collateral ligament
Annular ligament
Radius
Ulna
Ilium
Posterior sacroiliac ligament
Iliofemoral ligament
Ischiofemoral ligament
Sacrotuberous ligament
Metacarpals
Phalanges
Medial epicondyle
Lateral epicondyle
Head of radius
Olecranon of ulna
Posterior superior iliac spine
Sacrum
Greater sciatic notch
Head of femur
Greater trochanter
Key to Carpal Bones:
A Lunate
B Triquetrum
C Hamate
D Capitate
E Scaphoid
F Trapezium
G Trapezoid
Tibial colateral ligament
Medial meniscus
Anterior cruciate ligament
Fibular collateral ligament
Lateral meniscus
Posterior cruciate ligament
Interosseous membrane
Medial epicondyle
Lateral epicondyle
Lateral condyles
Head of fibula
Medial condyles
Tibia
Fibula
Medial malleolus
Lateral malleolus
Metatarsals
Talus
Calcaneus
Posterior tibiofibular ligament
Posterior talofibular ligament
Calcaneal (Achilles) tendon

© Fairman Studios, LLC, 2002. All Rights Reserved.

Joints

Joints, also called articulations, are points of contact between bones or between cartilage and bones. Joints are classified into three principle kinds based on their anatomy which also determines the type and degree of movement. These include:

- Fibrous joints
- Cartilaginous joints
- Synovial joints

Knee joint

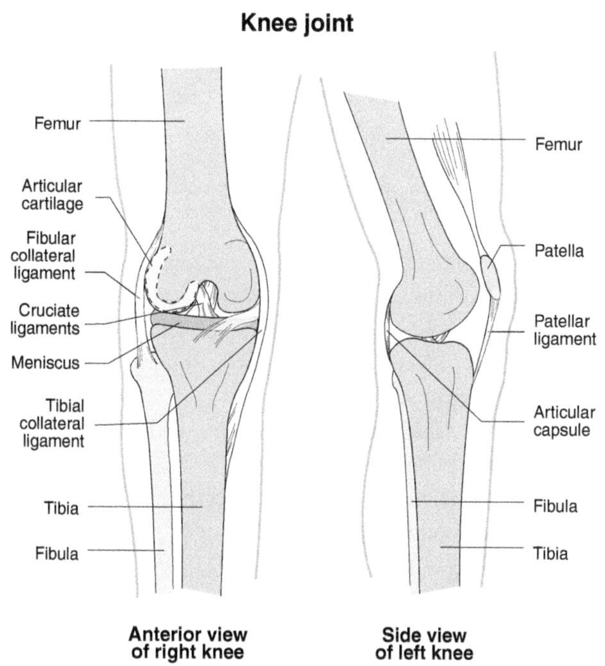

Fibrous Joints

Characteristics of fibrous joints are:

- Little or no movement
- Lack of a joint cavity
- Tightly joined by fibrous tissue

Fibrous joints are divided into two subcategories, sutures and syndesmoses. Sutures are located between the bones of the skull and may be composed of interlocking margins of jagged bone that fit together like a jigsaw puzzle or they may be composed of overlapping bone segments. In both types of suture, the bones are joined by a thin layer of fibrous tissue. The articulation between the tibia and fibula is an example of a syndesmosis. In a syndesmosis the bones are a little farther apart than a suture which allows a slight amount of movement, but the bones are still tightly joined by fibrous tissue.

Cartilaginous Joints

Characteristics of cartilaginous joints are:

- Lack of a joint cavity
- Tightly joined by cartilage
- Slight movement

Cartilaginous joints are divided into two categories, synchondroses and symphyses. A synchondrosis is a temporary joint found in the epiphyseal plate between the epiphysis and diaphysis of growing bones. It is composed of hyaline cartilage that will be replaced by bone when the bone has reached its adult length. A symphysis is composed of a broad, flat disc of cartilage. The intervertebral discs of the spine and the pubic symphysis are examples of this type of joint.

Cartilaginous joint

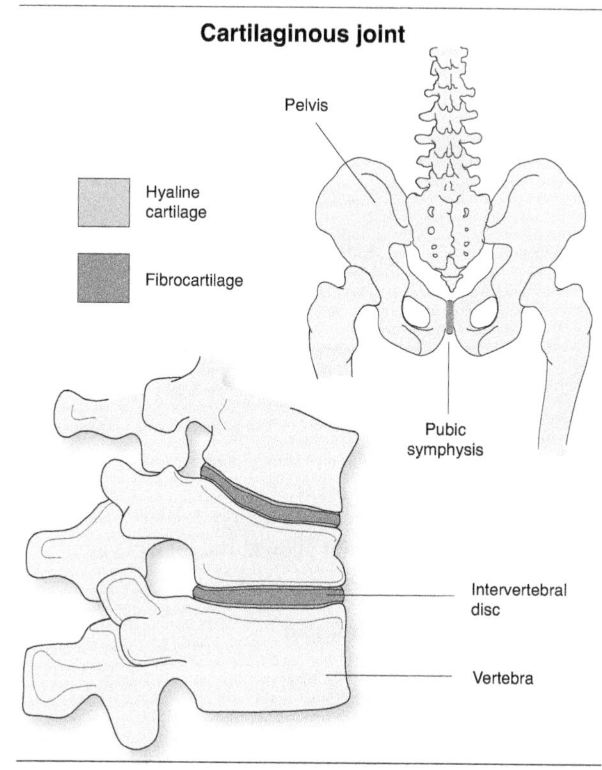

Synovial Joints

The shoulders, elbows, hips, and knees as well as smaller joints such as the carpal joints and interphalangeal joints are examples of synovial joints. Synovial joints possess the following characteristics:

- A joint cavity
- A layer of hyaline cartilage that covers the ends of the bones forming the articulation, also called articular cartilage
- A synovial membrane that lines the walls of the joint cavity and secretes synovial fluid to lubricate the joint
- Held together by ligaments which are bands of collagenous fibers
- Movement that is determined by the location of ligaments, muscles, tendons, and other bones that limit or obstruct movement in a particular direction

Synovial joints may also contain bursae. Bursae are sac-like structures formed by connective tissue and lined with a synovial membrane. They are filled with synovial fluid which provides a cushion. Bursae are found between skin and bones, tendons and bones, muscles and bones, and ligaments and bones.

Synovial joint

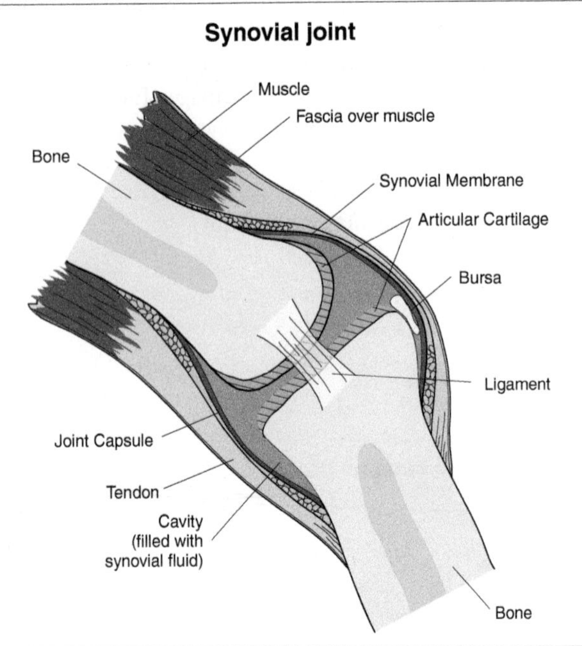

Synovial joints are subdivided into six types based primarily on the type of movement the joint allows. The six types are

- Ball and socket
- Condyloid, also called ellipsoid
- Gliding
- Hinge
- Pivot
- Saddle

Shoulder joint anatomy

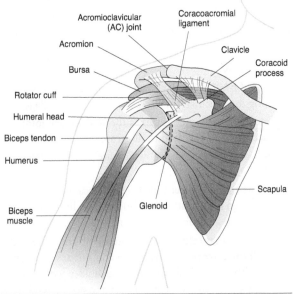

Ligaments are another important anatomic structure in the joint. A ligament is composed of bands of fibrous connective tissue. These bands are elastic and connect two bones together providing stability to the joint. Generally, the ligaments are named for the bones they connect. Injures to ligaments are called sprains.

Muscular System

Motion is an essential function that is made possible by the muscles of the body. Muscles work together with bones that form the framework of the body and joints that provide leverage for movement. Motion is accomplished by contraction of the muscles.

Muscles provide the body with the ability to move in obvious ways, such as walking or grasping a knife and fork, as well as less obvious ways which include beating of the heart and movement of food through the digestive tract. In addition to movement, muscles also maintain posture, provide the ability to sit or stand, stabilize joints, produce heat, and protect underlying structures.

Cells

Muscles are composed of highly specialized cells called fibers with four characteristics:

- Irritability which provides muscle tissue with the ability to respond to stimuli
- Contractility which provides muscles with the ability to shorten and thicken causing contraction of muscle tissue when a sufficient stimulus is received
- Extensibility which provides muscles with the ability to stretch when pulled
- Elasticity which provides muscles with the ability to return to their original shape after contraction or extension

There are three types of muscle fibers:

- Skeletal – cylindrical, multinucleated, striated fibers under voluntary control
- Smooth – spindle-shaped fibers with a single, centrally located nucleus that lack striations
- Cardiac – branching fibers with a single nucleus, striations, and intercalated discs

Skeletal and cardiac muscle fibers are covered by a plasma membrane called the sarcolemma.

Tissue

The three types of muscle tissue are all characterized by the ability of the tissue to contract. Two proteins present in muscle, actin and myosin, are contractile proteins that provide muscle with this ability. Muscle tissue is composed of tightly packed fibers. The fibers are usually arranged in bundles that are surrounded by connective tissue. Muscle tissue is also well supplied with nerves and blood vessels.

Skeletal Muscle Tissue

Skeletal muscle is attached to bone and is named for its location.

Skeletal muscles are wrapped in a fibrous connective tissue called epimysium. Extensions of the epimysium called perimysium divide the muscle tissue into bundles. Extensions of the perimysium called endomysium separate each muscle fiber. The epimysium, perimysium, and endomysium are continuous with the connective tissue that connects the muscle to bone, such as a tendon or aponeurosis. A tendon is a cord of connective tissue that attaches muscle to the periosteum of the bone and an aponeurosis is a broad, flat sheet of connective tissue that attaches

ICD-10-CM Anatomy & Physiology

to the periosteum or another muscle. These two structures work with the muscle to facilitate movement.

Skeletal muscles are heavily infiltrated with nerves and blood vessels which are necessary for muscle function, the primary one being contraction. Nerve cells provide the stimulus to contract. Blood vessels provide the nutrients and oxygen needed for muscle to have enough energy to contract. Blood vessels also carry away waste products that are eliminated when muscle energy is expended.

Smooth Muscle Tissue

There are two types of smooth muscle, visceral and multiunit. Visceral muscle is composed of sheets that form part of the walls of hollow organs, also called viscera. Examples include the stomach, intestines, uterus, and urinary bladder. The function of smooth muscle tissue is to contract and relax in a wave-like fashion as impulses spread along the tissue in an organized manner. When a single visceral muscle fiber is stimulated to contract by a nerve impulse, the impulse travels over adjacent fibers. The arrangement of the tightly bound muscle fibers in a branching pattern that form a continuous network facilitates the wave-like contraction. Multiunit smooth muscle consists of individual muscle fibers each with its own motor-nerve endings. Stimulation of a single multiunit fiber causes contraction of only that fiber. Multiunit smooth muscle is located in the walls of blood vessels, in erector muscles attached to hair follicles, and in intrinsic muscles of the eye, such as the iris.

Cardiac Muscle Tissue

Cardiac muscle tissue forms the walls of the heart and is classified as striated involuntary muscle tissue. Cardiac muscle tissue is composed of individual fibers that are covered by a plasma membrane called the sarcolemma. The fibers have internal myofibrils that overlap to form the microscopic protein myofilaments that give cardiac muscle a striated or striped appearance. Each fiber is separated by an intercalated disc that strengthens the cardiac tissue and enhances the conduction of nerve impulses from one cell to another. The function of cardiac muscle tissue is to contract and relax rhythmically in response to electrical stimulation from specialized conducting tissue within the heart.

Skeletal Muscles

Skeletal muscles produce movement by pulling on tendons, aponeuroses, or other connective tissue structures which in turn pull on bones or other muscles. Most skeletal muscles cover at least one joint and are attached to the articulating bones that form the joint. When bones articulate, one bone or set of bones usually moves more than the other bone or set of bones forming the joint. The place where a muscle/tendon attaches to the more stationary bone is called the origin and the attachment to the more movable bone is called the insertion. Usually the muscle/tendon origin is the more proximal point of attachment and the insertion is the more distal. The fleshy part of the muscle between the two bones is called the belly or gaster. The extension of the muscle attaching it to bone is the tendon. Tendons have a poor blood supply and are therefore slow to heal when injured or inflamed. Tendons attach muscle to bone and with the muscle provide motion to the joint, unlike ligaments which provide stability.

There are nearly 700 skeletal muscles in the human body. These muscles are named based on one or more of the following criteria:

- Direction of muscle fibers, such as rectus, transverse, oblique
- Location, such as temporalis, tibialis
- Size, such as maximus, minimus, brevis, longus
- Number of origins, such as biceps, triceps, quadriceps
- Site of origin and insertion, such as brachioradialis
- Shape, such as deltoid, trapezius
- Action, such as flexor, extensor, abductor, adductor

When learning the names of the muscles, it is helpful to subdivide them into groups, such as location and function or action. A table follows listing some of the most common muscles/tendons, their origin, insertion and action.

For diagnosis coding, it is important to know the general location of muscles and their action since diseases, disorders, and injuries of the muscles are generally reported using the site of the disorder and the action (flexor/extensor) rather than the specific muscle. For example, a muscle contracture is reported by laterality (right or left side) and by general region (shoulder, upper arm, forearm, hand, thigh, lower leg, ankle, foot).

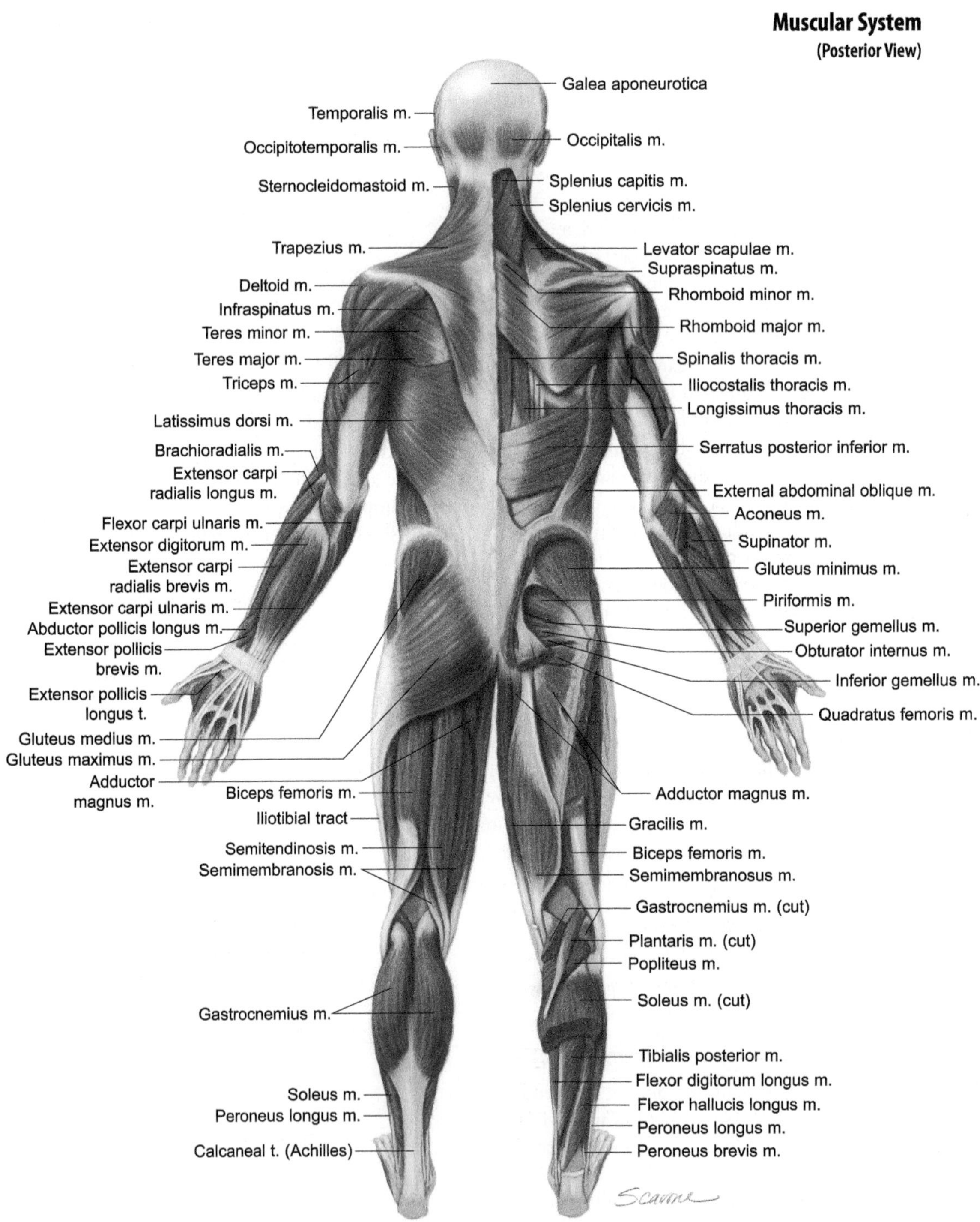
Muscular System
(Posterior View)
Galea aponeurotica
Temporalis m.
Occipitotemporalis m.
Occipitalis m.
Sternocleidomastoid m.
Splenius capitis m.
Splenius cervicis m.
Trapezius m.
Levator scapulae m.
Supraspinatus m.
Deltoid m.
Rhomboid minor m.
Infraspinatus m.
Teres minor m.
Rhomboid major m.
Teres major m.
Spinalis thoracis m.
Triceps m.
Iliocostalis thoracis m.
Longissimus thoracis m.
Latissimus dorsi m.
Brachioradialis m.
Serratus posterior inferior m.
Extensor carpi radialis longus m.
External abdominal oblique m.
Aconeus m.
Flexor carpi ulnaris m.
Extensor digitorum m.
Supinator m.
Extensor carpi radialis brevis m.
Gluteus minimus m.
Extensor carpi ulnaris m.
Piriformis m.
Abductor pollicis longus m.
Superior gemellus m.
Extensor pollicis brevis m.
Obturator internus m.
Inferior gemellus m.
Extensor pollicis longus t.
Quadratus femoris m.
Gluteus medius m.
Gluteus maximus m.
Adductor magnus m.
Biceps femoris m.
Adductor magnus m.
Iliotibial tract
Gracilis m.
Semitendinosis m.
Biceps femoris m.
Semimembranosis m.
Semimembranosus m.
Gastrocnemius m. (cut)
Plantaris m. (cut)
Popliteus m.
Soleus m. (cut)
Gastrocnemius m.
Tibialis posterior m.
Flexor digitorum longus m.
Soleus m.
Flexor hallucis longus m.
Peroneus longus m.
Peroneus longus m.
Calcaneal t. (Achilles)
Peroneus brevis m.
Scavone

© Fairman Studios, LLC, 2002. All Rights Reserved.

Muscular System
(Anterior View)

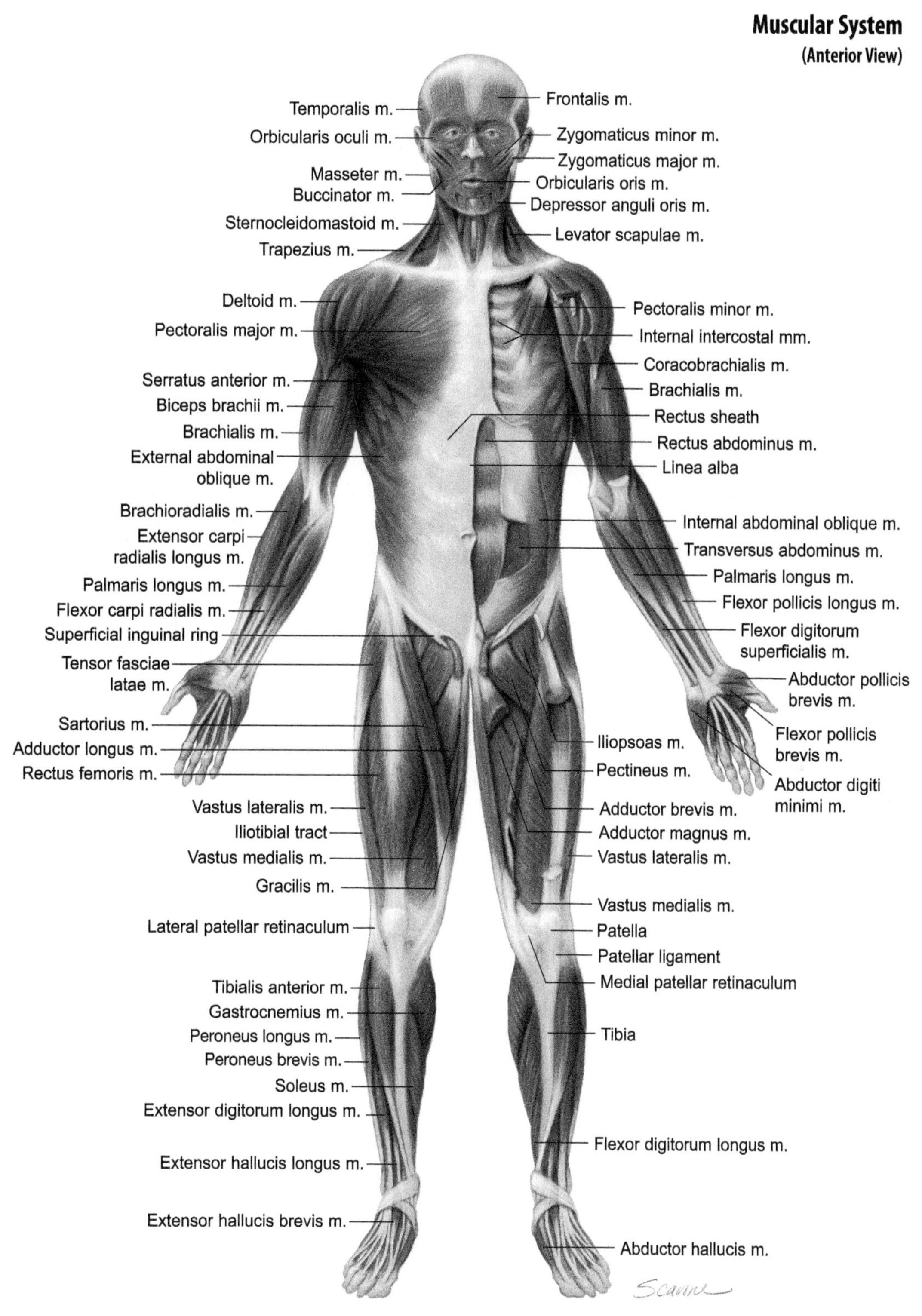
Temporalis m.
Frontalis m.
Orbicularis oculi m.
Zygomaticus minor m.
Zygomaticus major m.
Masseter m.
Buccinator m.
Orbicularis oris m.
Depressor anguli oris m.
Sternocleidomastoid m.
Levator scapulae m.
Trapezius m.
Deltoid m.
Pectoralis minor m.
Pectoralis major m.
Internal intercostal mm.
Coracobrachialis m.
Serratus anterior m.
Brachialis m.
Biceps brachii m.
Rectus sheath
Brachialis m.
Rectus abdominus m.
External abdominal oblique m.
Linea alba
Brachioradialis m.
Internal abdominal oblique m.
Extensor carpi radialis longus m.
Transversus abdominus m.
Palmaris longus m.
Palmaris longus m.
Flexor pollicis longus m.
Flexor carpi radialis m.
Superficial inguinal ring
Flexor digitorum superficialis m.
Tensor fasciae latae m.
Abductor pollicis brevis m.
Sartorius m.
Flexor pollicis brevis m.
Iliopsoas m.
Adductor longus m.
Pectineus m.
Rectus femoris m.
Abductor digiti minimi m.
Vastus lateralis m.
Adductor brevis m.
Iliotibial tract
Adductor magnus m.
Vastus medialis m.
Vastus lateralis m.
Gracilis m.
Vastus medialis m.
Lateral patellar retinaculum
Patella
Patellar ligament
Tibialis anterior m.
Medial patellar retinaculum
Gastrocnemius m.
Peroneus longus m.
Tibia
Peroneus brevis m.
Soleus m.
Extensor digitorum longus m.
Flexor digitorum longus m.
Extensor hallucis longus m.
Extensor hallucis brevis m.
Abductor hallucis m.

© Fairman Studios, LLC, 2002. All Rights Reserved.

ICD-10-CM Anatomy & Physiology

Muscle/Tendon	Location	Origin (O)/Insertion (I)	Action
Abductor pollicis brevis	Wrist/Hand/Thumb	O: Transverse carpal ligament and the tubercle of the scaphoid bone or (occasionally) the tubercle of the trapezium I: Base of the proximal phalanx of the thumb	Abducts the thumb and with muscles of the thenar eminence, acts to oppose the thumb
Abductor pollicis longus (APL)	Forearm/Thumb/Hand/Wrist	O: Posterior radius, posterior ulna and interosseous membrane I: Base 1st metacarpal Combined with the extensor pollicis brevis makes the anatomic snuff box.	Abducts and extends thumb at CMC joint; assists wrist abduction (radial deviation)
Achilles tendon	Lower Leg	O: Joins the gastrocnemius and soleus muscles I: Calcaneus	Flexor tendon – plantar flexes foot
Anconeus	Elbow	O: Lateral epicondyle humerus I: Posterior olecranon	Extends forearm
Brachialis	Elbow	O: Distal ½ anterior humeral shaft I: Coronoid process and ulnar tuberosity	Flexes forearm
Biceps brachii	Shoulder/Upper Arm	Long Head: O: Supraglenoid tubercle of the scapula to join the biceps tendon, short head in the middle of the humerus forming the biceps muscle belly Short Head: O: Coracoid process at the top of the scapula I: Radial tuberosity Long head and short head join in the middle of the humerus forming the biceps muscle belly	Flexes elbow Supinates forearm Weakly assists shoulder with forward flexion (long head) Short head provides horizontal adduction to stabilize shoulder joint and resist dislocation. With elbow flexed becomes a powerful supinator
Common flexor tendon 1. Pronator teres 2. Flexor carpi radialis (FCR) 3. Palmaris longus 4. Flexor digitorum superficialis (sublimis) (FDS) 5. Flexor carpi ulnaris (FCU)	Forearm/Hand	Common flexor tendon formed by 5 muscles of the forearm. There are slight variations in the site of origin and insertion 1. O: Medial epicondyle humerus and coronoid process of the ulna. I: Mid-lateral surface radial shaft 2. O: Medial epicondyle humerus. I: Base of 2nd and 3rd metacarpal 3. O: Medial epicondyle humerus. I: Palmar aponeurosis and flexor retinaculum 4. O: Medial epicondyle humerus, coronoid process ulna and anterior oblique line of radius. I: shaft middle phalanx digits 2-5 5. O: Medial epicondyle of the humerus, olecranon and posterior border ulna I: Pisiform, hook of hamate and 5th metacarpal.	1. Pronator Teres-pronation of forearm; assists elbow flexion 2. FCR- flexion and abduction of wrist (radial deviation) 3. Palmaris longus-assists wrist flexion 4. FDS- flexion middle phalanx PIP joint digits 2-4; assists wrist flexion 5. FCU- flexes and adducts hand at the wrist
Coracobrachialis	Shoulder/Upper Arm	O: Coracoid process I: Midshaft of humerus	Adducts & flexes shoulder
Deltoid	Shoulder/Upper Arm	O: Lateral 1/3 of clavicle, acromion and spine of scapula I: Deltoid tuberosity of humerus Large triangular shaped muscle composed of three parts	Anterior-Flex & medially rotate shoulder; Middle-assist w/abduction of humerus at shoulder; Posterior-extend & laterally rotate humerus
Extensor carpi radialis longus (ECRL)	Forearm/Hand	O: Lateral epicondyle humerus I: Dorsal surface 2nd metacarpal	Extends and abducts wrist; active during fist clenching
Extensor (digitorum) communis (EDC)	Forearm/Wrist/Hand/Finger	O: Lateral epicondyle humerus terminates into 4 tendons in the hand I: On the lateral and dorsal surfaces of digits 2-5 (fingers)	Extends the metacarpophalangeal (MCP), proximal interphalangeal (PIP) and distal interphalangeal (DIP) joints of 2nd-5th fingers and wrist
Extensor digitorum longus (EDL)	Lower Leg/Ankle/Foot	O: Lateral condyle tibia, proximal 2/3 anterior fibula shaft and interosseous membrane I: Middle and distal phalanx toes 2-5	Extension lateral 4 digits at metatarsophalangeal joint; assists dorsiflexion of foot at ankle

Muscle/Tendon	Location	Origin (O)/Insertion (I)	Action
Extensor hallicus longus (EHL)	Lower Leg/Ankle/Foot	O: Middle part anterior surface fibula and interosseous membrane I: Dorsal aspect base distal phalanx great toe	Extends great toe; assists dorsiflexion of foot at ankle; weak invertor
Extensor pollicis brevis (EPB)	Wrist/Hand/Thumb	O: Distal radius (dorsal surface) and interosseous membrane I: Base proximal phalanx thumb Combined with the abductor pollicis longus makes the anatomic snuff box	Extends the thumb at metacarpophalangeal joint (MCPJ)
Extensor pollicis longus (EPL)	Wrist/Hand/Thumb	O: Dorsal surface of the ulna and interosseous membrane I: Base distal phalanx thumb	Extends distal phalanx thumb at IP joint; assists wrist abduction
Flexor digitorum longus (FDL)	Lower Leg/Ankle/Foot	O: Medial posterior tibia shaft I: Base distal phalanx digits 2-5	Flexes digits 2-5; plantar flex ankle; supports longitudinal arch of foot
Flexor digitorum profundus (FDP)	Forearm/Wrist/Hand	O: Proximal 1/3 anterior-medial surface ulna and interosseous membrane; in the hand splits into 4 tendons I: Base of the distal phalanx, digits 2-5 (fingers)	Flexes the distal phalanx, digits 2-5 (fingers)
Flexor hallucis longus (FHL)	Lower Leg/Ankle/Foot	O: Inferior 2/3 posterior fibula; inferior interosseous membrane I: Base distal phalanx great toe (hallux)	Flexes great toe at all joints; weakly plantar flexes ankle; supports medial longitudinal arches of foot
Flexor pollicis brevis (FPB)	Wrist/Hand/Thumb	O: Distal edge of the transverse carpal ligament and the tubercle of the trapezium I: Proximal phalanx of the thumb	Flexes the thumb at the metacarpophalangeal (MCPJ) and carpometacarpal (CMC) joint
Flexor pollicis longus (FPL)	Forearm/Wrist/Hand/Thumb	O: Below the radial tuberosity on the anterior surface of the radius and interosseous membrane I: Base distal phalanx thumb	Flexes the thumb at the metacarpophalangeal (MCPJ) and interphalangeal (IPJ) joint
Hamstring	Upper Leg/Knee	Composed of three muscles 1. Semitendinosus O: Ischial tuberosity I: Anterior proximal tibial shaft Semimembranosus O: Ischial tuberosity I: Posterior medial tibial condyle 2. Biceps femoris O: Long head ischial tuberosity; short head linea aspera femoral shaft and lateral supracondylar line I: Head of fibula	1. Semitendinosus and Semimembranosus- Flexes leg at knee, when knee flexed medially rotates tibia; thigh extensor at hip joint; when hip & knee both flexed, extends trunk 2. Biceps femoris-Flexes leg and rotates laterally when knee flexed; extends thigh
Intrinsics of hand hypothenar 1. Abductor digiti minimi 2. Flexor digiti minimi brevis 3. Opponens digiti minimi	Wrist/Hand/Finger	1. O: Pisiform I: Medial side of base proximal phalanx 5th finger 2. O: Hook of hamate & flexor retinaculum I: Medial side of base proximal phalanx 5th finger 3. O: Hook of hamate and transverse carpal ligament I: Uulnar aspect shaft 5th metacarpal	1. Abducts 5th finger; assists flexion proximal phalanx 2. Flexes proximal phalanx 5th finger 3. Rotates the 5th metacarpal bone forward

Muscle/Tendon	Location	Origin (O)/Insertion (I)	Action
Intrinsics of hand short 1. Dorsal interossei 1-4 2. Dorsal interossei 1-3 3. Lumbricals 1st & 2nd 4. Lumbricals 3rd & 4th	Wrist/Hand	1. O: Adjacent sides of 2 MC I: Bases of proximal phalanges; extensor expansions of 2-4 fingers 2. O: Palmar surface 2nd, 4th & 5th MC I: Bases of proximal phalanges; extensor expansions of 2nd, 4th & 5th fingers 3. O: Lateral two tendons of FDP I: Lateral sides of extensor expansion of 2nd-5th 4. O: Medial 3 tendons of FDP I: Lateral sides of extensor expansion of 2nd-5th	1. Abduct 2-4 fingers from axial line; acts w/lumbricals to flex MCP jt and extend IP jt 2. Adduct 2nd, 4th, 5th fingers from axial line; assist lumbricals to flex MCP jt and extend IP jt; extensor expansions of 2nd-4th fingers 3. Flex MCP jt; extend IP joint 2-5 4. Flex MCP jt; extend IP joint 2-5
Intrinsics of hand thenar 1. Abductor pollicis brevis 2. Adductor pollicis 3. Flexor pollicis brevis 4. Opponens pollicis	Wrist/Hand/Thumb	1. O: Flexor retinaculum & tubercle scaphoid & trapezium I: :Lateral side of base of proximal phalanx thumb 2. O: Oblique head base 2nd & 3rd MC, capitate, adjacent carpals and transverse head anterior surface shaft 3rd MC I: Medial side base of proximal phalanx thumb 3. O: Flexor retinaculum & tubercle scaphoid & trapezium I: Lateral side of base of proximal phalanx thumb 4. O: Transverse carpal ligament and the tubercle of the trapezium I: Lateral border shaft 1st metacarpal	1. Abducts thumb; helps w/opposition 2. Adducts thumb toward lateral border of palm 3. Flexes thumb 4. Rotates the thumb in opposition with fingers
Lumbricals (foot)	Foot	O: Lumbricals-flexor digitorum longus tendon I: Medial side base proximal phalanges 2-5	Assist in joint movement between metatarsals
Patellar tendon	Knee/Lower Leg	Connects the bottom of the patella to the top of the tibia The tendon is actually a ligament because it joins bone to bone	Works with the quadriceps tendon to bend and straighten the knee
Pectoralis major	Chest/Upper Arm	O: Clavicle, sternum, ribs 2-6 I: Upper shaft of humerus	Adducts, flexes, medially rotates humerus
Peroneus (fibularis) brevis	Lower Leg/Ankle/Foot	O: Distal 2/3 lateral shaft fibula I: Becomes a tendon midcalf that runs behind the lateral malleolus inserts on tuberosity base 5th metatarsal	Eversion of foot; assists with plantar flexion of foot at ankle
Peroneus (fibularis) longus	Lower Leg/Ankle/Foot	O: Head and upper 2/3 lateral surface fibula I: Becomes a long tendon midcalf that runs behind the lateral malleolus and crosses obliquely on plantar surface of foot inserts on base 1st metatarsal and medial cuneiform	Eversion of foot; weak plantar flexion foot at ankle
Peroneus (fibularis) tertius	Lower Leg/Ankle/Foot	O: Inferior 1/3 anterior surface fibula and interosseous membrane I: Dorsum base 5th metatarsal	Dorsiflexes ankle and aids inversion of foot
Quadratus plantae	Foot	O: Calcaneus I: Flexor digitorum tendons	Assists flexor muscles

Muscle/Tendon	Location	Origin (O)/Insertion (I)	Action
Quadriceps femoris	Upper Leg/Knee	Composed of four muscles: Rectus femoris O: Anterior inferior iliac spine and ilium superior to acetabulum I: Combines to form quadriceps tendon; inserts base of patella and tibial tuberosity via patellar ligament Vastus lateralis O: Greater trochanter and lateral aspect femoral shaft I: Lateral patella and tendon of rectus femoris Vastus medialis O: Intertrochanteric line and medial aspect femoral shaft I: Medial border of quadriceps tendon and medial aspect of patella; tibial tuberosity via patellar ligament Vastus intermedius: O: Anterior and lateral surface femoral shaft I: Posterior surface upper border of patella; tibial tuberosity via patellar ligament	Extends leg at knee joint; rectus femoris with iliopsoas helps flex thigh and stabilized hip joint
Quadriceps tendon	Upper Leg/Knee	Fibrous band of tissue that connects the quadriceps muscle of the anterior thigh to the patella (kneecap)	Holds the patella (kneecap) in the patellofemoral groove of the femur enabling it to act as a fulcrum and provide power to bend and straighten the knee
Rotator cuff tendons:	Shoulder/Upper Arm	Rotator cuff tendons are formed by 4 muscles of the shoulder/upper arm. They all originate from the scapula and insert (terminate) on the humerus:	
1. Supraspinatus		1. O: Supraspinous fossa of scapula. I: Superior facet greater tuberosity humerus.	1. Initiates abduction of shoulder joint (completed by deltoid)
2. Infraspinatus		2. O: Infraspinous fossa of scapula. I: Middle facet greater tuberosity humerus.	2. Externally rotates the arm; helps hold humeral head in glenoid cavity
3. Teres minor		3. O: Middle half of the lateral border of the scapula. I: Inferior facet greater tuberosity humerus	3. Externally rotates the arm; helps hold humeral head in glenoid cavity
4. Subscapularis		4. O: Subscapular fossa of scapula. I: Either the lesser tuberosity humerus or the humeral neck.	4. Internally rotates and adducts the humerus; helps hold humeral head in glenoid cavity
Tibialis anterior	Lower Leg/Ankle/Foot	O: Lateral condyle and superior half lateral tibia I: Base 1st metatarsal, plantar surface medial cuneiform	Dorsiflexion ankle, foot inversion at subtalar and midtarsal joints
Tibialis posterior	Lower Leg/Ankle/Foot	O: Interosseus membrane; posterior surface of tibia and fibula I: Tuberosity of tarsal navicula, cuneiform and cuboid and bases of 2nd, 3rd and 4th metatarsals	Plantar flexes ankle; inverts foot
Triceps	Shoulder/Upper Arm	Long head: O: Infraglenoid tubercle of scapula; Lateral head: O: Upper half of posterior surface shaft of humerus Medial head O: Lower half of posterior surface shaft of humerus I: Olecranon process Only muscle on the back of the arm	Extends elbow joint; long head can adduct humerus and extend it from flexed position; stabilizes shoulder joint

Musculoskeletal System Coding Guidelines

Disorders of the musculoskeletal system are primarily contained in Chapter 13. Injuries affecting the musculoskeletal system such as fractures, dislocations, sprains and strains are found in Chapter 19. The guidelines for Chapter 13 as well codes for traumatic musculoskeletal injuries from Chapter 19 are included in the tables below. Refer to the ICD-1Ø-CM manual for general guidelines affecting all body systems such as infections, neoplasms and congenital anomalies and guidelines regarding complications of care.

- Instructions on coding for site and laterality
- Clarifications are given for assigning a code for the joint affected versus the specific bone affected
- Acute traumatic versus chronic or recurrent conditions are defined and coding instructions are provided
- Instructions are provided for coding pathologic fractures which now require a 7th digit extension to identify episode of care
- Osteoporosis is defined with coding instructions provided
- Codes for gout have been moved from Chapter 3 Endocrine, Nutritional and Metabolic Diseases to Chapter 13 Musculoskeletal System
- Instructions for coding of traumatic fractures and injuries are provided.
- Instructions for the proper application of the 7th character for injuries and traumatic fractures.
- Instructions for coding for complications of care.

ICD-10-CM – Chapter 13: Diseases of Musculoskeletal and Connective Tissue (M00-M99)

1. Site and laterality

Most of the codes within Chapter 13 have site and laterality designations. The site represents either the bone, joint or the muscle involved. For some conditions where more than one bone, joint or muscle is usually involved, such as osteoarthritis, there is a "multiple sites" code available. For categories where no multiple site code is provided and more than one bone, joint or muscle is involved, multiple codes should be used to indicate the different sites involved.

a. Bone versus joint

For certain conditions, the bone may be affected at the upper or lower end, (e.g., avascular necrosis of bone, M87, Osteoporosis, M80, M81). Though the portion of the bone affected may be at the joint, the site designation will be the bone, not the joint.

2. Acute traumatic versus chronic or recurrent musculoskeletal conditions

Many musculoskeletal conditions are a result of previous injury or trauma to a site, or are recurrent conditions. Bone, joint or muscle conditions that are the result of a healed injury are usually found in chapter 13. Recurrent bone, joint or muscle conditions are also usually found in chapter 13. Any current, acute injury should be coded to the appropriate injury code from chapter 19. Chronic or recurrent conditions should generally be coded with a code from chapter 13. If it is difficult to determine from the documentation in the record which code is best to describe a condition, query the provider.

3. Coding of Pathologic Fractures

7th character A is for use as long as the patient is receiving active treatment for the fracture. While the patient may be seen by a new or different provider over the course of treatment for a pathological fracture, assignment of the 7th character is based on whether the patient is undergoing active treatment and not whether the provider is seeing the patient for the first time.

7th character D is to be used for encounters after the patient has completed active treatment. The other 7th characters, listed under each subcategory in the Tabular List, are to be used for subsequent encounters for routine care of fractures during the healing and recovery phase as well as treatment of problems associated with the healing, such as malunions, nonunions, and sequelae.

Care for complications of surgical treatment for fracture repairs during the healing or recovery phase should be coded with the appropriate complication codes.

See Section I.C.19. Coding of traumatic fractures

4. Osteoporosis

Osteoporosis is a systemic condition, meaning that all bones of the musculoskeletal system are affected. Therefore, site is not a component of the codes under category M81, Osteoporosis without current pathological fracture. The site codes under category M80, Osteoporosis with current pathological fracture, identify the site of the fracture, not the osteoporosis.

a. Osteoporosis without pathological fracture

Category M81, Osteoporosis without current pathological fracture, is for use for patients with osteoporosis who do not currently have a pathologic fracture due to the osteoporosis, even if they have had a fracture in the past. For patients with a history of osteoporosis fractures, status code Z87.310, Personal history of (healed) osteoporosis fracture, should follow the code from M81.

b. Osteoporosis with current pathological fracture

Category M80, Osteoporosis with current pathological fracture, is for patients who have a current pathologic fracture at the time of an encounter. The codes under M80 identify the site of the fracture. A code from category M80, not a traumatic fracture code, should be used for any patient with known osteoporosis who suffers a fracture, even if the patient had a minor fall or trauma, if that fall or trauma would not usually break a normal, healthy bone.

ICD-10-CM – Chapter 19: Injury, poisoning, and certain other consequences of external causes (S00-T88)

5. Application of 7th Characters in Chapter 19

Most categories in chapter 19 have a 7th character requirement for each applicable code. Most categories in this chapter have three 7th character values (with the exception of fractures): A, initial encounter, D, subsequent encounter and S, sequela. Categories for traumatic fractures have additional 7th character values. While the patient may be seen by a new or different provider over the course of treatment for an injury, assignment of the 7th character is based on whether the patient is undergoing active treatment and not whether the provider is seeing the patient for the first time.

For complication codes, active treatment refers to treatment for the condition described by the code, even though it may be related to an earlier precipitating problem. For example, code T84.50XA, Infection and inflammatory reaction due to unspecified internal joint prosthesis, initial encounter, is used when active treatment is provided for the infection, even though the condition relates to the prosthetic device, implant or graft that was placed at a previous encounter.

7th character "A," initial encounter is used for each encounter where the patient is receiving active treatment for the condition.

7th character "D" subsequent encounter is used for encounters after the patient has completed active treatment of the condition and is receiving routine care for the condition during the healing or recovery phase.

The aftercare Z codes should not be used for aftercare for conditions such as injuries or poisonings, where 7th characters are provided to identify subsequent care. For example, for aftercare of an injury, assign the acute injury code with the 7th character "D" (subsequent encounter).

7th character "S," sequela, is for use for complications or conditions that arise as a direct result of a condition, such as scar formation after a burn. The scars are a sequela of the burn. When using the 7th character "S," it is necessary to use both the injury code that precipitated the sequela and the code for the sequela itself. The "S" is added only to the injury code, not the sequela code. The 7th character "S" identifies the injury responsible for the sequela. The specific type of sequela (e.g. scar) is sequenced first, followed by the injury code.

6. Coding of Injures

When coding injuries, assign separate codes for each injury unless a combination code is provided, in which case the combination code is assigned. Code T07, Unspecified multiple injuries should not be assigned in the inpatient setting unless information for a more specific code is not available. Traumatic injury codes (S00-T14.9) are not to be used for normal healing surgical wounds or to identify complications of surgical wounds.

The code for the most serious injury, as determined by the provider and the focus of treatment, is sequenced first.

a. Superficial injuries

Superficial injuries such as abrasions or contusions are not coded when associated with more severe injuries at the same site.

b. Primary injury with damage to nerves/blood vessels

When a primary injury results in minor damage to peripheral nerves or blood vessel, the primary injury is sequenced first with the additional code(s) for injuries to nerves and spinal cord (such as category S04), and/or injury to blood vessels or nerves, that injury should be sequenced first.

7. Coding of Traumatic Fractures

The principles of multiple coding of injuries should be followed in coding fractures. Fractures of specified sites are coded individually by site in accordance with both the provisions within categories S02, S12, S22, S32, S42, S49, S52, S59, S62, S72, S79, S82, S89, S92 and the level of detail furnished by medical record content.

A fracture not indicated as open or closed should be coded to closed. A fracture not indicated whether displaced or not displaced should be coded to displaced.

More specific guidelines are as follows:

a. Initial vs. Subsequent Encounter for Fractures

Traumatic fractures are coded using the appropriate 7th character for initial encounter (A, B, C) while the patient is receiving active treatment for the fracture. Examples of active treatment are: surgical treatment, emergence department encounter, and evaluation and continuing (ongoing) treatment by the same or different physician. The appropriate 7th character for initial encounter should also be assigned for a patient who delayed seeing treatment for the fracture or nonunion.

Fractures are coded using the appropriate 7th character for subsequent care for encounters after the patient has completed active treatment for the fracture and is receiving routine care for the fracture during the healing or recovery phase. Examples of fracture aftercare are: cast change or removal, an x-ray to check healing status of fracture, removal of external or internal fixation device, medication adjustment, and follow-up visits following fracture treatment.

Care for complications of surgical treatment for fracture repairs during the healing or recovery phase should be coded with the appropriate complication codes.

Care of complications of fractures, such as Malunion and nonunion, should be assigned for a patient who delayed seeking treatment for the fracture or nonunion (K, M, N) or subsequent care with Malunion (P, Q, R).

Malunion/nonunion: The appropriate 7th character for initial encounter should also be assigned for a patient who delayed seeking treatment for the fracture or nonunion.

The open fracture designations in the assignment of the 7th character for fractures of the forearm, femur and lower leg, including ankle are based on the Gustilo open fracture classification. When the Gustilo classification type is not specified for an open fracture, the 7th character for open fracture type I or II should be assigned (B, E, H, M, Q).

A code from category M80, not a traumatic fracture code, should be used for any patient with a known osteoporosis who suffers a fracture, even if the patient had a minor fall or trauma, if that fall or trauma would not usually break a normal, healthy bone.

See Section I.C.13. Osteoporosis

The aftercare Z codes should not be used for aftercare for traumatic fractures. For aftercare of traumatic fracture, assign the acute fracture code with the appropriate 7th character.

b. Multiple fractures sequencing

Multiple fractures are sequenced in accordance with the severity of the fracture

Documentation Elements of Musculoskeletal System

Key documentation elements for musculoskeletal system coding include:

- Fractures
  - Fracture codes require documentation of the type of fracture as displaced or nondisplaced
  - More specific information is required on the fracture type. Examples:
    - » Codes for fracture of the surgical neck of the humerus are specific as to whether the fracture is a 2, 3, or 4-part fracture
    - » Codes for fracture of the humeral shaft are specific as to whether the fracture is greenstick, transverse, oblique, spiral, comminuted, segmental, other, or unspecified
  - Seventh digit characters are required to identify:
    - » The episode of care as initial, subsequent, or sequela with subsequent episode of care further subcategorized as with routine healing, with delayed healing, nonunion, or malunion
    - » The fracture as closed or open
    - » Further classification of open fractures using the Gustilo open fracture classification system which identifies fractures as type I, II, IIIA, IIIB, IIIC

Diseases, Disorders, Injuries and Other Conditions of Musculoskeletal System

This section of the chapter looks at a variety of diseases, disorders, injuries, and other conditions involving the musculoskeletal system. The information presented in the anatomy and physiology section is expanded here to provide a better understanding regarding the part of the musculoskeletal system that is affected and how these conditions affect musculoskeletal system function. Specific information is provided for examples of conditions involving the musculoskeletal system.

Following the discussion of the various diseases, disease processes, disorders, injuries, and conditions, some diagnostic statements are provided with examples of coding in ICD-10-CM. The coding practice is followed by questions to help reinforce the student's knowledge of anatomy, physiology, and coding concepts. Answers to the coding questions can be found by reviewing the text or referring to the ICD-10-CM coding book.

Section 2.1 – Infectious/Parasitic Diseases

Most codes related to infectious and parasitic diseases that affect the musculoskeletal system are found in Chapter 13. Codes from *Chapter 1* – Certain Infectious and Parasitic Diseases are used primarily to report the infectious agent causing the musculoskeletal infection.

Osteomyelitis

Osteomyelitis is an infection of the bone that may be acute, subacute, or chronic. It can be caused by bacteria or fungi. The most common infecting organism is Staphylococcus aureus. Common causes of osteomyelitis include:

- An acute open injury, such as a laceration or open fracture
- A chronic open wound or soft tissue infection that eventually extends into deeper tissues including the bone
- A closed injury such as a hematoma or closed fracture that causes a blood clot near the bone that gets seeded with pathogenic bacteria
- An infection at a separate site that has spread through the blood to the bone

Osteomyelitis affects both adults and children. In adults, the bones of the vertebrae and pelvis are most often affected. In children, the ends of the long bones are more commonly affected.

Osteomyelitis resulting from an injury is reported as a sequela of the injury with the osteomyelitis code sequenced first. The injury code is also reported with the 7th digit extension 'S' to indicate that the osteomyelitis is a sequela of the injury.

Pyogenic Arthritis

Pyogenic arthritis may also be referred to as septic or infectious arthritis. It results when a pathogenic microorganism invades the joint either through the blood stream or through direct contamination of the joint from an open wound, surgical wound, or injection. Some of the more common infectious agents include, staphylococcus, hemophilus influenza, streptococcus, gonococcus, and other gram negative bacilli.

Infectious Myositis

Infectious myositis refers to an acute, subacute, or chronic infection of muscle tissue. It is found most often in individuals with other underlying health issues, such as diabetes, HIV infection, or malignant neoplasm.

Section 2.1 Coding Practice

Condition	ICD-10-CM
Acute osteomyelitis due to open comminuted fracture, right tibial shaft. Infecting organism S. aureus	M86.161, B95.7, S82.251S
Septic arthritis of the left knee. Culture positive for gram negative bacilli	M00.862, B96.89
Infective myositis of the quadriceps muscle, left leg due to Streptococcus viridans	M60.052, B95.4

Section 2.1 Questions

Are there any combination codes in ICD-10-CM for infectious/parasitic diseases of the musculoskeletal system? More specifically, can any infectious/parasitic diseases be reported with either a single code from the infectious/parasitic diseases chapter or from the musculoskeletal system chapter?

____

____

Is the code for gram negative bacilli a specific or nonspecific code?

____

____

Where is the quadriceps muscle located?

____

____

Can the correct code for Streptococcus viridans be found under the main term 'Infection' in the ICD-1Ø-CM Alphabetic Index? If not, under what term(s) is the correct code found?

____

____

See end of chapter for Coding Practice answers.

Section 2.2 – Neoplasms

Neoplasms of the musculoskeletal system like all neoplasms are abnormal tissues in which the cells grow and divide more rapidly than that of normal tissue. Musculoskeletal system neoplasms may be benign, malignant, or of uncertain behavior. Malignant neoplasms may be primary malignancies originating in cells and tissue in the musculoskeletal system or they may be secondary malignancies originating in a remote site and metastasizing to the bone. Understanding terminology as it related to neoplasms will often help with understanding the code selection. The suffix –oma indicates a benign neoplasm. Conversely, the suffix –sarcoma indicates a malignant process. In general, the prefix will be related to the tissue type. Musculoskeletal neoplasms are found in Chapter 2 CØØ-D49 in ICD-1Ø-CM.

Malignant Neoplasms

Compared to neoplasms of other tissues and sites, primary neoplasms of the muscles, bones, and other connective tissues of the musculoskeletal system are relatively rare. Musculoskeletal cancers may be divided into two broad categories which include those involving the muscles, bones, and joints, and myeloma which affects the bone marrow. See *Chapter 1* – Blood and Blood Forming Organs for a discussion of myeloma.

The most common primary malignancies of the musculoskeletal system include:

- Osteosarcoma
- Ewing's sarcoma
- Chondrosarcoma
- Soft tissue sarcoma

Osteosarcoma is the most common bone cancer and occurs most frequently in teenagers and young adults, but may also occur in children and older adults. Osteosarcoma arises in osteoblasts which are the cells that form new bone matrix. The most common sites for osteosarcoma are near the ends of the long bones where bone growth occurs.

Ewing's sarcoma occurs most frequently in children, usually affecting the shafts of long bones or the pelvis. The tumor may also involve the muscle and soft tissue around the tumor site. Ewing's sarcoma is one of the more aggressive types of bone cancer and can metastasize to remote sites including the bone marrow, lungs, kidneys, heart, adrenal glands, and other soft tissues.

Chondrosarcomas are a group of tumors that arise from cartilage cells. These tumors have diverse characteristics and behaviors ranging from slow-growing tumors that rarely metastasize to highly aggressive tumors that frequently spread to other sites. Chondrosarcomas primarily affect the elderly although they are also found in children and younger adults, particularly those with enchondrosis syndromes such as Ollier disease and Maffucci syndrome.

Rhabdomyosarcoma is a malignant tumor of skeletal muscle tissue. These tumors typically affect muscles of the arms or legs, but are not limited to these sites and may begin in any skeletal muscle tissue in the body. Rhabdomyosarcoma is more common in children than adults.

Soft tissue sarcomas affect muscle tissue as well as surrounding structures such as nerves, blood vessels, fibrous joint tissues, fat, and subcutaneous tissues. There are a number of different types of soft tissue sarcomas. The most common types are malignant fibrous histiosarcoma, liposarcoma, and synovial sarcoma. As their names imply, these three sarcomas affect the fibrous tissues, fat, and synovial tissues respectively. Most sarcomas are treated using a combination of excision or resection of the tumor and radiation therapy. Some types are also treated with chemotherapy.

The musculoskeletal system, particularly bone, is a common site of secondary malignant or metastatic tumors. Common neoplasms metastasizing to bone include cancers of the breast and prostate.

Benign Neoplasms

There are many different types of benign neoplasms of the musculoskeletal system. Some types require treatment while others do not. Some types include:

- Chondroblastoma
- Enchondroma
- Giant cell tumor
- Osteochondroma

Chondroblastomas are a rare type of cartilage tumor that originate in chondroblasts which are the cells that form new cartilage. These benign tumors most often affect the ends of the long bones in the arms and legs.

Enchondromas are benign tumors composed of cartilage that form in the intramedullary canal of bones. Enchondromas occur most often in childhood while bones are still growing. They typically do not require treatment unless they cause complications such as fracture at the site of the lesion.

Giant cell tumors may affect bone or soft tissues. Giant cell tumors of bone are relatively rare tumors that grow rapidly. They are composed of giant cells which are individual bone cells that fuse to form the giant cells. While most textbooks classify the tumor as benign, in ICD-1Ø-CM, a diagnosis of giant cell tumor that is not more specifically identified as chondromatous or benign is classified as a neoplasm of uncertain behavior. In rare instances, giant cell tumors do metastasize to the lungs in which case they are classified as malignant neoplasms. The most common site of giant cell bone tumors is the distal end of the femur. Common sites of giant cell tumors of the soft tissues are the tendon sheaths in the hand.

Osteochondromas are the most common types of benign bone tumors. They are caused by an overgrowth of cartilage and bone and are sometimes called osteocartilaginous exostoses. The most common sites are in the long bones near the epiphyseal plates. These tumors typically occur during the period of greatest skeletal growth which is between the ages of 10 and 25.

Section 2.2 Coding Practice

Condition	ICD-10-CM
Ewing's sarcoma, right ilium	C41.4
Osteochondroma, distal left femur	D16.22
Rhabdomyosarcoma, left deltoid muscle	C49.12

Section 2.2 Questions

Is code C41.4 specific to Ewing's sarcoma of the ilium?

What documentation is required to select the most specific diagnosis code for many neoplasms of the bone and muscle?

Where is the deltoid muscle located?

See end of chapter for Coding Practice answers.

Section 2.3 – Arthropathies

The term arthropathy refers to any disease that affects a joint. Conditions listed under arthropathies refer to conditions affecting the peripheral joints. Arthropathies of the vertebral joints are listed under the category Spondylopathies. Common arthropathies of the peripheral joints include:

- Infectious which can be direct or indirect infection
- Inflammatory polyarthropathies such as
  - Rheumatoid arthritis
  - Enteropathic arthropathies
  - Gout and other crystalline arthropathies
  - Villonodular synovitis
- Osteoarthritis
- Other joint disorders such as
  - Acquired deformities
  - Old injuries
  - Non-traumatic dislocation

Rheumatoid Arthritis

Rheumatoid arthritis is an autoimmune disorder affecting connective tissue. It causes chronic inflammation of the joints, particularly those in the hands and feet. It differs from other types of arthritis in that it affects the joint lining causing painful swelling that can eventually result in joint deformity. Rheumatoid arthritis, like other autoimmune disorders, is a systemic disease that can also cause systemic symptoms such as fever and fatigue. Because it affects connective tissue it can also have other organ system manifestations such as vasculitis and neuropathy. Rheumatoid arthritis is classified as sero-negative or sero-positive based on whether the patient tests negative or positive for rheumatoid factor in the blood. Sero-negative rheumatoid arthritis is generally less severe and less disabling than the sero-positive type.

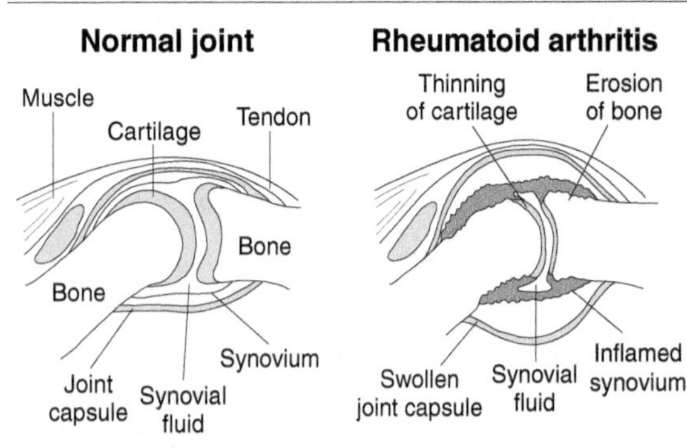

Enteropathic Arthropathies

Enteropathic arthropathies are diseases of the joints associated with or linked to gastrointestinal tract inflammation. The affected joints become inflamed and tender. Enteropathic arthropathies may occur as a result of or in conjunction with a gastrointestinal bacterial or parasitic infection as well as inflammatory diseases that are noninfectious in nature such as inflammatory bowel disease, Crohn's disease, or ulcerative colitis.

Gout

Gout is a form of arthritis caused by the deposition of urate crystals around one or more joints. These crystals cause inflammation of the joint. Gout usually presents suddenly and causes severe inflammation and pain around the affected joints. The tissue around the joints may appear red and swollen.

Villonodular synovitis

Villonodular synovitis, also called pigmented villonodular synovitis (PVNS), affects only joints lined with synovial tissue. PVNS may be diffuse or localized. The diffuse type is the most common and affects the entire synovial lining including the bursa and tendons of the joint. Diffuse PVNS occurs most frequently in the large joints. The less common localized type affects primarily the small joints of the hands and feet and often originates in the tendon sheath. PVNS is characterized by thickened synovium with projections that resemble villi or nodules that may be coarse or fine with either a shag carpet or fernlike appearance. The nodules may be sessile or pedunculated and occur most often on the tendons or as extra-articular lesions. PVNS usually presents as swelling of the joint with mild to moderate pain.

Osteoarthritis

Osteoarthritis, also referred to as degenerative arthritis or degenerative joint disease, is the most common form of inflammatory joint disease. It is caused by deterioration of the cartilage that covers the ends of the bones. This deterioration typically occurs slowly over a long time period. As the cartilage deteriorates, it becomes rough and causes irritation of the joint. As deterioration continues, the bone itself becomes exposed and eventually joint movement results in bone rubbing against bone, causing pain and damage to the bone itself.

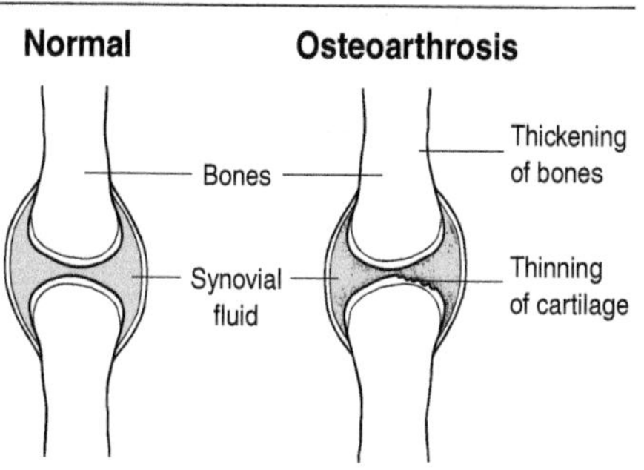

Acquired Deformities

Acquired deformities are those that occur or develop after birth and include conditions that are the result of old injuries. Acquired deformities may affect the bones, joints, muscles, tendons, ligaments, or other structures of the musculoskeletal system. Examples include acquired flexion deformities, limb length discrepancies, and hallux valgus or varus of the feet.

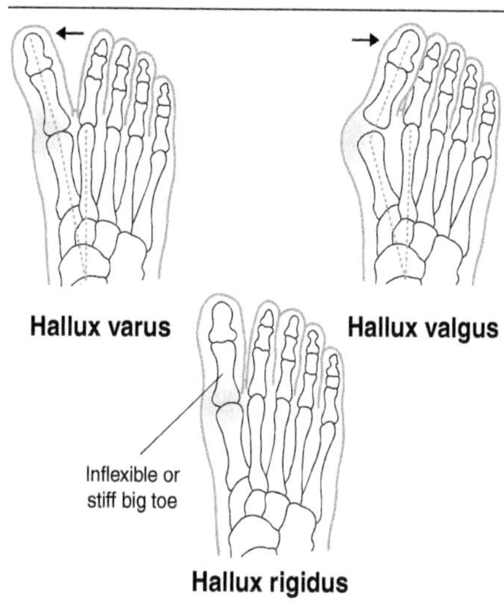

Old Injuries

Internal derangement of the knee is a common type of old injury. Injuries are classified as cystic, derangements due to old tear or injury, or other specified types. The old injury may affect the menisci and/or ligaments of the knee. Loose bodies in the joint, joint instability secondary to old ligament injury, and articular cartilage disorders are other conditions classified under internal derangement.

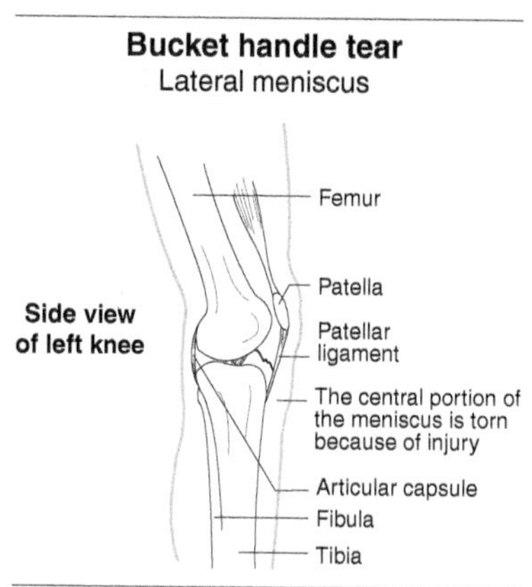

Non-traumatic Joint Dislocation

Pathologic dislocation is one type of non-traumatic dislocation. It occurs as a result of a disease process that affects the integrity of the joint. Non-traumatic dislocation can also occur in patients with excessive laxity in connective tissues at one or more joints. Individuals with some types of connective tissue disorders are more prone to non-traumatic dislocations. Old injuries can also damage the joint structures causing recurrent joint dislocation.

Other Joint Disorders

This category includes a variety of conditions affecting the joint, including: blood in the joint (hemarthrosis), joint fistula, joint instability not classified elsewhere, joint effusion, pain and stiffness, and osteophytes (bone spurs).

Section 2.3 Coding Practice

Condition	ICD-10-CM
Sero-negative rheumatoid arthritis affecting the joints of both hands	M06.041, M06.042
PVNS, left knee	M12.262
Old bucket handle tear lateral meniscus, right knee	M23.261
Recurrent dislocation, right shoulder	M24.411
Loose body, left elbow	M24.022

Section 2.3 Questions

What information is required to assign the most specific code for rheumatoid arthritis?

____

____

How is an old bucket handle tear of the meniscus classified in ICD-1Ø-CM?

____

____

Why isn't code S83.25- used for an old bucket handle tear?

____

____

See end of chapter for Coding Practice answers.

Section 2.4 – Systemic Connective Tissue Disorders

Connective tissues are a diverse group of tissues that include subcutaneous tissue, fascia, tendons, ligaments, cartilage, and bone, as well as blood and vascular structures. Systemic disorders are defined as those that affect multiple organs and/or multiple connective tissues. Conditions classified in this section include systemic autoimmune and systemic collagen vascular diseases.

Some disorders classified here include:

- Polyarteritis nodosa
- Systemic lupus erythematosus
- Systemic sclerosis, also referred to as systemic scleroderma
- Sicca syndrome

Polyarteritis Nodosa

Polyarteritis nodosa is a systemic inflammation of medium and small arteries primarily affecting those that supply the muscles. Inflammatory lesions usually begin at bifurcations or branch points in the arteries. These lesions begin in the inner layer of the vessel and then spread until the entire arterial wall is involved. This causes destruction of the internal and external elastic tissue resulting in microaneurysms that may rupture and hemorrhage. In addition, thrombi may form at the sites of inflammation. As inflammatory lesions increase in size, vessel obstruction from thrombi occurs, causing ischemia and eventually necrosis of affected tissue or organs. Sites and organs most often affected include the skin, joints, kidneys, gastrointestinal tract, heart, and eyes.

Systemic Lupus Erythematosus

Systemic lupus erythematosus (SLE) is an autoimmune disorder that affects many different tissues and organs of the body. Body systems and organs most often affected include the musculoskeletal system, cardiovascular system, nervous system, digestive system, eyes, lungs, kidneys, and blood forming organs. In the musculoskeletal system, SLE causes joint and muscle pain. Muscles may become inflamed which in turn causes muscle weakness and fatigue.

Systemic Sclerosis

Systemic sclerosis, also referred to as systemic scleroderma, is a chronic autoimmune disease that affects multiple body systems. The systemic type of the disease is characterized by fibrosis of the tissues and organs. The extent of the disease and the body systems affected vary significantly from one person to the next but the systemic type always affects internal organs. Sites and organs most often affected include musculoskeletal system, digestive system, nervous system, blood vessels, skin, lungs, heart, kidneys, and thyroid. Systemic sclerosis is subdivided into limited and diffuse types based on the extent of skin tightening. Skin tightening in the limited type is confined to the fingers, hands, and forearms distal to the elbow. The skin of the feet and lower leg distal to the knee may also be involved. The limited type is sometimes referred to as CRST or CREST syndrome, which describes a combination of symptoms including calcinosis, Raynaud's phenomenon, esophageal dysfunction, sclerodactyly, and telangiectasia. In the diffuse type, skin tightening extends into the trunk and proximal extremities.

Sicca Syndrome

Sicca syndrome, also referred to as sicca complex or Sjögren's disease, is a chronic autoimmune disease characterized by dry mouth, dry eyes, and lymphocytic infiltration of the exocrine glands. The extent and severity of the disease varies significantly. While virtually all organs can be affected, it more commonly affects the eyes, mouth, parotid glands, lungs, kidneys, skin, and nervous system. While symptoms vary depending on what organs are affected, approximately 60% of individuals with sicca syndrome report musculoskeletal symptoms including joint and muscle pain.

Section 2.4 Coding Practice

Condition	ICD-10-CM
Churg-Strauss syndrome	M30.1
Systemic lupus erythematosus	M32.10
CREST syndrome	M34.1
Sicca syndrome with arthralgia and myalgia	M35.03

Section 2.4 Questions

Can the code for polyarteritis with lung involvement be found under the term polyarteritis?

____

____

Can the code for Churg-Strauss syndrome be found under the term 'polyarteritis'?

____

____

Are Wegener's granulomatosis and Churg-Strauss syndrome reported with the same code?

____

____

For a patient with CREST syndrome with Raynaud's phenomenon, would the Raynaud's be reported as an additional code?

____

____

What is the code descriptor for M32.10? Does this code descriptor identify the specific organ(s) affected?

____

____

Systemic sclerosis is reported with codes from the musculoskeletal system chapter. Where are codes for isolated, also called circumscribed, scleroderma found?

____

____

Why is Sicca syndrome with arthralgia and myalgia reported with the code for Sicca syndrome with myopathy?

See end of chapter for Coding Practice answers.

Section 2.5 – Dorsopathies

The term dorsopathy refers to conditions affecting the back or spine. Dorsopathy is a very general term and covers a wide variety of diseases, disorders, and other conditions that affect the spine. Conditions classified under dorsopathy include:

- Deforming dorsopathies
  - Kyphosis
  - Lordosis
  - Scoliosis
- Spondylopathies
  - Ankylosing spondylitis and other inflammatory spondylopathies
  - Spondylosis
  - Spinal stenosis
  - Fatigue or stress fractures of the vertebrae
  - Collapsed vertebrae
- Other dorsopathies
  - Intervertebral disc disorders
  - Back pain including radiculopathy, cervicalgia, and sciatica

Kyphosis

Kyphosis refers to an abnormal convex or outward curvature of the spine, usually in the thoracic or thoracolumbar region. The curvature often gives the back a hunchback or humpback appearance. Kyphosis may be postural or structural. Postural kyphosis is due simply to poor posture and can be corrected using exercises. Structural kyphosis is caused by an abnormality in one or more structural components of the spine which include bone, intervertebral discs, nerves, ligaments, and muscles. Structural kyphosis may be acquired or congenital.

Lordosis

Lordosis refers to an inward curvature of the spine usually in the lumbar region and may also be called swayback. It is often a result of poor posture but may also be due to another disease of the spine such as discitis, osteoporosis, or spondylolisthesis.

Scoliosis

Scoliosis is an abnormal curvature of the spine to the left and/or right with the curve being shaped like a C or an S. It can also cause the spine to twist. When the twist occurs in the thoracic region, the rib cage also rotates out of normal position. Scoliosis usually becomes apparent in childhood or early adolescence but may be present at birth, occur from neurologic or other disease or have an adult onset. The severity is determined by the degree of the curvature. Idiopathic scoliosis is classified by age. Infantile codes are used for onset between birth through age 4; juvenile codes are used for ages 5 through 1Ø, adolescent codes are used for ages 11 through 17. Codes for congenital scoliosis are found in Chapter 17 Congenital Malformations, Deformations and Chromosomal Abnormalities

Scoliosis

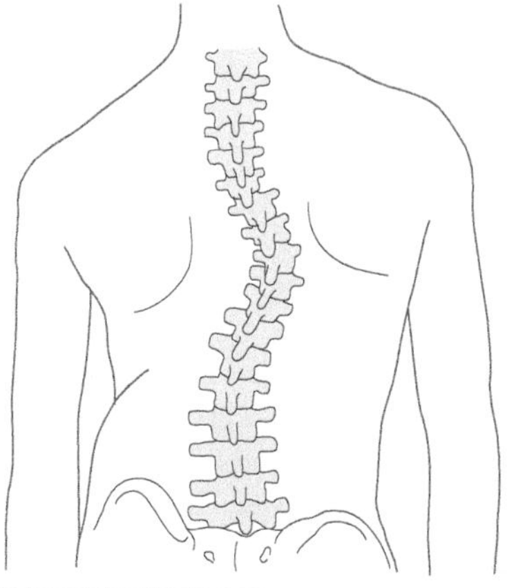

Spondylolysis, Spondylolisthesis, and Spondylitis

Spondy, spondyl, and spondylo are root words meaning vertebrae. Spondylolysis is a degenerative or developmental anomaly of a portion of the vertebra, usually the pars interarticularis, which is a segment of bone in the posterior aspect of the vertebra between the superior and inferior articular facets. Spondylolysis can lead to spondylolisthesis, a condition where there is forward movement of a vertebra in relation to the vertebra beneath it. Spondylitis is an inflammation of one or more vertebrae.

Spinal Stenosis

Spinal stenosis is a narrowing of the spinal canal that occurs most often in the cervical or lumbar region. The narrowing can put pressure on spinal nerves causing inflammation and pain. In the lumbar region, the nerve compression can also result in neurogenic claudication producing weakness, cramping, and pain in one or both legs after walking or standing but without quick relief with rest. Neurogenic claudication does not have a vascular origin. There will not be skin changes, hair loss or diminished pulses. Relief is often noted with bending forward.

Fatigue Fractures

Fatigue fractures, also called stress fractures, are overuse injuries of the bone. Overuse stresses the bone causing it to crack. Fatigue fractures are minute fractures that cause pain and can lead to more severe injury if overuse continues.

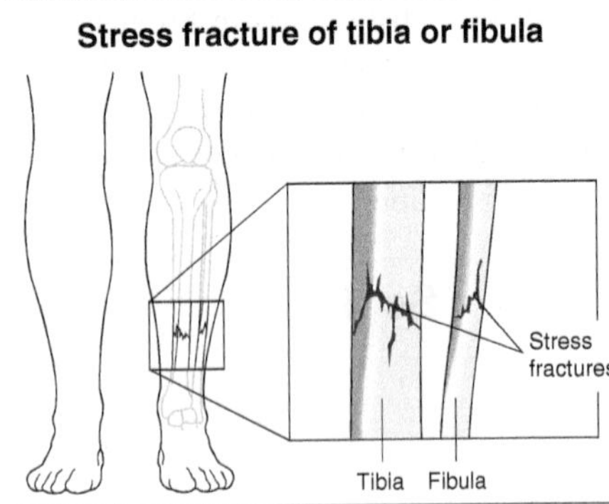

Collapsed Vertebrae

Collapsed vertebrae are also called compression or crush fractures. Just as the name implies, this condition is caused by the collapse of one or more vertebrae resulting in compression of underlying structures including spinal nerves. These types of fractures occur in the course of normal daily activity as opposed to overuse or trauma.

Intervertebral Disc Disorders

The intervertebral discs are composed of an inner gel-like substance called the nucleus pulposus which is enclosed in a tough fibrous tissue layer called the annulus pulposus. This disc is what allows the spinal column to move and it also serves as a shock absorber. There are a number of conditions that can affect the intervertebral discs, including displacement or degenerative disease. These conditions may occur with or without myelopathy at all levels and with or without radiculopathy at the cervical levels. Myelopathy is a general term used to describe any disorder of the spinal cord. In the case of a disc disorder with myelopathy, the spinal cord disorder is directly related to the disc disorder. Radiculopathy refers to changes in sensory, motor, or reflex functions as a result of compression on a spinal nerve.

Displacement of disc

Cervical vertebrae
Thoracic vertebrae
Lumbar vertebrae
Spinal cord
Interior herniates through annulus
Spinal nerve
Nucleus pulposus
Annulus
Cross-section

Section 2.5 Coding Practice

Condition	ICD-10-CM
Structural kyphosis of the thoracic spine due to Gibbus deformity	M40.294
Idiopathic kyphoscoliosis, thoracolumbar spine in a 9-year-old patient	M41.115
Subsequent encounter for evaluation of fatigue fracture of thoracolumbar spine with delayed healing	M48.45XG
Herniated nucleus pulposus L3-4 with myelopathy	M51.06

Section 2.5 Questions

Why is kyphosis in the example above coded as other kyphosis rather than unspecified kyphosis?

____

____

Why is kyphoscoliosis reported with a scoliosis code rather than a kyphosis code or a code from both categories?

____

____

Is congenital scoliosis coded under category M41 Scoliosis?

____

____

What does the term 'idiopathic' mean?

____

____

What documentation is required to assign the most specific code for fatigue fractures and collapsed vertebrae?

____

____

Herniated nucleus pulposus is synonymous with displacement of an intervertebral disc. In the example, why is it coded to disc disorder with myelopathy rather than to disc displacement?

____

____

See end of chapter for Coding Practice answers.

Section 2.6 – Soft Tissue Disorders

Soft tissues are found in muscle, tendon, synovium, and bursa. Disorders affecting these structures include:

- Infections
- Inflammation including noninfectious myositis, tendonitis, tenosynovitis, synovitis, bursitis
- Muscle disorders
  - Nontraumatic muscle separation
  - Muscle contracture
  - Muscle wasting and atrophy
- Tendon and synovial disorders

- Trigger finger
- Nontraumatic rupture of tendons
- Ganglion
- Other soft tissue disorders
  - Bursitis
  - Pain and pain syndromes including fibromyalgia

Myositis

Inflammation of muscle tissue is called myositis. The inflammation may be caused by an infection or be due to a noninfectious cause. Some types of myositis, such as polymyositis and dermatomyositis, are classified as systemic diseases since they affect more than one body system. Other types affect only the connective tissue of the musculoskeletal system. Some noninfectious types include:

- Interstitial myositis
- Myositis ossificans traumatica
- Myositis ossificans progressiva

Interstitial myositis is a rare disorder that primarily affects striated muscle tissue, although cardiac muscle is sometimes affected. This disorder causes fibrous degeneration of the affected muscles.

Myositis ossificans traumatica is characterized by calcification of muscle tissue at the site of an injury. Areas of calcification range from small asymptomatic masses in the muscle to moderate or large calcified masses that may be tender and cause temporary disability. The body usually absorbs moderate to large calcifications within 12 months of the injury. An exception is when an injury occurs near a joint. In these cases, the calcifications are sometimes complicated by ankylosis of the joint, reduction in range of motion, and failure of the body to absorb the calcified mass.

Myositis ossifications (traumatic)

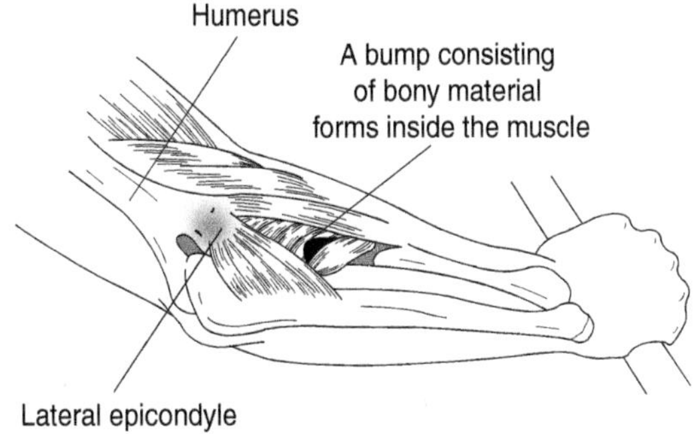

Myositis ossificans progressiva, also called fibrodysplasia ossificans, is a rare disabling genetic condition that results in ossification of soft connective tissues, including skeletal muscle, fascia, tendons, and ligaments. Initial symptoms usually appear by the age of 10 as painful lesions or masses. The soft connective tissue lesions eventually transform into bone. The disease causes severe disability with most individuals confined to a wheelchair by the age of 30.

Tendonitis, Tenosynovitis, Synovitis, and Bursitis

Tendons, synovial tissues, and bursae can become inflamed, causing pain. Tendonitis is an inflammation of the tough fibrous tissue of the tendon itself. Tenosynovitis is an inflammation of the protective synovial sheath that covers the tendon. Synovitis is an inflammation of the synovial membrane that lines articular joints. The cause of tendonitis, tenosynovitis, and synovitis is often the result of overuse or repetitive movements. Some sites are more prone to irritation and inflammation, such as the wrist in the region of the radial styloid. This is the location of a condition known as de Quervain's tenosynovitis. Bursitis is an inflammation of a fluid filled sac found in synovial joints.

Patellar tendinitis

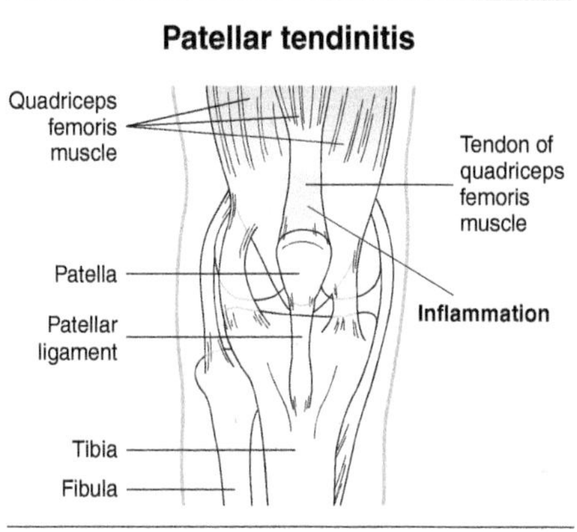

Muscle Disorders

Some of the more common muscle disorders include:

- Nontraumatic separation
- Contracture
- Wasting

Nontraumatic muscle separation or rupture refers to spontaneous separation or rupture. These conditions usually occur in elderly individuals with muscle degeneration. Separation, also referred to as muscle diastasis, refers to the separation of muscle fibers longitudinally along the length of the muscle, while rupture refers to a horizontal disruption of the muscle.

Muscle contracture is defined as a persistent, involuntary shortening of the muscle.

Muscle wasting and atrophy refers to the loss of muscle tissue which is usually due to disuse of the involved muscles and/or poor nutrition. Disuse may be due to an injury or illness that prevents exercise.

Tendon Disorders

Two of the more common tendon disorders are **trigger finger** and **ganglion cysts**. Trigger finger is the result of narrowing of the tendon sheath in the palm of an affected thumb or finger. This causes the affected digit to get caught in a bent position. Sometimes it is possible to straighten the finger which may cause a snapping sound and is what gives the condition its name. Sometimes the finger gets permanently stuck in the bent position. A ganglion cyst is a benign sac filled with a clear jelly-like material generally found near joints or located on the tendon sheath.

Fibromyalgia

Fibromyalgia is a chronic condition characterized by pain in the muscles, ligaments, and tendons throughout the body as well as tender points where even slight touch causes pain. The condition may also cause extreme fatigue. The cause is unknown. One theory is that people with fibromyalgia have an increased sensitivity to pain due to brain changes that cause the brain to become more sensitive to neurotransmitters for pain.

Section 2.6 Coding Practice

Condition	ICD-10-CM
Trigger finger of left index finger	M65.322
Adhesive tenosynovitis, right shoulder	M75.01
Myositis ossificans traumatica right thigh	M61.051

Section 2.6 Questions

What information is needed to code for trigger finger disorders?

In ICD-10-CM, is the code for adhesive tenosynovitis of the shoulder listed under 'Tenosynovitis' in the Alphabetic Index? If not, under what term is this condition listed?

See end of chapter for Coding Practice answers.

Section 10. 7 – Osteopathies and Chondropathies

The term osteopathy refers to any disorder of the bone; however, for coding purposes only disorders of the appendicular skeleton are included in this section of ICD-10-CM. The term chondropathy refers to disorders of the cartilage.

Disorders of Bone Density and Structure

A few of the more common disorders of bone density and structure include osteoporosis, pathologic fractures, fibrous dysplasia, and bone cysts.

Osteoporosis refers to a loss of bone mass and density. Bones become porous and lack the normal osseous architecture that gives them their strength. This causes bones to fracture more easily. The most common sites of fracture are the vertebrae, hips, and wrists.

Atypical femoral fracture is an insufficiency fracture of the subtrochanteric or diaphyseal region of the femur that occurs primarily in patients who have been treated with biphosphonates.

Pathologic fractures are those that occur in bone that has become weakened due to another disease process, such as malignancy, infection, or certain inherited bone disorders. Pathological fractures are not caused by trauma. Instead, they occur during the course of normal activities because the weakened bone is no longer able to sustain normal day-to-day stresses and suddenly fractures.

Pathological fracture of spine

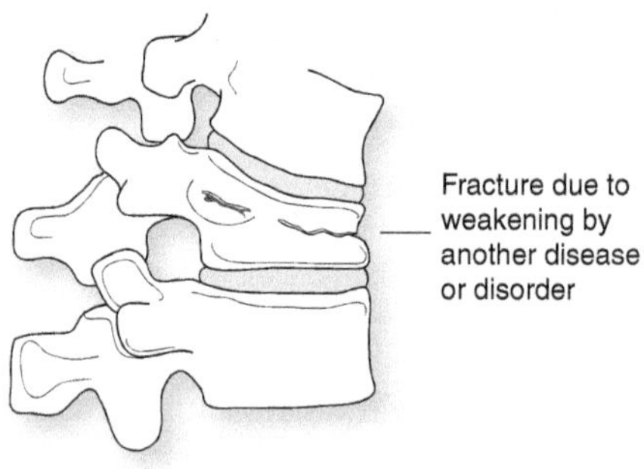

Fibrous dysplasia is a condition in which fibrous tissue is deposited instead of normal osseous tissue in a bone that is still growing. This fibrous tissue is not as strong as bone and can result in fracture or deformity.

Bone cysts are fluid filled cavities in the bone. A unicameral bone cyst is the most common type. These are solitary lesions that affect a single bone. They occur most often in children.

While they can occur at any site, bone cysts are more common in the proximal humerus and proximal femur. Aneurysmal bone cysts are blood filled fibrous masses that are classified as benign bone tumors. Even though they are classified as benign, aneurysmal bone cysts are locally destructive to both bone and surrounding tissue if left untreated. They can recur following removal.

Cartilage Disorders

Cartilage disorders are called chondropathies. Two disorders that affect cartilage are nontraumatic slipped epiphysis and osteochondritis dissecans.

A **slipped epiphysis** may result from trauma in which case it is called a physeal fracture or it may occur spontaneously without a concomitant traumatic injury. Physeal fractures are covered later in the chapter. A nontraumatic slipped epiphysis occurs when the growth plate slips out of its normal position causing displacement in relation to the diaphysis of the bone. Normally this is a gradual slippage but it may also occur suddenly. It usually occurs in preteenage children and most commonly in the hip prior to closure of the growth plate. Whether gradual or sudden, when the degree of slippage reaches a certain point, the joint becomes painful and range of motion may be affected. When it affects the hip this condition is commonly known by the acronym SCFE (slipped capital femoral epiphysis)

Osteochondritis dissecans is a condition that affects both bone and cartilage in the ossification centers at the proximal and distal ends of long bones. This disorder occurs most often in bones that have not attained full growth and is characterized by separation of joint cartilage from the underlying bone. This causes a loss of blood supply to the loose cartilage which in turn causes aseptic necrosis. The loose body may remain in place or become dislodged and migrate into the joint space. This can cause pain and instability of the joint. The most common sites of osteochondritis dissecans are the knees and elbows.

Section 2.7 Coding Practice

Condition	ICD-10-CM
Chronic slipped epiphysis upper right femur	M93.021
Senile osteoporosis	M81.0
Senile osteoporosis with fracture of vertebra, initial encounter	M80.08xA

Section 2.7 Questions

What term is 'slipped epiphysis of a site other than the upper femur' listed under in the Alphabetic Index?

____

____

What information is needed in order to properly code for a slipped epiphysis?

____

____

In ICD-10-CM, what term is used instead of 'senile' to describe osteoporosis in older individuals?

____

____

See end of chapter for Coding Practice answers.

Conditions Affecting Newborns

The primary conditions affecting the musculoskeletal system are birth injuries including fracture of the bones of the skull, clavicle, femur, and other long bones.

Section 2.8 – Congenital Malformations and Deformations of the Musculoskeletal System

Some of the more common congenital malformations affecting the musculoskeletal system include:

- Congenital hip dislocation
- Deformities of the feet
- Polydactyly
- Syndactyly

Congenital Hip Dysplasia and Dislocation

Hip dysplasia, also referred to as developmental dysplasia of the hip, is a condition in which the patient is born with an unstable hip joint. Congenital hip dislocation is a form of hip dysplasia in which the femoral head is not properly positioned in the acetabulum, which is critical for normal development of the acetabulum. Infants are examined at birth for hip dysplasia and dislocation. Undiagnosed hip dysplasia results in failure of the acetabulum to develop properly with resulting abnormal and painful gait and leg length discrepancies. Early diagnosis often allows treatment with a brace alone, while later diagnosis may require closed or open reduction of the hip, traction, and/or femoral shortening.

Deformities of the Feet

There are a number of congenital deformities that affect the soft tissues, joints, and/or bones of the feet. These are usually divided into those affecting three different regions. Deformities of the hind foot or rear foot involve the talus and calcaneus and related joints and soft tissues. Those in the midfoot affect other tarsal bones including the navicular, cuboid, and cuneiform bones and related joints and soft tissues. Those in the forefoot affect the metatarsals and phalanges and related joints and soft tissues. Two of the more common deformities are clubfoot, also referred to as talipes equinovarus, and calcaneovalgus.

Clubfoot is a complex anomaly that is either classified as extrinsic, which is a supple, soft tissue deformity, or intrinsic, which is a rigid deformity. Extrinsic clubfoot is typically treated with serial casting. Intrinsic clubfoot is also initially treated with serial casting but may require surgical interventions if casting does not result in adequate correction of the deformity.

Calcaneovalgus is a hyperextension deformity that originates in the tibiotalar joint. Depending on the severity of the deformity, the condition may be treated with stretching exercises, splinting, or serial casting.

Polydactyly

Polydactyly, also referred to as supernumerary digits, is a condition where there are more than five digits of the hands or feet. The condition usually involves an additional digit next to the fifth digit that may be composed only of soft tissue or it may be a completely duplicated digit composed of bones, tendons, vascular structures, and a nail.

Syndactyly

Syndactyly, also referred to as webbing, may affect the fingers or toes. It may be limited to soft tissue fusion or it may involve fusion of bones as well. Treatment depends on the extent of the fusion. Webbing of the toes usually does not cause any functional limitations and is not treated. Webbed fingers are more often treated by surgical separation.

Section 2.8 Coding Practice

Condition	ICD-10-CM
Congenital hip dislocation, right hip	Q65.01
Talipes equinovarus	Q66.0
Ulnar polydactyly, bilateral, soft tissue only	Q69.0

Section 2.8 Questions

What information is needed to accurately assign a code for congenital deformities of the hip?

____

____

What term(s) in the description of polydactyly above affect the code assignment in ICD-10-CM?

____

____

See end of chapter for Coding Practice answers.

Symptoms, Signs, and Abnormal Findings

The majority of symptoms and signs involving the musculoskeletal system are included with those involving the nervous system and were covered in Chapter 3 Nervous System of this book. There are only a limited number of codes for abnormal findings specific to the musculoskeletal system. These include:

- Abnormal findings in specimens of other body fluids and substances, such as synovial fluid or wound secretions
- Abnormal findings on diagnostic imaging of the limbs
- Abnormal findings on diagnostic imaging of other parts of the musculoskeletal system
- Abnormal results of function studies of peripheral nervous system

Section 2.9 – Injuries, Poisonings, and Other Consequences of External Causes

Specific documentation is required to allow capture of the most specific injury code. In addition, codes are organized first by the body area of the injury and then by the type of injury.

Body areas of injury as they relate to the musculoskeletal system are organized as follows:

- Head
- Neck
- Thorax
- Abdomen, lower back, lumbar spine, pelvis
- Shoulder and upper arm
- Elbow and forearm
- Wrist and Hand
- Hip and thigh
- Knee and lower leg
- Ankle and foot

Within each of the body areas, injuries are then organized by type beginning with more superficial injuries and ending with injuries involving deeper body structures. Types of musculoskeletal injuries covered in this section include:

- Contusions
- Open wounds
- Fractures
- Dislocations and sprains
- Nerve and blood vessel injuries
- Muscle, fascia, and tendon injuries
- Crush injuries
- Traumatic amputations
- Physeal fractures
- Other injuries to muscle, fascia, tendon, ligaments, bone or other tissues of the musculoskeletal system

Fractures

Coding of fractures in ICD-10-CM involves detailed documentation of the location, type of fracture (open vs. closed), the fracture configuration, displacement and like the majority of musculoskeletal conditions, laterality. Documentation for fractures that can be coded to the highest level of includes the following:

- Specific site of the fracture
- Specific bone and location on the bone such as proximal, shaft, distal
- Laterality, i.e. identification of the injury as right or left side
- Designation of general characteristics of fracture type
  - Displaced or nondisplaced
  - Open or closed
- Fracture configuration
  - Comminuted, transverse, oblique, 4-part, Greenstick, intraarticular, etc.
- Identification of some specific fracture patterns
- Maisonneuve, Barton's, Monteggia
- Seventh character extensions that provide additional information as follows:
  - Episode of care as initial, subsequent, or sequela
  - Status of fracture as open or closed
    - » Gustilo classification for some types of open fractures
  - Status of bone healing as routine, delayed, nonunion, or malunion
- Fractures of the epiphysis are categorized using the Salter-Harris classification.

Gustilo Open Fracture Classification

The Gustilo open fracture classification groups open fractures into three main categories designated as Type I, Type II and Type III with Type III injuries being further divided into Type IIIA, Type IIIB, and Type IIIC subcategories. The categories are defined by three characteristics which include:

- Mechanism of injury
- Extent of soft tissue damage
- Degree of bone injury or involvement

The specific characteristics for each type are as follows:

- *Type I*
  - Wound < 1 cm
  - Minimal soft tissue damage
  - Wound bed is clean
  - Typically low-energy type injury
  - Fracture type is typically one of the following:
    - » Simple transverse
    - » Short oblique
    - » Minimally comminuted
- *Type II*
  - Wound > 1 cm
  - Moderate soft tissue damage/crush injury
  - Wound bed moderately contamination
  - Typically low-energy type injury often a direct blow to the limb
  - Fracture type is typically one of the following:
    - » Simple transverse
    - » Short oblique
    - » Mildly comminuted

- *Type III*
  - Wound > 1 cm
  - Extensive soft tissue damage
  - Highly contaminated wound bed
  - Typically a high-energy type injury
  - Highly unstable fractures often with multiple bone fragments
  - Mechanism of injury farmyard injuries, gunshot wounds, high velocity crushing injuries
  - Injury patterns resulting in fractures always classified to this category include:
    - » Open segmental fracture regardless of wound size
    - » Diaphyseal fractures with segmental bone loss
    - » Open fractures with any type of vascular involvement
    - » Farmyard injuries or severely contaminated open fractures
    - » High velocity gunshot wound
    - » Fracture caused by crushing force from fast moving vehicle
    - » Open fractures with delayed treatment (over 8 hours)
- *Type IIIA*
  - Wound <10cm with crushed tissue and contamination
  - Adequate soft tissue coverage
  - No local or distant flap coverage required
  - Fracture may be open segmental or severely comminuted and still be subclassified as Type IIIA
- *Type IIIB*
  - Wound >10cm with crushed tissue, massive contamination and extensive soft tissue loss
  - Local or distant flap coverage required
  - Wound bed contamination requiring serial irrigation and debridement to clean the open fracture site
- *Type IIIC*
  - Major arterial injury requiring repair regardless of size of wound
  - Extensive repair usually requiring the skills of a vascular surgeon for limb salvage
  - Fractures classified using the Mangled Extremity Severity Score

Fracture Types

As stated above, fractures are first generally classified based upon the location of the fracture, the bone and the portion of the bone involved (i.e. whether the fracture is at the proximal or distal end or along the shaft and even whether it is described more specifically as the head, neck, tuberosity, etc.). They are then further classified as to whether they are displaced or nondisplaced and whether they are open or closed. Whether the fracture is open or closed is not defined by the fracture code itself but by the seventh character extender. If the documentation does not specify whether the fracture is displaced or nondisplaced, it is coded as displaced. If the documentation does not specify whether the fracture is opened or closed, it is coded as closed.

Many fracture codes require additional documentation as to the specific configuration or type which can vary based on what bone is fractured and the exact site of the fracture. Definitions for some of the specific types of fractures identified with codes in ICD-1Ø-CM are as follows:

Comminuted. A fracture in which the bone is broken in more than two pieces or fragments.

Greenstick. An incomplete fracture that occurs in children where one side of the bone breaks and the other side bends.

Oblique. A fracture line that runs at a diagonal along the long axis of the bone with the bone cortices of both fragments in the same plane.

Segmental. Several large fractures of the same bone where the larger fragments are nonadjacent segments. Occurs in the shaft of long bones.

Spiral. A fracture caused by twisting or rotation forces with a fracture line that twists or spirals along the long axis of the bone'

Torus. A bending or buckling of the bone without a complete fracture that occurs only in children due to the softness of the bone.

Transverse. A fracture line that is straight across the long axis of the bone.

Fractures

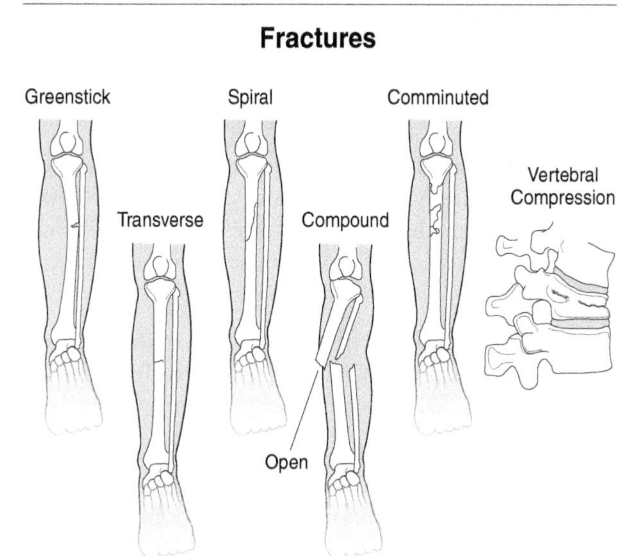

Additional Fracture Types

Fractures of some locations have characteristics unique to the location. Often the way a bone fractures is a function of the specific structure of the bone or joint. Some sites of the humerus, ulna, radius and patella have specific characteristics and fractures with these specific characteristics are assigned specific codes. In addition, traumatic physeal fractures, which are fractures involving the growth plate of the bone, are coded based on the specific characteristics of the growth plate fracture. Some of these specific fracture types are described below.

Proximal humerus. Fractures of the proximal or upper end of the humerus are classified using the Neer system. The proximal humerus is divided into four parts, the humeral head (surgical and anatomic neck), greater tubercle, lesser tubercle, and diaphysis or shaft. These four parts are separated by epiphyseal lines, also called growth plates when the bones are still growing during the developmental years. The anatomic neck is the section of the humerus above the tubercles. The surgical neck is at the narrowest aspect of the humerus just below the tubercles. When the proximal humerus is fractured, it typically occurs at the surgical neck and along one or more of the three epiphyseal lines. The proximal humerus may fracture into 2, 3, or 4 parts at the surgical neck which is why surgical neck fractures are designated as 2-, 3-, or 4-part fractures.

The classification of the fracture is based upon the number of fragments and whether there is separation or angulation of the fragments. A fracture part is considered displaced if it is angulated more than 45° or displaced greater than 1 cm. A fracture that is not displaced <1cm and angulated < 45° regardless of how many pieces is considered a one-part fracture. All other Neer classifications are based upon the total number of fractures and the number of fractures that are displaced or angulated. For example, a 2-part fracture can be 2-4 parts with one of those parts being displaced or angulated. A three-part fracture can be 3-4 parts with two of the parts being displaced or angulated.

Monteggia's fracture of ulna. A fracture of the middle third of the ulna in association with dislocation of the radial head.

Galeazzi's fracture of radius. A solitary fracture of the radial shaft at the junction of the middle and distal thirds with an accompanying subluxation or dislocation of the distal radioulnar joint (DRUJ).

Colles' fracture of distal radius. A fracture of the distal radius through the metaphysis approximately 4 cm proximal to the articular surface of the radius with dorsal displacement of the distal bone fragments. Deformity noted with these fractures is often referred to as a silver-fork deformity.

Smith's fracture of distal radius. A fracture of the distal radius 1-2 cm above the wrist with volar displacement of the distal bone fragments. Also called a reverse Colles'.

Osteochondral fracture of patella. A fracture as a result of a direct blow and/or dislocation of the patella. The fracture occurs at the point of contact and the fracture fragment contains articular cartilage, subchondral bone, and trabecular bone. The fragment may be displaced in the intra-articular region of the knee joint or it may be nondisplaced.

Longitudinal fracture of patella. A vertical (top to bottom) fracture of the patella.

Maisonneuve fracture. A spiral fracture of the proximal fibula near the neck with a tear of the anterior tibiofibular ligament.

Physeal fractures. These are also referred to as Salter-Harris fractures or traumatic epiphyseal separations and are listed under the category other and unspecified injuries. These fractures occur along the epiphyseal (growth) plates in bones that have not reached their full growth and in which the plates are still open and filled with cartilaginous tissue. They are listed in the Alphabetic Index under the main term 'Fracture' and then by site under the term 'physeal'.

Salter-Harris fractures are classified into nine types according to the amount of injury to the epiphysis and other involvement of bone. Documentation as to type is required to assign the most specific code. Types I-IV have specific codes for most sites. Types V-IX are reported under other physeal fracture. If no type is specified, the code is reported with an unspecified code.

Types I-IV are the most common types of physeal injuries and have the following characteristics:

- Type I – Epiphyseal separation with displacement of the epiphysis from the metaphysis at the growth plate. Fracture is generally nondisplaced. Usually occurs in young children where the growth plate is thick.
- Type II – Fracture through the growth plate and a portion of the metaphysis without fracture of the epiphysis. Most common type. Usually occurs in children after age 10.
- Type III – Fracture through the growth plate and a portion of the epiphysis which damages the reproductive layer of the physis. Occurs in children after age 10. Most common in the tibia.
- Type IV – Fracture through the epiphysis, across the growth plate and into the metaphysis causing damage to the reproductive layer of the physis. Requires reduction to prevent interruption of growth. May occur at any age. Most common in the distal humerus.
- Types V-IX are less common types of physeal injuries:
- Type V – A crush or compression injuring involving the growth plate without fracture of the metaphysis or epiphysis. Limb length inequality and angular deformities are common complications. Most common in the knee and ankle.
- Type VI – A rare injury with a portion of the epiphysis, metaphysis and growth plate missing. Generally occurs with an open fracture. Common causes farm equipment, lawnmowers, snow blowers, snowmobiles and gunshot wounds. Will result in growth disturbances.
- Type VII – An isolated injury of the epiphyseal plate
- Type VIII – An isolated injury to the metaphysis with potential complications related to endochondral ossification
- Type IX – An injury to the periosteum that may interfere with membranous growth

Section 2.9 Coding Practice

Condition	ICD-10-CM
Emergency department encounter for traumatic fracture of the medial malleolus right ankle	S82.51XA
Admission for traumatic open, displaced, severely comminuted, left femoral shaft fracture. Soft tissue loss minimal. No flaps or grafts required to repair the soft tissue.	S72.352C
Nonunion distal right humerus fracture	S42.401K

Condition	ICD-10-CM
Colles' fracture, left radius. Follow-up visit for cast removal.	S52.532D
Emergency department encounter for closed transverse fracture of the right radial and ulnar shafts sustained in a fall while skateboarding on school grounds	S52.221A, S52.321A, V00.131A, Y92.219, Y93.51
Partial growth plate arrest of distal right femur following traumatic Salter-Harris Type II fracture of distal femoral epiphysis sustained 1 year ago	M89.157, S79.121S

Section 2.9 Questions

Why is the medial malleolus fracture described above reported with the code for a displaced fracture?

____

____

What does the seventh character extension 'D' indicate for code S52.532D? Does the seventh character 'D' have the same meaning for all types of fractures?

____

____

Why are the fractures of the radial and ulnar shafts reported with two codes? What additional information about the injury is needed in ICD-1Ø-CM?

____

____

See end of chapter for Coding Practice answers.

Section 2.10 – Dislocations and Sprains

Dislocations are joint injuries that involve movement of the bones that form the joint into abnormal or disarranged positions. In a complete dislocation there is disruption and loss of contact between the articular surfaces of the involved bones. A partial or incomplete dislocation is referred to as subluxation and is characterized by an altered relationship between the bones without loss of contact between the articular surfaces. Dislocations may also be characterized by the direction of the dislocation as anterior, posterior, inferior, or other direction.

Some dislocation sites require additional information as to the extent of the injury or displacement. For example, dislocation of the acromioclavicular (AC) joint requires information on the extent of the displacement of the clavicle as a displacement of 1ØØ%-2ØØ% or > 2ØØ%. Most providers document AC joint injury by grade.

The Rockwood Classification of AC joint injuries are classified by grade:

Grade I: the acromioclavicular ligaments are stretched but not torn. The coracoclavicular ligaments are intact. The joint is not separated. Grade I would be equivalent to a sprain. S43.5-

Grade II: the acromioclavicular ligaments are ruptured and the joint separated; the coracoclavicular ligaments are intact. Grade II is equivalent to a subluxation. S43.11-

Grade III: the acromioclavicular and coracoclavicular ligaments are torn with wide separation of the joint. The coracoclavicular interspace is 25%-1ØØ% greater than the normal shoulder. Grade III is equivalent to a dislocation. Grade III is equivalent to S43.1Ø- unspecified dislocation of AC joint because the coracoclavicular interspace is less than 1ØØ% when compared to the normal shoulder

Grade IV: disruption of AC ligament, joint capsule, and coracoacromial ligament. Clavicle is completely displaced posteriorly through the trapezius muscle. Grade IV is equivalent to S43.15- posterior dislocation of AC joint.

Grade V: marked displacement of acromion and clavicle; clavicle displaced superiorly. Grade V is equivalent to either S43.12- dislocation of AC joint, 1ØØ%-2ØØ% displacement or subcategory S43.13- dislocation of AC joint, greater than 2ØØ% displacement. If the amount of displacement as compared to the normal shoulder is not specified, query the physician

Grade VI: clavicle lies inferior to the coracoid. Grade VI is equivalent to S43.14- inferior dislocation of AC joint.

Sprains are injuries to ligaments that help stabilize the joint but do not involve a dislocation or fracture. Sprains may also be referred to as tears. Sprains result from an abnormal or excessive force on the joint, such as twisting or a blow to the joint. Sprains in general are categorized in ICD-1Ø-CM either by the joint or ligament involved. Sprains are classified by grade based upon the amount of disruption to the ligament. Although the codes for sprains are not defined by grade, it helpful to understand what level of injury is involved.

- Grade 1-stretched beyond their normal range with some microscopic damage to the fibers but no tearing
- Grade 2-partial tearing affecting some but not all of the fibers; may have some loss of function and joint laxity
- Grade 3-nearly complete tear/rupture with gross instability

Dislocations

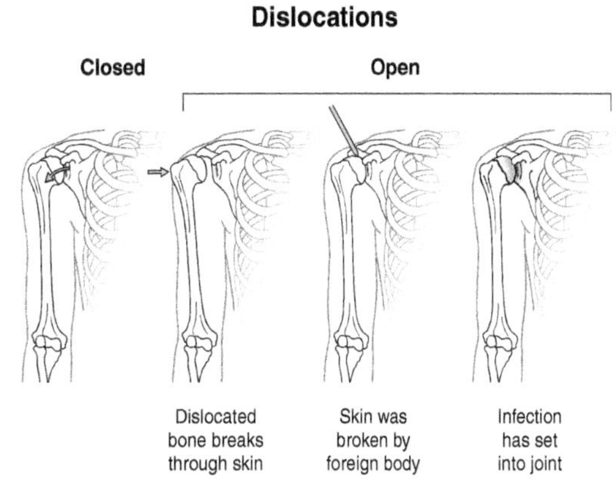

Section 2.10 Coding Practice

Condition	ICD-10-CM
Initial evaluation of right acromioclavicular (AC) joint separation with displacement of 150%	S43.121A
Torn anterior cruciate ligament (ACL) left knee, current injury	S83.512A
Subluxation proximal interphalangeal joint right index finger, new injury	S63.230A

Section 2.10 Questions

Is an acromioclavicular (AC) joint separation without documentation of open or closed status reported as an open or closed injury?

Is the code for the ACL injury specific to the anterior cruciate?

What external cause codes should be reported with the injury codes listed in the Coding Practice when additional information is available on the circumstances surrounding the injury?

Why are all Coding Practices reported with the 7th digit extension A?

See end of chapter for Coding Practice answers.

Section 2.11 – Muscle, Fascia, and Tendon Injuries

Injuries of muscle, fascia, and tendons in this category include strains, lacerations, other specified types of injuries that are not more specifically classified elsewhere, and unspecified injuries to these structures.

Strains are differentiated from sprains in that strains involve muscle, fascia, and tendons, while sprains typically involve ligaments. Strains are often an overuse type of injury.

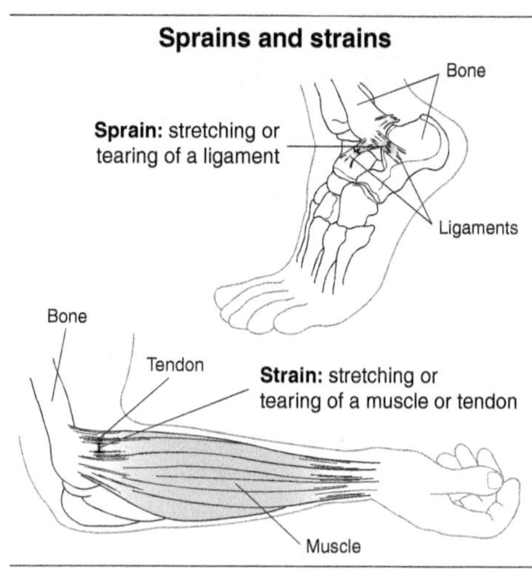

Crush Injuries

Crush injuries are severe types of injuries to soft tissues and most often involve the extremities. They are usually the result of the body part being trapped between two objects complicated by extreme force or pressure on the involved body part. Crush injuries result in muscle injury and muscle cell death. There are three mechanisms of injury to the cells:

1. Immediate muscle cell disruption and damage caused by the force of the crush
2. Continued direct pressure on the cells causing the cells to become ischemic
3. Vascular compromise due to compression of blood vessels and loss of blood supply to the muscle tissue

Traumatic Amputations

Traumatic amputation refers to the loss of part or all of a body part as a result of an accident or trauma. Amputations are classified by site and extent (partial or complete) and require the identification of the side of the body as right or left for assignment of the most specific code.

Section 2.11 Coding Practice

Condition	ICD-10-CM
Initial evaluation by hand surgeon regarding laceration of the flexor tendon of left index finger	S66.121A S61.211A
Initial evaluation for Dog bite right index finger with intact nail	S61.250A, W54.0XXA
Encounter for physical rehabilitation services for crush injury to right lower leg sustained in an automobile accident.	S87.81XD, V89.2XXD

Section 2.11 Questions

When coding for tendon lacerations what information is required to properly assign a code?

What information is needed when coding for open wounds?

See end of chapter for Coding Practice answers.

Terminology

Aponeurosis – The expansion at the end of a muscle that forms a tendon connecting the muscle with the parts that it moves.

Arthro- – Relating to a joint

Common tendon – A tendon that serves more than one muscle. Examples include the Achilles and Hamstring tendons.

Compound fracture – Open fracture

Diaphysis – The shaft of a long bone

Dorso- – Relating to the spine

Epiphysis – The distal or proximal end of a long bone that develops from a secondary ossification center distinct from the shaft, and that remains separated from the shaft by a layer of cartilage called the physis or epiphyseal cartilage until full bone growth is achieved

Idiopathic – Of unknown origin

Metaphysis – The section of bone between the epiphysis and diaphysis of a long bone

Myelopathy – Compression of the spinal cord as a result of disease or trauma May also be a disorder of bone marrow.

Osteochondral fracture – A break or tear in the articular cartilage along with a fracture of the bone.

Physis – Synonymous with epiphyseal cartilage, epiphyseal plate, or growth plate

Polyarthropathy – Arthropathy affecting more than five joints.

Radiculopathy – Disease of the spinal nerve roots due to compression from a disc or inflammation of the nerve root causing pain, weakness, numbness.

Spondylo – Referring to the vertebrae

Quiz— Section 2. Musculoskeletal System

1. There are three types of joints in the human body. Which term below does NOT describe a type of joint?
   a. Hyaline
   b. Fibrous
   c. Cartilaginous
   d. Synovial

2. Non-striated muscle fibers are found in what type of muscle tissue?
   a. Smooth
   b. Cardiac
   c. Skeletal
   d. Smooth and skeletal

3. Osteocytes are bone cells that:
   a. Make collagen and hydroxyapatite which are part of the intercellular tissue needed for new bone formation
   b. Secrete acids that dissolve hydroxyapatite so that the bone matrix can be resorbed and removed
   c. Make collagenase, an enzyme that breaks down collagen
   d. Occupy small cavities present in osseous tissue which are called lacunae

4. Irritability is a characteristic of muscle tissue that allows it to:
   a. Contract
   b. Respond to stimuli
   c. Stretch when pulled
   d. Return to its original shape

5. Which type of bone tumor listed below is a malignant neoplasm that arises in osteoblasts?
   a. Osteosarcoma
   b. Osteochondroma
   c. Chondrosarcoma
   d. Ewing's sarcoma

6. How are old injuries of the joints, such as an internal derangement of the knee reported?
   a. With an injury code and the seventh digit extension S to indicate a sequela
   b. With an injury code and the seventh digit extension D to indicate aftercare
   c. With a code from the musculoskeletal system chapter (M code) and an injury code and the seventh digit extension S to indicate a sequela
   d. With a code from the musculoskeletal system chapter (M code)

7. Subluxation is defined as:
   a. A tear in one of the ligaments that helps stabilize the joint
   b. A partial or incomplete dislocation
   c. A posterior dislocation
   d. Complete loss of contact of the bones in the joint

8. The patient sustained a segmental fracture of the right humeral shaft when he hit a patch of gravel while riding his bike at high speed down a steep hill causing him to fall when the bike skidded out of control. The humerus penetrated the skin and there was a large open wound that was contaminated with dirt and gravel. Soft tissue damage was moderate. The wound was extensively irrigated and debrided to remove the road debris. Open reduction and internal fixation was performed. Soft tissue rearrangement was performed to provide full coverage of the wound bed. Using the Gustilo classification system for open fractures, the fracture described above is classified as:
   a. Type II
   b. Type IIIa
   c. Type IIIb
   d. Type IIIc

9. A Salter-Harris fracture is:
   a. A traumatic fracture of the epiphyseal growth plate of a long bone
   b. A traumatic fracture of the distal femur
   c. A non-traumatic injury to the epiphyseal growth plate of a long bone
   d. A separation of the epiphyseal growth plate by either a traumatic or nontraumatic event

10. Which condition is NOT classified as a disorder of bone density or structure:
   a. Pathological fracture
   b. Osteonecrosis
   c. Fibrous dysplasia
   d. Bone cyst

See next page for answers.

Quiz Answers—Section 2: Musculoskeletal System

1. There are three types of joints in the human body. Which term below does NOT describe a type of joint?

   a. Hyaline

2. Non-striated muscle fibers are found in what type of muscle tissue?

   a. Smooth

3. Osteocytes are bone cells that:

   d. Occupy small cavities present in osseous tissue which are called lacunae

4. Irritability is a characteristic of muscle tissue that allows it to:

   b. Respond to stimuli

5. Which type of bone tumor listed below is a malignant neoplasm that arises in osteoblasts:

   a. Osteosarcoma

6. How are old injuries of the joints, such as an internal derangement of the knee reported?

   d. With a code from the musculoskeletal system chapter (M code)

7. Subluxation is defined as:

   b. A partial or incomplete dislocation

8. The patient sustained a segmental fracture of the right humeral shaft when he hit a patch of gravel while riding his bike at high speed down a steep hill causing him to fall when the bike skidded out of control. The humerus penetrated the skin and there was a large open wound that was contaminated with dirt and gravel. Soft tissue damage was moderate. The wound was extensively irrigated and debrided to remove the road debris. Open reduction and internal fixation was performed. Soft tissue rearrangement was performed to provide full coverage of the wound bed. Using the Gustilo classification system for open fractures, the fracture described above is classified as:

   c. Type IIIb

9. A Salter-Harris fracture is:

   a. A traumatic fracture of the epiphyseal growth plate of a long bone

10. Which condition is NOT classified as a disorder of bone density or structure:

    b. Osteonecrosis

Coding Practice Answers: Section 1. Nervous System

Section 1.1a Coding Practice

Question: Can the code for West Nile encephalitis be found under the term 'Infection' or 'Encephalitis'? If not, what term in the Alphabetic Index is used to locate the correct code for West Nile encephalitis?

Answer: The code for West Nile encephalitis can be found under 'Virus, West Nile, with, encephalitis'. The entry for 'Infection, West Nile' refers the coder to 'see Virus, West Nile'. The entry for 'Infection, brain' refers 'see also Encephalitis'; however West Nile is not listed under 'Encephalitis, viral, arthropod-borne, mosquito-borne'.

Question: Why is the vaccine coded in addition to the encephalitis when the vaccine is determined to be the cause of the encephalitis?

Answer: The vaccine is coded in addition to the postimmunization encephalitis because coding instructions state to identify the vaccine with an additional code.

Question: Which diagnosis listed above is reported with an unspecified or NOS code?

Answer: Idiopathic encephalitis is coded to an unspecified code.

Question: Which diagnosis listed above is reported using an NEC code?

Answer: Rasmussen encephalitis is coded to an 'other specified' or 'not elsewhere classified' code.

Question: What additional information is provided in the ICD-10-CM code when coding an adverse effect of vaccine?

Answer: Coding an adverse effect of vaccine also provides information about the intent (accidental, intentional, assault, undetermined as well as whether it is an initial or subsequent encounter or sequela

Section 1.1b Coding Practice

Question: What part of the nervous system is affected in herpes zoster encephalitis? In herpes zoster meningitis?

Answer: The brain is affected in herpes zoster encephalitis while the membranous coverings of the brain and/or spinal cord are affected in herpes zoster meningitis.

Question: Which codes report an uncomplicated herpes zoster infection?

Answer: B02.9 reports an uncomplicated herpes zoster infection.

Question: Which diagnoses report complications of herpes zoster?

Answer: The codes for herpes zoster encephalitis, meningitis, geniculate ganglionitis, myelitis, polyneuropathy, and trigeminal neuralgia all report nervous system complications of herpes zoster.

Question: Which codes report post-herpetic outbreak conditions?

Answer: Code B02.22 for trigeminal neuralgia and B02.29 other postherpetic nervous system involvement for neuralgia NEC report a post-herpetic outbreak condition. This is a condition that occurs as a second outbreak of the herpes zoster virus.

Question: How is post-herpetic radiculopathy reported?

Answer: B02.29 Other postherpetic nervous system involvement

Section 1.1c Coding Practice

Question: Why is only one code required for reporting meningitis due to Lyme disease?

Answer: Only one code is required to report meningitis due to Lyme disease because A69.21 is a combination code that clearly identifies the two conditions documented in the diagnosis.

Question: Which conditions listed above are reported using unspecified or NOS codes?

Answer: Spinal meningitis is reported with unspecified code G03.9, as the causative agent is not identified. Viral meningitis is also reported with an unspecified code, A87.9, since there is no further information specifying the virus.

Question: Why are two codes reported for meningitis due to Streptococcus pneumoniae infection?

Answer: Code G00.2 Streptococcal meningitis has a use additional code notation to further identify the organism. While Streptococcus is an organism it has multiple forms therefore the code is not specific to the organism. B95-B97.89 are codes for organisms as the cause of diseases listed elsewhere.

Section 1.2 Coding Practice

Question: Why is neurofibromatosis type 1 reported with a code from Chapter 17, Congenital Malformations, Deformations, and Chromosomal Abnormalities?

Answer: Neurofibromatosis type 1 is coded within the congenital malformations chapter because this is a genetic disease process that causes the growth of benign, tumor-like masses along nervous tissue as well as causing deformities of skin and bone. These tumor-like masses are not coded as individual morphologic neoplasms.

Question: What information is provided in the ICD-10-CM code for malignant schwannoma of the left sciatic nerve?

Answer: The ICD-10-CM code for a malignant schwannoma of the left sciatic nerve provides information regarding the type of connective and soft tissue affected being a peripheral nerve, and the lower limb on the left side.

Question: How are malignant neoplasms of peripheral nerves classified?

Answer: Malignant neoplasms of peripheral nerves are classified under a category provided specifically for peripheral nerves and autonomic nervous system and further identified by body area (head/neck/face, upper limb, lower limb, thorax, etc.) as well as laterality when appropriate.

Question: Even though meningothelial meningioma is not specifically described as a benign tumor, it is reported with a code for a benign neoplasm. Why?

Answer: Although most meningiomas are benign, do not assume the meningothelial meningioma is benign and reference the morphology in the index, which refers to 'see Neoplasm, meninges, benign'.

Section 1.3 Coding Practice

Question: What terms in the Alphabetic Index are used to identify the code for continuous ventilator support?

Answer: The code for continuous ventilator support, Z99.11, can be found under the index entry for 'Dependence, on, respirator' or Dependence, on, ventilator'.

Question: What is another term for juvenile spinal muscle atrophy III?

Answer: Kugelberg-Welander disease

Section 1.4 Coding Practice

Question: Why is the adverse effect code reported first?

Answer: Adverse effect codes from categories T36-T65 are combination codes that include the substance involved as well as the external cause and no additional external cause code is required. Because of this structure, the adverse effect code is sequenced first, followed by the code(s) that specify the exact nature or manifestation of the adverse effect, e.g. the neuroleptic-induced Parkinsonism.

Question: How is Parkinson's disease with related dementia coded?

Answer: Assign G20 for the Parkinson's disease and F02.80 or F02.81 for dementia in other diseases classified elsewhere with/without behavioral disturbances. Do not code as G31.83 dementia with Parkinsonism. Parkinsonism is a disorder that is a combination of multiple disorders that result in Parkinson like traits but not all patients with Parkinsonism have Parkinson's disease.

Section 1.5 Coding Practice

Question: What instruction for coding alcoholic encephalopathy is present in ICD-10-CM?

Answer: Instructions for coding alcoholic encephalopathy include a note to 'code also the associated alcoholism' from category F10-.

Question: Under what term is the code for Alzheimer's disease found in the Alphabetic Index?

Answer: In the Alphabetic Index, the code for Alzheimer's disease is found under the entry 'Disease, Alzheimer's'.

Question: How is Alzheimer's disease differ classified in ICD-10-CM?

Answer: Alzheimer's disease is as being early onset (G30.0), late onset (G30.1), other specified (G30.8), and unspecified (G30.9). Codes for delirium (F05), and dementia with (F02.81) or without (F02.80) behavioral disturbance are also coded.

Section 1.6 Coding Practice

Question: In addition to Multiple Sclerosis, what other code categories are available for demyelinating diseases of the central nervous system?

Answer: There are three code categories of diagnosis codes for demyelinating diseases of the central nervous system in ICD-10-CM:

G35 Multiple sclerosis

G36 Other acute disseminated demyelination

G37 Other demyelinating diseases of central nervous system

For other than multiple sclerosis these categories are further subdivided into the following subcategories:

G36.0 Neuromyelitis optica [Devic]

G36.1 Acute and subacute hemorrhagic leukoencephalitis (Hurst)

G36.8 Other specified acute disseminated demyelination

G36.9 Acute disseminated demyelination, unspecified

G37.0 Diffuse sclerosis of central nervous system

G37.1 Central demyelination of corpus callosum

G37.2 Central pontine myelinolysis

G37.3 Acute transverse myelitis in demyelinating disease of central nervous system

G37.4 Subacute necrotizing myelitis of central nervous system

G37.5 Concentric sclerosis [Balo] of central nervous system

G37.8 Other specified demyelinating diseases of central nervous system

G37.9 Demyelinating disease of central nervous system, unspecified

Question: How is Schilder's disease coded?

Answer: Schilder's disease is coded as G37.0 Diffuse sclerosis of central nervous system. Schilder's disease is listed as an inclusion term under G37.0. When referencing the Alphabetic Index, the look-up is Schilder disease which directs to code G37.0.

Question: How is multiple sclerosis with acute transverse myelitis coded?

Answer: How this would be coded would be based upon the presenting reason for the encounter. There is an Excludes 1 note under G37.3 Acute transverse myelitis in demyelinating diseases of the central nervous system excluding reporting of G35.0 multiple sclerosis with G37.3. If a patient with MS is presenting for management of the acute transverse myelitis, only the acute transverse myelitis should be coded.

Section 1.7 Coding Practice

Question: How is epilepsy with intractable seizures and status epilepticus coded?

Answer: Combination codes are used in ICD-10-CM to identify the type of epilepsy, the level of seizure control, and whether or not seizures present with status epilepticus. Each type is coded as either 'intractable' or 'not intractable' and further specified as either 'with status epilepticus' or 'without status epilepticus' and all four possible combinations are an inclusive part of the code description.

Question: Why is seizure NOS coded as a sign or symptom and not as epilepsy?

Answer: Seizure is coded as a sign or symptom and not as epilepsy because a seizure or convulsion is a sign of another, causative condition. Having a seizure does not automatically mean a person actually has a diagnosis of epilepsy. A seizure may also occur with other medical conditions without having epilepsy.

Section 1.8 Coding Practice

Question: When coding for migraine what types of information needs to be documented?

Answer: The type of migraine, the presence/absence of aura, the level of control and whether or not it presents with status migrainosus. Each type is coded as either 'intractable' or 'not intractable' and further specified as either 'with status migrainosus' or 'without status migrainosus' and These are combination codes with each term being an inclusive part of the code description.

Question: How are migraine variants coded in ICD-10-CM?

Answer: Each type of migraine variant is coded within its own subcategory which is even further subdivided. Cyclical vomiting, ophthalmoplegic migraine, periodic headache syndromes in child or adolescent, and abdominal migraine each have their own subcategory and are coded as combination codes to state the level of control, and whether or not it presents with status migrainosus. Each type is coded as either 'intractable' or 'not intractable' and further specified as either 'with status migrainosus' or 'without status migrainosus' and these combinations are an inclusive part of the code description.

Section 1.9 Coding Practice

Question: Why are transient ischemic attacks and related artery syndromes coded in the nervous system chapter instead of the circulatory system chapter?

Answer: Transient ischemic attacks, basilar and carotid artery syndromes, and transient global amnesia are coded in the nervous system chapter because these conditions involve the brain or a temporary loss or obstruction of blood flow to areas of the brain, causing neurological pathology.

Question: How is cerebral artery spasm coded?

Answer: Cerebral artery spasm is an inclusion term listed under G45.9 Transient cerebral ischemic attack, unspecified. Alphabetic Index look-up of Spasm, cerebral (arterial) (venous) directs to G45.9.

Section 1.10 Coding Practice

Question: Neuralgia NOS is reported with a code from the musculoskeletal system chapter. Why is it listed in the musculoskeletal system chapter and not in the nervous system chapter?

Answer: Neuralgia or neuritis NOS is coded in the musculoskeletal system chapter because unspecified pain is considered a general soft tissue disorder and not a disorder of a specific nerve, nerve root, or nerve plexus.

Question: How is clonic hemifacial spasm coded?

Answer: Clonic hemifacial spasm is coded using G51.3. Look-up in the Alphabetic Index is Spasm, hemifacial (clonic), G51.3.

Section 1.11 Coding Practice

Question: What information is necessary to code amputation status accurately in ICD-10-CM?

Answer: Level of amputation (upper arm, lower leg, above elbow, below knee, etc.) and laterality.

Question: What terminology is used for diagnoses of brachial or lumbosacral plexus lesions and nerve root lesions?

Answer: The diagnostic terminology of brachial or lumbosacral plexus disorders and nerve root disorders is used in the Tabular Index.

Question: How is compression of a nerve plexus coded when it is caused by another condition?

Answer: When a nerve plexus or root is compressed due to another underlying condition, it is coded to the specific plexus or root lesion in addition to the underlying condition. A separate, valid, three-digit category code is available for reporting all nerve root and plexus compressions in diseases classified elsewhere.

Section 1.12 Coding Practice

Question: How is myasthenia gravis without documentation of exacerbation coded?

Answer: When separate codes exist for with or without a specified manifestation/condition and it is not documented as with or without, the default is without.

Question: Is thyrotoxicosis the same thing as a thyrotoxic storm? If not, what is the difference?

Answer: Thyrotoxicosis is not the same thing as a thyrotoxic storm or crisis. Thyrotoxicosis is a clinically morbid condition caused by excessive amounts of thyroid hormones in the body, which may be caused from overactivity of the thyroid gland or ingestion of exogenous hormones. A thyrotoxic crisis or storm is a life-threatening condition that develops from an extremely exacerbated state of untreated or poorly treated hyperthyroidism. One can have thyrotoxicosis without thyrotoxic storm.

Question: How is initial encounter for accidental mercury induced myoneural disorder coded?

Answer: Mercury induced myoneural disorder, accidental T56.1X1A and G70.1. ICD-10-CM coding instructions for G70.1 toxic myoneural disorders state to code first the T code (T51-T65) to identify the toxic agent. The T codes for toxic effects further require causation such as accidental, intentional (self-harm), assault and undetermined. Causation is defined in the 6th character. The Official ICD-10-CM guidelines direct to assign causation as undetermined when it is unknown. In addition to causation, these codes require a 7th character to define the stage of care.

Section 1.13 Coding Practice

Question: Hereditary spastic paraplegia is not included in this code category. Where is it found and why is it listed in another category?

Answer: Hereditary spastic paraplegia is coded to G11.4. This is an inherited systemic disease that causes atrophy. It is classified with hereditary ataxias and coded in the same grouping with Huntington's disease and other inherited muscular atrophies affecting the central nervous system.

Question: What does the term diplegic mean?

Answer: Diplegic means paralysis of the corresponding (symmetrical) parts on either side of the body.

Question: When hemiplegia is the result of a cerebral infarction, is a separate code required to describe the hemiplegia?

Answer: When hemiplegia is the result of a cerebral infarction, a separate code is not required to describe the hemiplegia, because combination codes are available that classify the specific sequela as following a cerebral infarction.

Section 1.14 Coding Practice

Question: What type of nervous system disorder is carotid sinus syndrome?

Answer: Carotid sinus syndrome is an idiopathic neuropathy affecting the peripheral autonomic nervous system. It causes syncope or a brief loss of consciousness when pressure sensors in the carotid artery are stimulated.

Question: What term is used to find the correct code for Arnold-Chiari malformation type 1?

Answer: Arnold-Chiari malformation type I is found under the term 'Compression, brain (stem)' or 'Chiari's, malformation, type 1' Looking under 'Arnold-Chiari disease, obstruction, or syndrome' provides the codes for type II and type IV, with a 'see Encephalocele' reference for type III.

Question: Why is a complication code from the nervous system chapter used to report encephalopathy following CABG?

Answer: A complication code from the nervous system chapter is used to report encephalopathy following CABG because it is a complication of a surgical procedure affecting the nervous system. Codes for intra- and postprocedural complications affecting a particular system are located within the specific chapter.

Question: Where are intraoperative and post-procedural complications affecting the nervous system found?

Answer: Intraoperative and post-procedural complications affecting the nervous system are found in Chapter 6 Diseases of the Nervous System under category G97.

Section 1.15 Coding Practice

Question: Myasthenia gravis in adults is classified as a myoneural disorder. How is transient neonatal myasthenia gravis classified?

Answer: Transient neonatal myasthenia gravis is classified as an endocrine and metabolic disturbance specific to the fetus or newborn. It is classified as a disorder of muscle tone of the newborn.

Section 1.16 Coding Practice

Question: Why is spina bifida occulta listed under congenital malformation of the spine instead of under congenital malformations of the nervous system?

Answer: Spina bifida occulta is listed under congenital malformation of the spine instead of congenital malformation of the nervous system because it is a condition involving the spinal column, or vertebrae, which protect the spinal cord. Normal vertebral bone anatomy is affected. Radiography shows abnormal spinous processes and neural arches, but it usually does not cause nervous system problems because the spinal cord and nerves are rarely affected.

Section 1.17 Coding Practice

Question: What types of malaise and fatigue are identified in ICD-10-CM?

Answer: Weakness or asthenia NOS (R53.1), neoplastic (malignant) related fatigue (R53.0), other malaise (R53.81), and other fatigue (R53.83).

Section 1.18 Coding Practice

Question: What are the time frames regarding the loss of consciousness related to head trauma?

Answer: Time frames for loss of consciousness are an inherent part of the code description:

Without loss of consciousness

With loss of consciousness of 30 min or less

With loss of consciousness of 31 min to 59 min

With loss of consciousness of 1 hour to 5 hours 59 min

With loss of consciousness of 6 hours to 24 hours

With loss of consciousness greater than 24 hours with return to pre-existing conscious level with patient surviving

With loss of consciousness greater than 24 hours without return to pre-existing conscious level with patient surviving

With loss of consciousness of any duration with death due to brain injury prior to regaining consciousness

With loss of consciousness of any duration with death due to other cause prior to regaining consciousness

With loss of consciousness of unspecified duration

Question: Which codes listed in the practice examples above are external cause codes?

Answer: Only the codes that begin with W and Y in the coding practice examples above are external causes of morbidity codes.

Question: Which types of external cause codes require a 7th character extension to identify the episode of care?

Answer: Almost all categories of external cause codes require the 7th character extension except complications of medical and surgical care (Y62-Y84), blood alcohol levels (Y90), and place of occurrence codes (Y92).

Question: What does the 7th character extension for the external cause codes specify?

Answer: The 7th character for the external cause codes specifies the initial or subsequent encounter, or sequela.

Coding Practice 1.19

Question: Is F02.80 ever reported as the primary (first listed) diagnosis code?

Answer: Code F02.80 and F02.81 are manifestation codes and will never be reported as the first listed, primary diagnosis. Coding instructions require that the underlying physiological condition must be coded first.

Question: Why are two codes required to report post-concussion syndrome?

Answer: Two codes are required to report postconcussion syndrome per coding instructions for category F07 where postconcussion syndrome is classified. The underlying physiological condition must be coded first, so the appropriate concussion code with loss of consciousness is reported with a 7th digit denoting sequela, and the postconcussion syndrome code is listed next.

Question: Why is code Y90.1 used in conjunction with F10.920 in the example above?

Answer: Code Y90.1 in used in conjunction with F10.920 in the example above because an additional code is needed for the blood alcohol level, if applicable.

Coding Practice Answers: Section 2. Musculoskeletal System

Section 2.1 Coding Practice

Question: Are there any combined codes in ICD-10-CM for infectious/parasitic diseases of the musculoskeletal system? More specifically, can any infectious/parasitic diseases be reported with either a single code from the infectious/parasitic diseases chapter or from the musculoskeletal system chapter?

Answer: Yes. Pneumococcal arthritis is reported with a code from M00.1-.

Question: Is the code for gram negative bacilli a specific or nonspecific code?

Answer: Code B96.89 is a nonspecific 'other specified' code.

Question: Where is the quadriceps muscle located?

Answer: The quadriceps is a group of four muscles in the anterior thigh and includes the vastus lateralis, vastus medialis, vastus intermedius, and rectus femoris.

Question: Can the correct code for streptococcus viridans be found under the main term 'Infection' in the ICD-10-CM Alphabetic Index? If not, under what term(s) is the correct code found?

Answer: Yes. However, because only streptococcus A, B, D, and pneumoniae have specific codes, the correct code is designated by the term 'other specified.' In addition, the correct code can be found under the main term 'Streptococcus.'

Section 2.2 Coding Practice

Question: Is code C41.4 specific to Ewing's sarcoma of the ilium?

Answer: No. The code indicates only that the patient has a malignant neoplasm of the pelvic bones, sacrum and/or coccyx.

Question: What documentation is required to select the most specific code for many neoplasms of the bone and muscle?

Answer: Laterality should be documented.

Question: Where is the deltoid muscle located?

Answer: The deltoid is located in the shoulder.

Section 2.3 Coding Practice

Question: What information is required to assign the most specific code for rheumatoid arthritis?

Answer: In order to assign the most specific code, documentation must indicate whether there is other organ or system involvement, whether or not the rheumatoid arthritis is sero-positive or -negative (i.e. whether the patient tests positive for rheumatoid factor), the specific joint(s) affected, and laterality.

Question: How is an old bucket handle tear of the meniscus classified in ICD-10-CM

Answer: In the Alphabetic Index look-up under tear, torn-meniscus-old there is an instructional note to see Derangement, knee, meniscus, due to old tear. Derangement, knee, meniscus, due to old tear or injury defaults to M23.20. In the Tabular Index, old bucket handle tears are classified under the code category M23.2 Derangement of meniscus due to old tear or injury. There is an inclusion note under the category for old bucket handle tear. Subcategories are classified base upon medial or lateral meniscus, anterior horn, posterior horn, other and unspecified and laterality. Since the type of tear is identified as bucket handle an old bucket handle tear would be classified under subcategory M23.23 for medial meniscus and M23.26 for lateral meniscus.

Question: Why isn't code S83.25- used for an old bucket handle tear?

Answer: S83.25- identifies a current injury, not an old injury.

Section 2.4 Coding Practice

Question: Can the code for polyarteritis with lung involvement be found under the term polyarteritis?

Answer: Yes, polyarteritis can be found in the Alphabetic Index with the subcategory of 'with lung involvement'.

Question: In ICD-10-CM, are Wegener's granulomatosis and Churg-Strauss syndrome reported with the same code?

Answer: No. These two conditions have been assigned different codes.

Question: For a patient with CREST syndrome with Raynaud's phenomenon, would the Raynaud's be reported as an additional code?

Answer: No. CREST syndrome includes calcinosis, Raynaud's phenomenon, esophageal dysfunction, sclerodactyly and telangiectasia as part of the syndrome.

Question: What is the code descriptor for M32.10? Does this code descriptor identify the specific organ(s) affected?

Answer: Systemic lupus erythematosus (SLE), organ or system involvement unspecified. There are more specific codes for SLE, but these require documentation of the specific organ or system affected.

Question: Systemic sclerosis is reported with codes from the musculoskeletal system chapter. Where are codes for isolated, also called circumscribed, scleroderma found?

Answer: Isolated or circumscribed sclerodermas are found in Chapter 12, Diseases of the Skin and Subcutaneous tissue.

Question: Why is Sicca syndrome with arthralgia and myalgia reported with the code for Sicca syndrome with myopathy?

Answer: The term 'myopathy' refers to a disorder of the muscle tissue, which is a more general term than myalgia (muscle pain). Arthralgia is another symptom of Sicca syndrome but does not have a specific code; it is encompassed by the code for Sicca syndrome with myopathy.

Section 2.5 Coding Practice

Question: Why is kyphosis in the example above coded as other kyphosis rather than unspecified kyphosis?

Answer: An 'other specified' code is used because structural kyphosis is a specified type of kyphosis that does not have a more specific code. Whenever a condition is a specified type and there is not a specific code for that condition, the 'other specified' code should be used unless there is an excludes note or other coding instruction indicating that another code should be used.

Question: Why is kyphoscoliosis reported with a scoliosis code rather than a kyphosis code or a code from both categories?

Answer: The Alphabetic Index refers to the scoliosis codes and under category M41, there is an Includes note for kyphoscoliosis.

Question: Is congenital scoliosis coded under category M41 Scoliosis?

Answer: No, there is an Excludes 1 instruction under category M41 directing to code congenital scoliosis NOS as Q67.5 and congenital scoliosis due to bony malformation as category Q76.3.

Question: What does the term 'idiopathic' mean?

Answer: Idiopathic means the cause of the condition is unknown.

Question: What documentation is required to assign the most specific code for fatigue fractures and collapsed vertebrae?

Answer: Fatigue fractures require a 7th character to identify episode of care and whether the fatigue fracture is healing as expected. Episode of care codes include A for initial encounter, D for subsequent encounter with routine healing, G for subsequent encounter with delayed healing, and S for sequela.

Question: Herniated nucleus pulposus is synonymous with displacement of an intervertebral disc. In the example, why is it coded to disc disorder with myelopathy rather than to disc displacement?

Answer: In the Alphabetic Index under 'Herniation nucleus pulposus' there is an instruction to see Displacement, intervertebral disc, but under Displacement intervertebral disc with myelopathy, there is another instruction to see Disorder, disc, with myelopathy

Section 2.6 Coding Practice

Question: What information is needed to code for trigger finger disorders?

Answer: Laterality and which of the five fingers is affected.

Question: In ICD-10-CM, is the code for adhesive tenosynovitis of the shoulder listed under 'Tenosynovitis' in the Alphabetic Index? If not, under what term is this condition listed?

Answer: No. The code is listed under Capsulitis, adhesive.

Section 2.7 Coding Practice

Question: What term is slipped epiphysis of a site other than the upper femur listed under in the Alphabetic Index?

Answer: Slipped epiphysis of a site other than the upper femur may found under 'Osteochondropathy, specified type NEC'. A current traumatic slipped epiphysis is listed by site under fracture.

Question: What information is needed in order to properly code for a slipped epiphysis?

Answer: Whether the condition is traumatic or nontraumatic, location (upper femur or other site), laterality acute, chronic or acute on chronic.

Question: In ICD-10-CM what term is used instead of 'senile' to describe osteoporosis in older individuals?

Answer: The term used in ICD-10-CM is 'age-related' osteoporosis.

Section 2.8 Coding Practice

Question: What information is needed to accurately assign a code for congenital deformities of the hip?

Answer: In ICD-10-CM, the descriptors for congenital deformities of the hip include the type of deformity such as dislocation and valgus and varus deformities. Dislocation codes require documentation of partial or complete as well as laterality. A separate code exists for bilateral dislocations.

Question: What term(s) in the description of polydactyly above affect the code assignment in ICD-10-CM?

Answer: Since ICD-10-CM distinguishes between an accessory finger, accessory thumb, and accessory toe, the term ulnar is the key to identifying the correct code. The term ulnar polydactyly indicates that the accessory digit is on the ulnar side. This indicates that it is the hand and means that it would be classified as an accessory finger as opposed to an accessory thumb. Radial polydactyly refers to an accessory thumb.

Section 2.9 Coding Practice

Question: Why is the medial malleolus fracture described above reported with the code for a displaced fracture?

Answer: According to the Official Coding Guidelines, if the fracture is not specified as displaced or nondisplaced, the default is displaced.

Question: What does the seventh character extension 'D' indicate for code S52.532D? Does the seventh character 'D' have the same meaning for all types of injuries?

Answer: The seventh character 'D' indicates a subsequent encounter for closed fracture with routine healing. No, it does not. For all injuries, the seventh character 'D' means subsequent encounter. For certain traumatic fractures (Greenstick, Torus, physeal) the 'D' indicates a subsequent encounter for a fracture with routine healing. These types of fractures do not present as open injuries.

Question: Why are the fractures of the radial and ulnar shafts reported with two codes? What additional information about the injury is needed?

Answer: In ICD-10-CM, there is no code for radius with ulna so the fracture of each bone is reported separately. In addition to the specific bone and location on the bone, the fracture configuration/type (Greenstick, oblique, spiral, comminuted, segmental, transverse, bent bone, Galeazzi, Monteggia) and displacement is also needed for specificity in coding.

Section 2.10 Coding Practice

Question: Is an acromioclavicular (AC) joint separation without documentation of open or closed status reported as an open or closed injury?

Answer: ICD-10-CM does not differentiate between an open or closed dislocation in the dislocation code. However, if the patient has an open dislocation, a separate code is required for the open wound. An open wound would not be assumed so if the dislocation is not specified as open or closed, the default is closed.

Question: Is the code for the ACL injury specific to the anterior cruciate?

Answer: Yes.

Question: What external cause codes should be reported with the injury codes listed in the Coding Practice when additional information is available on the circumstances surrounding the injury?

Answer: External cause codes would be assigned for how the injury happened (cause), the intent (unintentional or accidental; intentional, such as suicide or assault), the place of occurrence, the activity the patient was participating in and work status. Place of occurrence, activity and status are only reported with the initial encounter.

Question: Why are all Coding Practices reported with the 7th digit extension A?

Answer: All conditions have qualifiers such as initial, current injury or new injury, indicating that care is being provided for the acute phase of the injury.

Section 2.11 Coding Practice

Question: When coding for tendon lacerations what information is required to properly assign a code?

Answer: Location and for fingers which finger, laterality, action of tendon (flexor, extensor, intrinsic). There is also an instructional note to code also

Question: What information is needed when coding for open wounds in the hand?

Answer: Laterality; type of open wound: laceration, puncture, bite, unspecified; presence of a foreign body; location including which finger; damage to the nail.

ICD-10-CM Documentation

Section 1. Nervous System

Diseases of the nervous system include disorders of the central nervous system that affect the brain and spinal cord, such as cerebral degeneration or Parkinson's disease, and diseases of the peripheral nervous system, such as polyneuropathy, myasthenia gravis, and muscular dystrophy. Some of the more commonly treated pain diagnoses are also classified as diseases of the nervous system, including: migraine and other headache syndromes, causalgia, complex regional pain syndrome I (CRPS I), neuralgia, and pain not elsewhere classified. Diseases of the nervous system are classified in Chapter 6.

Physician documentation is the basis for code assignment and the importance of proper documentation is imperative. ICD-1Ø-CM captures a greater level of specificity than in previous systems which will require more precise clinical information documented in the medical record. Updated and standardized clinical terminology is used in ICD-1Ø-CM to be consistent with the current standards providers use when diagnosing and treating nervous system disorders. Clinical terms such as commonly used synonyms for "intractable" migraine and more current terminology for epilepsy are found in the code descriptions.

For example, the terms "epilepsy" and "seizure disorder" describe central nervous system disorders characterized by sudden-onset seizures and muscle contractions. Seizure disorders and recurrent seizures are classified with epilepsy; however, convulsions, seizures not otherwise specified, febrile seizures, and hysterical seizures are classified as non-epileptic. So, a detailed description of the seizure is needed in order to differentiate between epilepsy and other seizures and to distinguish between seizure types.

Many nervous system conditions are manifestations of other diseases and dual coding is often required to report both the underlying condition and the manifestation. Dual coding is frequently required for infectious diseases of the central nervous system and precise documentation is needed in order to determine whether the condition is coded to the nervous system or to an infectious disease combination code.

Combination codes for common etiologies and symptoms or manifestations (e.g., dementia with Parkinsonism) are common in Chapter 6. The codes provide specific information and clinical detail. This places an even greater emphasis on the provider's documentation of the association between conditions, such as documenting the condition as "due to" a specified disease process.

Many diseases and conditions of the nervous system have additional elements which are captured in the code. For instance, providers routinely document the side of the body where disease or injury occurs (right, left, or bilateral), and laterality is included in many of the nervous system code description. Representative examples of documentation requirements are provided in this chapter and checklists are provided in Appendix A to help identify documentation deficiencies so that physicians and coders are aware of the specificity needed for proper code assignment.

There are 11 code blocks for the central and peripheral nervous system. The table below shows the category blocks for nervous system disorders.

ICD-10-CM Code Blocks	
G00-G09	Inflammatory Diseases of the Central Nervous System
G10-G14	Systemic Atrophies Primarily Affecting the Central Nervous System
G20-G26	Extrapyramidal and Movement Disorders
G30-G32	Other Degenerative Diseases of the Nervous System
G35-G37	Demyelinating Diseases of the Central Nervous System
G40-G47	Episodic and Paroxysmal Disorders
G50-G59	Nerve, Nerve Root and Plexus Disorders
G60-G65	Polyneuropathies and other Disorders of the Peripheral Nervous System
G70-G73	Diseases of Myoneural Junction and Muscle
G80-G83	Cerebral Palsy and Other Paralytic Syndromes
G89-G99	Other Disorders of the Nervous System

The organization of nervous system diseases in ICD-1Ø-CM includes:

- Hereditary and degenerative diseases of the central nervous system subdivided into four code blocks
  - G1Ø-G14 Systemic Atrophies Primarily Affecting the Central Nervous System
  - G2Ø-G26 Extrapyramidal and Movement Disorders
  - G3Ø-G32 Other Degenerative Diseases of the Nervous System
  - G35-G37 Demyelinating Diseases of the Central Nervous System
- Pain not elsewhere classified found in category G89 and of code block G89-G99 Other Disorders of the Nervous System
- Other headache syndromes classified in category G44 in code block G4Ø-G47 Episodic and Paroxysmal Disorders which also includes epilepsy (G4Ø), migraine (G43), transient cerebral ischemic attacks and related syndromes (G45), vascular syndromes of brain in cerebrovascular diseases (G46), and sleep disorders (G47)
- Disorders of the peripheral nervous system subdivided into three code blocks
  - G5Ø-G59 Nerve, Nerve Root and Plexus Disorders

- G6Ø-G65 Polyneuropathies and other Disorders of the Peripheral Nervous System
- G7Ø-G73 Diseases of Myoneural Junction and Muscle

- Intraoperative and postprocedural complications specific to the nervous system classified in Chapter 6 in code block G89-G99 Other Disorders of the Nervous System

Sleep apnea is located with diseases of the nervous system in Chapter 6. Nonspecific neuralgia and neuritis are not classified to the nervous system chapter; rather, these nonspecific diagnoses are located in the musculoskeletal chapter.

Because many underlying conditions can cause nervous system disorders, including infectious diseases, circulatory disorders, and external causes such as injury or drugs, careful review of the medical record documentation is needed in order to determine whether the condition is coded to the nervous system chapter or to another chapter.

Exclusions

There are no Excludes1 notes, but there are a number of Excludes2.

ICD-10-CM Excludes1	ICD-10-CM Excludes2
None	• Certain conditions originating in the perinatal period (P04-P96) • Certain infectious and parasitic diseases (A00-B99) • Complications of pregnancy, childbirth and the puerperium (O00-O9A) • Congenital malformations, deformations, and chromosomal abnormalities (Q00-Q99) • Endocrine, nutritional and metabolic diseases (E00-E88) • Injury, poisoning and certain other consequences of external causes (S00-T88) • Neoplasms (C00-D49) • Symptoms, signs and abnormal clinical and laboratory findings, not elsewhere classified (R00-R94)

Chapter Guidelines

Detailed guidelines are provided for coding certain conditions classified in Chapter 6 including:

- Dominant/nondominant side
- Pain not elsewhere classified

Dominant/Nondominant Side

The side of the body affected (right, left) is a component of the code for conditions that affect one side of the body. Codes such as hemiplegia and hemiparesis (category G81) and monoplegia of the upper limb (G83.2), and lower limb (G83.1) or unspecified monoplegia (G83.3) also identify whether the side affected is the dominant or nondominant side. When the documentation provides laterality but fails to identify the side affected as dominant or nondominant, and the classification system does not indicate a default, ICD-1Ø-CM provides the following guidelines:

- For ambidextrous patients, the default should be dominant
- If the left side is affected, the default is non-dominant
- If the right side is affected, the default is dominant

Pain Not Elsewhere Classified (G89)

According to the guidelines, the pain codes in category G89 Pain, not elsewhere classified, are used in conjunction with codes from other categories and chapters to provide more detail about acute or chronic pain and neoplasm-related pain. However, if the pain is not specified in the provider documentation as acute or chronic, post-thoracotomy, postprocedural, or neoplasm-related, codes from category G89 are not assigned.

Codes from category G89 are not assigned when the underlying or definitive diagnosis is known, unless the reason for the encounter is pain management rather than management of the underlying condition. When an admission or encounter is for treatment of the underlying condition, a code for the underlying condition is assigned as the principal diagnosis and no code from category G89 is assigned. For example, when a patient is admitted for spinal fusion to treat a vertebral fracture, the code for the vertebral fracture would be assigned as the principal diagnosis but no pain code is assigned.

Category G89 in Conjunction with Site-Specific Pain Codes

Guidelines for assigning pain codes as the principal or first-listed diagnosis when pain control or pain management is the reason for the admission/encounter direct the user to assign a code for the underlying cause of the pain as an additional diagnosis. A case example would be a patient with nerve impingement and severe back pain seen for a spinal canal steroid injection or a patient admitted for insertion of a neurostimulator for pain control; the appropriate pain code would be assigned as the principal or first-listed diagnosis. On the other hand, when an admission or encounter is for treatment of the underlying condition and a neurostimulator is also inserted for pain control during the same episode of care, the underlying condition is the principal diagnosis and the appropriate pain code should be assigned as a secondary diagnosis.

Pain codes from category G89 may be used in conjunction with site-specific pain codes that identify the site of pain (including codes from chapter 18) if the category G89 code provides additional diagnostic information such as describing whether the pain is acute or chronic. The sequencing of codes is dependent on the circumstances of the admission/encounter for example:

- The category G89 code is sequenced first followed by the code identifying the specific site of pain when the encounter is for pain control or pain management
- If the encounter is for any other reason and a related definitive diagnosis has not been confirmed in the provider's documentation, the specific site of the pain is coded first, followed by the category G89 code.

Postoperative Pain

Coding of postoperative pain is driven by the provider's documentation. For post-thoracotomy and other postoperative pain that is not specified as acute or chronic, the code for the acute form is the default.

Routine or expected postoperative pain immediately after surgery is not coded, but severe or an unexpected level of postoperative pain not associated with a specific postoperative complication is assigned to the appropriate postoperative pain code in category G89. Postoperative pain associated with a specific postoperative complication (e.g., painful wire sutures) is coded to Chapter 19 Injury, poisoning, and certain other consequences of external causes with an additional code from category G89 to identify acute or chronic pain.

Chronic Pain

Codes in category G89 differentiate between acute and chronic pain. There is no time frame defining when pain becomes chronic pain so, the provider's documentation directs the use of these codes. When chronic pain is documented, it is coded to subcategory G89.2. It is important to note that central pain syndrome (G89.Ø) and chronic pain syndrome (G89.4) are not the same as "chronic pain," so these codes should only be used when the provider has specifically documented these conditions.

Neoplasm Related Pain

Code G89.3 is assigned when the patient's pain is documented as being related to, associated with, or due to cancer, primary or secondary malignancy, or tumor. The code for neoplasm-related pain is assigned regardless of whether the pain is documented as acute or chronic. When the reason for the admission/encounter is documented as pain control/pain management, G89.3 is assigned as the principal or first-listed code with the underlying neoplasm reported as an additional diagnosis. When the admission/encounter is for management of the neoplasm and the pain associated with the neoplasm is also documented, code G89.3 may be assigned as an additional diagnosis. It is not necessary to assign an additional code for the site of the pain.

General Documentation Requirements

General documentation requirements differ depending on the particular nervous system disease or disorder. In general, specificity of the type and cause of the nervous system disorder is required and must be documented in the medical record. Some of the general documentation requirements are discussed here, but greater detail for some of the more common diseases and conditions of the nervous system will be provided in the next section.

According to the *ICD-1Ø-CM Official Guidelines for Coding and Reporting*, complete and accurate code assignment requires a joint effort between the provider and the coder. Without consistent, complete documentation in the medical record, accurate coding cannot be achieved. Much of the detail captured in the ICD-1Ø-CM codes is routinely documented by providers, such as the severity or status of the disease in terms of acuity, the etiology (e.g., neoplasm-related pain), and the significance of related diagnostic findings (e.g., EEG confirms a seizure disorder). Beyond these basic medical record documentation requirements, specifically describing the site, such as the specific nerve (e.g., lesion of medial popliteal nerve, right lower limb) rather than a general anatomical site will ensure optimal code assignment for nervous system disorders.

Documentation in the patient's record should clearly specify the cause-and-effect relationship between a symptom, manifestation, or complication and a disease or a medical intervention. For example, documentation should specify whether a complication occurred intraoperatively, as in intraoperative hemorrhage, or postoperatively.

In addition to these general documentation requirements, there are specific diseases and disorders that require greater detail in documentation to ensure optimal code assignment.

Code-Specific Documentation Requirements

In this section, the ICD-1Ø-CM code categories, subcategories, and subclassifications for some of the more commonly reported diseases and conditions of the nervous system are reviewed along with documentation requirements. The focus is on frequently reported conditions with specific clinical documentation requirements. Though not all of the codes with documentation requirements are discussed, this section will provide a representative sample of the type of additional documentation required for diseases of the nervous system. The section is organized alphabetically by the code category, subcategory, or subclassification, depending on whether the documentation affects only a single code or an entire subcategory or category.

Alzheimer's Disease

Alzheimer's disease is the most common form of dementia. The progressive degeneration of nerve cells in Alzheimer's disease manifests mental changes ranging from mild memory impairment to loss of cognitive function with dementia. Accurate code assignment of Alzheimer's disease, with or without associated dementia, requires comprehensive provider documentation that clearly distinguishes Alzheimer's dementia from senile dementia, senile degeneration, or senility.

Codes include more specificity so a diagnosis of Alzheimer's disease without further description of the onset (e.g., early onset, late onset) and the type of symptoms (e.g., depression, delusions) will not support optimal code assignment. It is essential that the provider documentation clarify dementia related to other conditions. Alzheimer's disease may also be associated with delirium or behavioral disturbances, so it is equally important to document these conditions when they are present.

Coding and Documentation Requirements

Identify type/onset of Alzheimer's disease:

- Early onset
- Late onset
- Other Alzheimer's disease
- Unspecified Alzheimer's disease

Use additional code when Alzheimer's disease is associated with:

- Delirium (FØ5)
- Dementia with behavioral disturbance (FØ2.81)
- Dementia without behavioral disturbance (FØ2.8Ø)

ICD-10-CM Code/Documentation	
G30.0	Alzheimer's disease with early onset
G30.1	Alzheimer's disease with late onset
G30.8	Other Alzheimer's disease
G30.9	Alzheimer's disease, unspecified

Documentation and Coding Example

A 77-year-old woman was brought for neurological evaluation by her husband because of a 6 month history of increasing memory impairment. Her husband began noticing a gradual worsening in her memory and increased difficulty finding words. He also noted a decline in social activity which he describes as "extremely out of character" for his wife. She appeared to be in a chronic state of confusion and was unable to converse in a logical or coherent manner, and her responses to questions were frequently inappropriate. Her confusion and memory problems became even more pronounced and her husband reported she was not sleeping at night.

The patient is well-groomed, alert, and friendly with no specific complaints. She worked in a secretarial position until her retirement at age 65. Her past medical history is significant for hysterectomy and although elevated blood pressure was documented on several occasions, she was never diagnosed with or medicated for HTN. All of her recent evaluations, including a CT scan, were reported as normal.

General medical and neurological exams were normal. She scored 15 out of a possible 3Ø on the mini mental state examination MMSE. Her speech was highly paraphasic. She couldn't remember what she had for breakfast. She was able to provide her name, but when asked about her current age, she incorrectly stated her birth month, but then became aware of this and became very angry. She was unable to give the current year, or the name of the current president.

Formal testing was conducted and she scored well below average in all cognitive domains on the Wechsler Memory scale, the Wechsler Adult Intelligence Scale, the Visuo-spatial Construction, and the Graphomotor Alternation Test. The results of the evaluation indicate that she meets clinical criteria for **Alzheimer's disease**. Patient was started on an empirical trial of neurotransmitters therapy, discharged home with daily home health care assistance.

Diagnosis: **Dementia in late onset Alzheimer's disease**

Diagnosis Code(s)

G3Ø.1 Alzheimer's disease with late onset

FØ2.8Ø Dementia in other diseases classified elsewhere without behavioral disturbance

Coding Note(s)

Alzheimer's disease with dementia requires dual coding with the underlying condition (Alzheimer's disease) coded first followed by a code for dementia with or without behavioral disturbance. Late onset Alzheimer's disease is coded to G3Ø.1. When Alzheimer's associated dementia is present, code FØ2.8- is assigned as an additional code.

Causalgia

Causalgia, also referred to as complex regional pain syndrome type II (CRPS II), is a type of neuropathic pain that occurs following a distinct nerve injury, usually to a peripheral nerve in an extremity. Symptoms include continuous burning or throbbing pain along the peripheral nerve; sensitivity to cold and/or touch; changes in skin temperature, color, and/or texture; hair and nail changes; joint stiffness and muscle spasms; and weakness and/or atrophy.

Codes for causalgia are specified by upper and lower limb and laterality. Causalgia of the upper limb is reported with codes in subcategory G56.4. Causalgia of the lower limb is reported with codes from subcategory G57.7. Fifth characters for both the upper and lower limbs identify laterality as unspecified (Ø), right (1), left (2), or bilateral (3).

Coding and Documentation Requirements

Identify site:

- Upper limb
  - Right
  - Left
  - Bilateral
  - Unspecified
- Lower limb
  - Right
  - Left
  - Bilateral
  - Unspecified

ICD-10-CM Code/Documentation	
G56.40	Causalgia of unspecified upper limb (complex regional pain syndrome II)
G56.41	Causalgia of right upper limb (complex regional pain syndrome II)
G56.42	Causalgia of left upper limb (complex regional pain syndrome II)
G56.43	Causalgia of bilateral upper limbs (complex regional pain syndrome II)
G57.70	Causalgia of unspecified lower limb (complex regional pain syndrome II)
G57.71	Causalgia of right lower limb (complex regional pain syndrome II)
G57.72	Causalgia of left lower limb (complex regional pain syndrome II)
G57.73	Causalgia of bilateral lower limbs (complex regional pain syndrome II)

Documentation and Coding Example

Patient is a 12-year-old Caucasian male referred to orthopedics by his pediatrician for evaluation of right foot pain and weakness. He is non-weight bearing on right lower extremity with use of crutches. The patient is accompanied to the appointment by his father. PMH includes seasonal allergies controlled with Cetirizine. Immunizations are up to date for age. Patient sustained a displaced fracture of the right fibula approximately two months ago complicated by right peroneal nerve injury while **racing on a BMX course**. He came over a jump, **lost control of the bike**

and landed hard on his right leg. No other riders were involved. The accident occurred out of town and he was initially seen in an Urgent Care Center where X-rays showed a displaced fracture of the proximal fibular shaft with peroneal nerve compression. He underwent an ORIF with decompression of the peroneal nerve. He was placed in a hinged knee brace, given crutches to use, and told to follow up with PMD or orthopedist when he returned home. He was able to ambulate without pain initially but started noticing some weakness in his right foot two weeks after discontinuing the brace. As the weakness increased he also began to have numbness and tingling on the top of the right foot. Walking and wearing shoes now cause unbearable pain. He denies any knee pain or loss of mobility. On examination, this is an anxious appearing, well nourished, thin, adolescent male. WT 84 lbs. (37th%) HT 62 in. (86th%). Cranial nerves grossly intact. Upper extremities are normal in strength, sensation, and movement. Cervical, thoracic, and lumbar spine all normal in appearance and movement. Hips and knees in good alignment with range of motion intact. Upper leg strength normal bilaterally. Left lower extremity has normal strength, sensation, and movement. Right lower extremity feels significantly warmer to touch than left and skin color is unusually red beginning 1Ø cm above ankle and extending though toes. He has hyperalgesia and marked allodynia on dorsal surface of right foot when skin is lightly stroked by examiners fingers. Hyperhidrosis is not appreciated. There is no muscle wasting noted but he has marked ankle weakness and right foot drop with attempted dorsiflexion. His is able to tolerate only a few steps weight bearing and he is noted to have a slapping gait with toe drag. Comprehensive x-rays obtained of right lower extremity including AP, lateral, and oblique views of knee; AP, lateral, and mortise views of the ankle; AP and lateral views of the tibia/fibula shafts which are negative for Maisonneuve injury but show **good calcification at the site of the transverse fracture of proximal fibula.**

Impression: **S/P right fibula fracture with secondary causalgia due to common peroneal nerve injury.**

Plan: MRI to include right knee, lower leg, and foot. Consider referral to neurology for EMG and pain management.

Diagnosis Code(s)

G57.71 Causalgia of right lower limb

S82.831S Other fracture of upper and lower end of right fibula, sequela

S84.11XS Injury of peroneal nerve at lower leg level, right leg, sequela

V18.ØXXS Pedal cycle driver injured in noncollision transport accident in nontraffic accident, sequela

Coding Note(s)

The causalgia of the right leg is a sequela of a fracture resulting in a nerve injury of the upper end of the fibula. The causalgia is the first listed diagnosis code. Laterality is a component of the causalgia code. The code identifying the injury that resulted in the sequela is listed next. The patient had a transverse fracture of the upper end of the fibula with compression of the peroneal nerve. Both injuries are coded with 7th character S to indicate a sequela (late effect). While there are codes specific to transverse fracture of the shaft of the fibula, there is not a specific code for transverse fracture of the upper end so the code for other fracture of upper and lower end of the right fibula is reported. In this case, the use of "and" means "and/or" in the code descriptor for code S82.831S. The physician has also documented that there is good calcification at the fracture site which indicates that the fracture has healed normally. The code for the nerve injury is specific to the peroneal nerve. Laterality is also a component of both the fracture and nerve injury codes. The BMX rider was involved in a noncollision, nontraffic accident which is reported with the 7th character S to indicate that the patient is being treated for a sequela of the BMX accident.

Complex Regional Pain Syndrome I

Reflex sympathetic dystrophy (RSD) is now more commonly referred to as complex regional pain syndrome I (CRPS I). CRPS I is a type of severe, debilitating neuropathic pain that usually results from an injury, but in CRPS I there is no direct injury to the nerve itself. The precipitating injury may range from major to relatively minor trauma. It can also occur following an illness or it can occur without any known cause. Intense pain of the affected region can result even from light touch. Other symptoms related to abnormal function of the sympathetic nervous system may also be evident including abnormal circulation, temperature, and sweating. If not promptly diagnosed and treated there can be loss of function in the affected limb followed by muscle atrophy and even changes in hair and skin.

CRPS I is reported with codes from subcategory G9Ø.5. Codes are specific to the upper or lower limbs and laterality is also a component of the codes.

Coding and Documentation Requirements

Identify the site:

- Upper limb
  - Right
  - Left
  - Bilateral
  - Unspecified side
- Lower limb
  - Right
  - Left
  - Bilateral
  - Unspecified side
- Other specified site
- Unspecified site

ICD-10-CM Code/Documentation	
G90.50	Complex regional pain syndrome I, unspecified
G90.511	Complex regional pain syndrome I of right upper limb
G90.512	Complex regional pain syndrome I of left upper limb
G90.513	Complex regional pain syndrome I of upper limb, bilateral
G90.519	Complex regional pain syndrome I of unspecified upper limb
G90.521	Complex regional pain syndrome I of right lower limb
G90.522	Complex regional pain syndrome I of left lower limb
G90.523	Complex regional pain syndrome I of lower limb, bilateral
G90.529	Complex regional pain syndrome I of unspecified lower limb
G90.59	Complex regional pain syndrome I of other specified site

Documentation and Coding Example

Seventy-one-year-old Asian female presents to PMD with **pain and swelling in both arms**. The patient was in her usual state of good health until one month ago when she was the **victim of an attempted purse snatching** outside a local restaurant. She held onto her purse which was looped over her left forearm, elbow bent, but she felt her **shoulder wrench and elbow twist** during the altercation. She declined medical attention at the time and treated her injury conservatively with heat and Aleve. She states the **left arm pain** has progressed from mild tingling to a continuous burning sensation extending from shoulder to fingertips. The initial **bruising on her left forearm** resolved within a week but swelling around the elbow has increased and now extends into the wrist and hand. She has difficulty with movement especially elbow extension. What is most concerning to her is that **in the past week her right arm, which was not injured at the time, has developed a tingling type pain and yesterday she noticed swelling in the wrist**. Temperature 94.2 HR 84 RR 16 BP 140/82. Current medications include Aleve, Os-Cal, and a multivitamin. On examination, this is a thin, athletic appearing woman who looks significantly younger than her stated age. Cranial nerves are grossly intact. PERRLA. Eyes are clear, nares patent, mucous membranes moist and pink. Neck supple without lymphadenopathy. HR regular, without bruits or rubs, Grade II, S1 ejection murmur is present. Breath sounds clear, equal bilaterally. Abdomen soft, non-distended with active bowel sounds. Lower extremities are completely benign with intact circulation, sensation, and movement. Right upper extremity has no bruising or discoloration noted. Shoulder is freely mobile without swelling or pain. Right elbow is not swollen but gentle manipulation elicits complaint of pain and obvious stiffness in the joint. Wrist is exquisitely tender and noticeably swollen over the carpal-metacarpal joint. Sensation is normal, skin warm, dry to touch. Examination of left upper extremity is difficult due to pain. Hyperalgesia is present from just below shoulder through fingertips. Swelling is most notable in the elbow and wrist with muscle wasting in the upper arm and forearm. Skin is pale in color, cool and moist to touch.

Impression: **Complex regional pain disorder, Type I, of both upper extremities. Sequela of direct injury to muscles/tendons left upper arm. No known injury or direct cause on the right.**

Plan: Comprehensive radiographs of bilateral upper extremities to r/o fracture and bone scan of same to assess for decreased bone density. Referral made to neurologist. Patient is offered a trial of physical therapy but she declines, stating she would prefer to wait until after she has been evaluated by neurology.

Diagnosis Code(s)

G90.513 Complex regional pain syndrome I of upper limb, bilateral

S46.902S Unspecified injury of unspecified muscle, fascia and tendon at shoulder and upper arm level, left arm, sequela

Y04.8XXS Assault by other bodily force, sequela

Coding Note(s)

The code descriptor has been changed from reflex sympathetic dystrophy (RSD) to complex regional pain syndrome I (CRPS I) to reflect current terminology for the condition. Laterality is a component of the code which has been documented as bilateral. The CRPS I on the left is a sequela of the injury to the left arm so that should be coded additionally. There is no documented injury to the right arm, but CRPS I can also occur without a known cause. Sequela of injury is reported with an injury code with 7th character S. The site of the injury is documented as the muscles and tendons of the upper left arm, but the specific muscle(s)/tendon(s) are not identified and the specific type of injury is not documented so the code for unspecified injury of unspecified muscle/tendon is assigned. A code for the external cause is also assigned with 7th character S. The external cause is a pulling/wrenching injury in an attempt to snatch a purse which would be classified as an assault using bodily force. There is not a specific code for pulling/wrenching so the code for other bodily force is assigned.

Epilepsy and Recurrent Seizures

Epilepsy is a neurological condition characterized by recurrent seizures. The terms "epilepsy" and "seizure disorder" describe central nervous system disorders characterized by sudden-onset seizures and muscle contractions. Epileptic seizures may be classified as idiopathic or symptomatic. Idiopathic seizures do not have a known cause but in some cases there is a family history of epilepsy. Symptomatic epilepsy is due to a specific cause, such as head trauma, stroke, brain tumors, alcohol or drug withdrawal, and other conditions. Epileptic seizures can also be a manifestation of neurologic or metabolic diseases.

Different terminology may be used to describe epilepsy such as epileptic or epilepsia attack, convulsion, fit, and seizure; however, in the medical record documentation, epilepsy must be clearly differentiated from a diagnosis of seizure or convulsion which is reported with codes from the signs and symptoms chapter rather than a code for epilepsy from the nervous system chapter. This means that a clear distinction must be made between a patient who has one seizure and a patient with epilepsy. Due to legal consequences, a code of epilepsy cannot be assigned unless it is clearly diagnosed by the provider.

Accurate coding of epilepsy and recurrent seizures depends entirely on provider documentation. Current clinical terminology and codes that capture the required detail for the specific type of epilepsy and complications such as status epilepticus and intractability are found in the code options for epilepsy. In order to assign the most specific code, clinical terminology related to the different types of epilepsy must be understood. Below are definitions of the commonly used terms describing epilepsy and recurrent seizures.

Absence epileptic syndrome – A type of generalized epilepsy characterized by an alteration of consciousness of brief duration (usually less than 2Ø seconds) with sudden onset and termination. The alteration of consciousness may include impaired awareness and memory of ongoing events as evidenced by mental confusion, an inability to response to external stimuli, and amnesia. May also be referred to as absence petit mal seizure.

Cryptogenic epilepsy – Epilepsy that is likely due to a specific cause but the cause has not yet been identified.

Epilepsia partialis continua – Unique type of prolonged seizure consisting of prolonged simple partial (localized) motor seizures, now more commonly referred to as Kozhevnikoff's (Kojevnikoff's, Kojewnikoff's, Kojevnikov's, Kojevnikov's) epilepsy.

Epileptic spasms – Epilepsy syndrome that is clinically similar to infantile spasms, but of a broader clinical classification that captures this syndrome when onset occurs in later childhood. Note: Infantile spasms are classified to the more general code for epileptic spasms.

Focal epilepsy – Epilepsy that is localized or starts in one area of the brain (synonymous with partial epilepsy and localization related epilepsy).

Generalized epilepsy – Epilepsy that involves the entire brain at the same time.

Grand mal status – An obsolete term used to describe generalized tonic-clonic seizures.

Idiopathic epilepsy – Epilepsy with no known cause, and the person has no other signs of neurological disease.

Infantile spasms – Epilepsy syndrome of infancy and childhood also referred to as West Syndrome characterized by brief bobbing or bowing of the head followed by relaxation and a return of the head to a normal upright position. Infantile spasms are also associated with developmental regression and if not controlled can lead to mental retardation.

Juvenile myoclonic epilepsy – A type of generalized epilepsy with onset in childhood characterized by shock-like muscle contractions in a group of muscles usually in the arms or legs that result in a jerking motion and generalized tonic-clonic seizures. The patient may also experience absence seizures. May also be referred to as impulsive petit mal seizure

Localization-related epilepsy – Epilepsy that is localized or starts in one area of the brain (synonymous with focal epilepsy and partial epilepsy).

Lennox-Gastaut syndrome – Severe form of epilepsy usually beginning before age 4 and associated with impaired intellectual functioning, developmental delay, and behavioral disturbances. Seizure types vary but may include tonic, atonic, myoclonic, or absence seizures. The patient may experience periods of frequent seizures mixed with brief seizure-free periods. The cause is often identified with more common causes being brain malformations, perinatal asphyxia, severe head injury, central nervous system infection, and inherited degenerative or metabolic conditions. However, in about a third of all cases no cause is identified.

Partial epilepsy – Epilepsy that is localized or starts in one area of the brain (synonymous with focal epilepsy and localization related epilepsy).

Petit mal status – An obsolete term used to describe a type of generalized epilepsy that does not involve tonic-clonic movements.

Status epilepticus – Repeated or prolonged seizures usually lasing more than 3Ø minutes. May be tonic-clonic (convulsive) type or nonconvulsive (absence) type.

Symptomatic epilepsy – Epilepsy due to a known cause

Tonic-clonic seizures – Seizures characterized by an increase in muscle tone and rhythmic jerking of muscles in one part or all of the body.

In addition to the specific types of epilepsy and epileptic syndromes described above, epilepsy is also classified as intractable or not intractable. Intractable seizures are those that are not responding to treatment. Terms used to describe intractable seizures include: pharmacologically resistant, pharmacoresistant, poorly controlled, refractory, or treatment resistant. Seizures that are not intractable are responding to treatment. Documentation that supports classification as not intractable would be "under control," "well controlled," and "seizure-free."

Seizure disorders and recurrent seizures are classified with epilepsy; however, convulsions, new-onset seizure, single seizure, febrile seizure, or hysterical seizure are classified as non-epileptic. Thorough documentation of the seizure is needed in order to differentiate between epilepsy and other seizures and to distinguish seizure types.

For some specific types of epilepsy, a distinction is made between idiopathic and symptomatic epilepsy. Localization related epilepsy must be documented as idiopathic (G4Ø.Ø) or symptomatic (G4Ø.1, G4Ø.2). In addition, generalized epilepsy is specifically described as idiopathic (G4Ø.3). There is also a specific subcategory for epileptic seizure related to external causes such as alcohol, drugs, hormonal changes, sleep deprivation, or stress. In addition, all types of epilepsy must be documented as intractable or not intractable and as with status epilepticus or without status epilepticus. Documentation should also clearly differentiate epilepsy and recurrent seizures from the following conditions which are reported elsewhere:

- Conversion disorder with seizures (F44.5)
- Convulsions NOS (R56.9)
- Hippocampal sclerosis (G93.81)
- Mesial temporal sclerosis (G93.81)
- Post traumatic seizures (R56.1)
- Seizure (convulsive) NOS (R56.9)
- Seizure of newborn (P9Ø)

- Temporal sclerosis (G93.81)
- Todd's paralysis (G83.8)

Coding and Documentation Requirements

Identify type of epilepsy or recurrent seizures:

- Absence epileptic syndrome
- Due to external causes
- Generalized
  - Idiopathic
  - Other generalized type
- Juvenile myoclonic epilepsy (also known as impulsive petit mal)
- Localization-related (focal) (partial)
  - Idiopathic (with seizures of localized onset)
  - Symptomatic
    - » With complex partial seizures
    - » With simple partial seizures
- Other epilepsy and recurrent seizures
  - Epileptic spasms
  - Lennox-Gastaut syndrome
  - Other epilepsy
  - Other seizures
- Unspecified epilepsy

Identify response to treatment:

- With intractable epilepsy, which includes:
  - Pharmacoresistant or pharmacologically resistant
  - Poorly controlled
  - Treatment resistant
  - Refractory (medically)
  - Without intractable epilepsy

Identify as with/without status epilepticus

- With status epilepticus
- Without status epilepticus

ICD-10-CM Code/Documentation	
G40.001	Localization-related (focal) (partial) idiopathic epilepsy and epileptic syndromes with seizures of localized onset, not intractable, with status epilepticus
G40.009	Localization-related (focal) (partial) idiopathic epilepsy and epileptic syndromes with seizures of localized onset, not intractable, without status epilepticus
G40.011	Localization-related (focal) (partial) idiopathic epilepsy and epileptic syndromes with seizures of localized onset, intractable, with status epilepticus
G40.019	Localization-related (focal) (partial) idiopathic epilepsy and epileptic syndromes with seizures of localized onset, intractable, without status epilepticus
G40.101	Localization-related (focal) (partial) symptomatic epilepsy and epileptic syndromes with simple partial seizures, not intractable, with status epilepticus
G40.109	Localization-related (focal) (partial) symptomatic epilepsy and epileptic syndromes with simple partial seizures, not intractable, without status epilepticus
G40.111	Localization-related (focal) (partial) symptomatic epilepsy and epileptic syndromes with simple partial seizures, intractable, with status epilepticus
G40.119	Localization-related (focal) (partial) symptomatic epilepsy and epileptic syndromes with simple partial seizures, intractable, without status epilepticus
G40.201	Localization-related (focal) (partial) symptomatic epilepsy and epileptic syndromes with complex partial seizures, not intractable, with status epilepticus
G40.209	Localization-related (focal) (partial) symptomatic epilepsy and epileptic syndromes with complex partial seizures, not intractable, without status epilepticus
G40.211	Localization-related (focal) (partial) symptomatic epilepsy and epileptic syndromes with complex partial seizures, intractable, with status epilepticus
G40.219	Localization-related (focal) (partial) symptomatic epilepsy and epileptic syndromes with complex partial seizures, intractable, without status epilepticus
G40.301	Generalized idiopathic epilepsy and epileptic syndromes, not intractable, with status epilepticus
G40.309	Generalized idiopathic epilepsy and epileptic syndromes, not intractable, without status epilepticus
G40.311	Generalized idiopathic epilepsy and epileptic syndromes, intractable, with status epilepticus
G40.319	Generalized idiopathic epilepsy and epileptic syndromes, intractable, without status epilepticus
G40.A01	Absence epileptic syndrome, not intractable, with status epilepticus
G40.A09	Absence epileptic syndrome, not intractable, without status epilepticus
G40.A11	Absence epileptic syndrome, intractable, with status epilepticus
G40.A19	Absence epileptic syndrome, intractable, without status epilepticus
G40.B01	Juvenile myoclonic epilepsy, not intractable, with status epilepticus
G40.B09	Juvenile myoclonic epilepsy, not intractable, without status epilepticus
G40.B11	Juvenile myoclonic epilepsy, intractable, with status epilepticus
G40.B19	Juvenile myoclonic epilepsy, intractable, without status epilepticus

ICD-10-CM Code/Documentation
G40.401 Other generalized epilepsy and epileptic syndromes, not intractable, with status epilepticus
G40.409 Other generalized epilepsy and epileptic syndromes, not intractable, without status epilepticus
G40.411 Other generalized epilepsy and epileptic syndromes, intractable, with status epilepticus
G40.419 Other generalized epilepsy and epileptic syndromes, intractable, without status epilepticus
G40.501 Epileptic seizures related to external causes, not intractable, with status epilepticus
G40.509 Epileptic seizures related to external causes, not intractable, without status epilepticus
G40.801 Other epilepsy, not intractable, with status epilepticus
G40.802 Other epilepsy, not intractable, without status epilepticus
G40.803 Other epilepsy, intractable, with status epilepticus
G40.804 Other epilepsy, intractable, without status epilepticus
G40.811 Lennox-Gastaut syndrome, not intractable, with status epilepticus
G40.812 Lennox-Gastaut syndrome, not intractable, without status epilepticus
G40.813 Lennox-Gastaut syndrome, intractable, with status epilepticus
G40.814 Lennox-Gastaut syndrome, intractable, without status epilepticus
G40.821 Epileptic spasms, not intractable, with status epilepticus
G40.822 Epileptic spasms, not intractable, without status epilepticus
G40.823 Epileptic spasms, intractable, with status epilepticus
G40.824 Epileptic spasms, intractable, without status epilepticus
G40.89 Other seizures
G40.901 Epilepsy, unspecified, not intractable, with status epilepticus
G40.909 Epilepsy, unspecified, not intractable, without status epilepticus
G40.911 Epilepsy, unspecified, intractable, with status epilepticus
G40.919 Epilepsy, unspecified, intractable, without status epilepticus

Documentation and Coding Example

A previously healthy 9-year-old boy was admitted to the hospital from the Emergency Department following several episodes of vomiting over several days and then episodes of jerking movements of the left side of the body, predominantly the left leg, accompanied by an altered mental status. While in the ED, he had repeated episodes of generalized seizures and remained in status epilepticus despite treatment with intravenous pyridoxine (two doses, 1ØØ mg each) and consequently was admitted.

He had been born at term and his developmental milestones were normal. There was no family history of seizures or mental retardation. The diagnostic workup done on admission was negative and included serum pyruvate, serum amino acids, blood lead, copper, and mercury levels, Epstein Barr virus IgG, herpes simplex virus, polymerase chain reaction and encephalitis panel, leptospira, mycoplasma, and rabies titers. The CSF protein and glucose were normal.

Initial scalp EEG recording showed frequent centrotemporal EEG spikes. Continuous scalp EEG monitoring showed multiple electroclinical seizures beginning in the right central region and spreading to both hemispheres. MRI demonstrated abnormally thickened cortex in the high right parietal lobe. Patient was treated with pentobarbital infusion and the clinical manifestations disappeared.

Diagnosis: **Refractory focal seizures, status epilepticus.**

Diagnosis Code(s)

G4Ø.Ø11 Localization-related (focal) (partial) idiopathic epilepsy and epileptic syndromes with seizures of localized onset, intractable, with status epilepticus

Coding Note(s)

Refractory is listed as a synonym for intractable. ICD-1Ø-CM lists benign childhood epilepsy with centrotemporal EEG spikes under subcategory G4Ø.Ø.

Extrapyramidal Disease and Movement Disorders

There are two systems of neural pathways that affect movement – the pyramidal system which is the direct activation pathway and the extrapyramidal system which is the indirect activation pathway. The pyramidal system is responsible for voluntary movement of the head, neck, and limbs. The extrapyramidal system is a second motor pathway that is responsible for control of movements. The extrapyramidal system modifies neural impulses that originate in the cerebral cortex and is responsible for selective activation and suppression of movements, initiation of movements, rate and force of movements, and coordination. Damage to the extrapyramidal system results in movement disorders.

Code block G2Ø-G26 Extrapyramidal and Movement Disorders contains codes for reporting these conditions.

Many movement disorders present with similar extrapyramidal symptoms, such as akathisia, dyskinesias, and dystonias. These disorders often resemble Parkinson's disease, so it is important that the medical record documentation clearly describes extrapyramidal and movement disorders.

Specific and complete documentation is necessary to avoid confusion between disorders and ensure the most accurate code assignment. Tremors, for example, are commonly associated with Parkinson's disease, but essential tremor is the most common type of tremor and the two conditions differ. In addition, people with essential tremor sometimes develop other neurological signs and symptoms — such as an unsteady gait. Medical record documentation by the provider that clearly describes extrapyramidal and movement disorders is essential. Documentation should include characteristics of the specific disorder. The following list includes other types of extrapyramidal and movement disorders, such as tremor:

- Chorea
- Essential tremor
- Familial tremor
- Drug-induced movement disorder (identify drug)
  - Akathisia
  - Chorea
  - Tics
  - Tremor
  - Other
  - Unspecified

- Intention/Other tremor
- Myoclonus
  - Drug-induced myoclonus (identify drug)
  - Palatal myoclonus
- Other specified extrapyramidal and movement disorders
  - Benign shuddering attacks
  - Restless legs syndrome
  - Stiff-man syndrome
- Tics of organic origin
- Unspecified movement disorder

The table below shows of the range of codes in the categories for extrapyramidal diseases and movement disorders. Four coding examples follow the table.

ICD-10-CM Category	ICD-10-CM Code/Documentation	
G20 Parkinson's Disease		
G21 Secondary parkinsonism	G21.0	Malignant neurologic syndrome
	G21.11	Neuroleptic induced parkinsonism
	G21.19	Other drug induced secondary parkinsonism
	G21.2	Secondary parkinsonism due to other external agents
	G21.3	Postencephalitic parkinsonism
	G21.4	Vascular parkinsonism
	G21.8	Other secondary parkinsonism
	G21.9	Secondary parkinsonism, unspecified
G23 Other degenerative diseases of basal ganglia	G23.0	Hallervorden-Spatz disease
	G23.1	Progressive supranuclear ophthalmoplegia [Steele-Richardson-Olszewski]
	G23.2	Striatonigral degeneration
	G23.8	Other specified degenerative diseases of basal ganglia
	G23.9	Degenerative diseases of basal ganglia, unspecified
G24 Dystonia	G24.01	Drug-induced subacute dystonia
	G24.02	Drug induced acute dystonia
	G24.09	Other drug induced dystonia
	G24.1	Genetic torsion dystonia
	G24.2	Idiopathic nonfamilial dystonia
	G24.3	Spasmodic torticollis
	G24.4	Idiopathic orofacial dystonia
	G24.5	Blepharospasm
	G24.8	Other dystonia
	G24.9	Dystonia, unspecified
G25 Other extrapyramidal and movement disorders	G25.0	Essential tremor
	G25.1	Drug-induced tremor
	G25.2	Other specified forms of tremor
	G25.3	Myoclonus
	G25.4	Drug-induced chorea
	G25.5	Other chorea
	G25.61	Drug induced tics
	G25.69	Other tics of organic origin
	G25.70	Drug induced movement disorder, unspecified
	G25.71	Drug induced akathisia
	G25.79	Other drug induced movement disorders
	G25.81	Restless legs syndrome
	G25.82	Stiff-man syndrome
	G25.83	Benign shuddering attacks
	G25.89	Other specified extrapyramidal and movement disorders
	G25.9	Extrapyramidal and movement disorder unspecified
G26 Extrapyramidal and movement disorders in diseases classified elsewhere		

Example 1: Secondary Parkinsonism

Parkinson's disease is a common debilitating disease affecting one out of every 1ØØ people over the age of 6Ø. The symptoms of Parkinson's disease include tremors, rigidity, and akinesia. The term "parkinsonism" refers to any condition that involves the types of movement changes seen in Parkinson's disease. Coding of secondary parkinsonism requires a clear understanding of the difference between Parkinson's disease and secondary parkinsonism. Parkinson's disease, also referred to as idiopathic parkinsonism, primary Parkinson's disease or primary parkinsonism, is not due to or caused by another underlying condition or external agent such as a drug. In contrast, secondary parkinsonism is always caused by an underlying condition or external agent, such as chemical or environmental toxins, drugs, encephalitis, cerebrovascular disease, or another physiological condition.

In the medical record documentation, secondary parkinsonism must be clearly differentiated from primary Parkinson's disease and the documentation must indicate the underlying cause of secondary parkinsonism. Parkinson's disease and secondary parkinsonism may also be associated with mental disorders such as dementia, depression, delirium, or behavioral disturbance. To ensure assignment of the most specific code, the documentation must specify the cause of secondary parkinsonism and indicate when the condition is associated with dementia, depression, delirium, or a behavioral disturbance.

Parkinson's disease and secondary parkinsonism codes are found under Extrapyramidal and movement disorders, categories G2Ø-G21.

Coding and Documentation Requirements

Identify the cause of secondary parkinsonism:

- Drug-induced
  - Malignant neuroleptic syndrome
  - Neuroleptic induced parkinsonism
  - Other drug induced secondary parkinsonism
- Due to other external agents
- Postencephalitic
- Vascular
- Other specified cause
- Unspecified cause

For drug or external agent induced secondary parkinsonism, use an additional code to identify the substance.

ICD-10-CM Code/Documentation	
G21.0	Malignant neuroleptic syndrome
G21.11	Neuroleptic induced parkinsonism
G21.19	Other drug induced secondary Parkinsonism
G21.2	Secondary parkinsonism due to other external agents
G21.3	Postencephalitic parkinsonism
G21.4	Vascular parkinsonism
G21.8	Other secondary parkinsonism
G21.9	Secondary parkinsonism, unspecified

Documentation and Coding Example

Follow-up visit for evaluation of **parkinsonism due to adverse effect of metoclopramide**.

History and Physical: This otherwise healthy 55-year-old man was given **metoclopramide** to treat symptomatic gastroesophageal reflux. Six months later he developed severe parkinsonism exhibiting tremors, limited movements, rigidity, and postural instability. He was started on L-dopa because his primary care physician did not realize the parkinsonism was drug-induced, and the metoclopramide was continued. The patient was referred to me six months ago for evaluation of parkinsonism after one year of taking both drugs. At that time, it was recognized that **the parkinsonism was drug-induced**. The metoclopramide was stopped and the patient has been slowly withdrawn from the L-dopa over the past six-months. On exam today, the patient's parkinsonism has resolved completely.

Diagnosis: **Drug-induced secondary parkinsonism** has resolved completely

Plan: Patient is to return to the care of his primary care physician.

Diagnosis Code(s)

G21.19 Other drug induced secondary parkinsonism

T45.ØX5D Adverse effect of antiallergic and antiemetic drugs, subsequent encounter

Coding Note(s)

An additional code is used to identify the drug responsible for the adverse effect. Metoclopramide is not classified as a neuroleptic drug, so the code for other drug induced secondary parkinsonism is assigned. An additional code is assigned for the adverse effect. The drug responsible for the adverse effect is identified with a code from categories T36-T5Ø with fifth or sixth character of 5. Adverse effect codes in ICD-1Ø-CM include a seventh character to indicate the episode of care (e.g., initial encounter, subsequent encounter, or sequela). This is a follow-up encounter so 7th character D is assigned for subsequent encounter.

Example 2: Other Degenerative Diseases of Basal Ganglia

Included in the extrapyramidal and movement disorders category block are other degenerative diseases of the basal ganglia. Degenerative diseases are characterized by progressive neuron degeneration. The basal ganglia are nerve cells located within the brain involved in the initiation of voluntary movement. Damage to the basal ganglia causes muscle stiffness or spasticity and tremors. Because the deficits are primarily in motor function, the extrapyramidal system and basal ganglia have been associated with movement disorders.

Many different degenerative diseases affect the brain and produce similar symptoms, so specific documentation is necessary to avoid confusion between disorders. For example, progressive supranuclear palsy is sometimes mistaken for Parkinson's disease, because both conditions are associated with stiffness, frequent falls, slurred speech, difficulty swallowing, and decreased spontaneous movement. Provider documentation in the medical record must clearly distinguish degenerative diseases of the basal ganglia from other degenerative diseases of the brain that are characterized by motor, cognitive, and psychiatric manifestations. To ensure assignment of the most specific code for degenerative diseases of the basal ganglia, provider documentation should describe:

- Etiology
- Location (e.g., the brainstem, basal ganglia, cerebellum)
- Clinical features
- Course of the disease

Coding and Documentation Requirements

Identify the type of basal ganglia degenerative disease:

- Hallervorden-Spatz disease
- Progressive supranuclear ophthalmoplegia [Steele-Richardson-Olszewski]
- Striatonigral degeneration
- Other specified basal ganglia degenerative disease, which includes:
  - Calcification of basal ganglia
- Unspecified basal ganglia degenerative disease

ICD-10-CM Code/Documentation	
G23.0	Hallervorden-Spatz disease
G23.1	Progressive supranuclear ophthalmoplegia [Steele-Richardson-Olszewski]
G23.2	Striatonigral degeneration
G23.8	Other specified degenerative diseases of basal ganglia
G23.9	Degenerative disease of basal ganglia, unspecified

Documentation and Coding Example

Follow-up Visit History: A 63-year-old male with a year-long history of headaches, dizziness, and progressive unsteadiness and stiffening of the left side of his body presented after experiencing several falls. There was no evidence of encephalitis or of previous ingestion of neuroleptic drugs, and no family history of Parkinson's. MRI scans of the brain ruled out stroke or hydrocephalus. On examination, there was akinesia and rigidity of all limbs, more pronounced on the left, and no tremor. Deep tendon reflexes were brisk, the plantar flexor sensation was intact. Command and pursuit eye movements were grossly impaired in all directions but Doll's eye movements were normal. Optokinetic nystagmus was markedly reduced in lateral gaze to either side and absent in the vertical plane, as was convergence, but the pupillary reactions were normal. There was no ptosis, nystagmus, oculomasticatory myorhythmia, or myoclonus. A diagnosis of **progressive supranuclear palsy** was considered based on the association of a supranuclear ophthalmoplegia and Parkinsonism, and the neuro-ophthalmic findings were consistent with a diagnosis of supranuclear ophthalmoplegia. He was started on trimethoprim 160 mg with sulphamethoxazole 800 mg twice daily and levodopa 100 mg with carbidopa 10 mg four times a day. There was rapid improvement in his eye movements with minimal residual restriction in upward gaze and gradual improvement in his other symptoms by day seven.

Diagnosis: **Progressive supranuclear ophthalmoplegia** responding well to current drug regimen.

Diagnosis Code(s)

G23.1 Progressive supranuclear ophthalmoplegia [Steele-Richardson-Olszewski]

Coding Note(s)

Progressive supranuclear ophthalmoplegia has a distinct code (G23.1).

Example 3: Tremor

There are three codes that describe specific types of tremors, G25.0 Essential tremor, G25.1 Drug-induced tremor, and G25.2 Other specified forms of tremor which includes intention tremor. It should be noted that a diagnosis of tremor that is not more specifically described in the documentation is reported with a symptom code, R25.1 Tremor unspecified. These codes are also found under the extrapyramidal and other movement disorders category.

Coding and Documentation Requirements

Identify the form of tremor:

- Drug-induced
- Essential/Familial
- Other specified form (includes intention tremor)

ICD-10-CM Code/Documentation	
G25.0	Essential tremor
G25.1	Drug-induced tremor
G25.2	Other specified forms of tremor

Documentation and Coding Example

Patient is a 64-year-old Caucasian female referred to Neurology by PMD for worsening tremor in her hands and head. PMH is significant for tremor that started in her hands at least twenty years ago and progressed slowly to arms and head/neck. Patient reports that most members of her family have the problem in varying degrees. She states that her symptoms have not interfered with ADLs or exercise. Her husband is a retired architect. She has not been employed outside the home in more than 40 years. The couple moved about 1 year ago from a relatively moist/cool coastal town to a warm/dry inland area to be closer to their children/grandchildren, and it was after the move that she noticed her tremor worsening. She states she spends 4-5 months of the year in England with family, and symptoms were less severe while she was there, but exacerbated upon her return home. This is a pleasant, impeccably groomed, thin but muscular woman who looks younger than her stated age. Her head nods continuously in yes/yes pattern, her voice quality is somewhat soft but she is easily understood, arm tremor is noted when she extends her right arm for a handshake, but not when her hands are resting in her lap. She states the tremor does seem to worsen when she is anxious or acutely ill. Her general health is good. She had laser surgery for acute glaucoma 10 years ago, uses Pilocarpine 2% eye gtts daily. Last eye exam was 6 weeks ago. She currently takes multivitamin and calcium supplements, but no other medications. On examination, WT 136 lbs., HT 67 inches, T 98.4, P 70, R 14, BP 130/78. PERRLA, eyes clear without redness or excessive tearing. TMs normal. Cranial nerves grossly intact. Upper extremities are negative for muscle atrophy, fasciculation, weakness, or tenderness. There is no drift, rigidity, or resistance. Reflexes are 2+, tone 4/5. Normal sensation to pin prick, temperature, and vibration. Lower extremities are the same with 3+ reflexes and 5/5 tone. Appendicular coordination normal, gait grossly normal. She has some stiffness in her left hip with a barely discernible limp which she states is residual injury from being struck by a car while walking across a street 13 years ago. Her tremor is limited to a gentle yes/yes nod of the head when upright and abates when she reclines and her head/neck is supported on a pillow. Her hand/arm tremor is characterized by a gentle, rhythmic shaking movement with all voluntary movement. It is quite pronounced when arms are extended out from the midline either forward or to the sides. She is able to hold a cup of water, bring it up to her mouth and drink using one hand but prefers to use both, especially with hot beverages to avoid spilling and possible burns. Pencil grip is normal and writing is legible but she performs the task slowly. She states she prefers to use a keyboard/computer. Using the small keyboard on her phone is laborious and she will voice activate most frequently called numbers and no longer does text messaging.

Impression: **Benign essential tremor** possibly exacerbated by move to warm climate. Discussed medication options including benefits and side effects and she agrees to a trial of propranolol. She is given samples of Inderal 40 mg to take BID and will return to clinic in 2 weeks for follow-up.

Diagnosis Code(s)

G25.0 Essential tremor

Coding Note(s)

There is a specific code for essential tremor, also referred to as benign essential tremor or familial tremor. Essential tremor is classified with other extrapyramidal and movement disorders in category G25.

Example 4: Restless Leg Syndrome (RLS)

Restless leg syndrome (RLS) is characterized by an irresistible need to move the legs due to uncomfortable sensations in them, such as creeping, crawling, tingling, or bubbling. However, movement does relieve the discomfort. Restless leg syndrome usually manifests at night or when sitting for long periods of time. The sensations are most often felt in the lower leg between the knee and ankle but can also be located in the upper leg or arms. RLS occurs most often in middle age or older adults and stress can exacerbate the condition.

Coding and Documentation Requirements

None.

ICD-10-CM Code/Documentation	
G25.81	Restless leg syndrome

Documentation and Coding Example

A 45-year-old woman presents to the office complaining of insomnia. She states she has had trouble falling asleep for many years, but the problem is worsening. In bed she feels an unbearable discomfort in the legs. She has also noticed this urge on long car rides. The problem is worse at night. She initially described the leg sensations as a "tingling" in her bones radiating from the ankles to the thighs, accompanied by the irresistible need to move her legs. Her symptoms improve when she gets up and walks around. The tingling sensation is now more like electrical shocks accompanied with involuntary, symmetrical limb jerks with restlessness occurring earlier (at 7 pm) and chronic insomnia.

Assessment/Plan: **Restless legs syndrome**. Start with small doses of pramipexole twice daily - Ø.Ø9 mg. at 6 pm and Ø.18 mg at 1Ø pm.

Diagnosis Code(s)

G25.81 Restless legs syndrome

Coding Note(s)

There is a distinct code to report restless legs syndrome. The syndrome includes the characteristic symptoms which are not separately reported. There is no laterality requirement for this code.

Hemiplegia and Hemiparesis

The terms hemiplegia and hemiparesis are often used interchangeably, but the two conditions are not the same. Hemiplegia is paralysis of one side of the body while hemiparesis is weakness on one side of the body. Hemiparesis is less severe than hemiplegia and both are a common side effect of stroke or cerebrovascular accident. Hemiplegia and hemiparesis must be clearly differentiated in the medical record documentation. Disability in these cases is determined by the underlying diagnosis, whether the paralysis is temporary or permanent, the extent of paralysis (monoplegia, hemiplegia, paraplegia, quadriplegia), and the body parts affected.

Hemiplegia and hemiparesis are frequently sequelae of cerebrovascular disease; however, cervical spinal cord diseases, peripheral nervous system diseases, and other conditions may manifest as hemiplegia. Precise, detailed provider documentation in the medical record is key to correct code assignment.

These conditions are reported with codes in category G81. There is a note indicating that codes in these categories are used only when hemiplegia or hemiparesis is documented without further specification, or is documented as old or longstanding of unspecified cause. The hemiplegia and hemiparesis codes may also be used in multiple coding scenarios to identify the specified types of hemiplegia resulting from any cause.

In hemiplegia and hemiparesis cases, the documentation needs to identify whether the dominant or nondominant side is affected. If the affected side is documented but not specified as dominant or nondominant, Code selection for a specified side without documentation of which side is dominant is reported as follows:

- If the left side is affected, the default is non-dominant
- If the right side is affected, the default is dominant
- In ambidextrous patients, the default is dominant

It should be noted that hemiplegia documented as congenital or infantile, or due to sequela of a cerebrovascular accident or disease is not reported with codes from these categories. Congenital hemiplegia is used to describe hemiplegia demonstrated at birth while infantile hemiplegia refers to hemiplegia that develops in infancy or within the first few years of life. Congenital or infantile hemiplegia is reported with a code from category G8Ø. Hemiplegia and hemiparesis due to sequelae of cerebrovascular disease is reported with codes from subcategories I69.Ø5, I69.15, I69.25, I69.35, I69.85, and I69.95.

To assign the most specific code for hemiplegia or hemiparesis, the correct category must first be identified. Documentation should be reviewed for the following descriptors:

- Congenital or infantile
- Due to late effect of cerebrovascular accident
- Not otherwise specified

For hemiplegia or hemiparesis of long-standing duration, or not specified as to cause, or to report hemiplegia or hemiparesis in a multiple coding scenario, the type of hemiplegia or hemiparesis must be identified along with the side which should be specified as dominant or nondominant.

Coding and Documentation Requirements

Identify the type of hemiplegia or hemiparesis:

- Flaccid
- Spastic
- Unspecified

Identify the side affected:

- Right
  - Dominant side
  - Nondominant side
- Left
  - Dominant side
  - Nondominant side
- Unspecified side

ICD-10-CM Code/Documentation	
G81.00	Flaccid hemiplegia affecting unspecified side
G81.01	Flaccid hemiplegia affecting right dominant side
G81.02	Flaccid hemiplegia affecting left dominant side
G81.03	Flaccid hemiplegia affecting right nondominant side
G81.04	Flaccid hemiplegia affecting left nondominant side
G81.10	Spastic hemiplegia affecting unspecified side
G81.11	Spastic hemiplegia affecting right dominant side
G81.12	Spastic hemiplegia affecting left dominant side
G81.13	Spastic hemiplegia affecting right nondominant side
G81.14	Spastic hemiplegia affecting left nondominant side
G81.90	Hemiplegia, unspecified affecting unspecified side
G81.91	Hemiplegia, unspecified affecting right dominant side
G81.92	Hemiplegia, unspecified affecting left dominant side
G81.93	Hemiplegia, unspecified affecting right nondominant side
G81.94	Hemiplegia, unspecified affecting left nondominant side

Documentation and Coding Example

Patient is a 78-year-old, **right-handed female with longstanding flaccid hemiplegia of unspecified cause affecting her left side.** On admission to the SNF, the patient is experiencing a largely flaccid hemiplegia with Chedoke McMaster Staging scores on the left side of 1/7 in the hand and arm, 1/7 in the leg and 1/7 in the foot, and 1/7 for posture. There were no sensory problems noted. The patient uses a manual wheelchair with a lap tray for mobility. She was able to complete a 2-person pivot transfer despite problems with her balance. She requires set-up assistance with her meals and one person to assist her with dressing, grooming, and bathing. Due to her poor recovery prognosis, the plan of care will focus on minimizing contractures and palliation of pain. Ensure the flaccid arm is continuously supported when the patient is sitting or transferring—use lap tray or arm sling. Very gentle range of motion exercises with physiotherapy.

Diagnosis: **Left-sided flaccid hemiplegia**

Diagnosis Code(s)

G81.04 Flaccid hemiplegia affecting left nondominant side

Coding Note(s)

This case is coded as flaccid hemiplegia of the nondominant side because the documentation describes the patient as right-handed, so the right side is the dominant side.

Migraine

Migraine is a common neurological disorder that often manifests as a headache. Usually unilateral and pulsating in nature, the headache results from abnormal brain activity along nerve pathways and brain chemical (neurotransmitter) changes. These affect blood flow in the brain and surrounding tissue and may trigger an "aura" or warning sign (visual, sensory, language, motor) before the onset of pain. Migraine headache is frequently accompanied by autonomic nervous system symptoms (nausea, vomiting, and sensitivity to light and/or sound). Triggers can include caffeine withdrawal, stress, lack of sleep. The various types of migraines are reported with codes in category G43. All migraines must be documented as intractable or not intractable. Terms that describe intractable migraine include: pharmacoresistant or pharmacologically resistant, treatment resistant, refractory, and poorly controlled. All migraines except cyclical vomiting (G43.A-), ophthalmoplegic (G43.B-), periodic headache syndromes child/adult (G43.C-) and abdominal migraines (G43.D-) must be documented as with status or without status migrainosus. Status migrainosus refers to a migraine that has lasted more than 72 hours.

Coding and Documentation Requirements

Identify migraine type:

- Abdominal
- Chronic without aura
- Cyclical vomiting
- Hemiplegic
- Menstrual
- Ophthalmoplegic
- Periodic headache syndromes child/adult
- Persistent aura
  - With cerebral infarction
  - Without cerebral infarction
- With aura
- Without aura
- Other migraine
- Unspecified

Identify presence/absence of intractability:

- Intractable
- Not intractable

Identify presence/absence of status migrainosus:

- With status migrainosus
- Without status migrainosus

Note – Status migrainosus is not required for migraines documented as abdominal, cyclical vomiting, ophthalmoplegic, or periodic head syndromes in child/adult.

Chronic Migraine without Aura

ICD-10-CM Code/Documentation	
G43.709	Chronic migraine without aura, not intractable, without status migrainosus
G43.719	Chronic migraine without aura, intractable, without status migrainosus
G43.701	Chronic migraine without aura, not intractable, with status migrainosus
G43.711	Chronic migraine without aura, intractable, with status migrainosus

Documentation and Coding Example

Presenting Complaint: Thirty-two-year-old Caucasian female is referred to Pain Management Clinic by her PMD for evaluation and treatment of **chronic migraine headache**.

History: PMH is significant for onset of migraines at age 13-14, typically associated with menstruation for 4-5 years and then becoming more frequent and unpredictable. Patient states her headaches are significantly worse in winter and summer since moving to the NE from Hawaii five years ago. She was initially treated with rizatriptan and ibuprofen for periodic pain management and when headaches became more frequent she was started on daily propranolol. She experienced symptomatic hypotension on propanolol and was switched to amitriptyline which worked well for a few years with headache days numbering 4-5 per month. Gradually her headache days increased and she was switched to topiramate daily, with dose now at 50 mg BID and Treximet taken as needed on acute pain days. She reports **15-20 pain days per month** on these medications for the past 6 months. Headaches are negative for aura, usually bilateral in the supraorbital and/or temporal area with a pulsating quality. She typically experiences photophobia and nausea without vomiting. Patient is married with a 2-year-old son and works part time as a middle school guidance counselor.

Physical Examination: Temperature 97.9 HR 74 RR 14 BP 102/60 WT 122.5 lbs. On examination, this is a pleasant, well-nourished but tired appearing young woman who looks her stated age. At this time, she is experiencing a pulsating headache of moderate intensity, location bilateral with focal area temporal on the right and temporal-supraorbital on the left. She awoke with pain this morning and it has been ongoing for the past 3 days. She denies photophobia or nausea. She has taken topiramate as prescribed but has not taken Treximet in over a week because she ran out. Cranial nerves grossly intact. Both upper and lower extremities have normal strength, movement, and sensation. PERRLA, eyes negative for conjunctival injection and excess tearing. There is no evidence of ptosis or eyelid edema. No lymphadenopathy present. Oral mucosa normal, throat benign. Nares patent without rhinorrhea or congestion. HR regular without bruits, rubs, or murmur. Breath sounds clear, equal bilaterally. Abdomen soft and non-distended, bowel sounds present all quadrants. Liver is palpated at RCM, spleen is not palpated.

Impression: **Intractable chronic migraine headache syndrome not responsive to drug therapy**. Patient is a good candidate for OnabotulinumtoxinA (Botox) therapy. The procedure was explained to patient, questions answered and informed consent obtained.

Procedure Note: Skin over treatment area prepped with alcohol. Vacuum dried powdered Botox 200 units was reconstituted with 4 ml preservative free 0.9% sodium chloride per manufacturers specification. Using a 30 gauge 0.5 inch needle, a total of 155 units (0.1 ml=5 units) of Botox was injected at 31 points including corrugator muscle (10 units/2 sites), procerus muscle (5 units/1 site), frontalis muscle (20 units/4 sites), temporalis muscle (40 units/8 sites), occipitalis muscle (30 units/6 sites), cervical paraspinal muscle group (20 units/4 sites), and trapezius muscle (30 units/6 sites). Patient tolerated the procedure well. She has some mild ptosis noted in left eyelid but it does not obstruct vision.

Plan: Patient is advised to continue current medications as prescribed and that she may experience headache, tenderness at injection site, and mild muscle weakness in the next few days. She should call if she develops any other symptoms or problems. Return to clinic in 5 days for recheck.

Diagnosis Code(s)

G43.719 Chronic migraine without aura, intractable, without status migrainosus

Coding Note(s)

Use of the code for intractable migraine requires documentation that the migraine has not responded to treatment. In this case the patient has been referred to pain medicine because of intractable migraine and that is the stated diagnosis of the pain medicine specialist. The physician has also documented a diagnosis of chronic migraine. Chronic migraine is typically defined as 15 or more headache days per month. The documentation indicates that the patient experiences 15-20 headache days per month which further supports the diagnosis of chronic migraine. Status migrainosus refers to a migraine that has lasted for more than 72 hours. There is no documentation to support status migrainosus so the code for without status migrainosus is assigned.

Migraine Variant

Migraine variant refers to a migraine that manifests in a form other than head pain. Migraine variants may be characterized by episodes of atypical sensory, motor, or visual aura, confusion, dysarthria, focal neurologic deficits, and other constitutional symptoms, with or without a headache. The provider documentation in the medical record must include enough detail to differentiate migraine variants from other migraines and other headache disorders.

The diagnosis of migraine variant is determined by the provider's documentation. Typically, there is a history of paroxysmal signs and symptoms with or without cephalgia and without other disorders that may contribute to the symptoms. Many patients have a family history of migraine.

In the medical record documentation, migraine variants must be clearly differentiated from other headache disorders such as trigeminal autonomic cephalgias (cluster headaches), stabbing headache, thunderclap headaches, hypnic headaches and hemicrania continua, and headache syndromes associated with physical activity (e.g., exertional headaches). Chronic migraine and status migrainosus are not considered migraine variants.

Coding and Documentation Requirements

Identify migraine variant:

- Abdominal migraine
- Cyclical vomiting
- Ophthalmoplegic migraine
- Periodic headache syndromes in child/adult
- Other migraine

Identify response to treatment:

- Intractable
- Not intractable

For migraine variants classified under other migraine, identify any status migrainosus:

- With status migrainosus
- Without status migrainosus

ICD-10-CM Code/Documentation	
G43.A0	Cyclical vomiting, not intractable
G43.A1	Cyclical vomiting, intractable
G43.B0	Ophthalmoplegic migraine, not intractable
G43.B1	Ophthalmoplegic migraine, intractable
G43.C0	Periodic headache syndromes in child or adult, not intractable
G43.C1	Periodic headache syndromes in child or adult, intractable
G43.D0	Abdominal migraine, not intractable
G43.D1	Abdominal migraine, intractable
G43.801	Other migraine, not intractable, with status migrainosus
G43.809	Other migraine, not intractable, without status migrainosus
G43.811	Other migraine, intractable, with status migrainosus
G43.819	Other migraine, intractable, without status migrainosus

Documentation and Coding Example

A 7-year-old girl presented with complete right oculomotor palsy. She complained the previous day of a headache in the orbital region, severe and throbbing in nature. She was given children's Tylenol and went to bed early. She awakened the following morning with complete ptosis of the right upper lid, periorbital pain, and blurred vision. On examination, the right pupil was 6 mm and slightly reactive to light. The neurologic examination and skull x-rays were normal; diagnostic workup including the glucose tolerance test was all negative. MRI and magnetic resonance angiography ruled out aneurysm, tumor, and sphenoid sinus mucocele. Intermittent angle-closure glaucoma with mydriasis was also excluded on gonioscopy. She experienced near complete resolution of her symptoms following treatment with NSAIDs.

Diagnosis: **Ophthalmoplegic migraine**

Diagnosis Code(s)

G43.BØ Ophthalmoplegic migraine, not intractable

Coding Note(s)

Ophthalmoplegic migraine is specified as intractable (with refractory migraine) or not intractable (without refractory migraine). The documentation does not mention intractable migraine or refractory migraine. An intractable or refractory migraine is any migraine that is impossible to manage or resistant to usual therapies.

Other Headache Syndromes

A complaint of headache is a common reason for seeking medical care. Headaches have many causes and while most headaches are benign, a headache may also be a symptom of another underlying disease such as cerebral hemorrhage. A diagnosis of headache that is not further qualified as a specific type, such as tension or migraine, is reported with a symptom code. Other headache syndromes is a broad category that includes many specific headache types with the exception of migraine which has its own category. Below are characteristics of the various types of headaches classified under other headache syndromes.

Cluster headache – Headache characterized by a cyclical pattern of intense, usually unilateral pain with a rapid onset. They are vascular in origin, caused by the sudden dilatation of one or more blood vessels around the trigeminal nerve. The pain often centers behind or around the eye (retro-orbital, orbital, supraorbital) or in the temporal area and has a boring/drilling quality. The pain may be accompanied by one (or more) cranial autonomic nervous system symptoms. Cluster headaches are benign, but can be quite disabling. Individuals may have a genetic predisposition for this type of headache Disorders of the hypothalamus, smoking, and traumatic brain injury may also be causative factors. Cluster headaches are subclassified as episodic or chronic. Episodic cluster headaches typically occur at least once per day, often at the same time of day for several weeks. The headaches are followed by weeks, months, or years that are completely pain free. Chronic cluster headaches may have "high" or "low" cycles in the frequency or intensity of pain but no real remission.

Drug induced headache (medication overuse headache, analgesic rebound headache) – A serious and disabling condition that can occur when medication is taken daily for tension, migraine, or other acute or chronic headache or other pain. As the medication wears off, the pain returns and more medication is needed. This creates a cycle of pain, medicating to relieve the pain, and more intense pain. The condition is more common in women, typically between the ages of 3Ø-4Ø, but it can occur at any age. Pain is often described as a constant dull ache that is worse in the morning and after exercise. Medications associated with this rebound headache phenomena include: acetaminophen, ibuprofen, naproxen, aspirin, codeine, hydrocodone, tramadol, and ergotamine. Triptans (sumatriptan) used for vascular headaches can also induce these headaches. To stop the pain cycle, medication must be discontinued, preferably abruptly and entirely, but slow withdrawal may be necessary in certain situations. This often results in withdrawal symptoms including headache, anxiety, insomnia, and gastrointestinal upset (nausea, vomiting). Withdrawal symptoms can last as long as 12 weeks but typically subside in 7-1Ø days. Non-steroidal anti-inflammatory drugs (ibuprofen, naproxen) may be given to help relieve rebound headache phenomena when these drugs have not been used previously by the patient to treat the primary headache.

Hemicrania continua – A chronic, persistent, primary headache that often varies in severity as it cycles over a 24 period. It is most often unilateral in location and does not change sides. The incidence is somewhat higher in women with age of onset in early adulthood. There can be migrainous qualities including: pulsating/throbbing pain, nausea and vomiting, photophobia (light sensitivity), and phonophobia (noise sensitivity) along with autonomic nervous system symptoms. The most striking definitive characteristic of hemicrania continua is that it responds almost immediately to treatment with the drug indomethacin.

New daily persistent headache (NDPH) – A distinct, primary headache syndrome with symptoms that can mimic chronic migraine and tension-type headaches. The onset of NDPH is typically abrupt and reaches peak intensity within 3 days. Most individuals can recall the exact day/time of onset of the headache. In some instances, the pain will follow an infection or flu-like illness, surgery, or stressful life event. Autoimmune and/or inflammatory conditions and hypermobility of the cervical spine may also be contributing factors. The pain can be self-limiting (pain ends after a few months) or unrelenting (pain lasts for years) and is often unresponsive to standard therapy.

Paroxysmal hemicranias – Rare type of headache, more common in women, that usually begins during adulthood. The pain is similar to cluster headaches, but is distinguished by greater frequency and shorter duration of the individual episodes, presence of one or more cranial autonomic nervous system symptoms, and a favorable response to the drug indomethacin. Pain is unilateral (always on the same side) and severe, with a throbbing/boring quality behind or around the eye (retro-orbital, orbital, supraorbital) and/or in the temporal area. There can be localized dull pain or soreness in these areas between episodes of acute pain. Occasionally pain may radiate to the ipsilateral (same side) shoulder, arm, or neck. One or more cranial autonomic nervous system symptoms usually accompanies the pain, such as lacrimation (eye tearing), conjunctival injection (eye redness), nasal congestion, rhinorrhea (runny nose), miosis (constricted pupil), ptosis (eyelid drooping), or eyelid edema (swelling). Cause is not known and there is no familial tendency. Paroxysmal hemicranias are subclassified as episodic or chronic. Episodic paroxysmal hemicranias are less severe and less frequent. In some individuals, this non-chronic phase will be a "pass though" to chronic paroxysmal hemicranias. Chronic paroxysmal hemicranias, also referred to as Sjaastad syndrome, is more common than episodic paroxysmal hemicranias and is characterized by more severe and more frequent episodes.

P**ost-traumatic headache** – Headache that occurs following a closed head injury or trauma to the neck area. It is a fairly common and self-limiting condition and may have characteristics of both tension and migrainous pain. The headache rarely occurs in isolation and accompanying symptoms can include: cervical (neck) pain, cognitive, behavioral, and/or somatic problems. Individuals with chronic pain disorders (other than headache), pre-existing headaches, and affective disorders are at greater risk for developing both acute and chronic post traumatic headache. The cycle of pain can be difficult to interrupt once it has been established and overuse of analgesics frequently results in rebound phenomena. This can lead to co-morbid psychiatric disorders, post-traumatic stress disorder, insomnia, substance abuse, and depression. Acute post-traumatic headache (APTH) can begin immediately or anytime in the 2 months following injury. Acute post-traumatic headache becomes chronic post-traumatic headache when the pain continues for longer than 2 months following injury.

Primary thunderclap headache – Relatively uncommon type of headache characterized by a dramatic, sudden, severe onset of pain anywhere in the head or neck area that peaks within 6Ø seconds and begins to fade in 1 hour. Residual pain/discomfort may be present for up to 1Ø days. The sympathetic nervous system is believed to be involved and nausea and vomiting may occur with the pain; however, the headache usually cannot be attributed to any specific disorder. Thunderclap headache may signal a potentially life threatening condition including: subarachnoid hemorrhage, cerebral venous sinus thrombosis, and cervical artery (carotid, vertebral artery) dissection.

Short-lasting unilateral neuralgiform headache with conjunctival injection and tearing (SUNCT) – A rare type of primary headache belonging to a group referred to as trigeminal autonomic cephalalgia (TAC). This headache is triggered by the cranial autonomic nervous system at the trigeminal (5th cranial) nerve. Pain is usually described as moderate to severe with a burning, piercing, or stabbing quality. It is unilateral, centered in or around the eye (retro-orbital, orbital, supraorbital) and/or the temporal area. It is characterized by bursts of pain, lasting from a few seconds to 5-6 minutes and can occur up to 2ØØ times per day (most commonly 5-6 times per hour). Cranial autonomic nervous system symptoms that accompany the pain include eye tearing (lacrimation) and conjunctival injection (eye redness). Nasal congestion, runny nose (rhinorrhea), constricted pupil (miosis), eyelid drooping (ptosis), or swelling (edema) may also occur. Men are affected more often than women with onset most commonly occurring after age 5Ø. Pain may radiate to the teeth, neck, and around the ears. It is more common during daytime hours and can occur at regular or irregular intervals without a distinct refractory period.

Tension-type headache (muscle contraction headache, stress headache) – Characterized by pain that encircles the head without a throbbing or pulsating quality. Nausea/vomiting, disruption in normal activities, photophobia (light sensitivity) and phonophobia (sound sensitivity) are not normally associated with the condition. Onset is typically gradual, often in the middle of the day and pain can be exacerbated by fatigue, poor posture, emotions, and mental stress (including depression). This headache is more common in women and no familial tendency has been identified. Tension or stress headaches are the most common type of headaches among adults. The terms tension headache and tension-type headache are considered synonymous. Tension-type headache is subclassified as episodic or chronic. Episodic and chronic tension-type headaches are differentiated from each other by the frequency with which the headache occurs with episodic being defined as greater than 1Ø but less than 15 headache days per month and chronic being defined as more than 15 days per month. Episodic tension headaches occur randomly and are often the result of temporary stress, anxiety, or fatigue.

Vascular headache – A broad or generalized term that includes cluster headache, migraine headache, and toxic (fever, chemical) headache. For coding purposes, headaches described as vascular but without more specific information as to type are reported with the code for vascular headache not elsewhere classified. Vascular headaches all involve changes in blood flow or in the vascular (blood vessel) system of the brain which trigger head pain and other neurological symptoms. These symptoms can include nausea and vomiting, vertigo (dizziness), photophobia (light sensitivity), phonophobia (noise sensitivity), visual disturbances, numbness and tingling (in any area of the body), problems with speech, and muscle weakness.

Other headache syndromes are reported with codes from category G44 and include: cluster headaches, vascular headache not elsewhere classified, tension-type headaches, post-traumatic headaches, drug-induced headaches as well as others. Response to treatment is a component of many codes in category G44. Cluster headache, paroxysmal hemicranias, short lasting unilateral neuralgiform headache with conjunctival injection and tearing (SUNCT), other trigeminal autonomic cephalgias (TAC), tension-type headache, post-traumatic headache, and drug-induced headache must be specified as intractable or not intractable. Intractable refers to headache syndromes that are not responding to treatment. Terms that describe intractable migraine include: pharmacoresistant or pharmacologically resistant, treatment resistant, refractory, and poorly controlled. Not intractable describes a headache that is responsive to and well controlled with treatment. In addition, vascular headache not elsewhere classified is also classified in the nervous system chapter with other headache syndromes and is reported with code G44.1.

Differentiation between the various types of headache can be difficult and patients often experience overlapping types of headache, so clearly documenting the type or types of headache the patient is experiencing is crucial to accurate diagnosis and appropriate treatment. This documentation is also needed for coding headache disorders.

Coding and Documentation Requirements

Identify the specific headache syndrome:

- Cluster headache syndrome
  - Chronic
  - Episodic
  - Unspecified
- Complicated headache syndromes
  - Hemicrania continua
  - New daily persistent headache (NDPH)
  - Primary thunderclap headache
  - Other complicated headache syndrome
- Drug induced headache, not elsewhere classified
- Other headache syndromes
  - Headache associated with sexual activity
  - Hypnic headache
  - Primary cough headache
  - Primary exertional headache
  - Primary stabbing headache
  - Other specified headache syndrome
- Other trigeminal autonomic cephalgias (TAC)
- Paroxysmal hemicranias
  - Chronic
  - Episodic
- Post-traumatic headache
  - Acute
  - Chronic
  - Unspecified
- Short lasting unilateral neuralgiform headache with conjunctival injection and tearing (SUNCT)
- Tension type headache
  - Chronic
  - Episodic
  - Unspecified
- Vascular headache, not elsewhere classified

Identify response to treatment for the following types: cluster, paroxysmal hemicranias, SUNCT, other TAC, tension-type, post-traumatic, and drug-induced:

- Intractable
- Not intractable

Cluster Headache Syndrome

ICD-10-CM Code/Documentation	
G44.001	Cluster headache syndrome, unspecified, intractable
G44.009	Cluster headache syndrome, unspecified, not intractable
G44.011	Episodic cluster headache, intractable
G44.019	Episodic cluster headache, not intractable
G44.021	Chronic cluster headache, intractable
G44.029	Chronic cluster headache, not intractable

Documentation and Coding Example 1

Thirty-seven-year-old Black male is referred to Pain Management Clinic by PCP for treatment of headaches. Patient is an attorney, working in a private, four-person firm focused on family law. He is in a committed relationship with his partner of 6 years and they are expecting a baby girl with a surrogate in 2 months. PMH is significant for being struck in the left temple/eye area by a baseball ten months ago during a recreational game with friends. He had no loss of consciousness or visual changes, but significant pain and swelling of the face and eye. He was evaluated in the ED, where ophthalmology exam, x-rays, and a CT scan showed no eye damage, facial/skull fracture, or intracranial bleeding. The first headache occurred 2 months after this injury and woke him from sleep with intense stabbing pain in the left eye, accompanied by tearing and eye redness. The pain subsided in about 15 minutes only to reoccur twice in the next few hours. He was seen emergently by his ophthalmologist and the exam was entirely benign. The headaches continued, usually awakening him from sleep with a stabbing sensation in his left eye that lasted 30-60 minutes. When the acute pain abated he often had residual aching in the periorbital area and stabbing pain again within a few hours. His PCP advised taking ibuprofen which was not helpful, prescribed Toradol which was also not helpful and finally Percodan which patient states caused nausea and hallucinations. Patient has researched alternative treatment options and has tried acupuncture, melatonin, and removing foods containing tyramine and MSG from his diet. He estimates headache days were 1-3 per week at the beginning, gradually decreasing until he had a 6 week period that was pain free. The headaches began again one week ago and patient requested a referral to pain specialist. On examination this is a soft spoken, slightly built young black male who looks his stated age. HT 69 inches, WT 150 lbs. T 96.8, P 58, R 14, BP 138/88. PERRLA, left eye has increased lacrimation, conjunctival injection and mild ptosis of the upper lid. Both nares are patent and the left naris has thin, clear mucus drainage. Oral mucosa moist and pink. Neck supple, without masses. Cranial nerves grossly intact. Upper extremities have brisk reflexes and good tone. Muscles are without atrophy, weakness, rigidity or tenderness. Heart rate regular, without bruit, murmur or rub. Breath sounds clear and equal bilaterally. Abdomen soft and non-tender with active bowel sounds in all quadrants. No evidence of hernia, normal male genitalia. Lower extremities have normal reflexes and good tone, no muscle atrophy, weakness, rigidity, or tenderness appreciated. Gait is normal. EKG is obtained and shows NSR. Impression: **Episodic cluster headache, poorly controlled with current medications**. Consider a trial of verapamil for headache prophylaxis and sumatriptan nasal spray for acute headache.

Patient is commended for his diligence in seeking alternative treatment options and is assured that the pain management team will listen and work closely with him to ensure that his headaches are managed in a way that allows him to fully participate in and enjoy life. Treatment options discussed and patient agrees to try verapamil 40 mg PO BID for 2 weeks and RTC for re-evaluation. He declines sumatriptan nasal spray at this time. He is, however, interested in oxygen therapy and we will discuss that at his next visit.

Diagnosis Code(s)

G44.011 Episodic cluster headache, intractable

Coding Note(s)

Codes require identification of the headache syndrome as intractable or not intractable. These terms describe the response to treatment. Intractable indicates that the episodic cluster headache is not responding to current treatment. This is documented using the term 'poorly controlled' which, according to coding notes, is a term that is considered the equivalent of intractable.

Tension-Type Headaches

ICD-10-CM Code/Documentation	
G44.201	Tension-type headache, unspecified, intractable
G44.209	Tension-type headache, unspecified, not intractable
G44.211	Episodic tension-type headache, intractable
G44.219	Episodic tension-type headache, not intractable
G44.221	Chronic tension-type headache, intractable
G44.229	Chronic tension-type headache, not intractable

Documentation and Coding Example 2

HPI: This 36-year-old female complains of **headaches several times per week for several months, usually at the end of the day**. The headaches are reportedly worse after increased time at the computer. The pain starts at the base of the neck and moves up to her forehead. The patient has tried regulating eating and sleeping, drinking more water and decreasing caffeine intake, without relief. OTC headache medications have provided "little to no" relief. The only thing that helps is to lie down and close her eyes.

On examination, her neck muscles are very tight and tender. There are multiple trigger points in the sub-occipital muscles and in the sternocleidomastoid on the right. Pressure on the sub-occipital trigger points reproduces the headache. Range of motion is decreased in neck flexion and right rotation. Other testing for nerve, muscle, and joint involvement was negative and the temporomandibular joint (TMJ) is not contributory.

Assessment/Plan: **Classic tension headache**. Poor posture and fatigue causes excess tension in the posterior neck muscles, especially the sub-occipital muscle group. Treatment to include massage therapy to release the muscle tension and patient education on proper posture and ergonomics.

Diagnosis Code(s)

G44.209 Tension-type headache, unspecified, not intractable

Coding Note(s)

Under the main term Headache, the Alphabetical Index lists tension (-type) as a subterm. Tension headache NOS is listed as an inclusion term in the Tabular for tension-type headache. All types of tension headache are classified in Chapter 6 Diseases of the Nervous System, under other headache syndromes, in the subcategory G44.2. This subcategory includes: tension headache, tension-type headache, episodic tension-type headache, and chronic tension-type headache. Psychological factors affecting physical conditions (F54) has an Excludes2 note listing tension-type headache (G44.2). Headache frequency and the type and severity of symptoms should be described in the clinical documentation. Detailed documentation of the etiology and any associated mental or organic illness also is necessary. Documentation of tension headache should also describe the response to treatment.

Monoplegia of Lower/Upper Limb

Monoplegia is also known as paralysis of one limb or monoplegia disorder. Sensory loss is typically more prominent in the distal segments of the limbs. It is important that the provider clearly document the etiology or underlying cause as there are many possible causes and the underlying cause can affect code assignment. Examples of causes include:

- Cerebral palsy
- Stroke

- Brain tumor
- Multiple sclerosis
- Motor neuron disease
- Nerve trauma, impingement, or inflammation
- Mononeuritis multiplex

Like hemiplegia and hemiparesis, monoplegia of a limb is frequently due to sequela of cerebrovascular disease, cervical spinal cord diseases, or peripheral nervous system diseases. The specific type of monoplegia should be clearly described in the provider documentation. For example, congenital monoplegia (demonstrated at birth) and infantile monoplegia (develops within the first few years of life) are classified to other categories, as is monoplegia due to late effect (sequela) of cerebrovascular disease/accident. Clear, complete provider documentation in the medical record of the type and cause of the monoplegia is essential for correct code assignment.

Monoplegia is classified in the category for other paralytic syndromes. Monoplegia is also classified by whether the upper (G83.2) or limb lower (G83.1) is affected; the side of the body affected; and whether the side affected is dominant or nondominant.

There is a note indicating that codes in these categories are used only when the paralytic syndrome, in this case monoplegia, is documented without further specification, or is documented as old or longstanding of unspecified cause. The monoplegia codes may also be used in multiple coding scenarios to identify the specified types of monoplegia resulting from any cause.

For monoplegia cases, the documentation needs to identify whether the dominant or nondominant side is affected. If the affected side is documented but not specified as dominant or nondominant, Code selection for a specified side without documentation of which side is dominant is reported the same as hemiplegia:

- If the left side is affected, the default is non-dominant
- If the right side is affected, the default is dominant
- In ambidextrous patients, the default is dominant

Coding and Documentation Requirements

Identify the affected limb:

- Lower
- Upper
- Unspecified

Identify the side affected:

- Right
  - Dominant side
  - Nondominant side
- Left
  - Dominant side
  - Nondominant side
- Unspecified side

Monoplegia of Lower Limb

ICD-10-CM Code/Documentation	
G83.10	Monoplegia of lower limb affecting unspecified side
G83.11	Monoplegia of lower limb affecting right dominant side
G83.12	Monoplegia of lower limb affecting left dominant side
G83.13	Monoplegia of lower limb affecting right nondominant side
G83.14	Monoplegia of lower limb affecting left nondominant side

Documentation and Coding Example 1

A 46-year-old male patient presented with complaints of neck pain, numbing sensation, and right leg weakness. The physical examination showed monoplegia of right leg, with intact sensory function. The other extremities had no neurologic deficits. MR imaging showed spinal cord compression and high signal intensity of spinal cord at C6-7. Therefore, the cause of monoplegia of the leg was thought to be the spinal cord ischemia.

Diagnosis: **Monoplegia, right leg, due to spinal cord ischemia.**

Diagnosis Code(s)

G95.11 Acute infarction of spinal cord (embolic) (nonembolic)

G83.11 Monoplegia of lower limb affecting right dominant side

Coding Note(s)

In this case, the affected side is documented but not specified as dominant or nondominant. ICD-10-CM code selection hierarchy states that if the right side is affected, the default is dominant. It should also be noted that this is a multiple coding scenario, requiring a code for the spinal cord ischemia, which is listed first, and a second code identifying the monoplegia.

Monoplegia of Upper Limb

ICD-10-CM Code/Documentation	
G83.20	Monoplegia of upper limb affecting unspecified side
G83.21	Monoplegia of upper limb affecting right dominant side
G83.22	Monoplegia of upper limb affecting left dominant side
G83.23	Monoplegia of upper limb affecting right nondominant side
G83.24	Monoplegia of upper limb affecting left nondominant side

Documentation and Coding Example 2

A 75-year-old female presented to the emergency department with sudden onset right upper limb weakness and altered sensation. The patient was previously well with an unremarkable medical history. On examination, she was apyrexial, normotensive and normoglycemic with a GCS of 15/15. Neurological examination revealed right upper limb hypotonia and power of Ø/5 in all hand and wrist muscle groups, 2/5 power in biceps and triceps, and 3/5 power in the shoulder girdle. Hypoesthesia was noted throughout the right upper limb. The remainder of the neurological examination did not reveal any other deficits. Baseline labs were normal. On brain MRI, mild ischemic change was noted throughout the cerebral white matter in the absence of infarcts within the basal ganglia, brainstem or cerebellum and cerebral venography was not suggestive of a recent thrombosis. Collectively the imaging studies were indicative of an acute parenchymal event with evidence of previous superficial bleeds. Following little improvement in right arm function after neurorehabilitation, the patient was discharged home.

Diagnosis: **Spontaneous right arm monoplegia secondary to probable cerebral amyloid angiopathy.**

Diagnosis Code(s)

G83.21 Monoplegia of upper limb affecting right dominant side

Coding Note(s)

Here again, the affected side is documented but not specified as dominant or nondominant. According to the code selection hierarchy in ICD-10-CM, the right side is affected so the default is dominant. ICD-10-CM Coding and Reporting Guidelines for Outpatient Services direct the user not to code diagnoses documented as "probable," "suspected," "questionable," "rule out," "working diagnosis," or other similar terms indicating uncertainty; therefore, no code is assigned for "probable cerebral amyloid angiopathy."

Section 1. Nervous System Summary

ICD-10-CM classifies diseases of the nervous system by the type of disease and by the cause of the disease or disorder, such as intraoperative and postprocedural complications or drug-induced. Documentation of the severity and/or status of the disease in terms of acute or chronic, as well as the site, etiology, and any secondary disease process are basic documentation requirements. Physician documentation of diagnostic test findings or confirmation of any diagnosis found in diagnostic test reports is also required documentation.

Nervous system coding requires a significant level of specificity, which makes the provider's medical 0record documentation particularly important. Precise clinical information will need to be documented in the medical record to accurately report the codes.

Section 1. Nervous System Resources

Documentation checklists are available in Appendix B for

- Headache syndromes
- Migraine
- Seizures

Section 1. Nervous System Quiz

1. CRPS II is
   a. severe neuropathic pain that may be a result of an illness or injury with intense pain to light touch, abnormal circulation, temperature and sweating
   b. usually occurs at night with an irresistible urge to move the legs due to unusual sensations such as tingling, creeping and crawling
   c. a type of neuropathic pain the occurs following a peripheral nerve injury resulting in burning or throbbing pain along the nerve, sensitivity to cold and touch, changes in skin color, temperature, texture, hair and nails
   d. Disease or damage to peripheral nerves resulting in impaired sensation, movement, gland or organ dysfunction.

2. How are seizure disorders and recurrent seizures classified?
   a. Seizure disorders and recurrent seizures are classified with epilepsy
   b. Seizure disorders and recurrent seizures are classified as non-epileptic
   c. Seizure disorders and recurrent seizures are classified as signs and symptoms
   d. None of the above

3. Which of the following is an alternate term for "intractable" migraine?
   a. Pharmacoresistant
   b. Refractory (medically)
   c. Poorly controlled
   d. All of the above

4. Where are coding and sequencing guidelines for diseases of the nervous system and complications due to the treatment of the diseases and conditions of the nervous system found?
   a. In the ICD-1Ø-CM Official Guidelines for Coding and Reporting chapter specific guidelines for Chapter 6
   b. In the Alphabetic Index and the Tabular List and the chapter specific guidelines for Chapter 6
   c. In other chapter specific guidelines in the ICD-1Ø-CM Official Guidelines for Coding and Reporting
   d. All of the above

5. What is the correct code assignment for an encounter for treatment of a condition causing pain?
   a. A code for the underlying condition is assigned as the principal diagnosis and a code from category G89 is assigned as an additional diagnosis.
   b. A code from category G89 is assigned as the principal diagnosis and no code is assigned for the underlying condition.
   c. A code for the underlying condition is assigned as the principal diagnosis and no code from category G89 is assigned.
   d. A code from category G89 is assigned as the principal diagnosis and a code for the underlying condition is assigned as an additional diagnosis.

6. Which of the following documentation is required for accurate coding of epilepsy?
   a. With or without intractable epilepsy
   b. Type of epilepsy
   c. With or without status epilepticus
   d. All of the above

7. When an admission is for treatment of an underlying condition and a neurostimulator is also inserted for pain control during the same episode of care, what is the correct code assignment?
   a. The underlying condition is the principal diagnosis and the appropriate pain code should be assigned as a secondary diagnosis.
   b. A code for the underlying condition is assigned as the principal diagnosis and no pain code is assigned as an additional diagnosis.
   c. A pain code is assigned as the principal diagnosis and a code for the underlying condition is assigned as an additional diagnosis.
   d. A code for insertion of a neurostimulator for pain control is assigned as the principal diagnosis and a pain code is assigned as an additional diagnosis.

8. Alzheimer's disease with dementia requires dual coding. What is the proper sequencing for Alzheimer's disease with dementia?
   a. The dementia is coded first with or without behavioral disturbance followed by a code for the underlying condition (Alzheimer's disease).
   b. Only the Alzheimer's disease is coded
   c. The Alzheimer's disease is coded first followed by a code for dementia with or without behavioral disturbance.
   d. The Alzheimer's disease is coded with an additional code for any behavioral disturbance.

9. In patients with hemiplegia, if the affected side is documented but not specified as dominant or nondominant, how is this coded?
    a. When the left side is affected, the default is non-dominant
    b. When the right side is affected, the default is dominant
    c. When the patient is ambidextrous, the default is dominant
    d. All of the above

10. What is the correct coding of a diagnosis documented as post-thoracotomy pain without further specification as acute or chronic?
    a. A code from Chapter 19 Injury, poisoning, and certain other consequences of external causes, is assigned
    b. Post-thoracotomy pain is routine postoperative pain and is not coded
    c. The code for acute post-thoracotomy pain is the default
    d. The code for chronic post-thoracotomy pain is the default

See end of chapter for answers and rationales.

Section 2. Musculoskeletal System

Codes for diseases of the musculoskeletal system and connective tissue are found in Chapter 13 in ICD-10-CM. Like many of the other chapters, the documentation needed to accurately code conditions of the musculoskeletal system require specificity and detail. For example, conditions affecting the cervical spine now require identification of the level as occipito-atlanto-axial or high cervical region, mid-cervical region identified by level C3-4, C4-5, C5-6 or cervicothoracic region. Laterality is also included for most musculoskeletal and connective tissue conditions affecting the extremities. For some conditions only right and left is provided, but for other conditions that frequently affect both sides, codes for bilateral are listed. Although not a new documentation requirement, physicians will need to clearly document whether the condition being treated is an acute traumatic condition, in which case it is reported with an injury code from Chapter 19, or an old or chronic condition, in which case it is reported with a code from Chapter 13. Pathologic fractures are reported based upon the causation such as due to neoplastic or other disease, location as well as episode of care. While episode of care is often clearly evident from the nature of the visit, (i.e. a follow-up visit to evaluate healing of a pathological fracture) current documentation should be reviewed to ensure that the initial episode of care is clearly differentiated from subsequent visits for routine healing, delayed healing, malunion, or nonunion of these fractures. If the condition is a sequela of a pathological fracture, that information should also be clearly noted in the medical record as this is also captured with the code for the pathological fracture. Additionally, each visit must be specific in defining the fracture. No longer can the providers merely state the patient is being seen for follow-up of a tibia fracture.

A good way to begin an analysis of documentation and coding requirements for each chapter is to be familiar with the chapter sections and ICD-10-CM chapter blocks. A table containing this information is provided below.

ICD-10-CM Blocks	
M00-M02	Infectious Arthropathies
M05-M14	Inflammatory Polyarthropathies
M15-M19	Osteoarthritis
M20-M25	Other Joint Disorders
M26-M27	Dentofacial Anomalies [Including Malocclusion] and Other Disorders of Jaw
M30-M36	Systemic Connective Tissue Disorders
M40-M43	Deforming Dorsopathies
M45-M49	Spondylopathies
M50-M54	Other Dorsopathies
M60-M63	Disorders of Muscles
M65-M67	Disorders of Synovium and Tendon
M70-M79	Other Soft Tissue Disorders
M80-M85	Disorders of Bone Density and Structure
M86-M90	Other Osteopathies
M91-M94	Chondropathies
M95	Other Disorders of the Musculoskeletal System and Connective Tissue
M96	Intraoperative and Postprocedural Complications and Disorders of Musculoskeletal System, Not Elsewhere Classified
M99	Biomechanical Lesions, Not Elsewhere Classified

The categories of codes for the various diseases of the musculoskeletal system and connective tissues have expanded from previous systems to allow for more specific classification. For example, arthropathies and related disorders are classified based upon causation such as infection, inflammatory diseases or wear and tear arthritis as well as other disorders of the joint.

Coding Note(s)

There is single chapter level coding instruction in ICD-10-CM, which instructs the coder to use an external cause code, if applicable, to identify the cause of the musculoskeletal condition. The external cause code is sequenced after the code for the musculoskeletal condition.

Exclusions

There are only Excludes2 chapter level exclusions notes for ICD-10-CM.

ICD-10-CM Excludes1	ICD-10-CM Excludes2
None	Arthropathic psoriasis (L40.5-) Certain conditions originating in the perinatal period (P04-P96) Certain infectious and parasitic diseases (A00-B99) Compartment syndrome (traumatic) (T79.A-) Complications of pregnancy, childbirth, and the puerperium (O00-O9A) Congenital malformations, deformations and chromosomal abnormalities (Q00-Q99) Endocrine, nutritional and metabolic diseases (E00-E88) Injury, poisoning and certain other consequences of external causes (S00-T88) Neoplasms (C00-D49) Symptoms, signs, and abnormal clinical and laboratory findings, not elsewhere classified (R00-R94)

Chapter Guidelines

Chapter specific guidelines are provided for musculoskeletal system and connective tissue coding. In ICD-10-CM, guidelines are listed for pathological fractures as well as the following:

- Site and laterality
- Acute traumatic versus chronic or recurrent musculoskeletal conditions
- Coding of pathologic fractures
- Osteoporosis

Site and Laterality

Most codes in Chapter 13 have site and laterality designations.

Site

- Site represents either the bone, joint, or the muscle involved
- For some conditions where more than one bone, joint, or muscle is usually involved, such as osteoarthritis, there is a "multiple sites" code available
- For categories where no multiple site code is provided and more than one bone, joint, or muscle is involved, multiple codes should be used to indicate the different sites involved
- Bone Versus Joint – For certain conditions, the bone may be affected at the upper or lower end, (e.g., avascular necrosis of bone, M87; osteoporosis, M80-M81). Though the portion of the bone affected may be at the joint, the site designation will be the bone, not the joint

Laterality

- Most conditions involving the extremities require documentation of right or left in addition to the specific site
- If laterality is not documented, there are codes for unspecified side; however, unspecified codes particularly those defining laterality should be used only in rare circumstances.

Acute Traumatic Versus Chronic or Recurrent Musculoskeletal Conditions

Many musculoskeletal conditions are a result of a previous injury or trauma to a site, or are recurrent conditions. Musculoskeletal conditions are classified either in Chapter 13 Diseases of the Musculoskeletal System and Connective tissue or in Chapter 19 Injury, Poisoning, and Certain Other Consequences of External Causes as follows:

- Healed injury – Bone, joint, or muscle conditions that are a result of a healed injury are usually found in Chapter 13
- Recurrent condition – Recurrent bone, joint, or muscle conditions are usually found in Chapter 13
- Chronic or other recurrent conditions – Conditions are generally reported with a code from Chapter 13
- Current acute injury – Current, acute injuries are coded to the appropriate injury code in Chapter 19

If it is difficult to determine from the available documentation whether the condition should be reported with a code from Chapter 13 or Chapter 19, the provider should be queried.

Coding of Pathologic Fractures

ICD-10-CM contains chapter guidelines for reporting pathologic fractures. These guidelines are primarily defining the use of the 7th character extension to define the episode of care. It is important that these guidelines be understood before coding for pathologic and stress fractures. Guidelines for use of the 7th character extension for coding pathologic fractures in ICD-10-CM are as follows:

- Initial encounter for fracture – The 7th character 'A' for initial episode of care is used for as long as the patient is receiving active treatment for the pathologic fracture. Examples of active treatment are:
  - Surgical treatment
  - Emergency department encounter
  - Evaluation and continuing treatment by the same or different physician
- Subsequent encounter for fracture with routine healing – The 7th character 'D' for subsequent encounter with routine fracture healing is used for encounters after the patient has completed active treatment and when the fracture is healing normally.
- Subsequent encounter for fracture with delayed healing – The 7th character 'G' for subsequent encounter for fracture with delayed healing is reported when the physician has documented that healing is delayed or is not occurring as rapidly as normally expected.
- Subsequent encounter for fracture with nonunion – The 7th character 'K' is reported when the physician has documented that there is nonunion of the fracture or that the fracture has failed to heal. This is a serious fracture complication that requires additional intervention and treatment by the physician.
- Subsequent encounter for fracture with malunion – The 7th character 'P' is reported when the fracture has healed in an abnormal or nonanatomic position. This is a serious fracture complication that requires additional intervention and treatment by the physician.
- Sequela – The 7th character 'S' is reported for complications or conditions that arise as a direct result of the pathological fracture, such as a leg length discrepancy following pathological fracture of the femur. The specific type of sequela is sequenced first followed by the pathological fracture code.

Care for complications of surgical treatment for pathological fracture repairs during the healing or recovery phase should be coded with the appropriate complication codes. See section I.C.19 of the Official Guidelines for information on coding of traumatic fractures.

Osteoporosis

Osteoporosis is a systemic condition, meaning that all bones of the musculoskeletal system are affected. Therefore, site is not a component of the codes under category M81 *Osteoporosis without current pathological fracture.* The site codes under M80 *Osteoporosis with current pathological fracture* identify the site of the fracture not the osteoporosis. Additional guidelines for osteoporosis are as follows:

- Osteoporosis without pathological fracture
  - Category M81 *Osteoporosis without current pathological fracture* is for use for patients with osteoporosis who do not currently have a pathological fracture due to the osteoporosis, even if they had a fracture in the past

  - For a patient with a history of osteoporosis fractures, status code Z87.31, *Personal history of osteoporosis fracture* should follow the code from M81
- Osteoporosis with current pathological fracture
  - Category M80 *Osteoporosis with current pathological fracture* is for patients who have a current pathologic fracture at the time of an encounter
  - The codes under M80 identify the site of the fracture
  - A code from category M80, not a traumatic fracture code, should be used for any patient with known osteoporosis who suffers a fracture, even if the patient had a minor fall or trauma, if that fall or trauma would not usually break a normal, healthy bone

General Documentation Requirements

When documenting diseases of the musculoskeletal system and connective tissue there are a number of general documentation requirements of which providers should be aware. The introduction and guidelines in the previous sections of this chapter identify some of the documentation requirements related to musculoskeletal and connective tissue diseases including more specific site designations and laterality. Documentation of episode of care is required for pathologic and stress fractures. The documentation must also clearly differentiate conditions that are acute traumatic conditions and those that are chronic or recurrent. Understanding documentation requirements for intraoperative and postprocedural complications will require a careful review of category M96 to ensure that the complication is described in sufficient detail to assign the most specific complication code. There are also combination codes that capture two or more related conditions, etiology and manifestations of certain conditions, or a disease process and common symptoms of the disease. Familiarity with the combination codes is needed to ensure that documentation is sufficient to capture any related conditions, both the etiology and manifestation, and/or any related symptoms for the condition being reported. A few examples of each of these general coding and documentation requirements are provided here. For those familiar with the former diagnosis system, ICD-10-CM has reclassified some conditions moving them into a different section. Such is the case of gout which was previously classified in Chapter 3 Endocrine, Nutritional, and Metabolic Diseases in ICD-9-CM but is now classified in Chapter 13 Diseases of the Musculoskeletal System and Connective Tissue.

Site

Site specificity is an important component of musculoskeletal system and connective tissue codes. Dorsopathies, which are conditions affecting the spine and intervertebral joints, provide a good example of site specificity. Codes for ankylosis (fusion) of the spine (M43.2-) are specific to the spine level and the ankylosis should be specified as affecting the occipito-atlanto-axial region, cervical region, cervicothoracic region, thoracic region, thoracolumbar region, lumbar region, lumbosacral region, or sacral and sacrococcygeal region.

Laterality

Laterality is required for the vast majority of musculoskeletal and connective tissue diseases and other conditions affecting the extremities. For example, trigger finger requires documentation of the specific finger (thumb, index finger, middle finger, ring finger, or little finger) and laterality (right, left). While there are also unspecified codes for unspecified finger and unspecified laterality, these codes should rarely be used because the affected finger and laterality should always be documented. Omission of this level of detail indicates to the health plan that the patient was not examined. An example of a condition where codes are available for bilateral conditions as well as for right and left is osteoarthritis of the hip (M16), knee (M17), and first carpometacarpal joints (M18). So, if a patient has primary arthritis of the knee, the physician must document both the condition and the site specific location: right, left or bilateral. For osteoarthritis affecting other joints, there are codes for right and left but not for bilateral. If both joints of one of these sites is affected, two codes—one for the right and one for the left, are assigned.

Episode of Care

Documentation of episode of care is required for pathologic and stress fractures which include: fatigue fractures of the vertebra (M48.4), collapsed vertebra (M48.5-), osteoporosis with pathological fracture (M80.-), stress fracture (M84.3-), pathologic fracture not elsewhere classified (M84,.4-), pathological fracture in neoplastic disease (M84.5-), and pathologic fracture in other disease (M84.6-). For these conditions, a 7th character extension is required identifying the episode of care as:

A	Initial encounter for fracture
D	Subsequent encounter for fracture with routine healing
G	Subsequent encounter for fracture with delayed healing
K	Subsequent encounter for fracture with nonunion
P	Subsequent encounter for fracture with malunion
S	Sequela

The physician must clearly document the episode of care and for subsequent encounters must identify whether the healing is routine or delayed or whether it is complicated by nonunion or malunion. Documentation of the fracture type (stress, pathologic and cause), location (femur, humerus, etc.) and laterality must be documented for each encounter where the patient is being seen for the condition. Codes cannot be assigned based upon prior detailed documentation. Any conditions resulting from a previous pathological fracture must also be clearly documented as sequela so the appropriate pathological fracture sequela code can be assigned in addition to the condition being treated.

Acute Traumatic Versus Old or Chronic Conditions

Acute traumatic and old or chronic conditions must be clearly differentiated in the documentation. Acute traumatic conditions are reported with codes from Chapter 19 Injury, Poisoning and Certain Other Consequences of External Causes, while old or chronic conditions are reported with codes from Chapter 13. For example, an old bucket handle tear of the knee is reported with a code from subcategory M23.2 *Derangement of meniscus due to old tear or injury*, whereas an acute current bucket handle tear is reported with a code from subcategory S83.2 *Tear of meniscus, current injury*.

Intraoperative and Postprocedural Complications NEC

Many codes for intraoperative and postprocedural complications and disorders of the musculoskeletal system are found at the end of Chapter 13 in category M96. This category contains codes for conditions such as postlaminectomy syndrome, postradiation kyphosis and scoliosis, and pseudoarthrosis after surgical fusion or arthrodesis. It also contains codes for intraoperative hemorrhage and hematoma, accidental puncture or laceration, and postprocedural hemorrhage or hematoma of musculoskeletal system structures, which all require documentation of the procedure as a musculoskeletal procedure or a procedure on another body system.

Combination Codes

Combination codes may capture two or more related conditions, etiology and manifestations of certain conditions, or a disease process and common symptoms of the disease. Combination codes that capture two related conditions can be found in category M16 Osteoarthritis of the hip which defines the condition of osteoarthritis resulting from dysplasia (M16.2, M16.3-). An example of a combination code that captures a disease process and a common symptom of that disease is found in category M47 Spondylosis. Here codes are provided for spondylosis (disease process) with radiculopathy (symptom).

Code-Specific Documentation Requirements

In this section, ICD-10-CM code categories, subcategories, and subclassifications for some of the more frequently reported diseases of the musculoskeletal system and connective tissue are reviewed along with specific documentation requirements identified. The focus is on conditions with more specific clinical documentation requirements. Although not all codes with significant documentation requirements are discussed, this section will provide a representative sample of the type of additional documentation needed for diseases of the musculoskeletal system and connective tissue. The section is organized alphabetically by the ICD10-CM code category, subcategory, or subclassification depending on whether the documentation affects only a single code or an entire subcategory or category.

Contracture Tendon Sheath

A muscle contracture is a shortening of the muscle and/or tendon sheath which prevents normal movement and flexibility. Causes can include: prolonged immobilization, scarring (trauma, burns), paralysis (stroke, spinal cord injuries), ischemia (e.g., Volkmann's contracture), cerebral palsy, and degenerative diseases affecting the muscles (e.g., muscular dystrophy).

A muscle spasm is a sudden, involuntary contraction of a single muscle or a muscle group. This condition is usually benign and self-limiting. The contraction of the muscle is temporary. Causes include abnormal or malfunctioning nerve signals, muscle fatigue (overuse, exertion), dehydration, electrolyte imbalance, decreased blood supply, and certain medications.

In ICD-10-CM, tendon and muscle contractures and muscle spasms are found under the section of soft tissue disorders. Subcategory M62.4 Contracture of muscle contains the alternate term contracture of tendon sheath, so a code from this subcategory is reported for either diagnosis. Codes in this subcategory are specific to site and documentation of laterality is also required. Muscle spasm is found under subcategory M62.83 and is further subdivided by muscle spasm of the back calf and other. Documentation requirements and clinical documentation for muscle or tendon contracture follows.

Coding and Documentation Requirements

Identify the site of the muscle or tendon contracture:

- Upper extremity
  - Shoulder
  - Upper arm
  - Forearm
  - Hand
- Lower extremity
  - Thigh
  - Lower leg
  - Ankle/Foot
- Other site
- Multiple sites
- Unspecified site

For muscle/tendon contracture of extremity, identify laterality:

- Right
- Left
- Unspecified

ICD-10-CM Code/Documentation	
M62.40	Contracture of muscle unspecified site
M62.411	Contracture of muscle, right shoulder
M62.412	Contracture of muscle, left shoulder
M62.419	Contracture of muscle, unspecified shoulder
M62.421	Contracture of muscle, right upper arm
M62.422	Contracture of muscle, left upper arm
M62.429	Contracture of muscle, unspecified upper arm
M62.431	Contracture of muscle, right forearm
M62.432	Contracture of muscle, left forearm
M62.439	Contracture of muscle, unspecified forearm
M62.441	Contracture of muscle, right hand
M62.442	Contracture of muscle, left hand
M62.449	Contracture of muscle, unspecified hand
M62.451	Contracture of muscle, right thigh
M62.452	Contracture of muscle, left thigh
M62.459	Contracture of muscle, unspecified thigh
M62.461	Contracture of muscle, right lower leg

ICD-10-CM Code/Documentation	
M62.462	Contracture of muscle, left lower leg
M62.469	Contracture of muscle, unspecified lower leg
M62.471	Contracture of muscle, right ankle and foot
M62.472	Contracture of muscle, left ankle and foot
M62.479	Contracture of muscle, unspecified ankle and foot
M62.48	Contracture of muscle, other site
M62.49	Contracture of muscle, multiple sites

Documentation and Coding Example

Fourteen-year-old Black male presents to Orthopedic Clinic with an interesting **deformity to his right wrist**. He is right hand dominant. Patient and mother give a history of a skateboard accident 1Ø months ago where he slammed into a metal pole causing a **soft tissue injury to his right forearm. He developed an infected hematoma** that was incised and drained and ultimately healed. ROM to elbow is intact. He is able to supinate and pronate fully. There is a moderate amount of ulnar deviation in the right wrist, causing focal disability. He has difficulty performing a pincher grasp, holding utensils and is unable to hold a small half-filled water bottle for more than a minute. X-rays of elbow, forearm, wrist unremarkable.

Impression: **Contracture of right extensor carpi ulnaris tendon causing deformity and functional disability of the wrist and hand due to old soft tissue injury**.

Plan: Occupational Therapy evaluation and authorization for 12 visits if approved by patient's insurance company. RTC in one month.

Diagnosis Code(s)

M62.431 Contracture of muscle, right forearm

S56.5Ø1S Unspecified injury of other extensor muscle, fascia and tendon at forearm level, sequela

VØØ.132S Skateboarder colliding with stationary object, sequela

Coding Note(s)

The extensor carpi ulnaris muscle is a muscle in the forearm, so the code for contracture of the right forearm muscle is reported. Contracture of tendon is reported with the same code as contracture of muscle. Based upon the documentation, the tendon/muscle contracture is a sequela of a soft tissue injury so an injury code with 7th character 'S' should also be reported. Coding of sequela will be covered in Chapter 19 of this book. The external cause of the sequela (late effect) is specific to a skateboarder colliding with a stationary object.

Gouty Arthropathy

Gout is an arthritis-like condition caused by an accumulation of uric acid in the blood which leads to inflammation of the joints. Acute gout typically affects one joint. Chronic gout is characterized by repeated episodes of pain and inflammation in one or more joints. Following repeated episodes of gout, some individuals develop chronic tophaceous gout. This condition is characterized by solid deposits of monosodium urate (MSU) crystals, called tophi in the joints, cartilage, bones, and other areas of the body. In some cases, tophi break through the skin and appear as white or yellowish-white, chalky nodules on the skin.

Even though gout is often considered a metabolic disorder in its origins, ICD-1Ø-CM classifies gout as a disease of the musculoskeletal system and connective tissue within two categories—M1Ø Gout and M1A Chronic gout. Gout may be due to toxic effects of lead or other drugs, renal impairment, other medical conditions, or an unknown cause (idiopathic). Category M1Ø includes gout due to any cause specified as acute gout, gout attack, gout flare, and other gout not specified as chronic. Subcategories identify the specific cause of the gout as idiopathic, lead-induced, drug-induced, due to renal impairment, due to other causes, or unspecified. Category M1A includes gout due to any cause specified as chronic.

Coding and Documentation Requirements

Identify type of gout:

- Chronic
- Other/unspecified, which includes:
  - Acute gout
  - Gout attack
  - Gout flare
  - Gout not otherwise specified
  - Podagra

Identify cause:

- Drug-induced
- Idiopathic
- Lead-induced
- Renal impairment
- Other secondary gout
- Unspecified

Identify site:

- Lower extremity
  - Ankle/foot
  - Hip
  - Knee
- Upper extremity
  - Elbow
  - Hand
  - Shoulder
  - Wrist
- Vertebrae
- Multiple sites
- Unspecified site

Identify laterality for extremities:

- Right
- Left
- Unspecified

For chronic gout, use a 7th character to identify any tophus:

- With tophus (1)
- Without tophus (0)

ICD-10-CM Code/Documentation	
M10.00	Idiopathic gout, unspecified site
M10.011	Idiopathic gout, right shoulder
M10.012	Idiopathic gout, left shoulder
M10.019	Idiopathic gout, unspecified shoulder
M10.021	Idiopathic gout, right elbow
M10.022	Idiopathic gout, left elbow
M10.029	Idiopathic gout, unspecified elbow
M10.031	Idiopathic gout, right wrist
M10.032	Idiopathic gout, left wrist
M10.039	Idiopathic gout, unspecified wrist
M10.041	Idiopathic gout, right hand
M10.042	Idiopathic gout, left hand
M10.049	Idiopathic gout, unspecified hand
M10.051	Idiopathic gout, right hip
M10.052	Idiopathic gout, left hip
M10.059	Idiopathic gout, unspecified hip
M10.061	Idiopathic gout, right knee
M10.062	Idiopathic gout, left knee
M10.069	Idiopathic gout, unspecified knee
M10.071	Idiopathic gout, right ankle and foot
M10.072	Idiopathic gout, left ankle and foot
M10.079	Idiopathic gout, unspecified ankle and foot
M10.08	Idiopathic gout, vertebrae
M10.09	Idiopathic gout, multiple sites

Documentation and Coding Example

Fifty-two-year-old Caucasian male presents to PMD with complaints of gout flare. PMH is significant for hypertension, seasonal allergies, and gout. Current medications include lisinopril, allopurinol, ASA, enzyme CoQ1Ø, loratadine, and Nasonex® spray. His only complaint is a **swollen great toe which he attributes to a gout flare**.

Temperature 97.4, HR 84, RR 14, BP 14Ø/78, Wt. 189. On examination, this is a well-groomed, well-nourished male who looks his stated age. Skin is tan and he has a few scattered seborrheic keratoses lesions present on face and back. He is reminded to use sunscreen and a hat when outdoors. Peripheral pulses full. Right leg is unremarkable. Left knee and ankle normal. **Left great toe is red, swollen, and tender to touch**. He is advised to take OTC ibuprofen or naproxen for his toe pain and to avoid alcohol, limit meat for a few weeks. He will return in 1 week for a recheck of his great toe.

Diagnosis: **Primary gout with gout flare left great toe**.

Diagnosis Code(s)

M1Ø.Ø72 Idiopathic gout, left ankle and foot

Coding Note(s)

The patient has a history of gout and is being seen for a gout flare. The inclusion terms under M1Ø Gout includes gout flare. Reporting a code for chronic gout requires specific documentation of the gout as a chronic condition. In addition, if the patient has chronic gout and a gout flare, report only the code for the gout flare. There is an Excludes1 note indicating that chronic gout (category M1A) is never reported with acute gout (category M1Ø).

Intervertebral Disc Disorders

Intervertebral disc disorders include conditions such as displacement, Schmorl's nodes, degenerative disc disease, intervertebral disc disorders, postlaminectomy syndrome, and other and unspecified disc disorders. Like spondylosis, several combination codes exist to define the disc disorder as well as associated symptoms of radiculopathy or myelopathy. Displacement of an intervertebral disc may also be referred to as ruptured or herniated intervertebral disc or herniated nucleus pulposus (HNP). This is because displacement occurs when the inner gel-like substance (nucleus pulposus) of the intervertebral disc bulges out from or herniates through the outer fibrous ring and into the spinal canal. The herniated or displaced nucleus pulposus may then press on spinal nerves causing pain or other sensory disturbances, such as tingling or numbness, as well as changes in motor function and reflexes.

In ICD-1Ø-CM, category M5Ø contains codes for cervical disc disorders with sites specific to the high cervical region, midcervical region redefined for October 1, 2Ø16 by disc space level (C4-C5, C5-C6, C6-C7), and cervicothoracic region. Category M51 contains codes for disc disorders of the thoracic, thoracolumbar, lumbar, and lumbosacral regions. In addition to codes specific to these sites, combination codes identify disc disorders as with myelopathy or with radiculopathy. There are also codes for other disc displacement, other disc degeneration, other cervical disc disorders, and unspecified disc disorders. Documentation must clearly describe the specific condition and any associated myelopathy or radiculopathy to ensure that the most specific code is assigned.

Coding and Documentation Requirements

Identify condition:

- Disc disorder
  - Identify symptom
    - » with myelopathy
    - » with radiculopathy
- Other disc displacement
- Other disc degeneration
- Other disc disorders
- Schmorl's nodes
- Unspecified disc disorder

Identify site:

- Cervical
  - Identify level
    - » High cervical (C2-C4)
    - » C4-5, C5-6, C6-7
    - » Cervicothoracic (C7-T1)
- Thoracic region
- Thoracolumbar region (T10-L1)
- Lumbar region

- Lumbosacral region
- Unspecified site

Note: In ICD-10-CM, codes for "other" disc displacement, degeneration, disorder are used for the specified condition when there is no documentation of either myelopathy or radiculopathy. If disc displacement, degeneration, or disorder are documented as with myelopathy or with radiculopathy, the codes for disc disorder with myelopathy or disc disorder with radiculopathy are reported.

Cervical Intervertebral Disc Disorders

ICD-10-CM Code/Documentation	
M50.20	Other cervical disc displacement, unspecified cervical region
M50.21	Other cervical disc displacement, high cervical region
M50.22	Other cervical disc displacement, mid-cervical region
M50.23	Other cervical disc displacement, cervicothoracic region
M50.30	Other cervical disc degeneration, unspecified cervical region
M50.31	Other cervical disc degeneration, high cervical region
M50.32	Other cervical disc degeneration, mid-cervical region
M50.33	Other cervical disc degeneration, cervicothoracic region
M50.00	Cervical disc disorder with myelopathy, unspecified cervical region
M50.01	Cervical disc disorder with myelopathy, high cervical region
M50.02	Cervical disc disorder with myelopathy, mid-cervical region
M50.03	Cervical disc disorder with myelopathy, cervicothoracic region
M50.80	Other cervical disc disorders, unspecified cervical region
M50.81	Other cervical disc disorders, high cervical region
M50.82	Other cervical disc disorders, mid-cervical region
M50.83	Other cervical disc disorders, cervicothoracic region
M50.90	Cervical disc disorder, unspecified, unspecified cervical region
M50.91	Cervical disc disorder, unspecified, high cervical region
M50.92	Cervical disc disorder, unspecified, mid-cervical region
M50.93	Cervical disc disorder, unspecified, cervicothoracic region
M50.10	Cervical disc disorder with radiculopathy, unspecified cervical region
M50.11	Cervical disc disorder with radiculopathy, high cervical region
M50.12	Cervical disc disorder with radiculopathy, mid-cervical region
M50.13	Cervical disc disorder with radiculopathy, cervicothoracic region
M54.11	Radiculopathy, occipito-atlanto-axial cervical region
M54.12	Radiculopathy, cervical region
M54.13	Radiculopathy, cervicothoracic region

Documentation and Coding Example

Thirty-three-year-old Caucasian female is referred to Neurology Clinic by PMD for right arm pain and weakness. Patient is a NICU RN working 3-5 twelve hour shifts/wk. primarily with premature infants. She can recall no injury to her neck or arm but simply awoke two weeks ago with a sharp pain that radiated through her shoulder, down her right arm to the tip of her thumb. She is left hand dominant. The pain is resolving but she continues to have weakness, numbness, and tingling in the arm. She treated her symptoms with rest, heat, and ibuprofen during 2 regularly scheduled days off and was able to return to work for her next scheduled shift. She was concerned about the residual weakness in her arm and called her PMD who ordered cervical spine films and an **MRI which showed disc displacement/ protrusion at C5-C6**. He prescribed oral steroids and Tramadol for pain, Lunesta for sleep and referred her to Neurology. On examination, this is a moderately obese woman who looks her stated age. PERRL, there is stiffness and decreased ROM in her neck, cranial nerves grossly intact. Exam of left upper extremity is unremarkable with intact pulses, reflexes, ROM and strength. Exam of right arm is significant for moderate weakness in the right bicep muscle and wrist extensor muscles. Sensation to both dull and sharp stimuli is decreased along the anterior right arm beginning at shoulder to mid forearm level. Pincher grasp is weak on the right. Pulses are intact as are reflexes. MRI is reviewed with patient and she does indeed have a **small herniation of the disc at C5-C6 space which is most likely the cause of her current myelopathy**. She is advised to stop taking the Lunesta and Tramadol and is prescribed Celebrex and acetaminophen for pain. PT agrees to see her this afternoon for initial evaluation, possible soft cervical collar. She is cleared to work as long as she does not lift more than 10 lbs. RTC in 2 weeks for recheck.

Diagnosis Code(s)

M50.022 Cervical disc disorder at C5-C6 level with myelopathy

Coding Note(s)

To identify the correct code, instructions in the Alphabetic Index are followed. Under Displacement, intervertebral disc, with myelopathy there is an instruction, see Disorder, disc, cervical, with myelopathy. Code M50.022 is identified as the correct code for Disorder, disc, with myelopathy, C5-C6.

Limb Pain

The cause of pain in a limb may not be readily evident. Often several conditions must be worked up and ruled out before a definitive diagnosis can be made. In the outpatient setting, conditions that are documented as possible or to be ruled-out cannot be listed as confirmed diagnoses. A non-specific symptom code is reported until the underlying cause of the pain has been diagnosed. Codes for limb pain refer to pain that is not located in the joint. There are more specific codes for joint pain. Limb pain would not be assigned if a known cause exists such as mononeuritis or neuralgia which would be reported with codes from the nervous system chapter. Limb pain is captured by codes in subcategory M79.6. The pain needs to be defined by the specific site and laterality. Details of documentation requirements are listed below.

Coding and Documentation Requirements

Identify site of pain:

- Upper extremity
  - Upper arm
  - Forearm
  - Hand
  - Finger(s)

  - Site not specified
- Lower extremity
  - Thigh
  - Lower leg
  - Foot
  - Toe(s)
  - Site not specified
- Unspecified limb

For upper and lower extremity, identify laterality

- Right
- Left
- Unspecified

There are codes for unspecified limb (not specified as upper or lower); unspecified arm (site not specified and not specified as right or left); unspecified leg (site not specified and laterality not specified). There are also codes for specified site but unspecified laterality for upper arm, forearm, hand, fingers, thigh, lower leg, foot, and toes. However, even though codes for unspecified limb and unspecified laterality are provided, they should be avoided as the specific limb affected and laterality should always be documented.

ICD-10-CM Code/Documentation	
Pain in Limb, Unspecified	
M79.601	Pain in right arm
M79.602	Pain in left arm
M79.603	Pain in arm, unspecified
M79.604	Pain in right leg
M79.605	Pain in left leg
M79.606	Pain in leg, unspecified
M79.609	Pain in unspecified limb
Pain in Upper Arm/Forearm/Hand/Fingers	
M79.621	Pain in right upper arm
M79.622	Pain in left upper arm
M79.629	Pain in unspecified upper arm
M79.631	Pain in right forearm
M79.632	Pain in left forearm
M79.639	Pain in unspecified forearm
M79.641	Pain in right hand
M79.642	Pain in left hand
M79.643	Pain in unspecified hand
M79.644	Pain in right finger(s)
M79.645	Pain in left finger(s)
M79.646	Pain in unspecified fingers
Pain in Thigh/Lower Leg/Foot/Toes	
M79.651	Pain in right thigh
M79.652	Pain in left thigh
M79.659	Pain in unspecified thigh
M79.661	Pain in right lower leg
M79.662	Pain in left lower leg
M79.669	Pain in unspecified lower leg
M79.671	Pain in right foot
M79.672	Pain in left foot
M79.673	Pain in unspecified foot
M79.674	Pain in right toe(s)
M79.675	Pain in left toes(s)
M79.676	Pain in unspecified toe(s)

Documentation and Coding Example

Twenty-five-year-old Hispanic male presents to Urgent Care Clinic with a four-day history of pain and swelling in left forearm. Patient is in good health and does not have a PMD, the last time he sought medical care was in college. He is employed full time developing computer software. He works from home most of the time, flying into the company's central office for a few days each month. His arm pain started on the last day of a 5-day trip to the central office. He can recall no injury although he did engage in daily, strenuous physical activities including ultimate Frisbee, volleyball, and basketball. Pain began as a dull ache in the inner arm midway between elbow and wrist. Upon returning home, he continues to experience a dull ache in the forearm which varies in intensity but is always present. He has applied ice to the area off and on for the past 2 days. This morning the remains achy so he seeks medical attention. On examination, this is a well groomed, well nourished, somewhat anxious young man. T 98.5, P 6Ø, R 12, BP 1Ø4/54, O2 Sat 99% on RA. Eyes clear, PERRLA. Nares patent, mucous membranes moist and pink, TMs normal. Neck supple without masses or lymphadenopathy. Cranial nerves grossly intact. Heart rate regular, breath sounds clear, equal bilaterally. Abdomen soft, nontender with active bowel sounds. No evidence of hernia, normal male genitalia. Examination of lower extremities is completely benign. Right upper extremity has normal strength, sensation and movement. Left upper arm has normal tone, strength, reflexes, sensation and circulation. The left elbow is unremarkable with normal ROM. The inner forearm is palpated. No mass or other signs of abnormality are noted other than the dull aching pain. Negative for Raynaud phenomena. Circulation and sensation intact through fingers. Supination and pronation exacerbates the pain as does fist clenching. X-ray of forearm is obtained and is negative for fracture.

Impression: **Pain left forearm of unknown etiology**.

Plan: Blood drawn for CBC w/diff, ESR, CRP, Quantitative Immunoglobulin levels, comprehensive metabolic panel. Results will be forwarded to Internal Medicine Department where he has an appointment scheduled in 3 days. He is fitted with a sling to be used PRN for comfort. He is advised to use ibuprofen for pain and to return to Urgent Care Clinic if symptoms worsen before his appointment with Internist.

Diagnosis Code(s)

M79.632 Pain in left forearm

Coding Note(s)

Pain of unknown etiology is specific to site and laterality.

Lumbago/Sciatica

Lumbago refers to non-specific pain in the lower back region. The condition is very common and may be acute, subacute, or chronic in nature. Lumbago is generally a symptom of benign musculoskeletal strain or sprain with no underlying disease or syndrome.

Sciatica is a set of symptoms characterized by pain, paresthesia (shock like pain in the arms and/or legs), and/or weakness in the low back, buttocks, or lower extremities. Symptoms result from compression of one or more spinal nerves (L4, L5, S1, S2, S3) that form the sciatic nerve (right and left branches). Causes can include herniated discs, spinal stenosis, pregnancy, injury or tumors.

In ICD-1Ø-CM, there is a code for lumbago alone designated by the descriptor low back pain (M54.5). There are also codes for sciatica alone (M54.3-) and a combination code for lumbago with sciatica (M54.4-). Codes for sciatica require documentation of laterality to identify the side of the sciatic nerve pain.

Coding and Documentation Requirements

Identify the low back pain/sciatica:

- Low back pain
  - With sciatica
    - Right side
    - Left side
    - Unspecified side
  - Without sciatica
- Sciatica
  - Right side
  - Left side
  - Unspecified side

ICD-10-CM Code/Documentation	
M54.5	Low back pain
M54.30	Sciatica, unspecified side
M54.31	Sciatica, right side
M54.32	Sciatica, left side
M54.40	Lumbago with sciatica, unspecified side
M54.41	Lumbago with sciatica, right side
M54.42	Lumbago with sciatica, left side

Documentation and Coding Example

Forty-two-year-old female presents to PMD with ongoing **sharp pain in her left buttocks radiating down the back of her left leg**. She states the pain began suddenly about 1 week ago as she was preparing and planting her Spring garden. She does not recall any specific injury only that she was hauling bags of soil and compost mix, bending a lot and on her knees weeding and planting. On examination, this is a very pleasant, quite tan, well developed, well-nourished woman who looks older than her stated age. She states she loves to be outdoors and never applies sunscreen, believing that sun exposure is healthy for her body. Cranial nerves grossly intact. Neurovascular exam of upper extremities is unremarkable. Thoracic spine is straight without swelling or tenderness to palpation. There is mild tenderness with palpation of her lumbar spine and moderate muscle spasm with deep palpation of her left buttocks. Forward bending elicits pain at the thoracolumbar junction. Leg lifts also elicit pain on the left. Patient states pain and stiffness is worse on rising in the morning, decreases when lying down and changes from sharp pain to dull ache when sitting. Patient declines x-ray of her spine as she believes radiation is harmful to her body. She declines prescriptions for pain medication, muscle relaxant, or NSAIDs. She is using topical arnica gel and an oral homeopathic for inflammation. She is agreeable to physical therapy for muscle flexibility and strengthening exercises. She is given a written prescription for PT because she would like to do some research and find a therapist who would be a good fit for her. RTC in 6 weeks, sooner if needed.

Impression: **Left sciatica with low back pain.**

Diagnosis Code(s)

M54.42 Lumbago with sciatica, left side

Coding Note(s)

There is a combination code for lumbago with sciatica is reported. Codes for sciatica and lumbago with sciatica are specific to the side of the sciatic pain. The physician has documented that the patient is experiencing left-sided sciatica.

Osteoarthritis

There are multiple codes in multiple code categories for osteoarthritis (M15, M16, M17, M18, and M19). These codes are to be used for osteoarthritis of extremity joints. Codes for osteoarthritis of the spine will be located in category M47. There are specific codes for primary and secondary arthritis with the codes for secondary arthritis being specific for post-traumatic osteoarthritis and other secondary osteoarthritis. It is important to note that there are also codes for post-traumatic arthritis, M12.5- that are not osteoarthritis. It is imperative that the documentation specifies whether the arthritis resulting from trauma is post-traumatic degenerative which is usually a result of trauma surrounding the joint such as following multiple ankle sprains vs. post-traumatic which is due to trauma involving the joint surface such as following a tibial pilon fracture. For secondary osteoarthritis of the hip there is also a specific code for osteoarthritis resulting from hip dysplasia. Codes for specific types of osteoarthritis require laterality (right, left). For the hip, knee and first CMC joint there are also bilateral codes. Codes for other secondary arthritis of the hip and knee must be specified as either bilateral or unilateral, but there are not specific codes for right and left. Unspecified osteoarthritis does not require any information on laterality. An additional category is available for polyosteoarthritis, category M15. This involved osteoarthritis of more than five joints and includes such disorders as Heberden's nodes and Bouchard's notes of the hands as well as primary generalized osteoarthritis. Bilateral osteoarthritis of a single joint should not be coded as polyosteoarthritis or generalized osteoarthritis.

Coding and documentation requirements for osteoarthritis are provided followed by a clinical example for osteoarthritis of the hip.

Coding and Documentation Requirements

Identify type of osteoarthritis:

- Primary
- Secondary
  - Post-traumatic
  - Resulting from hip dysplasia (hip only)
  - Other specified secondary osteoarthritis
  - Unspecified

Identify site:

- Hip
- Knee
- First carpometacarpal joint
- Shoulder
- Elbow
- Wrist
- Hand
- Ankle and foot

Identify laterality:

- Right
- Left
- Unspecified

Osteoarthritis Hip

ICD-10-CM Code/Documentation	
M16.0	Bilateral primary osteoarthritis of hip
M16.10	Unilateral primary osteoarthritis, unspecified hip
M16.11	Unilateral primary osteoarthritis, right hip
M16.12	Unilateral primary osteoarthritis, left hip
M16.2	Bilateral osteoarthritis of hip resulting from hip dysplasia
M16.30	Unilateral osteoarthritis of hip resulting from hip dysplasia, unspecified hip
M16.31	Unilateral osteoarthritis of hip resulting from hip dysplasia, right hip
M16.32	Unilateral osteoarthritis of hip resulting from hip dysplasia, left hip
M16.4	Bilateral post-traumatic osteoarthritis of hip
M16.50	Unilateral post-traumatic osteoarthritis, unspecified hip
M16.51	Unilateral post-traumatic osteoarthritis, right hip
M16.52	Unilateral post-traumatic osteoarthritis, left hip
M16.6	Other bilateral secondary osteoarthritis of hip
M16.7	Other unilateral secondary osteoarthritis of hip
M16.9	Osteoarthritis of hip, unspecified

Documentation and Coding Example

Sixty-one-year-old Caucasian female is referred to orthopedic clinic by PMD for ongoing right hip pain and stiffness. Patient sustained a **soft tissue injury to her right hip and leg 6 years ago** in a bicycle accident. X-rays at the time showed no fracture and she was treated conservatively with rest, ice and ibuprofen. She was able to return to her usual active lifestyle within a few weeks but over the years she has noticed increased stiffness, especially in the morning and she is taking acetaminophen for pain 4-5 times a week. On examination, this is a trim, fit appearing woman who looks younger than her stated age. Gait is normal. There is no evidence of osteophytic changes to small joints. Patient denies fatigue, weight loss or fevers. Cranial nerves grossly intact, neuromuscular exam of upper extremities is unremarkable. Muscle strength equal in lower extremities, there is marked tenderness with palpation of the right hip, no swelling, muscle wasting or crepitus. X-ray obtained of bilateral hips for comparison. Left hip x-ray and exam is relatively benign. Radiograph of right hip is significant for sclerosis of the superior aspect of the acetabulum along with single Egger cyst. Findings are consistent with **post-traumatic osteoarthritis of the hip**. Treatment options discussed with patient and she prefers a conservative plan at this time. She is referred to physical therapy 3 x week for 4 weeks and advised to take Naproxen sodium 22Ø mg BID. RTC in one month for re-evaluation.

Diagnosis Code

M16.51 Unilateral post-traumatic osteoarthritis, right hip

Coding Note(s)

The ICD-1Ø-CM code identifies the secondary osteoarthritis as post-traumatic and is also specific to site (hip) and laterality (right).

An external cause code is not required but if the documentation was sufficient on the circumstances of the accident an external cause code could also be reported to identify the cause of the post-traumatic osteoarthritis as a bicycle accident.

Osteoporosis

Osteoporosis is a systemic disease that affects previously constructed bone tissue. It is characterized by decreased bone density, weakness, and brittleness, making the bone more susceptible to fracture. Primary type 1 (postmenopausal) osteoporosis typically affects women after menopause. Primary type 2 (senile) osteoporosis is identified in both men and women after the age of 75. Secondary osteoporosis can occur in either sex and at any age. It arises from an underlying medical condition, prolonged immobilization or the use of certain drugs that affect mineral balance in the bones. With any type of osteoporosis, the most common bones affected are vertebrae, ribs, pelvis, and upper extremities. The condition is often asymptomatic until a fracture occurs.

In ICD-1Ø-CM, there are two categories for osteoporosis. Codes from category M8Ø are reported for osteoporosis with a current pathological fracture and codes from M81 are reported for osteoporosis without a current pathological fracture. Osteoporosis with or without pathological fracture is then subclassified as age-related or other specified type, which includes drug-induced, disuse, idiopathic, post-oophorectomy, postsurgical malabsorption, and post-traumatic osteoporosis. There is no code for unspecified osteoporosis. If documentation does not identify a specific type or cause of osteoporosis, the Alphabetic Index directs to 'age-related'. If the osteoporosis is associated with a current fracture, the fracture site and laterality must be documented. In addition, osteoporosis codes with a current pathological fracture require a 7th character to identify the episode of care.

The applicable 7th character extensions for osteoporosis with pathological fracture are as follows:

A Initial encounter for fracture

D Subsequent encounter for fracture with routine healing

G Subsequent encounter for fracture with delayed healing

K Subsequent encounter for fracture with nonunion

P Subsequent encounter for fracture with malunion

S Sequela

Coding and Documentation Requirements

Identify osteoporosis as with or without current pathological fracture:

- With current pathological fracture
- Without current pathological fracture

Identify type/cause of osteoporosis:

- Age-related
- Localized
- Other

For osteoporosis with current pathological fracture, identify site of fracture:

- Shoulder
- Humerus
- Forearm
- Hand
- Femur
- Lower leg
- Ankle/foot
- Vertebra(e)

Identify episode of care:

- Initial encounter
- Subsequent encounter
  - With routine healing
  - With delayed healing
  - With nonunion
  - With malunion
- Sequela

Senile/Age-Related Osteoporosis with Current Pathological Fracture of Forearm/Wrist

ICD-10-CM Code/Documentation	
M80.031-	Age related osteoporosis with current pathological fracture, right forearm
M80.032-	Age related osteoporosis with current pathological fracture, left forearm
M80.039-	Age related osteoporosis with current pathological fracture, unspecified forearm
Note: Requires 7th character to identify episode of care.	

Documentation and Coding Example

Fifty-nine-year-old Caucasian female returns to Orthopedic Clinic for a second postoperative visit. She is now five weeks S/P **fall at home** where she sustained a **fracture of the distal right radius**. She presented initially to the ED with pain, swelling and deformity of the right wrist and forearm with tenderness and swelling of the distal radius. Radiographs showed a **distal radial fracture and severe osteoporosis** of the radius and ulna. She underwent an ORIF that same day with application of soft cast/splint. She had a hard cast applied at her first PO visit 3 weeks ago. Patient states she is doing well and has no complaints. Bruising and swelling have subsided in her fingers and she has good ROM and neurovascular checks. She admits to mild pain, usually associated with over use, that is relieved with acetaminophen. X-ray in plaster shows the **fracture to be in good alignment with increased callus size when compared to previous film**. She is taking a Calcium supplement, Vitamin D 6000 units, Vitamin C 1000 mg daily and a multivitamin/mineral tablet. Patient is advised to continue with her present supplements. RTC in 3 weeks for x-ray out of plaster and application of splint. Patient is due for annual physical exam with her PCP in 3 months. She is advised to discuss having a DEXA scan to assess bone density since it has been 6 years since her last one and she has now entered menopause. Once they have those results she may need to consider more aggressive therapy for her osteoporosis.

Impression: **Healing distal radial fracture right forearm. Fracture due to postmenopausal osteoporosis**. S/P ORIF.

Diagnosis Code(s)

M80.031D Age related osteoporosis with current pathological fracture, right forearm, subsequent encounter for fracture with routine healing

W19.XXXD Unspecified fall, subsequent encounter

Coding Note(s)

Even though the fracture was sustained in a fall, ICD-10-CM coding guidelines state, "A code from category M80, not a traumatic fracture code, should be used for any patient with known osteoporosis who suffers a fracture, even if the patient had a minor fall or trauma, if that fall or trauma would not usually break a normal, healthy bone." An external cause code may be reported additionally to identify the pathological fracture as due to a fall. An unspecified fall is reported because the documentation does not provide any information on circumstances surrounding the fall, such as a fall due to tripping or a fall from one level to another. The 7th character D is assigned to identify this encounter as a subsequent visit for aftercare.

Radiculopathy

Neuritis is a general term for inflammation of a nerve or group of nerves. Symptoms will vary depending on the area of the body and the nerve(s) that are inflamed. Symptoms may include pain, tingling (paresthesia), weakness (paresis), numbness (hypoesthesia), paralysis, loss of reflexes, and muscle wasting. Causes can include injury, infection, disease, exposure to chemicals or toxins, and nutritional deficiencies.

Radiculitis is a term used to describe pain that radiates along the dermatome (sensory pathway) of a nerve or group of nerves and is caused by inflammation or irritation of the nerve root(s) near the spinal cord. Symptoms vary depending on the exact nerve root(s) affected, but can include pain with a sharp, stabbing, shooting or burning quality; tingling (paresthesia); numbness (hypoesthesia); weakness (paresis); loss of reflexes; and muscle wasting. Causes can include injury, anatomic abnormality (e.g., bone spur), degenerative disease, and bulging or ruptured intervertebral disc.

Neuralgia, neuritis, and radiculitis of unknown cause are reported with "not otherwise specified" codes. There are two subcategories, M54.1 Radiculopathy, which is specific to neuritis and radiculitis of a specific spinal level and M79.2 Neuralgia and neuritis unspecified.

Coding and Documentation Requirements

Identify site of neuritis/radiculitis:

- Occipito-atlanto-axial region
- Cervical region
- Cervicothoracic region
- Thoracic region
- Thoracolumbar region
- Lumbar region
- Lumbosacral region
- Sacral/sacrococcygeal region
- Unspecified site
  - Radiculitis
  - Neuritis/neuralgia

ICD-10-CM Code/Documentation	
M54.11	Radiculopathy, occipito-atlanto-axial region
M54.12	Radiculopathy, cervical region
M54.13	Radiculopathy, cervicothoracic region
M54.14	Radiculopathy, thoracic region
M54.15	Radiculopathy, thoracolumbar region
M54.18	Radiculopathy, lumbar region
M54.17	Radiculopathy, lumbosacral region
M54.10	Radiculopathy, site unspecified
M54.18	Radiculopathy, sacral and sacrococcygeal region
M79.2	Neuralgia and neuritis, unspecified

Documentation and Coding Example

Fifty-five-year-old Caucasian female presents to PMD with tingling and numbness in the labia/perineal area, right buttocks and back of right thigh X 2 months with weakness in the right leg for the past few days. Patient is divorced, her youngest son is living with his father and older son has moved out of state to attend school. She continues to work part time as an office assistant. She sits a lot for her job but is quite active outside of work. She regularly hikes and bikes, plays softball, bowls and swims. She can recall no injury or trauma to her back or legs, simply noticed tingling and numbness sitting on the seat of her bike one day. HT 7Ø inches, WT 138, T 99, P 66, R 14, BP 124/62. On examination, this is a pleasant, thin, athletic appearing woman who looks her stated age. Eyes clear, PERRLA. TMs normal, nares patent without drainage. Oral mucosa moist and pink. Neck supple without lymphadenopathy. Cranial nerves grossly intact. Upper extremities normal. HR regular without bruit, rub or murmur. Breath sounds clear and equal bilaterally. Abdomen soft with active bowel sounds. Last gynecological exam was 8 months ago and completely normal. LMP 14 days ago, periods are for the most part regular at an interval of 23-24 days. She is S/P left salpingectomy for ectopic pregnancy 15 years ago with tubal ligation on the right at the time of that surgery. Patient is sexually active with her boyfriend and reports no change in libido or diminished pleasure from intercourse. There have been no changes in her bowel or bladder habits. She has trouble discerning both sharp and dull sensation on the labia from the level of the urethral meatus through the perineum and anus, extending to the right buttocks and mid posterior right thigh. Tone is 5/5 on left leg, 4/5 on right with 3+ reflexes on left and 2+ on right. Mild, intermittent muscle fasciculation noted in right buttocks. No muscle atrophy, rigidity, resistance or tenderness noted in lower extremities. She has difficulty maintaining leg lift on right with very mild drift from midline. Gait is normal.

Impression: **Radiculitis, sacral region.**

Plan: MRI of lumbar spine and sacrum is scheduled. Patient is instructed to have fasting blood drawn for CBC w/diff, comprehensive metabolic panel, Thyroid panel, Lipid panel, Vitamin D3, Vitamin B panel. Follow up appointment in 1 week to review test results. Consider referral to neurologist for EMG at that time.

Diagnosis Code(s)

M54.18 Radiculopathy, sacral and sacrococcygeal region

Coding Note(s)

To identify radiculitis, instructions in the Alphabetic Index under radiculitis state to see radiculopathy. Under radiculopathy, the code is found based upon the location or causation. There is a specific code for radiculopathy of the sacral and sacrococcygeal region.

Rupture of Tendon, Nontraumatic

Nontraumatic ruptures of tendons occur most often in the elderly, particularly in patients with other risk factors such as corticosteroid use and/or use of certain antibiotics, particularly quinolones. Codes are specific to site, such as shoulder, upper arm, forearm, hand, thigh, lower leg, ankle and foot; and to action such as extensor, flexor, and other tendon. Because physicians may name the tendon, such as Achilles, and not the specific site and action such as lower leg flexor tendon, coders must become familiar with the muscles and tendons of the extremities and their action in order to assign the nontraumatic tendon rupture to the correct code. Muscles and tendon names are frequently based upon their action and location. Some of the terms related to muscles and tendons are listed below.

Abductor/Abduction – Abductor muscle(s) work to move a body part away from the midline (e.g., raising the arm).

Adductor/Adduction – Adductor muscle(s) work to bring a body part closer to the midline.

Circumduction – Circular or conical motion movement of a joint due to a composite action of flexion, abduction, extension and adduction in that order.

Dorsiflexion – Muscle(s) work to tip the upper surface of the foot (dorsum) toward the anterior leg, decreasing the angle between the foot and leg.

Elevation/Depression – Muscle(s) work to raise (elevate) a body part to a more superior level (shoulder shrug), then lower that body part to a more inferior position (depression).

Eversion/Inversion – Muscles work to obliquely rotate the foot along the medial side of the heel to the lateral side of the mid foot. With inversion, the sole of the foot is turned inward toward the opposite foot and in eversion, the sole of the foot is turned outward and away from the midline.

Extensor/Extension – An extensor muscle works to increase the angle between bones that converge at a joint. For example: straightening the elbow or knee and bending the wrist or spine backward. Muscles of the hand and foot often contain this function in their name (example: extensor digitorum).

Flexor/Flexion – A flexor muscle works to decrease the angle between bones that converge at a joint, for example bending the elbow or knee. Muscles of the hand and foot may contain this function in their name (example: flexor carpi radialis, flexor hallucis longus).

Insertion – Attachment of the muscle or tendon to the skeletal area that the muscle moves when it contracts. The location is usually more distal on the bone with greater mobility and less mass when compared to the muscle origin point.

Opposition – Special muscle action of the hand in which the carpal/metacarpal bones in the thumb and fingers allow them to come together at their fingertips.

Origin – Muscle origin is the fixed attachment of muscle to bone. The location is usually more proximal on the bone with greater stability and mass when compared to the muscle insertion site allowing the muscle to exert power when it contracts.

Plantar Flexion – Muscle(s) work to tip the lower surface of the foot (sole, plantar area) downward, increasing the angle between the foot and anterior leg.

Pronation/Supination – Special muscle action of the forearm in which the radius crosses over the ulna resulting in the dorsal surface of the hand turning forward or prone (pronation, palm down). When the radius uncrosses, the palmer surface of the hand returns to its normal supine forward position (supination, palm up).

Protraction/Retraction – Muscle(s) work to move a body part forward (protraction), for example hunching of shoulders, then backward (retraction) when shoulders are squared.

Rotation – A movement that occurs around the vertical or longitudinal axis moving the body part toward or away from the center axis. Lateral/external rotation moves the anterior surface away from the midline. Medial/internal rotation moves the anterior surface toward the midline of the body.

The table that follows identifies a number of specific muscles and tendons of the extremities, the location of the muscle (e.g., upper/lower extremity, upper/lower leg, upper/lower arm), a brief description of the muscle or tendon, the origin and insertion, and the action. When coding it is important to know the location of the rupture since many muscles/tendons cover multiple sites. The table is organized alphabetically by tendon/muscle. Following the table is a documentation and coding example.

Muscle/Tendon	Location	Origin (O)/Insertion (I)	Action
Abductor pollicis brevis	Wrist/Hand/Thumb	O: Transverse carpal ligament and the tubercle of the scaphoid bone or (occasionally) the tubercle of the trapezium I: Base of the proximal phalanx of the thumb	Abducts the thumb and with muscles of the thenar eminence, acts to oppose the thumb
Abductor pollicis longus (APL)	Forearm/Thumb/Hand/Wrist	O: Posterior radius, posterior ulna and interosseous membrane I: Base 1st metacarpal Combined with the extensor pollicis brevis makes the anatomic snuff box.	Abducts and extends thumb at CMC joint; assists wrist abduction (radial deviation)
Achilles tendon	Lower Leg	O: Joins the gastrocnemius and soleus muscles I: Calcaneus	Flexor tendon – plantar flexes foot
Anconeus	Elbow	O: Lateral epicondyle humerus I: Posterior olecranon	Extends forearm
Brachialis	Elbow	O: Distal ½ anterior humeral shaft I: Coronoid process and ulnar tuberosity	Flexes forearm
Biceps brachii	Shoulder/Upper Arm	Long Head: O: Supraglenoid tubercle of the scapula to join the biceps tendon, short head in the middle of the humerus forming the biceps muscle belly Short Head: O: Coracoid process at the top of the scapula I: Radial tuberosity Long head and short head join in the middle of the humerus forming the biceps muscle belly	Flexes elbow Supinates forearm Weakly assists shoulder with forward flexion (long head) Short head provides horizontal adduction to stabilize shoulder joint and resist dislocation. With elbow flexed becomes a powerful supinator
Common flexor tendon 1. Pronator teres 2. Flexor carpi radialis (FCR) 3. Palmaris longus 4. Flexor digitorum superficialis (sublimis) (FDS) 5. Flexor carpi ulnaris (FCU)	Forearm/Hand	Common flexor tendon formed by 5 muscles of the forearm. There are slight variations in the site of origin and insertion 1. O: Medial epicondyle humerus and coronoid process of the ulna. I: Mid-lateral surface radial shaft 2. O: Medial epicondyle humerus. I: Base of 2nd and 3rd metacarpal 3. O: Medial epicondyle humerus. I: Palmar aponeurosis and flexor retinaculum 4. O: Medial epicondyle humerus, coronoid process ulna and anterior oblique line of radius. I: shaft middle phalanx digits 2-5 5. O: Medial epicondyle of the humerus, olecranon and posterior border ulna I: Pisiform, hook of hamate and 5th metacarpal.	1. Pronator Teres-pronation of forearm; assists elbow flexion 2. FCR- flexion and abduction of wrist (radial deviation) 3. Palmaris longus-assists wrist flexion 4. FDS- flexion middle phalanx PIP joint digits 2-4; assists wrist flexion 5. FCU- flexes and adducts hand at the wrist
Coracobrachialis	Shoulder/Upper Arm	O: Coracoid process I: Midshaft of humerus	Adducts & flexes shoulder
Deltoid	Shoulder/Upper Arm	O: Lateral 1/3 of clavicle, acromion and spine of scapula I: Deltoid tuberosity of humerus Large triangular shaped muscle composed of three parts	Anterior-Flex & medially rotate shoulder; Middle-assist w/abduction of humerus at shoulder; Posterior-extend & laterally rotate humerus
Extensor carpi radialis longus (ECRL)	Forearm/Hand	O: Lateral epicondyle humerus I: Dorsal surface 2nd metacarpal	Extends and abducts wrist; active during fist clenching
Extensor (digitorum) communis (EDC)	Forearm/Wrist/Hand/Finger	O: Lateral epicondyle humerus terminates into 4 tendons in the hand I: On the lateral and dorsal surfaces of digits 2-5 (fingers)	Extends the metacarpophalangeal (MCP), proximal interphalangeal (PIP) and distal interphalangeal (DIP) joints of 2nd-5th fingers and wrist

Muscle/Tendon	Location	Origin (O)/Insertion (I)	Action
Extensor digitorum longus (EDL)	Lower Leg/Ankle/Foot	O: Lateral condyle tibia, proximal 2/3 anterior fibula shaft and interosseous membrane I: Middle and distal phalanx toes 2-5	Extension lateral 4 digits at metatarsophalangeal joint; assists dorsiflexion of foot at ankle
Extensor hallicus longus (EHL)	Lower Leg/Ankle/Foot	O: Middle part anterior surface fibula and interosseous membrane I: Dorsal aspect base distal phalanx great toe	Extends great toe; assists dorsiflexion of foot at ankle; weak invertor
Extensor pollicis brevis (EPB)	Wrist/Hand/Thumb	O: Distal radius (dorsal surface) and interosseous membrane I: Base proximal phalanx thumb Combined with the abductor pollicis longus makes the anatomic snuff box	Extends the thumb at metacarpophalangeal joint (MCPJ)
Extensor pollicis longus (EPL)	Wrist/Hand/Thumb	O: Dorsal surface of the ulna and interosseous membrane I: Base distal phalanx thumb	Extends distal phalanx thumb at IP joint; assists wrist abduction
Flexor digitorum longus (FDL)	Lower Leg/Ankle/Foot	O: Medial posterior tibia shaft I: Base distal phalanx digits 2-5	Flexes digits 2-5; plantar flex ankle; supports longitudinal arch of foot
Flexor digitorum profundus (FDP)	Forearm/Wrist/Hand	O: Proximal 1/3 anterior-medial surface ulna and interosseous membrane; in the hand splits into 4 tendons I: Base of the distal phalanx, digits 2-5 (fingers)	Flexes the distal phalanx, digits 2-5 (fingers)
Flexor hallucis longus (FHL)	Lower Leg/Ankle/Foot	O: Inferior 2/3 posterior fibula; inferior interosseous membrane I: Base distal phalanx great toe (hallux)	Flexes great toe at all joints; weakly plantar flexes ankle; supports medial longitudinal arches of foot
Flexor pollicis brevis (FPB)	Wrist/Hand/Thumb	O: Distal edge of the transverse carpal ligament and the tubercle of the trapezium I: Proximal phalanx of the thumb	Flexes the thumb at the metacarpophalangeal (MCPJ) and carpometacarpal (CMC) joint
Flexor pollicis longus (FPL)	Forearm/Wrist/Hand/Thumb	O: Below the radial tuberosity on the anterior surface of the radius and interosseous membrane I: Base distal phalanx thumb	Flexes the thumb at the metacarpophalangeal (MCPJ) and interphalangeal (IPJ) joint
Hamstring	Upper Leg/Knee	Composed of three muscles 1. Semitendinosus O: Ischial tuberosity I: Anterior proximal tibial shaft Semimembranosus O: Ischial tuberosity I: Posterior medial tibial condyle 2. Biceps femoris O: Long head ischial tuberosity; short head linea aspera femoral shaft and lateral supracondylar line I: Head of fibula	1. Semitendinosus and Semimembranosus- Flexes leg at knee, when knee flexed medially rotates tibia; thigh extensor at hip joint; when hip & knee both flexed, extends trunk 2. Biceps femoris-Flexes leg and rotates laterally when knee flexed; extends thigh
Intrinsics of hand hypothenar 1. Abductor digiti minimi 2. Flexor digiti minimi brevis 3. Opponens digiti minimi	Wrist/Hand/Finger	1. O: Pisiform I: Medial side of base proximal phalanx 5th finger 2. O: Hook of hamate & flexor retinaculum I: Medial side of base proximal phalanx 5th finger 3. O: Hook of hamate and transverse carpal ligament I: Uulnar aspect shaft 5th metacarpal	1. Abducts 5th finger; assists flexion proximal phalanx 2. Flexes proximal phalanx 5th finger 3. Rotates the 5th metacarpal bone forward

Muscle/Tendon	Location	Origin (O)/Insertion (I)	Action
Intrinsics of hand short 1. Dorsal interossei 1-4 2. Dorsal interossei 1-3 3. Lumbricals 1st & 2nd 4. Lumbricals 3rd & 4th	Wrist/Hand	1. O: Adjacent sides of 2 MC I: Bases of proximal phalanges; extensor expansions of 2-4 fingers 2. O: Palmar surface 2nd, 4th & 5th MC I: Bases of proximal phalanges; extensor expansions of 2nd, 4th & 5th fingers 3. O: Lateral two tendons of FDP I: Lateral sides of extensor expansion of 2nd-5th 4. O: Medial 3 tendons of FDP I: Lateral sides of extensor expansion of 2nd-5th	1. Abduct 2-4 fingers from axial line; acts w/lumbricals to flex MCP jt and extend IP jt 2. Adduct 2nd, 4th, 5th fingers from axial line; assist lumbricals to flex MCP jt and extend IP jt; extensor expansions of 2nd-4th fingers 3. Flex MCP jt; extend IP joint 2-5 4. Flex MCP jt; extend IP joint 2-5
Intrinsics of hand thenar 1. Abductor pollicis brevis 2. Adductor pollicis 3. Flexor pollicis brevis 4. Opponens pollicis	Wrist/Hand/Thumb	1. O: Flexor retinaculum & tubercle scaphoid & trapezium I: :Lateral side of base of proximal phalanx thumb 2. O: Oblique head base 2nd & 3rd MC, capitate, adjacent carpals and transverse head anterior surface shaft 3rd MC I: Medial side base of proximal phalanx thumb 3. O: Flexor retinaculum & tubercle scaphoid & trapezium I: Lateral side of base of proximal phalanx thumb 4. O: Transverse carpal ligament and the tubercle of the trapezium I: Lateral border shaft 1st metacarpal	1. Abducts thumb; helps w/opposition 2. Adducts thumb toward lateral border of palm 3. Flexes thumb 4. Rotates the thumb in opposition with fingers
Lumbricals (foot)	Foot	O: Lumbricals-flexor digitorum longus tendon I: Medial side base proximal phalanges 2-5	Assist in joint movement between metatarsals
Patellar tendon	Knee/Lower Leg	Connects the bottom of the patella to the top of the tibia The tendon is actually a ligament because it joins bone to bone	Works with the quadriceps tendon to bend and straighten the knee
Pectoralis major	Chest/Upper Arm	O: Clavicle, sternum, ribs 2-6 I: Upper shaft of humerus	Adducts, flexes, medially rotates humerus
Peroneus (fibularis) brevis	Lower Leg/Ankle/Foot	O: Distal 2/3 lateral shaft fibula I: Becomes a tendon midcalf that runs behind the lateral malleolus inserts on tuberosity base 5th metatarsal	Eversion of foot; assists with plantar flexion of foot at ankle
Peroneus (fibularis) longus	Lower Leg/Ankle/Foot	O: Head and upper 2/3 lateral surface fibula I: Becomes a long tendon midcalf that runs behind the lateral malleolus and crosses obliquely on plantar surface of foot inserts on base 1st metatarsal and medial cuneiform	Eversion of foot; weak plantar flexion foot at ankle
Peroneus (fibularis) tertius	Lower Leg/Ankle/Foot	O: Inferior 1/3 anterior surface fibula and interosseous membrane I: Dorsum base 5th metatarsal	Dorsiflexes ankle and aids inversion of foot
Quadratus plantae	Foot	O: Calcaneus I: Flexor digitorum tendons	Assists flexor muscles

Muscle/Tendon	Location	Origin (O)/Insertion (I)	Action
Quadriceps femoris	Upper Leg/Knee	Composed of four muscles: Rectus femoris O: Anterior inferior iliac spine and ilium superior to acetabulum I: Combines to form quadriceps tendon; inserts base of patella and tibial tuberosity via patellar ligament Vastus lateralis O: Greater trochanter and lateral aspect femoral shaft I: Lateral patella and tendon of rectus femoris Vastus medialis O: Intertrochanteric line and medial aspect femoral shaft I: Medial border of quadriceps tendon and medial aspect of patella; tibial tuberosity via patellar ligament Vastus intermedius: O: Anterior and lateral surface femoral shaft I: Posterior surface upper border of patella; tibial tuberosity via patellar ligament	Extends leg at knee joint; rectus femoris with iliopsoas helps flex thigh and stabilized hip joint
Quadriceps tendon	Upper Leg/Knee	Fibrous band of tissue that connects the quadriceps muscle of the anterior thigh to the patella (kneecap)	Holds the patella (kneecap) in the patellofemoral groove of the femur enabling it to act as a fulcrum and provide power to bend and straighten the knee
Rotator cuff tendons: 1. Supraspinatus 2. Infraspinatus 3. Teres minor 4. Subscapularis	Shoulder/Upper Arm	Rotator cuff tendons are formed by 4 muscles of the shoulder/upper arm. They all originate from the scapula and insert (terminate) on the humerus: 1. O: Supraspinous fossa of scapula. I: Superior facet greater tuberosity humerus. 2. O: Infraspinous fossa of scapula. I: Middle facet greater tuberosity humerus. 3. O: Middle half of the lateral border of the scapula. I: Inferior facet greater tuberosity humerus 4. O: Subscapular fossa of scapula. I: Either the lesser tuberosity humerus or the humeral neck.	1. Initiates abduction of shoulder joint (completed by deltoid) 2. Externally rotates the arm; helps hold humeral head in glenoid cavity 3. Externally rotates the arm; helps hold humeral head in glenoid cavity 4. Internally rotates and adducts the humerus; helps hold humeral head in glenoid cavity
Tibialis anterior	Lower Leg/Ankle/Foot	O: Lateral condyle and superior half lateral tibia I: Base 1st metatarsal, plantar surface medial cuneiform	Dorsiflexion ankle, foot inversion at subtalar and midtarsal joints
Tibialis posterior	Lower Leg/Ankle/Foot	O: Interosseus membrane; posterior surface of tibia and fibula I: Tuberosity of tarsal navicula, cuneiform and cuboid and bases of 2nd, 3rd and 4th metatarsals	Plantar flexes ankle; inverts foot
Triceps	Shoulder/Upper Arm	Long head: O: Infraglenoid tubercle of scapula; Lateral head: O: Upper half of posterior surface shaft of humerus Medial head O: Lower half of posterior surface shaft of humerus I: Olecranon process Only muscle on the back of the arm	Extends elbow joint; long head can adduct humerus and extend it from flexed position; stabilizes shoulder joint

Except for nontraumatic tears of the rotator cuff which are captured in subcategory M75.1, codes for nontraumatic tendon tears are found in subcategories M66.2-M66.8 and are defined as spontaneous rupture.

Coding and Documentation Requirements

Identify rupture as not related to injury or trauma.

Identify site of nontraumatic tendon rupture:

- Upper extremity
  - Shoulder
  - Upper arm
  - Forearm
  - Hand
- Lower extremity
  - Thigh
  - Lower leg
  - Ankle/foot
- Other site
- Multiple sites
- Unspecified tendon

Identify action of tendon:

- Extensor
- Flexor
- Other

ICD-10-CM Code/Documentation	
M66.221	Spontaneous rupture of extensor tendons, right upper arm
M66.222	Spontaneous rupture of extensor tendons, left upper arm
M66.229	Spontaneous rupture of extensor tendons, unspecified upper arm
M66.311	Spontaneous rupture of flexor tendons, right shoulder
M66.312	Spontaneous rupture of flexor tendons, left shoulder
M66.319	Spontaneous rupture of flexor tendons, unspecified shoulder
M66.321	Spontaneous rupture of flexor tendons, right upper arm
M66.322	Spontaneous rupture of flexor tendons, left upper arm
M66.329	Spontaneous rupture of flexor tendons, left upper arm
M66.231	Spontaneous rupture of extensor tendons, right forearm
M66.232	Spontaneous rupture of extensor tendons, left forearm
M66.239	Spontaneous rupture of extensor tendons, unspecified forearm
M66.241	Spontaneous rupture of extensor tendons, right hand
M66.242	Spontaneous rupture of extensor tendons, left hand
M22.249	Spontaneous rupture of extensor tendons, unspecified hand
M66.331	Spontaneous rupture of flexor tendons, right forearm
M66.332	Spontaneous rupture of flexor tendons, left forearm
M66.339	Spontaneous rupture of flexor tendons, unspecified forearm
M66.341	Spontaneous rupture of flexor tendons, right hand
M66.342	Spontaneous rupture of flexor tendons, left hand
M66.349	Spontaneous rupture of flexor tendons, unspecified hand

ICD-10-CM Code/Documentation	
M66.251	Spontaneous rupture of extensor tendons, right thigh
M66.252	Spontaneous rupture of extensor tendons, left thigh
M66.259	Spontaneous rupture of extensor tendons, unspecified thigh
M66.261	Spontaneous rupture of extensor tendons, right lower leg
M66.262	Spontaneous rupture of extensor tendons, left lower leg
M66.269	Spontaneous rupture of extensor tendons, unspecified lower leg
M66.361	Spontaneous rupture flexor tendons, right lower leg
M66.362	Spontaneous rupture flexor tendons, left lower leg
M66.369	Spontaneous rupture flexor tendons, unspecified lower leg
M66.271	Spontaneous rupture of extensor tendons, right ankle and foot
M66.272	Spontaneous rupture of extensor tendons, left ankle and foot
M66.279	Spontaneous rupture of extensor tendons, unspecified ankle and foot
M66.371	Spontaneous rupture of flexor tendons, right ankle and foot
M66.372	Spontaneous rupture of flexor tendons, left ankle and foot
M66.379	Spontaneous rupture of flexor tendons, unspecified ankle and foot
M66.28	Spontaneous rupture of extensor tendons, other site
M66.29	Spontaneous rupture of extensor tendons, multiple sites
M66.351	Spontaneous rupture of flexor tendons, right thigh
M66.352	Spontaneous rupture of flexor tendons, left thigh
M66.359	Spontaneous rupture of flexor tendons, unspecified thigh
M66.38	Spontaneous rupture of flexor tendons, other site
M66.39	Spontaneous rupture of flexor tendons, multiple sites

Documentation and Coding Example

Eighty-one-year-old Caucasian female is brought into ED by EMS after she awoke this morning with bilateral ankle swelling and pain that prevented her from getting out of bed. Patient resides alone and is able to drive and care completely for herself. She was in her usual state of good health until approximately two weeks ago when she became acutely ill with fever, malaise, and cough. She is fastidious about obtaining an annual flu vaccine so she attributed her symptoms to a summer cold. When her cough became productive and was accompanied by wheezing, she visited her PMD who obtained a CXR which showed left lower lobe infiltrates and was subsequently prescribed Advair Inhaler BID, Levaquin 5ØØ mg BID, and albuterol inhaler prn. She has been on these medications for 6 days and is just beginning to have some energy. She saw her PMD yesterday and a repeat CXR showed improvement. She noticed some stiffness in her right ankle last evening and dismissed it as simply muscle disuse but was dismayed this morning when both ankles were swollen and painful and she was unable to walk. She called her daughter who came right over and PMD advised transfer to ED by EMS. On examination, this is an anxious but pleasant octogenarian who looks younger than her stated age. She is alert and oriented x 3 and an excellent historian. T 96.1, P 8Ø, R 18, BP 114/84 O2 Sat on RA is 96%. She states she is widowed x 2Ø years. Her husband was in the diplomatic service and they traveled extensively. After his death she become somewhat of a celebrity by authoring a series of books on cooking and culinary adventure. Travel immunizations are current and her last trip was 3 months ago to Belize. She swims and/or walks daily and has had no recent injuries that she can recall. Heart rate shows SR on monitor with occasional benign PVCs. No audible murmur, bruit, or rubs are appreciated. Breath sounds have scattered wheezes with slightly decreased sounds in the left base. Abdomen soft, non-distended. Cranial nerves grossly intact and upper extremities WNL. Hips and knees are without swelling or pain and ROM is intact. There is a moderate amount of circumferential swelling in each ankle. No redness, bruising, or discoloration noted. Unable to adequately palpate along the Achilles tendon due to swelling and discomfort but a gap may be present 3-4 cm above heel on the right. Neurovascular status of feet and toes is unremarkable. Passive ROM to ankles elicits considerable pain and she is unable to actively plantar flex. Thompson's sign is positive as is Homan's. Given her recent illness and immobility, venous Doppler study is performed and DVT is ruled out. **MRI of bilateral ankles was obtained which is significant for Achilles rupture 4.5 cm proximal to calcaneal insertion site on the right and 6 cm proximal on the left.** There is no evidence of pre-existing tendinopathy in either extremity.

Impression: **Non-traumatic bilateral Achilles tendon rupture** possibly due to fluoroquinolone and steroid use.

Plan: Discontinue Levaquin® and Advair® and admit to orthopedic service.

Diagnosis Code(s)

M66.361 Spontaneous rupture flexor tendons right lower leg

M66.362 Spontaneous rupture flexor tendons left lower leg

Coding Note(s)

Nontraumatic ruptures of the tendon are defined by their action, not the specific tendon. The Achilles tendon is a flexor tendon in the lower leg. Laterality is a component of the code and so separate codes for right and left are reported since there is not a bilateral code. The documentation states that the tendon ruptures are "possibly" due to the fluoroquinolone and steroid use. Because the qualifier "possibly" is used, this would not be coded as an adverse effect for the ED encounter; however, it may be appropriate to code the adverse effect if the discharge summary also lists these medications as the cause or possible cause of the tendon ruptures.

Scoliosis

Scoliosis is an abnormal sideways curvature in the spine. The condition may be congenital (present at birth) or develop later in life, usually around the time of puberty. Congenital scoliosis is usually caused by vertebral anomalies. Other causes can include neuromuscular disorders (cerebral palsy, spinal muscular atrophy), trauma, and certain syndromes (Marfan's, Prader-Willi). In the majority of cases, no cause can be found and the condition is termed idiopathic. Scoliosis can decrease lung capacity, place pressure on the heart and large blood vessels in the chest, and may restrict physical activity.

Codes for scoliosis are listed in category M41. Codes are classified as idiopathic, thoracogenic, neuromuscular, other secondary scoliosis, other forms of scoliosis, and unspecified scoliosis. Codes for idiopathic scoliosis are categorized based on age at diagnosis as infantile (from birth through age 4), juvenile (ages 5 through 9 years), and adolescent (ages 11 through 17 years). There is also a subcategory for other idiopathic scoliosis. In addition, the site of curvature must be documented as cervical, cervicothoracic, thoracic, thoracolumbar, lumbar, or lumbosacral. These codes are not reported for congenital scoliosis which is reported with a code from Chapter 17 Congenital Malformations, Deformations, and Chromosomal Abnormalities.

Coding and Documentation Requirements

Identify type of scoliosis:

- Idiopathic
  - Infantile
  - Juvenile
  - Adolescent
  - Other
- Secondary
  - Neuromuscular
  - Other
- Thoracogenic
- Other form
- Unspecified

Identify site:

- Cervical
- Cervicothoracic
- Thoracic
- Thoracolumbar
- Lumbar
- Lumbosacral
- Sacral/sacrococcygeal (only applies to infantile idiopathic scoliosis)
- Site unspecified

Idiopathic Scoliosis

ICD-10-CM Code/Documentation	
Juvenile	
M41.112	Juvenile idiopathic scoliosis, cervical region
M41.113	Juvenile idiopathic scoliosis, cervicothoracic region
M41.114	Juvenile idiopathic scoliosis, thoracic region
M41.115	Juvenile idiopathic scoliosis, thoracolumbar region
M41.116	Juvenile idiopathic scoliosis, lumbar region
M41.117	Juvenile idiopathic scoliosis, lumbosacral region
M41.119	Juvenile idiopathic scoliosis, site unspecified
Adolescent	
M41.122	Adolescent idiopathic scoliosis, cervical region
M41.123	Adolescent idiopathic scoliosis, cervicothoracic region

M41.124	Adolescent idiopathic scoliosis, thoracic region
M41.125	Adolescent idiopathic scoliosis, thoracolumbar region
M41.126	Adolescent idiopathic scoliosis, lumbar region
M41.127	Adolescent idiopathic scoliosis, lumbosacral region
M41.129	Adolescent idiopathic scoliosis, site unspecified
Other	
M41.20	Other idiopathic scoliosis, site unspecified
M41.22	Other idiopathic scoliosis, cervical region
M41.23	Other idiopathic scoliosis, cervicothoracic region
M41.24	Other idiopathic scoliosis, thoracic region
M41.25	Other idiopathic scoliosis, thoracolumbar region
M41.26	Other idiopathic scoliosis, lumbar region
M41.27	Other idiopathic scoliosis, lumbosacral region
Infantile	
M41.00	Infantile idiopathic scoliosis, site unspecified
M41.02	Infantile idiopathic scoliosis, cervical region
M41.03	Infantile idiopathic scoliosis, cervicothoracic region
M41.04	Infantile idiopathic scoliosis, thoracic region
M41.05	Infantile idiopathic scoliosis, thoracolumbar region
M41.06	Infantile idiopathic scoliosis, lumbar region
M41.07	Infantile idiopathic scoliosis, lumbosacral region
M41.08	Infantile idiopathic scoliosis, sacral and sacrococcygeal region

Documentation and Coding Example

Twelve-year-old Hispanic female is referred to Pediatric Orthopedic Clinic by PMD for suspected scoliosis. She was initially noted to have a **right thoracic curve of 7 degrees** during routine screening by her school nurse. Patient was subsequently seen by her **pediatrician who examined her and obtained x-rays that indeed supported the school screening results.** PMH is significant for allergies and asthma well controlled with Singulair 5 mg daily, Xopenex inhaler only occasionally for symptoms. She also uses topical hydrocortisone for eczema PRN. On examination, this is a thin but well-nourished adolescent female, developmentally a Tanner II-III. Upper and lower reflexes intact, abdominal reflex pattern normal. Right shoulder is rotated forward and medial border of right scapula protrudes posteriorly. Examination of lower extremities shows negative hamstring tightness and a 1 cm length discrepancy. No ataxia and negative Romberg. Radiographs viewed on computer with parent and patient and are significant for a **30 degree right thoracic curve.** Diagnosis and treatment options discussed and questions answered. Patient will be fitted with a brace to be worn 16 hours a day. RTC in 3 months for repeat x-rays and examination.

Diagnosis Code(s)

M41.124 Adolescent idiopathic scoliosis, thoracic region

Coding Note(s)

In order to assign the most specific code for idiopathic scoliosis, the age of the patient and the site of the curvature must be documented.

Spondylosis

Spondylosis is stiffening or fixation of the vertebral joint(s) with fibrous or bony union across the joint resulting from age or a disease process. Spondylosis affects the vertebrae, intervertebral disc, and soft tissues of the spine. The condition may be complicated by spinal cord dysfunction, also referred to as myelopathy, resulting from narrowing of the spinal column and compression of the spinal cord. Spondylosis may also cause radiculopathy which is a general term for pain resulting from compression of a nerve. There are a number of very similar terms for conditions affecting the spine. Do not confuse spondylosis with spondylosis which is a degenerative or developmental deficiency of a portion of the vertebra, commonly involving the pars interarticularis. Careful review of the documentation is required to ensure that the correct code is assigned.

Category M47 contains codes for spondylosis. This category includes conditions documented as arthrosis or osteoarthritis of the spine and degeneration of the facet joints. There are subcategories for anterior spinal artery compression syndromes (M47.Ø1) and vertebral artery compression syndromes (M47.Ø2). Combination codes exist for spondylosis with myelopathy (M47.1-) and with radiculopathy (M47.2-). Spondylosis without myelopathy or radiculopathy is reported with codes from subcategory (M47.81-). There is also a subcategory for other specified spondylosis (M47.89) and a single code for spondylosis unspecified (M47.9). Codes are specific to the following regions of the spine: occipito-atlanto-axial (occiput to 2nd cervical), cervical, cervicothoracic (6th cervical to 1st thoracic), thoracic, thoracolumbar (1Øth thoracic to 1st lumbar), lumbar, lumbosacral (5 lumbar and 5 sacral), and sacral/sacrococcygeal.

Coding and Documentation Requirements

Identify condition:

- Anterior spinal artery compression syndrome
- Vertebral artery compression syndrome
- Spondylosis
  - with myelopathy
  - with radiculopathy
  - without myelopathy or radiculopathy
  - Other specified type
  - Unspecified

Identify site:

- Occipito-atlanto-axial region
- Cervical region
- Cervicothoracic region
- Thoracic region
- Thoracolumbar region

- Lumbar region
- Lumbosacral region
- Sacral/sacrococcygeal region
- Unspecified site

ICD-10-CM Code/Documentation	
M47.016	Anterior spinal artery compression syndromes, lumbar region
M47.26	Other spondylosis with radiculopathy, lumbar region
M47.27	Other spondylosis with radiculopathy, lumbosacral region
M47.28	Other spondylosis with radiculopathy, sacral and sacrococcygeal region
M47.816	Spondylosis without myelopathy or radiculopathy, lumbar region
M47.817	Spondylosis without myelopathy or radiculopathy, lumbosacral region
M47.818	Spondylosis without myelopathy or radiculopathy, sacral and sacrococcygeal region
M47.896	Other spondylosis, lumbar region
M47.897	Other spondylosis, lumbosacral region
M47.898	Other spondylosis, sacral and sacrococcygeal region
M47.16	Other spondylosis with myelopathy, lumbar region

Documentation and Coding Example

Fifty-eight-year-old Caucasian male presents to Occupational Medicine for routine physical. Patient is a long distance truck driver x 2Ø years. His only complaints are more frequent need to urinate and some mild low back pain and paresthesia in his left thigh. T 98.8, P 78, R 14, BP 138/88, Ht. 7Ø inches, Wt. 155 lbs. Vision is 2Ø/3Ø with glasses. Hearing by audiometry is WNL. EKG shows NSR without ectopy. On examination, PERRL, neck supple without lymphadenopathy. Nares patent, oral mucosa, pharynx moist and pink. Cranial nerves grossly intact. Neuromuscular exam of upper extremities unremarkable. Heart rate regular without bruit, rub, murmur. Breath sounds clear, equal bilaterally. Spinal column straight with mild tenderness in lumbar/sacral area. Abdomen soft, active bowel sounds. No evidence of hernia, testicles smooth. Circumcised penis is without discharge. Good sphincter tone on rectal exam, smooth, slightly enlarged prostate. Good ROM in lower extremities. Gait normal. Reflexes intact. Leg lifts do not produce pain. Sensation, both dull and sharp is reduced from lateral aspect to midline anterior of left thigh starting 4 cm below the hip ending 2 cm above the knee. He describes a prickling or tingling sensation at times over that entire area. Radiographs of spine obtained and reveal bony overgrowth on vertebral bodies L1-L4 and mild narrowing of the disc space. No disc protrusion is seen.

Impression: **Lumbar spondylosis with radiculopathy involving L1-L4.**

Plan: Occupational/Physical therapy evaluation and 12 treatments authorized. Risk management to evaluate his truck drivers seat for possible modifications after he is seen by OT/PT and recommendations are made. RTC in 4 weeks, sooner if symptoms worsen.

Diagnosis Code(s)

M47.26 Other spondylosis with radiculopathy, lumbar region

Coding Note(s)

There is a combination code that captures spondylosis, which is the disease process, and radiculopathy which is a common symptom of spondylosis.

Stress Fracture

A stress fracture is a small crack or break in a bone that arises from unusual or repeated force or overuse in an area of the body, most commonly the lower legs and feet. Symptoms include generalized pain and tenderness. When a stress fracture occurs in the lower extremity, pain and tenderness may increase with weight bearing. The pain may also be more pronounced at the beginning of exercise, decrease during the activity, and then increase again at the end of the workout.

There are specific codes for stress fractures of the pelvis and extremities as well as for stress fractures of the vertebrae. Stress fractures of the vertebrae are referred to as fatigue fractures with the alternate term stress fracture also listed. Fatigue fractures of the vertebrae are located in subcategory M48.4 and codes are specific to the region of the spine. There is also a subcategory (M48.5) for collapsed vertebra which may also be documented as wedging of vertebra. Codes for collapsed vertebra are not used to report fatigue fractures, pathological fractures due to neoplasm, osteoporosis or other pathological condition, or for traumatic fractures. Codes for stress fractures of other sites are located in subcategory M84.3 and codes are specific to site and also require documentation of laterality.

Coding and Documentation Requirements

For stress fracture of pelvis/extremity identify:

- Site
  - Lower extremity
    - Femur
    - Tibia
    - Fibula
    - Ankle
    - Foot
    - Toe(s)
  - Pelvis
  - Upper extremity
    - Shoulder
    - Humerus
    - Radius
    - Ulna
    - Hand
    - Finger(s)
- Laterality (not required for pelvis)
  - Right
  - Left
  - Unspecified

- Episode of care
  - Initial encounter
  - Subsequent encounter
    - » With routine healing
    - » With delayed healing
    - » With nonunion
    - » With malunion
  - Sequela

For fatigue fracture/collapsed vertebra, identify:

- Type
  - Fatigue fracture
  - Collapsed vertebra (wedging)
- Site/region of spine
  - Occipito-atlanto-axial region
  - Cervical
  - Cervicothoracic
  - Thoracic
  - Thoracolumbar
  - Lumbar
  - Lumbosacral
  - Sacral/sacrococcygeal
  - Unspecified site
- Episode of care
  - Initial encounter
  - Subsequent encounter
    - » With routine healing
    - » With delayed healing
  - Sequela

Stress Fracture Ankle/Foot/Toes

ICD-10-CM Code/Documentation	
M84.371-	Stress fracture, right ankle
M84.372-	Stress fracture, left ankle
M84.373-	Stress fracture, unspecified ankle
M84.374-	Stress fracture, right foot
M84.375-	Stress fracture, left foot
M84.376-	Stress fracture, unspecified foot
M84.377-	Stress fracture, right toe(s)
M84.378-	Stress fracture, left toe(s)
M84.379-	Stress fracture, unspecified toe(s)

Documentation and Coding Example

Patient is a twenty-eight-year-old Asian female who presents to Physiatrist with c/o right foot pain. She is well known to this practice as a member of a professional ballet company that we consult for. This petite, well nourished, graceful young woman is 3 months postdelivery of her first child. She retired from performing 2 years ago but has been teaching in the ballet school. She remained active during her pregnancy by taking ballet, Pilates, or yoga classes almost daily. She returned to teaching 2 months ago, usually assigned to upper level students 4 days a week. She noticed right mid-foot pain that radiated along the medial longitudinal arch one week after she returned to teaching. The pain increases with exercise and usually goes away with rest. For the past week she has noticed her shoes feel tight over that area but she has not noticed bruising or obvious swelling. On examination, there is mild dorsal foot swelling, pain with passive eversion and active inversion. Point tenderness is present at the mid medial arch and proximal to the dorsal portion of the navicular bone. X-ray obtained using a coned-down AP radiograph centered on the tarsal navicular which reveals a **small lateral fragment of the tarsal navicular bone.**

Impression: **Stress fracture of the right navicular.**

Plan: Walking boot x 6 weeks. Patient is advised to do non-weight bearing exercise only. RTC in 6 weeks for repeat x-ray and referral to PT.

Diagnosis Code(s)

M84.374A Stress fracture, right foot, initial encounter

Coding Note(s)

The tarsal navicular bone is one of the 7 tarsal bones of the foot. Under Fracture, traumatic, stress, tarsus in the Alphabetic Index, code M84.374- is identified as the correct code.

Section 2. Musculoskeletal System Summary

For the majority of connective tissue conditions and diseases of the musculoskeletal system specific documentation is required related to anatomic site and laterality. Episode of care is required for nontraumatic fractures (stress, pathologic and fractures related to osteoporosis). In addition, the need to clearly differentiate acute traumatic conditions from old or chronic conditions must be specified.

Section 2. Musculoskeletal System Resources

Documentation checklists are available in Appendix B for the following conditions:

- Burns, Corrosions, and Frostbite
- Diabetes Mellitus
- Fractures
- Gout
- Rheumatoid arthritis

Section 2. Musculoskeletal System Quiz

1. What condition below does not require documentation of episode of care?
   a. Collapsed vertebra
   b. Fatigue fracture of vertebra
   c. Unspecified disorder of bone continuity
   d. Stress fracture of foot

2. The ED physician has documented that an 82-year-old patient with severe senile osteoporosis sustained a left hip fracture from a same level fall on a carpeted surface. What code is reported for the fracture?
   a. M80.052A Age-related osteoporosis with current pathological fracture, left femur, initial encounter
   b. M80.852A Other osteoporosis with current pathological fracture, left femur, initial visit
   c. S72.002A Fracture of unspecified part of neck of left femur, initial encounter for closed fracture
   d. S72.065A Nondisplaced articular fracture of head of left femur, initial encounter for closed fracture

3. Identify which condition affecting the musculoskeletal system would generally not be reported with a code from Chapter 13.
   a. Healed injury
   b. Recurrent bone, joint or muscle condition
   c. Chronic conditions
   d. Current acute injury

4. The physician has documented that the patient has idiopathic osteonecrosis of the right femoral head. Since this condition affects the joint, what site is reported?
   a. The site is the joint
   b. The site is the bone
   c. The site is a combination code for the joint and the bone
   d. Two sites are reported identifying the bone and the joint

5. What condition is not reported with a code from Chapter 13?
   a. Arthropathic psoriasis
   b. Drug-induced gout
   c. Adhesive capsulitis of the shoulder
   d. Nontraumatic compartment syndrome

6. What condition would be reported with a code from subcategory M48.5- Collapsed vertebra?
   a. Current injury due to fatigue fracture
   b. New pathological fracture of vertebra due to neoplasm
   c. Wedging of vertebra
   d. Traumatic vertebral fracture

7. What information is NOT required to assign the most specific code for idiopathic scoliosis?
   a. Age of the patient at onset of the condition
   b. Location of the curve
   c. Affected region of the spine
   d. The specific form of scoliosis

8. Codes for osteoporosis in category M80 are specific to site. What does the site designate?
   a. The site of the osteoporosis and fracture
   b. The site of the osteoporosis
   c. The site of the fracture
   d. None of the above

9. Code M61.371 Calcification and ossification of muscles associated with burns, right ankle and foot is an example of what type of code?
   a. An injury code
   b. A combination code
   c. An episode of care code
   d. None of the above

10. What descriptor is not an example of site specificity?
    a. Mid-cervical region
    b. Achilles tendon
    c. Synovium
    d. First carpometacarpal joints

11. What information must be documented to assign the most specific code in category M1A Chronic gout that is not required for codes in category M10 Gout?
    a. With or without tophus
    b. Site
    c. Laterality
    d. All of the above

See end of chapter for answers and rationales.

Section 1. Nervous System Quiz Answers and Rationales

1. CRPS II is

   c. a type of neuropathic pain the occurs following a peripheral nerve injury resulting in burning or throbbing pain along the nerve, sensitivity to cold and touch, changes in skin color, temperature, texture, hair and nails

   Rationale: CRPS II or chronic regional pain syndrome is pain as a result of a direct injury to a nerve vs. RSD or CRPS I do not have to have a direct injury to a nerve. B is the definition for restless leg syndrome and d is the definition for neuropathy. For both CRPS I and CRPS II documentation of upper or lower extremity as well as laterality is required.

2. How are seizure disorders and recurrent seizures classified?

   a. Seizure disorders and recurrent seizures are classified with epilepsy

   Rationale: The Index entry for seizure disorder directs the user to see Epilepsy. Both Seizure disorder and recurrent seizures are indexed to G4Ø.9Ø9 Epilepsy, unspecified.

3. Which of the following is an alternate term for "intractable" migraine?

   d. All of the above

   Rationale: According to the instructional note under category G4Ø, the following terms are to be considered equivalent to intractable: pharmacoresistant (pharmacologically resistant), treatment resistant, refractory (medically), and poorly controlled.

4. Where are coding and sequencing guidelines for diseases of the nervous system and complications due to the treatment of the diseases and conditions of the nervous system found?

   b. In the Alphabetic Index and the Tabular List and the chapter specific guidelines for Chapter 6

   Rationale: the conventions and instructions of the classification along with the general and chapter-specific coding guidelines govern the selection and sequencing of ICD-1Ø-CM codes. According to Section I.A of the ICD-1Ø-CM coding guidelines, the conventions are the general rules for use of the classification independent of the guidelines. These conventions are incorporated within the Alphabetic Index and Tabular List of the ICD-1Ø-CM as instructional notes.

5. What is the correct code assignment for an encounter for treatment of a condition causing pain?

   c. A code for the underlying condition is assigned as the principal diagnosis and no code from category G89 is assigned.

   Rationale: According to the chapter specific coding guidelines for Chapter 6 of ICD-1Ø-CM, when an admission or encounter is for a procedure aimed at treating the underlying condition, a code for the underlying condition should be assigned as the principal diagnosis and no code from category G89 should be assigned.

6. Which of the following documentation is required for accurate coding of epilepsy?

   d. All of the above

   Rationale: Epilepsy is classified by the specific type and then as intractable or not intractable, and with or without status epilepticus. A note in lists the terms pharmacoresistant, pharmacologically resistant, poorly controlled, refractory, or treatment resistant as synonyms for intractable.

7. When an admission is for treatment of an underlying condition and a neurostimulator is also inserted for pain control during the same episode of care, what is the correct code assignment?

   a. The underlying condition is the principal diagnosis and the appropriate pain code should be assigned as a secondary diagnosis.

   Rationale: Section I.B.1.a of the ICD-1Ø-CM coding guidelines provides specific direction on coding Category G89 codes as principal diagnosis or the first-listed code. According to these guidelines, when a patient is admitted for a procedure aimed at treating the underlying condition and a neurostimulator is inserted for pain control during the same admission/encounter, a code for the underlying condition should be assigned as the principal diagnosis and the appropriate pain code should be assigned as a secondary diagnosis.

8. What is the proper sequencing for Alzheimer's disease with dementia?

   c. The Alzheimer's disease is coded first followed by a code for dementia with or without behavioral disturbance.

   Rationale: An instructional note at category G3Ø directs the coder to use an additional code to identify delirium, dementia with or without behavioral disturbance.

9. In patients with hemiplegia, if the affected side is documented but not specified as dominant or nondominant, how is this coded?

   d. All of the above

   Rationale: Section I.C.6.a of the ICD-1Ø-CM coding guidelines provides specific direction for cases where the affected side is documented, but not specified as dominant or nondominant. According to these guidelines, the default code is dominant for ambidextrous patients, nondominant when the left side is affected and dominant when the right side is affected.

10. What is the correct coding of a diagnosis documented as post-thoracotomy pain without further specification as acute or chronic?

    c. **The code for acute post-thoracotomy pain is the default**

    Rationale: According to Section I.C.6.b.3 of the ICD-10-CM coding guidelines, the default is the code for the acute form for post-thoracotomy pain when not specified as acute or chronic.

Section 2. Musculoskeletal System Quiz Answers and Rationales

1. What condition does not require documentation of episode of care?

    c. **Unspecified disorder of bone continuity**

    Rationale: Collapsed vertebra (M48.5-), fatigue fracture of vertebra (M48.4), and stress fracture of foot (M84.37-) all require documentation of episode of care. Unspecified disorder of bone continuity, even though it is also classified in category M84, does not require documentation episode of care.

2. The ED physician has documented that an 82-year-old patient with severe senile osteoporosis sustained a left hip fracture when he sustained a same level fall on a carpeted surface. What code is reported for the fracture?

    a. **M80.052A Age-related osteoporosis with current pathological fracture, left femur, initial encounter**

    Rationale: A code from category M80, not a traumatic fracture code, should be used for any patient with known osteoporosis who suffers a fracture, even if the patient had a minor fall or trauma, if that fall or trauma would not usually break a normal, healthy bone. The physician has documented that the patient has senile osteoporosis which is a reported with the code for age-related osteoporosis.

3. Identify which condition affecting the musculoskeletal system would generally not be reported with a code from Chapter 13.

    d. **Current acute injury**

    Rationale: Chapter guidelines identify healed, recurrent injuries and chronic conditions affecting the musculoskeletal system as conditions that are usually reported with codes from Chapter 13. Current acute injuries are usually reported with codes from Chapter 19.

4. The physician has documented that the patient has idiopathic osteonecrosis of the right femoral head. Since this condition affects the joint, what site is reported?

    b. **The site is the bone**

    Rationale: Coding guidelines related to site state the following: For certain conditions, the bone may be affected at the upper or lower end, (e.g., avascular necrosis of bone, M87; osteoporosis, M80-M81). Though the portion of the bone affected may be at the joint, the site designation will be the bone, not the joint.

5. What condition is not reported with a code from Chapter 13?

    a. **Arthropathic psoriasis**

    Rationale: The chapter level Excludes2 note identifies arthropathic psoriasis (L40.5-) as a condition that is not reported with a code from Chapter 13.

6. What condition would be reported with a code from subcategory M48.5- Collapsed vertebra?

    c. **Wedging of vertebra**

    Rationale: Subcategory (M48.5) is reported for collapsed vertebra, which may also be documented as wedging of vertebra. Codes for collapsed vertebra are not used to report a current injury due to fatigue fracture, pathological fractures due to neoplasm, osteoporosis or other pathological condition, or for traumatic fractures.

7. What information is NOT required to assign the most specific code for idiopathic scoliosis?

    d. **The specific form of scoliosis**

    Rationale: Idiopathic scoliosis is a specific form of scoliosis. It identifies the condition as being of unknown cause. Other forms are thoracogenic, neuromuscular, other secondary and other specified forms. The age of the patient is required in order to correctly classify the condition as infantile, juvenile, or adolescent. The location of the curve must be identified which may be documented as involving the either by the vertebra (T5-T10) involved or the region of the spine (thoracic).

8. Codes for osteoporosis in category M80 are specific to site. What does the site designate?

    c. **The site of the fracture**

    Rationale: Osteoporosis is a systemic condition, meaning that all bones of the musculoskeletal system are affected. Therefore, site is not a component of the codes under category M81 Osteoporosis without current pathological fracture. The site codes under M80 Osteoporosis with current pathological fracture identify the site of the fracture not the osteoporosis.

9. Code M61.371 Calcification and ossification of muscles associated with burns, right ankle and foot is an example of what type of code?

    b. A combination code

    Rationale: This is an example of a combination code. It captures the disease, disorder or other condition which is calcification and ossification of the muscles and the cause or etiology of the condition which is the burn.

10. What descriptor is not an example of site specificity?

    c. Synovium

    Rationale: Synovium is a type of tissue in the joints not a specific site in the musculoskeletal system. The site would be a specific joint such as the shoulder, wrist, or knee.

11. What information must be documented to assign the most specific code in category M1A Chronic gout that is not required for codes in category M10 Gout?

    a. With or without tophus

    Rationale: A 7th character is required for chronic gout to identify the condition as with or without tophus.

CPT® Procedural Coding

Introduction

Current Procedural Terminology (CPT) codes are published by the American Medical Association (AMA). The purpose of this coding system is to provide a uniform language for reporting services provided to patients.

A Category 1 CPT code is a five-digit numeric code used to describe medical, surgical, radiological, laboratory, Anesthesia, and evaluation/management services performed by physicians and other health care providers or entities. There are over 8,000 CPT codes ranging from 00100 through 99607. Beginning in 2002, the AMA added Category III (emerging technology) codes. In 2004, the AMA introduced Category II (supplemental tracking) codes. Both Category II and III codes are five-digit alphanumeric codes.

The entire family of procedure codes acceptable to Medicare is referred to as HCPCS, which is an acronym for:

H Healthcare

C Common

P Procedure

C Coding

S System

This family is comprised of two distinct parts or levels: Level I and Level II.

HCPCS Level I Codes (CPT)

HCPCS Level I codes consist of the five-digit codes listed in the *CPT®* published by the American Medical Association. These are the most frequently used codes to report services and procedures, since the codebook mainly consists of physician procedures. The codes are updated annually, and the new codes for the upcoming year are available at the end of the preceding year for use on January 1.

HCPCS Level II Codes

HCPCS Level II codes consist of five-digit alphanumeric codes utilizing letters A-V, and were developed specifically by the Centers for Medicare and Medicaid Services (CMS) to report services and supplies not found in Level I. HCPCS Level II is a standardized coding system that is used primarily to identify products; supplies; drugs and biologicals; durable medical equipment, prosthetics, orthotics, and supplies (DMEPOS); quality reporting measures; some physician and non-physician provider services; and other services, such as ambulance services. HCPCS Level II codes are recognized by Medicare and many other third-party payers.

The CPT Codebook

This coding reference book, which is updated annually, is organized into nine sections, sixteen appendices, and an alphabetic index. There are specific guidelines listed in the CPT codebook in the front of each section. These guidelines indicate interpretations and appropriate reporting of codes contained in that particular section. The guidelines should be reviewed prior to using any code in that section. The sections include:

- **Introduction and Illustrated Anatomical and Procedural Review** — Contains basic instructions for using the CPT codebook and reviews basic medical terminology and anatomy with additional information, references, and illustrations.
- **Evaluation and Management** — Provides the codes and guidelines for reporting patient evaluation and management services, most of which are face-to-face with the provider and based on established or new patient status. The codes are broadly grouped into place of service such as office, hospital, outpatient or ambulatory surgical center, emergency department, nursing home or other residential facility and/or type of service such as observation, consultations, critical care, newborn care, and preventive care.
- **Anesthesia** — Provides guidelines, codes, and modifiers for reporting services involving the administration of anesthesia for different types of procedures and on various locations of the body.
- **Surgery** — Identifies surgical procedures performed across all specialties and body systems. The procedure normally includes the necessary, related services in the surgical package without being stated as part of the code description.
- **Radiology** — Lists codes for diagnostic imaging, ultrasound, radiological guidance, radiation oncology, and nuclear medicine. Procedures in this section include x-ray, fluoroscopy, computed tomography, magnetic resonance imaging, angiography, lymphangiography, mammography, radiological supervision and interpretation for therapeutic transcatheter procedures, bone studies, radiation treatment and planning for cancer, brachytherapy, and radiopharmaceutical procedures.
- **Pathology and Laboratory** — Contains codes for reporting procedures and services processed in a laboratory facility. Tests include organ or disease panels, drug assays, urinalysis, chemistry profiles, microorganism identification, immunoassays, pathological examination of surgical samples, and reproductive-related procedures.
- **Medicine** — Identifies procedures that usually do not require operating room services. The medicine codes provided in this section cover a wide spectrum of specialties and include both diagnostic and therapeutic procedures. This section includes procedures such as neuromuscular testing, cardiac

catheterization, acupuncture, dialysis, chemotherapy, vaccine administration, and psychiatric services.

- **Category II Codes** — Lists supplemental, optional tracking codes composed of four digits and the letter F, used for performance measurement according to the CMS Physician Quality Reporting System (PQRS). These codes are intended to reduce the need for record abstraction and chart review and facilitate data collection by those seeking to measure quality of patient care.
- **Category III Codes** — Provide temporary codes composed of four digits and the letter T, established for reporting and tracking data for emerging technology, services, and procedures. When a Category III code is available, it must be used rather than reporting an unlisted code. These codes may or may not be assigned a Category I code at a future date.

The appendices include:

- **Appendix A – Modifiers** — Lists all the applicable modifiers for the CPT codes to identify when a service or procedure was altered by a specific circumstance or to provide additional information about the procedure performed. This includes anesthesia physical status modifiers, CPT Level I modifiers approved for ambulatory surgical centers and hospital outpatient departments, Category II modifiers and Level II HCPCS National modifiers.
- **Appendix B – Summary of Additions, Deletions, and Revisions** — Shows the current year's changes that were made to the codes.
- **Appendix C – Clinical Examples** — Gives real-life clinical scenarios and examples of patient evaluation and management encounters to help medical offices in reporting services provided to the patient.
- **Appendix D – Summary of CPT Add-on Codes** — Lists in numerical sequence all the codes designated in CPT as add-on codes. The add-on codes are only to be assigned in addition to the principal procedure and never stand alone. Add-on codes are also not subject to modifier 51 rules. These codes are additionally identified with a ✚ symbol. For guidance on reporting codes formerly listed in Appendix G, refer to the guidelines for code 99151-99153, and 99155-99157.
- **Appendix E – Summary of CPT Codes Exempt from Modifier 51** – Lists in numerical sequence all the CPT codes designated as exempt from the use of modifier 51 that have not been identified as add-on procedures or services. These codes are additionally identified with a ⊘ symbol.
- **Appendix F – Summary of CPT Codes Exempt from Modifier 63** — Lists in numerical sequence all the CPT codes designated as exempt from the use of modifier 63. These codes are additionally identified with a parenthetical instruction.
- **Appendix G – Summary of CPT Codes That Include Moderate (Conscious) Sedation** — The summary of CPT codes that include moderate (conscious) sedation (formerly Appendix G) has been removed from the CPT code set. The codes that were previously included were revised to remove the moderate (conscious) sedation symbol. For guidance on reporting codes formerly listed in Appendix G, refer to the guidelines for codes 99151-99153 and 99155-99157.
- **Appendix H – Alphabetical Clinical Topics Listing** — The Alphabetical Clinical Topics Listing (formerly Appendix H) has been removed from the CPT codebook. Since performance measures are subject to change each year, the alphabetic index to performance measures is now maintained on the AMA website at www.ama-assn.org/go/cpt. The online version will continue to provide PQRS measures in table format listed alphabetically by the disease or condition and crosswalked to the Category II codes used to report the quality measure.
- **Appendix I – Genetic Testing Code Modifiers** — The list of Genetic Testing Code Modifiers (formerly Appendix I) has been removed from the CPT code set. The addition of hundreds of molecular pathology codes resulted in the deletion of the stacking codes to which these modifiers applied. For the most current updates for molecular pathology coding in the CPT code set, see the AMA CPT website at www.ama-assn.org/go/cpt.
- **Appendix J – Electrodiagnostic Medicine Listing of Sensory, Motor, and Mixed Nerves** — Assigns each sensory, motor, and mixed nerve with its proper nerve conduction study code in order to improve accurate reporting of codes 95907-95913.
- **Appendix K – Product Pending FDA Approval** — Identifies vaccines that have already been assigned Category I codes that are still awaiting FDA approval. These are identified with the symbol ✗.
- **Appendix L – Vascular Families** — Outlines the tree of vascular families and identifies first-, second-, and third-order branches, assuming the beginning point was the aorta.
- **Appendix M – Renumbered CPT Codes – Citations Crosswalk** — This listing identifies codes that were deleted and renumbered from 2007 to 2009, and their crosswalk to current year code(s).
- **Appendix N – Summary of Resequenced CPT Codes** — This list identifies codes that do not appear in numeric sequence. Instead of deleting and renumbering existing codes that need to be moved, the existing codes are now being moved to the correct location without being renumbered. Resequenced codes are relocated to appear with codes for the appropriate code concept. The CPT codebook lists the code in numeric sequence without the code description. Instead, a parenthetical note is listed referencing the range of codes in which the resequenced code appears. The resequenced code is identified with a # symbol, and the full code description is listed for the resequenced code.
- **Appendix O – Multianalyte Assays with Algorithmic Analyses** — This list identifies codes for Multianalyte Assays with Algorithmic Analyses (MAAA) procedures that utilize multiple results derived from various types of assays (e.g., molecular pathology assays, non-nucleic acid based assays) that are typically unique to a single clinical laboratory or manufacturer.

- **Appendix P – CPT Codes That May Be Used For Synchronous Telemedicine Services** — This appendix first appeared in 2017 to list codes that may be used for reporting real-time telemedicine services when appended by modifier 95. These procedures include interactive electronic communication using audio-visual telecommunications equipment. These are identified with the symbol ☉.

Locating a CPT Code

Once familiar with the CPT codebook, identifying appropriate codes becomes less of a task. The numbers at the top of each page are for easy reference and give the range of codes located on that particular page.

Most sections list the sequence of codes in the following order:

- Top to bottom of body (head to toe)
- Central to peripheral in some subsections (i.e., cardiovascular and nervous system codes)
- Outside to inside of body (incision/excision)

There are two ways to locate a code in the CPT codebook:

- By anatomical site (numerically)
- The Index (alphabetically)

A code can be located simply by knowing the site or body system. For example, if a patient had an EKG performed in the emergency department, the user should try to locate a code through the Index. Alternatively, the coder could rationalize that a medicine service was performed to monitor the patient's heart which is part of the cardiovascular system. Since those medicine codes are found in the 93000 series of codes, the coder could then look in this section of the CPT codebook to locate the appropriate code.

The Index is organized by main terms, shown in bold typeface. There are four primary classes of main entries:

- Procedure or service – e.g., Cardiac Catheterization, Angioplasty
- Organ or other anatomic site – e.g., Heart, Chest, Abdomen
- Condition – e.g., Angina, Myocardial Infarction
- Synonyms, eponyms, and abbreviations – e.g., EKG, EMG, DXA

The main term is divided into specific sub-terms that help in selecting the appropriate code.

Whenever more than one code applies to a given index entry, a code range is listed. If two or more nonsequential codes apply, they will be separated by a comma. For example:

Electrocardiography

Evaluation ... 0178T-0180T, 93000, 93010, 93660

If more than one sequential code applies, they will be separated by a hyphen. For example:

Office and/or Other Outpatient Services

Established patient ... 99211-99215

A cross-reference provides instructions to the user on where to look when entries are listed under another heading.

See directs the user to refer to the term listed. This is used primarily for synonyms, eponyms, and abbreviations, such as:

Ear Canal

See Auditory Canal

The alphabetic index is not a substitute for the main text of CPT. The user must always refer to the main text to ensure that the code selection is accurate and not assign any codes from the index entry alone.

CPT Symbols

In addition to understanding the layout of CPT and knowing how to reference the book, the user must also understand symbols and their meanings.

● Indicates a new code has been added to the edition the coder is referencing. For example:

● 62380 Endoscopic decompression of spinal cord, nerve root(s), including laminotomy, partial facetectomy, foraminotomy, discectomy and/or excision of herniated intervertebral disc, 1 interspace, lumbar

▲ Indicates the code number is the same, but the definition or description has changed since the last edition

▲ 77003 Fluoroscopic guidance and localization of needle or catheter tip for spine or paraspinous diagnostic or therapeutic injection procedures (epidural or subarachnoid) (List separately in addition to code for primary procedure)

; Indicates a selection of suffixes that append to the main portion (prefix) of the code. For example:

96372 Therapeutic, prophylactic, or diagnostic injection (specify substance or drug); subcutaneous or intramuscular

96373 Therapeutic, prophylactic, or diagnostic injection (specify substance or drug); intra-arterial

96374 Therapeutic, prophylactic, or diagnostic injection (specify substance or drug); intravenous push, single or initial substance/drug

⊘ Identifies codes that are exempt from the use of modifier 51, but have not been designated as add-on procedures/ services.

⊘ 31500 Intubation, endotracheal, emergency procedure

Note: For more information on modifier 51, see the Modifier chapter.

☉ Identifies telemedicine codes.

☉ 90832 Psychotherapy, 30 minutes with patient

✗ Identifies codes that have been created for vaccines that are pending FDA approval (at the time of the publication of that year's CPT).

✗ 90739 Hepatitis B vaccine (HepB), adult dosage, 2 dose schedule, for intramuscular use

Add-on Codes

Add-on procedures or services are ones that are performed in addition to the primary procedure/service. In the CPT codebook, a ✚ indicates a CPT add-on code.

99291 Critical care, evaluation and management of the critically ill or critically injured patient; first 30-74 minutes

✚99292 each additional 30 minutes (List separately in addition to code for primary service)

The add-on procedure is performed on the same day by the same provider that performed the primary procedure/service. These codes should never be reported alone and should not be reported with modifier 51.

Modifiers

Modifiers consist of two numeric or alphanumeric digits appended to a code to indicate when a service or procedure that still fits the code description was altered by a specific circumstance or when additional information about the procedure performed needs to be provided.

Unlisted Procedure or Service

The procedure performed may not always be found with a designated code assignment in the CPT codebook. Unlisted procedure codes are provided in every section to be used in these cases. An accompanying operative report or other visit documentation is required when reporting unlisted codes in order for the payer to identify what the procedure entailed and determine its eligibility for reimbursement. An unlisted procedure code should not be used when a Category III code best describes the procedure performed.

Surgical Package

The concept of a global fee for surgical procedures is a long-established concept under which a single fee is billed that pays for all necessary services normally furnished by the surgeon before, during, and after the procedure. Since the fee schedule is based on uniform national relative values, it is necessary to have a uniform national definition of global surgery to assure that equivalent payment is made for the same amount of work and resources.

The following items are included in the global package reimbursement:

- Local anesthesia, digital block, or topical anesthesia
- After the decision for surgery is made, one E/M service one day before or the day of surgery
- Postoperative care that occurs directly after the procedure
- Examining the patient in the recovery area
- Any postoperative care occurring during the designated postoperative period

To assist in this uniform implementation, the CPT Editorial Panel created five modifiers (24, 25, 59, 78, and 79) to identify a service or procedure furnished during a global period that is not a part of the global surgery fee, such as a service unrelated to the condition requiring surgery or for treating the underlying condition and not for normal recovery from the surgery. Use of these modifiers allows such services to be reported in addition to the global fee.

Category II Codes

The Category II section of CPT contains a set of supplemental tracking codes that can be used for performance measurement. This section of codes was implemented in 2004 to facilitate data collection about the quality of care rendered for specific conditions. These codes report certain services and test results that support nationally established performance measures with evidence of contributing to increased quality patient care. It is not required for providers to report these codes; the use of these codes is optional.

Category II codes consist of five-digit alphanumeric codes that end in an F, and the following categories are included in this code set:

- Composite Codes
- Patient Management
- Patient History
- Physical Examination
- Diagnostic/Screening Processes or Results
- Therapeutic, Preventive, or Other Interventions
- Follow-up or Other Outcomes
- Patient Safety
- Structural Measures
- Nonmeasure Code Listing

Category III Codes

Category III codes are temporary codes that identify emerging technologies, services, and procedures and allow for data collection to determine clinical efficacy, utilization, and outcomes. They are alphanumeric codes that consist of four numbers, followed by the letter T.

A Category III code should be reported instead of an unlisted code whenever it accurately describes the procedure that was performed. These temporary codes may or may not be assigned a Category I CPT code in the future.

2019 CPT Codes and Crosswalks

The 2019 Anesthesia and Pain Management CPT codes and crosswalks begin following the Anesthesia and Surgery Guidelines section. Each code includes official CPT descriptions, official AMA Guidelines, Plain English Descriptions (PED), ICD-10-CM crosswalks, and Medicare-related information including: Base units, RVUs, Modifiers, and CCI edits (also known as NCCI).

Note: This Anesthesia and Pain Management coding book is not intended to replace the AMA's CPT codebook. Use this book in conjunction with the official AMA 2019 CPT codebook.

Anesthesia and Surgery Guidelines

Anesthesia Guidelines

Services involving administration of anesthesia are reported by the use of the anesthesia five-digit procedure code (00100-01999) plus modifier codes (defined under "Anesthesia Modifiers" later in these Guidelines).

The reporting of anesthesia services is appropriate by or under the responsible supervision of a physician. These services may include but are not limited to general, regional, supplementation of local anesthesia, or other supportive services in order to afford the patient the anesthesia care deemed optimal by the anesthesiologist during any procedure. These services include the usual preoperative and postoperative visits, the anesthesia care during the procedure, the administration of fluids and/or blood and the usual monitoring services (eg, ECG, temperature, blood pressure, oximetry, capnography, and mass spectrometry). Unusual forms of monitoring (eg, intra-arterial, central venous, and Swan-Ganz) are not included.

Items used by all physicians in reporting their services are presented in the **Introduction.** Some of the commonalities are repeated in this section for the convenience of those physicians referring to this section on **Anesthesia.** Other definitions and items unique to anesthesia are also listed.

To report moderate (conscious) sedation provided by a physician also performing the service for which conscious sedation is being provided, see codes 99151, 99152, 99153.

When a second physician other than the health care professional performing the diagnostic or therapeutic services provides moderate (conscious) sedation in the facility setting (eg, hospital, outpatient hospital/ambulatory surgery center, skilled nursing facility), the second physician reports the associated moderate sedation procedure/service 99155, 99156, 99157; when these services are performed by the second physician in the nonfacility setting (eg, physician office, freestanding imaging center), codes 99155, 99156, 99157 would not be reported. Moderate sedation does not include minimal sedation (anxiolysis), deep sedation, or monitored anesthesia care (00100-01999).

To report regional or general anesthesia provided by a physician also performing the services for which the anesthesia is being provided, see modifier 47 in Appendix A.

Time Reporting

Time for anesthesia procedures may be reported as is customary in the local area. Anesthesia time begins when the anesthesiologist begins to prepare the patient for the induction of anesthesia in the operating room (or in an equivalent area) and ends when the anesthesiologist is no longer in personal attendance, that is, when the patient may be safely placed under postoperative supervision.

Anesthesia Services

Services rendered in the office, home, or hospital; consultation; and other medical services are listed in the **Evaluation and Management Services** section (99201-99499 series) on page 11. "Special Services and Reporting" (99000-99091 series) are listed in the **Medicine** section.

Supplied Materials

Supplies and materials provided (eg, sterile trays, drugs) over and above those usually included with the office visit or other services rendered may be listed separately. Drugs, tray supplies, and materials provided should be listed and identified with 99070 or the appropriate supply code.

Separate or Multiple Procedures

When multiple surgical procedures are performed during a single anesthetic administration, the anesthesia code representing the most complex procedure is reported. The time reported is the combined total for all procedures.

▶Unlisted Service or Procedure◀

▶A service or procedure may be provided that is not listed in this edition of the CPT codebook. When reporting such a service, the appropriate "Unlisted Procedure" code may be used to indicate the service, identifying it by "Special Report" as discussed in the section below. The "Unlisted Procedures" and accompanying code for Anesthesia is as follows:◀

01999 Unlisted anesthesia procedure(s)

Special Report

A service that is rarely provided, unusual, variable, or new may require a special report. Pertinent information should include an adequate definition or description of the nature, extent, and need for the procedure and the time, effort, and equipment necessary to provide the service.

Anesthesia Modifiers

All anesthesia services are reported by use of the anesthesia five-digit procedure code (00100-01999) plus the addition of a physical status modifier. The use of other optional modifiers may be appropriate.

Physical Status Modifiers

Physical Status modifiers are represented by the initial letter 'P' followed by a single digit from 1 to 6 as defined in the following list:

P1: A normal healthy patient

P2: A patient with mild systemic disease

P3: A patient with severe systemic disease

P4: A patient with severe systemic disease that is a constant threat to life

CPT © 2018 American Medical Association. All rights reserved.

P5: A moribund patient who is not expected to survive without the operation

P6: A declared brain-dead patient whose organs are being removed for donor purposes

These six levels are consistent with the American Society of Anesthesiologists (ASA) ranking of patient physical status. Physical status is included in the CPT codebook to distinguish among various levels of complexity of the anesthesia service provided.

Example: 00100-P1

Qualifying Circumstances

More than one qualifying circumstance may be selected.

Many anesthesia services are provided under particularly difficult circumstances, depending on factors such as extraordinary condition of patient, notable operative conditions, and/or unusual risk factors. This section includes a list of important qualifying circumstances that significantly affect the character of the anesthesia service provided. These procedures would not be reported alone but would be reported as additional procedure numbers qualifying an anesthesia procedure or service.

✚ **99100** Anesthesia for patient of extreme age, younger than 1 year and older than 70 (List separately in addition to code for primary anesthesia procedure)

✚ **99116** Anesthesia complicated by utilization of total body hypothermia

(List separately in addition to code for primary anesthesia procedure)

✚ **99135** Anesthesia complicated by utilization of controlled hypotension

(List separately in addition to code for primary anesthesia procedure)

✚ **99140** Anesthesia complicated by emergency conditions (specify)

(An emergency is defined as existing when delay in treatment of the patient would lead to a significant increase in the threat to life or body part)

Surgery Guidelines

Guidelines to direct general reporting of services are presented in the **Introduction**. Some of the commonalities are repeated here for the convenience of those referring to this section on Surgery. Other definitions and items unique to **Surgery** are also listed.

Services

Services rendered in the office, home, or hospital, consultations, and other medical services are listed in the **Evaluation and Management Services** section (99201-99499) beginning on page 11.* "Special Services and Reports" (99000-99091) are listed in the **Medicine** section.

CPT Surgical Package Definition

By their very nature, the services to any patient are variable. The CPT codes that represent a readily identifiable surgical procedure thereby include, on a procedure-by-procedure basis, a variety of services. In defining the specific services "included" in a given CPT surgical code, the following services related to the surgery when furnished by the physician or other qualified health care professional who performs the surgery are included in addition to the operation per se:

- Evaluation and Management (E/M) service(s) subsequent to the decision for surgery on the day before and/or day of surgery (including history and physical)
- Local infiltration, metacarpal/metatarsal/digital block or topical anesthesia
- Immediate postoperative care, including dictating operative notes, talking with the family and other physicians or other qualified health care professionals
- Writing orders
- Evaluating the patient in the postanesthesia recovery area
- Typical postoperative follow-up care

Follow-Up Care for Diagnostic Procedures

Follow-up care for diagnostic procedures (eg, endoscopy, arthroscopy, injection procedures for radiography) includes only that care related to recovery from the diagnostic procedure itself. Care of the condition for which the diagnostic procedure was performed or of other concomitant conditions is not included and may be listed separately.

Follow-Up Care for Therapeutic Surgical Procedures

Follow-up care for therapeutic surgical procedures includes only that care which is usually a part of the surgical service. Complications, exacerbations, recurrence, or the presence of other diseases or injuries requiring additional services should be separately reported.

Supplied Materials

Supplies and materials (eg, sterile trays/drugs), over and above those usually included with the procedure(s) rendered are reported separately. List drugs, trays, supplies, and materials provided. Identify as 99070 or specific supply code.

Reporting More Than One Procedure/Service

When more than one procedure/service is performed on the same date, same session or during a post-operative period (subject to the "surgical package" concept), several CPT modifiers may apply (see Appendix A* for definition).

* Pages in this section refer to the AMA *CPT® 2019 Professional Edition.*

CPT © 2018 American Medical Association. All rights reserved

Separate Procedure

Some of the procedures or services listed in the CPT codebook that are commonly carried out as an integral component of a total service or procedure have been identified by the inclusion of the term "separate procedure." The codes designated as "separate procedure" should not be reported in addition to the code for the total procedure or service of which it is considered an integral component.

However, when a procedure or service that is designated as a "separate procedure" is carried out independently or considered to be unrelated or distinct from other procedures/services provided at that time, it may be reported by itself, or in addition to other procedures/services by appending modifier 59 to the specific "separate procedure" code to indicate that the procedure is not considered to be a component of another procedure, but is a distinct, independent procedure. This may represent a different session, different procedure or surgery, different site or organ system, separate incision/excision, separate lesion, or separate injury (or area of injury in extensive injuries).

Unlisted Service or Procedure

A service or procedure may be provided that is not listed in this edition of the CPT codebook. When reporting such a service, the appropriate "Unlisted Procedure" code may be used to indicate the service, identifying it by "Special Report" as discussed in the section below. The "Unlisted Procedures" and accompanying codes for **Surgery** are as follows:

15999	Unlisted procedure, excision pressure ulcer
17999	Unlisted procedure, skin, mucous membrane and subcutaneous tissue
19499	Unlisted procedure, breast
20999	Unlisted procedure, musculoskeletal system, general
21089	Unlisted maxillofacial prosthetic procedure
21299	Unlisted craniofacial and maxillofacial procedure
21499	Unlisted musculoskeletal procedure, head
21899	Unlisted procedure, neck or thorax
22899	Unlisted procedure, spine
22999	Unlisted procedure, abdomen, musculoskeletal system
23929	Unlisted procedure, shoulder
24999	Unlisted procedure, humerus or elbow
25999	Unlisted procedure, forearm or wrist
26989	Unlisted procedure, hands or fingers
27299	Unlisted procedure, pelvis or hip joint
27599	Unlisted procedure, femur or knee
27899	Unlisted procedure, leg or ankle
28899	Unlisted procedure, foot or toes
29799	Unlisted procedure, casting or strapping
29999	Unlisted procedure, arthroscopy
30999	Unlisted procedure, nose
31299	Unlisted procedure, accessory sinuses
31599	Unlisted procedure, larynx
31899	Unlisted procedure, trachea, bronchi
32999	Unlisted procedure, lungs and pleura
33999	Unlisted procedure, cardiac surgery
36299	Unlisted procedure, vascular injection
37501	Unlisted vascular endoscopy procedure
37799	Unlisted procedure, vascular surgery
38129	Unlisted laparoscopy procedure, spleen
38589	Unlisted laparoscopy procedure, lymphatic system
38999	Unlisted procedure, hemic or lymphatic system
39499	Unlisted procedure, mediastinum
39599	Unlisted procedure, diaphragm
40799	Unlisted procedure, lips
40899	Unlisted procedure, vestibule of mouth
41599	Unlisted procedure, tongue, floor of mouth
41899	Unlisted procedure, dentoalveolar structures
42299	Unlisted procedure, palate, uvula
42699	Unlisted procedure, salivary glands or ducts
42999	Unlisted procedure, pharynx, adenoids, or tonsils
43289	Unlisted laparoscopy procedure, esophagus
43499	Unlisted procedure, esophagus
43659	Unlisted laparoscopy procedure, stomach
43999	Unlisted procedure, stomach
44238	Unlisted laparoscopy procedure, intestine (except rectum)
44799	Unlisted procedure, small intestine
44899	Unlisted procedure, Meckel's diverticulum and the mesentery
44979	Unlisted laparoscopy procedure, appendix
45399	Unlisted procedure, colon
45499	Unlisted laparoscopy procedure, rectum
45999	Unlisted procedure, rectum
46999	Unlisted procedure, anus
47379	Unlisted laparoscopic procedure, liver
47399	Unlisted procedure, liver
47579	Unlisted laparoscopy procedure, biliary tract
47999	Unlisted procedure, biliary tract
48999	Unlisted procedure, pancreas
49329	Unlisted laparoscopy procedure, abdomen, peritoneum and omentum
49659	Unlisted laparoscopy procedure, hernioplasty, herniorrhaphy, herniotomy

Guidelines

CPT © 2018 American Medical Association. All rights reserved.

Guidelines

49999	Unlisted procedure, abdomen, peritoneum and omentum
50549	Unlisted laparoscopy procedure, renal
50949	Unlisted laparoscopy procedure, ureter
51999	Unlisted laparoscopy procedure, bladder
53899	Unlisted procedure, urinary system
54699	Unlisted laparoscopy procedure, testis
55559	Unlisted laparoscopy procedure, spermatic cord
55899	Unlisted procedure, male genital system
58578	Unlisted laparoscopy procedure, uterus
58579	Unlisted hysteroscopy procedure, uterus
58679	Unlisted laparoscopy procedure, oviduct, ovary
58999	Unlisted procedure, female genital system (nonobstetrical)
59897	Unlisted fetal invasive procedure, including ultrasound guidance, when performed
59898	Unlisted laparoscopy procedure, maternity care and delivery
59899	Unlisted procedure, maternity care and delivery
60659	Unlisted laparoscopy procedure, endocrine system
60699	Unlisted procedure, endocrine system
64999	Unlisted procedure, nervous system
66999	Unlisted procedure, anterior segment of eye
67299	Unlisted procedure, posterior segment
67399	Unlisted procedure, extraocular muscle
67599	Unlisted procedure, orbit
67999	Unlisted procedure, eyelids
68399	Unlisted procedure, conjunctiva
68899	Unlisted procedure, lacrimal system
69399	Unlisted procedure, external ear
69799	Unlisted procedure, middle ear
69949	Unlisted procedure, inner ear
69979	Unlisted procedure, temporal bone, middle fossa approach

Special Report

A service that is rarely provided, unusual, variable, or new may require a special report. Pertinent information should include an adequate definition or description of the nature, extent, and need for the procedure, and the time, effort, and equipment necessary to provide the service.

Imaging Guidance

▶When imaging guidance or imaging supervision and interpretation is included in a surgical procedure, guidelines for image documentation and report, included in the guidelines for Radiology (Including Nuclear Medicine and Diagnostic Ultrasound), will apply. Imaging guidance should not be reported for use of a nonimaging-guided tracking or localizing system (eg, radar signals, electromagnetic signals). Imaging guidance should only be reported when an imaging modality (eg, radiography, fluoroscopy, ultrasonography, magnetic resonance imaging, computed tomography, or nuclear medicine) is used and is appropriately documented.◀

Surgical Destruction

Surgical destruction is a part of a surgical procedure and different methods of destruction are not ordinarily listed separately unless the technique substantially alters the standard management of a problem or condition. Exceptions under special circumstances are provided for by separate code numbers.

* Pages in this section refer to the AMA *CPT® 2019 Professional Edition.*

CPT © 2018 American Medical Association. All rights reserved

Surgical Procedures on the Musculoskeletal System

Cast and strapping procedures appear at the end of this section.

The services listed below include the application and removal of the first cast or traction device only. Subsequent replacement of cast and/or traction device may require an additional listing.

Definitions

The terms "closed treatment," "open treatment," and "percutaneous skeletal fixation" have been carefully chosen to accurately reflect current orthopaedic procedural treatments.

Closed treatment specifically means that the fracture site is not surgically opened (exposed to the external environment and directly visualized). This terminology is used to describe procedures that treat fractures by three methods: (1) without manipulation; (2) with manipulation; or (3) with or without traction.

Open treatment is used when the fractured bone is either: (1) surgically opened (exposed to the external environment) and the fracture (bone ends) visualized and internal fixation may be used; or (2) the fractured bone is opened remote from the fracture site in order to insert an intramedullary nail across the fracture site (the fracture site is not opened and visualized).

Percutaneous skeletal fixation describes fracture treatment which is neither open nor closed. In this procedure, the fracture fragments are not visualized, but fixation (eg, pins) is placed across the fracture site, usually under X-ray imaging.

The type of fracture (eg, open, compound, closed) does not have any coding correlation with the type of treatment (eg, closed, open, or percutaneous) provided.

The codes for treatment of fractures and joint injuries (dislocations) are categorized by the type of manipulation (reduction) and stabilization (fixation or immobilization). These codes can apply to either open (compound) or closed fractures or joint injuries.

Skeletal traction is the application of a force (distracting or traction force) to a limb segment through a wire, pin, screw, or clamp that is attached (eg, penetrates) to bone.

Skin traction is the application of a force (longitudinal) to a limb using felt or strapping applied directly to skin only.

External fixation is the usage of skeletal pins plus an attaching mechanism/device used for temporary or definitive treatment of acute or chronic bony deformity.

Codes for obtaining autogenous bone grafts, cartilage, tendon, fascia lata grafts or other tissues through separate incisions are to be used only when the graft is not already listed as part of the basic procedure.

Re-reduction of a fracture and/or dislocation performed by the primary physician or other qualified health care professional may be identified by the addition of modifier 76 to the usual procedure number to indicate "Repeat Procedure or Service by Same Physician or Other Qualified Health Care Professional." (See Appendix A* guidelines.)

Codes for external fixation are to be used only when external fixation is not already listed as part of the basic procedure.

Manipulation is used throughout the musculoskeletal fracture and dislocation subsections to specifically mean the attempted reduction or restoration of a fracture or joint dislocation to its normal anatomic alignment by the application of manually applied forces.

Excision of subcutaneous soft connective tissue tumors (including simple or intermediate repair) involves the simple or marginal resection of tumors confined to subcutaneous tissue below the skin but above the deep fascia. These tumors are usually benign and are resected without removing a significant amount of surrounding normal tissue. Code selection is based on the location and size of the tumor. Code selection is determined by measuring the greatest diameter of the tumor plus that margin required for complete excision of the tumor. The margins refer to the most narrow margin required to adequately excise the tumor, based on the physician's judgment. The measurement of the tumor plus margin is made at the time of the excision. Appreciable vessel exploration and/or neuroplasty should be reported separately. Extensive undermining or other techniques to close a defect created by skin excision may require a complex repair which should be reported separately. Dissection or elevation of tissue planes to permit resection of the tumor is included in the excision. For excision of benign lesions of cutaneous origin (eg, sebaceous cyst), see 11400-11446.

Excision of fascial or subfascial soft tissue tumors (including simple or intermediate repair) involves the resection of tumors confined to the tissue within or below the deep fascia, but not involving the bone. These tumors are usually benign, are often intramuscular, and are resected without removing a significant amount of surrounding normal tissue. Code selection is based on size and location of the tumor. Code selection is determined by measuring the greatest diameter of the tumor plus that margin required for complete excision of the tumor. The margins refer to the most narrow margin required to adequately excise the tumor, based on individual judgment. The measurement of the tumor plus margin is made at the time of the excision. Appreciable vessel exploration and/ or neuroplasty should be reported separately. Extensive undermining or other techniques to close a defect created by skin excision may require a complex repair which should be reported separately. Dissection or elevation of tissue planes to permit resection of the tumor is included in the excision.

Digital (ie, fingers and toes) subfascial tumors are defined as those tumors involving the tendons, tendon sheaths, or joints of the digit. Tumors which simply abut but do not breach the tendon, tendon sheath, or joint capsule are considered subcutaneous soft tissue tumors.

Radical resection of soft connective tissue tumors (including simple or intermediate repair) involves the resection of the tumor with wide margins of normal tissue. Appreciable vessel exploration and/or neuroplasty repair or reconstruction (eg, adjacent tissue transfer[s], flap[s]) should be reported separately. Extensive undermining or other techniques to close a defect created by skin excision may require a complex repair which should be

CPT © 2018 American Medical Association. All rights reserved.

* Pages in this section refer to the AMA *CPT® 2019 Professional Edition.*

reported separately. Dissection or elevation of tissue planes to permit resection of the tumor is included in the excision. Although these tumors may be confined to a specific layer (eg, subcutaneous, subfascial), radical resection may involve removal of tissue from one or more layers. Radical resection of soft tissue tumors is most commonly used for malignant connective tissue tumors or very aggressive benign connective tissue tumors. Code selection is based on size and location of the tumor. Code selection is determined by measuring the greatest diameter of the tumor plus that margin required for complete excision of the tumor. The margins refer to the most narrow margin required to adequately excise the tumor, based on individual judgment. The measurement of the tumor plus margin is made at the time of the excision. For radical resection of tumor(s) of cutaneous origin (eg, melanoma), see 11600- 11646.

Radical resection of bone tumors (including simple or intermediate repair) involves the resection of the tumor with wide margins of normal tissue. Appreciable vessel exploration and/or neuroplasty and complex bone repair or reconstruction (eg, adjacent tissue transfer[s], flap[s]) should be reported separately. Extensive undermining or other techniques to close a defect created by skin excision may require a complex repair which should be reported separately. Dissection or elevation of tissue planes to permit resection of the tumor is included in the excision. It may require removal of the entire bone if tumor growth is extensive (eg, clavicle). Radical resection of bone tumors is usually performed for malignant tumors or very aggressive benign tumors. If surrounding soft tissue is removed during these procedures, the radical resection of soft tissue tumor codes should not be reported separately. Code selection is based solely on the location of the tumor, **not** on the size of the tumor or whether the tumor is benign or malignant, primary or metastatic.

Surgical Procedures on the Cardiovascular System

Selective vascular catheterizations should be coded to include introduction and all lesser order selective catheterizations used in the approach (eg, the description for a selective right middle cerebral artery catheterization includes the introduction and placement catheterization of the right common and internal carotid arteries).

Additional second and/or third order arterial catheterizations within the same family of arteries supplied by a single first order artery should be expressed by 36218 or 36248. Additional first order or higher catheterizations in vascular families supplied by a first order vessel different from a previously selected and coded family should be separately coded using the conventions described above.

(For monitoring, operation of pump and other nonsurgical services, see 99190-99192, 99291, 99292, 99354-99360)

(For other medical or laboratory related services, see appropriate section)

(For radiological supervision and interpretation, see 75600-75970)

* Pages in this section refer to the AMA *CPT® 2019 Professional Edition.*

CPT © 2018 American Medical Association. All rights reserved

00100

00100 Anesthesia for procedures on salivary glands, including biopsy

AMA *CPT Assistant*

00100: Feb 97: 4, Nov 99: 6, Feb 06: 9, Mar 06: 15, Nov 07: 8, Oct 11: 3, Jul 12: 13, Aug 14: 6, Dec 17: 8

ICD-10-CM Diagnostic Codes

C07	Malignant neoplasm of parotid gland
C08.0	Malignant neoplasm of submandibular gland
C08.1	Malignant neoplasm of sublingual gland
C08.9	Malignant neoplasm of major salivary gland, unspecified
D00.0	Carcinoma in situ of lip, oral cavity and pharynx
D10.2	Benign neoplasm of floor of mouth
D11.0	Benign neoplasm of parotid gland
D11.7	Benign neoplasm of other major salivary glands
D11.9	Benign neoplasm of major salivary gland, unspecified
D37.030	Neoplasm of uncertain behavior of the parotid salivary glands
D37.031	Neoplasm of uncertain behavior of the sublingual salivary glands
D37.032	Neoplasm of uncertain behavior of the submandibular salivary glands
D37.039	Neoplasm of uncertain behavior of the major salivary glands, unspecified
K11.4	Fistula of salivary gland
K11.5	Sialolithiasis
K11.6	Mucocele of salivary gland
K11.7	Disturbances of salivary secretion
K11.8	Other diseases of salivary glands
K11.9	Disease of salivary gland, unspecified
Q38.4	Congenital malformations of salivary glands and ducts
R68.2	Dry mouth, unspecified

CCI Edits

Refer to Appendix A for CCI edits.

Pub 100

00100: Pub 100-04, 12, 140.5, Pub 100-04, 12, 50, Pub 100-04, 12, 90.4.5

Base Units

Global: XXX

Code	Base Units
00100	5

Modifiers (PAR)

Code	Mod 50	Mod 51	Mod 62	Mod 80
00100	9	9	9	9

CPT © 2018 American Medical Association. All Rights Reserved.

00102

00102 Anesthesia for procedures involving plastic repair of cleft lip

AMA *CPT Assistant* ▯

00102: Nov 99: 6

ICD-10-CM Diagnostic Codes

Q36.0	Cleft lip, bilateral
Q36.1	Cleft lip, median
Q36.9	Cleft lip, unilateral
Q37.0	Cleft hard palate with bilateral cleft lip
Q37.1	Cleft hard palate with unilateral cleft lip
Q37.2	Cleft soft palate with bilateral cleft lip
Q37.3	Cleft soft palate with unilateral cleft lip
Q37.4	Cleft hard and soft palate with bilateral cleft lip
Q37.5	Cleft hard and soft palate with unilateral cleft lip
Q37.8	Unspecified cleft palate with bilateral cleft lip
Q37.9	Unspecified cleft palate with unilateral cleft lip
Q38.5	Congenital malformations of palate, not elsewhere classified

CCI Edits

Refer to Appendix A for CCI edits.

Pub 100

00102: Pub 100-04, 12, 140.5, Pub 100-04, 12, 50, Pub 100-04, 12, 90.4.5

Base Units

Global: XXX

Code	Base Units
00102	6

Modifiers (PAR)

Code	Mod 50	Mod 51	Mod 62	Mod 80
00102	9	9	9	9

CPT © 2018 American Medical Association. All Rights Reserved.

00103

00103 Anesthesia for reconstructive procedures of eyelid (eg, blepharoplasty, ptosis surgery)

AMA *CPT Assistant* ▢

00103: Nov 99: 6

ICD-10-CM Diagnostic Codes

⇄ C43.111 Malignant melanoma of right upper eyelid, including canthus
⇄ C43.112 Malignant melanoma of right lower eyelid, including canthus
⇄ C43.121 Malignant melanoma of left upper eyelid, including canthus
⇄ C43.122 Malignant melanoma of left lower eyelid, including canthus
⇄ C44.1021 Unspecified malignant neoplasm of skin of right upper eyelid, including canthus
⇄ C44.1022 Unspecified malignant neoplasm of skin of right lower eyelid, including canthus
⇄ C44.1091 Unspecified malignant neoplasm of skin of left upper eyelid, including canthus
⇄ C44.1092 Unspecified malignant neoplasm of skin of left lower eyelid, including canthus
⇄ C44.1121 Basal cell carcinoma of skin of right upper eyelid, including canthus
⇄ C44.1122 Basal cell carcinoma of skin of right lower eyelid, including canthus
⇄ C44.1191 Basal cell carcinoma of skin of left upper eyelid, including canthus
⇄ C44.1192 Basal cell carcinoma of skin of left lower eyelid, including canthus
⇄ C44.1221 Squamous cell carcinoma of skin of right upper eyelid, including canthus
⇄ C44.1222 Squamous cell carcinoma of skin of right lower eyelid, including canthus
⇄ C44.1291 Squamous cell carcinoma of skin of left upper eyelid, including canthus
⇄ C44.1292 Squamous cell carcinoma of skin of left lower eyelid, including canthus
⇄ C44.1321 Sebaceous cell carcinoma of skin of right upper eyelid, including canthus
⇄ C44.1322 Sebaceous cell carcinoma of skin of right lower eyelid, including canthus
⇄ C44.1391 Sebaceous cell carcinoma of skin of left upper eyelid, including canthus
⇄ C44.1392 Sebaceous cell carcinoma of skin of left lower eyelid, including canthus
⇄ C44.1921 Other specified malignant neoplasm of skin of right upper eyelid, including canthus
⇄ C44.1922 Other specified malignant neoplasm of skin of right lower eyelid, including canthus
⇄ C44.1991 Other specified malignant neoplasm of skin of left upper eyelid, including canthus
⇄ C44.1992 Other specified malignant neoplasm of skin of left lower eyelid, including canthus
⇄ C4A.111 Merkel cell carcinoma of right upper eyelid, including canthus
⇄ C4A.112 Merkel cell carcinoma of right lower eyelid, including canthus
⇄ C4A.121 Merkel cell carcinoma of left upper eyelid, including canthus
⇄ C4A.122 Merkel cell carcinoma of left lower eyelid, including canthus
⇄ D03.111 Melanoma in situ of right upper eyelid, including canthus
⇄ D03.112 Melanoma in situ of right lower eyelid, including canthus
⇄ D03.121 Melanoma in situ of left upper eyelid, including canthus
⇄ D03.122 Melanoma in situ of left lower eyelid, including canthus
⇄ D04.111 Carcinoma in situ of skin of right upper eyelid, including canthus
⇄ D04.112 Carcinoma in situ of skin of right lower eyelid, including canthus
⇄ D04.121 Carcinoma in situ of skin of left upper eyelid, including canthus
⇄ D04.122 Carcinoma in situ of skin of left lower eyelid, including canthus
⇄ D22.111 Melanocytic nevi of right upper eyelid, including canthus
⇄ D22.112 Melanocytic nevi of right lower eyelid, including canthus
⇄ D22.121 Melanocytic nevi of left upper eyelid, including canthus
⇄ D22.122 Melanocytic nevi of left lower eyelid, including canthus
⇄ D23.111 Other benign neoplasm of skin of right upper eyelid, including canthus
⇄ D23.112 Other benign neoplasm of skin of right lower eyelid, including canthus
⇄ D23.121 Other benign neoplasm of skin of left upper eyelid, including canthus
⇄ D23.122 Other benign neoplasm of skin of left lower eyelid, including canthus
⇄ H02.001 Unspecified entropion of right upper eyelid
⇄ H02.002 Unspecified entropion of right lower eyelid
⇄ H02.004 Unspecified entropion of left upper eyelid
⇄ H02.005 Unspecified entropion of left lower eyelid
⇄ H02.011 Cicatricial entropion of right upper eyelid
⇄ H02.012 Cicatricial entropion of right lower eyelid
⇄ H02.014 Cicatricial entropion of left upper eyelid
⇄ H02.015 Cicatricial entropion of left lower eyelid
⇄ H02.021 Mechanical entropion of right upper eyelid
⇄ H02.022 Mechanical entropion of right lower eyelid
⇄ H02.024 Mechanical entropion of left upper eyelid
⇄ H02.025 Mechanical entropion of left lower eyelid
⇄ H02.031 Senile entropion of right upper eyelid
⇄ H02.032 Senile entropion of right lower eyelid
⇄ H02.034 Senile entropion of left upper eyelid
⇄ H02.035 Senile entropion of left lower eyelid
⇄ H02.041 Spastic entropion of right upper eyelid
⇄ H02.042 Spastic entropion of right lower eyelid
⇄ H02.044 Spastic entropion of left upper eyelid
⇄ H02.045 Spastic entropion of left lower eyelid
⇄ H02.101 Unspecified ectropion of right upper eyelid
⇄ H02.102 Unspecified ectropion of right lower eyelid
⇄ H02.104 Unspecified ectropion of left upper eyelid
⇄ H02.105 Unspecified ectropion of left lower eyelid
⇄ H02.111 Cicatricial ectropion of right upper eyelid
⇄ H02.112 Cicatricial ectropion of right lower eyelid
⇄ H02.114 Cicatricial ectropion of left upper eyelid
⇄ H02.115 Cicatricial ectropion of left lower eyelid
⇄ H02.121 Mechanical ectropion of right upper eyelid
⇄ H02.122 Mechanical ectropion of right lower eyelid
⇄ H02.124 Mechanical ectropion of left upper eyelid
⇄ H02.125 Mechanical ectropion of left lower eyelid
⇄ H02.131 Senile ectropion of right upper eyelid
⇄ H02.132 Senile ectropion of right lower eyelid
⇄ H02.134 Senile ectropion of left upper eyelid
⇄ H02.135 Senile ectropion of left lower eyelid
⇄ H02.141 Spastic ectropion of right upper eyelid
⇄ H02.142 Spastic ectropion of right lower eyelid
⇄ H02.144 Spastic ectropion of left upper eyelid
⇄ H02.145 Spastic ectropion of left lower eyelid
⇄ H02.151 Paralytic ectropion of right upper eyelid
⇄ H02.152 Paralytic ectropion of right lower eyelid
⇄ H02.154 Paralytic ectropion of left upper eyelid
⇄ H02.155 Paralytic ectropion of left lower eyelid
⇄ H02.201 Unspecified lagophthalmos right upper eyelid

CPT © 2018 American Medical Association. All Rights Reserved.

⇄ H02.202 Unspecified lagophthalmos right lower eyelid
⇄ H02.204 Unspecified lagophthalmos left upper eyelid
⇄ H02.205 Unspecified lagophthalmos left lower eyelid
⇄ H02.20A Unspecified lagophthalmos right eye, upper and lower eyelids
⇄ H02.20B Unspecified lagophthalmos left eye, upper and lower eyelids
⇄ H02.20C Unspecified lagophthalmos, bilateral, upper and lower eyelids
⇄ H02.211 Cicatricial lagophthalmos right upper eyelid
⇄ H02.212 Cicatricial lagophthalmos right lower eyelid
⇄ H02.214 Cicatricial lagophthalmos left upper eyelid
⇄ H02.215 Cicatricial lagophthalmos left lower eyelid
⇄ H02.21A Cicatricial lagophthalmos right eye, upper and lower eyelids
⇄ H02.21B Cicatricial lagophthalmos left eye, upper and lower eyelids
⇄ H02.21C Cicatricial lagophthalmos, bilateral, upper and lower eyelids
⇄ H02.221 Mechanical lagophthalmos right upper eyelid
⇄ H02.222 Mechanical lagophthalmos right lower eyelid
⇄ H02.224 Mechanical lagophthalmos left upper eyelid
⇄ H02.225 Mechanical lagophthalmos left lower eyelid
⇄ H02.22A Mechanical lagophthalmos right eye, upper and lower eyelids
⇄ H02.22B Mechanical lagophthalmos left eye, upper and lower eyelids
⇄ H02.22C Mechanical lagophthalmos, bilateral, upper and lower eyelids
⇄ H02.231 Paralytic lagophthalmos right upper eyelid
⇄ H02.232 Paralytic lagophthalmos right lower eyelid
⇄ H02.234 Paralytic lagophthalmos left upper eyelid
⇄ H02.235 Paralytic lagophthalmos left lower eyelid
⇄ H02.23A Paralytic lagophthalmos right eye, upper and lower eyelids
⇄ H02.23B Paralytic lagophthalmos left eye, upper and lower eyelids
⇄ H02.23C Paralytic lagophthalmos, bilateral, upper and lower eyelids
⇄ H02.31 Blepharochalasis right upper eyelid
⇄ H02.32 Blepharochalasis right lower eyelid
⇄ H02.34 Blepharochalasis left upper eyelid
⇄ H02.35 Blepharochalasis left lower eyelid
⇄ H02.401 Unspecified ptosis of right eyelid
⇄ H02.402 Unspecified ptosis of left eyelid
⇄ H02.403 Unspecified ptosis of bilateral eyelids
⇄ H02.411 Mechanical ptosis of right eyelid
⇄ H02.412 Mechanical ptosis of left eyelid
⇄ H02.413 Mechanical ptosis of bilateral eyelids
⇄ H02.421 Myogenic ptosis of right eyelid
⇄ H02.422 Myogenic ptosis of left eyelid
⇄ H02.423 Myogenic ptosis of bilateral eyelids
⇄ H02.431 Paralytic ptosis of right eyelid
⇄ H02.432 Paralytic ptosis of left eyelid
⇄ H02.433 Paralytic ptosis of bilateral eyelids
⇄ H02.831 Dermatochalasis of right upper eyelid
⇄ H02.832 Dermatochalasis of right lower eyelid
⇄ H02.834 Dermatochalasis of left upper eyelid
⇄ H02.835 Dermatochalasis of left lower eyelid
⇄ H04.521 Eversion of right lacrimal punctum
⇄ H04.522 Eversion of left lacrimal punctum
⇄ H04.523 Eversion of bilateral lacrimal punctum
Q10.0 Congenital ptosis
Q10.1 Congenital ectropion
Q10.2 Congenital entropion
Q10.3 Other congenital malformations of eyelid
❼⇄ S01.101 Unspecified open wound of right eyelid and periocular area
❼⇄ S01.102 Unspecified open wound of left eyelid and periocular area
❼⇄ S01.111 Laceration without foreign body of right eyelid and periocular area
❼⇄ S01.112 Laceration without foreign body of left eyelid and periocular area
❼⇄ S01.121 Laceration with foreign body of right eyelid and periocular area
❼⇄ S01.122 Laceration with foreign body of left eyelid and periocular area
❼⇄ S01.131 Puncture wound without foreign body of right eyelid and periocular area
❼⇄ S01.132 Puncture wound without foreign body of left eyelid and periocular area
❼⇄ S01.141 Puncture wound with foreign body of right eyelid and periocular area
❼⇄ S01.142 Puncture wound with foreign body of left eyelid and periocular area
❼⇄ S01.151 Open bite of right eyelid and periocular area
❼⇄ S01.152 Open bite of left eyelid and periocular area
❼ T20.39 Burn of third degree of multiple sites of head, face, and neck
❼ T20.79 Corrosion of third degree of multiple sites of head, face, and neck
❼⇄ T26.01 Burn of right eyelid and periocular area
❼⇄ T26.02 Burn of left eyelid and periocular area
❼⇄ T26.51 Corrosion of right eyelid and periocular area
❼⇄ T26.52 Corrosion of left eyelid and periocular area

ICD-10-CM Coding Notes

For codes requiring a 7th character extension, refer to your ICD-10-CM book. Review the character descriptions and coding guidelines for proper selection. For some procedures, only certain characters will apply.

CCI Edits

Refer to Appendix A for CCI edits.

Pub 100

00103: Pub 100-04, 12, 140.5, Pub 100-04, 12, 50, Pub 100-04, 12, 90.4.5

Base Units

Global: XXX

Code	Base Units
00103	5

Modifiers (PAR)

Code	Mod 50	Mod 51	Mod 62	Mod 80
00103	9	9	9	9

CPT © 2018 American Medical Association. All Rights Reserved.

00104

00104 Anesthesia for electroconvulsive therapy

ICD-10-CM Diagnostic Codes

F20.0	Paranoid schizophrenia
F20.1	Disorganized schizophrenia
F20.2	Catatonic schizophrenia
F20.3	Undifferentiated schizophrenia
F20.5	Residual schizophrenia
F20.81	Schizophreniform disorder
F20.89	Other schizophrenia
F25.1	Schizoaffective disorder, depressive type
F30.13	Manic episode, severe, without psychotic symptoms
F30.2	Manic episode, severe with psychotic symptoms
F31.13	Bipolar disorder, current episode manic without psychotic features, severe
F31.2	Bipolar disorder, current episode manic severe with psychotic features
F31.4	Bipolar disorder, current episode depressed, severe, without psychotic features
F31.5	Bipolar disorder, current episode depressed, severe, with psychotic features
F31.63	Bipolar disorder, current episode mixed, severe, without psychotic features
F31.64	Bipolar disorder, current episode mixed, severe, with psychotic features
F32.2	Major depressive disorder, single episode, severe without psychotic features
F32.3	Major depressive disorder, single episode, severe with psychotic features
F33.2	Major depressive disorder, recurrent severe without psychotic features
F33.3	Major depressive disorder, recurrent, severe with psychotic symptoms
F60.3	Borderline personality disorder
G20	Parkinson's disease

CCI Edits

Refer to Appendix A for CCI edits.

Pub 100

00104: Pub 100-04, 12, 140.5, Pub 100-04, 12, 50, Pub 100-04, 12, 90.4.5

Base Units

Global: XXX

Code	Base Units
00104	4

Modifiers (PAR)

Code	Mod 50	Mod 51	Mod 62	Mod 80
00104	9	9	9	9

CPT © 2018 American Medical Association. All Rights Reserved.

00120

00120 Anesthesia for procedures on external, middle, and inner ear including biopsy; not otherwise specified

ICD-10-CM Diagnostic Codes

⇄	H61.311	Acquired stenosis of right external ear canal secondary to trauma
⇄	H61.312	Acquired stenosis of left external ear canal secondary to trauma
⇄	H61.321	Acquired stenosis of right external ear canal secondary to inflammation and infection
⇄	H61.322	Acquired stenosis of left external ear canal secondary to inflammation and infection
⇄	H68.111	Osseous obstruction of Eustachian tube, right ear
⇄	H68.112	Osseous obstruction of Eustachian tube, left ear
⇄	H68.113	Osseous obstruction of Eustachian tube, bilateral
⇄	H70.11	Chronic mastoiditis, right ear
⇄	H70.12	Chronic mastoiditis, left ear
⇄	H70.13	Chronic mastoiditis, bilateral
⇄	H71.01	Cholesteatoma of attic, right ear
⇄	H71.02	Cholesteatoma of attic, left ear
⇄	H71.03	Cholesteatoma of attic, bilateral
⇄	H71.11	Cholesteatoma of tympanum, right ear
⇄	H71.12	Cholesteatoma of tympanum, left ear
⇄	H71.13	Cholesteatoma of tympanum, bilateral
⇄	H72.01	Central perforation of tympanic membrane, right ear
⇄	H72.02	Central perforation of tympanic membrane, left ear
⇄	H72.11	Attic perforation of tympanic membrane, right ear
⇄	H72.12	Attic perforation of tympanic membrane, left ear
⇄	H72.811	Multiple perforations of tympanic membrane, right ear
⇄	H72.812	Multiple perforations of tympanic membrane, left ear
⇄	H72.821	Total perforations of tympanic membrane, right ear
⇄	H72.822	Total perforations of tympanic membrane, left ear
⇄	H72.91	Unspecified perforation of tympanic membrane, right ear
⇄	H72.92	Unspecified perforation of tympanic membrane, left ear
⇄	H74.01	Tympanosclerosis, right ear
⇄	H74.02	Tympanosclerosis, left ear
⇄	H74.03	Tympanosclerosis, bilateral
⇄	H74.311	Ankylosis of ear ossicles, right ear
⇄	H74.312	Ankylosis of ear ossicles, left ear
⇄	H74.313	Ankylosis of ear ossicles, bilateral
⇄	H74.321	Partial loss of ear ossicles, right ear
⇄	H74.322	Partial loss of ear ossicles, left ear
⇄	H74.323	Partial loss of ear ossicles, bilateral
⇄	H74.41	Polyp of right middle ear
⇄	H74.42	Polyp of left middle ear
⇄	H74.8X9	Other specified disorders of middle ear and mastoid, unspecified ear
⇄	H80.21	Cochlear otosclerosis, right ear
⇄	H80.22	Cochlear otosclerosis, left ear
⇄	H80.23	Cochlear otosclerosis, bilateral
⇄	H81.01	Ménière's disease, right ear
⇄	H81.02	Ménière's disease, left ear
⇄	H81.03	Ménière's disease, bilateral
	H90.0	Conductive hearing loss, bilateral
⇄	H90.11	Conductive hearing loss, unilateral, right ear, with unrestricted hearing on the contralateral side
⇄	H90.12	Conductive hearing loss, unilateral, left ear, with unrestricted hearing on the contralateral side
	H90.2	Conductive hearing loss, unspecified
❼⇄	S09.311	Primary blast injury of right ear
❼⇄	S09.312	Primary blast injury of left ear
❼⇄	S09.313	Primary blast injury of ear, bilateral
❼⇄	S09.391	Other specified injury of right middle and inner ear
❼⇄	S09.392	Other specified injury of left middle and inner ear

ICD-10-CM Coding Notes

For codes requiring a 7th character extension, refer to your ICD-10-CM book. Review the character descriptions and coding guidelines for proper selection. For some procedures, only certain characters will apply.

CCI Edits

Refer to Appendix A for CCI edits.

Pub 100

00120: Pub 100-04, 12, 140.5, Pub 100-04, 12, 50, Pub 100-04, 12, 90.4.5

Base Units

Global: XXX

Code	Base Units
00120	5

Modifiers (PAR)

Code	Mod 50	Mod 51	Mod 62	Mod 80
00120	9	9	9	9

CPT © 2018 American Medical Association. All Rights Reserved.

00124

00124 Anesthesia for procedures on external, middle, and inner ear including biopsy; otoscopy

AMA *CPT Assistant* □

00124: Nov 99: 7

ICD-10-CM Diagnostic Codes

⇄	H60.311	Diffuse otitis externa, right ear
⇄	H60.312	Diffuse otitis externa, left ear
⇄	H60.313	Diffuse otitis externa, bilateral
⇄	H60.41	Cholesteatoma of right external ear
⇄	H60.42	Cholesteatoma of left external ear
⇄	H60.43	Cholesteatoma of external ear, bilateral
⇄	H61.21	Impacted cerumen, right ear
⇄	H61.22	Impacted cerumen, left ear
⇄	H61.23	Impacted cerumen, bilateral
⇄	H61.311	Acquired stenosis of right external ear canal secondary to trauma
⇄	H61.312	Acquired stenosis of left external ear canal secondary to trauma
⇄	H61.313	Acquired stenosis of external ear canal secondary to trauma, bilateral
⇄	H61.321	Acquired stenosis of right external ear canal secondary to inflammation and infection
⇄	H61.322	Acquired stenosis of left external ear canal secondary to inflammation and infection
⇄	H61.323	Acquired stenosis of external ear canal secondary to inflammation and infection, bilateral
⇄	H61.811	Exostosis of right external canal
⇄	H61.812	Exostosis of left external canal
⇄	H61.813	Exostosis of external canal, bilateral
⇄	H72.01	Central perforation of tympanic membrane, right ear
⇄	H72.02	Central perforation of tympanic membrane, left ear
⇄	H72.03	Central perforation of tympanic membrane, bilateral
⇄	H72.11	Attic perforation of tympanic membrane, right ear
⇄	H72.12	Attic perforation of tympanic membrane, left ear
⇄	H72.13	Attic perforation of tympanic membrane, bilateral
⇄	H72.2X1	Other marginal perforations of tympanic membrane, right ear
⇄	H72.2X2	Other marginal perforations of tympanic membrane, left ear
⇄	H72.2X3	Other marginal perforations of tympanic membrane, bilateral
⇄	H72.811	Multiple perforations of tympanic membrane, right ear
⇄	H72.812	Multiple perforations of tympanic membrane, left ear
⇄	H72.813	Multiple perforations of tympanic membrane, bilateral
⇄	H72.821	Total perforations of tympanic membrane, right ear
⇄	H72.822	Total perforations of tympanic membrane, left ear
⇄	H72.823	Total perforations of tympanic membrane, bilateral
⇄	H92.01	Otalgia, right ear
⇄	H92.02	Otalgia, left ear
⇄	H92.03	Otalgia, bilateral
⇄	H92.11	Otorrhea, right ear
⇄	H92.12	Otorrhea, left ear
⇄	H92.13	Otorrhea, bilateral
⇄	H92.21	Otorrhagia, right ear
⇄	H92.22	Otorrhagia, left ear
⇄	H92.23	Otorrhagia, bilateral
❼⇄	T16.1	Foreign body in right ear
❼⇄	T16.2	Foreign body in left ear

ICD-10-CM Coding Notes

For codes requiring a 7th character extension, refer to your ICD-10-CM book. Review the character descriptions and coding guidelines for proper selection. For some procedures, only certain characters will apply.

CCI Edits

Refer to Appendix A for CCI edits.

Pub 100

00124: Pub 100-04, 12, 140.5, Pub 100-04, 12, 50, Pub 100-04, 12, 90.4.5

Base Units

Global: XXX

Code	Base Units
00124	4

Modifiers (PAR)

Code	Mod 50	Mod 51	Mod 62	Mod 80
00124	9	9	9	9

CPT © 2018 American Medical Association. All Rights Reserved.

00126

00126 Anesthesia for procedures on external, middle, and inner ear including biopsy; tympanotomy

ICD-10-CM Diagnostic Codes

⇄	H65.31	Chronic mucoid otitis media, right ear
⇄	H65.32	Chronic mucoid otitis media, left ear
⇄	H65.33	Chronic mucoid otitis media, bilateral
⇄	H66.004	Acute suppurative otitis media without spontaneous rupture of ear drum, recurrent, right ear
⇄	H66.005	Acute suppurative otitis media without spontaneous rupture of ear drum, recurrent, left ear
⇄	H66.006	Acute suppurative otitis media without spontaneous rupture of ear drum, recurrent, bilateral
⇄	H66.3X1	Other chronic suppurative otitis media, right ear
⇄	H66.3X2	Other chronic suppurative otitis media, left ear
⇄	H66.3X3	Other chronic suppurative otitis media, bilateral
⇄	H68.021	Chronic Eustachian salpingitis, right ear
⇄	H68.022	Chronic Eustachian salpingitis, left ear
⇄	H68.023	Chronic Eustachian salpingitis, bilateral
⇄	H69.81	Other specified disorders of Eustachian tube, right ear
⇄	H69.82	Other specified disorders of Eustachian tube, left ear
⇄	H69.83	Other specified disorders of Eustachian tube, bilateral
⇄	H71.01	Cholesteatoma of attic, right ear
⇄	H71.02	Cholesteatoma of attic, left ear
⇄	H71.03	Cholesteatoma of attic, bilateral
⇄	H71.11	Cholesteatoma of tympanum, right ear
⇄	H71.12	Cholesteatoma of tympanum, left ear
⇄	H71.13	Cholesteatoma of tympanum, bilateral
⇄	H71.91	Unspecified cholesteatoma, right ear
⇄	H71.92	Unspecified cholesteatoma, left ear
⇄	H71.93	Unspecified cholesteatoma, bilateral
	H90.0	Conductive hearing loss, bilateral
⇄	H90.11	Conductive hearing loss, unilateral, right ear, with unrestricted hearing on the contralateral side
⇄	H90.12	Conductive hearing loss, unilateral, left ear, with unrestricted hearing on the contralateral side
	H90.2	Conductive hearing loss, unspecified
⇄	H93.8X1	Other specified disorders of right ear
⇄	H93.8X2	Other specified disorders of left ear
⇄	H93.8X3	Other specified disorders of ear, bilateral
❼⇄	T16.1	Foreign body in right ear
❼⇄	T16.2	Foreign body in left ear

ICD-10-CM Coding Notes

For codes requiring a 7th character extension, refer to your ICD-10-CM book. Review the character descriptions and coding guidelines for proper selection. For some procedures, only certain characters will apply.

CCI Edits

Refer to Appendix A for CCI edits.

Pub 100

00126: Pub 100-04, 12, 140.5, Pub 100-04, 12, 50, Pub 100-04, 12, 90.4.5

Base Units

Global: XXX

Code	Base Units
00126	4

Modifiers (PAR)

Code	Mod 50	Mod 51	Mod 62	Mod 80
00126	9	9	9	9

CPT © 2018 American Medical Association. All Rights Reserved.

00140

00140 Anesthesia for procedures on eye; not otherwise specified

ICD-10-CM Diagnostic Codes

⇄	C69.01	Malignant neoplasm of right conjunctiva
⇄	C69.02	Malignant neoplasm of left conjunctiva
⇄	C69.11	Malignant neoplasm of right cornea
⇄	C69.12	Malignant neoplasm of left cornea
⇄	C69.41	Malignant neoplasm of right ciliary body
⇄	C69.42	Malignant neoplasm of left ciliary body
⇄	C69.51	Malignant neoplasm of right lacrimal gland and duct
⇄	C69.52	Malignant neoplasm of left lacrimal gland and duct
⇄	D31.01	Benign neoplasm of right conjunctiva
⇄	D31.02	Benign neoplasm of left conjunctiva
⇄	D31.11	Benign neoplasm of right cornea
⇄	D31.12	Benign neoplasm of left cornea
⇄	D31.41	Benign neoplasm of right ciliary body
⇄	D31.42	Benign neoplasm of left ciliary body
⇄	D31.51	Benign neoplasm of right lacrimal gland and duct
⇄	D31.52	Benign neoplasm of left lacrimal gland and duct
⇄	D31.61	Benign neoplasm of unspecified site of right orbit
⇄	D31.62	Benign neoplasm of unspecified site of left orbit
⇄	H04.551	Acquired stenosis of right nasolacrimal duct
⇄	H04.552	Acquired stenosis of left nasolacrimal duct
⇄	H04.553	Acquired stenosis of bilateral nasolacrimal duct
⇄	H11.221	Conjunctival granuloma, right eye
⇄	H11.222	Conjunctival granuloma, left eye
⇄	H11.223	Conjunctival granuloma, bilateral
⇄	H16.071	Perforated corneal ulcer, right eye
⇄	H16.072	Perforated corneal ulcer, left eye
⇄	H16.073	Perforated corneal ulcer, bilateral
❼⇄	S05.51	Penetrating wound with foreign body of right eyeball
❼⇄	S05.52	Penetrating wound with foreign body of left eyeball

ICD-10-CM Coding Notes

For codes requiring a 7th character extension, refer to your ICD-10-CM book. Review the character descriptions and coding guidelines for proper selection. For some procedures, only certain characters will apply.

CCI Edits

Refer to Appendix A for CCI edits.

Pub 100

00140: Pub 100-04, 12, 140.5, Pub 100-04, 12, 50, Pub 100-04, 12, 90.4.5

Base Units

Global: XXX

Code	Base Units
00140	5

Modifiers (PAR)

Code	Mod 50	Mod 51	Mod 62	Mod 80
00140	9	9	9	9

CPT © 2018 American Medical Association. All Rights Reserved.

00142

00142 Anesthesia for procedures on eye; lens surgery

ICD-10-CM Diagnostic Codes

	E08.36	Diabetes mellitus due to underlying condition with diabetic cataract
	E09.36	Drug or chemical induced diabetes mellitus with diabetic cataract
	E10.36	Type 1 diabetes mellitus with diabetic cataract
	E11.36	Type 2 diabetes mellitus with diabetic cataract
	E13.36	Other specified diabetes mellitus with diabetic cataract
⇄	H25.011	Cortical age-related cataract, right eye
⇄	H25.012	Cortical age-related cataract, left eye
⇄	H25.013	Cortical age-related cataract, bilateral
⇄	H25.041	Posterior subcapsular polar age-related cataract, right eye
⇄	H25.042	Posterior subcapsular polar age-related cataract, left eye
⇄	H25.043	Posterior subcapsular polar age-related cataract, bilateral
⇄	H25.11	Age-related nuclear cataract, right eye
⇄	H25.12	Age-related nuclear cataract, left eye
⇄	H25.13	Age-related nuclear cataract, bilateral
⇄	H26.031	Infantile and juvenile nuclear cataract, right eye
⇄	H26.032	Infantile and juvenile nuclear cataract, left eye
⇄	H26.033	Infantile and juvenile nuclear cataract, bilateral
⇄	H26.111	Localized traumatic opacities, right eye
⇄	H26.112	Localized traumatic opacities, left eye
⇄	H26.113	Localized traumatic opacities, bilateral
⇄	H26.211	Cataract with neovascularization, right eye
⇄	H26.212	Cataract with neovascularization, left eye
⇄	H26.213	Cataract with neovascularization, bilateral
⇄	H26.221	Cataract secondary to ocular disorders (degenerative) (inflammatory), right eye
⇄	H26.222	Cataract secondary to ocular disorders (degenerative) (inflammatory), left eye
⇄	H26.223	Cataract secondary to ocular disorders (degenerative) (inflammatory), bilateral
⇄	H26.31	Drug-induced cataract, right eye
⇄	H26.32	Drug-induced cataract, left eye
⇄	H26.33	Drug-induced cataract, bilateral
⇄	H27.111	Subluxation of lens, right eye
⇄	H27.112	Subluxation of lens, left eye
⇄	H27.121	Anterior dislocation of lens, right eye
⇄	H27.122	Anterior dislocation of lens, left eye
⇄	H27.131	Posterior dislocation of lens, right eye
⇄	H27.132	Posterior dislocation of lens, left eye
⇄	H59.021	Cataract (lens) fragments in eye following cataract surgery, right eye
⇄	H59.022	Cataract (lens) fragments in eye following cataract surgery, left eye
⇄	H59.023	Cataract (lens) fragments in eye following cataract surgery, bilateral
❼⇄	S05.8X1	Other injuries of right eye and orbit
❼⇄	S05.8X2	Other injuries of left eye and orbit

ICD-10-CM Coding Notes

For codes requiring a 7th character extension, refer to your ICD-10-CM book. Review the character descriptions and coding guidelines for proper selection. For some procedures, only certain characters will apply.

CCI Edits

Refer to Appendix A for CCI edits.

Pub 100

00142: Pub 100-04, 12, 140.5, Pub 100-04, 12, 50, Pub 100-04, 12, 90.4.5

Base Units

Global: XXX

Code	Base Units
00142	4

Modifiers (PAR)

Code	Mod 50	Mod 51	Mod 62	Mod 80
00142	9	9	9	9

● New ▲ Revised ✚ Add On ⊘Modifier 51 Exempt ★Telemedicine ▯ CPT QuickRef ⁄FDA Pending ⇄ Laterality ❼ Seventh Character ♂Male ♀Female

CPT © 2018 American Medical Association. All Rights Reserved.

00144

00144 Anesthesia for procedures on eye; corneal transplant

ICD-10-CM Diagnostic Codes

	B00.52	Herpesviral keratitis
	B02.33	Zoster keratitis
⇄	H16.011	Central corneal ulcer, right eye
⇄	H16.012	Central corneal ulcer, left eye
⇄	H16.013	Central corneal ulcer, bilateral
⇄	H16.071	Perforated corneal ulcer, right eye
⇄	H16.072	Perforated corneal ulcer, left eye
⇄	H16.073	Perforated corneal ulcer, bilateral
⇄	H16.441	Deep vascularization of cornea, right eye
⇄	H16.442	Deep vascularization of cornea, left eye
⇄	H16.443	Deep vascularization of cornea, bilateral
	H16.8	Other keratitis
⇄	H17.01	Adherent leukoma, right eye
⇄	H17.02	Adherent leukoma, left eye
⇄	H17.03	Adherent leukoma, bilateral
⇄	H17.11	Central corneal opacity, right eye
⇄	H17.12	Central corneal opacity, left eye
⇄	H17.13	Central corneal opacity, bilateral
	H17.89	Other corneal scars and opacities
⇄	H18.211	Corneal edema secondary to contact lens, right eye
⇄	H18.212	Corneal edema secondary to contact lens, left eye
⇄	H18.213	Corneal edema secondary to contact lens, bilateral
	H18.51	Endothelial corneal dystrophy
	H18.52	Epithelial (juvenile) corneal dystrophy
⇄	H18.621	Keratoconus, unstable, right eye
⇄	H18.622	Keratoconus, unstable, left eye
⇄	H18.623	Keratoconus, unstable, bilateral
	Q13.3	Congenital corneal opacity
	Q13.4	Other congenital corneal malformations
⑦⇄	S05.01	Injury of conjunctiva and corneal abrasion without foreign body, right eye
⑦⇄	S05.02	Injury of conjunctiva and corneal abrasion without foreign body, left eye
⑦⇄	S05.31	Ocular laceration without prolapse or loss of intraocular tissue, right eye
⑦⇄	S05.32	Ocular laceration without prolapse or loss of intraocular tissue, left eye
	T86.840	Corneal transplant rejection
	T86.841	Corneal transplant failure

ICD-10-CM Coding Notes

For codes requiring a 7th character extension, refer to your ICD-10-CM book. Review the character descriptions and coding guidelines for proper selection. For some procedures, only certain characters will apply.

CCI Edits

Refer to Appendix A for CCI edits.

Pub 100

00144: Pub 100-04, 12, 140.5, Pub 100-04, 12, 50, Pub 100-04, 12, 90.4.5

Base Units

Global: XXX

Code	Base Units
00144	6

Modifiers (PAR)

Code	Mod 50	Mod 51	Mod 62	Mod 80
00144	9	9	9	9

CPT © 2018 American Medical Association. All Rights Reserved.

00145

00145 Anesthesia for procedures on eye; vitreoretinal surgery

ICD-10-CM Diagnostic Codes

➐⇄	E08.351	Diabetes mellitus due to underlying condition with proliferative diabetic retinopathy with macular edema
➐⇄	E08.359	Diabetes mellitus due to underlying condition with proliferative diabetic retinopathy without macular edema
➐⇄	E09.351	Drug or chemical induced diabetes mellitus with proliferative diabetic retinopathy with macular edema
➐⇄	E09.359	Drug or chemical induced diabetes mellitus with proliferative diabetic retinopathy without macular edema
➐⇄	E10.351	Type 1 diabetes mellitus with proliferative diabetic retinopathy with macular edema
➐⇄	E10.359	Type 1 diabetes mellitus with proliferative diabetic retinopathy without macular edema
➐⇄	E11.351	Type 2 diabetes mellitus with proliferative diabetic retinopathy with macular edema
➐⇄	E11.359	Type 2 diabetes mellitus with proliferative diabetic retinopathy without macular edema
➐⇄	E13.351	Other specified diabetes mellitus with proliferative diabetic retinopathy with macular edema
➐⇄	E13.359	Other specified diabetes mellitus with proliferative diabetic retinopathy without macular edema
⇄	H33.011	Retinal detachment with single break, right eye
⇄	H33.012	Retinal detachment with single break, left eye
⇄	H33.021	Retinal detachment with multiple breaks, right eye
⇄	H33.022	Retinal detachment with multiple breaks, left eye
⇄	H33.031	Retinal detachment with giant retinal tear, right eye
⇄	H33.032	Retinal detachment with giant retinal tear, left eye
⇄	H33.041	Retinal detachment with retinal dialysis, right eye
⇄	H33.042	Retinal detachment with retinal dialysis, left eye
⇄	H33.051	Total retinal detachment, right eye
⇄	H33.052	Total retinal detachment, left eye
⇄	H33.21	Serous retinal detachment, right eye
⇄	H33.22	Serous retinal detachment, left eye
⇄	H33.311	Horseshoe tear of retina without detachment, right eye
⇄	H33.312	Horseshoe tear of retina without detachment, left eye
⇄	H33.41	Traction detachment of retina, right eye
⇄	H33.42	Traction detachment of retina, left eye
⇄	H35.141	Retinopathy of prematurity, stage 3, right eye
⇄	H35.142	Retinopathy of prematurity, stage 3, left eye
⇄	H35.143	Retinopathy of prematurity, stage 3, bilateral
⇄	H35.151	Retinopathy of prematurity, stage 4, right eye
⇄	H35.152	Retinopathy of prematurity, stage 4, left eye
⇄	H35.153	Retinopathy of prematurity, stage 4, bilateral
⇄	H35.161	Retinopathy of prematurity, stage 5, right eye
⇄	H35.162	Retinopathy of prematurity, stage 5, left eye
⇄	H35.163	Retinopathy of prematurity, stage 5, bilateral
⇄	H35.21	Other non-diabetic proliferative retinopathy, right eye
⇄	H35.22	Other non-diabetic proliferative retinopathy, left eye
⇄	H35.3111	Nonexudative age-related macular degeneration, right eye, early dry stage
⇄	H35.3112	Nonexudative age-related macular degeneration, right eye, intermediate dry stage
⇄	H35.3113	Nonexudative age-related macular degeneration, right eye, advanced atrophic without subfoveal involvement
⇄	H35.3114	Nonexudative age-related macular degeneration, right eye, advanced atrophic with subfoveal involvement
⇄	H35.3121	Nonexudative age-related macular degeneration, left eye, early dry stage
⇄	H35.3122	Nonexudative age-related macular degeneration, left eye, intermediate dry stage
⇄	H35.3123	Nonexudative age-related macular degeneration, left eye, advanced atrophic without subfoveal involvement
⇄	H35.3124	Nonexudative age-related macular degeneration, left eye, advanced atrophic with subfoveal involvement
⇄	H35.3131	Nonexudative age-related macular degeneration, bilateral, early dry stage
⇄	H35.3132	Nonexudative age-related macular degeneration, bilateral, intermediate dry stage
⇄	H35.3133	Nonexudative age-related macular degeneration, bilateral, advanced atrophic without subfoveal involvement
⇄	H35.3134	Nonexudative age-related macular degeneration, bilateral, advanced atrophic with subfoveal involvement
⇄	H35.3211	Exudative age-related macular degeneration, right eye, with active choroidal neovascularization
⇄	H35.3212	Exudative age-related macular degeneration, right eye, with inactive choroidal neovascularization
⇄	H35.3213	Exudative age-related macular degeneration, right eye, with inactive scar
⇄	H35.3221	Exudative age-related macular degeneration, left eye, with active choroidal neovascularization
⇄	H35.3222	Exudative age-related macular degeneration, left eye, with inactive choroidal neovascularization
⇄	H35.3223	Exudative age-related macular degeneration, left eye, with inactive scar
⇄	H35.3231	Exudative age-related macular degeneration, bilateral, with active choroidal neovascularization
⇄	H35.3232	Exudative age-related macular degeneration, bilateral, with inactive choroidal neovascularization
⇄	H35.3233	Exudative age-related macular degeneration, bilateral, with inactive scar
⇄	H35.341	Macular cyst, hole, or pseudohole, right eye
⇄	H35.342	Macular cyst, hole, or pseudohole, left eye
⇄	H35.371	Puckering of macula, right eye
⇄	H35.372	Puckering of macula, left eye
	H35.81	Retinal edema
⇄	H59.211	Accidental puncture and laceration of right eye and adnexa during an ophthalmic procedure
⇄	H59.212	Accidental puncture and laceration of left eye and adnexa during an ophthalmic procedure

ICD-10-CM Coding Notes

For codes requiring a 7th character extension, refer to your ICD-10-CM book. Review the character descriptions and coding guidelines for proper selection. For some procedures, only certain characters will apply.

CCI Edits

Refer to Appendix A for CCI edits.

Pub 100

00145: Pub 100-04, 12, 140.5, Pub 100-04, 12, 50, Pub 100-04, 12, 90.4.5

Base Units

Global: XXX

Code	Base Units
00145	6

Modifiers (PAR)

Code	Mod 50	Mod 51	Mod 62	Mod 80
00145	9	9	9	9

CPT © 2018 American Medical Association. All Rights Reserved.

00147

00147 Anesthesia for procedures on eye; iridectomy

ICD-10-CM Diagnostic Codes

	H21.82	Plateau iris syndrome (post-iridectomy) (postprocedural)
⇄	H27.111	Subluxation of lens, right eye
⇄	H27.112	Subluxation of lens, left eye
⇄	H27.113	Subluxation of lens, bilateral
⇄	H27.121	Anterior dislocation of lens, right eye
⇄	H27.122	Anterior dislocation of lens, left eye
⇄	H27.123	Anterior dislocation of lens, bilateral
⇄	H27.131	Posterior dislocation of lens, right eye
⇄	H27.132	Posterior dislocation of lens, left eye
⇄	H27.133	Posterior dislocation of lens, bilateral
❼⇄	H40.131	Pigmentary glaucoma, right eye
❼⇄	H40.132	Pigmentary glaucoma, left eye
❼⇄	H40.133	Pigmentary glaucoma, bilateral
⇄	H40.211	Acute angle-closure glaucoma, right eye
⇄	H40.212	Acute angle-closure glaucoma, left eye
⇄	H40.213	Acute angle-closure glaucoma, bilateral
❼⇄	H40.221	Chronic angle-closure glaucoma, right eye
❼⇄	H40.222	Chronic angle-closure glaucoma, left eye
❼⇄	H40.223	Chronic angle-closure glaucoma, bilateral
⇄	H40.231	Intermittent angle-closure glaucoma, right eye
⇄	H40.232	Intermittent angle-closure glaucoma, left eye
⇄	H40.233	Intermittent angle-closure glaucoma, bilateral
⇄	H40.241	Residual stage of angle-closure glaucoma, right eye
⇄	H40.242	Residual stage of angle-closure glaucoma, left eye
⇄	H40.243	Residual stage of angle-closure glaucoma, bilateral
❼⇄	H40.31	Glaucoma secondary to eye trauma, right eye
❼⇄	H40.32	Glaucoma secondary to eye trauma, left eye
❼⇄	H40.33	Glaucoma secondary to eye trauma, bilateral
❼⇄	H40.41	Glaucoma secondary to eye inflammation, right eye
❼⇄	H40.42	Glaucoma secondary to eye inflammation, left eye
❼⇄	H40.43	Glaucoma secondary to eye inflammation, bilateral
❼⇄	H40.51	Glaucoma secondary to other eye disorders, right eye
❼⇄	H40.52	Glaucoma secondary to other eye disorders, left eye
❼⇄	H40.53	Glaucoma secondary to other eye disorders, bilateral
❼⇄	H40.61	Glaucoma secondary to drugs, right eye
❼⇄	H40.62	Glaucoma secondary to drugs, left eye
❼⇄	H40.63	Glaucoma secondary to drugs, bilateral
	Q13.2	Other congenital malformations of iris
❼⇄	S05.11	Contusion of eyeball and orbital tissues, right eye
❼⇄	S05.12	Contusion of eyeball and orbital tissues, left eye
❼⇄	S05.21	Ocular laceration and rupture with prolapse or loss of intraocular tissue, right eye
❼⇄	S05.22	Ocular laceration and rupture with prolapse or loss of intraocular tissue, left eye
❼⇄	S05.31	Ocular laceration without prolapse or loss of intraocular tissue, right eye
❼⇄	S05.32	Ocular laceration without prolapse or loss of intraocular tissue, left eye
❼⇄	S05.41	Penetrating wound of orbit with or without foreign body, right eye
❼⇄	S05.42	Penetrating wound of orbit with or without foreign body, left eye
❼⇄	S05.51	Penetrating wound with foreign body of right eyeball
❼⇄	S05.52	Penetrating wound with foreign body of left eyeball
❼⇄	S05.61	Penetrating wound without foreign body of right eyeball
❼⇄	S05.62	Penetrating wound without foreign body of left eyeball
❼⇄	S05.8X1	Other injuries of right eye and orbit
❼⇄	S05.8X2	Other injuries of left eye and orbit

ICD-10-CM Coding Notes

For codes requiring a 7th character extension, refer to your ICD-10-CM book. Review the character descriptions and coding guidelines for proper selection. For some procedures, only certain characters will apply.

CCI Edits

Refer to Appendix A for CCI edits.

Pub 100

00147: Pub 100-04, 12, 140.5, Pub 100-04, 12, 50, Pub 100-04, 12, 90.4.5

Base Units

Global: XXX

Code	Base Units
00147	4

Modifiers (PAR)

Code	Mod 50	Mod 51	Mod 62	Mod 80
00147	9	9	9	9

CPT © 2018 American Medical Association. All Rights Reserved.

00148

00148 Anesthesia for procedures on eye; ophthalmoscopy

ICD-10-CM Diagnostic Codes

⇄	H16.391	Other interstitial and deep keratitis, right eye
⇄	H16.392	Other interstitial and deep keratitis, left eye
⇄	H16.393	Other interstitial and deep keratitis, bilateral
⇄	H21.231	Degeneration of iris (pigmentary), right eye
⇄	H21.232	Degeneration of iris (pigmentary), left eye
⇄	H21.233	Degeneration of iris (pigmentary), bilateral
⇄	H21.41	Pupillary membranes, right eye
⇄	H21.42	Pupillary membranes, left eye
⇄	H21.43	Pupillary membranes, bilateral
⇄	H33.191	Other retinoschisis and retinal cysts, right eye
⇄	H33.192	Other retinoschisis and retinal cysts, left eye
⇄	H33.193	Other retinoschisis and retinal cysts, bilateral
⇄	H35.20	Other non-diabetic proliferative retinopathy, unspecified eye
⇄	H35.21	Other non-diabetic proliferative retinopathy, right eye
⇄	H35.22	Other non-diabetic proliferative retinopathy, left eye
⇄	H35.3111	Nonexudative age-related macular degeneration, right eye, early dry stage
⇄	H35.3112	Nonexudative age-related macular degeneration, right eye, intermediate dry stage
⇄	H35.3113	Nonexudative age-related macular degeneration, right eye, advanced atrophic without subfoveal involvement
⇄	H35.3114	Nonexudative age-related macular degeneration, right eye, advanced atrophic with subfoveal involvement
⇄	H35.3121	Nonexudative age-related macular degeneration, left eye, early dry stage
⇄	H35.3122	Nonexudative age-related macular degeneration, left eye, intermediate dry stage
⇄	H35.3123	Nonexudative age-related macular degeneration, left eye, advanced atrophic without subfoveal involvement
⇄	H35.3124	Nonexudative age-related macular degeneration, left eye, advanced atrophic with subfoveal involvement
⇄	H35.3131	Nonexudative age-related macular degeneration, bilateral, early dry stage
⇄	H35.3132	Nonexudative age-related macular degeneration, bilateral, intermediate dry stage
⇄	H35.3133	Nonexudative age-related macular degeneration, bilateral, advanced atrophic without subfoveal involvement
⇄	H35.3134	Nonexudative age-related macular degeneration, bilateral, advanced atrophic with subfoveal involvement
⇄	H35.3211	Exudative age-related macular degeneration, right eye, with active choroidal neovascularization
⇄	H35.3212	Exudative age-related macular degeneration, right eye, with inactive choroidal neovascularization
⇄	H35.3213	Exudative age-related macular degeneration, right eye, with inactive scar
⇄	H35.3221	Exudative age-related macular degeneration, left eye, with active choroidal neovascularization
⇄	H35.3222	Exudative age-related macular degeneration, left eye, with inactive choroidal neovascularization
⇄	H35.3223	Exudative age-related macular degeneration, left eye, with inactive scar
⇄	H35.3231	Exudative age-related macular degeneration, bilateral, with active choroidal neovascularization
⇄	H35.3232	Exudative age-related macular degeneration, bilateral, with inactive choroidal neovascularization
⇄	H35.3233	Exudative age-related macular degeneration, bilateral, with inactive scar
	H35.33	Angioid streaks of macula
	H35.81	Retinal edema
⇄	H43.01	Vitreous prolapse, right eye
⇄	H43.02	Vitreous prolapse, left eye
⇄	H43.03	Vitreous prolapse, bilateral
⇄	H43.11	Vitreous hemorrhage, right eye
⇄	H43.12	Vitreous hemorrhage, left eye
⇄	H43.13	Vitreous hemorrhage, bilateral
⇄	H44.111	Panuveitis, right eye
⇄	H44.112	Panuveitis, left eye
⇄	H44.113	Panuveitis, bilateral
⇄	H46.01	Optic papillitis, right eye
⇄	H46.02	Optic papillitis, left eye
⇄	H46.03	Optic papillitis, bilateral
⇄	H53.121	Transient visual loss, right eye
⇄	H53.122	Transient visual loss, left eye
⇄	H53.123	Transient visual loss, bilateral
⇄	H53.131	Sudden visual loss, right eye
⇄	H53.132	Sudden visual loss, left eye
⇄	H53.133	Sudden visual loss, bilateral
⇄	H53.141	Visual discomfort, right eye
⇄	H53.142	Visual discomfort, left eye
⇄	H53.143	Visual discomfort, bilateral
	H53.2	Diplopia
⇄	H53.481	Generalized contraction of visual field, right eye
⇄	H53.482	Generalized contraction of visual field, left eye
⇄	H53.483	Generalized contraction of visual field, bilateral
	H53.60	Unspecified night blindness
	H53.8	Other visual disturbances
❼⇄	S05.51	Penetrating wound with foreign body of right eyeball
❼⇄	S05.52	Penetrating wound with foreign body of left eyeball
❼⇄	S05.61	Penetrating wound without foreign body of right eyeball
❼⇄	S05.62	Penetrating wound without foreign body of left eyeball

ICD-10-CM Coding Notes

For codes requiring a 7th character extension, refer to your ICD-10-CM book. Review the character descriptions and coding guidelines for proper selection. For some procedures, only certain characters will apply.

CCI Edits

Refer to Appendix A for CCI edits.

Pub 100

00148: Pub 100-04, 12, 140.5, Pub 100-04, 12, 50, Pub 100-04, 12, 90.4.5

Base Units

Global: XXX

Code	Base Units
00148	4

Modifiers (PAR)

Code	Mod 50	Mod 51	Mod 62	Mod 80
00148	9	9	9	9

CPT © 2018 American Medical Association. All Rights Reserved.

00160

00160 Anesthesia for procedures on nose and accessory sinuses; not otherwise specified

ICD-10-CM Diagnostic Codes

⇄	H04.531	Neonatal obstruction of right nasolacrimal duct
⇄	H04.532	Neonatal obstruction of left nasolacrimal duct
⇄	H04.533	Neonatal obstruction of bilateral nasolacrimal duct
	J01.00	Acute maxillary sinusitis, unspecified
	J01.01	Acute recurrent maxillary sinusitis
	J01.10	Acute frontal sinusitis, unspecified
	J01.11	Acute recurrent frontal sinusitis
	J01.20	Acute ethmoidal sinusitis, unspecified
	J01.21	Acute recurrent ethmoidal sinusitis
	J01.30	Acute sphenoidal sinusitis, unspecified
	J01.31	Acute recurrent sphenoidal sinusitis
	J01.40	Acute pansinusitis, unspecified
	J01.41	Acute recurrent pansinusitis
	J01.80	Other acute sinusitis
	J01.81	Other acute recurrent sinusitis
	J01.90	Acute sinusitis, unspecified
	J01.91	Acute recurrent sinusitis, unspecified
	J32.0	Chronic maxillary sinusitis
	J32.1	Chronic frontal sinusitis
	J32.2	Chronic ethmoidal sinusitis
	J32.3	Chronic sphenoidal sinusitis
	J32.4	Chronic pansinusitis
	J32.8	Other chronic sinusitis
	J32.9	Chronic sinusitis, unspecified
	J33.0	Polyp of nasal cavity
	J33.1	Polypoid sinus degeneration
	J33.8	Other polyp of sinus
	J34.0	Abscess, furuncle and carbuncle of nose
	J34.1	Cyst and mucocele of nose and nasal sinus
	J34.2	Deviated nasal septum
	J34.81	Nasal mucositis (ulcerative)
	J34.89	Other specified disorders of nose and nasal sinuses
	R04.0	Epistaxis
❼	S01.20	Unspecified open wound of nose
❼	S01.21	Laceration without foreign body of nose
❼	S01.22	Laceration with foreign body of nose
❼	S01.23	Puncture wound without foreign body of nose
❼	S01.24	Puncture wound with foreign body of nose
❼	S01.25	Open bite of nose
❼	S02.2	Fracture of nasal bones
❼	T17.0	Foreign body in nasal sinus
❼	T17.1	Foreign body in nostril

ICD-10-CM Coding Notes

For codes requiring a 7th character extension, refer to your ICD-10-CM book. Review the character descriptions and coding guidelines for proper selection. For some procedures, only certain characters will apply.

CCI Edits

Refer to Appendix A for CCI edits.

Pub 100

00160: Pub 100-04, 12, 140.5, Pub 100-04, 12, 50, Pub 100-04, 12, 90.4.5

Base Units

Global: XXX

Code	Base Units
00160	5

Modifiers (PAR)

Code	Mod 50	Mod 51	Mod 62	Mod 80
00160	9	9	9	9

CPT © 2018 American Medical Association. All Rights Reserved.

00162

00162 Anesthesia for procedures on nose and accessory sinuses; radical surgery

ICD-10-CM Diagnostic Codes

C30.0	Malignant neoplasm of nasal cavity
C31.0	Malignant neoplasm of maxillary sinus
C31.1	Malignant neoplasm of ethmoidal sinus
C31.2	Malignant neoplasm of frontal sinus
C31.3	Malignant neoplasm of sphenoid sinus
C31.8	Malignant neoplasm of overlapping sites of accessory sinuses
C31.9	Malignant neoplasm of accessory sinus, unspecified
C43.31	Malignant melanoma of nose
C44.301	Unspecified malignant neoplasm of skin of nose
C44.311	Basal cell carcinoma of skin of nose
C44.321	Squamous cell carcinoma of skin of nose
C44.391	Other specified malignant neoplasm of skin of nose
C4A.31	Merkel cell carcinoma of nose
J01.00	Acute maxillary sinusitis, unspecified
J01.01	Acute recurrent maxillary sinusitis
J01.10	Acute frontal sinusitis, unspecified
J01.11	Acute recurrent frontal sinusitis
J01.20	Acute ethmoidal sinusitis, unspecified
J01.21	Acute recurrent ethmoidal sinusitis
J01.30	Acute sphenoidal sinusitis, unspecified
J01.31	Acute recurrent sphenoidal sinusitis
J01.40	Acute pansinusitis, unspecified
J01.41	Acute recurrent pansinusitis
J01.80	Other acute sinusitis
J01.81	Other acute recurrent sinusitis
J01.90	Acute sinusitis, unspecified
J01.91	Acute recurrent sinusitis, unspecified
J32.0	Chronic maxillary sinusitis
J32.1	Chronic frontal sinusitis
J32.2	Chronic ethmoidal sinusitis
J32.3	Chronic sphenoidal sinusitis
J32.4	Chronic pansinusitis
J32.8	Other chronic sinusitis
J32.9	Chronic sinusitis, unspecified
J33.0	Polyp of nasal cavity
J33.1	Polypoid sinus degeneration
J33.8	Other polyp of sinus
J34.0	Abscess, furuncle and carbuncle of nose
J34.1	Cyst and mucocele of nose and nasal sinus
J34.2	Deviated nasal septum
J34.3	Hypertrophy of nasal turbinates
J34.81	Nasal mucositis (ulcerative)
J34.89	Other specified disorders of nose and nasal sinuses
R04.0	Epistaxis
❼ S01.21	Laceration without foreign body of nose
❼ S01.22	Laceration with foreign body of nose
❼ S01.23	Puncture wound without foreign body of nose
❼ S01.24	Puncture wound with foreign body of nose
❼ S01.25	Open bite of nose
❼ S02.2	Fracture of nasal bones
❼ T17.0	Foreign body in nasal sinus
❼ T17.1	Foreign body in nostril

ICD-10-CM Coding Notes

For codes requiring a 7th character extension, refer to your ICD-10-CM book. Review the character descriptions and coding guidelines for proper selection. For some procedures, only certain characters will apply.

CCI Edits

Refer to Appendix A for CCI edits.

Pub 100

00162: Pub 100-04, 12, 140.5, Pub 100-04, 12, 50, Pub 100-04, 12, 90.4.5

Base Units

Global: XXX

Code	Base Units
00162	7

Modifiers (PAR)

Code	Mod 50	Mod 51	Mod 62	Mod 80
00162	9	9	9	9

CPT © 2018 American Medical Association. All Rights Reserved.

00164

00164 Anesthesia for procedures on nose and accessory sinuses; biopsy, soft tissue

ICD-10-CM Diagnostic Codes

C11.3	Malignant neoplasm of anterior wall of nasopharynx
C30.0	Malignant neoplasm of nasal cavity
C31.0	Malignant neoplasm of maxillary sinus
C31.1	Malignant neoplasm of ethmoidal sinus
C31.2	Malignant neoplasm of frontal sinus
C31.3	Malignant neoplasm of sphenoid sinus
C31.8	Malignant neoplasm of overlapping sites of accessory sinuses
C31.9	Malignant neoplasm of accessory sinus, unspecified
C43.31	Malignant melanoma of nose
C44.301	Unspecified malignant neoplasm of skin of nose
C44.311	Basal cell carcinoma of skin of nose
C44.321	Squamous cell carcinoma of skin of nose
C44.391	Other specified malignant neoplasm of skin of nose
C4A.31	Merkel cell carcinoma of nose
C76.0	Malignant neoplasm of head, face and neck
C78.39	Secondary malignant neoplasm of other respiratory organs
C79.89	Secondary malignant neoplasm of other specified sites
D02.3	Carcinoma in situ of other parts of respiratory system
D09.8	Carcinoma in situ of other specified sites
D10.6	Benign neoplasm of nasopharynx
D14.0	Benign neoplasm of middle ear, nasal cavity and accessory sinuses
D36.7	Benign neoplasm of other specified sites
D37.05	Neoplasm of uncertain behavior of pharynx
D38.5	Neoplasm of uncertain behavior of other respiratory organs
D48.7	Neoplasm of uncertain behavior of other specified sites
D49.1	Neoplasm of unspecified behavior of respiratory system
J33.0	Polyp of nasal cavity
J33.1	Polypoid sinus degeneration
J33.8	Other polyp of sinus
J33.9	Nasal polyp, unspecified
J34.0	Abscess, furuncle and carbuncle of nose
J34.3	Hypertrophy of nasal turbinates
J34.81	Nasal mucositis (ulcerative)
J34.89	Other specified disorders of nose and nasal sinuses

CCI Edits

Refer to Appendix A for CCI edits.

Pub 100

00164: Pub 100-04, 12, 140.5, Pub 100-04, 12, 50, Pub 100-04, 12, 90.4.5

Base Units

Global: XXX

Code	Base Units
00164	4

Modifiers (PAR)

Code	Mod 50	Mod 51	Mod 62	Mod 80
00164	9	9	9	9

CPT © 2018 American Medical Association. All Rights Reserved.

00170

00170 Anesthesia for intraoral procedures, including biopsy; not otherwise specified

ICD-10-CM Diagnostic Codes

C02.0	Malignant neoplasm of dorsal surface of tongue
C02.1	Malignant neoplasm of border of tongue
C02.2	Malignant neoplasm of ventral surface of tongue
C02.4	Malignant neoplasm of lingual tonsil
C02.8	Malignant neoplasm of overlapping sites of tongue
C03.0	Malignant neoplasm of upper gum
C03.1	Malignant neoplasm of lower gum
C04.0	Malignant neoplasm of anterior floor of mouth
C04.1	Malignant neoplasm of lateral floor of mouth
C04.8	Malignant neoplasm of overlapping sites of floor of mouth
C05.0	Malignant neoplasm of hard palate
C05.1	Malignant neoplasm of soft palate
C05.2	Malignant neoplasm of uvula
C06.0	Malignant neoplasm of cheek mucosa
C06.1	Malignant neoplasm of vestibule of mouth
C06.89	Malignant neoplasm of overlapping sites of other parts of mouth
C09.0	Malignant neoplasm of tonsillar fossa
C09.1	Malignant neoplasm of tonsillar pillar (anterior) (posterior)
C10.1	Malignant neoplasm of anterior surface of epiglottis
C10.2	Malignant neoplasm of lateral wall of oropharynx
C10.3	Malignant neoplasm of posterior wall of oropharynx
D00.02	Carcinoma in situ of buccal mucosa
D00.04	Carcinoma in situ of soft palate
D00.05	Carcinoma in situ of hard palate
D00.06	Carcinoma in situ of floor of mouth
D00.07	Carcinoma in situ of tongue
D00.08	Carcinoma in situ of pharynx
D10.4	Benign neoplasm of tonsil
D10.5	Benign neoplasm of other parts of oropharynx
D37.09	Neoplasm of uncertain behavior of other specified sites of the oral cavity
D49.0	Neoplasm of unspecified behavior of digestive system
J03.01	Acute recurrent streptococcal tonsillitis
J05.11	Acute epiglottitis with obstruction
J35.01	Chronic tonsillitis
J35.02	Chronic adenoiditis
J35.03	Chronic tonsillitis and adenoiditis
J35.1	Hypertrophy of tonsils
J35.2	Hypertrophy of adenoids
J35.3	Hypertrophy of tonsils with hypertrophy of adenoids
J35.8	Other chronic diseases of tonsils and adenoids
J35.9	Chronic disease of tonsils and adenoids, unspecified
J36	Peritonsillar abscess
J39.0	Retropharyngeal and parapharyngeal abscess
K09.8	Other cysts of oral region, not elsewhere classified
K09.9	Cyst of oral region, unspecified
K13.21	Leukoplakia of oral mucosa, including tongue
K13.4	Granuloma and granuloma-like lesions of oral mucosa
K13.79	Other lesions of oral mucosa
R04.1	Hemorrhage from throat
➐ S01.512	Laceration without foreign body of oral cavity
➐ S01.522	Laceration with foreign body of oral cavity
➐ S01.532	Puncture wound without foreign body of oral cavity
➐ S01.542	Puncture wound with foreign body of oral cavity
➐ S01.552	Open bite of oral cavity

ICD-10-CM Coding Notes

For codes requiring a 7th character extension, refer to your ICD-10-CM book. Review the character descriptions and coding guidelines for proper selection. For some procedures, only certain characters will apply.

CCI Edits

Refer to Appendix A for CCI edits.

Pub 100

00170: Pub 100-04, 12, 140.5, Pub 100-04, 12, 50, Pub 100-04, 12, 90.4.5

Base Units

Global: XXX

Code	Base Units
00170	5

Modifiers (PAR)

Code	Mod 50	Mod 51	Mod 62	Mod 80
00170	9	9	9	9

CPT © 2018 American Medical Association. All Rights Reserved.

00172

00172 Anesthesia for intraoral procedures, including biopsy; repair of cleft palate

ICD-10-CM Diagnostic Codes

Q35.1	Cleft hard palate
Q35.3	Cleft soft palate
Q35.5	Cleft hard palate with cleft soft palate
Q35.7	Cleft uvula
Q35.9	Cleft palate, unspecified
Q37.0	Cleft hard palate with bilateral cleft lip
Q37.1	Cleft hard palate with unilateral cleft lip
Q37.2	Cleft soft palate with bilateral cleft lip
Q37.3	Cleft soft palate with unilateral cleft lip
Q37.4	Cleft hard and soft palate with bilateral cleft lip
Q37.5	Cleft hard and soft palate with unilateral cleft lip
Q37.8	Unspecified cleft palate with bilateral cleft lip
Q37.9	Unspecified cleft palate with unilateral cleft lip

CCI Edits

Refer to Appendix A for CCI edits.

Pub 100

00172: Pub 100-04, 12, 140.5, Pub 100-04, 12, 50, Pub 100-04, 12, 90.4.5

Base Units

Global: XXX

Code	Base Units
00172	6

Modifiers (PAR)

Code	Mod 50	Mod 51	Mod 62	Mod 80
00172	9	9	9	9

CPT © 2018 American Medical Association. All Rights Reserved.

00174

00174 Anesthesia for intraoral procedures, including biopsy; excision of retropharyngeal tumor

ICD-10-CM Diagnostic Codes

C01	Malignant neoplasm of base of tongue
C09.0	Malignant neoplasm of tonsillar fossa
C09.1	Malignant neoplasm of tonsillar pillar (anterior) (posterior)
C09.8	Malignant neoplasm of overlapping sites of tonsil
C09.9	Malignant neoplasm of tonsil, unspecified
C10.0	Malignant neoplasm of vallecula
C10.1	Malignant neoplasm of anterior surface of epiglottis
C10.2	Malignant neoplasm of lateral wall of oropharynx
C10.3	Malignant neoplasm of posterior wall of oropharynx
C10.4	Malignant neoplasm of branchial cleft
C10.8	Malignant neoplasm of overlapping sites of oropharynx
C10.9	Malignant neoplasm of oropharynx, unspecified
C11.0	Malignant neoplasm of superior wall of nasopharynx
C11.1	Malignant neoplasm of posterior wall of nasopharynx
C11.2	Malignant neoplasm of lateral wall of nasopharynx
C11.3	Malignant neoplasm of anterior wall of nasopharynx
C11.8	Malignant neoplasm of overlapping sites of nasopharynx
C11.9	Malignant neoplasm of nasopharynx, unspecified
C12	Malignant neoplasm of pyriform sinus
C13.0	Malignant neoplasm of postcricoid region
C13.1	Malignant neoplasm of aryepiglottic fold, hypopharyngeal aspect
C13.2	Malignant neoplasm of posterior wall of hypopharynx
C13.8	Malignant neoplasm of overlapping sites of hypopharynx
C13.9	Malignant neoplasm of hypopharynx, unspecified
C14.0	Malignant neoplasm of pharynx, unspecified
C14.2	Malignant neoplasm of Waldeyer's ring
C14.8	Malignant neoplasm of overlapping sites of lip, oral cavity and pharynx
C76.0	Malignant neoplasm of head, face and neck
C79.89	Secondary malignant neoplasm of other specified sites
D00.07	Carcinoma in situ of tongue
D00.08	Carcinoma in situ of pharynx
D10.1	Benign neoplasm of tongue
D10.4	Benign neoplasm of tonsil
D10.5	Benign neoplasm of other parts of oropharynx
D10.6	Benign neoplasm of nasopharynx
D10.7	Benign neoplasm of hypopharynx
D10.9	Benign neoplasm of pharynx, unspecified
D37.02	Neoplasm of uncertain behavior of tongue
D37.05	Neoplasm of uncertain behavior of pharynx
D49.0	Neoplasm of unspecified behavior of digestive system
J38.1	Polyp of vocal cord and larynx
J39.2	Other diseases of pharynx
R22.1	Localized swelling, mass and lump, neck

CCI Edits

Refer to Appendix A for CCI edits.

Pub 100

00174: Pub 100-04, 12, 140.5, Pub 100-04, 12, 50, Pub 100-04, 12, 90.4.5

Base Units

Global: XXX

Code	Base Units
00174	6

Modifiers (PAR)

Code	Mod 50	Mod 51	Mod 62	Mod 80
00174	9	9	9	9

CPT © 2018 American Medical Association. All Rights Reserved.

00176

00176 Anesthesia for intraoral procedures, including biopsy; radical surgery

ICD-10-CM Diagnostic Codes

C01	Malignant neoplasm of base of tongue
C02.0	Malignant neoplasm of dorsal surface of tongue
C02.1	Malignant neoplasm of border of tongue
C02.2	Malignant neoplasm of ventral surface of tongue
C02.3	Malignant neoplasm of anterior two-thirds of tongue, part unspecified
C02.4	Malignant neoplasm of lingual tonsil
C02.8	Malignant neoplasm of overlapping sites of tongue
C02.9	Malignant neoplasm of tongue, unspecified
C03.0	Malignant neoplasm of upper gum
C03.1	Malignant neoplasm of lower gum
C03.9	Malignant neoplasm of gum, unspecified
C04.0	Malignant neoplasm of anterior floor of mouth
C04.1	Malignant neoplasm of lateral floor of mouth
C04.8	Malignant neoplasm of overlapping sites of floor of mouth
C04.9	Malignant neoplasm of floor of mouth, unspecified
C05.0	Malignant neoplasm of hard palate
C05.1	Malignant neoplasm of soft palate
C05.2	Malignant neoplasm of uvula
C05.8	Malignant neoplasm of overlapping sites of palate
C05.9	Malignant neoplasm of palate, unspecified
C06.0	Malignant neoplasm of cheek mucosa
C06.1	Malignant neoplasm of vestibule of mouth
C06.2	Malignant neoplasm of retromolar area
C06.80	Malignant neoplasm of overlapping sites of unspecified parts of mouth
C06.89	Malignant neoplasm of overlapping sites of other parts of mouth
C06.9	Malignant neoplasm of mouth, unspecified
C07	Malignant neoplasm of parotid gland
C08.0	Malignant neoplasm of submandibular gland
C08.1	Malignant neoplasm of sublingual gland
C08.9	Malignant neoplasm of major salivary gland, unspecified
C09.0	Malignant neoplasm of tonsillar fossa
C09.1	Malignant neoplasm of tonsillar pillar (anterior) (posterior)
C09.8	Malignant neoplasm of overlapping sites of tonsil
C09.9	Malignant neoplasm of tonsil, unspecified
C10.0	Malignant neoplasm of vallecula
C10.1	Malignant neoplasm of anterior surface of epiglottis
C10.2	Malignant neoplasm of lateral wall of oropharynx
C10.3	Malignant neoplasm of posterior wall of oropharynx
C10.4	Malignant neoplasm of branchial cleft
C10.8	Malignant neoplasm of overlapping sites of oropharynx
C10.9	Malignant neoplasm of oropharynx, unspecified
C11.0	Malignant neoplasm of superior wall of nasopharynx
C11.1	Malignant neoplasm of posterior wall of nasopharynx
C11.2	Malignant neoplasm of lateral wall of nasopharynx
C11.3	Malignant neoplasm of anterior wall of nasopharynx
C11.8	Malignant neoplasm of overlapping sites of nasopharynx
C11.9	Malignant neoplasm of nasopharynx, unspecified
C12	Malignant neoplasm of pyriform sinus
C13.0	Malignant neoplasm of postcricoid region
C13.1	Malignant neoplasm of aryepiglottic fold, hypopharyngeal aspect
C13.2	Malignant neoplasm of posterior wall of hypopharynx
C13.8	Malignant neoplasm of overlapping sites of hypopharynx
C13.9	Malignant neoplasm of hypopharynx, unspecified
C14.0	Malignant neoplasm of pharynx, unspecified
C14.2	Malignant neoplasm of Waldeyer's ring
C14.8	Malignant neoplasm of overlapping sites of lip, oral cavity and pharynx
C47.0	Malignant neoplasm of peripheral nerves of head, face and neck
C49.0	Malignant neoplasm of connective and soft tissue of head, face and neck
C76.0	Malignant neoplasm of head, face and neck
C77.0	Secondary and unspecified malignant neoplasm of lymph nodes of head, face and neck
C79.89	Secondary malignant neoplasm of other specified sites
K06.010	Localized gingival recession, unspecified
K06.011	Localized gingival recession, minimal
K06.012	Localized gingival recession, moderate
K06.013	Localized gingival recession, severe
K06.020	Generalized gingival recession, unspecified
K06.021	Generalized gingival recession, minimal
K06.022	Generalized gingival recession, moderate
K06.023	Generalized gingival recession, severe

CCI Edits

Refer to Appendix A for CCI edits.

Pub 100

00176: Pub 100-04, 12, 140.5, Pub 100-04, 12, 50, Pub 100-04, 12, 90.4.5

Base Units

Global: XXX

Code	Base Units
00176	7

Modifiers (PAR)

Code	Mod 50	Mod 51	Mod 62	Mod 80
00176	9	9	9	9

CPT © 2018 American Medical Association. All Rights Reserved.

00190

00190 Anesthesia for procedures on facial bones or skull; not otherwise specified

ICD-10-CM Diagnostic Codes

	D16.4	Benign neoplasm of bones of skull and face
	D16.5	Benign neoplasm of lower jaw bone
	M26.07	Excessive tuberosity of jaw
	M26.53	Deviation in opening and closing of the mandible
	M27.40	Unspecified cyst of jaw
	M27.49	Other cysts of jaw
	M89.38	Hypertrophy of bone, other site
	M89.8X8	Other specified disorders of bone, other site
❼	S02.0	Fracture of vault of skull
❼⇄	S02.101	Fracture of base of skull, right side
❼⇄	S02.102	Fracture of base of skull, left side
❼⇄	S02.11A	Type I occipital condyle fracture, right side
❼⇄	S02.11B	Type I occipital condyle fracture, left side
❼⇄	S02.11C	Type II occipital condyle fracture, right side
❼⇄	S02.11D	Type II occipital condyle fracture, left side
❼⇄	S02.11E	Type III occipital condyle fracture, right side
❼⇄	S02.11F	Type III occipital condyle fracture, left side
❼⇄	S02.11G	Other fracture of occiput, right side
❼⇄	S02.11H	Other fracture of occiput, left side
❼	S02.19	Other fracture of base of skull
❼	S02.2	Fracture of nasal bones
❼⇄	S02.31	Fracture of orbital floor, right side
❼⇄	S02.32	Fracture of orbital floor, left side
❼⇄	S02.40A	Malar fracture, right side
❼⇄	S02.40B	Malar fracture, left side
❼⇄	S02.40C	Maxillary fracture, right side
❼⇄	S02.40D	Maxillary fracture, left side
❼⇄	S02.40E	Zygomatic fracture, right side
❼⇄	S02.40F	Zygomatic fracture, left side
❼	S02.42	Fracture of alveolus of maxilla
❼⇄	S02.611	Fracture of condylar process of right mandible
❼⇄	S02.612	Fracture of condylar process of left mandible
❼⇄	S02.621	Fracture of subcondylar process of right mandible
❼⇄	S02.622	Fracture of subcondylar process of left mandible
❼⇄	S02.631	Fracture of coronoid process of right mandible
❼⇄	S02.632	Fracture of coronoid process of left mandible
❼⇄	S02.641	Fracture of ramus of right mandible
❼⇄	S02.642	Fracture of ramus of left mandible
❼⇄	S02.651	Fracture of angle of right mandible
❼⇄	S02.652	Fracture of angle of left mandible
❼	S02.66	Fracture of symphysis of mandible
❼⇄	S02.671	Fracture of alveolus of right mandible
❼⇄	S02.672	Fracture of alveolus of left mandible
❼	S02.69	Fracture of mandible of other specified site
❼⇄	S02.81	Fracture of other specified skull and facial bones, right side
❼⇄	S02.82	Fracture of other specified skull and facial bones, left side
❼⇄	S03.01	Dislocation of jaw, right side
❼⇄	S03.02	Dislocation of jaw, left side
❼⇄	S03.03	Dislocation of jaw, bilateral

ICD-10-CM Coding Notes

For codes requiring a 7th character extension, refer to your ICD-10-CM book. Review the character descriptions and coding guidelines for proper selection. For some procedures, only certain characters will apply.

CCI Edits

Refer to Appendix A for CCI edits.

Pub 100

00190: Pub 100-04, 12, 140.5, Pub 100-04, 12, 50, Pub 100-04, 12, 90.4.5

Base Units

Global: XXX

Code	Base Units
00190	5

Modifiers (PAR)

Code	Mod 50	Mod 51	Mod 62	Mod 80
00190	9	9	9	9

CPT © 2018 American Medical Association. All Rights Reserved.

00192

00192 Anesthesia for procedures on facial bones or skull; radical surgery (including prognathism)

ICD-10-CM Diagnostic Codes

	C41.0	Malignant neoplasm of bones of skull and face
	C41.1	Malignant neoplasm of mandible
	C79.89	Secondary malignant neoplasm of other specified sites
	D16.4	Benign neoplasm of bones of skull and face
	D16.5	Benign neoplasm of lower jaw bone
	D48.0	Neoplasm of uncertain behavior of bone and articular cartilage
	D49.2	Neoplasm of unspecified behavior of bone, soft tissue, and skin
	H05.30	Unspecified deformity of orbit
	M26.19	Other specified anomalies of jaw-cranial base relationship
	M26.71	Alveolar maxillary hyperplasia
	M26.72	Alveolar mandibular hyperplasia
	M26.73	Alveolar maxillary hypoplasia
	M26.74	Alveolar mandibular hypoplasia
	M26.9	Dentofacial anomaly, unspecified
	M27.0	Developmental disorders of jaws
	M27.1	Giant cell granuloma, central
	Q67.0	Congenital facial asymmetry
	Q75.0	Craniosynostosis
	Q75.1	Craniofacial dysostosis
	Q75.2	Hypertelorism
	Q75.4	Mandibulofacial dysostosis
	Q75.5	Oculomandibular dysostosis
	Q75.8	Other specified congenital malformations of skull and face bones
	Q87.0	Congenital malformation syndromes predominantly affecting facial appearance
❼	S02.0	Fracture of vault of skull
❼ ⇄	S02.101	Fracture of base of skull, right side
❼ ⇄	S02.102	Fracture of base of skull, left side
❼ ⇄	S02.11A	Type I occipital condyle fracture, right side
❼ ⇄	S02.11B	Type I occipital condyle fracture, left side
❼ ⇄	S02.11C	Type II occipital condyle fracture, right side
❼ ⇄	S02.11D	Type II occipital condyle fracture, left side
❼ ⇄	S02.11E	Type III occipital condyle fracture, right side
❼ ⇄	S02.11F	Type III occipital condyle fracture, left side
❼ ⇄	S02.11G	Other fracture of occiput, right side
❼ ⇄	S02.11H	Other fracture of occiput, left side
❼	S02.19	Other fracture of base of skull
❼	S02.2	Fracture of nasal bones
❼ ⇄	S02.31	Fracture of orbital floor, right side
❼ ⇄	S02.32	Fracture of orbital floor, left side
❼ ⇄	S02.40A	Malar fracture, right side
❼ ⇄	S02.40B	Malar fracture, left side
❼ ⇄	S02.40C	Maxillary fracture, right side
❼ ⇄	S02.40D	Maxillary fracture, left side
❼ ⇄	S02.40E	Zygomatic fracture, right side
❼ ⇄	S02.40F	Zygomatic fracture, left side
❼	S02.411	LeFort I fracture
❼	S02.412	LeFort II fracture
❼	S02.413	LeFort III fracture
❼	S02.42	Fracture of alveolus of maxilla
❼ ⇄	S02.611	Fracture of condylar process of right mandible
❼ ⇄	S02.612	Fracture of condylar process of left mandible
❼ ⇄	S02.621	Fracture of subcondylar process of right mandible
❼ ⇄	S02.622	Fracture of subcondylar process of left mandible
❼ ⇄	S02.631	Fracture of coronoid process of right mandible
❼ ⇄	S02.632	Fracture of coronoid process of left mandible
❼ ⇄	S02.641	Fracture of ramus of right mandible
❼ ⇄	S02.642	Fracture of ramus of left mandible
❼ ⇄	S02.651	Fracture of angle of right mandible
❼ ⇄	S02.652	Fracture of angle of left mandible
❼	S02.66	Fracture of symphysis of mandible
	S02.67	Fracture of alveolus of mandible
❼ ⇄	S02.671	Fracture of alveolus of right mandible
❼ ⇄	S02.672	Fracture of alveolus of left mandible
❼	S02.69	Fracture of mandible of other specified site
❼ ⇄	S02.81	Fracture of other specified skull and facial bones, right side
❼ ⇄	S02.82	Fracture of other specified skull and facial bones, left side

ICD-10-CM Coding Notes

For codes requiring a 7th character extension, refer to your ICD-10-CM book. Review the character descriptions and coding guidelines for proper selection. For some procedures, only certain characters will apply.

CCI Edits

Refer to Appendix A for CCI edits.

Pub 100

00192: Pub 100-04, 12, 140.5, Pub 100-04, 12, 50, Pub 100-04, 12, 90.4.5

Base Units

Global: XXX

Code	Base Units
00192	7

Modifiers (PAR)

Code	Mod 50	Mod 51	Mod 62	Mod 80
00192	9	9	9	9

CPT © 2018 American Medical Association. All Rights Reserved.

00210

00210 Anesthesia for intracranial procedures; not otherwise specified

ICD-10-CM Diagnostic Codes

C70.0	Malignant neoplasm of cerebral meninges
C71.0	Malignant neoplasm of cerebrum, except lobes and ventricles
C71.1	Malignant neoplasm of frontal lobe
C71.2	Malignant neoplasm of temporal lobe
C71.3	Malignant neoplasm of parietal lobe
C71.4	Malignant neoplasm of occipital lobe
C71.5	Malignant neoplasm of cerebral ventricle
C71.6	Malignant neoplasm of cerebellum
C71.7	Malignant neoplasm of brain stem
C71.8	Malignant neoplasm of overlapping sites of brain
C75.1	Malignant neoplasm of pituitary gland
C79.31	Secondary malignant neoplasm of brain
C79.32	Secondary malignant neoplasm of cerebral meninges
D32.0	Benign neoplasm of cerebral meninges
D33.0	Benign neoplasm of brain, supratentorial
D33.1	Benign neoplasm of brain, infratentorial
D33.3	Benign neoplasm of cranial nerves
G20	Parkinson's disease
G40.011	Localization-related (focal) (partial) idiopathic epilepsy and epileptic syndromes with seizures of localized onset, intractable, with status epilepticus
G40.019	Localization-related (focal) (partial) idiopathic epilepsy and epileptic syndromes with seizures of localized onset, intractable, without status epilepticus
G40.111	Localization-related (focal) (partial) symptomatic epilepsy and epileptic syndromes with simple partial seizures, intractable, with status epilepticus
G40.119	Localization-related (focal) (partial) symptomatic epilepsy and epileptic syndromes with simple partial seizures, intractable, without status epilepticus
G40.211	Localization-related (focal) (partial) symptomatic epilepsy and epileptic syndromes with complex partial seizures, intractable, with status epilepticus
G40.219	Localization-related (focal) (partial) symptomatic epilepsy and epileptic syndromes with complex partial seizures, intractable, without status epilepticus
G40.301	Generalized idiopathic epilepsy and epileptic syndromes, not intractable, with status epilepticus
G40.309	Generalized idiopathic epilepsy and epileptic syndromes, not intractable, without status epilepticus
G40.311	Generalized idiopathic epilepsy and epileptic syndromes, intractable, with status epilepticus
G40.319	Generalized idiopathic epilepsy and epileptic syndromes, intractable, without status epilepticus
G40.411	Other generalized epilepsy and epileptic syndromes, intractable, with status epilepticus
G40.419	Other generalized epilepsy and epileptic syndromes, intractable, without status epilepticus
G40.911	Epilepsy, unspecified, intractable, with status epilepticus
G40.919	Epilepsy, unspecified, intractable, without status epilepticus
G40.A11	Absence epileptic syndrome, intractable, with status epilepticus
G40.A19	Absence epileptic syndrome, intractable, without status epilepticus
G40.B11	Juvenile myoclonic epilepsy, intractable, with status epilepticus
G40.B19	Juvenile myoclonic epilepsy, intractable, without status epilepticus
❼ T85.110	Breakdown (mechanical) of implanted electronic neurostimulator of brain electrode (lead)
❼ T85.120	Displacement of implanted electronic neurostimulator of brain electrode (lead)
❼ T85.190	Other mechanical complication of implanted electronic neurostimulator of brain electrode (lead)
❼ T85.731	Infection and inflammatory reaction due to implanted electronic neurostimulator of brain, electrode (lead)
❼ T85.810	Embolism due to nervous system prosthetic devices, implants and grafts
❼ T85.820	Fibrosis due to nervous system prosthetic devices, implants and grafts
❼ T85.830	Hemorrhage due to nervous system prosthetic devices, implants and grafts
❼ T85.840	Pain due to nervous system prosthetic devices, implants and grafts
❼ T85.850	Stenosis due to nervous system prosthetic devices, implants and grafts
❼ T85.860	Thrombosis due to nervous system prosthetic devices, implants and grafts
❼ T85.890	Other specified complication of nervous system prosthetic devices, implants and grafts
Z45.42	Encounter for adjustment and management of neuropacemaker (brain) (peripheral nerve) (spinal cord)

ICD-10-CM Coding Notes

For codes requiring a 7th character extension, refer to your ICD-10-CM book. Review the character descriptions and coding guidelines for proper selection. For some procedures, only certain characters will apply.

CCI Edits

Refer to Appendix A for CCI edits.

Pub 100

00210: Pub 100-04, 12, 140.5, Pub 100-04, 12, 50, Pub 100-04, 12, 90.4.5

Base Units

Global: XXX

Code	Base Units
00210	11

Modifiers (PAR)

Code	Mod 50	Mod 51	Mod 62	Mod 80
00210	9	9	9	9

CPT © 2018 American Medical Association. All Rights Reserved.

00211

00211 Anesthesia for intracranial procedures; craniotomy or craniectomy for evacuation of hematoma

ICD-10-CM Diagnostic Codes

- ➆⇄ S06.340 Traumatic hemorrhage of right cerebrum without loss of consciousness
- ➆⇄ S06.349 Traumatic hemorrhage of right cerebrum with loss of consciousness of unspecified duration
- ➆⇄ S06.350 Traumatic hemorrhage of left cerebrum without loss of consciousness
- ➆⇄ S06.359 Traumatic hemorrhage of left cerebrum with loss of consciousness of unspecified duration
- ➆ S06.360 Traumatic hemorrhage of cerebrum, unspecified, without loss of consciousness
- ➆ S06.369 Traumatic hemorrhage of cerebrum, unspecified, with loss of consciousness of unspecified duration
- ➆ S06.370 Contusion, laceration, and hemorrhage of cerebellum without loss of consciousness
- ➆ S06.379 Contusion, laceration, and hemorrhage of cerebellum with loss of consciousness of unspecified duration
- ➆ S06.380 Contusion, laceration, and hemorrhage of brainstem without loss of consciousness
- ➆ S06.389 Contusion, laceration, and hemorrhage of brainstem with loss of consciousness of unspecified duration
- ➆ S06.4X0 Epidural hemorrhage without loss of consciousness
- ➆ S06.4X9 Epidural hemorrhage with loss of consciousness of unspecified duration
- ➆ S06.5X0 Traumatic subdural hemorrhage without loss of consciousness
- ➆ S06.5X1 Traumatic subdural hemorrhage with loss of consciousness of 30 minutes or less
- ➆ S06.5X2 Traumatic subdural hemorrhage with loss of consciousness of 31 minutes to 59 minutes
- ➆ S06.5X3 Traumatic subdural hemorrhage with loss of consciousness of 1 hour to 5 hours 59 minutes
- ➆ S06.5X4 Traumatic subdural hemorrhage with loss of consciousness of 6 hours to 24 hours
- ➆ S06.5X5 Traumatic subdural hemorrhage with loss of consciousness greater than 24 hours with return to pre-existing conscious level
- ➆ S06.5X6 Traumatic subdural hemorrhage with loss of consciousness greater than 24 hours without return to pre-existing conscious level with patient surviving
- ➆ S06.5X9 Traumatic subdural hemorrhage with loss of consciousness of unspecified duration
- ➆ S06.6X0 Traumatic subarachnoid hemorrhage without loss of consciousness
- ➆ S06.6X1 Traumatic subarachnoid hemorrhage with loss of consciousness of 30 minutes or less
- ➆ S06.6X2 Traumatic subarachnoid hemorrhage with loss of consciousness of 31 minutes to 59 minutes
- ➆ S06.6X3 Traumatic subarachnoid hemorrhage with loss of consciousness of 1 hour to 5 hours 59 minutes
- ➆ S06.6X4 Traumatic subarachnoid hemorrhage with loss of consciousness of 6 hours to 24 hours
- ➆ S06.6X5 Traumatic subarachnoid hemorrhage with loss of consciousness greater than 24 hours with return to pre-existing conscious level
- ➆ S06.6X6 Traumatic subarachnoid hemorrhage with loss of consciousness greater than 24 hours without return to pre-existing conscious level with patient surviving
- ➆ S06.6X9 Traumatic subarachnoid hemorrhage with loss of consciousness of unspecified duration

ICD-10-CM Coding Notes

For codes requiring a 7th character extension, refer to your ICD-10-CM book. Review the character descriptions and coding guidelines for proper selection. For some procedures, only certain characters will apply.

CCI Edits

Refer to Appendix A for CCI edits.

Pub 100

00211: Pub 100-04, 12, 140.5, Pub 100-04, 12, 50, Pub 100-04, 12, 90.4.5

Base Units

Global: XXX

Code	Base Units
00211	10

Modifiers (PAR)

Code	Mod 50	Mod 51	Mod 62	Mod 80
00211	9	9	9	9

CPT © 2018 American Medical Association. All Rights Reserved.

00212

00212 Anesthesia for intracranial procedures; subdural taps

ICD-10-CM Diagnostic Codes

	G03.9	Meningitis, unspecified
	G06.0	Intracranial abscess and granuloma
⇄	G81.91	Hemiplegia, unspecified affecting right dominant side
⇄	G81.92	Hemiplegia, unspecified affecting left dominant side
⇄	G81.93	Hemiplegia, unspecified affecting right nondominant side
⇄	G81.94	Hemiplegia, unspecified affecting left nondominant side
	G91.1	Obstructive hydrocephalus
	G91.2	(Idiopathic) normal pressure hydrocephalus
	G91.3	Post-traumatic hydrocephalus, unspecified
	G91.9	Hydrocephalus, unspecified
	G93.6	Cerebral edema
	I62.00	Nontraumatic subdural hemorrhage, unspecified
	I62.1	Nontraumatic extradural hemorrhage
	I62.9	Nontraumatic intracranial hemorrhage, unspecified
	P52.0	Intraventricular (nontraumatic) hemorrhage, grade 1, of newborn
	P52.1	Intraventricular (nontraumatic) hemorrhage, grade 2, of newborn
	P52.21	Intraventricular (nontraumatic) hemorrhage, grade 3, of newborn
	P52.22	Intraventricular (nontraumatic) hemorrhage, grade 4, of newborn
	P52.3	Unspecified intraventricular (nontraumatic) hemorrhage of newborn
	P52.4	Intracerebral (nontraumatic) hemorrhage of newborn
	P52.5	Subarachnoid (nontraumatic) hemorrhage of newborn
	P52.6	Cerebellar (nontraumatic) and posterior fossa hemorrhage of newborn
	P52.8	Other intracranial (nontraumatic) hemorrhages of newborn
	P52.9	Intracranial (nontraumatic) hemorrhage of newborn, unspecified
	Q03.0	Malformations of aqueduct of Sylvius
	Q03.1	Atresia of foramina of Magendie and Luschka
	Q03.8	Other congenital hydrocephalus
	Q03.9	Congenital hydrocephalus, unspecified
	R40.0	Somnolence
	R40.20	Unspecified coma
	R51	Headache
	R56.9	Unspecified convulsions
➐	S06.1X0	Traumatic cerebral edema without loss of consciousness
➐	S06.1X1	Traumatic cerebral edema with loss of consciousness of 30 minutes or less
➐	S06.1X2	Traumatic cerebral edema with loss of consciousness of 31 minutes to 59 minutes
➐	S06.1X3	Traumatic cerebral edema with loss of consciousness of 1 hour to 5 hours 59 minutes
➐	S06.1X4	Traumatic cerebral edema with loss of consciousness of 6 hours to 24 hours
➐	S06.1X5	Traumatic cerebral edema with loss of consciousness greater than 24 hours with return to pre-existing conscious level
➐	S06.1X6	Traumatic cerebral edema with loss of consciousness greater than 24 hours without return to pre-existing conscious level with patient surviving
➐	S06.1X7	Traumatic cerebral edema with loss of consciousness of any duration with death due to brain injury prior to regaining consciousness
➐	S06.1X8	Traumatic cerebral edema with loss of consciousness of any duration with death due to other cause prior to regaining consciousness
➐	S06.1X9	Traumatic cerebral edema with loss of consciousness of unspecified duration
➐	S06.9X0	Unspecified intracranial injury without loss of consciousness
➐	S06.9X1	Unspecified intracranial injury with loss of consciousness of 30 minutes or less
➐	S06.9X2	Unspecified intracranial injury with loss of consciousness of 31 minutes to 59 minutes
➐	S06.9X3	Unspecified intracranial injury with loss of consciousness of 1 hour to 5 hours 59 minutes
➐	S06.9X4	Unspecified intracranial injury with loss of consciousness of 6 hours to 24 hours
➐	S06.9X5	Unspecified intracranial injury with loss of consciousness greater than 24 hours with return to pre-existing conscious level
➐	S06.9X6	Unspecified intracranial injury with loss of consciousness greater than 24 hours without return to pre-existing conscious level with patient surviving
➐	S06.9X9	Unspecified intracranial injury with loss of consciousness of unspecified duration

ICD-10-CM Coding Notes

For codes requiring a 7th character extension, refer to your ICD-10-CM book. Review the character descriptions and coding guidelines for proper selection. For some procedures, only certain characters will apply.

CCI Edits

Refer to Appendix A for CCI edits.

Pub 100

00212: Pub 100-04, 12, 140.5, Pub 100-04, 12, 50, Pub 100-04, 12, 90.4.5

Base Units

Global: XXX

Code	Base Units
00212	5

Modifiers (PAR)

Code	Mod 50	Mod 51	Mod 62	Mod 80
00212	9	9	9	9

CPT © 2018 American Medical Association. All Rights Reserved.

00214

00214 Anesthesia for intracranial procedures; burr holes, including ventriculography

AMA *CPT Assistant*

00214: Nov 99: 7

ICD-10-CM Diagnostic Codes

	G93.5	Compression of brain
➐	S06.4X0	Epidural hemorrhage without loss of consciousness
➐	S06.4X1	Epidural hemorrhage with loss of consciousness of 30 minutes or less
➐	S06.4X2	Epidural hemorrhage with loss of consciousness of 31 minutes to 59 minutes
➐	S06.4X3	Epidural hemorrhage with loss of consciousness of 1 hour to 5 hours 59 minutes
➐	S06.4X4	Epidural hemorrhage with loss of consciousness of 6 hours to 24 hours
➐	S06.4X5	Epidural hemorrhage with loss of consciousness greater than 24 hours with return to pre-existing conscious level
➐	S06.4X6	Epidural hemorrhage with loss of consciousness greater than 24 hours without return to pre-existing conscious level with patient surviving
➐	S06.4X9	Epidural hemorrhage with loss of consciousness of unspecified duration
➐	S06.5X0	Traumatic subdural hemorrhage without loss of consciousness
➐	S06.5X1	Traumatic subdural hemorrhage with loss of consciousness of 30 minutes or less
➐	S06.5X2	Traumatic subdural hemorrhage with loss of consciousness of 31 minutes to 59 minutes
➐	S06.5X3	Traumatic subdural hemorrhage with loss of consciousness of 1 hour to 5 hours 59 minutes
➐	S06.5X4	Traumatic subdural hemorrhage with loss of consciousness of 6 hours to 24 hours
➐	S06.5X5	Traumatic subdural hemorrhage with loss of consciousness greater than 24 hours with return to pre-existing conscious level
➐	S06.5X6	Traumatic subdural hemorrhage with loss of consciousness greater than 24 hours without return to pre-existing conscious level with patient surviving
➐	S06.5X9	Traumatic subdural hemorrhage with loss of consciousness of unspecified duration
➐	S06.6X0	Traumatic subarachnoid hemorrhage without loss of consciousness
➐	S06.6X9	Traumatic subarachnoid hemorrhage with loss of consciousness of unspecified duration

ICD-10-CM Coding Notes

For codes requiring a 7th character extension, refer to your ICD-10-CM book. Review the character descriptions and coding guidelines for proper selection. For some procedures, only certain characters will apply.

CCI Edits

Refer to Appendix A for CCI edits.

Pub 100

00214: Pub 100-04, 12, 140.5, Pub 100-04, 12, 50, Pub 100-04, 12, 90.4.5

Base Units

Global: XXX

Code	Base Units
00214	9

Modifiers (PAR)

Code	Mod 50	Mod 51	Mod 62	Mod 80
00214	9	9	9	9

CPT © 2018 American Medical Association. All Rights Reserved.

00215

00215 Anesthesia for intracranial procedures; cranioplasty or elevation of depressed skull fracture, extradural (simple or compound)

ICD-10-CM Diagnostic Codes

	C41.0	Malignant neoplasm of bones of skull and face
	Q75.0	Craniosynostosis
	Q75.1	Craniofacial dysostosis
	Q75.2	Hypertelorism
	Q75.3	Macrocephaly
	Q75.8	Other specified congenital malformations of skull and face bones
	Q87.0	Congenital malformation syndromes predominantly affecting facial appearance
⑦	S02.0	Fracture of vault of skull
⑦⇄	S02.101	Fracture of base of skull, right side
⑦⇄	S02.102	Fracture of base of skull, left side
⑦⇄	S02.11A	Type I occipital condyle fracture, right side
⑦⇄	S02.11B	Type I occipital condyle fracture, left side
⑦⇄	S02.11C	Type II occipital condyle fracture, right side
⑦⇄	S02.11D	Type II occipital condyle fracture, left side
⑦⇄	S02.11E	Type III occipital condyle fracture, right side
⑦⇄	S02.11F	Type III occipital condyle fracture, left side
⑦⇄	S02.11G	Other fracture of occiput, right side
⑦⇄	S02.11H	Other fracture of occiput, left side
⑦	S02.19	Other fracture of base of skull
⑦	S02.2	Fracture of nasal bones
⑦⇄	S02.81	Fracture of other specified skull and facial bones, right side
⑦⇄	S02.82	Fracture of other specified skull and facial bones, left side

ICD-10-CM Coding Notes

For codes requiring a 7th character extension, refer to your ICD-10-CM book. Review the character descriptions and coding guidelines for proper selection. For some procedures, only certain characters will apply.

CCI Edits

Refer to Appendix A for CCI edits.

Pub 100

00215: Pub 100-04, 12, 140.5, Pub 100-04, 12, 50, Pub 100-04, 12, 90.4.5

Base Units

Global: XXX

Code	Base Units
00215	9

Modifiers (PAR)

Code	Mod 50	Mod 51	Mod 62	Mod 80
00215	9	9	9	9

CPT © 2018 American Medical Association. All Rights Reserved.

00216

00216 Anesthesia for intracranial procedures; vascular procedures

ICD-10-CM Diagnostic Codes

⇄	I60.01	Nontraumatic subarachnoid hemorrhage from right carotid siphon and bifurcation
⇄	I60.02	Nontraumatic subarachnoid hemorrhage from left carotid siphon and bifurcation
⇄	I60.11	Nontraumatic subarachnoid hemorrhage from right middle cerebral artery
⇄	I60.12	Nontraumatic subarachnoid hemorrhage from left middle cerebral artery
	I60.2	Nontraumatic subarachnoid hemorrhage from anterior communicating artery
⇄	I60.31	Nontraumatic subarachnoid hemorrhage from right posterior communicating artery
⇄	I60.32	Nontraumatic subarachnoid hemorrhage from left posterior communicating artery
	I60.4	Nontraumatic subarachnoid hemorrhage from basilar artery
⇄	I60.51	Nontraumatic subarachnoid hemorrhage from right vertebral artery
⇄	I60.52	Nontraumatic subarachnoid hemorrhage from left vertebral artery
	I60.6	Nontraumatic subarachnoid hemorrhage from other intracranial arteries
	I60.7	Nontraumatic subarachnoid hemorrhage from unspecified intracranial artery
	I60.8	Other nontraumatic subarachnoid hemorrhage
	I60.9	Nontraumatic subarachnoid hemorrhage, unspecified
	I61.0	Nontraumatic intracerebral hemorrhage in hemisphere, subcortical
	I61.1	Nontraumatic intracerebral hemorrhage in hemisphere, cortical
	I61.3	Nontraumatic intracerebral hemorrhage in brain stem
	I61.4	Nontraumatic intracerebral hemorrhage in cerebellum
	I61.5	Nontraumatic intracerebral hemorrhage, intraventricular
	I61.6	Nontraumatic intracerebral hemorrhage, multiple localized
	I61.8	Other nontraumatic intracerebral hemorrhage
	I61.9	Nontraumatic intracerebral hemorrhage, unspecified
	I62.01	Nontraumatic acute subdural hemorrhage
	I62.02	Nontraumatic subacute subdural hemorrhage
	I62.03	Nontraumatic chronic subdural hemorrhage
	I67.0	Dissection of cerebral arteries, nonruptured
	I67.1	Cerebral aneurysm, nonruptured
	I67.2	Cerebral atherosclerosis
	Q28.2	Arteriovenous malformation of cerebral vessels
	Q28.3	Other malformations of cerebral vessels
❼⇄	S06.810	Injury of right internal carotid artery, intracranial portion, not elsewhere classified without loss of consciousness
❼⇄	S06.819	Injury of right internal carotid artery, intracranial portion, not elsewhere classified with loss of consciousness of unspecified duration
❼⇄	S06.820	Injury of left internal carotid artery, intracranial portion, not elsewhere classified without loss of consciousness
❼⇄	S06.829	Injury of left internal carotid artery, intracranial portion, not elsewhere classified with loss of consciousness of unspecified duration

ICD-10-CM Coding Notes

For codes requiring a 7th character extension, refer to your ICD-10-CM book. Review the character descriptions and coding guidelines for proper selection. For some procedures, only certain characters will apply.

CCI Edits

Refer to Appendix A for CCI edits.

Pub 100

00216: Pub 100-04, 12, 140.5, Pub 100-04, 12, 50, Pub 100-04, 12, 90.4.5

Base Units

Global: XXX

Code	Base Units
00216	15

Modifiers (PAR)

Code	Mod 50	Mod 51	Mod 62	Mod 80
00216	9	9	9	9

CPT © 2018 American Medical Association. All Rights Reserved.

00218

00218 Anesthesia for intracranial procedures; procedures in sitting position

ICD-10-CM Diagnostic Codes

	C70.0	Malignant neoplasm of cerebral meninges
	C70.1	Malignant neoplasm of spinal meninges
	C71.0	Malignant neoplasm of cerebrum, except lobes and ventricles
	C71.1	Malignant neoplasm of frontal lobe
	C71.2	Malignant neoplasm of temporal lobe
	C71.3	Malignant neoplasm of parietal lobe
	C71.4	Malignant neoplasm of occipital lobe
	C71.5	Malignant neoplasm of cerebral ventricle
	C71.6	Malignant neoplasm of cerebellum
	C71.7	Malignant neoplasm of brain stem
	C71.8	Malignant neoplasm of overlapping sites of brain
	C79.31	Secondary malignant neoplasm of brain
	C79.32	Secondary malignant neoplasm of cerebral meninges
	D18.02	Hemangioma of intracranial structures
	D32.0	Benign neoplasm of cerebral meninges
	D32.1	Benign neoplasm of spinal meninges
	D33.0	Benign neoplasm of brain, supratentorial
	D33.1	Benign neoplasm of brain, infratentorial
	D33.3	Benign neoplasm of cranial nerves
	G91.1	Obstructive hydrocephalus
	G91.2	(Idiopathic) normal pressure hydrocephalus
	G91.3	Post-traumatic hydrocephalus, unspecified
	G91.8	Other hydrocephalus
	G93.0	Cerebral cysts
⑦⇄	S02.101	Fracture of base of skull, right side
⑦⇄	S02.102	Fracture of base of skull, left side

ICD-10-CM Coding Notes

For codes requiring a 7th character extension, refer to your ICD-10-CM book. Review the character descriptions and coding guidelines for proper selection. For some procedures, only certain characters will apply.

CCI Edits

Refer to Appendix A for CCI edits.

Pub 100

00218: Pub 100-04, 12, 140.5, Pub 100-04, 12, 50, Pub 100-04, 12, 90.4.5

Base Units

Global: XXX

Code	Base Units
00218	13

Modifiers (PAR)

Code	Mod 50	Mod 51	Mod 62	Mod 80
00218	9	9	9	9

CPT © 2018 American Medical Association. All Rights Reserved.

00220

00220 Anesthesia for intracranial procedures; cerebrospinal fluid shunting procedures

ICD-10-CM Diagnostic Codes

	G91.0	Communicating hydrocephalus
	G91.1	Obstructive hydrocephalus
	G91.2	(Idiopathic) normal pressure hydrocephalus
	G91.3	Post-traumatic hydrocephalus, unspecified
	G91.4	Hydrocephalus in diseases classified elsewhere
	G91.8	Other hydrocephalus
	G91.9	Hydrocephalus, unspecified
	Q03.0	Malformations of aqueduct of Sylvius
	Q03.1	Atresia of foramina of Magendie and Luschka
	Q03.8	Other congenital hydrocephalus
	Q03.9	Congenital hydrocephalus, unspecified
	Q05.0	Cervical spina bifida with hydrocephalus
	Q05.1	Thoracic spina bifida with hydrocephalus
	Q05.2	Lumbar spina bifida with hydrocephalus
	Q05.3	Sacral spina bifida with hydrocephalus
	Q05.4	Unspecified spina bifida with hydrocephalus
7	T85.01	Breakdown (mechanical) of ventricular intracranial (communicating) shunt
7	T85.02	Displacement of ventricular intracranial (communicating) shunt
7	T85.03	Leakage of ventricular intracranial (communicating) shunt
7	T85.09	Other mechanical complication of ventricular intracranial (communicating) shunt
7	T85.730	Infection and inflammatory reaction due to ventricular intracranial (communicating) shunt
7	T85.810	Embolism due to nervous system prosthetic devices, implants and grafts
7	T85.820	Fibrosis due to nervous system prosthetic devices, implants and grafts
7	T85.830	Hemorrhage due to nervous system prosthetic devices, implants and grafts
7	T85.840	Pain due to nervous system prosthetic devices, implants and grafts
7	T85.850	Stenosis due to nervous system prosthetic devices, implants and grafts
7	T85.860	Thrombosis due to nervous system prosthetic devices, implants and grafts
7	T85.890	Other specified complication of nervous system prosthetic devices, implants and grafts
	Z45.41	Encounter for adjustment and management of cerebrospinal fluid drainage device

ICD-10-CM Coding Notes

For codes requiring a 7th character extension, refer to your ICD-10-CM book. Review the character descriptions and coding guidelines for proper selection. For some procedures, only certain characters will apply.

CCI Edits

Refer to Appendix A for CCI edits.

Pub 100

00220: Pub 100-04, 12, 140.5, Pub 100-04, 12, 50, Pub 100-04, 12, 90.4.5

Base Units

Global: XXX

Code	Base Units
00220	10

Modifiers (PAR)

Code	Mod 50	Mod 51	Mod 62	Mod 80
00220	9	9	9	9

CPT © 2018 American Medical Association. All Rights Reserved.

00222

00222 Anesthesia for intracranial procedures; electrocoagulation of intracranial nerve

AMA *CPT Assistant*

00222: Jul 12: 13

ICD-10-CM Diagnostic Codes

⇄	C72.21	Malignant neoplasm of right olfactory nerve
⇄	C72.22	Malignant neoplasm of left olfactory nerve
⇄	C72.31	Malignant neoplasm of right optic nerve
⇄	C72.32	Malignant neoplasm of left optic nerve
⇄	C72.41	Malignant neoplasm of right acoustic nerve
⇄	C72.42	Malignant neoplasm of left acoustic nerve
	C72.50	Malignant neoplasm of unspecified cranial nerve
	C72.59	Malignant neoplasm of other cranial nerves
	C79.49	Secondary malignant neoplasm of other parts of nervous system
	D33.3	Benign neoplasm of cranial nerves
	D43.3	Neoplasm of uncertain behavior of cranial nerves
	D49.7	Neoplasm of unspecified behavior of endocrine glands and other parts of nervous system
	G50.0	Trigeminal neuralgia
	G50.1	Atypical facial pain
	G50.8	Other disorders of trigeminal nerve
	G50.9	Disorder of trigeminal nerve, unspecified
	G51.1	Geniculate ganglionitis
⇄	G51.31	Clonic hemifacial spasm, right
⇄	G51.32	Clonic hemifacial spasm, left
⇄	G51.33	Clonic hemifacial spasm, bilateral
⇄	G51.39	Clonic hemifacial spasm, unspecified
	G51.4	Facial myokymia
	G51.8	Other disorders of facial nerve
	G51.9	Disorder of facial nerve, unspecified
	G52.0	Disorders of olfactory nerve
	G52.1	Disorders of glossopharyngeal nerve
	G52.2	Disorders of vagus nerve
	G52.3	Disorders of hypoglossal nerve
	G52.7	Disorders of multiple cranial nerves
	G52.8	Disorders of other specified cranial nerves
	G52.9	Cranial nerve disorder, unspecified
	G53	Cranial nerve disorders in diseases classified elsewhere

CCI Edits

Refer to Appendix A for CCI edits.

Pub 100

00222: Pub 100-04, 12, 140.5, Pub 100-04, 12, 50, Pub 100-04, 12, 90.4.5

Base Units

Global: XXX

Code	Base Units
00222	6

Modifiers (PAR)

Code	Mod 50	Mod 51	Mod 62	Mod 80
00222	9	9	9	9

CPT © 2018 American Medical Association. All Rights Reserved.

00300

00300 Anesthesia for all procedures on the integumentary system, muscles and nerves of head, neck, and posterior trunk, not otherwise specified

AMA *CPT Assistant* ▯

00300: Nov 99: 7, Mar 06: 15, Oct 11: 3, Jul 12: 13

ICD-10-CM Diagnostic Codes

	B02.21	Postherpetic geniculate ganglionitis
	B02.22	Postherpetic trigeminal neuralgia
	C43.4	Malignant melanoma of scalp and neck
	C43.59	Malignant melanoma of other part of trunk
	C4A.4	Merkel cell carcinoma of scalp and neck
	C4A.59	Merkel cell carcinoma of other part of trunk
	E08.622	Diabetes mellitus due to underlying condition with other skin ulcer
	E09.622	Drug or chemical induced diabetes mellitus with other skin ulcer
	E10.622	Type 1 diabetes mellitus with other skin ulcer
	E11.622	Type 2 diabetes mellitus with other skin ulcer
	E13.622	Other specified diabetes mellitus with other skin ulcer
	G50.0	Trigeminal neuralgia
	G50.1	Atypical facial pain
	G51.1	Geniculate ganglionitis
	G51.8	Other disorders of facial nerve
⇄	L89.114	Pressure ulcer of right upper back, stage 4
⇄	L89.119	Pressure ulcer of right upper back, unspecified stage
⇄	L89.124	Pressure ulcer of left upper back, stage 4
⇄	L89.129	Pressure ulcer of left upper back, unspecified stage
⇄	L89.134	Pressure ulcer of right lower back, stage 4
⇄	L89.139	Pressure ulcer of right lower back, unspecified stage
⇄	L89.144	Pressure ulcer of left lower back, stage 4
⇄	L89.149	Pressure ulcer of left lower back, unspecified stage
	L89.154	Pressure ulcer of sacral region, stage 4
	L89.159	Pressure ulcer of sacral region, unspecified stage
⇄	L89.214	Pressure ulcer of right hip, stage 4
⇄	L89.219	Pressure ulcer of right hip, unspecified stage
⇄	L89.224	Pressure ulcer of left hip, stage 4
⇄	L89.229	Pressure ulcer of left hip, unspecified stage
	L89.304	Pressure ulcer of unspecified buttock, stage 4
	L89.309	Pressure ulcer of unspecified buttock, unspecified stage
⇄	L89.314	Pressure ulcer of right buttock, stage 4
⇄	L89.319	Pressure ulcer of right buttock, unspecified stage
⇄	L89.324	Pressure ulcer of left buttock, stage 4
⇄	L89.329	Pressure ulcer of left buttock, unspecified stage
	L98.413	Non-pressure chronic ulcer of buttock with necrosis of muscle
	L98.415	Non-pressure chronic ulcer of buttock with muscle involvement without evidence of necrosis
	L98.419	Non-pressure chronic ulcer of buttock with unspecified severity
	L98.423	Non-pressure chronic ulcer of back with necrosis of muscle
	L98.425	Non-pressure chronic ulcer of back with muscle involvement without evidence of necrosis
	L98.429	Non-pressure chronic ulcer of back with unspecified severity
	M60.08	Infective myositis, other site
❼⇄	S21.211	Laceration without foreign body of right back wall of thorax without penetration into thoracic cavity
❼⇄	S21.212	Laceration without foreign body of left back wall of thorax without penetration into thoracic cavity
❼⇄	S21.231	Puncture wound without foreign body of right back wall of thorax without penetration into thoracic cavity
❼⇄	S21.232	Puncture wound without foreign body of left back wall of thorax without penetration into thoracic cavity
❼⇄	S21.251	Open bite of right back wall of thorax without penetration into thoracic cavity
❼⇄	S21.252	Open bite of left back wall of thorax without penetration into thoracic cavity
❼	S29.022	Laceration of muscle and tendon of back wall of thorax
❼	S31.010	Laceration without foreign body of lower back and pelvis without penetration into retroperitoneum
❼	S31.030	Puncture wound without foreign body of lower back and pelvis without penetration into retroperitoneum
❼	S31.050	Open bite of lower back and pelvis without penetration into retroperitoneum
❼⇄	S31.811	Laceration without foreign body of right buttock
❼⇄	S31.813	Puncture wound without foreign body of right buttock
❼⇄	S31.815	Open bite of right buttock
❼⇄	S31.821	Laceration without foreign body of left buttock
❼⇄	S31.823	Puncture wound without foreign body of left buttock
❼⇄	S31.825	Open bite of left buttock

ICD-10-CM Coding Notes

For codes requiring a 7th character extension, refer to your ICD-10-CM book. Review the character descriptions and coding guidelines for proper selection. For some procedures, only certain characters will apply.

CCI Edits

Refer to Appendix A for CCI edits.

Pub 100

00300: Pub 100-04, 12, 140.5, Pub 100-04, 12, 50, Pub 100-04, 12, 90.4.5

Base Units

Global: XXX

Code	Base Units
00300	5

Modifiers (PAR)

Code	Mod 50	Mod 51	Mod 62	Mod 80
00300	9	9	9	9

CPT © 2018 American Medical Association. All Rights Reserved.

00320

00320 Anesthesia for all procedures on esophagus, thyroid, larynx, trachea and lymphatic system of neck; not otherwise specified, age 1 year or older

ICD-10-CM Diagnostic Codes

C15.3	Malignant neoplasm of upper third of esophagus
C32.0	Malignant neoplasm of glottis
C32.1	Malignant neoplasm of supraglottis
C32.2	Malignant neoplasm of subglottis
C32.3	Malignant neoplasm of laryngeal cartilage
C32.8	Malignant neoplasm of overlapping sites of larynx
C32.9	Malignant neoplasm of larynx, unspecified
C33	Malignant neoplasm of trachea
C73	Malignant neoplasm of thyroid gland
C76.0	Malignant neoplasm of head, face and neck
C77.0	Secondary and unspecified malignant neoplasm of lymph nodes of head, face and neck

CCI Edits

Refer to Appendix A for CCI edits.

Pub 100

00320: Pub 100-04, 12, 140.5, Pub 100-04, 12, 50, Pub 100-04, 12, 90.4.5

Base Units

Global: XXX

Code	Base Units
00320	6

Modifiers (PAR)

Code	Mod 50	Mod 51	Mod 62	Mod 80
00320	9	9	9	9

CPT © 2018 American Medical Association. All Rights Reserved.

00322

00322 Anesthesia for all procedures on esophagus, thyroid, larynx, trachea and lymphatic system of neck; needle biopsy of thyroid

(For procedures on cervical spine and cord, see 00600, 00604, 00670)

ICD-10-CM Diagnostic Codes

C73	Malignant neoplasm of thyroid gland
C79.89	Secondary malignant neoplasm of other specified sites
D09.3	Carcinoma in situ of thyroid and other endocrine glands
D34	Benign neoplasm of thyroid gland
D44.0	Neoplasm of uncertain behavior of thyroid gland
D49.7	Neoplasm of unspecified behavior of endocrine glands and other parts of nervous system
E04.0	Nontoxic diffuse goiter
E04.1	Nontoxic single thyroid nodule
E04.2	Nontoxic multinodular goiter
E04.8	Other specified nontoxic goiter
E04.9	Nontoxic goiter, unspecified
E05.00	Thyrotoxicosis with diffuse goiter without thyrotoxic crisis or storm
E05.01	Thyrotoxicosis with diffuse goiter with thyrotoxic crisis or storm
E05.10	Thyrotoxicosis with toxic single thyroid nodule without thyrotoxic crisis or storm
E05.11	Thyrotoxicosis with toxic single thyroid nodule with thyrotoxic crisis or storm
E05.20	Thyrotoxicosis with toxic multinodular goiter without thyrotoxic crisis or storm
E05.21	Thyrotoxicosis with toxic multinodular goiter with thyrotoxic crisis or storm
E05.30	Thyrotoxicosis from ectopic thyroid tissue without thyrotoxic crisis or storm
E05.31	Thyrotoxicosis from ectopic thyroid tissue with thyrotoxic crisis or storm
E05.40	Thyrotoxicosis factitia without thyrotoxic crisis or storm
E05.41	Thyrotoxicosis factitia with thyrotoxic crisis or storm
E05.80	Other thyrotoxicosis without thyrotoxic crisis or storm
E05.81	Other thyrotoxicosis with thyrotoxic crisis or storm
E05.90	Thyrotoxicosis, unspecified without thyrotoxic crisis or storm
E05.91	Thyrotoxicosis, unspecified with thyrotoxic crisis or storm
E06.0	Acute thyroiditis
E06.1	Subacute thyroiditis
E06.2	Chronic thyroiditis with transient thyrotoxicosis
E06.3	Autoimmune thyroiditis
E06.5	Other chronic thyroiditis
E06.9	Thyroiditis, unspecified
R22.1	Localized swelling, mass and lump, neck

CCI Edits

Refer to Appendix A for CCI edits.

Pub 100

00322: Pub 100-04, 12, 140.5, Pub 100-04, 12, 50, Pub 100-04, 12, 90.4.5

Base Units

Global: XXX

Code	Base Units
00322	3

Modifiers (PAR)

Code	Mod 50	Mod 51	Mod 62	Mod 80
00322	9	9	9	9

CPT © 2018 American Medical Association. All Rights Reserved.

00326

00326 Anesthesia for all procedures on the larynx and trachea in children younger than 1 year of age

(Do not report 00326 in conjunction with 99100)

AMA *CPT Assistant*

00326: Dec 17: 8

ICD-10-CM Diagnostic Codes

	J04.11	Acute tracheitis with obstruction
	J04.2	Acute laryngotracheitis
	J04.31	Supraglottitis, unspecified, with obstruction
	J05.11	Acute epiglottitis with obstruction
	J06.0	Acute laryngopharyngitis
	J37.1	Chronic laryngotracheitis
	J38.7	Other diseases of larynx
	P22.0	Respiratory distress syndrome of newborn
	P22.8	Other respiratory distress of newborn
	P22.9	Respiratory distress of newborn, unspecified
	P24.01	Meconium aspiration with respiratory symptoms
	P24.11	Neonatal aspiration of (clear) amniotic fluid and mucus with respiratory symptoms
	P24.21	Neonatal aspiration of blood with respiratory symptoms
	P24.31	Neonatal aspiration of milk and regurgitated food with respiratory symptoms
	P24.81	Other neonatal aspiration with respiratory symptoms
	P28.2	Cyanotic attacks of newborn
	Q31.0	Web of larynx
	Q31.1	Congenital subglottic stenosis
	Q31.2	Laryngeal hypoplasia
	Q31.3	Laryngocele
	Q31.5	Congenital laryngomalacia
	Q31.8	Other congenital malformations of larynx
	Q31.9	Congenital malformation of larynx, unspecified
	Q32.0	Congenital tracheomalacia
	Q32.1	Other congenital malformations of trachea
	Q39.1	Atresia of esophagus with tracheo-esophageal fistula
	Q39.2	Congenital tracheo-esophageal fistula without atresia
❼	T17.300	Unspecified foreign body in larynx causing asphyxiation
❼	T17.308	Unspecified foreign body in larynx causing other injury
❼	T17.310	Gastric contents in larynx causing asphyxiation
❼	T17.318	Gastric contents in larynx causing other injury
❼	T17.320	Food in larynx causing asphyxiation
❼	T17.328	Food in larynx causing other injury
❼	T17.390	Other foreign object in larynx causing asphyxiation
❼	T17.398	Other foreign object in larynx causing other injury
❼	T17.400	Unspecified foreign body in trachea causing asphyxiation
❼	T17.408	Unspecified foreign body in trachea causing other injury
❼	T17.410	Gastric contents in trachea causing asphyxiation
❼	T17.418	Gastric contents in trachea causing other injury
❼	T17.420	Food in trachea causing asphyxiation
❼	T17.428	Food in trachea causing other injury
❼	T17.490	Other foreign object in trachea causing asphyxiation
❼	T17.498	Other foreign object in trachea causing other injury

ICD-10-CM Coding Notes

For codes requiring a 7th character extension, refer to your ICD-10-CM book. Review the character descriptions and coding guidelines for proper selection. For some procedures, only certain characters will apply.

CCI Edits

Refer to Appendix A for CCI edits.

Pub 100

00326: Pub 100-04, 12, 140.5, Pub 100-04, 12, 50, Pub 100-04, 12, 90.4.5

Base Units

Global: XXX

Code	Base Units
00326	7

Modifiers (PAR)

Code	Mod 50	Mod 51	Mod 62	Mod 80
00326	9	9	9	9

CPT © 2018 American Medical Association. All Rights Reserved.

00350

00350 Anesthesia for procedures on major vessels of neck; not otherwise specified

ICD-10-CM Diagnostic Codes

⇄	I63.211	Cerebral infarction due to unspecified occlusion or stenosis of right vertebral artery
⇄	I63.212	Cerebral infarction due to unspecified occlusion or stenosis of left vertebral artery
⇄	I63.213	Cerebral infarction due to unspecified occlusion or stenosis of bilateral vertebral arteries
	I63.22	Cerebral infarction due to unspecified occlusion or stenosis of basilar artery
⇄	I63.231	Cerebral infarction due to unspecified occlusion or stenosis of right carotid arteries
⇄	I63.232	Cerebral infarction due to unspecified occlusion or stenosis of left carotid arteries
⇄	I63.233	Cerebral infarction due to unspecified occlusion or stenosis of bilateral carotid arteries
	I63.29	Cerebral infarction due to unspecified occlusion or stenosis of other precerebral arteries
	I63.81	Other cerebral infarction due to occlusion or stenosis of small artery
	I63.89	Other cerebral infarction
⇄	I65.01	Occlusion and stenosis of right vertebral artery
⇄	I65.02	Occlusion and stenosis of left vertebral artery
⇄	I65.03	Occlusion and stenosis of bilateral vertebral arteries
	I65.1	Occlusion and stenosis of basilar artery
⇄	I65.21	Occlusion and stenosis of right carotid artery
⇄	I65.22	Occlusion and stenosis of left carotid artery
⇄	I65.23	Occlusion and stenosis of bilateral carotid arteries
	I65.8	Occlusion and stenosis of other precerebral arteries
	I65.9	Occlusion and stenosis of unspecified precerebral artery
	I67.2	Cerebral atherosclerosis
	I67.82	Cerebral ischemia
	I67.850	Cerebral autosomal dominant arteriopathy with subcortical infarcts and leukoencephalopathy
	I67.858	Other hereditary cerebrovascular disease
	I72.0	Aneurysm of carotid artery
	I77.1	Stricture of artery
	I77.2	Rupture of artery
	I77.71	Dissection of carotid artery
	I97.42	Intraoperative hemorrhage and hematoma of a circulatory system organ or structure complicating other procedure
	I97.51	Accidental puncture and laceration of a circulatory system organ or structure during a circulatory system procedure
	I97.52	Accidental puncture and laceration of a circulatory system organ or structure during other procedure
	I97.811	Intraoperative cerebrovascular infarction during other surgery
	I97.821	Postprocedural cerebrovascular infarction following other surgery
	R41.82	Altered mental status, unspecified
	R42	Dizziness and giddiness
	R55	Syncope and collapse
❼⇄	S15.011	Minor laceration of right carotid artery
❼⇄	S15.012	Minor laceration of left carotid artery
❼⇄	S15.021	Major laceration of right carotid artery
❼⇄	S15.022	Major laceration of left carotid artery
❼⇄	S15.091	Other specified injury of right carotid artery
❼⇄	S15.092	Other specified injury of left carotid artery
❼⇄	S15.111	Minor laceration of right vertebral artery
❼⇄	S15.112	Minor laceration of left vertebral artery
❼⇄	S15.121	Major laceration of right vertebral artery
❼⇄	S15.122	Major laceration of left vertebral artery
❼⇄	S15.191	Other specified injury of right vertebral artery
❼⇄	S15.192	Other specified injury of left vertebral artery
❼⇄	S15.211	Minor laceration of right external jugular vein
❼⇄	S15.212	Minor laceration of left external jugular vein
❼⇄	S15.221	Major laceration of right external jugular vein
❼⇄	S15.222	Major laceration of left external jugular vein
❼⇄	S15.291	Other specified injury of right external jugular vein
❼⇄	S15.292	Other specified injury of left external jugular vein
❼⇄	S15.311	Minor laceration of right internal jugular vein
❼⇄	S15.312	Minor laceration of left internal jugular vein
❼⇄	S15.321	Major laceration of right internal jugular vein
❼⇄	S15.322	Major laceration of left internal jugular vein
❼⇄	S15.391	Other specified injury of right internal jugular vein
❼⇄	S15.392	Other specified injury of left internal jugular vein
❼	S15.8	Injury of other specified blood vessels at neck level
❼	S15.9	Injury of unspecified blood vessel at neck level

ICD-10-CM Coding Notes

For codes requiring a 7th character extension, refer to your ICD-10-CM book. Review the character descriptions and coding guidelines for proper selection. For some procedures, only certain characters will apply.

CCI Edits

Refer to Appendix A for CCI edits.

Pub 100

00350: Pub 100-04, 12, 140.5, Pub 100-04, 12, 50, Pub 100-04, 12, 90.4.5

Base Units

Global: XXX

Code	Base Units
00350	10

Modifiers (PAR)

Code	Mod 50	Mod 51	Mod 62	Mod 80
00350	9	9	9	9

CPT © 2018 American Medical Association. All Rights Reserved.

00352

00352 Anesthesia for procedures on major vessels of neck; simple ligation

(For arteriography, use 01916)

AMA *CPT Assistant* □

00352: Nov 07: 8, Jul 12: 13

ICD-10-CM Diagnostic Codes

	D18.00	Hemangioma unspecified site
	D18.02	Hemangioma of intracranial structures
	I72.0	Aneurysm of carotid artery
	I77.0	Arteriovenous fistula, acquired
	I77.2	Rupture of artery
	Q27.30	Arteriovenous malformation, site unspecified
	Q27.39	Arteriovenous malformation, other site
	Q28.0	Arteriovenous malformation of precerebral vessels
	Q28.2	Arteriovenous malformation of cerebral vessels
➐⇄	S15.011	Minor laceration of right carotid artery
➐⇄	S15.012	Minor laceration of left carotid artery
➐⇄	S15.021	Major laceration of right carotid artery
➐⇄	S15.022	Major laceration of left carotid artery
➐⇄	S15.091	Other specified injury of right carotid artery
➐⇄	S15.092	Other specified injury of left carotid artery
➐⇄	S15.111	Minor laceration of right vertebral artery
➐⇄	S15.112	Minor laceration of left vertebral artery
➐⇄	S15.191	Other specified injury of right vertebral artery
➐⇄	S15.192	Other specified injury of left vertebral artery
➐⇄	S15.211	Minor laceration of right external jugular vein
➐⇄	S15.212	Minor laceration of left external jugular vein
➐⇄	S15.221	Major laceration of right external jugular vein
➐⇄	S15.222	Major laceration of left external jugular vein
➐⇄	S15.291	Other specified injury of right external jugular vein
➐⇄	S15.292	Other specified injury of left external jugular vein
➐⇄	S15.311	Minor laceration of right internal jugular vein
➐⇄	S15.312	Minor laceration of left internal jugular vein
➐⇄	S15.321	Major laceration of right internal jugular vein
➐⇄	S15.322	Major laceration of left internal jugular vein
➐⇄	S15.391	Other specified injury of right internal jugular vein
➐⇄	S15.392	Other specified injury of left internal jugular vein
➐	S15.8	Injury of other specified blood vessels at neck level
➐	S15.9	Injury of unspecified blood vessel at neck level

ICD-10-CM Coding Notes

For codes requiring a 7th character extension, refer to your ICD-10-CM book. Review the character descriptions and coding guidelines for proper selection. For some procedures, only certain characters will apply.

CCI Edits

Refer to Appendix A for CCI edits.

Pub 100

00352: Pub 100-04, 12, 140.5, Pub 100-04, 12, 50, Pub 100-04, 12, 90.4.5

Base Units

Global: XXX

Code	Base Units
00352	5

Modifiers (PAR)

Code	Mod 50	Mod 51	Mod 62	Mod 80
00352	9	9	9	9

CPT © 2018 American Medical Association. All Rights Reserved.

00400

00400 Anesthesia for procedures on the integumentary system on the extremities, anterior trunk and perineum; not otherwise specified

AMA *CPT Assistant* ▯

00400: Mar 06: 15, Nov 07: 8, Oct 11: 3, Jul 12: 13

ICD-10-CM Diagnostic Codes

	C43.52	Malignant melanoma of skin of breast
	C43.59	Malignant melanoma of other part of trunk
⇄	C43.61	Malignant melanoma of right upper limb, including shoulder
⇄	C43.62	Malignant melanoma of left upper limb, including shoulder
⇄	C43.71	Malignant melanoma of right lower limb, including hip
⇄	C43.72	Malignant melanoma of left lower limb, including hip
⇄	C50.011	Malignant neoplasm of nipple and areola, right female breast ♀
⇄	C50.012	Malignant neoplasm of nipple and areola, left female breast ♀
⇄	C50.111	Malignant neoplasm of central portion of right female breast ♀
⇄	C50.112	Malignant neoplasm of central portion of left female breast ♀
⇄	C50.211	Malignant neoplasm of upper-inner quadrant of right female breast ♀
⇄	C50.212	Malignant neoplasm of upper-inner quadrant of left female breast ♀
⇄	C50.311	Malignant neoplasm of lower-inner quadrant of right female breast ♀
⇄	C50.312	Malignant neoplasm of lower-inner quadrant of left female breast ♀
⇄	C50.411	Malignant neoplasm of upper-outer quadrant of right female breast ♀
⇄	C50.412	Malignant neoplasm of upper-outer quadrant of left female breast ♀
⇄	C50.511	Malignant neoplasm of lower-outer quadrant of right female breast ♀
⇄	C50.512	Malignant neoplasm of lower-outer quadrant of left female breast ♀
⇄	C50.611	Malignant neoplasm of axillary tail of right female breast ♀
⇄	C50.612	Malignant neoplasm of axillary tail of left female breast ♀
⇄	C50.811	Malignant neoplasm of overlapping sites of right female breast ♀
⇄	C50.812	Malignant neoplasm of overlapping sites of left female breast ♀
⇄	D05.01	Lobular carcinoma in situ of right breast
⇄	D05.02	Lobular carcinoma in situ of left breast
⇄	D05.11	Intraductal carcinoma in situ of right breast
⇄	D05.12	Intraductal carcinoma in situ of left breast
⇄	D05.81	Other specified type of carcinoma in situ of right breast
⇄	D05.82	Other specified type of carcinoma in situ of left breast
⇄	D05.91	Unspecified type of carcinoma in situ of right breast
⇄	D05.92	Unspecified type of carcinoma in situ of left breast
⇄	L97.111	Non-pressure chronic ulcer of right thigh limited to breakdown of skin
⇄	L97.112	Non-pressure chronic ulcer of right thigh with fat layer exposed
⇄	L97.115	Non-pressure chronic ulcer of right thigh with muscle involvement without evidence of necrosis
⇄	L97.118	Non-pressure chronic ulcer of right thigh with other specified severity
⇄	L97.121	Non-pressure chronic ulcer of left thigh limited to breakdown of skin
⇄	L97.122	Non-pressure chronic ulcer of left thigh with fat layer exposed
⇄	L97.125	Non-pressure chronic ulcer of left thigh with muscle involvement without evidence of necrosis
⇄	L97.128	Non-pressure chronic ulcer of left thigh with other specified severity
⇄	L97.211	Non-pressure chronic ulcer of right calf limited to breakdown of skin
⇄	L97.212	Non-pressure chronic ulcer of right calf with fat layer exposed
⇄	L97.215	Non-pressure chronic ulcer of right calf with muscle involvement without evidence of necrosis
⇄	L97.218	Non-pressure chronic ulcer of right calf with other specified severity
⇄	L97.221	Non-pressure chronic ulcer of left calf limited to breakdown of skin
⇄	L97.222	Non-pressure chronic ulcer of left calf with fat layer exposed
⇄	L97.225	Non-pressure chronic ulcer of left calf with muscle involvement without evidence of necrosis
⇄	L97.311	Non-pressure chronic ulcer of right ankle limited to breakdown of skin
⇄	L97.312	Non-pressure chronic ulcer of right ankle with fat layer exposed
⇄	L97.321	Non-pressure chronic ulcer of left ankle limited to breakdown of skin
⇄	L97.322	Non-pressure chronic ulcer of left ankle with fat layer exposed
⇄	L97.411	Non-pressure chronic ulcer of right heel and midfoot limited to breakdown of skin
⇄	L97.412	Non-pressure chronic ulcer of right heel and midfoot with fat layer exposed
⇄	L97.421	Non-pressure chronic ulcer of left heel and midfoot limited to breakdown of skin
⇄	L97.422	Non-pressure chronic ulcer of left heel and midfoot with fat layer exposed
⇄	N60.21	Fibroadenosis of right breast
⇄	N60.22	Fibroadenosis of left breast
⇄	N63.10	Unspecified lump in the right breast, unspecified quadrant
⇄	N63.11	Unspecified lump in the right breast, upper outer quadrant
⇄	N63.12	Unspecified lump in the right breast, upper inner quadrant
⇄	N63.13	Unspecified lump in the right breast, lower outer quadrant
⇄	N63.14	Unspecified lump in the right breast, lower inner quadrant
⇄	N63.21	Unspecified lump in the left breast, upper outer quadrant
⇄	N63.22	Unspecified lump in the left breast, upper inner quadrant
⇄	N63.23	Unspecified lump in the left breast, lower outer quadrant
⇄	N63.24	Unspecified lump in the left breast, lower inner quadrant
⇄	N63.31	Unspecified lump in axillary tail of the right breast
⇄	N63.32	Unspecified lump in axillary tail of the left breast
⇄	N63.41	Unspecified lump in right breast, subareolar
⇄	N63.42	Unspecified lump in left breast, subareolar

CCI Edits

Refer to Appendix A for CCI edits.

Pub 100

00400: Pub 100-04, 12, 140.5, Pub 100-04, 12, 50, Pub 100-04, 12, 90.4.5

Base Units

Global: XXX

Code	Base Units
00400	3

Modifiers (PAR)

Code	Mod 50	Mod 51	Mod 62	Mod 80
00400	9	9	9	9

CPT © 2018 American Medical Association. All Rights Reserved.

00402

00402 Anesthesia for procedures on the integumentary system on the extremities, anterior trunk and perineum; reconstructive procedures on breast (eg, reduction or augmentation mammoplasty, muscle flaps)

ICD-10-CM Diagnostic Codes

⇄ C50.011 Malignant neoplasm of nipple and areola, right female breast ♀
⇄ C50.012 Malignant neoplasm of nipple and areola, left female breast ♀
⇄ C50.111 Malignant neoplasm of central portion of right female breast ♀
⇄ C50.112 Malignant neoplasm of central portion of left female breast ♀
⇄ C50.211 Malignant neoplasm of upper-inner quadrant of right female breast ♀
⇄ C50.212 Malignant neoplasm of upper-inner quadrant of left female breast ♀
⇄ C50.311 Malignant neoplasm of lower-inner quadrant of right female breast ♀
⇄ C50.312 Malignant neoplasm of lower-inner quadrant of left female breast ♀
⇄ C50.411 Malignant neoplasm of upper-outer quadrant of right female breast ♀
⇄ C50.412 Malignant neoplasm of upper-outer quadrant of left female breast ♀
⇄ C50.511 Malignant neoplasm of lower-outer quadrant of right female breast ♀
⇄ C50.512 Malignant neoplasm of lower-outer quadrant of left female breast ♀
⇄ C50.611 Malignant neoplasm of axillary tail of right female breast ♀
⇄ C50.612 Malignant neoplasm of axillary tail of left female breast ♀
⇄ C50.811 Malignant neoplasm of overlapping sites of right female breast ♀
⇄ C50.812 Malignant neoplasm of overlapping sites of left female breast ♀
⇄ C50.911 Malignant neoplasm of unspecified site of right female breast ♀
⇄ C50.912 Malignant neoplasm of unspecified site of left female breast ♀
N62 Hypertrophy of breast
N64.81 Ptosis of breast
N64.82 Hypoplasia of breast
N65.0 Deformity of reconstructed breast
N65.1 Disproportion of reconstructed breast
Q83.0 Congenital absence of breast with absent nipple
Q83.2 Absent nipple
Q83.8 Other congenital malformations of breast
➐ T85.41 Breakdown (mechanical) of breast prosthesis and implant
➐ T85.42 Displacement of breast prosthesis and implant
➐ T85.43 Leakage of breast prosthesis and implant
➐ T85.44 Capsular contracture of breast implant
➐ T85.49 Other mechanical complication of breast prosthesis and implant
➐ T85.79 Infection and inflammatory reaction due to other internal prosthetic devices, implants and grafts
➐ T85.828 Fibrosis due to other internal prosthetic devices, implants and grafts
➐ T85.838 Hemorrhage due to other internal prosthetic devices, implants and grafts
➐ T85.848 Pain due to other internal prosthetic devices, implants and grafts
➐ T85.898 Other specified complication of other internal prosthetic devices, implants and grafts
Z40.01 Encounter for prophylactic removal of breast
Z41.1 Encounter for cosmetic surgery
Z42.1 Encounter for breast reconstruction following mastectomy
⇄ Z45.811 Encounter for adjustment or removal of right breast implant
⇄ Z45.812 Encounter for adjustment or removal of left breast implant
Z85.3 Personal history of malignant neoplasm of breast
⇄ Z90.11 Acquired absence of right breast and nipple
⇄ Z90.12 Acquired absence of left breast and nipple
⇄ Z90.13 Acquired absence of bilateral breasts and nipples

ICD-10-CM Coding Notes

For codes requiring a 7th character extension, refer to your ICD-10-CM book. Review the character descriptions and coding guidelines for proper selection. For some procedures, only certain characters will apply.

CCI Edits

Refer to Appendix A for CCI edits.

Pub 100

00402: Pub 100-04, 12, 140.5, Pub 100-04, 12, 50, Pub 100-04, 12, 90.4.5

Base Units

Global: XXX

Code	Base Units
00402	5

Modifiers (PAR)

Code	Mod 50	Mod 51	Mod 62	Mod 80
00402	9	9	9	9

CPT © 2018 American Medical Association. All Rights Reserved.

00404

00404 Anesthesia for procedures on the integumentary system on the extremities, anterior trunk and perineum; radical or modified radical procedures on breast

ICD-10-CM Diagnostic Codes

⇄ C50.011 Malignant neoplasm of nipple and areola, right female breast ♀
⇄ C50.012 Malignant neoplasm of nipple and areola, left female breast ♀
⇄ C50.019 Malignant neoplasm of nipple and areola, unspecified female breast ♀
⇄ C50.021 Malignant neoplasm of nipple and areola, right male breast ♂
⇄ C50.022 Malignant neoplasm of nipple and areola, left male breast ♂
⇄ C50.029 Malignant neoplasm of nipple and areola, unspecified male breast ♂
⇄ C50.111 Malignant neoplasm of central portion of right female breast ♀
⇄ C50.112 Malignant neoplasm of central portion of left female breast ♀
⇄ C50.119 Malignant neoplasm of central portion of unspecified female breast ♀
⇄ C50.121 Malignant neoplasm of central portion of right male breast ♂
⇄ C50.122 Malignant neoplasm of central portion of left male breast ♂
⇄ C50.129 Malignant neoplasm of central portion of unspecified male breast ♂
⇄ C50.211 Malignant neoplasm of upper-inner quadrant of right female breast ♀
⇄ C50.212 Malignant neoplasm of upper-inner quadrant of left female breast ♀
⇄ C50.219 Malignant neoplasm of upper-inner quadrant of unspecified female breast ♀
⇄ C50.221 Malignant neoplasm of upper-inner quadrant of right male breast ♂
⇄ C50.222 Malignant neoplasm of upper-inner quadrant of left male breast ♂
⇄ C50.229 Malignant neoplasm of upper-inner quadrant of unspecified male breast ♂
⇄ C50.311 Malignant neoplasm of lower-inner quadrant of right female breast ♀
⇄ C50.312 Malignant neoplasm of lower-inner quadrant of left female breast ♀
⇄ C50.319 Malignant neoplasm of lower-inner quadrant of unspecified female breast ♀
⇄ C50.321 Malignant neoplasm of lower-inner quadrant of right male breast ♂
⇄ C50.322 Malignant neoplasm of lower-inner quadrant of left male breast ♂
⇄ C50.329 Malignant neoplasm of lower-inner quadrant of unspecified male breast ♂
⇄ C50.411 Malignant neoplasm of upper-outer quadrant of right female breast ♀
⇄ C50.412 Malignant neoplasm of upper-outer quadrant of left female breast ♀
⇄ C50.419 Malignant neoplasm of upper-outer quadrant of unspecified female breast ♀
⇄ C50.421 Malignant neoplasm of upper-outer quadrant of right male breast ♂
⇄ C50.422 Malignant neoplasm of upper-outer quadrant of left male breast ♂
⇄ C50.429 Malignant neoplasm of upper-outer quadrant of unspecified male breast ♂
⇄ C50.511 Malignant neoplasm of lower-outer quadrant of right female breast ♀
⇄ C50.512 Malignant neoplasm of lower-outer quadrant of left female breast ♀
⇄ C50.519 Malignant neoplasm of lower-outer quadrant of unspecified female breast ♀
⇄ C50.521 Malignant neoplasm of lower-outer quadrant of right male breast ♂
⇄ C50.522 Malignant neoplasm of lower-outer quadrant of left male breast ♂
⇄ C50.529 Malignant neoplasm of lower-outer quadrant of unspecified male breast ♂
⇄ C50.611 Malignant neoplasm of axillary tail of right female breast ♀
⇄ C50.612 Malignant neoplasm of axillary tail of left female breast ♀
⇄ C50.619 Malignant neoplasm of axillary tail of unspecified female breast ♀
⇄ C50.621 Malignant neoplasm of axillary tail of right male breast ♂
⇄ C50.622 Malignant neoplasm of axillary tail of left male breast ♂
⇄ C50.629 Malignant neoplasm of axillary tail of unspecified male breast ♂
⇄ C50.811 Malignant neoplasm of overlapping sites of right female breast ♀
⇄ C50.812 Malignant neoplasm of overlapping sites of left female breast ♀
⇄ C50.819 Malignant neoplasm of overlapping sites of unspecified female breast ♀
⇄ C50.821 Malignant neoplasm of overlapping sites of right male breast ♂
⇄ C50.822 Malignant neoplasm of overlapping sites of left male breast ♂
⇄ C50.829 Malignant neoplasm of overlapping sites of unspecified male breast ♂
⇄ C50.911 Malignant neoplasm of unspecified site of right female breast ♀
⇄ C50.912 Malignant neoplasm of unspecified site of left female breast ♀
⇄ C50.919 Malignant neoplasm of unspecified site of unspecified female breast ♀
⇄ C50.921 Malignant neoplasm of unspecified site of right male breast ♂
⇄ C50.922 Malignant neoplasm of unspecified site of left male breast ♂
⇄ C50.929 Malignant neoplasm of unspecified site of unspecified male breast ♂
C77.3 Secondary and unspecified malignant neoplasm of axilla and upper limb lymph nodes
C79.81 Secondary malignant neoplasm of breast
Z17.0 Estrogen receptor positive status [ER+]
Z17.1 Estrogen receptor negative status [ER-]

CCI Edits

Refer to Appendix A for CCI edits.

Pub 100

00404: Pub 100-04, 12, 140.5, Pub 100-04, 12, 50, Pub 100-04, 12, 90.4.5

Base Units

Global: XXX

Code	Base Units
00404	5

Modifiers (PAR)

Code	Mod 50	Mod 51	Mod 62	Mod 80
00404	9	9	9	9

CPT © 2018 American Medical Association. All Rights Reserved.

00406

00406 Anesthesia for procedures on the integumentary system on the extremities, anterior trunk and perineum; radical or modified radical procedures on breast with internal mammary node dissection

ICD-10-CM Diagnostic Codes

⇄ C50.011 Malignant neoplasm of nipple and areola, right female breast ♀
⇄ C50.012 Malignant neoplasm of nipple and areola, left female breast ♀
⇄ C50.019 Malignant neoplasm of nipple and areola, unspecified female breast ♀
⇄ C50.021 Malignant neoplasm of nipple and areola, right male breast ♂
⇄ C50.022 Malignant neoplasm of nipple and areola, left male breast ♂
⇄ C50.029 Malignant neoplasm of nipple and areola, unspecified male breast ♂
⇄ C50.111 Malignant neoplasm of central portion of right female breast ♀
⇄ C50.112 Malignant neoplasm of central portion of left female breast ♀
⇄ C50.119 Malignant neoplasm of central portion of unspecified female breast ♀
⇄ C50.121 Malignant neoplasm of central portion of right male breast ♂
⇄ C50.122 Malignant neoplasm of central portion of left male breast ♂
⇄ C50.129 Malignant neoplasm of central portion of unspecified male breast ♂
⇄ C50.211 Malignant neoplasm of upper-inner quadrant of right female breast ♀
⇄ C50.212 Malignant neoplasm of upper-inner quadrant of left female breast ♀
⇄ C50.219 Malignant neoplasm of upper-inner quadrant of unspecified female breast ♀
⇄ C50.221 Malignant neoplasm of upper-inner quadrant of right male breast ♂
⇄ C50.222 Malignant neoplasm of upper-inner quadrant of left male breast ♂
⇄ C50.229 Malignant neoplasm of upper-inner quadrant of unspecified male breast ♂
⇄ C50.311 Malignant neoplasm of lower-inner quadrant of right female breast ♀
⇄ C50.312 Malignant neoplasm of lower-inner quadrant of left female breast ♀
⇄ C50.319 Malignant neoplasm of lower-inner quadrant of unspecified female breast ♀
⇄ C50.321 Malignant neoplasm of lower-inner quadrant of right male breast ♂
⇄ C50.322 Malignant neoplasm of lower-inner quadrant of left male breast ♂
⇄ C50.329 Malignant neoplasm of lower-inner quadrant of unspecified male breast ♂
⇄ C50.411 Malignant neoplasm of upper-outer quadrant of right female breast ♀
⇄ C50.412 Malignant neoplasm of upper-outer quadrant of left female breast ♀
⇄ C50.419 Malignant neoplasm of upper-outer quadrant of unspecified female breast ♀
⇄ C50.421 Malignant neoplasm of upper-outer quadrant of right male breast ♂
⇄ C50.422 Malignant neoplasm of upper-outer quadrant of left male breast ♂
⇄ C50.429 Malignant neoplasm of upper-outer quadrant of unspecified male breast ♂
⇄ C50.511 Malignant neoplasm of lower-outer quadrant of right female breast ♀
⇄ C50.512 Malignant neoplasm of lower-outer quadrant of left female breast ♀
⇄ C50.519 Malignant neoplasm of lower-outer quadrant of unspecified female breast ♀
⇄ C50.521 Malignant neoplasm of lower-outer quadrant of right male breast ♂
⇄ C50.522 Malignant neoplasm of lower-outer quadrant of left male breast ♂
⇄ C50.529 Malignant neoplasm of lower-outer quadrant of unspecified male breast ♂
⇄ C50.611 Malignant neoplasm of axillary tail of right female breast ♀
⇄ C50.612 Malignant neoplasm of axillary tail of left female breast ♀
⇄ C50.619 Malignant neoplasm of axillary tail of unspecified female breast ♀
⇄ C50.621 Malignant neoplasm of axillary tail of right male breast ♂
⇄ C50.622 Malignant neoplasm of axillary tail of left male breast ♂
⇄ C50.629 Malignant neoplasm of axillary tail of unspecified male breast ♂
⇄ C50.811 Malignant neoplasm of overlapping sites of right female breast ♀
⇄ C50.812 Malignant neoplasm of overlapping sites of left female breast ♀
⇄ C50.819 Malignant neoplasm of overlapping sites of unspecified female breast ♀
⇄ C50.821 Malignant neoplasm of overlapping sites of right male breast ♂
⇄ C50.822 Malignant neoplasm of overlapping sites of left male breast ♂
⇄ C50.829 Malignant neoplasm of overlapping sites of unspecified male breast ♂
⇄ C50.911 Malignant neoplasm of unspecified site of right female breast ♀
⇄ C50.912 Malignant neoplasm of unspecified site of left female breast ♀
⇄ C50.919 Malignant neoplasm of unspecified site of unspecified female breast ♀
⇄ C50.921 Malignant neoplasm of unspecified site of right male breast ♂
⇄ C50.922 Malignant neoplasm of unspecified site of left male breast ♂
⇄ C50.929 Malignant neoplasm of unspecified site of unspecified male breast ♂
C77.3 Secondary and unspecified malignant neoplasm of axilla and upper limb lymph nodes
C79.81 Secondary malignant neoplasm of breast
Z17.0 Estrogen receptor positive status [ER+]
Z17.1 Estrogen receptor negative status [ER-]

CCI Edits

Refer to Appendix A for CCI edits.

Pub 100

00406: Pub 100-04, 12, 140.5, Pub 100-04, 12, 50, Pub 100-04, 12, 90.4.5

Base Units

Global: XXX

Code	Base Units
00406	13

Modifiers (PAR)

Code	Mod 50	Mod 51	Mod 62	Mod 80
00406	9	9	9	9

CPT © 2018 American Medical Association. All Rights Reserved.

00410

00410 Anesthesia for procedures on the integumentary system on the extremities, anterior trunk and perineum; electrical conversion of arrhythmias

ICD-10-CM Diagnostic Codes

I47.0	Re-entry ventricular arrhythmia
I47.1	Supraventricular tachycardia
I47.2	Ventricular tachycardia
I47.9	Paroxysmal tachycardia, unspecified
I48.0	Paroxysmal atrial fibrillation
I48.1	Persistent atrial fibrillation
I48.2	Chronic atrial fibrillation
I48.3	Typical atrial flutter
I48.4	Atypical atrial flutter
I48.91	Unspecified atrial fibrillation
I48.92	Unspecified atrial flutter
I49.01	Ventricular fibrillation
I49.02	Ventricular flutter
I49.1	Atrial premature depolarization
I49.2	Junctional premature depolarization
I49.3	Ventricular premature depolarization
I49.40	Unspecified premature depolarization
I49.49	Other premature depolarization
I49.5	Sick sinus syndrome
I49.8	Other specified cardiac arrhythmias
I49.9	Cardiac arrhythmia, unspecified

CCI Edits

Refer to Appendix A for CCI edits.

Pub 100

00410: Pub 100-04, 12, 140.5, Pub 100-04, 12, 50, Pub 100-04, 12, 90.4.5

Base Units

Global: XXX

Code	Base Units
00410	4

Modifiers (PAR)

Code	Mod 50	Mod 51	Mod 62	Mod 80
00410	9	9	9	9

CPT © 2018 American Medical Association. All Rights Reserved.

00450

00450 Anesthesia for procedures on clavicle and scapula; not otherwise specified

ICD-10-CM Diagnostic Codes

⇄ M71.311 Other bursal cyst, right shoulder
⇄ M71.312 Other bursal cyst, left shoulder
⇄ M85.411 Solitary bone cyst, right shoulder
⇄ M85.412 Solitary bone cyst, left shoulder
⇄ M85.511 Aneurysmal bone cyst, right shoulder
⇄ M85.512 Aneurysmal bone cyst, left shoulder
⇄ M85.611 Other cyst of bone, right shoulder
⇄ M85.612 Other cyst of bone, left shoulder
❼⇄ S42.001 Fracture of unspecified part of right clavicle
❼⇄ S42.002 Fracture of unspecified part of left clavicle
❼⇄ S42.011 Anterior displaced fracture of sternal end of right clavicle
❼⇄ S42.012 Anterior displaced fracture of sternal end of left clavicle
❼⇄ S42.014 Posterior displaced fracture of sternal end of right clavicle
❼⇄ S42.015 Posterior displaced fracture of sternal end of left clavicle
❼⇄ S42.017 Nondisplaced fracture of sternal end of right clavicle
❼⇄ S42.018 Nondisplaced fracture of sternal end of left clavicle
❼⇄ S42.021 Displaced fracture of shaft of right clavicle
❼⇄ S42.022 Displaced fracture of shaft of left clavicle
❼⇄ S42.024 Nondisplaced fracture of shaft of right clavicle
❼⇄ S42.025 Nondisplaced fracture of shaft of left clavicle
❼⇄ S42.031 Displaced fracture of lateral end of right clavicle
❼⇄ S42.032 Displaced fracture of lateral end of left clavicle
❼⇄ S42.034 Nondisplaced fracture of lateral end of right clavicle
❼⇄ S42.035 Nondisplaced fracture of lateral end of left clavicle
❼⇄ S42.101 Fracture of unspecified part of scapula, right shoulder
❼⇄ S42.102 Fracture of unspecified part of scapula, left shoulder
❼⇄ S42.111 Displaced fracture of body of scapula, right shoulder
❼⇄ S42.112 Displaced fracture of body of scapula, left shoulder
❼⇄ S42.114 Nondisplaced fracture of body of scapula, right shoulder
❼⇄ S42.115 Nondisplaced fracture of body of scapula, left shoulder
❼⇄ S42.121 Displaced fracture of acromial process, right shoulder
❼⇄ S42.122 Displaced fracture of acromial process, left shoulder
❼⇄ S42.124 Nondisplaced fracture of acromial process, right shoulder
❼⇄ S42.125 Nondisplaced fracture of acromial process, left shoulder
❼⇄ S42.131 Displaced fracture of coracoid process, right shoulder
❼⇄ S42.132 Displaced fracture of coracoid process, left shoulder
❼⇄ S42.134 Nondisplaced fracture of coracoid process, right shoulder
❼⇄ S42.135 Nondisplaced fracture of coracoid process, left shoulder
❼⇄ S42.141 Displaced fracture of glenoid cavity of scapula, right shoulder
❼⇄ S42.142 Displaced fracture of glenoid cavity of scapula, left shoulder
❼⇄ S42.144 Nondisplaced fracture of glenoid cavity of scapula, right shoulder
❼⇄ S42.145 Nondisplaced fracture of glenoid cavity of scapula, left shoulder
❼⇄ S42.151 Displaced fracture of neck of scapula, right shoulder
❼⇄ S42.152 Displaced fracture of neck of scapula, left shoulder
❼⇄ S42.154 Nondisplaced fracture of neck of scapula, right shoulder
❼⇄ S42.155 Nondisplaced fracture of neck of scapula, left shoulder
❼⇄ S42.191 Fracture of other part of scapula, right shoulder
❼⇄ S42.192 Fracture of other part of scapula, left shoulder
❼⇄ S43.101 Unspecified dislocation of right acromioclavicular joint
❼⇄ S43.102 Unspecified dislocation of left acromioclavicular joint
❼⇄ S43.111 Subluxation of right acromioclavicular joint
❼⇄ S43.112 Subluxation of left acromioclavicular joint
❼⇄ S43.121 Dislocation of right acromioclavicular joint, 100%-200% displacement
❼⇄ S43.122 Dislocation of left acromioclavicular joint, 100%-200% displacement
❼⇄ S43.131 Dislocation of right acromioclavicular joint, greater than 200% displacement
❼⇄ S43.132 Dislocation of left acromioclavicular joint, greater than 200% displacement
❼⇄ S43.141 Inferior dislocation of right acromioclavicular joint
❼⇄ S43.142 Inferior dislocation of left acromioclavicular joint
❼⇄ S43.151 Posterior dislocation of right acromioclavicular joint
❼⇄ S43.152 Posterior dislocation of left acromioclavicular joint
❼⇄ S43.201 Unspecified subluxation of right sternoclavicular joint
❼⇄ S43.202 Unspecified subluxation of left sternoclavicular joint
❼⇄ S43.204 Unspecified dislocation of right sternoclavicular joint
❼⇄ S43.205 Unspecified dislocation of left sternoclavicular joint
❼⇄ S43.211 Anterior subluxation of right sternoclavicular joint
❼⇄ S43.212 Anterior subluxation of left sternoclavicular joint
❼⇄ S43.214 Anterior dislocation of right sternoclavicular joint
❼⇄ S43.215 Anterior dislocation of left sternoclavicular joint
❼⇄ S43.221 Posterior subluxation of right sternoclavicular joint
❼⇄ S43.222 Posterior subluxation of left sternoclavicular joint
❼⇄ S43.224 Posterior dislocation of right sternoclavicular joint
❼⇄ S43.225 Posterior dislocation of left sternoclavicular joint
❼⇄ S43.311 Subluxation of right scapula
❼⇄ S43.312 Subluxation of left scapula
❼⇄ S43.314 Dislocation of right scapula
❼⇄ S43.315 Dislocation of left scapula

ICD-10-CM Coding Notes

For codes requiring a 7th character extension, refer to your ICD-10-CM book. Review the character descriptions and coding guidelines for proper selection. For some procedures, only certain characters will apply.

CCI Edits

Refer to Appendix A for CCI edits.

Pub 100

00450: Pub 100-04, 12, 140.5, Pub 100-04, 12, 50, Pub 100-04, 12, 90.4.5

Base Units

Global: XXX

Code	Base Units
00450	5

Modifiers (PAR)

Code	Mod 50	Mod 51	Mod 62	Mod 80
00450	9	9	9	9

CPT © 2018 American Medical Association. All Rights Reserved.

00454

00454 Anesthesia for procedures on clavicle and scapula; biopsy of clavicle

ICD-10-CM Diagnostic Codes

	C41.3	Malignant neoplasm of ribs, sternum and clavicle
	C79.51	Secondary malignant neoplasm of bone
	D16.7	Benign neoplasm of ribs, sternum and clavicle
	D48.0	Neoplasm of uncertain behavior of bone and articular cartilage
	D49.2	Neoplasm of unspecified behavior of bone, soft tissue, and skin
⇄	M25.511	Pain in right shoulder
⇄	M25.512	Pain in left shoulder
⇄	M85.411	Solitary bone cyst, right shoulder
⇄	M85.412	Solitary bone cyst, left shoulder
⇄	M85.511	Aneurysmal bone cyst, right shoulder
⇄	M85.611	Other cyst of bone, right shoulder
⇄	M85.612	Other cyst of bone, left shoulder
⇄	M85.811	Other specified disorders of bone density and structure, right shoulder
⇄	M85.812	Other specified disorders of bone density and structure, left shoulder
⇄	M86.011	Acute hematogenous osteomyelitis, right shoulder
⇄	M86.012	Acute hematogenous osteomyelitis, left shoulder
⇄	M86.111	Other acute osteomyelitis, right shoulder
⇄	M86.112	Other acute osteomyelitis, left shoulder
⇄	M86.211	Subacute osteomyelitis, right shoulder
⇄	M86.212	Subacute osteomyelitis, left shoulder
⇄	M86.311	Chronic multifocal osteomyelitis, right shoulder
⇄	M86.312	Chronic multifocal osteomyelitis, left shoulder
⇄	M86.411	Chronic osteomyelitis with draining sinus, right shoulder
⇄	M86.412	Chronic osteomyelitis with draining sinus, left shoulder
⇄	M86.511	Other chronic hematogenous osteomyelitis, right shoulder
⇄	M86.512	Other chronic hematogenous osteomyelitis, left shoulder
⇄	M86.611	Other chronic osteomyelitis, right shoulder
⇄	M86.612	Other chronic osteomyelitis, left shoulder
	M86.8X1	Other osteomyelitis, shoulder
⇄	M87.011	Idiopathic aseptic necrosis of right shoulder
⇄	M87.012	Idiopathic aseptic necrosis of left shoulder
⇄	M88.811	Osteitis deformans of right shoulder
⇄	M88.812	Osteitis deformans of left shoulder
⇄	M89.211	Other disorders of bone development and growth, right shoulder
⇄	M89.212	Other disorders of bone development and growth, left shoulder
⇄	M89.311	Hypertrophy of bone, right shoulder
⇄	M89.312	Hypertrophy of bone, left shoulder
⇄	M89.411	Other hypertrophic osteoarthropathy, right shoulder
⇄	M89.412	Other hypertrophic osteoarthropathy, left shoulder
⇄	M89.511	Osteolysis, right shoulder
⇄	M89.512	Osteolysis, left shoulder
⇄	M89.711	Major osseous defect, right shoulder region
⇄	M89.712	Major osseous defect, left shoulder region
	M89.8X1	Other specified disorders of bone, shoulder

CCI Edits

Refer to Appendix A for CCI edits.

Pub 100

00454: Pub 100-04, 12, 140.5, Pub 100-04, 12, 50, Pub 100-04, 12, 90.4.5

Base Units

Global: XXX

Code	Base Units
00454	3

Modifiers (PAR)

Code	Mod 50	Mod 51	Mod 62	Mod 80
00454	9	9	9	9

CPT © 2018 American Medical Association. All Rights Reserved.

00470

00470 Anesthesia for partial rib resection; not otherwise specified

ICD-10-CM Diagnostic Codes

	C41.3	Malignant neoplasm of ribs, sternum and clavicle
	C79.51	Secondary malignant neoplasm of bone
	D16.7	Benign neoplasm of ribs, sternum and clavicle
	D48.0	Neoplasm of uncertain behavior of bone and articular cartilage
	D49.2	Neoplasm of unspecified behavior of bone, soft tissue, and skin
	J86.0	Pyothorax with fistula
	J86.9	Pyothorax without fistula
	M86.38	Chronic multifocal osteomyelitis, other site
	M86.48	Chronic osteomyelitis with draining sinus, other site
	M86.58	Other chronic hematogenous osteomyelitis, other site
	M86.68	Other chronic osteomyelitis, other site
	M86.8X8	Other osteomyelitis, other site
	Q76.5	Cervical rib
	Q76.6	Other congenital malformations of ribs
➐⇄	S22.31	Fracture of one rib, right side
➐⇄	S22.32	Fracture of one rib, left side
➐⇄	S22.41	Multiple fractures of ribs, right side
➐⇄	S22.42	Multiple fractures of ribs, left side
➐⇄	S22.43	Multiple fractures of ribs, bilateral
➐	S22.5	Flail chest
➐	S28.0	Crushed chest
➐⇄	S32.311	Displaced avulsion fracture of right ilium
➐⇄	S32.312	Displaced avulsion fracture of left ilium
➐	T81.49	Infection following a procedure, other surgical site

ICD-10-CM Coding Notes

For codes requiring a 7th character extension, refer to your ICD-10-CM book. Review the character descriptions and coding guidelines for proper selection. For some procedures, only certain characters will apply.

CCI Edits

Refer to Appendix A for CCI edits.

Pub 100

00470: Pub 100-04, 12, 140.5, Pub 100-04, 12, 50, Pub 100-04, 12, 90.4.5

Base Units

Global: XXX

Code	Base Units
00470	6

Modifiers (PAR)

Code	Mod 50	Mod 51	Mod 62	Mod 80
00470	9	9	9	9

CPT © 2018 American Medical Association. All Rights Reserved.

00472

00472 Anesthesia for partial rib resection; thoracoplasty (any type)

ICD-10-CM Diagnostic Codes

	A15.0	Tuberculosis of lung
	A15.4	Tuberculosis of intrathoracic lymph nodes
	A15.5	Tuberculosis of larynx, trachea and bronchus
	A15.6	Tuberculous pleurisy
	A15.7	Primary respiratory tuberculosis
	A15.8	Other respiratory tuberculosis
	A15.9	Respiratory tuberculosis unspecified
	B59	Pneumocystosis
⇄	C34.01	Malignant neoplasm of right main bronchus
⇄	C34.02	Malignant neoplasm of left main bronchus
⇄	C34.11	Malignant neoplasm of upper lobe, right bronchus or lung
⇄	C34.12	Malignant neoplasm of upper lobe, left bronchus or lung
	C34.2	Malignant neoplasm of middle lobe, bronchus or lung
⇄	C34.31	Malignant neoplasm of lower lobe, right bronchus or lung
⇄	C34.32	Malignant neoplasm of lower lobe, left bronchus or lung
⇄	C34.81	Malignant neoplasm of overlapping sites of right bronchus and lung
⇄	C34.82	Malignant neoplasm of overlapping sites of left bronchus and lung
⇄	C34.91	Malignant neoplasm of unspecified part of right bronchus or lung
⇄	C34.92	Malignant neoplasm of unspecified part of left bronchus or lung
	C41.3	Malignant neoplasm of ribs, sternum and clavicle
⇄	C78.0	Secondary malignant neoplasm of lung
	J65	Pneumoconiosis associated with tuberculosis
	J82	Pulmonary eosinophilia, not elsewhere classified
	J84.81	Lymphangioleiomyomatosis
	J85.1	Abscess of lung with pneumonia
	J85.2	Abscess of lung without pneumonia
	J86.0	Pyothorax with fistula
	J86.9	Pyothorax without fistula
	J92.9	Pleural plaque without asbestos
	J93.12	Secondary spontaneous pneumothorax
	J93.81	Chronic pneumothorax
	J93.82	Other air leak
	J93.83	Other pneumothorax
	J93.9	Pneumothorax, unspecified
	K22.3	Perforation of esophagus
	Q87.4	Marfan's syndrome
❼⇄	S21.301	Unspecified open wound of right front wall of thorax with penetration into thoracic cavity
❼⇄	S21.302	Unspecified open wound of left front wall of thorax with penetration into thoracic cavity
❼⇄	S21.401	Unspecified open wound of right back wall of thorax with penetration into thoracic cavity
❼⇄	S21.402	Unspecified open wound of left back wall of thorax with penetration into thoracic cavity
❼	S22.20	Unspecified fracture of sternum
❼	S22.21	Fracture of manubrium
❼	S22.22	Fracture of body of sternum
❼	S22.23	Sternal manubrial dissociation
❼	S22.24	Fracture of xiphoid process
❼⇄	S22.31	Fracture of one rib, right side
❼⇄	S22.32	Fracture of one rib, left side
❼⇄	S22.39	Fracture of one rib, unspecified side
❼⇄	S22.41	Multiple fractures of ribs, right side
❼⇄	S22.42	Multiple fractures of ribs, left side
❼⇄	S22.43	Multiple fractures of ribs, bilateral
❼⇄	S22.49	Multiple fractures of ribs, unspecified side
❼	S22.5	Flail chest
❼	S27.0	Traumatic pneumothorax
❼	S27.1	Traumatic hemothorax
	S27.3	Other and unspecified injuries of lung
❼	S28.0	Crushed chest
❼	T81.49	Infection following a procedure, other surgical site
	Z90.2	Acquired absence of lung [part of]

ICD-10-CM Coding Notes

For codes requiring a 7th character extension, refer to your ICD-10-CM book. Review the character descriptions and coding guidelines for proper selection. For some procedures, only certain characters will apply.

CCI Edits

Refer to Appendix A for CCI edits.

Pub 100

00472: Pub 100-04, 12, 140.5, Pub 100-04, 12, 50, Pub 100-04, 12, 90.4.5

Base Units

Global: XXX

Code	Base Units
00472	10

Modifiers (PAR)

Code	Mod 50	Mod 51	Mod 62	Mod 80
00472	9	9	9	9

CPT © 2018 American Medical Association. All Rights Reserved.

00474

00474 Anesthesia for partial rib resection; radical procedures (eg, pectus excavatum)

AMA *CPT Assistant*

00474: Nov 07: 8, Jul 12: 13

ICD-10-CM Diagnostic Codes

	C41.3	Malignant neoplasm of ribs, sternum and clavicle
	C49.3	Malignant neoplasm of connective and soft tissue of thorax
	C76.1	Malignant neoplasm of thorax
	C79.51	Secondary malignant neoplasm of bone
	C79.89	Secondary malignant neoplasm of other specified sites
	J86.0	Pyothorax with fistula
	J86.9	Pyothorax without fistula
	Q67.6	Pectus excavatum
	Q67.7	Pectus carinatum
	Q67.8	Other congenital deformities of chest
	Q87.4	Marfan's syndrome
⑦	S28.0	Crushed chest
⑦	T81.43	Infection following a procedure, organ and space surgical site
⑦	T81.49	Infection following a procedure, other surgical site

ICD-10-CM Coding Notes

For codes requiring a 7th character extension, refer to your ICD-10-CM book. Review the character descriptions and coding guidelines for proper selection. For some procedures, only certain characters will apply.

CCI Edits

Refer to Appendix A for CCI edits.

Pub 100

00474: Pub 100-04, 12, 140.5, Pub 100-04, 12, 50, Pub 100-04, 12, 90.4.5

Base Units

Global: XXX

Code	Base Units
00474	13

Modifiers (PAR)

Code	Mod 50	Mod 51	Mod 62	Mod 80
00474	9	9	9	9

CPT © 2018 American Medical Association. All Rights Reserved.

00500

00500 Anesthesia for all procedures on esophagus

AMA *CPT Assistant* ☐

00500: Mar 06: 15, Nov 07: 8, Oct 11: 3, Jul 12: 13

ICD-10-CM Diagnostic Codes

	C15.3	Malignant neoplasm of upper third of esophagus
	C15.4	Malignant neoplasm of middle third of esophagus
	C15.5	Malignant neoplasm of lower third of esophagus
	C15.8	Malignant neoplasm of overlapping sites of esophagus
	D00.1	Carcinoma in situ of esophagus
	D13.0	Benign neoplasm of esophagus
	K20.8	Other esophagitis
	K20.9	Esophagitis, unspecified
	K21.0	Gastro-esophageal reflux disease with esophagitis
	K21.9	Gastro-esophageal reflux disease without esophagitis
	K22.0	Achalasia of cardia
	K22.10	Ulcer of esophagus without bleeding
	K22.11	Ulcer of esophagus with bleeding
	K22.2	Esophageal obstruction
	K22.3	Perforation of esophagus
	K22.4	Dyskinesia of esophagus
	K22.5	Diverticulum of esophagus, acquired
	K22.6	Gastro-esophageal laceration-hemorrhage syndrome
	K22.710	Barrett's esophagus with low grade dysplasia
	K22.711	Barrett's esophagus with high grade dysplasia
	K22.719	Barrett's esophagus with dysplasia, unspecified
	K22.8	Other specified diseases of esophagus
	K92.0	Hematemesis
	K94.31	Esophagostomy hemorrhage
	K94.32	Esophagostomy infection
	K94.33	Esophagostomy malfunction
	K94.39	Other complications of esophagostomy
	P78.83	Newborn esophageal reflux
	P92.01	Bilious vomiting of newborn
	P92.09	Other vomiting of newborn
	Q39.0	Atresia of esophagus without fistula
	Q39.1	Atresia of esophagus with tracheo-esophageal fistula
	Q39.2	Congenital tracheo-esophageal fistula without atresia
	Q39.3	Congenital stenosis and stricture of esophagus
	Q39.4	Esophageal web
➐	S27.813	Laceration of esophagus (thoracic part)
➐	S27.818	Other injury of esophagus (thoracic part)
➐	T18.120	Food in esophagus causing compression of trachea
➐	T18.128	Food in esophagus causing other injury
➐	T18.190	Other foreign object in esophagus causing compression of trachea
➐	T18.198	Other foreign object in esophagus causing other injury

ICD-10-CM Coding Notes

For codes requiring a 7th character extension, refer to your ICD-10-CM book. Review the character descriptions and coding guidelines for proper selection. For some procedures, only certain characters will apply.

CCI Edits

Refer to Appendix A for CCI edits.

Pub 100

00500: Pub 100-04, 12, 140.5, Pub 100-04, 12, 50, Pub 100-04, 12, 90.4.5

Base Units

Global: XXX

Code	Base Units
00500	15

Modifiers (PAR)

Code	Mod 50	Mod 51	Mod 62	Mod 80
00500	9	9	9	9

CPT © 2018 American Medical Association. All Rights Reserved.

00520

00520 Anesthesia for closed chest procedures; (including bronchoscopy) not otherwise specified

AMA *CPT Assistant*

00520: Nov 99: 7

ICD-10-CM Diagnostic Codes

⇄	C34.01	Malignant neoplasm of right main bronchus
⇄	C34.02	Malignant neoplasm of left main bronchus
⇄	C34.11	Malignant neoplasm of upper lobe, right bronchus or lung
⇄	C34.12	Malignant neoplasm of upper lobe, left bronchus or lung
	C34.2	Malignant neoplasm of middle lobe, bronchus or lung
⇄	C34.31	Malignant neoplasm of lower lobe, right bronchus or lung
⇄	C34.32	Malignant neoplasm of lower lobe, left bronchus or lung
⇄	C34.81	Malignant neoplasm of overlapping sites of right bronchus and lung
⇄	C34.82	Malignant neoplasm of overlapping sites of left bronchus and lung
⇄	C34.91	Malignant neoplasm of unspecified part of right bronchus or lung
⇄	C34.92	Malignant neoplasm of unspecified part of left bronchus or lung
⇄	D02.21	Carcinoma in situ of right bronchus and lung
⇄	D02.22	Carcinoma in situ of left bronchus and lung
⇄	D14.31	Benign neoplasm of right bronchus and lung
⇄	D14.32	Benign neoplasm of left bronchus and lung
	D38.1	Neoplasm of uncertain behavior of trachea, bronchus and lung
	D49.1	Neoplasm of unspecified behavior of respiratory system
	J15.9	Unspecified bacterial pneumonia
	J18.0	Bronchopneumonia, unspecified organism
	J18.1	Lobar pneumonia, unspecified organism
	J18.2	Hypostatic pneumonia, unspecified organism
	J18.8	Other pneumonia, unspecified organism
	J18.9	Pneumonia, unspecified organism
	J80	Acute respiratory distress syndrome
	J96.01	Acute respiratory failure with hypoxia
	J96.02	Acute respiratory failure with hypercapnia
	J96.91	Respiratory failure, unspecified with hypoxia
	J96.92	Respiratory failure, unspecified with hypercapnia
	R04.2	Hemoptysis
	R05	Cough
	R06.00	Dyspnea, unspecified
	R06.01	Orthopnea
	R06.02	Shortness of breath
	R06.09	Other forms of dyspnea
	R06.1	Stridor
	R07.1	Chest pain on breathing
	R84.6	Abnormal cytological findings in specimens from respiratory organs and thorax
	R84.7	Abnormal histological findings in specimens from respiratory organs and thorax
	R91.1	Solitary pulmonary nodule
	R91.8	Other nonspecific abnormal finding of lung field
	R94.2	Abnormal results of pulmonary function studies

CCI Edits

Refer to Appendix A for CCI edits.

Pub 100

00520: Pub 100-04, 12, 140.5, Pub 100-04, 12, 50, Pub 100-04, 12, 90.4.5

Base Units

Global: XXX

Code	Base Units
00520	6

Modifiers (PAR)

Code	Mod 50	Mod 51	Mod 62	Mod 80
00520	9	9	9	9

CPT © 2018 American Medical Association. All Rights Reserved.

00522

00522 Anesthesia for closed chest procedures; needle biopsy of pleura

ICD-10-CM Diagnostic Codes

⇄	C34.01	Malignant neoplasm of right main bronchus
⇄	C34.02	Malignant neoplasm of left main bronchus
⇄	C34.11	Malignant neoplasm of upper lobe, right bronchus or lung
⇄	C34.12	Malignant neoplasm of upper lobe, left bronchus or lung
	C34.2	Malignant neoplasm of middle lobe, bronchus or lung
⇄	C34.31	Malignant neoplasm of lower lobe, right bronchus or lung
⇄	C34.32	Malignant neoplasm of lower lobe, left bronchus or lung
⇄	C34.81	Malignant neoplasm of overlapping sites of right bronchus and lung
⇄	C34.82	Malignant neoplasm of overlapping sites of left bronchus and lung
⇄	C34.91	Malignant neoplasm of unspecified part of right bronchus or lung
⇄	C34.92	Malignant neoplasm of unspecified part of left bronchus or lung
	C38.0	Malignant neoplasm of heart
	C38.2	Malignant neoplasm of posterior mediastinum
	C38.3	Malignant neoplasm of mediastinum, part unspecified
	C38.4	Malignant neoplasm of pleura
	C38.8	Malignant neoplasm of overlapping sites of heart, mediastinum and pleura
	C45.0	Mesothelioma of pleura
	C76.1	Malignant neoplasm of thorax
	C78.2	Secondary malignant neoplasm of pleura
	C7A.090	Malignant carcinoid tumor of the bronchus and lung
	D19.0	Benign neoplasm of mesothelial tissue of pleura
	D38.2	Neoplasm of uncertain behavior of pleura
	D49.1	Neoplasm of unspecified behavior of respiratory system
	J86.0	Pyothorax with fistula
	J86.9	Pyothorax without fistula
	J90	Pleural effusion, not elsewhere classified
	J91.0	Malignant pleural effusion
	J91.8	Pleural effusion in other conditions classified elsewhere
	J92.0	Pleural plaque with presence of asbestos
	J92.9	Pleural plaque without asbestos
	J93.0	Spontaneous tension pneumothorax
	J93.11	Primary spontaneous pneumothorax
	J93.12	Secondary spontaneous pneumothorax
	J93.81	Chronic pneumothorax
	J93.82	Other air leak
	J93.83	Other pneumothorax
	J94.0	Chylous effusion
	J94.1	Fibrothorax
	J94.2	Hemothorax
	J94.8	Other specified pleural conditions
	J94.9	Pleural condition, unspecified
	R22.2	Localized swelling, mass and lump, trunk
	Z85.110	Personal history of malignant carcinoid tumor of bronchus and lung
	Z85.118	Personal history of other malignant neoplasm of bronchus and lung
	Z85.3	Personal history of malignant neoplasm of breast

CCI Edits

Refer to Appendix A for CCI edits.

Pub 100

00522: Pub 100-04, 12, 140.5, Pub 100-04, 12, 50, Pub 100-04, 12, 90.4.5

Base Units

Global: XXX

Code	Base Units
00522	4

Modifiers (PAR)

Code	Mod 50	Mod 51	Mod 62	Mod 80
00522	9	9	9	9

CPT © 2018 American Medical Association. All Rights Reserved.

00524

00524 Anesthesia for closed chest procedures; pneumocentesis

ICD-10-CM Diagnostic Codes

⇄	C34.01	Malignant neoplasm of right main bronchus
⇄	C34.02	Malignant neoplasm of left main bronchus
⇄	C34.11	Malignant neoplasm of upper lobe, right bronchus or lung
⇄	C34.12	Malignant neoplasm of upper lobe, left bronchus or lung
	C34.2	Malignant neoplasm of middle lobe, bronchus or lung
⇄	C34.31	Malignant neoplasm of lower lobe, right bronchus or lung
⇄	C34.32	Malignant neoplasm of lower lobe, left bronchus or lung
⇄	C34.81	Malignant neoplasm of overlapping sites of right bronchus and lung
⇄	C34.82	Malignant neoplasm of overlapping sites of left bronchus and lung
⇄	C34.91	Malignant neoplasm of unspecified part of right bronchus or lung
⇄	C34.92	Malignant neoplasm of unspecified part of left bronchus or lung
⇄	C78.01	Secondary malignant neoplasm of right lung
⇄	C78.02	Secondary malignant neoplasm of left lung
	C7A.090	Malignant carcinoid tumor of the bronchus and lung
	J18.0	Bronchopneumonia, unspecified organism
	J18.1	Lobar pneumonia, unspecified organism
	J18.2	Hypostatic pneumonia, unspecified organism
	J18.8	Other pneumonia, unspecified organism
	J18.9	Pneumonia, unspecified organism
	J81.0	Acute pulmonary edema
	J81.1	Chronic pulmonary edema
	R22.2	Localized swelling, mass and lump, trunk

CCI Edits

Refer to Appendix A for CCI edits.

Pub 100

00524: Pub 100-04, 12, 140.5, Pub 100-04, 12, 50, Pub 100-04, 12, 90.4.5

Base Units

Global: XXX

Code	Base Units
00524	4

Modifiers (PAR)

Code	Mod 50	Mod 51	Mod 62	Mod 80
00524	9	9	9	9

CPT © 2018 American Medical Association. All Rights Reserved.

00528

00528 Anesthesia for closed chest procedures; mediastinoscopy and diagnostic thoracoscopy not utilizing 1 lung ventilation

(For tracheobronchial reconstruction, use 00539)

AMA *CPT Assistant* ▯

00528: Nov 99: 7

ICD-10-CM Diagnostic Codes

C37	Malignant neoplasm of thymus
C38.0	Malignant neoplasm of heart
C38.1	Malignant neoplasm of anterior mediastinum
C38.2	Malignant neoplasm of posterior mediastinum
C38.4	Malignant neoplasm of pleura
C38.8	Malignant neoplasm of overlapping sites of heart, mediastinum and pleura
C76.1	Malignant neoplasm of thorax
C77.1	Secondary and unspecified malignant neoplasm of intrathoracic lymph nodes
C78.1	Secondary malignant neoplasm of mediastinum
C79.89	Secondary malignant neoplasm of other specified sites
C7A.091	Malignant carcinoid tumor of the thymus
C7B.1	Secondary Merkel cell carcinoma
D09.3	Carcinoma in situ of thyroid and other endocrine glands
D15.0	Benign neoplasm of thymus
D15.2	Benign neoplasm of mediastinum
D38.3	Neoplasm of uncertain behavior of mediastinum
D38.4	Neoplasm of uncertain behavior of thymus
D49.89	Neoplasm of unspecified behavior of other specified sites
E32.0	Persistent hyperplasia of thymus
E32.8	Other diseases of thymus
E32.9	Disease of thymus, unspecified
I88.1	Chronic lymphadenitis, except mesenteric
J85.3	Abscess of mediastinum
J98.51	Mediastinitis
J98.59	Other diseases of mediastinum, not elsewhere classified
L04.1	Acute lymphadenitis of trunk
R22.2	Localized swelling, mass and lump, trunk
R59.0	Localized enlarged lymph nodes

CCI Edits

Refer to Appendix A for CCI edits.

Pub 100

00528: Pub 100-04, 12, 140.5, Pub 100-04, 12, 50, Pub 100-04, 12, 90.4.5

Base Units

Global: XXX

Code	Base Units
00528	8

Modifiers (PAR)

Code	Mod 50	Mod 51	Mod 62	Mod 80
00528	9	9	9	9

CPT © 2018 American Medical Association. All Rights Reserved.

00529

00529 Anesthesia for closed chest procedures; mediastinoscopy and diagnostic thoracoscopy utilizing 1 lung ventilation

AMA *CPT Assistant* □

00529: Jun 04: 3

ICD-10-CM Diagnostic Codes

C37	Malignant neoplasm of thymus
C38.1	Malignant neoplasm of anterior mediastinum
C38.2	Malignant neoplasm of posterior mediastinum
C38.4	Malignant neoplasm of pleura
C38.8	Malignant neoplasm of overlapping sites of heart, mediastinum and pleura
C76.1	Malignant neoplasm of thorax
C77.1	Secondary and unspecified malignant neoplasm of intrathoracic lymph nodes
C78.1	Secondary malignant neoplasm of mediastinum
C79.89	Secondary malignant neoplasm of other specified sites
C7A.091	Malignant carcinoid tumor of the thymus
C7B.1	Secondary Merkel cell carcinoma
D09.3	Carcinoma in situ of thyroid and other endocrine glands
D15.0	Benign neoplasm of thymus
D15.2	Benign neoplasm of mediastinum
D38.3	Neoplasm of uncertain behavior of mediastinum
D38.4	Neoplasm of uncertain behavior of thymus
D49.89	Neoplasm of unspecified behavior of other specified sites
E32.0	Persistent hyperplasia of thymus
E32.8	Other diseases of thymus
E32.9	Disease of thymus, unspecified
I88.1	Chronic lymphadenitis, except mesenteric
J85.3	Abscess of mediastinum
J98.51	Mediastinitis
J98.59	Other diseases of mediastinum, not elsewhere classified
L04.1	Acute lymphadenitis of trunk
R22.2	Localized swelling, mass and lump, trunk
R59.0	Localized enlarged lymph nodes

CCI Edits

Refer to Appendix A for CCI edits.

Pub 100

00529: Pub 100-04, 12, 140.5, Pub 100-04, 12, 50, Pub 100-04, 12, 90.4.5

Base Units

Global: XXX

Code	Base Units
00529	11

Modifiers (PAR)

Code	Mod 50	Mod 51	Mod 62	Mod 80
00529	9	9	9	9

CPT © 2018 American Medical Association. All Rights Reserved.

00530

00530 Anesthesia for permanent transvenous pacemaker insertion

ICD-10-CM Diagnostic Codes

I44.0	Atrioventricular block, first degree
I44.1	Atrioventricular block, second degree
I44.2	Atrioventricular block, complete
I44.30	Unspecified atrioventricular block
I44.39	Other atrioventricular block
I44.4	Left anterior fascicular block
I44.5	Left posterior fascicular block
I44.60	Unspecified fascicular block
I44.69	Other fascicular block
I44.7	Left bundle-branch block, unspecified
I45.0	Right fascicular block
I45.10	Unspecified right bundle-branch block
I45.19	Other right bundle-branch block
I45.2	Bifascicular block
I45.3	Trifascicular block
I45.4	Nonspecific intraventricular block
I45.5	Other specified heart block
I45.6	Pre-excitation syndrome
I45.81	Long QT syndrome
I45.89	Other specified conduction disorders
I47.0	Re-entry ventricular arrhythmia
I47.1	Supraventricular tachycardia
I47.2	Ventricular tachycardia
I47.9	Paroxysmal tachycardia, unspecified
I48.0	Paroxysmal atrial fibrillation
I48.1	Persistent atrial fibrillation
I48.2	Chronic atrial fibrillation
I48.3	Typical atrial flutter
I48.4	Atypical atrial flutter
I48.91	Unspecified atrial fibrillation
I48.92	Unspecified atrial flutter
I49.02	Ventricular flutter
I49.1	Atrial premature depolarization
I49.2	Junctional premature depolarization
I49.3	Ventricular premature depolarization
I49.40	Unspecified premature depolarization
I49.49	Other premature depolarization
I49.5	Sick sinus syndrome
I49.8	Other specified cardiac arrhythmias
I49.9	Cardiac arrhythmia, unspecified
R00.1	Bradycardia, unspecified
R55	Syncope and collapse

CCI Edits

Refer to Appendix A for CCI edits.

Pub 100

00530: Pub 100-04, 12, 140.5, Pub 100-04, 12, 50, Pub 100-04, 12, 90.4.5

Base Units

Global: XXX

Code	Base Units
00530	4

Modifiers (PAR)

Code	Mod 50	Mod 51	Mod 62	Mod 80
00530	9	9	9	9

CPT © 2018 American Medical Association. All Rights Reserved.

00532

00532 Anesthesia for access to central venous circulation

ICD-10-CM Diagnostic Codes

There are too many ICD-10-CM codes to list. Refer to ICD-10-CM code book for associated diagnostic codes.

CCI Edits

Refer to Appendix A for CCI edits.

Pub 100

00532: Pub 100-04, 12, 140.5, Pub 100-04, 12, 50, Pub 100-04, 12, 90.4.5

Base Units

Global: XXX

Code	Base Units
00532	4

Modifiers (PAR)

Code	Mod 50	Mod 51	Mod 62	Mod 80
00532	9	9	9	9

CPT © 2018 American Medical Association. All Rights Reserved.

00534

00534 Anesthesia for transvenous insertion or replacement of pacing cardioverter-defibrillator

(For transthoracic approach, use 00560)

ICD-10-CM Diagnostic Codes

	I44.0	Atrioventricular block, first degree
	I44.1	Atrioventricular block, second degree
	I44.2	Atrioventricular block, complete
	I44.30	Unspecified atrioventricular block
	I44.39	Other atrioventricular block
	I44.4	Left anterior fascicular block
	I44.5	Left posterior fascicular block
	I44.60	Unspecified fascicular block
	I44.69	Other fascicular block
	I44.7	Left bundle-branch block, unspecified
	I45.0	Right fascicular block
	I45.10	Unspecified right bundle-branch block
	I45.19	Other right bundle-branch block
	I45.2	Bifascicular block
	I45.3	Trifascicular block
	I45.4	Nonspecific intraventricular block
	I45.5	Other specified heart block
	I45.6	Pre-excitation syndrome
	I45.81	Long QT syndrome
	I45.89	Other specified conduction disorders
	I45.9	Conduction disorder, unspecified
	I47.0	Re-entry ventricular arrhythmia
	I47.1	Supraventricular tachycardia
	I47.2	Ventricular tachycardia
	I47.9	Paroxysmal tachycardia, unspecified
	I48.0	Paroxysmal atrial fibrillation
	I48.1	Persistent atrial fibrillation
	I48.2	Chronic atrial fibrillation
	I48.3	Typical atrial flutter
	I48.4	Atypical atrial flutter
	I48.9	Unspecified atrial fibrillation and atrial flutter
	I49.0	Ventricular fibrillation and flutter
	I49.1	Atrial premature depolarization
	I49.2	Junctional premature depolarization
	I49.3	Ventricular premature depolarization
	I49.40	Unspecified premature depolarization
	I49.49	Other premature depolarization
	I49.5	Sick sinus syndrome
	I49.8	Other specified cardiac arrhythmias
	I49.9	Cardiac arrhythmia, unspecified
❼	T82.110	Breakdown (mechanical) of cardiac electrode
❼	T82.111	Breakdown (mechanical) of cardiac pulse generator (battery)
❼	T82.118	Breakdown (mechanical) of other cardiac electronic device
❼	T82.120	Displacement of cardiac electrode
❼	T82.121	Displacement of cardiac pulse generator (battery)
❼	T82.128	Displacement of other cardiac electronic device
❼	T82.190	Other mechanical complication of cardiac electrode
❼	T82.191	Other mechanical complication of cardiac pulse generator (battery)
❼	T82.198	Other mechanical complication of other cardiac electronic device

ICD-10-CM Coding Notes

For codes requiring a 7th character extension, refer to your ICD-10-CM book. Review the character descriptions and coding guidelines for proper selection. For some procedures, only certain characters will apply.

CCI Edits

Refer to Appendix A for CCI edits.

Pub 100

00534: Pub 100-04, 12, 140.5, Pub 100-04, 12, 50, Pub 100-04, 12, 90.4.5

Base Units

Global: XXX

Code	Base Units
00534	7

Modifiers (PAR)

Code	Mod 50	Mod 51	Mod 62	Mod 80
00534	9	9	9	9

CPT © 2018 American Medical Association. All Rights Reserved.

00537

00537 Anesthesia for cardiac electrophysiologic procedures including radiofrequency ablation

ICD-10-CM Diagnostic Codes

I45.6	Pre-excitation syndrome
I45.89	Other specified conduction disorders
I45.9	Conduction disorder, unspecified
I47.0	Re-entry ventricular arrhythmia
I47.1	Supraventricular tachycardia
I47.2	Ventricular tachycardia
I48.0	Paroxysmal atrial fibrillation
I48.1	Persistent atrial fibrillation
I48.2	Chronic atrial fibrillation
I48.3	Typical atrial flutter
I48.4	Atypical atrial flutter
I48.91	Unspecified atrial fibrillation
I48.92	Unspecified atrial flutter
I49.01	Ventricular fibrillation
I49.02	Ventricular flutter
I49.1	Atrial premature depolarization
I49.2	Junctional premature depolarization
I49.3	Ventricular premature depolarization
I49.40	Unspecified premature depolarization
I49.49	Other premature depolarization
I49.8	Other specified cardiac arrhythmias
I49.9	Cardiac arrhythmia, unspecified

CCI Edits

Refer to Appendix A for CCI edits.

Pub 100

00537: Pub 100-04, 12, 140.5, Pub 100-04, 12, 50, Pub 100-04, 12, 90.4.5

Base Units

Global: XXX

Code	Base Units
00537	7

Modifiers (PAR)

Code	Mod 50	Mod 51	Mod 62	Mod 80
00537	9	9	9	9

CPT © 2018 American Medical Association. All Rights Reserved.

00539

00539 Anesthesia for tracheobronchial reconstruction

ICD-10-CM Diagnostic Codes

	C33	Malignant neoplasm of trachea
⇄	C34.01	Malignant neoplasm of right main bronchus
⇄	C34.02	Malignant neoplasm of left main bronchus
⇄	C34.11	Malignant neoplasm of upper lobe, right bronchus or lung
⇄	C34.12	Malignant neoplasm of upper lobe, left bronchus or lung
	C34.2	Malignant neoplasm of middle lobe, bronchus or lung
⇄	C34.31	Malignant neoplasm of lower lobe, right bronchus or lung
⇄	C34.32	Malignant neoplasm of lower lobe, left bronchus or lung
⇄	C34.81	Malignant neoplasm of overlapping sites of right bronchus and lung
⇄	C34.82	Malignant neoplasm of overlapping sites of left bronchus and lung
⇄	C34.91	Malignant neoplasm of unspecified part of right bronchus or lung
⇄	C34.92	Malignant neoplasm of unspecified part of left bronchus or lung
	C7A.090	Malignant carcinoid tumor of the bronchus and lung
	D02.1	Carcinoma in situ of trachea
⇄	D02.21	Carcinoma in situ of right bronchus and lung
⇄	D02.22	Carcinoma in situ of left bronchus and lung
	D14.2	Benign neoplasm of trachea
⇄	D14.31	Benign neoplasm of right bronchus and lung
⇄	D14.32	Benign neoplasm of left bronchus and lung
	D38.1	Neoplasm of uncertain behavior of trachea, bronchus and lung
	D49.1	Neoplasm of unspecified behavior of respiratory system
	J38.6	Stenosis of larynx
	J38.7	Other diseases of larynx
	J39.8	Other specified diseases of upper respiratory tract
	J95.02	Infection of tracheostomy stoma
	J95.03	Malfunction of tracheostomy stoma
	J95.04	Tracheo-esophageal fistula following tracheostomy
	J95.09	Other tracheostomy complication
	Q32.1	Other congenital malformations of trachea
	Q32.3	Congenital stenosis of bronchus
❼	S11.021	Laceration without foreign body of trachea
❼	S11.022	Laceration with foreign body of trachea
❼	S11.023	Puncture wound without foreign body of trachea
❼	S11.024	Puncture wound with foreign body of trachea
❼	S11.025	Open bite of trachea
❼	S11.029	Unspecified open wound of trachea
❼⇄	S21.309	Unspecified open wound of unspecified front wall of thorax with penetration into thoracic cavity
❼	S27.431	Laceration of bronchus, unilateral
❼	S27.432	Laceration of bronchus, bilateral
❼	S27.491	Other injury of bronchus, unilateral
❼	S27.492	Other injury of bronchus, bilateral
❼	S27.53	Laceration of thoracic trachea
❼	S27.59	Other injury of thoracic trachea
❼	T27.0	Burn of larynx and trachea
❼	T27.1	Burn involving larynx and trachea with lung
❼	T27.4	Corrosion of larynx and trachea
❼	T27.5	Corrosion involving larynx and trachea with lung
	Z93.0	Tracheostomy status

ICD-10-CM Coding Notes

For codes requiring a 7th character extension, refer to your ICD-10-CM book. Review the character descriptions and coding guidelines for proper selection. For some procedures, only certain characters will apply.

CCI Edits

Refer to Appendix A for CCI edits.

Pub 100

00539: Pub 100-04, 12, 140.5, Pub 100-04, 12, 50, Pub 100-04, 12, 90.4.5

Base Units

Global: XXX

Code	Base Units
00539	18

Modifiers (PAR)

Code	Mod 50	Mod 51	Mod 62	Mod 80
00539	9	9	9	9

CPT © 2018 American Medical Association. All Rights Reserved.

00540

00540 Anesthesia for thoracotomy procedures involving lungs, pleura, diaphragm, and mediastinum (including surgical thoracoscopy); not otherwise specified

ICD-10-CM Diagnostic Codes

⇄	C34.11	Malignant neoplasm of upper lobe, right bronchus or lung
⇄	C34.12	Malignant neoplasm of upper lobe, left bronchus or lung
	C34.2	Malignant neoplasm of middle lobe, bronchus or lung
⇄	C34.31	Malignant neoplasm of lower lobe, right bronchus or lung
⇄	C34.32	Malignant neoplasm of lower lobe, left bronchus or lung
⇄	C34.81	Malignant neoplasm of overlapping sites of right bronchus and lung
⇄	C34.82	Malignant neoplasm of overlapping sites of left bronchus and lung
⇄	C34.91	Malignant neoplasm of unspecified part of right bronchus or lung
⇄	C34.92	Malignant neoplasm of unspecified part of left bronchus or lung
	C38.1	Malignant neoplasm of anterior mediastinum
	C38.2	Malignant neoplasm of posterior mediastinum
	C38.3	Malignant neoplasm of mediastinum, part unspecified
	C38.4	Malignant neoplasm of pleura
	C38.8	Malignant neoplasm of overlapping sites of heart, mediastinum and pleura
	C7A.090	Malignant carcinoid tumor of the bronchus and lung
	J43.9	Emphysema, unspecified
	J85.1	Abscess of lung with pneumonia
	J85.2	Abscess of lung without pneumonia
	J85.3	Abscess of mediastinum
	J86.0	Pyothorax with fistula
	J86.9	Pyothorax without fistula
	J91.0	Malignant pleural effusion
	J91.8	Pleural effusion in other conditions classified elsewhere
	J93.0	Spontaneous tension pneumothorax
	J93.11	Primary spontaneous pneumothorax
	J93.12	Secondary spontaneous pneumothorax
	J93.81	Chronic pneumothorax
	J93.82	Other air leak
	J93.83	Other pneumothorax
	J94.1	Fibrothorax
	J94.2	Hemothorax
	J94.8	Other specified pleural conditions
	J98.51	Mediastinitis
	J98.59	Other diseases of mediastinum, not elsewhere classified
	J98.6	Disorders of diaphragm
	Q33.0	Congenital cystic lung
	Q33.8	Other congenital malformations of lung
	Q34.0	Anomaly of pleura
	Q34.1	Congenital cyst of mediastinum
	Q34.8	Other specified congenital malformations of respiratory system

CCI Edits

Refer to Appendix A for CCI edits.

Pub 100

00540: Pub 100-04, 12, 140.5, Pub 100-04, 12, 50, Pub 100-04, 12, 90.4.5

Base Units

Global: XXX

Code	Base Units
00540	12

Modifiers (PAR)

Code	Mod 50	Mod 51	Mod 62	Mod 80
00540	9	9	9	9

CPT © 2018 American Medical Association. All Rights Reserved.

00541

00541 Anesthesia for thoracotomy procedures involving lungs, pleura, diaphragm, and mediastinum (including surgical thoracoscopy); utilizing 1 lung ventilation

(For thoracic spine and cord anesthesia procedures via an anterior transthoracic approach, see 00625-00626)

ICD-10-CM Diagnostic Codes

⇄ C34.10 Malignant neoplasm of upper lobe, unspecified bronchus or lung
⇄ C34.11 Malignant neoplasm of upper lobe, right bronchus or lung
⇄ C34.12 Malignant neoplasm of upper lobe, left bronchus or lung
C34.2 Malignant neoplasm of middle lobe, bronchus or lung
⇄ C34.31 Malignant neoplasm of lower lobe, right bronchus or lung
⇄ C34.32 Malignant neoplasm of lower lobe, left bronchus or lung
⇄ C34.81 Malignant neoplasm of overlapping sites of right bronchus and lung
⇄ C34.82 Malignant neoplasm of overlapping sites of left bronchus and lung
⇄ C34.91 Malignant neoplasm of unspecified part of right bronchus or lung
⇄ C34.92 Malignant neoplasm of unspecified part of left bronchus or lung
C38.1 Malignant neoplasm of anterior mediastinum
C38.2 Malignant neoplasm of posterior mediastinum
C38.3 Malignant neoplasm of mediastinum, part unspecified
C38.8 Malignant neoplasm of overlapping sites of heart, mediastinum and pleura
C7A.090 Malignant carcinoid tumor of the bronchus and lung
J43.9 Emphysema, unspecified
J85.1 Abscess of lung with pneumonia
J85.2 Abscess of lung without pneumonia
J85.3 Abscess of mediastinum
J86.0 Pyothorax with fistula
J86.9 Pyothorax without fistula
J91.0 Malignant pleural effusion
J91.8 Pleural effusion in other conditions classified elsewhere
J93.0 Spontaneous tension pneumothorax
J93.11 Primary spontaneous pneumothorax
J93.12 Secondary spontaneous pneumothorax
J93.81 Chronic pneumothorax
J93.82 Other air leak
J93.83 Other pneumothorax
J93.9 Pneumothorax, unspecified
J94.1 Fibrothorax
J94.2 Hemothorax
J94.8 Other specified pleural conditions
J98.51 Mediastinitis
J98.59 Other diseases of mediastinum, not elsewhere classified
J98.6 Disorders of diaphragm
J98.8 Other specified respiratory disorders
Q33.0 Congenital cystic lung
Q33.8 Other congenital malformations of lung
Q33.9 Congenital malformation of lung, unspecified
Q34.0 Anomaly of pleura
Q34.1 Congenital cyst of mediastinum
Q34.8 Other specified congenital malformations of respiratory system
Q34.9 Congenital malformation of respiratory system, unspecified
Q79.0 Congenital diaphragmatic hernia
Q79.1 Other congenital malformations of diaphragm
Q79.3 Gastroschisis

CCI Edits

Refer to Appendix A for CCI edits.

Pub 100

00541: Pub 100-04, 12, 140.5, Pub 100-04, 12, 50, Pub 100-04, 12, 90.4.5

Base Units

Global: XXX

Code	Base Units
00541	15

Modifiers (PAR)

Code	Mod 50	Mod 51	Mod 62	Mod 80
00541	9	9	9	9

CPT © 2018 American Medical Association. All Rights Reserved.

00542

00542 Anesthesia for thoracotomy procedures involving lungs, pleura, diaphragm, and mediastinum (including surgical thoracoscopy); decortication

ICD-10-CM Diagnostic Codes

J92.0	Pleural plaque with presence of asbestos
J92.9	Pleural plaque without asbestos
J94.1	Fibrothorax
J94.8	Other specified pleural conditions
J96.11	Chronic respiratory failure with hypoxia
J96.12	Chronic respiratory failure with hypercapnia
J96.21	Acute and chronic respiratory failure with hypoxia
J96.22	Acute and chronic respiratory failure with hypercapnia
J96.91	Respiratory failure, unspecified with hypoxia
J96.92	Respiratory failure, unspecified with hypercapnia
J98.4	Other disorders of lung
R06.00	Dyspnea, unspecified
R06.01	Orthopnea
R06.02	Shortness of breath
R06.09	Other forms of dyspnea
R09.1	Pleurisy

CCI Edits

Refer to Appendix A for CCI edits.

Pub 100

00542: Pub 100-04, 12, 140.5, Pub 100-04, 12, 50, Pub 100-04, 12, 90.4.5

Base Units

Global: XXX

Code	Base Units
00542	15

Modifiers (PAR)

Code	Mod 50	Mod 51	Mod 62	Mod 80
00542	9	9	9	9

CPT © 2018 American Medical Association. All Rights Reserved.

00546

00546 Anesthesia for thoracotomy procedures involving lungs, pleura, diaphragm, and mediastinum (including surgical thoracoscopy); pulmonary resection with thoracoplasty

ICD-10-CM Diagnostic Codes

	A15.0	Tuberculosis of lung
	A15.5	Tuberculosis of larynx, trachea and bronchus
	A15.7	Primary respiratory tuberculosis
	A15.8	Other respiratory tuberculosis
	A15.9	Respiratory tuberculosis unspecified
⇄	C34.01	Malignant neoplasm of right main bronchus
⇄	C34.02	Malignant neoplasm of left main bronchus
⇄	C34.11	Malignant neoplasm of upper lobe, right bronchus or lung
⇄	C34.12	Malignant neoplasm of upper lobe, left bronchus or lung
	C34.2	Malignant neoplasm of middle lobe, bronchus or lung
⇄	C34.31	Malignant neoplasm of lower lobe, right bronchus or lung
⇄	C34.32	Malignant neoplasm of lower lobe, left bronchus or lung
⇄	C34.81	Malignant neoplasm of overlapping sites of right bronchus and lung
⇄	C34.82	Malignant neoplasm of overlapping sites of left bronchus and lung
⇄	C34.91	Malignant neoplasm of unspecified part of right bronchus or lung
⇄	C34.92	Malignant neoplasm of unspecified part of left bronchus or lung
	C38.1	Malignant neoplasm of anterior mediastinum
	C38.2	Malignant neoplasm of posterior mediastinum
	C38.3	Malignant neoplasm of mediastinum, part unspecified
	C38.4	Malignant neoplasm of pleura
	C38.8	Malignant neoplasm of overlapping sites of heart, mediastinum and pleura
	C41.3	Malignant neoplasm of ribs, sternum and clavicle
	C76.1	Malignant neoplasm of thorax
⇄	C78.01	Secondary malignant neoplasm of right lung
⇄	C78.02	Secondary malignant neoplasm of left lung
	C78.1	Secondary malignant neoplasm of mediastinum
	C78.2	Secondary malignant neoplasm of pleura
	C7A.090	Malignant carcinoid tumor of the bronchus and lung
	J86.0	Pyothorax with fistula
	J86.9	Pyothorax without fistula
❼⇄	S21.301	Unspecified open wound of right front wall of thorax with penetration into thoracic cavity
❼⇄	S21.302	Unspecified open wound of left front wall of thorax with penetration into thoracic cavity
❼⇄	S21.311	Laceration without foreign body of right front wall of thorax with penetration into thoracic cavity
❼⇄	S21.312	Laceration without foreign body of left front wall of thorax with penetration into thoracic cavity
❼⇄	S21.321	Laceration with foreign body of right front wall of thorax with penetration into thoracic cavity
❼⇄	S21.322	Laceration with foreign body of left front wall of thorax with penetration into thoracic cavity
❼⇄	S21.401	Unspecified open wound of right back wall of thorax with penetration into thoracic cavity
❼⇄	S21.402	Unspecified open wound of left back wall of thorax with penetration into thoracic cavity
❼⇄	S21.411	Laceration without foreign body of right back wall of thorax with penetration into thoracic cavity
❼⇄	S21.412	Laceration without foreign body of left back wall of thorax with penetration into thoracic cavity
❼⇄	S21.421	Laceration with foreign body of right back wall of thorax with penetration into thoracic cavity
❼⇄	S21.422	Laceration with foreign body of left back wall of thorax with penetration into thoracic cavity
❼	S27.311	Primary blast injury of lung, unilateral
❼	S27.312	Primary blast injury of lung, bilateral
❼	S27.331	Laceration of lung, unilateral
❼	S27.332	Laceration of lung, bilateral
❼	S27.411	Primary blast injury of bronchus, unilateral
❼	S27.412	Primary blast injury of bronchus, bilateral
❼	S27.431	Laceration of bronchus, unilateral
❼	S27.432	Laceration of bronchus, bilateral
❼	S28.0	Crushed chest
❼	S28.1	Traumatic amputation (partial) of part of thorax, except breast

ICD-10-CM Coding Notes

For codes requiring a 7th character extension, refer to your ICD-10-CM book. Review the character descriptions and coding guidelines for proper selection. For some procedures, only certain characters will apply.

CCI Edits

Refer to Appendix A for CCI edits.

Pub 100

00546: Pub 100-04, 12, 140.5, Pub 100-04, 12, 50, Pub 100-04, 12, 90.4.5

Base Units

Global: XXX

Code	Base Units
00546	15

Modifiers (PAR)

Code	Mod 50	Mod 51	Mod 62	Mod 80
00546	9	9	9	9

CPT © 2018 American Medical Association. All Rights Reserved.

00548

00548 Anesthesia for thoracotomy procedures involving lungs, pleura, diaphragm, and mediastinum (including surgical thoracoscopy); intrathoracic procedures on the trachea and bronchi

AMA *CPT Assistant*

00548: Nov 97: 10

ICD-10-CM Diagnostic Codes

	C33	Malignant neoplasm of trachea
⇄	C34.01	Malignant neoplasm of right main bronchus
⇄	C34.02	Malignant neoplasm of left main bronchus
⇄	C34.11	Malignant neoplasm of upper lobe, right bronchus or lung
⇄	C34.12	Malignant neoplasm of upper lobe, left bronchus or lung
	C34.2	Malignant neoplasm of middle lobe, bronchus or lung
⇄	C34.31	Malignant neoplasm of lower lobe, right bronchus or lung
⇄	C34.32	Malignant neoplasm of lower lobe, left bronchus or lung
⇄	C34.81	Malignant neoplasm of overlapping sites of right bronchus and lung
⇄	C34.82	Malignant neoplasm of overlapping sites of left bronchus and lung
⇄	C34.91	Malignant neoplasm of unspecified part of right bronchus or lung
⇄	C34.92	Malignant neoplasm of unspecified part of left bronchus or lung
➐	S11.021	Laceration without foreign body of trachea
➐	S11.022	Laceration with foreign body of trachea
➐	S11.023	Puncture wound without foreign body of trachea
➐	S11.024	Puncture wound with foreign body of trachea
➐	S11.025	Open bite of trachea
➐	S11.029	Unspecified open wound of trachea
➐⇄	S21.301	Unspecified open wound of right front wall of thorax with penetration into thoracic cavity
➐⇄	S21.302	Unspecified open wound of left front wall of thorax with penetration into thoracic cavity
➐⇄	S21.311	Laceration without foreign body of right front wall of thorax with penetration into thoracic cavity
➐⇄	S21.312	Laceration without foreign body of left front wall of thorax with penetration into thoracic cavity
➐⇄	S21.321	Laceration with foreign body of right front wall of thorax with penetration into thoracic cavity
➐⇄	S21.322	Laceration with foreign body of left front wall of thorax with penetration into thoracic cavity
➐⇄	S21.331	Puncture wound without foreign body of right front wall of thorax with penetration into thoracic cavity
➐⇄	S21.332	Puncture wound without foreign body of left front wall of thorax with penetration into thoracic cavity
➐⇄	S21.341	Puncture wound with foreign body of right front wall of thorax with penetration into thoracic cavity
➐⇄	S21.342	Puncture wound with foreign body of left front wall of thorax with penetration into thoracic cavity
➐⇄	S21.351	Open bite of right front wall of thorax with penetration into thoracic cavity
➐⇄	S21.352	Open bite of left front wall of thorax with penetration into thoracic cavity
➐⇄	S21.401	Unspecified open wound of right back wall of thorax with penetration into thoracic cavity
➐⇄	S21.402	Unspecified open wound of left back wall of thorax with penetration into thoracic cavity
➐⇄	S21.411	Laceration without foreign body of right back wall of thorax with penetration into thoracic cavity
➐⇄	S21.412	Laceration without foreign body of left back wall of thorax with penetration into thoracic cavity
➐⇄	S21.421	Laceration with foreign body of right back wall of thorax with penetration into thoracic cavity
➐⇄	S21.422	Laceration with foreign body of left back wall of thorax with penetration into thoracic cavity
➐⇄	S21.431	Puncture wound without foreign body of right back wall of thorax with penetration into thoracic cavity
➐⇄	S21.432	Puncture wound without foreign body of left back wall of thorax with penetration into thoracic cavity
➐⇄	S21.441	Puncture wound with foreign body of right back wall of thorax with penetration into thoracic cavity
➐⇄	S21.442	Puncture wound with foreign body of left back wall of thorax with penetration into thoracic cavity
➐⇄	S21.451	Open bite of right back wall of thorax with penetration into thoracic cavity
➐⇄	S21.452	Open bite of left back wall of thorax with penetration into thoracic cavity
➐	S27.401	Unspecified injury of bronchus, unilateral
➐	S27.402	Unspecified injury of bronchus, bilateral
➐	S27.411	Primary blast injury of bronchus, unilateral
➐	S27.412	Primary blast injury of bronchus, bilateral
➐	S27.431	Laceration of bronchus, unilateral
➐	S27.432	Laceration of bronchus, bilateral
➐	S27.51	Primary blast injury of thoracic trachea
➐	S27.53	Laceration of thoracic trachea
➐	T17.520	Food in bronchus causing asphyxiation
➐	T17.528	Food in bronchus causing other injury
➐	T17.590	Other foreign object in bronchus causing asphyxiation
➐	T17.598	Other foreign object in bronchus causing other injury

ICD-10-CM Coding Notes

For codes requiring a 7th character extension, refer to your ICD-10-CM book. Review the character descriptions and coding guidelines for proper selection. For some procedures, only certain characters will apply.

CCI Edits

Refer to Appendix A for CCI edits.

Pub 100

00548: Pub 100-04, 12, 140.5, Pub 100-04, 12, 50, Pub 100-04, 12, 90.4.5

Base Units

Global: XXX

Code	Base Units
00548	17

Modifiers (PAR)

Code	Mod 50	Mod 51	Mod 62	Mod 80
00548	9	9	9	9

● New ▲ Revised ✚ Add On ⊘Modifier 51 Exempt ★Telemedicine ▯ CPT QuickRef ⁄⁄ FDA Pending ⇄ Laterality ➐ Seventh Character ♂Male ♀Female

CPT © 2018 American Medical Association. All Rights Reserved.

00550

00550 Anesthesia for sternal debridement

ICD-10-CM Diagnostic Codes

	J85.3	Abscess of mediastinum
	J98.51	Mediastinitis
	J98.59	Other diseases of mediastinum, not elsewhere classified
➐⇄	S21.101	Unspecified open wound of right front wall of thorax without penetration into thoracic cavity
➐⇄	S21.102	Unspecified open wound of left front wall of thorax without penetration into thoracic cavity
➐⇄	S21.121	Laceration with foreign body of right front wall of thorax without penetration into thoracic cavity
➐⇄	S21.122	Laceration with foreign body of left front wall of thorax without penetration into thoracic cavity
➐	S22.21	Fracture of manubrium
➐	S22.22	Fracture of body of sternum
➐	S22.23	Sternal manubrial dissociation
➐	S22.24	Fracture of xiphoid process
➐	S29.021	Laceration of muscle and tendon of front wall of thorax
➐	T81.32	Disruption of internal operation (surgical) wound, not elsewhere classified
➐	T81.33	Disruption of traumatic injury wound repair
➐	T81.49	Infection following a procedure, other surgical site

ICD-10-CM Coding Notes

For codes requiring a 7th character extension, refer to your ICD-10-CM book. Review the character descriptions and coding guidelines for proper selection. For some procedures, only certain characters will apply.

CCI Edits

Refer to Appendix A for CCI edits.

Pub 100

00550: Pub 100-04, 12, 140.5, Pub 100-04, 12, 50, Pub 100-04, 12, 90.4.5

Base Units

Global: XXX

Code	Base Units
00550	10

Modifiers (PAR)

Code	Mod 50	Mod 51	Mod 62	Mod 80
00550	9	9	9	9

CPT © 2018 American Medical Association. All Rights Reserved.

00560

00560 Anesthesia for procedures on heart, pericardial sac, and great vessels of chest; without pump oxygenator

ICD-10-CM Diagnostic Codes

I21.01	ST elevation (STEMI) myocardial infarction involving left main coronary artery
I21.02	ST elevation (STEMI) myocardial infarction involving left anterior descending coronary artery
I21.09	ST elevation (STEMI) myocardial infarction involving other coronary artery of anterior wall
I21.11	ST elevation (STEMI) myocardial infarction involving right coronary artery
I21.19	ST elevation (STEMI) myocardial infarction involving other coronary artery of inferior wall
I21.21	ST elevation (STEMI) myocardial infarction involving left circumflex coronary artery
I21.29	ST elevation (STEMI) myocardial infarction involving other sites
I21.3	ST elevation (STEMI) myocardial infarction of unspecified site
I21.4	Non-ST elevation (NSTEMI) myocardial infarction
I22.0	Subsequent ST elevation (STEMI) myocardial infarction of anterior wall
I22.1	Subsequent ST elevation (STEMI) myocardial infarction of inferior wall
I22.2	Subsequent non-ST elevation (NSTEMI) myocardial infarction
I22.8	Subsequent ST elevation (STEMI) myocardial infarction of other sites
I22.9	Subsequent ST elevation (STEMI) myocardial infarction of unspecified site
I25.10	Atherosclerotic heart disease of native coronary artery without angina pectoris
I25.110	Atherosclerotic heart disease of native coronary artery with unstable angina pectoris
I25.111	Atherosclerotic heart disease of native coronary artery with angina pectoris with documented spasm
I25.118	Atherosclerotic heart disease of native coronary artery with other forms of angina pectoris
I25.119	Atherosclerotic heart disease of native coronary artery with unspecified angina pectoris
I27.20	Pulmonary hypertension, unspecified
I27.21	Secondary pulmonary arterial hypertension
I27.22	Pulmonary hypertension due to left heart disease
I27.23	Pulmonary hypertension due to lung diseases and hypoxia
I27.24	Chronic thromboembolic pulmonary hypertension
I27.29	Other secondary pulmonary hypertension
I27.83	Eisenmenger's syndrome
I31.1	Chronic constrictive pericarditis
I31.3	Pericardial effusion (noninflammatory)
I31.4	Cardiac tamponade
I50.810	Right heart failure, unspecified
I50.811	Acute right heart failure
I50.812	Chronic right heart failure
I50.813	Acute on chronic right heart failure
I50.814	Right heart failure due to left heart failure
I50.82	Biventricular heart failure
I50.83	High output heart failure
I50.84	End stage heart failure
I50.89	Other heart failure

CCI Edits

Refer to Appendix A for CCI edits.

Pub 100

00560: Pub 100-04, 12, 140.5, Pub 100-04, 12, 50, Pub 100-04, 12, 90.4.5

Base Units

Global: XXX

Code	Base Units
00560	15

Modifiers (PAR)

Code	Mod 50	Mod 51	Mod 62	Mod 80
00560	9	9	9	9

CPT © 2018 American Medical Association. All Rights Reserved.

00561

00561 Anesthesia for procedures on heart, pericardial sac, and great vessels of chest; with pump oxygenator, younger than 1 year of age

(Do not report 00561 in conjunction with 99100, 99116, and 99135)

AMA *CPT Assistant* ▯

00561: Dec 17: 8

ICD-10-CM Diagnostic Codes

I27.20	Pulmonary hypertension, unspecified
I27.21	Secondary pulmonary arterial hypertension
I27.22	Pulmonary hypertension due to left heart disease
I27.23	Pulmonary hypertension due to lung diseases and hypoxia
I27.24	Chronic thromboembolic pulmonary hypertension
I27.29	Other secondary pulmonary hypertension
I27.83	Eisenmenger's syndrome
Q20.0	Common arterial trunk
Q20.1	Double outlet right ventricle
Q20.2	Double outlet left ventricle
Q20.4	Double inlet ventricle
Q21.0	Ventricular septal defect
Q21.1	Atrial septal defect
Q21.2	Atrioventricular septal defect
Q21.4	Aortopulmonary septal defect
Q22.0	Pulmonary valve atresia
Q22.1	Congenital pulmonary valve stenosis
Q22.2	Congenital pulmonary valve insufficiency
Q22.3	Other congenital malformations of pulmonary valve
Q22.4	Congenital tricuspid stenosis
Q22.5	Ebstein's anomaly
Q22.6	Hypoplastic right heart syndrome
Q23.0	Congenital stenosis of aortic valve
Q23.1	Congenital insufficiency of aortic valve
Q23.2	Congenital mitral stenosis
Q23.3	Congenital mitral insufficiency
Q24.3	Pulmonary infundibular stenosis
Q25.0	Patent ductus arteriosus
Q25.1	Coarctation of aorta
Q25.2	Atresia of aorta
Q25.3	Supravalvular aortic stenosis
Q25.5	Atresia of pulmonary artery
Q25.6	Stenosis of pulmonary artery
Q25.71	Coarctation of pulmonary artery
Q25.72	Congenital pulmonary arteriovenous malformation
Q26.2	Total anomalous pulmonary venous connection
Q26.3	Partial anomalous pulmonary venous connection

CCI Edits

Refer to Appendix A for CCI edits.

Pub 100

00561: Pub 100-04, 12, 140.5, Pub 100-04, 12, 50, Pub 100-04, 12, 90.4.5

Base Units

Global: XXX

Code	Base Units
00561	25

Modifiers (PAR)

Code	Mod 50	Mod 51	Mod 62	Mod 80
00561	9	9	9	9

CPT © 2018 American Medical Association. All Rights Reserved.

00562

00562 Anesthesia for procedures on heart, pericardial sac, and great vessels of chest; with pump oxygenator, age 1 year or older, for all noncoronary bypass procedures (eg, valve procedures) or for re-operation for coronary bypass more than 1 month after original operation

ICD-10-CM Diagnostic Codes

I25.710	Atherosclerosis of autologous vein coronary artery bypass graft(s) with unstable angina pectoris
I25.711	Atherosclerosis of autologous vein coronary artery bypass graft(s) with angina pectoris with documented spasm
I25.718	Atherosclerosis of autologous vein coronary artery bypass graft(s) with other forms of angina pectoris
I25.719	Atherosclerosis of autologous vein coronary artery bypass graft(s) with unspecified angina pectoris
I25.720	Atherosclerosis of autologous artery coronary artery bypass graft(s) with unstable angina pectoris
I25.721	Atherosclerosis of autologous artery coronary artery bypass graft(s) with angina pectoris with documented spasm
I25.728	Atherosclerosis of autologous artery coronary artery bypass graft(s) with other forms of angina pectoris
I25.729	Atherosclerosis of autologous artery coronary artery bypass graft(s) with unspecified angina pectoris
I27.20	Pulmonary hypertension, unspecified
I27.21	Secondary pulmonary arterial hypertension
I27.22	Pulmonary hypertension due to left heart disease
I27.23	Pulmonary hypertension due to lung diseases and hypoxia
I27.24	Chronic thromboembolic pulmonary hypertension
I27.29	Other secondary pulmonary hypertension
I27.83	Eisenmenger's syndrome
I34.0	Nonrheumatic mitral (valve) insufficiency
I34.1	Nonrheumatic mitral (valve) prolapse
I34.2	Nonrheumatic mitral (valve) stenosis
I34.8	Other nonrheumatic mitral valve disorders
I35.0	Nonrheumatic aortic (valve) stenosis
I35.1	Nonrheumatic aortic (valve) insufficiency
I35.2	Nonrheumatic aortic (valve) stenosis with insufficiency
I35.8	Other nonrheumatic aortic valve disorders
I36.0	Nonrheumatic tricuspid (valve) stenosis
I36.1	Nonrheumatic tricuspid (valve) insufficiency
I36.2	Nonrheumatic tricuspid (valve) stenosis with insufficiency
I36.8	Other nonrheumatic tricuspid valve disorders
I37.0	Nonrheumatic pulmonary valve stenosis
I37.1	Nonrheumatic pulmonary valve insufficiency
I37.2	Nonrheumatic pulmonary valve stenosis with insufficiency
I37.8	Other nonrheumatic pulmonary valve disorders

CCI Edits

Refer to Appendix A for CCI edits.

Pub 100

00562: Pub 100-04, 12, 140.5, Pub 100-04, 12, 50, Pub 100-04, 12, 90.4.5

Base Units

Global: XXX

Code	Base Units
00562	20

Modifiers (PAR)

Code	Mod 50	Mod 51	Mod 62	Mod 80
00562	9	9	9	9

CPT © 2018 American Medical Association. All Rights Reserved.

00563

00563 Anesthesia for procedures on heart, pericardial sac, and great vessels of chest; with pump oxygenator with hypothermic circulatory arrest

ICD-10-CM Diagnostic Codes

I23.1	Atrial septal defect as current complication following acute myocardial infarction
I23.2	Ventricular septal defect as current complication following acute myocardial infarction
I23.3	Rupture of cardiac wall without hemopericardium as current complication following acute myocardial infarction
I23.4	Rupture of chordae tendineae as current complication following acute myocardial infarction
I23.5	Rupture of papillary muscle as current complication following acute myocardial infarction
I23.6	Thrombosis of atrium, auricular appendage, and ventricle as current complications following acute myocardial infarction
I25.3	Aneurysm of heart
I27.20	Pulmonary hypertension, unspecified
I27.21	Secondary pulmonary arterial hypertension
I27.22	Pulmonary hypertension due to left heart disease
I27.23	Pulmonary hypertension due to lung diseases and hypoxia
I27.24	Chronic thromboembolic pulmonary hypertension
I27.29	Other secondary pulmonary hypertension
I27.83	Eisenmenger's syndrome
I42.1	Obstructive hypertrophic cardiomyopathy
I42.2	Other hypertrophic cardiomyopathy
I42.5	Other restrictive cardiomyopathy
I51.0	Cardiac septal defect, acquired
I71.01	Dissection of thoracic aorta
I71.2	Thoracic aortic aneurysm, without rupture
Q20.1	Double outlet right ventricle
Q20.2	Double outlet left ventricle
Q21.0	Ventricular septal defect
Q21.1	Atrial septal defect
Q21.2	Atrioventricular septal defect
Q21.3	Tetralogy of Fallot
Q21.4	Aortopulmonary septal defect
Q21.8	Other congenital malformations of cardiac septa
Q22.0	Pulmonary valve atresia
Q22.5	Ebstein's anomaly
Q22.6	Hypoplastic right heart syndrome
Q24.2	Cor triatriatum
Q24.4	Congenital subaortic stenosis
Q25.1	Coarctation of aorta
Q25.2	Atresia of aorta
Q25.3	Supravalvular aortic stenosis
Q25.4	Other congenital malformations of aorta
Q25.5	Atresia of pulmonary artery
Q26.2	Total anomalous pulmonary venous connection
Q26.3	Partial anomalous pulmonary venous connection

CCI Edits

Refer to Appendix A for CCI edits.

Pub 100

00563: Pub 100-04, 12, 140.5, Pub 100-04, 12, 50, Pub 100-04, 12, 90.4.5

Base Units

Global: XXX

Code	Base Units
00563	25

Modifiers (PAR)

Code	Mod 50	Mod 51	Mod 62	Mod 80
00563	9	9	9	9

CPT © 2018 American Medical Association. All Rights Reserved.

00566

00566 Anesthesia for direct coronary artery bypass grafting; without pump oxygenator

ICD-10-CM Diagnostic Codes

I21.01	ST elevation (STEMI) myocardial infarction involving left main coronary artery
I21.02	ST elevation (STEMI) myocardial infarction involving left anterior descending coronary artery
I21.09	ST elevation (STEMI) myocardial infarction involving other coronary artery of anterior wall
I21.11	ST elevation (STEMI) myocardial infarction involving right coronary artery
I21.19	ST elevation (STEMI) myocardial infarction involving other coronary artery of inferior wall
I21.21	ST elevation (STEMI) myocardial infarction involving left circumflex coronary artery
I21.29	ST elevation (STEMI) myocardial infarction involving other sites
I21.3	ST elevation (STEMI) myocardial infarction of unspecified site
I21.4	Non-ST elevation (NSTEMI) myocardial infarction
I22.0	Subsequent ST elevation (STEMI) myocardial infarction of anterior wall
I22.1	Subsequent ST elevation (STEMI) myocardial infarction of inferior wall
I22.2	Subsequent non-ST elevation (NSTEMI) myocardial infarction
I22.8	Subsequent ST elevation (STEMI) myocardial infarction of other sites
I22.9	Subsequent ST elevation (STEMI) myocardial infarction of unspecified site
I25.110	Atherosclerotic heart disease of native coronary artery with unstable angina pectoris
I25.111	Atherosclerotic heart disease of native coronary artery with angina pectoris with documented spasm
I25.118	Atherosclerotic heart disease of native coronary artery with other forms of angina pectoris
I25.119	Atherosclerotic heart disease of native coronary artery with unspecified angina pectoris
I25.41	Coronary artery aneurysm
I25.42	Coronary artery dissection
I25.811	Atherosclerosis of native coronary artery of transplanted heart without angina pectoris
I25.82	Chronic total occlusion of coronary artery
I25.83	Coronary atherosclerosis due to lipid rich plaque
I25.84	Coronary atherosclerosis due to calcified coronary lesion
Q24.5	Malformation of coronary vessels

CCI Edits

Refer to Appendix A for CCI edits.

Pub 100

00566: Pub 100-04, 12, 140.5, Pub 100-04, 12, 50, Pub 100-04, 12, 90.4.5

Base Units

Global: XXX

Code	Base Units
00566	25

Modifiers (PAR)

Code	Mod 50	Mod 51	Mod 62	Mod 80
00566	9	9	9	9

CPT © 2018 American Medical Association. All Rights Reserved.

00567

00567 Anesthesia for direct coronary artery bypass grafting; with pump oxygenator

ICD-10-CM Diagnostic Codes

I21.01	ST elevation (STEMI) myocardial infarction involving left main coronary artery
I21.02	ST elevation (STEMI) myocardial infarction involving left anterior descending coronary artery
I21.09	ST elevation (STEMI) myocardial infarction involving other coronary artery of anterior wall
I21.11	ST elevation (STEMI) myocardial infarction involving right coronary artery
I21.19	ST elevation (STEMI) myocardial infarction involving other coronary artery of inferior wall
I21.21	ST elevation (STEMI) myocardial infarction involving left circumflex coronary artery
I21.29	ST elevation (STEMI) myocardial infarction involving other sites
I21.3	ST elevation (STEMI) myocardial infarction of unspecified site
I21.4	Non-ST elevation (NSTEMI) myocardial infarction
I22.0	Subsequent ST elevation (STEMI) myocardial infarction of anterior wall
I22.1	Subsequent ST elevation (STEMI) myocardial infarction of inferior wall
I22.2	Subsequent non-ST elevation (NSTEMI) myocardial infarction
I22.8	Subsequent ST elevation (STEMI) myocardial infarction of other sites
I22.9	Subsequent ST elevation (STEMI) myocardial infarction of unspecified site
I25.110	Atherosclerotic heart disease of native coronary artery with unstable angina pectoris
I25.111	Atherosclerotic heart disease of native coronary artery with angina pectoris with documented spasm
I25.118	Atherosclerotic heart disease of native coronary artery with other forms of angina pectoris
I25.119	Atherosclerotic heart disease of native coronary artery with unspecified angina pectoris
I25.41	Coronary artery aneurysm
I25.42	Coronary artery dissection
I25.811	Atherosclerosis of native coronary artery of transplanted heart without angina pectoris
I25.82	Chronic total occlusion of coronary artery
I25.83	Coronary atherosclerosis due to lipid rich plaque
I25.84	Coronary atherosclerosis due to calcified coronary lesion
Q24.5	Malformation of coronary vessels

CCI Edits

Refer to Appendix A for CCI edits.

Pub 100

00567: Pub 100-04, 12, 140.5, Pub 100-04, 12, 50, Pub 100-04, 12, 90.4.5

Base Units

Global: XXX

Code	Base Units
00567	18

Modifiers (PAR)

Code	Mod 50	Mod 51	Mod 62	Mod 80
00567	9	9	9	9

CPT © 2018 American Medical Association. All Rights Reserved.

00580

00580 Anesthesia for heart transplant or heart/lung transplant

AMA *CPT Assistant*

00580: Nov 07: 8, Jul 12: 13

ICD-10-CM Diagnostic Codes

B33.24	Viral cardiomyopathy
D86.0	Sarcoidosis of lung
D86.85	Sarcoid myocarditis
I21.9	Acute myocardial infarction, unspecified
I21.A1	Myocardial infarction type 2
I21.A9	Other myocardial infarction type
I25.3	Aneurysm of heart
I25.5	Ischemic cardiomyopathy
I25.9	Chronic ischemic heart disease, unspecified
I27.0	Primary pulmonary hypertension
I27.2	Other secondary pulmonary hypertension
I27.20	Pulmonary hypertension, unspecified
I27.21	Secondary pulmonary arterial hypertension
I27.22	Pulmonary hypertension due to left heart disease
I27.23	Pulmonary hypertension due to lung diseases and hypoxia
I27.24	Chronic thromboembolic pulmonary hypertension
I27.29	Other secondary pulmonary hypertension
I27.83	Eisenmenger's syndrome
I27.89	Other specified pulmonary heart diseases
I27.9	Pulmonary heart disease, unspecified
I42.0	Dilated cardiomyopathy
I42.7	Cardiomyopathy due to drug and external agent
I43	Cardiomyopathy in diseases classified elsewhere
I50.1	Left ventricular failure, unspecified
I50.810	Right heart failure, unspecified
I50.811	Acute right heart failure
I50.812	Chronic right heart failure
I50.813	Acute on chronic right heart failure
I50.814	Right heart failure due to left heart failure
I50.82	Biventricular heart failure
I50.83	High output heart failure
I50.84	End stage heart failure
I50.89	Other heart failure
I50.9	Heart failure, unspecified

CCI Edits

Refer to Appendix A for CCI edits.

Pub 100

00580: Pub 100-04, 12, 140.5, Pub 100-04, 12, 50, Pub 100-04, 12, 90.4.5

Base Units

Global: XXX

Code	Base Units
00580	20

Modifiers (PAR)

Code	Mod 50	Mod 51	Mod 62	Mod 80
00580	9	9	9	9

CPT © 2018 American Medical Association. All Rights Reserved.

00600

00600 Anesthesia for procedures on cervical spine and cord; not otherwise specified

(For percutaneous image-guided spine and spinal cord anesthesia procedures, see 01935, 01936)

AMA *CPT Assistant*

00600: Mar 06: 15, May 07: 9, Nov 07: 8, Oct 11: 3, Jul 12: 13

ICD-10-CM Diagnostic Codes

	M50.01	Cervical disc disorder with myelopathy, high cervical region
	M50.021	Cervical disc disorder at C4-C5 level with myelopathy
	M50.022	Cervical disc disorder at C5-C6 level with myelopathy
	M50.023	Cervical disc disorder at C6-C7 level with myelopathy
	M50.03	Cervical disc disorder with myelopathy, cervicothoracic region
	M50.11	Cervical disc disorder with radiculopathy, high cervical region
	M50.121	Cervical disc disorder at C4-C5 level with radiculopathy
	M50.122	Cervical disc disorder at C5-C6 level with radiculopathy
	M50.123	Cervical disc disorder at C6-C7 level with radiculopathy
	M50.13	Cervical disc disorder with radiculopathy, cervicothoracic region
	M50.21	Other cervical disc displacement, high cervical region
	M50.221	Other cervical disc displacement at C4-C5 level
	M50.222	Other cervical disc displacement at C5-C6 level
	M50.223	Other cervical disc displacement at C6-C7 level
	M50.23	Other cervical disc displacement, cervicothoracic region
	M53.1	Cervicobrachial syndrome
	M53.2X1	Spinal instabilities, occipito-atlanto-axial region
	M53.2X2	Spinal instabilities, cervical region
	M53.2X3	Spinal instabilities, cervicothoracic region
	M99.11	Subluxation complex (vertebral) of cervical region
	Q05.5	Cervical spina bifida without hydrocephalus
❼	S12.14	Type III traumatic spondylolisthesis of second cervical vertebra
❼	S12.44	Type III traumatic spondylolisthesis of fifth cervical vertebra
❼	S12.450	Other traumatic displaced spondylolisthesis of fifth cervical vertebra
❼	S12.451	Other traumatic nondisplaced spondylolisthesis of fifth cervical vertebra
❼	S12.54	Type III traumatic spondylolisthesis of sixth cervical vertebra
❼	S12.550	Other traumatic displaced spondylolisthesis of sixth cervical vertebra
❼	S12.551	Other traumatic nondisplaced spondylolisthesis of sixth cervical vertebra
❼	S13.0	Traumatic rupture of cervical intervertebral disc
❼	S14.102	Unspecified injury at C2 level of cervical spinal cord
❼	S14.105	Unspecified injury at C5 level of cervical spinal cord
❼	S14.106	Unspecified injury at C6 level of cervical spinal cord

ICD-10-CM Coding Notes

For codes requiring a 7th character extension, refer to your ICD-10-CM book. Review the character descriptions and coding guidelines for proper selection. For some procedures, only certain characters will apply.

CCI Edits

Refer to Appendix A for CCI edits.

Pub 100

00600: Pub 100-04, 12, 140.5, Pub 100-04, 12, 50, Pub 100-04, 12, 90.4.5

Base Units

Global: XXX

Code	Base Units
00600	10

Modifiers (PAR)

Code	Mod 50	Mod 51	Mod 62	Mod 80
00600	9	9	9	9

CPT © 2018 American Medical Association. All Rights Reserved.

00604

00604 Anesthesia for procedures on cervical spine and cord; procedures with patient in the sitting position

ICD-10-CM Diagnostic Codes

M43.01 Spondylolysis, occipito-atlanto-axial region
M43.02 Spondylolysis, cervical region
M43.03 Spondylolysis, cervicothoracic region
M43.11 Spondylolisthesis, occipito-atlanto-axial region
M43.12 Spondylolisthesis, cervical region
M43.13 Spondylolisthesis, cervicothoracic region
M48.01 Spinal stenosis, occipito-atlanto-axial region
M48.02 Spinal stenosis, cervical region
M48.03 Spinal stenosis, cervicothoracic region
M50.01 Cervical disc disorder with myelopathy, high cervical region
M50.021 Cervical disc disorder at C4-C5 level with myelopathy
M50.022 Cervical disc disorder at C5-C6 level with myelopathy
M50.023 Cervical disc disorder at C6-C7 level with myelopathy
M50.03 Cervical disc disorder with myelopathy, cervicothoracic region
M50.11 Cervical disc disorder with radiculopathy, high cervical region
M50.121 Cervical disc disorder at C4-C5 level with radiculopathy
M50.122 Cervical disc disorder at C5-C6 level with radiculopathy
M50.123 Cervical disc disorder at C6-C7 level with radiculopathy
M50.13 Cervical disc disorder with radiculopathy, cervicothoracic region
M50.21 Other cervical disc displacement, high cervical region
M50.221 Other cervical disc displacement at C4-C5 level
M50.222 Other cervical disc displacement at C5-C6 level
M50.223 Other cervical disc displacement at C6-C7 level
M50.23 Other cervical disc displacement, cervicothoracic region
M50.31 Other cervical disc degeneration, high cervical region
M50.321 Other cervical disc degeneration at C4-C5 level
M50.322 Other cervical disc degeneration at C5-C6 level
M50.323 Other cervical disc degeneration at C6-C7 level
M50.33 Other cervical disc degeneration, cervicothoracic region
M53.1 Cervicobrachial syndrome
M53.2X2 Spinal instabilities, cervical region
M54.2 Cervicalgia
M54.81 Occipital neuralgia
➐ S12.100 Unspecified displaced fracture of second cervical vertebra
➐ S12.101 Unspecified nondisplaced fracture of second cervical vertebra
➐ S12.110 Anterior displaced Type II dens fracture
➐ S12.111 Posterior displaced Type II dens fracture
➐ S12.112 Nondisplaced Type II dens fracture
➐ S12.190 Other displaced fracture of second cervical vertebra
➐ S12.191 Other nondisplaced fracture of second cervical vertebra
➐ S12.44 Type III traumatic spondylolisthesis of fifth cervical vertebra
➐ S12.450 Other traumatic displaced spondylolisthesis of fifth cervical vertebra
➐ S12.451 Other traumatic nondisplaced spondylolisthesis of fifth cervical vertebra
➐ S12.54 Type III traumatic spondylolisthesis of sixth cervical vertebra
➐ S12.550 Other traumatic displaced spondylolisthesis of sixth cervical vertebra
➐ S12.551 Other traumatic nondisplaced spondylolisthesis of sixth cervical vertebra

ICD-10-CM Coding Notes

For codes requiring a 7th character extension, refer to your ICD-10-CM book. Review the character descriptions and coding guidelines for proper selection. For some procedures, only certain characters will apply.

CCI Edits

Refer to Appendix A for CCI edits.

Pub 100

00604: Pub 100-04, 12, 140.5, Pub 100-04, 12, 50, Pub 100-04, 12, 90.4.5

Base Units

Global: XXX

Code	Base Units
00604	13

Modifiers (PAR)

Code	Mod 50	Mod 51	Mod 62	Mod 80
00604	9	9	9	9

CPT © 2018 American Medical Association. All Rights Reserved.

00625

00625 Anesthesia for procedures on the thoracic spine and cord, via an anterior transthoracic approach; not utilizing 1 lung ventilation

AMA *CPT Assistant* ☐

00625: Mar 07: 9

ICD-10-CM Diagnostic Codes

	M40.14	Other secondary kyphosis, thoracic region
	M40.15	Other secondary kyphosis, thoracolumbar region
	M40.204	Unspecified kyphosis, thoracic region
	M40.205	Unspecified kyphosis, thoracolumbar region
	M40.294	Other kyphosis, thoracic region
	M40.295	Other kyphosis, thoracolumbar region
	M41.04	Infantile idiopathic scoliosis, thoracic region
	M41.05	Infantile idiopathic scoliosis, thoracolumbar region
	M41.114	Juvenile idiopathic scoliosis, thoracic region
	M41.115	Juvenile idiopathic scoliosis, thoracolumbar region
	M41.124	Adolescent idiopathic scoliosis, thoracic region
	M41.125	Adolescent idiopathic scoliosis, thoracolumbar region
	M41.24	Other idiopathic scoliosis, thoracic region
	M41.25	Other idiopathic scoliosis, thoracolumbar region
	M41.34	Thoracogenic scoliosis, thoracic region
	M41.35	Thoracogenic scoliosis, thoracolumbar region
	M43.14	Spondylolisthesis, thoracic region
	M43.15	Spondylolisthesis, thoracolumbar region
	M48.34	Traumatic spondylopathy, thoracic region
	M48.35	Traumatic spondylopathy, thoracolumbar region
	M51.04	Intervertebral disc disorders with myelopathy, thoracic region
	M51.14	Intervertebral disc disorders with radiculopathy, thoracic region
	M51.24	Other intervertebral disc displacement, thoracic region
	M51.34	Other intervertebral disc degeneration, thoracic region
➐	M84.58	Pathological fracture in neoplastic disease, other specified site
➐	S22.010	Wedge compression fracture of first thoracic vertebra
➐	S22.012	Unstable burst fracture of first thoracic vertebra
➐	S22.020	Wedge compression fracture of second thoracic vertebra
➐	S22.022	Unstable burst fracture of second thoracic vertebra
➐	S22.030	Wedge compression fracture of third thoracic vertebra
➐	S22.032	Unstable burst fracture of third thoracic vertebra
➐	S22.040	Wedge compression fracture of fourth thoracic vertebra
➐	S22.042	Unstable burst fracture of fourth thoracic vertebra
➐	S22.050	Wedge compression fracture of T5-T6 vertebra
➐	S22.052	Unstable burst fracture of T5-T6 vertebra
➐	S22.060	Wedge compression fracture of T7-T8 vertebra
➐	S22.062	Unstable burst fracture of T7-T8 vertebra
➐	S22.070	Wedge compression fracture of T9-T10 vertebra
➐	S22.072	Unstable burst fracture of T9-T10 vertebra
➐	S22.080	Wedge compression fracture of T11-T12 vertebra
➐	S22.082	Unstable burst fracture of T11-T12 vertebra
➐	S24.151	Other incomplete lesion at T1 level of thoracic spinal cord
➐	S24.152	Other incomplete lesion at T2-T6 level of thoracic spinal cord
➐	S24.153	Other incomplete lesion at T7-T10 level of thoracic spinal cord
➐	S24.154	Other incomplete lesion at T11-T12 level of thoracic spinal cord

ICD-10-CM Coding Notes

For codes requiring a 7th character extension, refer to your ICD-10-CM book. Review the character descriptions and coding guidelines for proper selection. For some procedures, only certain characters will apply.

CCI Edits

Refer to Appendix A for CCI edits.

Pub 100

00625: Pub 100-04, 12, 140.5, Pub 100-04, 12, 50, Pub 100-04, 12, 90.4.5

Base Units

Global: XXX

Code	Base Units
00625	13

Modifiers (PAR)

Code	Mod 50	Mod 51	Mod 62	Mod 80
00625	9	9	9	9

CPT © 2018 American Medical Association. All Rights Reserved.

00626

00626 Anesthesia for procedures on the thoracic spine and cord, via an anterior transthoracic approach; utilizing 1 lung ventilation

(For anesthesia for thoracotomy procedures other than spinal, see 00540-00541)

AMA *CPT Assistant*

00626: Mar 07: 9

ICD-10-CM Diagnostic Codes

M40.14	Other secondary kyphosis, thoracic region
M40.15	Other secondary kyphosis, thoracolumbar region
M40.204	Unspecified kyphosis, thoracic region
M40.205	Unspecified kyphosis, thoracolumbar region
M40.294	Other kyphosis, thoracic region
M40.295	Other kyphosis, thoracolumbar region
M41.04	Infantile idiopathic scoliosis, thoracic region
M41.05	Infantile idiopathic scoliosis, thoracolumbar region
M41.114	Juvenile idiopathic scoliosis, thoracic region
M41.115	Juvenile idiopathic scoliosis, thoracolumbar region
M41.124	Adolescent idiopathic scoliosis, thoracic region
M41.125	Adolescent idiopathic scoliosis, thoracolumbar region
M41.24	Other idiopathic scoliosis, thoracic region
M41.25	Other idiopathic scoliosis, thoracolumbar region
M41.34	Thoracogenic scoliosis, thoracic region
M41.35	Thoracogenic scoliosis, thoracolumbar region
M43.14	Spondylolisthesis, thoracic region
M43.15	Spondylolisthesis, thoracolumbar region
M48.34	Traumatic spondylopathy, thoracic region
M48.35	Traumatic spondylopathy, thoracolumbar region
M51.04	Intervertebral disc disorders with myelopathy, thoracic region
M51.05	Intervertebral disc disorders with myelopathy, thoracolumbar region
M51.14	Intervertebral disc disorders with radiculopathy, thoracic region
M51.15	Intervertebral disc disorders with radiculopathy, thoracolumbar region
M51.24	Other intervertebral disc displacement, thoracic region
M51.25	Other intervertebral disc displacement, thoracolumbar region
M51.34	Other intervertebral disc degeneration, thoracic region
M51.35	Other intervertebral disc degeneration, thoracolumbar region
M51.84	Other intervertebral disc disorders, thoracic region
M51.85	Other intervertebral disc disorders, thoracolumbar region
❼ S22.010	Wedge compression fracture of first thoracic vertebra
❼ S22.020	Wedge compression fracture of second thoracic vertebra
❼ S22.030	Wedge compression fracture of third thoracic vertebra
❼ S22.040	Wedge compression fracture of fourth thoracic vertebra
❼ S22.050	Wedge compression fracture of T5-T6 vertebra
❼ S22.060	Wedge compression fracture of T7-T8 vertebra
❼ S22.070	Wedge compression fracture of T9-T10 vertebra
❼ S22.080	Wedge compression fracture of T11-T12 vertebra
❼ S23.0	Traumatic rupture of thoracic intervertebral disc
❼ S24.111	Complete lesion at T1 level of thoracic spinal cord
❼ S24.112	Complete lesion at T2-T6 level of thoracic spinal cord
❼ S24.113	Complete lesion at T7-T10 level of thoracic spinal cord
❼ S24.114	Complete lesion at T11-T12 level of thoracic spinal cord
❼ S24.151	Other incomplete lesion at T1 level of thoracic spinal cord
❼ S24.152	Other incomplete lesion at T2-T6 level of thoracic spinal cord
❼ S24.153	Other incomplete lesion at T7-T10 level of thoracic spinal cord
❼ S24.154	Other incomplete lesion at T11-T12 level of thoracic spinal cord

ICD-10-CM Coding Notes

For codes requiring a 7th character extension, refer to your ICD-10-CM book. Review the character descriptions and coding guidelines for proper selection. For some procedures, only certain characters will apply.

CCI Edits

Refer to Appendix A for CCI edits.

Pub 100

00626: Pub 100-04, 12, 140.5, Pub 100-04, 12, 50, Pub 100-04, 12, 90.4.5

Base Units

Global: XXX

Code	Base Units
00626	15

Modifiers (PAR)

Code	Mod 50	Mod 51	Mod 62	Mod 80
00626	9	9	9	9

CPT © 2018 American Medical Association. All Rights Reserved.

00630

00630 Anesthesia for procedures in lumbar region; not otherwise specified

ICD-10-CM Diagnostic Codes

	M41.06	Infantile idiopathic scoliosis, lumbar region
	M41.07	Infantile idiopathic scoliosis, lumbosacral region
	M41.116	Juvenile idiopathic scoliosis, lumbar region
	M41.117	Juvenile idiopathic scoliosis, lumbosacral region
	M41.126	Adolescent idiopathic scoliosis, lumbar region
	M41.127	Adolescent idiopathic scoliosis, lumbosacral region
	M41.26	Other idiopathic scoliosis, lumbar region
	M41.27	Other idiopathic scoliosis, lumbosacral region
	M41.86	Other forms of scoliosis, lumbar region
	M41.87	Other forms of scoliosis, lumbosacral region
	M43.16	Spondylolisthesis, lumbar region
	M43.17	Spondylolisthesis, lumbosacral region
	M48.061	Spinal stenosis, lumbar region without neurogenic claudication
	M48.062	Spinal stenosis, lumbar region with neurogenic claudication
	M48.07	Spinal stenosis, lumbosacral region
	M48.36	Traumatic spondylopathy, lumbar region
	M48.37	Traumatic spondylopathy, lumbosacral region
	M51.06	Intervertebral disc disorders with myelopathy, lumbar region
	M51.07	Intervertebral disc disorders with myelopathy, lumbosacral region
	M51.16	Intervertebral disc disorders with radiculopathy, lumbar region
	M51.17	Intervertebral disc disorders with radiculopathy, lumbosacral region
	M51.26	Other intervertebral disc displacement, lumbar region
	M51.27	Other intervertebral disc displacement, lumbosacral region
	M51.36	Other intervertebral disc degeneration, lumbar region
	M51.37	Other intervertebral disc degeneration, lumbosacral region
	M51.46	Schmorl's nodes, lumbar region
	M51.47	Schmorl's nodes, lumbosacral region
	M51.86	Other intervertebral disc disorders, lumbar region
	M51.87	Other intervertebral disc disorders, lumbosacral region
➐	S32.010	Wedge compression fracture of first lumbar vertebra
➐	S32.012	Unstable burst fracture of first lumbar vertebra
➐	S32.020	Wedge compression fracture of second lumbar vertebra
➐	S32.022	Unstable burst fracture of second lumbar vertebra
➐	S32.030	Wedge compression fracture of third lumbar vertebra
➐	S32.032	Unstable burst fracture of third lumbar vertebra
➐	S32.040	Wedge compression fracture of fourth lumbar vertebra
➐	S32.042	Unstable burst fracture of fourth lumbar vertebra
➐	S32.050	Wedge compression fracture of fifth lumbar vertebra
➐	S32.052	Unstable burst fracture of fifth lumbar vertebra
➐	S34.111	Complete lesion of L1 level of lumbar spinal cord
➐	S34.112	Complete lesion of L2 level of lumbar spinal cord
➐	S34.113	Complete lesion of L3 level of lumbar spinal cord
➐	S34.114	Complete lesion of L4 level of lumbar spinal cord
➐	S34.115	Complete lesion of L5 level of lumbar spinal cord
➐	S34.121	Incomplete lesion of L1 level of lumbar spinal cord
➐	S34.122	Incomplete lesion of L2 level of lumbar spinal cord
➐	S34.123	Incomplete lesion of L3 level of lumbar spinal cord
➐	S34.124	Incomplete lesion of L4 level of lumbar spinal cord
➐	S34.125	Incomplete lesion of L5 level of lumbar spinal cord

ICD-10-CM Coding Notes

For codes requiring a 7th character extension, refer to your ICD-10-CM book. Review the character descriptions and coding guidelines for proper selection. For some procedures, only certain characters will apply.

CCI Edits

Refer to Appendix A for CCI edits.

Pub 100

00630: Pub 100-04, 12, 140.5, Pub 100-04, 12, 50, Pub 100-04, 12, 90.4.5

Base Units

Global: XXX

Code	Base Units
00630	8

Modifiers (PAR)

Code	Mod 50	Mod 51	Mod 62	Mod 80
00630	9	9	9	9

CPT © 2018 American Medical Association. All Rights Reserved.

00632

00632 Anesthesia for procedures in lumbar region; lumbar sympathectomy

ICD-10-CM Diagnostic Codes

⇄	G57.71	Causalgia of right lower limb
⇄	G57.72	Causalgia of left lower limb
⇄	G90.521	Complex regional pain syndrome I of right lower limb
⇄	G90.522	Complex regional pain syndrome I of left lower limb
⇄	G90.523	Complex regional pain syndrome I of lower limb, bilateral
⇄	I70.211	Atherosclerosis of native arteries of extremities with intermittent claudication, right leg
⇄	I70.212	Atherosclerosis of native arteries of extremities with intermittent claudication, left leg
⇄	I70.213	Atherosclerosis of native arteries of extremities with intermittent claudication, bilateral legs
⇄	I70.221	Atherosclerosis of native arteries of extremities with rest pain, right leg
⇄	I70.222	Atherosclerosis of native arteries of extremities with rest pain, left leg
⇄	I70.223	Atherosclerosis of native arteries of extremities with rest pain, bilateral legs
⇄	I70.311	Atherosclerosis of unspecified type of bypass graft(s) of the extremities with intermittent claudication, right leg
⇄	I70.312	Atherosclerosis of unspecified type of bypass graft(s) of the extremities with intermittent claudication, left leg
⇄	I70.313	Atherosclerosis of unspecified type of bypass graft(s) of the extremities with intermittent claudication, bilateral legs
⇄	I70.321	Atherosclerosis of unspecified type of bypass graft(s) of the extremities with rest pain, right leg
⇄	I70.322	Atherosclerosis of unspecified type of bypass graft(s) of the extremities with rest pain, left leg
⇄	I70.323	Atherosclerosis of unspecified type of bypass graft(s) of the extremities with rest pain, bilateral legs
⇄	I70.411	Atherosclerosis of autologous vein bypass graft(s) of the extremities with intermittent claudication, right leg
⇄	I70.412	Atherosclerosis of autologous vein bypass graft(s) of the extremities with intermittent claudication, left leg
⇄	I70.413	Atherosclerosis of autologous vein bypass graft(s) of the extremities with intermittent claudication, bilateral legs
⇄	I70.421	Atherosclerosis of autologous vein bypass graft(s) of the extremities with rest pain, right leg
⇄	I70.422	Atherosclerosis of autologous vein bypass graft(s) of the extremities with rest pain, left leg
⇄	I70.423	Atherosclerosis of autologous vein bypass graft(s) of the extremities with rest pain, bilateral legs
⇄	I70.511	Atherosclerosis of nonautologous biological bypass graft(s) of the extremities with intermittent claudication, right leg
⇄	I70.512	Atherosclerosis of nonautologous biological bypass graft(s) of the extremities with intermittent claudication, left leg
⇄	I70.513	Atherosclerosis of nonautologous biological bypass graft(s) of the extremities with intermittent claudication, bilateral legs
⇄	I70.521	Atherosclerosis of nonautologous biological bypass graft(s) of the extremities with rest pain, right leg
⇄	I70.522	Atherosclerosis of nonautologous biological bypass graft(s) of the extremities with rest pain, left leg
⇄	I70.523	Atherosclerosis of nonautologous biological bypass graft(s) of the extremities with rest pain, bilateral legs
⇄	I70.611	Atherosclerosis of nonbiological bypass graft(s) of the extremities with intermittent claudication, right leg
⇄	I70.612	Atherosclerosis of nonbiological bypass graft(s) of the extremities with intermittent claudication, left leg
⇄	I70.613	Atherosclerosis of nonbiological bypass graft(s) of the extremities with intermittent claudication, bilateral legs
⇄	I70.621	Atherosclerosis of nonbiological bypass graft(s) of the extremities with rest pain, right leg
⇄	I70.622	Atherosclerosis of nonbiological bypass graft(s) of the extremities with rest pain, left leg
⇄	I70.623	Atherosclerosis of nonbiological bypass graft(s) of the extremities with rest pain, bilateral legs
⇄	I70.711	Atherosclerosis of other type of bypass graft(s) of the extremities with intermittent claudication, right leg
⇄	I70.712	Atherosclerosis of other type of bypass graft(s) of the extremities with intermittent claudication, left leg
⇄	I70.713	Atherosclerosis of other type of bypass graft(s) of the extremities with intermittent claudication, bilateral legs
⇄	I70.721	Atherosclerosis of other type of bypass graft(s) of the extremities with rest pain, right leg
⇄	I70.722	Atherosclerosis of other type of bypass graft(s) of the extremities with rest pain, left leg
⇄	I70.723	Atherosclerosis of other type of bypass graft(s) of the extremities with rest pain, bilateral legs
	I73.00	Raynaud's syndrome without gangrene
	I73.9	Peripheral vascular disease, unspecified

CCI Edits

Refer to Appendix A for CCI edits.

Pub 100

00632: Pub 100-04, 12, 140.5, Pub 100-04, 12, 50, Pub 100-04, 12, 90.4.5

Base Units

Global: XXX

Code	Base Units
00632	7

Modifiers (PAR)

Code	Mod 50	Mod 51	Mod 62	Mod 80
00632	9	9	9	9

CPT © 2018 American Medical Association. All Rights Reserved.

00635

00635 Anesthesia for procedures in lumbar region; diagnostic or therapeutic lumbar puncture

ICD-10-CM Diagnostic Codes

A39.0	Meningococcal meningitis
A39.81	Meningococcal encephalitis
A83.6	Rocio virus disease
A83.8	Other mosquito-borne viral encephalitis
A83.9	Mosquito-borne viral encephalitis, unspecified
A92.31	West Nile virus infection with encephalitis
B00.4	Herpesviral encephalitis
B01.11	Varicella encephalitis and encephalomyelitis
B10.01	Human herpesvirus 6 encephalitis
B10.09	Other human herpesvirus encephalitis
C91.00	Acute lymphoblastic leukemia not having achieved remission
C91.02	Acute lymphoblastic leukemia, in relapse
C92.00	Acute myeloblastic leukemia, not having achieved remission
C92.02	Acute myeloblastic leukemia, in relapse
G00.0	Hemophilus meningitis
G00.1	Pneumococcal meningitis
G00.2	Streptococcal meningitis
G00.3	Staphylococcal meningitis
G00.8	Other bacterial meningitis
G00.9	Bacterial meningitis, unspecified
G01	Meningitis in bacterial diseases classified elsewhere
G02	Meningitis in other infectious and parasitic diseases classified elsewhere
G03.1	Chronic meningitis
G03.8	Meningitis due to other specified causes
G03.9	Meningitis, unspecified
G04.00	Acute disseminated encephalitis and encephalomyelitis, unspecified
G04.01	Postinfectious acute disseminated encephalitis and encephalomyelitis (postinfectious ADEM)
G04.2	Bacterial meningoencephalitis and meningomyelitis, not elsewhere classified
G04.30	Acute necrotizing hemorrhagic encephalopathy, unspecified
G04.81	Other encephalitis and encephalomyelitis
G04.90	Encephalitis and encephalomyelitis, unspecified
G04.91	Myelitis, unspecified
G05.3	Encephalitis and encephalomyelitis in diseases classified elsewhere
G05.4	Myelitis in diseases classified elsewhere
G11.1	Early-onset cerebellar ataxia
G12.20	Motor neuron disease, unspecified
G12.29	Other motor neuron disease
G37.3	Acute transverse myelitis in demyelinating disease of central nervous system
G37.4	Subacute necrotizing myelitis of central nervous system
G44.52	New daily persistent headache (NDPH)
I60.8	Other nontraumatic subarachnoid hemorrhage
I60.9	Nontraumatic subarachnoid hemorrhage, unspecified
P10.3	Subarachnoid hemorrhage due to birth injury
R51	Headache

CCI Edits

Refer to Appendix A for CCI edits.

Pub 100

00635: Pub 100-04, 12, 140.5, Pub 100-04, 12, 50, Pub 100-04, 12, 90.4.5

Base Units

Global: XXX

Code	Base Units
00635	4

Modifiers (PAR)

Code	Mod 50	Mod 51	Mod 62	Mod 80
00635	9	9	9	9

CPT © 2018 American Medical Association. All Rights Reserved.

00640

00640 Anesthesia for manipulation of the spine or for closed procedures on the cervical, thoracic or lumbar spine

ICD-10-CM Diagnostic Codes

⓻	M80.08	Age-related osteoporosis with current pathological fracture, vertebra(e)
⓻	S12.290	Other displaced fracture of third cervical vertebra
⓻	S12.390	Other displaced fracture of fourth cervical vertebra
⓻	S12.490	Other displaced fracture of fifth cervical vertebra
⓻	S12.590	Other displaced fracture of sixth cervical vertebra
⓻	S12.690	Other displaced fracture of seventh cervical vertebra
⓻	S13.140	Subluxation of C3/C4 cervical vertebrae
⓻	S13.141	Dislocation of C3/C4 cervical vertebrae
⓻	S13.150	Subluxation of C4/C5 cervical vertebrae
⓻	S13.151	Dislocation of C4/C5 cervical vertebrae
⓻	S13.160	Subluxation of C5/C6 cervical vertebrae
⓻	S13.161	Dislocation of C5/C6 cervical vertebrae
⓻	S13.170	Subluxation of C6/C7 cervical vertebrae
⓻	S13.171	Dislocation of C6/C7 cervical vertebrae
⓻	S13.180	Subluxation of C7/T1 cervical vertebrae
⓻	S13.181	Dislocation of C7/T1 cervical vertebrae
⓻	S22.010	Wedge compression fracture of first thoracic vertebra
⓻	S22.020	Wedge compression fracture of second thoracic vertebra
⓻	S22.030	Wedge compression fracture of third thoracic vertebra
⓻	S22.040	Wedge compression fracture of fourth thoracic vertebra
⓻	S22.050	Wedge compression fracture of T5-T6 vertebra
⓻	S22.060	Wedge compression fracture of T7-T8 vertebra
⓻	S22.070	Wedge compression fracture of T9-T10 vertebra
⓻	S22.080	Wedge compression fracture of T11-T12 vertebra
⓻	S23.110	Subluxation of T1/T2 thoracic vertebra
⓻	S23.111	Dislocation of T1/T2 thoracic vertebra
⓻	S23.120	Subluxation of T2/T3 thoracic vertebra
⓻	S23.121	Dislocation of T2/T3 thoracic vertebra
⓻	S23.122	Subluxation of T3/T4 thoracic vertebra
⓻	S23.123	Dislocation of T3/T4 thoracic vertebra
⓻	S23.130	Subluxation of T4/T5 thoracic vertebra
⓻	S23.131	Dislocation of T4/T5 thoracic vertebra
⓻	S23.132	Subluxation of T5/T6 thoracic vertebra
⓻	S23.133	Dislocation of T5/T6 thoracic vertebra
⓻	S23.140	Subluxation of T6/T7 thoracic vertebra
⓻	S23.141	Dislocation of T6/T7 thoracic vertebra
⓻	S23.142	Subluxation of T7/T8 thoracic vertebra
⓻	S23.143	Dislocation of T7/T8 thoracic vertebra
⓻	S23.150	Subluxation of T8/T9 thoracic vertebra
⓻	S23.151	Dislocation of T8/T9 thoracic vertebra
⓻	S23.152	Subluxation of T9/T10 thoracic vertebra
⓻	S23.153	Dislocation of T9/T10 thoracic vertebra
⓻	S23.160	Subluxation of T10/T11 thoracic vertebra
⓻	S23.161	Dislocation of T10/T11 thoracic vertebra
⓻	S23.162	Subluxation of T11/T12 thoracic vertebra
⓻	S23.163	Dislocation of T11/T12 thoracic vertebra
⓻	S23.170	Subluxation of T12/L1 thoracic vertebra
⓻	S23.171	Dislocation of T12/L1 thoracic vertebra
⓻	S32.010	Wedge compression fracture of first lumbar vertebra
⓻	S32.020	Wedge compression fracture of second lumbar vertebra
⓻	S32.030	Wedge compression fracture of third lumbar vertebra
⓻	S32.040	Wedge compression fracture of fourth lumbar vertebra
⓻	S32.050	Wedge compression fracture of fifth lumbar vertebra
⓻	S33.110	Subluxation of L1/L2 lumbar vertebra
⓻	S33.111	Dislocation of L1/L2 lumbar vertebra
⓻	S33.120	Subluxation of L2/L3 lumbar vertebra
⓻	S33.121	Dislocation of L2/L3 lumbar vertebra
⓻	S33.130	Subluxation of L3/L4 lumbar vertebra
⓻	S33.131	Dislocation of L3/L4 lumbar vertebra
⓻	S33.140	Subluxation of L4/L5 lumbar vertebra
⓻	S33.141	Dislocation of L4/L5 lumbar vertebra

ICD-10-CM Coding Notes

For codes requiring a 7th character extension, refer to your ICD-10-CM book. Review the character descriptions and coding guidelines for proper selection. For some procedures, only certain characters will apply.

CCI Edits

Refer to Appendix A for CCI edits.

Pub 100

00640: Pub 100-04, 12, 140.5, Pub 100-04, 12, 50, Pub 100-04, 12, 90.4.5

Base Units

Global: XXX

Code	Base Units
00640	3

Modifiers (PAR)

Code	Mod 50	Mod 51	Mod 62	Mod 80
00640	9	9	9	9

CPT © 2018 American Medical Association. All Rights Reserved.

00670

00670 Anesthesia for extensive spine and spinal cord procedures (eg, spinal instrumentation or vascular procedures)

AMA *CPT Assistant*

00670: Nov 07: 8, Jul 12: 13

ICD-10-CM Diagnostic Codes

C41.2	Malignant neoplasm of vertebral column
C72.0	Malignant neoplasm of spinal cord
M40.12	Other secondary kyphosis, cervical region
M40.13	Other secondary kyphosis, cervicothoracic region
M40.14	Other secondary kyphosis, thoracic region
M40.15	Other secondary kyphosis, thoracolumbar region
M40.292	Other kyphosis, cervical region
M40.293	Other kyphosis, cervicothoracic region
M40.294	Other kyphosis, thoracic region
M40.295	Other kyphosis, thoracolumbar region
M41.02	Infantile idiopathic scoliosis, cervical region
M41.03	Infantile idiopathic scoliosis, cervicothoracic region
M41.04	Infantile idiopathic scoliosis, thoracic region
M41.05	Infantile idiopathic scoliosis, thoracolumbar region
M41.06	Infantile idiopathic scoliosis, lumbar region
M41.07	Infantile idiopathic scoliosis, lumbosacral region
M41.08	Infantile idiopathic scoliosis, sacral and sacrococcygeal region
M41.112	Juvenile idiopathic scoliosis, cervical region
M41.113	Juvenile idiopathic scoliosis, cervicothoracic region
M41.114	Juvenile idiopathic scoliosis, thoracic region
M41.115	Juvenile idiopathic scoliosis, thoracolumbar region
M41.116	Juvenile idiopathic scoliosis, lumbar region
M41.117	Juvenile idiopathic scoliosis, lumbosacral region
M41.122	Adolescent idiopathic scoliosis, cervical region
M41.123	Adolescent idiopathic scoliosis, cervicothoracic region
M41.124	Adolescent idiopathic scoliosis, thoracic region
M41.125	Adolescent idiopathic scoliosis, thoracolumbar region
M41.126	Adolescent idiopathic scoliosis, lumbar region
M41.127	Adolescent idiopathic scoliosis, lumbosacral region
Q05.0	Cervical spina bifida with hydrocephalus
Q05.1	Thoracic spina bifida with hydrocephalus
Q05.2	Lumbar spina bifida with hydrocephalus
Q05.5	Cervical spina bifida without hydrocephalus
Q05.6	Thoracic spina bifida without hydrocephalus
Q05.7	Lumbar spina bifida without hydrocephalus
Q76.2	Congenital spondylolisthesis
Q76.3	Congenital scoliosis due to congenital bony malformation
Q76.411	Congenital kyphosis, occipito-atlanto-axial region
Q76.412	Congenital kyphosis, cervical region
Q76.413	Congenital kyphosis, cervicothoracic region
Q76.414	Congenital kyphosis, thoracic region

CCI Edits

Refer to Appendix A for CCI edits.

Pub 100

00670: Pub 100-04, 12, 140.5, Pub 100-04, 12, 50, Pub 100-04, 12, 90.4.5

Base Units

Global: XXX

Code	Base Units
00670	13

Modifiers (PAR)

Code	Mod 50	Mod 51	Mod 62	Mod 80
00670	9	9	9	9

CPT © 2018 American Medical Association. All Rights Reserved.

00700

00700 Anesthesia for procedures on upper anterior abdominal wall; not otherwise specified

AMA *CPT Assistant*

00700: Mar 06: 15, Nov 07: 8, Oct 11: 3, Jul 12: 13

ICD-10-CM Diagnostic Codes

	C49.4	Malignant neoplasm of connective and soft tissue of abdomen
	C79.89	Secondary malignant neoplasm of other specified sites
	D17.39	Benign lipomatous neoplasm of skin and subcutaneous tissue of other sites
	D17.9	Benign lipomatous neoplasm, unspecified
	D21.4	Benign neoplasm of connective and other soft tissue of abdomen
	D48.1	Neoplasm of uncertain behavior of connective and other soft tissue
	D49.2	Neoplasm of unspecified behavior of bone, soft tissue, and skin
➐⇄	S31.100	Unspecified open wound of abdominal wall, right upper quadrant without penetration into peritoneal cavity
➐⇄	S31.101	Unspecified open wound of abdominal wall, left upper quadrant without penetration into peritoneal cavity
➐⇄	S31.102	Unspecified open wound of abdominal wall, epigastric region without penetration into peritoneal cavity
➐⇄	S31.105	Unspecified open wound of abdominal wall, periumbilic region without penetration into peritoneal cavity
➐⇄	S31.110	Laceration without foreign body of abdominal wall, right upper quadrant without penetration into peritoneal cavity
➐⇄	S31.111	Laceration without foreign body of abdominal wall, left upper quadrant without penetration into peritoneal cavity
➐⇄	S31.112	Laceration without foreign body of abdominal wall, epigastric region without penetration into peritoneal cavity
➐⇄	S31.115	Laceration without foreign body of abdominal wall, periumbilic region without penetration into peritoneal cavity
➐⇄	S31.120	Laceration of abdominal wall with foreign body, right upper quadrant without penetration into peritoneal cavity
➐⇄	S31.121	Laceration of abdominal wall with foreign body, left upper quadrant without penetration into peritoneal cavity
➐⇄	S31.122	Laceration of abdominal wall with foreign body, epigastric region without penetration into peritoneal cavity
➐⇄	S31.125	Laceration of abdominal wall with foreign body, periumbilic region without penetration into peritoneal cavity
➐⇄	S31.130	Puncture wound of abdominal wall without foreign body, right upper quadrant without penetration into peritoneal cavity
➐⇄	S31.131	Puncture wound of abdominal wall without foreign body, left upper quadrant without penetration into peritoneal cavity
➐⇄	S31.132	Puncture wound of abdominal wall without foreign body, epigastric region without penetration into peritoneal cavity
➐⇄	S31.135	Puncture wound of abdominal wall without foreign body, periumbilic region without penetration into peritoneal cavity
➐⇄	S31.140	Puncture wound of abdominal wall with foreign body, right upper quadrant without penetration into peritoneal cavity
➐⇄	S31.141	Puncture wound of abdominal wall with foreign body, left upper quadrant without penetration into peritoneal cavity
➐⇄	S31.142	Puncture wound of abdominal wall with foreign body, epigastric region without penetration into peritoneal cavity
➐⇄	S31.145	Puncture wound of abdominal wall with foreign body, periumbilic region without penetration into peritoneal cavity
➐⇄	S31.150	Open bite of abdominal wall, right upper quadrant without penetration into peritoneal cavity
➐⇄	S31.151	Open bite of abdominal wall, left upper quadrant without penetration into peritoneal cavity
➐⇄	S31.152	Open bite of abdominal wall, epigastric region without penetration into peritoneal cavity
➐⇄	S31.155	Open bite of abdominal wall, periumbilic region without penetration into peritoneal cavity
➐	S39.021	Laceration of muscle, fascia and tendon of abdomen

ICD-10-CM Coding Notes

For codes requiring a 7th character extension, refer to your ICD-10-CM book. Review the character descriptions and coding guidelines for proper selection. For some procedures, only certain characters will apply.

CCI Edits

Refer to Appendix A for CCI edits.

Pub 100

00700: Pub 100-04, 12, 140.5, Pub 100-04, 12, 50, Pub 100-04, 12, 90.4.5

Base Units

Global: XXX

Code	Base Units
00700	4

Modifiers (PAR)

Code	Mod 50	Mod 51	Mod 62	Mod 80
00700	9	9	9	9

CPT © 2018 American Medical Association. All Rights Reserved.

00702

00702 Anesthesia for procedures on upper anterior abdominal wall; percutaneous liver biopsy

ICD-10-CM Diagnostic Codes

C22.0	Liver cell carcinoma
C22.1	Intrahepatic bile duct carcinoma
C22.2	Hepatoblastoma
C22.3	Angiosarcoma of liver
C22.4	Other sarcomas of liver
C22.7	Other specified carcinomas of liver
C22.8	Malignant neoplasm of liver, primary, unspecified as to type
C22.9	Malignant neoplasm of liver, not specified as primary or secondary
C24.0	Malignant neoplasm of extrahepatic bile duct
C78.7	Secondary malignant neoplasm of liver and intrahepatic bile duct
C78.89	Secondary malignant neoplasm of other digestive organs
D01.5	Carcinoma in situ of liver, gallbladder and bile ducts
D13.4	Benign neoplasm of liver
D37.6	Neoplasm of uncertain behavior of liver, gallbladder and bile ducts
D49.0	Neoplasm of unspecified behavior of digestive system
D86.89	Sarcoidosis of other sites
E83.01	Wilson's disease
E83.110	Hereditary hemochromatosis
E83.111	Hemochromatosis due to repeated red blood cell transfusions
E83.118	Other hemochromatosis
E83.119	Hemochromatosis, unspecified
K71.0	Toxic liver disease with cholestasis
K73.0	Chronic persistent hepatitis, not elsewhere classified
K74.0	Hepatic fibrosis
K74.60	Unspecified cirrhosis of liver
K74.69	Other cirrhosis of liver
K75.2	Nonspecific reactive hepatitis
K75.3	Granulomatous hepatitis, not elsewhere classified
K75.4	Autoimmune hepatitis
K75.81	Nonalcoholic steatohepatitis (NASH)
K75.89	Other specified inflammatory liver diseases
K75.9	Inflammatory liver disease, unspecified
K76.89	Other specified diseases of liver
R16.0	Hepatomegaly, not elsewhere classified
R16.2	Hepatomegaly with splenomegaly, not elsewhere classified
R17	Unspecified jaundice
⇄ R19.01	Right upper quadrant abdominal swelling, mass and lump
R94.5	Abnormal results of liver function studies
Z94.4	Liver transplant status

CCI Edits

Refer to Appendix A for CCI edits.

Pub 100

00702: Pub 100-04, 12, 140.5, Pub 100-04, 12, 50, Pub 100-04, 12, 90.4.5

Base Units

Global: XXX

Code	Base Units
00702	4

Modifiers (PAR)

Code	Mod 50	Mod 51	Mod 62	Mod 80
00702	9	9	9	9

CPT © 2018 American Medical Association. All Rights Reserved.

00730

00730 Anesthesia for procedures on upper posterior abdominal wall

ICD-10-CM Diagnostic Codes

	C49.6	Malignant neoplasm of connective and soft tissue of trunk, unspecified
	C79.89	Secondary malignant neoplasm of other specified sites
	D17.39	Benign lipomatous neoplasm of skin and subcutaneous tissue of other sites
	D17.9	Benign lipomatous neoplasm, unspecified
	D21.6	Benign neoplasm of connective and other soft tissue of trunk, unspecified
	D48.1	Neoplasm of uncertain behavior of connective and other soft tissue
	D49.2	Neoplasm of unspecified behavior of bone, soft tissue, and skin
➐⇄	S31.110	Laceration without foreign body of abdominal wall, right upper quadrant without penetration into peritoneal cavity
➐⇄	S31.111	Laceration without foreign body of abdominal wall, left upper quadrant without penetration into peritoneal cavity
➐⇄	S31.120	Laceration of abdominal wall with foreign body, right upper quadrant without penetration into peritoneal cavity
➐⇄	S31.121	Laceration of abdominal wall with foreign body, left upper quadrant without penetration into peritoneal cavity
➐⇄	S31.130	Puncture wound of abdominal wall without foreign body, right upper quadrant without penetration into peritoneal cavity
➐⇄	S31.131	Puncture wound of abdominal wall without foreign body, left upper quadrant without penetration into peritoneal cavity
➐⇄	S31.140	Puncture wound of abdominal wall with foreign body, right upper quadrant without penetration into peritoneal cavity
➐⇄	S31.141	Puncture wound of abdominal wall with foreign body, left upper quadrant without penetration into peritoneal cavity
➐⇄	S31.150	Open bite of abdominal wall, right upper quadrant without penetration into peritoneal cavity
➐⇄	S31.151	Open bite of abdominal wall, left upper quadrant without penetration into peritoneal cavity
➐	S39.021	Laceration of muscle, fascia and tendon of abdomen

ICD-10-CM Coding Notes

For codes requiring a 7th character extension, refer to your ICD-10-CM book. Review the character descriptions and coding guidelines for proper selection. For some procedures, only certain characters will apply.

CCI Edits

Refer to Appendix A for CCI edits.

Pub 100

00730: Pub 100-04, 12, 140.5, Pub 100-04, 12, 50, Pub 100-04, 12, 90.4.5

Base Units

Global: XXX

Code	Base Units
00730	5

Modifiers (PAR)

Code	Mod 50	Mod 51	Mod 62	Mod 80
00730	9	9	9	9

CPT © 2018 American Medical Association. All Rights Reserved.

00731-00732

00731 Anesthesia for upper gastrointestinal endoscopic procedures, endoscope introduced proximal to duodenum; not otherwise specified

00732 Anesthesia for upper gastrointestinal endoscopic procedures, endoscope introduced proximal to duodenum; endoscopic retrograde cholangiopancreatography (ERCP)

(For combined upper and lower gastrointestinal endoscopic procedures, use 00813)

AMA *CPT Assistant* ☐

00731: Dec 17: 8
00732: Dec 17: 8

ICD-10-CM Diagnostic Codes

K21.0	Gastro-esophageal reflux disease with esophagitis
K22.0	Achalasia of cardia
K22.710	Barrett's esophagus with low grade dysplasia
K22.711	Barrett's esophagus with high grade dysplasia
K22.8	Other specified diseases of esophagus
K25.4	Chronic or unspecified gastric ulcer with hemorrhage
K25.5	Chronic or unspecified gastric ulcer with perforation
K25.6	Chronic or unspecified gastric ulcer with both hemorrhage and perforation
K25.7	Chronic gastric ulcer without hemorrhage or perforation
K25.9	Gastric ulcer, unspecified as acute or chronic, without hemorrhage or perforation
K56.50	Intestinal adhesions [bands], unspecified as to partial versus complete obstruction
K56.51	Intestinal adhesions [bands], with partial obstruction
K56.52	Intestinal adhesions [bands] with complete obstruction
K56.600	Partial intestinal obstruction, unspecified as to cause
K56.601	Complete intestinal obstruction, unspecified as to cause
K56.609	Unspecified intestinal obstruction, unspecified as to partial versus complete obstruction
K56.690	Other partial intestinal obstruction
K56.691	Other complete intestinal obstruction
K56.699	Other intestinal obstruction unspecified as to partial versus complete obstruction
K90.0	Celiac disease
K91.30	Postprocedural intestinal obstruction, unspecified as to partial versus complete
K91.31	Postprocedural partial intestinal obstruction
K91.32	Postprocedural complete intestinal obstruction
K92.0	Hematemesis
K92.2	Gastrointestinal hemorrhage, unspecified
P54.0	Neonatal hematemesis
P92.09	Other vomiting of newborn
⇄ R10.11	Right upper quadrant pain
⇄ R10.12	Left upper quadrant pain
R10.13	Epigastric pain
R11.11	Vomiting without nausea
R11.12	Projectile vomiting
R11.13	Vomiting of fecal matter
R11.2	Nausea with vomiting, unspecified
R12	Heartburn
R13.0	Aphagia
R13.14	Dysphagia, pharyngoesophageal phase
R63.4	Abnormal weight loss

CCI Edits

Refer to Appendix A for CCI edits.

Pub 100

00731: Pub 100-04, 12, 140.5, Pub 100-04, 12, 50, Pub 100-04, 12, 90.4.5, Pub 100-04, 6, 20.6
00732: Pub 100-04, 12, 140.5, Pub 100-04, 12, 50, Pub 100-04, 12, 90.4.5, Pub 100-04, 6, 20.6

Base Units

Global: XXX

Code	Base Units
00731	5
00732	6

Modifiers (PAR)

Code	Mod 50	Mod 51	Mod 62	Mod 80
00731	9	9	9	9
00732	9	9	9	9

CPT © 2018 American Medical Association. All Rights Reserved.

00750

00750 Anesthesia for hernia repairs in upper abdomen; not otherwise specified

ICD-10-CM Diagnostic Codes

K42.0	Umbilical hernia with obstruction, without gangrene
K42.1	Umbilical hernia with gangrene
K42.9	Umbilical hernia without obstruction or gangrene
K45.0	Other specified abdominal hernia with obstruction, without gangrene
K45.1	Other specified abdominal hernia with gangrene
K45.8	Other specified abdominal hernia without obstruction or gangrene
K46.0	Unspecified abdominal hernia with obstruction, without gangrene
K46.1	Unspecified abdominal hernia with gangrene
K46.9	Unspecified abdominal hernia without obstruction or gangrene

CCI Edits

Refer to Appendix A for CCI edits.

Pub 100

00750: Pub 100-04, 12, 140.5, Pub 100-04, 12, 50, Pub 100-04, 12, 90.4.5

Base Units

Global: XXX

Code	Base Units
00750	4

Modifiers (PAR)

Code	Mod 50	Mod 51	Mod 62	Mod 80
00750	9	9	9	9

CPT © 2018 American Medical Association. All Rights Reserved.

00752

00752 Anesthesia for hernia repairs in upper abdomen; lumbar and ventral (incisional) hernias and/or wound dehiscence

ICD-10-CM Diagnostic Codes

	K43.0	Incisional hernia with obstruction, without gangrene
	K43.1	Incisional hernia with gangrene
	K43.2	Incisional hernia without obstruction or gangrene
	K43.3	Parastomal hernia with obstruction, without gangrene
	K43.4	Parastomal hernia with gangrene
	K43.5	Parastomal hernia without obstruction or gangrene
	K43.6	Other and unspecified ventral hernia with obstruction, without gangrene
	K43.7	Other and unspecified ventral hernia with gangrene
	K43.9	Ventral hernia without obstruction or gangrene
	K45.0	Other specified abdominal hernia with obstruction, without gangrene
	K45.1	Other specified abdominal hernia with gangrene
	K45.8	Other specified abdominal hernia without obstruction or gangrene
	O90.0	Disruption of cesarean delivery wound ♀
⓻	T81.30	Disruption of wound, unspecified
⓻	T81.31	Disruption of external operation (surgical) wound, not elsewhere classified
⓻	T81.32	Disruption of internal operation (surgical) wound, not elsewhere classified
⓻	T81.33	Disruption of traumatic injury wound repair

ICD-10-CM Coding Notes

For codes requiring a 7th character extension, refer to your ICD-10-CM book. Review the character descriptions and coding guidelines for proper selection. For some procedures, only certain characters will apply.

CCI Edits

Refer to Appendix A for CCI edits.

Pub 100

00752: Pub 100-04, 12, 140.5, Pub 100-04, 12, 50, Pub 100-04, 12, 90.4.5

Base Units

Global: XXX

Code	Base Units
00752	6

Modifiers (PAR)

Code	Mod 50	Mod 51	Mod 62	Mod 80
00752	9	9	9	9

● New ▲ Revised ✚ Add On ⊘Modifier 51 Exempt ★Telemedicine ▯ CPT QuickRef ⁄FDA Pending ⇄ Laterality ⓻ Seventh Character ♂Male ♀Female

CPT © 2018 American Medical Association. All Rights Reserved.

00754

00754 Anesthesia for hernia repairs in upper abdomen; omphalocele

ICD-10-CM Diagnostic Codes

Q79.2	Exomphalos
Q79.59	Other congenital malformations of abdominal wall

CCI Edits

Refer to Appendix A for CCI edits.

Pub 100

00754: Pub 100-04, 12, 140.5, Pub 100-04, 12, 50, Pub 100-04, 12, 90.4.5

Base Units

Global: XXX

Code	Base Units
00754	7

Modifiers (PAR)

Code	Mod 50	Mod 51	Mod 62	Mod 80
00754	9	9	9	9

CPT © 2018 American Medical Association. All Rights Reserved.

00756

00756 Anesthesia for hernia repairs in upper abdomen; transabdominal repair of diaphragmatic hernia

ICD-10-CM Diagnostic Codes

K44.0	Diaphragmatic hernia with obstruction, without gangrene
K44.1	Diaphragmatic hernia with gangrene
K44.9	Diaphragmatic hernia without obstruction or gangrene
Q40.1	Congenital hiatus hernia
Q79.0	Congenital diaphragmatic hernia

CCI Edits

Refer to Appendix A for CCI edits.

Pub 100

00756: Pub 100-04, 12, 140.5, Pub 100-04, 12, 50, Pub 100-04, 12, 90.4.5

Base Units

Global: XXX

Code	Base Units
00756	7

Modifiers (PAR)

Code	Mod 50	Mod 51	Mod 62	Mod 80
00756	9	9	9	9

CPT © 2018 American Medical Association. All Rights Reserved.

00770

00770 Anesthesia for all procedures on major abdominal blood vessels

ICD-10-CM Diagnostic Codes

	I70.0	Atherosclerosis of aorta
	I70.1	Atherosclerosis of renal artery
	I71.02	Dissection of abdominal aorta
	I71.4	Abdominal aortic aneurysm, without rupture
	I72.2	Aneurysm of renal artery
	I72.3	Aneurysm of iliac artery
	I74.01	Saddle embolus of abdominal aorta
	I74.09	Other arterial embolism and thrombosis of abdominal aorta
	I77.72	Dissection of iliac artery
	I77.73	Dissection of renal artery
	I79.0	Aneurysm of aorta in diseases classified elsewhere
	I82.220	Acute embolism and thrombosis of inferior vena cava
	I82.221	Chronic embolism and thrombosis of inferior vena cava
⇄	I82.421	Acute embolism and thrombosis of right iliac vein
⇄	I82.422	Acute embolism and thrombosis of left iliac vein
⇄	I82.423	Acute embolism and thrombosis of iliac vein, bilateral
	I97.410	Intraoperative hemorrhage and hematoma of a circulatory system organ or structure complicating a cardiac catheterization
	I97.51	Accidental puncture and laceration of a circulatory system organ or structure during a circulatory system procedure
	I97.52	Accidental puncture and laceration of a circulatory system organ or structure during other procedure
	I97.610	Postprocedural hemorrhage of a circulatory system organ or structure following a cardiac catheterization
❼	S35.01	Minor laceration of abdominal aorta
❼	S35.02	Major laceration of abdominal aorta
❼	S35.11	Minor laceration of inferior vena cava
❼	S35.12	Major laceration of inferior vena cava
❼	S35.211	Minor laceration of celiac artery
❼	S35.212	Major laceration of celiac artery
❼	S35.221	Minor laceration of superior mesenteric artery
❼	S35.222	Major laceration of superior mesenteric artery
❼	S35.231	Minor laceration of inferior mesenteric artery
❼	S35.232	Major laceration of inferior mesenteric artery
❼	S35.311	Laceration of portal vein
❼	S35.321	Laceration of splenic vein
❼	S35.331	Laceration of superior mesenteric vein
❼	S35.341	Laceration of inferior mesenteric vein
❼⇄	S35.411	Laceration of right renal artery
❼⇄	S35.412	Laceration of left renal artery
❼⇄	S35.414	Laceration of right renal vein
❼⇄	S35.415	Laceration of left renal vein
❼⇄	S35.511	Injury of right iliac artery
❼⇄	S35.512	Injury of left iliac artery
❼⇄	S35.514	Injury of right iliac vein
❼⇄	S35.515	Injury of left iliac vein
❼	S35.8X1	Laceration of other blood vessels at abdomen, lower back and pelvis level

ICD-10-CM Coding Notes

For codes requiring a 7th character extension, refer to your ICD-10-CM book. Review the character descriptions and coding guidelines for proper selection. For some procedures, only certain characters will apply.

CCI Edits

Refer to Appendix A for CCI edits.

Pub 100

00770: Pub 100-04, 12, 140.5, Pub 100-04, 12, 50, Pub 100-04, 12, 90.4.5

Base Units

Global: XXX

Code	Base Units
00770	15

Modifiers (PAR)

Code	Mod 50	Mod 51	Mod 62	Mod 80
00770	9	9	9	9

CPT © 2018 American Medical Association. All Rights Reserved.

00790

00790 Anesthesia for intraperitoneal procedures in upper abdomen including laparoscopy; not otherwise specified

ICD-10-CM Diagnostic Codes

C15.5	Malignant neoplasm of lower third of esophagus
C16.0	Malignant neoplasm of cardia
C16.1	Malignant neoplasm of fundus of stomach
C16.2	Malignant neoplasm of body of stomach
C16.3	Malignant neoplasm of pyloric antrum
C16.4	Malignant neoplasm of pylorus
C16.5	Malignant neoplasm of lesser curvature of stomach, unspecified
C16.6	Malignant neoplasm of greater curvature of stomach, unspecified
C16.8	Malignant neoplasm of overlapping sites of stomach
C17.0	Malignant neoplasm of duodenum
K25.0	Acute gastric ulcer with hemorrhage
K25.1	Acute gastric ulcer with perforation
K25.2	Acute gastric ulcer with both hemorrhage and perforation
K25.4	Chronic or unspecified gastric ulcer with hemorrhage
K25.5	Chronic or unspecified gastric ulcer with perforation
K25.6	Chronic or unspecified gastric ulcer with both hemorrhage and perforation
K50.012	Crohn's disease of small intestine with intestinal obstruction
K50.013	Crohn's disease of small intestine with fistula
K50.014	Crohn's disease of small intestine with abscess
K57.00	Diverticulitis of small intestine with perforation and abscess without bleeding
K57.01	Diverticulitis of small intestine with perforation and abscess with bleeding
K66.0	Peritoneal adhesions (postprocedural) (postinfection)
K80.01	Calculus of gallbladder with acute cholecystitis with obstruction
K80.11	Calculus of gallbladder with chronic cholecystitis with obstruction
K80.13	Calculus of gallbladder with acute and chronic cholecystitis with obstruction
K80.19	Calculus of gallbladder with other cholecystitis with obstruction
K80.33	Calculus of bile duct with acute cholangitis with obstruction
K80.35	Calculus of bile duct with chronic cholangitis with obstruction
K80.37	Calculus of bile duct with acute and chronic cholangitis with obstruction
K80.43	Calculus of bile duct with acute cholecystitis with obstruction
K80.45	Calculus of bile duct with chronic cholecystitis with obstruction
K80.47	Calculus of bile duct with acute and chronic cholecystitis with obstruction
K82.0	Obstruction of gallbladder
K82.2	Perforation of gallbladder
K82.A1	Gangrene of gallbladder in cholecystitis
K82.A2	Perforation of gallbladder in cholecystitis
K83.2	Perforation of bile duct
K91.31	Postprocedural partial intestinal obstruction
K91.32	Postprocedural complete intestinal obstruction
Q41.0	Congenital absence, atresia and stenosis of duodenum
Q44.2	Atresia of bile ducts
Q44.3	Congenital stenosis and stricture of bile ducts
Q44.5	Other congenital malformations of bile ducts

CCI Edits

Refer to Appendix A for CCI edits.

Pub 100

00790: Pub 100-04, 12, 140.5, Pub 100-04, 12, 50, Pub 100-04, 12, 90.4.5

Base Units

Global: XXX

Code	Base Units
00790	7

Modifiers (PAR)

Code	Mod 50	Mod 51	Mod 62	Mod 80
00790	9	9	9	9

CPT © 2018 American Medical Association. All Rights Reserved.

00792

00792 Anesthesia for intraperitoneal procedures in upper abdomen including laparoscopy; partial hepatectomy or management of liver hemorrhage (excluding liver biopsy)

ICD-10-CM Diagnostic Codes

	C22.0	Liver cell carcinoma
	C22.1	Intrahepatic bile duct carcinoma
	C22.2	Hepatoblastoma
	C22.3	Angiosarcoma of liver
	C22.4	Other sarcomas of liver
	C22.7	Other specified carcinomas of liver
	C22.8	Malignant neoplasm of liver, primary, unspecified as to type
	C22.9	Malignant neoplasm of liver, not specified as primary or secondary
	C24.0	Malignant neoplasm of extrahepatic bile duct
	C78.7	Secondary malignant neoplasm of liver and intrahepatic bile duct
	D01.5	Carcinoma in situ of liver, gallbladder and bile ducts
	D13.4	Benign neoplasm of liver
	D37.6	Neoplasm of uncertain behavior of liver, gallbladder and bile ducts
	D49.0	Neoplasm of unspecified behavior of digestive system
	K91.61	Intraoperative hemorrhage and hematoma of a digestive system organ or structure complicating a digestive system procedure
	K91.62	Intraoperative hemorrhage and hematoma of a digestive system organ or structure complicating other procedure
	K91.71	Accidental puncture and laceration of a digestive system organ or structure during a digestive system procedure
	K91.72	Accidental puncture and laceration of a digestive system organ or structure during other procedure
	K91.840	Postprocedural hemorrhage of a digestive system organ or structure following a digestive system procedure
	K91.841	Postprocedural hemorrhage of a digestive system organ or structure following other procedure
➐	S36.113	Laceration of liver, unspecified degree
➐	S36.114	Minor laceration of liver
➐	S36.115	Moderate laceration of liver
➐	S36.116	Major laceration of liver
➐	S36.118	Other injury of liver

ICD-10-CM Coding Notes

For codes requiring a 7th character extension, refer to your ICD-10-CM book. Review the character descriptions and coding guidelines for proper selection. For some procedures, only certain characters will apply.

CCI Edits

Refer to Appendix A for CCI edits.

Pub 100

00792: Pub 100-04, 12, 140.5, Pub 100-04, 12, 50, Pub 100-04, 12, 90.4.5

Base Units

Global: XXX

Code	Base Units
00792	13

Modifiers (PAR)

Code	Mod 50	Mod 51	Mod 62	Mod 80
00792	9	9	9	9

CPT © 2018 American Medical Association. All Rights Reserved.

00794

00794 Anesthesia for intraperitoneal procedures in upper abdomen including laparoscopy; pancreatectomy, partial or total (eg, Whipple procedure)

ICD-10-CM Diagnostic Codes

	C25.0	Malignant neoplasm of head of pancreas
	C25.1	Malignant neoplasm of body of pancreas
	C25.2	Malignant neoplasm of tail of pancreas
	C25.3	Malignant neoplasm of pancreatic duct
	C25.4	Malignant neoplasm of endocrine pancreas
	C25.7	Malignant neoplasm of other parts of pancreas
	C25.8	Malignant neoplasm of overlapping sites of pancreas
	C25.9	Malignant neoplasm of pancreas, unspecified
	C78.89	Secondary malignant neoplasm of other digestive organs
	D01.7	Carcinoma in situ of other specified digestive organs
	D13.6	Benign neoplasm of pancreas
	D37.8	Neoplasm of uncertain behavior of other specified digestive organs
	K85.02	Idiopathic acute pancreatitis with infected necrosis
	K85.12	Biliary acute pancreatitis with infected necrosis
	K85.22	Alcohol induced acute pancreatitis with infected necrosis
	K85.32	Drug induced acute pancreatitis with infected necrosis
	K86.2	Cyst of pancreas
	K86.3	Pseudocyst of pancreas
	K86.89	Other specified diseases of pancreas
❼	S36.260	Major laceration of head of pancreas
❼	S36.261	Major laceration of body of pancreas
❼	S36.262	Major laceration of tail of pancreas
❼	S36.269	Major laceration of unspecified part of pancreas
❼	S36.290	Other injury of head of pancreas
❼	S36.291	Other injury of body of pancreas
❼	S36.292	Other injury of tail of pancreas
❼	S36.299	Other injury of unspecified part of pancreas

ICD-10-CM Coding Notes

For codes requiring a 7th character extension, refer to your ICD-10-CM book. Review the character descriptions and coding guidelines for proper selection. For some procedures, only certain characters will apply.

CCI Edits

Refer to Appendix A for CCI edits.

Pub 100

00794: Pub 100-04, 12, 140.5, Pub 100-04, 12, 50, Pub 100-04, 12, 90.4.5

Base Units

Global: XXX

Code	Base Units
00794	8

Modifiers (PAR)

Code	Mod 50	Mod 51	Mod 62	Mod 80
00794	9	9	9	9

CPT © 2018 American Medical Association. All Rights Reserved.

00796

00796 Anesthesia for intraperitoneal procedures in upper abdomen including laparoscopy; liver transplant (recipient)

(For harvesting of liver, use 01990)

ICD-10-CM Diagnostic Codes

B16.0	Acute hepatitis B with delta-agent with hepatic coma
B16.1	Acute hepatitis B with delta-agent without hepatic coma
B16.2	Acute hepatitis B without delta-agent with hepatic coma
B17.8	Other specified acute viral hepatitis
B18.0	Chronic viral hepatitis B with delta-agent
B18.1	Chronic viral hepatitis B without delta-agent
B18.2	Chronic viral hepatitis C
B18.8	Other chronic viral hepatitis
C22.0	Liver cell carcinoma
E70.21	Tyrosinemia
E83.01	Wilson's disease
E83.110	Hereditary hemochromatosis
E83.118	Other hemochromatosis
E88.01	Alpha-1-antitrypsin deficiency
K70.30	Alcoholic cirrhosis of liver without ascites
K70.31	Alcoholic cirrhosis of liver with ascites
K71.10	Toxic liver disease with hepatic necrosis, without coma
K71.11	Toxic liver disease with hepatic necrosis, with coma
K71.2	Toxic liver disease with acute hepatitis
K71.3	Toxic liver disease with chronic persistent hepatitis
K71.50	Toxic liver disease with chronic active hepatitis without ascites
K71.51	Toxic liver disease with chronic active hepatitis with ascites
K71.6	Toxic liver disease with hepatitis, not elsewhere classified
K71.7	Toxic liver disease with fibrosis and cirrhosis of liver
K72.00	Acute and subacute hepatic failure without coma
K72.01	Acute and subacute hepatic failure with coma
K72.10	Chronic hepatic failure without coma
K72.11	Chronic hepatic failure with coma
K73.0	Chronic persistent hepatitis, not elsewhere classified
K73.2	Chronic active hepatitis, not elsewhere classified
K73.8	Other chronic hepatitis, not elsewhere classified
K74.3	Primary biliary cirrhosis
K74.4	Secondary biliary cirrhosis
K74.60	Unspecified cirrhosis of liver
K74.69	Other cirrhosis of liver
K83.01	Primary sclerosing cholangitis
K83.09	Other cholangitis
Q44.2	Atresia of bile ducts
Q44.6	Cystic disease of liver

CCI Edits

Refer to Appendix A for CCI edits.

Pub 100

00796: Pub 100-04, 12, 140.5, Pub 100-04, 12, 50, Pub 100-04, 12, 90.4.5

Base Units

Global: XXX

Code	Base Units
00796	30

Modifiers (PAR)

Code	Mod 50	Mod 51	Mod 62	Mod 80
00796	9	9	9	9

CPT © 2018 American Medical Association. All Rights Reserved.

00797

00797 Anesthesia for intraperitoneal procedures in upper abdomen including laparoscopy; gastric restrictive procedure for morbid obesity

AMA *CPT Assistant*

00797: Nov 07: 8, Jul 12: 13

ICD-10-CM Diagnostic Codes

- E11.21 Type 2 diabetes mellitus with diabetic nephropathy
- E11.22 Type 2 diabetes mellitus with diabetic chronic kidney disease
- E11.29 Type 2 diabetes mellitus with other diabetic kidney complication
- E11.41 Type 2 diabetes mellitus with diabetic mononeuropathy
- E11.42 Type 2 diabetes mellitus with diabetic polyneuropathy
- E11.43 Type 2 diabetes mellitus with diabetic autonomic (poly) neuropathy
- E11.44 Type 2 diabetes mellitus with diabetic amyotrophy
- E11.49 Type 2 diabetes mellitus with other diabetic neurological complication
- E11.51 Type 2 diabetes mellitus with diabetic peripheral angiopathy without gangrene
- E11.59 Type 2 diabetes mellitus with other circulatory complications
- E11.65 Type 2 diabetes mellitus with hyperglycemia
- E11.69 Type 2 diabetes mellitus with other specified complication
- E66.01 Morbid (severe) obesity due to excess calories
- E66.09 Other obesity due to excess calories
- E66.2 Morbid (severe) obesity with alveolar hypoventilation
- K76.0 Fatty (change of) liver, not elsewhere classified
- Z68.35 Body mass index (BMI) 35.0-35.9, adult
- Z68.36 Body mass index (BMI) 36.0-36.9, adult
- Z68.37 Body mass index (BMI) 37.0-37.9, adult
- Z68.38 Body mass index (BMI) 38.0-38.9, adult
- Z68.39 Body mass index (BMI) 39.0-39.9, adult
- Z68.41 Body mass index (BMI) 40.0-44.9, adult
- Z68.42 Body mass index (BMI) 45.0-49.9, adult
- Z68.43 Body mass index (BMI) 50-59.9, adult
- Z68.44 Body mass index (BMI) 60.0-69.9, adult
- Z68.45 Body mass index (BMI) 70 or greater, adult

CCI Edits

Refer to Appendix A for CCI edits.

Pub 100

00797: Pub 100-04, 12, 140.5, Pub 100-04, 12, 50, Pub 100-04, 12, 90.4.5

Base Units

Global: XXX

Code	Base Units
00797	11

Modifiers (PAR)

Code	Mod 50	Mod 51	Mod 62	Mod 80
00797	9	9	9	9

CPT © 2018 American Medical Association. All Rights Reserved.

00800

00800 Anesthesia for procedures on lower anterior abdominal wall; not otherwise specified

AMA *CPT Assistant* □

00800: Mar 06: 15, Nov 07: 8, Oct 11: 3, Jul 12: 13

ICD-10-CM Diagnostic Codes

	C49.4	Malignant neoplasm of connective and soft tissue of abdomen
	C49.5	Malignant neoplasm of connective and soft tissue of pelvis
	C49.6	Malignant neoplasm of connective and soft tissue of trunk, unspecified
	C49.8	Malignant neoplasm of overlapping sites of connective and soft tissue
	C79.89	Secondary malignant neoplasm of other specified sites
	D21.4	Benign neoplasm of connective and other soft tissue of abdomen
	D21.6	Benign neoplasm of connective and other soft tissue of trunk, unspecified
	D48.1	Neoplasm of uncertain behavior of connective and other soft tissue
	D49.2	Neoplasm of unspecified behavior of bone, soft tissue, and skin
	K94.00	Colostomy complication, unspecified
	K94.01	Colostomy hemorrhage
	K94.02	Colostomy infection
	K94.03	Colostomy malfunction
	K94.09	Other complications of colostomy
	K94.10	Enterostomy complication, unspecified
	K94.11	Enterostomy hemorrhage
	K94.12	Enterostomy infection
	K94.13	Enterostomy malfunction
	K94.19	Other complications of enterostomy
	L02.211	Cutaneous abscess of abdominal wall
	L02.221	Furuncle of abdominal wall
	L02.231	Carbuncle of abdominal wall
	N99.510	Cystostomy hemorrhage
	N99.511	Cystostomy infection
	N99.512	Cystostomy malfunction
	N99.518	Other cystostomy complication
	Q79.59	Other congenital malformations of abdominal wall
⑦⇄	S31.113	Laceration without foreign body of abdominal wall, right lower quadrant without penetration into peritoneal cavity
⑦⇄	S31.114	Laceration without foreign body of abdominal wall, left lower quadrant without penetration into peritoneal cavity
⑦⇄	S31.115	Laceration without foreign body of abdominal wall, periumbilic region without penetration into peritoneal cavity
⑦⇄	S31.123	Laceration of abdominal wall with foreign body, right lower quadrant without penetration into peritoneal cavity
⑦⇄	S31.124	Laceration of abdominal wall with foreign body, left lower quadrant without penetration into peritoneal cavity
⑦⇄	S31.125	Laceration of abdominal wall with foreign body, periumbilic region without penetration into peritoneal cavity
⑦⇄	S31.133	Puncture wound of abdominal wall without foreign body, right lower quadrant without penetration into peritoneal cavity
⑦⇄	S31.134	Puncture wound of abdominal wall without foreign body, left lower quadrant without penetration into peritoneal cavity
⑦⇄	S31.135	Puncture wound of abdominal wall without foreign body, periumbilic region without penetration into peritoneal cavity
⑦⇄	S31.143	Puncture wound of abdominal wall with foreign body, right lower quadrant without penetration into peritoneal cavity
⑦⇄	S31.144	Puncture wound of abdominal wall with foreign body, left lower quadrant without penetration into peritoneal cavity
⑦⇄	S31.145	Puncture wound of abdominal wall with foreign body, periumbilic region without penetration into peritoneal cavity
⑦⇄	S31.153	Open bite of abdominal wall, right lower quadrant without penetration into peritoneal cavity
⑦⇄	S31.154	Open bite of abdominal wall, left lower quadrant without penetration into peritoneal cavity
⑦⇄	S31.155	Open bite of abdominal wall, periumbilic region without penetration into peritoneal cavity
⑦	T85.611	Breakdown (mechanical) of intraperitoneal dialysis catheter
⑦	T85.621	Displacement of intraperitoneal dialysis catheter
⑦	T85.691	Other mechanical complication of intraperitoneal dialysis catheter
⑦	T85.71	Infection and inflammatory reaction due to peritoneal dialysis catheter

ICD-10-CM Coding Notes

For codes requiring a 7th character extension, refer to your ICD-10-CM book. Review the character descriptions and coding guidelines for proper selection. For some procedures, only certain characters will apply.

CCI Edits

Refer to Appendix A for CCI edits.

Pub 100

00800: Pub 100-04, 12, 140.5, Pub 100-04, 12, 50, Pub 100-04, 12, 90.4.5

Base Units

Global: XXX

Code	Base Units
00800	4

Modifiers (PAR)

Code	Mod 50	Mod 51	Mod 62	Mod 80
00800	9	9	9	9

CPT © 2018 American Medical Association. All Rights Reserved.

00802

00802 Anesthesia for procedures on lower anterior abdominal wall; panniculectomy

ICD-10-CM Diagnostic Codes

E65	Localized adiposity
L91.8	Other hypertrophic disorders of the skin
L91.9	Hypertrophic disorder of the skin, unspecified
M79.3	Panniculitis, unspecified
Z98.84	Bariatric surgery status

CCI Edits

Refer to Appendix A for CCI edits.

Pub 100

00802: Pub 100-04, 12, 140.5, Pub 100-04, 12, 50, Pub 100-04, 12, 90.4.5

Base Units

Global: XXX

Code	Base Units
00802	5

Modifiers (PAR)

Code	Mod 50	Mod 51	Mod 62	Mod 80
00802	9	9	9	9

CPT © 2018 American Medical Association. All Rights Reserved.

00811-00812

00811 Anesthesia for lower intestinal endoscopic procedures, endoscope introduced distal to duodenum; not otherwise specified

00812 Anesthesia for lower intestinal endoscopic procedures, endoscope introduced distal to duodenum; screening colonoscopy

(Report 00812 to describe anesthesia for any screening colonoscopy regardless of ultimate findings)

AMA *CPT Assistant*

00811: Dec 17: 8
00812: Dec 17: 8

ICD-10-CM Diagnostic Codes

C18.0	Malignant neoplasm of cecum
C18.2	Malignant neoplasm of ascending colon
C18.3	Malignant neoplasm of hepatic flexure
C18.4	Malignant neoplasm of transverse colon
C18.5	Malignant neoplasm of splenic flexure
C18.6	Malignant neoplasm of descending colon
C18.7	Malignant neoplasm of sigmoid colon
C18.8	Malignant neoplasm of overlapping sites of colon
C18.9	Malignant neoplasm of colon, unspecified
C19	Malignant neoplasm of rectosigmoid junction
C20	Malignant neoplasm of rectum
C21.0	Malignant neoplasm of anus, unspecified
C21.8	Malignant neoplasm of overlapping sites of rectum, anus and anal canal
D01.0	Carcinoma in situ of colon
D01.1	Carcinoma in situ of rectosigmoid junction
D01.2	Carcinoma in situ of rectum
D01.3	Carcinoma in situ of anus and anal canal
D12.0	Benign neoplasm of cecum
D12.2	Benign neoplasm of ascending colon
D12.3	Benign neoplasm of transverse colon
D12.4	Benign neoplasm of descending colon
D12.5	Benign neoplasm of sigmoid colon
D12.6	Benign neoplasm of colon, unspecified
D12.7	Benign neoplasm of rectosigmoid junction
D12.8	Benign neoplasm of rectum
D12.9	Benign neoplasm of anus and anal canal
D50.0	Iron deficiency anemia secondary to blood loss (chronic)
K50.111	Crohn's disease of large intestine with rectal bleeding
K50.112	Crohn's disease of large intestine with intestinal obstruction
K50.113	Crohn's disease of large intestine with fistula
K50.114	Crohn's disease of large intestine with abscess
K50.118	Crohn's disease of large intestine with other complication
K50.119	Crohn's disease of large intestine with unspecified complications
K51.00	Ulcerative (chronic) pancolitis without complications
K51.011	Ulcerative (chronic) pancolitis with rectal bleeding
K51.012	Ulcerative (chronic) pancolitis with intestinal obstruction
K51.013	Ulcerative (chronic) pancolitis with fistula
K51.014	Ulcerative (chronic) pancolitis with abscess
K51.018	Ulcerative (chronic) pancolitis with other complication
K51.019	Ulcerative (chronic) pancolitis with unspecified complications
K51.20	Ulcerative (chronic) proctitis without complications
K51.211	Ulcerative (chronic) proctitis with rectal bleeding
K51.212	Ulcerative (chronic) proctitis with intestinal obstruction
K51.213	Ulcerative (chronic) proctitis with fistula
K51.214	Ulcerative (chronic) proctitis with abscess
K51.218	Ulcerative (chronic) proctitis with other complication
K51.219	Ulcerative (chronic) proctitis with unspecified complications
K51.30	Ulcerative (chronic) rectosigmoiditis without complications
K51.40	Inflammatory polyps of colon without complications
K51.50	Left sided colitis without complications
K51.80	Other ulcerative colitis without complications
K51.90	Ulcerative colitis, unspecified, without complications
K52.9	Noninfective gastroenteritis and colitis, unspecified
K56.1	Intussusception
K56.2	Volvulus
K57.30	Diverticulosis of large intestine without perforation or abscess without bleeding
K57.31	Diverticulosis of large intestine without perforation or abscess with bleeding
K57.32	Diverticulitis of large intestine without perforation or abscess without bleeding
K57.33	Diverticulitis of large intestine without perforation or abscess with bleeding
K57.90	Diverticulosis of intestine, part unspecified, without perforation or abscess without bleeding
K57.91	Diverticulosis of intestine, part unspecified, without perforation or abscess with bleeding
K57.92	Diverticulitis of intestine, part unspecified, without perforation or abscess without bleeding
K57.93	Diverticulitis of intestine, part unspecified, without perforation or abscess with bleeding
K58.0	Irritable bowel syndrome with diarrhea
K58.9	Irritable bowel syndrome without diarrhea
K59.00	Constipation, unspecified
K59.01	Slow transit constipation
K59.02	Outlet dysfunction constipation
K59.9	Functional intestinal disorder, unspecified
K62.1	Rectal polyp
K63.5	Polyp of colon
K64.0	First degree hemorrhoids
K64.1	Second degree hemorrhoids
K64.2	Third degree hemorrhoids
K64.3	Fourth degree hemorrhoids
K64.8	Other hemorrhoids
R19.4	Change in bowel habit
R19.5	Other fecal abnormalities
Z12.11	Encounter for screening for malignant neoplasm of colon

CCI Edits

Refer to Appendix A for CCI edits.

Pub 100

00811: Pub 100-04, 12, 140.5, Pub 100-04, 12, 50, Pub 100-04, 12, 90.4.5, Pub 100-04, 18, 1.2, Pub 100-04, 18, 60.1.1, Pub 100-04, 6, 20.6
00812: Pub 100-04, 12, 140.5, Pub 100-04, 12, 50, Pub 100-04, 12, 90.4.5, Pub 100-04, 18, 1.2, Pub 100-04, 18, 60.1.1, Pub 100-04, 6, 20.6

Base Units

Global: XXX

Code	Base Units
00811	4
00812	3

Modifiers (PAR)

Code	Mod 50	Mod 51	Mod 62	Mod 80
00811	9	9	9	9
00812	9	9	9	9

CPT © 2018 American Medical Association. All Rights Reserved.

00813

00813 Anesthesia for combined upper and lower gastrointestinal endoscopic procedures, endoscope introduced both proximal to and distal to the duodenum

AMA *CPT Assistant*

00813: Dec 17: 8

ICD-10-CM Diagnostic Codes

C16.0	Malignant neoplasm of cardia
C16.1	Malignant neoplasm of fundus of stomach
C16.2	Malignant neoplasm of body of stomach
C16.3	Malignant neoplasm of pyloric antrum
C16.4	Malignant neoplasm of pylorus
C16.5	Malignant neoplasm of lesser curvature of stomach, unspecified
C16.8	Malignant neoplasm of overlapping sites of stomach
C17.0	Malignant neoplasm of duodenum
C17.1	Malignant neoplasm of jejunum
C17.2	Malignant neoplasm of ileum
C17.3	Meckel's diverticulum, malignant
C17.8	Malignant neoplasm of overlapping sites of small intestine
C18.0	Malignant neoplasm of cecum
C18.2	Malignant neoplasm of ascending colon
C18.3	Malignant neoplasm of hepatic flexure
C18.4	Malignant neoplasm of transverse colon
C18.5	Malignant neoplasm of splenic flexure
C18.6	Malignant neoplasm of descending colon
C18.7	Malignant neoplasm of sigmoid colon
C18.8	Malignant neoplasm of overlapping sites of colon
C19	Malignant neoplasm of rectosigmoid junction
C20	Malignant neoplasm of rectum
C21.1	Malignant neoplasm of anal canal
C21.2	Malignant neoplasm of cloacogenic zone
C21.8	Malignant neoplasm of overlapping sites of rectum, anus and anal canal
D01.0	Carcinoma in situ of colon
D01.1	Carcinoma in situ of rectosigmoid junction
D01.2	Carcinoma in situ of rectum
D01.3	Carcinoma in situ of anus and anal canal
D12.0	Benign neoplasm of cecum
D12.2	Benign neoplasm of ascending colon
D12.3	Benign neoplasm of transverse colon
D12.4	Benign neoplasm of descending colon
D12.5	Benign neoplasm of sigmoid colon
D12.7	Benign neoplasm of rectosigmoid junction
D12.8	Benign neoplasm of rectum
D12.9	Benign neoplasm of anus and anal canal
D50.0	Iron deficiency anemia secondary to blood loss (chronic)
K21.0	Gastro-esophageal reflux disease with esophagitis
K22.0	Achalasia of cardia
K22.710	Barrett's esophagus with low grade dysplasia
K22.711	Barrett's esophagus with high grade dysplasia
K22.8	Other specified diseases of esophagus
K25.4	Chronic or unspecified gastric ulcer with hemorrhage
K25.5	Chronic or unspecified gastric ulcer with perforation
K25.6	Chronic or unspecified gastric ulcer with both hemorrhage and perforation
K25.7	Chronic gastric ulcer without hemorrhage or perforation
K25.9	Gastric ulcer, unspecified as acute or chronic, without hemorrhage or perforation
K26.4	Chronic or unspecified duodenal ulcer with hemorrhage
K26.5	Chronic or unspecified duodenal ulcer with perforation
K26.6	Chronic or unspecified duodenal ulcer with both hemorrhage and perforation
K26.7	Chronic duodenal ulcer without hemorrhage or perforation
K26.9	Duodenal ulcer, unspecified as acute or chronic, without hemorrhage or perforation
K28.4	Chronic or unspecified gastrojejunal ulcer with hemorrhage
K28.5	Chronic or unspecified gastrojejunal ulcer with perforation
K28.6	Chronic or unspecified gastrojejunal ulcer with both hemorrhage and perforation
K28.7	Chronic gastrojejunal ulcer without hemorrhage or perforation
K28.9	Gastrojejunal ulcer, unspecified as acute or chronic, without hemorrhage or perforation
K50.80	Crohn's disease of both small and large intestine without complications
K50.812	Crohn's disease of both small and large intestine with intestinal obstruction
K50.813	Crohn's disease of both small and large intestine with fistula
K50.814	Crohn's disease of both small and large intestine with abscess
K50.818	Crohn's disease of both small and large intestine with other complication
K50.819	Crohn's disease of both small and large intestine with unspecified complications
K51.00	Ulcerative (chronic) pancolitis without complications
K51.011	Ulcerative (chronic) pancolitis with rectal bleeding
K51.012	Ulcerative (chronic) pancolitis with intestinal obstruction
K51.013	Ulcerative (chronic) pancolitis with fistula
K51.014	Ulcerative (chronic) pancolitis with abscess
K51.018	Ulcerative (chronic) pancolitis with other complication
K51.019	Ulcerative (chronic) pancolitis with unspecified complications
K51.20	Ulcerative (chronic) proctitis without complications
K51.211	Ulcerative (chronic) proctitis with rectal bleeding
K51.212	Ulcerative (chronic) proctitis with intestinal obstruction
K51.213	Ulcerative (chronic) proctitis with fistula
K51.214	Ulcerative (chronic) proctitis with abscess
K51.218	Ulcerative (chronic) proctitis with other complication
K51.219	Ulcerative (chronic) proctitis with unspecified complications
K51.30	Ulcerative (chronic) rectosigmoiditis without complications
K51.311	Ulcerative (chronic) rectosigmoiditis with rectal bleeding
K51.312	Ulcerative (chronic) rectosigmoiditis with intestinal obstruction
K51.313	Ulcerative (chronic) rectosigmoiditis with fistula
K51.314	Ulcerative (chronic) rectosigmoiditis with abscess
K51.318	Ulcerative (chronic) rectosigmoiditis with other complication
K51.319	Ulcerative (chronic) rectosigmoiditis with unspecified complications
K51.40	Inflammatory polyps of colon without complications
K51.411	Inflammatory polyps of colon with rectal bleeding
K51.412	Inflammatory polyps of colon with intestinal obstruction
K51.413	Inflammatory polyps of colon with fistula
K51.414	Inflammatory polyps of colon with abscess
K51.418	Inflammatory polyps of colon with other complication
K51.419	Inflammatory polyps of colon with unspecified complications
K51.50	Left sided colitis without complications
K51.511	Left sided colitis with rectal bleeding
K51.512	Left sided colitis with intestinal obstruction
K51.513	Left sided colitis with fistula
K51.514	Left sided colitis with abscess
K51.518	Left sided colitis with other complication
K51.519	Left sided colitis with unspecified complications

CPT © 2018 American Medical Association. All Rights Reserved.

K51.80 Other ulcerative colitis without complications
K51.811 Other ulcerative colitis with rectal bleeding
K51.812 Other ulcerative colitis with intestinal obstruction
K51.813 Other ulcerative colitis with fistula
K51.814 Other ulcerative colitis with abscess
K51.818 Other ulcerative colitis with other complication
K51.819 Other ulcerative colitis with unspecified complications
K52.9 Noninfective gastroenteritis and colitis, unspecified
K56.1 Intussusception
K56.2 Volvulus
K56.50 Intestinal adhesions [bands], unspecified as to partial versus complete obstruction
K56.51 Intestinal adhesions [bands], with partial obstruction
K56.52 Intestinal adhesions [bands] with complete obstruction
K56.600 Partial intestinal obstruction, unspecified as to cause
K56.601 Complete intestinal obstruction, unspecified as to cause
K56.609 Unspecified intestinal obstruction, unspecified as to partial versus complete obstruction
K56.690 Other partial intestinal obstruction
K56.691 Other complete intestinal obstruction
K56.699 Other intestinal obstruction unspecified as to partial versus complete obstruction
K57.40 Diverticulitis of both small and large intestine with perforation and abscess without bleeding
K57.41 Diverticulitis of both small and large intestine with perforation and abscess with bleeding
K57.50 Diverticulosis of both small and large intestine without perforation or abscess without bleeding
K57.51 Diverticulosis of both small and large intestine without perforation or abscess with bleeding
K57.52 Diverticulitis of both small and large intestine without perforation or abscess without bleeding
K57.53 Diverticulitis of both small and large intestine without perforation or abscess with bleeding
K58.0 Irritable bowel syndrome with diarrhea
K58.9 Irritable bowel syndrome without diarrhea
K59.00 Constipation, unspecified
K59.01 Slow transit constipation
K59.02 Outlet dysfunction constipation
K59.9 Functional intestinal disorder, unspecified
K62.1 Rectal polyp
K63.0 Abscess of intestine
K63.2 Fistula of intestine
K63.3 Ulcer of intestine
K63.5 Polyp of colon
K63.81 Dieulafoy lesion of intestine
K64.0 First degree hemorrhoids
K64.1 Second degree hemorrhoids
K64.2 Third degree hemorrhoids
K64.3 Fourth degree hemorrhoids
K64.8 Other hemorrhoids
K90.0 Celiac disease
K91.30 Postprocedural intestinal obstruction, unspecified as to partial versus complete
K91.31 Postprocedural partial intestinal obstruction
K91.32 Postprocedural complete intestinal obstruction
K92.0 Hematemesis
K92.2 Gastrointestinal hemorrhage, unspecified
P54.0 Neonatal hematemesis
P92.09 Other vomiting of newborn
R10.10 Upper abdominal pain, unspecified
⇄ R10.11 Right upper quadrant pain
⇄ R10.12 Left upper quadrant pain
R10.13 Epigastric pain
R10.30 Lower abdominal pain, unspecified
⇄ R10.31 Right lower quadrant pain
⇄ R10.32 Left lower quadrant pain
R10.33 Periumbilical pain
R10.84 Generalized abdominal pain
R11.11 Vomiting without nausea
R11.12 Projectile vomiting
R11.13 Vomiting of fecal matter
R11.2 Nausea with vomiting, unspecified
R12 Heartburn
R13.0 Aphagia
R13.14 Dysphagia, pharyngoesophageal phase
R19.4 Change in bowel habit
R19.5 Other fecal abnormalities
R63.4 Abnormal weight loss
Z12.11 Encounter for screening for malignant neoplasm of colon

CCI Edits

Refer to Appendix A for CCI edits.

Pub 100

00813: Pub 100-04, 12, 140.5, Pub 100-04, 12, 50, Pub 100-04, 12, 90.4.5, Pub 100-04, 6, 20.6

Base Units

Global: XXX

Code	Base Units
00813	5

Modifiers (PAR)

Code	Mod 50	Mod 51	Mod 62	Mod 80
00813	9	9	9	9

CPT © 2018 American Medical Association. All Rights Reserved.

00820

00820 Anesthesia for procedures on lower posterior abdominal wall

ICD-10-CM Diagnostic Codes

	C47.6	Malignant neoplasm of peripheral nerves of trunk, unspecified
	C49.6	Malignant neoplasm of connective and soft tissue of trunk, unspecified
	C79.89	Secondary malignant neoplasm of other specified sites
	D21.6	Benign neoplasm of connective and other soft tissue of trunk, unspecified
	D36.17	Benign neoplasm of peripheral nerves and autonomic nervous system of trunk, unspecified
	D48.1	Neoplasm of uncertain behavior of connective and other soft tissue
	D48.2	Neoplasm of uncertain behavior of peripheral nerves and autonomic nervous system
	D49.2	Neoplasm of unspecified behavior of bone, soft tissue, and skin
	L02.212	Cutaneous abscess of back [any part, except buttock]
	L02.222	Furuncle of back [any part, except buttock]
	L02.232	Carbuncle of back [any part, except buttock]
⇄	L89.130	Pressure ulcer of right lower back, unstageable
⇄	L89.133	Pressure ulcer of right lower back, stage 3
⇄	L89.134	Pressure ulcer of right lower back, stage 4
⇄	L89.140	Pressure ulcer of left lower back, unstageable
⇄	L89.143	Pressure ulcer of left lower back, stage 3
⇄	L89.144	Pressure ulcer of left lower back, stage 4
	L98.422	Non-pressure chronic ulcer of back with fat layer exposed
	L98.423	Non-pressure chronic ulcer of back with necrosis of muscle
❼	S31.010	Laceration without foreign body of lower back and pelvis without penetration into retroperitoneum
❼	S31.020	Laceration with foreign body of lower back and pelvis without penetration into retroperitoneum
❼	S31.030	Puncture wound without foreign body of lower back and pelvis without penetration into retroperitoneum
❼	S31.040	Puncture wound with foreign body of lower back and pelvis without penetration into retroperitoneum
❼	S31.050	Open bite of lower back and pelvis without penetration into retroperitoneum

ICD-10-CM Coding Notes

For codes requiring a 7th character extension, refer to your ICD-10-CM book. Review the character descriptions and coding guidelines for proper selection. For some procedures, only certain characters will apply.

CCI Edits

Refer to Appendix A for CCI edits.

Pub 100

00820: Pub 100-04, 12, 140.5, Pub 100-04, 12, 50, Pub 100-04, 12, 90.4.5

Base Units

Global: XXX

Code	Base Units
00820	5

Modifiers (PAR)

Code	Mod 50	Mod 51	Mod 62	Mod 80
00820	9	9	9	9

CPT © 2018 American Medical Association. All Rights Reserved.

00830

00830 Anesthesia for hernia repairs in lower abdomen; not otherwise specified

ICD-10-CM Diagnostic Codes

K40.00	Bilateral inguinal hernia, with obstruction, without gangrene, not specified as recurrent
K40.01	Bilateral inguinal hernia, with obstruction, without gangrene, recurrent
K40.10	Bilateral inguinal hernia, with gangrene, not specified as recurrent
K40.11	Bilateral inguinal hernia, with gangrene, recurrent
K40.20	Bilateral inguinal hernia, without obstruction or gangrene, not specified as recurrent
K40.21	Bilateral inguinal hernia, without obstruction or gangrene, recurrent
K40.30	Unilateral inguinal hernia, with obstruction, without gangrene, not specified as recurrent
K40.31	Unilateral inguinal hernia, with obstruction, without gangrene, recurrent
K40.40	Unilateral inguinal hernia, with gangrene, not specified as recurrent
K40.41	Unilateral inguinal hernia, with gangrene, recurrent
K40.90	Unilateral inguinal hernia, without obstruction or gangrene, not specified as recurrent
K40.91	Unilateral inguinal hernia, without obstruction or gangrene, recurrent
K41.00	Bilateral femoral hernia, with obstruction, without gangrene, not specified as recurrent
K41.01	Bilateral femoral hernia, with obstruction, without gangrene, recurrent
K41.10	Bilateral femoral hernia, with gangrene, not specified as recurrent
K41.11	Bilateral femoral hernia, with gangrene, recurrent
K41.20	Bilateral femoral hernia, without obstruction or gangrene, not specified as recurrent
K41.21	Bilateral femoral hernia, without obstruction or gangrene, recurrent
K41.30	Unilateral femoral hernia, with obstruction, without gangrene, not specified as recurrent
K41.31	Unilateral femoral hernia, with obstruction, without gangrene, recurrent
K41.40	Unilateral femoral hernia, with gangrene, not specified as recurrent
K41.41	Unilateral femoral hernia, with gangrene, recurrent
K41.90	Unilateral femoral hernia, without obstruction or gangrene, not specified as recurrent
K41.91	Unilateral femoral hernia, without obstruction or gangrene, recurrent
K42.0	Umbilical hernia with obstruction, without gangrene
K42.1	Umbilical hernia with gangrene
K42.9	Umbilical hernia without obstruction or gangrene
K45.0	Other specified abdominal hernia with obstruction, without gangrene
K45.1	Other specified abdominal hernia with gangrene
K45.8	Other specified abdominal hernia without obstruction or gangrene
N43.0	Encysted hydrocele ♂
N43.1	Infected hydrocele ♂
N43.2	Other hydrocele ♂
N43.3	Hydrocele, unspecified ♂
P83.5	Congenital hydrocele ♂

CCI Edits

Refer to Appendix A for CCI edits.

Pub 100

00830: Pub 100-04, 12, 140.5, Pub 100-04, 12, 50, Pub 100-04, 12, 90.4.5

Base Units

Global: XXX

Code	Base Units
00830	4

Modifiers (PAR)

Code	Mod 50	Mod 51	Mod 62	Mod 80
00830	9	9	9	9

CPT © 2018 American Medical Association. All Rights Reserved.

00832

00832 Anesthesia for hernia repairs in lower abdomen; ventral and incisional hernias

(For hernia repairs in the infant 1 year of age or younger, see 00834, 00836)

ICD-10-CM Diagnostic Codes

K43.0	Incisional hernia with obstruction, without gangrene
K43.1	Incisional hernia with gangrene
K43.2	Incisional hernia without obstruction or gangrene
K43.3	Parastomal hernia with obstruction, without gangrene
K43.4	Parastomal hernia with gangrene
K43.5	Parastomal hernia without obstruction or gangrene
K43.6	Other and unspecified ventral hernia with obstruction, without gangrene
K43.7	Other and unspecified ventral hernia with gangrene
K43.9	Ventral hernia without obstruction or gangrene

CCI Edits

Refer to Appendix A for CCI edits.

Pub 100

00832: Pub 100-04, 12, 140.5, Pub 100-04, 12, 50, Pub 100-04, 12, 90.4.5

Base Units

Global: XXX

Code	Base Units
00832	6

Modifiers (PAR)

Code	Mod 50	Mod 51	Mod 62	Mod 80
00832	9	9	9	9

CPT © 2018 American Medical Association. All Rights Reserved.

00834

00834 Anesthesia for hernia repairs in the lower abdomen not otherwise specified, younger than 1 year of age

(Do not report 00834 in conjunction with 99100)

AMA *CPT Assistant*

00834: Dec 17: 8

ICD-10-CM Diagnostic Codes

K40.00	Bilateral inguinal hernia, with obstruction, without gangrene, not specified as recurrent
K40.01	Bilateral inguinal hernia, with obstruction, without gangrene, recurrent
K40.10	Bilateral inguinal hernia, with gangrene, not specified as recurrent
K40.11	Bilateral inguinal hernia, with gangrene, recurrent
K40.20	Bilateral inguinal hernia, without obstruction or gangrene, not specified as recurrent
K40.21	Bilateral inguinal hernia, without obstruction or gangrene, recurrent
K40.30	Unilateral inguinal hernia, with obstruction, without gangrene, not specified as recurrent
K40.31	Unilateral inguinal hernia, with obstruction, without gangrene, recurrent
K40.40	Unilateral inguinal hernia, with gangrene, not specified as recurrent
K40.41	Unilateral inguinal hernia, with gangrene, recurrent
K40.90	Unilateral inguinal hernia, without obstruction or gangrene, not specified as recurrent
K40.91	Unilateral inguinal hernia, without obstruction or gangrene, recurrent
K41.00	Bilateral femoral hernia, with obstruction, without gangrene, not specified as recurrent
K41.01	Bilateral femoral hernia, with obstruction, without gangrene, recurrent
K41.10	Bilateral femoral hernia, with gangrene, not specified as recurrent
K41.11	Bilateral femoral hernia, with gangrene, recurrent
K41.20	Bilateral femoral hernia, without obstruction or gangrene, not specified as recurrent
K41.21	Bilateral femoral hernia, without obstruction or gangrene, recurrent
K41.30	Unilateral femoral hernia, with obstruction, without gangrene, not specified as recurrent
K41.31	Unilateral femoral hernia, with obstruction, without gangrene, recurrent
K41.40	Unilateral femoral hernia, with gangrene, not specified as recurrent
K41.41	Unilateral femoral hernia, with gangrene, recurrent
K41.90	Unilateral femoral hernia, without obstruction or gangrene, not specified as recurrent
K41.91	Unilateral femoral hernia, without obstruction or gangrene, recurrent
K42.0	Umbilical hernia with obstruction, without gangrene
K42.1	Umbilical hernia with gangrene
K42.9	Umbilical hernia without obstruction or gangrene
K45.0	Other specified abdominal hernia with obstruction, without gangrene
K45.1	Other specified abdominal hernia with gangrene
K45.8	Other specified abdominal hernia without obstruction or gangrene
P83.5	Congenital hydrocele ♂

CCI Edits

Refer to Appendix A for CCI edits.

Pub 100

00834: Pub 100-04, 12, 140.5, Pub 100-04, 12, 50, Pub 100-04, 12, 90.4.5

Base Units

Global: XXX

Code	Base Units
00834	5

Modifiers (PAR)

Code	Mod 50	Mod 51	Mod 62	Mod 80
00834	9	9	9	9

CPT © 2018 American Medical Association. All Rights Reserved.

00836

00836 Anesthesia for hernia repairs in the lower abdomen not otherwise specified, infants younger than 37 weeks gestational age at birth and younger than 50 weeks gestational age at time of surgery

(Do not report 00836 in conjunction with 99100)

AMA *CPT Assistant* □

00836: Dec 17: 8

ICD-10-CM Diagnostic Codes

K40.00	Bilateral inguinal hernia, with obstruction, without gangrene, not specified as recurrent
K40.01	Bilateral inguinal hernia, with obstruction, without gangrene, recurrent
K40.10	Bilateral inguinal hernia, with gangrene, not specified as recurrent
K40.11	Bilateral inguinal hernia, with gangrene, recurrent
K40.20	Bilateral inguinal hernia, without obstruction or gangrene, not specified as recurrent
K40.21	Bilateral inguinal hernia, without obstruction or gangrene, recurrent
K40.30	Unilateral inguinal hernia, with obstruction, without gangrene, not specified as recurrent
K40.31	Unilateral inguinal hernia, with obstruction, without gangrene, recurrent
K40.40	Unilateral inguinal hernia, with gangrene, not specified as recurrent
K40.41	Unilateral inguinal hernia, with gangrene, recurrent
K40.90	Unilateral inguinal hernia, without obstruction or gangrene, not specified as recurrent
K40.91	Unilateral inguinal hernia, without obstruction or gangrene, recurrent
K41.00	Bilateral femoral hernia, with obstruction, without gangrene, not specified as recurrent
K41.01	Bilateral femoral hernia, with obstruction, without gangrene, recurrent
K41.10	Bilateral femoral hernia, with gangrene, not specified as recurrent
K41.11	Bilateral femoral hernia, with gangrene, recurrent
K41.20	Bilateral femoral hernia, without obstruction or gangrene, not specified as recurrent
K41.21	Bilateral femoral hernia, without obstruction or gangrene, recurrent
K41.30	Unilateral femoral hernia, with obstruction, without gangrene, not specified as recurrent
K41.31	Unilateral femoral hernia, with obstruction, without gangrene, recurrent
K41.40	Unilateral femoral hernia, with gangrene, not specified as recurrent
K41.41	Unilateral femoral hernia, with gangrene, recurrent
K41.90	Unilateral femoral hernia, without obstruction or gangrene, not specified as recurrent
K41.91	Unilateral femoral hernia, without obstruction or gangrene, recurrent
K42.0	Umbilical hernia with obstruction, without gangrene
K42.1	Umbilical hernia with gangrene
K42.9	Umbilical hernia without obstruction or gangrene
K45.0	Other specified abdominal hernia with obstruction, without gangrene
K45.1	Other specified abdominal hernia with gangrene
K45.8	Other specified abdominal hernia without obstruction or gangrene
P83.5	Congenital hydrocele ♂

CCI Edits

Refer to Appendix A for CCI edits.

Pub 100

00836: Pub 100-04, 12, 140.5, Pub 100-04, 12, 50, Pub 100-04, 12, 90.4.5

Base Units

Global: XXX

Code	Base Units
00836	6

Modifiers (PAR)

Code	Mod 50	Mod 51	Mod 62	Mod 80
00836	9	9	9	9

CPT © 2018 American Medical Association. All Rights Reserved.

00840

00840 Anesthesia for intraperitoneal procedures in lower abdomen including laparoscopy; not otherwise specified

ICD-10-CM Diagnostic Codes

	C18.7	Malignant neoplasm of sigmoid colon
	C18.8	Malignant neoplasm of overlapping sites of colon
	C18.9	Malignant neoplasm of colon, unspecified
	C19	Malignant neoplasm of rectosigmoid junction
	C20	Malignant neoplasm of rectum
	C21.8	Malignant neoplasm of overlapping sites of rectum, anus and anal canal
	C53.0	Malignant neoplasm of endocervix ♀
	C53.1	Malignant neoplasm of exocervix ♀
	C53.8	Malignant neoplasm of overlapping sites of cervix uteri ♀
	C54.0	Malignant neoplasm of isthmus uteri ♀
	C54.1	Malignant neoplasm of endometrium ♀
	C54.2	Malignant neoplasm of myometrium ♀
	C54.3	Malignant neoplasm of fundus uteri ♀
	C54.8	Malignant neoplasm of overlapping sites of corpus uteri ♀
⇄	C56.1	Malignant neoplasm of right ovary ♀
⇄	C56.2	Malignant neoplasm of left ovary ♀
	C57.8	Malignant neoplasm of overlapping sites of female genital organs ♀
	D25.0	Submucous leiomyoma of uterus ♀
	D25.1	Intramural leiomyoma of uterus ♀
	D25.2	Subserosal leiomyoma of uterus ♀
	K35.20	Acute appendicitis with generalized peritonitis, without abscess
	K35.21	Acute appendicitis with generalized peritonitis, with abscess
	K35.30	Acute appendicitis with localized peritonitis, without perforation or gangrene
	K35.31	Acute appendicitis with localized peritonitis and gangrene, without perforation
	K35.32	Acute appendicitis with perforation and localized peritonitis, without abscess
	K35.33	Acute appendicitis with perforation and localized peritonitis, with abscess
	K35.890	Other acute appendicitis without perforation or gangrene
	K35.891	Other acute appendicitis without perforation, with gangrene
	K50.112	Crohn's disease of large intestine with intestinal obstruction
	K50.113	Crohn's disease of large intestine with fistula
	K50.114	Crohn's disease of large intestine with abscess
	K50.812	Crohn's disease of both small and large intestine with intestinal obstruction
	K50.813	Crohn's disease of both small and large intestine with fistula
	K50.814	Crohn's disease of both small and large intestine with abscess
	K56.0	Paralytic ileus
	K56.1	Intussusception
	K56.2	Volvulus
	K56.50	Intestinal adhesions [bands], unspecified as to partial versus complete obstruction
	K56.51	Intestinal adhesions [bands], with partial obstruction
	K56.52	Intestinal adhesions [bands] with complete obstruction
	K56.690	Other partial intestinal obstruction
	K56.691	Other complete intestinal obstruction
	K56.699	Other intestinal obstruction unspecified as to partial versus complete obstruction
	K66.0	Peritoneal adhesions (postprocedural) (postinfection)
	K91.30	Postprocedural intestinal obstruction, unspecified as to partial versus complete
	K91.31	Postprocedural partial intestinal obstruction
	K91.32	Postprocedural complete intestinal obstruction
	N80.0	Endometriosis of uterus ♀
	N80.1	Endometriosis of ovary ♀
	N80.2	Endometriosis of fallopian tube ♀
	N80.3	Endometriosis of pelvic peritoneum ♀
	N80.5	Endometriosis of intestine ♀
	N80.8	Other endometriosis ♀
	N81.2	Incomplete uterovaginal prolapse ♀
	N81.3	Complete uterovaginal prolapse ♀
⇄	N83.01	Follicular cyst of right ovary ♀
⇄	N83.02	Follicular cyst of left ovary ♀
⇄	N83.11	Corpus luteum cyst of right ovary ♀
⇄	N83.12	Corpus luteum cyst of left ovary ♀
⇄	N83.291	Other ovarian cyst, right side ♀
⇄	N83.292	Other ovarian cyst, left side ♀
⇄	N83.311	Acquired atrophy of right ovary ♀
⇄	N83.312	Acquired atrophy of left ovary ♀
⇄	N83.321	Acquired atrophy of right fallopian tube ♀
⇄	N83.322	Acquired atrophy of left fallopian tube ♀
⇄	N83.331	Acquired atrophy of right ovary and fallopian tube ♀
⇄	N83.332	Acquired atrophy of left ovary and fallopian tube ♀
⇄	N83.41	Prolapse and hernia of right ovary and fallopian tube ♀
⇄	N83.42	Prolapse and hernia of left ovary and fallopian tube ♀
⇄	N83.511	Torsion of right ovary and ovarian pedicle ♀
⇄	N83.512	Torsion of left ovary and ovarian pedicle ♀
⇄	N83.521	Torsion of right fallopian tube ♀
⇄	N83.522	Torsion of left fallopian tube ♀
	N85.02	Endometrial intraepithelial neoplasia [EIN] ♀
	N85.2	Hypertrophy of uterus ♀
	N95.0	Postmenopausal bleeding ♀
	N97.1	Female infertility of tubal origin ♀

CCI Edits

Refer to Appendix A for CCI edits.

Pub 100

00840: Pub 100-04, 12, 140.5, Pub 100-04, 12, 50, Pub 100-04, 12, 90.4.5

Base Units

Global: XXX

Code	Base Units
00840	6

Modifiers (PAR)

Code	Mod 50	Mod 51	Mod 62	Mod 80
00840	9	9	9	9

CPT © 2018 American Medical Association. All Rights Reserved.

00842

00842 Anesthesia for intraperitoneal procedures in lower abdomen including laparoscopy; amniocentesis

ICD-10-CM Diagnostic Codes

	O09.511	Supervision of elderly primigravida, first trimester ♀
	O09.512	Supervision of elderly primigravida, second trimester ♀
	O09.513	Supervision of elderly primigravida, third trimester ♀
	O09.521	Supervision of elderly multigravida, first trimester ♀
	O09.522	Supervision of elderly multigravida, second trimester ♀
	O09.523	Supervision of elderly multigravida, third trimester ♀
	O28.0	Abnormal hematological finding on antenatal screening of mother ♀
	O28.1	Abnormal biochemical finding on antenatal screening of mother ♀
	O28.2	Abnormal cytological finding on antenatal screening of mother ♀
	O28.3	Abnormal ultrasonic finding on antenatal screening of mother ♀
	O28.4	Abnormal radiological finding on antenatal screening of mother ♀
	O28.5	Abnormal chromosomal and genetic finding on antenatal screening of mother ♀
	O28.8	Other abnormal findings on antenatal screening of mother ♀
➐	O35.0	Maternal care for (suspected) central nervous system malformation in fetus
➐	O35.1	Maternal care for (suspected) chromosomal abnormality in fetus
➐	O35.2	Maternal care for (suspected) hereditary disease in fetus
➐	O35.3	Maternal care for (suspected) damage to fetus from viral disease in mother
➐	O35.7	Maternal care for (suspected) damage to fetus by other medical procedures
➐	O35.8	Maternal care for other (suspected) fetal abnormality and damage
➐	O36.011	Maternal care for anti-D [Rh] antibodies, first trimester
➐	O36.012	Maternal care for anti-D [Rh] antibodies, second trimester
➐	O36.013	Maternal care for anti-D [Rh] antibodies, third trimester
➐	O36.091	Maternal care for other rhesus isoimmunization, first trimester
➐	O36.092	Maternal care for other rhesus isoimmunization, second trimester
➐	O36.093	Maternal care for other rhesus isoimmunization, third trimester
➐	O36.111	Maternal care for Anti-A sensitization, first trimester
➐	O36.112	Maternal care for Anti-A sensitization, second trimester
➐	O36.113	Maternal care for Anti-A sensitization, third trimester
➐	O36.191	Maternal care for other isoimmunization, first trimester
➐	O36.192	Maternal care for other isoimmunization, second trimester
➐	O36.193	Maternal care for other isoimmunization, third trimester
➐	O40.1	Polyhydramnios, first trimester
➐	O40.2	Polyhydramnios, second trimester
➐	O40.3	Polyhydramnios, third trimester
➐	O41.101	Infection of amniotic sac and membranes, unspecified, first trimester
➐	O41.102	Infection of amniotic sac and membranes, unspecified, second trimester
➐	O41.103	Infection of amniotic sac and membranes, unspecified, third trimester
➐	O41.121	Chorioamnionitis, first trimester
➐	O41.122	Chorioamnionitis, second trimester
➐	O41.123	Chorioamnionitis, third trimester
➐	O41.141	Placentitis, first trimester
➐	O41.142	Placentitis, second trimester
➐	O41.143	Placentitis, third trimester
➐	O41.8X1	Other specified disorders of amniotic fluid and membranes, first trimester
➐	O41.8X2	Other specified disorders of amniotic fluid and membranes, second trimester
➐	O41.8X3	Other specified disorders of amniotic fluid and membranes, third trimester
➐	O41.91	Disorder of amniotic fluid and membranes, unspecified, first trimester
➐	O41.92	Disorder of amniotic fluid and membranes, unspecified, second trimester
➐	O41.93	Disorder of amniotic fluid and membranes, unspecified, third trimester
	O48.0	Post-term pregnancy ♀
	O48.1	Prolonged pregnancy ♀
	Z03.73	Encounter for suspected fetal anomaly ruled out ♀
	Z36	Encounter for antenatal screening of mother ♀

ICD-10-CM Coding Notes

For codes requiring a 7th character extension, refer to your ICD-10-CM book. Review the character descriptions and coding guidelines for proper selection. For some procedures, only certain characters will apply.

CCI Edits

Refer to Appendix A for CCI edits.

Pub 100

00842: Pub 100-04, 12, 140.5, Pub 100-04, 12, 50, Pub 100-04, 12, 90.4.5

Base Units

Global: XXX

Code	Base Units
00842	4

Modifiers (PAR)

Code	Mod 50	Mod 51	Mod 62	Mod 80
00842	9	9	9	9

CPT © 2018 American Medical Association. All Rights Reserved.

00844

00844 Anesthesia for intraperitoneal procedures in lower abdomen including laparoscopy; abdominoperineal resection

ICD-10-CM Diagnostic Codes

C18.7	Malignant neoplasm of sigmoid colon
C18.8	Malignant neoplasm of overlapping sites of colon
C19	Malignant neoplasm of rectosigmoid junction
C20	Malignant neoplasm of rectum
C21.0	Malignant neoplasm of anus, unspecified
C21.1	Malignant neoplasm of anal canal
C21.2	Malignant neoplasm of cloacogenic zone
C21.8	Malignant neoplasm of overlapping sites of rectum, anus and anal canal

CCI Edits

Refer to Appendix A for CCI edits.

Pub 100

00844: Pub 100-04, 12, 140.5, Pub 100-04, 12, 50, Pub 100-04, 12, 90.4.5

Base Units

Global: XXX

Code	Base Units
00844	7

Modifiers (PAR)

Code	Mod 50	Mod 51	Mod 62	Mod 80
00844	9	9	9	9

CPT © 2018 American Medical Association. All Rights Reserved.

00846

00846 Anesthesia for intraperitoneal procedures in lower abdomen including laparoscopy; radical hysterectomy

ICD-10-CM Diagnostic Codes

C53.0	Malignant neoplasm of endocervix ♀
C53.1	Malignant neoplasm of exocervix ♀
C53.8	Malignant neoplasm of overlapping sites of cervix uteri ♀
C53.9	Malignant neoplasm of cervix uteri, unspecified ♀
C54.0	Malignant neoplasm of isthmus uteri ♀
C54.1	Malignant neoplasm of endometrium ♀
C54.2	Malignant neoplasm of myometrium ♀
C54.3	Malignant neoplasm of fundus uteri ♀
C54.8	Malignant neoplasm of overlapping sites of corpus uteri ♀
C54.9	Malignant neoplasm of corpus uteri, unspecified ♀
C77.4	Secondary and unspecified malignant neoplasm of inguinal and lower limb lymph nodes
C77.5	Secondary and unspecified malignant neoplasm of intrapelvic lymph nodes
C77.8	Secondary and unspecified malignant neoplasm of lymph nodes of multiple regions

CCI Edits

Refer to Appendix A for CCI edits.

Pub 100

00846: Pub 100-04, 12, 140.5, Pub 100-04, 12, 50, Pub 100-04, 12, 90.4.5

Base Units

Global: XXX

Code	Base Units
00846	8

Modifiers (PAR)

Code	Mod 50	Mod 51	Mod 62	Mod 80
00846	9	9	9	9

CPT © 2018 American Medical Association. All Rights Reserved.

00848

00848 Anesthesia for intraperitoneal procedures in lower abdomen including laparoscopy; pelvic exenteration

ICD-10-CM Diagnostic Codes

	C18.6	Malignant neoplasm of descending colon
	C18.7	Malignant neoplasm of sigmoid colon
	C18.8	Malignant neoplasm of overlapping sites of colon
	C18.9	Malignant neoplasm of colon, unspecified
	C19	Malignant neoplasm of rectosigmoid junction
	C20	Malignant neoplasm of rectum
	C21.0	Malignant neoplasm of anus, unspecified
	C21.1	Malignant neoplasm of anal canal
	C21.2	Malignant neoplasm of cloacogenic zone
	C21.8	Malignant neoplasm of overlapping sites of rectum, anus and anal canal
	C48.1	Malignant neoplasm of specified parts of peritoneum
	C48.2	Malignant neoplasm of peritoneum, unspecified
	C53.0	Malignant neoplasm of endocervix ♀
	C53.1	Malignant neoplasm of exocervix ♀
	C53.8	Malignant neoplasm of overlapping sites of cervix uteri ♀
	C53.9	Malignant neoplasm of cervix uteri, unspecified ♀
	C54.0	Malignant neoplasm of isthmus uteri ♀
	C54.1	Malignant neoplasm of endometrium ♀
	C54.2	Malignant neoplasm of myometrium ♀
	C54.3	Malignant neoplasm of fundus uteri ♀
	C54.8	Malignant neoplasm of overlapping sites of corpus uteri ♀
	C54.9	Malignant neoplasm of corpus uteri, unspecified ♀
	C55	Malignant neoplasm of uterus, part unspecified ♀
⇄	C56.1	Malignant neoplasm of right ovary ♀
⇄	C56.2	Malignant neoplasm of left ovary ♀
⇄	C56.9	Malignant neoplasm of unspecified ovary ♀
⇄	C57.00	Malignant neoplasm of unspecified fallopian tube ♀
⇄	C57.01	Malignant neoplasm of right fallopian tube ♀
⇄	C57.02	Malignant neoplasm of left fallopian tube ♀
⇄	C57.10	Malignant neoplasm of unspecified broad ligament ♀
⇄	C57.11	Malignant neoplasm of right broad ligament ♀
⇄	C57.12	Malignant neoplasm of left broad ligament ♀
⇄	C57.20	Malignant neoplasm of unspecified round ligament ♀
⇄	C57.21	Malignant neoplasm of right round ligament ♀
⇄	C57.22	Malignant neoplasm of left round ligament ♀
	C57.3	Malignant neoplasm of parametrium ♀
	C57.4	Malignant neoplasm of uterine adnexa, unspecified ♀
	C57.7	Malignant neoplasm of other specified female genital organs ♀
	C57.8	Malignant neoplasm of overlapping sites of female genital organs ♀
	C57.9	Malignant neoplasm of female genital organ, unspecified ♀
	C76.3	Malignant neoplasm of pelvis
	C77.4	Secondary and unspecified malignant neoplasm of inguinal and lower limb lymph nodes
	C77.5	Secondary and unspecified malignant neoplasm of intrapelvic lymph nodes
	C77.8	Secondary and unspecified malignant neoplasm of lymph nodes of multiple regions
	C78.5	Secondary malignant neoplasm of large intestine and rectum
	C78.6	Secondary malignant neoplasm of retroperitoneum and peritoneum
	C79.10	Secondary malignant neoplasm of unspecified urinary organs
	C79.11	Secondary malignant neoplasm of bladder
	C79.19	Secondary malignant neoplasm of other urinary organs
⇄	C79.60	Secondary malignant neoplasm of unspecified ovary ♀
⇄	C79.61	Secondary malignant neoplasm of right ovary ♀
⇄	C79.62	Secondary malignant neoplasm of left ovary ♀
	C79.82	Secondary malignant neoplasm of genital organs
	C7A.024	Malignant carcinoid tumor of the descending colon
	C7A.025	Malignant carcinoid tumor of the sigmoid colon
	C7A.026	Malignant carcinoid tumor of the rectum
	C7A.029	Malignant carcinoid tumor of the large intestine, unspecified portion
	C7B.04	Secondary carcinoid tumors of peritoneum

CCI Edits

Refer to Appendix A for CCI edits.

Pub 100

00848: Pub 100-04, 12, 140.5, Pub 100-04, 12, 50, Pub 100-04, 12, 90.4.5

Base Units

Global: XXX

Code	Base Units
00848	8

Modifiers (PAR)

Code	Mod 50	Mod 51	Mod 62	Mod 80
00848	9	9	9	9

CPT © 2018 American Medical Association. All Rights Reserved.

00851

00851 Anesthesia for intraperitoneal procedures in lower abdomen including laparoscopy; tubal ligation/transection

AMA *CPT Assistant*

00851: Oct 14: 14

ICD-10-CM Diagnostic Codes

Z30.2	Encounter for sterilization
Z98.51	Tubal ligation status ♀

CCI Edits

Refer to Appendix A for CCI edits.

Pub 100

00851: Pub 100-04, 12, 140.5, Pub 100-04, 12, 50, Pub 100-04, 12, 90.4.5

Base Units

Global: XXX

Code	Base Units
00851	6

Modifiers (PAR)

Code	Mod 50	Mod 51	Mod 62	Mod 80
00851	9	9	9	9

CPT © 2018 American Medical Association. All Rights Reserved.

00860

00860 Anesthesia for extraperitoneal procedures in lower abdomen, including urinary tract; not otherwise specified

ICD-10-CM Diagnostic Codes

⇄	C66.1	Malignant neoplasm of right ureter
⇄	C66.2	Malignant neoplasm of left ureter
	C67.0	Malignant neoplasm of trigone of bladder
	C67.1	Malignant neoplasm of dome of bladder
	C67.2	Malignant neoplasm of lateral wall of bladder
	C67.3	Malignant neoplasm of anterior wall of bladder
	C67.4	Malignant neoplasm of posterior wall of bladder
	C67.5	Malignant neoplasm of bladder neck
	C67.6	Malignant neoplasm of ureteric orifice
	C67.8	Malignant neoplasm of overlapping sites of bladder
	C67.9	Malignant neoplasm of bladder, unspecified
	N13.1	Hydronephrosis with ureteral stricture, not elsewhere classified
	N13.2	Hydronephrosis with renal and ureteral calculous obstruction
	N13.9	Obstructive and reflux uropathy, unspecified
	N20.1	Calculus of ureter
	N32.0	Bladder-neck obstruction
	N32.3	Diverticulum of bladder
	N39.3	Stress incontinence (female) (male)
	N39.41	Urge incontinence
	N39.42	Incontinence without sensory awareness
	N39.43	Post-void dribbling
	N39.44	Nocturnal enuresis
	N39.45	Continuous leakage
	N39.46	Mixed incontinence
	N39.490	Overflow incontinence
	N39.498	Other specified urinary incontinence
	N40.1	Benign prostatic hyperplasia with lower urinary tract symptoms ♂
	N40.3	Nodular prostate with lower urinary tract symptoms ♂
	N42.31	Prostatic intraepithelial neoplasia ♂
	N42.32	Atypical small acinar proliferation of prostate ♂
	N42.39	Other dysplasia of prostate ♂
	N81.11	Cystocele, midline ♀
	N81.12	Cystocele, lateral ♀
	N81.5	Vaginal enterocele ♀
	N81.6	Rectocele ♀
	N81.81	Perineocele ♀
	N81.82	Incompetence or weakening of pubocervical tissue ♀
	N81.83	Incompetence or weakening of rectovaginal tissue ♀
	N81.85	Cervical stump prolapse ♀
	N81.89	Other female genital prolapse ♀
	N82.0	Vesicovaginal fistula ♀
	N82.5	Female genital tract-skin fistulae ♀
	N82.8	Other female genital tract fistulae ♀
	Q62.12	Congenital occlusion of ureterovesical orifice
	Q62.62	Displacement of ureter
	Q62.63	Anomalous implantation of ureter
	Q62.7	Congenital vesico-uretero-renal reflux
	R33.8	Other retention of urine
	R35.0	Frequency of micturition
	R35.1	Nocturia
	R39.15	Urgency of urination
	R39.16	Straining to void
➐	S37.23	Laceration of bladder
➐	S37.33	Laceration of urethra

ICD-10-CM Coding Notes

For codes requiring a 7th character extension, refer to your ICD-10-CM book. Review the character descriptions and coding guidelines for proper selection. For some procedures, only certain characters will apply.

CCI Edits

Refer to Appendix A for CCI edits.

Pub 100

00860: Pub 100-04, 12, 140.5, Pub 100-04, 12, 50, Pub 100-04, 12, 90.4.5

Base Units

Global: XXX

Code	Base Units
00860	6

Modifiers (PAR)

Code	Mod 50	Mod 51	Mod 62	Mod 80
00860	9	9	9	9

CPT © 2018 American Medical Association. All Rights Reserved.

00862

00862 Anesthesia for extraperitoneal procedures in lower abdomen, including urinary tract; renal procedures, including upper one-third of ureter, or donor nephrectomy

ICD-10-CM Diagnostic Codes

⇄	C64.1	Malignant neoplasm of right kidney, except renal pelvis
⇄	C64.2	Malignant neoplasm of left kidney, except renal pelvis
⇄	C65.1	Malignant neoplasm of right renal pelvis
⇄	C65.2	Malignant neoplasm of left renal pelvis
⇄	C66.1	Malignant neoplasm of right ureter
⇄	C66.2	Malignant neoplasm of left ureter
⇄	D30.01	Benign neoplasm of right kidney
⇄	D30.02	Benign neoplasm of left kidney
⇄	D30.11	Benign neoplasm of right renal pelvis
⇄	D30.12	Benign neoplasm of left renal pelvis
⇄	D30.21	Benign neoplasm of right ureter
⇄	D30.22	Benign neoplasm of left ureter
	N13.1	Hydronephrosis with ureteral stricture, not elsewhere classified
	N13.2	Hydronephrosis with renal and ureteral calculous obstruction
	N13.30	Unspecified hydronephrosis
	N13.39	Other hydronephrosis
	N13.4	Hydroureter
	N13.6	Pyonephrosis
	N15.1	Renal and perinephric abscess
	N20.0	Calculus of kidney
	N20.1	Calculus of ureter
	N20.2	Calculus of kidney with calculus of ureter
	N28.1	Cyst of kidney, acquired
	N99.71	Accidental puncture and laceration of a genitourinary system organ or structure during a genitourinary system procedure
	N99.72	Accidental puncture and laceration of a genitourinary system organ or structure during other procedure
	Q61.01	Congenital single renal cyst
	Q61.02	Congenital multiple renal cysts
	Q61.11	Cystic dilatation of collecting ducts
	Q61.19	Other polycystic kidney, infantile type
	Q61.2	Polycystic kidney, adult type
	Q61.4	Renal dysplasia
	Q61.5	Medullary cystic kidney
	Q61.8	Other cystic kidney diseases
	Q62.0	Congenital hydronephrosis
	Q62.11	Congenital occlusion of ureteropelvic junction
	Q62.2	Congenital megaureter
	Q62.39	Other obstructive defects of renal pelvis and ureter
	Q62.69	Other malposition of ureter
	Q62.7	Congenital vesico-uretero-renal reflux
	Q63.8	Other specified congenital malformations of kidney
❼⇄	S37.051	Moderate laceration of right kidney
❼⇄	S37.052	Moderate laceration of left kidney
❼⇄	S37.061	Major laceration of right kidney
❼⇄	S37.062	Major laceration of left kidney
❼	S37.13	Laceration of ureter
	Z52.4	Kidney donor

ICD-10-CM Coding Notes

For codes requiring a 7th character extension, refer to your ICD-10-CM book. Review the character descriptions and coding guidelines for proper selection. For some procedures, only certain characters will apply.

CCI Edits

Refer to Appendix A for CCI edits.

Pub 100

00862: Pub 100-04, 12, 140.5, Pub 100-04, 12, 50, Pub 100-04, 12, 90.4.5

Base Units

Global: XXX

Code	Base Units
00862	7

Modifiers (PAR)

Code	Mod 50	Mod 51	Mod 62	Mod 80
00862	9	9	9	9

CPT © 2018 American Medical Association. All Rights Reserved.

00864

00864 Anesthesia for extraperitoneal procedures in lower abdomen, including urinary tract; total cystectomy

ICD-10-CM Diagnostic Codes

C67.0	Malignant neoplasm of trigone of bladder
C67.1	Malignant neoplasm of dome of bladder
C67.2	Malignant neoplasm of lateral wall of bladder
C67.3	Malignant neoplasm of anterior wall of bladder
C67.4	Malignant neoplasm of posterior wall of bladder
C67.5	Malignant neoplasm of bladder neck
C67.6	Malignant neoplasm of ureteric orifice
C67.7	Malignant neoplasm of urachus
C67.8	Malignant neoplasm of overlapping sites of bladder
C67.9	Malignant neoplasm of bladder, unspecified
C79.11	Secondary malignant neoplasm of bladder
D41.4	Neoplasm of uncertain behavior of bladder

CCI Edits

Refer to Appendix A for CCI edits.

Pub 100

00864: Pub 100-04, 12, 140.5, Pub 100-04, 12, 50, Pub 100-04, 12, 90.4.5

Base Units

Global: XXX

Code	Base Units
00864	8

Modifiers (PAR)

Code	Mod 50	Mod 51	Mod 62	Mod 80
00864	9	9	9	9

CPT © 2018 American Medical Association. All Rights Reserved.

00865

00865 Anesthesia for extraperitoneal procedures in lower abdomen, including urinary tract; radical prostatectomy (suprapubic, retropubic)

ICD-10-CM Diagnostic Codes

C61	Malignant neoplasm of prostate ♂
C77.4	Secondary and unspecified malignant neoplasm of inguinal and lower limb lymph nodes
C77.5	Secondary and unspecified malignant neoplasm of intrapelvic lymph nodes
C79.82	Secondary malignant neoplasm of genital organs
D07.5	Carcinoma in situ of prostate ♂
D40.0	Neoplasm of uncertain behavior of prostate ♂

CCI Edits

Refer to Appendix A for CCI edits.

Pub 100

00865: Pub 100-04, 12, 140.5, Pub 100-04, 12, 50, Pub 100-04, 12, 90.4.5

Base Units

Global: XXX

Code	Base Units
00865	7

Modifiers (PAR)

Code	Mod 50	Mod 51	Mod 62	Mod 80
00865	9	9	9	9

CPT © 2018 American Medical Association. All Rights Reserved.

00866

00866 Anesthesia for extraperitoneal procedures in lower abdomen, including urinary tract; adrenalectomy

ICD-10-CM Diagnostic Codes

⇄	C74.01	Malignant neoplasm of cortex of right adrenal gland
⇄	C74.02	Malignant neoplasm of cortex of left adrenal gland
⇄	C74.11	Malignant neoplasm of medulla of right adrenal gland
⇄	C74.12	Malignant neoplasm of medulla of left adrenal gland
⇄	C74.91	Malignant neoplasm of unspecified part of right adrenal gland
⇄	C74.92	Malignant neoplasm of unspecified part of left adrenal gland
⇄	C79.71	Secondary malignant neoplasm of right adrenal gland
⇄	C79.72	Secondary malignant neoplasm of left adrenal gland
	D09.3	Carcinoma in situ of thyroid and other endocrine glands
⇄	D35.01	Benign neoplasm of right adrenal gland
⇄	D35.02	Benign neoplasm of left adrenal gland
⇄	D44.11	Neoplasm of uncertain behavior of right adrenal gland
⇄	D44.12	Neoplasm of uncertain behavior of left adrenal gland
	D49.7	Neoplasm of unspecified behavior of endocrine glands and other parts of nervous system
	E24.8	Other Cushing's syndrome
	E24.9	Cushing's syndrome, unspecified
	E26.01	Conn's syndrome
	E26.09	Other primary hyperaldosteronism
	E26.89	Other hyperaldosteronism
	E27.8	Other specified disorders of adrenal gland
	Q89.1	Congenital malformations of adrenal gland

CCI Edits

Refer to Appendix A for CCI edits.

Pub 100

00866: Pub 100-04, 12, 140.5, Pub 100-04, 12, 50, Pub 100-04, 12, 90.4.5

Base Units

Global: XXX

Code	Base Units
00866	10

Modifiers (PAR)

Code	Mod 50	Mod 51	Mod 62	Mod 80
00866	9	9	9	9

CPT © 2018 American Medical Association. All Rights Reserved.

00868

00868 Anesthesia for extraperitoneal procedures in lower abdomen, including urinary tract; renal transplant (recipient)

(For donor nephrectomy, use 00862)

(For harvesting kidney from brain-dead patient, use 01990)

ICD-10-CM Diagnostic Codes

⇄	C64.1	Malignant neoplasm of right kidney, except renal pelvis
⇄	C64.2	Malignant neoplasm of left kidney, except renal pelvis
⇄	C65.1	Malignant neoplasm of right renal pelvis
⇄	C65.2	Malignant neoplasm of left renal pelvis
	C7A.093	Malignant carcinoid tumor of the kidney
	D59.3	Hemolytic-uremic syndrome
	E08.22	Diabetes mellitus due to underlying condition with diabetic chronic kidney disease
	E09.22	Drug or chemical induced diabetes mellitus with diabetic chronic kidney disease
	E10.22	Type 1 diabetes mellitus with diabetic chronic kidney disease
	E11.22	Type 2 diabetes mellitus with diabetic chronic kidney disease
	E13.22	Other specified diabetes mellitus with diabetic chronic kidney disease
	I12.0	Hypertensive chronic kidney disease with stage 5 chronic kidney disease or end stage renal disease
	I13.11	Hypertensive heart and chronic kidney disease without heart failure, with stage 5 chronic kidney disease, or end stage renal disease
	I13.2	Hypertensive heart and chronic kidney disease with heart failure and with stage 5 chronic kidney disease, or end stage renal disease
	N18.5	Chronic kidney disease, stage 5
	N18.6	End stage renal disease
	N28.1	Cyst of kidney, acquired
	Q61.02	Congenital multiple renal cysts
	Q61.1	Polycystic kidney, infantile type
	Q61.2	Polycystic kidney, adult type
	Q61.3	Polycystic kidney, unspecified
	Q61.4	Renal dysplasia
	Q61.5	Medullary cystic kidney
	Q61.8	Other cystic kidney diseases
	Q61.9	Cystic kidney disease, unspecified
	T86.11	Kidney transplant rejection
	T86.12	Kidney transplant failure
	Z94.0	Kidney transplant status
	Z99.2	Dependence on renal dialysis

CCI Edits

Refer to Appendix A for CCI edits.

Pub 100

00868: Pub 100-04, 12, 140.5, Pub 100-04, 12, 50, Pub 100-04, 12, 90.4.5

Base Units

Global: XXX

Code	Base Units
00868	10

Modifiers (PAR)

Code	Mod 50	Mod 51	Mod 62	Mod 80
00868	9	9	9	9

CPT © 2018 American Medical Association. All Rights Reserved.

00870

00870 Anesthesia for extraperitoneal procedures in lower abdomen, including urinary tract; cystolithotomy

ICD-10-CM Diagnostic Codes

N21.0	Calculus in bladder
N21.1	Calculus in urethra
N21.8	Other lower urinary tract calculus
N21.9	Calculus of lower urinary tract, unspecified

CCI Edits

Refer to Appendix A for CCI edits.

Pub 100

00870: Pub 100-04, 12, 140.5, Pub 100-04, 12, 50, Pub 100-04, 12, 90.4.5

Base Units

Global: XXX

Code	Base Units
00870	5

Modifiers (PAR)

Code	Mod 50	Mod 51	Mod 62	Mod 80
00870	9	9	9	9

CPT © 2018 American Medical Association. All Rights Reserved.

00872

00872 Anesthesia for lithotripsy, extracorporeal shock wave; with water bath

ICD-10-CM Diagnostic Codes

N20.0	Calculus of kidney
N20.1	Calculus of ureter
N20.2	Calculus of kidney with calculus of ureter
N20.9	Urinary calculus, unspecified
N21.0	Calculus in bladder
N21.1	Calculus in urethra
N21.8	Other lower urinary tract calculus
N21.9	Calculus of lower urinary tract, unspecified
N22	Calculus of urinary tract in diseases classified elsewhere

CCI Edits

Refer to Appendix A for CCI edits.

Pub 100

00872: Pub 100-04, 12, 140.5, Pub 100-04, 12, 50, Pub 100-04, 12, 90.4.5

Base Units

Global: XXX

Code	Base Units
00872	7

Modifiers (PAR)

Code	Mod 50	Mod 51	Mod 62	Mod 80
00872	9	9	9	9

CPT © 2018 American Medical Association. All Rights Reserved.

00873

00873 Anesthesia for lithotripsy, extracorporeal shock wave; without water bath

ICD-10-CM Diagnostic Codes

N20.0	Calculus of kidney
N20.1	Calculus of ureter
N20.2	Calculus of kidney with calculus of ureter
N20.9	Urinary calculus, unspecified
N21.0	Calculus in bladder
N21.1	Calculus in urethra
N21.8	Other lower urinary tract calculus
N21.9	Calculus of lower urinary tract, unspecified
N22	Calculus of urinary tract in diseases classified elsewhere

CCI Edits

Refer to Appendix A for CCI edits.

Pub 100

00873: Pub 100-04, 12, 140.5, Pub 100-04, 12, 50, Pub 100-04, 12, 90.4.5

Base Units

Global: XXX

Code	Base Units
00873	5

Modifiers (PAR)

Code	Mod 50	Mod 51	Mod 62	Mod 80
00873	9	9	9	9

CPT © 2018 American Medical Association. All Rights Reserved.

00880

00880 Anesthesia for procedures on major lower abdominal vessels; not otherwise specified

ICD-10-CM Diagnostic Codes

	I71.02	Dissection of abdominal aorta
	I71.3	Abdominal aortic aneurysm, ruptured
	I71.4	Abdominal aortic aneurysm, without rupture
	I72.3	Aneurysm of iliac artery
	I72.8	Aneurysm of other specified arteries
	I74.01	Saddle embolus of abdominal aorta
	I74.09	Other arterial embolism and thrombosis of abdominal aorta
	I74.5	Embolism and thrombosis of iliac artery
	I74.8	Embolism and thrombosis of other arteries
	I75.89	Atheroembolism of other site
	I76	Septic arterial embolism
	I77.0	Arteriovenous fistula, acquired
	I77.1	Stricture of artery
	I77.2	Rupture of artery
	I77.3	Arterial fibromuscular dysplasia
	I77.5	Necrosis of artery
	I77.72	Dissection of iliac artery
	I77.79	Dissection of other specified artery
	I77.811	Abdominal aortic ectasia
	I77.89	Other specified disorders of arteries and arterioles
	I79.0	Aneurysm of aorta in diseases classified elsewhere
	I82.220	Acute embolism and thrombosis of inferior vena cava
	I82.221	Chronic embolism and thrombosis of inferior vena cava
	I82.890	Acute embolism and thrombosis of other specified veins
	I82.891	Chronic embolism and thrombosis of other specified veins
	Q27.39	Arteriovenous malformation, other site
	Q27.8	Other specified congenital malformations of peripheral vascular system
➐	S35.01	Minor laceration of abdominal aorta
➐	S35.02	Major laceration of abdominal aorta
➐	S35.09	Other injury of abdominal aorta
➐	S35.231	Minor laceration of inferior mesenteric artery
➐	S35.232	Major laceration of inferior mesenteric artery
➐	S35.238	Other injury of inferior mesenteric artery
➐⇄	S35.511	Injury of right iliac artery
➐⇄	S35.512	Injury of left iliac artery
➐⇄	S35.514	Injury of right iliac vein
➐⇄	S35.515	Injury of left iliac vein
➐⇄	S35.531	Injury of right uterine artery
➐⇄	S35.532	Injury of left uterine artery
➐⇄	S35.534	Injury of right uterine vein
➐⇄	S35.535	Injury of left uterine vein
➐	S35.59	Injury of other iliac blood vessels
➐	S35.8X1	Laceration of other blood vessels at abdomen, lower back and pelvis level
➐	S35.8X8	Other specified injury of other blood vessels at abdomen, lower back and pelvis level

ICD-10-CM Coding Notes

For codes requiring a 7th character extension, refer to your ICD-10-CM book. Review the character descriptions and coding guidelines for proper selection. For some procedures, only certain characters will apply.

CCI Edits

Refer to Appendix A for CCI edits.

Pub 100

00880: Pub 100-04, 12, 140.5, Pub 100-04, 12, 50, Pub 100-04, 12, 90.4.5

Base Units

Global: XXX

Code	Base Units
00880	15

Modifiers (PAR)

Code	Mod 50	Mod 51	Mod 62	Mod 80
00880	9	9	9	9

CPT © 2018 American Medical Association. All Rights Reserved.

00882

00882 Anesthesia for procedures on major lower abdominal vessels; inferior vena cava ligation

ICD-10-CM Diagnostic Codes

⇄	I80.11	Phlebitis and thrombophlebitis of right femoral vein
⇄	I80.12	Phlebitis and thrombophlebitis of left femoral vein
⇄	I80.13	Phlebitis and thrombophlebitis of femoral vein, bilateral
⇄	I80.211	Phlebitis and thrombophlebitis of right iliac vein
⇄	I80.212	Phlebitis and thrombophlebitis of left iliac vein
⇄	I80.213	Phlebitis and thrombophlebitis of iliac vein, bilateral
⇄	I80.291	Phlebitis and thrombophlebitis of other deep vessels of right lower extremity
⇄	I80.292	Phlebitis and thrombophlebitis of other deep vessels of left lower extremity
⇄	I80.293	Phlebitis and thrombophlebitis of other deep vessels of lower extremity, bilateral
⇄	I82.411	Acute embolism and thrombosis of right femoral vein
⇄	I82.412	Acute embolism and thrombosis of left femoral vein
⇄	I82.413	Acute embolism and thrombosis of femoral vein, bilateral
⇄	I82.421	Acute embolism and thrombosis of right iliac vein
⇄	I82.422	Acute embolism and thrombosis of left iliac vein
⇄	I82.423	Acute embolism and thrombosis of iliac vein, bilateral
⇄	I82.4Y1	Acute embolism and thrombosis of unspecified deep veins of right proximal lower extremity
⇄	I82.4Y2	Acute embolism and thrombosis of unspecified deep veins of left proximal lower extremity
⇄	I82.4Y3	Acute embolism and thrombosis of unspecified deep veins of proximal lower extremity, bilateral

CCI Edits

Refer to Appendix A for CCI edits.

Pub 100

00882: Pub 100-04, 12, 140.5, Pub 100-04, 12, 50, Pub 100-04, 12, 90.4.5

Base Units

Global: XXX

Code	Base Units
00882	10

Modifiers (PAR)

Code	Mod 50	Mod 51	Mod 62	Mod 80
00882	9	9	9	9

CPT © 2018 American Medical Association. All Rights Reserved.

00902

00902 Anesthesia for; anorectal procedure

AMA Coding Notes

Anesthesia for Procedures on the Perineum

(For perineal procedures on integumentary system, muscles and nerves, see 00300, 00400)

AMA *CPT Assistant*

00902: Mar 06: 15, Oct 11: 3, Jul 12: 13

ICD-10-CM Diagnostic Codes

	C20	Malignant neoplasm of rectum
	C21.0	Malignant neoplasm of anus, unspecified
	C21.1	Malignant neoplasm of anal canal
	C21.2	Malignant neoplasm of cloacogenic zone
	C21.8	Malignant neoplasm of overlapping sites of rectum, anus and anal canal
	C78.5	Secondary malignant neoplasm of large intestine and rectum
	C7A.026	Malignant carcinoid tumor of the rectum
	D01.2	Carcinoma in situ of rectum
	D01.3	Carcinoma in situ of anus and anal canal
	D12.8	Benign neoplasm of rectum
	D37.5	Neoplasm of uncertain behavior of rectum
	D37.8	Neoplasm of uncertain behavior of other specified digestive organs
	D3A.026	Benign carcinoid tumor of the rectum
	D49.0	Neoplasm of unspecified behavior of digestive system
	K51.211	Ulcerative (chronic) proctitis with rectal bleeding
	K51.212	Ulcerative (chronic) proctitis with intestinal obstruction
	K51.213	Ulcerative (chronic) proctitis with fistula
	K51.214	Ulcerative (chronic) proctitis with abscess
	K51.218	Ulcerative (chronic) proctitis with other complication
	K51.219	Ulcerative (chronic) proctitis with unspecified complications
	K60.1	Chronic anal fissure
	K60.3	Anal fistula
	K60.4	Rectal fistula
	K60.5	Anorectal fistula
	K61.0	Anal abscess
	K61.1	Rectal abscess
	K61.2	Anorectal abscess
	K61.31	Horseshoe abscess
	K61.39	Other ischiorectal abscess
	K61.4	Intrasphincteric abscess
	K61.5	Supralevator abscess
	K62.0	Anal polyp
	K62.1	Rectal polyp
	K62.2	Anal prolapse
	K62.3	Rectal prolapse
	K62.4	Stenosis of anus and rectum
	K62.82	Dysplasia of anus
	K62.89	Other specified diseases of anus and rectum
	R15.9	Full incontinence of feces
⑦	S36.61	Primary blast injury of rectum
⑦	S36.62	Contusion of rectum
⑦	S36.63	Laceration of rectum
⑦	S36.69	Other injury of rectum

ICD-10-CM Coding Notes

For codes requiring a 7th character extension, refer to your ICD-10-CM book. Review the character descriptions and coding guidelines for proper selection. For some procedures, only certain characters will apply.

CCI Edits

Refer to Appendix A for CCI edits.

Pub 100

00902: Pub 100-04, 12, 140.5, Pub 100-04, 12, 50, Pub 100-04, 12, 90.4.5

Base Units

Global: XXX

Code	Base Units
00902	5

Modifiers (PAR)

Code	Mod 50	Mod 51	Mod 62	Mod 80
00902	9	9	9	9

CPT © 2018 American Medical Association. All Rights Reserved.

00904

00904 Anesthesia for; radical perineal procedure

AMA Coding Notes

Anesthesia for Procedures on the Perineum

(For perineal procedures on integumentary system, muscles and nerves, see 00300, 00400)

ICD-10-CM Diagnostic Codes

	C51.0	Malignant neoplasm of labium majus ♀
	C51.1	Malignant neoplasm of labium minus ♀
	C51.2	Malignant neoplasm of clitoris ♀
	C51.8	Malignant neoplasm of overlapping sites of vulva ♀
	C51.9	Malignant neoplasm of vulva, unspecified ♀
	C52	Malignant neoplasm of vagina ♀
	C79.82	Secondary malignant neoplasm of genital organs
	D07.1	Carcinoma in situ of vulva ♀
	D07.30	Carcinoma in situ of unspecified female genital organs ♀
	D07.39	Carcinoma in situ of other female genital organs ♀
	D39.8	Neoplasm of uncertain behavior of other specified female genital organs ♀
	N42.89	Other specified disorders of prostate ♂
⑦	S31.41	Laceration without foreign body of vagina and vulva
⑦	S31.42	Laceration with foreign body of vagina and vulva
⑦	S31.43	Puncture wound without foreign body of vagina and vulva
⑦	S31.44	Puncture wound with foreign body of vagina and vulva
⑦	S31.45	Open bite of vagina and vulva
⑦	S38.03	Crushing injury of vulva

ICD-10-CM Coding Notes

For codes requiring a 7th character extension, refer to your ICD-10-CM book. Review the character descriptions and coding guidelines for proper selection. For some procedures, only certain characters will apply.

CCI Edits

Refer to Appendix A for CCI edits.

Pub 100

00904: Pub 100-04, 12, 140.5, Pub 100-04, 12, 50, Pub 100-04, 12, 90.4.5

Base Units

Global: XXX

Code	Base Units
00904	7

Modifiers (PAR)

Code	Mod 50	Mod 51	Mod 62	Mod 80
00904	9	9	9	9

CPT © 2018 American Medical Association. All Rights Reserved.

00906

00906 Anesthesia for; vulvectomy

AMA Coding Notes

Anesthesia for Procedures on the Perineum

(For perineal procedures on integumentary system, muscles and nerves, see 00300, 00400)

ICD-10-CM Diagnostic Codes

C51.0	Malignant neoplasm of labium majus ♀
C51.1	Malignant neoplasm of labium minus ♀
C51.2	Malignant neoplasm of clitoris ♀
C51.8	Malignant neoplasm of overlapping sites of vulva ♀
C51.9	Malignant neoplasm of vulva, unspecified ♀
C79.82	Secondary malignant neoplasm of genital organs

CCI Edits

Refer to Appendix A for CCI edits.

Pub 100

00906: Pub 100-04, 12, 140.5, Pub 100-04, 12, 50, Pub 100-04, 12, 90.4.5

Base Units

Global: XXX

Code	Base Units
00906	4

Modifiers (PAR)

Code	Mod 50	Mod 51	Mod 62	Mod 80
00906	9	9	9	9

CPT © 2018 American Medical Association. All Rights Reserved.

00908

00908 Anesthesia for; perineal prostatectomy

AMA Coding Notes

Anesthesia for Procedures on the Perineum

(For perineal procedures on integumentary system, muscles and nerves, see 00300, 00400)

ICD-10-CM Diagnostic Codes

C61	Malignant neoplasm of prostate ♂
C79.82	Secondary malignant neoplasm of genital organs
D29.1	Benign neoplasm of prostate ♂
D40.0	Neoplasm of uncertain behavior of prostate ♂
N13.8	Other obstructive and reflux uropathy
N39.3	Stress incontinence (female) (male)
N39.41	Urge incontinence
N39.42	Incontinence without sensory awareness
N39.43	Post-void dribbling
N39.44	Nocturnal enuresis
N39.45	Continuous leakage
N39.46	Mixed incontinence
N39.490	Overflow incontinence
N39.498	Other specified urinary incontinence
N40.1	Benign prostatic hyperplasia with lower urinary tract symptoms ♂
N40.3	Nodular prostate with lower urinary tract symptoms ♂
N41.2	Abscess of prostate ♂
N41.4	Granulomatous prostatitis ♂
N41.8	Other inflammatory diseases of prostate ♂
N42.0	Calculus of prostate ♂
N42.1	Congestion and hemorrhage of prostate ♂
N42.31	Prostatic intraepithelial neoplasia ♂
N42.32	Atypical small acinar proliferation of prostate ♂
N42.39	Other dysplasia of prostate ♂
N42.83	Cyst of prostate ♂
R33.8	Other retention of urine
R35.0	Frequency of micturition
R35.1	Nocturia
R39.11	Hesitancy of micturition
R39.12	Poor urinary stream
R39.14	Feeling of incomplete bladder emptying
R39.15	Urgency of urination
R39.16	Straining to void

CCI Edits

Refer to Appendix A for CCI edits.

Pub 100

00908: Pub 100-04, 12, 140.5, Pub 100-04, 12, 50, Pub 100-04, 12, 90.4.5

Base Units

Global: XXX

Code	Base Units
00908	6

Modifiers (PAR)

Code	Mod 50	Mod 51	Mod 62	Mod 80
00908	9	9	9	9

CPT © 2018 American Medical Association. All Rights Reserved.

00910

00910 Anesthesia for transurethral procedures (including urethrocystoscopy); not otherwise specified

AMA Coding Notes

Anesthesia for Procedures on the Perineum

(For perineal procedures on integumentary system, muscles and nerves, see 00300, 00400)

ICD-10-CM Diagnostic Codes

C61	Malignant neoplasm of prostate ♂
C67.8	Malignant neoplasm of overlapping sites of bladder
D07.5	Carcinoma in situ of prostate ♂
D09.0	Carcinoma in situ of bladder
N13.1	Hydronephrosis with ureteral stricture, not elsewhere classified
N13.39	Other hydronephrosis
N13.4	Hydroureter
N13.71	Vesicoureteral-reflux without reflux nephropathy
N13.721	Vesicoureteral-reflux with reflux nephropathy without hydroureter, unilateral
N13.722	Vesicoureteral-reflux with reflux nephropathy without hydroureter, bilateral
N13.731	Vesicoureteral-reflux with reflux nephropathy with hydroureter, unilateral
N13.732	Vesicoureteral-reflux with reflux nephropathy with hydroureter, bilateral
N13.8	Other obstructive and reflux uropathy
N30.10	Interstitial cystitis (chronic) without hematuria
N30.11	Interstitial cystitis (chronic) with hematuria
N32.0	Bladder-neck obstruction
N35.010	Post-traumatic urethral stricture, male, meatal ♂
N35.011	Post-traumatic bulbous urethral stricture ♂
N35.012	Post-traumatic membranous urethral stricture ♂
N35.013	Post-traumatic anterior urethral stricture ♂
N35.016	Post-traumatic urethral stricture, male, overlapping sites ♂
N35.021	Urethral stricture due to childbirth ♀
N35.028	Other post-traumatic urethral stricture, female ♀
N35.111	Postinfective urethral stricture, not elsewhere classified, male, meatal ♂
N35.112	Postinfective bulbous urethral stricture, not elsewhere classified, male ♂
N35.113	Postinfective membranous urethral stricture, not elsewhere classified, male ♂
N35.114	Postinfective anterior urethral stricture, not elsewhere classified, male ♂
N35.116	Postinfective urethral stricture, not elsewhere classified, male, overlapping sites ♂
N35.12	Postinfective urethral stricture, not elsewhere classified, female ♀
N35.811	Other urethral stricture, male, meatal ♂
N35.812	Other urethral bulbous stricture, male ♂
N35.813	Other membranous urethral stricture, male ♂
N35.814	Other anterior urethral stricture, male, anterior ♂
N35.816	Other urethral stricture, male, overlapping sites ♂
N35.82	Other urethral stricture, female ♀
N35.911	Unspecified urethral stricture, male, meatal ♂
N35.912	Unspecified bulbous urethral stricture, male ♂
N35.913	Unspecified membranous urethral stricture, male ♂
N35.914	Unspecified anterior urethral stricture, male ♂
N35.916	Unspecified urethral stricture, male, overlapping sites ♂
N35.92	Unspecified urethral stricture, female ♀
N36.0	Urethral fistula
N36.1	Urethral diverticulum
N36.2	Urethral caruncle
N39.3	Stress incontinence (female) (male)
N40.0	Benign prostatic hyperplasia without lower urinary tract symptoms ♂
N40.1	Benign prostatic hyperplasia with lower urinary tract symptoms ♂
N40.2	Nodular prostate without lower urinary tract symptoms ♂
N40.3	Nodular prostate with lower urinary tract symptoms ♂
N41.2	Abscess of prostate ♂
N42.31	Prostatic intraepithelial neoplasia ♂
N42.32	Atypical small acinar proliferation of prostate ♂
N42.39	Other dysplasia of prostate ♂
N81.0	Urethrocele ♀
N99.111	Postprocedural bulbous urethral stricture, male ♂
N99.112	Postprocedural membranous urethral stricture, male ♂
N99.113	Postprocedural anterior bulbous urethral stricture, male ♂
N99.115	Postprocedural fossa navicularis urethral stricture ♂
N99.116	Postprocedural urethral stricture, male, overlapping sites ♂
Q62.0	Congenital hydronephrosis
Q62.11	Congenital occlusion of ureteropelvic junction
Q62.12	Congenital occlusion of ureterovesical orifice
Q62.63	Anomalous implantation of ureter
Q62.7	Congenital vesico-uretero-renal reflux
Q64.2	Congenital posterior urethral valves
Q64.31	Congenital bladder neck obstruction
Q64.32	Congenital stricture of urethra
Q64.39	Other atresia and stenosis of urethra and bladder neck
Q64.70	Unspecified congenital malformation of bladder and urethra
Q64.71	Congenital prolapse of urethra
Q64.72	Congenital prolapse of urinary meatus
Q64.74	Double urethra
Q64.75	Double urinary meatus
Q64.79	Other congenital malformations of bladder and urethra
R31.0	Gross hematuria
R31.1	Benign essential microscopic hematuria
R31.21	Asymptomatic microscopic hematuria
R31.29	Other microscopic hematuria

CCI Edits

Refer to Appendix A for CCI edits.

Pub 100

00910: Pub 100-04, 12, 140.5, Pub 100-04, 12, 50, Pub 100-04, 12, 90.4.5

Base Units

Global: XXX

Code	Base Units
00910	3

Modifiers (PAR)

Code	Mod 50	Mod 51	Mod 62	Mod 80
00910	9	9	9	9

CPT © 2018 American Medical Association. All Rights Reserved.

00912

00912 Anesthesia for transurethral procedures (including urethrocystoscopy); transurethral resection of bladder tumor(s)

AMA Coding Notes

Anesthesia for Procedures on the Perineum

(For perineal procedures on integumentary system, muscles and nerves, see 00300, 00400)

ICD-10-CM Diagnostic Codes

C67.0	Malignant neoplasm of trigone of bladder
C67.1	Malignant neoplasm of dome of bladder
C67.2	Malignant neoplasm of lateral wall of bladder
C67.3	Malignant neoplasm of anterior wall of bladder
C67.4	Malignant neoplasm of posterior wall of bladder
C67.5	Malignant neoplasm of bladder neck
C67.6	Malignant neoplasm of ureteric orifice
C67.7	Malignant neoplasm of urachus
C67.8	Malignant neoplasm of overlapping sites of bladder
C67.9	Malignant neoplasm of bladder, unspecified
C79.11	Secondary malignant neoplasm of bladder
D09.0	Carcinoma in situ of bladder
D30.3	Benign neoplasm of bladder
D41.4	Neoplasm of uncertain behavior of bladder
D49.4	Neoplasm of unspecified behavior of bladder

CCI Edits

Refer to Appendix A for CCI edits.

Pub 100

00912: Pub 100-04, 12, 140.5, Pub 100-04, 12, 50, Pub 100-04, 12, 90.4.5

Base Units

Global: XXX

Code	Base Units
00912	5

Modifiers (PAR)

Code	Mod 50	Mod 51	Mod 62	Mod 80
00912	9	9	9	9

CPT © 2018 American Medical Association. All Rights Reserved.

00914

00914 Anesthesia for transurethral procedures (including urethrocystoscopy); transurethral resection of prostate

AMA Coding Notes

Anesthesia for Procedures on the Perineum

(For perineal procedures on integumentary system, muscles and nerves, see 00300, 00400)

ICD-10-CM Diagnostic Codes

C61	Malignant neoplasm of prostate ♂
C79.82	Secondary malignant neoplasm of genital organs
D07.5	Carcinoma in situ of prostate ♂
D29.1	Benign neoplasm of prostate ♂
D40.0	Neoplasm of uncertain behavior of prostate ♂
N39.41	Urge incontinence
N39.42	Incontinence without sensory awareness
N39.43	Post-void dribbling
N39.44	Nocturnal enuresis
N39.45	Continuous leakage
N39.46	Mixed incontinence
N39.490	Overflow incontinence
N39.498	Other specified urinary incontinence
N40.1	Benign prostatic hyperplasia with lower urinary tract symptoms ♂
N40.3	Nodular prostate with lower urinary tract symptoms ♂
N41.4	Granulomatous prostatitis ♂
N42.31	Prostatic intraepithelial neoplasia ♂
N42.32	Atypical small acinar proliferation of prostate ♂
N42.39	Other dysplasia of prostate ♂
R33.8	Other retention of urine
R35.0	Frequency of micturition
R35.1	Nocturia
R39.11	Hesitancy of micturition
R39.12	Poor urinary stream
R39.14	Feeling of incomplete bladder emptying
R39.15	Urgency of urination
R39.16	Straining to void

CCI Edits

Refer to Appendix A for CCI edits.

Pub 100

00914: Pub 100-04, 12, 140.5, Pub 100-04, 12, 50, Pub 100-04, 12, 90.4.5

Base Units

Global: XXX

Code	Base Units
00914	5

Modifiers (PAR)

Code	Mod 50	Mod 51	Mod 62	Mod 80
00914	9	9	9	9

CPT © 2018 American Medical Association. All Rights Reserved.

00916

00916 Anesthesia for transurethral procedures (including urethrocystoscopy); post-transurethral resection bleeding

AMA Coding Notes

Anesthesia for Procedures on the Perineum

(For perineal procedures on integumentary system, muscles and nerves, see 00300, 00400)

ICD-10-CM Diagnostic Codes

N99.820 Postprocedural hemorrhage of a genitourinary system organ or structure following a genitourinary system procedure

CCI Edits

Refer to Appendix A for CCI edits.

Pub 100

00916: Pub 100-04, 12, 140.5, Pub 100-04, 12, 50, Pub 100-04, 12, 90.4.5

Base Units

Global: XXX

Code	Base Units
00916	5

Modifiers (PAR)

Code	Mod 50	Mod 51	Mod 62	Mod 80
00916	9	9	9	9

CPT © 2018 American Medical Association. All Rights Reserved.

00918

00918 Anesthesia for transurethral procedures (including urethrocystoscopy); with fragmentation, manipulation and/or removal of ureteral calculus

AMA Coding Notes

Anesthesia for Procedures on the Perineum

(For perineal procedures on integumentary system, muscles and nerves, see 00300, 00400)

AMA *CPT Assistant*

00918: Nov 99: 8, Apr 09: 8

ICD-10-CM Diagnostic Codes

N13.2	Hydronephrosis with renal and ureteral calculous obstruction
N13.6	Pyonephrosis
N20.1	Calculus of ureter
N20.2	Calculus of kidney with calculus of ureter

CCI Edits

Refer to Appendix A for CCI edits.

Pub 100

00918: Pub 100-04, 12, 140.5, Pub 100-04, 12, 50, Pub 100-04, 12, 90.4.5

Base Units

Global: XXX

Code	Base Units
00918	5

Modifiers (PAR)

Code	Mod 50	Mod 51	Mod 62	Mod 80
00918	9	9	9	9

CPT © 2018 American Medical Association. All Rights Reserved.

00920

00920 Anesthesia for procedures on male genitalia (including open urethral procedures); not otherwise specified

AMA Coding Notes

Anesthesia for Procedures on the Perineum

(For perineal procedures on integumentary system, muscles and nerves, see 00300, 00400)

AMA *CPT Assistant* ▯

00920: Sep 12: 16

ICD-10-CM Diagnostic Codes

	I86.1	Scrotal varices ♂
	N43.0	Encysted hydrocele ♂
	N43.1	Infected hydrocele ♂
	N43.2	Other hydrocele ♂
	N43.41	Spermatocele of epididymis, single ♂
	N43.42	Spermatocele of epididymis, multiple ♂
	N44.01	Extravaginal torsion of spermatic cord ♂
	N44.1	Cyst of tunica albuginea testis ♂
	N44.2	Benign cyst of testis ♂
	N45.4	Abscess of epididymis or testis ♂
	N47.0	Adherent prepuce, newborn ♂
	N47.1	Phimosis ♂
	N47.5	Adhesions of prepuce and glans penis ♂
	N48.21	Abscess of corpus cavernosum and penis ♂
	N50.3	Cyst of epididymis ♂
⇄	N50.811	Right testicular pain ♂
⇄	N50.812	Left testicular pain ♂
	N50.82	Scrotal pain ♂
	N50.89	Other specified disorders of the male genital organs ♂
	Q54.0	Hypospadias, balanic ♂
	Q54.1	Hypospadias, penile ♂
	Q54.2	Hypospadias, penoscrotal ♂
	Q54.3	Hypospadias, perineal ♂
	Q54.4	Congenital chordee ♂
	Q54.8	Other hypospadias ♂
	Q64.0	Epispadias
❼	S31.31	Laceration without foreign body of scrotum and testes
❼	S31.33	Puncture wound without foreign body of scrotum and testes
❼	S31.35	Open bite of scrotum and testes
❼	S38.231	Complete traumatic amputation of scrotum and testis

ICD-10-CM Coding Notes

For codes requiring a 7th character extension, refer to your ICD-10-CM book. Review the character descriptions and coding guidelines for proper selection. For some procedures, only certain characters will apply.

CCI Edits

Refer to Appendix A for CCI edits.

Pub 100

00920: Pub 100-04, 12, 140.5, Pub 100-04, 12, 50, Pub 100-04, 12, 90.4.5

Base Units

Global: XXX

Code	Base Units
00920	3

Modifiers (PAR)

Code	Mod 50	Mod 51	Mod 62	Mod 80
00920	9	9	9	9

CPT © 2018 American Medical Association. All Rights Reserved.

00921

00921 Anesthesia for procedures on male genitalia (including open urethral procedures); vasectomy, unilateral or bilateral

AMA Coding Notes

Anesthesia for Procedures on the Perineum

(For perineal procedures on integumentary system, muscles and nerves, see 00300, 00400)

ICD-10-CM Diagnostic Codes

Z30.2 Encounter for sterilization

CCI Edits

Refer to Appendix A for CCI edits.

Pub 100

00921: Pub 100-04, 12, 140.5, Pub 100-04, 12, 50, Pub 100-04, 12, 90.4.5

Base Units

Global: XXX

Code	Base Units
00921	3

Modifiers (PAR)

Code	Mod 50	Mod 51	Mod 62	Mod 80
00921	9	9	9	9

CPT © 2018 American Medical Association. All Rights Reserved.

00922

00922 Anesthesia for procedures on male genitalia (including open urethral procedures); seminal vesicles

AMA Coding Notes

Anesthesia for Procedures on the Perineum

(For perineal procedures on integumentary system, muscles and nerves, see 00300, 00400)

ICD-10-CM Diagnostic Codes

N49.0	Inflammatory disorders of seminal vesicle ♂
N50.82	Scrotal pain ♂
N50.89	Other specified disorders of the male genital organs ♂
Q55.4	Other congenital malformations of vas deferens, epididymis, seminal vesicles and prostate ♂

CCI Edits

Refer to Appendix A for CCI edits.

Pub 100

00922: Pub 100-04, 12, 140.5, Pub 100-04, 12, 50, Pub 100-04, 12, 90.4.5

Base Units

Global: XXX

Code	Base Units
00922	6

Modifiers (PAR)

Code	Mod 50	Mod 51	Mod 62	Mod 80
00922	9	9	9	9

CPT © 2018 American Medical Association. All Rights Reserved.

00924

00924 Anesthesia for procedures on male genitalia (including open urethral procedures); undescended testis, unilateral or bilateral

AMA Coding Notes

Anesthesia for Procedures on the Perineum

(For perineal procedures on integumentary system, muscles and nerves, see 00300, 00400)

ICD-10-CM Diagnostic Codes

Q53.00	Ectopic testis, unspecified ♂
Q53.01	Ectopic testis, unilateral ♂
Q53.02	Ectopic testes, bilateral ♂
Q53.10	Unspecified undescended testicle, unilateral ♂
Q53.111	Unilateral intraabdominal testis ♂
Q53.112	Unilateral inguinal testis ♂
Q53.12	Ectopic perineal testis, unilateral ♂
Q53.13	Unilateral high scrotal testis ♂
Q53.20	Undescended testicle, unspecified, bilateral ♂
Q53.211	Bilateral intraabdominal testes ♂
Q53.212	Bilateral inguinal testes ♂
Q53.22	Ectopic perineal testis, bilateral ♂
Q53.9	Undescended testicle, unspecified ♂

CCI Edits

Refer to Appendix A for CCI edits.

Pub 100

00924: Pub 100-04, 12, 140.5, Pub 100-04, 12, 50, Pub 100-04, 12, 90.4.5

Base Units

Global: XXX

Code	Base Units
00924	4

Modifiers (PAR)

Code	Mod 50	Mod 51	Mod 62	Mod 80
00924	9	9	9	9

CPT © 2018 American Medical Association. All Rights Reserved.

00926

00926 Anesthesia for procedures on male genitalia (including open urethral procedures); radical orchiectomy, inguinal

AMA Coding Notes

Anesthesia for Procedures on the Perineum

(For perineal procedures on integumentary system, muscles and nerves, see 00300, 00400)

ICD-10-CM Diagnostic Codes

⇄	C62.00	Malignant neoplasm of unspecified undescended testis ♂
⇄	C62.01	Malignant neoplasm of undescended right testis ♂
⇄	C62.02	Malignant neoplasm of undescended left testis ♂
⇄	C62.10	Malignant neoplasm of unspecified descended testis ♂
⇄	C62.11	Malignant neoplasm of descended right testis ♂
⇄	C62.12	Malignant neoplasm of descended left testis ♂
⇄	C62.90	Malignant neoplasm of unspecified testis, unspecified whether descended or undescended ♂
⇄	C62.91	Malignant neoplasm of right testis, unspecified whether descended or undescended ♂
⇄	C62.92	Malignant neoplasm of left testis, unspecified whether descended or undescended ♂
	C79.82	Secondary malignant neoplasm of genital organs
⇄	D40.10	Neoplasm of uncertain behavior of unspecified testis ♂
⇄	D40.11	Neoplasm of uncertain behavior of right testis ♂
⇄	D40.12	Neoplasm of uncertain behavior of left testis ♂

CCI Edits

Refer to Appendix A for CCI edits.

Pub 100

00926: Pub 100-04, 12, 140.5, Pub 100-04, 12, 50, Pub 100-04, 12, 90.4.5

Base Units

Global: XXX

Code	Base Units
00926	4

Modifiers (PAR)

Code	Mod 50	Mod 51	Mod 62	Mod 80
00926	9	9	9	9

CPT © 2018 American Medical Association. All Rights Reserved.

00928

00928 Anesthesia for procedures on male genitalia (including open urethral procedures); radical orchiectomy, abdominal

AMA Coding Notes

Anesthesia for Procedures on the Perineum

(For perineal procedures on integumentary system, muscles and nerves, see 00300, 00400)

ICD-10-CM Diagnostic Codes

⇄	C62.00	Malignant neoplasm of unspecified undescended testis ♂
⇄	C62.01	Malignant neoplasm of undescended right testis ♂
⇄	C62.02	Malignant neoplasm of undescended left testis ♂
⇄	C62.10	Malignant neoplasm of unspecified descended testis ♂
⇄	C62.11	Malignant neoplasm of descended right testis ♂
⇄	C62.12	Malignant neoplasm of descended left testis ♂
⇄	C62.90	Malignant neoplasm of unspecified testis, unspecified whether descended or undescended ♂
⇄	C62.91	Malignant neoplasm of right testis, unspecified whether descended or undescended ♂
⇄	C62.92	Malignant neoplasm of left testis, unspecified whether descended or undescended ♂
	C79.82	Secondary malignant neoplasm of genital organs
	D07.69	Carcinoma in situ of other male genital organs ♂
⇄	D40.10	Neoplasm of uncertain behavior of unspecified testis ♂
⇄	D40.11	Neoplasm of uncertain behavior of right testis ♂
⇄	D40.12	Neoplasm of uncertain behavior of left testis ♂

CCI Edits

Refer to Appendix A for CCI edits.

Pub 100

00928: Pub 100-04, 12, 140.5, Pub 100-04, 12, 50, Pub 100-04, 12, 90.4.5

Base Units

Global: XXX

Code	Base Units
00928	6

Modifiers (PAR)

Code	Mod 50	Mod 51	Mod 62	Mod 80
00928	9	9	9	9

CPT © 2018 American Medical Association. All Rights Reserved.

00930

00930 Anesthesia for procedures on male genitalia (including open urethral procedures); orchiopexy, unilateral or bilateral

AMA Coding Notes

Anesthesia for Procedures on the Perineum

(For perineal procedures on integumentary system, muscles and nerves, see 00300, 00400)

ICD-10-CM Diagnostic Codes

N44.00	Torsion of testis, unspecified ♂
N44.01	Extravaginal torsion of spermatic cord ♂
N44.02	Intravaginal torsion of spermatic cord ♂
N44.03	Torsion of appendix testis ♂
N44.04	Torsion of appendix epididymis ♂
Q53.00	Ectopic testis, unspecified ♂
Q53.01	Ectopic testis, unilateral ♂
Q53.02	Ectopic testes, bilateral ♂
Q53.10	Unspecified undescended testicle, unilateral ♂
Q53.12	Ectopic perineal testis, unilateral ♂
Q53.20	Undescended testicle, unspecified, bilateral ♂
Q53.22	Ectopic perineal testis, bilateral ♂
Q53.9	Undescended testicle, unspecified ♂

CCI Edits

Refer to Appendix A for CCI edits.

Pub 100

00930: Pub 100-04, 12, 140.5, Pub 100-04, 12, 50, Pub 100-04, 12, 90.4.5

Base Units

Global: XXX

Code	Base Units
00930	4

Modifiers (PAR)

Code	Mod 50	Mod 51	Mod 62	Mod 80
00930	9	9	9	9

CPT © 2018 American Medical Association. All Rights Reserved.

00932

00932 Anesthesia for procedures on male genitalia (including open urethral procedures); complete amputation of penis

AMA Coding Notes

Anesthesia for Procedures on the Perineum

(For perineal procedures on integumentary system, muscles and nerves, see 00300, 00400)

ICD-10-CM Diagnostic Codes

	C60.0	Malignant neoplasm of prepuce ♂
	C60.1	Malignant neoplasm of glans penis ♂
	C60.2	Malignant neoplasm of body of penis ♂
	C60.8	Malignant neoplasm of overlapping sites of penis ♂
	C60.9	Malignant neoplasm of penis, unspecified ♂
	C79.82	Secondary malignant neoplasm of genital organs
❼	S31.21	Laceration without foreign body of penis
❼	S31.22	Laceration with foreign body of penis
❼	S31.25	Open bite of penis
❼	S38.01	Crushing injury of penis
❼	T21.06	Burn of unspecified degree of male genital region
❼	T21.26	Burn of second degree of male genital region
❼	T21.36	Burn of third degree of male genital region

ICD-10-CM Coding Notes

For codes requiring a 7th character extension, refer to your ICD-10-CM book. Review the character descriptions and coding guidelines for proper selection. For some procedures, only certain characters will apply.

CCI Edits

Refer to Appendix A for CCI edits.

Pub 100

00932: Pub 100-04, 12, 140.5, Pub 100-04, 12, 50, Pub 100-04, 12, 90.4.5

Base Units

Global: XXX

Code	Base Units
00932	4

Modifiers (PAR)

Code	Mod 50	Mod 51	Mod 62	Mod 80
00932	9	9	9	9

CPT © 2018 American Medical Association. All Rights Reserved.

00934

00934 Anesthesia for procedures on male genitalia (including open urethral procedures); radical amputation of penis with bilateral inguinal lymphadenectomy

AMA Coding Notes

Anesthesia for Procedures on the Perineum

(For perineal procedures on integumentary system, muscles and nerves, see 00300, 00400)

ICD-10-CM Diagnostic Codes

C60.0	Malignant neoplasm of prepuce ♂
C60.1	Malignant neoplasm of glans penis ♂
C60.2	Malignant neoplasm of body of penis ♂
C60.8	Malignant neoplasm of overlapping sites of penis ♂
C60.9	Malignant neoplasm of penis, unspecified ♂
C77.4	Secondary and unspecified malignant neoplasm of inguinal and lower limb lymph nodes
C79.82	Secondary malignant neoplasm of genital organs

CCI Edits

Refer to Appendix A for CCI edits.

Pub 100

00934: Pub 100-04, 12, 140.5, Pub 100-04, 12, 50, Pub 100-04, 12, 90.4.5

Base Units

Global: XXX

Code	Base Units
00934	6

Modifiers (PAR)

Code	Mod 50	Mod 51	Mod 62	Mod 80
00934	9	9	9	9

CPT © 2018 American Medical Association. All Rights Reserved.

00936

00936 Anesthesia for procedures on male genitalia (including open urethral procedures); radical amputation of penis with bilateral inguinal and iliac lymphadenectomy

AMA Coding Notes

Anesthesia for Procedures on the Perineum

(For perineal procedures on integumentary system, muscles and nerves, see 00300, 00400)

ICD-10-CM Diagnostic Codes

C60.0	Malignant neoplasm of prepuce ♂
C60.1	Malignant neoplasm of glans penis ♂
C60.2	Malignant neoplasm of body of penis ♂
C60.8	Malignant neoplasm of overlapping sites of penis ♂
C60.9	Malignant neoplasm of penis, unspecified ♂
C77.4	Secondary and unspecified malignant neoplasm of inguinal and lower limb lymph nodes
C77.5	Secondary and unspecified malignant neoplasm of intrapelvic lymph nodes
C79.82	Secondary malignant neoplasm of genital organs

CCI Edits

Refer to Appendix A for CCI edits.

Pub 100

00936: Pub 100-04, 12, 140.5, Pub 100-04, 12, 50, Pub 100-04, 12, 90.4.5

Base Units

Global: XXX

Code	Base Units
00936	8

Modifiers (PAR)

Code	Mod 50	Mod 51	Mod 62	Mod 80
00936	9	9	9	9

CPT © 2018 American Medical Association. All Rights Reserved.

00938

00938 Anesthesia for procedures on male genitalia (including open urethral procedures); insertion of penile prosthesis (perineal approach)

AMA Coding Notes

Anesthesia for Procedures on the Perineum

(For perineal procedures on integumentary system, muscles and nerves, see 00300, 00400)

ICD-10-CM Diagnostic Codes

N52.01	Erectile dysfunction due to arterial insufficiency ♂
N52.02	Corporo-venous occlusive erectile dysfunction ♂
N52.03	Combined arterial insufficiency and corporo-venous occlusive erectile dysfunction ♂
N52.1	Erectile dysfunction due to diseases classified elsewhere ♂
N52.2	Drug-induced erectile dysfunction ♂
N52.31	Erectile dysfunction following radical prostatectomy ♂
N52.32	Erectile dysfunction following radical cystectomy ♂
N52.33	Erectile dysfunction following urethral surgery ♂
N52.34	Erectile dysfunction following simple prostatectomy ♂
N52.39	Other and unspecified postprocedural erectile dysfunction ♂
N52.8	Other male erectile dysfunction ♂
N52.9	Male erectile dysfunction, unspecified ♂

CCI Edits

Refer to Appendix A for CCI edits.

Pub 100

00938: Pub 100-04, 12, 140.5, Pub 100-04, 12, 50, Pub 100-04, 12, 90.4.5

Base Units

Global: XXX

Code	Base Units
00938	4

Modifiers (PAR)

Code	Mod 50	Mod 51	Mod 62	Mod 80
00938	9	9	9	9

CPT © 2018 American Medical Association. All Rights Reserved.

00940

00940 Anesthesia for vaginal procedures (including biopsy of labia, vagina, cervix or endometrium); not otherwise specified

AMA Coding Notes

Anesthesia for Procedures on the Perineum

(For perineal procedures on integumentary system, muscles and nerves, see 00300, 00400)

ICD-10-CM Diagnostic Codes

C51.0	Malignant neoplasm of labium majus ♀
C51.1	Malignant neoplasm of labium minus ♀
C51.2	Malignant neoplasm of clitoris ♀
C51.8	Malignant neoplasm of overlapping sites of vulva ♀
C51.9	Malignant neoplasm of vulva, unspecified ♀
C52	Malignant neoplasm of vagina ♀
C54.1	Malignant neoplasm of endometrium ♀
C79.82	Secondary malignant neoplasm of genital organs
D06.0	Carcinoma in situ of endocervix ♀
D06.1	Carcinoma in situ of exocervix ♀
D06.7	Carcinoma in situ of other parts of cervix ♀
D06.9	Carcinoma in situ of cervix, unspecified ♀
D07.0	Carcinoma in situ of endometrium ♀
D07.1	Carcinoma in situ of vulva ♀
D07.2	Carcinoma in situ of vagina ♀
D26.0	Other benign neoplasm of cervix uteri ♀
D26.1	Other benign neoplasm of corpus uteri ♀
D28.0	Benign neoplasm of vulva ♀
D28.1	Benign neoplasm of vagina ♀
N75.0	Cyst of Bartholin's gland ♀
N75.1	Abscess of Bartholin's gland ♀
N76.4	Abscess of vulva ♀
N80.0	Endometriosis of uterus ♀
N80.4	Endometriosis of rectovaginal septum and vagina ♀
N82.5	Female genital tract-skin fistulae ♀
N84.1	Polyp of cervix uteri ♀
N84.2	Polyp of vagina ♀
N84.3	Polyp of vulva ♀
N85.02	Endometrial intraepithelial neoplasia [EIN] ♀
N86	Erosion and ectropion of cervix uteri ♀
N87.1	Moderate cervical dysplasia ♀
N88.0	Leukoplakia of cervix uteri ♀
N88.2	Stricture and stenosis of cervix uteri ♀
N88.3	Incompetence of cervix uteri ♀
N89.1	Moderate vaginal dysplasia ♀
N89.4	Leukoplakia of vagina ♀
N89.5	Stricture and atresia of vagina ♀
N90.1	Moderate vulvar dysplasia ♀
N90.4	Leukoplakia of vulva ♀
N90.7	Vulvar cyst ♀
O71.3	Obstetric laceration of cervix ♀
O71.4	Obstetric high vaginal laceration alone ♀
Q52.10	Doubling of vagina, unspecified ♀
Q52.11	Transverse vaginal septum ♀
Q52.12	Longitudinal vaginal septum ♀
Q52.3	Imperforate hymen ♀
Q52.5	Fusion of labia ♀

CCI Edits

Refer to Appendix A for CCI edits.

Pub 100

00940: Pub 100-04, 12, 140.5, Pub 100-04, 12, 50, Pub 100-04, 12, 90.4.5

Base Units

Global: XXX

Code	Base Units
00940	3

Modifiers (PAR)

Code	Mod 50	Mod 51	Mod 62	Mod 80
00940	9	9	9	9

CPT © 2018 American Medical Association. All Rights Reserved.

CPT® Procedural Coding

00942

00942 Anesthesia for vaginal procedures (including biopsy of labia, vagina, cervix or endometrium); colpotomy, vaginectomy, colporrhaphy, and open urethral procedures

AMA Coding Notes

Anesthesia for Procedures on the Perineum

(For perineal procedures on integumentary system, muscles and nerves, see 00300, 00400)

ICD-10-CM Diagnostic Codes

	C52	Malignant neoplasm of vagina ♀
	C53.0	Malignant neoplasm of endocervix ♀
	C53.1	Malignant neoplasm of exocervix ♀
	C53.8	Malignant neoplasm of overlapping sites of cervix uteri ♀
	C53.9	Malignant neoplasm of cervix uteri, unspecified ♀
	C68.0	Malignant neoplasm of urethra
	C79.82	Secondary malignant neoplasm of genital organs
	D06.0	Carcinoma in situ of endocervix ♀
	D06.1	Carcinoma in situ of exocervix ♀
	D06.7	Carcinoma in situ of other parts of cervix ♀
	D06.9	Carcinoma in situ of cervix, unspecified ♀
	D07.2	Carcinoma in situ of vagina ♀
	D09.19	Carcinoma in situ of other urinary organs
	D26.0	Other benign neoplasm of cervix uteri ♀
	D28.1	Benign neoplasm of vagina ♀
	D39.8	Neoplasm of uncertain behavior of other specified female genital organs ♀
	N36.0	Urethral fistula
	N36.1	Urethral diverticulum
	N36.2	Urethral caruncle
	N36.5	Urethral false passage
	N39.3	Stress incontinence (female) (male)
	N81.0	Urethrocele ♀
	N81.10	Cystocele, unspecified ♀
	N81.11	Cystocele, midline ♀
	N81.12	Cystocele, lateral ♀
	N81.5	Vaginal enterocele ♀
	N81.6	Rectocele ♀
	N81.83	Incompetence or weakening of rectovaginal tissue ♀
	N81.85	Cervical stump prolapse ♀
	N81.89	Other female genital prolapse ♀
	N82.1	Other female urinary-genital tract fistulae ♀
	R87.611	Atypical squamous cells cannot exclude high grade squamous intraepithelial lesion on cytologic smear of cervix (ASC-H) ♀
	R87.613	High grade squamous intraepithelial lesion on cytologic smear of cervix (HGSIL) ♀
	R87.614	Cytologic evidence of malignancy on smear of cervix ♀
	R87.623	High grade squamous intraepithelial lesion on cytologic smear of vagina (HGSIL) ♀
	R87.624	Cytologic evidence of malignancy on smear of vagina ♀
	R87.810	Cervical high risk human papillomavirus (HPV) DNA test positive ♀
❼	S31.40	Unspecified open wound of vagina and vulva
❼	S31.41	Laceration without foreign body of vagina and vulva
❼	S31.42	Laceration with foreign body of vagina and vulva
❼	S31.43	Puncture wound without foreign body of vagina and vulva
❼	S31.44	Puncture wound with foreign body of vagina and vulva
❼	S31.45	Open bite of vagina and vulva
❼	T19.2	Foreign body in vulva and vagina

ICD-10-CM Coding Notes

For codes requiring a 7th character extension, refer to your ICD-10-CM book. Review the character descriptions and coding guidelines for proper selection. For some procedures, only certain characters will apply.

CCI Edits

Refer to Appendix A for CCI edits.

Pub 100

00942: Pub 100-04, 12, 140.5, Pub 100-04, 12, 50, Pub 100-04, 12, 90.4.5

Base Units

Global: XXX

Code	Base Units
00942	4

Modifiers (PAR)

Code	Mod 50	Mod 51	Mod 62	Mod 80
00942	9	9	9	9

CPT © 2018 American Medical Association. All Rights Reserved.

00944

00944 Anesthesia for vaginal procedures (including biopsy of labia, vagina, cervix or endometrium); vaginal hysterectomy

AMA Coding Notes

Anesthesia for Procedures on the Perineum

(For perineal procedures on integumentary system, muscles and nerves, see 00300, 00400)

ICD-10-CM Diagnostic Codes

C53.0	Malignant neoplasm of endocervix ♀
C53.1	Malignant neoplasm of exocervix ♀
C53.8	Malignant neoplasm of overlapping sites of cervix uteri ♀
C53.9	Malignant neoplasm of cervix uteri, unspecified ♀
C54.0	Malignant neoplasm of isthmus uteri ♀
C54.1	Malignant neoplasm of endometrium ♀
C54.2	Malignant neoplasm of myometrium ♀
C54.3	Malignant neoplasm of fundus uteri ♀
C54.8	Malignant neoplasm of overlapping sites of corpus uteri ♀
C54.9	Malignant neoplasm of corpus uteri, unspecified ♀
C55	Malignant neoplasm of uterus, part unspecified ♀
C79.82	Secondary malignant neoplasm of genital organs
D06.0	Carcinoma in situ of endocervix ♀
D06.1	Carcinoma in situ of exocervix ♀
D06.7	Carcinoma in situ of other parts of cervix ♀
D06.9	Carcinoma in situ of cervix, unspecified ♀
D07.0	Carcinoma in situ of endometrium ♀
D25.0	Submucous leiomyoma of uterus ♀
D25.1	Intramural leiomyoma of uterus ♀
D25.2	Subserosal leiomyoma of uterus ♀
D26.0	Other benign neoplasm of cervix uteri ♀
D26.1	Other benign neoplasm of corpus uteri ♀
D26.7	Other benign neoplasm of other parts of uterus ♀
D26.9	Other benign neoplasm of uterus, unspecified ♀
D39.0	Neoplasm of uncertain behavior of uterus ♀
D39.8	Neoplasm of uncertain behavior of other specified female genital organs ♀
N80.0	Endometriosis of uterus ♀
N81.2	Incomplete uterovaginal prolapse ♀
N81.3	Complete uterovaginal prolapse ♀
N81.4	Uterovaginal prolapse, unspecified ♀
N85.00	Endometrial hyperplasia, unspecified ♀
N85.01	Benign endometrial hyperplasia ♀
N85.02	Endometrial intraepithelial neoplasia [EIN] ♀
N85.2	Hypertrophy of uterus ♀
N87.0	Mild cervical dysplasia ♀
N87.1	Moderate cervical dysplasia ♀
N87.9	Dysplasia of cervix uteri, unspecified ♀
N92.4	Excessive bleeding in the premenopausal period ♀
N95.0	Postmenopausal bleeding ♀
Z40.03	Encounter for prophylactic removal of fallopian tube(s) ♀

CCI Edits

Refer to Appendix A for CCI edits.

Pub 100

00944: Pub 100-04, 12, 140.5, Pub 100-04, 12, 50, Pub 100-04, 12, 90.4.5

Base Units

Global: XXX

Code	Base Units
00944	6

Modifiers (PAR)

Code	Mod 50	Mod 51	Mod 62	Mod 80
00944	9	9	9	9

CPT © 2018 American Medical Association. All Rights Reserved.

00948

00948 Anesthesia for vaginal procedures (including biopsy of labia, vagina, cervix or endometrium); cervical cerclage

AMA Coding Notes

Anesthesia for Procedures on the Perineum

(For perineal procedures on integumentary system, muscles and nerves, see 00300, 00400)

ICD-10-CM Diagnostic Codes

O34.30	Maternal care for cervical incompetence, unspecified trimester ♀
O34.31	Maternal care for cervical incompetence, first trimester ♀
O34.32	Maternal care for cervical incompetence, second trimester ♀
O34.33	Maternal care for cervical incompetence, third trimester ♀
O34.40	Maternal care for other abnormalities of cervix, unspecified trimester ♀
O34.41	Maternal care for other abnormalities of cervix, first trimester ♀
O34.42	Maternal care for other abnormalities of cervix, second trimester ♀
O34.43	Maternal care for other abnormalities of cervix, third trimester ♀

CCI Edits

Refer to Appendix A for CCI edits.

Pub 100

00948: Pub 100-04, 12, 140.5, Pub 100-04, 12, 50, Pub 100-04, 12, 90.4.5

Base Units

Global: XXX

Code	Base Units
00948	4

Modifiers (PAR)

Code	Mod 50	Mod 51	Mod 62	Mod 80
00948	9	9	9	9

CPT © 2018 American Medical Association. All Rights Reserved.

00950

00950 Anesthesia for vaginal procedures (including biopsy of labia, vagina, cervix or endometrium); culdoscopy

AMA Coding Notes

Anesthesia for Procedures on the Perineum

(For perineal procedures on integumentary system, muscles and nerves, see 00300, 00400)

ICD-10-CM Diagnostic Codes

	N70.11	Chronic salpingitis ♀
	N70.12	Chronic oophoritis ♀
	N70.13	Chronic salpingitis and oophoritis ♀
	N80.1	Endometriosis of ovary ♀
	N80.2	Endometriosis of fallopian tube ♀
⇄	N83.01	Follicular cyst of right ovary ♀
⇄	N83.02	Follicular cyst of left ovary ♀
⇄	N83.11	Corpus luteum cyst of right ovary ♀
⇄	N83.12	Corpus luteum cyst of left ovary ♀
⇄	N83.291	Other ovarian cyst, right side ♀
⇄	N83.292	Other ovarian cyst, left side ♀
⇄	N83.511	Torsion of right ovary and ovarian pedicle ♀
⇄	N83.512	Torsion of left ovary and ovarian pedicle ♀
⇄	N83.521	Torsion of right fallopian tube ♀
⇄	N83.522	Torsion of left fallopian tube ♀
	N83.53	Torsion of ovary, ovarian pedicle and fallopian tube ♀
	N83.6	Hematosalpinx ♀
	N97.1	Female infertility of tubal origin ♀
	O00.00	Abdominal pregnancy without intrauterine pregnancy ♀
	O00.01	Abdominal pregnancy with intrauterine pregnancy ♀
⇄	O00.101	Right tubal pregnancy without intrauterine pregnancy ♀
⇄	O00.102	Left tubal pregnancy without intrauterine pregnancy ♀
⇄	O00.112	Left tubal pregnancy with intrauterine pregnancy ♀
⇄	O00.201	Right ovarian pregnancy without intrauterine pregnancy ♀
⇄	O00.211	Right ovarian pregnancy with intrauterine pregnancy ♀
⇄	O00.212	Left ovarian pregnancy with intrauterine pregnancy ♀
	O00.80	Other ectopic pregnancy without intrauterine pregnancy ♀
	O00.81	Other ectopic pregnancy with intrauterine pregnancy ♀
	R10.2	Pelvic and perineal pain
⇄	R19.03	Right lower quadrant abdominal swelling, mass and lump
⇄	R19.04	Left lower quadrant abdominal swelling, mass and lump
	Z30.2	Encounter for sterilization

CCI Edits

Refer to Appendix A for CCI edits.

Pub 100

00950: Pub 100-04, 12, 140.5, Pub 100-04, 12, 50, Pub 100-04, 12, 90.4.5

Base Units

Global: XXX

Code	Base Units
00950	5

Modifiers (PAR)

Code	Mod 50	Mod 51	Mod 62	Mod 80
00950	9	9	9	9

CPT © 2018 American Medical Association. All Rights Reserved.

00952

00952 Anesthesia for vaginal procedures (including biopsy of labia, vagina, cervix or endometrium); hysteroscopy and/or hysterosalpingography

AMA Coding Notes

Anesthesia for Procedures on the Perineum

(For perineal procedures on integumentary system, muscles and nerves, see 00300, 00400)

AMA *CPT Assistant*

00952: Nov 99: 8, Jul 12: 13

ICD-10-CM Diagnostic Codes

	D06.0	Carcinoma in situ of endocervix ♀
	D06.7	Carcinoma in situ of other parts of cervix ♀
	D07.0	Carcinoma in situ of endometrium ♀
	D25.0	Submucous leiomyoma of uterus ♀
	D25.1	Intramural leiomyoma of uterus ♀
	D26.0	Other benign neoplasm of cervix uteri ♀
	D26.1	Other benign neoplasm of corpus uteri ♀
	D26.7	Other benign neoplasm of other parts of uterus ♀
	N80.0	Endometriosis of uterus ♀
	N80.2	Endometriosis of fallopian tube ♀
	N80.8	Other endometriosis ♀
	N84.0	Polyp of corpus uteri ♀
	N84.1	Polyp of cervix uteri ♀
	N84.8	Polyp of other parts of female genital tract ♀
	N85.00	Endometrial hyperplasia, unspecified ♀
	N85.01	Benign endometrial hyperplasia ♀
	N85.02	Endometrial intraepithelial neoplasia [EIN] ♀
	N85.6	Intrauterine synechiae ♀
	N92.0	Excessive and frequent menstruation with regular cycle ♀
	N92.1	Excessive and frequent menstruation with irregular cycle ♀
	N92.4	Excessive bleeding in the premenopausal period ♀
	N97.1	Female infertility of tubal origin ♀
	N97.2	Female infertility of uterine origin ♀
	Q51.20	Other doubling of uterus, unspecified ♀
	Q51.21	Other complete doubling of uterus ♀
	Q51.22	Other partial doubling of uterus ♀
	Q51.28	Other doubling of uterus, other specified ♀
⑦	T83.31	Breakdown (mechanical) of intrauterine contraceptive device
⑦	T83.32	Displacement of intrauterine contraceptive device
⑦	T83.39	Other mechanical complication of intrauterine contraceptive device
⑦	T83.69	Infection and inflammatory reaction due to other prosthetic device, implant and graft in genital tract
⑦	T83.89	Other specified complication of genitourinary prosthetic devices, implants and grafts
	Z30.2	Encounter for sterilization

ICD-10-CM Coding Notes

For codes requiring a 7th character extension, refer to your ICD-10-CM book. Review the character descriptions and coding guidelines for proper selection. For some procedures, only certain characters will apply.

CCI Edits

Refer to Appendix A for CCI edits.

Pub 100

00952: Pub 100-04, 12, 140.5, Pub 100-04, 12, 50, Pub 100-04, 12, 90.4.5

Base Units

Global: XXX

Code	Base Units
00952	4

Modifiers (PAR)

Code	Mod 50	Mod 51	Mod 62	Mod 80
00952	9	9	9	9

CPT © 2018 American Medical Association. All Rights Reserved.

01112

01112 Anesthesia for bone marrow aspiration and/or biopsy, anterior or posterior iliac crest

AMA *CPT Assistant* ☐

01112: Mar 06: 15, Oct 11: 3, Jul 12: 13

ICD-10-CM Diagnostic Codes

C79.52	Secondary malignant neoplasm of bone marrow
C81.90	Hodgkin lymphoma, unspecified, unspecified site
C81.99	Hodgkin lymphoma, unspecified, extranodal and solid organ sites
C85.90	Non-Hodgkin lymphoma, unspecified, unspecified site
C85.99	Non-Hodgkin lymphoma, unspecified, extranodal and solid organ sites
C90.00	Multiple myeloma not having achieved remission
C91.00	Acute lymphoblastic leukemia not having achieved remission
C92.00	Acute myeloblastic leukemia, not having achieved remission
C92.40	Acute promyelocytic leukemia, not having achieved remission
C92.50	Acute myelomonocytic leukemia, not having achieved remission
C92.60	Acute myeloid leukemia with 11q23-abnormality not having achieved remission
C92.A0	Acute myeloid leukemia with multilineage dysplasia, not having achieved remission
C95.00	Acute leukemia of unspecified cell type not having achieved remission
D46.9	Myelodysplastic syndrome, unspecified
D47.1	Chronic myeloproliferative disease
D61.81	Pancytopenia
D64.9	Anemia, unspecified
D69.6	Thrombocytopenia, unspecified
D70.9	Neutropenia, unspecified
D72.819	Decreased white blood cell count, unspecified
D72.829	Elevated white blood cell count, unspecified
R16.1	Splenomegaly, not elsewhere classified
R16.2	Hepatomegaly with splenomegaly, not elsewhere classified
R50.9	Fever, unspecified

CCI Edits

Refer to Appendix A for CCI edits.

Pub 100

01112: Pub 100-04, 12, 140.5, Pub 100-04, 12, 50, Pub 100-04, 12, 90.4.5

Base Units

Global: XXX

Code	Base Units
01112	5

Modifiers (PAR)

Code	Mod 50	Mod 51	Mod 62	Mod 80
01112	9	9	9	9

CPT © 2018 American Medical Association. All Rights Reserved.

01120

01120 Anesthesia for procedures on bony pelvis

ICD-10-CM Diagnostic Codes

	C41.4	Malignant neoplasm of pelvic bones, sacrum and coccyx
	C79.51	Secondary malignant neoplasm of bone
	D16.8	Benign neoplasm of pelvic bones, sacrum and coccyx
	D48.0	Neoplasm of uncertain behavior of bone and articular cartilage
	D49.2	Neoplasm of unspecified behavior of bone, soft tissue, and skin
	M85.48	Solitary bone cyst, other site
	M85.58	Aneurysmal bone cyst, other site
	M85.68	Other cyst of bone, other site
	M86.38	Chronic multifocal osteomyelitis, other site
	M86.48	Chronic osteomyelitis with draining sinus, other site
	M86.58	Other chronic hematogenous osteomyelitis, other site
	M86.68	Other chronic osteomyelitis, other site
⇄	M87.050	Idiopathic aseptic necrosis of pelvis
⇄	M87.150	Osteonecrosis due to drugs, pelvis
⇄	M87.350	Other secondary osteonecrosis, pelvis
⇄	M87.850	Other osteonecrosis, pelvis
❼⇄	S32.311	Displaced avulsion fracture of right ilium
❼⇄	S32.312	Displaced avulsion fracture of left ilium
❼⇄	S32.314	Nondisplaced avulsion fracture of right ilium
❼⇄	S32.315	Nondisplaced avulsion fracture of left ilium
❼⇄	S32.391	Other fracture of right ilium
❼⇄	S32.392	Other fracture of left ilium
❼⇄	S32.412	Displaced fracture of anterior wall of left acetabulum
❼⇄	S32.511	Fracture of superior rim of right pubis
❼⇄	S32.591	Other specified fracture of right pubis
❼⇄	S32.592	Other specified fracture of left pubis
❼⇄	S32.611	Displaced avulsion fracture of right ischium
❼⇄	S32.612	Displaced avulsion fracture of left ischium
❼⇄	S32.614	Nondisplaced avulsion fracture of right ischium
❼⇄	S32.615	Nondisplaced avulsion fracture of left ischium
❼⇄	S32.691	Other specified fracture of right ischium
❼⇄	S32.692	Other specified fracture of left ischium
❼	S32.89	Fracture of other parts of pelvis
❼	S33.2	Dislocation of sacroiliac and sacrococcygeal joint

ICD-10-CM Coding Notes

For codes requiring a 7th character extension, refer to your ICD-10-CM book. Review the character descriptions and coding guidelines for proper selection. For some procedures, only certain characters will apply.

CCI Edits

Refer to Appendix A for CCI edits.

Pub 100

01120: Pub 100-04, 12, 140.5, Pub 100-04, 12, 50, Pub 100-04, 12, 90.4.5

Base Units

Global: XXX

Code	Base Units
01120	6

Modifiers (PAR)

Code	Mod 50	Mod 51	Mod 62	Mod 80
01120	9	9	9	9

CPT © 2018 American Medical Association. All Rights Reserved.

01130

01130 Anesthesia for body cast application or revision

ICD-10-CM Diagnostic Codes

M40.13 Other secondary kyphosis, cervicothoracic region
M40.14 Other secondary kyphosis, thoracic region
M40.15 Other secondary kyphosis, thoracolumbar region
M40.293 Other kyphosis, cervicothoracic region
M40.294 Other kyphosis, thoracic region
M40.295 Other kyphosis, thoracolumbar region
M41.03 Infantile idiopathic scoliosis, cervicothoracic region
M41.04 Infantile idiopathic scoliosis, thoracic region
M41.05 Infantile idiopathic scoliosis, thoracolumbar region
M41.06 Infantile idiopathic scoliosis, lumbar region
M41.07 Infantile idiopathic scoliosis, lumbosacral region
M41.08 Infantile idiopathic scoliosis, sacral and sacrococcygeal region
M41.113 Juvenile idiopathic scoliosis, cervicothoracic region
M41.114 Juvenile idiopathic scoliosis, thoracic region
M41.115 Juvenile idiopathic scoliosis, thoracolumbar region
M41.116 Juvenile idiopathic scoliosis, lumbar region
M41.117 Juvenile idiopathic scoliosis, lumbosacral region
M41.123 Adolescent idiopathic scoliosis, cervicothoracic region
M41.124 Adolescent idiopathic scoliosis, thoracic region
M41.125 Adolescent idiopathic scoliosis, thoracolumbar region
M41.126 Adolescent idiopathic scoliosis, lumbar region
M41.127 Adolescent idiopathic scoliosis, lumbosacral region
M41.23 Other idiopathic scoliosis, cervicothoracic region
M41.24 Other idiopathic scoliosis, thoracic region
M41.25 Other idiopathic scoliosis, thoracolumbar region
M41.26 Other idiopathic scoliosis, lumbar region
M41.27 Other idiopathic scoliosis, lumbosacral region
M41.34 Thoracogenic scoliosis, thoracic region
M41.35 Thoracogenic scoliosis, thoracolumbar region
Q05.1 Thoracic spina bifida with hydrocephalus
Q05.2 Lumbar spina bifida with hydrocephalus
Q05.6 Thoracic spina bifida without hydrocephalus
Q05.8 Sacral spina bifida without hydrocephalus
Q67.5 Congenital deformity of spine
⑦ S22.012 Unstable burst fracture of first thoracic vertebra
⑦ S22.018 Other fracture of first thoracic vertebra
⑦ S22.022 Unstable burst fracture of second thoracic vertebra
⑦ S22.028 Other fracture of second thoracic vertebra
⑦ S22.032 Unstable burst fracture of third thoracic vertebra
⑦ S22.038 Other fracture of third thoracic vertebra
⑦ S22.042 Unstable burst fracture of fourth thoracic vertebra
⑦ S22.048 Other fracture of fourth thoracic vertebra
⑦ S22.052 Unstable burst fracture of T5-T6 vertebra
⑦ S22.058 Other fracture of T5-T6 vertebra
⑦ S22.062 Unstable burst fracture of T7-T8 vertebra
⑦ S22.068 Other fracture of T7-T8 thoracic vertebra
⑦ S22.072 Unstable burst fracture of T9-T10 vertebra
⑦ S22.078 Other fracture of T9-T10 vertebra
⑦ S22.082 Unstable burst fracture of T11-T12 vertebra
⑦ S22.088 Other fracture of T11-T12 vertebra
⑦⇄ S22.41 Multiple fractures of ribs, right side
⑦⇄ S22.42 Multiple fractures of ribs, left side
⑦⇄ S22.43 Multiple fractures of ribs, bilateral
⑦ S22.5 Flail chest
⑦ S32.002 Unstable burst fracture of unspecified lumbar vertebra
⑦ S32.012 Unstable burst fracture of first lumbar vertebra
⑦ S32.018 Other fracture of first lumbar vertebra
⑦ S32.022 Unstable burst fracture of second lumbar vertebra
⑦ S32.028 Other fracture of second lumbar vertebra
⑦ S32.032 Unstable burst fracture of third lumbar vertebra
⑦ S32.038 Other fracture of third lumbar vertebra
⑦ S32.042 Unstable burst fracture of fourth lumbar vertebra
⑦ S32.048 Other fracture of fourth lumbar vertebra
⑦ S32.052 Unstable burst fracture of fifth lumbar vertebra
⑦ S32.058 Other fracture of fifth lumbar vertebra
⑦ S32.810 Multiple fractures of pelvis with stable disruption of pelvic ring
⑦ S32.811 Multiple fractures of pelvis with unstable disruption of pelvic ring
⑦ S32.82 Multiple fractures of pelvis without disruption of pelvic ring
⑦ S32.9 Fracture of unspecified parts of lumbosacral spine and pelvis

ICD-10-CM Coding Notes

For codes requiring a 7th character extension, refer to your ICD-10-CM book. Review the character descriptions and coding guidelines for proper selection. For some procedures, only certain characters will apply.

CCI Edits

Refer to Appendix A for CCI edits.

Pub 100

01130: Pub 100-04, 12, 140.5, Pub 100-04, 12, 50, Pub 100-04, 12, 90.4.5

Base Units

Global: XXX

Code	Base Units
01130	3

Modifiers (PAR)

Code	Mod 50	Mod 51	Mod 62	Mod 80
01130	9	9	9	9

CPT © 2018 American Medical Association. All Rights Reserved.

01140

01140 Anesthesia for interpelviabdominal (hindquarter) amputation

ICD-10-CM Diagnostic Codes

⇄	C40.21	Malignant neoplasm of long bones of right lower limb
⇄	C40.22	Malignant neoplasm of long bones of left lower limb
	C41.4	Malignant neoplasm of pelvic bones, sacrum and coccyx
⇄	C47.21	Malignant neoplasm of peripheral nerves of right lower limb, including hip
⇄	C47.22	Malignant neoplasm of peripheral nerves of left lower limb, including hip
	C47.5	Malignant neoplasm of peripheral nerves of pelvis
⇄	C49.21	Malignant neoplasm of connective and soft tissue of right lower limb, including hip
⇄	C49.22	Malignant neoplasm of connective and soft tissue of left lower limb, including hip
	C49.5	Malignant neoplasm of connective and soft tissue of pelvis
	C79.51	Secondary malignant neoplasm of bone
	C79.89	Secondary malignant neoplasm of other specified sites
❼⇄	S77.01	Crushing injury of right hip
❼⇄	S77.02	Crushing injury of left hip
❼⇄	S77.21	Crushing injury of right hip with thigh
❼⇄	S77.22	Crushing injury of left hip with thigh
❼⇄	S78.021	Partial traumatic amputation at right hip joint
❼⇄	S78.022	Partial traumatic amputation at left hip joint

ICD-10-CM Coding Notes

For codes requiring a 7th character extension, refer to your ICD-10-CM book. Review the character descriptions and coding guidelines for proper selection. For some procedures, only certain characters will apply.

CCI Edits

Refer to Appendix A for CCI edits.

Pub 100

01140: Pub 100-04, 12, 140.5, Pub 100-04, 12, 50, Pub 100-04, 12, 90.4.5

Base Units

Global: XXX

Code	Base Units
01140	15

Modifiers (PAR)

Code	Mod 50	Mod 51	Mod 62	Mod 80
01140	9	9	9	9

CPT © 2018 American Medical Association. All Rights Reserved.

01150

01150 Anesthesia for radical procedures for tumor of pelvis, except hindquarter amputation

ICD-10-CM Diagnostic Codes

C41.4	Malignant neoplasm of pelvic bones, sacrum and coccyx
C47.5	Malignant neoplasm of peripheral nerves of pelvis
C49.5	Malignant neoplasm of connective and soft tissue of pelvis
C79.51	Secondary malignant neoplasm of bone
C79.89	Secondary malignant neoplasm of other specified sites

CCI Edits

Refer to Appendix A for CCI edits.

Pub 100

01150: Pub 100-04, 12, 140.5, Pub 100-04, 12, 50, Pub 100-04, 12, 90.4.5

Base Units

Global: XXX

Code	Base Units
01150	10

Modifiers (PAR)

Code	Mod 50	Mod 51	Mod 62	Mod 80
01150	9	9	9	9

CPT © 2018 American Medical Association. All Rights Reserved.

01160

01160 Anesthesia for closed procedures involving symphysis pubis or sacroiliac joint

ICD-10-CM Diagnostic Codes

⇄	M07.651	Enteropathic arthropathies, right hip
⇄	M07.652	Enteropathic arthropathies, left hip
⇄	M12.551	Traumatic arthropathy, right hip
⇄	M12.552	Traumatic arthropathy, left hip
⇄	M12.851	Other specific arthropathies, not elsewhere classified, right hip
⇄	M12.852	Other specific arthropathies, not elsewhere classified, left hip
⇄	M13.151	Monoarthritis, not elsewhere classified, right hip
⇄	M13.152	Monoarthritis, not elsewhere classified, left hip
⇄	M13.851	Other specified arthritis, right hip
⇄	M13.852	Other specified arthritis, left hip
	M16.0	Bilateral primary osteoarthritis of hip
⇄	M16.11	Unilateral primary osteoarthritis, right hip
⇄	M16.12	Unilateral primary osteoarthritis, left hip
	M16.4	Bilateral post-traumatic osteoarthritis of hip
⇄	M16.51	Unilateral post-traumatic osteoarthritis, right hip
⇄	M16.52	Unilateral post-traumatic osteoarthritis, left hip
	M16.6	Other bilateral secondary osteoarthritis of hip
	M16.7	Other unilateral secondary osteoarthritis of hip
⇄	M25.551	Pain in right hip
⇄	M25.552	Pain in left hip
	M46.1	Sacroiliitis, not elsewhere classified
❼⇄	M84.350	Stress fracture, pelvis
❼⇄	M84.454	Pathological fracture, pelvis
❼⇄	M84.550	Pathological fracture in neoplastic disease, pelvis
⇄	M84.851	Other disorders of continuity of bone, right pelvic region and thigh
⇄	M84.852	Other disorders of continuity of bone, left pelvic region and thigh
❼	S32.89	Fracture of other parts of pelvis
❼	S33.2	Dislocation of sacroiliac and sacrococcygeal joint
❼	S33.39	Dislocation of other parts of lumbar spine and pelvis
❼	S33.4	Traumatic rupture of symphysis pubis
❼	S33.6	Sprain of sacroiliac joint

ICD-10-CM Coding Notes

For codes requiring a 7th character extension, refer to your ICD-10-CM book. Review the character descriptions and coding guidelines for proper selection. For some procedures, only certain characters will apply.

CCI Edits

Refer to Appendix A for CCI edits.

Pub 100

01160: Pub 100-04, 12, 140.5, Pub 100-04, 12, 50, Pub 100-04, 12, 90.4.5

Base Units

Global: XXX

Code	Base Units
01160	4

Modifiers (PAR)

Code	Mod 50	Mod 51	Mod 62	Mod 80
01160	9	9	9	9

CPT © 2018 American Medical Association. All Rights Reserved.

01170

01170 Anesthesia for open procedures involving symphysis pubis or sacroiliac joint

ICD-10-CM Diagnostic Codes

⇄	M25.751	Osteophyte, right hip
⇄	M25.752	Osteophyte, left hip
➐⇄	M84.350	Stress fracture, pelvis
➐⇄	M84.454	Pathological fracture, pelvis
➐⇄	M84.550	Pathological fracture in neoplastic disease, pelvis
⇄	M84.851	Other disorders of continuity of bone, right pelvic region and thigh
⇄	M84.852	Other disorders of continuity of bone, left pelvic region and thigh
➐	S32.89	Fracture of other parts of pelvis
➐	S33.2	Dislocation of sacroiliac and sacrococcygeal joint
➐	S33.39	Dislocation of other parts of lumbar spine and pelvis
➐	S33.4	Traumatic rupture of symphysis pubis
➐	S33.6	Sprain of sacroiliac joint

ICD-10-CM Coding Notes

For codes requiring a 7th character extension, refer to your ICD-10-CM book. Review the character descriptions and coding guidelines for proper selection. For some procedures, only certain characters will apply.

CCI Edits

Refer to Appendix A for CCI edits.

Pub 100

01170: Pub 100-04, 12, 140.5, Pub 100-04, 12, 50, Pub 100-04, 12, 90.4.5

Base Units

Global: XXX

Code	Base Units
01170	8

Modifiers (PAR)

Code	Mod 50	Mod 51	Mod 62	Mod 80
01170	9	9	9	9

CPT © 2018 American Medical Association. All Rights Reserved.

01173

01173 Anesthesia for open repair of fracture disruption of pelvis or column fracture involving acetabulum

AMA *CPT Assistant*

01173: Jun 04: 3, 4

ICD-10-CM Diagnostic Codes

⑦	S32.110	Nondisplaced Zone I fracture of sacrum
⑦	S32.111	Minimally displaced Zone I fracture of sacrum
⑦	S32.112	Severely displaced Zone I fracture of sacrum
⑦	S32.120	Nondisplaced Zone II fracture of sacrum
⑦	S32.121	Minimally displaced Zone II fracture of sacrum
⑦	S32.122	Severely displaced Zone II fracture of sacrum
⑦	S32.130	Nondisplaced Zone III fracture of sacrum
⑦	S32.131	Minimally displaced Zone III fracture of sacrum
⑦	S32.132	Severely displaced Zone III fracture of sacrum
⑦	S32.14	Type 1 fracture of sacrum
⑦	S32.15	Type 2 fracture of sacrum
⑦	S32.16	Type 3 fracture of sacrum
⑦	S32.17	Type 4 fracture of sacrum
⑦	S32.19	Other fracture of sacrum
⑦⇄	S32.411	Displaced fracture of anterior wall of right acetabulum
⑦⇄	S32.412	Displaced fracture of anterior wall of left acetabulum
⑦⇄	S32.414	Nondisplaced fracture of anterior wall of right acetabulum
⑦⇄	S32.415	Nondisplaced fracture of anterior wall of left acetabulum
⑦⇄	S32.421	Displaced fracture of posterior wall of right acetabulum
⑦⇄	S32.422	Displaced fracture of posterior wall of left acetabulum
⑦⇄	S32.424	Nondisplaced fracture of posterior wall of right acetabulum
⑦⇄	S32.425	Nondisplaced fracture of posterior wall of left acetabulum
⑦⇄	S32.431	Displaced fracture of anterior column [iliopubic] of right acetabulum
⑦⇄	S32.432	Displaced fracture of anterior column [iliopubic] of left acetabulum
⑦⇄	S32.434	Nondisplaced fracture of anterior column [iliopubic] of right acetabulum
⑦⇄	S32.435	Nondisplaced fracture of anterior column [iliopubic] of left acetabulum
⑦⇄	S32.441	Displaced fracture of posterior column [ilioischial] of right acetabulum
⑦⇄	S32.442	Displaced fracture of posterior column [ilioischial] of left acetabulum
⑦⇄	S32.444	Nondisplaced fracture of posterior column [ilioischial] of right acetabulum
⑦⇄	S32.445	Nondisplaced fracture of posterior column [ilioischial] of left acetabulum
⑦⇄	S32.451	Displaced transverse fracture of right acetabulum
⑦⇄	S32.452	Displaced transverse fracture of left acetabulum
⑦⇄	S32.454	Nondisplaced transverse fracture of right acetabulum
⑦⇄	S32.455	Nondisplaced transverse fracture of left acetabulum
⑦⇄	S32.461	Displaced associated transverse-posterior fracture of right acetabulum
⑦⇄	S32.462	Displaced associated transverse-posterior fracture of left acetabulum
⑦⇄	S32.464	Nondisplaced associated transverse-posterior fracture of right acetabulum
⑦⇄	S32.465	Nondisplaced associated transverse-posterior fracture of left acetabulum
⑦⇄	S32.471	Displaced fracture of medial wall of right acetabulum
⑦⇄	S32.472	Displaced fracture of medial wall of left acetabulum
⑦⇄	S32.474	Nondisplaced fracture of medial wall of right acetabulum
⑦⇄	S32.475	Nondisplaced fracture of medial wall of left acetabulum
⑦⇄	S32.481	Displaced dome fracture of right acetabulum
⑦⇄	S32.482	Displaced dome fracture of left acetabulum
⑦⇄	S32.484	Nondisplaced dome fracture of right acetabulum
⑦⇄	S32.485	Nondisplaced dome fracture of left acetabulum
⑦⇄	S32.491	Other specified fracture of right acetabulum
⑦⇄	S32.492	Other specified fracture of left acetabulum
⑦	S32.810	Multiple fractures of pelvis with stable disruption of pelvic ring
⑦	S32.811	Multiple fractures of pelvis with unstable disruption of pelvic ring
⑦	S32.82	Multiple fractures of pelvis without disruption of pelvic ring
⑦	S32.89	Fracture of other parts of pelvis

ICD-10-CM Coding Notes

For codes requiring a 7th character extension, refer to your ICD-10-CM book. Review the character descriptions and coding guidelines for proper selection. For some procedures, only certain characters will apply.

CCI Edits

Refer to Appendix A for CCI edits.

Pub 100

01173: Pub 100-04, 12, 140.5, Pub 100-04, 12, 50, Pub 100-04, 12, 90.4.5

Base Units

Global: XXX

Code	Base Units
01173	12

Modifiers (PAR)

Code	Mod 50	Mod 51	Mod 62	Mod 80
01173	9	9	9	9

CPT © 2018 American Medical Association. All Rights Reserved.

01200

01200 Anesthesia for all closed procedures involving hip joint

AMA *CPT Assistant* ☐

01200: Mar 06: 15, Nov 07: 8, Jul 12: 13

ICD-10-CM Diagnostic Codes

⇄	C40.21	Malignant neoplasm of long bones of right lower limb
⇄	C40.22	Malignant neoplasm of long bones of left lower limb
	C79.51	Secondary malignant neoplasm of bone
⇄	D16.21	Benign neoplasm of long bones of right lower limb
⇄	D16.22	Benign neoplasm of long bones of left lower limb
	D48.0	Neoplasm of uncertain behavior of bone and articular cartilage
	D49.2	Neoplasm of unspecified behavior of bone, soft tissue, and skin
⇄	M00.051	Staphylococcal arthritis, right hip
⇄	M00.052	Staphylococcal arthritis, left hip
⇄	M00.151	Pneumococcal arthritis, right hip
⇄	M00.152	Pneumococcal arthritis, left hip
⇄	M00.251	Other streptococcal arthritis, right hip
⇄	M00.252	Other streptococcal arthritis, left hip
⇄	M00.851	Arthritis due to other bacteria, right hip
⇄	M00.852	Arthritis due to other bacteria, left hip
	M00.9	Pyogenic arthritis, unspecified
⇄	M24.351	Pathological dislocation of right hip, not elsewhere classified
⇄	M24.352	Pathological dislocation of left hip, not elsewhere classified
⇄	M24.451	Recurrent dislocation, right hip
⇄	M24.452	Recurrent dislocation, left hip
⇄	Q65.01	Congenital dislocation of right hip, unilateral
⇄	Q65.02	Congenital dislocation of left hip, unilateral
	Q65.1	Congenital dislocation of hip, bilateral
⇄	Q65.31	Congenital partial dislocation of right hip, unilateral
⇄	Q65.32	Congenital partial dislocation of left hip, unilateral
	Q65.4	Congenital partial dislocation of hip, bilateral
❼⇄	S73.011	Posterior subluxation of right hip
❼⇄	S73.012	Posterior subluxation of left hip
❼⇄	S73.014	Posterior dislocation of right hip
❼⇄	S73.015	Posterior dislocation of left hip
❼⇄	S73.021	Obturator subluxation of right hip
❼⇄	S73.022	Obturator subluxation of left hip
❼⇄	S73.024	Obturator dislocation of right hip
❼⇄	S73.025	Obturator dislocation of left hip
❼⇄	S73.031	Other anterior subluxation of right hip
❼⇄	S73.032	Other anterior subluxation of left hip
❼⇄	S73.041	Central subluxation of right hip
❼⇄	S73.042	Central subluxation of left hip
❼⇄	S73.045	Central dislocation of left hip
❼⇄	T84.020	Dislocation of internal right hip prosthesis
❼⇄	T84.021	Dislocation of internal left hip prosthesis
❼⇄	T84.51	Infection and inflammatory reaction due to internal right hip prosthesis
❼⇄	T84.52	Infection and inflammatory reaction due to internal left hip prosthesis

ICD-10-CM Coding Notes

For codes requiring a 7th character extension, refer to your ICD-10-CM book. Review the character descriptions and coding guidelines for proper selection. For some procedures, only certain characters will apply.

CCI Edits

Refer to Appendix A for CCI edits.

Pub 100

01200: Pub 100-04, 12, 140.5, Pub 100-04, 12, 50, Pub 100-04, 12, 90.4.5

Base Units

Global: XXX

Code	Base Units
01200	4

Modifiers (PAR)

Code	Mod 50	Mod 51	Mod 62	Mod 80
01200	9	9	9	9

CPT © 2018 American Medical Association. All Rights Reserved.

01202

01202 Anesthesia for arthroscopic procedures of hip joint

ICD-10-CM Diagnostic Codes

⇄ M00.051 Staphylococcal arthritis, right hip
⇄ M00.052 Staphylococcal arthritis, left hip
⇄ M00.151 Pneumococcal arthritis, right hip
⇄ M00.152 Pneumococcal arthritis, left hip
⇄ M00.251 Other streptococcal arthritis, right hip
⇄ M00.252 Other streptococcal arthritis, left hip
⇄ M00.851 Arthritis due to other bacteria, right hip
⇄ M00.852 Arthritis due to other bacteria, left hip
⇄ M12.251 Villonodular synovitis (pigmented), right hip
⇄ M12.252 Villonodular synovitis (pigmented), left hip
⇄ M12.551 Traumatic arthropathy, right hip
⇄ M12.552 Traumatic arthropathy, left hip
⇄ M12.851 Other specific arthropathies, not elsewhere classified, right hip
⇄ M12.852 Other specific arthropathies, not elsewhere classified, left hip
M16.0 Bilateral primary osteoarthritis of hip
⇄ M16.11 Unilateral primary osteoarthritis, right hip
⇄ M16.12 Unilateral primary osteoarthritis, left hip
M16.2 Bilateral osteoarthritis resulting from hip dysplasia
⇄ M16.31 Unilateral osteoarthritis resulting from hip dysplasia, right hip
⇄ M16.32 Unilateral osteoarthritis resulting from hip dysplasia, left hip
M16.4 Bilateral post-traumatic osteoarthritis of hip
⇄ M16.51 Unilateral post-traumatic osteoarthritis, right hip
⇄ M16.52 Unilateral post-traumatic osteoarthritis, left hip
M16.6 Other bilateral secondary osteoarthritis of hip
M16.7 Other unilateral secondary osteoarthritis of hip
⇄ M24.051 Loose body in right hip
⇄ M24.052 Loose body in left hip
⇄ M24.151 Other articular cartilage disorders, right hip
⇄ M24.152 Other articular cartilage disorders, left hip
⇄ M24.251 Disorder of ligament, right hip
⇄ M24.252 Disorder of ligament, left hip
⇄ M25.451 Effusion, right hip
⇄ M25.452 Effusion, left hip
⇄ M25.751 Osteophyte, right hip
⇄ M25.752 Osteophyte, left hip
⇄ M25.851 Other specified joint disorders, right hip
⇄ M25.852 Other specified joint disorders, left hip
⇄ M67.851 Other specified disorders of synovium, right hip
⇄ M67.852 Other specified disorders of synovium, left hip
⇄ M70.61 Trochanteric bursitis, right hip
⇄ M70.62 Trochanteric bursitis, left hip
⇄ M70.71 Other bursitis of hip, right hip
⇄ M70.72 Other bursitis of hip, left hip
⇄ M71.351 Other bursal cyst, right hip
⇄ M71.352 Other bursal cyst, left hip
⇄ M85.351 Osteitis condensans, right thigh
⇄ M85.352 Osteitis condensans, left thigh
⇄ M85.451 Solitary bone cyst, right pelvis
⇄ M85.452 Solitary bone cyst, left pelvis

CCI Edits

Refer to Appendix A for CCI edits.

Pub 100

01202: Pub 100-04, 12, 140.5, Pub 100-04, 12, 50, Pub 100-04, 12, 90.4.5

Base Units

Global: XXX

Code	Base Units
01202	4

Modifiers (PAR)

Code	Mod 50	Mod 51	Mod 62	Mod 80
01202	9	9	9	9

CPT © 2018 American Medical Association. All Rights Reserved.

01210

01210 Anesthesia for open procedures involving hip joint; not otherwise specified

ICD-10-CM Diagnostic Codes

⇄	M00.051	Staphylococcal arthritis, right hip
⇄	M00.052	Staphylococcal arthritis, left hip
⇄	M00.151	Pneumococcal arthritis, right hip
⇄	M00.152	Pneumococcal arthritis, left hip
⇄	M00.251	Other streptococcal arthritis, right hip
⇄	M00.252	Other streptococcal arthritis, left hip
⇄	M00.851	Arthritis due to other bacteria, right hip
⇄	M00.852	Arthritis due to other bacteria, left hip
❼⇄	M80.051	Age-related osteoporosis with current pathological fracture, right femur
❼⇄	M80.052	Age-related osteoporosis with current pathological fracture, left femur
❼⇄	M80.851	Other osteoporosis with current pathological fracture, right femur
❼⇄	M84.451	Pathological fracture, right femur
❼⇄	M84.452	Pathological fracture, left femur
❼⇄	M84.551	Pathological fracture in neoplastic disease, right femur
❼⇄	M84.552	Pathological fracture in neoplastic disease, left femur
⇄	Q65.01	Congenital dislocation of right hip, unilateral
⇄	Q65.02	Congenital dislocation of left hip, unilateral
	Q65.1	Congenital dislocation of hip, bilateral
	Q65.2	Congenital dislocation of hip, unspecified
⇄	Q65.31	Congenital partial dislocation of right hip, unilateral
⇄	Q65.32	Congenital partial dislocation of left hip, unilateral
	Q65.4	Congenital partial dislocation of hip, bilateral
	Q65.5	Congenital partial dislocation of hip, unspecified
❼⇄	S72.021	Displaced fracture of epiphysis (separation) (upper) of right femur
❼⇄	S72.022	Displaced fracture of epiphysis (separation) (upper) of left femur
❼⇄	S72.024	Nondisplaced fracture of epiphysis (separation) (upper) of right femur
❼⇄	S72.025	Nondisplaced fracture of epiphysis (separation) (upper) of left femur
❼⇄	S72.031	Displaced midcervical fracture of right femur
❼⇄	S72.032	Displaced midcervical fracture of left femur
❼⇄	S72.034	Nondisplaced midcervical fracture of right femur
❼⇄	S72.035	Nondisplaced midcervical fracture of left femur
❼⇄	S72.041	Displaced fracture of base of neck of right femur
❼⇄	S72.042	Displaced fracture of base of neck of left femur
❼⇄	S72.044	Nondisplaced fracture of base of neck of right femur
❼⇄	S72.045	Nondisplaced fracture of base of neck of left femur
❼⇄	S72.061	Displaced articular fracture of head of right femur
❼⇄	S72.062	Displaced articular fracture of head of left femur
❼⇄	S72.064	Nondisplaced articular fracture of head of right femur
❼⇄	S72.065	Nondisplaced articular fracture of head of left femur
❼⇄	S72.091	Other fracture of head and neck of right femur
❼⇄	S72.092	Other fracture of head and neck of left femur

ICD-10-CM Coding Notes

For codes requiring a 7th character extension, refer to your ICD-10-CM book. Review the character descriptions and coding guidelines for proper selection. For some procedures, only certain characters will apply.

CCI Edits

Refer to Appendix A for CCI edits.

Pub 100

01210: Pub 100-04, 12, 140.5, Pub 100-04, 12, 50, Pub 100-04, 12, 90.4.5

Base Units

Global: XXX

Code	Base Units
01210	6

Modifiers (PAR)

Code	Mod 50	Mod 51	Mod 62	Mod 80
01210	9	9	9	9

CPT © 2018 American Medical Association. All Rights Reserved.

01212

01212 Anesthesia for open procedures involving hip joint; hip disarticulation

ICD-10-CM Diagnostic Codes

⇄	C40.21	Malignant neoplasm of long bones of right lower limb
⇄	C40.22	Malignant neoplasm of long bones of left lower limb
⇄	C47.21	Malignant neoplasm of peripheral nerves of right lower limb, including hip
⇄	C47.22	Malignant neoplasm of peripheral nerves of left lower limb, including hip
⇄	C49.21	Malignant neoplasm of connective and soft tissue of right lower limb, including hip
⇄	C49.22	Malignant neoplasm of connective and soft tissue of left lower limb, including hip
	C79.51	Secondary malignant neoplasm of bone
	C79.89	Secondary malignant neoplasm of other specified sites
❼⇄	S77.11	Crushing injury of right thigh
❼⇄	S77.12	Crushing injury of left thigh
❼⇄	S78.011	Complete traumatic amputation at right hip joint
❼⇄	S78.012	Complete traumatic amputation at left hip joint
❼⇄	S78.021	Partial traumatic amputation at right hip joint
❼⇄	S78.022	Partial traumatic amputation at left hip joint
❼⇄	T24.391	Burn of third degree of multiple sites of right lower limb, except ankle and foot
❼⇄	T24.392	Burn of third degree of multiple sites of left lower limb, except ankle and foot

ICD-10-CM Coding Notes

For codes requiring a 7th character extension, refer to your ICD-10-CM book. Review the character descriptions and coding guidelines for proper selection. For some procedures, only certain characters will apply.

CCI Edits

Refer to Appendix A for CCI edits.

Pub 100

01212: Pub 100-04, 12, 140.5, Pub 100-04, 12, 50, Pub 100-04, 12, 90.4.5

Base Units

Global: XXX

Code	Base Units
01212	10

Modifiers (PAR)

Code	Mod 50	Mod 51	Mod 62	Mod 80
01212	9	9	9	9

● New ▲ Revised ✚ Add On ⊘Modifier 51 Exempt ★Telemedicine ▯ CPT QuickRef ✗FDA Pending ⇄ Laterality ❼ Seventh Character ♂Male ♀Female

CPT © 2018 American Medical Association. All Rights Reserved.

01214

01214 Anesthesia for open procedures involving hip joint; total hip arthroplasty

ICD-10-CM Diagnostic Codes

⇄	M12.051	Chronic postrheumatic arthropathy [Jaccoud], right hip
⇄	M12.052	Chronic postrheumatic arthropathy [Jaccoud], left hip
⇄	M12.551	Traumatic arthropathy, right hip
⇄	M12.552	Traumatic arthropathy, left hip
⇄	M12.851	Other specific arthropathies, not elsewhere classified, right hip
⇄	M12.852	Other specific arthropathies, not elsewhere classified, left hip
⇄	M13.151	Monoarthritis, not elsewhere classified, right hip
⇄	M13.152	Monoarthritis, not elsewhere classified, left hip
⇄	M13.851	Other specified arthritis, right hip
⇄	M13.852	Other specified arthritis, left hip
	M16.0	Bilateral primary osteoarthritis of hip
⇄	M16.11	Unilateral primary osteoarthritis, right hip
⇄	M16.12	Unilateral primary osteoarthritis, left hip
	M16.2	Bilateral osteoarthritis resulting from hip dysplasia
⇄	M16.31	Unilateral osteoarthritis resulting from hip dysplasia, right hip
⇄	M16.32	Unilateral osteoarthritis resulting from hip dysplasia, left hip
	M16.4	Bilateral post-traumatic osteoarthritis of hip
⇄	M16.51	Unilateral post-traumatic osteoarthritis, right hip
⇄	M16.52	Unilateral post-traumatic osteoarthritis, left hip
	M16.6	Other bilateral secondary osteoarthritis of hip
	M16.7	Other unilateral secondary osteoarthritis of hip
⇄	M25.251	Flail joint, right hip
⇄	M25.252	Flail joint, left hip
⇄	M25.351	Other instability, right hip
⇄	M25.352	Other instability, left hip
❼⇄	M80.051	Age-related osteoporosis with current pathological fracture, right femur
❼⇄	M80.052	Age-related osteoporosis with current pathological fracture, left femur
❼⇄	M80.851	Other osteoporosis with current pathological fracture, right femur
❼⇄	M80.852	Other osteoporosis with current pathological fracture, left femur
❼⇄	M84.451	Pathological fracture, right femur
❼⇄	M84.452	Pathological fracture, left femur
❼⇄	M84.551	Pathological fracture in neoplastic disease, right femur
❼⇄	M84.552	Pathological fracture in neoplastic disease, left femur
❼⇄	M84.651	Pathological fracture in other disease, right femur
❼⇄	M84.652	Pathological fracture in other disease, left femur
❼⇄	S72.021	Displaced fracture of epiphysis (separation) (upper) of right femur
❼⇄	S72.022	Displaced fracture of epiphysis (separation) (upper) of left femur
❼⇄	S72.031	Displaced midcervical fracture of right femur
❼⇄	S72.032	Displaced midcervical fracture of left femur
❼⇄	S72.041	Displaced fracture of base of neck of right femur
❼⇄	S72.042	Displaced fracture of base of neck of left femur
❼⇄	S72.061	Displaced articular fracture of head of right femur
❼⇄	S72.21	Displaced subtrochanteric fracture of right femur
❼⇄	S72.22	Displaced subtrochanteric fracture of left femur

ICD-10-CM Coding Notes

For codes requiring a 7th character extension, refer to your ICD-10-CM book. Review the character descriptions and coding guidelines for proper selection. For some procedures, only certain characters will apply.

CCI Edits

Refer to Appendix A for CCI edits.

Pub 100

01214: Pub 100-04, 12, 140.5, Pub 100-04, 12, 50, Pub 100-04, 12, 90.4.5

Base Units

Global: XXX

Code	Base Units
01214	8

Modifiers (PAR)

Code	Mod 50	Mod 51	Mod 62	Mod 80
01214	9	9	9	9

CPT © 2018 American Medical Association. All Rights Reserved.

01215

01215 Anesthesia for open procedures involving hip joint; revision of total hip arthroplasty

ICD-10-CM Diagnostic Codes

7 ⇄	M97.01	Periprosthetic fracture around internal prosthetic right hip joint
7 ⇄	M97.02	Periprosthetic fracture around internal prosthetic left hip joint
7 ⇄	T84.010	Broken internal right hip prosthesis
7 ⇄	T84.011	Broken internal left hip prosthesis
7 ⇄	T84.020	Dislocation of internal right hip prosthesis
7 ⇄	T84.021	Dislocation of internal left hip prosthesis
7 ⇄	T84.030	Mechanical loosening of internal right hip prosthetic joint
7 ⇄	T84.031	Mechanical loosening of internal left hip prosthetic joint
7 ⇄	T84.050	Periprosthetic osteolysis of internal prosthetic right hip joint
7 ⇄	T84.051	Periprosthetic osteolysis of internal prosthetic left hip joint
7 ⇄	T84.060	Wear of articular bearing surface of internal prosthetic right hip joint
7 ⇄	T84.061	Wear of articular bearing surface of internal prosthetic left hip joint
7 ⇄	T84.090	Other mechanical complication of internal right hip prosthesis
7 ⇄	T84.091	Other mechanical complication of internal left hip prosthesis
7 ⇄	T84.51	Infection and inflammatory reaction due to internal right hip prosthesis
7 ⇄	T84.52	Infection and inflammatory reaction due to internal left hip prosthesis
7	T84.81	Embolism due to internal orthopedic prosthetic devices, implants and grafts
7	T84.82	Fibrosis due to internal orthopedic prosthetic devices, implants and grafts
7	T84.83	Hemorrhage due to internal orthopedic prosthetic devices, implants and grafts
7	T84.84	Pain due to internal orthopedic prosthetic devices, implants and grafts
7	T84.85	Stenosis due to internal orthopedic prosthetic devices, implants and grafts
7	T84.86	Thrombosis due to internal orthopedic prosthetic devices, implants and grafts
7	T84.89	Other specified complication of internal orthopedic prosthetic devices, implants and grafts

ICD-10-CM Coding Notes

For codes requiring a 7th character extension, refer to your ICD-10-CM book. Review the character descriptions and coding guidelines for proper selection. For some procedures, only certain characters will apply.

CCI Edits

Refer to Appendix A for CCI edits.

Pub 100

01215: Pub 100-04, 12, 140.5, Pub 100-04, 12, 50, Pub 100-04, 12, 90.4.5

Base Units

Global: XXX

Code	Base Units
01215	10

Modifiers (PAR)

Code	Mod 50	Mod 51	Mod 62	Mod 80
01215	9	9	9	9

CPT © 2018 American Medical Association. All Rights Reserved.

01220

01220 Anesthesia for all closed procedures involving upper two-thirds of femur

ICD-10-CM Diagnostic Codes

⇄	C40.21	Malignant neoplasm of long bones of right lower limb
⇄	C40.22	Malignant neoplasm of long bones of left lower limb
	C79.51	Secondary malignant neoplasm of bone
⇄	D16.21	Benign neoplasm of long bones of right lower limb
⇄	D16.22	Benign neoplasm of long bones of left lower limb
➐⇄	M84.751	Incomplete atypical femoral fracture, right leg
➐⇄	M84.752	Incomplete atypical femoral fracture, left leg
⇄	M85.551	Aneurysmal bone cyst, right thigh
⇄	M85.552	Aneurysmal bone cyst, left thigh
⇄	M85.651	Other cyst of bone, right thigh
⇄	M85.652	Other cyst of bone, left thigh
⇄	M85.851	Other specified disorders of bone density and structure, right thigh
⇄	M85.852	Other specified disorders of bone density and structure, left thigh
⇄	M89.351	Hypertrophy of bone, right femur
⇄	M89.352	Hypertrophy of bone, left femur
➐⇄	S72.111	Displaced fracture of greater trochanter of right femur
➐⇄	S72.112	Displaced fracture of greater trochanter of left femur
➐⇄	S72.114	Nondisplaced fracture of greater trochanter of right femur
➐⇄	S72.115	Nondisplaced fracture of greater trochanter of left femur
➐⇄	S72.121	Displaced fracture of lesser trochanter of right femur
➐⇄	S72.122	Displaced fracture of lesser trochanter of left femur
➐⇄	S72.124	Nondisplaced fracture of lesser trochanter of right femur
➐⇄	S72.125	Nondisplaced fracture of lesser trochanter of left femur
➐⇄	S72.141	Displaced intertrochanteric fracture of right femur
➐⇄	S72.142	Displaced intertrochanteric fracture of left femur
➐⇄	S72.144	Nondisplaced intertrochanteric fracture of right femur
➐⇄	S72.145	Nondisplaced intertrochanteric fracture of left femur
➐⇄	S72.21	Displaced subtrochanteric fracture of right femur
➐⇄	S72.22	Displaced subtrochanteric fracture of left femur
➐⇄	S72.24	Nondisplaced subtrochanteric fracture of right femur
➐⇄	S72.25	Nondisplaced subtrochanteric fracture of left femur
➐⇄	S72.321	Displaced transverse fracture of shaft of right femur
➐⇄	S72.322	Displaced transverse fracture of shaft of left femur
➐⇄	S72.324	Nondisplaced transverse fracture of shaft of right femur
➐⇄	S72.325	Nondisplaced transverse fracture of shaft of left femur
➐⇄	S72.331	Displaced oblique fracture of shaft of right femur
➐⇄	S72.332	Displaced oblique fracture of shaft of left femur
➐⇄	S72.334	Nondisplaced oblique fracture of shaft of right femur
➐⇄	S72.335	Nondisplaced oblique fracture of shaft of left femur
➐⇄	S72.391	Other fracture of shaft of right femur
➐⇄	S72.392	Other fracture of shaft of left femur

ICD-10-CM Coding Notes

For codes requiring a 7th character extension, refer to your ICD-10-CM book. Review the character descriptions and coding guidelines for proper selection. For some procedures, only certain characters will apply.

CCI Edits

Refer to Appendix A for CCI edits.

Pub 100

01220: Pub 100-04, 12, 140.5, Pub 100-04, 12, 50, Pub 100-04, 12, 90.4.5

Base Units

Global: XXX

Code	Base Units
01220	4

Modifiers (PAR)

Code	Mod 50	Mod 51	Mod 62	Mod 80
01220	9	9	9	9

CPT © 2018 American Medical Association. All Rights Reserved.

01230

01230 Anesthesia for open procedures involving upper two-thirds of femur; not otherwise specified

ICD-10-CM Diagnostic Codes

⇄	C40.21	Malignant neoplasm of long bones of right lower limb
⇄	C40.22	Malignant neoplasm of long bones of left lower limb
	C79.51	Secondary malignant neoplasm of bone
⇄	D16.21	Benign neoplasm of long bones of right lower limb
⇄	D16.22	Benign neoplasm of long bones of left lower limb
➐⇄	M80.051	Age-related osteoporosis with current pathological fracture, right femur
➐⇄	M80.851	Other osteoporosis with current pathological fracture, right femur
➐⇄	M80.852	Other osteoporosis with current pathological fracture, left femur
➐⇄	M84.451	Pathological fracture, right femur
➐⇄	M84.452	Pathological fracture, left femur
➐⇄	M84.551	Pathological fracture in neoplastic disease, right femur
➐⇄	M84.552	Pathological fracture in neoplastic disease, left femur
➐⇄	M84.651	Pathological fracture in other disease, right femur
➐⇄	M84.652	Pathological fracture in other disease, left femur
➐⇄	M84.751	Incomplete atypical femoral fracture, right leg
➐⇄	M84.752	Incomplete atypical femoral fracture, left leg
➐⇄	M84.754	Complete transverse atypical femoral fracture, right leg
➐⇄	M84.755	Complete transverse atypical femoral fracture, left leg
➐⇄	M84.757	Complete oblique atypical femoral fracture, right leg
➐⇄	M84.758	Complete oblique atypical femoral fracture, left leg
⇄	M85.551	Aneurysmal bone cyst, right thigh
⇄	M85.552	Aneurysmal bone cyst, left thigh
⇄	M85.651	Other cyst of bone, right thigh
⇄	M85.652	Other cyst of bone, left thigh
⇄	M86.651	Other chronic osteomyelitis, right thigh
⇄	M86.652	Other chronic osteomyelitis, left thigh
➐⇄	S72.031	Displaced midcervical fracture of right femur
➐⇄	S72.032	Displaced midcervical fracture of left femur
➐⇄	S72.041	Displaced fracture of base of neck of right femur
➐⇄	S72.042	Displaced fracture of base of neck of left femur
➐⇄	S72.21	Displaced subtrochanteric fracture of right femur
➐⇄	S72.22	Displaced subtrochanteric fracture of left femur
➐⇄	S72.321	Displaced transverse fracture of shaft of right femur
➐⇄	S72.322	Displaced transverse fracture of shaft of left femur
➐⇄	S72.325	Nondisplaced transverse fracture of shaft of left femur
➐⇄	S72.331	Displaced oblique fracture of shaft of right femur
➐⇄	S72.332	Displaced oblique fracture of shaft of left femur
➐⇄	S72.341	Displaced spiral fracture of shaft of right femur
➐⇄	S72.342	Displaced spiral fracture of shaft of left femur
➐⇄	S72.351	Displaced comminuted fracture of shaft of right femur
➐⇄	S72.352	Displaced comminuted fracture of shaft of left femur
➐⇄	S72.361	Displaced segmental fracture of shaft of right femur
➐⇄	S72.362	Displaced segmental fracture of shaft of left femur
➐⇄	S72.391	Other fracture of shaft of right femur
➐⇄	S72.392	Other fracture of shaft of left femur
➐⇄	S79.091	Other physeal fracture of upper end of right femur
➐⇄	S79.092	Other physeal fracture of upper end of left femur

ICD-10-CM Coding Notes

For codes requiring a 7th character extension, refer to your ICD-10-CM book. Review the character descriptions and coding guidelines for proper selection. For some procedures, only certain characters will apply.

CCI Edits

Refer to Appendix A for CCI edits.

Pub 100

01230: Pub 100-04, 12, 140.5, Pub 100-04, 12, 50, Pub 100-04, 12, 90.4.5

Base Units

Global: XXX

Code	Base Units
01230	6

Modifiers (PAR)

Code	Mod 50	Mod 51	Mod 62	Mod 80
01230	9	9	9	9

CPT © 2018 American Medical Association. All Rights Reserved.

01232

01232 Anesthesia for open procedures involving upper two-thirds of femur; amputation

ICD-10-CM Diagnostic Codes

⇄	C40.21	Malignant neoplasm of long bones of right lower limb
⇄	C40.22	Malignant neoplasm of long bones of left lower limb
⇄	C47.21	Malignant neoplasm of peripheral nerves of right lower limb, including hip
⇄	C47.22	Malignant neoplasm of peripheral nerves of left lower limb, including hip
⇄	C49.21	Malignant neoplasm of connective and soft tissue of right lower limb, including hip
⇄	C49.22	Malignant neoplasm of connective and soft tissue of left lower limb, including hip
	C79.89	Secondary malignant neoplasm of other specified sites
	E08.51	Diabetes mellitus due to underlying condition with diabetic peripheral angiopathy without gangrene
	E08.52	Diabetes mellitus due to underlying condition with diabetic peripheral angiopathy with gangrene
	E08.622	Diabetes mellitus due to underlying condition with other skin ulcer
	E09.51	Drug or chemical induced diabetes mellitus with diabetic peripheral angiopathy without gangrene
	E09.52	Drug or chemical induced diabetes mellitus with diabetic peripheral angiopathy with gangrene
	E09.622	Drug or chemical induced diabetes mellitus with other skin ulcer
	E10.51	Type 1 diabetes mellitus with diabetic peripheral angiopathy without gangrene
	E10.52	Type 1 diabetes mellitus with diabetic peripheral angiopathy with gangrene
	E10.622	Type 1 diabetes mellitus with other skin ulcer
	E11.51	Type 2 diabetes mellitus with diabetic peripheral angiopathy without gangrene
	E11.52	Type 2 diabetes mellitus with diabetic peripheral angiopathy with gangrene
	E11.622	Type 2 diabetes mellitus with other skin ulcer
	E13.51	Other specified diabetes mellitus with diabetic peripheral angiopathy without gangrene
	E13.52	Other specified diabetes mellitus with diabetic peripheral angiopathy with gangrene
	E13.622	Other specified diabetes mellitus with other skin ulcer
⇄	I70.231	Atherosclerosis of native arteries of right leg with ulceration of thigh
⇄	I70.241	Atherosclerosis of native arteries of left leg with ulceration of thigh
⇄	I70.261	Atherosclerosis of native arteries of extremities with gangrene, right leg
⇄	I70.262	Atherosclerosis of native arteries of extremities with gangrene, left leg
⇄	I70.263	Atherosclerosis of native arteries of extremities with gangrene, bilateral legs
⇄	L97.113	Non-pressure chronic ulcer of right thigh with necrosis of muscle
⇄	L97.114	Non-pressure chronic ulcer of right thigh with necrosis of bone
⇄	L97.123	Non-pressure chronic ulcer of left thigh with necrosis of muscle
⇄	L97.124	Non-pressure chronic ulcer of left thigh with necrosis of bone
❼⇄	S77.11	Crushing injury of right thigh
❼⇄	S77.12	Crushing injury of left thigh
❼⇄	S78.111	Complete traumatic amputation at level between right hip and knee
❼⇄	S78.112	Complete traumatic amputation at level between left hip and knee
❼⇄	S78.121	Partial traumatic amputation at level between right hip and knee
❼⇄	S78.122	Partial traumatic amputation at level between left hip and knee
❼⇄	T24.391	Burn of third degree of multiple sites of right lower limb, except ankle and foot
❼⇄	T24.392	Burn of third degree of multiple sites of left lower limb, except ankle and foot
⇄	T87.33	Neuroma of amputation stump, right lower extremity
⇄	T87.34	Neuroma of amputation stump, left lower extremity
⇄	T87.43	Infection of amputation stump, right lower extremity
⇄	T87.53	Necrosis of amputation stump, right lower extremity
⇄	T87.54	Necrosis of amputation stump, left lower extremity

ICD-10-CM Coding Notes

For codes requiring a 7th character extension, refer to your ICD-10-CM book. Review the character descriptions and coding guidelines for proper selection. For some procedures, only certain characters will apply.

CCI Edits

Refer to Appendix A for CCI edits.

Pub 100

01232: Pub 100-04, 12, 140.5, Pub 100-04, 12, 50, Pub 100-04, 12, 90.4.5

Base Units

Global: XXX

Code	Base Units
01232	5

Modifiers (PAR)

Code	Mod 50	Mod 51	Mod 62	Mod 80
01232	9	9	9	9

CPT © 2018 American Medical Association. All Rights Reserved.

01234

01234 Anesthesia for open procedures involving upper two-thirds of femur; radical resection

ICD-10-CM Diagnostic Codes

⇄	C40.21	Malignant neoplasm of long bones of right lower limb
⇄	C40.22	Malignant neoplasm of long bones of left lower limb
⇄	C47.21	Malignant neoplasm of peripheral nerves of right lower limb, including hip
⇄	C47.22	Malignant neoplasm of peripheral nerves of left lower limb, including hip
⇄	C49.21	Malignant neoplasm of connective and soft tissue of right lower limb, including hip
⇄	C49.22	Malignant neoplasm of connective and soft tissue of left lower limb, including hip
	C79.51	Secondary malignant neoplasm of bone
	C79.89	Secondary malignant neoplasm of other specified sites

CCI Edits

Refer to Appendix A for CCI edits.

Pub 100

01234: Pub 100-04, 12, 140.5, Pub 100-04, 12, 50, Pub 100-04, 12, 90.4.5

Base Units

Global: XXX

Code	Base Units
01234	8

Modifiers (PAR)

Code	Mod 50	Mod 51	Mod 62	Mod 80
01234	9	9	9	9

CPT © 2018 American Medical Association. All Rights Reserved.

01250

01250 Anesthesia for all procedures on nerves, muscles, tendons, fascia, and bursae of upper leg

ICD-10-CM Diagnostic Codes

	G80.0	Spastic quadriplegic cerebral palsy
	G80.1	Spastic diplegic cerebral palsy
	G80.2	Spastic hemiplegic cerebral palsy
⇄	M62.051	Separation of muscle (nontraumatic), right thigh
⇄	M62.052	Separation of muscle (nontraumatic), left thigh
⇄	M62.151	Other rupture of muscle (nontraumatic), right thigh
⇄	M62.152	Other rupture of muscle (nontraumatic), left thigh
⇄	M62.451	Contracture of muscle, right thigh
⇄	M62.452	Contracture of muscle, left thigh
⇄	M65.051	Abscess of tendon sheath, right thigh
⇄	M65.052	Abscess of tendon sheath, left thigh
⇄	M66.251	Spontaneous rupture of extensor tendons, right thigh
⇄	M66.252	Spontaneous rupture of extensor tendons, left thigh
⇄	M66.351	Spontaneous rupture of flexor tendons, right thigh
⇄	M66.352	Spontaneous rupture of flexor tendons, left thigh
⇄	M66.851	Spontaneous rupture of other tendons, right thigh
⇄	M66.852	Spontaneous rupture of other tendons, left thigh
⇄	M79.A21	Nontraumatic compartment syndrome of right lower extremity
⇄	M79.A22	Nontraumatic compartment syndrome of left lower extremity
❼⇄	S71.111	Laceration without foreign body, right thigh
❼⇄	S71.112	Laceration without foreign body, left thigh
❼⇄	S71.121	Laceration with foreign body, right thigh
❼⇄	S71.122	Laceration with foreign body, left thigh
❼⇄	S71.141	Puncture wound with foreign body, right thigh
❼⇄	S71.142	Puncture wound with foreign body, left thigh
❼⇄	S71.151	Open bite, right thigh
❼⇄	S71.152	Open bite, left thigh
❼⇄	S74.01	Injury of sciatic nerve at hip and thigh level, right leg
❼⇄	S74.02	Injury of sciatic nerve at hip and thigh level, left leg
❼⇄	S74.11	Injury of femoral nerve at hip and thigh level, right leg
❼⇄	S74.12	Injury of femoral nerve at hip and thigh level, left leg
❼⇄	S76.121	Laceration of right quadriceps muscle, fascia and tendon
❼⇄	S76.122	Laceration of left quadriceps muscle, fascia and tendon
❼⇄	S76.191	Other specified injury of right quadriceps muscle, fascia and tendon
❼⇄	S76.192	Other specified injury of left quadriceps muscle, fascia and tendon
❼⇄	S76.221	Laceration of adductor muscle, fascia and tendon of right thigh
❼⇄	S76.222	Laceration of adductor muscle, fascia and tendon of left thigh
❼⇄	S76.291	Other injury of adductor muscle, fascia and tendon of right thigh
❼⇄	S76.292	Other injury of adductor muscle, fascia and tendon of left thigh
❼⇄	S76.321	Laceration of muscle, fascia and tendon of the posterior muscle group at thigh level, right thigh
❼⇄	S76.322	Laceration of muscle, fascia and tendon of the posterior muscle group at thigh level, left thigh
❼⇄	S76.391	Other specified injury of muscle, fascia and tendon of the posterior muscle group at thigh level, right thigh
❼⇄	S76.392	Other specified injury of muscle, fascia and tendon of the posterior muscle group at thigh level, left thigh
❼⇄	S76.821	Laceration of other specified muscles, fascia and tendons at thigh level, right thigh
❼⇄	S76.822	Laceration of other specified muscles, fascia and tendons at thigh level, left thigh
❼⇄	S76.891	Other injury of other specified muscles, fascia and tendons at thigh level, right thigh
❼⇄	S76.892	Other injury of other specified muscles, fascia and tendons at thigh level, left thigh
❼⇄	T79.A21	Traumatic compartment syndrome of right lower extremity
❼⇄	T79.A22	Traumatic compartment syndrome of left lower extremity

ICD-10-CM Coding Notes

For codes requiring a 7th character extension, refer to your ICD-10-CM book. Review the character descriptions and coding guidelines for proper selection. For some procedures, only certain characters will apply.

CCI Edits

Refer to Appendix A for CCI edits.

Pub 100

01250: Pub 100-04, 12, 140.5, Pub 100-04, 12, 50, Pub 100-04, 12, 90.4.5

Base Units

Global: XXX

Code	Base Units
01250	4

Modifiers (PAR)

Code	Mod 50	Mod 51	Mod 62	Mod 80
01250	9	9	9	9

CPT © 2018 American Medical Association. All Rights Reserved.

01260

01260 Anesthesia for all procedures involving veins of upper leg, including exploration

ICD-10-CM Diagnostic Codes

⇄ I80.01 Phlebitis and thrombophlebitis of superficial vessels of right lower extremity
⇄ I80.02 Phlebitis and thrombophlebitis of superficial vessels of left lower extremity
⇄ I80.11 Phlebitis and thrombophlebitis of right femoral vein
⇄ I80.12 Phlebitis and thrombophlebitis of left femoral vein
⇄ I80.13 Phlebitis and thrombophlebitis of femoral vein, bilateral
⇄ I80.201 Phlebitis and thrombophlebitis of unspecified deep vessels of right lower extremity
⇄ I80.202 Phlebitis and thrombophlebitis of unspecified deep vessels of left lower extremity
⇄ I80.203 Phlebitis and thrombophlebitis of unspecified deep vessels of lower extremities, bilateral
⇄ I80.291 Phlebitis and thrombophlebitis of other deep vessels of right lower extremity
⇄ I80.292 Phlebitis and thrombophlebitis of other deep vessels of left lower extremity
⇄ I80.293 Phlebitis and thrombophlebitis of other deep vessels of lower extremity, bilateral
⇄ I82.411 Acute embolism and thrombosis of right femoral vein
⇄ I82.412 Acute embolism and thrombosis of left femoral vein
⇄ I82.413 Acute embolism and thrombosis of femoral vein, bilateral
⇄ I82.492 Acute embolism and thrombosis of other specified deep vein of left lower extremity
⇄ I82.493 Acute embolism and thrombosis of other specified deep vein of lower extremity, bilateral
⇄ I82.4Y2 Acute embolism and thrombosis of unspecified deep veins of left proximal lower extremity
⇄ I82.4Y3 Acute embolism and thrombosis of unspecified deep veins of proximal lower extremity, bilateral
⇄ I83.011 Varicose veins of right lower extremity with ulcer of thigh
⇄ I83.021 Varicose veins of left lower extremity with ulcer of thigh
⇄ I83.11 Varicose veins of right lower extremity with inflammation
⇄ I83.12 Varicose veins of left lower extremity with inflammation
⇄ I83.211 Varicose veins of right lower extremity with both ulcer of thigh and inflammation
⇄ I83.221 Varicose veins of left lower extremity with both ulcer of thigh and inflammation
⇄ I83.811 Varicose veins of right lower extremity with pain
⇄ I83.812 Varicose veins of left lower extremity with pain
⇄ I83.813 Varicose veins of bilateral lower extremities with pain
⇄ I83.891 Varicose veins of right lower extremity with other complications
⇄ I83.892 Varicose veins of left lower extremity with other complications
⇄ I83.893 Varicose veins of bilateral lower extremities with other complications
⇄ I87.011 Postthrombotic syndrome with ulcer of right lower extremity
⇄ I87.012 Postthrombotic syndrome with ulcer of left lower extremity
⇄ I87.013 Postthrombotic syndrome with ulcer of bilateral lower extremity
⇄ I87.021 Postthrombotic syndrome with inflammation of right lower extremity
⇄ I87.022 Postthrombotic syndrome with inflammation of left lower extremity
⇄ I87.023 Postthrombotic syndrome with inflammation of bilateral lower extremity
⇄ I87.031 Postthrombotic syndrome with ulcer and inflammation of right lower extremity
⇄ I87.032 Postthrombotic syndrome with ulcer and inflammation of left lower extremity
⇄ I87.033 Postthrombotic syndrome with ulcer and inflammation of bilateral lower extremity
⇄ I87.091 Postthrombotic syndrome with other complications of right lower extremity
⇄ I87.092 Postthrombotic syndrome with other complications of left lower extremity
⇄ I87.093 Postthrombotic syndrome with other complications of bilateral lower extremity
I87.2 Venous insufficiency (chronic) (peripheral)
⇄ I87.311 Chronic venous hypertension (idiopathic) with ulcer of right lower extremity
⇄ I87.312 Chronic venous hypertension (idiopathic) with ulcer of left lower extremity
⇄ I87.313 Chronic venous hypertension (idiopathic) with ulcer of bilateral lower extremity
⇄ I87.321 Chronic venous hypertension (idiopathic) with inflammation of right lower extremity
⇄ I87.322 Chronic venous hypertension (idiopathic) with inflammation of left lower extremity
⇄ I87.323 Chronic venous hypertension (idiopathic) with inflammation of bilateral lower extremity
⇄ I87.331 Chronic venous hypertension (idiopathic) with ulcer and inflammation of right lower extremity
⇄ I87.332 Chronic venous hypertension (idiopathic) with ulcer and inflammation of left lower extremity
⇄ I87.333 Chronic venous hypertension (idiopathic) with ulcer and inflammation of bilateral lower extremity
⇄ I87.391 Chronic venous hypertension (idiopathic) with other complications of right lower extremity
⇄ I87.392 Chronic venous hypertension (idiopathic) with other complications of left lower extremity
⇄ I87.393 Chronic venous hypertension (idiopathic) with other complications of bilateral lower extremity
Q27.32 Arteriovenous malformation of vessel of lower limb
Q27.8 Other specified congenital malformations of peripheral vascular system
➐⇄ S75.111 Minor laceration of femoral vein at hip and thigh level, right leg
➐⇄ S75.112 Minor laceration of femoral vein at hip and thigh level, left leg
➐⇄ S75.121 Major laceration of femoral vein at hip and thigh level, right leg
➐⇄ S75.122 Major laceration of femoral vein at hip and thigh level, left leg
➐⇄ S75.191 Other specified injury of femoral vein at hip and thigh level, right leg
➐⇄ S75.192 Other specified injury of femoral vein at hip and thigh level, left leg
➐⇄ S75.211 Minor laceration of greater saphenous vein at hip and thigh level, right leg
➐⇄ S75.212 Minor laceration of greater saphenous vein at hip and thigh level, left leg
➐⇄ S75.221 Major laceration of greater saphenous vein at hip and thigh level, right leg
➐⇄ S75.222 Major laceration of greater saphenous vein at hip and thigh level, left leg
➐⇄ S75.291 Other specified injury of greater saphenous vein at hip and thigh level, right leg
➐⇄ S75.292 Other specified injury of greater saphenous vein at hip and thigh level, left leg
➐⇄ S75.811 Laceration of other blood vessels at hip and thigh level, right leg
➐⇄ S75.812 Laceration of other blood vessels at hip and thigh level, left leg
➐⇄ S75.891 Other specified injury of other blood vessels at hip and thigh level, right leg
➐⇄ S75.892 Other specified injury of other blood vessels at hip and thigh level, left leg
➐ T82.318 Breakdown (mechanical) of other vascular grafts
➐ T82.328 Displacement of other vascular grafts
➐ T82.338 Leakage of other vascular grafts

CPT © 2018 American Medical Association. All Rights Reserved.

- ➐ T82.398 Other mechanical complication of other vascular grafts
- ➐ T82.7 Infection and inflammatory reaction due to other cardiac and vascular devices, implants and grafts
- ➐ T82.818 Embolism due to vascular prosthetic devices, implants and grafts
- ➐ T82.828 Fibrosis due to vascular prosthetic devices, implants and grafts
- ➐ T82.838 Hemorrhage due to vascular prosthetic devices, implants and grafts
- ➐ T82.848 Pain due to vascular prosthetic devices, implants and grafts
- ➐ T82.858 Stenosis of other vascular prosthetic devices, implants and grafts
- ➐ T82.868 Thrombosis due to vascular prosthetic devices, implants and grafts
- ➐ T82.898 Other specified complication of vascular prosthetic devices, implants and grafts

ICD-10-CM Coding Notes

For codes requiring a 7th character extension, refer to your ICD-10-CM book. Review the character descriptions and coding guidelines for proper selection. For some procedures, only certain characters will apply.

CCI Edits

Refer to Appendix A for CCI edits.

Pub 100

01260: Pub 100-04, 12, 140.5, Pub 100-04, 12, 50, Pub 100-04, 12, 90.4.5

Base Units

Global: XXX

Code	Base Units
01260	3

Modifiers (PAR)

Code	Mod 50	Mod 51	Mod 62	Mod 80
01260	9	9	9	9

CPT © 2018 American Medical Association. All Rights Reserved.

01270

01270 Anesthesia for procedures involving arteries of upper leg, including bypass graft; not otherwise specified

ICD-10-CM Diagnostic Codes

⇄	I70.211	Atherosclerosis of native arteries of extremities with intermittent claudication, right leg
⇄	I70.212	Atherosclerosis of native arteries of extremities with intermittent claudication, left leg
⇄	I70.213	Atherosclerosis of native arteries of extremities with intermittent claudication, bilateral legs
⇄	I70.221	Atherosclerosis of native arteries of extremities with rest pain, right leg
⇄	I70.222	Atherosclerosis of native arteries of extremities with rest pain, left leg
⇄	I70.223	Atherosclerosis of native arteries of extremities with rest pain, bilateral legs
⇄	I70.231	Atherosclerosis of native arteries of right leg with ulceration of thigh
⇄	I70.232	Atherosclerosis of native arteries of right leg with ulceration of calf
⇄	I70.233	Atherosclerosis of native arteries of right leg with ulceration of ankle
⇄	I70.234	Atherosclerosis of native arteries of right leg with ulceration of heel and midfoot
⇄	I70.235	Atherosclerosis of native arteries of right leg with ulceration of other part of foot
⇄	I70.238	Atherosclerosis of native arteries of right leg with ulceration of other part of lower right leg
⇄	I70.241	Atherosclerosis of native arteries of left leg with ulceration of thigh
⇄	I70.242	Atherosclerosis of native arteries of left leg with ulceration of calf
⇄	I70.243	Atherosclerosis of native arteries of left leg with ulceration of ankle
⇄	I70.244	Atherosclerosis of native arteries of left leg with ulceration of heel and midfoot
⇄	I70.245	Atherosclerosis of native arteries of left leg with ulceration of other part of foot
⇄	I70.248	Atherosclerosis of native arteries of left leg with ulceration of other part of lower left leg
⇄	I70.261	Atherosclerosis of native arteries of extremities with gangrene, right leg
⇄	I70.262	Atherosclerosis of native arteries of extremities with gangrene, left leg
⇄	I70.263	Atherosclerosis of native arteries of extremities with gangrene, bilateral legs
⇄	I70.291	Other atherosclerosis of native arteries of extremities, right leg
⇄	I70.292	Other atherosclerosis of native arteries of extremities, left leg
⇄	I70.293	Other atherosclerosis of native arteries of extremities, bilateral legs
	I72.4	Aneurysm of artery of lower extremity
	I74.3	Embolism and thrombosis of arteries of the lower extremities
⇄	I75.021	Atheroembolism of right lower extremity
⇄	I75.022	Atheroembolism of left lower extremity
⇄	I75.023	Atheroembolism of bilateral lower extremities
	I77.1	Stricture of artery
	I77.2	Rupture of artery
	I77.5	Necrosis of artery
❼⇄	S75.011	Minor laceration of femoral artery, right leg
❼⇄	S75.012	Minor laceration of femoral artery, left leg
❼⇄	S75.021	Major laceration of femoral artery, right leg
❼⇄	S75.022	Major laceration of femoral artery, left leg
❼⇄	S75.091	Other specified injury of femoral artery, right leg
❼⇄	S75.092	Other specified injury of femoral artery, left leg
❼⇄	S75.811	Laceration of other blood vessels at hip and thigh level, right leg
❼⇄	S75.812	Laceration of other blood vessels at hip and thigh level, left leg
❼⇄	S75.891	Other specified injury of other blood vessels at hip and thigh level, right leg
❼⇄	S75.892	Other specified injury of other blood vessels at hip and thigh level, left leg
❼	T82.312	Breakdown (mechanical) of femoral arterial graft (bypass)
❼	T82.318	Breakdown (mechanical) of other vascular grafts
❼	T82.322	Displacement of femoral arterial graft (bypass)
❼	T82.328	Displacement of other vascular grafts
❼	T82.332	Leakage of femoral arterial graft (bypass)
❼	T82.338	Leakage of other vascular grafts
❼	T82.392	Other mechanical complication of femoral arterial graft (bypass)
❼	T82.398	Other mechanical complication of other vascular grafts
❼	T82.518	Breakdown (mechanical) of other cardiac and vascular devices and implants
❼	T82.528	Displacement of other cardiac and vascular devices and implants
❼	T82.538	Leakage of other cardiac and vascular devices and implants
❼	T82.598	Other mechanical complication of other cardiac and vascular devices and implants
❼	T82.7	Infection and inflammatory reaction due to other cardiac and vascular devices, implants and grafts
❼	T82.818	Embolism due to vascular prosthetic devices, implants and grafts
❼	T82.828	Fibrosis due to vascular prosthetic devices, implants and grafts
❼	T82.838	Hemorrhage due to vascular prosthetic devices, implants and grafts
❼	T82.848	Pain due to vascular prosthetic devices, implants and grafts
❼	T82.858	Stenosis of other vascular prosthetic devices, implants and grafts
❼	T82.868	Thrombosis due to vascular prosthetic devices, implants and grafts
❼	T82.898	Other specified complication of vascular prosthetic devices, implants and grafts

ICD-10-CM Coding Notes

For codes requiring a 7th character extension, refer to your ICD-10-CM book. Review the character descriptions and coding guidelines for proper selection. For some procedures, only certain characters will apply.

CCI Edits

Refer to Appendix A for CCI edits.

Pub 100

01270: Pub 100-04, 12, 140.5, Pub 100-04, 12, 50, Pub 100-04, 12, 90.4.5

Base Units

Global: XXX

Code	Base Units
01270	8

Modifiers (PAR)

Code	Mod 50	Mod 51	Mod 62	Mod 80
01270	9	9	9	9

CPT © 2018 American Medical Association. All Rights Reserved.

01272

01272 Anesthesia for procedures involving arteries of upper leg, including bypass graft; femoral artery ligation

ICD-10-CM Diagnostic Codes

⇄	C49.21	Malignant neoplasm of connective and soft tissue of right lower limb, including hip
⇄	C49.22	Malignant neoplasm of connective and soft tissue of left lower limb, including hip
⇄	C76.51	Malignant neoplasm of right lower limb
⇄	C76.52	Malignant neoplasm of left lower limb
❼⇄	S78.111	Complete traumatic amputation at level between right hip and knee
❼⇄	S78.112	Complete traumatic amputation at level between left hip and knee
❼⇄	S78.121	Partial traumatic amputation at level between right hip and knee
❼⇄	S78.122	Partial traumatic amputation at level between left hip and knee

ICD-10-CM Coding Notes

For codes requiring a 7th character extension, refer to your ICD-10-CM book. Review the character descriptions and coding guidelines for proper selection. For some procedures, only certain characters will apply.

CCI Edits

Refer to Appendix A for CCI edits.

Pub 100

01272: Pub 100-04, 12, 140.5, Pub 100-04, 12, 50, Pub 100-04, 12, 90.4.5

Base Units

Global: XXX

Code	Base Units
01272	4

Modifiers (PAR)

Code	Mod 50	Mod 51	Mod 62	Mod 80
01272	9	9	9	9

CPT © 2018 American Medical Association. All Rights Reserved.

01274

01274 Anesthesia for procedures involving arteries of upper leg, including bypass graft; femoral artery embolectomy

AMA *CPT Assistant* ▯

01274: Nov 07: 8, Jul 12: 13

ICD-10-CM Diagnostic Codes

	I74.3	Embolism and thrombosis of arteries of the lower extremities
⇄	I75.021	Atheroembolism of right lower extremity
⇄	I75.022	Atheroembolism of left lower extremity

CCI Edits

Refer to Appendix A for CCI edits.

Pub 100

01274: Pub 100-04, 12, 140.5, Pub 100-04, 12, 50, Pub 100-04, 12, 90.4.5

Base Units

Global: XXX

Code	Base Units
01274	6

Modifiers (PAR)

Code	Mod 50	Mod 51	Mod 62	Mod 80
01274	9	9	9	9

CPT © 2018 American Medical Association. All Rights Reserved.

01320

01320 Anesthesia for all procedures on nerves, muscles, tendons, fascia, and bursae of knee and/or popliteal area

AMA *CPT Assistant* ☐

01320: Mar 06: 15, Nov 07: 8, Oct 11: 3, Jul 12: 13

ICD-10-CM Diagnostic Codes

⇄ M23.611 Other spontaneous disruption of anterior cruciate ligament of right knee
⇄ M23.612 Other spontaneous disruption of anterior cruciate ligament of left knee
⇄ M23.621 Other spontaneous disruption of posterior cruciate ligament of right knee
⇄ M23.622 Other spontaneous disruption of posterior cruciate ligament of left knee
⇄ M23.631 Other spontaneous disruption of medial collateral ligament of right knee
⇄ M23.632 Other spontaneous disruption of medial collateral ligament of left knee
⇄ M23.641 Other spontaneous disruption of lateral collateral ligament of right knee
⇄ M23.642 Other spontaneous disruption of lateral collateral ligament of left knee
⇄ M23.671 Other spontaneous disruption of capsular ligament of right knee
⇄ M23.672 Other spontaneous disruption of capsular ligament of left knee
⇄ M65.861 Other synovitis and tenosynovitis, right lower leg
⇄ M65.862 Other synovitis and tenosynovitis, left lower leg
⇄ M66.251 Spontaneous rupture of extensor tendons, right thigh
⇄ M66.252 Spontaneous rupture of extensor tendons, left thigh
⇄ M67.461 Ganglion, right knee
⇄ M67.462 Ganglion, left knee
⇄ M67.51 Plica syndrome, right knee
⇄ M67.52 Plica syndrome, left knee
⇄ M67.863 Other specified disorders of tendon, right knee
⇄ M67.864 Other specified disorders of tendon, left knee
⇄ M70.41 Prepatellar bursitis, right knee
⇄ M70.42 Prepatellar bursitis, left knee
⇄ M70.51 Other bursitis of knee, right knee
⇄ M70.52 Other bursitis of knee, left knee
⇄ M71.061 Abscess of bursa, right knee
⇄ M71.062 Abscess of bursa, left knee
⇄ M71.161 Other infective bursitis, right knee
⇄ M71.162 Other infective bursitis, left knee
⇄ M71.21 Synovial cyst of popliteal space [Baker], right knee
⇄ M71.22 Synovial cyst of popliteal space [Baker], left knee
⇄ M71.561 Other bursitis, not elsewhere classified, right knee
⇄ M71.562 Other bursitis, not elsewhere classified, left knee
⇄ M71.861 Other specified bursopathies, right knee
⇄ M71.862 Other specified bursopathies, left knee
⇄ M76.51 Patellar tendinitis, right knee
⇄ M76.52 Patellar tendinitis, left knee
➐⇄ S83.411 Sprain of medial collateral ligament of right knee
➐⇄ S83.412 Sprain of medial collateral ligament of left knee
➐⇄ S83.421 Sprain of lateral collateral ligament of right knee
➐⇄ S83.422 Sprain of lateral collateral ligament of left knee
➐⇄ S83.511 Sprain of anterior cruciate ligament of right knee
➐⇄ S83.512 Sprain of anterior cruciate ligament of left knee
➐⇄ S83.521 Sprain of posterior cruciate ligament of right knee
➐⇄ S83.522 Sprain of posterior cruciate ligament of left knee
➐⇄ S83.61 Sprain of the superior tibiofibular joint and ligament, right knee
➐⇄ S83.62 Sprain of the superior tibiofibular joint and ligament, left knee
➐⇄ S83.8X1 Sprain of other specified parts of right knee
➐⇄ S83.8X2 Sprain of other specified parts of left knee

ICD-10-CM Coding Notes

For codes requiring a 7th character extension, refer to your ICD-10-CM book. Review the character descriptions and coding guidelines for proper selection. For some procedures, only certain characters will apply.

CCI Edits

Refer to Appendix A for CCI edits.

Pub 100

01320: Pub 100-04, 12, 140.5, Pub 100-04, 12, 50, Pub 100-04, 12, 90.4.5

Base Units

Global: XXX

Code	Base Units
01320	4

Modifiers (PAR)

Code	Mod 50	Mod 51	Mod 62	Mod 80
01320	9	9	9	9

CPT © 2018 American Medical Association. All Rights Reserved.

01340

01340 Anesthesia for all closed procedures on lower one-third of femur

ICD-10-CM Diagnostic Codes

⇄	C40.21	Malignant neoplasm of long bones of right lower limb
⇄	C40.22	Malignant neoplasm of long bones of left lower limb
	C79.51	Secondary malignant neoplasm of bone
⇄	D16.21	Benign neoplasm of long bones of right lower limb
⇄	D16.22	Benign neoplasm of long bones of left lower limb
⇄	M85.551	Aneurysmal bone cyst, right thigh
⇄	M85.552	Aneurysmal bone cyst, left thigh
⇄	M85.651	Other cyst of bone, right thigh
⇄	M85.652	Other cyst of bone, left thigh
⇄	M85.851	Other specified disorders of bone density and structure, right thigh
⇄	M85.852	Other specified disorders of bone density and structure, left thigh
⇄	M89.351	Hypertrophy of bone, right femur
⇄	M89.352	Hypertrophy of bone, left femur
❼⇄	S72.421	Displaced fracture of lateral condyle of right femur
❼⇄	S72.422	Displaced fracture of lateral condyle of left femur
❼⇄	S72.424	Nondisplaced fracture of lateral condyle of right femur
❼⇄	S72.425	Nondisplaced fracture of lateral condyle of left femur
❼⇄	S72.431	Displaced fracture of medial condyle of right femur
❼⇄	S72.432	Displaced fracture of medial condyle of left femur
❼⇄	S72.434	Nondisplaced fracture of medial condyle of right femur
❼⇄	S72.435	Nondisplaced fracture of medial condyle of left femur
❼⇄	S72.441	Displaced fracture of lower epiphysis (separation) of right femur
❼⇄	S72.442	Displaced fracture of lower epiphysis (separation) of left femur
❼⇄	S72.444	Nondisplaced fracture of lower epiphysis (separation) of right femur
❼⇄	S72.445	Nondisplaced fracture of lower epiphysis (separation) of left femur
❼⇄	S72.451	Displaced supracondylar fracture without intracondylar extension of lower end of right femur
❼⇄	S72.452	Displaced supracondylar fracture without intracondylar extension of lower end of left femur
❼⇄	S72.454	Nondisplaced supracondylar fracture without intracondylar extension of lower end of right femur
❼⇄	S72.455	Nondisplaced supracondylar fracture without intracondylar extension of lower end of left femur
❼⇄	S72.461	Displaced supracondylar fracture with intracondylar extension of lower end of right femur
❼⇄	S72.462	Displaced supracondylar fracture with intracondylar extension of lower end of left femur
❼⇄	S72.464	Nondisplaced supracondylar fracture with intracondylar extension of lower end of right femur
❼⇄	S72.465	Nondisplaced supracondylar fracture with intracondylar extension of lower end of left femur
❼⇄	S72.471	Torus fracture of lower end of right femur
❼⇄	S72.472	Torus fracture of lower end of left femur
❼⇄	S72.491	Other fracture of lower end of right femur
❼⇄	S72.492	Other fracture of lower end of left femur
❼⇄	S72.8X1	Other fracture of right femur
❼⇄	S72.8X2	Other fracture of left femur

ICD-10-CM Coding Notes

For codes requiring a 7th character extension, refer to your ICD-10-CM book. Review the character descriptions and coding guidelines for proper selection. For some procedures, only certain characters will apply.

CCI Edits

Refer to Appendix A for CCI edits.

Pub 100

01340: Pub 100-04, 12, 140.5, Pub 100-04, 12, 50, Pub 100-04, 12, 90.4.5

Base Units

Global: XXX

Code	Base Units
01340	4

Modifiers (PAR)

Code	Mod 50	Mod 51	Mod 62	Mod 80
01340	9	9	9	9

CPT © 2018 American Medical Association. All Rights Reserved.

01360

01360 Anesthesia for all open procedures on lower one-third of femur

ICD-10-CM Diagnostic Codes

⇄ D16.21 Benign neoplasm of long bones of right lower limb
⇄ D16.22 Benign neoplasm of long bones of left lower limb
⇄ M85.551 Aneurysmal bone cyst, right thigh
⇄ M85.552 Aneurysmal bone cyst, left thigh
⇄ M85.651 Other cyst of bone, right thigh
⇄ M85.652 Other cyst of bone, left thigh
⇄ M85.851 Other specified disorders of bone density and structure, right thigh
⇄ M85.852 Other specified disorders of bone density and structure, left thigh
⇄ Q72.811 Congenital shortening of right lower limb
⇄ Q72.812 Congenital shortening of left lower limb
❼⇄ S72.411 Displaced unspecified condyle fracture of lower end of right femur
❼⇄ S72.412 Displaced unspecified condyle fracture of lower end of left femur
❼⇄ S72.414 Nondisplaced unspecified condyle fracture of lower end of right femur
❼⇄ S72.415 Nondisplaced unspecified condyle fracture of lower end of left femur
❼⇄ S72.421 Displaced fracture of lateral condyle of right femur
❼⇄ S72.422 Displaced fracture of lateral condyle of left femur
❼⇄ S72.424 Nondisplaced fracture of lateral condyle of right femur
❼⇄ S72.425 Nondisplaced fracture of lateral condyle of left femur
❼⇄ S72.431 Displaced fracture of medial condyle of right femur
❼⇄ S72.432 Displaced fracture of medial condyle of left femur
❼⇄ S72.434 Nondisplaced fracture of medial condyle of right femur
❼⇄ S72.435 Nondisplaced fracture of medial condyle of left femur
❼⇄ S72.441 Displaced fracture of lower epiphysis (separation) of right femur
❼⇄ S72.442 Displaced fracture of lower epiphysis (separation) of left femur
❼⇄ S72.444 Nondisplaced fracture of lower epiphysis (separation) of right femur
❼⇄ S72.445 Nondisplaced fracture of lower epiphysis (separation) of left femur
❼⇄ S72.451 Displaced supracondylar fracture without intracondylar extension of lower end of right femur
❼⇄ S72.452 Displaced supracondylar fracture without intracondylar extension of lower end of left femur
❼⇄ S72.454 Nondisplaced supracondylar fracture without intracondylar extension of lower end of right femur
❼⇄ S72.455 Nondisplaced supracondylar fracture without intracondylar extension of lower end of left femur
❼⇄ S72.461 Displaced supracondylar fracture with intracondylar extension of lower end of right femur
❼⇄ S72.462 Displaced supracondylar fracture with intracondylar extension of lower end of left femur
❼⇄ S72.464 Nondisplaced supracondylar fracture with intracondylar extension of lower end of right femur
❼⇄ S72.465 Nondisplaced supracondylar fracture with intracondylar extension of lower end of left femur
❼⇄ S72.471 Torus fracture of lower end of right femur
❼⇄ S72.472 Torus fracture of lower end of left femur
❼⇄ S72.491 Other fracture of lower end of right femur
❼⇄ S72.492 Other fracture of lower end of left femur
❼⇄ S72.8X1 Other fracture of right femur
❼⇄ S72.8X2 Other fracture of left femur

ICD-10-CM Coding Notes

For codes requiring a 7th character extension, refer to your ICD-10-CM book. Review the character descriptions and coding guidelines for proper selection. For some procedures, only certain characters will apply.

CCI Edits

Refer to Appendix A for CCI edits.

Pub 100

01360: Pub 100-04, 12, 140.5, Pub 100-04, 12, 50, Pub 100-04, 12, 90.4.5

Base Units

Global: XXX

Code	Base Units
01360	5

Modifiers (PAR)

Code	Mod 50	Mod 51	Mod 62	Mod 80
01360	9	9	9	9

CPT © 2018 American Medical Association. All Rights Reserved.

01380

01380 Anesthesia for all closed procedures on knee joint

ICD-10-CM Diagnostic Codes

⇄	M22.01	Recurrent dislocation of patella, right knee
⇄	M22.02	Recurrent dislocation of patella, left knee
⇄	M22.11	Recurrent subluxation of patella, right knee
⇄	M22.12	Recurrent subluxation of patella, left knee
⇄	M23.211	Derangement of anterior horn of medial meniscus due to old tear or injury, right knee
⇄	M23.212	Derangement of anterior horn of medial meniscus due to old tear or injury, left knee
⇄	M23.311	Other meniscus derangements, anterior horn of medial meniscus, right knee
⇄	M23.312	Other meniscus derangements, anterior horn of medial meniscus, left knee
⇄	M24.361	Pathological dislocation of right knee, not elsewhere classified
⇄	M24.362	Pathological dislocation of left knee, not elsewhere classified
⇄	M24.461	Recurrent dislocation, right knee
⇄	M24.462	Recurrent dislocation, left knee
⇄	M65.161	Other infective (teno)synovitis, right knee
⇄	M65.162	Other infective (teno)synovitis, left knee
⇄	M65.861	Other synovitis and tenosynovitis, right lower leg
⇄	M65.862	Other synovitis and tenosynovitis, left lower leg
⇄	M67.261	Synovial hypertrophy, not elsewhere classified, right lower leg
⇄	M67.262	Synovial hypertrophy, not elsewhere classified, left lower leg
⇄	M67.51	Plica syndrome, right knee
⇄	M67.52	Plica syndrome, left knee
⇄	M67.861	Other specified disorders of synovium, right knee
⇄	M67.862	Other specified disorders of synovium, left knee
	Q68.2	Congenital deformity of knee
❼⇄	S83.011	Lateral subluxation of right patella
❼⇄	S83.012	Lateral subluxation of left patella
❼⇄	S83.014	Lateral dislocation of right patella
❼⇄	S83.015	Lateral dislocation of left patella
❼⇄	S83.091	Other subluxation of right patella
❼⇄	S83.092	Other subluxation of left patella
❼⇄	S83.094	Other dislocation of right patella
❼⇄	S83.095	Other dislocation of left patella
❼⇄	S83.111	Anterior subluxation of proximal end of tibia, right knee
❼⇄	S83.112	Anterior subluxation of proximal end of tibia, left knee
❼⇄	S83.114	Anterior dislocation of proximal end of tibia, right knee
❼⇄	S83.115	Anterior dislocation of proximal end of tibia, left knee
❼⇄	S83.121	Posterior subluxation of proximal end of tibia, right knee
❼⇄	S83.122	Posterior subluxation of proximal end of tibia, left knee
❼⇄	S83.124	Posterior dislocation of proximal end of tibia, right knee
❼⇄	S83.125	Posterior dislocation of proximal end of tibia, left knee
❼⇄	S83.131	Medial subluxation of proximal end of tibia, right knee
❼⇄	S83.132	Medial subluxation of proximal end of tibia, left knee
❼⇄	S83.134	Medial dislocation of proximal end of tibia, right knee
❼⇄	S83.135	Medial dislocation of proximal end of tibia, left knee
❼⇄	S83.141	Lateral subluxation of proximal end of tibia, right knee
❼⇄	S83.142	Lateral subluxation of proximal end of tibia, left knee
❼⇄	S83.144	Lateral dislocation of proximal end of tibia, right knee
❼⇄	S83.145	Lateral dislocation of proximal end of tibia, left knee
❼⇄	S83.191	Other subluxation of right knee
❼⇄	S83.192	Other subluxation of left knee
❼⇄	S83.194	Other dislocation of right knee
❼⇄	S83.195	Other dislocation of left knee

ICD-10-CM Coding Notes

For codes requiring a 7th character extension, refer to your ICD-10-CM book. Review the character descriptions and coding guidelines for proper selection. For some procedures, only certain characters will apply.

CCI Edits

Refer to Appendix A for CCI edits.

Pub 100

01380: Pub 100-04, 12, 140.5, Pub 100-04, 12, 50, Pub 100-04, 12, 90.4.5

Base Units

Global: XXX

Code	Base Units
01380	3

Modifiers (PAR)

Code	Mod 50	Mod 51	Mod 62	Mod 80
01380	9	9	9	9

CPT © 2018 American Medical Association. All Rights Reserved.

01382

01382 Anesthesia for diagnostic arthroscopic procedures of knee joint

ICD-10-CM Diagnostic Codes

⇄	M00.061	Staphylococcal arthritis, right knee
⇄	M00.062	Staphylococcal arthritis, left knee
⇄	M00.161	Pneumococcal arthritis, right knee
⇄	M00.162	Pneumococcal arthritis, left knee
⇄	M00.261	Other streptococcal arthritis, right knee
⇄	M00.262	Other streptococcal arthritis, left knee
⇄	M00.861	Arthritis due to other bacteria, right knee
⇄	M00.862	Arthritis due to other bacteria, left knee
	M17.0	Bilateral primary osteoarthritis of knee
⇄	M17.11	Unilateral primary osteoarthritis, right knee
⇄	M17.12	Unilateral primary osteoarthritis, left knee
⇄	M17.31	Unilateral post-traumatic osteoarthritis, right knee
⇄	M17.32	Unilateral post-traumatic osteoarthritis, left knee
	M17.4	Other bilateral secondary osteoarthritis of knee
	M17.5	Other unilateral secondary osteoarthritis of knee
⇄	M22.01	Recurrent dislocation of patella, right knee
⇄	M22.02	Recurrent dislocation of patella, left knee
⇄	M22.11	Recurrent subluxation of patella, right knee
⇄	M22.12	Recurrent subluxation of patella, left knee
⇄	M22.2X1	Patellofemoral disorders, right knee
⇄	M22.2X2	Patellofemoral disorders, left knee
⇄	M22.41	Chondromalacia patellae, right knee
⇄	M22.42	Chondromalacia patellae, left knee
⇄	M22.8X1	Other disorders of patella, right knee
⇄	M22.8X2	Other disorders of patella, left knee
⇄	M23.011	Cystic meniscus, anterior horn of medial meniscus, right knee
⇄	M23.012	Cystic meniscus, anterior horn of medial meniscus, left knee
⇄	M23.021	Cystic meniscus, posterior horn of medial meniscus, right knee
⇄	M23.022	Cystic meniscus, posterior horn of medial meniscus, left knee
⇄	M23.031	Cystic meniscus, other medial meniscus, right knee
⇄	M23.032	Cystic meniscus, other medial meniscus, left knee
⇄	M23.041	Cystic meniscus, anterior horn of lateral meniscus, right knee
⇄	M23.042	Cystic meniscus, anterior horn of lateral meniscus, left knee
⇄	M23.051	Cystic meniscus, posterior horn of lateral meniscus, right knee
⇄	M23.052	Cystic meniscus, posterior horn of lateral meniscus, left knee
⇄	M23.061	Cystic meniscus, other lateral meniscus, right knee
⇄	M23.062	Cystic meniscus, other lateral meniscus, left knee
⇄	M23.51	Chronic instability of knee, right knee
⇄	M23.52	Chronic instability of knee, left knee
⇄	M23.8X1	Other internal derangements of right knee
⇄	M23.8X2	Other internal derangements of left knee
⇄	M25.061	Hemarthrosis, right knee
⇄	M25.062	Hemarthrosis, left knee
⇄	M25.361	Other instability, right knee
⇄	M25.362	Other instability, left knee
⇄	M25.461	Effusion, right knee
⇄	M25.462	Effusion, left knee
⇄	M25.561	Pain in right knee
⇄	M25.562	Pain in left knee
⇄	M25.661	Stiffness of right knee, not elsewhere classified
⇄	M25.662	Stiffness of left knee, not elsewhere classified

CCI Edits

Refer to Appendix A for CCI edits.

Pub 100

01382: Pub 100-04, 12, 140.5, Pub 100-04, 12, 50, Pub 100-04, 12, 90.4.5

Base Units

Global: XXX

Code	Base Units
01382	3

Modifiers (PAR)

Code	Mod 50	Mod 51	Mod 62	Mod 80
01382	9	9	9	9

CPT © 2018 American Medical Association. All Rights Reserved.

01390

01390 Anesthesia for all closed procedures on upper ends of tibia, fibula, and/or patella

ICD-10-CM Diagnostic Codes

⇄ C40.21 Malignant neoplasm of long bones of right lower limb
C79.51 Secondary malignant neoplasm of bone
⇄ D16.21 Benign neoplasm of long bones of right lower limb
⇄ D16.22 Benign neoplasm of long bones of left lower limb
➐⇄ M84.461 Pathological fracture, right tibia
➐⇄ M84.462 Pathological fracture, left tibia
➐⇄ M84.463 Pathological fracture, right fibula
➐⇄ M84.464 Pathological fracture, left fibula
➐⇄ M84.561 Pathological fracture in neoplastic disease, right tibia
➐⇄ M84.562 Pathological fracture in neoplastic disease, left tibia
➐⇄ M84.563 Pathological fracture in neoplastic disease, right fibula
➐⇄ M84.564 Pathological fracture in neoplastic disease, left fibula
➐⇄ M84.661 Pathological fracture in other disease, right tibia
➐⇄ M84.662 Pathological fracture in other disease, left tibia
➐⇄ M84.663 Pathological fracture in other disease, right fibula
➐⇄ M84.664 Pathological fracture in other disease, left fibula
⇄ M89.361 Hypertrophy of bone, right tibia
⇄ M89.362 Hypertrophy of bone, left tibia
⇄ M89.363 Hypertrophy of bone, right fibula
⇄ M89.364 Hypertrophy of bone, left fibula
➐⇄ S82.011 Displaced osteochondral fracture of right patella
➐⇄ S82.012 Displaced osteochondral fracture of left patella
➐⇄ S82.014 Nondisplaced osteochondral fracture of right patella
➐⇄ S82.015 Nondisplaced osteochondral fracture of left patella
➐⇄ S82.021 Displaced longitudinal fracture of right patella
➐⇄ S82.022 Displaced longitudinal fracture of left patella
➐⇄ S82.024 Nondisplaced longitudinal fracture of right patella
➐⇄ S82.025 Nondisplaced longitudinal fracture of left patella
➐⇄ S82.031 Displaced transverse fracture of right patella
➐⇄ S82.032 Displaced transverse fracture of left patella
➐⇄ S82.034 Nondisplaced transverse fracture of right patella
➐⇄ S82.035 Nondisplaced transverse fracture of left patella
➐⇄ S82.041 Displaced comminuted fracture of right patella
➐⇄ S82.042 Displaced comminuted fracture of left patella
➐⇄ S82.044 Nondisplaced comminuted fracture of right patella
➐⇄ S82.045 Nondisplaced comminuted fracture of left patella
➐⇄ S82.091 Other fracture of right patella
➐⇄ S82.092 Other fracture of left patella
➐⇄ S82.111 Displaced fracture of right tibial spine
➐⇄ S82.112 Displaced fracture of left tibial spine
➐⇄ S82.114 Nondisplaced fracture of right tibial spine
➐⇄ S82.115 Nondisplaced fracture of left tibial spine
➐⇄ S82.121 Displaced fracture of lateral condyle of right tibia
➐⇄ S82.122 Displaced fracture of lateral condyle of left tibia
➐⇄ S82.124 Nondisplaced fracture of lateral condyle of right tibia
➐⇄ S82.125 Nondisplaced fracture of lateral condyle of left tibia
➐⇄ S82.131 Displaced fracture of medial condyle of right tibia
➐⇄ S82.132 Displaced fracture of medial condyle of left tibia
➐⇄ S82.134 Nondisplaced fracture of medial condyle of right tibia
➐⇄ S82.135 Nondisplaced fracture of medial condyle of left tibia
➐⇄ S82.141 Displaced bicondylar fracture of right tibia
➐⇄ S82.142 Displaced bicondylar fracture of left tibia
➐⇄ S82.144 Nondisplaced bicondylar fracture of right tibia
➐⇄ S82.145 Nondisplaced bicondylar fracture of left tibia
➐⇄ S82.151 Displaced fracture of right tibial tuberosity
➐⇄ S82.152 Displaced fracture of left tibial tuberosity
➐⇄ S82.154 Nondisplaced fracture of right tibial tuberosity
➐⇄ S82.155 Nondisplaced fracture of left tibial tuberosity
➐⇄ S82.161 Torus fracture of upper end of right tibia
➐⇄ S82.162 Torus fracture of upper end of left tibia
➐⇄ S82.191 Other fracture of upper end of right tibia
➐⇄ S82.192 Other fracture of upper end of left tibia

ICD-10-CM Coding Notes

For codes requiring a 7th character extension, refer to your ICD-10-CM book. Review the character descriptions and coding guidelines for proper selection. For some procedures, only certain characters will apply.

CCI Edits

Refer to Appendix A for CCI edits.

Pub 100

01390: Pub 100-04, 12, 140.5, Pub 100-04, 12, 50, Pub 100-04, 12, 90.4.5

Base Units

Global: XXX

Code	Base Units
01390	3

Modifiers (PAR)

Code	Mod 50	Mod 51	Mod 62	Mod 80
01390	9	9	9	9

CPT © 2018 American Medical Association. All Rights Reserved.

01392

01392 Anesthesia for all open procedures on upper ends of tibia, fibula, and/or patella

ICD-10-CM Diagnostic Codes

⇄ C40.21 Malignant neoplasm of long bones of right lower limb
⇄ C40.22 Malignant neoplasm of long bones of left lower limb
⇄ D16.21 Benign neoplasm of long bones of right lower limb
⇄ D16.22 Benign neoplasm of long bones of left lower limb
⇄ M85.361 Osteitis condensans, right lower leg
⇄ M85.362 Osteitis condensans, left lower leg
⇄ M85.461 Solitary bone cyst, right tibia and fibula
⇄ M85.462 Solitary bone cyst, left tibia and fibula
⇄ M85.562 Aneurysmal bone cyst, left lower leg
⇄ M85.661 Other cyst of bone, right lower leg
⇄ M85.662 Other cyst of bone, left lower leg
⇄ M85.861 Other specified disorders of bone density and structure, right lower leg
⇄ M85.862 Other specified disorders of bone density and structure, left lower leg
⇄ M86.461 Chronic osteomyelitis with draining sinus, right tibia and fibula
⇄ M86.462 Chronic osteomyelitis with draining sinus, left tibia and fibula
⇄ M86.561 Other chronic hematogenous osteomyelitis, right tibia and fibula
⇄ M86.562 Other chronic hematogenous osteomyelitis, left tibia and fibula
⇄ M86.661 Other chronic osteomyelitis, right tibia and fibula
⇄ M86.662 Other chronic osteomyelitis, left tibia and fibula
⇄ M89.160 Complete physeal arrest, right proximal tibia
⇄ M89.161 Complete physeal arrest, left proximal tibia
⇄ M89.162 Partial physeal arrest, right proximal tibia
⇄ M89.163 Partial physeal arrest, left proximal tibia
❼⇄ S82.011 Displaced osteochondral fracture of right patella
❼⇄ S82.012 Displaced osteochondral fracture of left patella
❼⇄ S82.014 Nondisplaced osteochondral fracture of right patella
❼⇄ S82.015 Nondisplaced osteochondral fracture of left patella
❼⇄ S82.021 Displaced longitudinal fracture of right patella
❼⇄ S82.022 Displaced longitudinal fracture of left patella
❼⇄ S82.024 Nondisplaced longitudinal fracture of right patella
❼⇄ S82.025 Nondisplaced longitudinal fracture of left patella
❼⇄ S82.031 Displaced transverse fracture of right patella
❼⇄ S82.032 Displaced transverse fracture of left patella
❼⇄ S82.034 Nondisplaced transverse fracture of right patella
❼⇄ S82.035 Nondisplaced transverse fracture of left patella
❼⇄ S82.041 Displaced comminuted fracture of right patella
❼⇄ S82.042 Displaced comminuted fracture of left patella
❼⇄ S82.044 Nondisplaced comminuted fracture of right patella
❼⇄ S82.045 Nondisplaced comminuted fracture of left patella
❼⇄ S82.091 Other fracture of right patella
❼⇄ S82.092 Other fracture of left patella
❼⇄ S82.111 Displaced fracture of right tibial spine
❼⇄ S82.112 Displaced fracture of left tibial spine
❼⇄ S82.114 Nondisplaced fracture of right tibial spine
❼⇄ S82.115 Nondisplaced fracture of left tibial spine
❼⇄ S82.121 Displaced fracture of lateral condyle of right tibia
❼⇄ S82.122 Displaced fracture of lateral condyle of left tibia
❼⇄ S82.124 Nondisplaced fracture of lateral condyle of right tibia
❼⇄ S82.125 Nondisplaced fracture of lateral condyle of left tibia
❼⇄ S82.131 Displaced fracture of medial condyle of right tibia
❼⇄ S82.132 Displaced fracture of medial condyle of left tibia
❼⇄ S82.134 Nondisplaced fracture of medial condyle of right tibia
❼⇄ S82.135 Nondisplaced fracture of medial condyle of left tibia
❼⇄ S82.141 Displaced bicondylar fracture of right tibia
❼⇄ S82.142 Displaced bicondylar fracture of left tibia
❼⇄ S82.144 Nondisplaced bicondylar fracture of right tibia
❼⇄ S82.145 Nondisplaced bicondylar fracture of left tibia
❼⇄ S82.151 Displaced fracture of right tibial tuberosity
❼⇄ S82.152 Displaced fracture of left tibial tuberosity
❼⇄ S82.154 Nondisplaced fracture of right tibial tuberosity
❼⇄ S82.155 Nondisplaced fracture of left tibial tuberosity
❼⇄ S82.161 Torus fracture of upper end of right tibia
❼⇄ S82.162 Torus fracture of upper end of left tibia
❼⇄ S82.191 Other fracture of upper end of right tibia
❼⇄ S82.192 Other fracture of upper end of left tibia

ICD-10-CM Coding Notes

For codes requiring a 7th character extension, refer to your ICD-10-CM book. Review the character descriptions and coding guidelines for proper selection. For some procedures, only certain characters will apply.

CCI Edits

Refer to Appendix A for CCI edits.

Pub 100

01392: Pub 100-04, 12, 140.5, Pub 100-04, 12, 50, Pub 100-04, 12, 90.4.5

Base Units

Global: XXX

Code	Base Units
01392	4

Modifiers (PAR)

Code	Mod 50	Mod 51	Mod 62	Mod 80
01392	9	9	9	9

CPT © 2018 American Medical Association. All Rights Reserved.

01400

01400 Anesthesia for open or surgical arthroscopic procedures on knee joint; not otherwise specified

ICD-10-CM Diagnostic Codes

⇄	M00.061	Staphylococcal arthritis, right knee
⇄	M00.062	Staphylococcal arthritis, left knee
⇄	M12.261	Villonodular synovitis (pigmented), right knee
⇄	M12.262	Villonodular synovitis (pigmented), left knee
	M17.0	Bilateral primary osteoarthritis of knee
⇄	M17.11	Unilateral primary osteoarthritis, right knee
⇄	M17.12	Unilateral primary osteoarthritis, left knee
	M17.2	Bilateral post-traumatic osteoarthritis of knee
⇄	M17.31	Unilateral post-traumatic osteoarthritis, right knee
⇄	M17.32	Unilateral post-traumatic osteoarthritis, left knee
	M17.4	Other bilateral secondary osteoarthritis of knee
	M17.5	Other unilateral secondary osteoarthritis of knee
⇄	M22.01	Recurrent dislocation of patella, right knee
⇄	M22.02	Recurrent dislocation of patella, left knee
⇄	M22.2X1	Patellofemoral disorders, right knee
⇄	M22.2X2	Patellofemoral disorders, left knee
⇄	M22.41	Chondromalacia patellae, right knee
⇄	M22.42	Chondromalacia patellae, left knee
⇄	M23.211	Derangement of anterior horn of medial meniscus due to old tear or injury, right knee
⇄	M23.212	Derangement of anterior horn of medial meniscus due to old tear or injury, left knee
⇄	M23.221	Derangement of posterior horn of medial meniscus due to old tear or injury, right knee
⇄	M23.222	Derangement of posterior horn of medial meniscus due to old tear or injury, left knee
⇄	M23.231	Derangement of other medial meniscus due to old tear or injury, right knee
⇄	M23.232	Derangement of other medial meniscus due to old tear or injury, left knee
⇄	M23.241	Derangement of anterior horn of lateral meniscus due to old tear or injury, right knee
⇄	M23.242	Derangement of anterior horn of lateral meniscus due to old tear or injury, left knee
⇄	M23.251	Derangement of posterior horn of lateral meniscus due to old tear or injury, right knee
⇄	M23.252	Derangement of posterior horn of lateral meniscus due to old tear or injury, left knee
⇄	M23.261	Derangement of other lateral meniscus due to old tear or injury, right knee
⇄	M23.41	Loose body in knee, right knee
⇄	M23.42	Loose body in knee, left knee
⇄	M23.51	Chronic instability of knee, right knee
⇄	M23.52	Chronic instability of knee, left knee
⇄	M23.611	Other spontaneous disruption of anterior cruciate ligament of right knee
⇄	M23.612	Other spontaneous disruption of anterior cruciate ligament of left knee
⇄	M23.621	Other spontaneous disruption of posterior cruciate ligament of right knee
⇄	M23.622	Other spontaneous disruption of posterior cruciate ligament of left knee
⇄	M23.631	Other spontaneous disruption of medial collateral ligament of right knee
⇄	M23.632	Other spontaneous disruption of medial collateral ligament of left knee
⇄	M23.641	Other spontaneous disruption of lateral collateral ligament of right knee
⇄	M23.642	Other spontaneous disruption of lateral collateral ligament of left knee
⇄	M23.671	Other spontaneous disruption of capsular ligament of right knee
⇄	M23.672	Other spontaneous disruption of capsular ligament of left knee
⇄	M23.8X1	Other internal derangements of right knee
⇄	M23.8X2	Other internal derangements of left knee
⇄	M93.261	Osteochondritis dissecans, right knee
⇄	M93.262	Osteochondritis dissecans, left knee
❼⇄	S82.111	Displaced fracture of right tibial spine
❼⇄	S82.112	Displaced fracture of left tibial spine
❼⇄	S82.114	Nondisplaced fracture of right tibial spine
❼⇄	S82.115	Nondisplaced fracture of left tibial spine
❼⇄	S82.141	Displaced bicondylar fracture of right tibia
❼⇄	S82.142	Displaced bicondylar fracture of left tibia
❼⇄	S82.144	Nondisplaced bicondylar fracture of right tibia
❼⇄	S82.145	Nondisplaced bicondylar fracture of left tibia

ICD-10-CM Coding Notes

For codes requiring a 7th character extension, refer to your ICD-10-CM book. Review the character descriptions and coding guidelines for proper selection. For some procedures, only certain characters will apply.

CCI Edits

Refer to Appendix A for CCI edits.

Pub 100

01400: Pub 100-04, 12, 140.5, Pub 100-04, 12, 50, Pub 100-04, 12, 90.4.5

Base Units

Global: XXX

Code	Base Units
01400	4

Modifiers (PAR)

Code	Mod 50	Mod 51	Mod 62	Mod 80
01400	9	9	9	9

CPT © 2018 American Medical Association. All Rights Reserved.

01402

01402 Anesthesia for open or surgical arthroscopic procedures on knee joint; total knee arthroplasty

ICD-10-CM Diagnostic Codes

	M17.0	Bilateral primary osteoarthritis of knee
⇄	M17.11	Unilateral primary osteoarthritis, right knee
⇄	M17.12	Unilateral primary osteoarthritis, left knee
	M17.2	Bilateral post-traumatic osteoarthritis of knee
⇄	M17.31	Unilateral post-traumatic osteoarthritis, right knee
⇄	M17.32	Unilateral post-traumatic osteoarthritis, left knee
	M17.4	Other bilateral secondary osteoarthritis of knee
	M17.5	Other unilateral secondary osteoarthritis of knee
⇄	M21.061	Valgus deformity, not elsewhere classified, right knee
⇄	M21.062	Valgus deformity, not elsewhere classified, left knee
⇄	M25.261	Flail joint, right knee
⇄	M25.262	Flail joint, left knee
⇄	M25.361	Other instability, right knee
⇄	M25.362	Other instability, left knee
⇄	M25.461	Effusion, right knee
⇄	M25.462	Effusion, left knee
⇄	M25.561	Pain in right knee
⇄	M25.562	Pain in left knee
➐⇄	M97.11	Periprosthetic fracture around internal prosthetic right knee joint
➐⇄	M97.12	Periprosthetic fracture around internal prosthetic left knee joint
➐⇄	T84.012	Broken internal right knee prosthesis
➐⇄	T84.013	Broken internal left knee prosthesis
➐⇄	T84.022	Instability of internal right knee prosthesis
➐⇄	T84.023	Instability of internal left knee prosthesis
➐⇄	T84.032	Mechanical loosening of internal right knee prosthetic joint
➐⇄	T84.033	Mechanical loosening of internal left knee prosthetic joint
➐⇄	T84.052	Periprosthetic osteolysis of internal prosthetic right knee joint
➐⇄	T84.053	Periprosthetic osteolysis of internal prosthetic left knee joint
➐⇄	T84.062	Wear of articular bearing surface of internal prosthetic right knee joint
➐⇄	T84.063	Wear of articular bearing surface of internal prosthetic left knee joint
➐⇄	T84.092	Other mechanical complication of internal right knee prosthesis
➐⇄	T84.093	Other mechanical complication of internal left knee prosthesis
➐⇄	T84.53	Infection and inflammatory reaction due to internal right knee prosthesis
➐⇄	T84.54	Infection and inflammatory reaction due to internal left knee prosthesis
➐	T85.828	Fibrosis due to other internal prosthetic devices, implants and grafts
➐	T85.838	Hemorrhage due to other internal prosthetic devices, implants and grafts
➐	T85.848	Pain due to other internal prosthetic devices, implants and grafts
➐	T85.898	Other specified complication of other internal prosthetic devices, implants and grafts

ICD-10-CM Coding Notes

For codes requiring a 7th character extension, refer to your ICD-10-CM book. Review the character descriptions and coding guidelines for proper selection. For some procedures, only certain characters will apply.

CCI Edits

Refer to Appendix A for CCI edits.

Pub 100

01402: Pub 100-04, 12, 140.5, Pub 100-04, 12, 50, Pub 100-04, 12, 90.4.5

Base Units

Global: XXX

Code	Base Units
01402	7

Modifiers (PAR)

Code	Mod 50	Mod 51	Mod 62	Mod 80
01402	9	9	9	9

CPT © 2018 American Medical Association. All Rights Reserved.

01404

01404 Anesthesia for open or surgical arthroscopic procedures on knee joint; disarticulation at knee

ICD-10-CM Diagnostic Codes

⇄	C40.21	Malignant neoplasm of long bones of right lower limb
⇄	C40.22	Malignant neoplasm of long bones of left lower limb
⇄	C47.21	Malignant neoplasm of peripheral nerves of right lower limb, including hip
⇄	C47.22	Malignant neoplasm of peripheral nerves of left lower limb, including hip
⇄	C49.21	Malignant neoplasm of connective and soft tissue of right lower limb, including hip
⇄	C49.22	Malignant neoplasm of connective and soft tissue of left lower limb, including hip
	E10.51	Type 1 diabetes mellitus with diabetic peripheral angiopathy without gangrene
	E10.52	Type 1 diabetes mellitus with diabetic peripheral angiopathy with gangrene
	E10.621	Type 1 diabetes mellitus with foot ulcer
	E10.622	Type 1 diabetes mellitus with other skin ulcer
	E11.51	Type 2 diabetes mellitus with diabetic peripheral angiopathy without gangrene
	E11.52	Type 2 diabetes mellitus with diabetic peripheral angiopathy with gangrene
	E11.621	Type 2 diabetes mellitus with foot ulcer
	E11.622	Type 2 diabetes mellitus with other skin ulcer
⇄	I70.232	Atherosclerosis of native arteries of right leg with ulceration of calf
⇄	I70.233	Atherosclerosis of native arteries of right leg with ulceration of ankle
⇄	I70.235	Atherosclerosis of native arteries of right leg with ulceration of other part of foot
⇄	I70.242	Atherosclerosis of native arteries of left leg with ulceration of calf
⇄	I70.243	Atherosclerosis of native arteries of left leg with ulceration of ankle
⇄	I70.244	Atherosclerosis of native arteries of left leg with ulceration of heel and midfoot
⇄	I70.262	Atherosclerosis of native arteries of extremities with gangrene, left leg
⇄	L97.213	Non-pressure chronic ulcer of right calf with necrosis of muscle
⇄	L97.214	Non-pressure chronic ulcer of right calf with necrosis of bone
⇄	L97.223	Non-pressure chronic ulcer of left calf with necrosis of muscle
⇄	L97.224	Non-pressure chronic ulcer of left calf with necrosis of bone
❼⇄	S87.81	Crushing injury of right lower leg
❼⇄	S87.82	Crushing injury of left lower leg
❼⇄	S88.011	Complete traumatic amputation at knee level, right lower leg
❼⇄	S88.012	Complete traumatic amputation at knee level, left lower leg
❼⇄	S88.021	Partial traumatic amputation at knee level, right lower leg
❼⇄	S88.022	Partial traumatic amputation at knee level, left lower leg
❼⇄	S88.111	Complete traumatic amputation at level between knee and ankle, right lower leg
❼⇄	S88.112	Complete traumatic amputation at level between knee and ankle, left lower leg
❼⇄	S88.121	Partial traumatic amputation at level between knee and ankle, right lower leg
❼⇄	S88.122	Partial traumatic amputation at level between knee and ankle, left lower leg
❼⇄	T24.391	Burn of third degree of multiple sites of right lower limb, except ankle and foot
❼⇄	T24.392	Burn of third degree of multiple sites of left lower limb, except ankle and foot
⇄	T87.33	Neuroma of amputation stump, right lower extremity
⇄	T87.34	Neuroma of amputation stump, left lower extremity
⇄	T87.43	Infection of amputation stump, right lower extremity
⇄	T87.44	Infection of amputation stump, left lower extremity
⇄	T87.53	Necrosis of amputation stump, right lower extremity
⇄	T87.54	Necrosis of amputation stump, left lower extremity

ICD-10-CM Coding Notes

For codes requiring a 7th character extension, refer to your ICD-10-CM book. Review the character descriptions and coding guidelines for proper selection. For some procedures, only certain characters will apply.

CCI Edits

Refer to Appendix A for CCI edits.

Pub 100

01404: Pub 100-04, 12, 140.5, Pub 100-04, 12, 50, Pub 100-04, 12, 90.4.5

Base Units

Global: XXX

Code	Base Units
01404	5

Modifiers (PAR)

Code	Mod 50	Mod 51	Mod 62	Mod 80
01404	9	9	9	9

CPT © 2018 American Medical Association. All Rights Reserved.

01420

01420 Anesthesia for all cast applications, removal, or repair involving knee joint

ICD-10-CM Diagnostic Codes

⇄	M66.261	Spontaneous rupture of extensor tendons, right lower leg
⇄	M66.262	Spontaneous rupture of extensor tendons, left lower leg
➐⇄	S76.111	Strain of right quadriceps muscle, fascia and tendon
➐⇄	S76.112	Strain of left quadriceps muscle, fascia and tendon
➐⇄	S82.011	Displaced osteochondral fracture of right patella
➐⇄	S82.012	Displaced osteochondral fracture of left patella
➐⇄	S82.014	Nondisplaced osteochondral fracture of right patella
➐⇄	S82.015	Nondisplaced osteochondral fracture of left patella
➐⇄	S82.021	Displaced longitudinal fracture of right patella
➐⇄	S82.022	Displaced longitudinal fracture of left patella
➐⇄	S82.024	Nondisplaced longitudinal fracture of right patella
➐⇄	S82.025	Nondisplaced longitudinal fracture of left patella
➐⇄	S82.031	Displaced transverse fracture of right patella
➐⇄	S82.032	Displaced transverse fracture of left patella
➐⇄	S82.034	Nondisplaced transverse fracture of right patella
➐⇄	S82.035	Nondisplaced transverse fracture of left patella
➐⇄	S82.041	Displaced comminuted fracture of right patella
➐⇄	S82.042	Displaced comminuted fracture of left patella
➐⇄	S82.044	Nondisplaced comminuted fracture of right patella
➐⇄	S82.045	Nondisplaced comminuted fracture of left patella
➐⇄	S82.091	Other fracture of right patella
➐⇄	S82.092	Other fracture of left patella
➐⇄	S83.011	Lateral subluxation of right patella
➐⇄	S83.012	Lateral subluxation of left patella
➐⇄	S83.014	Lateral dislocation of right patella
➐⇄	S83.015	Lateral dislocation of left patella
➐⇄	S83.091	Other subluxation of right patella
➐⇄	S83.092	Other subluxation of left patella
➐⇄	S83.094	Other dislocation of right patella
➐⇄	S83.095	Other dislocation of left patella
➐⇄	S83.61	Sprain of the superior tibiofibular joint and ligament, right knee
➐⇄	S83.62	Sprain of the superior tibiofibular joint and ligament, left knee
➐⇄	S83.8X1	Sprain of other specified parts of right knee
➐⇄	S83.8X2	Sprain of other specified parts of left knee
➐⇄	S89.021	Salter-Harris Type II physeal fracture of upper end of right tibia
➐⇄	S89.022	Salter-Harris Type II physeal fracture of upper end of left tibia
➐⇄	S89.031	Salter-Harris Type III physeal fracture of upper end of right tibia
➐⇄	S89.032	Salter-Harris Type III physeal fracture of upper end of left tibia
➐⇄	S89.041	Salter-Harris Type IV physeal fracture of upper end of right tibia
➐⇄	S89.042	Salter-Harris Type IV physeal fracture of upper end of left tibia
➐⇄	S89.091	Other physeal fracture of upper end of right tibia
➐⇄	S89.092	Other physeal fracture of upper end of left tibia

ICD-10-CM Coding Notes

For codes requiring a 7th character extension, refer to your ICD-10-CM book. Review the character descriptions and coding guidelines for proper selection. For some procedures, only certain characters will apply.

CCI Edits

Refer to Appendix A for CCI edits.

Pub 100

01420: Pub 100-04, 12, 140.5, Pub 100-04, 12, 50, Pub 100-04, 12, 90.4.5

Base Units

Global: XXX

Code	Base Units
01420	3

Modifiers (PAR)

Code	Mod 50	Mod 51	Mod 62	Mod 80
01420	9	9	9	9

CPT © 2018 American Medical Association. All Rights Reserved.

01430

01430 Anesthesia for procedures on veins of knee and popliteal area; not otherwise specified

ICD-10-CM Diagnostic Codes

⇄ I80.221 Phlebitis and thrombophlebitis of right popliteal vein
⇄ I80.222 Phlebitis and thrombophlebitis of left popliteal vein
⇄ I80.223 Phlebitis and thrombophlebitis of popliteal vein, bilateral
⇄ I80.291 Phlebitis and thrombophlebitis of other deep vessels of right lower extremity
⇄ I80.292 Phlebitis and thrombophlebitis of other deep vessels of left lower extremity
⇄ I80.293 Phlebitis and thrombophlebitis of other deep vessels of lower extremity, bilateral
⇄ I82.431 Acute embolism and thrombosis of right popliteal vein
⇄ I82.432 Acute embolism and thrombosis of left popliteal vein
⇄ I82.433 Acute embolism and thrombosis of popliteal vein, bilateral
⇄ I82.531 Chronic embolism and thrombosis of right popliteal vein
⇄ I82.532 Chronic embolism and thrombosis of left popliteal vein
⇄ I82.533 Chronic embolism and thrombosis of popliteal vein, bilateral
⇄ I82.591 Chronic embolism and thrombosis of other specified deep vein of right lower extremity
⇄ I82.592 Chronic embolism and thrombosis of other specified deep vein of left lower extremity
⇄ I82.593 Chronic embolism and thrombosis of other specified deep vein of lower extremity, bilateral
⇄ I83.012 Varicose veins of right lower extremity with ulcer of calf
⇄ I83.022 Varicose veins of left lower extremity with ulcer of calf
⇄ I83.11 Varicose veins of right lower extremity with inflammation
⇄ I83.12 Varicose veins of left lower extremity with inflammation
⇄ I83.212 Varicose veins of right lower extremity with both ulcer of calf and inflammation
⇄ I83.222 Varicose veins of left lower extremity with both ulcer of calf and inflammation
⇄ I83.811 Varicose veins of right lower extremity with pain
⇄ I83.812 Varicose veins of left lower extremity with pain
⇄ I83.813 Varicose veins of bilateral lower extremities with pain
⇄ I83.891 Varicose veins of right lower extremity with other complications
⇄ I83.892 Varicose veins of left lower extremity with other complications
⇄ I83.893 Varicose veins of bilateral lower extremities with other complications
⇄ I87.011 Postthrombotic syndrome with ulcer of right lower extremity
⇄ I87.012 Postthrombotic syndrome with ulcer of left lower extremity
⇄ I87.013 Postthrombotic syndrome with ulcer of bilateral lower extremity
⇄ I87.021 Postthrombotic syndrome with inflammation of right lower extremity
⇄ I87.022 Postthrombotic syndrome with inflammation of left lower extremity
⇄ I87.023 Postthrombotic syndrome with inflammation of bilateral lower extremity
⇄ I87.031 Postthrombotic syndrome with ulcer and inflammation of right lower extremity
⇄ I87.032 Postthrombotic syndrome with ulcer and inflammation of left lower extremity
⇄ I87.033 Postthrombotic syndrome with ulcer and inflammation of bilateral lower extremity
⇄ I87.091 Postthrombotic syndrome with other complications of right lower extremity
⇄ I87.092 Postthrombotic syndrome with other complications of left lower extremity
⇄ I87.093 Postthrombotic syndrome with other complications of bilateral lower extremity
I87.1 Compression of vein
I87.2 Venous insufficiency (chronic) (peripheral)
⇄ I87.311 Chronic venous hypertension (idiopathic) with ulcer of right lower extremity
⇄ I87.312 Chronic venous hypertension (idiopathic) with ulcer of left lower extremity
⇄ I87.313 Chronic venous hypertension (idiopathic) with ulcer of bilateral lower extremity
⇄ I87.321 Chronic venous hypertension (idiopathic) with inflammation of right lower extremity
⇄ I87.322 Chronic venous hypertension (idiopathic) with inflammation of left lower extremity
⇄ I87.323 Chronic venous hypertension (idiopathic) with inflammation of bilateral lower extremity
⇄ I87.331 Chronic venous hypertension (idiopathic) with ulcer and inflammation of right lower extremity
⇄ I87.332 Chronic venous hypertension (idiopathic) with ulcer and inflammation of left lower extremity
⇄ I87.333 Chronic venous hypertension (idiopathic) with ulcer and inflammation of bilateral lower extremity
➐⇄ S85.311 Laceration of greater saphenous vein at lower leg level, right leg
➐⇄ S85.312 Laceration of greater saphenous vein at lower leg level, left leg
➐⇄ S85.391 Other specified injury of greater saphenous vein at lower leg level, right leg
➐⇄ S85.392 Other specified injury of greater saphenous vein at lower leg level, left leg
➐⇄ S85.411 Laceration of lesser saphenous vein at lower leg level, right leg
➐⇄ S85.412 Laceration of lesser saphenous vein at lower leg level, left leg
➐⇄ S85.491 Other specified injury of lesser saphenous vein at lower leg level, right leg
➐⇄ S85.492 Other specified injury of lesser saphenous vein at lower leg level, left leg
➐⇄ S85.511 Laceration of popliteal vein, right leg
➐⇄ S85.512 Laceration of popliteal vein, left leg
➐⇄ S85.591 Other specified injury of popliteal vein, right leg
➐⇄ S85.592 Other specified injury of popliteal vein, left leg
➐⇄ S85.811 Laceration of other blood vessels at lower leg level, right leg
➐⇄ S85.812 Laceration of other blood vessels at lower leg level, left leg
➐⇄ S85.891 Other specified injury of other blood vessels at lower leg level, right leg
➐⇄ S85.892 Other specified injury of other blood vessels at lower leg level, left leg

ICD-10-CM Coding Notes

For codes requiring a 7th character extension, refer to your ICD-10-CM book. Review the character descriptions and coding guidelines for proper selection. For some procedures, only certain characters will apply.

CCI Edits

Refer to Appendix A for CCI edits.

Pub 100

01430: Pub 100-04, 12, 140.5, Pub 100-04, 12, 50, Pub 100-04, 12, 90.4.5

Base Units

Global: XXX

Code	Base Units
01430	3

Modifiers (PAR)

Code	Mod 50	Mod 51	Mod 62	Mod 80
01430	9	9	9	9

CPT © 2018 American Medical Association. All Rights Reserved.

01432

01432 Anesthesia for procedures on veins of knee and popliteal area; arteriovenous fistula

ICD-10-CM Diagnostic Codes

	I77.0	Arteriovenous fistula, acquired
	Q27.32	Arteriovenous malformation of vessel of lower limb
⑦⇄	S85.091	Other specified injury of popliteal artery, right leg
⑦⇄	S85.092	Other specified injury of popliteal artery, left leg
⑦⇄	S85.591	Other specified injury of popliteal vein, right leg
⑦⇄	S85.592	Other specified injury of popliteal vein, left leg

ICD-10-CM Coding Notes

For codes requiring a 7th character extension, refer to your ICD-10-CM book. Review the character descriptions and coding guidelines for proper selection. For some procedures, only certain characters will apply.

CCI Edits

Refer to Appendix A for CCI edits.

Pub 100

01432: Pub 100-04, 12, 140.5, Pub 100-04, 12, 50, Pub 100-04, 12, 90.4.5

Base Units

Global: XXX

Code	Base Units
01432	6

Modifiers (PAR)

Code	Mod 50	Mod 51	Mod 62	Mod 80
01432	9	9	9	9

CPT © 2018 American Medical Association. All Rights Reserved.

01440

01440 Anesthesia for procedures on arteries of knee and popliteal area; not otherwise specified

ICD-10-CM Diagnostic Codes

⇄ I70.211 Atherosclerosis of native arteries of extremities with intermittent claudication, right leg
⇄ I70.212 Atherosclerosis of native arteries of extremities with intermittent claudication, left leg
⇄ I70.213 Atherosclerosis of native arteries of extremities with intermittent claudication, bilateral legs
⇄ I70.221 Atherosclerosis of native arteries of extremities with rest pain, right leg
⇄ I70.222 Atherosclerosis of native arteries of extremities with rest pain, left leg
⇄ I70.223 Atherosclerosis of native arteries of extremities with rest pain, bilateral legs
⇄ I70.231 Atherosclerosis of native arteries of right leg with ulceration of thigh
⇄ I70.232 Atherosclerosis of native arteries of right leg with ulceration of calf
⇄ I70.233 Atherosclerosis of native arteries of right leg with ulceration of ankle
⇄ I70.234 Atherosclerosis of native arteries of right leg with ulceration of heel and midfoot
⇄ I70.235 Atherosclerosis of native arteries of right leg with ulceration of other part of foot
⇄ I70.238 Atherosclerosis of native arteries of right leg with ulceration of other part of lower right leg
⇄ I70.241 Atherosclerosis of native arteries of left leg with ulceration of thigh
⇄ I70.242 Atherosclerosis of native arteries of left leg with ulceration of calf
⇄ I70.243 Atherosclerosis of native arteries of left leg with ulceration of ankle
⇄ I70.244 Atherosclerosis of native arteries of left leg with ulceration of heel and midfoot
⇄ I70.245 Atherosclerosis of native arteries of left leg with ulceration of other part of foot
⇄ I70.248 Atherosclerosis of native arteries of left leg with ulceration of other part of lower left leg
⇄ I70.261 Atherosclerosis of native arteries of extremities with gangrene, right leg
⇄ I70.262 Atherosclerosis of native arteries of extremities with gangrene, left leg
⇄ I70.263 Atherosclerosis of native arteries of extremities with gangrene, bilateral legs
⇄ I70.291 Other atherosclerosis of native arteries of extremities, right leg
⇄ I70.292 Other atherosclerosis of native arteries of extremities, left leg
⇄ I70.293 Other atherosclerosis of native arteries of extremities, bilateral legs
I73.9 Peripheral vascular disease, unspecified
I74.3 Embolism and thrombosis of arteries of the lower extremities
⇄ I75.021 Atheroembolism of right lower extremity
⇄ I75.022 Atheroembolism of left lower extremity
⇄ I75.023 Atheroembolism of bilateral lower extremities
I77.0 Arteriovenous fistula, acquired
I77.1 Stricture of artery
I77.2 Rupture of artery
I77.5 Necrosis of artery
➐⇄ S85.011 Laceration of popliteal artery, right leg
➐⇄ S85.012 Laceration of popliteal artery, left leg
➐⇄ S85.091 Other specified injury of popliteal artery, right leg
➐⇄ S85.092 Other specified injury of popliteal artery, left leg
➐ T82.318 Breakdown (mechanical) of other vascular grafts
➐ T82.328 Displacement of other vascular grafts
➐ T82.338 Leakage of other vascular grafts
➐ T82.518 Breakdown (mechanical) of other cardiac and vascular devices and implants
➐ T82.528 Displacement of other cardiac and vascular devices and implants
➐ T82.538 Leakage of other cardiac and vascular devices and implants
➐ T82.598 Other mechanical complication of other cardiac and vascular devices and implants
➐ T82.7 Infection and inflammatory reaction due to other cardiac and vascular devices, implants and grafts
➐ T82.818 Embolism due to vascular prosthetic devices, implants and grafts
➐ T82.828 Fibrosis due to vascular prosthetic devices, implants and grafts
➐ T82.838 Hemorrhage due to vascular prosthetic devices, implants and grafts
➐ T82.848 Pain due to vascular prosthetic devices, implants and grafts
➐ T82.858 Stenosis of other vascular prosthetic devices, implants and grafts
➐ T82.868 Thrombosis due to vascular prosthetic devices, implants and grafts

ICD-10-CM Coding Notes

For codes requiring a 7th character extension, refer to your ICD-10-CM book. Review the character descriptions and coding guidelines for proper selection. For some procedures, only certain characters will apply.

CCI Edits

Refer to Appendix A for CCI edits.

Pub 100

01440: Pub 100-04, 12, 140.5, Pub 100-04, 12, 50, Pub 100-04, 12, 90.4.5

Base Units

Global: XXX

Code	Base Units
01440	8

Modifiers (PAR)

Code	Mod 50	Mod 51	Mod 62	Mod 80
01440	9	9	9	9

CPT © 2018 American Medical Association. All Rights Reserved.

01442

01442 Anesthesia for procedures on arteries of knee and popliteal area; popliteal thromboendarterectomy, with or without patch graft

ICD-10-CM Diagnostic Codes

⇄	I70.201	Unspecified atherosclerosis of native arteries of extremities, right leg
⇄	I70.202	Unspecified atherosclerosis of native arteries of extremities, left leg
⇄	I70.203	Unspecified atherosclerosis of native arteries of extremities, bilateral legs
⇄	I70.211	Atherosclerosis of native arteries of extremities with intermittent claudication, right leg
⇄	I70.212	Atherosclerosis of native arteries of extremities with intermittent claudication, left leg
⇄	I70.213	Atherosclerosis of native arteries of extremities with intermittent claudication, bilateral legs
⇄	I70.221	Atherosclerosis of native arteries of extremities with rest pain, right leg
⇄	I70.222	Atherosclerosis of native arteries of extremities with rest pain, left leg
⇄	I70.223	Atherosclerosis of native arteries of extremities with rest pain, bilateral legs
⇄	I70.231	Atherosclerosis of native arteries of right leg with ulceration of thigh
⇄	I70.232	Atherosclerosis of native arteries of right leg with ulceration of calf
⇄	I70.233	Atherosclerosis of native arteries of right leg with ulceration of ankle
⇄	I70.234	Atherosclerosis of native arteries of right leg with ulceration of heel and midfoot
⇄	I70.235	Atherosclerosis of native arteries of right leg with ulceration of other part of foot
⇄	I70.241	Atherosclerosis of native arteries of left leg with ulceration of thigh
⇄	I70.242	Atherosclerosis of native arteries of left leg with ulceration of calf
⇄	I70.243	Atherosclerosis of native arteries of left leg with ulceration of ankle
⇄	I70.244	Atherosclerosis of native arteries of left leg with ulceration of heel and midfoot
⇄	I70.245	Atherosclerosis of native arteries of left leg with ulceration of other part of foot
⇄	I70.261	Atherosclerosis of native arteries of extremities with gangrene, right leg
⇄	I70.262	Atherosclerosis of native arteries of extremities with gangrene, left leg
⇄	I70.263	Atherosclerosis of native arteries of extremities with gangrene, bilateral legs
⇄	I70.291	Other atherosclerosis of native arteries of extremities, right leg
⇄	I70.292	Other atherosclerosis of native arteries of extremities, left leg
⇄	I70.293	Other atherosclerosis of native arteries of extremities, bilateral legs
	I73.9	Peripheral vascular disease, unspecified
	I74.3	Embolism and thrombosis of arteries of the lower extremities
⇄	I75.021	Atheroembolism of right lower extremity
⇄	I75.022	Atheroembolism of left lower extremity
⇄	I75.023	Atheroembolism of bilateral lower extremities

CCI Edits

Refer to Appendix A for CCI edits.

Pub 100

01442: Pub 100-04, 12, 140.5, Pub 100-04, 12, 50, Pub 100-04, 12, 90.4.5

Base Units

Global: XXX

Code	Base Units
01442	8

Modifiers (PAR)

Code	Mod 50	Mod 51	Mod 62	Mod 80
01442	9	9	9	9

CPT © 2018 American Medical Association. All Rights Reserved.

01444

01444 Anesthesia for procedures on arteries of knee and popliteal area; popliteal excision and graft or repair for occlusion or aneurysm

AMA *CPT Assistant*

01444: Nov 07: 8, Jul 12: 13

ICD-10-CM Diagnostic Codes

⇄ I70.211 Atherosclerosis of native arteries of extremities with intermittent claudication, right leg
⇄ I70.212 Atherosclerosis of native arteries of extremities with intermittent claudication, left leg
⇄ I70.213 Atherosclerosis of native arteries of extremities with intermittent claudication, bilateral legs
⇄ I70.221 Atherosclerosis of native arteries of extremities with rest pain, right leg
⇄ I70.222 Atherosclerosis of native arteries of extremities with rest pain, left leg
⇄ I70.223 Atherosclerosis of native arteries of extremities with rest pain, bilateral legs
⇄ I70.231 Atherosclerosis of native arteries of right leg with ulceration of thigh
⇄ I70.232 Atherosclerosis of native arteries of right leg with ulceration of calf
⇄ I70.233 Atherosclerosis of native arteries of right leg with ulceration of ankle
⇄ I70.234 Atherosclerosis of native arteries of right leg with ulceration of heel and midfoot
⇄ I70.235 Atherosclerosis of native arteries of right leg with ulceration of other part of foot
⇄ I70.238 Atherosclerosis of native arteries of right leg with ulceration of other part of lower right leg
⇄ I70.241 Atherosclerosis of native arteries of left leg with ulceration of thigh
⇄ I70.242 Atherosclerosis of native arteries of left leg with ulceration of calf
⇄ I70.243 Atherosclerosis of native arteries of left leg with ulceration of ankle
⇄ I70.244 Atherosclerosis of native arteries of left leg with ulceration of heel and midfoot
⇄ I70.245 Atherosclerosis of native arteries of left leg with ulceration of other part of foot
⇄ I70.248 Atherosclerosis of native arteries of left leg with ulceration of other part of lower left leg
⇄ I70.261 Atherosclerosis of native arteries of extremities with gangrene, right leg
⇄ I70.262 Atherosclerosis of native arteries of extremities with gangrene, left leg
⇄ I70.263 Atherosclerosis of native arteries of extremities with gangrene, bilateral legs
⇄ I70.291 Other atherosclerosis of native arteries of extremities, right leg
⇄ I70.292 Other atherosclerosis of native arteries of extremities, left leg
⇄ I70.293 Other atherosclerosis of native arteries of extremities, bilateral legs
I72.4 Aneurysm of artery of lower extremity
I74.3 Embolism and thrombosis of arteries of the lower extremities
⇄ I75.021 Atheroembolism of right lower extremity
⇄ I75.022 Atheroembolism of left lower extremity
⇄ I75.023 Atheroembolism of bilateral lower extremities
I77.79 Dissection of other specified artery

CCI Edits

Refer to Appendix A for CCI edits.

Pub 100

01444: Pub 100-04, 12, 140.5, Pub 100-04, 12, 50, Pub 100-04, 12, 90.4.5

Base Units

Global: XXX

Code	Base Units
01444	8

Modifiers (PAR)

Code	Mod 50	Mod 51	Mod 62	Mod 80
01444	9	9	9	9

CPT © 2018 American Medical Association. All Rights Reserved.

01462

01462 Anesthesia for all closed procedures on lower leg, ankle, and foot

AMA *CPT Assistant* ☐

01462: Mar 06: 15, Nov 07: 8, Oct 11: 3, Jul 12: 13

ICD-10-CM Diagnostic Codes

➐⇄	S82.421	Displaced transverse fracture of shaft of right fibula
➐⇄	S82.422	Displaced transverse fracture of shaft of left fibula
➐⇄	S82.431	Displaced oblique fracture of shaft of right fibula
➐⇄	S82.432	Displaced oblique fracture of shaft of left fibula
➐⇄	S82.441	Displaced spiral fracture of shaft of right fibula
➐⇄	S82.442	Displaced spiral fracture of shaft of left fibula
➐⇄	S82.451	Displaced comminuted fracture of shaft of right fibula
➐⇄	S82.452	Displaced comminuted fracture of shaft of left fibula
➐⇄	S82.461	Displaced segmental fracture of shaft of right fibula
➐⇄	S82.462	Displaced segmental fracture of shaft of left fibula
➐⇄	S82.491	Other fracture of shaft of right fibula
➐⇄	S82.492	Other fracture of shaft of left fibula
➐⇄	S82.51	Displaced fracture of medial malleolus of right tibia
➐⇄	S82.52	Displaced fracture of medial malleolus of left tibia
➐⇄	S82.61	Displaced fracture of lateral malleolus of right fibula
➐⇄	S82.62	Displaced fracture of lateral malleolus of left fibula
➐⇄	S82.831	Other fracture of upper and lower end of right fibula
➐⇄	S82.832	Other fracture of upper and lower end of left fibula
➐⇄	S82.841	Displaced bimalleolar fracture of right lower leg
➐⇄	S82.842	Displaced bimalleolar fracture of left lower leg
➐⇄	S82.851	Displaced trimalleolar fracture of right lower leg
➐⇄	S82.852	Displaced trimalleolar fracture of left lower leg
➐⇄	S82.861	Displaced Maisonneuve's fracture of right leg
➐⇄	S82.862	Displaced Maisonneuve's fracture of left leg
➐⇄	S82.871	Displaced pilon fracture of right tibia
➐⇄	S82.872	Displaced pilon fracture of left tibia
➐⇄	S92.011	Displaced fracture of body of right calcaneus
➐⇄	S92.012	Displaced fracture of body of left calcaneus
➐⇄	S92.121	Displaced fracture of body of right talus
➐⇄	S92.122	Displaced fracture of body of left talus
➐⇄	S92.211	Displaced fracture of cuboid bone of right foot
➐⇄	S92.212	Displaced fracture of cuboid bone of left foot
➐⇄	S92.221	Displaced fracture of lateral cuneiform of right foot
➐⇄	S92.222	Displaced fracture of lateral cuneiform of left foot
➐⇄	S92.231	Displaced fracture of intermediate cuneiform of right foot
➐⇄	S92.232	Displaced fracture of intermediate cuneiform of left foot
➐⇄	S92.241	Displaced fracture of medial cuneiform of right foot
➐⇄	S92.242	Displaced fracture of medial cuneiform of left foot
➐⇄	S92.251	Displaced fracture of navicular [scaphoid] of right foot
➐⇄	S92.252	Displaced fracture of navicular [scaphoid] of left foot
➐⇄	S92.811	Other fracture of right foot
➐⇄	S92.812	Other fracture of left foot
➐⇄	S93.01	Subluxation of right ankle joint
➐⇄	S93.02	Subluxation of left ankle joint
➐⇄	S93.04	Dislocation of right ankle joint
➐⇄	S93.05	Dislocation of left ankle joint
➐⇄	S93.311	Subluxation of tarsal joint of right foot
➐⇄	S93.312	Subluxation of tarsal joint of left foot
➐⇄	S93.314	Dislocation of tarsal joint of right foot
➐⇄	S93.315	Dislocation of tarsal joint of left foot
➐⇄	S93.321	Subluxation of tarsometatarsal joint of right foot
➐⇄	S93.322	Subluxation of tarsometatarsal joint of left foot
➐⇄	S93.324	Dislocation of tarsometatarsal joint of right foot
➐⇄	S93.325	Dislocation of tarsometatarsal joint of left foot

ICD-10-CM Coding Notes

For codes requiring a 7th character extension, refer to your ICD-10-CM book. Review the character descriptions and coding guidelines for proper selection. For some procedures, only certain characters will apply.

CCI Edits

Refer to Appendix A for CCI edits.

Pub 100

01462: Pub 100-04, 12, 140.5, Pub 100-04, 12, 50, Pub 100-04, 12, 90.4.5

Base Units

Global: XXX

Code	Base Units
01462	3

Modifiers (PAR)

Code	Mod 50	Mod 51	Mod 62	Mod 80
01462	9	9	9	9

CPT © 2018 American Medical Association. All Rights Reserved.

01464

01464 Anesthesia for arthroscopic procedures of ankle and/or foot

ICD-10-CM Diagnostic Codes

⇄ M12.271 Villonodular synovitis (pigmented), right ankle and foot
⇄ M12.272 Villonodular synovitis (pigmented), left ankle and foot
⇄ M19.071 Primary osteoarthritis, right ankle and foot
⇄ M19.072 Primary osteoarthritis, left ankle and foot
⇄ M19.171 Post-traumatic osteoarthritis, right ankle and foot
⇄ M19.172 Post-traumatic osteoarthritis, left ankle and foot
⇄ M19.271 Secondary osteoarthritis, right ankle and foot
⇄ M19.272 Secondary osteoarthritis, left ankle and foot
⇄ M24.071 Loose body in right ankle
⇄ M24.072 Loose body in left ankle
⇄ M24.171 Other articular cartilage disorders, right ankle
⇄ M24.172 Other articular cartilage disorders, left ankle
⇄ M24.271 Disorder of ligament, right ankle
⇄ M24.272 Disorder of ligament, left ankle
⇄ M24.371 Pathological dislocation of right ankle, not elsewhere classified
⇄ M24.372 Pathological dislocation of left ankle, not elsewhere classified
⇄ M24.471 Recurrent dislocation, right ankle
⇄ M24.472 Recurrent dislocation, left ankle
⇄ M24.571 Contracture, right ankle
⇄ M24.572 Contracture, left ankle
⇄ M25.371 Other instability, right ankle
⇄ M25.372 Other instability, left ankle
⇄ M25.471 Effusion, right ankle
⇄ M25.472 Effusion, left ankle
⇄ M25.571 Pain in right ankle and joints of right foot
⇄ M25.572 Pain in left ankle and joints of left foot
⇄ M25.671 Stiffness of right ankle, not elsewhere classified
⇄ M25.672 Stiffness of left ankle, not elsewhere classified
⇄ M25.771 Osteophyte, right ankle
⇄ M25.772 Osteophyte, left ankle
⇄ M25.871 Other specified joint disorders, right ankle and foot
⇄ M25.872 Other specified joint disorders, left ankle and foot
⇄ M65.871 Other synovitis and tenosynovitis, right ankle and foot
⇄ M65.872 Other synovitis and tenosynovitis, left ankle and foot
M72.2 Plantar fascial fibromatosis
⇄ M77.51 Other enthesopathy of right foot
⇄ M92.61 Juvenile osteochondrosis of tarsus, right ankle
⇄ M92.62 Juvenile osteochondrosis of tarsus, left ankle
⇄ M92.71 Juvenile osteochondrosis of metatarsus, right foot
⇄ M92.72 Juvenile osteochondrosis of metatarsus, left foot
⇄ M93.271 Osteochondritis dissecans, right ankle and joints of right foot
⇄ M93.272 Osteochondritis dissecans, left ankle and joints of left foot
⇄ M93.871 Other specified osteochondropathies, right ankle and foot
⇄ M93.971 Osteochondropathy, unspecified, right ankle and foot
⇄ M93.972 Osteochondropathy, unspecified, left ankle and foot
⇄ M94.271 Chondromalacia, right ankle and joints of right foot
⇄ M94.272 Chondromalacia, left ankle and joints of left foot
M94.8X7 Other specified disorders of cartilage, ankle and foot
❼⇄ S82.871 Displaced pilon fracture of right tibia
❼⇄ S82.872 Displaced pilon fracture of left tibia
❼⇄ S82.874 Nondisplaced pilon fracture of right tibia
❼⇄ S82.875 Nondisplaced pilon fracture of left tibia
❼⇄ S92.141 Displaced dome fracture of right talus
❼⇄ S92.142 Displaced dome fracture of left talus
❼⇄ S92.144 Nondisplaced dome fracture of right talus
❼⇄ S92.145 Nondisplaced dome fracture of left talus

ICD-10-CM Coding Notes

For codes requiring a 7th character extension, refer to your ICD-10-CM book. Review the character descriptions and coding guidelines for proper selection. For some procedures, only certain characters will apply.

CCI Edits

Refer to Appendix A for CCI edits.

Pub 100

01464: Pub 100-04, 12, 140.5, Pub 100-04, 12, 50, Pub 100-04, 12, 90.4.5

Base Units

Global: XXX

Code	Base Units
01464	3

Modifiers (PAR)

Code	Mod 50	Mod 51	Mod 62	Mod 80
01464	9	9	9	9

CPT © 2018 American Medical Association. All Rights Reserved.

01470

01470 Anesthesia for procedures on nerves, muscles, tendons, and fascia of lower leg, ankle, and foot; not otherwise specified

ICD-10-CM Diagnostic Codes

	E08.621	Diabetes mellitus due to underlying condition with foot ulcer
	E08.622	Diabetes mellitus due to underlying condition with other skin ulcer
	E09.621	Drug or chemical induced diabetes mellitus with foot ulcer
	E09.622	Drug or chemical induced diabetes mellitus with other skin ulcer
	E10.621	Type 1 diabetes mellitus with foot ulcer
	E10.622	Type 1 diabetes mellitus with other skin ulcer
	E11.621	Type 2 diabetes mellitus with foot ulcer
	E11.622	Type 2 diabetes mellitus with other skin ulcer
	E13.621	Other specified diabetes mellitus with foot ulcer
	E13.622	Other specified diabetes mellitus with other skin ulcer
⇄	G57.51	Tarsal tunnel syndrome, right lower limb
⇄	G57.52	Tarsal tunnel syndrome, left lower limb
⇄	G57.61	Lesion of plantar nerve, right lower limb
⇄	G57.62	Lesion of plantar nerve, left lower limb
	I73.9	Peripheral vascular disease, unspecified
⇄	L89.513	Pressure ulcer of right ankle, stage 3
⇄	L89.514	Pressure ulcer of right ankle, stage 4
⇄	L89.523	Pressure ulcer of left ankle, stage 3
⇄	L89.524	Pressure ulcer of left ankle, stage 4
⇄	L89.613	Pressure ulcer of right heel, stage 3
⇄	L89.614	Pressure ulcer of right heel, stage 4
⇄	L89.623	Pressure ulcer of left heel, stage 3
⇄	L89.624	Pressure ulcer of left heel, stage 4
⇄	L97.213	Non-pressure chronic ulcer of right calf with necrosis of muscle
⇄	L97.223	Non-pressure chronic ulcer of left calf with necrosis of muscle
⇄	L97.313	Non-pressure chronic ulcer of right ankle with necrosis of muscle
⇄	L97.323	Non-pressure chronic ulcer of left ankle with necrosis of muscle
⇄	L97.413	Non-pressure chronic ulcer of right heel and midfoot with necrosis of muscle
⇄	L97.423	Non-pressure chronic ulcer of left heel and midfoot with necrosis of muscle
⇄	L97.513	Non-pressure chronic ulcer of other part of right foot with necrosis of muscle
⇄	L97.523	Non-pressure chronic ulcer of other part of left foot with necrosis of muscle
⇄	M65.861	Other synovitis and tenosynovitis, right lower leg
⇄	M65.862	Other synovitis and tenosynovitis, left lower leg
⇄	M65.871	Other synovitis and tenosynovitis, right ankle and foot
⇄	M65.872	Other synovitis and tenosynovitis, left ankle and foot
⇄	M67.471	Ganglion, right ankle and foot
⇄	M67.472	Ganglion, left ankle and foot
	M72.2	Plantar fascial fibromatosis
➐⇄	S84.01	Injury of tibial nerve at lower leg level, right leg
➐⇄	S84.02	Injury of tibial nerve at lower leg level, left leg
➐⇄	S84.21	Injury of cutaneous sensory nerve at lower leg level, right leg
➐⇄	S84.22	Injury of cutaneous sensory nerve at lower leg level, left leg
➐⇄	S86.121	Laceration of other muscle(s) and tendon(s) of posterior muscle group at lower leg level, right leg
➐⇄	S86.122	Laceration of other muscle(s) and tendon(s) of posterior muscle group at lower leg level, left leg
➐⇄	S86.221	Laceration of muscle(s) and tendon(s) of anterior muscle group at lower leg level, right leg
➐⇄	S86.222	Laceration of muscle(s) and tendon(s) of anterior muscle group at lower leg level, left leg
➐⇄	S86.321	Laceration of muscle(s) and tendon(s) of peroneal muscle group at lower leg level, right leg
➐⇄	S86.322	Laceration of muscle(s) and tendon(s) of peroneal muscle group at lower leg level, left leg
➐⇄	S86.821	Laceration of other muscle(s) and tendon(s) at lower leg level, right leg
➐⇄	S86.822	Laceration of other muscle(s) and tendon(s) at lower leg level, left leg
➐⇄	S94.21	Injury of deep peroneal nerve at ankle and foot level, right leg
➐⇄	S94.22	Injury of deep peroneal nerve at ankle and foot level, left leg
➐⇄	S94.31	Injury of cutaneous sensory nerve at ankle and foot level, right leg
➐⇄	S94.32	Injury of cutaneous sensory nerve at ankle and foot level, left leg
➐⇄	S94.8X1	Injury of other nerves at ankle and foot level, right leg
➐⇄	S94.8X2	Injury of other nerves at ankle and foot level, left leg

ICD-10-CM Coding Notes

For codes requiring a 7th character extension, refer to your ICD-10-CM book. Review the character descriptions and coding guidelines for proper selection. For some procedures, only certain characters will apply.

CCI Edits

Refer to Appendix A for CCI edits.

Pub 100

01470: Pub 100-04, 12, 140.5, Pub 100-04, 12, 50, Pub 100-04, 12, 90.4.5

Base Units

Global: XXX

Code	Base Units
01470	3

Modifiers (PAR)

Code	Mod 50	Mod 51	Mod 62	Mod 80
01470	9	9	9	9

CPT® Procedural Coding

CPT © 2018 American Medical Association. All Rights Reserved.

01472

01472 Anesthesia for procedures on nerves, muscles, tendons, and fascia of lower leg, ankle, and foot; repair of ruptured Achilles tendon, with or without graft

ICD-10-CM Diagnostic Codes

⇄	M66.361	Spontaneous rupture of flexor tendons, right lower leg
⇄	M66.362	Spontaneous rupture of flexor tendons, left lower leg
⇄	M66.861	Spontaneous rupture of other tendons, right lower leg
⇄	M66.862	Spontaneous rupture of other tendons, left lower leg
❼⇄	S86.011	Strain of right Achilles tendon
❼⇄	S86.012	Strain of left Achilles tendon
❼⇄	S86.021	Laceration of right Achilles tendon
❼⇄	S86.022	Laceration of left Achilles tendon

ICD-10-CM Coding Notes

For codes requiring a 7th character extension, refer to your ICD-10-CM book. Review the character descriptions and coding guidelines for proper selection. For some procedures, only certain characters will apply.

CCI Edits

Refer to Appendix A for CCI edits.

Pub 100

01472: Pub 100-04, 12, 140.5, Pub 100-04, 12, 50, Pub 100-04, 12, 90.4.5

Base Units

Global: XXX

Code	Base Units
01472	5

Modifiers (PAR)

Code	Mod 50	Mod 51	Mod 62	Mod 80
01472	9	9	9	9

CPT © 2018 American Medical Association. All Rights Reserved.

01474

01474 Anesthesia for procedures on nerves, muscles, tendons, and fascia of lower leg, ankle, and foot; gastrocnemius recession (eg, Strayer procedure)

ICD-10-CM Diagnostic Codes

	G80.0	Spastic quadriplegic cerebral palsy
	G80.1	Spastic diplegic cerebral palsy
	G80.2	Spastic hemiplegic cerebral palsy
	G80.8	Other cerebral palsy
⇄	M21.6X1	Other acquired deformities of right foot
⇄	M21.6X2	Other acquired deformities of left foot
⇄	M62.461	Contracture of muscle, right lower leg
⇄	M62.462	Contracture of muscle, left lower leg

CCI Edits

Refer to Appendix A for CCI edits.

Pub 100

01474: Pub 100-04, 12, 140.5, Pub 100-04, 12, 50, Pub 100-04, 12, 90.4.5

Base Units

Global: XXX

Code	Base Units
01474	5

Modifiers (PAR)

Code	Mod 50	Mod 51	Mod 62	Mod 80
01474	9	9	9	9

CPT © 2018 American Medical Association. All Rights Reserved.

01480

01480 Anesthesia for open procedures on bones of lower leg, ankle, and foot; not otherwise specified

ICD-10-CM Diagnostic Codes

⇄ L97.116 Non-pressure chronic ulcer of right thigh with bone involvement without evidence of necrosis
⇄ L97.126 Non-pressure chronic ulcer of left thigh with bone involvement without evidence of necrosis
⇄ L97.216 Non-pressure chronic ulcer of right calf with bone involvement without evidence of necrosis
⇄ L97.226 Non-pressure chronic ulcer of left calf with bone involvement without evidence of necrosis
⇄ L97.316 Non-pressure chronic ulcer of right ankle with bone involvement without evidence of necrosis
⇄ L97.326 Non-pressure chronic ulcer of left ankle with bone involvement without evidence of necrosis
⇄ L97.416 Non-pressure chronic ulcer of right heel and midfoot with bone involvement without evidence of necrosis
⇄ L97.426 Non-pressure chronic ulcer of left heel and midfoot with bone involvement without evidence of necrosis
⇄ L97.516 Non-pressure chronic ulcer of other part of right foot with bone involvement without evidence of necrosis
⇄ L97.526 Non-pressure chronic ulcer of other part of left foot with bone involvement without evidence of necrosis
⇄ L97.816 Non-pressure chronic ulcer of other part of right lower leg with bone involvement without evidence of necrosis
⇄ L97.826 Non-pressure chronic ulcer of other part of left lower leg with bone involvement without evidence of necrosis
⇄ M20.11 Hallux valgus (acquired), right foot
⇄ M20.12 Hallux valgus (acquired), left foot
⇄ M20.21 Hallux rigidus, right foot
⇄ M20.22 Hallux rigidus, left foot
⇄ M20.41 Other hammer toe(s) (acquired), right foot
⇄ M20.42 Other hammer toe(s) (acquired), left foot
⇄ M20.5X1 Other deformities of toe(s) (acquired), right foot
⇄ M20.5X2 Other deformities of toe(s) (acquired), left foot
⇄ M21.611 Bunion of right foot
⇄ M21.612 Bunion of left foot
⇄ M21.621 Bunionette of right foot
⇄ M21.622 Bunionette of left foot
Q66.0 Congenital talipes equinovarus
Q66.1 Congenital talipes calcaneovarus
Q66.21 Congenital metatarsus primus varus
Q66.3 Other congenital varus deformities of feet
Q66.4 Congenital talipes calcaneovalgus
⑦⇄ S82.221 Displaced transverse fracture of shaft of right tibia
⑦⇄ S82.222 Displaced transverse fracture of shaft of left tibia
⑦⇄ S82.231 Displaced oblique fracture of shaft of right tibia
⑦⇄ S82.232 Displaced oblique fracture of shaft of left tibia
⑦⇄ S82.241 Displaced spiral fracture of shaft of right tibia
⑦⇄ S82.242 Displaced spiral fracture of shaft of left tibia
⑦⇄ S82.251 Displaced comminuted fracture of shaft of right tibia
⑦⇄ S82.252 Displaced comminuted fracture of shaft of left tibia
⑦⇄ S82.261 Displaced segmental fracture of shaft of right tibia
⑦⇄ S82.262 Displaced segmental fracture of shaft of left tibia
⑦⇄ S82.391 Other fracture of lower end of right tibia
⑦⇄ S82.392 Other fracture of lower end of left tibia
⑦⇄ S82.451 Displaced comminuted fracture of shaft of right fibula
⑦⇄ S82.452 Displaced comminuted fracture of shaft of left fibula
⑦⇄ S82.51 Displaced fracture of medial malleolus of right tibia
⑦⇄ S82.52 Displaced fracture of medial malleolus of left tibia
⑦⇄ S82.61 Displaced fracture of lateral malleolus of right fibula
⑦⇄ S82.62 Displaced fracture of lateral malleolus of left fibula
⑦⇄ S82.831 Other fracture of upper and lower end of right fibula
⑦⇄ S82.832 Other fracture of upper and lower end of left fibula
⑦⇄ S82.841 Displaced bimalleolar fracture of right lower leg
⑦⇄ S82.842 Displaced bimalleolar fracture of left lower leg
⑦⇄ S82.851 Displaced trimalleolar fracture of right lower leg
⑦⇄ S82.852 Displaced trimalleolar fracture of left lower leg
⑦⇄ S82.861 Displaced Maisonneuve's fracture of right leg
⑦⇄ S82.862 Displaced Maisonneuve's fracture of left leg
⑦⇄ S92.011 Displaced fracture of body of right calcaneus
⑦⇄ S92.012 Displaced fracture of body of left calcaneus
⑦⇄ S92.051 Displaced other extraarticular fracture of right calcaneus
⑦⇄ S92.052 Displaced other extraarticular fracture of left calcaneus
⑦⇄ S92.061 Displaced intraarticular fracture of right calcaneus
⑦⇄ S92.062 Displaced intraarticular fracture of left calcaneus
⑦⇄ S92.111 Displaced fracture of neck of right talus
⑦⇄ S92.112 Displaced fracture of neck of left talus
⑦⇄ S92.121 Displaced fracture of body of right talus
⑦⇄ S92.122 Displaced fracture of body of left talus
⑦⇄ S92.141 Displaced dome fracture of right talus
⑦⇄ S92.142 Displaced dome fracture of left talus
⑦⇄ S92.251 Displaced fracture of navicular [scaphoid] of right foot
⑦⇄ S92.252 Displaced fracture of navicular [scaphoid] of left foot
⑦⇄ S92.811 Other fracture of right foot
⑦⇄ S92.812 Other fracture of left foot
⑦⇄ S99.031 Salter-Harris Type III physeal fracture of right calcaneus
⑦⇄ S99.032 Salter-Harris Type III physeal fracture of left calcaneus
⑦⇄ S99.041 Salter-Harris Type IV physeal fracture of right calcaneus
⑦⇄ S99.042 Salter-Harris Type IV physeal fracture of left calcaneus
S99.13 Salter-Harris Type III physeal fracture of metatarsal
⑦⇄ S99.131 Salter-Harris Type III physeal fracture of right metatarsal
⑦⇄ S99.132 Salter-Harris Type III physeal fracture of left metatarsal
⑦⇄ S99.141 Salter-Harris Type IV physeal fracture of right metatarsal
⑦⇄ S99.142 Salter-Harris Type IV physeal fracture of left metatarsal
⑦⇄ S99.221 Salter-Harris Type II physeal fracture of phalanx of right toe
⑦⇄ S99.222 Salter-Harris Type II physeal fracture of phalanx of left toe
⑦⇄ S99.231 Salter-Harris Type III physeal fracture of phalanx of right toe
⑦⇄ S99.232 Salter-Harris Type III physeal fracture of phalanx of left toe
⑦⇄ S99.241 Salter-Harris Type IV physeal fracture of phalanx of right toe
⑦⇄ S99.242 Salter-Harris Type IV physeal fracture of phalanx of left toe

ICD-10-CM Coding Notes

For codes requiring a 7th character extension, refer to your ICD-10-CM book. Review the character descriptions and coding guidelines for proper selection. For some procedures, only certain characters will apply.

CCI Edits

Refer to Appendix A for CCI edits.

Pub 100

01480: Pub 100-04, 12, 140.5, Pub 100-04, 12, 50, Pub 100-04, 12, 90.4.5

CPT © 2018 American Medical Association. All Rights Reserved.

Base Units

Global: XXX

Code	Base Units
01480	3

Modifiers (PAR)

Code	Mod 50	Mod 51	Mod 62	Mod 80
01480	9	9	9	9

CPT © 2018 American Medical Association. All Rights Reserved.

01482

01482 Anesthesia for open procedures on bones of lower leg, ankle, and foot; radical resection (including below knee amputation)

ICD-10-CM Diagnostic Codes

⇄ C40.21 Malignant neoplasm of long bones of right lower limb
⇄ C40.22 Malignant neoplasm of long bones of left lower limb
⇄ C47.21 Malignant neoplasm of peripheral nerves of right lower limb, including hip
⇄ C47.22 Malignant neoplasm of peripheral nerves of left lower limb, including hip
⇄ C49.21 Malignant neoplasm of connective and soft tissue of right lower limb, including hip
⇄ C49.22 Malignant neoplasm of connective and soft tissue of left lower limb, including hip
E10.51 Type 1 diabetes mellitus with diabetic peripheral angiopathy without gangrene
E10.52 Type 1 diabetes mellitus with diabetic peripheral angiopathy with gangrene
E10.59 Type 1 diabetes mellitus with other circulatory complications
E11.51 Type 2 diabetes mellitus with diabetic peripheral angiopathy without gangrene
E11.52 Type 2 diabetes mellitus with diabetic peripheral angiopathy with gangrene
E11.59 Type 2 diabetes mellitus with other circulatory complications
⇄ I70.231 Atherosclerosis of native arteries of right leg with ulceration of thigh
⇄ I70.232 Atherosclerosis of native arteries of right leg with ulceration of calf
⇄ I70.233 Atherosclerosis of native arteries of right leg with ulceration of ankle
⇄ I70.234 Atherosclerosis of native arteries of right leg with ulceration of heel and midfoot
⇄ I70.235 Atherosclerosis of native arteries of right leg with ulceration of other part of foot
⇄ I70.238 Atherosclerosis of native arteries of right leg with ulceration of other part of lower right leg
⇄ I70.242 Atherosclerosis of native arteries of left leg with ulceration of calf
⇄ I70.243 Atherosclerosis of native arteries of left leg with ulceration of ankle
⇄ I70.244 Atherosclerosis of native arteries of left leg with ulceration of heel and midfoot
⇄ I70.245 Atherosclerosis of native arteries of left leg with ulceration of other part of foot
⇄ I70.248 Atherosclerosis of native arteries of left leg with ulceration of other part of lower left leg
⇄ I70.261 Atherosclerosis of native arteries of extremities with gangrene, right leg
⇄ I70.262 Atherosclerosis of native arteries of extremities with gangrene, left leg
⇄ I70.263 Atherosclerosis of native arteries of extremities with gangrene, bilateral legs
I73.9 Peripheral vascular disease, unspecified
⇄ L97.213 Non-pressure chronic ulcer of right calf with necrosis of muscle
⇄ L97.214 Non-pressure chronic ulcer of right calf with necrosis of bone
⇄ L97.223 Non-pressure chronic ulcer of left calf with necrosis of muscle
⇄ L97.224 Non-pressure chronic ulcer of left calf with necrosis of bone
⇄ L97.313 Non-pressure chronic ulcer of right ankle with necrosis of muscle
⇄ L97.314 Non-pressure chronic ulcer of right ankle with necrosis of bone
⇄ L97.323 Non-pressure chronic ulcer of left ankle with necrosis of muscle
⇄ L97.324 Non-pressure chronic ulcer of left ankle with necrosis of bone
⇄ L97.413 Non-pressure chronic ulcer of right heel and midfoot with necrosis of muscle
⇄ L97.414 Non-pressure chronic ulcer of right heel and midfoot with necrosis of bone
⇄ L97.423 Non-pressure chronic ulcer of left heel and midfoot with necrosis of muscle
⇄ L97.424 Non-pressure chronic ulcer of left heel and midfoot with necrosis of bone
⇄ L97.513 Non-pressure chronic ulcer of other part of right foot with necrosis of muscle
⇄ L97.514 Non-pressure chronic ulcer of other part of right foot with necrosis of bone
⇄ L97.523 Non-pressure chronic ulcer of other part of left foot with necrosis of muscle
⇄ L97.524 Non-pressure chronic ulcer of other part of left foot with necrosis of bone
➐⇄ S87.81 Crushing injury of right lower leg
➐⇄ S87.82 Crushing injury of left lower leg
➐⇄ S88.111 Complete traumatic amputation at level between knee and ankle, right lower leg
➐⇄ S88.112 Complete traumatic amputation at level between knee and ankle, left lower leg
➐⇄ S88.121 Partial traumatic amputation at level between knee and ankle, right lower leg
➐⇄ S88.122 Partial traumatic amputation at level between knee and ankle, left lower leg
➐⇄ S97.01 Crushing injury of right ankle
➐⇄ S97.02 Crushing injury of left ankle
➐⇄ S97.81 Crushing injury of right foot
➐⇄ S97.82 Crushing injury of left foot
➐⇄ S98.011 Complete traumatic amputation of right foot at ankle level
➐⇄ S98.012 Complete traumatic amputation of left foot at ankle level
➐⇄ S98.021 Partial traumatic amputation of right foot at ankle level
➐⇄ S98.022 Partial traumatic amputation of left foot at ankle level
➐⇄ S98.311 Complete traumatic amputation of right midfoot
➐⇄ S98.312 Complete traumatic amputation of left midfoot
➐⇄ S98.321 Partial traumatic amputation of right midfoot
➐⇄ S98.322 Partial traumatic amputation of left midfoot

ICD-10-CM Coding Notes

For codes requiring a 7th character extension, refer to your ICD-10-CM book. Review the character descriptions and coding guidelines for proper selection. For some procedures, only certain characters will apply.

CCI Edits

Refer to Appendix A for CCI edits.

Pub 100

01482: Pub 100-04, 12, 140.5, Pub 100-04, 12, 50, Pub 100-04, 12, 90.4.5

Base Units

Global: XXX

Code	Base Units
01482	4

Modifiers (PAR)

Code	Mod 50	Mod 51	Mod 62	Mod 80
01482	9	9	9	9

CPT © 2018 American Medical Association. All Rights Reserved.

01484

01484 Anesthesia for open procedures on bones of lower leg, ankle, and foot; osteotomy or osteoplasty of tibia and/or fibula

ICD-10-CM Diagnostic Codes

⇄	M19.071	Primary osteoarthritis, right ankle and foot
⇄	M19.072	Primary osteoarthritis, left ankle and foot
⇄	M19.171	Post-traumatic osteoarthritis, right ankle and foot
⇄	M19.172	Post-traumatic osteoarthritis, left ankle and foot
⇄	M19.271	Secondary osteoarthritis, right ankle and foot
⇄	M19.272	Secondary osteoarthritis, left ankle and foot
⇄	M21.761	Unequal limb length (acquired), right tibia
⇄	M21.762	Unequal limb length (acquired), left tibia
⇄	M21.763	Unequal limb length (acquired), right fibula
⇄	M21.764	Unequal limb length (acquired), left fibula
⇄	Q72.51	Longitudinal reduction defect of right tibia
⇄	Q72.52	Longitudinal reduction defect of left tibia
⇄	Q72.53	Longitudinal reduction defect of tibia, bilateral
⇄	Q72.61	Longitudinal reduction defect of right fibula
⇄	Q72.62	Longitudinal reduction defect of left fibula
⇄	Q72.63	Longitudinal reduction defect of fibula, bilateral

CCI Edits

Refer to Appendix A for CCI edits.

Pub 100

01484: Pub 100-04, 12, 140.5, Pub 100-04, 12, 50, Pub 100-04, 12, 90.4.5

Base Units

Global: XXX

Code	Base Units
01484	4

Modifiers (PAR)

Code	Mod 50	Mod 51	Mod 62	Mod 80
01484	9	9	9	9

CPT © 2018 American Medical Association. All Rights Reserved.

01486

01486 Anesthesia for open procedures on bones of lower leg, ankle, and foot; total ankle replacement

ICD-10-CM Diagnostic Codes

	Code	Description
⇄	M19.071	Primary osteoarthritis, right ankle and foot
⇄	M19.072	Primary osteoarthritis, left ankle and foot
⇄	M19.171	Post-traumatic osteoarthritis, right ankle and foot
⇄	M19.172	Post-traumatic osteoarthritis, left ankle and foot
⇄	M19.271	Secondary osteoarthritis, right ankle and foot
⇄	M19.272	Secondary osteoarthritis, left ankle and foot

CCI Edits

Refer to Appendix A for CCI edits.

Pub 100

01486: Pub 100-04, 12, 140.5, Pub 100-04, 12, 50, Pub 100-04, 12, 90.4.5

Base Units

Global: XXX

Code	Base Units
01486	7

Modifiers (PAR)

Code	Mod 50	Mod 51	Mod 62	Mod 80
01486	9	9	9	9

CPT © 2018 American Medical Association. All Rights Reserved.

01490

01490 Anesthesia for lower leg cast application, removal, or repair

ICD-10-CM Diagnostic Codes

⇄ M66.271 Spontaneous rupture of extensor tendons, right ankle and foot
⇄ M66.272 Spontaneous rupture of extensor tendons, left ankle and foot
⇄ M66.371 Spontaneous rupture of flexor tendons, right ankle and foot
⇄ M66.372 Spontaneous rupture of flexor tendons, left ankle and foot
⇄ M66.871 Spontaneous rupture of other tendons, right ankle and foot
⇄ M66.872 Spontaneous rupture of other tendons, left ankle and foot
Q66.0 Congenital talipes equinovarus
Q66.7 Congenital pes cavus
❼⇄ S82.311 Torus fracture of lower end of right tibia
❼⇄ S82.312 Torus fracture of lower end of left tibia
❼⇄ S82.391 Other fracture of lower end of right tibia
❼⇄ S82.392 Other fracture of lower end of left tibia
❼⇄ S82.54 Nondisplaced fracture of medial malleolus of right tibia
❼⇄ S82.55 Nondisplaced fracture of medial malleolus of left tibia
❼⇄ S82.64 Nondisplaced fracture of lateral malleolus of right fibula
❼⇄ S82.65 Nondisplaced fracture of lateral malleolus of left fibula
❼⇄ S82.821 Torus fracture of lower end of right fibula
❼⇄ S82.822 Torus fracture of lower end of left fibula
❼⇄ S82.844 Nondisplaced bimalleolar fracture of right lower leg
❼⇄ S82.845 Nondisplaced bimalleolar fracture of left lower leg
❼⇄ S82.854 Nondisplaced trimalleolar fracture of right lower leg
❼⇄ S82.855 Nondisplaced trimalleolar fracture of left lower leg
❼⇄ S82.891 Other fracture of right lower leg
❼⇄ S82.892 Other fracture of left lower leg
❼⇄ S86.021 Laceration of right Achilles tendon
❼⇄ S86.022 Laceration of left Achilles tendon
❼⇄ S86.121 Laceration of other muscle(s) and tendon(s) of posterior muscle group at lower leg level, right leg
❼⇄ S86.122 Laceration of other muscle(s) and tendon(s) of posterior muscle group at lower leg level, left leg
❼⇄ S86.221 Laceration of muscle(s) and tendon(s) of anterior muscle group at lower leg level, right leg
❼⇄ S86.222 Laceration of muscle(s) and tendon(s) of anterior muscle group at lower leg level, left leg
❼⇄ S86.321 Laceration of muscle(s) and tendon(s) of peroneal muscle group at lower leg level, right leg
❼⇄ S86.322 Laceration of muscle(s) and tendon(s) of peroneal muscle group at lower leg level, left leg

ICD-10-CM Coding Notes

For codes requiring a 7th character extension, refer to your ICD-10-CM book. Review the character descriptions and coding guidelines for proper selection. For some procedures, only certain characters will apply.

CCI Edits

Refer to Appendix A for CCI edits.

Pub 100

01490: Pub 100-04, 12, 140.5, Pub 100-04, 12, 50, Pub 100-04, 12, 90.4.5

Base Units

Global: XXX

Code	Base Units
01490	3

Modifiers (PAR)

Code	Mod 50	Mod 51	Mod 62	Mod 80
01490	9	9	9	9

CPT © 2018 American Medical Association. All Rights Reserved.

01500

01500 Anesthesia for procedures on arteries of lower leg, including bypass graft; not otherwise specified

ICD-10-CM Diagnostic Codes

	Code	Description
	E10.51	Type 1 diabetes mellitus with diabetic peripheral angiopathy without gangrene
	E10.52	Type 1 diabetes mellitus with diabetic peripheral angiopathy with gangrene
	E10.59	Type 1 diabetes mellitus with other circulatory complications
	E11.51	Type 2 diabetes mellitus with diabetic peripheral angiopathy without gangrene
	E11.52	Type 2 diabetes mellitus with diabetic peripheral angiopathy with gangrene
	E11.59	Type 2 diabetes mellitus with other circulatory complications
⇄	I70.211	Atherosclerosis of native arteries of extremities with intermittent claudication, right leg
⇄	I70.212	Atherosclerosis of native arteries of extremities with intermittent claudication, left leg
⇄	I70.213	Atherosclerosis of native arteries of extremities with intermittent claudication, bilateral legs
⇄	I70.221	Atherosclerosis of native arteries of extremities with rest pain, right leg
⇄	I70.222	Atherosclerosis of native arteries of extremities with rest pain, left leg
⇄	I70.223	Atherosclerosis of native arteries of extremities with rest pain, bilateral legs
⇄	I70.231	Atherosclerosis of native arteries of right leg with ulceration of thigh
⇄	I70.232	Atherosclerosis of native arteries of right leg with ulceration of calf
⇄	I70.233	Atherosclerosis of native arteries of right leg with ulceration of ankle
⇄	I70.234	Atherosclerosis of native arteries of right leg with ulceration of heel and midfoot
⇄	I70.235	Atherosclerosis of native arteries of right leg with ulceration of other part of foot
⇄	I70.238	Atherosclerosis of native arteries of right leg with ulceration of other part of lower right leg
⇄	I70.241	Atherosclerosis of native arteries of left leg with ulceration of thigh
⇄	I70.242	Atherosclerosis of native arteries of left leg with ulceration of calf
⇄	I70.243	Atherosclerosis of native arteries of left leg with ulceration of ankle
⇄	I70.244	Atherosclerosis of native arteries of left leg with ulceration of heel and midfoot
⇄	I70.245	Atherosclerosis of native arteries of left leg with ulceration of other part of foot
⇄	I70.248	Atherosclerosis of native arteries of left leg with ulceration of other part of lower left leg
⇄	I70.261	Atherosclerosis of native arteries of extremities with gangrene, right leg
⇄	I70.262	Atherosclerosis of native arteries of extremities with gangrene, left leg
⇄	I70.263	Atherosclerosis of native arteries of extremities with gangrene, bilateral legs
⇄	I70.291	Other atherosclerosis of native arteries of extremities, right leg
⇄	I70.292	Other atherosclerosis of native arteries of extremities, left leg
⇄	I70.293	Other atherosclerosis of native arteries of extremities, bilateral legs
	I72.4	Aneurysm of artery of lower extremity
	I73.9	Peripheral vascular disease, unspecified
	I77.79	Dissection of other specified artery
➐⇄	S85.011	Laceration of popliteal artery, right leg
➐⇄	S85.012	Laceration of popliteal artery, left leg
➐⇄	S85.141	Laceration of anterior tibial artery, right leg
➐⇄	S85.142	Laceration of anterior tibial artery, left leg
➐⇄	S85.171	Laceration of posterior tibial artery, right leg
➐⇄	S85.172	Laceration of posterior tibial artery, left leg
➐⇄	S85.211	Laceration of peroneal artery, right leg
➐⇄	S85.212	Laceration of peroneal artery, left leg

ICD-10-CM Coding Notes

For codes requiring a 7th character extension, refer to your ICD-10-CM book. Review the character descriptions and coding guidelines for proper selection. For some procedures, only certain characters will apply.

CCI Edits

Refer to Appendix A for CCI edits.

Pub 100

01500: Pub 100-04, 12, 140.5, Pub 100-04, 12, 50, Pub 100-04, 12, 90.4.5

Base Units

Global: XXX

Code	Base Units
01500	8

Modifiers (PAR)

Code	Mod 50	Mod 51	Mod 62	Mod 80
01500	9	9	9	9

CPT © 2018 American Medical Association. All Rights Reserved.

01502

01502 Anesthesia for procedures on arteries of lower leg, including bypass graft; embolectomy, direct or with catheter

ICD-10-CM Diagnostic Codes

⇄	I70.211	Atherosclerosis of native arteries of extremities with intermittent claudication, right leg
⇄	I70.212	Atherosclerosis of native arteries of extremities with intermittent claudication, left leg
⇄	I70.213	Atherosclerosis of native arteries of extremities with intermittent claudication, bilateral legs
⇄	I70.221	Atherosclerosis of native arteries of extremities with rest pain, right leg
⇄	I70.222	Atherosclerosis of native arteries of extremities with rest pain, left leg
⇄	I70.223	Atherosclerosis of native arteries of extremities with rest pain, bilateral legs
⇄	I70.231	Atherosclerosis of native arteries of right leg with ulceration of thigh
⇄	I70.232	Atherosclerosis of native arteries of right leg with ulceration of calf
⇄	I70.233	Atherosclerosis of native arteries of right leg with ulceration of ankle
⇄	I70.234	Atherosclerosis of native arteries of right leg with ulceration of heel and midfoot
⇄	I70.235	Atherosclerosis of native arteries of right leg with ulceration of other part of foot
⇄	I70.238	Atherosclerosis of native arteries of right leg with ulceration of other part of lower right leg
⇄	I70.241	Atherosclerosis of native arteries of left leg with ulceration of thigh
⇄	I70.242	Atherosclerosis of native arteries of left leg with ulceration of calf
⇄	I70.243	Atherosclerosis of native arteries of left leg with ulceration of ankle
⇄	I70.244	Atherosclerosis of native arteries of left leg with ulceration of heel and midfoot
⇄	I70.245	Atherosclerosis of native arteries of left leg with ulceration of other part of foot
⇄	I70.248	Atherosclerosis of native arteries of left leg with ulceration of other part of lower left leg
⇄	I70.261	Atherosclerosis of native arteries of extremities with gangrene, right leg
⇄	I70.262	Atherosclerosis of native arteries of extremities with gangrene, left leg
⇄	I70.263	Atherosclerosis of native arteries of extremities with gangrene, bilateral legs
⇄	I70.268	Atherosclerosis of native arteries of extremities with gangrene, other extremity
⇄	I70.291	Other atherosclerosis of native arteries of extremities, right leg
⇄	I70.292	Other atherosclerosis of native arteries of extremities, left leg
⇄	I70.293	Other atherosclerosis of native arteries of extremities, bilateral legs
	I73.9	Peripheral vascular disease, unspecified
	I74.3	Embolism and thrombosis of arteries of the lower extremities
⇄	I75.021	Atheroembolism of right lower extremity
⇄	I75.022	Atheroembolism of left lower extremity
⇄	I75.023	Atheroembolism of bilateral lower extremities
❼	T82.818	Embolism due to vascular prosthetic devices, implants and grafts

ICD-10-CM Coding Notes

For codes requiring a 7th character extension, refer to your ICD-10-CM book. Review the character descriptions and coding guidelines for proper selection. For some procedures, only certain characters will apply.

CCI Edits

Refer to Appendix A for CCI edits.

Pub 100

01502: Pub 100-04, 12, 140.5, Pub 100-04, 12, 50, Pub 100-04, 12, 90.4.5

Base Units

Global: XXX

Code	Base Units
01502	6

Modifiers (PAR)

Code	Mod 50	Mod 51	Mod 62	Mod 80
01502	9	9	9	9

CPT © 2018 American Medical Association. All Rights Reserved.

01520

01520 Anesthesia for procedures on veins of lower leg; not otherwise specified

ICD-10-CM Diagnostic Codes

	Code	Description
	I73.9	Peripheral vascular disease, unspecified
⇄	I80.01	Phlebitis and thrombophlebitis of superficial vessels of right lower extremity
⇄	I80.02	Phlebitis and thrombophlebitis of superficial vessels of left lower extremity
⇄	I80.231	Phlebitis and thrombophlebitis of right tibial vein
⇄	I80.232	Phlebitis and thrombophlebitis of left tibial vein
⇄	I80.233	Phlebitis and thrombophlebitis of tibial vein, bilateral
⇄	I80.291	Phlebitis and thrombophlebitis of other deep vessels of right lower extremity
⇄	I80.292	Phlebitis and thrombophlebitis of other deep vessels of left lower extremity
⇄	I80.293	Phlebitis and thrombophlebitis of other deep vessels of lower extremity, bilateral
⇄	I82.441	Acute embolism and thrombosis of right tibial vein
⇄	I82.442	Acute embolism and thrombosis of left tibial vein
⇄	I82.443	Acute embolism and thrombosis of tibial vein, bilateral
⇄	I82.491	Acute embolism and thrombosis of other specified deep vein of right lower extremity
⇄	I82.492	Acute embolism and thrombosis of other specified deep vein of left lower extremity
⇄	I82.493	Acute embolism and thrombosis of other specified deep vein of lower extremity, bilateral
⇄	I83.012	Varicose veins of right lower extremity with ulcer of calf
⇄	I83.013	Varicose veins of right lower extremity with ulcer of ankle
⇄	I83.014	Varicose veins of right lower extremity with ulcer of heel and midfoot
⇄	I83.015	Varicose veins of right lower extremity with ulcer other part of foot
⇄	I83.018	Varicose veins of right lower extremity with ulcer other part of lower leg
⇄	I83.022	Varicose veins of left lower extremity with ulcer of calf
⇄	I83.023	Varicose veins of left lower extremity with ulcer of ankle
⇄	I83.024	Varicose veins of left lower extremity with ulcer of heel and midfoot
⇄	I83.025	Varicose veins of left lower extremity with ulcer other part of foot
⇄	I83.028	Varicose veins of left lower extremity with ulcer other part of lower leg
⇄	I83.11	Varicose veins of right lower extremity with inflammation
⇄	I83.12	Varicose veins of left lower extremity with inflammation
⇄	I83.212	Varicose veins of right lower extremity with both ulcer of calf and inflammation
⇄	I83.214	Varicose veins of right lower extremity with both ulcer of heel and midfoot and inflammation
⇄	I83.215	Varicose veins of right lower extremity with both ulcer other part of foot and inflammation
⇄	I83.218	Varicose veins of right lower extremity with both ulcer of other part of lower extremity and inflammation
⇄	I83.222	Varicose veins of left lower extremity with both ulcer of calf and inflammation
⇄	I83.223	Varicose veins of left lower extremity with both ulcer of ankle and inflammation
⇄	I83.224	Varicose veins of left lower extremity with both ulcer of heel and midfoot and inflammation
⇄	I83.225	Varicose veins of left lower extremity with both ulcer other part of foot and inflammation
⇄	I83.228	Varicose veins of left lower extremity with both ulcer of other part of lower extremity and inflammation
⇄	I83.811	Varicose veins of right lower extremity with pain
⇄	I83.812	Varicose veins of left lower extremity with pain
⇄	I83.813	Varicose veins of bilateral lower extremities with pain
⇄	I83.891	Varicose veins of right lower extremity with other complications
⇄	I83.892	Varicose veins of left lower extremity with other complications
⇄	I83.893	Varicose veins of bilateral lower extremities with other complications
⇄	I87.001	Postthrombotic syndrome without complications of right lower extremity
⇄	I87.002	Postthrombotic syndrome without complications of left lower extremity
⇄	I87.003	Postthrombotic syndrome without complications of bilateral lower extremity
⇄	I87.011	Postthrombotic syndrome with ulcer of right lower extremity
⇄	I87.012	Postthrombotic syndrome with ulcer of left lower extremity
⇄	I87.013	Postthrombotic syndrome with ulcer of bilateral lower extremity
⇄	I87.021	Postthrombotic syndrome with inflammation of right lower extremity
⇄	I87.022	Postthrombotic syndrome with inflammation of left lower extremity
⇄	I87.023	Postthrombotic syndrome with inflammation of bilateral lower extremity
⇄	I87.031	Postthrombotic syndrome with ulcer and inflammation of right lower extremity
⇄	I87.032	Postthrombotic syndrome with ulcer and inflammation of left lower extremity
⇄	I87.033	Postthrombotic syndrome with ulcer and inflammation of bilateral lower extremity
⇄	I87.091	Postthrombotic syndrome with other complications of right lower extremity
⇄	I87.092	Postthrombotic syndrome with other complications of left lower extremity
⇄	I87.093	Postthrombotic syndrome with other complications of bilateral lower extremity
⇄	I87.311	Chronic venous hypertension (idiopathic) with ulcer of right lower extremity
⇄	I87.312	Chronic venous hypertension (idiopathic) with ulcer of left lower extremity
⇄	I87.313	Chronic venous hypertension (idiopathic) with ulcer of bilateral lower extremity
⇄	I87.321	Chronic venous hypertension (idiopathic) with inflammation of right lower extremity
⇄	I87.322	Chronic venous hypertension (idiopathic) with inflammation of left lower extremity
⇄	I87.323	Chronic venous hypertension (idiopathic) with inflammation of bilateral lower extremity
⇄	I87.331	Chronic venous hypertension (idiopathic) with ulcer and inflammation of right lower extremity
⇄	I87.332	Chronic venous hypertension (idiopathic) with ulcer and inflammation of left lower extremity
⇄	I87.333	Chronic venous hypertension (idiopathic) with ulcer and inflammation of bilateral lower extremity
⇄	I87.391	Chronic venous hypertension (idiopathic) with other complications of right lower extremity
⇄	I87.392	Chronic venous hypertension (idiopathic) with other complications of left lower extremity
⇄	I87.393	Chronic venous hypertension (idiopathic) with other complications of bilateral lower extremity
❼⇄	S85.311	Laceration of greater saphenous vein at lower leg level, right leg
❼⇄	S85.312	Laceration of greater saphenous vein at lower leg level, left leg
❼⇄	S85.411	Laceration of lesser saphenous vein at lower leg level, right leg

CPT © 2018 American Medical Association. All Rights Reserved.

➐⇄ S85.412	Laceration of lesser saphenous vein at lower leg level, left leg
➐⇄ S85.511	Laceration of popliteal vein, right leg
➐⇄ S85.512	Laceration of popliteal vein, left leg
➐⇄ S85.811	Laceration of other blood vessels at lower leg level, right leg
➐⇄ S85.812	Laceration of other blood vessels at lower leg level, left leg

ICD-10-CM Coding Notes

For codes requiring a 7th character extension, refer to your ICD-10-CM book. Review the character descriptions and coding guidelines for proper selection. For some procedures, only certain characters will apply.

CCI Edits

Refer to Appendix A for CCI edits.

Pub 100

01520: Pub 100-04, 12, 140.5, Pub 100-04, 12, 50, Pub 100-04, 12, 90.4.5

Base Units

Global: XXX

Code	Base Units
01520	3

Modifiers (PAR)

Code	Mod 50	Mod 51	Mod 62	Mod 80
01520	9	9	9	9

CPT © 2018 American Medical Association. All Rights Reserved.

01522

01522 Anesthesia for procedures on veins of lower leg; venous thrombectomy, direct or with catheter

AMA *CPT Assistant* ☐

01522: Nov 07: 8, Jul 12: 13

ICD-10-CM Diagnostic Codes

⇄	I82.441	Acute embolism and thrombosis of right tibial vein
⇄	I82.442	Acute embolism and thrombosis of left tibial vein
⇄	I82.443	Acute embolism and thrombosis of tibial vein, bilateral
⇄	I82.491	Acute embolism and thrombosis of other specified deep vein of right lower extremity
⇄	I82.492	Acute embolism and thrombosis of other specified deep vein of left lower extremity
⇄	I82.493	Acute embolism and thrombosis of other specified deep vein of lower extremity, bilateral
➐	T82.818	Embolism due to vascular prosthetic devices, implants and grafts
➐	T82.868	Thrombosis due to vascular prosthetic devices, implants and grafts

ICD-10-CM Coding Notes

For codes requiring a 7th character extension, refer to your ICD-10-CM book. Review the character descriptions and coding guidelines for proper selection. For some procedures, only certain characters will apply.

CCI Edits

Refer to Appendix A for CCI edits.

Pub 100

01522: Pub 100-04, 12, 140.5, Pub 100-04, 12, 50, Pub 100-04, 12, 90.4.5

Base Units

Global: XXX

Code	Base Units
01522	5

Modifiers (PAR)

Code	Mod 50	Mod 51	Mod 62	Mod 80
01522	9	9	9	9

CPT © 2018 American Medical Association. All Rights Reserved.

01610

01610 Anesthesia for all procedures on nerves, muscles, tendons, fascia, and bursae of shoulder and axilla

AMA Coding Guideline

Anesthesia for Procedures on the Shoulder and Axilla

Includes humeral head and neck, sternoclavicular joint, acromioclavicular joint, and shoulder joint.

AMA *CPT Assistant* ☐

01610: Mar 06: 15, Nov 07: 8, Oct 11: 3, Jul 12: 13

ICD-10-CM Diagnostic Codes

⇄ C43.61 Malignant melanoma of right upper limb, including shoulder
⇄ C43.62 Malignant melanoma of left upper limb, including shoulder
⇄ C47.11 Malignant neoplasm of peripheral nerves of right upper limb, including shoulder
⇄ C47.12 Malignant neoplasm of peripheral nerves of left upper limb, including shoulder
⇄ C49.11 Malignant neoplasm of connective and soft tissue of right upper limb, including shoulder
⇄ C49.12 Malignant neoplasm of connective and soft tissue of left upper limb, including shoulder
⇄ C4A.61 Merkel cell carcinoma of right upper limb, including shoulder
⇄ C4A.62 Merkel cell carcinoma of left upper limb, including shoulder
C79.89 Secondary malignant neoplasm of other specified sites
⇄ D21.11 Benign neoplasm of connective and other soft tissue of right upper limb, including shoulder
⇄ D21.12 Benign neoplasm of connective and other soft tissue of left upper limb, including shoulder
D36.12 Benign neoplasm of peripheral nerves and autonomic nervous system, upper limb, including shoulder
D48.1 Neoplasm of uncertain behavior of connective and other soft tissue
D48.2 Neoplasm of uncertain behavior of peripheral nerves and autonomic nervous system
D49.2 Neoplasm of unspecified behavior of bone, soft tissue, and skin
G54.0 Brachial plexus disorders
G54.5 Neuralgic amyotrophy
⇄ M75.01 Adhesive capsulitis of right shoulder
⇄ M75.02 Adhesive capsulitis of left shoulder
⇄ M75.111 Incomplete rotator cuff tear or rupture of right shoulder, not specified as traumatic
⇄ M75.112 Incomplete rotator cuff tear or rupture of left shoulder, not specified as traumatic
⇄ M75.121 Complete rotator cuff tear or rupture of right shoulder, not specified as traumatic
⇄ M75.122 Complete rotator cuff tear or rupture of left shoulder, not specified as traumatic
⇄ M75.21 Bicipital tendinitis, right shoulder
⇄ M75.22 Bicipital tendinitis, left shoulder
⇄ M75.31 Calcific tendinitis of right shoulder
⇄ M75.32 Calcific tendinitis of left shoulder
⇄ M75.51 Bursitis of right shoulder
⇄ M75.52 Bursitis of left shoulder
⇄ M75.81 Other shoulder lesions, right shoulder
⇄ M75.82 Other shoulder lesions, left shoulder
❼⇄ S46.011 Strain of muscle(s) and tendon(s) of the rotator cuff of right shoulder
❼⇄ S46.012 Strain of muscle(s) and tendon(s) of the rotator cuff of left shoulder
❼⇄ S46.021 Laceration of muscle(s) and tendon(s) of the rotator cuff of right shoulder
❼⇄ S46.022 Laceration of muscle(s) and tendon(s) of the rotator cuff of left shoulder
❼⇄ S46.091 Other injury of muscle(s) and tendon(s) of the rotator cuff of right shoulder
❼⇄ S46.092 Other injury of muscle(s) and tendon(s) of the rotator cuff of left shoulder
❼⇄ S46.111 Strain of muscle, fascia and tendon of long head of biceps, right arm
❼⇄ S46.112 Strain of muscle, fascia and tendon of long head of biceps, left arm
❼⇄ S46.121 Laceration of muscle, fascia and tendon of long head of biceps, right arm
❼⇄ S46.122 Laceration of muscle, fascia and tendon of long head of biceps, left arm
❼⇄ S46.191 Other injury of muscle, fascia and tendon of long head of biceps, right arm
❼⇄ S46.192 Other injury of muscle, fascia and tendon of long head of biceps, left arm
❼⇄ S46.211 Strain of muscle, fascia and tendon of other parts of biceps, right arm
❼⇄ S46.212 Strain of muscle, fascia and tendon of other parts of biceps, left arm
❼⇄ S46.221 Laceration of muscle, fascia and tendon of other parts of biceps, right arm
❼⇄ S46.222 Laceration of muscle, fascia and tendon of other parts of biceps, left arm
❼⇄ S46.291 Other injury of muscle, fascia and tendon of other parts of biceps, right arm
❼⇄ S46.292 Other injury of muscle, fascia and tendon of other parts of biceps, left arm
❼⇄ S46.311 Strain of muscle, fascia and tendon of triceps, right arm
❼⇄ S46.312 Strain of muscle, fascia and tendon of triceps, left arm
❼⇄ S46.321 Laceration of muscle, fascia and tendon of triceps, right arm
❼⇄ S46.322 Laceration of muscle, fascia and tendon of triceps, left arm
❼⇄ S46.391 Other injury of muscle, fascia and tendon of triceps, right arm
❼⇄ S46.392 Other injury of muscle, fascia and tendon of triceps, left arm
❼⇄ S46.811 Strain of other muscles, fascia and tendons at shoulder and upper arm level, right arm
❼⇄ S46.812 Strain of other muscles, fascia and tendons at shoulder and upper arm level, left arm
❼⇄ S46.821 Laceration of other muscles, fascia and tendons at shoulder and upper arm level, right arm
❼⇄ S46.822 Laceration of other muscles, fascia and tendons at shoulder and upper arm level, left arm
❼⇄ S46.891 Other injury of other muscles, fascia and tendons at shoulder and upper arm level, right arm
❼⇄ S46.892 Other injury of other muscles, fascia and tendons at shoulder and upper arm level, left arm

ICD-10-CM Coding Notes

For codes requiring a 7th character extension, refer to your ICD-10-CM book. Review the character descriptions and coding guidelines for proper selection. For some procedures, only certain characters will apply.

CCI Edits

Refer to Appendix A for CCI edits.

Pub 100

01610: Pub 100-04, 12, 140.5, Pub 100-04, 12, 50, Pub 100-04, 12, 90.4.5

Base Units

Global: XXX

Code	Base Units
01610	5

Modifiers (PAR)

Code	Mod 50	Mod 51	Mod 62	Mod 80
01610	9	9	9	9

CPT © 2018 American Medical Association. All Rights Reserved.

01620

01620 Anesthesia for all closed procedures on humeral head and neck, sternoclavicular joint, acromioclavicular joint, and shoulder joint

AMA Coding Guideline

Anesthesia for Procedures on the Shoulder and Axilla

Includes humeral head and neck, sternoclavicular joint, acromioclavicular joint, and shoulder joint.

ICD-10-CM Diagnostic Codes

⇄	M24.311	Pathological dislocation of right shoulder, not elsewhere classified
⇄	M24.312	Pathological dislocation of left shoulder, not elsewhere classified
⇄	M24.411	Recurrent dislocation, right shoulder
⇄	M24.412	Recurrent dislocation, left shoulder
❼⇄	S42.221	2-part displaced fracture of surgical neck of right humerus
❼⇄	S42.222	2-part displaced fracture of surgical neck of left humerus
❼⇄	S42.224	2-part nondisplaced fracture of surgical neck of right humerus
❼⇄	S42.225	2-part nondisplaced fracture of surgical neck of left humerus
❼⇄	S42.231	3-part fracture of surgical neck of right humerus
❼⇄	S42.232	3-part fracture of surgical neck of left humerus
❼⇄	S42.241	4-part fracture of surgical neck of right humerus
❼⇄	S42.242	4-part fracture of surgical neck of left humerus
❼⇄	S42.251	Displaced fracture of greater tuberosity of right humerus
❼⇄	S42.252	Displaced fracture of greater tuberosity of left humerus
❼⇄	S42.254	Nondisplaced fracture of greater tuberosity of right humerus
❼⇄	S42.255	Nondisplaced fracture of greater tuberosity of left humerus
❼⇄	S42.261	Displaced fracture of lesser tuberosity of right humerus
❼⇄	S42.262	Displaced fracture of lesser tuberosity of left humerus
❼⇄	S42.264	Nondisplaced fracture of lesser tuberosity of right humerus
❼⇄	S42.265	Nondisplaced fracture of lesser tuberosity of left humerus
❼⇄	S42.271	Torus fracture of upper end of right humerus
❼⇄	S42.272	Torus fracture of upper end of left humerus
❼⇄	S42.291	Other displaced fracture of upper end of right humerus
❼⇄	S42.292	Other displaced fracture of upper end of left humerus
❼⇄	S42.294	Other nondisplaced fracture of upper end of right humerus
❼⇄	S42.295	Other nondisplaced fracture of upper end of left humerus
❼⇄	S43.011	Anterior subluxation of right humerus
❼⇄	S43.012	Anterior subluxation of left humerus
❼⇄	S43.014	Anterior dislocation of right humerus
❼⇄	S43.015	Anterior dislocation of left humerus
❼⇄	S43.021	Posterior subluxation of right humerus
❼⇄	S43.022	Posterior subluxation of left humerus
❼⇄	S43.024	Posterior dislocation of right humerus
❼⇄	S43.025	Posterior dislocation of left humerus
❼⇄	S43.031	Inferior subluxation of right humerus
❼⇄	S43.032	Inferior subluxation of left humerus
❼⇄	S43.034	Inferior dislocation of right humerus
❼⇄	S43.035	Inferior dislocation of left humerus
❼⇄	S43.081	Other subluxation of right shoulder joint
❼⇄	S43.082	Other subluxation of left shoulder joint
❼⇄	S43.084	Other dislocation of right shoulder joint
❼⇄	S43.085	Other dislocation of left shoulder joint
❼⇄	S43.111	Subluxation of right acromioclavicular joint
❼⇄	S43.112	Subluxation of left acromioclavicular joint
❼⇄	S43.121	Dislocation of right acromioclavicular joint, 100%-200% displacement
❼⇄	S43.122	Dislocation of left acromioclavicular joint, 100%-200% displacement
❼⇄	S43.131	Dislocation of right acromioclavicular joint, greater than 200% displacement
❼⇄	S43.132	Dislocation of left acromioclavicular joint, greater than 200% displacement
❼⇄	S43.141	Inferior dislocation of right acromioclavicular joint
❼⇄	S43.142	Inferior dislocation of left acromioclavicular joint
❼⇄	S43.151	Posterior dislocation of right acromioclavicular joint
❼⇄	S43.152	Posterior dislocation of left acromioclavicular joint
❼⇄	S43.211	Anterior subluxation of right sternoclavicular joint
❼⇄	S43.212	Anterior subluxation of left sternoclavicular joint
❼⇄	S43.214	Anterior dislocation of right sternoclavicular joint
❼⇄	S43.215	Anterior dislocation of left sternoclavicular joint
❼⇄	S43.221	Posterior subluxation of right sternoclavicular joint
❼⇄	S43.222	Posterior subluxation of left sternoclavicular joint
❼⇄	S43.224	Posterior dislocation of right sternoclavicular joint
❼⇄	S43.225	Posterior dislocation of left sternoclavicular joint

ICD-10-CM Coding Notes

For codes requiring a 7th character extension, refer to your ICD-10-CM book. Review the character descriptions and coding guidelines for proper selection. For some procedures, only certain characters will apply.

CCI Edits

Refer to Appendix A for CCI edits.

Pub 100

01620: Pub 100-04, 12, 140.5, Pub 100-04, 12, 50, Pub 100-04, 12, 90.4.5

Base Units

Global: XXX

Code	Base Units
01620	4

Modifiers (PAR)

Code	Mod 50	Mod 51	Mod 62	Mod 80
01620	9	9	9	9

CPT © 2018 American Medical Association. All Rights Reserved.

01622

01622 Anesthesia for diagnostic arthroscopic procedures of shoulder joint

AMA Coding Guideline

Anesthesia for Procedures on the Shoulder and Axilla

Includes humeral head and neck, sternoclavicular joint, acromioclavicular joint, and shoulder joint.

ICD-10-CM Diagnostic Codes

- ⇄ M00.111 Pneumococcal arthritis, right shoulder
- ⇄ M00.112 Pneumococcal arthritis, left shoulder
- ⇄ M00.211 Other streptococcal arthritis, right shoulder
- ⇄ M00.212 Other streptococcal arthritis, left shoulder
- ⇄ M00.811 Arthritis due to other bacteria, right shoulder
- ⇄ M00.812 Arthritis due to other bacteria, left shoulder
- ⇄ M05.711 Rheumatoid arthritis with rheumatoid factor of right shoulder without organ or systems involvement
- ⇄ M05.712 Rheumatoid arthritis with rheumatoid factor of left shoulder without organ or systems involvement
- ⇄ M06.011 Rheumatoid arthritis without rheumatoid factor, right shoulder
- ⇄ M06.012 Rheumatoid arthritis without rheumatoid factor, left shoulder
- ⇄ M06.211 Rheumatoid bursitis, right shoulder
- ⇄ M06.212 Rheumatoid bursitis, left shoulder
- ⇄ M06.311 Rheumatoid nodule, right shoulder
- ⇄ M06.312 Rheumatoid nodule, left shoulder
- ⇄ M12.211 Villonodular synovitis (pigmented), right shoulder
- ⇄ M12.212 Villonodular synovitis (pigmented), left shoulder
- ⇄ M12.311 Palindromic rheumatism, right shoulder
- ⇄ M12.312 Palindromic rheumatism, left shoulder
- ⇄ M12.411 Intermittent hydrarthrosis, right shoulder
- ⇄ M12.412 Intermittent hydrarthrosis, left shoulder
- ⇄ M12.511 Traumatic arthropathy, right shoulder
- ⇄ M12.512 Traumatic arthropathy, left shoulder
- ⇄ M12.811 Other specific arthropathies, not elsewhere classified, right shoulder
- ⇄ M12.812 Other specific arthropathies, not elsewhere classified, left shoulder
- ⇄ M19.011 Primary osteoarthritis, right shoulder
- ⇄ M19.012 Primary osteoarthritis, left shoulder
- ⇄ M19.111 Post-traumatic osteoarthritis, right shoulder
- ⇄ M19.112 Post-traumatic osteoarthritis, left shoulder
- ⇄ M19.211 Secondary osteoarthritis, right shoulder
- ⇄ M19.222 Secondary osteoarthritis, left elbow
- ⇄ M24.011 Loose body in right shoulder
- ⇄ M24.012 Loose body in left shoulder
- ⇄ M24.111 Other articular cartilage disorders, right shoulder
- ⇄ M24.112 Other articular cartilage disorders, left shoulder
- ⇄ M25.011 Hemarthrosis, right shoulder
- ⇄ M25.012 Hemarthrosis, left shoulder
- ⇄ M25.311 Other instability, right shoulder
- ⇄ M25.312 Other instability, left shoulder
- ⇄ M25.411 Effusion, right shoulder
- ⇄ M25.412 Effusion, left shoulder
- ⇄ M25.511 Pain in right shoulder
- ⇄ M25.512 Pain in left shoulder
- ⇄ M25.611 Stiffness of right shoulder, not elsewhere classified
- ⇄ M25.612 Stiffness of left shoulder, not elsewhere classified

CCI Edits

Refer to Appendix A for CCI edits.

Pub 100

01622: Pub 100-04, 12, 140.5, Pub 100-04, 12, 50, Pub 100-04, 12, 90.4.5

Base Units

Global: XXX

Code	Base Units
01622	4

Modifiers (PAR)

Code	Mod 50	Mod 51	Mod 62	Mod 80
01622	9	9	9	9

CPT © 2018 American Medical Association. All Rights Reserved.

01630

01630 Anesthesia for open or surgical arthroscopic procedures on humeral head and neck, sternoclavicular joint, acromioclavicular joint, and shoulder joint; not otherwise specified

AMA Coding Guideline

Anesthesia for Procedures on the Shoulder and Axilla

Includes humeral head and neck, sternoclavicular joint, acromioclavicular joint, and shoulder joint.

ICD-10-CM Diagnostic Codes

⇄ M12.211 Villonodular synovitis (pigmented), right shoulder
⇄ M12.212 Villonodular synovitis (pigmented), left shoulder
⇄ M12.511 Traumatic arthropathy, right shoulder
⇄ M12.512 Traumatic arthropathy, left shoulder
⇄ M19.011 Primary osteoarthritis, right shoulder
⇄ M19.012 Primary osteoarthritis, left shoulder
⇄ M19.111 Post-traumatic osteoarthritis, right shoulder
⇄ M19.112 Post-traumatic osteoarthritis, left shoulder
⇄ M19.211 Secondary osteoarthritis, right shoulder
⇄ M19.212 Secondary osteoarthritis, left shoulder
⇄ M24.411 Recurrent dislocation, right shoulder
⇄ M24.412 Recurrent dislocation, left shoulder
⇄ M25.711 Osteophyte, right shoulder
⇄ M25.712 Osteophyte, left shoulder
⇄ M75.01 Adhesive capsulitis of right shoulder
⇄ M75.02 Adhesive capsulitis of left shoulder
⇄ M75.111 Incomplete rotator cuff tear or rupture of right shoulder, not specified as traumatic
⇄ M75.112 Incomplete rotator cuff tear or rupture of left shoulder, not specified as traumatic
⇄ M75.121 Complete rotator cuff tear or rupture of right shoulder, not specified as traumatic
⇄ M75.122 Complete rotator cuff tear or rupture of left shoulder, not specified as traumatic
⇄ M75.21 Bicipital tendinitis, right shoulder
⇄ M75.22 Bicipital tendinitis, left shoulder
⇄ M75.31 Calcific tendinitis of right shoulder
⇄ M75.32 Calcific tendinitis of left shoulder
⇄ M75.41 Impingement syndrome of right shoulder
⇄ M75.42 Impingement syndrome of left shoulder
⇄ M75.51 Bursitis of right shoulder
⇄ M75.52 Bursitis of left shoulder
⇄ M75.81 Other shoulder lesions, right shoulder
⇄ M75.82 Other shoulder lesions, left shoulder
❼⇄ S42.031 Displaced fracture of lateral end of right clavicle
❼⇄ S42.032 Displaced fracture of lateral end of left clavicle
❼⇄ S42.121 Displaced fracture of acromial process, right shoulder
❼⇄ S42.122 Displaced fracture of acromial process, left shoulder
❼⇄ S42.131 Displaced fracture of coracoid process, right shoulder
❼⇄ S42.132 Displaced fracture of coracoid process, left shoulder
❼⇄ S42.141 Displaced fracture of glenoid cavity of scapula, right shoulder
❼⇄ S42.142 Displaced fracture of glenoid cavity of scapula, left shoulder
❼⇄ S42.144 Nondisplaced fracture of glenoid cavity of scapula, right shoulder
❼⇄ S42.145 Nondisplaced fracture of glenoid cavity of scapula, left shoulder
❼⇄ S42.221 2-part displaced fracture of surgical neck of right humerus
❼⇄ S42.222 2-part displaced fracture of surgical neck of left humerus
❼⇄ S42.224 2-part nondisplaced fracture of surgical neck of right humerus
❼⇄ S42.225 2-part nondisplaced fracture of surgical neck of left humerus
❼⇄ S42.231 3-part fracture of surgical neck of right humerus
❼⇄ S42.232 3-part fracture of surgical neck of left humerus
❼⇄ S42.241 4-part fracture of surgical neck of right humerus
❼⇄ S42.242 4-part fracture of surgical neck of left humerus
❼⇄ S42.251 Displaced fracture of greater tuberosity of right humerus
❼⇄ S42.252 Displaced fracture of greater tuberosity of left humerus
❼⇄ S42.254 Nondisplaced fracture of greater tuberosity of right humerus
❼⇄ S42.255 Nondisplaced fracture of greater tuberosity of left humerus
❼⇄ S42.261 Displaced fracture of lesser tuberosity of right humerus
❼⇄ S42.262 Displaced fracture of lesser tuberosity of left humerus
❼⇄ S42.264 Nondisplaced fracture of lesser tuberosity of right humerus
❼⇄ S42.265 Nondisplaced fracture of lesser tuberosity of left humerus
❼⇄ S42.271 Torus fracture of upper end of right humerus
❼⇄ S42.272 Torus fracture of upper end of left humerus
❼⇄ S42.291 Other displaced fracture of upper end of right humerus
❼⇄ S42.292 Other displaced fracture of upper end of left humerus
❼⇄ S42.294 Other nondisplaced fracture of upper end of right humerus
❼⇄ S42.295 Other nondisplaced fracture of upper end of left humerus
❼⇄ S43.411 Sprain of right coracohumeral (ligament)
❼⇄ S43.412 Sprain of left coracohumeral (ligament)
❼⇄ S43.421 Sprain of right rotator cuff capsule
❼⇄ S43.422 Sprain of left rotator cuff capsule
❼⇄ S43.431 Superior glenoid labrum lesion of right shoulder
❼⇄ S43.432 Superior glenoid labrum lesion of left shoulder
❼⇄ S43.491 Other sprain of right shoulder joint
❼⇄ S43.492 Other sprain of left shoulder joint
❼⇄ S43.51 Sprain of right acromioclavicular joint
❼⇄ S43.52 Sprain of left acromioclavicular joint
❼⇄ S43.61 Sprain of right sternoclavicular joint
❼⇄ S43.62 Sprain of left sternoclavicular joint
❼⇄ S43.81 Sprain of other specified parts of right shoulder girdle
❼⇄ S43.82 Sprain of other specified parts of left shoulder girdle

ICD-10-CM Coding Notes

For codes requiring a 7th character extension, refer to your ICD-10-CM book. Review the character descriptions and coding guidelines for proper selection. For some procedures, only certain characters will apply.

CCI Edits

Refer to Appendix A for CCI edits.

Pub 100

01630: Pub 100-04, 12, 140.5, Pub 100-04, 12, 50, Pub 100-04, 12, 90.4.5

Base Units

Global: XXX

Code	Base Units
01630	5

Modifiers (PAR)

Code	Mod 50	Mod 51	Mod 62	Mod 80
01630	9	9	9	9

● New ▲ Revised ✚ Add On ⊘Modifier 51 Exempt ★Telemedicine ▯ CPT QuickRef ⁄⁄FDA Pending ⇄ Laterality ❼ Seventh Character ♂Male ♀Female

CPT © 2018 American Medical Association. All Rights Reserved.

01634

01634 Anesthesia for open or surgical arthroscopic procedures on humeral head and neck, sternoclavicular joint, acromioclavicular joint, and shoulder joint; shoulder disarticulation

AMA Coding Guideline

Anesthesia for Procedures on the Shoulder and Axilla

Includes humeral head and neck, sternoclavicular joint, acromioclavicular joint, and shoulder joint.

ICD-10-CM Diagnostic Codes

⇄	C40.01	Malignant neoplasm of scapula and long bones of right upper limb
⇄	C40.02	Malignant neoplasm of scapula and long bones of left upper limb
⇄	C47.11	Malignant neoplasm of peripheral nerves of right upper limb, including shoulder
⇄	C47.12	Malignant neoplasm of peripheral nerves of left upper limb, including shoulder
⇄	C49.11	Malignant neoplasm of connective and soft tissue of right upper limb, including shoulder
⇄	C49.12	Malignant neoplasm of connective and soft tissue of left upper limb, including shoulder
❼⇄	S41.011	Laceration without foreign body of right shoulder
❼⇄	S41.012	Laceration without foreign body of left shoulder
❼⇄	S41.021	Laceration with foreign body of right shoulder
❼⇄	S41.022	Laceration with foreign body of left shoulder
❼⇄	S41.051	Open bite of right shoulder
❼⇄	S41.052	Open bite of left shoulder
❼⇄	S46.091	Other injury of muscle(s) and tendon(s) of the rotator cuff of right shoulder
❼⇄	S46.092	Other injury of muscle(s) and tendon(s) of the rotator cuff of left shoulder
❼⇄	S46.191	Other injury of muscle, fascia and tendon of long head of biceps, right arm
❼⇄	S46.192	Other injury of muscle, fascia and tendon of long head of biceps, left arm
❼⇄	S46.291	Other injury of muscle, fascia and tendon of other parts of biceps, right arm
❼⇄	S46.292	Other injury of muscle, fascia and tendon of other parts of biceps, left arm
❼⇄	S46.391	Other injury of muscle, fascia and tendon of triceps, right arm
❼⇄	S46.392	Other injury of muscle, fascia and tendon of triceps, left arm
❼⇄	S46.991	Other injury of unspecified muscle, fascia and tendon at shoulder and upper arm level, right arm
❼⇄	S46.992	Other injury of unspecified muscle, fascia and tendon at shoulder and upper arm level, left arm
❼⇄	S47.1	Crushing injury of right shoulder and upper arm
❼⇄	S47.2	Crushing injury of left shoulder and upper arm
❼⇄	S48.011	Complete traumatic amputation at right shoulder joint
❼⇄	S48.012	Complete traumatic amputation at left shoulder joint
❼⇄	S48.021	Partial traumatic amputation at right shoulder joint
❼⇄	S48.022	Partial traumatic amputation at left shoulder joint
❼⇄	S48.111	Complete traumatic amputation at level between right shoulder and elbow
❼⇄	S48.112	Complete traumatic amputation at level between left shoulder and elbow
❼⇄	S48.121	Partial traumatic amputation at level between right shoulder and elbow
❼⇄	S48.122	Partial traumatic amputation at level between left shoulder and elbow

ICD-10-CM Coding Notes

For codes requiring a 7th character extension, refer to your ICD-10-CM book. Review the character descriptions and coding guidelines for proper selection. For some procedures, only certain characters will apply.

CCI Edits

Refer to Appendix A for CCI edits.

Pub 100

01634: Pub 100-04, 12, 140.5, Pub 100-04, 12, 50, Pub 100-04, 12, 90.4.5

Base Units

Global: XXX

Code	Base Units
01634	9

Modifiers (PAR)

Code	Mod 50	Mod 51	Mod 62	Mod 80
01634	9	9	9	9

CPT © 2018 American Medical Association. All Rights Reserved.

01636

01636 Anesthesia for open or surgical arthroscopic procedures on humeral head and neck, sternoclavicular joint, acromioclavicular joint, and shoulder joint; interthoracoscapular (forequarter) amputation

AMA Coding Guideline

Anesthesia for Procedures on the Shoulder and Axilla

Includes humeral head and neck, sternoclavicular joint, acromioclavicular joint, and shoulder joint.

ICD-10-CM Diagnostic Codes

⇄	C40.01	Malignant neoplasm of scapula and long bones of right upper limb
⇄	C40.02	Malignant neoplasm of scapula and long bones of left upper limb
	C41.3	Malignant neoplasm of ribs, sternum and clavicle
⇄	C47.11	Malignant neoplasm of peripheral nerves of right upper limb, including shoulder
⇄	C47.12	Malignant neoplasm of peripheral nerves of left upper limb, including shoulder
⇄	C49.11	Malignant neoplasm of connective and soft tissue of right upper limb, including shoulder
⇄	C49.12	Malignant neoplasm of connective and soft tissue of left upper limb, including shoulder
❼	S28.0	Crushed chest
❼⇄	S47.1	Crushing injury of right shoulder and upper arm
❼⇄	S47.2	Crushing injury of left shoulder and upper arm
❼⇄	S48.011	Complete traumatic amputation at right shoulder joint
❼⇄	S48.012	Complete traumatic amputation at left shoulder joint
❼⇄	S48.021	Partial traumatic amputation at right shoulder joint
❼⇄	S48.022	Partial traumatic amputation at left shoulder joint

ICD-10-CM Coding Notes

For codes requiring a 7th character extension, refer to your ICD-10-CM book. Review the character descriptions and coding guidelines for proper selection. For some procedures, only certain characters will apply.

CCI Edits

Refer to Appendix A for CCI edits.

Pub 100

01636: Pub 100-04, 12, 140.5, Pub 100-04, 12, 50, Pub 100-04, 12, 90.4.5

Base Units

Global: XXX

Code	Base Units
01636	15

Modifiers (PAR)

Code	Mod 50	Mod 51	Mod 62	Mod 80
01636	9	9	9	9

CPT © 2018 American Medical Association. All Rights Reserved.

01638

01638 Anesthesia for open or surgical arthroscopic procedures on humeral head and neck, sternoclavicular joint, acromioclavicular joint, and shoulder joint; total shoulder replacement

AMA Coding Guideline

Anesthesia for Procedures on the Shoulder and Axilla

Includes humeral head and neck, sternoclavicular joint, acromioclavicular joint, and shoulder joint.

ICD-10-CM Diagnostic Codes

⇄	M05.711	Rheumatoid arthritis with rheumatoid factor of right shoulder without organ or systems involvement
⇄	M05.712	Rheumatoid arthritis with rheumatoid factor of left shoulder without organ or systems involvement
⇄	M06.011	Rheumatoid arthritis without rheumatoid factor, right shoulder
⇄	M06.012	Rheumatoid arthritis without rheumatoid factor, left shoulder
⇄	M12.51	Traumatic arthropathy, shoulder
⇄	M19.011	Primary osteoarthritis, right shoulder
⇄	M19.012	Primary osteoarthritis, left shoulder
⇄	M19.111	Post-traumatic osteoarthritis, right shoulder
⇄	M19.112	Post-traumatic osteoarthritis, left shoulder
⇄	M19.211	Secondary osteoarthritis, right shoulder
⇄	M19.212	Secondary osteoarthritis, left shoulder
⇄	M75.121	Complete rotator cuff tear or rupture of right shoulder, not specified as traumatic
⇄	M75.122	Complete rotator cuff tear or rupture of left shoulder, not specified as traumatic
❼⇄	M80.011	Age-related osteoporosis with current pathological fracture, right shoulder
❼⇄	M80.012	Age-related osteoporosis with current pathological fracture, left shoulder
❼⇄	M80.811	Other osteoporosis with current pathological fracture, right shoulder
❼⇄	M80.812	Other osteoporosis with current pathological fracture, left shoulder
❼⇄	M84.411	Pathological fracture, right shoulder
❼⇄	M84.412	Pathological fracture, left shoulder
❼⇄	M84.511	Pathological fracture in neoplastic disease, right shoulder
❼⇄	M84.512	Pathological fracture in neoplastic disease, left shoulder
⇄	M87.011	Idiopathic aseptic necrosis of right shoulder
⇄	M87.012	Idiopathic aseptic necrosis of left shoulder
⇄	M87.211	Osteonecrosis due to previous trauma, right shoulder
⇄	M87.212	Osteonecrosis due to previous trauma, left shoulder
❼⇄	M97.31	Periprosthetic fracture around internal prosthetic right shoulder joint
❼⇄	M97.32	Periprosthetic fracture around internal prosthetic left shoulder joint
❼⇄	S42.141	Displaced fracture of glenoid cavity of scapula, right shoulder
❼⇄	S42.142	Displaced fracture of glenoid cavity of scapula, left shoulder
❼⇄	S42.241	4-part fracture of surgical neck of right humerus
❼⇄	S42.242	4-part fracture of surgical neck of left humerus
❼⇄	S42.291	Other displaced fracture of upper end of right humerus
❼⇄	S42.292	Other displaced fracture of upper end of left humerus
❼	T84.018	Broken internal joint prosthesis, other site
❼⇄	T84.028	Dislocation of other internal joint prosthesis
❼⇄	T84.038	Mechanical loosening of other internal prosthetic joint
❼⇄	T84.068	Wear of articular bearing surface of other internal prosthetic joint
❼⇄	T84.098	Other mechanical complication of other internal joint prosthesis
⇄	Z96.611	Presence of right artificial shoulder joint
⇄	Z96.612	Presence of left artificial shoulder joint

ICD-10-CM Coding Notes

For codes requiring a 7th character extension, refer to your ICD-10-CM book. Review the character descriptions and coding guidelines for proper selection. For some procedures, only certain characters will apply.

CCI Edits

Refer to Appendix A for CCI edits.

Pub 100

01638: Pub 100-04, 12, 140.5, Pub 100-04, 12, 50, Pub 100-04, 12, 90.4.5

Base Units

Global: XXX

Code	Base Units
01638	10

Modifiers (PAR)

Code	Mod 50	Mod 51	Mod 62	Mod 80
01638	9	9	9	9

CPT © 2018 American Medical Association. All Rights Reserved.

01650

01650 Anesthesia for procedures on arteries of shoulder and axilla; not otherwise specified

AMA Coding Guideline

Anesthesia for Procedures on the Shoulder and Axilla

Includes humeral head and neck, sternoclavicular joint, acromioclavicular joint, and shoulder joint.

ICD-10-CM Diagnostic Codes

⇄ I70.218 Atherosclerosis of native arteries of extremities with intermittent claudication, other extremity
⇄ I70.228 Atherosclerosis of native arteries of extremities with rest pain, other extremity
⇄ I70.25 Atherosclerosis of native arteries of other extremities with ulceration
⇄ I70.268 Atherosclerosis of native arteries of extremities with gangrene, other extremity
⇄ I70.298 Other atherosclerosis of native arteries of extremities, other extremity
⇄ I70.318 Atherosclerosis of unspecified type of bypass graft(s) of the extremities with intermittent claudication, other extremity
⇄ I70.328 Atherosclerosis of unspecified type of bypass graft(s) of the extremities with rest pain, other extremity
⇄ I70.35 Atherosclerosis of unspecified type of bypass graft(s) of other extremity with ulceration
⇄ I70.368 Atherosclerosis of unspecified type of bypass graft(s) of the extremities with gangrene, other extremity
⇄ I70.398 Other atherosclerosis of unspecified type of bypass graft(s) of the extremities, other extremity
⇄ I70.418 Atherosclerosis of autologous vein bypass graft(s) of the extremities with intermittent claudication, other extremity
⇄ I70.428 Atherosclerosis of autologous vein bypass graft(s) of the extremities with rest pain, other extremity
⇄ I70.45 Atherosclerosis of autologous vein bypass graft(s) of other extremity with ulceration
⇄ I70.468 Atherosclerosis of autologous vein bypass graft(s) of the extremities with gangrene, other extremity
⇄ I70.498 Other atherosclerosis of autologous vein bypass graft(s) of the extremities, other extremity
⇄ I70.518 Atherosclerosis of nonautologous biological bypass graft(s) of the extremities with intermittent claudication, other extremity
⇄ I70.528 Atherosclerosis of nonautologous biological bypass graft(s) of the extremities with rest pain, other extremity
⇄ I70.55 Atherosclerosis of nonautologous biological bypass graft(s) of other extremity with ulceration
⇄ I70.568 Atherosclerosis of nonautologous biological bypass graft(s) of the extremities with gangrene, other extremity
⇄ I70.598 Other atherosclerosis of nonautologous biological bypass graft(s) of the extremities, other extremity
⇄ I70.618 Atherosclerosis of nonbiological bypass graft(s) of the extremities with intermittent claudication, other extremity
⇄ I70.628 Atherosclerosis of nonbiological bypass graft(s) of the extremities with rest pain, other extremity
⇄ I70.65 Atherosclerosis of nonbiological bypass graft(s) of other extremity with ulceration
⇄ I70.668 Atherosclerosis of nonbiological bypass graft(s) of the extremities with gangrene, other extremity
⇄ I70.698 Other atherosclerosis of nonbiological bypass graft(s) of the extremities, other extremity
⇄ I70.718 Atherosclerosis of other type of bypass graft(s) of the extremities with intermittent claudication, other extremity
⇄ I70.728 Atherosclerosis of other type of bypass graft(s) of the extremities with rest pain, other extremity
⇄ I70.75 Atherosclerosis of other type of bypass graft(s) of other extremity with ulceration
⇄ I70.768 Atherosclerosis of other type of bypass graft(s) of the extremities with gangrene, other extremity
⇄ I70.798 Other atherosclerosis of other type of bypass graft(s) of the extremities, other extremity
I74.2 Embolism and thrombosis of arteries of the upper extremities
⇄ I75.011 Atheroembolism of right upper extremity
⇄ I75.012 Atheroembolism of left upper extremity
I77.0 Arteriovenous fistula, acquired
I77.1 Stricture of artery
I77.2 Rupture of artery
I77.5 Necrosis of artery
➐⇄ S45.011 Laceration of axillary artery, right side
➐⇄ S45.012 Laceration of axillary artery, left side
➐⇄ S45.091 Other specified injury of axillary artery, right side
➐⇄ S45.092 Other specified injury of axillary artery, left side
➐⇄ S45.811 Laceration of other specified blood vessels at shoulder and upper arm level, right arm
➐⇄ S45.812 Laceration of other specified blood vessels at shoulder and upper arm level, left arm
➐⇄ S45.891 Other specified injury of other specified blood vessels at shoulder and upper arm level, right arm
➐⇄ S45.892 Other specified injury of other specified blood vessels at shoulder and upper arm level, left arm
➐ T80.1 Vascular complications following infusion, transfusion and therapeutic injection
➐ T82.318 Breakdown (mechanical) of other vascular grafts
➐ T82.328 Displacement of other vascular grafts
➐ T82.338 Leakage of other vascular grafts
➐ T82.398 Other mechanical complication of other vascular grafts
➐ T82.7 Infection and inflammatory reaction due to other cardiac and vascular devices, implants and grafts
➐ T82.818 Embolism due to vascular prosthetic devices, implants and grafts
➐ T82.828 Fibrosis due to vascular prosthetic devices, implants and grafts
➐ T82.838 Hemorrhage due to vascular prosthetic devices, implants and grafts
➐ T82.848 Pain due to vascular prosthetic devices, implants and grafts
➐ T82.858 Stenosis of other vascular prosthetic devices, implants and grafts
➐ T82.868 Thrombosis due to vascular prosthetic devices, implants and grafts
➐ T82.898 Other specified complication of vascular prosthetic devices, implants and grafts

ICD-10-CM Coding Notes

For codes requiring a 7th character extension, refer to your ICD-10-CM book. Review the character descriptions and coding guidelines for proper selection. For some procedures, only certain characters will apply.

CCI Edits

Refer to Appendix A for CCI edits.

Pub 100

01650: Pub 100-04, 12, 140.5, Pub 100-04, 12, 50, Pub 100-04, 12, 90.4.5

Base Units

Global: XXX

Code	Base Units
01650	6

Modifiers (PAR)

Code	Mod 50	Mod 51	Mod 62	Mod 80
01650	9	9	9	9

CPT © 2018 American Medical Association. All Rights Reserved.

01652

01652 Anesthesia for procedures on arteries of shoulder and axilla; axillary-brachial aneurysm

AMA Coding Guideline

Anesthesia for Procedures on the Shoulder and Axilla

Includes humeral head and neck, sternoclavicular joint, acromioclavicular joint, and shoulder joint.

ICD-10-CM Diagnostic Codes

⇄	I70.218	Atherosclerosis of native arteries of extremities with intermittent claudication, other extremity
⇄	I70.228	Atherosclerosis of native arteries of extremities with rest pain, other extremity
⇄	I70.25	Atherosclerosis of native arteries of other extremities with ulceration
⇄	I70.268	Atherosclerosis of native arteries of extremities with gangrene, other extremity
⇄	I70.298	Other atherosclerosis of native arteries of extremities, other extremity
	I72.1	Aneurysm of artery of upper extremity
	I74.2	Embolism and thrombosis of arteries of the upper extremities
⇄	I75.011	Atheroembolism of right upper extremity
⇄	I75.012	Atheroembolism of left upper extremity
⇄	I75.013	Atheroembolism of bilateral upper extremities
	I77.79	Dissection of other specified artery
	Q27.8	Other specified congenital malformations of peripheral vascular system
➐⇄	S45.091	Other specified injury of axillary artery, right side
➐⇄	S45.092	Other specified injury of axillary artery, left side
➐⇄	S45.191	Other specified injury of brachial artery, right side
➐⇄	S45.192	Other specified injury of brachial artery, left side

ICD-10-CM Coding Notes

For codes requiring a 7th character extension, refer to your ICD-10-CM book. Review the character descriptions and coding guidelines for proper selection. For some procedures, only certain characters will apply.

CCI Edits

Refer to Appendix A for CCI edits.

Pub 100

01652: Pub 100-04, 12, 140.5, Pub 100-04, 12, 50, Pub 100-04, 12, 90.4.5

Base Units

Global: XXX

Code	Base Units
01652	10

Modifiers (PAR)

Code	Mod 50	Mod 51	Mod 62	Mod 80
01652	9	9	9	9

CPT © 2018 American Medical Association. All Rights Reserved.

01654

01654 Anesthesia for procedures on arteries of shoulder and axilla; bypass graft

AMA Coding Guideline

Anesthesia for Procedures on the Shoulder and Axilla

Includes humeral head and neck, sternoclavicular joint, acromioclavicular joint, and shoulder joint.

ICD-10-CM Diagnostic Codes

	G45.2	Multiple and bilateral precerebral artery syndromes
⇄	I70.218	Atherosclerosis of native arteries of extremities with intermittent claudication, other extremity
⇄	I70.228	Atherosclerosis of native arteries of extremities with rest pain, other extremity
⇄	I70.25	Atherosclerosis of native arteries of other extremities with ulceration
⇄	I70.268	Atherosclerosis of native arteries of extremities with gangrene, other extremity
⇄	I70.298	Other atherosclerosis of native arteries of extremities, other extremity
⇄	I70.318	Atherosclerosis of unspecified type of bypass graft(s) of the extremities with intermittent claudication, other extremity
⇄	I70.328	Atherosclerosis of unspecified type of bypass graft(s) of the extremities with rest pain, other extremity
⇄	I70.35	Atherosclerosis of unspecified type of bypass graft(s) of other extremity with ulceration
⇄	I70.368	Atherosclerosis of unspecified type of bypass graft(s) of the extremities with gangrene, other extremity
⇄	I70.398	Other atherosclerosis of unspecified type of bypass graft(s) of the extremities, other extremity
⇄	I70.418	Atherosclerosis of autologous vein bypass graft(s) of the extremities with intermittent claudication, other extremity
⇄	I70.428	Atherosclerosis of autologous vein bypass graft(s) of the extremities with rest pain, other extremity
⇄	I70.45	Atherosclerosis of autologous vein bypass graft(s) of other extremity with ulceration
⇄	I70.468	Atherosclerosis of autologous vein bypass graft(s) of the extremities with gangrene, other extremity
⇄	I70.498	Other atherosclerosis of autologous vein bypass graft(s) of the extremities, other extremity
⇄	I70.518	Atherosclerosis of nonautologous biological bypass graft(s) of the extremities with intermittent claudication, other extremity
⇄	I70.528	Atherosclerosis of nonautologous biological bypass graft(s) of the extremities with rest pain, other extremity
⇄	I70.55	Atherosclerosis of nonautologous biological bypass graft(s) of other extremity with ulceration
⇄	I70.568	Atherosclerosis of nonautologous biological bypass graft(s) of the extremities with gangrene, other extremity
⇄	I70.598	Other atherosclerosis of nonautologous biological bypass graft(s) of the extremities, other extremity
⇄	I70.618	Atherosclerosis of nonbiological bypass graft(s) of the extremities with intermittent claudication, other extremity
⇄	I70.628	Atherosclerosis of nonbiological bypass graft(s) of the extremities with rest pain, other extremity
⇄	I70.65	Atherosclerosis of nonbiological bypass graft(s) of other extremity with ulceration
⇄	I70.668	Atherosclerosis of nonbiological bypass graft(s) of the extremities with gangrene, other extremity
⇄	I70.698	Other atherosclerosis of nonbiological bypass graft(s) of the extremities, other extremity
⇄	I70.718	Atherosclerosis of other type of bypass graft(s) of the extremities with intermittent claudication, other extremity
⇄	I70.728	Atherosclerosis of other type of bypass graft(s) of the extremities with rest pain, other extremity
⇄	I70.75	Atherosclerosis of other type of bypass graft(s) of other extremity with ulceration
⇄	I70.768	Atherosclerosis of other type of bypass graft(s) of the extremities with gangrene, other extremity
⇄	I70.798	Other atherosclerosis of other type of bypass graft(s) of the extremities, other extremity
	I74.2	Embolism and thrombosis of arteries of the upper extremities
⇄	I75.011	Atheroembolism of right upper extremity
⇄	I75.012	Atheroembolism of left upper extremity
⇄	I75.013	Atheroembolism of bilateral upper extremities
	I77.1	Stricture of artery
	I77.2	Rupture of artery
	I77.5	Necrosis of artery
⑦⇄	S41.011	Laceration without foreign body of right shoulder
⑦⇄	S41.012	Laceration without foreign body of left shoulder
⑦⇄	S41.031	Puncture wound without foreign body of right shoulder
⑦⇄	S41.032	Puncture wound without foreign body of left shoulder
⑦⇄	S41.051	Open bite of right shoulder
⑦⇄	S41.052	Open bite of left shoulder
⑦⇄	S41.111	Laceration without foreign body of right upper arm
⑦⇄	S41.112	Laceration without foreign body of left upper arm
⑦⇄	S41.131	Puncture wound without foreign body of right upper arm
⑦⇄	S41.132	Puncture wound without foreign body of left upper arm
⑦⇄	S41.151	Open bite of right upper arm
⑦⇄	S41.152	Open bite of left upper arm
⑦⇄	S45.011	Laceration of axillary artery, right side
⑦⇄	S45.012	Laceration of axillary artery, left side
⑦⇄	S45.091	Other specified injury of axillary artery, right side
⑦⇄	S45.092	Other specified injury of axillary artery, left side
⑦⇄	S45.111	Laceration of brachial artery, right side
⑦⇄	S45.112	Laceration of brachial artery, left side
⑦⇄	S45.191	Other specified injury of brachial artery, right side
⑦⇄	S45.192	Other specified injury of brachial artery, left side
⑦⇄	S45.811	Laceration of other specified blood vessels at shoulder and upper arm level, right arm
⑦⇄	S45.819	Laceration of other specified blood vessels at shoulder and upper arm level, unspecified arm
⑦⇄	S45.891	Other specified injury of other specified blood vessels at shoulder and upper arm level, right arm
⑦⇄	S45.892	Other specified injury of other specified blood vessels at shoulder and upper arm level, left arm

ICD-10-CM Coding Notes

For codes requiring a 7th character extension, refer to your ICD-10-CM book. Review the character descriptions and coding guidelines for proper selection. For some procedures, only certain characters will apply.

CCI Edits

Refer to Appendix A for CCI edits.

Pub 100

01654: Pub 100-04, 12, 140.5, Pub 100-04, 12, 50, Pub 100-04, 12, 90.4.5

Base Units

Global: XXX

Code	Base Units
01654	8

Modifiers (PAR)

Code	Mod 50	Mod 51	Mod 62	Mod 80
01654	9	9	9	9

CPT © 2018 American Medical Association. All Rights Reserved.

01656

01656 Anesthesia for procedures on arteries of shoulder and axilla; axillary-femoral bypass graft

AMA Coding Guideline

Anesthesia for Procedures on the Shoulder and Axilla

Includes humeral head and neck, sternoclavicular joint, acromioclavicular joint, and shoulder joint.

ICD-10-CM Diagnostic Codes

	E10.51	Type 1 diabetes mellitus with diabetic peripheral angiopathy without gangrene
	E10.52	Type 1 diabetes mellitus with diabetic peripheral angiopathy with gangrene
	E10.59	Type 1 diabetes mellitus with other circulatory complications
	E11.51	Type 2 diabetes mellitus with diabetic peripheral angiopathy without gangrene
	E11.52	Type 2 diabetes mellitus with diabetic peripheral angiopathy with gangrene
	E11.59	Type 2 diabetes mellitus with other circulatory complications
	F17.210	Nicotine dependence, cigarettes, uncomplicated
	F17.211	Nicotine dependence, cigarettes, in remission
	F17.213	Nicotine dependence, cigarettes, with withdrawal
	F17.218	Nicotine dependence, cigarettes, with other nicotine-induced disorders
	F17.219	Nicotine dependence, cigarettes, with unspecified nicotine-induced disorders
⇄	I70.211	Atherosclerosis of native arteries of extremities with intermittent claudication, right leg
⇄	I70.212	Atherosclerosis of native arteries of extremities with intermittent claudication, left leg
⇄	I70.221	Atherosclerosis of native arteries of extremities with rest pain, right leg
⇄	I70.222	Atherosclerosis of native arteries of extremities with rest pain, left leg
⇄	I70.231	Atherosclerosis of native arteries of right leg with ulceration of thigh
⇄	I70.232	Atherosclerosis of native arteries of right leg with ulceration of calf
⇄	I70.233	Atherosclerosis of native arteries of right leg with ulceration of ankle
⇄	I70.234	Atherosclerosis of native arteries of right leg with ulceration of heel and midfoot
⇄	I70.235	Atherosclerosis of native arteries of right leg with ulceration of other part of foot
⇄	I70.238	Atherosclerosis of native arteries of right leg with ulceration of other part of lower right leg
⇄	I70.241	Atherosclerosis of native arteries of left leg with ulceration of thigh
⇄	I70.242	Atherosclerosis of native arteries of left leg with ulceration of calf
⇄	I70.243	Atherosclerosis of native arteries of left leg with ulceration of ankle
⇄	I70.244	Atherosclerosis of native arteries of left leg with ulceration of heel and midfoot
⇄	I70.245	Atherosclerosis of native arteries of left leg with ulceration of other part of foot
⇄	I70.248	Atherosclerosis of native arteries of left leg with ulceration of other part of lower left leg
⇄	I70.291	Other atherosclerosis of native arteries of extremities, right leg
⇄	I70.292	Other atherosclerosis of native arteries of extremities, left leg
	I73.9	Peripheral vascular disease, unspecified
	I77.1	Stricture of artery
	I77.2	Rupture of artery
	I77.79	Dissection of other specified artery
	Z72.0	Tobacco use
	Z87.891	Personal history of nicotine dependence

CCI Edits

Refer to Appendix A for CCI edits.

Pub 100

01656: Pub 100-04, 12, 140.5, Pub 100-04, 12, 50, Pub 100-04, 12, 90.4.5

Base Units

Global: XXX

Code	Base Units
01656	10

Modifiers (PAR)

Code	Mod 50	Mod 51	Mod 62	Mod 80
01656	9	9	9	9

CPT © 2018 American Medical Association. All Rights Reserved.

01670

01670 Anesthesia for all procedures on veins of shoulder and axilla

AMA Coding Guideline

Anesthesia for Procedures on the Shoulder and Axilla

Includes humeral head and neck, sternoclavicular joint, acromioclavicular joint, and shoulder joint.

ICD-10-CM Diagnostic Codes

	I73.9	Peripheral vascular disease, unspecified
	I80.8	Phlebitis and thrombophlebitis of other sites
⇄	I82.621	Acute embolism and thrombosis of deep veins of right upper extremity
⇄	I82.622	Acute embolism and thrombosis of deep veins of left upper extremity
⇄	I82.623	Acute embolism and thrombosis of deep veins of upper extremity, bilateral
⇄	I82.721	Chronic embolism and thrombosis of deep veins of right upper extremity
⇄	I82.722	Chronic embolism and thrombosis of deep veins of left upper extremity
⇄	I82.723	Chronic embolism and thrombosis of deep veins of upper extremity, bilateral
⇄	I82.A11	Acute embolism and thrombosis of right axillary vein
⇄	I82.A12	Acute embolism and thrombosis of left axillary vein
⇄	I82.A13	Acute embolism and thrombosis of axillary vein, bilateral
⇄	I82.A21	Chronic embolism and thrombosis of right axillary vein
⇄	I82.A22	Chronic embolism and thrombosis of left axillary vein
⇄	I82.A23	Chronic embolism and thrombosis of axillary vein, bilateral
⇄	I82.B11	Acute embolism and thrombosis of right subclavian vein
⇄	I82.B12	Acute embolism and thrombosis of left subclavian vein
⇄	I82.B13	Acute embolism and thrombosis of subclavian vein, bilateral
⇄	I82.B21	Chronic embolism and thrombosis of right subclavian vein
⇄	I82.B22	Chronic embolism and thrombosis of left subclavian vein
⇄	I82.B23	Chronic embolism and thrombosis of subclavian vein, bilateral
	I87.1	Compression of vein
	Q27.9	Congenital malformation of peripheral vascular system, unspecified
❼⇄	S45.211	Laceration of axillary or brachial vein, right side
❼⇄	S45.212	Laceration of axillary or brachial vein, left side
❼⇄	S45.291	Other specified injury of axillary or brachial vein, right side
❼⇄	S45.292	Other specified injury of axillary or brachial vein, left side
❼⇄	S45.311	Laceration of superficial vein at shoulder and upper arm level, right arm
❼⇄	S45.312	Laceration of superficial vein at shoulder and upper arm level, left arm
❼⇄	S45.391	Other specified injury of superficial vein at shoulder and upper arm level, right arm
❼⇄	S45.392	Other specified injury of superficial vein at shoulder and upper arm level, left arm
❼⇄	S45.811	Laceration of other specified blood vessels at shoulder and upper arm level, right arm
❼⇄	S45.812	Laceration of other specified blood vessels at shoulder and upper arm level, left arm
❼⇄	S45.891	Other specified injury of other specified blood vessels at shoulder and upper arm level, right arm
❼⇄	S45.892	Other specified injury of other specified blood vessels at shoulder and upper arm level, left arm

ICD-10-CM Coding Notes

For codes requiring a 7th character extension, refer to your ICD-10-CM book. Review the character descriptions and coding guidelines for proper selection. For some procedures, only certain characters will apply.

CCI Edits

Refer to Appendix A for CCI edits.

Pub 100

01670: Pub 100-04, 12, 140.5, Pub 100-04, 12, 50, Pub 100-04, 12, 90.4.5

Base Units

Global: XXX

Code	Base Units
01670	4

Modifiers (PAR)

Code	Mod 50	Mod 51	Mod 62	Mod 80
01670	9	9	9	9

CPT © 2018 American Medical Association. All Rights Reserved.

01680

01680 Anesthesia for shoulder cast application, removal or repair, not otherwise specified

AMA Coding Guideline

Anesthesia for Procedures on the Shoulder and Axilla

Includes humeral head and neck, sternoclavicular joint, acromioclavicular joint, and shoulder joint.

ICD-10-CM Diagnostic Codes

- ➐⇄ S42.221 2-part displaced fracture of surgical neck of right humerus
- ➐⇄ S42.222 2-part displaced fracture of surgical neck of left humerus
- ➐⇄ S42.224 2-part nondisplaced fracture of surgical neck of right humerus
- ➐⇄ S42.225 2-part nondisplaced fracture of surgical neck of left humerus
- ➐⇄ S42.231 3-part fracture of surgical neck of right humerus
- ➐⇄ S42.232 3-part fracture of surgical neck of left humerus
- ➐⇄ S42.241 4-part fracture of surgical neck of right humerus
- ➐⇄ S42.242 4-part fracture of surgical neck of left humerus
- ➐⇄ S42.251 Displaced fracture of greater tuberosity of right humerus
- ➐⇄ S42.252 Displaced fracture of greater tuberosity of left humerus
- ➐⇄ S42.254 Nondisplaced fracture of greater tuberosity of right humerus
- ➐⇄ S42.255 Nondisplaced fracture of greater tuberosity of left humerus
- ➐⇄ S42.261 Displaced fracture of lesser tuberosity of right humerus
- ➐⇄ S42.262 Displaced fracture of lesser tuberosity of left humerus
- ➐⇄ S42.264 Nondisplaced fracture of lesser tuberosity of right humerus
- ➐⇄ S42.265 Nondisplaced fracture of lesser tuberosity of left humerus
- ➐⇄ S42.271 Torus fracture of upper end of right humerus
- ➐⇄ S42.272 Torus fracture of upper end of left humerus
- ➐⇄ S42.291 Other displaced fracture of upper end of right humerus
- ➐⇄ S42.292 Other displaced fracture of upper end of left humerus
- ➐⇄ S42.294 Other nondisplaced fracture of upper end of right humerus
- ➐⇄ S42.295 Other nondisplaced fracture of upper end of left humerus
- ➐⇄ S42.311 Greenstick fracture of shaft of humerus, right arm
- ➐⇄ S42.312 Greenstick fracture of shaft of humerus, left arm
- ➐⇄ S42.321 Displaced transverse fracture of shaft of humerus, right arm
- ➐⇄ S42.322 Displaced transverse fracture of shaft of humerus, left arm
- ➐⇄ S42.324 Nondisplaced transverse fracture of shaft of humerus, right arm
- ➐⇄ S42.325 Nondisplaced transverse fracture of shaft of humerus, left arm
- ➐⇄ S42.331 Displaced oblique fracture of shaft of humerus, right arm
- ➐⇄ S42.342 Displaced spiral fracture of shaft of humerus, left arm
- ➐⇄ S42.344 Nondisplaced spiral fracture of shaft of humerus, right arm
- ➐⇄ S42.345 Nondisplaced spiral fracture of shaft of humerus, left arm
- ➐⇄ S42.351 Displaced comminuted fracture of shaft of humerus, right arm
- ➐⇄ S42.352 Displaced comminuted fracture of shaft of humerus, left arm
- ➐⇄ S42.354 Nondisplaced comminuted fracture of shaft of humerus, right arm
- ➐⇄ S42.355 Nondisplaced comminuted fracture of shaft of humerus, left arm
- ➐⇄ S42.361 Displaced segmental fracture of shaft of humerus, right arm
- ➐⇄ S42.362 Displaced segmental fracture of shaft of humerus, left arm
- ➐⇄ S42.364 Nondisplaced segmental fracture of shaft of humerus, right arm
- ➐⇄ S42.365 Nondisplaced segmental fracture of shaft of humerus, left arm
- ➐⇄ S42.391 Other fracture of shaft of right humerus
- ➐⇄ S42.392 Other fracture of shaft of left humerus
- ➐⇄ S49.031 Salter-Harris Type III physeal fracture of upper end of humerus, right arm
- ➐⇄ S49.032 Salter-Harris Type III physeal fracture of upper end of humerus, left arm
- ➐⇄ S49.041 Salter-Harris Type IV physeal fracture of upper end of humerus, right arm
- ➐⇄ S49.042 Salter-Harris Type IV physeal fracture of upper end of humerus, left arm
- ➐⇄ S49.091 Other physeal fracture of upper end of humerus, right arm
- ➐⇄ S49.092 Other physeal fracture of upper end of humerus, left arm

ICD-10-CM Coding Notes

For codes requiring a 7th character extension, refer to your ICD-10-CM book. Review the character descriptions and coding guidelines for proper selection. For some procedures, only certain characters will apply.

CCI Edits

Refer to Appendix A for CCI edits.

Pub 100

01680: Pub 100-04, 12, 140.5, Pub 100-04, 12, 50, Pub 100-04, 12, 90.4.5

Base Units

Global: XXX

Code	Base Units
01680	3

Modifiers (PAR)

Code	Mod 50	Mod 51	Mod 62	Mod 80
01680	9	9	9	9

CPT © 2018 American Medical Association. All Rights Reserved.

01710

01710 Anesthesia for procedures on nerves, muscles, tendons, fascia, and bursae of upper arm and elbow; not otherwise specified

AMA *CPT Assistant* ▯

01710: Mar 06: 15, Nov 07: 8, Oct 11: 3, Jul 12: 13

ICD-10-CM Diagnostic Codes

⇄	G56.11	Other lesions of median nerve, right upper limb
⇄	G56.12	Other lesions of median nerve, left upper limb
⇄	G56.13	Other lesions of median nerve, bilateral upper limbs
⇄	G56.21	Lesion of ulnar nerve, right upper limb
⇄	G56.22	Lesion of ulnar nerve, left upper limb
⇄	G56.23	Lesion of ulnar nerve, bilateral upper limbs
⇄	G56.31	Lesion of radial nerve, right upper limb
⇄	G56.32	Lesion of radial nerve, left upper limb
⇄	G56.33	Lesion of radial nerve, bilateral upper limbs
⇄	G56.81	Other specified mononeuropathies of right upper limb
⇄	G56.82	Other specified mononeuropathies of left upper limb
⇄	G56.83	Other specified mononeuropathies of bilateral upper limbs
⇄	M62.021	Separation of muscle (nontraumatic), right upper arm
⇄	M62.022	Separation of muscle (nontraumatic), left upper arm
⇄	M62.121	Other rupture of muscle (nontraumatic), right upper arm
⇄	M62.122	Other rupture of muscle (nontraumatic), left upper arm
⇄	M62.421	Contracture of muscle, right upper arm
⇄	M62.422	Contracture of muscle, left upper arm
⇄	M65.021	Abscess of tendon sheath, right upper arm
⇄	M65.022	Abscess of tendon sheath, left upper arm
⇄	M66.221	Spontaneous rupture of extensor tendons, right upper arm
⇄	M66.222	Spontaneous rupture of extensor tendons, left upper arm
⇄	M66.321	Spontaneous rupture of flexor tendons, right upper arm
⇄	M66.322	Spontaneous rupture of flexor tendons, left upper arm
⇄	M70.21	Olecranon bursitis, right elbow
⇄	M70.22	Olecranon bursitis, left elbow
⇄	M70.31	Other bursitis of elbow, right elbow
⇄	M70.32	Other bursitis of elbow, left elbow
⇄	M71.021	Abscess of bursa, right elbow
⇄	M71.022	Abscess of bursa, left elbow
⇄	M79.A11	Nontraumatic compartment syndrome of right upper extremity
⇄	M79.A12	Nontraumatic compartment syndrome of left upper extremity
⑦⇄	S41.111	Laceration without foreign body of right upper arm
⑦⇄	S41.112	Laceration without foreign body of left upper arm
⑦⇄	S41.121	Laceration with foreign body of right upper arm
⑦⇄	S41.122	Laceration with foreign body of left upper arm
⑦⇄	S41.151	Open bite of right upper arm
⑦⇄	S41.152	Open bite of left upper arm
⑦⇄	S44.11	Injury of median nerve at upper arm level, right arm
⑦⇄	S44.12	Injury of median nerve at upper arm level, left arm
⑦⇄	S44.21	Injury of radial nerve at upper arm level, right arm
⑦⇄	S44.22	Injury of radial nerve at upper arm level, left arm
⑦⇄	S44.41	Injury of musculocutaneous nerve, right arm
⑦⇄	S44.42	Injury of musculocutaneous nerve, left arm
⑦⇄	S44.51	Injury of cutaneous sensory nerve at shoulder and upper arm level, right arm
⑦⇄	S44.52	Injury of cutaneous sensory nerve at shoulder and upper arm level, left arm
⑦⇄	S46.211	Strain of muscle, fascia and tendon of other parts of biceps, right arm
⑦⇄	S46.212	Strain of muscle, fascia and tendon of other parts of biceps, left arm
⑦⇄	S46.221	Laceration of muscle, fascia and tendon of other parts of biceps, right arm
⑦⇄	S46.222	Laceration of muscle, fascia and tendon of other parts of biceps, left arm
⑦⇄	S46.311	Strain of muscle, fascia and tendon of triceps, right arm
⑦⇄	S46.312	Strain of muscle, fascia and tendon of triceps, left arm
⑦⇄	S46.321	Laceration of muscle, fascia and tendon of triceps, right arm
⑦⇄	S46.322	Laceration of muscle, fascia and tendon of triceps, left arm
⑦⇄	S46.811	Strain of other muscles, fascia and tendons at shoulder and upper arm level, right arm
⑦⇄	S46.812	Strain of other muscles, fascia and tendons at shoulder and upper arm level, left arm
⑦⇄	S46.821	Laceration of other muscles, fascia and tendons at shoulder and upper arm level, right arm
⑦⇄	S46.822	Laceration of other muscles, fascia and tendons at shoulder and upper arm level, left arm
⑦⇄	T79.A11	Traumatic compartment syndrome of right upper extremity
⑦⇄	T79.A12	Traumatic compartment syndrome of left upper extremity

ICD-10-CM Coding Notes

For codes requiring a 7th character extension, refer to your ICD-10-CM book. Review the character descriptions and coding guidelines for proper selection. For some procedures, only certain characters will apply.

CCI Edits

Refer to Appendix A for CCI edits.

Pub 100

01710: Pub 100-04, 12, 140.5, Pub 100-04, 12, 50, Pub 100-04, 12, 90.4.5

Base Units

Global: XXX

Code	Base Units
01710	3

Modifiers (PAR)

Code	Mod 50	Mod 51	Mod 62	Mod 80
01710	9	9	9	9

CPT © 2018 American Medical Association. All Rights Reserved.

01712

01712 Anesthesia for procedures on nerves, muscles, tendons, fascia, and bursae of upper arm and elbow; tenotomy, elbow to shoulder, open

ICD-10-CM Diagnostic Codes

⇄ M21.221 Flexion deformity, right elbow
⇄ M21.222 Flexion deformity, left elbow
⇄ M25.321 Other instability, right elbow
⇄ M25.322 Other instability, left elbow
⇄ M62.421 Contracture of muscle, right upper arm
⇄ M62.422 Contracture of muscle, left upper arm
⇄ M65.021 Abscess of tendon sheath, right upper arm
⇄ M65.022 Abscess of tendon sheath, left upper arm
⇄ M65.121 Other infective (teno)synovitis, right elbow
⇄ M65.122 Other infective (teno)synovitis, left elbow
⇄ M65.221 Calcific tendinitis, right upper arm
⇄ M65.222 Calcific tendinitis, left upper arm
⇄ M65.821 Other synovitis and tenosynovitis, right upper arm
⇄ M65.822 Other synovitis and tenosynovitis, left upper arm
⇄ M67.823 Other specified disorders of tendon, right elbow
⇄ M67.824 Other specified disorders of tendon, left elbow

CCI Edits

Refer to Appendix A for CCI edits.

Pub 100

01712: Pub 100-04, 12, 140.5, Pub 100-04, 12, 50, Pub 100-04, 12, 90.4.5

Base Units

Global: XXX

Code	Base Units
01712	5

Modifiers (PAR)

Code	Mod 50	Mod 51	Mod 62	Mod 80
01712	9	9	9	9

CPT © 2018 American Medical Association. All Rights Reserved.

01714

01714 Anesthesia for procedures on nerves, muscles, tendons, fascia, and bursae of upper arm and elbow; tenoplasty, elbow to shoulder

ICD-10-CM Diagnostic Codes

	G54.0	Brachial plexus disorders
	P14.0	Erb's paralysis due to birth injury
	P14.1	Klumpke's paralysis due to birth injury
	P14.3	Other brachial plexus birth injuries
❼	S14.3	Injury of brachial plexus

ICD-10-CM Coding Notes

For codes requiring a 7th character extension, refer to your ICD-10-CM book. Review the character descriptions and coding guidelines for proper selection. For some procedures, only certain characters will apply.

CCI Edits

Refer to Appendix A for CCI edits.

Pub 100

01714: Pub 100-04, 12, 140.5, Pub 100-04, 12, 50, Pub 100-04, 12, 90.4.5

Base Units

Global: XXX

Code	Base Units
01714	5

Modifiers (PAR)

Code	Mod 50	Mod 51	Mod 62	Mod 80
01714	9	9	9	9

CPT © 2018 American Medical Association. All Rights Reserved.

01716

01716 Anesthesia for procedures on nerves, muscles, tendons, fascia, and bursae of upper arm and elbow; tenodesis, rupture of long tendon of biceps

ICD-10-CM Diagnostic Codes

⇄	M62.011	Separation of muscle (nontraumatic), right shoulder
⇄	M62.012	Separation of muscle (nontraumatic), left shoulder
⇄	M62.111	Other rupture of muscle (nontraumatic), right shoulder
⇄	M62.112	Other rupture of muscle (nontraumatic), left shoulder
⇄	M75.21	Bicipital tendinitis, right shoulder
⇄	M75.22	Bicipital tendinitis, left shoulder
⇄	M75.31	Calcific tendinitis of right shoulder
⇄	M75.32	Calcific tendinitis of left shoulder
⇄	M75.41	Impingement syndrome of right shoulder
⇄	M75.42	Impingement syndrome of left shoulder
➐⇄	S46.111	Strain of muscle, fascia and tendon of long head of biceps, right arm
➐⇄	S46.112	Strain of muscle, fascia and tendon of long head of biceps, left arm

ICD-10-CM Coding Notes

For codes requiring a 7th character extension, refer to your ICD-10-CM book. Review the character descriptions and coding guidelines for proper selection. For some procedures, only certain characters will apply.

CCI Edits

Refer to Appendix A for CCI edits.

Pub 100

01716: Pub 100-04, 12, 140.5, Pub 100-04, 12, 50, Pub 100-04, 12, 90.4.5

Base Units

Global: XXX

Code	Base Units
01716	5

Modifiers (PAR)

Code	Mod 50	Mod 51	Mod 62	Mod 80
01716	9	9	9	9

CPT © 2018 American Medical Association. All Rights Reserved.

01730

01730 Anesthesia for all closed procedures on humerus and elbow

ICD-10-CM Diagnostic Codes

⇄ M70.31 Other bursitis of elbow, right elbow
⇄ M70.32 Other bursitis of elbow, left elbow
⇄ M77.01 Medial epicondylitis, right elbow
⇄ M77.02 Medial epicondylitis, left elbow
➐⇄ S42.411 Displaced simple supracondylar fracture without intercondylar fracture of right humerus
➐⇄ S42.412 Displaced simple supracondylar fracture without intercondylar fracture of left humerus
➐⇄ S42.421 Displaced comminuted supracondylar fracture without intercondylar fracture of right humerus
➐⇄ S42.422 Displaced comminuted supracondylar fracture without intercondylar fracture of left humerus
➐⇄ S42.431 Displaced fracture (avulsion) of lateral epicondyle of right humerus
➐⇄ S42.432 Displaced fracture (avulsion) of lateral epicondyle of left humerus
➐⇄ S42.441 Displaced fracture (avulsion) of medial epicondyle of right humerus
➐⇄ S42.442 Displaced fracture (avulsion) of medial epicondyle of left humerus
➐⇄ S42.444 Nondisplaced fracture (avulsion) of medial epicondyle of right humerus
➐⇄ S42.445 Nondisplaced fracture (avulsion) of medial epicondyle of left humerus
➐⇄ S42.447 Incarcerated fracture (avulsion) of medial epicondyle of right humerus
➐⇄ S42.448 Incarcerated fracture (avulsion) of medial epicondyle of left humerus
➐⇄ S42.451 Displaced fracture of lateral condyle of right humerus
➐⇄ S42.452 Displaced fracture of lateral condyle of left humerus
➐⇄ S42.461 Displaced fracture of medial condyle of right humerus
➐⇄ S42.462 Displaced fracture of medial condyle of left humerus
➐⇄ S42.464 Nondisplaced fracture of medial condyle of right humerus
➐⇄ S42.465 Nondisplaced fracture of medial condyle of left humerus
➐⇄ S42.471 Displaced transcondylar fracture of right humerus
➐⇄ S42.472 Displaced transcondylar fracture of left humerus
➐⇄ S42.491 Other displaced fracture of lower end of right humerus
➐⇄ S42.492 Other displaced fracture of lower end of left humerus
➐⇄ S52.021 Displaced fracture of olecranon process without intraarticular extension of right ulna
➐⇄ S52.022 Displaced fracture of olecranon process without intraarticular extension of left ulna
➐⇄ S52.031 Displaced fracture of olecranon process with intraarticular extension of right ulna
➐⇄ S52.032 Displaced fracture of olecranon process with intraarticular extension of left ulna
➐⇄ S52.041 Displaced fracture of coronoid process of right ulna
➐⇄ S52.042 Displaced fracture of coronoid process of left ulna
➐⇄ S52.091 Other fracture of upper end of right ulna
➐⇄ S52.092 Other fracture of upper end of left ulna
➐⇄ S52.121 Displaced fracture of head of right radius
➐⇄ S52.122 Displaced fracture of head of left radius
➐⇄ S52.131 Displaced fracture of neck of right radius
➐⇄ S52.132 Displaced fracture of neck of left radius
➐⇄ S52.181 Other fracture of upper end of right radius
➐⇄ S52.182 Other fracture of upper end of left radius
➐⇄ S53.011 Anterior subluxation of right radial head
➐⇄ S53.012 Anterior subluxation of left radial head
➐⇄ S53.014 Anterior dislocation of right radial head
➐⇄ S53.015 Anterior dislocation of left radial head
➐⇄ S53.021 Posterior subluxation of right radial head
➐⇄ S53.022 Posterior subluxation of left radial head
➐⇄ S53.024 Posterior dislocation of right radial head
➐⇄ S53.025 Posterior dislocation of left radial head
➐⇄ S53.111 Anterior subluxation of right ulnohumeral joint
➐⇄ S53.112 Anterior subluxation of left ulnohumeral joint
➐⇄ S53.114 Anterior dislocation of right ulnohumeral joint
➐⇄ S53.115 Anterior dislocation of left ulnohumeral joint
➐⇄ S53.121 Posterior subluxation of right ulnohumeral joint
➐⇄ S53.122 Posterior subluxation of left ulnohumeral joint
➐⇄ S53.124 Posterior dislocation of right ulnohumeral joint
➐⇄ S53.125 Posterior dislocation of left ulnohumeral joint
➐⇄ S53.131 Medial subluxation of right ulnohumeral joint
➐⇄ S53.132 Medial subluxation of left ulnohumeral joint
➐⇄ S53.134 Medial dislocation of right ulnohumeral joint
➐⇄ S53.135 Medial dislocation of left ulnohumeral joint
➐⇄ S53.141 Lateral subluxation of right ulnohumeral joint
➐⇄ S53.142 Lateral subluxation of left ulnohumeral joint
➐⇄ S53.144 Lateral dislocation of right ulnohumeral joint
➐⇄ S53.145 Lateral dislocation of left ulnohumeral joint

ICD-10-CM Coding Notes

For codes requiring a 7th character extension, refer to your ICD-10-CM book. Review the character descriptions and coding guidelines for proper selection. For some procedures, only certain characters will apply.

CCI Edits

Refer to Appendix A for CCI edits.

Pub 100

01730: Pub 100-04, 12, 140.5, Pub 100-04, 12, 50, Pub 100-04, 12, 90.4.5

Base Units

Global: XXX

Code	Base Units
01730	3

Modifiers (PAR)

Code	Mod 50	Mod 51	Mod 62	Mod 80
01730	9	9	9	9

CPT © 2018 American Medical Association. All Rights Reserved.

01732

01732 Anesthesia for diagnostic arthroscopic procedures of elbow joint

ICD-10-CM Diagnostic Codes

⇄ M05.721 Rheumatoid arthritis with rheumatoid factor of right elbow without organ or systems involvement
⇄ M05.722 Rheumatoid arthritis with rheumatoid factor of left elbow without organ or systems involvement
⇄ M05.821 Other rheumatoid arthritis with rheumatoid factor of right elbow
⇄ M05.822 Other rheumatoid arthritis with rheumatoid factor of left elbow
⇄ M06.021 Rheumatoid arthritis without rheumatoid factor, right elbow
⇄ M06.022 Rheumatoid arthritis without rheumatoid factor, left elbow
⇄ M06.321 Rheumatoid nodule, right elbow
⇄ M06.322 Rheumatoid nodule, left elbow
⇄ M08.221 Juvenile rheumatoid arthritis with systemic onset, right elbow
⇄ M08.222 Juvenile rheumatoid arthritis with systemic onset, left elbow
⇄ M08.421 Pauciarticular juvenile rheumatoid arthritis, right elbow
⇄ M08.422 Pauciarticular juvenile rheumatoid arthritis, left elbow
⇄ M08.821 Other juvenile arthritis, right elbow
⇄ M08.822 Other juvenile arthritis, left elbow
⇄ M12.221 Villonodular synovitis (pigmented), right elbow
⇄ M12.222 Villonodular synovitis (pigmented), left elbow
⇄ M12.521 Traumatic arthropathy, right elbow
⇄ M12.522 Traumatic arthropathy, left elbow
⇄ M12.821 Other specific arthropathies, not elsewhere classified, right elbow
⇄ M12.822 Other specific arthropathies, not elsewhere classified, left elbow
⇄ M13.121 Monoarthritis, not elsewhere classified, right elbow
⇄ M13.122 Monoarthritis, not elsewhere classified, left elbow
⇄ M19.021 Primary osteoarthritis, right elbow
⇄ M19.022 Primary osteoarthritis, left elbow
⇄ M19.121 Post-traumatic osteoarthritis, right elbow
⇄ M19.122 Post-traumatic osteoarthritis, left elbow
⇄ M24.121 Other articular cartilage disorders, right elbow
⇄ M24.122 Other articular cartilage disorders, left elbow
⇄ M24.221 Disorder of ligament, right elbow
⇄ M24.222 Disorder of ligament, left elbow
⇄ M67.821 Other specified disorders of synovium, right elbow
⇄ M67.822 Other specified disorders of synovium, left elbow
⇄ M77.01 Medial epicondylitis, right elbow
⇄ M77.02 Medial epicondylitis, left elbow
⇄ M77.11 Lateral epicondylitis, right elbow
⇄ M77.12 Lateral epicondylitis, left elbow
⇄ M93.221 Osteochondritis dissecans, right elbow
⇄ M93.222 Osteochondritis dissecans, left elbow

CCI Edits

Refer to Appendix A for CCI edits.

Pub 100

01732: Pub 100-04, 12, 140.5, Pub 100-04, 12, 50, Pub 100-04, 12, 90.4.5

Base Units

Global: XXX

Code	Base Units
01732	3

Modifiers (PAR)

Code	Mod 50	Mod 51	Mod 62	Mod 80
01732	9	9	9	9

CPT © 2018 American Medical Association. All Rights Reserved.

01740

01740 Anesthesia for open or surgical arthroscopic procedures of the elbow; not otherwise specified

ICD-10-CM Diagnostic Codes

⇄ M05.721 Rheumatoid arthritis with rheumatoid factor of right elbow without organ or systems involvement
⇄ M05.722 Rheumatoid arthritis with rheumatoid factor of left elbow without organ or systems involvement
⇄ M05.821 Other rheumatoid arthritis with rheumatoid factor of right elbow
⇄ M05.822 Other rheumatoid arthritis with rheumatoid factor of left elbow
⇄ M06.021 Rheumatoid arthritis without rheumatoid factor, right elbow
⇄ M06.022 Rheumatoid arthritis without rheumatoid factor, left elbow
⇄ M06.321 Rheumatoid nodule, right elbow
⇄ M06.322 Rheumatoid nodule, left elbow
⇄ M12.221 Villonodular synovitis (pigmented), right elbow
⇄ M12.222 Villonodular synovitis (pigmented), left elbow
⇄ M12.521 Traumatic arthropathy, right elbow
⇄ M12.522 Traumatic arthropathy, left elbow
⇄ M19.021 Primary osteoarthritis, right elbow
⇄ M19.022 Primary osteoarthritis, left elbow
⇄ M24.021 Loose body in right elbow
⇄ M24.022 Loose body in left elbow
⇄ M24.121 Other articular cartilage disorders, right elbow
⇄ M24.122 Other articular cartilage disorders, left elbow
⇄ M67.821 Other specified disorders of synovium, right elbow
⇄ M67.822 Other specified disorders of synovium, left elbow
⇄ M77.01 Medial epicondylitis, right elbow
⇄ M77.02 Medial epicondylitis, left elbow
⇄ M77.11 Lateral epicondylitis, right elbow
⇄ M77.12 Lateral epicondylitis, left elbow
⇄ M93.221 Osteochondritis dissecans, right elbow
⇄ M93.222 Osteochondritis dissecans, left elbow
❼⇄ S42.421 Displaced comminuted supracondylar fracture without intercondylar fracture of right humerus
❼⇄ S42.422 Displaced comminuted supracondylar fracture without intercondylar fracture of left humerus
❼⇄ S42.431 Displaced fracture (avulsion) of lateral epicondyle of right humerus
❼⇄ S42.432 Displaced fracture (avulsion) of lateral epicondyle of left humerus
❼⇄ S42.441 Displaced fracture (avulsion) of medial epicondyle of right humerus
❼⇄ S42.442 Displaced fracture (avulsion) of medial epicondyle of left humerus
❼⇄ S42.447 Incarcerated fracture (avulsion) of medial epicondyle of right humerus
❼⇄ S42.448 Incarcerated fracture (avulsion) of medial epicondyle of left humerus
❼⇄ S42.451 Displaced fracture of lateral condyle of right humerus
❼⇄ S42.452 Displaced fracture of lateral condyle of left humerus
❼⇄ S42.461 Displaced fracture of medial condyle of right humerus
❼⇄ S42.462 Displaced fracture of medial condyle of left humerus
❼⇄ S42.471 Displaced transcondylar fracture of right humerus
❼⇄ S42.472 Displaced transcondylar fracture of left humerus
❼⇄ S42.491 Other displaced fracture of lower end of right humerus
❼⇄ S42.492 Other displaced fracture of lower end of left humerus
❼⇄ S49.131 Salter-Harris Type III physeal fracture of lower end of humerus, right arm
❼⇄ S49.132 Salter-Harris Type III physeal fracture of lower end of humerus, left arm
❼⇄ S49.141 Salter-Harris Type IV physeal fracture of lower end of humerus, right arm
❼⇄ S49.142 Salter-Harris Type IV physeal fracture of lower end of humerus, left arm
❼⇄ S52.021 Displaced fracture of olecranon process without intraarticular extension of right ulna
❼⇄ S52.022 Displaced fracture of olecranon process without intraarticular extension of left ulna
❼⇄ S52.031 Displaced fracture of olecranon process with intraarticular extension of right ulna
❼⇄ S52.032 Displaced fracture of olecranon process with intraarticular extension of left ulna
❼⇄ S52.041 Displaced fracture of coronoid process of right ulna
❼⇄ S52.042 Displaced fracture of coronoid process of left ulna
❼⇄ S52.121 Displaced fracture of head of right radius
❼⇄ S52.122 Displaced fracture of head of left radius
❼⇄ S52.131 Displaced fracture of neck of right radius
❼⇄ S52.132 Displaced fracture of neck of left radius
❼⇄ S52.271 Monteggia's fracture of right ulna
❼⇄ S52.272 Monteggia's fracture of left ulna
❼⇄ S53.014 Anterior dislocation of right radial head
❼⇄ S53.015 Anterior dislocation of left radial head
❼⇄ S53.024 Posterior dislocation of right radial head
❼⇄ S53.025 Posterior dislocation of left radial head
❼⇄ S53.094 Other dislocation of right radial head
❼⇄ S53.095 Other dislocation of left radial head
❼⇄ S53.114 Anterior dislocation of right ulnohumeral joint
❼⇄ S53.115 Anterior dislocation of left ulnohumeral joint
❼⇄ S53.124 Posterior dislocation of right ulnohumeral joint
❼⇄ S53.125 Posterior dislocation of left ulnohumeral joint
❼⇄ S53.134 Medial dislocation of right ulnohumeral joint
❼⇄ S53.135 Medial dislocation of left ulnohumeral joint
❼⇄ S53.144 Lateral dislocation of right ulnohumeral joint
❼⇄ S53.145 Lateral dislocation of left ulnohumeral joint
❼⇄ S53.194 Other dislocation of right ulnohumeral joint
❼⇄ S53.195 Other dislocation of left ulnohumeral joint
❼⇄ S53.21 Traumatic rupture of right radial collateral ligament
❼⇄ S53.22 Traumatic rupture of left radial collateral ligament
❼⇄ S53.31 Traumatic rupture of right ulnar collateral ligament
❼⇄ S53.32 Traumatic rupture of left ulnar collateral ligament

ICD-10-CM Coding Notes

For codes requiring a 7th character extension, refer to your ICD-10-CM book. Review the character descriptions and coding guidelines for proper selection. For some procedures, only certain characters will apply.

CCI Edits

Refer to Appendix A for CCI edits.

Pub 100

01740: Pub 100-04, 12, 140.5, Pub 100-04, 12, 50, Pub 100-04, 12, 90.4.5

Base Units

Global: XXX

Code	Base Units
01740	4

Modifiers (PAR)

Code	Mod 50	Mod 51	Mod 62	Mod 80
01740	9	9	9	9

● New ▲ Revised ✚ Add On ⊘Modifier 51 Exempt ★Telemedicine ☐ CPT QuickRef ⁄⁄FDA Pending ⇄ Laterality ❼ Seventh Character ♂Male ♀Female

CPT © 2018 American Medical Association. All Rights Reserved.

01742

01742 Anesthesia for open or surgical arthroscopic procedures of the elbow; osteotomy of humerus

ICD-10-CM Diagnostic Codes

⇄	C40.01	Malignant neoplasm of scapula and long bones of right upper limb
⇄	C40.02	Malignant neoplasm of scapula and long bones of left upper limb
⇄	D16.01	Benign neoplasm of scapula and long bones of right upper limb
⇄	D16.02	Benign neoplasm of scapula and long bones of left upper limb
	D48.0	Neoplasm of uncertain behavior of bone and articular cartilage
	D49.2	Neoplasm of unspecified behavior of bone, soft tissue, and skin
⇄	L89.014	Pressure ulcer of right elbow, stage 4
⇄	L89.024	Pressure ulcer of left elbow, stage 4
⇄	M19.021	Primary osteoarthritis, right elbow
⇄	M19.022	Primary osteoarthritis, left elbow
⇄	M19.121	Post-traumatic osteoarthritis, right elbow
⇄	M19.122	Post-traumatic osteoarthritis, left elbow
⇄	M21.021	Valgus deformity, not elsewhere classified, right elbow
⇄	M21.022	Valgus deformity, not elsewhere classified, left elbow
⇄	M21.121	Varus deformity, not elsewhere classified, right elbow
⇄	M21.122	Varus deformity, not elsewhere classified, left elbow
	Q68.8	Other specified congenital musculoskeletal deformities
	Q77.8	Other osteochondrodysplasia with defects of growth of tubular bones and spine
	Q78.4	Enchondromatosis
➐⇄	S42.421	Displaced comminuted supracondylar fracture without intercondylar fracture of right humerus
➐⇄	S42.422	Displaced comminuted supracondylar fracture without intercondylar fracture of left humerus
➐⇄	S42.431	Displaced fracture (avulsion) of lateral epicondyle of right humerus
➐⇄	S42.432	Displaced fracture (avulsion) of lateral epicondyle of left humerus
➐⇄	S42.441	Displaced fracture (avulsion) of medial epicondyle of right humerus
➐⇄	S42.442	Displaced fracture (avulsion) of medial epicondyle of left humerus
➐⇄	S42.451	Displaced fracture of lateral condyle of right humerus
➐⇄	S42.452	Displaced fracture of lateral condyle of left humerus
➐⇄	S42.461	Displaced fracture of medial condyle of right humerus
➐⇄	S42.462	Displaced fracture of medial condyle of left humerus
➐⇄	S42.471	Displaced transcondylar fracture of right humerus
➐⇄	S42.472	Displaced transcondylar fracture of left humerus
➐⇄	S42.491	Other displaced fracture of lower end of right humerus
➐⇄	S42.492	Other displaced fracture of lower end of left humerus

ICD-10-CM Coding Notes

For codes requiring a 7th character extension, refer to your ICD-10-CM book. Review the character descriptions and coding guidelines for proper selection. For some procedures, only certain characters will apply.

CCI Edits

Refer to Appendix A for CCI edits.

Pub 100

01742: Pub 100-04, 12, 140.5, Pub 100-04, 12, 50, Pub 100-04, 12, 90.4.5

Base Units

Global: XXX

Code	Base Units
01742	5

Modifiers (PAR)

Code	Mod 50	Mod 51	Mod 62	Mod 80
01742	9	9	9	9

CPT © 2018 American Medical Association. All Rights Reserved.

01744

01744 Anesthesia for open or surgical arthroscopic procedures of the elbow; repair of nonunion or malunion of humerus

ICD-10-CM Diagnostic Codes

- ➐⇄ M80.021 Age-related osteoporosis with current pathological fracture, right humerus
- ➐⇄ M80.022 Age-related osteoporosis with current pathological fracture, left humerus
- ➐⇄ M80.821 Other osteoporosis with current pathological fracture, right humerus
- ➐⇄ M80.822 Other osteoporosis with current pathological fracture, left humerus
- ➐⇄ M84.321 Stress fracture, right humerus
- ➐⇄ M84.322 Stress fracture, left humerus
- ➐⇄ M84.421 Pathological fracture, right humerus
- ➐⇄ M84.422 Pathological fracture, left humerus
- ➐⇄ M84.521 Pathological fracture in neoplastic disease, right humerus
- ➐⇄ M84.522 Pathological fracture in neoplastic disease, left humerus
- ➐⇄ S42.411 Displaced simple supracondylar fracture without intercondylar fracture of right humerus
- ➐⇄ S42.412 Displaced simple supracondylar fracture without intercondylar fracture of left humerus
- ➐⇄ S42.414 Nondisplaced simple supracondylar fracture without intercondylar fracture of right humerus
- ➐⇄ S42.415 Nondisplaced simple supracondylar fracture without intercondylar fracture of left humerus
- ➐⇄ S42.421 Displaced comminuted supracondylar fracture without intercondylar fracture of right humerus
- ➐⇄ S42.422 Displaced comminuted supracondylar fracture without intercondylar fracture of left humerus
- ➐⇄ S42.424 Nondisplaced comminuted supracondylar fracture without intercondylar fracture of right humerus
- ➐⇄ S42.425 Nondisplaced comminuted supracondylar fracture without intercondylar fracture of left humerus
- ➐⇄ S42.431 Displaced fracture (avulsion) of lateral epicondyle of right humerus
- ➐⇄ S42.432 Displaced fracture (avulsion) of lateral epicondyle of left humerus
- ➐⇄ S42.434 Nondisplaced fracture (avulsion) of lateral epicondyle of right humerus
- ➐⇄ S42.435 Nondisplaced fracture (avulsion) of lateral epicondyle of left humerus
- ➐⇄ S42.441 Displaced fracture (avulsion) of medial epicondyle of right humerus
- ➐⇄ S42.442 Displaced fracture (avulsion) of medial epicondyle of left humerus
- ➐⇄ S42.444 Nondisplaced fracture (avulsion) of medial epicondyle of right humerus
- ➐⇄ S42.445 Nondisplaced fracture (avulsion) of medial epicondyle of left humerus
- ➐⇄ S42.447 Incarcerated fracture (avulsion) of medial epicondyle of right humerus
- ➐⇄ S42.448 Incarcerated fracture (avulsion) of medial epicondyle of left humerus
- ➐⇄ S42.451 Displaced fracture of lateral condyle of right humerus
- ➐⇄ S42.452 Displaced fracture of lateral condyle of left humerus
- ➐⇄ S42.454 Nondisplaced fracture of lateral condyle of right humerus
- ➐⇄ S42.461 Displaced fracture of medial condyle of right humerus
- ➐⇄ S42.462 Displaced fracture of medial condyle of left humerus
- ➐⇄ S42.464 Nondisplaced fracture of medial condyle of right humerus
- ➐⇄ S42.465 Nondisplaced fracture of medial condyle of left humerus
- ➐⇄ S42.471 Displaced transcondylar fracture of right humerus
- ➐⇄ S42.472 Displaced transcondylar fracture of left humerus
- ➐⇄ S42.474 Nondisplaced transcondylar fracture of right humerus
- ➐⇄ S42.475 Nondisplaced transcondylar fracture of left humerus
- ➐⇄ S42.491 Other displaced fracture of lower end of right humerus
- ➐⇄ S42.492 Other displaced fracture of lower end of left humerus
- ➐⇄ S42.494 Other nondisplaced fracture of lower end of right humerus
- ➐⇄ S42.495 Other nondisplaced fracture of lower end of left humerus

ICD-10-CM Coding Notes

For codes requiring a 7th character extension, refer to your ICD-10-CM book. Review the character descriptions and coding guidelines for proper selection. For some procedures, only certain characters will apply.

CCI Edits

Refer to Appendix A for CCI edits.

Pub 100

01744: Pub 100-04, 12, 140.5, Pub 100-04, 12, 50, Pub 100-04, 12, 90.4.5

Base Units

Global: XXX

Code	Base Units
01744	5

Modifiers (PAR)

Code	Mod 50	Mod 51	Mod 62	Mod 80
01744	9	9	9	9

CPT © 2018 American Medical Association. All Rights Reserved.

01756

01756 Anesthesia for open or surgical arthroscopic procedures of the elbow; radical procedures

ICD-10-CM Diagnostic Codes

⇄	C40.01	Malignant neoplasm of scapula and long bones of right upper limb
⇄	C40.02	Malignant neoplasm of scapula and long bones of left upper limb
⇄	C47.11	Malignant neoplasm of peripheral nerves of right upper limb, including shoulder
⇄	C47.12	Malignant neoplasm of peripheral nerves of left upper limb, including shoulder
⇄	C49.11	Malignant neoplasm of connective and soft tissue of right upper limb, including shoulder
⇄	C49.12	Malignant neoplasm of connective and soft tissue of left upper limb, including shoulder
❼⇄	S57.01	Crushing injury of right elbow
❼⇄	S57.02	Crushing injury of left elbow
❼⇄	S58.011	Complete traumatic amputation at elbow level, right arm
❼⇄	S58.012	Complete traumatic amputation at elbow level, left arm
❼⇄	S58.021	Partial traumatic amputation at elbow level, right arm
❼⇄	S58.022	Partial traumatic amputation at elbow level, left arm
⇄	T87.0X1	Complications of reattached (part of) right upper extremity
⇄	T87.0X2	Complications of reattached (part of) left upper extremity
⇄	T87.31	Neuroma of amputation stump, right upper extremity
⇄	T87.32	Neuroma of amputation stump, left upper extremity
⇄	T87.41	Infection of amputation stump, right upper extremity
⇄	T87.42	Infection of amputation stump, left upper extremity
⇄	T87.51	Necrosis of amputation stump, right upper extremity
⇄	T87.52	Necrosis of amputation stump, left upper extremity

ICD-10-CM Coding Notes

For codes requiring a 7th character extension, refer to your ICD-10-CM book. Review the character descriptions and coding guidelines for proper selection. For some procedures, only certain characters will apply.

CCI Edits

Refer to Appendix A for CCI edits.

Pub 100

01756: Pub 100-04, 12, 140.5, Pub 100-04, 12, 50, Pub 100-04, 12, 90.4.5

Base Units

Global: XXX

Code	Base Units
01756	6

Modifiers (PAR)

Code	Mod 50	Mod 51	Mod 62	Mod 80
01756	9	9	9	9

CPT © 2018 American Medical Association. All Rights Reserved.

01758

01758 Anesthesia for open or surgical arthroscopic procedures of the elbow; excision of cyst or tumor of humerus

ICD-10-CM Diagnostic Codes

⇄	C40.01	Malignant neoplasm of scapula and long bones of right upper limb
⇄	C40.02	Malignant neoplasm of scapula and long bones of left upper limb
⇄	D16.01	Benign neoplasm of scapula and long bones of right upper limb
⇄	D16.02	Benign neoplasm of scapula and long bones of left upper limb
	D48.0	Neoplasm of uncertain behavior of bone and articular cartilage
	D49.2	Neoplasm of unspecified behavior of bone, soft tissue, and skin
⇄	M85.421	Solitary bone cyst, right humerus
⇄	M85.422	Solitary bone cyst, left humerus
⇄	M85.521	Aneurysmal bone cyst, right upper arm
⇄	M85.522	Aneurysmal bone cyst, left upper arm
⇄	M85.621	Other cyst of bone, right upper arm
⇄	M85.622	Other cyst of bone, left upper arm

CCI Edits

Refer to Appendix A for CCI edits.

Pub 100

01758: Pub 100-04, 12, 140.5, Pub 100-04, 12, 50, Pub 100-04, 12, 90.4.5

Base Units

Global: XXX

Code	Base Units
01758	5

Modifiers (PAR)

Code	Mod 50	Mod 51	Mod 62	Mod 80
01758	9	9	9	9

CPT © 2018 American Medical Association. All Rights Reserved.

01760

01760 Anesthesia for open or surgical arthroscopic procedures of the elbow; total elbow replacement

ICD-10-CM Diagnostic Codes

⇄	C40.01	Malignant neoplasm of scapula and long bones of right upper limb
⇄	C40.02	Malignant neoplasm of scapula and long bones of left upper limb
⇄	D16.01	Benign neoplasm of scapula and long bones of right upper limb
⇄	D16.02	Benign neoplasm of scapula and long bones of left upper limb
	D48.0	Neoplasm of uncertain behavior of bone and articular cartilage
	D49.2	Neoplasm of unspecified behavior of bone, soft tissue, and skin
⇄	M05.721	Rheumatoid arthritis with rheumatoid factor of right elbow without organ or systems involvement
⇄	M05.722	Rheumatoid arthritis with rheumatoid factor of left elbow without organ or systems involvement
⇄	M05.821	Other rheumatoid arthritis with rheumatoid factor of right elbow
⇄	M05.822	Other rheumatoid arthritis with rheumatoid factor of left elbow
⇄	M06.021	Rheumatoid arthritis without rheumatoid factor, right elbow
⇄	M06.022	Rheumatoid arthritis without rheumatoid factor, left elbow
⇄	M06.821	Other specified rheumatoid arthritis, right elbow
⇄	M06.822	Other specified rheumatoid arthritis, left elbow
⇄	M12.521	Traumatic arthropathy, right elbow
⇄	M12.522	Traumatic arthropathy, left elbow
⇄	M19.021	Primary osteoarthritis, right elbow
⇄	M19.022	Primary osteoarthritis, left elbow
⇄	M19.121	Post-traumatic osteoarthritis, right elbow
⇄	M19.122	Post-traumatic osteoarthritis, left elbow
⇄	M19.221	Secondary osteoarthritis, right elbow
⇄	M19.222	Secondary osteoarthritis, left elbow
⇄	M85.421	Solitary bone cyst, right humerus
⇄	M85.422	Solitary bone cyst, left humerus
⇄	M85.521	Aneurysmal bone cyst, right upper arm
⇄	M85.522	Aneurysmal bone cyst, left upper arm
⇄	M85.621	Other cyst of bone, right upper arm
⇄	M85.622	Other cyst of bone, left upper arm
⇄	M89.721	Major osseous defect, right humerus
⇄	M89.722	Major osseous defect, left humerus
❼⇄	S42.431	Displaced fracture (avulsion) of lateral epicondyle of right humerus
❼⇄	S42.432	Displaced fracture (avulsion) of lateral epicondyle of left humerus
❼⇄	S42.441	Displaced fracture (avulsion) of medial epicondyle of right humerus
❼⇄	S42.442	Displaced fracture (avulsion) of medial epicondyle of left humerus
❼⇄	S42.447	Incarcerated fracture (avulsion) of medial epicondyle of right humerus
❼⇄	S42.448	Incarcerated fracture (avulsion) of medial epicondyle of left humerus
❼⇄	S42.451	Displaced fracture of lateral condyle of right humerus
❼⇄	S42.452	Displaced fracture of lateral condyle of left humerus
❼⇄	S42.461	Displaced fracture of medial condyle of right humerus
❼⇄	S42.462	Displaced fracture of medial condyle of left humerus
❼⇄	S42.471	Displaced transcondylar fracture of right humerus
❼⇄	S42.472	Displaced transcondylar fracture of left humerus
❼⇄	S42.491	Other displaced fracture of lower end of right humerus
❼⇄	S42.492	Other displaced fracture of lower end of left humerus
❼⇄	S52.031	Displaced fracture of olecranon process with intraarticular extension of right ulna
❼⇄	S52.032	Displaced fracture of olecranon process with intraarticular extension of left ulna
❼⇄	S52.041	Displaced fracture of coronoid process of right ulna
❼⇄	S52.042	Displaced fracture of coronoid process of left ulna
❼⇄	S52.091	Other fracture of upper end of right ulna
❼⇄	S52.092	Other fracture of upper end of left ulna
❼⇄	S52.121	Displaced fracture of head of right radius
❼⇄	S52.122	Displaced fracture of head of left radius
❼⇄	S52.131	Displaced fracture of neck of right radius
❼⇄	S52.132	Displaced fracture of neck of left radius
❼⇄	S52.181	Other fracture of upper end of right radius
❼⇄	S52.182	Other fracture of upper end of left radius

ICD-10-CM Coding Notes

For codes requiring a 7th character extension, refer to your ICD-10-CM book. Review the character descriptions and coding guidelines for proper selection. For some procedures, only certain characters will apply.

CCI Edits

Refer to Appendix A for CCI edits.

Pub 100

01760: Pub 100-04, 12, 140.5, Pub 100-04, 12, 50, Pub 100-04, 12, 90.4.5

Base Units

Global: XXX

Code	Base Units
01760	7

Modifiers (PAR)

Code	Mod 50	Mod 51	Mod 62	Mod 80
01760	9	9	9	9

CPT © 2018 American Medical Association. All Rights Reserved.

01770

01770 Anesthesia for procedures on arteries of upper arm and elbow; not otherwise specified

ICD-10-CM Diagnostic Codes

⇄ I70.218 Atherosclerosis of native arteries of extremities with intermittent claudication, other extremity
⇄ I70.228 Atherosclerosis of native arteries of extremities with rest pain, other extremity
⇄ I70.25 Atherosclerosis of native arteries of other extremities with ulceration
⇄ I70.268 Atherosclerosis of native arteries of extremities with gangrene, other extremity
⇄ I70.298 Other atherosclerosis of native arteries of extremities, other extremity
⇄ I70.318 Atherosclerosis of unspecified type of bypass graft(s) of the extremities with intermittent claudication, other extremity
⇄ I70.328 Atherosclerosis of unspecified type of bypass graft(s) of the extremities with rest pain, other extremity
⇄ I70.35 Atherosclerosis of unspecified type of bypass graft(s) of other extremity with ulceration
⇄ I70.368 Atherosclerosis of unspecified type of bypass graft(s) of the extremities with gangrene, other extremity
⇄ I70.398 Other atherosclerosis of unspecified type of bypass graft(s) of the extremities, other extremity
⇄ I70.418 Atherosclerosis of autologous vein bypass graft(s) of the extremities with intermittent claudication, other extremity
⇄ I70.428 Atherosclerosis of autologous vein bypass graft(s) of the extremities with rest pain, other extremity
⇄ I70.45 Atherosclerosis of autologous vein bypass graft(s) of other extremity with ulceration
⇄ I70.468 Atherosclerosis of autologous vein bypass graft(s) of the extremities with gangrene, other extremity
⇄ I70.498 Other atherosclerosis of autologous vein bypass graft(s) of the extremities, other extremity
⇄ I70.518 Atherosclerosis of nonautologous biological bypass graft(s) of the extremities with intermittent claudication, other extremity
⇄ I70.528 Atherosclerosis of nonautologous biological bypass graft(s) of the extremities with rest pain, other extremity
⇄ I70.55 Atherosclerosis of nonautologous biological bypass graft(s) of other extremity with ulceration
⇄ I70.568 Atherosclerosis of nonautologous biological bypass graft(s) of the extremities with gangrene, other extremity
⇄ I70.598 Other atherosclerosis of nonautologous biological bypass graft(s) of the extremities, other extremity
⇄ I70.618 Atherosclerosis of nonbiological bypass graft(s) of the extremities with intermittent claudication, other extremity
⇄ I70.628 Atherosclerosis of nonbiological bypass graft(s) of the extremities with rest pain, other extremity
⇄ I70.65 Atherosclerosis of nonbiological bypass graft(s) of other extremity with ulceration
⇄ I70.668 Atherosclerosis of nonbiological bypass graft(s) of the extremities with gangrene, other extremity
⇄ I70.698 Other atherosclerosis of nonbiological bypass graft(s) of the extremities, other extremity
⇄ I70.718 Atherosclerosis of other type of bypass graft(s) of the extremities with intermittent claudication, other extremity
⇄ I70.728 Atherosclerosis of other type of bypass graft(s) of the extremities with rest pain, other extremity
⇄ I70.75 Atherosclerosis of other type of bypass graft(s) of other extremity with ulceration
⇄ I70.768 Atherosclerosis of other type of bypass graft(s) of the extremities with gangrene, other extremity
⇄ I70.798 Other atherosclerosis of other type of bypass graft(s) of the extremities, other extremity
I74.2 Embolism and thrombosis of arteries of the upper extremities
⇄ I75.011 Atheroembolism of right upper extremity
⇄ I75.012 Atheroembolism of left upper extremity
I77.0 Arteriovenous fistula, acquired
I77.1 Stricture of artery
I77.2 Rupture of artery
I77.5 Necrosis of artery
Q27.31 Arteriovenous malformation of vessel of upper limb
Q27.8 Other specified congenital malformations of peripheral vascular system
➐⇄ S45.111 Laceration of brachial artery, right side
➐⇄ S45.112 Laceration of brachial artery, left side
➐⇄ S45.191 Other specified injury of brachial artery, right side
➐⇄ S45.192 Other specified injury of brachial artery, left side
➐⇄ S45.811 Laceration of other specified blood vessels at shoulder and upper arm level, right arm
➐⇄ S45.812 Laceration of other specified blood vessels at shoulder and upper arm level, left arm
➐⇄ S45.891 Other specified injury of other specified blood vessels at shoulder and upper arm level, right arm
➐⇄ S45.892 Other specified injury of other specified blood vessels at shoulder and upper arm level, left arm
➐ T80.1 Vascular complications following infusion, transfusion and therapeutic injection
➐ T82.318 Breakdown (mechanical) of other vascular grafts
➐ T82.328 Displacement of other vascular grafts
➐ T82.338 Leakage of other vascular grafts
➐ T82.398 Other mechanical complication of other vascular grafts
➐ T82.7 Infection and inflammatory reaction due to other cardiac and vascular devices, implants and grafts
➐ T82.818 Embolism due to vascular prosthetic devices, implants and grafts
➐ T82.828 Fibrosis due to vascular prosthetic devices, implants and grafts
➐ T82.838 Hemorrhage due to vascular prosthetic devices, implants and grafts
➐ T82.848 Pain due to vascular prosthetic devices, implants and grafts
➐ T82.858 Stenosis of other vascular prosthetic devices, implants and grafts
➐ T82.868 Thrombosis due to vascular prosthetic devices, implants and grafts

ICD-10-CM Coding Notes

For codes requiring a 7th character extension, refer to your ICD-10-CM book. Review the character descriptions and coding guidelines for proper selection. For some procedures, only certain characters will apply.

CCI Edits

Refer to Appendix A for CCI edits.

Pub 100

01770: Pub 100-04, 12, 140.5, Pub 100-04, 12, 50, Pub 100-04, 12, 90.4.5

Base Units

Global: XXX

Code	Base Units
01770	6

Modifiers (PAR)

Code	Mod 50	Mod 51	Mod 62	Mod 80
01770	9	9	9	9

CPT © 2018 American Medical Association. All Rights Reserved.

01772

01772 Anesthesia for procedures on arteries of upper arm and elbow; embolectomy

ICD-10-CM Diagnostic Codes

⇄	I70.218	Atherosclerosis of native arteries of extremities with intermittent claudication, other extremity
⇄	I70.228	Atherosclerosis of native arteries of extremities with rest pain, other extremity
⇄	I70.25	Atherosclerosis of native arteries of other extremities with ulceration
⇄	I70.268	Atherosclerosis of native arteries of extremities with gangrene, other extremity
⇄	I70.298	Other atherosclerosis of native arteries of extremities, other extremity
	I74.2	Embolism and thrombosis of arteries of the upper extremities
⇄	I75.011	Atheroembolism of right upper extremity
⇄	I75.012	Atheroembolism of left upper extremity
❼	T82.818	Embolism due to vascular prosthetic devices, implants and grafts

ICD-10-CM Coding Notes

For codes requiring a 7th character extension, refer to your ICD-10-CM book. Review the character descriptions and coding guidelines for proper selection. For some procedures, only certain characters will apply.

CCI Edits

Refer to Appendix A for CCI edits.

Pub 100

01772: Pub 100-04, 12, 140.5, Pub 100-04, 12, 50, Pub 100-04, 12, 90.4.5

Base Units

Global: XXX

Code	Base Units
01772	6

Modifiers (PAR)

Code	Mod 50	Mod 51	Mod 62	Mod 80
01772	9	9	9	9

CPT © 2018 American Medical Association. All Rights Reserved.

01780

01780 Anesthesia for procedures on veins of upper arm and elbow; not otherwise specified

ICD-10-CM Diagnostic Codes

⇄	I82.611	Acute embolism and thrombosis of superficial veins of right upper extremity
⇄	I82.612	Acute embolism and thrombosis of superficial veins of left upper extremity
⇄	I82.613	Acute embolism and thrombosis of superficial veins of upper extremity, bilateral
⇄	I82.621	Acute embolism and thrombosis of deep veins of right upper extremity
⇄	I82.622	Acute embolism and thrombosis of deep veins of left upper extremity
⇄	I82.623	Acute embolism and thrombosis of deep veins of upper extremity, bilateral
⇄	I82.711	Chronic embolism and thrombosis of superficial veins of right upper extremity
⇄	I82.712	Chronic embolism and thrombosis of superficial veins of left upper extremity
⇄	I82.713	Chronic embolism and thrombosis of superficial veins of upper extremity, bilateral
⇄	I82.721	Chronic embolism and thrombosis of deep veins of right upper extremity
⇄	I82.722	Chronic embolism and thrombosis of deep veins of left upper extremity
⇄	I82.723	Chronic embolism and thrombosis of deep veins of upper extremity, bilateral
	I87.1	Compression of vein
	I87.2	Venous insufficiency (chronic) (peripheral)
	I87.8	Other specified disorders of veins
	Q27.8	Other specified congenital malformations of peripheral vascular system
❼⇄	S45.291	Other specified injury of axillary or brachial vein, right side
❼⇄	S45.292	Other specified injury of axillary or brachial vein, left side
❼⇄	S45.391	Other specified injury of superficial vein at shoulder and upper arm level, right arm
❼⇄	S45.392	Other specified injury of superficial vein at shoulder and upper arm level, left arm
❼⇄	S45.891	Other specified injury of other specified blood vessels at shoulder and upper arm level, right arm
❼⇄	S45.892	Other specified injury of other specified blood vessels at shoulder and upper arm level, left arm

ICD-10-CM Coding Notes

For codes requiring a 7th character extension, refer to your ICD-10-CM book. Review the character descriptions and coding guidelines for proper selection. For some procedures, only certain characters will apply.

CCI Edits

Refer to Appendix A for CCI edits.

Pub 100

01780: Pub 100-04, 12, 140.5, Pub 100-04, 12, 50, Pub 100-04, 12, 90.4.5

Base Units

Global: XXX

Code	Base Units
01780	3

Modifiers (PAR)

Code	Mod 50	Mod 51	Mod 62	Mod 80
01780	9	9	9	9

CPT © 2018 American Medical Association. All Rights Reserved.

01782

01782 Anesthesia for procedures on veins of upper arm and elbow; phleborrhaphy

AMA *CPT Assistant* ▯

01782: Nov 07: 8, Jul 12: 13

ICD-10-CM Diagnostic Codes

❼⇄	S41.111	Laceration without foreign body of right upper arm
❼⇄	S41.112	Laceration without foreign body of left upper arm
❼⇄	S41.121	Laceration with foreign body of right upper arm
❼⇄	S41.122	Laceration with foreign body of left upper arm
❼⇄	S41.131	Puncture wound without foreign body of right upper arm
❼⇄	S41.132	Puncture wound without foreign body of left upper arm
❼⇄	S41.141	Puncture wound with foreign body of right upper arm
❼⇄	S41.142	Puncture wound with foreign body of left upper arm
❼⇄	S41.151	Open bite of right upper arm
❼⇄	S41.152	Open bite of left upper arm
❼⇄	S45.211	Laceration of axillary or brachial vein, right side
❼⇄	S45.212	Laceration of axillary or brachial vein, left side
❼⇄	S45.291	Other specified injury of axillary or brachial vein, right side
❼⇄	S45.292	Other specified injury of axillary or brachial vein, left side
❼⇄	S45.311	Laceration of superficial vein at shoulder and upper arm level, right arm
❼⇄	S45.312	Laceration of superficial vein at shoulder and upper arm level, left arm
❼⇄	S45.391	Other specified injury of superficial vein at shoulder and upper arm level, right arm
❼⇄	S45.392	Other specified injury of superficial vein at shoulder and upper arm level, left arm
❼⇄	S45.811	Laceration of other specified blood vessels at shoulder and upper arm level, right arm
❼⇄	S45.812	Laceration of other specified blood vessels at shoulder and upper arm level, left arm
❼⇄	S45.891	Other specified injury of other specified blood vessels at shoulder and upper arm level, right arm
❼⇄	S45.892	Other specified injury of other specified blood vessels at shoulder and upper arm level, left arm

ICD-10-CM Coding Notes

For codes requiring a 7th character extension, refer to your ICD-10-CM book. Review the character descriptions and coding guidelines for proper selection. For some procedures, only certain characters will apply.

CCI Edits

Refer to Appendix A for CCI edits.

Pub 100

01782: Pub 100-04, 12, 140.5, Pub 100-04, 12, 50, Pub 100-04, 12, 90.4.5

Base Units

Global: XXX

Code	Base Units
01782	4

Modifiers (PAR)

Code	Mod 50	Mod 51	Mod 62	Mod 80
01782	9	9	9	9

CPT © 2018 American Medical Association. All Rights Reserved.

01810

01810 Anesthesia for all procedures on nerves, muscles, tendons, fascia, and bursae of forearm, wrist, and hand

AMA *CPT Assistant* ☐

01810: Mar 06: 15, Nov 07: 8, Oct 11: 3, Jul 12: 13

ICD-10-CM Diagnostic Codes

⇄	G56.01	Carpal tunnel syndrome, right upper limb
⇄	G56.02	Carpal tunnel syndrome, left upper limb
⇄	G56.03	Carpal tunnel syndrome, bilateral upper limbs
⇄	G56.11	Other lesions of median nerve, right upper limb
⇄	G56.12	Other lesions of median nerve, left upper limb
⇄	G56.13	Other lesions of median nerve, bilateral upper limbs
⇄	G56.21	Lesion of ulnar nerve, right upper limb
⇄	G56.22	Lesion of ulnar nerve, left upper limb
⇄	G56.23	Lesion of ulnar nerve, bilateral upper limbs
⇄	G56.31	Lesion of radial nerve, right upper limb
⇄	G56.32	Lesion of radial nerve, left upper limb
⇄	G56.33	Lesion of radial nerve, bilateral upper limbs
⇄	G56.81	Other specified mononeuropathies of right upper limb
⇄	G56.82	Other specified mononeuropathies of left upper limb
⇄	G56.83	Other specified mononeuropathies of bilateral upper limbs
⇄	M62.231	Nontraumatic ischemic infarction of muscle, right forearm
⇄	M62.232	Nontraumatic ischemic infarction of muscle, left forearm
⇄	M62.241	Nontraumatic ischemic infarction of muscle, right hand
⇄	M62.242	Nontraumatic ischemic infarction of muscle, left hand
⇄	M62.431	Contracture of muscle, right forearm
⇄	M62.432	Contracture of muscle, left forearm
⇄	M62.441	Contracture of muscle, right hand
⇄	M62.442	Contracture of muscle, left hand
⇄	M65.031	Abscess of tendon sheath, right forearm
⇄	M65.032	Abscess of tendon sheath, left forearm
⇄	M65.041	Abscess of tendon sheath, right hand
⇄	M65.042	Abscess of tendon sheath, left hand
⇄	M65.311	Trigger thumb, right thumb
⇄	M65.312	Trigger thumb, left thumb
⇄	M65.321	Trigger finger, right index finger
⇄	M65.322	Trigger finger, left index finger
⇄	M65.331	Trigger finger, right middle finger
⇄	M65.332	Trigger finger, left middle finger
⇄	M65.341	Trigger finger, right ring finger
⇄	M65.342	Trigger finger, left ring finger
⇄	M65.351	Trigger finger, right little finger
⇄	M65.352	Trigger finger, left little finger
	M65.4	Radial styloid tenosynovitis [de Quervain]
⇄	M65.831	Other synovitis and tenosynovitis, right forearm
⇄	M65.832	Other synovitis and tenosynovitis, left forearm
⇄	M65.841	Other synovitis and tenosynovitis, right hand
⇄	M65.842	Other synovitis and tenosynovitis, left hand
⇄	M67.341	Transient synovitis, right hand
⇄	M67.342	Transient synovitis, left hand
⇄	M67.431	Ganglion, right wrist
⇄	M67.432	Ganglion, left wrist
⇄	M67.441	Ganglion, right hand
⇄	M67.442	Ganglion, left hand
⇄	M70.11	Bursitis, right hand
⇄	M79.A11	Nontraumatic compartment syndrome of right upper extremity
⇄	M79.A12	Nontraumatic compartment syndrome of left upper extremity
❼⇄	S54.01	Injury of ulnar nerve at forearm level, right arm
❼⇄	S54.02	Injury of ulnar nerve at forearm level, left arm
❼⇄	S54.11	Injury of median nerve at forearm level, right arm
❼⇄	S54.12	Injury of median nerve at forearm level, left arm
❼⇄	S54.31	Injury of cutaneous sensory nerve at forearm level, right arm
❼⇄	S54.32	Injury of cutaneous sensory nerve at forearm level, left arm
❼⇄	S64.01	Injury of ulnar nerve at wrist and hand level of right arm
❼⇄	S64.02	Injury of ulnar nerve at wrist and hand level of left arm
❼⇄	S64.11	Injury of median nerve at wrist and hand level of right arm
❼⇄	S64.12	Injury of median nerve at wrist and hand level of left arm
❼⇄	T79.A11	Traumatic compartment syndrome of right upper extremity
❼⇄	T79.A12	Traumatic compartment syndrome of left upper extremity

ICD-10-CM Coding Notes

For codes requiring a 7th character extension, refer to your ICD-10-CM book. Review the character descriptions and coding guidelines for proper selection. For some procedures, only certain characters will apply.

CCI Edits

Refer to Appendix A for CCI edits.

Pub 100

01810: Pub 100-04, 12, 140.5, Pub 100-04, 12, 50, Pub 100-04, 12, 90.4.5

Base Units

Global: XXX

Code	Base Units
01810	3

Modifiers (PAR)

Code	Mod 50	Mod 51	Mod 62	Mod 80
01810	9	9	9	9

CPT © 2018 American Medical Association. All Rights Reserved.

01820

01820 Anesthesia for all closed procedures on radius, ulna, wrist, or hand bones

ICD-10-CM Diagnostic Codes

⑦⇄	S52.221	Displaced transverse fracture of shaft of right ulna
⑦⇄	S52.222	Displaced transverse fracture of shaft of left ulna
⑦⇄	S52.231	Displaced oblique fracture of shaft of right ulna
⑦⇄	S52.232	Displaced oblique fracture of shaft of left ulna
⑦⇄	S52.241	Displaced spiral fracture of shaft of ulna, right arm
⑦⇄	S52.242	Displaced spiral fracture of shaft of ulna, left arm
⑦⇄	S52.251	Displaced comminuted fracture of shaft of ulna, right arm
⑦⇄	S52.252	Displaced comminuted fracture of shaft of ulna, left arm
⑦⇄	S52.261	Displaced segmental fracture of shaft of ulna, right arm
⑦⇄	S52.262	Displaced segmental fracture of shaft of ulna, left arm
⑦⇄	S52.271	Monteggia's fracture of right ulna
⑦⇄	S52.272	Monteggia's fracture of left ulna
⑦⇄	S52.321	Displaced transverse fracture of shaft of right radius
⑦⇄	S52.322	Displaced transverse fracture of shaft of left radius
⑦⇄	S52.331	Displaced oblique fracture of shaft of right radius
⑦⇄	S52.332	Displaced oblique fracture of shaft of left radius
⑦⇄	S52.341	Displaced spiral fracture of shaft of radius, right arm
⑦⇄	S52.342	Displaced spiral fracture of shaft of radius, left arm
⑦⇄	S52.361	Displaced segmental fracture of shaft of radius, right arm
⑦⇄	S52.362	Displaced segmental fracture of shaft of radius, left arm
⑦⇄	S52.371	Galeazzi's fracture of right radius
⑦⇄	S52.372	Galeazzi's fracture of left radius
⑦⇄	S52.531	Colles' fracture of right radius
⑦⇄	S52.532	Colles' fracture of left radius
⑦⇄	S52.541	Smith's fracture of right radius
⑦⇄	S52.542	Smith's fracture of left radius
⑦⇄	S52.551	Other extraarticular fracture of lower end of right radius
⑦⇄	S52.552	Other extraarticular fracture of lower end of left radius
⑦⇄	S52.561	Barton's fracture of right radius
⑦⇄	S52.562	Barton's fracture of left radius
⑦⇄	S52.571	Other intraarticular fracture of lower end of right radius
⑦⇄	S52.572	Other intraarticular fracture of lower end of left radius
⑦⇄	S52.611	Displaced fracture of right ulna styloid process
⑦⇄	S52.612	Displaced fracture of left ulna styloid process
⑦⇄	S52.691	Other fracture of lower end of right ulna
⑦⇄	S52.692	Other fracture of lower end of left ulna
⑦⇄	S59.211	Salter-Harris Type I physeal fracture of lower end of radius, right arm
⑦⇄	S59.212	Salter-Harris Type I physeal fracture of lower end of radius, left arm
⑦⇄	S59.221	Salter-Harris Type II physeal fracture of lower end of radius, right arm
⑦⇄	S59.222	Salter-Harris Type II physeal fracture of lower end of radius, left arm
⑦⇄	S62.011	Displaced fracture of distal pole of navicular [scaphoid] bone of right wrist
⑦⇄	S62.012	Displaced fracture of distal pole of navicular [scaphoid] bone of left wrist
⑦⇄	S62.021	Displaced fracture of middle third of navicular [scaphoid] bone of right wrist
⑦⇄	S62.022	Displaced fracture of middle third of navicular [scaphoid] bone of left wrist
⑦⇄	S62.031	Displaced fracture of proximal third of navicular [scaphoid] bone of right wrist
⑦⇄	S62.032	Displaced fracture of proximal third of navicular [scaphoid] bone of left wrist

ICD-10-CM Coding Notes

For codes requiring a 7th character extension, refer to your ICD-10-CM book. Review the character descriptions and coding guidelines for proper selection. For some procedures, only certain characters will apply.

CCI Edits

Refer to Appendix A for CCI edits.

Pub 100

01820: Pub 100-04, 12, 140.5, Pub 100-04, 12, 50, Pub 100-04, 12, 90.4.5

Base Units

Global: XXX

Code	Base Units
01820	3

Modifiers (PAR)

Code	Mod 50	Mod 51	Mod 62	Mod 80
01820	9	9	9	9

CPT © 2018 American Medical Association. All Rights Reserved.

01829

01829 Anesthesia for diagnostic arthroscopic procedures on the wrist

ICD-10-CM Diagnostic Codes

⇄ G56.01 Carpal tunnel syndrome, right upper limb
⇄ G56.02 Carpal tunnel syndrome, left upper limb
⇄ G56.03 Carpal tunnel syndrome, bilateral upper limbs
⇄ G56.11 Other lesions of median nerve, right upper limb
⇄ G56.12 Other lesions of median nerve, left upper limb
⇄ G56.13 Other lesions of median nerve, bilateral upper limbs
⇄ G56.21 Lesion of ulnar nerve, right upper limb
⇄ G56.22 Lesion of ulnar nerve, left upper limb
⇄ G56.23 Lesion of ulnar nerve, bilateral upper limbs
⇄ G56.31 Lesion of radial nerve, right upper limb
⇄ G56.32 Lesion of radial nerve, left upper limb
⇄ G56.33 Lesion of radial nerve, bilateral upper limbs
⇄ M05.731 Rheumatoid arthritis with rheumatoid factor of right wrist without organ or systems involvement
⇄ M05.732 Rheumatoid arthritis with rheumatoid factor of left wrist without organ or systems involvement
⇄ M06.031 Rheumatoid arthritis without rheumatoid factor, right wrist
⇄ M06.032 Rheumatoid arthritis without rheumatoid factor, left wrist
⇄ M12.231 Villonodular synovitis (pigmented), right wrist
⇄ M12.232 Villonodular synovitis (pigmented), left wrist
⇄ M12.531 Traumatic arthropathy, right wrist
⇄ M12.532 Traumatic arthropathy, left wrist
⇄ M13.131 Monoarthritis, not elsewhere classified, right wrist
⇄ M13.132 Monoarthritis, not elsewhere classified, left wrist
⇄ M13.831 Other specified arthritis, right wrist
⇄ M13.832 Other specified arthritis, left wrist
⇄ M19.031 Primary osteoarthritis, right wrist
⇄ M19.032 Primary osteoarthritis, left wrist
⇄ M19.131 Post-traumatic osteoarthritis, right wrist
⇄ M19.132 Post-traumatic osteoarthritis, left wrist
⇄ M19.231 Secondary osteoarthritis, right wrist
⇄ M19.232 Secondary osteoarthritis, left wrist
⇄ M24.131 Other articular cartilage disorders, right wrist
⇄ M24.132 Other articular cartilage disorders, left wrist
⇄ M24.231 Disorder of ligament, right wrist
⇄ M24.232 Disorder of ligament, left wrist
⇄ M25.331 Other instability, right wrist
⇄ M25.332 Other instability, left wrist
⇄ M25.531 Pain in right wrist
⇄ M25.532 Pain in left wrist
⇄ M25.631 Stiffness of right wrist, not elsewhere classified
⇄ M25.632 Stiffness of left wrist, not elsewhere classified
⇄ M25.731 Osteophyte, right wrist
⇄ M25.732 Osteophyte, left wrist
⇄ M66.131 Rupture of synovium, right wrist
⇄ M66.132 Rupture of synovium, left wrist
⇄ M67.431 Ganglion, right wrist
⇄ M67.432 Ganglion, left wrist
⇄ M70.031 Crepitant synovitis (acute) (chronic), right wrist
⇄ M70.032 Crepitant synovitis (acute) (chronic), left wrist
⇄ M71.031 Abscess of bursa, right wrist
⇄ M71.032 Abscess of bursa, left wrist
⇄ M71.131 Other infective bursitis, right wrist
⇄ M71.132 Other infective bursitis, left wrist
⇄ M71.331 Other bursal cyst, right wrist
⇄ M71.332 Other bursal cyst, left wrist
⇄ M71.531 Other bursitis, not elsewhere classified, right wrist
⇄ M71.532 Other bursitis, not elsewhere classified, left wrist
❼⇄ S63.311 Traumatic rupture of collateral ligament of right wrist
❼⇄ S63.312 Traumatic rupture of collateral ligament of left wrist
❼⇄ S63.321 Traumatic rupture of right radiocarpal ligament
❼⇄ S63.322 Traumatic rupture of left radiocarpal ligament
❼⇄ S63.331 Traumatic rupture of right ulnocarpal (palmar) ligament
❼⇄ S63.332 Traumatic rupture of left ulnocarpal (palmar) ligament
❼⇄ S63.391 Traumatic rupture of other ligament of right wrist
❼⇄ S63.392 Traumatic rupture of other ligament of left wrist
❼⇄ S63.511 Sprain of carpal joint of right wrist
❼⇄ S63.512 Sprain of carpal joint of left wrist
❼⇄ S63.521 Sprain of radiocarpal joint of right wrist
❼⇄ S63.522 Sprain of radiocarpal joint of left wrist
❼⇄ S64.01 Injury of ulnar nerve at wrist and hand level of right arm
❼⇄ S64.02 Injury of ulnar nerve at wrist and hand level of left arm
❼⇄ S64.11 Injury of median nerve at wrist and hand level of right arm
❼⇄ S64.12 Injury of median nerve at wrist and hand level of left arm
❼⇄ S64.21 Injury of radial nerve at wrist and hand level of right arm
❼⇄ S64.22 Injury of radial nerve at wrist and hand level of left arm

ICD-10-CM Coding Notes

For codes requiring a 7th character extension, refer to your ICD-10-CM book. Review the character descriptions and coding guidelines for proper selection. For some procedures, only certain characters will apply.

CCI Edits

Refer to Appendix A for CCI edits.

Pub 100

01829: Pub 100-04, 12, 140.5, Pub 100-04, 12, 50, Pub 100-04, 12, 90.4.5

Base Units

Global: XXX

Code	Base Units
01829	3

Modifiers (PAR)

Code	Mod 50	Mod 51	Mod 62	Mod 80
01829	9	9	9	9

CPT © 2018 American Medical Association. All Rights Reserved.

01830

01830 Anesthesia for open or surgical arthroscopic/endoscopic procedures on distal radius, distal ulna, wrist, or hand joints; not otherwise specified

ICD-10-CM Diagnostic Codes

⇄	G56.01	Carpal tunnel syndrome, right upper limb
⇄	G56.02	Carpal tunnel syndrome, left upper limb
⇄	G56.03	Carpal tunnel syndrome, bilateral upper limbs
⇄	M05.731	Rheumatoid arthritis with rheumatoid factor of right wrist without organ or systems involvement
⇄	M05.732	Rheumatoid arthritis with rheumatoid factor of left wrist without organ or systems involvement
⇄	M06.031	Rheumatoid arthritis without rheumatoid factor, right wrist
⇄	M06.032	Rheumatoid arthritis without rheumatoid factor, left wrist
⇄	M12.231	Villonodular synovitis (pigmented), right wrist
⇄	M12.232	Villonodular synovitis (pigmented), left wrist
⇄	M12.531	Traumatic arthropathy, right wrist
⇄	M12.532	Traumatic arthropathy, left wrist
	M18.0	Bilateral primary osteoarthritis of first carpometacarpal joints
⇄	M18.11	Unilateral primary osteoarthritis of first carpometacarpal joint, right hand
⇄	M18.12	Unilateral primary osteoarthritis of first carpometacarpal joint, left hand
⇄	M19.031	Primary osteoarthritis, right wrist
⇄	M19.032	Primary osteoarthritis, left wrist
⇄	M24.431	Recurrent dislocation, right wrist
⇄	M24.432	Recurrent dislocation, left wrist
⇄	M25.731	Osteophyte, right wrist
⇄	M25.732	Osteophyte, left wrist
⇄	M71.031	Abscess of bursa, right wrist
⇄	M71.032	Abscess of bursa, left wrist
❼⇄	S52.531	Colles' fracture of right radius
❼⇄	S52.532	Colles' fracture of left radius
❼⇄	S52.541	Smith's fracture of right radius
❼⇄	S52.542	Smith's fracture of left radius
❼⇄	S52.561	Barton's fracture of right radius
❼⇄	S52.562	Barton's fracture of left radius
❼⇄	S52.571	Other intraarticular fracture of lower end of right radius
❼⇄	S52.572	Other intraarticular fracture of lower end of left radius
❼⇄	S62.011	Displaced fracture of distal pole of navicular [scaphoid] bone of right wrist
❼⇄	S62.012	Displaced fracture of distal pole of navicular [scaphoid] bone of left wrist
❼⇄	S62.021	Displaced fracture of middle third of navicular [scaphoid] bone of right wrist
❼⇄	S62.022	Displaced fracture of middle third of navicular [scaphoid] bone of left wrist
❼⇄	S62.031	Displaced fracture of proximal third of navicular [scaphoid] bone of right wrist
❼⇄	S62.032	Displaced fracture of proximal third of navicular [scaphoid] bone of left wrist
❼⇄	S62.211	Bennett's fracture, right hand
❼⇄	S62.212	Bennett's fracture, left hand
❼⇄	S62.221	Displaced Rolando's fracture, right hand
❼⇄	S62.222	Displaced Rolando's fracture, left hand
❼⇄	S62.511	Displaced fracture of proximal phalanx of right thumb
❼⇄	S62.512	Displaced fracture of proximal phalanx of left thumb
❼⇄	S62.521	Displaced fracture of distal phalanx of right thumb
❼⇄	S62.522	Displaced fracture of distal phalanx of left thumb
❼⇄	S62.630	Displaced fracture of distal phalanx of right index finger
❼⇄	S62.631	Displaced fracture of distal phalanx of left index finger
❼⇄	S62.632	Displaced fracture of distal phalanx of right middle finger
❼⇄	S62.633	Displaced fracture of distal phalanx of left middle finger
❼⇄	S62.634	Displaced fracture of distal phalanx of right ring finger
❼⇄	S62.635	Displaced fracture of distal phalanx of left ring finger
❼⇄	S62.636	Displaced fracture of distal phalanx of right little finger
❼⇄	S62.637	Displaced fracture of distal phalanx of left little finger
❼⇄	S63.311	Traumatic rupture of collateral ligament of right wrist
❼⇄	S63.312	Traumatic rupture of collateral ligament of left wrist
❼⇄	S63.321	Traumatic rupture of right radiocarpal ligament
❼⇄	S63.322	Traumatic rupture of left radiocarpal ligament
❼⇄	S63.331	Traumatic rupture of right ulnocarpal (palmar) ligament
❼⇄	S63.332	Traumatic rupture of left ulnocarpal (palmar) ligament
❼⇄	S63.391	Traumatic rupture of other ligament of right wrist
❼⇄	S63.392	Traumatic rupture of other ligament of left wrist

ICD-10-CM Coding Notes

For codes requiring a 7th character extension, refer to your ICD-10-CM book. Review the character descriptions and coding guidelines for proper selection. For some procedures, only certain characters will apply.

CCI Edits

Refer to Appendix A for CCI edits.

Pub 100

01830: Pub 100-04, 12, 140.5, Pub 100-04, 12, 50, Pub 100-04, 12, 90.4.5

Base Units

Global: XXX

Code	Base Units
01830	3

Modifiers (PAR)

Code	Mod 50	Mod 51	Mod 62	Mod 80
01830	9	9	9	9

CPT © 2018 American Medical Association. All Rights Reserved.

01832

01832 Anesthesia for open or surgical arthroscopic/endoscopic procedures on distal radius, distal ulna, wrist, or hand joints; total wrist replacement

ICD-10-CM Diagnostic Codes

⇄	M05.731	Rheumatoid arthritis with rheumatoid factor of right wrist without organ or systems involvement
⇄	M05.732	Rheumatoid arthritis with rheumatoid factor of left wrist without organ or systems involvement
⇄	M06.031	Rheumatoid arthritis without rheumatoid factor, right wrist
⇄	M06.032	Rheumatoid arthritis without rheumatoid factor, left wrist
⇄	M12.831	Other specific arthropathies, not elsewhere classified, right wrist
⇄	M12.832	Other specific arthropathies, not elsewhere classified, left wrist
⇄	M13.131	Monoarthritis, not elsewhere classified, right wrist
⇄	M13.132	Monoarthritis, not elsewhere classified, left wrist
⇄	M13.831	Other specified arthritis, right wrist
⇄	M13.832	Other specified arthritis, left wrist
⇄	M19.031	Primary osteoarthritis, right wrist
⇄	M19.032	Primary osteoarthritis, left wrist
⇄	M19.131	Post-traumatic osteoarthritis, right wrist
⇄	M19.132	Post-traumatic osteoarthritis, left wrist
⇄	M19.231	Secondary osteoarthritis, right wrist
⇄	M19.232	Secondary osteoarthritis, left wrist

CCI Edits

Refer to Appendix A for CCI edits.

Pub 100

01832: Pub 100-04, 12, 140.5, Pub 100-04, 12, 50, Pub 100-04, 12, 90.4.5

Base Units

Global: XXX

Code	Base Units
01832	6

Modifiers (PAR)

Code	Mod 50	Mod 51	Mod 62	Mod 80
01832	9	9	9	9

CPT © 2018 American Medical Association. All Rights Reserved.

01840

01840 Anesthesia for procedures on arteries of forearm, wrist, and hand; not otherwise specified

ICD-10-CM Diagnostic Codes

⇄ I70.218 Atherosclerosis of native arteries of extremities with intermittent claudication, other extremity
⇄ I70.228 Atherosclerosis of native arteries of extremities with rest pain, other extremity
⇄ I70.25 Atherosclerosis of native arteries of other extremities with ulceration
⇄ I70.268 Atherosclerosis of native arteries of extremities with gangrene, other extremity
⇄ I70.298 Other atherosclerosis of native arteries of extremities, other extremity
I72.1 Aneurysm of artery of upper extremity
I74.2 Embolism and thrombosis of arteries of the upper extremities
⇄ I75.011 Atheroembolism of right upper extremity
⇄ I75.012 Atheroembolism of left upper extremity
⇄ I75.013 Atheroembolism of bilateral upper extremities
I77.0 Arteriovenous fistula, acquired
I77.1 Stricture of artery
I77.2 Rupture of artery
I77.5 Necrosis of artery
I77.79 Dissection of other specified artery
N18.6 End stage renal disease
➐⇄ S55.011 Laceration of ulnar artery at forearm level, right arm
➐⇄ S55.012 Laceration of ulnar artery at forearm level, left arm
➐⇄ S55.091 Other specified injury of ulnar artery at forearm level, right arm
➐⇄ S55.092 Other specified injury of ulnar artery at forearm level, left arm
➐⇄ S55.111 Laceration of radial artery at forearm level, right arm
➐⇄ S55.112 Laceration of radial artery at forearm level, left arm
➐⇄ S55.191 Other specified injury of radial artery at forearm level, right arm
➐⇄ S55.192 Other specified injury of radial artery at forearm level, left arm
➐⇄ S55.811 Laceration of other blood vessels at forearm level, right arm
➐⇄ S55.812 Laceration of other blood vessels at forearm level, left arm
➐⇄ S55.891 Other specified injury of other blood vessels at forearm level, right arm
➐⇄ S55.892 Other specified injury of other blood vessels at forearm level, left arm
➐⇄ S65.011 Laceration of ulnar artery at wrist and hand level of right arm
➐⇄ S65.012 Laceration of ulnar artery at wrist and hand level of left arm
➐⇄ S65.091 Other specified injury of ulnar artery at wrist and hand level of right arm
➐⇄ S65.092 Other specified injury of ulnar artery at wrist and hand level of left arm
➐⇄ S65.111 Laceration of radial artery at wrist and hand level of right arm
➐⇄ S65.112 Laceration of radial artery at wrist and hand level of left arm
➐⇄ S65.191 Other specified injury of radial artery at wrist and hand level of right arm
➐⇄ S65.192 Other specified injury of radial artery at wrist and hand level of left arm
➐⇄ S65.211 Laceration of superficial palmar arch of right hand
➐⇄ S65.212 Laceration of superficial palmar arch of left hand
➐⇄ S65.291 Other specified injury of superficial palmar arch of right hand
➐⇄ S65.292 Other specified injury of superficial palmar arch of left hand
➐⇄ S65.311 Laceration of deep palmar arch of right hand
➐⇄ S65.312 Laceration of deep palmar arch of left hand
➐⇄ S65.391 Other specified injury of deep palmar arch of right hand
➐⇄ S65.392 Other specified injury of deep palmar arch of left hand
➐⇄ S65.411 Laceration of blood vessel of right thumb
➐⇄ S65.412 Laceration of blood vessel of left thumb
➐⇄ S65.491 Other specified injury of blood vessel of right thumb
➐⇄ S65.492 Other specified injury of blood vessel of left thumb
➐⇄ S65.510 Laceration of blood vessel of right index finger
➐⇄ S65.511 Laceration of blood vessel of left index finger
➐⇄ S65.512 Laceration of blood vessel of right middle finger
➐⇄ S65.513 Laceration of blood vessel of left middle finger
➐⇄ S65.514 Laceration of blood vessel of right ring finger
➐⇄ S65.515 Laceration of blood vessel of left ring finger
➐⇄ S65.516 Laceration of blood vessel of right little finger
➐⇄ S65.517 Laceration of blood vessel of left little finger
➐⇄ S65.590 Other specified injury of blood vessel of right index finger
➐⇄ S65.591 Other specified injury of blood vessel of left index finger
➐⇄ S65.592 Other specified injury of blood vessel of right middle finger
➐⇄ S65.593 Other specified injury of blood vessel of left middle finger
➐⇄ S65.594 Other specified injury of blood vessel of right ring finger
➐⇄ S65.595 Other specified injury of blood vessel of left ring finger
➐⇄ S65.596 Other specified injury of blood vessel of right little finger
➐⇄ S65.597 Other specified injury of blood vessel of left little finger
➐⇄ S65.811 Laceration of other blood vessels at wrist and hand level of right arm
➐⇄ S65.812 Laceration of other blood vessels at wrist and hand level of left arm
➐⇄ S65.891 Other specified injury of other blood vessels at wrist and hand level of right arm
➐⇄ S65.892 Other specified injury of other blood vessels at wrist and hand level of left arm

ICD-10-CM Coding Notes

For codes requiring a 7th character extension, refer to your ICD-10-CM book. Review the character descriptions and coding guidelines for proper selection. For some procedures, only certain characters will apply.

CCI Edits

Refer to Appendix A for CCI edits.

Pub 100

01840: Pub 100-04, 12, 140.5, Pub 100-04, 12, 50, Pub 100-04, 12, 90.4.5

Base Units

Global: XXX

Code	Base Units
01840	6

Modifiers (PAR)

Code	Mod 50	Mod 51	Mod 62	Mod 80
01840	9	9	9	9

CPT® Procedural Coding

CPT © 2018 American Medical Association. All Rights Reserved.

01842

01842 Anesthesia for procedures on arteries of forearm, wrist, and hand; embolectomy

ICD-10-CM Diagnostic Codes

⇄	I70.218	Atherosclerosis of native arteries of extremities with intermittent claudication, other extremity
⇄	I70.228	Atherosclerosis of native arteries of extremities with rest pain, other extremity
⇄	I70.25	Atherosclerosis of native arteries of other extremities with ulceration
⇄	I70.268	Atherosclerosis of native arteries of extremities with gangrene, other extremity
⇄	I70.298	Other atherosclerosis of native arteries of extremities, other extremity
	I74.2	Embolism and thrombosis of arteries of the upper extremities
⇄	I75.011	Atheroembolism of right upper extremity
⇄	I75.012	Atheroembolism of left upper extremity
⇄	I75.013	Atheroembolism of bilateral upper extremities
❼	T82.818	Embolism due to vascular prosthetic devices, implants and grafts
❼	T82.868	Thrombosis due to vascular prosthetic devices, implants and grafts

ICD-10-CM Coding Notes

For codes requiring a 7th character extension, refer to your ICD-10-CM book. Review the character descriptions and coding guidelines for proper selection. For some procedures, only certain characters will apply.

CCI Edits

Refer to Appendix A for CCI edits.

Pub 100

01842: Pub 100-04, 12, 140.5, Pub 100-04, 12, 50, Pub 100-04, 12, 90.4.5

Base Units

Global: XXX

Code	Base Units
01842	6

Modifiers (PAR)

Code	Mod 50	Mod 51	Mod 62	Mod 80
01842	9	9	9	9

CPT © 2018 American Medical Association. All Rights Reserved.

01844

01844 Anesthesia for vascular shunt, or shunt revision, any type (eg, dialysis)

ICD-10-CM Diagnostic Codes

	E08.22	Diabetes mellitus due to underlying condition with diabetic chronic kidney disease
	E09.22	Drug or chemical induced diabetes mellitus with diabetic chronic kidney disease
	E10.22	Type 1 diabetes mellitus with diabetic chronic kidney disease
	E11.22	Type 2 diabetes mellitus with diabetic chronic kidney disease
	E13.22	Other specified diabetes mellitus with diabetic chronic kidney disease
	I12.0	Hypertensive chronic kidney disease with stage 5 chronic kidney disease or end stage renal disease
	I13.11	Hypertensive heart and chronic kidney disease without heart failure, with stage 5 chronic kidney disease, or end stage renal disease
	I13.2	Hypertensive heart and chronic kidney disease with heart failure and with stage 5 chronic kidney disease, or end stage renal disease
	N03.2	Chronic nephritic syndrome with diffuse membranous glomerulonephritis
	N03.3	Chronic nephritic syndrome with diffuse mesangial proliferative glomerulonephritis
	N03.4	Chronic nephritic syndrome with diffuse endocapillary proliferative glomerulonephritis
	N03.5	Chronic nephritic syndrome with diffuse mesangiocapillary glomerulonephritis
	N03.6	Chronic nephritic syndrome with dense deposit disease
	N03.7	Chronic nephritic syndrome with diffuse crescentic glomerulonephritis
	N04.2	Nephrotic syndrome with diffuse membranous glomerulonephritis
	N04.3	Nephrotic syndrome with diffuse mesangial proliferative glomerulonephritis
	N04.4	Nephrotic syndrome with diffuse endocapillary proliferative glomerulonephritis
	N04.5	Nephrotic syndrome with diffuse mesangiocapillary glomerulonephritis
	N04.6	Nephrotic syndrome with dense deposit disease
	N04.7	Nephrotic syndrome with diffuse crescentic glomerulonephritis
	N18.6	End stage renal disease
❼	T82.510	Breakdown (mechanical) of surgically created arteriovenous fistula
❼	T82.511	Breakdown (mechanical) of surgically created arteriovenous shunt
❼	T82.520	Displacement of surgically created arteriovenous fistula
❼	T82.521	Displacement of surgically created arteriovenous shunt
❼	T82.530	Leakage of surgically created arteriovenous fistula
❼	T82.531	Leakage of surgically created arteriovenous shunt
❼	T82.590	Other mechanical complication of surgically created arteriovenous fistula
❼	T82.591	Other mechanical complication of surgically created arteriovenous shunt
❼	T82.7	Infection and inflammatory reaction due to other cardiac and vascular devices, implants and grafts
❼	T82.818	Embolism due to vascular prosthetic devices, implants and grafts
❼	T82.828	Fibrosis due to vascular prosthetic devices, implants and grafts
❼	T82.838	Hemorrhage due to vascular prosthetic devices, implants and grafts
❼	T82.848	Pain due to vascular prosthetic devices, implants and grafts
❼	T82.858	Stenosis of other vascular prosthetic devices, implants and grafts
❼	T82.868	Thrombosis due to vascular prosthetic devices, implants and grafts
❼	T82.898	Other specified complication of vascular prosthetic devices, implants and grafts

ICD-10-CM Coding Notes

For codes requiring a 7th character extension, refer to your ICD-10-CM book. Review the character descriptions and coding guidelines for proper selection. For some procedures, only certain characters will apply.

CCI Edits

Refer to Appendix A for CCI edits.

Pub 100

01844: Pub 100-04, 12, 140.5, Pub 100-04, 12, 50, Pub 100-04, 12, 90.4.5

Base Units

Global: XXX

Code	Base Units
01844	6

Modifiers (PAR)

Code	Mod 50	Mod 51	Mod 62	Mod 80
01844	9	9	9	9

CPT © 2018 American Medical Association. All Rights Reserved.

01850

01850 Anesthesia for procedures on veins of forearm, wrist, and hand; not otherwise specified

ICD-10-CM Diagnostic Codes

	Code	Description
⇄	I82.611	Acute embolism and thrombosis of superficial veins of right upper extremity
⇄	I82.612	Acute embolism and thrombosis of superficial veins of left upper extremity
⇄	I82.613	Acute embolism and thrombosis of superficial veins of upper extremity, bilateral
⇄	I82.621	Acute embolism and thrombosis of deep veins of right upper extremity
⇄	I82.622	Acute embolism and thrombosis of deep veins of left upper extremity
⇄	I82.623	Acute embolism and thrombosis of deep veins of upper extremity, bilateral
⇄	I82.711	Chronic embolism and thrombosis of superficial veins of right upper extremity
⇄	I82.712	Chronic embolism and thrombosis of superficial veins of left upper extremity
⇄	I82.713	Chronic embolism and thrombosis of superficial veins of upper extremity, bilateral
⇄	I82.721	Chronic embolism and thrombosis of deep veins of right upper extremity
⇄	I82.722	Chronic embolism and thrombosis of deep veins of left upper extremity
⇄	I82.723	Chronic embolism and thrombosis of deep veins of upper extremity, bilateral
	I87.1	Compression of vein
	I87.2	Venous insufficiency (chronic) (peripheral)
	I87.8	Other specified disorders of veins
	Q27.8	Other specified congenital malformations of peripheral vascular system
❼⇄	S55.211	Laceration of vein at forearm level, right arm
❼⇄	S55.212	Laceration of vein at forearm level, left arm
❼⇄	S55.291	Other specified injury of vein at forearm level, right arm
❼⇄	S55.292	Other specified injury of vein at forearm level, left arm
❼⇄	S65.411	Laceration of blood vessel of right thumb
❼⇄	S65.412	Laceration of blood vessel of left thumb
❼⇄	S65.491	Other specified injury of blood vessel of right thumb
❼⇄	S65.492	Other specified injury of blood vessel of left thumb
❼⇄	S65.510	Laceration of blood vessel of right index finger
❼⇄	S65.511	Laceration of blood vessel of left index finger
❼⇄	S65.512	Laceration of blood vessel of right middle finger
❼⇄	S65.513	Laceration of blood vessel of left middle finger
❼⇄	S65.514	Laceration of blood vessel of right ring finger
❼⇄	S65.515	Laceration of blood vessel of left ring finger
❼⇄	S65.516	Laceration of blood vessel of right little finger
❼⇄	S65.517	Laceration of blood vessel of left little finger
❼⇄	S65.590	Other specified injury of blood vessel of right index finger
❼⇄	S65.591	Other specified injury of blood vessel of left index finger
❼⇄	S65.592	Other specified injury of blood vessel of right middle finger
❼⇄	S65.593	Other specified injury of blood vessel of left middle finger
❼⇄	S65.594	Other specified injury of blood vessel of right ring finger
❼⇄	S65.595	Other specified injury of blood vessel of left ring finger
❼⇄	S65.596	Other specified injury of blood vessel of right little finger
❼⇄	S65.597	Other specified injury of blood vessel of left little finger
❼⇄	S65.811	Laceration of other blood vessels at wrist and hand level of right arm
❼⇄	S65.812	Laceration of other blood vessels at wrist and hand level of left arm
❼⇄	S65.891	Other specified injury of other blood vessels at wrist and hand level of right arm
❼⇄	S65.892	Other specified injury of other blood vessels at wrist and hand level of left arm

ICD-10-CM Coding Notes

For codes requiring a 7th character extension, refer to your ICD-10-CM book. Review the character descriptions and coding guidelines for proper selection. For some procedures, only certain characters will apply.

CCI Edits

Refer to Appendix A for CCI edits.

Pub 100

01850: Pub 100-04, 12, 140.5, Pub 100-04, 12, 50, Pub 100-04, 12, 90.4.5

Base Units

Global: XXX

Code	Base Units
01850	3

Modifiers (PAR)

Code	Mod 50	Mod 51	Mod 62	Mod 80
01850	9	9	9	9

CPT © 2018 American Medical Association. All Rights Reserved.

01852

01852 Anesthesia for procedures on veins of forearm, wrist, and hand; phleborrhaphy

ICD-10-CM Diagnostic Codes

	Code	Description
➐⇄	S55.211	Laceration of vein at forearm level, right arm
➐⇄	S55.212	Laceration of vein at forearm level, left arm
➐⇄	S65.411	Laceration of blood vessel of right thumb
➐⇄	S65.412	Laceration of blood vessel of left thumb
➐⇄	S65.510	Laceration of blood vessel of right index finger
➐⇄	S65.511	Laceration of blood vessel of left index finger
➐⇄	S65.512	Laceration of blood vessel of right middle finger
➐⇄	S65.513	Laceration of blood vessel of left middle finger
➐⇄	S65.514	Laceration of blood vessel of right ring finger
➐⇄	S65.515	Laceration of blood vessel of left ring finger
➐⇄	S65.516	Laceration of blood vessel of right little finger
➐⇄	S65.517	Laceration of blood vessel of left little finger
➐⇄	S65.811	Laceration of other blood vessels at wrist and hand level of right arm
➐⇄	S65.812	Laceration of other blood vessels at wrist and hand level of left arm

ICD-10-CM Coding Notes

For codes requiring a 7th character extension, refer to your ICD-10-CM book. Review the character descriptions and coding guidelines for proper selection. For some procedures, only certain characters will apply.

CCI Edits

Refer to Appendix A for CCI edits.

Pub 100

01852: Pub 100-04, 12, 140.5, Pub 100-04, 12, 50, Pub 100-04, 12, 90.4.5

Base Units

Global: XXX

Code	Base Units
01852	4

Modifiers (PAR)

Code	Mod 50	Mod 51	Mod 62	Mod 80
01852	9	9	9	9

CPT © 2018 American Medical Association. All Rights Reserved.

01860

01860 Anesthesia for forearm, wrist, or hand cast application, removal, or repair

AMA *CPT Assistant*

01860: Nov 07: 8, Jul 12: 13

ICD-10-CM Diagnostic Codes

	Code	Description
⇄	M24.841	Other specific joint derangements of right hand, not elsewhere classified
⇄	M24.842	Other specific joint derangements of left hand, not elsewhere classified
⇄	M25.241	Flail joint, right hand
⇄	M25.242	Flail joint, left hand
⇄	M25.341	Other instability, right hand
⇄	M25.342	Other instability, left hand
❼⇄	S52.531	Colles' fracture of right radius
❼⇄	S52.532	Colles' fracture of left radius
❼⇄	S52.541	Smith's fracture of right radius
❼⇄	S52.542	Smith's fracture of left radius
❼⇄	S52.551	Other extraarticular fracture of lower end of right radius
❼⇄	S52.552	Other extraarticular fracture of lower end of left radius
❼⇄	S52.561	Barton's fracture of right radius
❼⇄	S52.562	Barton's fracture of left radius
❼⇄	S52.571	Other intraarticular fracture of lower end of right radius
❼⇄	S52.572	Other intraarticular fracture of lower end of left radius
❼⇄	S52.591	Other fractures of lower end of right radius
❼⇄	S52.592	Other fractures of lower end of left radius
❼⇄	S59.021	Salter-Harris Type II physeal fracture of lower end of ulna, right arm
❼⇄	S59.022	Salter-Harris Type II physeal fracture of lower end of ulna, left arm
❼⇄	S59.031	Salter-Harris Type III physeal fracture of lower end of ulna, right arm
❼⇄	S59.032	Salter-Harris Type III physeal fracture of lower end of ulna, left arm
❼⇄	S59.041	Salter-Harris Type IV physeal fracture of lower end of ulna, right arm
❼⇄	S59.042	Salter-Harris Type IV physeal fracture of lower end of ulna, left arm
❼⇄	S59.091	Other physeal fracture of lower end of ulna, right arm
❼⇄	S59.092	Other physeal fracture of lower end of ulna, left arm
❼⇄	S59.221	Salter-Harris Type II physeal fracture of lower end of radius, right arm
❼⇄	S59.222	Salter-Harris Type II physeal fracture of lower end of radius, left arm
❼⇄	S59.231	Salter-Harris Type III physeal fracture of lower end of radius, right arm
❼⇄	S59.232	Salter-Harris Type III physeal fracture of lower end of radius, left arm
❼⇄	S59.241	Salter-Harris Type IV physeal fracture of lower end of radius, right arm
❼⇄	S59.242	Salter-Harris Type IV physeal fracture of lower end of radius, left arm
❼⇄	S59.291	Other physeal fracture of lower end of radius, right arm
❼⇄	S59.292	Other physeal fracture of lower end of radius, left arm
❼⇄	S62.011	Displaced fracture of distal pole of navicular [scaphoid] bone of right wrist
❼⇄	S62.012	Displaced fracture of distal pole of navicular [scaphoid] bone of left wrist
❼⇄	S62.014	Nondisplaced fracture of distal pole of navicular [scaphoid] bone of right wrist
❼⇄	S62.015	Nondisplaced fracture of distal pole of navicular [scaphoid] bone of left wrist
❼⇄	S62.021	Displaced fracture of middle third of navicular [scaphoid] bone of right wrist
❼⇄	S62.022	Displaced fracture of middle third of navicular [scaphoid] bone of left wrist
❼⇄	S62.024	Nondisplaced fracture of middle third of navicular [scaphoid] bone of right wrist
❼⇄	S62.025	Nondisplaced fracture of middle third of navicular [scaphoid] bone of left wrist
❼⇄	S62.031	Displaced fracture of proximal third of navicular [scaphoid] bone of right wrist
❼⇄	S62.032	Displaced fracture of proximal third of navicular [scaphoid] bone of left wrist
❼⇄	S62.034	Nondisplaced fracture of proximal third of navicular [scaphoid] bone of right wrist
❼⇄	S62.035	Nondisplaced fracture of proximal third of navicular [scaphoid] bone of left wrist
❼⇄	S63.061	Subluxation of metacarpal (bone), proximal end of right hand
❼⇄	S63.062	Subluxation of metacarpal (bone), proximal end of left hand
❼⇄	S63.064	Dislocation of metacarpal (bone), proximal end of right hand
❼⇄	S63.065	Dislocation of metacarpal (bone), proximal end of left hand

ICD-10-CM Coding Notes

For codes requiring a 7th character extension, refer to your ICD-10-CM book. Review the character descriptions and coding guidelines for proper selection. For some procedures, only certain characters will apply.

CCI Edits

Refer to Appendix A for CCI edits.

Pub 100

01860: Pub 100-04, 12, 140.5, Pub 100-04, 12, 50, Pub 100-04, 12, 90.4.5

Base Units

Global: XXX

Code	Base Units
01860	3

Modifiers (PAR)

Code	Mod 50	Mod 51	Mod 62	Mod 80
01860	9	9	9	9

CPT © 2018 American Medical Association. All Rights Reserved.

01916

01916 Anesthesia for diagnostic arteriography/venography

(Do not report 01916 in conjunction with therapeutic codes 01924-01926, 01930-01933)

AMA *CPT Assistant*

01916: Nov 07: 8, Oct 11: 3, Jul 12: 13

ICD-10-CM Diagnostic Codes

	Code	Description
	G45.0	Vertebro-basilar artery syndrome
	G45.1	Carotid artery syndrome (hemispheric)
	G45.2	Multiple and bilateral precerebral artery syndromes
	G45.3	Amaurosis fugax
	G45.8	Other transient cerebral ischemic attacks and related syndromes
	G45.9	Transient cerebral ischemic attack, unspecified
	I26.09	Other pulmonary embolism with acute cor pulmonale
	I26.99	Other pulmonary embolism without acute cor pulmonale
	I63.9	Cerebral infarction, unspecified
⇄	I65.01	Occlusion and stenosis of right vertebral artery
⇄	I65.02	Occlusion and stenosis of left vertebral artery
⇄	I65.03	Occlusion and stenosis of bilateral vertebral arteries
	I65.1	Occlusion and stenosis of basilar artery
⇄	I65.21	Occlusion and stenosis of right carotid artery
⇄	I65.22	Occlusion and stenosis of left carotid artery
⇄	I65.23	Occlusion and stenosis of bilateral carotid arteries
	I65.8	Occlusion and stenosis of other precerebral arteries
	I67.0	Dissection of cerebral arteries, nonruptured
	I67.1	Cerebral aneurysm, nonruptured
	I67.2	Cerebral atherosclerosis
	I71.01	Dissection of thoracic aorta
	I71.02	Dissection of abdominal aorta
	I71.03	Dissection of thoracoabdominal aorta
	I71.2	Thoracic aortic aneurysm, without rupture
	I71.4	Abdominal aortic aneurysm, without rupture
	I71.6	Thoracoabdominal aortic aneurysm, without rupture
	I72.0	Aneurysm of carotid artery
	I72.2	Aneurysm of renal artery
	I72.3	Aneurysm of iliac artery
	I74.01	Saddle embolus of abdominal aorta
	I74.09	Other arterial embolism and thrombosis of abdominal aorta
	I74.11	Embolism and thrombosis of thoracic aorta
	I74.2	Embolism and thrombosis of arteries of the upper extremities
	I74.3	Embolism and thrombosis of arteries of the lower extremities
	I74.5	Embolism and thrombosis of iliac artery
	I74.8	Embolism and thrombosis of other arteries
	I77.71	Dissection of carotid artery
	K55.011	Focal (segmental) acute (reversible) ischemia of small intestine
	K55.012	Diffuse acute (reversible) ischemia of small intestine
	K55.019	Acute (reversible) ischemia of small intestine, extent unspecified
	K55.021	Focal (segmental) acute infarction of small intestine
	K55.022	Diffuse acute infarction of small intestine
	K55.029	Acute infarction of small intestine, extent unspecified
	K55.031	Focal (segmental) acute (reversible) ischemia of large intestine
	K55.032	Diffuse acute (reversible) ischemia of large intestine
	K55.039	Acute (reversible) ischemia of large intestine, extent unspecified
	K55.041	Focal (segmental) acute infarction of large intestine
	K55.042	Diffuse acute infarction of large intestine
	K55.049	Acute infarction of large intestine, extent unspecified
	K55.051	Focal (segmental) acute (reversible) ischemia of intestine, part unspecified
	K55.052	Diffuse acute (reversible) ischemia of intestine, part unspecified
	K55.059	Acute (reversible) ischemia of intestine, part and extent unspecified
	K55.061	Focal (segmental) acute infarction of intestine, part unspecified
	K55.062	Diffuse acute infarction of intestine, part unspecified
	K55.069	Acute infarction of intestine, part and extent unspecified
	K55.1	Chronic vascular disorders of intestine
	Q28.0	Arteriovenous malformation of precerebral vessels
	Q28.1	Other malformations of precerebral vessels
	Q28.2	Arteriovenous malformation of cerebral vessels
	Q28.3	Other malformations of cerebral vessels
	Q28.8	Other specified congenital malformations of circulatory system
	Q28.9	Congenital malformation of circulatory system, unspecified
	R42	Dizziness and giddiness
	R55	Syncope and collapse

CCI Edits

Refer to Appendix A for CCI edits.

Pub 100

01916: Pub 100-04, 12, 140.5, Pub 100-04, 12, 50, Pub 100-04, 12, 90.4.5

Base Units

Global: XXX

Code	Base Units
01916	5

Modifiers (PAR)

Code	Mod 50	Mod 51	Mod 62	Mod 80
01916	9	9	9	9

CPT © 2018 American Medical Association. All Rights Reserved.

01920

01920 Anesthesia for cardiac catheterization including coronary angiography and ventriculography (not to include Swan-Ganz catheter)

ICD-10-CM Diagnostic Codes

I20.0 Unstable angina
I20.1 Angina pectoris with documented spasm
I20.8 Other forms of angina pectoris
I21.01 ST elevation (STEMI) myocardial infarction involving left main coronary artery
I21.02 ST elevation (STEMI) myocardial infarction involving left anterior descending coronary artery
I21.09 ST elevation (STEMI) myocardial infarction involving other coronary artery of anterior wall
I21.11 ST elevation (STEMI) myocardial infarction involving right coronary artery
I21.19 ST elevation (STEMI) myocardial infarction involving other coronary artery of inferior wall
I21.21 ST elevation (STEMI) myocardial infarction involving left circumflex coronary artery
I21.29 ST elevation (STEMI) myocardial infarction involving other sites
I21.3 ST elevation (STEMI) myocardial infarction of unspecified site
I21.4 Non-ST elevation (NSTEMI) myocardial infarction
I22.0 Subsequent ST elevation (STEMI) myocardial infarction of anterior wall
I22.1 Subsequent ST elevation (STEMI) myocardial infarction of inferior wall
I22.2 Subsequent non-ST elevation (NSTEMI) myocardial infarction
I22.8 Subsequent ST elevation (STEMI) myocardial infarction of other sites
I22.9 Subsequent ST elevation (STEMI) myocardial infarction of unspecified site
I23.0 Hemopericardium as current complication following acute myocardial infarction
I23.1 Atrial septal defect as current complication following acute myocardial infarction
I23.2 Ventricular septal defect as current complication following acute myocardial infarction
I23.3 Rupture of cardiac wall without hemopericardium as current complication following acute myocardial infarction
I23.4 Rupture of chordae tendineae as current complication following acute myocardial infarction
I23.5 Rupture of papillary muscle as current complication following acute myocardial infarction
I23.6 Thrombosis of atrium, auricular appendage, and ventricle as current complications following acute myocardial infarction
I23.7 Postinfarction angina
I23.8 Other current complications following acute myocardial infarction
I25.110 Atherosclerotic heart disease of native coronary artery with unstable angina pectoris
I25.111 Atherosclerotic heart disease of native coronary artery with angina pectoris with documented spasm
I25.118 Atherosclerotic heart disease of native coronary artery with other forms of angina pectoris
I25.119 Atherosclerotic heart disease of native coronary artery with unspecified angina pectoris
I25.41 Coronary artery aneurysm
I25.42 Coronary artery dissection
I25.82 Chronic total occlusion of coronary artery
I25.83 Coronary atherosclerosis due to lipid rich plaque
I25.84 Coronary atherosclerosis due to calcified coronary lesion
I34.0 Nonrheumatic mitral (valve) insufficiency
I34.1 Nonrheumatic mitral (valve) prolapse
I34.2 Nonrheumatic mitral (valve) stenosis
I34.8 Other nonrheumatic mitral valve disorders
I35.0 Nonrheumatic aortic (valve) stenosis
I35.1 Nonrheumatic aortic (valve) insufficiency
I35.2 Nonrheumatic aortic (valve) stenosis with insufficiency
I35.8 Other nonrheumatic aortic valve disorders
I36.0 Nonrheumatic tricuspid (valve) stenosis
I36.1 Nonrheumatic tricuspid (valve) insufficiency
I36.2 Nonrheumatic tricuspid (valve) stenosis with insufficiency
I36.8 Other nonrheumatic tricuspid valve disorders
I37.0 Nonrheumatic pulmonary valve stenosis
I37.1 Nonrheumatic pulmonary valve insufficiency
I37.2 Nonrheumatic pulmonary valve stenosis with insufficiency
I37.8 Other nonrheumatic pulmonary valve disorders
Q20.0 Common arterial trunk
Q20.1 Double outlet right ventricle
Q20.2 Double outlet left ventricle
Q20.3 Discordant ventriculoarterial connection
Q20.4 Double inlet ventricle
Q20.8 Other congenital malformations of cardiac chambers and connections
Q21.0 Ventricular septal defect
Q21.1 Atrial septal defect
Q21.2 Atrioventricular septal defect
Q21.3 Tetralogy of Fallot
Q21.4 Aortopulmonary septal defect
Q21.8 Other congenital malformations of cardiac septa
Q22.0 Pulmonary valve atresia
Q22.1 Congenital pulmonary valve stenosis
Q22.2 Congenital pulmonary valve insufficiency
Q22.3 Other congenital malformations of pulmonary valve
Q22.4 Congenital tricuspid stenosis
Q22.5 Ebstein's anomaly
Q22.6 Hypoplastic right heart syndrome
Q23.0 Congenital stenosis of aortic valve
Q23.1 Congenital insufficiency of aortic valve
Q23.2 Congenital mitral stenosis
Q23.3 Congenital mitral insufficiency
Q23.4 Hypoplastic left heart syndrome
Q24.3 Pulmonary infundibular stenosis
Q24.4 Congenital subaortic stenosis
Q24.5 Malformation of coronary vessels
Q25.0 Patent ductus arteriosus
Q25.1 Coarctation of aorta
Q25.3 Supravalvular aortic stenosis
Q25.71 Coarctation of pulmonary artery

CCI Edits

Refer to Appendix A for CCI edits.

Pub 100

01920: Pub 100-04, 12, 140.5, Pub 100-04, 12, 50, Pub 100-04, 12, 90.4.5

Base Units

Global: XXX

Code	Base Units
01920	7

Modifiers (PAR)

Code	Mod 50	Mod 51	Mod 62	Mod 80
01920	9	9	9	9

● New ▲ Revised ✚ Add On ⊘Modifier 51 Exempt ★Telemedicine ▢ CPT QuickRef ✗FDA Pending ⇄ Laterality ● Seventh Character ♂Male ♀Female

CPT © 2018 American Medical Association. All Rights Reserved.

01922

01922 Anesthesia for non-invasive imaging or radiation therapy

ICD-10-CM Diagnostic Codes

There are too many ICD-10-CM codes to list. Refer to ICD-10-CM code book for associated diagnostic codes.

CCI Edits

Refer to Appendix A for CCI edits.

Pub 100

01922: Pub 100-04, 12, 140.5, Pub 100-04, 12, 50, Pub 100-04, 12, 90.4.5

Base Units

Global: XXX

Code	Base Units
01922	7

Modifiers (PAR)

Code	Mod 50	Mod 51	Mod 62	Mod 80
01922	9	9	9	9

CPT © 2018 American Medical Association. All Rights Reserved.

01924

01924 Anesthesia for therapeutic interventional radiological procedures involving the arterial system; not otherwise specified

ICD-10-CM Diagnostic Codes

	Code	Description
	I70.1	Atherosclerosis of renal artery
⇄	I70.211	Atherosclerosis of native arteries of extremities with intermittent claudication, right leg
⇄	I70.212	Atherosclerosis of native arteries of extremities with intermittent claudication, left leg
⇄	I70.213	Atherosclerosis of native arteries of extremities with intermittent claudication, bilateral legs
⇄	I70.218	Atherosclerosis of native arteries of extremities with intermittent claudication, other extremity
⇄	I70.221	Atherosclerosis of native arteries of extremities with rest pain, right leg
⇄	I70.222	Atherosclerosis of native arteries of extremities with rest pain, left leg
⇄	I70.223	Atherosclerosis of native arteries of extremities with rest pain, bilateral legs
⇄	I70.228	Atherosclerosis of native arteries of extremities with rest pain, other extremity
⇄	I70.411	Atherosclerosis of autologous vein bypass graft(s) of the extremities with intermittent claudication, right leg
⇄	I70.412	Atherosclerosis of autologous vein bypass graft(s) of the extremities with intermittent claudication, left leg
⇄	I70.413	Atherosclerosis of autologous vein bypass graft(s) of the extremities with intermittent claudication, bilateral legs
⇄	I70.418	Atherosclerosis of autologous vein bypass graft(s) of the extremities with intermittent claudication, other extremity
⇄	I70.421	Atherosclerosis of autologous vein bypass graft(s) of the extremities with rest pain, right leg
⇄	I70.422	Atherosclerosis of autologous vein bypass graft(s) of the extremities with rest pain, left leg
⇄	I70.423	Atherosclerosis of autologous vein bypass graft(s) of the extremities with rest pain, bilateral legs
⇄	I70.428	Atherosclerosis of autologous vein bypass graft(s) of the extremities with rest pain, other extremity
	I72.1	Aneurysm of artery of upper extremity
	I72.2	Aneurysm of renal artery
	I72.3	Aneurysm of iliac artery
	I72.4	Aneurysm of artery of lower extremity
	I74.01	Saddle embolus of abdominal aorta
	I74.09	Other arterial embolism and thrombosis of abdominal aorta
	I74.2	Embolism and thrombosis of arteries of the upper extremities
	I74.3	Embolism and thrombosis of arteries of the lower extremities
	I74.5	Embolism and thrombosis of iliac artery
	I74.8	Embolism and thrombosis of other arteries
⇄	I75.011	Atheroembolism of right upper extremity
⇄	I75.012	Atheroembolism of left upper extremity
⇄	I75.013	Atheroembolism of bilateral upper extremities
⇄	I75.021	Atheroembolism of right lower extremity
⇄	I75.022	Atheroembolism of left lower extremity
⇄	I75.023	Atheroembolism of bilateral lower extremities
	I75.81	Atheroembolism of kidney
	I77.1	Stricture of artery
	I77.72	Dissection of iliac artery
	I77.73	Dissection of renal artery
	Q27.1	Congenital renal artery stenosis
	Q27.2	Other congenital malformations of renal artery
	Q27.31	Arteriovenous malformation of vessel of upper limb
	Q27.32	Arteriovenous malformation of vessel of lower limb
	Q27.33	Arteriovenous malformation of digestive system vessel
	Q27.34	Arteriovenous malformation of renal vessel
	Q27.39	Arteriovenous malformation, other site
	Q27.8	Other specified congenital malformations of peripheral vascular system
	Q28.8	Other specified congenital malformations of circulatory system

CCI Edits

Refer to Appendix A for CCI edits.

Pub 100

01924: Pub 100-04, 12, 140.5, Pub 100-04, 12, 50, Pub 100-04, 12, 90.4.5

Base Units

Global: XXX

Code	Base Units
01924	5

Modifiers (PAR)

Code	Mod 50	Mod 51	Mod 62	Mod 80
01924	9	9	9	9

CPT © 2018 American Medical Association. All Rights Reserved.

01925

01925 Anesthesia for therapeutic interventional radiological procedures involving the arterial system; carotid or coronary

ICD-10-CM Diagnostic Codes

I21.01 ST elevation (STEMI) myocardial infarction involving left main coronary artery
I21.02 ST elevation (STEMI) myocardial infarction involving left anterior descending coronary artery
I21.11 ST elevation (STEMI) myocardial infarction involving right coronary artery
I21.19 ST elevation (STEMI) myocardial infarction involving other coronary artery of inferior wall
I21.21 ST elevation (STEMI) myocardial infarction involving left circumflex coronary artery
I21.29 ST elevation (STEMI) myocardial infarction involving other sites
I21.3 ST elevation (STEMI) myocardial infarction of unspecified site
I21.4 Non-ST elevation (NSTEMI) myocardial infarction
I22.0 Subsequent ST elevation (STEMI) myocardial infarction of anterior wall
I22.1 Subsequent ST elevation (STEMI) myocardial infarction of inferior wall
I22.2 Subsequent non-ST elevation (NSTEMI) myocardial infarction
I22.8 Subsequent ST elevation (STEMI) myocardial infarction of other sites
I24.0 Acute coronary thrombosis not resulting in myocardial infarction
I24.8 Other forms of acute ischemic heart disease
I25.10 Atherosclerotic heart disease of native coronary artery without angina pectoris
I25.110 Atherosclerotic heart disease of native coronary artery with unstable angina pectoris
I25.111 Atherosclerotic heart disease of native coronary artery with angina pectoris with documented spasm
I25.118 Atherosclerotic heart disease of native coronary artery with other forms of angina pectoris
I25.119 Atherosclerotic heart disease of native coronary artery with unspecified angina pectoris
I25.41 Coronary artery aneurysm
I25.42 Coronary artery dissection
I25.6 Silent myocardial ischemia
I25.710 Atherosclerosis of autologous vein coronary artery bypass graft(s) with unstable angina pectoris
I25.711 Atherosclerosis of autologous vein coronary artery bypass graft(s) with angina pectoris with documented spasm
I25.718 Atherosclerosis of autologous vein coronary artery bypass graft(s) with other forms of angina pectoris
I25.719 Atherosclerosis of autologous vein coronary artery bypass graft(s) with unspecified angina pectoris
I25.720 Atherosclerosis of autologous artery coronary artery bypass graft(s) with unstable angina pectoris
I25.721 Atherosclerosis of autologous artery coronary artery bypass graft(s) with angina pectoris with documented spasm
I25.728 Atherosclerosis of autologous artery coronary artery bypass graft(s) with other forms of angina pectoris
I25.729 Atherosclerosis of autologous artery coronary artery bypass graft(s) with unspecified angina pectoris
I25.730 Atherosclerosis of nonautologous biological coronary artery bypass graft(s) with unstable angina pectoris
I25.731 Atherosclerosis of nonautologous biological coronary artery bypass graft(s) with angina pectoris with documented spasm
I25.738 Atherosclerosis of nonautologous biological coronary artery bypass graft(s) with other forms of angina pectoris
I25.739 Atherosclerosis of nonautologous biological coronary artery bypass graft(s) with unspecified angina pectoris
I25.790 Atherosclerosis of other coronary artery bypass graft(s) with unstable angina pectoris
I25.791 Atherosclerosis of other coronary artery bypass graft(s) with angina pectoris with documented spasm
I25.798 Atherosclerosis of other coronary artery bypass graft(s) with other forms of angina pectoris
I25.799 Atherosclerosis of other coronary artery bypass graft(s) with unspecified angina pectoris
I25.810 Atherosclerosis of coronary artery bypass graft(s) without angina pectoris
I25.82 Chronic total occlusion of coronary artery
I25.83 Coronary atherosclerosis due to lipid rich plaque
I25.84 Coronary atherosclerosis due to calcified coronary lesion
I25.89 Other forms of chronic ischemic heart disease
⇄ I63.031 Cerebral infarction due to thrombosis of right carotid artery
⇄ I63.032 Cerebral infarction due to thrombosis of left carotid artery
⇄ I63.033 Cerebral infarction due to thrombosis of bilateral carotid arteries
⇄ I63.131 Cerebral infarction due to embolism of right carotid artery
⇄ I63.132 Cerebral infarction due to embolism of left carotid artery
⇄ I63.133 Cerebral infarction due to embolism of bilateral carotid arteries
⇄ I63.231 Cerebral infarction due to unspecified occlusion or stenosis of right carotid arteries
⇄ I63.232 Cerebral infarction due to unspecified occlusion or stenosis of left carotid arteries
⇄ I63.233 Cerebral infarction due to unspecified occlusion or stenosis of bilateral carotid arteries
⇄ I65.21 Occlusion and stenosis of right carotid artery
⇄ I65.22 Occlusion and stenosis of left carotid artery
⇄ I65.23 Occlusion and stenosis of bilateral carotid arteries
I72.0 Aneurysm of carotid artery
I77.71 Dissection of carotid artery

CCI Edits

Refer to Appendix A for CCI edits.

Pub 100

01925: Pub 100-04, 12, 140.5, Pub 100-04, 12, 50, Pub 100-04, 12, 90.4.5

Base Units

Global: XXX

Code	Base Units
01925	7

Modifiers (PAR)

Code	Mod 50	Mod 51	Mod 62	Mod 80
01925	9	9	9	9

CPT © 2018 American Medical Association. All Rights Reserved.

01926

01926 Anesthesia for therapeutic interventional radiological procedures involving the arterial system; intracranial, intracardiac, or aortic

ICD-10-CM Diagnostic Codes

C70.0 Malignant neoplasm of cerebral meninges
C71.0 Malignant neoplasm of cerebrum, except lobes and ventricles
C71.1 Malignant neoplasm of frontal lobe
C71.2 Malignant neoplasm of temporal lobe
C71.3 Malignant neoplasm of parietal lobe
C71.4 Malignant neoplasm of occipital lobe
C71.5 Malignant neoplasm of cerebral ventricle
C71.6 Malignant neoplasm of cerebellum
C71.7 Malignant neoplasm of brain stem
C71.8 Malignant neoplasm of overlapping sites of brain
C79.31 Secondary malignant neoplasm of brain
C79.32 Secondary malignant neoplasm of cerebral meninges
D18.02 Hemangioma of intracranial structures
D33.0 Benign neoplasm of brain, supratentorial
D33.1 Benign neoplasm of brain, infratentorial
D43.1 Neoplasm of uncertain behavior of brain, infratentorial
D43.2 Neoplasm of uncertain behavior of brain, unspecified
D49.6 Neoplasm of unspecified behavior of brain
I34.2 Nonrheumatic mitral (valve) stenosis
I35.0 Nonrheumatic aortic (valve) stenosis
I36.0 Nonrheumatic tricuspid (valve) stenosis
I37.0 Nonrheumatic pulmonary valve stenosis
⇄ I66.01 Occlusion and stenosis of right middle cerebral artery
⇄ I66.02 Occlusion and stenosis of left middle cerebral artery
⇄ I66.03 Occlusion and stenosis of bilateral middle cerebral arteries
⇄ I66.11 Occlusion and stenosis of right anterior cerebral artery
⇄ I66.12 Occlusion and stenosis of left anterior cerebral artery
⇄ I66.13 Occlusion and stenosis of bilateral anterior cerebral arteries
⇄ I66.21 Occlusion and stenosis of right posterior cerebral artery
⇄ I66.22 Occlusion and stenosis of left posterior cerebral artery
⇄ I66.23 Occlusion and stenosis of bilateral posterior cerebral arteries
I66.3 Occlusion and stenosis of cerebellar arteries
I66.8 Occlusion and stenosis of other cerebral arteries
I71.02 Dissection of abdominal aorta
I71.4 Abdominal aortic aneurysm, without rupture
I74.01 Saddle embolus of abdominal aorta
I74.09 Other arterial embolism and thrombosis of abdominal aorta
Q22.1 Congenital pulmonary valve stenosis
Q22.4 Congenital tricuspid stenosis
Q23.0 Congenital stenosis of aortic valve
Q23.2 Congenital mitral stenosis
Q23.4 Hypoplastic left heart syndrome
Q28.2 Arteriovenous malformation of cerebral vessels
Q28.3 Other malformations of cerebral vessels

CCI Edits

Refer to Appendix A for CCI edits.

Pub 100

01926: Pub 100-04, 12, 140.5, Pub 100-04, 12, 50, Pub 100-04, 12, 90.4.5

Base Units

Global: XXX

Code	Base Units
01926	8

Modifiers (PAR)

Code	Mod 50	Mod 51	Mod 62	Mod 80
01926	9	9	9	9

CPT © 2018 American Medical Association. All Rights Reserved.

01930

01930 Anesthesia for therapeutic interventional radiological procedures involving the venous/lymphatic system (not to include access to the central circulation); not otherwise specified

ICD-10-CM Diagnostic Codes

⇄ I82.411 Acute embolism and thrombosis of right femoral vein
⇄ I82.412 Acute embolism and thrombosis of left femoral vein
⇄ I82.413 Acute embolism and thrombosis of femoral vein, bilateral
⇄ I82.421 Acute embolism and thrombosis of right iliac vein
⇄ I82.422 Acute embolism and thrombosis of left iliac vein
⇄ I82.423 Acute embolism and thrombosis of iliac vein, bilateral
⇄ I82.431 Acute embolism and thrombosis of right popliteal vein
⇄ I82.432 Acute embolism and thrombosis of left popliteal vein
⇄ I82.433 Acute embolism and thrombosis of popliteal vein, bilateral
⇄ I82.441 Acute embolism and thrombosis of right tibial vein
⇄ I82.442 Acute embolism and thrombosis of left tibial vein
⇄ I82.443 Acute embolism and thrombosis of tibial vein, bilateral
⇄ I82.491 Acute embolism and thrombosis of other specified deep vein of right lower extremity
⇄ I82.492 Acute embolism and thrombosis of other specified deep vein of left lower extremity
⇄ I82.493 Acute embolism and thrombosis of other specified deep vein of lower extremity, bilateral
⇄ I82.511 Chronic embolism and thrombosis of right femoral vein
⇄ I82.512 Chronic embolism and thrombosis of left femoral vein
⇄ I82.513 Chronic embolism and thrombosis of femoral vein, bilateral
⇄ I82.521 Chronic embolism and thrombosis of right iliac vein
⇄ I82.522 Chronic embolism and thrombosis of left iliac vein
⇄ I82.523 Chronic embolism and thrombosis of iliac vein, bilateral
⇄ I82.531 Chronic embolism and thrombosis of right popliteal vein
⇄ I82.532 Chronic embolism and thrombosis of left popliteal vein
⇄ I82.533 Chronic embolism and thrombosis of popliteal vein, bilateral
⇄ I82.541 Chronic embolism and thrombosis of right tibial vein
⇄ I82.542 Chronic embolism and thrombosis of left tibial vein
⇄ I82.543 Chronic embolism and thrombosis of tibial vein, bilateral
⇄ I82.591 Chronic embolism and thrombosis of other specified deep vein of right lower extremity
⇄ I82.592 Chronic embolism and thrombosis of other specified deep vein of left lower extremity
⇄ I82.593 Chronic embolism and thrombosis of other specified deep vein of lower extremity, bilateral
⇄ I82.621 Acute embolism and thrombosis of deep veins of right upper extremity
⇄ I82.622 Acute embolism and thrombosis of deep veins of left upper extremity
⇄ I82.623 Acute embolism and thrombosis of deep veins of upper extremity, bilateral
⇄ I82.721 Chronic embolism and thrombosis of deep veins of right upper extremity
⇄ I82.722 Chronic embolism and thrombosis of deep veins of left upper extremity
⇄ I82.723 Chronic embolism and thrombosis of deep veins of upper extremity, bilateral
⇄ I82.A11 Acute embolism and thrombosis of right axillary vein
⇄ I82.A12 Acute embolism and thrombosis of left axillary vein
⇄ I82.A13 Acute embolism and thrombosis of axillary vein, bilateral
⇄ I82.A21 Chronic embolism and thrombosis of right axillary vein
⇄ I82.A22 Chronic embolism and thrombosis of left axillary vein
⇄ I82.A23 Chronic embolism and thrombosis of axillary vein, bilateral
⇄ I83.11 Varicose veins of right lower extremity with inflammation
⇄ I83.12 Varicose veins of left lower extremity with inflammation
⇄ I83.811 Varicose veins of right lower extremity with pain
⇄ I83.812 Varicose veins of left lower extremity with pain
⇄ I83.813 Varicose veins of bilateral lower extremities with pain
⇄ I83.891 Varicose veins of right lower extremity with other complications
⇄ I83.892 Varicose veins of left lower extremity with other complications
⇄ I83.893 Varicose veins of bilateral lower extremities with other complications
⇄ I83.91 Asymptomatic varicose veins of right lower extremity
⇄ I83.92 Asymptomatic varicose veins of left lower extremity
⇄ I83.93 Asymptomatic varicose veins of bilateral lower extremities
I89.0 Lymphedema, not elsewhere classified
I89.1 Lymphangitis
I89.8 Other specified noninfective disorders of lymphatic vessels and lymph nodes
I89.9 Noninfective disorder of lymphatic vessels and lymph nodes, unspecified
N28.0 Ischemia and infarction of kidney
❼ T82.818 Embolism due to vascular prosthetic devices, implants and grafts
❼ T82.868 Thrombosis due to vascular prosthetic devices, implants and grafts

ICD-10-CM Coding Notes

For codes requiring a 7th character extension, refer to your ICD-10-CM book. Review the character descriptions and coding guidelines for proper selection. For some procedures, only certain characters will apply.

CCI Edits

Refer to Appendix A for CCI edits.

Pub 100

01930: Pub 100-04, 12, 140.5, Pub 100-04, 12, 50, Pub 100-04, 12, 90.4.5

Base Units

Global: XXX

Code	Base Units
01930	5

Modifiers (PAR)

Code	Mod 50	Mod 51	Mod 62	Mod 80
01930	9	9	9	9

CPT © 2018 American Medical Association. All Rights Reserved.

01931

01931 Anesthesia for therapeutic interventional radiological procedures involving the venous/lymphatic system (not to include access to the central circulation); intrahepatic or portal circulation (eg, transvenous intrahepatic portosystemic shunt[s] [TIPS])

AMA *CPT Assistant* ☐

01931: Apr 08: 3

ICD-10-CM Diagnostic Codes

B65.9	Schistosomiasis, unspecified
I82.0	Budd-Chiari syndrome
I85.00	Esophageal varices without bleeding
I85.01	Esophageal varices with bleeding
I85.10	Secondary esophageal varices without bleeding
I85.11	Secondary esophageal varices with bleeding
I86.4	Gastric varices
K31.89	Other diseases of stomach and duodenum
K70.30	Alcoholic cirrhosis of liver without ascites
K70.31	Alcoholic cirrhosis of liver with ascites
K71.50	Toxic liver disease with chronic active hepatitis without ascites
K71.51	Toxic liver disease with chronic active hepatitis with ascites
K71.7	Toxic liver disease with fibrosis and cirrhosis of liver
K74.4	Secondary biliary cirrhosis
K74.5	Biliary cirrhosis, unspecified
K74.60	Unspecified cirrhosis of liver
K74.69	Other cirrhosis of liver
K75.1	Phlebitis of portal vein
K76.5	Hepatic veno-occlusive disease
K76.6	Portal hypertension
K76.7	Hepatorenal syndrome
K76.81	Hepatopulmonary syndrome
K77	Liver disorders in diseases classified elsewhere
R18.0	Malignant ascites
R18.8	Other ascites

CCI Edits

Refer to Appendix A for CCI edits.

Pub 100

01931: Pub 100-04, 12, 140.5, Pub 100-04, 12, 50, Pub 100-04, 12, 90.4.5

Base Units

Global: XXX

Code	Base Units
01931	7

Modifiers (PAR)

Code	Mod 50	Mod 51	Mod 62	Mod 80
01931	9	9	9	9

CPT © 2018 American Medical Association. All Rights Reserved.

01932

01932 Anesthesia for therapeutic interventional radiological procedures involving the venous/ lymphatic system (not to include access to the central circulation); intrathoracic or jugular

ICD-10-CM Diagnostic Codes

	Code	Description
	I82.210	Acute embolism and thrombosis of superior vena cava
	I82.211	Chronic embolism and thrombosis of superior vena cava
	I82.220	Acute embolism and thrombosis of inferior vena cava
	I82.221	Chronic embolism and thrombosis of inferior vena cava
	I82.290	Acute embolism and thrombosis of other thoracic veins
	I82.291	Chronic embolism and thrombosis of other thoracic veins
⇄	I82.B11	Acute embolism and thrombosis of right subclavian vein
⇄	I82.B12	Acute embolism and thrombosis of left subclavian vein
⇄	I82.B13	Acute embolism and thrombosis of subclavian vein, bilateral
⇄	I82.B21	Chronic embolism and thrombosis of right subclavian vein
⇄	I82.B22	Chronic embolism and thrombosis of left subclavian vein
⇄	I82.B23	Chronic embolism and thrombosis of subclavian vein, bilateral
⇄	I82.C11	Acute embolism and thrombosis of right internal jugular vein
⇄	I82.C12	Acute embolism and thrombosis of left internal jugular vein
⇄	I82.C13	Acute embolism and thrombosis of internal jugular vein, bilateral
⇄	I82.C21	Chronic embolism and thrombosis of right internal jugular vein
⇄	I82.C22	Chronic embolism and thrombosis of left internal jugular vein
⇄	I82.C23	Chronic embolism and thrombosis of internal jugular vein, bilateral
	I87.1	Compression of vein
	I87.8	Other specified disorders of veins
	I88.1	Chronic lymphadenitis, except mesenteric
	I89.0	Lymphedema, not elsewhere classified
	I89.1	Lymphangitis
	I89.8	Other specified noninfective disorders of lymphatic vessels and lymph nodes
	I89.9	Noninfective disorder of lymphatic vessels and lymph nodes, unspecified
	Q26.0	Congenital stenosis of vena cava
	Q26.8	Other congenital malformations of great veins
	Q28.8	Other specified congenital malformations of circulatory system

CCI Edits

Refer to Appendix A for CCI edits.

Pub 100

01932: Pub 100-04, 12, 140.5, Pub 100-04, 12, 50, Pub 100-04, 12, 90.4.5

Base Units

Global: XXX

Code	Base Units
01932	6

Modifiers (PAR)

Code	Mod 50	Mod 51	Mod 62	Mod 80
01932	9	9	9	9

CPT © 2018 American Medical Association. All Rights Reserved.

01933

01933 Anesthesia for therapeutic interventional radiological procedures involving the venous/ lymphatic system (not to include access to the central circulation); intracranial

ICD-10-CM Diagnostic Codes

	Code	Description
	I63.6	Cerebral infarction due to cerebral venous thrombosis, nonpyogenic
	I67.6	Nonpyogenic thrombosis of intracranial venous system
	I67.89	Other cerebrovascular disease
⇄	I82.C11	Acute embolism and thrombosis of right internal jugular vein
⇄	I82.C12	Acute embolism and thrombosis of left internal jugular vein
⇄	I82.C13	Acute embolism and thrombosis of internal jugular vein, bilateral
⇄	I82.C21	Chronic embolism and thrombosis of right internal jugular vein
⇄	I82.C22	Chronic embolism and thrombosis of left internal jugular vein
⇄	I82.C23	Chronic embolism and thrombosis of internal jugular vein, bilateral
	Q28.3	Other malformations of cerebral vessels

CCI Edits

Refer to Appendix A for CCI edits.

Pub 100

01933: Pub 100-04, 12, 140.5, Pub 100-04, 12, 50, Pub 100-04, 12, 90.4.5

Base Units

Global: XXX

Code	Base Units
01933	7

Modifiers (PAR)

Code	Mod 50	Mod 51	Mod 62	Mod 80
01933	9	9	9	9

CPT © 2018 American Medical Association. All Rights Reserved.

01935

01935 Anesthesia for percutaneous image guided procedures on the spine and spinal cord; diagnostic

AMA *CPT Assistant*

01935: Apr 08: 3

ICD-10-CM Diagnostic Codes

	Code	Description
	G54.2	Cervical root disorders, not elsewhere classified
	G54.3	Thoracic root disorders, not elsewhere classified
	G54.4	Lumbosacral root disorders, not elsewhere classified
	G54.8	Other nerve root and plexus disorders
	M54.11	Radiculopathy, occipito-atlanto-axial region
	M54.12	Radiculopathy, cervical region
	M54.13	Radiculopathy, cervicothoracic region
	M54.14	Radiculopathy, thoracic region
	M54.15	Radiculopathy, thoracolumbar region
	M54.16	Radiculopathy, lumbar region
	M54.17	Radiculopathy, lumbosacral region
	M54.18	Radiculopathy, sacral and sacrococcygeal region
	M54.2	Cervicalgia
⇄	M54.31	Sciatica, right side
⇄	M54.32	Sciatica, left side
⇄	M54.41	Lumbago with sciatica, right side
⇄	M54.42	Lumbago with sciatica, left side
	M54.5	Low back pain
	M54.6	Pain in thoracic spine
	M54.89	Other dorsalgia

CCI Edits

Refer to Appendix A for CCI edits.

Pub 100

01935: Pub 100-04, 12, 140.5, Pub 100-04, 12, 50, Pub 100-04, 12, 90.4.5

Base Units

Global: XXX

Code	Base Units
01935	5

Modifiers (PAR)

Code	Mod 50	Mod 51	Mod 62	Mod 80
01935	9	9	9	9

CPT © 2018 American Medical Association. All Rights Reserved.

01936

01936 Anesthesia for percutaneous image guided procedures on the spine and spinal cord; therapeutic

AMA *CPT Assistant*

01936: Apr 08: 3, Jul 12: 13

ICD-10-CM Diagnostic Codes

G95.0	Syringomyelia and syringobulbia
G96.12	Meningeal adhesions (cerebral) (spinal)
G96.19	Other disorders of meninges, not elsewhere classified
M46.41	Discitis, unspecified, occipito-atlanto-axial region
M46.42	Discitis, unspecified, cervical region
M46.43	Discitis, unspecified, cervicothoracic region
M46.44	Discitis, unspecified, thoracic region
M46.45	Discitis, unspecified, thoracolumbar region
M46.46	Discitis, unspecified, lumbar region
M46.47	Discitis, unspecified, lumbosacral region
M46.48	Discitis, unspecified, sacral and sacrococcygeal region
M50.01	Cervical disc disorder with myelopathy, high cervical region
M50.021	Cervical disc disorder at C4-C5 level with myelopathy
M50.022	Cervical disc disorder at C5-C6 level with myelopathy
M50.023	Cervical disc disorder at C6-C7 level with myelopathy
M50.03	Cervical disc disorder with myelopathy, cervicothoracic region
M50.11	Cervical disc disorder with radiculopathy, high cervical region
M50.121	Cervical disc disorder at C4-C5 level with radiculopathy
M50.122	Cervical disc disorder at C5-C6 level with radiculopathy
M50.123	Cervical disc disorder at C6-C7 level with radiculopathy
M50.13	Cervical disc disorder with radiculopathy, cervicothoracic region
M50.21	Other cervical disc displacement, high cervical region
M50.221	Other cervical disc displacement at C4-C5 level
M50.222	Other cervical disc displacement at C5-C6 level
M50.223	Other cervical disc displacement at C6-C7 level
M50.23	Other cervical disc displacement, cervicothoracic region
M50.31	Other cervical disc degeneration, high cervical region
M50.321	Other cervical disc degeneration at C4-C5 level
M50.322	Other cervical disc degeneration at C5-C6 level
M50.323	Other cervical disc degeneration at C6-C7 level
M50.33	Other cervical disc degeneration, cervicothoracic region
M50.81	Other cervical disc disorders, high cervical region
M50.821	Other cervical disc disorders at C4-C5 level
M50.822	Other cervical disc disorders at C5-C6 level
M50.823	Other cervical disc disorders at C6-C7 level
M50.83	Other cervical disc disorders, cervicothoracic region
M51.04	Intervertebral disc disorders with myelopathy, thoracic region
M51.05	Intervertebral disc disorders with myelopathy, thoracolumbar region
M51.06	Intervertebral disc disorders with myelopathy, lumbar region
M51.07	Intervertebral disc disorders with myelopathy, lumbosacral region
M51.14	Intervertebral disc disorders with radiculopathy, thoracic region
M51.15	Intervertebral disc disorders with radiculopathy, thoracolumbar region
M51.16	Intervertebral disc disorders with radiculopathy, lumbar region
M51.17	Intervertebral disc disorders with radiculopathy, lumbosacral region
M51.24	Other intervertebral disc displacement, thoracic region
M51.25	Other intervertebral disc displacement, thoracolumbar region
M51.26	Other intervertebral disc displacement, lumbar region
M51.27	Other intervertebral disc displacement, lumbosacral region
M51.34	Other intervertebral disc degeneration, thoracic region
M51.35	Other intervertebral disc degeneration, thoracolumbar region
M51.36	Other intervertebral disc degeneration, lumbar region
M51.37	Other intervertebral disc degeneration, lumbosacral region
M51.44	Schmorl's nodes, thoracic region
M51.45	Schmorl's nodes, thoracolumbar region
M51.46	Schmorl's nodes, lumbar region
M51.47	Schmorl's nodes, lumbosacral region
M51.84	Other intervertebral disc disorders, thoracic region
M51.85	Other intervertebral disc disorders, thoracolumbar region
M51.86	Other intervertebral disc disorders, lumbar region
M51.87	Other intervertebral disc disorders, lumbosacral region
Q28.8	Other specified congenital malformations of circulatory system

CCI Edits

Refer to Appendix A for CCI edits.

Pub 100

01936: Pub 100-04, 12, 140.5, Pub 100-04, 12, 50, Pub 100-04, 12, 90.4.5

Base Units

Global: XXX

Code	Base Units
01936	5

Modifiers (PAR)

Code	Mod 50	Mod 51	Mod 62	Mod 80
01936	9	9	9	9

CPT © 2018 American Medical Association. All Rights Reserved.

01951

01951 Anesthesia for second- and third-degree burn excision or debridement with or without skin grafting, any site, for total body surface area (TBSA) treated during anesthesia and surgery; less than 4% total body surface area

AMA *CPT Assistant*

01951: Mar 06: 15, Oct 11: 3, Jul 12: 13

ICD-10-CM Diagnostic Codes

- ⑦⇄ T20.211 Burn of second degree of right ear [any part, except ear drum]
- ⑦⇄ T20.212 Burn of second degree of left ear [any part, except ear drum]
- ⑦ T20.22 Burn of second degree of lip(s)
- ⑦ T20.23 Burn of second degree of chin
- ⑦ T20.24 Burn of second degree of nose (septum)
- ⑦ T20.25 Burn of second degree of scalp [any part]
- ⑦ T20.26 Burn of second degree of forehead and cheek
- ⑦ T20.27 Burn of second degree of neck
- ⑦ T20.29 Burn of second degree of multiple sites of head, face, and neck
- ⑦⇄ T20.311 Burn of third degree of right ear [any part, except ear drum]
- ⑦⇄ T20.312 Burn of third degree of left ear [any part, except ear drum]
- ⑦ T20.32 Burn of third degree of lip(s)
- ⑦ T20.33 Burn of third degree of chin
- ⑦ T20.34 Burn of third degree of nose (septum)
- ⑦ T20.35 Burn of third degree of scalp [any part]
- ⑦ T20.36 Burn of third degree of forehead and cheek
- ⑦ T20.37 Burn of third degree of neck
- ⑦ T20.39 Burn of third degree of multiple sites of head, face, and neck
- ⑦ T21.21 Burn of second degree of chest wall
- ⑦ T21.22 Burn of second degree of abdominal wall
- ⑦ T21.23 Burn of second degree of upper back
- ⑦ T21.24 Burn of second degree of lower back
- ⑦ T21.25 Burn of second degree of buttock
- ⑦ T21.26 Burn of second degree of male genital region
- ⑦ T21.27 Burn of second degree of female genital region
- ⑦ T21.29 Burn of second degree of other site of trunk
- ⑦ T21.31 Burn of third degree of chest wall
- ⑦ T21.32 Burn of third degree of abdominal wall
- ⑦ T21.33 Burn of third degree of upper back
- ⑦ T21.34 Burn of third degree of lower back
- ⑦ T21.35 Burn of third degree of buttock
- ⑦ T21.36 Burn of third degree of male genital region
- ⑦ T21.37 Burn of third degree of female genital region
- ⑦ T21.39 Burn of third degree of other site of trunk
- ⑦⇄ T22.211 Burn of second degree of right forearm
- ⑦⇄ T22.212 Burn of second degree of left forearm
- ⑦⇄ T22.221 Burn of second degree of right elbow
- ⑦⇄ T22.222 Burn of second degree of left elbow
- ⑦⇄ T22.231 Burn of second degree of right upper arm
- ⑦⇄ T22.232 Burn of second degree of left upper arm
- ⑦⇄ T22.241 Burn of second degree of right axilla
- ⑦⇄ T22.242 Burn of second degree of left axilla
- ⑦⇄ T22.251 Burn of second degree of right shoulder
- ⑦⇄ T22.252 Burn of second degree of left shoulder
- ⑦⇄ T22.261 Burn of second degree of right scapular region
- ⑦⇄ T22.262 Burn of second degree of left scapular region
- ⑦⇄ T22.291 Burn of second degree of multiple sites of right shoulder and upper limb, except wrist and hand
- ⑦⇄ T22.292 Burn of second degree of multiple sites of left shoulder and upper limb, except wrist and hand
- ⑦⇄ T22.311 Burn of third degree of right forearm
- ⑦⇄ T22.312 Burn of third degree of left forearm
- ⑦⇄ T22.321 Burn of third degree of right elbow
- ⑦⇄ T22.322 Burn of third degree of left elbow
- ⑦⇄ T22.331 Burn of third degree of right upper arm
- ⑦⇄ T22.332 Burn of third degree of left upper arm
- ⑦⇄ T22.341 Burn of third degree of right axilla
- ⑦⇄ T22.342 Burn of third degree of left axilla
- ⑦⇄ T22.351 Burn of third degree of right shoulder
- ⑦⇄ T22.352 Burn of third degree of left shoulder
- ⑦⇄ T22.361 Burn of third degree of right scapular region
- ⑦⇄ T22.362 Burn of third degree of left scapular region
- ⑦⇄ T22.391 Burn of third degree of multiple sites of right shoulder and upper limb, except wrist and hand
- ⑦⇄ T22.392 Burn of third degree of multiple sites of left shoulder and upper limb, except wrist and hand
- ⑦⇄ T23.211 Burn of second degree of right thumb (nail)
- ⑦⇄ T23.212 Burn of second degree of left thumb (nail)
- ⑦⇄ T23.221 Burn of second degree of single right finger (nail) except thumb
- ⑦⇄ T23.222 Burn of second degree of single left finger (nail) except thumb
- ⑦⇄ T23.231 Burn of second degree of multiple right fingers (nail), not including thumb
- ⑦⇄ T23.232 Burn of second degree of multiple left fingers (nail), not including thumb
- ⑦⇄ T23.241 Burn of second degree of multiple right fingers (nail), including thumb
- ⑦⇄ T23.242 Burn of second degree of multiple left fingers (nail), including thumb
- ⑦⇄ T23.251 Burn of second degree of right palm
- ⑦⇄ T23.252 Burn of second degree of left palm
- ⑦⇄ T23.261 Burn of second degree of back of right hand
- ⑦⇄ T23.262 Burn of second degree of back of left hand
- ⑦⇄ T23.271 Burn of second degree of right wrist
- ⑦⇄ T23.272 Burn of second degree of left wrist
- ⑦⇄ T23.291 Burn of second degree of multiple sites of right wrist and hand
- ⑦⇄ T23.292 Burn of second degree of multiple sites of left wrist and hand
- ⑦⇄ T23.311 Burn of third degree of right thumb (nail)
- ⑦⇄ T23.312 Burn of third degree of left thumb (nail)
- ⑦⇄ T23.321 Burn of third degree of single right finger (nail) except thumb
- ⑦⇄ T23.322 Burn of third degree of single left finger (nail) except thumb
- ⑦⇄ T23.331 Burn of third degree of multiple right fingers (nail), not including thumb
- ⑦⇄ T23.332 Burn of third degree of multiple left fingers (nail), not including thumb
- ⑦⇄ T23.341 Burn of third degree of multiple right fingers (nail), including thumb
- ⑦⇄ T23.342 Burn of third degree of multiple left fingers (nail), including thumb
- ⑦⇄ T23.351 Burn of third degree of right palm
- ⑦⇄ T23.352 Burn of third degree of left palm
- ⑦⇄ T23.361 Burn of third degree of back of right hand
- ⑦⇄ T23.362 Burn of third degree of back of left hand
- ⑦⇄ T23.371 Burn of third degree of right wrist
- ⑦⇄ T23.372 Burn of third degree of left wrist
- ⑦⇄ T23.391 Burn of third degree of multiple sites of right wrist and hand
- ⑦⇄ T23.392 Burn of third degree of multiple sites of left wrist and hand
- ⑦⇄ T24.211 Burn of second degree of right thigh
- ⑦⇄ T24.212 Burn of second degree of left thigh
- ⑦⇄ T24.221 Burn of second degree of right knee
- ⑦⇄ T24.222 Burn of second degree of left knee
- ⑦⇄ T24.231 Burn of second degree of right lower leg
- ⑦⇄ T24.232 Burn of second degree of left lower leg
- ⑦⇄ T24.291 Burn of second degree of multiple sites of right lower limb, except ankle and foot
- ⑦⇄ T24.292 Burn of second degree of multiple sites of left lower limb, except ankle and foot
- ⑦⇄ T24.311 Burn of third degree of right thigh
- ⑦⇄ T24.312 Burn of third degree of left thigh
- ⑦⇄ T24.321 Burn of third degree of right knee

CPT © 2018 American Medical Association. All Rights Reserved.

➐⇄	T24.322	Burn of third degree of left knee
➐⇄	T24.331	Burn of third degree of right lower leg
➐⇄	T24.332	Burn of third degree of left lower leg
➐⇄	T24.391	Burn of third degree of multiple sites of right lower limb, except ankle and foot
➐⇄	T24.392	Burn of third degree of multiple sites of left lower limb, except ankle and foot
➐⇄	T25.211	Burn of second degree of right ankle
➐⇄	T25.212	Burn of second degree of left ankle
➐⇄	T25.221	Burn of second degree of right foot
➐⇄	T25.222	Burn of second degree of left foot
➐⇄	T25.231	Burn of second degree of right toe(s) (nail)
➐⇄	T25.232	Burn of second degree of left toe(s) (nail)
➐⇄	T25.291	Burn of second degree of multiple sites of right ankle and foot
➐⇄	T25.292	Burn of second degree of multiple sites of left ankle and foot
➐⇄	T25.311	Burn of third degree of right ankle
➐⇄	T25.312	Burn of third degree of left ankle
➐⇄	T25.321	Burn of third degree of right foot
➐⇄	T25.322	Burn of third degree of left foot
➐⇄	T25.331	Burn of third degree of right toe(s) (nail)
➐⇄	T25.332	Burn of third degree of left toe(s) (nail)
➐⇄	T25.391	Burn of third degree of multiple sites of right ankle and foot
➐⇄	T25.392	Burn of third degree of multiple sites of left ankle and foot
➐⇄	T26.01	Burn of right eyelid and periocular area
➐⇄	T26.02	Burn of left eyelid and periocular area
	T31.0	Burns involving less than 10% of body surface

ICD-10-CM Coding Notes

For codes requiring a 7th character extension, refer to your ICD-10-CM book. Review the character descriptions and coding guidelines for proper selection. For some procedures, only certain characters will apply.

CCI Edits

Refer to Appendix A for CCI edits.

Pub 100

01951: Pub 100-04, 12, 140.5, Pub 100-04, 12, 50, Pub 100-04, 12, 90.4.5

Base Units

Global: XXX

Code	Base Units
01951	3

Modifiers (PAR)

Code	Mod 50	Mod 51	Mod 62	Mod 80
01951	9	9	9	9

CPT © 2018 American Medical Association. All Rights Reserved.

01952

01952 Anesthesia for second- and third-degree burn excision or debridement with or without skin grafting, any site, for total body surface area (TBSA) treated during anesthesia and surgery; between 4% and 9% of total body surface area

ICD-10-CM Diagnostic Codes

	Code	Description
⑦⇄	T20.211	Burn of second degree of right ear [any part, except ear drum]
⑦⇄	T20.212	Burn of second degree of left ear [any part, except ear drum]
⑦	T20.22	Burn of second degree of lip(s)
⑦	T20.23	Burn of second degree of chin
⑦	T20.24	Burn of second degree of nose (septum)
⑦	T20.25	Burn of second degree of scalp [any part]
⑦	T20.26	Burn of second degree of forehead and cheek
⑦	T20.27	Burn of second degree of neck
⑦	T20.29	Burn of second degree of multiple sites of head, face, and neck
⑦⇄	T20.311	Burn of third degree of right ear [any part, except ear drum]
⑦⇄	T20.312	Burn of third degree of left ear [any part, except ear drum]
⑦	T20.32	Burn of third degree of lip(s)
⑦	T20.33	Burn of third degree of chin
⑦	T20.34	Burn of third degree of nose (septum)
⑦	T20.35	Burn of third degree of scalp [any part]
⑦	T20.36	Burn of third degree of forehead and cheek
⑦	T20.37	Burn of third degree of neck
⑦	T20.39	Burn of third degree of multiple sites of head, face, and neck
⑦	T21.21	Burn of second degree of chest wall
⑦	T21.22	Burn of second degree of abdominal wall
⑦	T21.23	Burn of second degree of upper back
⑦	T21.24	Burn of second degree of lower back
⑦	T21.25	Burn of second degree of buttock
⑦	T21.26	Burn of second degree of male genital region
⑦	T21.27	Burn of second degree of female genital region
⑦	T21.29	Burn of second degree of other site of trunk
⑦	T21.31	Burn of third degree of chest wall
⑦	T21.32	Burn of third degree of abdominal wall
⑦	T21.33	Burn of third degree of upper back
⑦	T21.34	Burn of third degree of lower back
⑦	T21.35	Burn of third degree of buttock
⑦	T21.36	Burn of third degree of male genital region
⑦	T21.37	Burn of third degree of female genital region
⑦	T21.39	Burn of third degree of other site of trunk
⑦⇄	T22.211	Burn of second degree of right forearm
⑦⇄	T22.212	Burn of second degree of left forearm
⑦⇄	T22.221	Burn of second degree of right elbow
⑦⇄	T22.222	Burn of second degree of left elbow
⑦⇄	T22.231	Burn of second degree of right upper arm
⑦⇄	T22.232	Burn of second degree of left upper arm
⑦⇄	T22.241	Burn of second degree of right axilla
⑦⇄	T22.242	Burn of second degree of left axilla
⑦⇄	T22.251	Burn of second degree of right shoulder
⑦⇄	T22.252	Burn of second degree of left shoulder
⑦⇄	T22.261	Burn of second degree of right scapular region
⑦⇄	T22.262	Burn of second degree of left scapular region
⑦⇄	T22.291	Burn of second degree of multiple sites of right shoulder and upper limb, except wrist and hand
⑦⇄	T22.292	Burn of second degree of multiple sites of left shoulder and upper limb, except wrist and hand
⑦⇄	T22.311	Burn of third degree of right forearm
⑦⇄	T22.312	Burn of third degree of left forearm
⑦⇄	T22.321	Burn of third degree of right elbow
⑦⇄	T22.322	Burn of third degree of left elbow
⑦⇄	T22.331	Burn of third degree of right upper arm
⑦⇄	T22.332	Burn of third degree of left upper arm
⑦⇄	T22.341	Burn of third degree of right axilla
⑦⇄	T22.342	Burn of third degree of left axilla
⑦⇄	T22.351	Burn of third degree of right shoulder
⑦⇄	T22.352	Burn of third degree of left shoulder
⑦⇄	T22.361	Burn of third degree of right scapular region
⑦⇄	T22.362	Burn of third degree of left scapular region
⑦⇄	T22.391	Burn of third degree of multiple sites of right shoulder and upper limb, except wrist and hand
⑦⇄	T22.392	Burn of third degree of multiple sites of left shoulder and upper limb, except wrist and hand
⑦⇄	T23.211	Burn of second degree of right thumb (nail)
⑦⇄	T23.212	Burn of second degree of left thumb (nail)
⑦⇄	T23.221	Burn of second degree of single right finger (nail) except thumb
⑦⇄	T23.222	Burn of second degree of single left finger (nail) except thumb
⑦⇄	T23.231	Burn of second degree of multiple right fingers (nail), not including thumb
⑦⇄	T23.232	Burn of second degree of multiple left fingers (nail), not including thumb
⑦⇄	T23.241	Burn of second degree of multiple right fingers (nail), including thumb
⑦⇄	T23.242	Burn of second degree of multiple left fingers (nail), including thumb
⑦⇄	T23.251	Burn of second degree of right palm
⑦⇄	T23.252	Burn of second degree of left palm
⑦⇄	T23.261	Burn of second degree of back of right hand
⑦⇄	T23.262	Burn of second degree of back of left hand
⑦⇄	T23.271	Burn of second degree of right wrist
⑦⇄	T23.272	Burn of second degree of left wrist
⑦⇄	T23.291	Burn of second degree of multiple sites of right wrist and hand
⑦⇄	T23.292	Burn of second degree of multiple sites of left wrist and hand
⑦⇄	T23.311	Burn of third degree of right thumb (nail)
⑦⇄	T23.312	Burn of third degree of left thumb (nail)
⑦⇄	T23.321	Burn of third degree of single right finger (nail) except thumb
⑦⇄	T23.322	Burn of third degree of single left finger (nail) except thumb
⑦⇄	T23.331	Burn of third degree of multiple right fingers (nail), not including thumb
⑦⇄	T23.332	Burn of third degree of multiple left fingers (nail), not including thumb
⑦⇄	T23.341	Burn of third degree of multiple right fingers (nail), including thumb
⑦⇄	T23.342	Burn of third degree of multiple left fingers (nail), including thumb
⑦⇄	T23.351	Burn of third degree of right palm
⑦⇄	T23.352	Burn of third degree of left palm
⑦⇄	T23.361	Burn of third degree of back of right hand
⑦⇄	T23.362	Burn of third degree of back of left hand
⑦⇄	T23.371	Burn of third degree of right wrist
⑦⇄	T23.372	Burn of third degree of left wrist
⑦⇄	T23.391	Burn of third degree of multiple sites of right wrist and hand
⑦⇄	T23.392	Burn of third degree of multiple sites of left wrist and hand
⑦⇄	T24.211	Burn of second degree of right thigh
⑦⇄	T24.212	Burn of second degree of left thigh
⑦⇄	T24.221	Burn of second degree of right knee
⑦⇄	T24.222	Burn of second degree of left knee
⑦⇄	T24.231	Burn of second degree of right lower leg
⑦⇄	T24.232	Burn of second degree of left lower leg
⑦⇄	T24.291	Burn of second degree of multiple sites of right lower limb, except ankle and foot
⑦⇄	T24.292	Burn of second degree of multiple sites of left lower limb, except ankle and foot
⑦⇄	T24.311	Burn of third degree of right thigh
⑦⇄	T24.312	Burn of third degree of left thigh
⑦⇄	T24.321	Burn of third degree of right knee

CPT © 2018 American Medical Association. All Rights Reserved.

➐⇄	T24.322	Burn of third degree of left knee
➐⇄	T24.331	Burn of third degree of right lower leg
➐⇄	T24.332	Burn of third degree of left lower leg
➐⇄	T24.391	Burn of third degree of multiple sites of right lower limb, except ankle and foot
➐⇄	T24.392	Burn of third degree of multiple sites of left lower limb, except ankle and foot
➐⇄	T25.211	Burn of second degree of right ankle
➐⇄	T25.212	Burn of second degree of left ankle
➐⇄	T25.221	Burn of second degree of right foot
➐⇄	T25.222	Burn of second degree of left foot
➐⇄	T25.231	Burn of second degree of right toe(s) (nail)
➐⇄	T25.232	Burn of second degree of left toe(s) (nail)
➐⇄	T25.291	Burn of second degree of multiple sites of right ankle and foot
➐⇄	T25.292	Burn of second degree of multiple sites of left ankle and foot
➐⇄	T25.311	Burn of third degree of right ankle
➐⇄	T25.312	Burn of third degree of left ankle
➐⇄	T25.321	Burn of third degree of right foot
➐⇄	T25.322	Burn of third degree of left foot
➐⇄	T25.331	Burn of third degree of right toe(s) (nail)
➐⇄	T25.332	Burn of third degree of left toe(s) (nail)
➐⇄	T25.391	Burn of third degree of multiple sites of right ankle and foot
➐⇄	T25.392	Burn of third degree of multiple sites of left ankle and foot
➐⇄	T26.01	Burn of right eyelid and periocular area
➐⇄	T26.02	Burn of left eyelid and periocular area
	T31.0	Burns involving less than 10% of body surface

ICD-10-CM Coding Notes

For codes requiring a 7th character extension, refer to your ICD-10-CM book. Review the character descriptions and coding guidelines for proper selection. For some procedures, only certain characters will apply.

CCI Edits

Refer to Appendix A for CCI edits.

Pub 100

01952: Pub 100-04, 12, 140.5, Pub 100-04, 12, 50, Pub 100-04, 12, 90.4.5

Base Units

Global: XXX

Code	Base Units
01952	5

Modifiers (PAR)

Code	Mod 50	Mod 51	Mod 62	Mod 80
01952	9	9	9	9

CPT © 2018 American Medical Association. All Rights Reserved.

01953

+ 01953 Anesthesia for second- and third-degree burn excision or debridement with or without skin grafting, any site, for total body surface area (TBSA) treated during anesthesia and surgery; each additional 9% total body surface area or part thereof (List separately in addition to code for primary procedure)

(Use 01953 in conjunction with 01952)

AMA *CPT Assistant*

01953: Jun 11: 13, Jul 12: 13

ICD-10-CM Diagnostic Codes

See Primary Procedure code for crosswalks.

CCI Edits

Refer to Appendix A for CCI edits.

Pub 100

01953: Pub 100-04, 12, 140.5, Pub 100-04, 12, 50, Pub 100-04, 12, 90.4.5

Base Units

Global: XXX

Code	Base Units
01953	1

Modifiers (PAR)

Code	Mod 50	Mod 51	Mod 62	Mod 80
01953	9	9	9	9

CPT © 2018 American Medical Association. All Rights Reserved.

01958

01958 Anesthesia for external cephalic version procedure

AMA *CPT Assistant*

01958: Jun 04: 5, 6, Oct 11: 3, Jul 12: 13

ICD-10-CM Diagnostic Codes

⑦	O32.0	Maternal care for unstable lie
⑦	O32.1	Maternal care for breech presentation
⑦	O32.2	Maternal care for transverse and oblique lie
⑦	O32.3	Maternal care for face, brow and chin presentation
⑦	O32.4	Maternal care for high head at term
⑦	O32.6	Maternal care for compound presentation
⑦	O32.8	Maternal care for other malpresentation of fetus
⑦	O32.9	Maternal care for malpresentation of fetus, unspecified

ICD-10-CM Coding Notes

For codes requiring a 7th character extension, refer to your ICD-10-CM book. Review the character descriptions and coding guidelines for proper selection. For some procedures, only certain characters will apply.

CCI Edits

Refer to Appendix A for CCI edits.

Pub 100

01958: Pub 100-04, 12, 140.5, Pub 100-04, 12, 50, Pub 100-04, 12, 90.4.5

Base Units

Global: XXX

Code	Base Units
01958	5

Modifiers (PAR)

Code	Mod 50	Mod 51	Mod 62	Mod 80
01958	9	9	9	9

CPT © 2018 American Medical Association. All Rights Reserved.

01960

01960 Anesthesia for vaginal delivery only

AMA *CPT Assistant* □

01960: Dec 01: 3

ICD-10-CM Diagnostic Codes

	Code	Description
	O42.011	Preterm premature rupture of membranes, onset of labor within 24 hours of rupture, first trimester ♀
	O42.012	Preterm premature rupture of membranes, onset of labor within 24 hours of rupture, second trimester ♀
	O42.013	Preterm premature rupture of membranes, onset of labor within 24 hours of rupture, third trimester ♀
	O42.02	Full-term premature rupture of membranes, onset of labor within 24 hours of rupture ♀
	O42.92	Full-term premature rupture of membranes, unspecified as to length of time between rupture and onset of labor ♀
❼	O60.12	Preterm labor second trimester with preterm delivery second trimester
❼	O60.13	Preterm labor second trimester with preterm delivery third trimester
❼	O60.14	Preterm labor third trimester with preterm delivery third trimester
❼	O60.22	Term delivery with preterm labor, second trimester
❼	O60.23	Term delivery with preterm labor, third trimester
	O62.0	Primary inadequate contractions ♀
	O62.1	Secondary uterine inertia ♀
	O62.2	Other uterine inertia ♀
	O62.8	Other abnormalities of forces of labor ♀
	O63.0	Prolonged first stage (of labor) ♀
	O63.1	Prolonged second stage (of labor) ♀
❼	O64.0	Obstructed labor due to incomplete rotation of fetal head
❼	O64.1	Obstructed labor due to breech presentation
❼	O64.2	Obstructed labor due to face presentation
❼	O64.3	Obstructed labor due to brow presentation
❼	O64.4	Obstructed labor due to shoulder presentation
❼	O64.5	Obstructed labor due to compound presentation
❼	O64.8	Obstructed labor due to other malposition and malpresentation
❼	O64.9	Obstructed labor due to malposition and malpresentation, unspecified
	O66.0	Obstructed labor due to shoulder dystocia ♀
	O68	Labor and delivery complicated by abnormality of fetal acid-base balance ♀
❼	O69.0	Labor and delivery complicated by prolapse of cord
❼	O69.1	Labor and delivery complicated by cord around neck, with compression
❼	O69.2	Labor and delivery complicated by other cord entanglement, with compression
❼	O69.3	Labor and delivery complicated by short cord
❼	O69.4	Labor and delivery complicated by vasa previa
❼	O69.5	Labor and delivery complicated by vascular lesion of cord
❼	O69.81	Labor and delivery complicated by cord around neck, without compression
❼	O69.82	Labor and delivery complicated by other cord entanglement, without compression
❼	O69.89	Labor and delivery complicated by other cord complications
❼	O69.9	Labor and delivery complicated by cord complication, unspecified
	O70.0	First degree perineal laceration during delivery ♀
	O70.1	Second degree perineal laceration during delivery ♀
	O70.2	Third degree perineal laceration during delivery ♀
	O70.3	Fourth degree perineal laceration during delivery ♀
	O70.4	Anal sphincter tear complicating delivery, not associated with third degree laceration ♀
	O70.9	Perineal laceration during delivery, unspecified ♀
	O71.3	Obstetric laceration of cervix ♀
	O71.4	Obstetric high vaginal laceration alone ♀
	O73.0	Retained placenta without hemorrhage ♀
	O73.1	Retained portions of placenta and membranes, without hemorrhage ♀
	O75.5	Delayed delivery after artificial rupture of membranes ♀
	O76	Abnormality in fetal heart rate and rhythm complicating labor and delivery ♀
	O77.0	Labor and delivery complicated by meconium in amniotic fluid ♀
	O77.8	Labor and delivery complicated by other evidence of fetal stress ♀
	O80	Encounter for full-term uncomplicated delivery ♀

ICD-10-CM Coding Notes

For codes requiring a 7th character extension, refer to your ICD-10-CM book. Review the character descriptions and coding guidelines for proper selection. For some procedures, only certain characters will apply.

CCI Edits

Refer to Appendix A for CCI edits.

Pub 100

01960: Pub 100-04, 12, 140.5, Pub 100-04, 12, 50, Pub 100-04, 12, 90.4.5

Base Units

Global: XXX

Code	Base Units
01960	5

Modifiers (PAR)

Code	Mod 50	Mod 51	Mod 62	Mod 80
01960	9	9	9	9

CPT © 2018 American Medical Association. All Rights Reserved.

01961

01961 Anesthesia for cesarean delivery only

ICD-10-CM Diagnostic Codes

	Code	Description
	O61.0	Failed medical induction of labor ♀
	O61.1	Failed instrumental induction of labor ♀
	O61.8	Other failed induction of labor ♀
	O62.0	Primary inadequate contractions ♀
	O62.1	Secondary uterine inertia ♀
	O62.2	Other uterine inertia ♀
	O62.4	Hypertonic, incoordinate, and prolonged uterine contractions ♀
❼	O64.0	Obstructed labor due to incomplete rotation of fetal head
❼	O64.1	Obstructed labor due to breech presentation
❼	O64.2	Obstructed labor due to face presentation
❼	O64.3	Obstructed labor due to brow presentation
❼	O64.4	Obstructed labor due to shoulder presentation
❼	O64.5	Obstructed labor due to compound presentation
❼	O64.8	Obstructed labor due to other malposition and malpresentation
❼	O64.9	Obstructed labor due to malposition and malpresentation, unspecified
	O65.0	Obstructed labor due to deformed pelvis ♀
	O65.1	Obstructed labor due to generally contracted pelvis ♀
	O65.2	Obstructed labor due to pelvic inlet contraction ♀
	O65.3	Obstructed labor due to pelvic outlet and mid-cavity contraction ♀
	O65.4	Obstructed labor due to fetopelvic disproportion, unspecified ♀
	O65.5	Obstructed labor due to abnormality of maternal pelvic organs ♀
	O65.8	Obstructed labor due to other maternal pelvic abnormalities ♀
	O66.0	Obstructed labor due to shoulder dystocia ♀
	O66.2	Obstructed labor due to unusually large fetus ♀
	O66.40	Failed trial of labor, unspecified ♀
	O66.41	Failed attempted vaginal birth after previous cesarean delivery ♀
	O66.6	Obstructed labor due to other multiple fetuses ♀
	O67.0	Intrapartum hemorrhage with coagulation defect ♀
	O67.8	Other intrapartum hemorrhage ♀
	O68	Labor and delivery complicated by abnormality of fetal acid-base balance ♀
	O71.02	Rupture of uterus before onset of labor, second trimester ♀
	O71.03	Rupture of uterus before onset of labor, third trimester ♀
	O71.1	Rupture of uterus during labor ♀
	O75.81	Maternal exhaustion complicating labor and delivery ♀
	O75.82	Onset (spontaneous) of labor after 37 completed weeks of gestation but before 39 completed weeks gestation, with delivery by (planned) cesarean section ♀
	O76	Abnormality in fetal heart rate and rhythm complicating labor and delivery ♀
	O77.8	Labor and delivery complicated by other evidence of fetal stress ♀
	O82	Encounter for cesarean delivery without indication ♀

ICD-10-CM Coding Notes

For codes requiring a 7th character extension, refer to your ICD-10-CM book. Review the character descriptions and coding guidelines for proper selection. For some procedures, only certain characters will apply.

CCI Edits

Refer to Appendix A for CCI edits.

Pub 100

01961: Pub 100-04, 12, 140.5, Pub 100-04, 12, 50, Pub 100-04, 12, 90.4.5

Base Units

Global: XXX

Code	Base Units
01961	7

Modifiers (PAR)

Code	Mod 50	Mod 51	Mod 62	Mod 80
01961	9	9	9	9

CPT © 2018 American Medical Association. All Rights Reserved.

01962

01962 Anesthesia for urgent hysterectomy following delivery

ICD-10-CM Diagnostic Codes

O43.212	Placenta accreta, second trimester ♀
O43.213	Placenta accreta, third trimester ♀
O43.222	Placenta increta, second trimester ♀
O43.223	Placenta increta, third trimester ♀
O43.232	Placenta percreta, second trimester ♀
O43.233	Placenta percreta, third trimester ♀
O72.0	Third-stage hemorrhage ♀
O72.1	Other immediate postpartum hemorrhage ♀

CCI Edits

Refer to Appendix A for CCI edits.

Pub 100

01962: Pub 100-04, 12, 140.5, Pub 100-04, 12, 50, Pub 100-04, 12, 90.4.5

Base Units

Global: XXX

Code	Base Units
01962	8

Modifiers (PAR)

Code	Mod 50	Mod 51	Mod 62	Mod 80
01962	9	9	9	9

CPT © 2018 American Medical Association. All Rights Reserved.

01963

01963 Anesthesia for cesarean hysterectomy without any labor analgesia/anesthesia care

ICD-10-CM Diagnostic Codes

C53.0	Malignant neoplasm of endocervix ♀
C53.1	Malignant neoplasm of exocervix ♀
C53.8	Malignant neoplasm of overlapping sites of cervix uteri ♀
C53.9	Malignant neoplasm of cervix uteri, unspecified ♀
C54.0	Malignant neoplasm of isthmus uteri ♀
C54.1	Malignant neoplasm of endometrium ♀
C54.2	Malignant neoplasm of myometrium ♀
C54.3	Malignant neoplasm of fundus uteri ♀
C54.8	Malignant neoplasm of overlapping sites of corpus uteri ♀
C54.9	Malignant neoplasm of corpus uteri, unspecified ♀
C55	Malignant neoplasm of uterus, part unspecified ♀
D25.0	Submucous leiomyoma of uterus ♀
D25.1	Intramural leiomyoma of uterus ♀
D25.2	Subserosal leiomyoma of uterus ♀
D25.9	Leiomyoma of uterus, unspecified ♀
O43.212	Placenta accreta, second trimester ♀
O43.213	Placenta accreta, third trimester ♀
O43.222	Placenta increta, second trimester ♀
O43.223	Placenta increta, third trimester ♀
O43.232	Placenta percreta, second trimester ♀
O43.233	Placenta percreta, third trimester ♀
O71.02	Rupture of uterus before onset of labor, second trimester ♀
O71.03	Rupture of uterus before onset of labor, third trimester ♀
O71.1	Rupture of uterus during labor ♀
O72.0	Third-stage hemorrhage ♀
O72.1	Other immediate postpartum hemorrhage ♀

CCI Edits

Refer to Appendix A for CCI edits.

Pub 100

01963: Pub 100-04, 12, 140.5, Pub 100-04, 12, 50, Pub 100-04, 12, 90.4.5

Base Units

Global: XXX

Code	Base Units
01963	8

Modifiers (PAR)

Code	Mod 50	Mod 51	Mod 62	Mod 80
01963	9	9	9	9

CPT © 2018 American Medical Association. All Rights Reserved.

01965

01965 Anesthesia for incomplete or missed abortion procedures

ICD-10-CM Diagnostic Codes

O02.1	Missed abortion ♀
O03.0	Genital tract and pelvic infection following incomplete spontaneous abortion ♀
O03.1	Delayed or excessive hemorrhage following incomplete spontaneous abortion ♀
O03.2	Embolism following incomplete spontaneous abortion ♀
O03.30	Unspecified complication following incomplete spontaneous abortion ♀
O03.31	Shock following incomplete spontaneous abortion ♀
O03.32	Renal failure following incomplete spontaneous abortion ♀
O03.33	Metabolic disorder following incomplete spontaneous abortion ♀
O03.34	Damage to pelvic organs following incomplete spontaneous abortion ♀
O03.35	Other venous complications following incomplete spontaneous abortion ♀
O03.36	Cardiac arrest following incomplete spontaneous abortion ♀
O03.37	Sepsis following incomplete spontaneous abortion ♀
O03.38	Urinary tract infection following incomplete spontaneous abortion ♀
O03.39	Incomplete spontaneous abortion with other complications ♀
O03.4	Incomplete spontaneous abortion without complication ♀

CCI Edits

Refer to Appendix A for CCI edits.

Pub 100

01965: Pub 100-04, 12, 140.5, Pub 100-04, 12, 50, Pub 100-04, 12, 90.4.5

Base Units

Global: XXX

Code	Base Units
01965	4

Modifiers (PAR)

Code	Mod 50	Mod 51	Mod 62	Mod 80
01965	9	9	9	9

CPT © 2018 American Medical Association. All Rights Reserved.

01966

01966 Anesthesia for induced abortion procedures

ICD-10-CM Diagnostic Codes

Z33.2	Encounter for elective termination of pregnancy ♀

CCI Edits

Refer to Appendix A for CCI edits.

Pub 100

01966: Pub 100-04, 12, 140.5, Pub 100-04, 12, 50, Pub 100-04, 12, 90.4.5

Base Units

Global: XXX

Code	Base Units
01966	4

Modifiers (PAR)

Code	Mod 50	Mod 51	Mod 62	Mod 80
01966	9	9	9	9

CPT © 2018 American Medical Association. All Rights Reserved.

01967

01967 Neuraxial labor analgesia/anesthesia for planned vaginal delivery (this includes any repeat subarachnoid needle placement and drug injection and/or any necessary replacement of an epidural catheter during labor)

AMA *CPT Assistant* ▢

01967: Dec 01: 3, Oct 14: 14

ICD-10-CM Diagnostic Codes

	Code	Description
➐	O60.12	Preterm labor second trimester with preterm delivery second trimester
➐	O60.13	Preterm labor second trimester with preterm delivery third trimester
➐	O60.14	Preterm labor third trimester with preterm delivery third trimester
➐	O60.22	Term delivery with preterm labor, second trimester
➐	O60.23	Term delivery with preterm labor, third trimester
	O62.0	Primary inadequate contractions ♀
	O62.1	Secondary uterine inertia ♀
	O62.2	Other uterine inertia ♀
	O62.3	Precipitate labor ♀
	O62.4	Hypertonic, incoordinate, and prolonged uterine contractions ♀
	O62.8	Other abnormalities of forces of labor ♀
	O63.9	Long labor, unspecified ♀
➐	O64.0	Obstructed labor due to incomplete rotation of fetal head
➐	O64.1	Obstructed labor due to breech presentation
➐	O64.2	Obstructed labor due to face presentation
➐	O64.3	Obstructed labor due to brow presentation
➐	O64.4	Obstructed labor due to shoulder presentation
➐	O64.5	Obstructed labor due to compound presentation
➐	O64.8	Obstructed labor due to other malposition and malpresentation
➐	O69.0	Labor and delivery complicated by prolapse of cord
➐	O69.1	Labor and delivery complicated by cord around neck, with compression
➐	O69.2	Labor and delivery complicated by other cord entanglement, with compression
➐	O69.81	Labor and delivery complicated by cord around neck, without compression
➐	O69.82	Labor and delivery complicated by other cord entanglement, without compression
➐	O69.89	Labor and delivery complicated by other cord complications
	O70.0	First degree perineal laceration during delivery ♀
	O70.1	Second degree perineal laceration during delivery ♀
	O70.2	Third degree perineal laceration during delivery ♀
	O70.3	Fourth degree perineal laceration during delivery ♀
	O70.4	Anal sphincter tear complicating delivery, not associated with third degree laceration ♀
	O75.5	Delayed delivery after artificial rupture of membranes ♀
	O75.89	Other specified complications of labor and delivery ♀
	O76	Abnormality in fetal heart rate and rhythm complicating labor and delivery ♀
	O77.0	Labor and delivery complicated by meconium in amniotic fluid ♀
	O77.1	Fetal stress in labor or delivery due to drug administration ♀
	O77.8	Labor and delivery complicated by other evidence of fetal stress ♀
	O77.9	Labor and delivery complicated by fetal stress, unspecified ♀
	O80	Encounter for full-term uncomplicated delivery ♀

ICD-10-CM Coding Notes

For codes requiring a 7th character extension, refer to your ICD-10-CM book. Review the character descriptions and coding guidelines for proper selection. For some procedures, only certain characters will apply.

CCI Edits

Refer to Appendix A for CCI edits.

Pub 100

01967: Pub 100-04, 12, 140.5, Pub 100-04, 12, 50, Pub 100-04, 12, 90.4.5

Base Units

Global: XXX

Code	Base Units
01967	5

Modifiers (PAR)

Code	Mod 50	Mod 51	Mod 62	Mod 80
01967	9	9	9	9

CPT © 2018 American Medical Association. All Rights Reserved.

01968

✚ **01968 Anesthesia for cesarean delivery following neuraxial labor analgesia/anesthesia (List separately in addition to code for primary procedure performed)**

(Use 01968 in conjunction with 01967)

AMA *CPT Assistant* ▯

01968: Dec 01: 3, Jun 11: 13, Oct 14: 14

ICD-10-CM Diagnostic Codes

See Primary Procedure code for crosswalks.

CCI Edits

Refer to Appendix A for CCI edits.

Pub 100

01968: Pub 100-04, 12, 140.5, Pub 100-04, 12, 50, Pub 100-04, 12, 90.4.5

Base Units

Global: XXX

Code	Base Units
01968	2

Modifiers (PAR)

Code	Mod 50	Mod 51	Mod 62	Mod 80
01968	9	9	9	9

CPT © 2018 American Medical Association. All Rights Reserved.

01969

✚ **01969 Anesthesia for cesarean hysterectomy following neuraxial labor analgesia/anesthesia (List separately in addition to code for primary procedure performed)**

(Use 01969 in conjunction with 01967)

AMA *CPT Assistant*

01969: Dec 01: 3, Jun 11: 13, Jul 12: 13

ICD-10-CM Diagnostic Codes

See Primary Procedure code for crosswalks.

CCI Edits

Refer to Appendix A for CCI edits.

Pub 100

01969: Pub 100-04, 12, 140.5, Pub 100-04, 12, 50, Pub 100-04, 12, 90.4.5

Base Units

Global: XXX

Code	Base Units
01969	5

Modifiers (PAR)

Code	Mod 50	Mod 51	Mod 62	Mod 80
01969	9	9	9	9

CPT © 2018 American Medical Association. All Rights Reserved.

01990

01990 Physiological support for harvesting of organ(s) from brain-dead patient

AMA *CPT Assistant*

01990: Mar 06: 15, Nov 07: 8, Oct 11: 3, Jul 12: 13

ICD-10-CM Diagnostic Codes

G93.82 Brain death

CCI Edits

Refer to Appendix A for CCI edits.

Pub 100

01990: Pub 100-04, 12, 140.5, Pub 100-04, 12, 50, Pub 100-04, 12, 90.4.5

Base Units

Global: XXX

Code	Base Units
01990	7

Modifiers (PAR)

Code	Mod 50	Mod 51	Mod 62	Mod 80
01990	9	9	9	9

CPT © 2018 American Medical Association. All Rights Reserved.

01991

01991 Anesthesia for diagnostic or therapeutic nerve blocks and injections (when block or injection is performed by a different physician or other qualified health care professional); other than the prone position

ICD-10-CM Diagnostic Codes

	Code	Description
	B02.21	Postherpetic geniculate ganglionitis
	B02.22	Postherpetic trigeminal neuralgia
	B02.23	Postherpetic polyneuropathy
	G50.0	Trigeminal neuralgia
	G50.1	Atypical facial pain
	G50.8	Other disorders of trigeminal nerve
	G51.0	Bell's palsy
	G51.1	Geniculate ganglionitis
⇄	G51.31	Clonic hemifacial spasm, right
⇄	G51.32	Clonic hemifacial spasm, left
⇄	G51.33	Clonic hemifacial spasm, bilateral
⇄	G51.39	Clonic hemifacial spasm, unspecified
	G51.8	Other disorders of facial nerve
⇄	G56.41	Causalgia of right upper limb
⇄	G56.42	Causalgia of left upper limb
⇄	G56.43	Causalgia of bilateral upper limbs
⇄	G56.81	Other specified mononeuropathies of right upper limb
⇄	G56.82	Other specified mononeuropathies of left upper limb
⇄	G57.71	Causalgia of right lower limb
⇄	G57.72	Causalgia of left lower limb
⇄	G57.81	Other specified mononeuropathies of right lower limb
⇄	G57.82	Other specified mononeuropathies of left lower limb
	G58.0	Intercostal neuropathy
	G89.11	Acute pain due to trauma
	G89.12	Acute post-thoracotomy pain
	G89.18	Other acute postprocedural pain
	G89.21	Chronic pain due to trauma
	G89.22	Chronic post-thoracotomy pain
	G89.28	Other chronic postprocedural pain
	G89.29	Other chronic pain
⇄	G90.511	Complex regional pain syndrome I of right upper limb
⇄	G90.512	Complex regional pain syndrome I of left upper limb
⇄	G90.513	Complex regional pain syndrome I of upper limb, bilateral
⇄	G90.521	Complex regional pain syndrome I of right lower limb
⇄	G90.522	Complex regional pain syndrome I of left lower limb
⇄	G90.523	Complex regional pain syndrome I of lower limb, bilateral

CCI Edits

Refer to Appendix A for CCI edits.

Pub 100

01991: Pub 100-04, 12, 140.5, Pub 100-04, 12, 50, Pub 100-04, 12, 90.4.5

Base Units

Global: XXX

Code	Base Units
01991	3

Modifiers (PAR)

Code	Mod 50	Mod 51	Mod 62	Mod 80
01991	9	9	9	9

CPT © 2018 American Medical Association. All Rights Reserved.

01992

01992 Anesthesia for diagnostic or therapeutic nerve blocks and injections (when block or injection is performed by a different physician or other qualified health care professional); prone position

(Do not report 01991 or 01992 in conjunction with 99151, 99152, 99153, 99155, 99156, 99157)

(When regional intravenous administration of local anesthetic agent or other medication in the upper or lower extremity is used as the anesthetic for a surgical procedure, report the appropriate anesthesia code. To report a Bier block for pain management, use 64999)

(For intra-arterial or intravenous therapy for pain management, see 96373, 96374)

ICD-10-CM Diagnostic Codes

	Code	Description
	G44.001	Cluster headache syndrome, unspecified, intractable
	G44.009	Cluster headache syndrome, unspecified, not intractable
	G44.011	Episodic cluster headache, intractable
	G44.019	Episodic cluster headache, not intractable
	G44.021	Chronic cluster headache, intractable
	G44.029	Chronic cluster headache, not intractable
	G44.031	Episodic paroxysmal hemicrania, intractable
	G44.039	Episodic paroxysmal hemicrania, not intractable
	G44.041	Chronic paroxysmal hemicrania, intractable
	G44.049	Chronic paroxysmal hemicrania, not intractable
	G44.89	Other headache syndrome
	G54.2	Cervical root disorders, not elsewhere classified
	G54.3	Thoracic root disorders, not elsewhere classified
	G54.4	Lumbosacral root disorders, not elsewhere classified
	G58.8	Other specified mononeuropathies
	G89.11	Acute pain due to trauma
	G89.12	Acute post-thoracotomy pain
	G89.18	Other acute postprocedural pain
	G89.21	Chronic pain due to trauma
	G89.22	Chronic post-thoracotomy pain
	G89.28	Other chronic postprocedural pain
	G89.3	Neoplasm related pain (acute) (chronic)
	G89.4	Chronic pain syndrome
➐	M48.51	Collapsed vertebra, not elsewhere classified, occipito-atlanto-axial region
➐	M48.52	Collapsed vertebra, not elsewhere classified, cervical region
➐	M48.53	Collapsed vertebra, not elsewhere classified, cervicothoracic region
➐	M48.54	Collapsed vertebra, not elsewhere classified, thoracic region
➐	M48.55	Collapsed vertebra, not elsewhere classified, thoracolumbar region
➐	M48.57	Collapsed vertebra, not elsewhere classified, lumbosacral region
➐	M48.58	Collapsed vertebra, not elsewhere classified, sacral and sacrococcygeal region
	M50.11	Cervical disc disorder with radiculopathy, high cervical region
	M50.120	Mid-cervical disc disorder, unspecified
	M50.121	Cervical disc disorder at C4-C5 level with radiculopathy
	M50.122	Cervical disc disorder at C5-C6 level with radiculopathy
	M50.123	Cervical disc disorder at C6-C7 level with radiculopathy
	M50.13	Cervical disc disorder with radiculopathy, cervicothoracic region
	M51.15	Intervertebral disc disorders with radiculopathy, thoracolumbar region
	M51.16	Intervertebral disc disorders with radiculopathy, lumbar region
	M51.17	Intervertebral disc disorders with radiculopathy, lumbosacral region
	M54.11	Radiculopathy, occipito-atlanto-axial region
	M54.12	Radiculopathy, cervical region
	M54.13	Radiculopathy, cervicothoracic region
	M54.14	Radiculopathy, thoracic region
	M54.15	Radiculopathy, thoracolumbar region
	M54.16	Radiculopathy, lumbar region
	M54.17	Radiculopathy, lumbosacral region
	M54.18	Radiculopathy, sacral and sacrococcygeal region
	M54.2	Cervicalgia
⇄	M54.31	Sciatica, right side
⇄	M54.32	Sciatica, left side
⇄	M54.41	Lumbago with sciatica, right side
⇄	M54.42	Lumbago with sciatica, left side
	M54.5	Low back pain
	M54.6	Pain in thoracic spine
	M54.81	Occipital neuralgia
	M54.89	Other dorsalgia
➐	S14.2	Injury of nerve root of cervical spine
➐	S24.2	Injury of nerve root of thoracic spine
➐	S34.21	Injury of nerve root of lumbar spine
➐	S34.22	Injury of nerve root of sacral spine

ICD-10-CM Coding Notes

For codes requiring a 7th character extension, refer to your ICD-10-CM book. Review the character descriptions and coding guidelines for proper selection. For some procedures, only certain characters will apply.

CCI Edits

Refer to Appendix A for CCI edits.

Pub 100

01992: Pub 100-04, 12, 140.5, Pub 100-04, 12, 50, Pub 100-04, 12, 90.4.5

Base Units

Global: XXX

Code	Base Units
01992	5

Modifiers (PAR)

Code	Mod 50	Mod 51	Mod 62	Mod 80
01992	9	9	9	9

CPT © 2018 American Medical Association. All Rights Reserved.

01996

01996 Daily hospital management of epidural or subarachnoid continuous drug administration

(Report code 01996 for daily hospital management of continuous epidural or subarachnoid drug administration performed after insertion of an epidural or subarachnoid catheter)

AMA *CPT Assistant*

01996: Feb 97: 5, Nov 97: 10, May 99: 6, Jul 12: 5, Oct 12: 14, May 15: 10

ICD-10-CM Diagnostic Codes

G89.0	Central pain syndrome
G89.11	Acute pain due to trauma
G89.12	Acute post-thoracotomy pain
G89.18	Other acute postprocedural pain
G89.21	Chronic pain due to trauma
G89.22	Chronic post-thoracotomy pain
G89.28	Other chronic postprocedural pain
G89.3	Neoplasm related pain (acute) (chronic)
G89.4	Chronic pain syndrome

CCI Edits

Refer to Appendix A for CCI edits.

Pub 100

01996: Pub 100-04, 12, 140.5, Pub 100-04, 12, 50, Pub 100-04, 12, 90.4.5

Base Units

Global: XXX

Code	Base Units
01996	3

Modifiers (PAR)

Code	Mod 50	Mod 51	Mod 62	Mod 80
01996	9	9	9	9

CPT © 2018 American Medical Association. All Rights Reserved.

20526

20526 Injection, therapeutic (eg, local anesthetic, corticosteroid), carpal tunnel

AMA Coding Guideline

Please see the Surgery Guidelines section for the following guidelines:

- *Surgical Procedures on the Musculoskeletal System*

AMA Coding Notes

General Introduction or Removal Procedures on the Musculoskeletal System

(For injection procedure for arthrography, see anatomical area)

(For injection of autologous adipose-derived regenerative cells, see 0489T, 0490T)

AMA *CPT Assistant* ☐

20526: Mar 02: 7

Plain English Description

A therapeutic injection using a local anesthetic or corticosteroid is performed to treat symptoms of carpal tunnel syndrome. This procedure is referred to as a carpal tunnel or median nerve injection. The flexor carpi radialis (FCR) and palmaris longus (PL) tendons are located. The skin over the planned needle insertion site is cleansed. The needle is inserted just proximal to the most proximal wrist crease and medial to the PL tendon. The needle is directed toward the ring finger and advanced until the PL tendon is encountered. The syringe is retraced to ensure that the needle is clear of all blood vessels. The local anesthetic or steroid solution is injected. The needle is removed and the local anesthetic or steroid is allowed to disperse distally using gravity and finger motion.

Carpal tunnel therapeutic injection

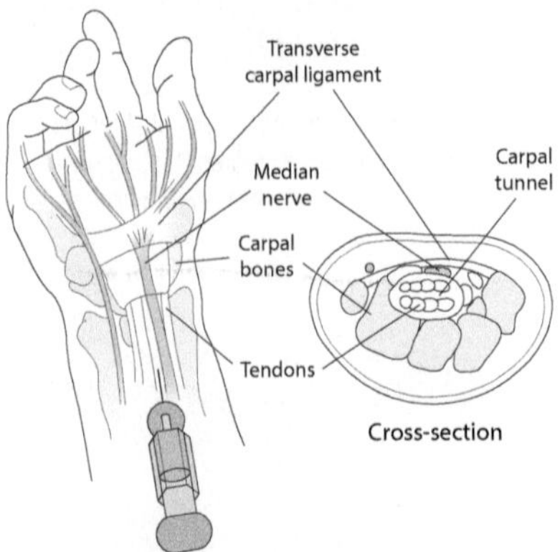

A therapeutic injection of corticosteroid or anesthetic is injected to help relieve the symptoms of carpal tunnel syndrome.

ICD-10-CM Diagnostic Codes

	Code	Description
⇄	G56.01	Carpal tunnel syndrome, right upper limb
⇄	G56.02	Carpal tunnel syndrome, left upper limb
⇄	G56.03	Carpal tunnel syndrome, bilateral upper limbs
⇄	G56.10	Other lesions of median nerve, unspecified upper limb
⇄	G56.11	Other lesions of median nerve, right upper limb
⇄	G56.12	Other lesions of median nerve, left upper limb
⇄	G56.13	Other lesions of median nerve, bilateral upper limbs
⇄	M25.531	Pain in right wrist
⇄	M25.532	Pain in left wrist
⇄	M25.539	Pain in unspecified wrist
⇄	M65.831	Other synovitis and tenosynovitis, right forearm
⇄	M65.832	Other synovitis and tenosynovitis, left forearm

CCI Edits

Refer to Appendix A for CCI edits.

Facility RVUs ☐

Code	Work	PE Facility	MP	Total Facility
20526	0.94	0.56	0.16	1.66

Non-facility RVUs ☐

Code	Work	PE Non-Facility	MP	Total Non-Facility
20526	0.94	1.10	0.16	2.20

Modifiers (PAR) ☐

Code	Mod 50	Mod 51	Mod 62	Mod 66	Mod 80
20526	1	2	0	0	1

Global Period

Code	Days
20526	000

CPT © 2018 American Medical Association. All Rights Reserved.

20550-20551

20550 Injection(s); single tendon sheath, or ligament, aponeurosis (eg, plantar "fascia")

(For injection of Morton's neuroma, see 64455, 64632)

20551 Injection(s); single tendon origin/ insertion

(Do not report 20550, 20551 in conjunction with 0232T, 0481T)

(For harvesting, preparation, and injection[s] of platelet-rich plasma, use 0232T)

AMA Coding Guideline

Please see the Surgery Guidelines section for the following guidelines:

- *Surgical Procedures on the Musculoskeletal System*

AMA Coding Notes

General Introduction or Removal Procedures on the Musculoskeletal System

(For injection procedure for arthrography, see anatomical area)

(For injection of autologous adipose-derived regenerative cells, see 0489T, 0490T)

AMA *CPT Assistant*

20550: Jan 96: 7, Jun 98: 10, Mar 02: 7, Aug 03: 14, Sep 03: 13, Dec 03: 11, Jan 09: 6, Jul 12: 14, Oct 14: 9

20551: Mar 02: 7, Sep 03: 13, Oct 14: 9, Dec 17: 16

Plain English Description

The physician injects a single tendon sheath, ligament, or aponeurosis (20550) or a single tendon origin or insertion (20551). In 20550, the site of maximum tenderness is identified by palpation. The needle is advanced into the tendon sheath, ligament, or aponeurosis and an anesthetic, steroid, or other therapeutic substance is injected. More than one injection to the same tendon sheath or ligament may be administered. In 20551, the tendon origin or insertion is located. A needle is advanced into the origin or insertion and an anesthetic, steroid, or other therapeutic substance is injected.

Injections

Plantar fascia
Achilles tendon
Aponeurosis
A therapeutic agent is injected into a single tendon sheath, ligament or aponeurosis.
A therapeutic agent is injected into a tendon origin or insertion point.

ICD-10-CM Diagnostic Codes

	Code	Description
	M54.2	Cervicalgia
⇄	M54.31	Sciatica, right side
⇄	M54.32	Sciatica, left side
⇄	M54.41	Lumbago with sciatica, right side
⇄	M54.42	Lumbago with sciatica, left side
	M54.5	Low back pain
	M54.6	Pain in thoracic spine
	M54.81	Occipital neuralgia
	M54.89	Other dorsalgia
	M65.4	Radial styloid tenosynovitis [de Quervain]
⇄	M65.811	Other synovitis and tenosynovitis, right shoulder
⇄	M65.812	Other synovitis and tenosynovitis, left shoulder
⇄	M65.821	Other synovitis and tenosynovitis, right upper arm
⇄	M65.822	Other synovitis and tenosynovitis, left upper arm
⇄	M65.831	Other synovitis and tenosynovitis, right forearm
⇄	M65.832	Other synovitis and tenosynovitis, left forearm
⇄	M65.841	Other synovitis and tenosynovitis, right hand
⇄	M65.842	Other synovitis and tenosynovitis, left hand
⇄	M65.851	Other synovitis and tenosynovitis, right thigh
⇄	M65.852	Other synovitis and tenosynovitis, left thigh
⇄	M65.861	Other synovitis and tenosynovitis, right lower leg
⇄	M65.862	Other synovitis and tenosynovitis, left lower leg
⇄	M65.871	Other synovitis and tenosynovitis, right ankle and foot
⇄	M65.872	Other synovitis and tenosynovitis, left ankle and foot
	M65.88	Other synovitis and tenosynovitis, other site
	M65.89	Other synovitis and tenosynovitis, multiple sites
⇄	M70.11	Bursitis, right hand
⇄	M70.12	Bursitis, left hand
⇄	M70.21	Olecranon bursitis, right elbow
⇄	M70.22	Olecranon bursitis, left elbow
⇄	M70.31	Other bursitis of elbow, right elbow
⇄	M70.32	Other bursitis of elbow, left elbow
⇄	M70.41	Prepatellar bursitis, right knee
⇄	M70.42	Prepatellar bursitis, left knee
⇄	M70.51	Other bursitis of knee, right knee
⇄	M70.61	Trochanteric bursitis, right hip
⇄	M70.62	Trochanteric bursitis, left hip
⇄	M70.71	Other bursitis of hip, right hip
⇄	M70.72	Other bursitis of hip, left hip
⇄	M71.52	Other bursitis, not elsewhere classified, elbow
⇄	M75.01	Adhesive capsulitis of right shoulder
⇄	M75.111	Incomplete rotator cuff tear or rupture of right shoulder, not specified as traumatic
⇄	M75.112	Incomplete rotator cuff tear or rupture of left shoulder, not specified as traumatic
⇄	M75.21	Bicipital tendinitis, right shoulder
⇄	M75.22	Bicipital tendinitis, left shoulder
⇄	M75.31	Calcific tendinitis of right shoulder
⇄	M75.32	Calcific tendinitis of left shoulder
⇄	M75.41	Impingement syndrome of right shoulder
⇄	M75.42	Impingement syndrome of left shoulder
⇄	M75.51	Bursitis of right shoulder
⇄	M75.52	Bursitis of left shoulder
⇄	M75.81	Other shoulder lesions, right shoulder
⇄	M75.82	Other shoulder lesions, left shoulder
⇄	M76.01	Gluteal tendinitis, right hip
⇄	M76.02	Gluteal tendinitis, left hip
⇄	M76.11	Psoas tendinitis, right hip
⇄	M76.12	Psoas tendinitis, left hip
⇄	M76.21	Iliac crest spur, right hip
⇄	M76.22	Iliac crest spur, left hip
⇄	M76.31	Iliotibial band syndrome, right leg
⇄	M76.32	Iliotibial band syndrome, left leg
⇄	M76.41	Tibial collateral bursitis [Pellegrini-Stieda], right leg
⇄	M76.42	Tibial collateral bursitis [Pellegrini-Stieda], left leg
⇄	M76.51	Patellar tendinitis, right knee
⇄	M76.52	Patellar tendinitis, left knee
⇄	M76.61	Achilles tendinitis, right leg
⇄	M76.62	Achilles tendinitis, left leg
⇄	M76.71	Peroneal tendinitis, right leg
⇄	M76.72	Peroneal tendinitis, left leg
⇄	M76.811	Anterior tibial syndrome, right leg
⇄	M76.812	Anterior tibial syndrome, left leg
⇄	M76.821	Posterior tibial tendinitis, right leg
⇄	M76.822	Posterior tibial tendinitis, left leg
⇄	M76.891	Other specified enthesopathies of right lower limb, excluding foot
⇄	M76.892	Other specified enthesopathies of left lower limb, excluding foot
⇄	M77.01	Medial epicondylitis, right elbow
⇄	M77.02	Medial epicondylitis, left elbow
⇄	M77.11	Lateral epicondylitis, right elbow
⇄	M77.12	Lateral epicondylitis, left elbow
⇄	M77.21	Periarthritis, right wrist
⇄	M77.22	Periarthritis, left wrist
⇄	M77.31	Calcaneal spur, right foot
⇄	M77.32	Calcaneal spur, left foot
⇄	M77.41	Metatarsalgia, right foot
⇄	M77.42	Metatarsalgia, left foot
⇄	M77.51	Other enthesopathy of right foot
⇄	M77.52	Other enthesopathy of left foot
⇄	M79.621	Pain in right upper arm
⇄	M79.622	Pain in left upper arm
⇄	M79.631	Pain in right forearm

CPT © 2018 American Medical Association. All Rights Reserved.

⇄	M79.632	Pain in left forearm
⇄	M79.641	Pain in right hand
⇄	M79.642	Pain in left hand
⇄	M79.651	Pain in right thigh
⇄	M79.652	Pain in left thigh
⇄	M79.661	Pain in right lower leg
⇄	M79.662	Pain in left lower leg
⇄	M79.671	Pain in right foot
⇄	M79.672	Pain in left foot
⇄	M79.674	Pain in right toe(s)
⇄	M79.675	Pain in left toe(s)
	M79.7	Fibromyalgia

CCI Edits

Refer to Appendix A for CCI edits.

Facility RVUs 🗋

Code	Work	PE Facility	MP	Total Facility
20550	0.75	0.29	0.09	1.13
20551	0.75	0.32	0.08	1.15

Non-facility RVUs 🗋

Code	Work	PE Non-Facility	MP	Total Non-Facility
20550	0.75	0.67	0.09	1.51
20551	0.75	0.70	0.08	1.53

Modifiers (PAR) 🗋

Code	Mod 50	Mod 51	Mod 62	Mod 66	Mod 80
20550	1	2	0	0	1
20551	0	2	0	0	1

Global Period

Code	Days
20550	000
20551	000

CPT © 2018 American Medical Association. All Rights Reserved.

20552-20553

20552 Injection(s); single or multiple trigger point(s), 1 or 2 muscle(s)

20553 Injection(s); single or multiple trigger point(s), 3 or more muscles

(If imaging guidance is performed, see 76942, 77002, 77021)

AMA Coding Guideline

Please see the Surgery Guidelines section for the following guidelines:

- *Surgical Procedures on the Musculoskeletal System*

AMA Coding Notes

General Introduction or Removal Procedures on the Musculoskeletal System

(For injection procedure for arthrography, see anatomical area)

(For injection of autologous adipose-derived regenerative cells, see 0489T, 0490T)

AMA *CPT Assistant* □

20552: Mar 02: 7, May 03: 19, Sep 03: 11, Feb 10: 9, Feb 11: 5, Jul 11: 16, Apr 12: 19, Oct 14: 9, Jun 17: 10, Dec 17: 16

20553: Mar 02: 7, May 03: 19, Sep 03: 11, Jun 08: 8, Feb 10: 9, Feb 11: 5, Jul 11: 16, Oct 14: 9, Jun 17: 10

Plain English Description

The physician injects a single or multiple trigger points in one or two muscles (20552) or three or more muscles (20553). Trigger points are tiny contraction knots that develop in a muscle when it is injured or overworked. The physician identifies the trigger points by palpating the muscle. The needle is advanced into the muscle and an anesthetic, steroid, or other therapeutic substance is injected. This is repeated until all trigger points on all involved muscles have been treated.

Injection

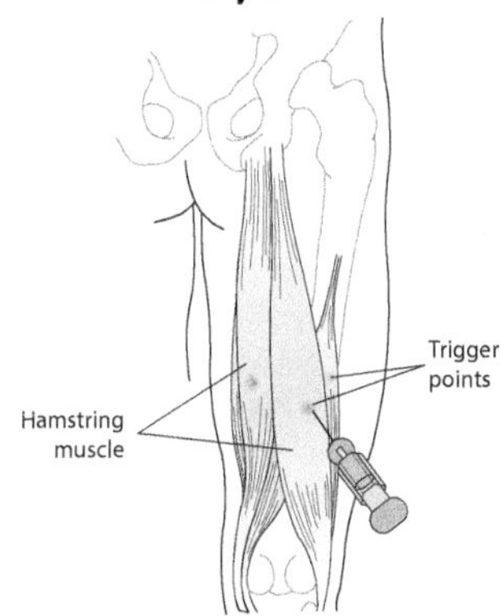

An anesthetic or therapeutic solution is injected into one or more trigger points in one or more muscles.

ICD-10-CM Diagnostic Codes

	Code	Description
	M43.6	Torticollis
	M54.2	Cervicalgia
	M54.5	Low back pain
	M54.9	Dorsalgia, unspecified
⇄	M60.811	Other myositis, right shoulder
⇄	M60.812	Other myositis, left shoulder
⇄	M60.821	Other myositis, right upper arm
⇄	M60.822	Other myositis, left upper arm
⇄	M60.831	Other myositis, right forearm
⇄	M60.832	Other myositis, left forearm
⇄	M60.841	Other myositis, right hand
⇄	M60.842	Other myositis, left hand
⇄	M60.851	Other myositis, right thigh
⇄	M60.852	Other myositis, left thigh
⇄	M60.861	Other myositis, right lower leg
⇄	M60.862	Other myositis, left lower leg
⇄	M60.871	Other myositis, right ankle and foot
⇄	M60.872	Other myositis, left ankle and foot
	M60.89	Other myositis, multiple sites
	M79.11	Myalgia of mastication muscle
	M79.12	Myalgia of auxiliary muscles, head and neck
	M79.18	Myalgia, other site
⇄	M79.621	Pain in right upper arm
⇄	M79.622	Pain in left upper arm
⇄	M79.631	Pain in right forearm
⇄	M79.632	Pain in left forearm
⇄	M79.644	Pain in right finger(s)
⇄	M79.645	Pain in left finger(s)
⇄	M79.651	Pain in right thigh
⇄	M79.652	Pain in left thigh
⇄	M79.661	Pain in right lower leg
⇄	M79.662	Pain in left lower leg
⇄	M79.671	Pain in right foot
⇄	M79.672	Pain in left foot
⇄	M79.674	Pain in right toe(s)
⇄	M79.675	Pain in left toe(s)
	M79.7	Fibromyalgia
	R68.84	Jaw pain

CCI Edits

Refer to Appendix A for CCI edits.

Facility RVUs □

Code	Work	PE Facility	MP	Total Facility
20552	0.66	0.36	0.07	1.09
20553	0.75	0.41	0.08	1.24

Non-facility RVUs □

Code	Work	PE Non-Facility	MP	Total Non-Facility
20552	0.66	0.84	0.07	1.57
20553	0.75	0.98	0.08	1.81

Modifiers (PAR) □

Code	Mod 50	Mod 51	Mod 62	Mod 66	Mod 80
20552	0	2	0	0	1
20553	0	2	0	0	1

Global Period

Code	Days
20552	000
20553	000

CPT © 2018 American Medical Association. All Rights Reserved.

20600-20604

20600 Arthrocentesis, aspiration and/or injection, small joint or bursa (eg, fingers, toes); without ultrasound guidance

20604 Arthrocentesis, aspiration and/or injection, small joint or bursa (eg, fingers, toes); with ultrasound guidance, with permanent recording and reporting

(Do not report 20600, 20604 in conjunction with 76942, 0489T, 0490T)

(If fluoroscopic, CT, or MRI guidance is performed, see 77002, 77012, 77021)

AMA Coding Guideline

Please see the Surgery Guidelines section for the following guidelines:

- *Surgical Procedures on the Musculoskeletal System*

AMA Coding Notes

General Introduction or Removal Procedures on the Musculoskeletal System

(For injection procedure for arthrography, see anatomical area)

(For injection of autologous adipose-derived regenerative cells, see 0489T, 0490T)

AMA *CPT Assistant* ◻

20600: Dec 07: 10, Feb 15: 6, Nov 15: 10, Aug 17: 9

20604: Feb 15: 6, Jul 15: 10

Plain English Description

Arthrocentesis and/or aspiration is performed to remove fluid from a joint or bursa in order to diagnose the cause of joint effusion and/or to reduce pain caused by the excess fluid. Injection of a joint or bursa may be performed in conjunction with the arthrocentesis procedure and is typically performed using an anti-inflammatory medication such as a steroid to reduce inflammation of the joint or bursa. The skin over the joint is cleansed. A local anesthetic is injected as needed. A needle with a syringe attached is inserted into the affected joint or bursa. Fluid is removed and sent for separately reportable laboratory analysis. This may be followed by a separate injection of medication into the joint or bursa. Use 20600 for arthrocentesis, aspiration and/or injection of a small joint or bursa, such as in the fingers or toes when no ultrasound guidance is used for needle placement. Report 20604 when ultrasonic guidance is used and a permanent recording is made with a report of the procedure.

Arthrocentesis

Fluid is aspirated and/or injected into a joint or bursa.
Bone
Ligament
Synovium
Tendon
Bone
Synovial fluid

Cross-section of joint

ICD-10-CM Diagnostic Codes

	Code	Description
⇄	M00.071	Staphylococcal arthritis, right ankle and foot
⇄	M00.072	Staphylococcal arthritis, left ankle and foot
⇄	M00.841	Arthritis due to other bacteria, right hand
⇄	M00.842	Arthritis due to other bacteria, left hand
⇄	M00.871	Arthritis due to other bacteria, right ankle and foot
⇄	M00.872	Arthritis due to other bacteria, left ankle and foot
	M00.9	Pyogenic arthritis, unspecified
⇄	M02.341	Reiter's disease, right hand
⇄	M02.342	Reiter's disease, left hand
⇄	M02.371	Reiter's disease, right ankle and foot
⇄	M02.372	Reiter's disease, left ankle and foot
⇄	M05.741	Rheumatoid arthritis with rheumatoid factor of right hand without organ or systems involvement
⇄	M05.742	Rheumatoid arthritis with rheumatoid factor of left hand without organ or systems involvement
⇄	M05.771	Rheumatoid arthritis with rheumatoid factor of right ankle and foot without organ or systems involvement
⇄	M05.772	Rheumatoid arthritis with rheumatoid factor of left ankle and foot without organ or systems involvement
⇄	M06.041	Rheumatoid arthritis without rheumatoid factor, right hand
⇄	M06.042	Rheumatoid arthritis without rheumatoid factor, left hand
⇄	M06.071	Rheumatoid arthritis without rheumatoid factor, right ankle and foot
⇄	M06.072	Rheumatoid arthritis without rheumatoid factor, left ankle and foot
⇄	M07.641	Enteropathic arthropathies, right hand
⇄	M07.642	Enteropathic arthropathies, left hand
⇄	M07.671	Enteropathic arthropathies, right ankle and foot
⇄	M07.672	Enteropathic arthropathies, left ankle and foot
⇄	M10.041	Idiopathic gout, right hand
⇄	M10.042	Idiopathic gout, left hand
⇄	M10.071	Idiopathic gout, right ankle and foot
⇄	M10.072	Idiopathic gout, left ankle and foot
⇄	M11.241	Other chondrocalcinosis, right hand
⇄	M11.242	Other chondrocalcinosis, left hand
⇄	M11.271	Other chondrocalcinosis, right ankle and foot
⇄	M11.272	Other chondrocalcinosis, left ankle and foot
⇄	M12.541	Traumatic arthropathy, right hand
⇄	M12.542	Traumatic arthropathy, left hand
⇄	M12.571	Traumatic arthropathy, right ankle and foot
⇄	M12.572	Traumatic arthropathy, left ankle and foot
⇄	M12.841	Other specific arthropathies, not elsewhere classified, right hand
⇄	M12.842	Other specific arthropathies, not elsewhere classified, left hand
⇄	M14.641	Charcôt's joint, right hand
⇄	M14.642	Charcôt's joint, left hand
⇄	M14.671	Charcôt's joint, right ankle and foot
⇄	M14.672	Charcôt's joint, left ankle and foot
⇄	M19.041	Primary osteoarthritis, right hand
⇄	M19.042	Primary osteoarthritis, left hand
⇄	M19.071	Primary osteoarthritis, right ankle and foot
⇄	M19.072	Primary osteoarthritis, left ankle and foot
⇄	M19.141	Post-traumatic osteoarthritis, right hand
⇄	M19.142	Post-traumatic osteoarthritis, left hand
⇄	M19.172	Post-traumatic osteoarthritis, left ankle and foot
⇄	M19.241	Secondary osteoarthritis, right hand
⇄	M19.242	Secondary osteoarthritis, left hand
⇄	M19.271	Secondary osteoarthritis, right ankle and foot
⇄	M19.272	Secondary osteoarthritis, left ankle and foot
❼⇄	M1A.041	Idiopathic chronic gout, right hand
❼⇄	M1A.042	Idiopathic chronic gout, left hand
❼⇄	M1A.071	Idiopathic chronic gout, right ankle and foot
❼⇄	M1A.072	Idiopathic chronic gout, left ankle and foot
❼	M1A.09	Idiopathic chronic gout, multiple sites
⇄	M25.041	Hemarthrosis, right hand
⇄	M25.042	Hemarthrosis, left hand
⇄	M25.441	Effusion, right hand
⇄	M25.442	Effusion, left hand
⇄	M25.474	Effusion, right foot
⇄	M25.475	Effusion, left foot
⇄	M25.541	Pain in joints of right hand
⇄	M25.542	Pain in joints of left hand
⇄	M25.571	Pain in right ankle and joints of right foot
⇄	M25.572	Pain in left ankle and joints of left foot
⇄	M65.841	Other synovitis and tenosynovitis, right hand

CPT © 2018 American Medical Association. All Rights Reserved.

⇄	M65.842	Other synovitis and tenosynovitis, left hand
⇄	M65.871	Other synovitis and tenosynovitis, right ankle and foot
⇄	M65.872	Other synovitis and tenosynovitis, left ankle and foot
⇄	M67.873	Other specified disorders of tendon, right ankle and foot
⇄	M67.874	Other specified disorders of tendon, left ankle and foot
⇄	M70.11	Bursitis, right hand
⇄	M70.12	Bursitis, left hand
⇄	M70.871	Other soft tissue disorders related to use, overuse and pressure, right ankle and foot
⇄	M70.872	Other soft tissue disorders related to use, overuse and pressure, left ankle and foot
⇄	M71.871	Other specified bursopathies, right ankle and foot
⇄	M71.872	Other specified bursopathies, left ankle and foot
⇄	M79.644	Pain in right finger(s)
⇄	M79.645	Pain in left finger(s)
⇄	M79.674	Pain in right toe(s)
⇄	M79.675	Pain in left toe(s)

ICD-10-CM Coding Notes

For codes requiring a 7th character extension, refer to your ICD-10-CM book. Review the character descriptions and coding guidelines for proper selection. For some procedures, only certain characters will apply.

CCI Edits

Refer to Appendix A for CCI edits.

Facility RVUs ☐

Code	Work	PE Facility	MP	Total Facility
20600	0.66	0.29	0.08	1.03
20604	0.89	0.35	0.10	1.34

Non-facility RVUs ☐

Code	Work	PE Non-Facility	MP	Total Non-Facility
20600	0.66	0.64	0.08	1.38
20604	0.89	1.11	0.10	2.10

Modifiers (PAR) ☐

Code	Mod 50	Mod 51	Mod 62	Mod 66	Mod 80
20600	1	2	0	0	1
20604	1	2	0	0	1

Global Period

Code	Days
20600	000
20604	000

CPT © 2018 American Medical Association. All Rights Reserved.

20605-20606

20605 Arthrocentesis, aspiration and/or injection, intermediate joint or bursa (eg, temporomandibular, acromioclavicular, wrist, elbow or ankle, olecranon bursa); without ultrasound guidance

20606 Arthrocentesis, aspiration and/or injection, intermediate joint or bursa (eg, temporomandibular, acromioclavicular, wrist, elbow or ankle, olecranon bursa); with ultrasound guidance, with permanent recording and reporting

(Do not report 20605, 20606 in conjunction with 76942)

(If fluoroscopic, CT, or MRI guidance is performed, see 77002, 77012, 77021)

AMA Coding Guideline

Please see the Surgery Guidelines section for the following guidelines:

- *Surgical Procedures on the Musculoskeletal System*

AMA Coding Notes

General Introduction or Removal Procedures on the Musculoskeletal System

(For injection procedure for arthrography, see anatomical area)

(For injection of autologous adipose-derived regenerative cells, see 0489T, 0490T)

AMA *CPT Assistant* ☐

20605: Dec 07: 10, Feb 15: 6, Nov 15: 10, Aug 17: 9

20606: Feb 15: 6, Jul 15: 10

Plain English Description

Arthrocentesis, or aspiration is performed to remove fluid from a joint or bursa in order to diagnose the cause of joint effusion and/or to reduce pain caused by the excess fluid. Injection of a joint or bursa may be performed in conjunction with the arthrocentesis procedure and is typically performed using an anti-inflammatory medication such as a steroid to reduce inflammation of the joint or bursa. The skin over the joint is cleansed. A local anesthetic is injected as needed. A needle with a syringe attached is inserted into the affected joint or bursa. Fluid is removed and sent for separately reportable laboratory analysis. This may be followed by a separate injection of medication into the joint or bursa. Use 20605 for an intermediate joint or bursa, such as the temporomandibular joint, acromioclavicular joint, wrist, elbow, or ankle joint, or the olecranon bursa when no ultrasound guidance is used for needle placement. Report 20606 when ultrasonic guidance is used and a permanent recording is made with a report of the procedure.

Arthrocentesis

Fluid is aspirated and/or injected into a joint or bursa.

Bone
Ligament
Synovium
Tendon
Bone
Synovial fluid

Cross-section of joint

ICD-10-CM Diagnostic Codes

⇄ M00.821 Arthritis due to other bacteria, right elbow
⇄ M00.822 Arthritis due to other bacteria, left elbow
⇄ M00.831 Arthritis due to other bacteria, right wrist
⇄ M00.832 Arthritis due to other bacteria, left wrist
⇄ M00.871 Arthritis due to other bacteria, right ankle and foot
⇄ M00.872 Arthritis due to other bacteria, left ankle and foot
M00.9 Pyogenic arthritis, unspecified
⇄ M02.321 Reiter's disease, right elbow
⇄ M02.322 Reiter's disease, left elbow
⇄ M02.331 Reiter's disease, right wrist
⇄ M02.332 Reiter's disease, left wrist
⇄ M02.371 Reiter's disease, right ankle and foot
⇄ M02.372 Reiter's disease, left ankle and foot
⇄ M05.721 Rheumatoid arthritis with rheumatoid factor of right elbow without organ or systems involvement
⇄ M05.722 Rheumatoid arthritis with rheumatoid factor of left elbow without organ or systems involvement
⇄ M05.731 Rheumatoid arthritis with rheumatoid factor of right wrist without organ or systems involvement
⇄ M05.732 Rheumatoid arthritis with rheumatoid factor of left wrist without organ or systems involvement
⇄ M05.771 Rheumatoid arthritis with rheumatoid factor of right ankle and foot without organ or systems involvement
⇄ M05.772 Rheumatoid arthritis with rheumatoid factor of left ankle and foot without organ or systems involvement
⇄ M06.021 Rheumatoid arthritis without rheumatoid factor, right elbow
⇄ M06.022 Rheumatoid arthritis without rheumatoid factor, left elbow
⇄ M06.031 Rheumatoid arthritis without rheumatoid factor, right wrist
⇄ M06.032 Rheumatoid arthritis without rheumatoid factor, left wrist
⇄ M06.071 Rheumatoid arthritis without rheumatoid factor, right ankle and foot
⇄ M06.072 Rheumatoid arthritis without rheumatoid factor, left ankle and foot
⇄ M07.621 Enteropathic arthropathies, right elbow
⇄ M07.622 Enteropathic arthropathies, left elbow
⇄ M07.631 Enteropathic arthropathies, right wrist
⇄ M07.632 Enteropathic arthropathies, left wrist
⇄ M07.671 Enteropathic arthropathies, right ankle and foot
⇄ M07.672 Enteropathic arthropathies, left ankle and foot
⇄ M10.171 Lead-induced gout, right ankle and foot
⇄ M10.172 Lead-induced gout, left ankle and foot
⇄ M10.271 Drug-induced gout, right ankle and foot
⇄ M10.272 Drug-induced gout, left ankle and foot
⇄ M10.371 Gout due to renal impairment, right ankle and foot
⇄ M10.372 Gout due to renal impairment, left ankle and foot
⇄ M10.471 Other secondary gout, right ankle and foot
⇄ M10.472 Other secondary gout, left ankle and foot
⇄ M11.221 Other chondrocalcinosis, right elbow
⇄ M11.222 Other chondrocalcinosis, left elbow
⇄ M11.231 Other chondrocalcinosis, right wrist
⇄ M11.232 Other chondrocalcinosis, left wrist
⇄ M11.271 Other chondrocalcinosis, right ankle and foot
⇄ M11.272 Other chondrocalcinosis, left ankle and foot
⇄ M12.521 Traumatic arthropathy, right elbow
⇄ M12.522 Traumatic arthropathy, left elbow
⇄ M12.531 Traumatic arthropathy, right wrist
⇄ M12.571 Traumatic arthropathy, right ankle and foot
⇄ M12.572 Traumatic arthropathy, left ankle and foot
⇄ M14.621 Charcôt's joint, right elbow
⇄ M14.622 Charcôt's joint, left elbow
⇄ M14.631 Charcôt's joint, right wrist
⇄ M14.632 Charcôt's joint, left wrist
⇄ M14.671 Charcôt's joint, right ankle and foot
⇄ M14.672 Charcôt's joint, left ankle and foot
⇄ M19.021 Primary osteoarthritis, right elbow
⇄ M19.022 Primary osteoarthritis, left elbow
⇄ M19.031 Primary osteoarthritis, right wrist
⇄ M19.032 Primary osteoarthritis, left wrist
⇄ M19.071 Primary osteoarthritis, right ankle and foot
⇄ M19.072 Primary osteoarthritis, left ankle and foot

CPT © 2018 American Medical Association. All Rights Reserved.

⇄ M19.121 Post-traumatic osteoarthritis, right elbow
⇄ M19.122 Post-traumatic osteoarthritis, left elbow
⇄ M19.131 Post-traumatic osteoarthritis, right wrist
⇄ M19.132 Post-traumatic osteoarthritis, left wrist
⇄ M19.171 Post-traumatic osteoarthritis, right ankle and foot
⇄ M19.172 Post-traumatic osteoarthritis, left ankle and foot
⇄ M19.221 Secondary osteoarthritis, right elbow
⇄ M19.222 Secondary osteoarthritis, left elbow
⇄ M19.231 Secondary osteoarthritis, right wrist
⇄ M19.232 Secondary osteoarthritis, left wrist
⇄ M19.271 Secondary osteoarthritis, right ankle and foot
⇄ M19.272 Secondary osteoarthritis, left ankle and foot
❼⇄ M1A.011 Idiopathic chronic gout, right shoulder
❼⇄ M1A.012 Idiopathic chronic gout, left shoulder
❼⇄ M1A.021 Idiopathic chronic gout, right elbow
❼⇄ M1A.022 Idiopathic chronic gout, left elbow
❼⇄ M1A.031 Idiopathic chronic gout, right wrist
❼⇄ M1A.032 Idiopathic chronic gout, left wrist
❼⇄ M1A.071 Idiopathic chronic gout, right ankle and foot
❼⇄ M1A.072 Idiopathic chronic gout, left ankle and foot
⇄ M25.021 Hemarthrosis, right elbow
⇄ M25.022 Hemarthrosis, left elbow
⇄ M25.031 Hemarthrosis, right wrist
⇄ M25.032 Hemarthrosis, left wrist
⇄ M25.071 Hemarthrosis, right ankle
⇄ M25.072 Hemarthrosis, left ankle
⇄ M25.431 Effusion, right wrist
⇄ M25.432 Effusion, left wrist
⇄ M25.471 Effusion, right ankle
⇄ M25.472 Effusion, left ankle
⇄ M25.521 Pain in right elbow
⇄ M25.522 Pain in left elbow
⇄ M25.531 Pain in right wrist
⇄ M25.532 Pain in left wrist
⇄ M25.571 Pain in right ankle and joints of right foot
⇄ M25.572 Pain in left ankle and joints of left foot
⇄ M26.601 Right temporomandibular joint disorder, unspecified
⇄ M26.602 Left temporomandibular joint disorder, unspecified
⇄ M26.603 Bilateral temporomandibular joint disorder, unspecified
⇄ M26.611 Adhesions and ankylosis of right temporomandibular joint
⇄ M26.612 Adhesions and ankylosis of left temporomandibular joint
⇄ M26.613 Adhesions and ankylosis of bilateral temporomandibular joint
⇄ M26.621 Arthralgia of right temporomandibular joint
⇄ M26.622 Arthralgia of left temporomandibular joint
⇄ M26.623 Arthralgia of bilateral temporomandibular joint
⇄ M26.631 Articular disc disorder of right temporomandibular joint
⇄ M26.632 Articular disc disorder of left temporomandibular joint
⇄ M26.633 Articular disc disorder of bilateral temporomandibular joint
⇄ M65.871 Other synovitis and tenosynovitis, right ankle and foot
⇄ M65.872 Other synovitis and tenosynovitis, left ankle and foot
⇄ M67.871 Other specified disorders of synovium, right ankle and foot
⇄ M67.872 Other specified disorders of synovium, left ankle and foot
⇄ M70.031 Crepitant synovitis (acute) (chronic), right wrist
⇄ M70.032 Crepitant synovitis (acute) (chronic), left wrist
⇄ M70.21 Olecranon bursitis, right elbow
⇄ M70.22 Olecranon bursitis, left elbow
⇄ M70.31 Other bursitis of elbow, right elbow
⇄ M70.32 Other bursitis of elbow, left elbow
⇄ M71.021 Abscess of bursa, right elbow
⇄ M71.022 Abscess of bursa, left elbow
⇄ M71.031 Abscess of bursa, right wrist
⇄ M71.032 Abscess of bursa, left wrist
⇄ M71.071 Abscess of bursa, right ankle and foot
⇄ M71.072 Abscess of bursa, left ankle and foot
⇄ M71.121 Other infective bursitis, right elbow
⇄ M71.122 Other infective bursitis, left elbow
⇄ M71.131 Other infective bursitis, right wrist
⇄ M71.132 Other infective bursitis, left wrist
⇄ M71.171 Other infective bursitis, right ankle and foot
⇄ M71.172 Other infective bursitis, left ankle and foot
⇄ M71.371 Other bursal cyst, right ankle and foot
⇄ M71.372 Other bursal cyst, left ankle and foot
⇄ M71.571 Other bursitis, not elsewhere classified, right ankle and foot
⇄ M71.572 Other bursitis, not elsewhere classified, left ankle and foot
⇄ M71.811 Other specified bursopathies, right shoulder
⇄ M71.812 Other specified bursopathies, left shoulder
⇄ M71.821 Other specified bursopathies, right elbow
⇄ M71.822 Other specified bursopathies, left elbow
⇄ M71.831 Other specified bursopathies, right wrist
⇄ M71.832 Other specified bursopathies, left wrist
⇄ M71.871 Other specified bursopathies, right ankle and foot
⇄ M71.872 Other specified bursopathies, left ankle and foot
⇄ M75.41 Impingement syndrome of right shoulder
⇄ M75.42 Impingement syndrome of left shoulder
⇄ M75.51 Bursitis of right shoulder
⇄ M75.52 Bursitis of left shoulder
⇄ M77.01 Medial epicondylitis, right elbow
⇄ M77.02 Medial epicondylitis, left elbow
⇄ M77.11 Lateral epicondylitis, right elbow
⇄ M77.12 Lateral epicondylitis, left elbow
⇄ M77.21 Periarthritis, right wrist
⇄ M77.22 Periarthritis, left wrist

ICD-10-CM Coding Notes

For codes requiring a 7th character extension, refer to your ICD-10-CM book. Review the character descriptions and coding guidelines for proper selection. For some procedures, only certain characters will apply.

CCI Edits

Refer to Appendix A for CCI edits.

Facility RVUs ▯

Code	Work	PE Facility	MP	Total Facility
20605	0.68	0.31	0.08	1.07
20606	1.00	0.41	0.12	1.53

Non-facility RVUs ▯

Code	Work	PE Non-Facility	MP	Total Non-Facility
20605	0.68	0.68	0.08	1.44
20606	1.00	1.20	0.12	2.32

Modifiers (PAR) ▯

Code	Mod 50	Mod 51	Mod 62	Mod 66	Mod 80
20605	1	2	0	0	1
20606	1	2	0	0	1

Global Period

Code	Days
20605	000
20606	000

CPT © 2018 American Medical Association. All Rights Reserved.

20610-20611

20610 Arthrocentesis, aspiration and/or injection, major joint or bursa (eg, shoulder, hip, knee, subacromial bursa); without ultrasound guidance

20611 Arthrocentesis, aspiration and/or injection, major joint or bursa (eg, shoulder, hip, knee, subacromial bursa); with ultrasound guidance, with permanent recording and reporting

(Do not report 20610, 20611 in conjunction with 27369, 76942)

(If fluoroscopic, CT, or MRI guidance is performed, see 77002, 77012, 77021)

AMA Coding Guideline

Please see the Surgery Guidelines section for the following guidelines:

- *Surgical Procedures on the Musculoskeletal System*

AMA Coding Notes

General Introduction or Removal Procedures on the Musculoskeletal System

(For injection procedure for arthrography, see anatomical area)

(For injection of autologous adipose-derived regenerative cells, see 0489T, 0490T)

AMA *CPT Assistant* ☐

20610: Spring 92: 8, Mar 01: 10, Apr 04: 15, Jul 06: 1, Dec 07: 10, Jul 08: 9, Mar 12: 6, Jun 12: 14, Dec 14: 18, Feb 15: 6, Aug 15: 6, Nov 15: 10, Apr 17: 10

20611: Feb 15: 6, Jul 15: 10, Aug 15: 6, Nov 15: 10

Plain English Description

Arthrocentesis, aspiration, and/or injection of a joint or bursa is performed. Arthrocentesis and aspiration is performed to remove fluid from a joint or bursa in order to diagnose the cause of joint effusion and/or to reduce pain caused by the excess fluid. Injection of a joint or bursa may be performed in conjunction with the arthrocentesis procedure and is typically performed using an anti-inflammatory medication such as a steroid to reduce inflammation of the joint or bursa. The skin over the joint is cleansed. A local anesthetic is injected as needed. A needle with a syringe attached is inserted into the affected joint or bursa. Fluid is removed and sent for separately reportable laboratory analysis. This may be followed by a separate injection of medication into the joint or bursa. Use 20610 for a major joint or bursa, such as the shoulder, knee, or hip joint, or the subacromial bursa when no ultrasound guidance is used for needle placement. Report 20611 when ultrasonic guidance is used and a permanent recording is made with a report of the procedure.

Arthrocentesis, aspiration and/or injection, major joint or bursa

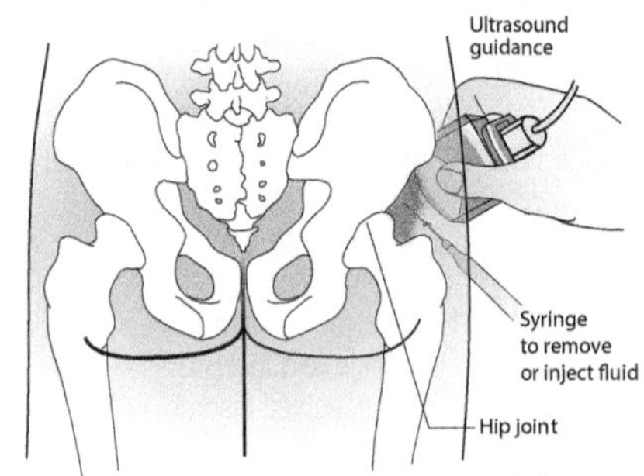

ICD-10-CM Diagnostic Codes

	Code	Description
⇄	M02.311	Reiter's disease, right shoulder
⇄	M02.312	Reiter's disease, left shoulder
⇄	M02.351	Reiter's disease, right hip
⇄	M02.352	Reiter's disease, left hip
⇄	M02.361	Reiter's disease, right knee
⇄	M02.362	Reiter's disease, left knee
⇄	M05.611	Rheumatoid arthritis of right shoulder with involvement of other organs and systems
⇄	M05.612	Rheumatoid arthritis of left shoulder with involvement of other organs and systems
⇄	M05.661	Rheumatoid arthritis of right knee with involvement of other organs and systems
⇄	M05.662	Rheumatoid arthritis of left knee with involvement of other organs and systems
⇄	M05.711	Rheumatoid arthritis with rheumatoid factor of right shoulder without organ or systems involvement
⇄	M05.712	Rheumatoid arthritis with rheumatoid factor of left shoulder without organ or systems involvement
⇄	M05.751	Rheumatoid arthritis with rheumatoid factor of right hip without organ or systems involvement
⇄	M05.752	Rheumatoid arthritis with rheumatoid factor of left hip without organ or systems involvement
⇄	M05.761	Rheumatoid arthritis with rheumatoid factor of right knee without organ or systems involvement
⇄	M05.762	Rheumatoid arthritis with rheumatoid factor of left knee without organ or systems involvement
⇄	M06.011	Rheumatoid arthritis without rheumatoid factor, right shoulder
⇄	M06.012	Rheumatoid arthritis without rheumatoid factor, left shoulder
⇄	M06.051	Rheumatoid arthritis without rheumatoid factor, right hip
⇄	M06.052	Rheumatoid arthritis without rheumatoid factor, left hip
⇄	M06.061	Rheumatoid arthritis without rheumatoid factor, right knee
⇄	M06.062	Rheumatoid arthritis without rheumatoid factor, left knee
⇄	M07.611	Enteropathic arthropathies, right shoulder
⇄	M07.612	Enteropathic arthropathies, left shoulder
⇄	M07.651	Enteropathic arthropathies, right hip
⇄	M07.652	Enteropathic arthropathies, left hip
⇄	M07.661	Enteropathic arthropathies, right knee
⇄	M07.662	Enteropathic arthropathies, left knee
⇄	M10.011	Idiopathic gout, right shoulder
⇄	M10.012	Idiopathic gout, left shoulder
⇄	M10.051	Idiopathic gout, right hip
⇄	M10.052	Idiopathic gout, left hip
⇄	M10.061	Idiopathic gout, right knee
⇄	M10.062	Idiopathic gout, left knee
⇄	M11.211	Other chondrocalcinosis, right shoulder
⇄	M11.212	Other chondrocalcinosis, left shoulder
⇄	M11.251	Other chondrocalcinosis, right hip
⇄	M11.252	Other chondrocalcinosis, left hip
⇄	M11.261	Other chondrocalcinosis, right knee
⇄	M11.262	Other chondrocalcinosis, left knee
⇄	M12.511	Traumatic arthropathy, right shoulder
⇄	M12.512	Traumatic arthropathy, left shoulder
⇄	M12.551	Traumatic arthropathy, right hip
⇄	M12.552	Traumatic arthropathy, left hip
⇄	M12.561	Traumatic arthropathy, right knee
⇄	M12.562	Traumatic arthropathy, left knee
⇄	M13.851	Other specified arthritis, right hip
⇄	M13.852	Other specified arthritis, left hip
⇄	M14.611	Charcôt's joint, right shoulder
⇄	M14.612	Charcôt's joint, left shoulder
⇄	M14.622	Charcôt's joint, left elbow
⇄	M14.651	Charcôt's joint, right hip
⇄	M14.652	Charcôt's joint, left hip
⇄	M14.661	Charcôt's joint, right knee
⇄	M14.662	Charcôt's joint, left knee
⇄	M14.811	Arthropathies in other specified diseases classified elsewhere, right shoulder
⇄	M14.812	Arthropathies in other specified diseases classified elsewhere, left shoulder
⇄	M14.821	Arthropathies in other specified diseases classified elsewhere, right elbow
⇄	M14.822	Arthropathies in other specified diseases classified elsewhere, left elbow
	M16.0	Bilateral primary osteoarthritis of hip
	M16.2	Bilateral osteoarthritis resulting from hip dysplasia
⇄	M16.31	Unilateral osteoarthritis resulting from hip dysplasia, right hip
⇄	M16.32	Unilateral osteoarthritis resulting from hip dysplasia, left hip
	M16.4	Bilateral post-traumatic osteoarthritis of hip
⇄	M16.51	Unilateral post-traumatic osteoarthritis, right hip
⇄	M16.52	Unilateral post-traumatic osteoarthritis, left hip

CPT © 2018 American Medical Association. All Rights Reserved.

	M16.6	Other bilateral secondary osteoarthritis of hip
	M16.7	Other unilateral secondary osteoarthritis of hip
	M17.0	Bilateral primary osteoarthritis of knee
⇄	M17.11	Unilateral primary osteoarthritis, right knee
⇄	M17.12	Unilateral primary osteoarthritis, left knee
	M17.2	Bilateral post-traumatic osteoarthritis of knee
⇄	M17.31	Unilateral post-traumatic osteoarthritis, right knee
⇄	M17.32	Unilateral post-traumatic osteoarthritis, left knee
	M17.4	Other bilateral secondary osteoarthritis of knee
	M17.5	Other unilateral secondary osteoarthritis of knee
⇄	M19.011	Primary osteoarthritis, right shoulder
⇄	M19.012	Primary osteoarthritis, left shoulder
⇄	M19.021	Primary osteoarthritis, right elbow
⇄	M19.022	Primary osteoarthritis, left elbow
⇄	M19.11	Post-traumatic osteoarthritis, shoulder
⇄	M19.111	Post-traumatic osteoarthritis, right shoulder
⇄	M19.112	Post-traumatic osteoarthritis, left shoulder
⇄	M19.211	Secondary osteoarthritis, right shoulder
⇄	M19.212	Secondary osteoarthritis, left shoulder
❼⇄	M1A.011	Idiopathic chronic gout, right shoulder
❼⇄	M1A.012	Idiopathic chronic gout, left shoulder
❼⇄	M1A.051	Idiopathic chronic gout, right hip
❼⇄	M1A.052	Idiopathic chronic gout, left hip
❼⇄	M1A.061	Idiopathic chronic gout, right knee
❼⇄	M1A.062	Idiopathic chronic gout, left knee
⇄	M25.011	Hemarthrosis, right shoulder
⇄	M25.012	Hemarthrosis, left shoulder
⇄	M25.052	Hemarthrosis, left hip
⇄	M25.061	Hemarthrosis, right knee
⇄	M25.411	Effusion, right shoulder
⇄	M25.412	Effusion, left shoulder
⇄	M25.451	Effusion, right hip
⇄	M25.462	Effusion, left knee
⇄	M25.511	Pain in right shoulder
⇄	M25.512	Pain in left shoulder
⇄	M25.551	Pain in right hip
⇄	M25.552	Pain in left hip
⇄	M25.561	Pain in right knee
⇄	M65.811	Other synovitis and tenosynovitis, right shoulder
⇄	M65.812	Other synovitis and tenosynovitis, left shoulder
⇄	M65.852	Other synovitis and tenosynovitis, left thigh
⇄	M65.861	Other synovitis and tenosynovitis, right lower leg
⇄	M70.41	Prepatellar bursitis, right knee
⇄	M70.52	Other bursitis of knee, left knee
⇄	M70.61	Trochanteric bursitis, right hip
⇄	M70.71	Other bursitis of hip, right hip
⇄	M71.851	Other specified bursopathies, right hip
⇄	M71.862	Other specified bursopathies, left knee
⇄	M75.01	Adhesive capsulitis of right shoulder
⇄	M75.02	Adhesive capsulitis of left shoulder
⇄	M75.111	Incomplete rotator cuff tear or rupture of right shoulder, not specified as traumatic
⇄	M75.112	Incomplete rotator cuff tear or rupture of left shoulder, not specified as traumatic
⇄	M75.121	Complete rotator cuff tear or rupture of right shoulder, not specified as traumatic
⇄	M75.122	Complete rotator cuff tear or rupture of left shoulder, not specified as traumatic
⇄	M75.51	Bursitis of right shoulder
⇄	M75.52	Bursitis of left shoulder

ICD-10-CM Coding Notes

For codes requiring a 7th character extension, refer to your ICD-10-CM book. Review the character descriptions and coding guidelines for proper selection. For some procedures, only certain characters will apply.

CCI Edits

Refer to Appendix A for CCI edits.

Facility RVUs □

Code	Work	PE Facility	MP	Total Facility
20610	0.79	0.41	0.12	1.32
20611	1.10	0.50	0.15	1.75

Non-facility RVUs □

Code	Work	PE Non-Facility	MP	Total Non-Facility
20610	0.79	0.80	0.12	1.71
20611	1.10	1.36	0.15	2.61

Modifiers (PAR) □

Code	Mod 50	Mod 51	Mod 62	Mod 66	Mod 80
20610	1	2	0	0	1
20611	1	2	0	0	1

Global Period

Code	Days
20610	000
20611	000

CPT © 2018 American Medical Association. All Rights Reserved.

27096

27096 Injection procedure for sacroiliac joint, anesthetic/steroid, with image guidance (fluoroscopy or CT) including arthrography when performed

(27096 is to be used only with CT or fluoroscopic imaging confirmation of intra-articular needle positioning)

(If CT or fluoroscopy imaging is not performed, use 20552)

(Code 27096 is a unilateral procedure. For bilateral procedure, use modifier 50)

AMA Coding Guideline

Surgical Procedures on the Pelvis and Hip Joint

Including head and neck of femur.

Please see the Surgery Guidelines section for the following guidelines:

- *Surgical Procedures on the Musculoskeletal System*

AMA *CPT Assistant* ▢

27096: Nov 99: 12, Apr 03: 8, Apr 04: 15, Jul 08: 9, Jan 12: 3, Aug 15: 6

Plain English Description

Injection of an anesthetic or steroid into the sacroiliac joint is performed with the use of fluoroscopic or CT guidance and joint arthrography as needed. The skin over the injection site is cleansed and a local anesthetic is injected. Using continuous fluoroscopic or CT guidance, a needle is inserted into the joint and fluid is aspirated as needed. If arthrography is performed, a radiopaque substance is injected into the sacroiliac joint. Once the radiopaque substance has been distributed throughout the joint, separately reportable radiographic images are obtained. An anesthetic or steroid injection is then administered.

Injection procedure for sacroiliac joint

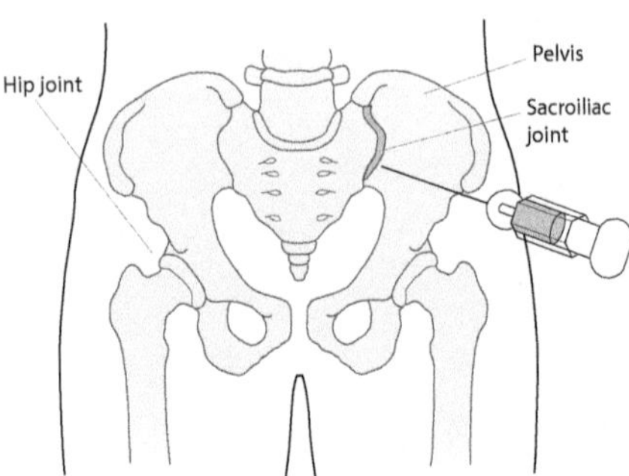

Using image guidance, anesthetic/steroid is injected into the sacroiliac joint. Includes arthrography.

ICD-10-CM Diagnostic Codes

	Code	Description
	M46.1	Sacroiliitis, not elsewhere classified
	M53.2X8	Spinal instabilities, sacral and sacrococcygeal region
	M53.3	Sacrococcygeal disorders, not elsewhere classified
	M53.88	Other specified dorsopathies, sacral and sacrococcygeal region
	M54.18	Radiculopathy, sacral and sacrococcygeal region
	M54.5	Low back pain
❼⇄	S32.391	Other fracture of right ilium
❼⇄	S32.392	Other fracture of left ilium
❼	S33.2	Dislocation of sacroiliac and sacrococcygeal joint
❼	S33.6	Sprain of sacroiliac joint

ICD-10-CM Coding Notes

For codes requiring a 7th character extension, refer to your ICD-10-CM book. Review the character descriptions and coding guidelines for proper selection. For some procedures, only certain characters will apply.

CCI Edits

Refer to Appendix A for CCI edits.

Facility RVUs ▢

Code	Work	PE Facility	MP	Total Facility
27096	1.48	0.78	0.12	2.38

Non-facility RVUs ▢

Code	Work	PE Non-Facility	MP	Total Non-Facility
27096	1.48	2.96	0.12	4.56

Modifiers (PAR) ▢

Code	Mod 50	Mod 51	Mod 62	Mod 66	Mod 80
27096	1	2	0	0	1

Global Period

Code	Days
27096	000

CPT © 2018 American Medical Association. All Rights Reserved.

28890

28890 Extracorporeal shock wave, high energy, performed by a physician or other qualified health care professional, requiring anesthesia other than local, including ultrasound guidance, involving the plantar fascia

(For extracorporeal shock wave therapy involving musculoskeletal system not otherwise specified, see 0101T, 0102T)

(For extracorporeal shock wave therapy involving integumentary system not otherwise specified, see 0512T, 0513T)

(Do not report 28890 in conjunction with 0512T, 06X2TX, when treating the same area)

AMA Coding Guideline

Please see the Surgery Guidelines section for the following guidelines:

- *Surgical Procedures on the Musculoskeletal System*

AMA *CPT Assistant* ▯

28890: Dec 05: 10, Mar 06: 1

Plain English Description

High energy extracorporeal shock wave (ESW) therapy requiring regional or general anesthesia is performed on the plantar fascia using ultrasound guidance. The foot is examined and the point of maximal heel tenderness is identified. The planned site of ESW therapy is marked. The heel is prepped and either a heel block (regional anesthesia) or general anesthesia is administered. High energy shock waves are then administered per the ESW manufacturer's instructions to the previously identified area of the heel.

Extracorporeal shock wave

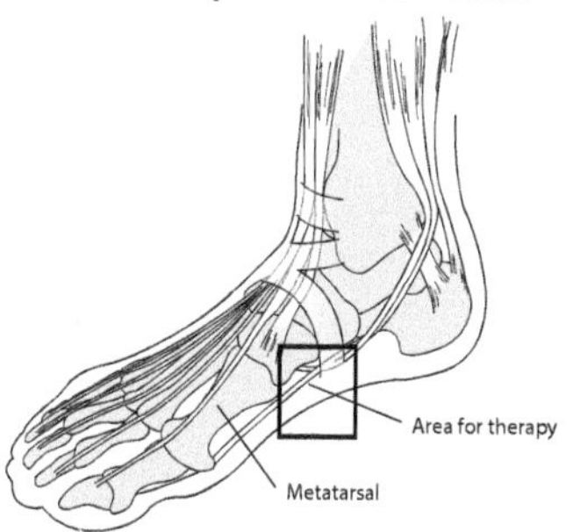

The physician uses shock wave therapy to treat an inflammation of the fibrous bands that hold the heel bone to the metatarsal bones of the foot.

ICD-10-CM Diagnostic Codes

M72.2 Plantar fascial fibromatosis

CCI Edits

Refer to Appendix A for CCI edits.

Facility RVUs ▯

Code	Work	PE Facility	MP	Total Facility
28890	3.45	2.68	0.27	6.40

Non-facility RVUs ▯

Code	Work	PE Non-Facility	MP	Total Non-Facility
28890	3.45	5.60	0.27	9.32

Modifiers (PAR) ▯

Code	Mod 50	Mod 51	Mod 62	Mod 66	Mod 80
28890	1	2	1	0	1

Global Period

Code	Days
28890	090

CPT © 2018 American Medical Association. All Rights Reserved.

36000

36000 Introduction of needle or intracatheter, vein

AMA Coding Guideline

Intravenous Vascular Introduction and Injection Procedures

An intracatheter is a sheathed combination of needle and short catheter.

Vascular Introduction and Injection Procedures

Listed services for injection procedures include necessary local anesthesia, introduction of needles or catheter, injection of contrast media with or without automatic power injection, and/or necessary pre- and postinjection care specifically related to the injection procedure.

Selective vascular catheterization should be coded to include introduction and all lesser order selective catheterization used in the approach (eg, the description for a selective right middle cerebral artery catheterization includes the introduction and placement catheterization of the right common and internal carotid arteries).

Additional second and/or third order arterial catheterization within the same family of arteries or veins supplied by a single first order vessel should be expressed by 36012, 36218, or 36248.

Additional first order or higher catheterization in vascular families supplied by a first order vessel different from a previously selected and coded family should be separately coded using the conventions described above.

Surgical Procedures on Arteries and Veins

Primary vascular procedure listings include establishing both inflow and outflow by whatever procedures necessary. Also included is that portion of the operative arteriogram performed by the surgeon, as indicated. Sympathectomy, when done, is included in the listed aortic procedures. For unlisted vascular procedure, use 37799.

Please see the Surgery Guidelines section for the following guidelines:

- *Surgical Procedures on the Cardiovascular System*

AMA Coding Notes

Vascular Introduction and Injection Procedures

(For radiological supervision and interpretation, see Radiology)

(For injection procedures in conjunction with cardiac catheterization, see 93452-93461, 93563-93568)

(For chemotherapy of malignant disease, see 96401-96549)

AMA *CPT Assistant* ◻

36000: Summer 95: 2, Apr 98: 1, 3, 7, Jul 98: 1, Apr 03: 26, Oct 03: 2, Jul 06: 4, Feb 07: 10, Jul 07: 1, Dec 08: 7, May 14: 4, Sep 14: 13, Oct 14: 6

Plain English Description

The physician may place a metal needle, such as a butterfly or scalp needle; a plastic catheter mounted on a metal needle, also referred to as a plastic needle; or an intracatheter, which is a catheter inserted through a needle. The planned puncture site is selected and cleansed. The selected device is then introduced into the vein. A butterfly needle can be introduced into smaller veins in the hand. The butterfly shape stabilizes the hub on the skin surface. If a plastic needle is used, the metal tip is introduced into the vein and then removed. The plastic catheter is advanced into the vein. If an intracatheter is used, the metal needle is used to puncture the vein. The catheter is then introduced through the needle into the vein. The needle or intracatheter is secured to the skin with tape.

Introduction of needle or intracatheter, vein

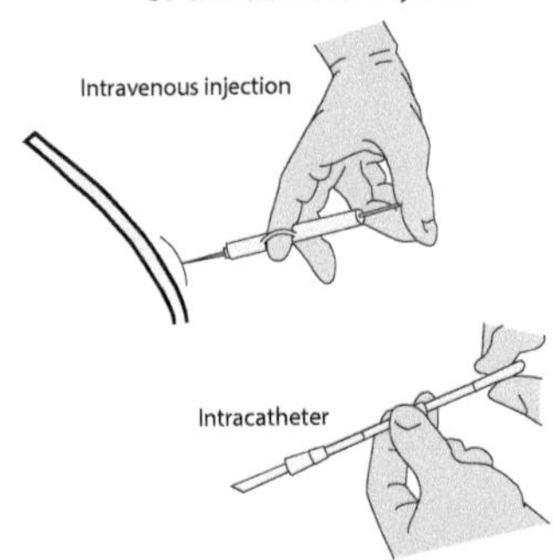

ICD-10-CM Diagnostic Codes

There are too many ICD-10-CM codes to list. Refer to ICD-10-CM code book for associated diagnostic codes.

CCI Edits

Refer to Appendix A for CCI edits.

Pub 100

36000: Pub 100-04, 12, 30.6.12

Facility RVUs ◻

Code	Work	PE Facility	MP	Total Facility
36000	0.18	0.07	0.02	0.27

Non-facility RVUs ◻

Code	Work	PE Non-Facility	MP	Total Non-Facility
36000	0.18	0.57	0.02	0.77

Modifiers (PAR) ◻

Code	Mod 50	Mod 51	Mod 62	Mod 66	Mod 80
36000	9	9	9	9	9

Global Period

Code	Days
36000	XXX

CPT © 2018 American Medical Association. All Rights Reserved

36010

36010 Introduction of catheter, superior or inferior vena cava

AMA Coding Guideline

Intravenous Vascular Introduction and Injection Procedures

An intracatheter is a sheathed combination of needle and short catheter.

Vascular Introduction and Injection Procedures

Listed services for injection procedures include necessary local anesthesia, introduction of needles or catheter, injection of contrast media with or without automatic power injection, and/or necessary pre- and postinjection care specifically related to the injection procedure.

Selective vascular catheterization should be coded to include introduction and all lesser order selective catheterization used in the approach (eg, the description for a selective right middle cerebral artery catheterization includes the introduction and placement catheterization of the right common and internal carotid arteries).

Additional second and/or third order arterial catheterization within the same family of arteries or veins supplied by a single first order vessel should be expressed by 36012, 36218, or 36248.

Additional first order or higher catheterization in vascular families supplied by a first order vessel different from a previously selected and coded family should be separately coded using the conventions described above.

Surgical Procedures on Arteries and Veins

Primary vascular procedure listings include establishing both inflow and outflow by whatever procedures necessary. Also included is that portion of the operative arteriogram performed by the surgeon, as indicated. Sympathectomy, when done, is included in the listed aortic procedures. For unlisted vascular procedure, use 37799.

Please see the Surgery Guidelines section for the following guidelines:

- *Surgical Procedures on the Cardiovascular System*

AMA Coding Notes

Vascular Introduction and Injection Procedures

(For radiological supervision and interpretation, see Radiology)

(For injection procedures in conjunction with cardiac catheterization, see 93452-93461, 93563-93568)

(For chemotherapy of malignant disease, see 96401-96549)

AMA *CPT Assistant* ☐

36010: Aug 96: 2, Apr 98: 7, Sep 00: 11, May 01: 10, Jul 03: 12, Oct 08: 11, Jan 09: 7, Apr 12: 4, Feb 17: 14

Plain English Description

Common access veins include the brachial and cephalic veins. A small incision is made over the planned puncture site and an introducer sheath placed in the vein. A guidewire is advanced through the access vein and into the superior or inferior vena cava. The catheter is then advanced over the guidewire into the superior or inferior vena cava. If the puncture site is the brachial or cephalic vein, the inferior vena cava is accessed by advancing the guidewire and catheter into the superior vena cava, through the right atrium and into the inferior vena cava. Injection of medication and/or radiopaque contrast is performed as needed.

Introduction of catheter, superior or inferior vena cava

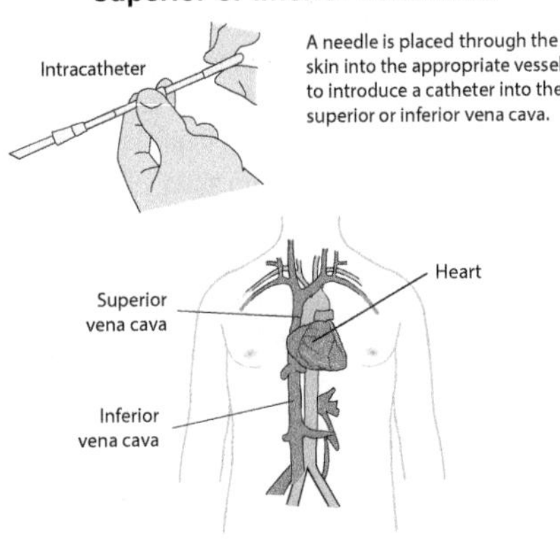
Intracatheter
A needle is placed through the skin into the appropriate vessel to introduce a catheter into the superior or inferior vena cava.
Superior vena cava
Heart
Inferior vena cava

ICD-10-CM Diagnostic Codes

There are too many ICD-10-CM codes to list. Refer to ICD-10-CM code book for associated diagnostic codes.

CCI Edits

Refer to Appendix A for CCI edits.

Facility RVUs ☐

Code	Work	PE Facility	MP	Total Facility
36010	2.18	0.64	0.37	3.19

Non-facility RVUs ☐

Code	Work	PE Non-Facility	MP	Total Non-Facility
36010	2.18	11.73	0.37	14.28

Modifiers (PAR) ☐

Code	Mod 50	Mod 51	Mod 62	Mod 66	Mod 80
36010	1	2	0	0	1

Global Period

Code	Days
36010	XXX

CPT © 2018 American Medical Association. All Rights Reserved.

36011-36012

36011 Selective catheter placement, venous system; first order branch (eg, renal vein, jugular vein)

36012 Selective catheter placement, venous system; second order, or more selective, branch (eg, left adrenal vein, petrosal sinus)

AMA Coding Guideline

Intravenous Vascular Introduction and Injection Procedures

An intracatheter is a sheathed combination of needle and short catheter.

Vascular Introduction and Injection Procedures

Listed services for injection procedures include necessary local anesthesia, introduction of needles or catheter, injection of contrast media with or without automatic power injection, and/or necessary pre- and postinjection care specifically related to the injection procedure.

Selective vascular catheterization should be coded to include introduction and all lesser order selective catheterization used in the approach (eg, the description for a selective right middle cerebral artery catheterization includes the introduction and placement catheterization of the right common and internal carotid arteries).

Additional second and/or third order arterial catheterization within the same family of arteries or veins supplied by a single first order vessel should be expressed by 36012, 36218, or 36248.

Additional first order or higher catheterization in vascular families supplied by a first order vessel different from a previously selected and coded family should be separately coded using the conventions described above.

Surgical Procedures on Arteries and Veins

Primary vascular procedure listings include establishing both inflow and outflow by whatever procedures necessary. Also included is that portion of the operative arteriogram performed by the surgeon, as indicated. Sympathectomy, when done, is included in the listed aortic procedures. For unlisted vascular procedure, use 37799.

Please see the Surgery Guidelines section for the following guidelines:

- *Surgical Procedures on the Cardiovascular System*

AMA Coding Notes

Vascular Introduction and Injection Procedures

(For radiological supervision and interpretation, see Radiology)

(For injection procedures in conjunction with cardiac catheterization, see 93452-93461, 93563-93568)

(For chemotherapy of malignant disease, see 96401-96549)

AMA *CPT Assistant* ☐

36011: Aug 96: 11, Apr 98: 7, Jul 03: 12, Dec 03: 2, Apr 12: 5

36012: Aug 96: 11, Sep 98: 7, Jul 03: 12, Apr 12: 5

Plain English Description

A selective venous catheterization procedure is performed. Common access veins include the brachial and cephalic veins. A small incision is made over the planned puncture site and an introducer sheath placed in the vein. From the brachial or cephalic vein, a guidewire is advanced through the access vein and into the superior vena cava. From there, the catheter is advanced into a venous branch off the superior vena cava, such as the jugular vein, or the catheter may be advanced through the right atrium and into the inferior vena cava and then into a branch off the inferior vena cava, such as the hepatic or renal vein. The catheter may remain in the first order branch which is any vein that drains directly into the vena cava or the catheter may be advanced into a second order or more selective branch, such as the petrosal sinus or left adrenal vein. Injection of medication and/or radiopaque contrast is performed as needed. Use 36011 for selective catheter placement in a first order vein branch and 36012 for a second order or more selective vein branch.

Selective catheter placement, venous system

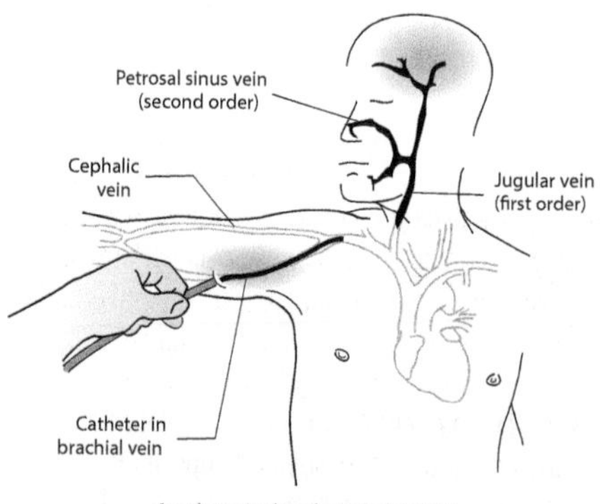

A catheter is placed into first (36011); second (36012) venous order branch.

ICD-10-CM Diagnostic Codes

There are too many ICD-10-CM codes to list. Refer to ICD-10-CM code book for associated diagnostic codes.

CCI Edits

Refer to Appendix A for CCI edits.

Facility RVUs ☐

Code	Work	PE Facility	MP	Total Facility
36011	3.14	0.94	0.46	4.54
36012	3.51	0.99	0.53	5.03

Non-facility RVUs ☐

Code	Work	PE Non-Facility	MP	Total Non-Facility
36011	3.14	20.42	0.46	24.02
36012	3.51	20.46	0.53	24.50

Modifiers (PAR) ☐

Code	Mod 50	Mod 51	Mod 62	Mod 66	Mod 80
36011	1	2	0	0	1
36012	1	2	0	0	1

Global Period

Code	Days
36011	XXX
36012	XXX

CPT © 2018 American Medical Association. All Rights Reserved.

36013-36015

36013 Introduction of catheter, right heart or main pulmonary artery

36014 Selective catheter placement, left or right pulmonary artery

36015 Selective catheter placement, segmental or subsegmental pulmonary artery

(For insertion of flow directed catheter (eg, Swan-Ganz), use 93503)

(For venous catheterization for selective organ blood sampling, use 36500)

AMA Coding Guideline

Intravenous Vascular Introduction and Injection Procedures

An intracatheter is a sheathed combination of needle and short catheter.

Vascular Introduction and Injection Procedures

Listed services for injection procedures include necessary local anesthesia, introduction of needles or catheter, injection of contrast media with or without automatic power injection, and/or necessary pre- and postinjection care specifically related to the injection procedure.

Selective vascular catheterization should be coded to include introduction and all lesser order selective catheterization used in the approach (eg, the description for a selective right middle cerebral artery catheterization includes the introduction and placement catheterization of the right common and internal carotid arteries).

Additional second and/or third order arterial catheterization within the same family of arteries or veins supplied by a single first order vessel should be expressed by 36012, 36218, or 36248.

Additional first order or higher catheterization in vascular families supplied by a first order vessel different from a previously selected and coded family should be separately coded using the conventions described above.

Surgical Procedures on Arteries and Veins

Primary vascular procedure listings include establishing both inflow and outflow by whatever procedures necessary. Also included is that portion of the operative arteriogram performed by the surgeon, as indicated. Sympathectomy, when done, is included in the listed aortic procedures. For unlisted vascular procedure, use 37799.

Please see the Surgery Guidelines section for the following guidelines:

- *Surgical Procedures on the Cardiovascular System*

AMA Coding Notes

Vascular Introduction and Injection Procedures

(For radiological supervision and interpretation, see Radiology)

(For injection procedures in conjunction with cardiac catheterization, see 93452-93461, 93563-93568)

(For chemotherapy of malignant disease, see 96401-96549)

AMA *CPT Assistant* □

36013: Aug 96: 11, Oct 08: 11, Jan 09: 7

36014: Aug 96: 11, Apr 98: 7

36015: Aug 96: 11, Sep 00: 11, Mar 12: 10

Plain English Description

A catheter is introduced into the right heart or main pulmonary artery (36013) or selective catheterization is performed with placement of the catheter in the left or right pulmonary artery (36014) or a segmental or subsegmental pulmonary artery (36015). The catheter is introduced into an extremity vein, with the preferred introduction site being the right femoral vein, although the left femoral vein or an upper extremity vein may also be used. A small skin incision is made over the planned venous insertion site. An introducer sheath is placed in the vein and a guidewire inserted. If the right femoral vein is used, the guidewire is manipulated through the femoral and iliac veins and into the inferior vena cava and advanced to the right atrium. A pigtail catheter with a tip deflecting wire is advanced over the guidewire and into the right atrium. The guidewire is removed. The catheter may remain in the right atrium or a tip deflecting wire may be used to advance the catheter into the right ventricle and main pulmonary artery. In 36014, selective catheterization of the left or right pulmonary artery is performed. The catheter is introduced into the right atrium, advanced into the right ventricle and then into the pulmonary artery as described above. The physician then selectively manipulates the catheter into the left or right pulmonary arteries. In 36015, selective catheterization of a segmental or subsegmental pulmonary artery is performed. The catheter is placed in the left or right pulmonary artery as described above and then manipulated into a segmental or subsegmental pulmonary artery. The segmental and subsegmental arteries are the branches that divide and subdivide within the lungs. Injection of medication and/or radiopaque contrast is performed as needed.

Introduction of catheter, right heart or main pulmonary artery

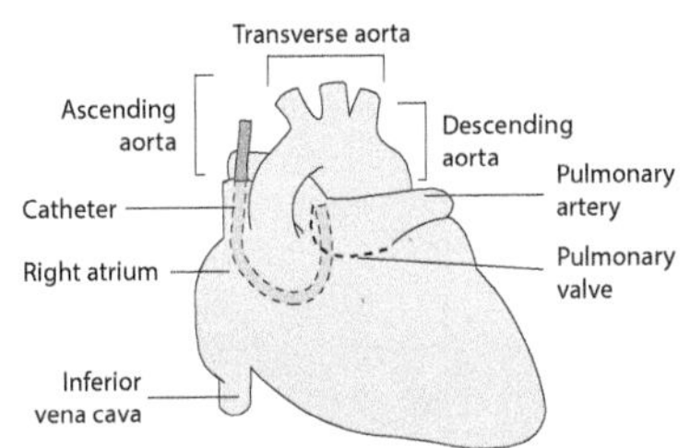

A needle is inserted through the skin into the appropriate vein to introduce a catheter into the right side of the heart or pulmonary artery.

ICD-10-CM Diagnostic Codes

I42.0	Dilated cardiomyopathy
I42.5	Other restrictive cardiomyopathy
I42.8	Other cardiomyopathies
I42.9	Cardiomyopathy, unspecified
I44.2	Atrioventricular block, complete
I44.7	Left bundle-branch block, unspecified
I47.0	Re-entry ventricular arrhythmia
I47.2	Ventricular tachycardia
I48.0	Paroxysmal atrial fibrillation
I48.2	Chronic atrial fibrillation
I49.5	Sick sinus syndrome
I50.1	Left ventricular failure, unspecified
I50.21	Acute systolic (congestive) heart failure
I50.22	Chronic systolic (congestive) heart failure
I50.23	Acute on chronic systolic (congestive) heart failure
I50.31	Acute diastolic (congestive) heart failure
I50.33	Acute on chronic diastolic (congestive) heart failure
I50.41	Acute combined systolic (congestive) and diastolic (congestive) heart failure
I50.42	Chronic combined systolic (congestive) and diastolic (congestive) heart failure
I50.43	Acute on chronic combined systolic (congestive) and diastolic (congestive) heart failure
I82.211	Chronic embolism and thrombosis of superior vena cava
I82.291	Chronic embolism and thrombosis of other thoracic veins
I82.890	Acute embolism and thrombosis of other specified veins
I82.90	Acute embolism and thrombosis of unspecified vein
J91.8	Pleural effusion in other conditions classified elsewhere
J96.01	Acute respiratory failure with hypoxia
J96.02	Acute respiratory failure with hypercapnia
Q25.5	Atresia of pulmonary artery
Q25.6	Stenosis of pulmonary artery
Q25.71	Coarctation of pulmonary artery
Q25.72	Congenital pulmonary arteriovenous malformation
Q25.79	Other congenital malformations of pulmonary artery
R00.0	Tachycardia, unspecified
R00.1	Bradycardia, unspecified
R06.02	Shortness of breath
R06.09	Other forms of dyspnea
R06.3	Periodic breathing
R07.9	Chest pain, unspecified

CCI Edits

Refer to Appendix A for CCI edits.

CPT © 2018 American Medical Association. All Rights Reserved.

Facility RVUs ☐

Code	Work	PE Facility	MP	Total Facility
36013	2.52	0.70	0.30	3.52
36014	3.02	0.94	0.42	4.38
36015	3.51	1.07	0.40	4.98

Non-facility RVUs ☐

Code	Work	PE Non-Facility	MP	Total Non-Facility
36013	2.52	19.02	0.30	21.84
36014	3.02	19.62	0.42	23.06
36015	3.51	21.07	0.40	24.98

Modifiers (PAR) ☐

Code	Mod 50	Mod 51	Mod 62	Mod 66	Mod 80
36013	0	2	0	0	1
36014	1	2	0	0	1
36015	1	2	0	0	1

Global Period

Code	Days
36013	XXX
36014	XXX
36015	XXX

CPT © 2018 American Medical Association. All Rights Reserved.

36100

36100 Introduction of needle or intracatheter, carotid or vertebral artery

(For bilateral procedure, report 36100 with modifier 50)

AMA Coding Guideline

Vascular Introduction and Injection Procedures

Listed services for injection procedures include necessary local anesthesia, introduction of needles or catheter, injection of contrast media with or without automatic power injection, and/or necessary pre- and postinjection care specifically related to the injection procedure.

Selective vascular catheterization should be coded to include introduction and all lesser order selective catheterization used in the approach (eg, the description for a selective right middle cerebral artery catheterization includes the introduction and placement catheterization of the right common and internal carotid arteries).

Additional second and/or third order arterial catheterization within the same family of arteries or veins supplied by a single first order vessel should be expressed by 36012, 36218, or 36248.

Additional first order or higher catheterization in vascular families supplied by a first order vessel different from a previously selected and coded family should be separately coded using the conventions described above.

Surgical Procedures on Arteries and Veins

Primary vascular procedure listings include establishing both inflow and outflow by whatever procedures necessary. Also included is that portion of the operative arteriogram performed by the surgeon, as indicated. Sympathectomy, when done, is included in the listed aortic procedures. For unlisted vascular procedure, use 37799.

Please see the Surgery Guidelines section for the following guidelines:

- *Surgical Procedures on the Cardiovascular System*

AMA Coding Notes

Intra-Arterial-Intra-Aortic Vascular Injection Procedures

(For radiological supervision and interpretation, see Radiology)

Vascular Introduction and Injection Procedures

(For radiological supervision and interpretation, see Radiology)

(For injection procedures in conjunction with cardiac catheterization, see 93452-93461, 93563-93568)

(For chemotherapy of malignant disease, see 96401-96549)

AMA *CPT Assistant*

36100: Aug 96: 11

Plain English Description

To place a needle or intracatheter in the carotid artery, the artery is first located by palpation. The carotid artery is stabilized between the index and middle fingers and the needle or intracatheter introduced through the skin, advanced toward the artery until the tip touches the artery wall, and the artery is then punctured. The needle or intracatheter is advanced in a cephalad direction taking care not to injure the carotid artery intima (inner lining). To place a needle or intracatheter in the vertebral artery, the vertebral artery is approached laterally and the needle or intracatheter advanced between one of the cervical interspaces. The skin of the neck is compressed against the cervical spine using the index and middle fingers. The skin is punctured and the needle or intracatheter advanced until it touches the intervertebral foramina at the anterior tubercle of the transverse process. The needle or intracatheter is advanced into the vertebral artery. Blood is aspirated to ensure that the needle or intracatheter is properly placed within the carotid or vertebral artery. Injection of medication and/or radiopaque contrast media is performed as needed.

Introduction of needle or intracatheter

Catheter is inserted into artery after needle and guidewire insertion.

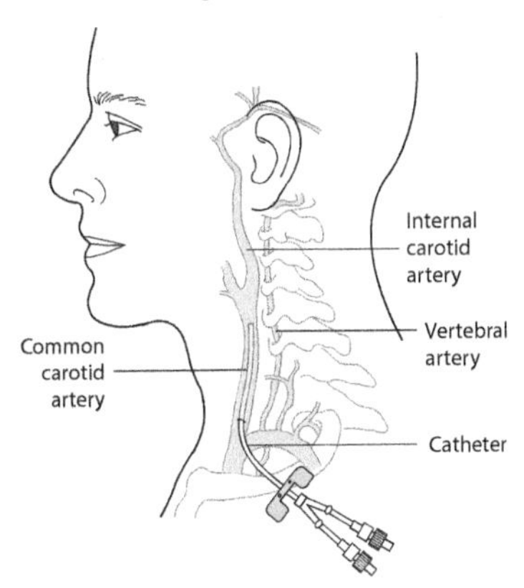

ICD-10-CM Diagnostic Codes

There are too many ICD-10-CM codes to list. Refer to ICD-10-CM code book for associated diagnostic codes.

CCI Edits

Refer to Appendix A for CCI edits.

Facility RVUs

Code	Work	PE Facility	MP	Total Facility
36100	3.02	0.82	0.70	4.54

Non-facility RVUs

Code	Work	PE Non-Facility	MP	Total Non-Facility
36100	3.02	11.09	0.70	14.81

Modifiers (PAR)

Code	Mod 50	Mod 51	Mod 62	Mod 66	Mod 80
36100	1	2	0	0	1

Global Period

Code	Days
36100	XXX

CPT © 2018 American Medical Association. All Rights Reserved.

36140

36140 Introduction of needle or intracatheter, upper or lower extremity artery

(For insertion of arteriovenous cannula, see 36810-36821)

AMA Coding Guideline

Vascular Introduction and Injection Procedures

Listed services for injection procedures include necessary local anesthesia, introduction of needles or catheter, injection of contrast media with or without automatic power injection, and/or necessary pre- and postinjection care specifically related to the injection procedure.

Selective vascular catheterization should be coded to include introduction and all lesser order selective catheterization used in the approach (eg, the description for a selective right middle cerebral artery catheterization includes the introduction and placement catheterization of the right common and internal carotid arteries).

Additional second and/or third order arterial catheterization within the same family of arteries or veins supplied by a single first order vessel should be expressed by 36012, 36218, or 36248.

Additional first order or higher catheterization in vascular families supplied by a first order vessel different from a previously selected and coded family should be separately coded using the conventions described above.

Surgical Procedures on Arteries and Veins

Primary vascular procedure listings include establishing both inflow and outflow by whatever procedures necessary. Also included is that portion of the operative arteriogram performed by the surgeon, as indicated. Sympathectomy, when done, is included in the listed aortic procedures. For unlisted vascular procedure, use 37799.

Please see the Surgery Guidelines section for the following guidelines:

- *Surgical Procedures on the Cardiovascular System*

AMA Coding Notes

Intra-Arterial-Intra-Aortic Vascular Injection Procedures

(For radiological supervision and interpretation, see Radiology)

Vascular Introduction and Injection Procedures

(For radiological supervision and interpretation, see Radiology)

(For injection procedures in conjunction with cardiac catheterization, see 93452-93461, 93563-93568)

(For chemotherapy of malignant disease, see 96401-96549)

AMA *CPT Assistant* ◻

36140: Fall 93: 16, Aug 96: 3, Nov 99: 32-33, Oct 03: 2, Jul 06: 4, 7, Jul 07: 1, Dec 07: 10-11, Jun 09: 10, Jul 11: 5

Plain English Description

A needle or intracatheter is introduced into an upper or lower extremity artery. To place a needle or intracatheter into a target artery, such as the brachial or radial artery, the artery may first be located by palpation and stabilized between the index and middle fingers or the access area over the target artery visualized. The needle or intracatheter is introduced through the skin, advanced toward the artery until the tip touches the arterial wall, and the artery is then punctured. The needle may be left within the artery or an intracatheter may be advanced through the artery. Injections, such as medication and/or radiopaque contrast can then be performed as needed.

Introduction of needle or intracatheter; extremity artery

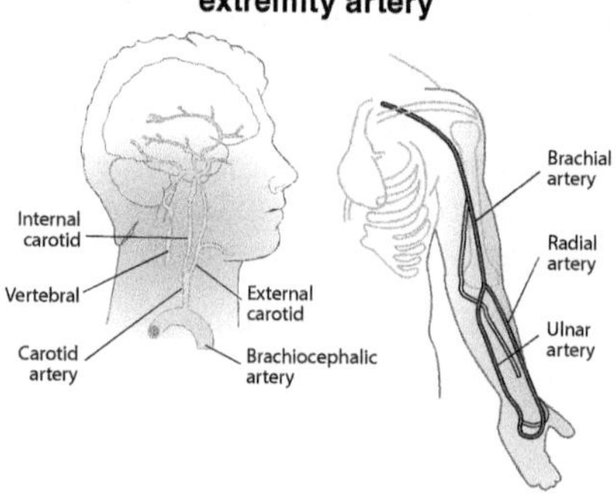

ICD-10-CM Diagnostic Codes

There are too many ICD-10-CM codes to list. Refer to ICD-10-CM code book for associated diagnostic codes.

CCI Edits

Refer to Appendix A for CCI edits.

Facility RVUs ◻

Code	Work	PE Facility	MP	Total Facility
36140	1.76	0.50	0.36	2.62

Non-facility RVUs ◻

Code	Work	PE Non-Facility	MP	Total Non-Facility
36140	1.76	10.61	0.36	12.73

Modifiers (PAR) ◻

Code	Mod 50	Mod 51	Mod 62	Mod 66	Mod 80
36140	0	2	0	0	1

Global Period

Code	Days
36140	XXX

CPT © 2018 American Medical Association. All Rights Reserved.

36400-36406

36400 Venipuncture, younger than age 3 years, necessitating the skill of a physician or other qualified health care professional, not to be used for routine venipuncture; femoral or jugular vein

36405 Venipuncture, younger than age 3 years, necessitating the skill of a physician or other qualified health care professional, not to be used for routine venipuncture; scalp vein

36406 Venipuncture, younger than age 3 years, necessitating the skill of a physician or other qualified health care professional, not to be used for routine venipuncture; other vein

AMA Coding Guideline

Venous Procedures

Venipuncture, needle or catheter for diagnostic study or intravenous therapy, percutaneous. These codes are also used to report the therapy as specified. For collection of a specimen from an established catheter, use 36592. For collection of a specimen from a completely implantable venous access device, use 36591.

Vascular Introduction and Injection Procedures

Listed services for injection procedures include necessary local anesthesia, introduction of needles or catheter, injection of contrast media with or without automatic power injection, and/or necessary pre- and postinjection care specifically related to the injection procedure.

Selective vascular catheterization should be coded to include introduction and all lesser order selective catheterization used in the approach (eg, the description for a selective right middle cerebral artery catheterization includes the introduction and placement catheterization of the right common and internal carotid arteries).

Additional second and/or third order arterial catheterization within the same family of arteries or veins supplied by a single first order vessel should be expressed by 36012, 36218, or 36248.

Additional first order or higher catheterization in vascular families supplied by a first order vessel different from a previously selected and coded family should be separately coded using the conventions described above.

Surgical Procedures on Arteries and Veins

Primary vascular procedure listings include establishing both inflow and outflow by whatever procedures necessary. Also included is that portion of the operative arteriogram performed by the surgeon, as indicated. Sympathectomy, when done, is included in the listed aortic procedures. For unlisted vascular procedure, use 37799.

Please see the Surgery Guidelines section for the following guidelines:

- *Surgical Procedures on the Cardiovascular System*

AMA Coding Notes

Vascular Introduction and Injection Procedures

(For radiological supervision and interpretation, see Radiology)

(For injection procedures in conjunction with cardiac catheterization, see 93452-93461, 93563-93568)

(For chemotherapy of malignant disease, see 96401-96549)

AMA *CPT Assistant*

36400: Jul 06: 4, Jul 07: 1, Dec 08: 7, May 14: 4
36405: Jul 06: 4, Jul 07: 1, Dec 08: 7, May 14: 4
36406: Jul 06: 4, Jul 07: 1, May 14: 4

Plain English Description

The most common sites for venipuncture in infants and young children include the scalp, external jugular, femoral, saphenous, dorsal veins of the hand, or dorsal arch of the foot. The circumstances necessitating the skill of a physician or other qualified health care professional for the venipuncture procedure are documented and the required consents obtained from the parent or guardian. The most appropriate site for the venipuncture is selected. The site is prepped for sterile entry. The selected vein is punctured and the necessary blood samples obtained for separately reportable laboratory studies. Use 36400 for venipuncture of a jugular or femoral vein, 36405 for a scalp vein, and 36406 for any other vein.

Venipuncture younger than age 3 years

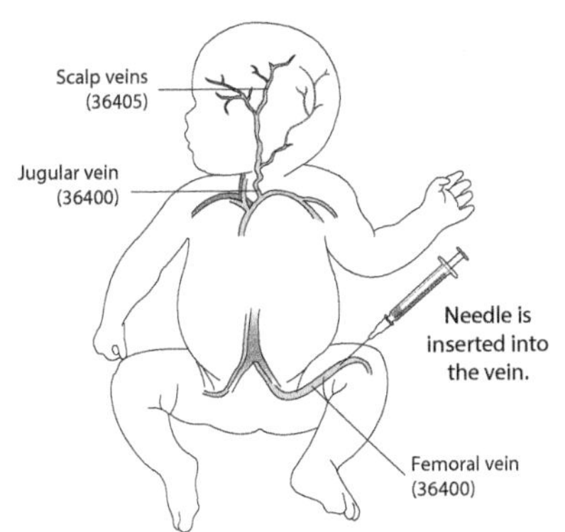

For other vein, use code 36406

ICD-10-CM Diagnostic Codes

There are too many ICD-10-CM codes to list. Refer to ICD-10-CM code book for associated diagnostic codes.

CCI Edits

Refer to Appendix A for CCI edits.

Facility RVUs

Code	Work	PE Facility	MP	Total Facility
36400	0.38	0.13	0.02	0.53
36405	0.31	0.11	0.02	0.44
36406	0.18	0.06	0.01	0.25

Non-facility RVUs

Code	Work	PE Non-Facility	MP	Total Non-Facility
36400	0.38	0.35	0.02	0.75
36405	0.31	0.33	0.02	0.66
36406	0.18	0.28	0.01	0.47

Modifiers (PAR)

Code	Mod 50	Mod 51	Mod 62	Mod 66	Mod 80
36400	0	2	0	0	1
36405	0	2	0	0	1
36406	0	2	0	0	1

Global Period

Code	Days
36400	XXX
36405	XXX
36406	XXX

CPT © 2018 American Medical Association. All Rights Reserved.

36410

36410 Venipuncture, age 3 years or older, necessitating the skill of a physician or other qualified health care professional (separate procedure), for diagnostic or therapeutic purposes (not to be used for routine venipuncture)

AMA Coding Guideline

Venous Procedures

Venipuncture, needle or catheter for diagnostic study or intravenous therapy, percutaneous. These codes are also used to report the therapy as specified. For collection of a specimen from an established catheter, use 36592. For collection of a specimen from a completely implantable venous access device, use 36591.

Vascular Introduction and Injection Procedures

Listed services for injection procedures include necessary local anesthesia, introduction of needles or catheter, injection of contrast media with or without automatic power injection, and/or necessary pre- and postinjection care specifically related to the injection procedure.

Selective vascular catheterization should be coded to include introduction and all lesser order selective catheterization used in the approach (eg, the description for a selective right middle cerebral artery catheterization includes the introduction and placement catheterization of the right common and internal carotid arteries).

Additional second and/or third order arterial catheterization within the same family of arteries or veins supplied by a single first order vessel should be expressed by 36012, 36218, or 36248.

Additional first order or higher catheterization in vascular families supplied by a first order vessel different from a previously selected and coded family should be separately coded using the conventions described above.

Surgical Procedures on Arteries and Veins

Primary vascular procedure listings include establishing both inflow and outflow by whatever procedures necessary. Also included is that portion of the operative arteriogram performed by the surgeon, as indicated. Sympathectomy, when done, is included in the listed aortic procedures. For unlisted vascular procedure, use 37799.

Please see the Surgery Guidelines section for the following guidelines:

- *Surgical Procedures on the Cardiovascular System*

AMA Coding Notes

Vascular Introduction and Injection Procedures

(For radiological supervision and interpretation, see Radiology)

(For injection procedures in conjunction with cardiac catheterization, see 93452-93461, 93563-93568)

(For chemotherapy of malignant disease, see 96401-96549)

AMA *CPT Assistant* □

36410: Jun 96: 10, May 01: 11, Aug 02: 2, Oct 03: 10, Feb 07: 10, Jul 07: 1, Dec 08: 7, Sep 13: 18, Oct 14: 6

Plain English Description

The circumstances necessitating the skill of a physician or other qualified health care professional for the venipuncture procedure are documented and the required consents obtained from the patient, parent or guardian. The most appropriate site for the venipuncture is selected. The site is prepped for sterile entry. The selected vein is punctured and the necessary blood samples obtained or medication administered. Blood specimens are sent to the laboratory for separately reportable laboratory studies.

Venipuncture, age 3 years or older

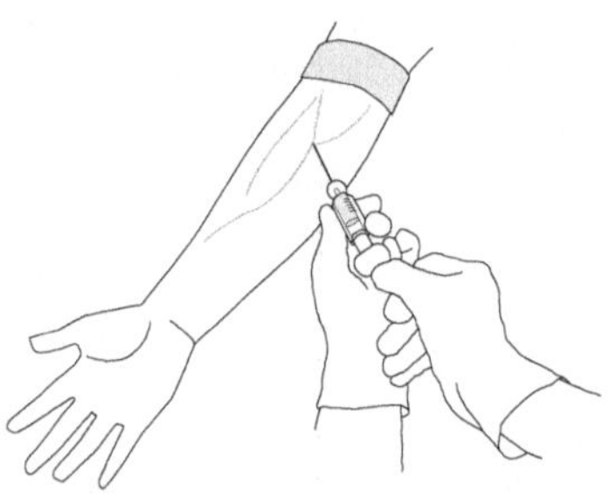

A needle is inserted through the skin into the vein of a patient over the age of three. The needle is withdrawn after the desired diagnostic or therapeutic procedure is completed.

ICD-10-CM Diagnostic Codes

There are too many ICD-10-CM codes to list. Refer to ICD-10-CM code book for associated diagnostic codes.

CCI Edits

Refer to Appendix A for CCI edits.

Pub 100

36410: Pub 100-04, 12, 30.6.12

Facility RVUs □

Code	Work	PE Facility	MP	Total Facility
36410	0.18	0.07	0.02	0.27

Non-facility RVUs □

Code	Work	PE Non-Facility	MP	Total Non-Facility
36410	0.18	0.29	0.02	0.49

Modifiers (PAR) □

Code	Mod 50	Mod 51	Mod 62	Mod 66	Mod 80
36410	0	2	0	0	1

Global Period

Code	Days
36410	XXX

CPT © 2018 American Medical Association. All Rights Reserved.

36415

36415 Collection of venous blood by venipuncture

(Do not report modifier 63 in conjunction with 36415)

AMA Coding Guideline

Venous Procedures

Venipuncture, needle or catheter for diagnostic study or intravenous therapy, percutaneous. These codes are also used to report the therapy as specified. For collection of a specimen from an established catheter, use 36592. For collection of a specimen from a completely implantable venous access device, use 36591.

Vascular Introduction and Injection Procedures

Listed services for injection procedures include necessary local anesthesia, introduction of needles or catheter, injection of contrast media with or without automatic power injection, and/or necessary pre- and postinjection care specifically related to the injection procedure.

Selective vascular catheterization should be coded to include introduction and all lesser order selective catheterization used in the approach (eg, the description for a selective right middle cerebral artery catheterization includes the introduction and placement catheterization of the right common and internal carotid arteries).

Additional second and/or third order arterial catheterization within the same family of arteries or veins supplied by a single first order vessel should be expressed by 36012, 36218, or 36248.

Additional first order or higher catheterization in vascular families supplied by a first order vessel different from a previously selected and coded family should be separately coded using the conventions described above.

Surgical Procedures on Arteries and Veins

Primary vascular procedure listings include establishing both inflow and outflow by whatever procedures necessary. Also included is that portion of the operative arteriogram performed by the surgeon, as indicated. Sympathectomy, when done, is included in the listed aortic procedures. For unlisted vascular procedure, use 37799.

Please see the Surgery Guidelines section for the following guidelines:

- *Surgical Procedures on the Cardiovascular System*

AMA Coding Notes

Vascular Introduction and Injection Procedures

(For radiological supervision and interpretation, see Radiology)

(For injection procedures in conjunction with cardiac catheterization, see 93452-93461, 93563-93568)

(For chemotherapy of malignant disease, see 96401-96549)

AMA *CPT Assistant* ☐

36415: Jun 96: 10, Mar 98: 10, Oct 99: 11, Aug 00: 2, Feb 07: 10, Jul 07: 1, Dec 08: 7, May 14: 4

Plain English Description

In 36415, an appropriate vein is selected, usually one of the larger antecubital veins such as the median cubital, basilic, or cephalic veins. A tourniquet is placed above the planned puncture site. The site is disinfected with an alcohol pad. A needle is attached to a hub and the vein is punctured. A Vacutainer tube is attached to the hub and the blood specimen is collected. The Vacutainer tube is removed. Depending on the specific blood tests required, multiple Vacutainers may be filled from the same puncture site. In 36416, a blood sample is obtained by capillary puncture usually performed on the fingertip, ear lobe, heel or toe. Heel and toe sites are typically used only on neonates and infants. The planned puncture site is cleaned with an alcohol pad. A lancet is used to puncture the skin. A drop of blood is allowed to form at the puncture site and is then touched with a capillary tube to collect the specimen.

Collection of venous blood by venipuncture

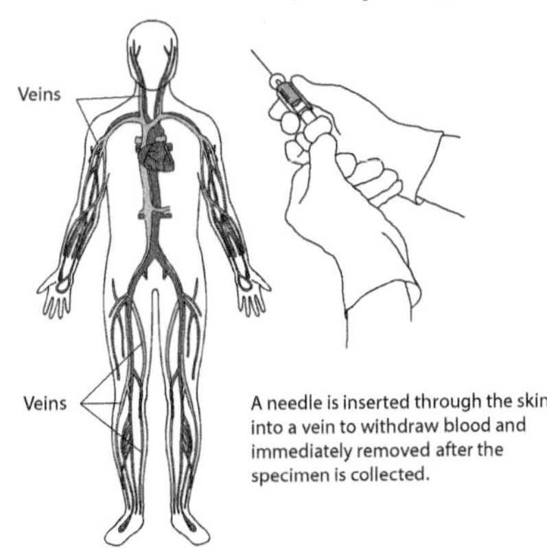

Veins
Veins
A needle is inserted through the skin into a vein to withdraw blood and immediately removed after the specimen is collected.

ICD-10-CM Diagnostic Codes

There are too many ICD-10-CM codes to list. Refer to ICD-10-CM code book for associated diagnostic codes.

CCI Edits

Refer to Appendix A for CCI edits.

Pub 100

36415: Pub 100-04, 12, 30.6.12, Pub 100-04, 16, 60.1.4

Facility RVUs ☐

Code	Work	PE Facility	MP	Total Facility
36415	0.00	0.00	0.00	0.00

Non-facility RVUs ☐

Code	Work	PE Non-Facility	MP	Total Non-Facility
36415	0.00	0.00	0.00	0.00

Modifiers (PAR) ☐

Code	Mod 50	Mod 51	Mod 62	Mod 66	Mod 80
36415	9	9	9	9	9

Global Period

Code	Days
36415	XXX

CPT © 2018 American Medical Association. All Rights Reserved.

36420-36425

36420 Venipuncture, cutdown; younger than age 1 year

(Do not report modifier 63 in conjunction with 36420)

36425 Venipuncture, cutdown; age 1 or over

(Do not report 36425 in conjunction with 36475, 36476, 36478)

AMA Coding Guideline

Venous Procedures

Venipuncture, needle or catheter for diagnostic study or intravenous therapy, percutaneous. These codes are also used to report the therapy as specified. For collection of a specimen from an established catheter, use 36592. For collection of a specimen from a completely implantable venous access device, use 36591.

Vascular Introduction and Injection Procedures

Listed services for injection procedures include necessary local anesthesia, introduction of needles or catheter, injection of contrast media with or without automatic power injection, and/or necessary pre- and postinjection care specifically related to the injection procedure.

Selective vascular catheterization should be coded to include introduction and all lesser order selective catheterization used in the approach (eg, the description for a selective right middle cerebral artery catheterization includes the introduction and placement catheterization of the right common and internal carotid arteries).

Additional second and/or third order arterial catheterization within the same family of arteries or veins supplied by a single first order vessel should be expressed by 36012, 36218, or 36248.

Additional first order or higher catheterization in vascular families supplied by a first order vessel different from a previously selected and coded family should be separately coded using the conventions described above.

Surgical Procedures on Arteries and Veins

Primary vascular procedure listings include establishing both inflow and outflow by whatever procedures necessary. Also included is that portion of the operative arteriogram performed by the surgeon, as indicated. Sympathectomy, when done, is included in the listed aortic procedures. For unlisted vascular procedure, use 37799.

Please see the Surgery Guidelines section for the following guidelines:

- *Surgical Procedures on the Cardiovascular System*

AMA Coding Notes

Vascular Introduction and Injection Procedures

(For radiological supervision and interpretation, see Radiology)

(For injection procedures in conjunction with cardiac catheterization, see 93452-93461, 93563-93568)

(For chemotherapy of malignant disease, see 96401-96549)

AMA *CPT Assistant* ☐

36420: Nov 99: 32-33, Aug 00: 2, Oct 03: 2, Jul 06: 4

36425: Oct 14: 6

Plain English Description

Venipuncture is accomplished using a cutdown procedure to access a deep or small vein. The site is prepped for sterile entry. The skin is nicked and the vein carefully exposed. A needle is inserted into the vein and the necessary blood samples obtained or medication administered. Use 36420 for a child younger than age 1. Use 36420 for patients age 1 or over.

Venipuncture

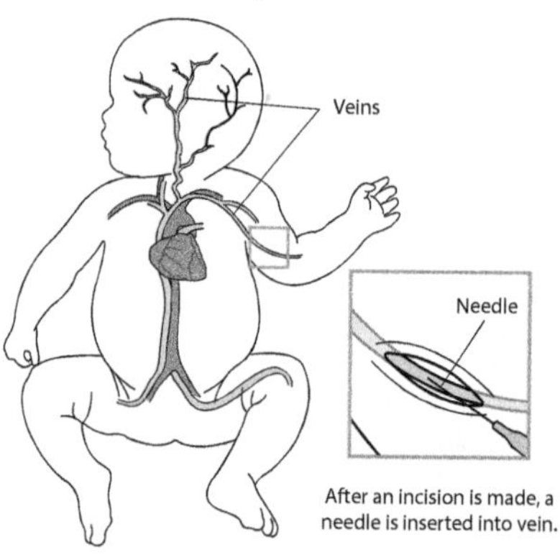

After an incision is made, a needle is inserted into vein.

ICD-10-CM Diagnostic Codes

There are too many ICD-10-CM codes to list. Refer to ICD-10-CM code book for associated diagnostic codes.

CCI Edits

Refer to Appendix A for CCI edits.

Pub 100

36425: Pub 100-04, 13, 70.2

Facility RVUs ☐

Code	Work	PE Facility	MP	Total Facility
36420	1.01	0.18	0.16	1.35
36425	0.76	0.30	0.10	1.16

Non-facility RVUs ☐

Code	Work	PE Non-Facility	MP	Total Non-Facility
36420	1.01	0.18	0.16	1.35
36425	0.76	0.30	0.10	1.16

Modifiers (PAR) ☐

Code	Mod 50	Mod 51	Mod 62	Mod 66	Mod 80
36420	0	2	0	0	0
36425	0	2	0	0	1

Global Period

Code	Days
36420	XXX
36425	XXX

CPT © 2018 American Medical Association. All Rights Reserved.

36430

36430 Transfusion, blood or blood components

(When a partial exchange transfusion is performed in a newborn, use 36456)

AMA Coding Guideline

Venous Procedures

Venipuncture, needle or catheter for diagnostic study or intravenous therapy, percutaneous. These codes are also used to report the therapy as specified. For collection of a specimen from an established catheter, use 36592. For collection of a specimen from a completely implantable venous access device, use 36591.

Vascular Introduction and Injection Procedures

Listed services for injection procedures include necessary local anesthesia, introduction of needles or catheter, injection of contrast media with or without automatic power injection, and/or necessary pre- and postinjection care specifically related to the injection procedure.

Selective vascular catheterization should be coded to include introduction and all lesser order selective catheterization used in the approach (eg, the description for a selective right middle cerebral artery catheterization includes the introduction and placement catheterization of the right common and internal carotid arteries).

Additional second and/or third order arterial catheterization within the same family of arteries or veins supplied by a single first order vessel should be expressed by 36012, 36218, or 36248.

Additional first order or higher catheterization in vascular families supplied by a first order vessel different from a previously selected and coded family should be separately coded using the conventions described above.

Surgical Procedures on Arteries and Veins

Primary vascular procedure listings include establishing both inflow and outflow by whatever procedures necessary. Also included is that portion of the operative arteriogram performed by the surgeon, as indicated. Sympathectomy, when done, is included in the listed aortic procedures. For unlisted vascular procedure, use 37799.

Please see the Surgery Guidelines section for the following guidelines:

- *Surgical Procedures on the Cardiovascular System*

AMA Coding Notes

Vascular Introduction and Injection Procedures

(For radiological supervision and interpretation, see Radiology)

(For injection procedures in conjunction with cardiac catheterization, see 93452-93461, 93563-93568)

(For chemotherapy of malignant disease, see 96401-96549)

AMA *CPT Assistant* ▯

36430: Aug 97: 18, Nov 99: 32-33, Aug 00: 2, Mar 01: 10, Oct 03: 2, Jul 06: 4, Jul 07: 1, Jul 17: 4

Plain English Description

Blood and blood components include whole blood, platelets, packed red blood cells, and plasma products. Transfusions are performed to replace blood that is lost or depleted due to an injury, surgery, sickle cell disease, or treatment for a malignant neoplasm. Red blood cells are given to increase the number of blood cells that transport oxygen and nutrients throughout the body, platelets to control bleeding and improve blood clotting, and plasma to replace total blood volume and provide blood factors that improve blood clotting. The skin is prepped over the planned transfusion site and an intravenous line inserted. Any medication ordered by the physician is administered prior to the transfusion. The blood and/or blood components are administered. The patient is monitored during the transfusion for any signs of adverse reaction.

Transfusion, blood or blood components

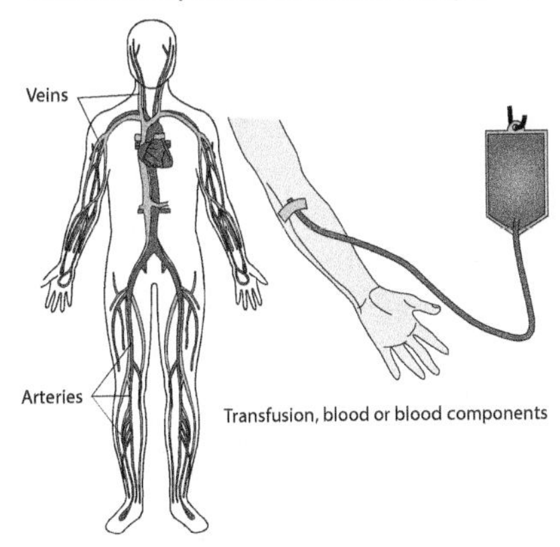

ICD-10-CM Diagnostic Codes

There are too many ICD-10-CM codes to list. Refer to ICD-10-CM code book for associated diagnostic codes.

CCI Edits

Refer to Appendix A for CCI edits.

Pub 100

36430: Pub 100-03, 1, 110.16, Pub 100-03, 1, 110.7, Pub 100-04, 4, 231.8

Facility RVUs ▯

Code	Work	PE Facility	MP	Total Facility
36430	0.00	0.97	0.02	0.99

Non-facility RVUs ▯

Code	Work	PE Non-Facility	MP	Total Non-Facility
36430	0.00	0.97	0.02	0.99

Modifiers (PAR) ▯

Code	Mod 50	Mod 51	Mod 62	Mod 66	Mod 80
36430	0	0	0	0	1

Global Period

Code	Days
36430	XXX

● New ▲ Revised ✚ Add On ⊘Modifier 51 Exempt ★Telemedicine ▯ CPT QuickRef ⁄⁄FDA Pending ⇄ Laterality ❼ Seventh Character ♂Male ♀Female

CPT © 2018 American Medical Association. All Rights Reserved.

36440

36440 Push transfusion, blood, 2 years or younger

(When a partial exchange transfusion is performed in a newborn, use 36456)

AMA Coding Guideline

Venous Procedures

Venipuncture, needle or catheter for diagnostic study or intravenous therapy, percutaneous. These codes are also used to report the therapy as specified. For collection of a specimen from an established catheter, use 36592. For collection of a specimen from a completely implantable venous access device, use 36591.

Vascular Introduction and Injection Procedures

Listed services for injection procedures include necessary local anesthesia, introduction of needles or catheter, injection of contrast media with or without automatic power injection, and/or necessary pre- and postinjection care specifically related to the injection procedure.

Selective vascular catheterization should be coded to include introduction and all lesser order selective catheterization used in the approach (eg, the description for a selective right middle cerebral artery catheterization includes the introduction and placement catheterization of the right common and internal carotid arteries).

Additional second and/or third order arterial catheterization within the same family of arteries or veins supplied by a single first order vessel should be expressed by 36012, 36218, or 36248.

Additional first order or higher catheterization in vascular families supplied by a first order vessel different from a previously selected and coded family should be separately coded using the conventions described above.

Surgical Procedures on Arteries and Veins

Primary vascular procedure listings include establishing both inflow and outflow by whatever procedures necessary. Also included is that portion of the operative arteriogram performed by the surgeon, as indicated. Sympathectomy, when done, is included in the listed aortic procedures. For unlisted vascular procedure, use 37799.

Please see the Surgery Guidelines section for the following guidelines:

- *Surgical Procedures on the Cardiovascular System*

AMA Coding Notes

Vascular Introduction and Injection Procedures

(For radiological supervision and interpretation, see Radiology)

(For injection procedures in conjunction with cardiac catheterization, see 93452-93461, 93563-93568)

(For chemotherapy of malignant disease, see 96401-96549)

AMA *CPT Assistant* ◻

36440: Aug 00: 2, Oct 03: 2, Jul 06: 4, Jul 07: 1, Jul 17: 4

Plain English Description

Transfusions are performed to replace blood that is lost or depleted due to an injury, surgery, sickle cell disease, or treatment for a malignant neoplasm. Push transfusion may be performed through a previously established intravenous line or a new intravenous line may be placed. Any medication ordered by the physician is administered prior to the transfusion. The blood is then administered using a push technique over a relatively short period of time, usually less than 15 minutes. The child is monitored during and after the transfusion for any signs of adverse reaction.

ICD-10-CM Diagnostic Codes

There are too many ICD-10-CM codes to list. Refer to ICD-10-CM code book for associated diagnostic codes.

CCI Edits

Refer to Appendix A for CCI edits.

Pub 100

36440: Pub 100-03, 1, 110.16, Pub 100-03, 1, 110.7, Pub 100-04, 4, 231.8

Facility RVUs ◻

Code	Work	PE Facility	MP	Total Facility
36440	1.03	0.36	0.07	1.46

Non-facility RVUs ◻

Code	Work	PE Non-Facility	MP	Total Non-Facility
36440	1.03	0.36	0.07	1.46

Modifiers (PAR) ◻

Code	Mod 50	Mod 51	Mod 62	Mod 66	Mod 80
36440	0	2	0	0	0

Global Period

Code	Days
36440	XXX

CPT © 2018 American Medical Association. All Rights Reserved.

36555-36556

36555 Insertion of non-tunneled centrally inserted central venous catheter; younger than 5 years of age

(For peripherally inserted non-tunneled central venous catheter, younger than 5 years of age, use 36568)

36556 Insertion of non-tunneled centrally inserted central venous catheter; age 5 years or older

(For peripherally inserted non-tunneled central venous catheter, age 5 years or older, use 36569)

AMA Coding Guideline

Insertion of Central Venous Access Device

Peripherally inserted central venous catheters (PICCs) may be placed or replaced with or without imaging guidance. When performed without imaging guidance, report using 36568 or 36569. When imaging guidance (eg, ultrasound, fluoroscopy) is used for PICC placement or repositioning, bundled service codes 36572, 36573, 36584 include all imaging necessary to complete the procedure, image documentation (representative images from all modalities used are stored to patient's permanent record), associated radiological supervision and interpretation, venography performed through the same venous puncture, and documentation of final central position of the catheter with imaging. Ultrasound guidance for PICC placement should include documentation of evaluation of the potential puncture sites, patency of the entry vein, and real-time ultrasound visualization of needle entry into the vein.

Codes 71045, 71046, 71047, 71048 should not be reported for the purpose of documenting the final catheter position on the same day of service as 36572, 36573, 36584. Codes 36572, 36573, 36584 include confirmation of catheter tip location. The physician or other qualified health care professional reporting image-guided PICC insertion cannot report confirmation of catheter tip location separately (eg, via X ray, ultrasound). Report 36572, 36573, 36584 with modifier 52 when performed without confirmation of catheter tip location.

"Midline" catheters by definition terminate in the peripheral venous system. They are not central venous access devices and may not be reported as a PICC service. Midline catheter placement may be reported with 36400, 36405, 36406, or 36410. PICCs placed using magnetic guidance or any other guidance modality that does not include imaging or image documentation are reported with 36568, 36569.

Central Venous Access Procedures

To qualify as a central venous access catheter or device, the tip of the catheter/device must terminate in the subclavian, brachiocephalic (innominate) or iliac veins, the superior or inferior vena cava, or the right atrium. The venous access device may be either centrally inserted (jugular, subclavian, femoral vein or inferior vena cava catheter entry site) or peripherally inserted (eg, basilic, cephalic, or saphenous vein entry site). The device may be accessed for use either via exposed catheter (external to the skin), via a subcutaneous port or via a subcutaneous pump.

The procedures involving these types of devices fall into five categories:

1. Insertion (placement of catheter through a newly established venous access)
2. Repair (fixing device without replacement of either catheter or port/pump, other than pharmacologic or mechanical correction of intracatheter or pericatheter occlusion [see 36595 or 36596])
3. Partial replacement of only the catheter component associated with a port/pump device, but not entire device
4. Complete replacement of entire device via same venous access site (complete exchange)
5. Removal of entire device.

There is no coding distinction between venous access achieved percutaneously versus by cutdown or based on catheter size.

For the repair, partial (catheter only) replacement, complete replacement, or removal of both catheters (placed from separate venous access sites) of a multi-catheter device, with or without subcutaneous ports/pumps, use the appropriate code describing the service with a frequency of two.

If an existing central venous access device is removed and a new one placed via a separate venous access site, appropriate codes for both procedures (removal of old, if code exists, and insertion of new device) should be reported.

When imaging guidance is used for centrally inserted central venous catheters, for gaining access to the venous entry site and/or for manipulating the catheter into final central position, imaging guidance codes (eg, 76937, 77001) may be reported separately. Do not use 76937, 77001 in conjunction with 36568, 36569, 36572, 36573, 36584.

Please see the Surgical Guidelines section for the following table: The Central Venous Access Procedures Table

Vascular Introduction and Injection Procedures

Listed services for injection procedures include necessary local anesthesia, introduction of needles or catheter, injection of contrast media with or without automatic power injection, and/or necessary pre- and postinjection care specifically related to the injection procedure.

Selective vascular catheterization should be coded to include introduction and all lesser order selective catheterization used in the approach (eg, the description for a selective right middle cerebral artery catheterization includes the introduction and placement catheterization of the right common and internal carotid arteries).

Additional second and/or third order arterial catheterization within the same family of arteries or veins supplied by a single first order vessel should be expressed by 36012, 36218, or 36248.

Additional first order or higher catheterization in vascular families supplied by a first order vessel different from a previously selected and coded family should be separately coded using the conventions described above.

Surgical Procedures on Arteries and VeinsPrimary vascular procedure listings include establishing both inflow and outflow by whatever procedures necessary. Also included is that portion of the operative arteriogram performed by the surgeon, as indicated. Sympathectomy, when done, is included in the listed aortic procedures. For unlisted vascular procedure, use 37799.

Please see the Surgery Guidelines section for the following guidelines:

- *Surgical Procedures on the Cardiovascular System*

AMA Coding Notes

Central Venous Access Procedures

(For refilling and maintenance of an implantable pump or reservoir for intravenous or intra-arterial drug delivery, use 96522)

Vascular Introduction and Injection Procedures

(For radiological supervision and interpretation, see Radiology)

(For injection procedures in conjunction with cardiac catheterization, see 93452-93461, 93563-93568)

(For chemotherapy of malignant disease, see 96401-96549)

AMA *CPT Assistant* ◻

36555: Dec 04: 7, Jul 06: 4, Jul 07: 1, Jun 08: 8

36556: Dec 04: 7, Jun 08: 8

Plain English Description

A non-tunneled centrally inserted central venous catheter (CVC) is placed. A CVC must terminate in the subclavian, brachiocephalic, or iliac veins, the superior or inferior vena cava, or right atrium. A non-tunneled CVC is placed directly into the jugular, subclavian, or femoral vein or the inferior vena cava. Separately reportable imaging guidance may be used to access the venous entry site and/or to manipulate the catheter tip to the final central position. Local anesthesia is administered at the planned puncture site. There are two techniques for insertion. Using a peel-away cannula technique, a cannula with a stylet is inserted into the selected

CPT © 2018 American Medical Association. All Rights Reserved.

vein. The stylet is removed. The catheter is advanced through the cannula into the vein and advanced into the brachiocephalic vein, subclavian vein, superior vena cava, or right atrium or the iliac vein or inferior vena cava. Using a Seldinger technique, the skin and vein are punctured with a needle. A guidewire is inserted through the needle and advanced several centimeters. An introducer sheath and dilator are advanced over the guidewire and the guidewire and dilator removed. The catheter is then advanced through the introducer sheath and into the brachiocephalic vein, subclavian vein, superior vena cava or right atrium, or iliac vein or inferior vena cava. Placement is checked by separately reportable radiographs. The CVC is secured with sutures and a dressing applied over the insertion site. Use 36555 for non-tunneled CVC placement in a child younger than age 5 and 36556 for a patient age 5 or older.

Insertion of non-tunneled centrally inserted central venous catheter

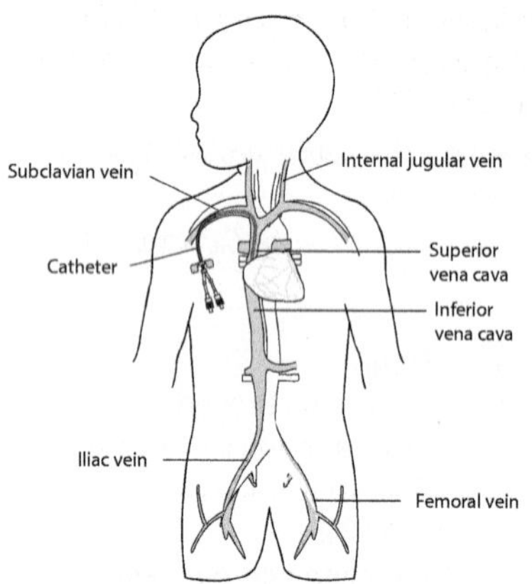

ICD-10-CM Diagnostic Codes

There are too many ICD-10-CM codes to list. Refer to ICD-10-CM code book for associated diagnostic codes.

CCI Edits

Refer to Appendix A for CCI edits.

Facility RVUs

Code	Work	PE Facility	MP	Total Facility
36555	1.93	0.38	0.15	2.46
36556	1.75	0.50	0.20	2.45

Non-facility RVUs

Code	Work	PE Non-Facility	MP	Total Non-Facility
36555	1.93	3.25	0.15	5.33
36556	1.75	4.04	0.20	5.99

Modifiers (PAR)

Code	Mod 50	Mod 51	Mod 62	Mod 66	Mod 80
36555	0	0	0	0	1
36556	0	0	0	0	1

Global Period

Code	Days
36555	000
36556	000

CPT © 2018 American Medical Association. All Rights Reserved.

36557-36558

36557 Insertion of tunneled centrally inserted central venous catheter, without subcutaneous port or pump; younger than 5 years of age

36558 Insertion of tunneled centrally inserted central venous catheter, without subcutaneous port or pump; age 5 years or older

(For peripherally inserted central venous catheter with port, 5 years or older, use 36571)

AMA Coding Guideline

Insertion of Central Venous Access Device

Peripherally inserted central venous catheters (PICCs) may be placed or replaced with or without imaging guidance. When performed without imaging guidance, report using 36568 or 36569. When imaging guidance (eg, ultrasound, fluoroscopy) is used for PICC placement or repositioning, bundled service codes 36572, 36573, 36584 include all imaging necessary to complete the procedure, image documentation (representative images from all modalities used are stored to patient's permanent record), associated radiological supervision and interpretation, venography performed through the same venous puncture, and documentation of final central position of the catheter with imaging. Ultrasound guidance for PICC placement should include documentation of evaluation of the potential puncture sites, patency of the entry vein, and real-time ultrasound visualization of needle entry into the vein.

Codes 71045, 71046, 71047, 71048 should not be reported for the purpose of documenting the final catheter position on the same day of service as 36572, 36573, 36584. Codes 36572, 36573, 36584 include confirmation of catheter tip location. The physician or other qualified health care professional reporting image-guided PICC insertion cannot report confirmation of catheter tip location separately (eg, via X ray, ultrasound). Report 36572, 36573, 36584 with modifier 52 when performed without confirmation of catheter tip location.

"Midline" catheters by definition terminate in the peripheral venous system. They are not central venous access devices and may not be reported as a PICC service. Midline catheter placement may be reported with 36400, 36405, 36406, or 36410. PICCs placed using magnetic guidance or any other guidance modality that does not include imaging or image documentation are reported with 36568, 36569.

Central Venous Access Procedures

To qualify as a central venous access catheter or device, the tip of the catheter/device must terminate in the subclavian, brachiocephalic (innominate) or iliac veins, the superior or inferior vena cava, or the right atrium. The venous access device may be either centrally inserted (jugular, subclavian, femoral vein or inferior vena cava catheter entry site) or peripherally inserted (eg, basilic, cephalic, or saphenous vein entry site). The device may be accessed for use either via exposed catheter (external to the skin), via a subcutaneous port or via a subcutaneous pump.

The procedures involving these types of devices fall into five categories:

1. Insertion (placement of catheter through a newly established venous access)
2. Repair (fixing device without replacement of either catheter or port/pump, other than pharmacologic or mechanical correction of intracatheter or pericatheter occlusion [see 36595 or 36596])
3. Partial replacement of only the catheter component associated with a port/pump device, but not entire device
4. Complete replacement of entire device via same venous access site (complete exchange)
5. Removal of entire device.

There is no coding distinction between venous access achieved percutaneously versus by cutdown or based on catheter size.

For the repair, partial (catheter only) replacement, complete replacement, or removal of both catheters (placed from separate venous access sites) of a multi-catheter device, with or without subcutaneous ports/pumps, use the appropriate code describing the service with a frequency of two.

If an existing central venous access device is removed and a new one placed via a separate venous access site, appropriate codes for both procedures (removal of old, if code exists, and insertion of new device) should be reported.

When imaging guidance is used for centrally inserted central venous catheters, for gaining access to the venous entry site and/or for manipulating the catheter into final central position, imaging guidance codes (eg, 76937, 77001) may be reported separately. Do not use 76937, 77001 in conjunction with 36568, 36569, 36572, 36573, 36584.

Please see the Surgical Guidelines section for the following table: The Central Venous Access Procedures Table

Vascular Introduction and Injection Procedures

Listed services for injection procedures include necessary local anesthesia, introduction of needles or catheter, injection of contrast media with or without automatic power injection, and/or necessary pre- and postinjection care specifically related to the injection procedure.

Selective vascular catheterization should be coded to include introduction and all lesser order selective catheterization used in the approach (eg, the description for a selective right middle cerebral artery catheterization includes the introduction and placement catheterization of the right common and internal carotid arteries).

Additional second and/or third order arterial catheterization within the same family of arteries or veins supplied by a single first order vessel should be expressed by 36012, 36218, or 36248.

Additional first order or higher catheterization in vascular families supplied by a first order vessel different from a previously selected and coded family should be separately coded using the conventions described above.

Surgical Procedures on Arteries and VeinsPrimary vascular procedure listings include establishing both inflow and outflow by whatever procedures necessary. Also included is that portion of the operative arteriogram performed by the surgeon, as indicated. Sympathectomy, when done, is included in the listed aortic procedures. For unlisted vascular procedure, use 37799.

Please see the Surgery Guidelines section for the following guidelines:

- *Surgical Procedures on the Cardiovascular System*

AMA Coding Notes

Central Venous Access Procedures

(For refilling and maintenance of an implantable pump or reservoir for intravenous or intra-arterial drug delivery, use 96522)

Vascular Introduction and Injection Procedures

(For radiological supervision and interpretation, see Radiology)

(For injection procedures in conjunction with cardiac catheterization, see 93452-93461, 93563-93568)

(For chemotherapy of malignant disease, see 96401-96549)

AMA *CPT Assistant* ☐

36557: Dec 04: 7, Jun 08: 8

36558: Dec 04: 7, Jun 08: 8, Jan 15: 13

Plain English Description

A tunneled centrally inserted central venous catheter (CVC) is placed. A CVC must terminate in the subclavian, brachiocephalic, or iliac veins, the superior or inferior vena cava, or right atrium. A tunneled CVC is placed through a subcutaneous tunnel into the jugular, subclavian, or femoral vein or the inferior vena cava with the most common venous access site for tunneled devices being the jugular vein. Separately reportable imaging guidance may be used to access the venous entry site and/or to manipulate the catheter tip to the final central position. Local anesthesia is

CPT © 2018 American Medical Association. All Rights Reserved.

administered at the planned puncture site. Using a Seldinger technique to access the jugular vein, the skin and vein are punctured with a needle. A guidewire is inserted through the needle and advanced several centimeters. An incision is made in the chest wall and a subcutaneous tunnel is created. An introducer sheath and dilator are advanced over the guidewire and the guidewire and dilator removed. The catheter is then advanced through the tunnel to the introducer sheath in the jugular vein and into the brachiocephalic vein, subclavian vein, superior vena cava or right atrium. Placement is checked by separately reportable radiographs. The CVC is secured with sutures, the incision in the chest wall closed with sutures, and a dressing applied over the insertion site. Use 36557 for tunneled CVC placement in a child younger than age 5 and 36558 for a patient age 5 or older.

Insertion of tunneled centrally inserted CVAD, without subcutaneous port or pump

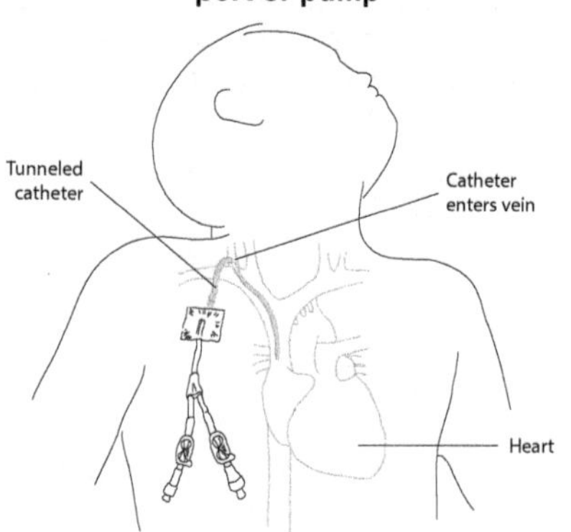

ICD-10-CM Diagnostic Codes

There are too many ICD-10-CM codes to list. Refer to ICD-10-CM code book for associated diagnostic codes.

CCI Edits

Refer to Appendix A for CCI edits.

Facility RVUs

Code	Work	PE Facility	MP	Total Facility
36557	4.89	3.13	1.16	9.18
36558	4.59	2.36	0.59	7.54

Non-facility RVUs

Code	Work	PE Non-Facility	MP	Total Non-Facility
36557	4.89	23.01	1.16	29.06
36558	4.59	16.52	0.59	21.70

Modifiers (PAR)

Code	Mod 50	Mod 51	Mod 62	Mod 66	Mod 80
36557	1	2	0	0	0
36558	1	2	0	0	0

Global Period

Code	Days
36557	010
36558	010

CPT © 2018 American Medical Association. All Rights Reserved.

36560-36561

36560 Insertion of tunneled centrally inserted central venous access device, with subcutaneous port; younger than 5 years of age

(For peripherally inserted central venous access device with subcutaneous port, younger than 5 years of age, use 36570)

36561 Insertion of tunneled centrally inserted central venous access device, with subcutaneous port; age 5 years or older

(For peripherally inserted central venous catheter with subcutaneous port, 5 years or older, use 36571)

AMA Coding Guideline

Insertion of Central Venous Access Device

Peripherally inserted central venous catheters (PICCs) may be placed or replaced with or without imaging guidance. When performed without imaging guidance, report using 36568 or 36569. When imaging guidance (eg, ultrasound, fluoroscopy) is used for PICC placement or repositioning, bundled service codes 36572, 36573, 36584 include all imaging necessary to complete the procedure, image documentation (representative images from all modalities used are stored to patient's permanent record), associated radiological supervision and interpretation, venography performed through the same venous puncture, and documentation of final central position of the catheter with imaging. Ultrasound guidance for PICC placement should include documentation of evaluation of the potential puncture sites, patency of the entry vein, and real-time ultrasound visualization of needle entry into the vein.

Codes 71045, 71046, 71047, 71048 should not be reported for the purpose of documenting the final catheter position on the same day of service as 36572, 36573, 36584. Codes 36572, 36573, 36584 include confirmation of catheter tip location. The physician or other qualified health care professional reporting image-guided PICC insertion cannot report confirmation of catheter tip location separately (eg, via X ray, ultrasound). Report 36572, 36573, 36584 with modifier 52 when performed without confirmation of catheter tip location.

"Midline" catheters by definition terminate in the peripheral venous system. They are not central venous access devices and may not be reported as a PICC service. Midline catheter placement may be reported with 36400, 36405, 36406, or 36410. PICCs placed using magnetic guidance or any other guidance modality that does not include imaging or image documentation are reported with 36568, 36569.

Central Venous Access Procedures

To qualify as a central venous access catheter or device, the tip of the catheter/device must terminate in the subclavian, brachiocephalic (innominate) or iliac veins, the superior or inferior vena cava, or the right atrium. The venous access device may be either centrally inserted (jugular, subclavian, femoral vein or inferior vena cava catheter entry site) or peripherally inserted (eg, basilic, cephalic, or saphenous vein entry site). The device may be accessed for use either via exposed catheter (external to the skin), via a subcutaneous port or via a subcutaneous pump.

The procedures involving these types of devices fall into five categories:

1. Insertion (placement of catheter through a newly established venous access)
2. Repair (fixing device without replacement of either catheter or port/pump, other than pharmacologic or mechanical correction of intracatheter or pericatheter occlusion [see 36595 or 36596])
3. Partial replacement of only the catheter component associated with a port/pump device, but not entire device
4. Complete replacement of entire device via same venous access site (complete exchange)
5. Removal of entire device.

There is no coding distinction between venous access achieved percutaneously versus by cutdown or based on catheter size.

For the repair, partial (catheter only) replacement, complete replacement, or removal of both catheters (placed from separate venous access sites) of a multi-catheter device, with or without subcutaneous ports/pumps, use the appropriate code describing the service with a frequency of two.

If an existing central venous access device is removed and a new one placed via a separate venous access site, appropriate codes for both procedures (removal of old, if code exists, and insertion of new device) should be reported.

When imaging guidance is used for centrally inserted central venous catheters, for gaining access to the venous entry site and/or for manipulating the catheter into final central position, imaging guidance codes (eg, 76937, 77001) may be reported separately. Do not use 76937, 77001 in conjunction with 36568, 36569, 36572, 36573, 36584.

Please see the Surgical Guidelines section for the following table: The Central Venous Access Procedures Table

Vascular Introduction and Injection Procedures

Listed services for injection procedures include necessary local anesthesia, introduction of needles or catheter, injection of contrast media with or without automatic power injection, and/or necessary pre- and postinjection care specifically related to the injection procedure.

Selective vascular catheterization should be coded to include introduction and all lesser order selective catheterization used in the approach (eg, the description for a selective right middle cerebral artery catheterization includes the introduction and placement catheterization of the right common and internal carotid arteries).

Additional second and/or third order arterial catheterization within the same family of arteries or veins supplied by a single first order vessel should be expressed by 36012, 36218, or 36248.

Additional first order or higher catheterization in vascular families supplied by a first order vessel different from a previously selected and coded family should be separately coded using the conventions described above.

Surgical Procedures on Arteries and VeinsPrimary vascular procedure listings include establishing both inflow and outflow by whatever procedures necessary. Also included is that portion of the operative arteriogram performed by the surgeon, as indicated. Sympathectomy, when done, is included in the listed aortic procedures. For unlisted vascular procedure, use 37799.

Please see the Surgery Guidelines section for the following guidelines:

- *Surgical Procedures on the Cardiovascular System*

AMA Coding Notes

Central Venous Access Procedures

(For refilling and maintenance of an implantable pump or reservoir for intravenous or intra-arterial drug delivery, use 96522)

Vascular Introduction and Injection Procedures

(For radiological supervision and interpretation, see Radiology)

(For injection procedures in conjunction with cardiac catheterization, see 93452-93461, 93563-93568)

(For chemotherapy of malignant disease, see 96401-96549)

AMA *CPT Assistant* ☐

36560: Dec 04: 7, Jun 08: 8, Dec 09: 11
36561: Dec 04: 7, Jun 08: 8, Dec 09: 11

Plain English Description

A tunneled centrally inserted central venous catheter (CVC) with a subcutaneous port is placed. A CVC must terminate in the subclavian, brachiocephalic, or iliac veins, the superior or inferior vena cava, or right atrium. A tunneled CVC is placed through a subcutaneous tunnel into the jugular, subclavian, or femoral vein or the inferior vena cava with the most common venous access site for tunneled devices being the jugular vein. Separately reportable imaging guidance may be used to access the venous entry site and/or to manipulate the catheter tip to the final central position. Local anesthesia is administered

CPT © 2018 American Medical Association. All Rights Reserved.

at the planned puncture site. Using a Seldinger technique to access the jugular vein, the skin and vein are punctured with a needle. A guidewire is inserted through the needle and advanced several centimeters. A subcutaneous pocket is then created for placement of the port. A subcutaneous tunnel is created from the venous access site to the subcutaneous pocket. An introducer sheath and dilator are advanced over the guidewire and the guidewire and dilator removed. The catheter is then advanced through the tunnel to the introducer sheath in the jugular vein and into the brachiocephalic vein, subclavian vein, superior vena cava or right atrium. Placement is checked by separately reportable radiographs. The catheter and port are connected and the port is placed in the subcutaneous pocket. The incision over the venous access site is closed. The port is sutured into place and the pocket is closed. Use 36560 for tunneled CVC placement with subcutaneous port in a child younger than age 5 and 36561 for a patient age 5 or older.

Insertion of tunneled centrally inserted central venous access device with subcutaneous port

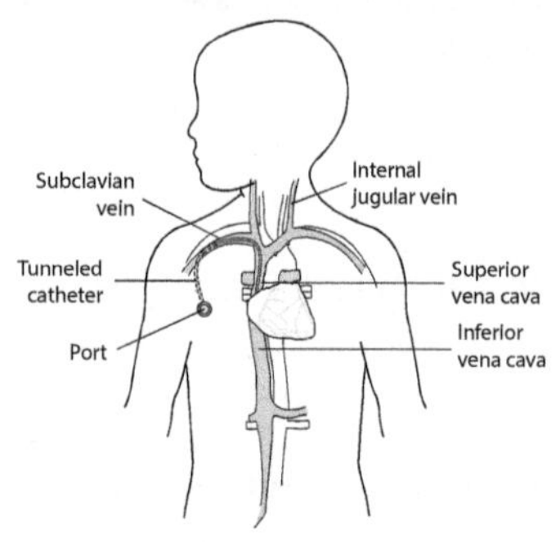

ICD-10-CM Diagnostic Codes

There are too many ICD-10-CM codes to list. Refer to ICD-10-CM code book for associated diagnostic codes.

CCI Edits

Refer to Appendix A for CCI edits.

Facility RVUs ☐

Code	Work	PE Facility	MP	Total Facility
36560	6.04	3.54	1.46	11.04
36561	5.79	3.01	0.94	9.74

Non-facility RVUs ☐

Code	Work	PE Non-Facility	MP	Total Non-Facility
36560	6.04	29.65	1.46	37.15
36561	5.79	23.88	0.94	30.61

Modifiers (PAR) ☐

Code	Mod 50	Mod 51	Mod 62	Mod 66	Mod 80
36560	1	2	0	0	0
36561	1	2	0	0	0

Global Period

Code	Days
36560	010
36561	010

CPT © 2018 American Medical Association. All Rights Reserved.

36563

36563 Insertion of tunneled centrally inserted central venous access device with subcutaneous pump

AMA Coding Guideline

Insertion of Central Venous Access Device

Peripherally inserted central venous catheters (PICCs) may be placed or replaced with or without imaging guidance. When performed without imaging guidance, report using 36568 or 36569. When imaging guidance (eg, ultrasound, fluoroscopy) is used for PICC placement or repositioning, bundled service codes 36572, 36573, 36584 include all imaging necessary to complete the procedure, image documentation (representative images from all modalities used are stored to patient's permanent record), associated radiological supervision and interpretation, venography performed through the same venous puncture, and documentation of final central position of the catheter with imaging. Ultrasound guidance for PICC placement should include documentation of evaluation of the potential puncture sites, patency of the entry vein, and real-time ultrasound visualization of needle entry into the vein.

Codes 71045, 71046, 71047, 71048 should not be reported for the purpose of documenting the final catheter position on the same day of service as 36572, 36573, 36584. Codes 36572, 36573, 36584 include confirmation of catheter tip location. The physician or other qualified health care professional reporting image-guided PICC insertion cannot report confirmation of catheter tip location separately (eg, via X ray, ultrasound). Report 36572, 36573, 36584 with modifier 52 when performed without confirmation of catheter tip location.

"Midline" catheters by definition terminate in the peripheral venous system. They are not central venous access devices and may not be reported as a PICC service. Midline catheter placement may be reported with 36400, 36405, 36406, or 36410. PICCs placed using magnetic guidance or any other guidance modality that does not include imaging or image documentation are reported with 36568, 36569.

Central Venous Access Procedures

To qualify as a central venous access catheter or device, the tip of the catheter/device must terminate in the subclavian, brachiocephalic (innominate) or iliac veins, the superior or inferior vena cava, or the right atrium. The venous access device may be either centrally inserted (jugular, subclavian, femoral vein or inferior vena cava catheter entry site) or peripherally inserted (eg, basilic, cephalic, or saphenous vein entry site). The device may be accessed for use either via exposed catheter (external to the skin), via a subcutaneous port or via a subcutaneous pump.

The procedures involving these types of devices fall into five categories:

1. Insertion (placement of catheter through a newly established venous access)
2. Repair (fixing device without replacement of either catheter or port/pump, other than pharmacologic or mechanical correction of intracatheter or pericatheter occlusion [see 36595 or 36596])
3. Partial replacement of only the catheter component associated with a port/pump device, but not entire device
4. Complete replacement of entire device via same venous access site (complete exchange)
5. Removal of entire device.

There is no coding distinction between venous access achieved percutaneously versus by cutdown or based on catheter size.

For the repair, partial (catheter only) replacement, complete replacement, or removal of both catheters (placed from separate venous access sites) of a multi-catheter device, with or without subcutaneous ports/pumps, use the appropriate code describing the service with a frequency of two.

If an existing central venous access device is removed and a new one placed via a separate venous access site, appropriate codes for both procedures (removal of old, if code exists, and insertion of new device) should be reported.

When imaging guidance is used for centrally inserted central venous catheters, for gaining access to the venous entry site and/or for manipulating the catheter into final central position, imaging guidance codes (eg, 76937, 77001) may be reported separately. Do not use 76937, 77001 in conjunction with 36568, 36569, 36572, 36573, 36584.

Please see the Surgical Guidelines section for the following table: The Central Venous Access Procedures Table

Vascular Introduction and Injection Procedures

Listed services for injection procedures include necessary local anesthesia, introduction of needles or catheter, injection of contrast media with or without automatic power injection, and/or necessary pre- and postinjection care specifically related to the injection procedure.

Selective vascular catheterization should be coded to include introduction and all lesser order selective catheterization used in the approach (eg, the description for a selective right middle cerebral artery catheterization includes the introduction and placement catheterization of the right common and internal carotid arteries).

Additional second and/or third order arterial catheterization within the same family of arteries or veins supplied by a single first order vessel should be expressed by 36012, 36218, or 36248. Additional first order or higher catheterization in vascular families supplied by a first order vessel different from a previously selected and coded family should be separately coded using the conventions described above.

Surgical Procedures on Arteries and VeinsPrimary vascular procedure listings include establishing both inflow and outflow by whatever procedures necessary. Also included is that portion of the operative arteriogram performed by the surgeon, as indicated. Sympathectomy, when done, is included in the listed aortic procedures. For unlisted vascular procedure, use 37799.

Please see the Surgery Guidelines section for the following guidelines:

- *Surgical Procedures on the Cardiovascular System*

AMA Coding Notes

Central Venous Access Procedures

(For refilling and maintenance of an implantable pump or reservoir for intravenous or intra-arterial drug delivery, use 96522)

Vascular Introduction and Injection Procedures

(For radiological supervision and interpretation, see Radiology)

(For injection procedures in conjunction with cardiac catheterization, see 93452-93461, 93563-93568)

(For chemotherapy of malignant disease, see 96401-96549)

AMA *CPT Assistant* ▯

36563: Dec 04: 8, Jun 08: 8

Plain English Description

A central venous catheter (CVC) must terminate in the subclavian, brachiocephalic, or iliac veins, the superior or inferior vena cava, or right atrium. A tunneled CVC is placed through a subcutaneous tunnel into the jugular, subclavian, or femoral vein or the inferior vena cava with the most common venous access site for tunneled devices being the jugular vein. Separately reportable imaging guidance may be used to access the venous entry site and/or to manipulate the catheter tip to the final central position. Local anesthesia is administered at the planned puncture site. Using a Seldinger technique to access the jugular vein, the skin and vein are punctured with a needle. A guidewire is inserted through the needle and advanced several centimeters. A subcutaneous pocket is then created for placement of the pump. A subcutaneous tunnel is created from the venous access site to the subcutaneous pocket. An introducer sheath and dilator are advanced over the guidewire and the guidewire and dilator removed. The catheter is then advanced through the tunnel to the introducer sheath in the jugular vein and into the brachiocephalic vein, subclavian vein, superior

CPT © 2018 American Medical Association. All Rights Reserved.

vena cava or right atrium. Placement is checked by separately reportable radiographs. The catheter and pump are connected and the pump placed in the subcutaneous pocket. The incision over the venous access site is closed. The pump is sutured into place and the pocket is closed.

Insertion of tunneled centrally inserted central venous access device

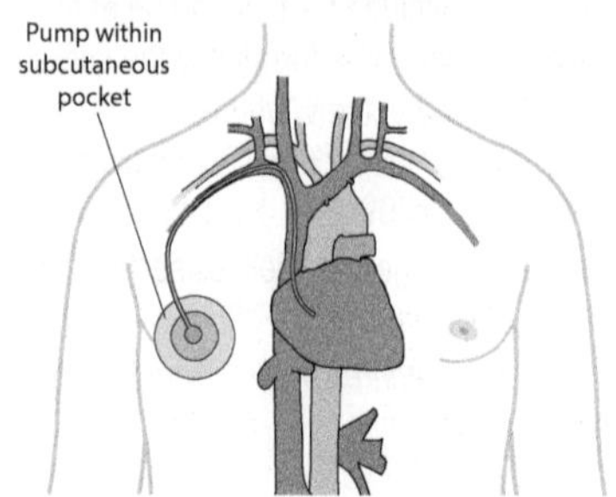

A tunneled centrally inserted central venous catheter (CVC) is positioned in the vena cava, subclavian, iliac, or brachiocephalic vein, or right atrium by creating a tunnel through the skin and subcutaneous tissue, usually from the jugular vein.

ICD-10-CM Diagnostic Codes

There are too many ICD-10-CM codes to list. Refer to ICD-10-CM code book for associated diagnostic codes.

CCI Edits

Refer to Appendix A for CCI edits.

Facility RVUs

Code	Work	PE Facility	MP	Total Facility
36563	5.99	3.28	1.33	10.60

Non-facility RVUs

Code	Work	PE Non-Facility	MP	Total Non-Facility
36563	5.99	27.15	1.33	34.47

Modifiers (PAR)

Code	Mod 50	Mod 51	Mod 62	Mod 66	Mod 80
36563	0	2	0	0	0

Global Period

Code	Days
36563	010

CPT © 2018 American Medical Association. All Rights Reserved.

36565-36566

36565 Insertion of tunneled centrally inserted central venous access device, requiring 2 catheters via 2 separate venous access sites; without subcutaneous port or pump (eg, Tesio type catheter)

36566 Insertion of tunneled centrally inserted central venous access device, requiring 2 catheters via 2 separate venous access sites; with subcutaneous port(s)

"Midline" catheters by definition terminate in the peripheral venous system. They are not central venous access devices and may not be reported as a PICC service. Midline catheter placement may be reported with 36400, 36405, 36406, or 36410. PICCs placed using magnetic guidance or any other guidance modality that does not include imaging or image documentation are reported with 36568, 36569.

AMA Coding Guideline

Insertion of Central Venous Access Device

Peripherally inserted central venous catheters (PICCs) may be placed or replaced with or without imaging guidance. When performed without imaging guidance, report using 36568 or 36569. When imaging guidance (eg, ultrasound, fluoroscopy) is used for PICC placement or repositioning, bundled service codes 36572, 36573, 36584 include all imaging necessary to complete the procedure, image documentation (representative images from all modalities used are stored to patient's permanent record), associated radiological supervision and interpretation, venography performed through the same venous puncture, and documentation of final central position of the catheter with imaging. Ultrasound guidance for PICC placement should include documentation of evaluation of the potential puncture sites, patency of the entry vein, and real-time ultrasound visualization of needle entry into the vein.

Codes 71045, 71046, 71047, 71048 should not be reported for the purpose of documenting the final catheter position on the same day of service as 36572, 36573, 36584. Codes 36572, 36573, 36584 include confirmation of catheter tip location. The physician or other qualified health care professional reporting image-guided PICC insertion cannot report confirmation of catheter tip location separately (eg, via X ray, ultrasound). Report 36572, 36573, 36584 with modifier 52 when performed without confirmation of catheter tip location.

"Midline" catheters by definition terminate in the peripheral venous system. They are not central venous access devices and may not be reported as a PICC service. Midline catheter placement may be reported with 36400, 36405, 36406, or 36410. PICCs placed using magnetic guidance or any other guidance modality that does not include imaging or image documentation are reported with 36568, 36569.

Central Venous Access Procedures

To qualify as a central venous access catheter or device, the tip of the catheter/device must terminate in the subclavian, brachiocephalic (innominate) or iliac veins, the superior or inferior vena cava, or the right atrium. The venous access device may be either centrally inserted (jugular, subclavian, femoral vein or inferior vena cava catheter entry site) or peripherally inserted (eg, basilic, cephalic, or saphenous vein entry site). The device may be accessed for use either via exposed catheter (external to the skin), via a subcutaneous port or via a subcutaneous pump.

The procedures involving these types of devices fall into five categories:

1. Insertion (placement of catheter through a newly established venous access)
2. Repair (fixing device without replacement of either catheter or port/pump, other than pharmacologic or mechanical correction of intracatheter or pericatheter occlusion [see 36595 or 36596])
3. Partial replacement of only the catheter component associated with a port/pump device, but not entire device
4. Complete replacement of entire device via same venous access site (complete exchange)
5. Removal of entire device.

There is no coding distinction between venous access achieved percutaneously versus by cutdown or based on catheter size.

For the repair, partial (catheter only) replacement, complete replacement, or removal of both catheters (placed from separate venous access sites) of a multi-catheter device, with or without subcutaneous ports/pumps, use the appropriate code describing the service with a frequency of two.

If an existing central venous access device is removed and a new one placed via a separate venous access site, appropriate codes for both procedures (removal of old, if code exists, and insertion of new device) should be reported.

When imaging guidance is used for centrally inserted central venous catheters, for gaining access to the venous entry site and/or for manipulating the catheter into final central position, imaging guidance codes (eg, 76937, 77001) may be reported separately. Do not use 76937, 77001 in conjunction with 36568, 36569, 36572, 36573, 36584.

Please see the Surgical Guidelines section for the following table: The Central Venous Access Procedures Table

Vascular Introduction and Injection Procedures

Listed services for injection procedures include necessary local anesthesia, introduction of needles or catheter, injection of contrast media with or without automatic power injection, and/or necessary pre- and postinjection care specifically related to the injection procedure.

Selective vascular catheterization should be coded to include introduction and all lesser order selective catheterization used in the approach (eg, the description for a selective right middle cerebral artery catheterization includes the introduction and placement catheterization of the right common and internal carotid arteries).

Additional second and/or third order arterial catheterization within the same family of arteries or veins supplied by a single first order vessel should be expressed by 36012, 36218, or 36248.

Additional first order or higher catheterization in vascular families supplied by a first order vessel different from a previously selected and coded family should be separately coded using the conventions described above.

Surgical Procedures on Arteries and VeinsPrimary vascular procedure listings include establishing both inflow and outflow by whatever procedures necessary. Also included is that portion of the operative arteriogram performed by the surgeon, as indicated. Sympathectomy, when done, is included in the listed aortic procedures. For unlisted vascular procedure, use 37799.

Please see the Surgery Guidelines section for the following guidelines:

- *Surgical Procedures on the Cardiovascular System*

AMA Coding Notes

Central Venous Access Procedures

(For refilling and maintenance of an implantable pump or reservoir for intravenous or intra-arterial drug delivery, use 96522)

Vascular Introduction and Injection Procedures

(For radiological supervision and interpretation, see Radiology)

(For injection procedures in conjunction with cardiac catheterization, see 93452-93461, 93563-93568)

(For chemotherapy of malignant disease, see 96401-96549)

AMA *CPT Assistant* ▢

36565: Dec 04: 8, Jun 08: 8
36566: Dec 04: 8, Jun 08: 8

CPT © 2018 American Medical Association. All Rights Reserved.

Plain English Description

Two tunneled centrally inserted central venous catheters (CVC) are placed via two separate venous access sites. A CVC must terminate in the subclavian, brachiocephalic, or iliac veins, the superior or inferior vena cava, or right atrium. A tunneled CVC is placed through a subcutaneous tunnel into the jugular, subclavian, or femoral vein or the inferior vena cava with the most common venous access site for tunneled devices being the jugular vein. Separately reportable imaging guidance may be used to access the venous entry site and/or to manipulate the catheter tip to the final central position. Local anesthesia is administered at the planned puncture site. In 36565, two tunneled CVCs are placed without connection to a subcutaneous port or pump. Using a Seldinger technique to access the jugular vein, the skin and vein are punctured with a needle. A guidewire is inserted through the needle and advanced several centimeters. An incision is made in the chest wall and a subcutaneous tunnel is created. An introducer sheath and dilator are advanced over the guidewire and the guidewire and dilator removed. The catheter is then advanced through the tunnel to the introducer sheath in the jugular vein and into the brachiocephalic vein, subclavian vein, superior vena cava or right atrium. Placement is checked by separately reportable radiographs. The CVC is secured with sutures, the incision in the chest wall closed with sutures, and a dressing applied over the insertion site. A second tunneled CVC is placed in the same manner via a separately venous access site. In 36566, two tunneled CVCs are placed with connection to a subcutaneous port. Placement of the tunneled catheter is performed as described above. A subcutaneous pocket is then created for placement of the port. A subcutaneous tunnel is created from the venous access site to the subcutaneous pocket. The catheter and port are connected and the port is placed in the subcutaneous pocket. The incision over the venous access site is closed. The port is sutured into place and the pocket is closed. A second catheter and port are placed in the same manner.

Insertion of tunneled centrally inserted central venous access device, requiring two catheters

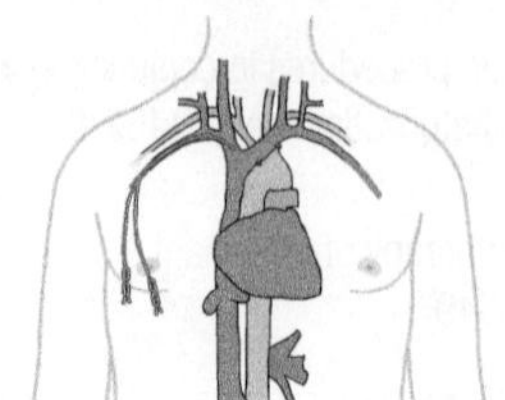

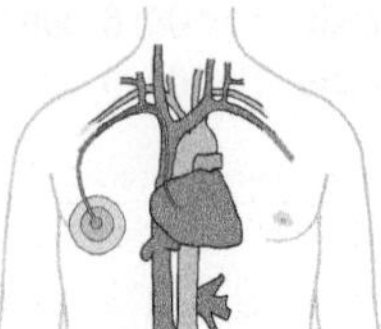

A CVC is introduced into the inferior vena cava or jugular, subclavian, or femoral vein by creating two separate tunnels through the skin and subcutaneous tissue. With (36566); without (36565) ports

ICD-10-CM Diagnostic Codes

There are too many ICD-10-CM codes to list. Refer to ICD-10-CM code book for associated diagnostic codes.

CCI Edits

Refer to Appendix A for CCI edits.

Facility RVUs 🗆

Code	Work	PE Facility	MP	Total Facility
36565	5.79	2.60	1.24	9.63
36566	6.29	2.94	1.23	10.46

Non-facility RVUs 🗆

Code	Work	PE Non-Facility	MP	Total Non-Facility
36565	5.79	17.82	1.24	24.85
36566	6.29	128.25	1.23	135.77

Modifiers (PAR) 🗆

Code	Mod 50	Mod 51	Mod 62	Mod 66	Mod 80
36565	1	2	0	0	0
36566	1	2	0	0	0

Global Period

Code	Days
36565	010
36566	010

CPT © 2018 American Medical Association. All Rights Reserved.

36568-36569

▲ **36568 Insertion of peripherally inserted central venous catheter (PICC), without subcutaneous port or pump, without imaging guidance; younger than 5 years of age**

(For placement of centrally inserted non-tunneled central venous catheter, without subcutaneous port or pump, younger than 5 years of age, use 36555)

(For placement of peripherally inserted non-tunneled central venous catheter, without subcutaneous port or pump, with imaging guidance, younger than 5 years of age, use 36572)

▲ **36569 Insertion of peripherally inserted central venous catheter (PICC), without subcutaneous port or pump, without imaging guidance; age 5 years or older**

(Do not report 36568, 36569 in conjunction with 76937, 77001)

(For placement of centrally inserted non-tunneled central venous catheter, without subcutaneous port or pump, age 5 years or older, use 36556)

(For placement of peripherally inserted non-tunneled central venous catheter, without subcutaneous port or pump, with imaging guidance, age 5 years or older, use 36573)

AMA Coding Guideline

Insertion of Central Venous Access Device

Peripherally inserted central venous catheters (PICCs) may be placed or replaced with or without imaging guidance. When performed without imaging guidance, report using 36568 or 36569. When imaging guidance (eg, ultrasound, fluoroscopy) is used for PICC placement or repositioning, bundled service codes 36572, 36573, 36584 include all imaging necessary to complete the procedure, image documentation (representative images from all modalities used are stored to patient's permanent record), associated radiological supervision and interpretation, venography performed through the same venous puncture, and documentation of final central position of the catheter with imaging. Ultrasound guidance for PICC placement should include documentation of evaluation of the potential puncture sites, patency of the entry vein, and real-time ultrasound visualization of needle entry into the vein.

Codes 71045, 71046, 71047, 71048 should not be reported for the purpose of documenting the final catheter position on the same day of service as 36572, 36573, 36584. Codes 36572, 36573, 36584 include confirmation of catheter tip location. The physician or other qualified health care professional reporting image-guided PICC insertion cannot report confirmation of catheter tip location separately (eg, via X ray, ultrasound). Report 36572, 36573, 36584 with modifier 52 when performed without confirmation of catheter tip location.

Central Venous Access Procedures

To qualify as a central venous access catheter or device, the tip of the catheter/device must terminate in the subclavian, brachiocephalic (innominate) or iliac veins, the superior or inferior vena cava, or the right atrium. The venous access device may be either centrally inserted (jugular, subclavian, femoral vein or inferior vena cava catheter entry site) or peripherally inserted (eg, basilic, cephalic, or saphenous vein entry site). The device may be accessed for use either via exposed catheter (external to the skin), via a subcutaneous port or via a subcutaneous pump.

The procedures involving these types of devices fall into five categories:

1. Insertion (placement of catheter through a newly established venous access)
2. Repair (fixing device without replacement of either catheter or port/pump, other than pharmacologic or mechanical correction of intracatheter or pericatheter occlusion [see 36595 or 36596])
3. Partial replacement of only the catheter component associated with a port/pump device, but not entire device
4. Complete replacement of entire device via same venous access site (complete exchange)
5. Removal of entire device.

There is no coding distinction between venous access achieved percutaneously versus by cutdown or based on catheter size.

For the repair, partial (catheter only) replacement, complete replacement, or removal of both catheters (placed from separate venous access sites) of a multi-catheter device, with or without subcutaneous ports/pumps, use the appropriate code describing the service with a frequency of two.

If an existing central venous access device is removed and a new one placed via a separate venous access site, appropriate codes for both procedures (removal of old, if code exists, and insertion of new device) should be reported.

When imaging guidance is used for centrally inserted central venous catheters, for gaining access to the venous entry site and/or for manipulating the catheter into final central position, imaging guidance codes (eg, 76937, 77001) may be reported separately. Do not use 76937, 77001 in conjunction with 36568, 36569, 36572, 36573, 36584.

Please see the Surgical Guidelines section for the following table: The Central Venous Access Procedures Table

Vascular Introduction and Injection Procedures

Listed services for injection procedures include necessary local anesthesia, introduction of needles or catheter, injection of contrast media with or without automatic power injection, and/or necessary pre- and postinjection care specifically related to the injection procedure.

Selective vascular catheterization should be coded to include introduction and all lesser order selective catheterization used in the approach (eg, the description for a selective right middle cerebral artery catheterization includes the introduction and placement catheterization of the right common and internal carotid arteries).

Additional second and/or third order arterial catheterization within the same family of arteries or veins supplied by a single first order vessel should be expressed by 36012, 36218, or 36248.

Additional first order or higher catheterization in vascular families supplied by a first order vessel different from a previously selected and coded family should be separately coded using the conventions described above.

Surgical Procedures on Arteries and VeinsPrimary vascular procedure listings include establishing both inflow and outflow by whatever procedures necessary. Also included is that portion of the operative arteriogram performed by the surgeon, as indicated. Sympathectomy, when done, is included in the listed aortic procedures. For unlisted vascular procedure, use 37799.

Please see the Surgery Guidelines section for the following guidelines:

- *Surgical Procedures on the Cardiovascular System*

AMA Coding Notes

Central Venous Access Procedures

(For refilling and maintenance of an implantable pump or reservoir for intravenous or intra-arterial drug delivery, use 96522)

Vascular Introduction and Injection Procedures

(For radiological supervision and interpretation, see Radiology)

(For injection procedures in conjunction with cardiac catheterization, see 93452-93461, 93563-93568)

(For chemotherapy of malignant disease, see 96401-96549)

AMA *CPT Assistant* ▯

36568: Oct 04: 14, Dec 04: 8, May 05: 13, Jun 08: 8, Nov 12: 14

36569: Oct 04: 14, Dec 04: 8, May 05: 13, Jun 08: 8, Nov 12: 14, Sep 13: 18, Sep 14: 13

Plain English Description

A peripherally inserted central venous catheter (PICC) is similar to an intravenous line and is used for the delivery of medication or fluids into the bloodstream over a prolonged period of time. A

CPT © 2018 American Medical Association. All Rights Reserved.

central venous catheter tip terminates in either the innominate, subclavian, or iliac veins, the vena cava, or the right atrium. For peripheral insertion, a suitable large vein in the arm is used, typically one of the deeper veins located above the elbow such as the basilic, cephalic, or brachial vein, or the saphenous vein in the leg. PICC line insertion done without imaging guidance is typically done at the bedside in a blind insertion manner. The planned inserted site is cleansed and a local anesthetic is injected. The catheter is then inserted into the selected venous access site and threaded into the deep vein of the upper arm through the central venous system until the distal tip is located in the lower third of the superior vena cava near the cavoatrial junction. Since catheter tip location must be confirmed prior to initiating IV therapy, a separately reportable chest x-ray is done for confirmation. Another method of insertion without using imaging guidance is the use of bedside magnetic navigation and EKG in adults with healthy heart function. A sensor is placed on the patient's chest before insertion site sterilization and two EKG electrodes are placed on the torso. A specially designed magnetic tipped catheter with an intravascular electrode in the lumen is then threaded to the cavoatrial junction while providing real time feedback on catheter tip location through passive magnetic guidance and cardiac electrical signal detection. This lowers the rate of malposition and removes the need for additional x-ray exposure and interpretation. The PICC is secured with sutures and a dressing is applied over the insertion site in the arm. Report 36568 for a (non-tunneled) PICC line insertion without using imaging guidance and without a subcutaneous port or pump (accessed via the exposed catheter external to the skin) in a patient younger than 5, and 36569 in a patient age 5 and older.

Insertion of peripherally inserted central venous catheter (PICC)

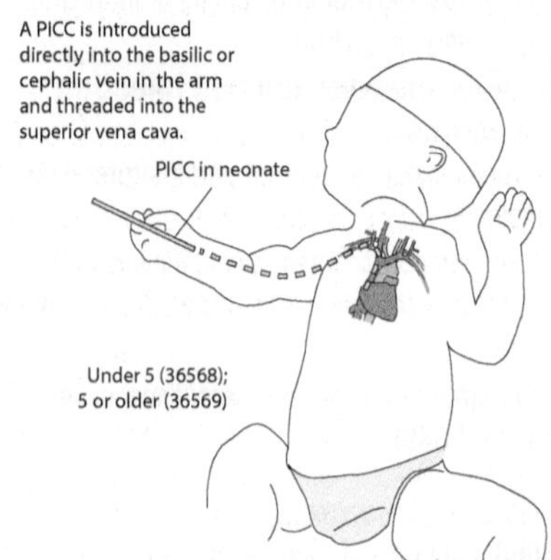
A PICC is introduced directly into the basilic or cephalic vein in the arm and threaded into the superior vena cava.
PICC in neonate
Under 5 (36568);
5 or older (36569)

ICD-10-CM Diagnostic Codes

There are too many ICD-10-CM codes to list. Refer to ICD-10-CM code book for associated diagnostic codes.

CCI Edits

Refer to Appendix A for CCI edits.

Facility RVUs

Code	Work	PE Facility	MP	Total Facility
36568	2.11	0.36	0.18	2.65
36569	1.90	0.65	0.17	2.72

Non-facility RVUs

Code	Work	PE Non-Facility	MP	Total Non-Facility
36568	2.11	0.36	0.18	2.65
36569	1.90	0.65	0.17	2.72

Modifiers (PAR)

Code	Mod 50	Mod 51	Mod 62	Mod 66	Mod 80
36568	0	0	0	0	1
36569	0	0	0	0	1

Global Period

Code	Days
36568	000
36569	000

CPT © 2018 American Medical Association. All Rights Reserved.

36570-36571

36570 Insertion of peripherally inserted central venous access device, with subcutaneous port; younger than 5 years of age

(For insertion of tunneled centrally inserted central venous access device with subcutaneous port, younger than 5 years of age, use 36560)

36571 Insertion of peripherally inserted central venous access device, with subcutaneous port; age 5 years or older

(For insertion of tunneled centrally inserted central venous access device with subcutaneous port, age 5 years or older, use 36561)

AMA Coding Guideline

Insertion of Central Venous Access Device

Peripherally inserted central venous catheters (PICCs) may be placed or replaced with or without imaging guidance. When performed without imaging guidance, report using 36568 or 36569. When imaging guidance (eg, ultrasound, fluoroscopy) is used for PICC placement or repositioning, bundled service codes 36572, 36573, 36584 include all imaging necessary to complete the procedure, image documentation (representative images from all modalities used are stored to patient's permanent record), associated radiological supervision and interpretation, venography performed through the same venous puncture, and documentation of final central position of the catheter with imaging. Ultrasound guidance for PICC placement should include documentation of evaluation of the potential puncture sites, patency of the entry vein, and real-time ultrasound visualization of needle entry into the vein.

Codes 71045, 71046, 71047, 71048 should not be reported for the purpose of documenting the final catheter position on the same day of service as 36572, 36573, 36584. Codes 36572, 36573, 36584 include confirmation of catheter tip location. The physician or other qualified health care professional reporting image-guided PICC insertion cannot report confirmation of catheter tip location separately (eg, via X ray, ultrasound). Report 36572, 36573, 36584 with modifier 52 when performed without confirmation of catheter tip location.

Central Venous Access Procedures

To qualify as a central venous access catheter or device, the tip of the catheter/device must terminate in the subclavian, brachiocephalic (innominate) or iliac veins, the superior or inferior vena cava, or the right atrium. The venous access device may be either centrally inserted (jugular, subclavian, femoral vein or inferior vena cava catheter entry site) or peripherally inserted (eg, basilic, cephalic, or saphenous vein entry site). The device may be accessed for use either via exposed catheter (external to the skin), via a subcutaneous port or via a subcutaneous pump.

The procedures involving these types of devices fall into five categories:

1. Insertion (placement of catheter through a newly established venous access)
2. Repair (fixing device without replacement of either catheter or port/pump, other than pharmacologic or mechanical correction of intracatheter or pericatheter occlusion [see 36595 or 36596])
3. Partial replacement of only the catheter component associated with a port/pump device, but not entire device
4. Complete replacement of entire device via same venous access site (complete exchange)
5. Removal of entire device.

There is no coding distinction between venous access achieved percutaneously versus by cutdown or based on catheter size.

For the repair, partial (catheter only) replacement, complete replacement, or removal of both catheters (placed from separate venous access sites) of a multi-catheter device, with or without subcutaneous ports/pumps, use the appropriate code describing the service with a frequency of two.

If an existing central venous access device is removed and a new one placed via a separate venous access site, appropriate codes for both procedures (removal of old, if code exists, and insertion of new device) should be reported.

When imaging guidance is used for centrally inserted central venous catheters, for gaining access to the venous entry site and/or for manipulating the catheter into final central position, imaging guidance codes (eg, 76937, 77001) may be reported separately. Do not use 76937, 77001 in conjunction with 36568, 36569, 36572, 36573, 36584.

Please see the Surgical Guidelines section for the following table: The Central Venous Access Procedures Table

Vascular Introduction and Injection Procedures

Listed services for injection procedures include necessary local anesthesia, introduction of needles or catheter, injection of contrast media with or without automatic power injection, and/or necessary pre- and postinjection care specifically related to the injection procedure.

Selective vascular catheterization should be coded to include introduction and all lesser order selective catheterization used in the approach (eg, the description for a selective right middle cerebral artery catheterization includes the introduction and placement catheterization of the right common and internal carotid arteries).

Additional second and/or third order arterial catheterization within the same family of arteries or veins supplied by a single first order vessel should be expressed by 36012, 36218, or 36248. Additional first order or higher catheterization in vascular families supplied by a first order vessel different from a previously selected and coded family should be separately coded using the conventions described above.

Surgical Procedures on Arteries and VeinsPrimary vascular procedure listings include establishing both inflow and outflow by whatever procedures necessary. Also included is that portion of the operative arteriogram performed by the surgeon, as indicated. Sympathectomy, when done, is included in the listed aortic procedures. For unlisted vascular procedure, use 37799.

Please see the Surgery Guidelines section for the following guidelines:

- *Surgical Procedures on the Cardiovascular System*

AMA Coding Notes

Central Venous Access Procedures

(For refilling and maintenance of an implantable pump or reservoir for intravenous or intra-arterial drug delivery, use 96522)

Vascular Introduction and Injection Procedures

(For radiological supervision and interpretation, see Radiology)

(For injection procedures in conjunction with cardiac catheterization, see 93452-93461, 93563-93568)

(For chemotherapy of malignant disease, see 96401-96549)

AMA *CPT Assistant* ☐

36570: Dec 04: 8, Jun 08: 8, Dec 09: 11

36571: Dec 04: 9, Jun 08: 8, Dec 09: 11

Plain English Description

This type of device includes a port inserted under the skin that is attached to a catheter placed in a peripheral vein and advanced into the superior vena cava. Ultrasound is used as needed to identify a suitable large vein in the arm. Typically, one of the deeper veins located above the elbow is used, such as the basilic, cephalic, or brachial vein. The planned catheter insertion site is incised and the selected vein exposed. Using a Seldinger technique, the vein is punctured with a needle. A guidewire is inserted through the needle and advanced several centimeters. An introducer sheath and dilator are advanced over the guidewire and the guidewire and dilator removed. The catheter is advanced through the introducer sheath and into the brachiocephalic vein, subclavian vein, or superior vena cava. Separately reportable radiographs check placement. The catheter is anchored in the subcutaneous tissue. A subcutaneous pocket is then created for placement of the port. The catheter is tunneled to the port and the catheter and port connected. The incision over the venous access site is closed. The port is sutured into place and

CPT © 2018 American Medical Association. All Rights Reserved.

the pocket is closed. Use 36570 for peripherally inserted central venous access device (VAD) with port placement in a child younger than age 5 and 36571 for a patient age 5 or older.

Insertion of PICC with port

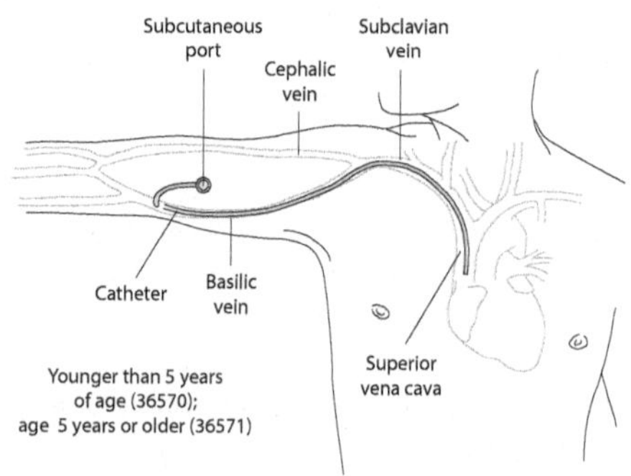

ICD-10-CM Diagnostic Codes

There are too many ICD-10-CM codes to list. Refer to ICD-10-CM code book for associated diagnostic codes.

CCI Edits

Refer to Appendix A for CCI edits.

Facility RVUs

Code	Work	PE Facility	MP	Total Facility
36570	5.11	3.21	1.24	9.56
36571	5.09	2.95	0.96	9.00

Non-facility RVUs

Code	Work	PE Non-Facility	MP	Total Non-Facility
36570	5.11	34.53	1.24	40.88
36571	5.09	29.83	0.96	35.88

Modifiers (PAR)

Code	Mod 50	Mod 51	Mod 62	Mod 66	Mod 80
36570	1	2	0	0	0
36571	1	2	0	0	0

Global Period

Code	Days
36570	010
36571	010

CPT © 2018 American Medical Association. All Rights Reserved.

36572-36573

● **36572 Insertion of peripherally inserted central venous catheter (PICC), without subcutaneous port or pump, including all imaging guidance, image documentation, and all associated radiological supervision and interpretation required to perform the insertion; younger than 5 years of age**

(For placement of centrally inserted non-tunneled central venous catheter, without subcutaneous port or pump, younger than 5 years of age, use 36555)

(For placement of peripherally inserted non-tunneled central venous catheter, without subcutaneous port or pump, without imaging guidance, younger than 5 years of age, use 36568)

● **36573 Insertion of peripherally inserted central venous catheter (PICC), without subcutaneous port or pump, including all imaging guidance, image documentation, and all associated radiological supervision and interpretation required to perform the insertion; age 5 years or older**

(For placement of centrally inserted non-tunneled central venous catheter, without subcutaneous port or pump, age 5 years or older, use 36556)

(For placement of peripherally inserted non-tunneled central venous catheter, without subcutaneous port or pump, without imaging guidance, age 5 years or older, use 36569)

(Do not report 36572, 36573 in conjunction with 76937, 77001)

AMA Coding Guideline

Insertion of Central Venous Access Device

Peripherally inserted central venous catheters (PICCs) may be placed or replaced with or without imaging guidance. When performed without imaging guidance, report using 36568 or 36569. When imaging guidance (eg, ultrasound, fluoroscopy) is used for PICC placement or repositioning, bundled service codes 36572, 36573, 36584 include all imaging necessary to complete the procedure, image documentation (representative images from all modalities used are stored to patient's permanent record), associated radiological supervision and interpretation, venography performed through the same venous puncture, and documentation of final central position of the catheter with imaging. Ultrasound guidance for PICC placement should include documentation of evaluation of the potential puncture sites, patency of the entry vein, and real-time ultrasound visualization of needle entry into the vein.

Codes 71045, 71046, 71047, 71048 should not be reported for the purpose of documenting the final catheter position on the same day of service as 36572, 36573, 36584. Codes 36572, 36573, 36584 include confirmation of catheter tip location. The physician or other qualified health care professional reporting image-guided PICC insertion cannot report confirmation of catheter tip location separately (eg, via X ray, ultrasound). Report 36572, 36573, 36584 with modifier 52 when performed without confirmation of catheter tip location.

Central Venous Access Procedures

To qualify as a central venous access catheter or device, the tip of the catheter/device must terminate in the subclavian, brachiocephalic (innominate) or iliac veins, the superior or inferior vena cava, or the right atrium. The venous access device may be either centrally inserted (jugular, subclavian, femoral vein or inferior vena cava catheter entry site) or peripherally inserted (eg, basilic, cephalic, or saphenous vein entry site). The device may be accessed for use either via exposed catheter (external to the skin), via a subcutaneous port or via a subcutaneous pump.

The procedures involving these types of devices fall into five categories:

1. Insertion (placement of catheter through a newly established venous access)
2. Repair (fixing device without replacement of either catheter or port/pump, other than pharmacologic or mechanical correction of intracatheter or pericatheter occlusion [see 36595 or 36596])
3. Partial replacement of only the catheter component associated with a port/pump device, but not entire device
4. Complete replacement of entire device via same venous access site (complete exchange)
5. Removal of entire device.

There is no coding distinction between venous access achieved percutaneously versus by cutdown or based on catheter size.

For the repair, partial (catheter only) replacement, complete replacement, or removal of both catheters (placed from separate venous access sites) of a multi-catheter device, with or without subcutaneous ports/pumps, use the appropriate code describing the service with a frequency of two.

If an existing central venous access device is removed and a new one placed via a separate venous access site, appropriate codes for both procedures (removal of old, if code exists, and insertion of new device) should be reported.

When imaging guidance is used for centrally inserted central venous catheters, for gaining access to the venous entry site and/or for manipulating the catheter into final central position, imaging guidance codes (eg, 76937, 77001) may be reported separately. Do not use 76937, 77001 in conjunction with 36568, 36569, 36572, 36573, 36584.

Please see the Surgical Guidelines section for the following table: The Central Venous Access Procedures Table

Vascular Introduction and Injection Procedures

Listed services for injection procedures include necessary local anesthesia, introduction of needles or catheter, injection of contrast media with or without automatic power injection, and/or necessary pre- and postinjection care specifically related to the injection procedure.

Selective vascular catheterization should be coded to include introduction and all lesser order selective catheterization used in the approach (eg, the description for a selective right middle cerebral artery catheterization includes the introduction and placement catheterization of the right common and internal carotid arteries).

Additional second and/or third order arterial catheterization within the same family of arteries or veins supplied by a single first order vessel should be expressed by 36012, 36218, or 36248.

Additional first order or higher catheterization in vascular families supplied by a first order vessel different from a previously selected and coded family should be separately coded using the conventions described above.

Surgical Procedures on Arteries and VeinsPrimary vascular procedure listings include establishing both inflow and outflow by whatever procedures necessary. Also included is that portion of the operative arteriogram performed by the surgeon, as indicated. Sympathectomy, when done, is included in the listed aortic procedures. For unlisted vascular procedure, use 37799.

Please see the Surgery Guidelines section for the following guidelines:

- *Surgical Procedures on the Cardiovascular System*

AMA Coding Notes

Central Venous Access Procedures

(For refilling and maintenance of an implantable pump or reservoir for intravenous or intra-arterial drug delivery, use 96522)

Vascular Introduction and Injection Procedures

(For radiological supervision and interpretation, see Radiology)

(For injection procedures in conjunction with cardiac catheterization, see 93452-93461, 93563-93568)

(For chemotherapy of malignant disease, see 96401-96549)

CPT © 2018 American Medical Association. All Rights Reserved.

Plain English Description

A peripherally inserted central venous catheter (PICC) is similar to an intravenous line and is used for the delivery of medication or fluids into the bloodstream over a prolonged period of time. A central venous catheter tip terminates in either the innominate, subclavian, or iliac veins, the vena cava, or the right atrium. For peripheral insertion, a suitable large vein in the arm is used, typically one of the deeper veins located above the elbow such as the basilic, cephalic, or brachial vein, or the saphenous vein in the leg. The planned inserted site is cleansed with bactericidal solution. A tourniquet is placed on the arm and a local anesthetic is injected at the planned insertion site. There are two techniques for insertion. Using a peel-away cannula technique, a cannula with a stylet is inserted into the selected vein. The stylet is removed. The PICC line is advanced through the cannula into the vein and advanced into the brachiocephalic vein, subclavian vein, or superior vena cava. Using a Seldinger technique, the skin and vein are punctured with a needle. A guidewire is inserted through the needle and advanced several centimeters. An introducer sheath and dilator are advanced over the guidewire and the guidewire and dilator are removed. The PICC line is then advanced through the introducer sheath and into the brachiocephalic vein, subclavian vein, or superior vena cava. The PICC is secured with sutures and a dressing is applied over the insertion site in the arm. These codes include all imaging guidance needed for completion of the procedure with documentation, interpretation, and confirmation of final catheter tip location. Report 36572 for (non-tunneled) PICC line placement without a subcutaneous port or pump (accessed via the exposed catheter external to the skin) in a patient younger than 5 and 36573 for a patient age 5 and older.

Insertion of PICC with port or pump

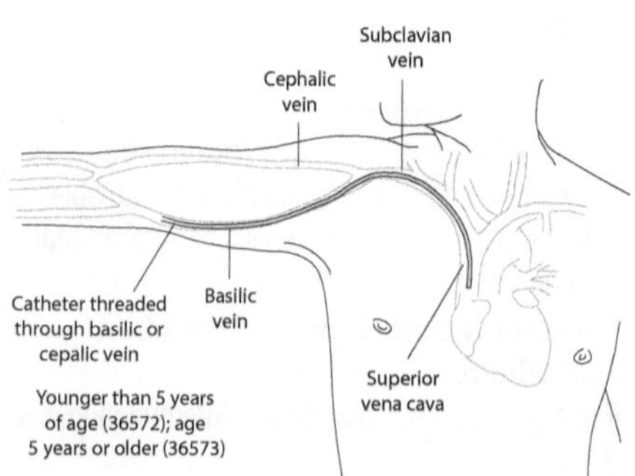

ICD-10-CM Diagnostic Codes

There are too many ICD-10-CM codes to list. Refer to ICD-10-CM code book for associated diagnostic codes.

CCI Edits

Refer to Appendix A for CCI edits.

Facility RVUs ☐

Code	Work	PE Facility	MP	Total Facility
36572	1.82	0.67	0.16	2.65
36573	1.70	0.57	0.18	2.45

Non-facility RVUs ☐

Code	Work	PE Non-Facility	MP	Total Non-Facility
36572	1.82	9.92	0.16	11.90
36573	1.70	9.32	0.18	11.20

Modifiers (PAR) ☐

Code	Mod 50	Mod 51	Mod 62	Mod 66	Mod 80
36572	0	0	0	0	1
36573	0	0	0	0	1

Global Period

Code	Days
36572	000
36573	000

CPT © 2018 American Medical Association. All Rights Reserved.

36575-36576

36575 Repair of tunneled or non-tunneled central venous access catheter, without subcutaneous port or pump, central or peripheral insertion site

36576 Repair of central venous access device, with subcutaneous port or pump, central or peripheral insertion site

AMA Coding Guideline

Central Venous Access Procedures

To qualify as a central venous access catheter or device, the tip of the catheter/device must terminate in the subclavian, brachiocephalic (innominate) or iliac veins, the superior or inferior vena cava, or the right atrium. The venous access device may be either centrally inserted (jugular, subclavian, femoral vein or inferior vena cava catheter entry site) or peripherally inserted (eg, basilic, cephalic, or saphenous vein entry site). The device may be accessed for use either via exposed catheter (external to the skin), via a subcutaneous port or via a subcutaneous pump.

The procedures involving these types of devices fall into five categories:

1. Insertion (placement of catheter through a newly established venous access)
2. Repair (fixing device without replacement of either catheter or port/pump, other than pharmacologic or mechanical correction of intracatheter or pericatheter occlusion [see 36595 or 36596])
3. Partial replacement of only the catheter component associated with a port/pump device, but not entire device
4. Complete replacement of entire device via same venous access site (complete exchange)
5. Removal of entire device.

There is no coding distinction between venous access achieved percutaneously versus by cutdown or based on catheter size.

For the repair, partial (catheter only) replacement, complete replacement, or removal of both catheters (placed from separate venous access sites) of a multi-catheter device, with or without subcutaneous ports/pumps, use the appropriate code describing the service with a frequency of two.

If an existing central venous access device is removed and a new one placed via a separate venous access site, appropriate codes for both procedures (removal of old, if code exists, and insertion of new device) should be reported.

When imaging guidance is used for centrally inserted central venous catheters, for gaining access to the venous entry site and/or for manipulating the catheter into final central position, imaging guidance codes (eg, 76937, 77001) may be reported separately. Do not use 76937, 77001 in conjunction with 36568, 36569, 36572, 36573, 36584.

Please see the Surgical Guidelines section for the following table: The Central Venous Access Procedures Table

Vascular Introduction and Injection Procedures

Listed services for injection procedures include necessary local anesthesia, introduction of needles or catheter, injection of contrast media with or without automatic power injection, and/or necessary pre- and postinjection care specifically related to the injection procedure.

Selective vascular catheterization should be coded to include introduction and all lesser order selective catheterization used in the approach (eg, the description for a selective right middle cerebral artery catheterization includes the introduction and placement catheterization of the right common and internal carotid arteries).

Additional second and/or third order arterial catheterization within the same family of arteries or veins supplied by a single first order vessel should be expressed by 36012, 36218, or 36248.

Additional first order or higher catheterization in vascular families supplied by a first order vessel different from a previously selected and coded family should be separately coded using the conventions described above.

Surgical Procedures on Arteries and Veins

Primary vascular procedure listings include establishing both inflow and outflow by whatever procedures necessary. Also included is that portion of the operative arteriogram performed by the surgeon, as indicated. Sympathectomy, when done, is included in the listed aortic procedures. For unlisted vascular procedure, use 37799.

Please see the Surgery Guidelines section for the following guidelines:

- *Surgical Procedures on the Cardiovascular System*

AMA Coding Notes

Repair of Central Venous Access Device

(For mechanical removal of pericatheter obstructive material, use 36595)

(For mechanical removal of intracatheter obstructive material, use 36596)

Central Venous Access Procedures

(For refilling and maintenance of an implantable pump or reservoir for intravenous or intra-arterial drug delivery, use 96522)

Vascular Introduction and Injection Procedures

(For radiological supervision and interpretation, see Radiology)

(For injection procedures in conjunction with cardiac catheterization, see 93452-93461, 93563-93568)

(For chemotherapy of malignant disease, see 96401-96549)

AMA *CPT Assistant* □

36576: Dec 04: 9, Jun 08: 8

Plain English Description

A previously placed tunneled or non-tunneled central venous access catheter is repaired. This procedure is performed when a portion of the catheter external to the vein is damaged. The repair may be performed on a peripherally or centrally placed catheter. In 36575, the damage to the catheter is evaluated. A non-tunneled catheter that has been cut can be repaired by trimming the remaining catheter and splicing a new catheter hub segment onto the existing catheter. The repair is then checked using an injection of intravenous fluid. A tunneled catheter may be repaired as described above if the external portion of catheter is damaged. If the catheter contained in the tunnel requires repair, the tunneled portion of the catheter may be exposed by incising the skin and subcutaneous tissue. The necessary catheter repairs are then completed and a new subcutaneous tunnel created as needed. The repaired catheter is secured with sutures. In 36576, a tunneled catheter with a subcutaneous port or pump is repaired. Repair of a catheter leak is one of the more common types of repairs. The port or pump pocket is opened. The catheter is disconnected and the damaged section identified. The damaged section of catheter is removed by trimming the catheter at a point proximal to the damage. The catheter is then reconnected to the port or pump. The repaired catheter is tested to ensure there are no leaks by injecting intravenous fluid. The port or pump is returned to the subcutaneous pocket and secured with sutures. The pocket is closed.

Repair of central venous access device

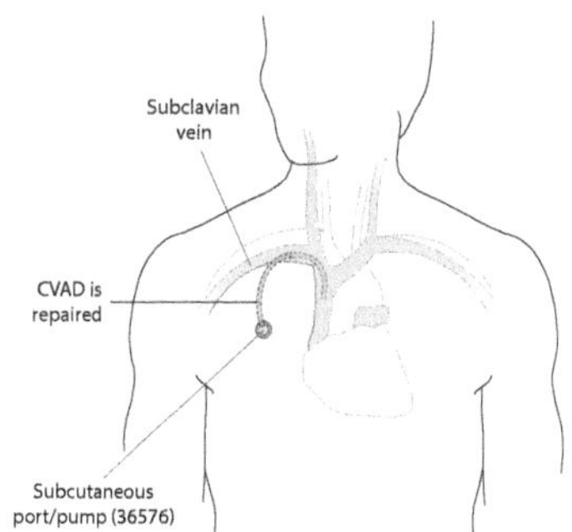

A tunneled/nontunneled CVAD without port/pump is repaired (36575); a CVAD with a port/pump is repaired (36576).

ICD-10-CM Diagnostic Codes

⑦	T82.518	Breakdown (mechanical) of other cardiac and vascular devices and implants
⑦	T82.598	Other mechanical complication of other cardiac and vascular devices and implants

CPT © 2018 American Medical Association. All Rights Reserved.

❼	T82.898	Other specified complication of vascular prosthetic devices, implants and grafts
❼	T82.9	Unspecified complication of cardiac and vascular prosthetic device, implant and graft
	Z45.2	Encounter for adjustment and management of vascular access device

ICD-10-CM Coding Notes

For codes requiring a 7th character extension, refer to your ICD-10-CM book. Review the character descriptions and coding guidelines for proper selection. For some procedures, only certain characters will apply.

CCI Edits

Refer to Appendix A for CCI edits.

Facility RVUs ▯

Code	Work	PE Facility	MP	Total Facility
36575	0.67	0.25	0.09	1.01
36576	2.99	1.79	0.55	5.33

Non-facility RVUs ▯

Code	Work	PE Non-Facility	MP	Total Non-Facility
36575	0.67	3.83	0.09	4.59
36576	2.99	5.77	0.55	9.31

Modifiers (PAR) ▯

Code	Mod 50	Mod 51	Mod 62	Mod 66	Mod 80
36575	0	2	0	0	0
36576	0	2	0	0	0

Global Period

Code	Days
36575	000
36576	010

CPT © 2018 American Medical Association. All Rights Reserved.

36578

36578 Replacement, catheter only, of central venous access device, with subcutaneous port or pump, central or peripheral insertion site

(For complete replacement of entire device through same venous access, use 36582 or 36583)

AMA Coding Guideline

Central Venous Access Procedures

To qualify as a central venous access catheter or device, the tip of the catheter/device must terminate in the subclavian, brachiocephalic (innominate) or iliac veins, the superior or inferior vena cava, or the right atrium. The venous access device may be either centrally inserted (jugular, subclavian, femoral vein or inferior vena cava catheter entry site) or peripherally inserted (eg, basilic, cephalic, or saphenous vein entry site). The device may be accessed for use either via exposed catheter (external to the skin), via a subcutaneous port or via a subcutaneous pump.

The procedures involving these types of devices fall into five categories:

1. Insertion (placement of catheter through a newly established venous access)
2. Repair (fixing device without replacement of either catheter or port/pump, other than pharmacologic or mechanical correction of intracatheter or pericatheter occlusion [see 36595 or 36596])
3. Partial replacement of only the catheter component associated with a port/pump device, but not entire device
4. Complete replacement of entire device via same venous access site (complete exchange)
5. Removal of entire device.

There is no coding distinction between venous access achieved percutaneously versus by cutdown or based on catheter size.

For the repair, partial (catheter only) replacement, complete replacement, or removal of both catheters (placed from separate venous access sites) of a multi-catheter device, with or without subcutaneous ports/pumps, use the appropriate code describing the service with a frequency of two.

If an existing central venous access device is removed and a new one placed via a separate venous access site, appropriate codes for both procedures (removal of old, if code exists, and insertion of new device) should be reported.

When imaging guidance is used for centrally inserted central venous catheters, for gaining access to the venous entry site and/or for manipulating the catheter into final central position, imaging guidance codes (eg, 76937, 77001) may be reported separately. Do not use 76937, 77001 in conjunction with 36568, 36569, 36572, 36573, 36584.

Please see the Surgical Guidelines section for the following table: The Central Venous Access Procedures Table

Vascular Introduction and Injection Procedures

Listed services for injection procedures include necessary local anesthesia, introduction of needles or catheter, injection of contrast media with or without automatic power injection, and/or necessary pre- and postinjection care specifically related to the injection procedure.

Selective vascular catheterization should be coded to include introduction and all lesser order selective catheterization used in the approach (eg, the description for a selective right middle cerebral artery catheterization includes the introduction and placement catheterization of the right common and internal carotid arteries).

Additional second and/or third order arterial catheterization within the same family of arteries or veins supplied by a single first order vessel should be expressed by 36012, 36218, or 36248.

Additional first order or higher catheterization in vascular families supplied by a first order vessel different from a previously selected and coded family should be separately coded using the conventions described above.

Surgical Procedures on Arteries and Veins

Primary vascular procedure listings include establishing both inflow and outflow by whatever procedures necessary. Also included is that portion of the operative arteriogram performed by the surgeon, as indicated. Sympathectomy, when done, is included in the listed aortic procedures. For unlisted vascular procedure, use 37799.

Please see the Surgery Guidelines section for the following guidelines:

- *Surgical Procedures on the Cardiovascular System*

AMA Coding Notes

Central Venous Access Procedures

(For refilling and maintenance of an implantable pump or reservoir for intravenous or intra-arterial drug delivery, use 96522)

Vascular Introduction and Injection Procedures

(For radiological supervision and interpretation, see Radiology)

(For injection procedures in conjunction with cardiac catheterization, see 93452-93461, 93563-93568)

(For chemotherapy of malignant disease, see 96401-96549)

AMA *CPT Assistant* □

36578: Dec 04: 10, Jun 08: 8

Plain English Description

Catheter replacement may be performed on a peripherally or centrally placed catheter. The subcutaneous pocket is opened and the port or pump examined to ensure proper function of that component. Separately reportable radiographs are obtained to verify that the tip of the existing PICC or CVC is correctly positioned. The catheter is then inspected and found to be occluded or damaged. A guidewire is placed through the existing catheter which is withdrawn over the guidewire. A new catheter is then advanced over the guidewire and the tip positioned in the subclavian, brachiocephalic, or iliac vein, the superior or inferior vena cava, or right atrium. The catheter is attached to the port or pump device and the connection checked for leaks using an injection of intravenous fluid. The port or pump is returned to the subcutaneous pocket and secured with sutures. The pocket is closed.

Replacement, catheter only, of central venous access device

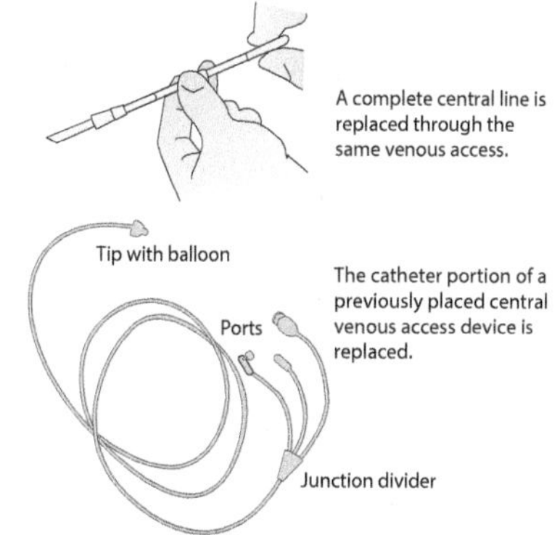
A complete central line is replaced through the same venous access.
Tip with balloon
Ports
The catheter portion of a previously placed central venous access device is replaced.
Junction divider

ICD-10-CM Diagnostic Codes

	Code	Description
➐	T82.518	Breakdown (mechanical) of other cardiac and vascular devices and implants
➐	T82.598	Other mechanical complication of other cardiac and vascular devices and implants
➐	T82.7	Infection and inflammatory reaction due to other cardiac and vascular devices, implants and grafts
➐	T82.898	Other specified complication of vascular prosthetic devices, implants and grafts
➐	T82.9	Unspecified complication of cardiac and vascular prosthetic device, implant and graft
	Z45.2	Encounter for adjustment and management of vascular access device

ICD-10-CM Coding Notes

For codes requiring a 7th character extension, refer to your ICD-10-CM book. Review the character descriptions and coding guidelines for proper selection. For some procedures, only certain characters will apply.

CCI Edits

Refer to Appendix A for CCI edits.

CPT © 2018 American Medical Association. All Rights Reserved.

Facility RVUs

Code	Work	PE Facility	MP	Total Facility
36578	3.29	2.03	0.54	5.86

Non-facility RVUs

Code	Work	PE Non-Facility	MP	Total Non-Facility
36578	3.29	9.23	0.54	13.06

Modifiers (PAR)

Code	Mod 50	Mod 51	Mod 62	Mod 66	Mod 80
36578	0	2	0	0	0

Global Period

Code	Days
36578	010

CPT © 2018 American Medical Association. All Rights Reserved.

36580-36581

36580 Replacement, complete, of a non-tunneled centrally inserted central venous catheter, without subcutaneous port or pump, through same venous access

36581 Replacement, complete, of a tunneled centrally inserted central venous catheter, without subcutaneous port or pump, through same venous access

AMA Coding Guideline

Central Venous Access Procedures

To qualify as a central venous access catheter or device, the tip of the catheter/device must terminate in the subclavian, brachiocephalic (innominate) or iliac veins, the superior or inferior vena cava, or the right atrium. The venous access device may be either centrally inserted (jugular, subclavian, femoral vein or inferior vena cava catheter entry site) or peripherally inserted (eg, basilic, cephalic, or saphenous vein entry site). The device may be accessed for use either via exposed catheter (external to the skin), via a subcutaneous port or via a subcutaneous pump.

The procedures involving these types of devices fall into five categories:

1. Insertion (placement of catheter through a newly established venous access)
2. Repair (fixing device without replacement of either catheter or port/pump, other than pharmacologic or mechanical correction of intracatheter or pericatheter occlusion [see 36595 or 36596])
3. Partial replacement of only the catheter component associated with a port/pump device, but not entire device
4. Complete replacement of entire device via same venous access site (complete exchange)
5. Removal of entire device.

There is no coding distinction between venous access achieved percutaneously versus by cutdown or based on catheter size.

For the repair, partial (catheter only) replacement, complete replacement, or removal of both catheters (placed from separate venous access sites) of a multi-catheter device, with or without subcutaneous ports/pumps, use the appropriate code describing the service with a frequency of two.

If an existing central venous access device is removed and a new one placed via a separate venous access site, appropriate codes for both procedures (removal of old, if code exists, and insertion of new device) should be reported.

When imaging guidance is used for centrally inserted central venous catheters, for gaining access to the venous entry site and/or for manipulating the catheter into final central position, imaging guidance codes (eg, 76937, 77001) may be reported separately. Do not use 76937, 77001 in conjunction with 36568, 36569, 36572, 36573, 36584.

Please see the Surgical Guidelines section for the following table: The Central Venous Access Procedures Table

Vascular Introduction and Injection Procedures

Listed services for injection procedures include necessary local anesthesia, introduction of needles or catheter, injection of contrast media with or without automatic power injection, and/or necessary pre- and postinjection care specifically related to the injection procedure.

Selective vascular catheterization should be coded to include introduction and all lesser order selective catheterization used in the approach (eg, the description for a selective right middle cerebral artery catheterization includes the introduction and placement catheterization of the right common and internal carotid arteries).

Additional second and/or third order arterial catheterization within the same family of arteries or veins supplied by a single first order vessel should be expressed by 36012, 36218, or 36248.

Additional first order or higher catheterization in vascular families supplied by a first order vessel different from a previously selected and coded family should be separately coded using the conventions described above.

Surgical Procedures on Arteries and Veins

Primary vascular procedure listings include establishing both inflow and outflow by whatever procedures necessary. Also included is that portion of the operative arteriogram performed by the surgeon, as indicated. Sympathectomy, when done, is included in the listed aortic procedures. For unlisted vascular procedure, use 37799.

Please see the Surgery Guidelines section for the following guidelines:

- *Surgical Procedures on the Cardiovascular System*

AMA Coding Notes

Central Venous Access Procedures

(For refilling and maintenance of an implantable pump or reservoir for intravenous or intra-arterial drug delivery, use 96522)

Vascular Introduction and Injection Procedures

(For radiological supervision and interpretation, see Radiology)

(For injection procedures in conjunction with cardiac catheterization, see 93452-93461, 93563-93568)

(For chemotherapy of malignant disease, see 96401-96549)

AMA *CPT Assistant* □

36580: Dec 04: 10, Jun 08: 8
36581: Dec 04: 10, Jun 08: 8

Plain English Description

Complete replacement of a centrally inserted central venous catheter (CVC) without a subcutaneous port or pump is performed through the same venous access site. Replacement is performed when a catheter becomes partially or completed obstructed or when another malfunction occurs. Separately reportable radiographs are obtained to verify that the tip of the CVC is correctly positioned. In 36580, a non-tunneled CVC is replaced. A guidewire is placed through the existing catheter which is withdrawn over the guidewire. A new catheter is then advanced over the guidewire and the tip positioned in the subclavian, brachiocephalic, or iliac vein, the superior or inferior vena cava, or right atrium. The new catheter is secured with sutures and flushed with heparin or attached to tubing for administration of intravenous fluids or medication. In 36581, a tunneled CVC is replaced. The indwelling catheter is dissected free of subcutaneous tissue. A guidewire is placed through the existing catheter which is withdrawn over the guidewire. A new catheter is then advanced over the guidewire and the tip positioned in the subclavian, brachiocephalic, or iliac vein, the superior or inferior vena cava, or right atrium. The new catheter is secured within the tunnel with sutures and flushed with heparin or attached to tubing for administration of intravenous fluids or medication.

Replacement, complete, of centrally inserted central venous catheter

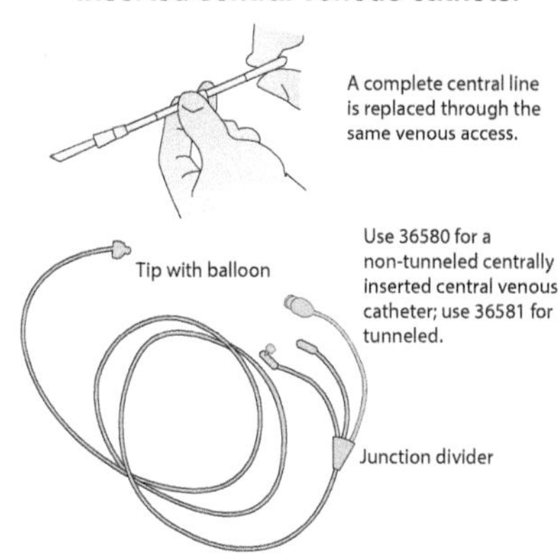
A complete central line is replaced through the same venous access.
Tip with balloon
Use 36580 for a non-tunneled centrally inserted central venous catheter; use 36581 for tunneled.
Junction divider

ICD-10-CM Diagnostic Codes

➐	T80.211	Bloodstream infection due to central venous catheter
➐	T80.212	Local infection due to central venous catheter
➐	T80.218	Other infection due to central venous catheter
➐	T80.219	Unspecified infection due to central venous catheter
➐	T82.518	Breakdown (mechanical) of other cardiac and vascular devices and implants
➐	T82.538	Leakage of other cardiac and vascular devices and implants
➐	T82.598	Other mechanical complication of other cardiac and vascular devices and implants

CPT © 2018 American Medical Association. All Rights Reserved.

❼	T82.898	Other specified complication of vascular prosthetic devices, implants and grafts
	Z45.2	Encounter for adjustment and management of vascular access device

ICD-10-CM Coding Notes

For codes requiring a 7th character extension, refer to your ICD-10-CM book. Review the character descriptions and coding guidelines for proper selection. For some procedures, only certain characters will apply.

CCI Edits

Refer to Appendix A for CCI edits.

Facility RVUs

Code	Work	PE Facility	MP	Total Facility
36580	1.31	0.46	0.15	1.92
36581	3.23	1.68	0.40	5.31

Non-facility RVUs

Code	Work	PE Non-Facility	MP	Total Non-Facility
36580	1.31	4.67	0.15	6.13
36581	3.23	17.85	0.40	21.48

Modifiers (PAR)

Code	Mod 50	Mod 51	Mod 62	Mod 66	Mod 80
36580	0	0	0	0	1
36581	0	2	0	0	0

Global Period

Code	Days
36580	000
36581	010

CPT © 2018 American Medical Association. All Rights Reserved.

36582-36583

36582 Replacement, complete, of a tunneled centrally inserted central venous access device, with subcutaneous port, through same venous access

36583 Replacement, complete, of a tunneled centrally inserted central venous access device, with subcutaneous pump, through same venous access

AMA Coding Guideline

Central Venous Access Procedures

To qualify as a central venous access catheter or device, the tip of the catheter/device must terminate in the subclavian, brachiocephalic (innominate) or iliac veins, the superior or inferior vena cava, or the right atrium. The venous access device may be either centrally inserted (jugular, subclavian, femoral vein or inferior vena cava catheter entry site) or peripherally inserted (eg, basilic, cephalic, or saphenous vein entry site). The device may be accessed for use either via exposed catheter (external to the skin), via a subcutaneous port or via a subcutaneous pump.

The procedures involving these types of devices fall into five categories:

1. Insertion (placement of catheter through a newly established venous access)
2. Repair (fixing device without replacement of either catheter or port/pump, other than pharmacologic or mechanical correction of intracatheter or pericatheter occlusion [see 36595 or 36596])
3. Partial replacement of only the catheter component associated with a port/pump device, but not entire device
4. Complete replacement of entire device via same venous access site (complete exchange)
5. Removal of entire device.

There is no coding distinction between venous access achieved percutaneously versus by cutdown or based on catheter size.

For the repair, partial (catheter only) replacement, complete replacement, or removal of both catheters (placed from separate venous access sites) of a multi-catheter device, with or without subcutaneous ports/pumps, use the appropriate code describing the service with a frequency of two.

If an existing central venous access device is removed and a new one placed via a separate venous access site, appropriate codes for both procedures (removal of old, if code exists, and insertion of new device) should be reported.

When imaging guidance is used for centrally inserted central venous catheters, for gaining access to the venous entry site and/or for manipulating the catheter into final central position, imaging guidance codes (eg, 76937, 77001) may be reported separately. Do not use 76937, 77001 in conjunction with 36568, 36569, 36572, 36573, 36584.

Please see the Surgical Guidelines section for the following table: The Central Venous Access Procedures Table

Vascular Introduction and Injection Procedures

Listed services for injection procedures include necessary local anesthesia, introduction of needles or catheter, injection of contrast media with or without automatic power injection, and/or necessary pre- and postinjection care specifically related to the injection procedure.

Selective vascular catheterization should be coded to include introduction and all lesser order selective catheterization used in the approach (eg, the description for a selective right middle cerebral artery catheterization includes the introduction and placement catheterization of the right common and internal carotid arteries).

Additional second and/or third order arterial catheterization within the same family of arteries or veins supplied by a single first order vessel should be expressed by 36012, 36218, or 36248.

Additional first order or higher catheterization in vascular families supplied by a first order vessel different from a previously selected and coded family should be separately coded using the conventions described above.

Surgical Procedures on Arteries and Veins

Primary vascular procedure listings include establishing both inflow and outflow by whatever procedures necessary. Also included is that portion of the operative arteriogram performed by the surgeon, as indicated. Sympathectomy, when done, is included in the listed aortic procedures. For unlisted vascular procedure, use 37799.

Please see the Surgery Guidelines section for the following guidelines:

- *Surgical Procedures on the Cardiovascular System*

AMA Coding Notes

Central Venous Access Procedures

(For refilling and maintenance of an implantable pump or reservoir for intravenous or intra-arterial drug delivery, use 96522)

Vascular Introduction and Injection Procedures

(For radiological supervision and interpretation, see Radiology)

(For injection procedures in conjunction with cardiac catheterization, see 93452-93461, 93563-93568)

(For chemotherapy of malignant disease, see 96401-96549)

AMA *CPT Assistant* ☐

36582: Dec 04: 10, Jun 08: 8
36583: Dec 04: 10-11, Jun 08: 8

Plain English Description

Complete replacement of a centrally inserted central venous catheter (CVC) with a subcutaneous port or pump is performed through the same venous access site. Replacement is performed when malfunction of the port or pump as well as the CVC occurs. Separately reportable radiographs are obtained to verify that the tip of the CVC is correctly positioned. The subcutaneous pocket is opened and the catheter separated from the port or pump. The port or pump are examined and determined to require replacement. The port or pump is removed. The catheter is also inspected and found to be occluded or damaged. A guidewire is placed through the existing catheter which is withdrawn over the guidewire. A new catheter is then advanced over the guidewire and the tip positioned in the subclavian, brachiocephalic, or iliac vein, the superior or inferior vena cava, or right atrium. A new port or pump is placed in the subcutaneous pocket. The new catheter is attached to the port or pump device and the connection checked for leaks using an injection of intravenous fluid. The pocket is closed. Use 36582 for complete replacement of a CVC and subcutaneous port and 36583 for complete replacement of a CVC and subcutaneous pump.

Complete replacement of a tunneled centrally inserted central venous catheter

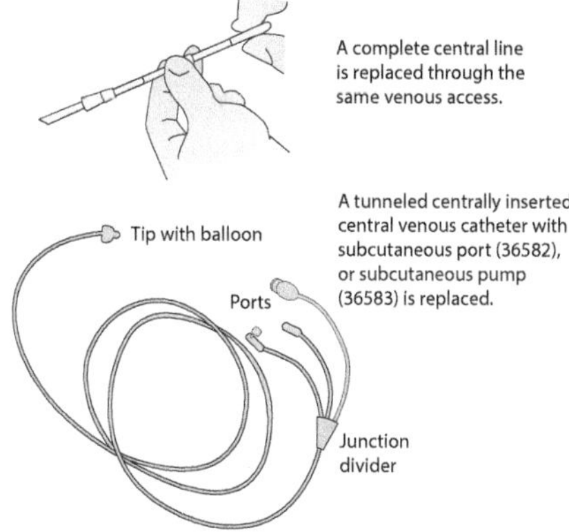
A complete central line is replaced through the same venous access.
A tunneled centrally inserted central venous catheter with subcutaneous port (36582), or subcutaneous pump (36583) is replaced.
Tip with balloon
Ports
Junction divider

ICD-10-CM Diagnostic Codes

➐	T80.211	Bloodstream infection due to central venous catheter
➐	T80.212	Local infection due to central venous catheter
➐	T80.218	Other infection due to central venous catheter
➐	T82.518	Breakdown (mechanical) of other cardiac and vascular devices and implants
➐	T82.538	Leakage of other cardiac and vascular devices and implants
➐	T82.598	Other mechanical complication of other cardiac and vascular devices and implants
➐	T82.898	Other specified complication of vascular prosthetic devices, implants and grafts
	Z45.2	Encounter for adjustment and management of vascular access device

CPT © 2018 American Medical Association. All Rights Reserved.

ICD-10-CM Coding Notes

For codes requiring a 7th character extension, refer to your ICD-10-CM book. Review the character descriptions and coding guidelines for proper selection. For some procedures, only certain characters will apply.

CCI Edits

Refer to Appendix A for CCI edits.

Facility RVUs

Code	Work	PE Facility	MP	Total Facility
36582	4.99	2.58	0.81	8.38
36583	5.04	3.19	1.21	9.44

Non-facility RVUs

Code	Work	PE Non-Facility	MP	Total Non-Facility
36582	4.99	22.55	0.81	28.35
36583	5.04	29.65	1.21	35.90

Modifiers (PAR)

Code	Mod 50	Mod 51	Mod 62	Mod 66	Mod 80
36582	0	2	0	0	0
36583	0	2	0	0	0

Global Period

Code	Days
36582	010
36583	010

CPT © 2018 American Medical Association. All Rights Reserved.

36584-36585

▲ **36584 Replacement, complete, of a peripherally inserted central venous catheter (PICC), without subcutaneous port or pump, through same venous access, including all imaging guidance, image documentation, and all associated radiological supervision and interpretation required to perform the replacement**

(For replacement of a peripherally inserted central venous catheter [PICC] without subcutaneous port or pump, through same venous access, without imaging guidance, use 37799)

(Do not report 36584 in conjunction with 76937, 77001)

36585 Replacement, complete, of a peripherally inserted central venous access device, with subcutaneous port, through same venous access

AMA Coding Guideline

Central Venous Access Procedures

To qualify as a central venous access catheter or device, the tip of the catheter/device must terminate in the subclavian, brachiocephalic (innominate) or iliac veins, the superior or inferior vena cava, or the right atrium. The venous access device may be either centrally inserted (jugular, subclavian, femoral vein or inferior vena cava catheter entry site) or peripherally inserted (eg, basilic, cephalic, or saphenous vein entry site). The device may be accessed for use either via exposed catheter (external to the skin), via a subcutaneous port or via a subcutaneous pump.

The procedures involving these types of devices fall into five categories:

1. Insertion (placement of catheter through a newly established venous access)
2. Repair (fixing device without replacement of either catheter or port/pump, other than pharmacologic or mechanical correction of intracatheter or pericatheter occlusion [see 36595 or 36596])
3. Partial replacement of only the catheter component associated with a port/pump device, but not entire device
4. Complete replacement of entire device via same venous access site (complete exchange)
5. Removal of entire device.

There is no coding distinction between venous access achieved percutaneously versus by cutdown or based on catheter size.

For the repair, partial (catheter only) replacement, complete replacement, or removal of both catheters (placed from separate venous access sites) of a multi-catheter device, with or without subcutaneous ports/pumps, use the appropriate code describing the service with a frequency of two.

If an existing central venous access device is removed and a new one placed via a separate venous access site, appropriate codes for both procedures (removal of old, if code exists, and insertion of new device) should be reported.

When imaging guidance is used for centrally inserted central venous catheters, for gaining access to the venous entry site and/or for manipulating the catheter into final central position, imaging guidance codes (eg, 76937, 77001) may be reported separately. Do not use 76937, 77001 in conjunction with 36568, 36569, 36572, 36573, 36584.

Please see the Surgical Guidelines section for the following table: The Central Venous Access Procedures Table

Vascular Introduction and Injection Procedures

Listed services for injection procedures include necessary local anesthesia, introduction of needles or catheter, injection of contrast media with or without automatic power injection, and/or necessary pre- and postinjection care specifically related to the injection procedure.

Selective vascular catheterization should be coded to include introduction and all lesser order selective catheterization used in the approach (eg, the description for a selective right middle cerebral artery catheterization includes the introduction and placement catheterization of the right common and internal carotid arteries).

Additional second and/or third order arterial catheterization within the same family of arteries or veins supplied by a single first order vessel should be expressed by 36012, 36218, or 36248.

Additional first order or higher catheterization in vascular families supplied by a first order vessel different from a previously selected and coded family should be separately coded using the conventions described above.

Surgical Procedures on Arteries and Veins

Primary vascular procedure listings include establishing both inflow and outflow by whatever procedures necessary. Also included is that portion of the operative arteriogram performed by the surgeon, as indicated. Sympathectomy, when done, is included in the listed aortic procedures. For unlisted vascular procedure, use 37799.

Please see the Surgery Guidelines section for the following guidelines:

- *Surgical Procedures on the Cardiovascular System*

AMA Coding Notes

Central Venous Access Procedures

(For refilling and maintenance of an implantable pump or reservoir for intravenous or intra-arterial drug delivery, use 96522)

Vascular Introduction and Injection Procedures

(For radiological supervision and interpretation, see Radiology)

(For injection procedures in conjunction with cardiac catheterization, see 93452-93461, 93563-93568)

(For chemotherapy of malignant disease, see 96401-96549)

AMA *CPT Assistant* □

36584: Dec 04: 11, Jun 08: 8
36585: Dec 04: 11, Jun 08: 8

Plain English Description

A peripherally inserted central venous catheter (PICC) is similar to an intravenous line and is used for the delivery of medication or fluids into the bloodstream over a prolonged period of time. For complete replacement, the existing venous access site is first inspected to ensure that it can be used. The site is cleansed and a local anesthetic is injected. The new catheter is primed with flush solution. The existing catheter is grasped and partially removed leaving several centimeters still within the vein. The existing catheter is trimmed leaving approximately 10 cm outside the vein. The existing catheter is secured with a hemostat to prevent catheter migration. The introducer is advanced into the vein over the trimmed end of the existing catheter. Once the introducer is in place, the existing catheter is completely removed from the vein. The new PICC line is then inserted through the introducer into the vein and advanced into the brachiocephalic vein, subclavian vein, or superior vena cava. The PICC is secured with sutures and a dressing is applied over the insertion site in the arm. This includes all imaging guidance needed for replacement with documentation, interpretation, and confirmation of final catheter tip location. For complete replacement with a subcutaneous port (36585), the subcutaneous pocket is opened and the port site is inspected. The port is separated from the catheter and the port is removed from the pocket. The existing catheter is dissected free of the subcutaneous tissue and the existing venous access site is exposed. The existing catheter is grasped and partially removed and the new PICC line is inserted as described above. Placement is checked by separately reportable radiographs. The new catheter is anchored in the subcutaneous tissue and the new port is placed in the subcutaneous pocket. The new catheter is tunneled to the new port and the two components are connected. The incision over the venous access site is closed. The port is sutured into place and the pocket is closed.

CPT © 2018 American Medical Association. All Rights Reserved.

Replacement, complete, of a peripherally inserted central venous catheter (PICC)
Without subcutaneous port or pump (36584); with subcutaneous port (36585)

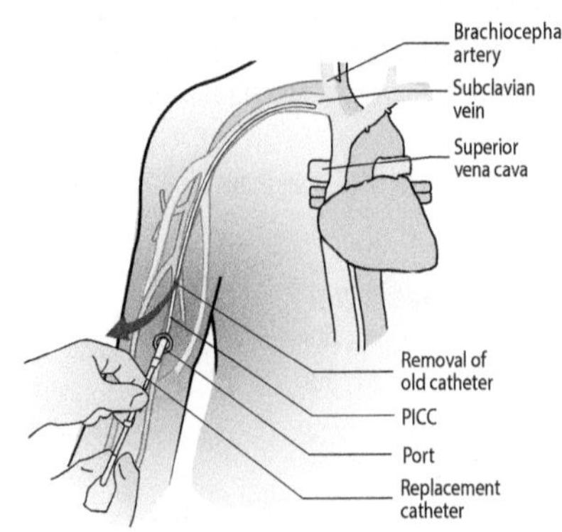

ICD-10-CM Diagnostic Codes

➐	T80.211	Bloodstream infection due to central venous catheter
➐	T80.212	Local infection due to central venous catheter
➐	T80.218	Other infection due to central venous catheter
➐	T82.518	Breakdown (mechanical) of other cardiac and vascular devices and implants
➐	T82.538	Leakage of other cardiac and vascular devices and implants
➐	T82.598	Other mechanical complication of other cardiac and vascular devices and implants
➐	T82.898	Other specified complication of vascular prosthetic devices, implants and grafts
	Z45.2	Encounter for adjustment and management of vascular access device

ICD-10-CM Coding Notes

For codes requiring a 7th character extension, refer to your ICD-10-CM book. Review the character descriptions and coding guidelines for proper selection. For some procedures, only certain characters will apply.

CCI Edits

Refer to Appendix A for CCI edits.

Facility RVUs ☐

Code	Work	PE Facility	MP	Total Facility
36584	1.20	0.42	0.11	1.73
36585	4.59	2.41	0.80	7.80

Non-facility RVUs ☐

Code	Work	PE Non-Facility	MP	Total Non-Facility
36584	1.20	8.47	0.11	9.78
36585	4.59	25.12	0.80	30.51

Modifiers (PAR) ☐

Code	Mod 50	Mod 51	Mod 62	Mod 66	Mod 80
36584	0	0	0	0	1
36585	0	2	0	0	0

Global Period

Code	Days
36584	000
36585	010

CPT © 2018 American Medical Association. All Rights Reserved.

36589-36590

36589 Removal of tunneled central venous catheter, without subcutaneous port or pump

36590 Removal of tunneled central venous access device, with subcutaneous port or pump, central or peripheral insertion

(Do not report 36589 or 36590 for removal of non-tunneled central venous catheters)

AMA Coding Guideline

Central Venous Access Procedures

To qualify as a central venous access catheter or device, the tip of the catheter/device must terminate in the subclavian, brachiocephalic (innominate) or iliac veins, the superior or inferior vena cava, or the right atrium. The venous access device may be either centrally inserted (jugular, subclavian, femoral vein or inferior vena cava catheter entry site) or peripherally inserted (eg, basilic, cephalic, or saphenous vein entry site). The device may be accessed for use either via exposed catheter (external to the skin), via a subcutaneous port or via a subcutaneous pump.

The procedures involving these types of devices fall into five categories:

1. Insertion (placement of catheter through a newly established venous access)
2. Repair (fixing device without replacement of either catheter or port/pump, other than pharmacologic or mechanical correction of intracatheter or pericatheter occlusion [see 36595 or 36596])
3. Partial replacement of only the catheter component associated with a port/pump device, but not entire device
4. Complete replacement of entire device via same venous access site (complete exchange)
5. Removal of entire device.

There is no coding distinction between venous access achieved percutaneously versus by cutdown or based on catheter size.

For the repair, partial (catheter only) replacement, complete replacement, or removal of both catheters (placed from separate venous access sites) of a multi-catheter device, with or without subcutaneous ports/pumps, use the appropriate code describing the service with a frequency of two.

If an existing central venous access device is removed and a new one placed via a separate venous access site, appropriate codes for both procedures (removal of old, if code exists, and insertion of new device) should be reported.

When imaging guidance is used for centrally inserted central venous catheters, for gaining access to the venous entry site and/or for manipulating the catheter into final central position, imaging guidance codes (eg, 76937, 77001) may be reported separately. Do not use 76937, 77001 in conjunction with 36568, 36569, 36572, 36573, 36584.

Please see the Surgical Guidelines section for the following table: The Central Venous Access Procedures Table

Vascular Introduction and Injection Procedures

Listed services for injection procedures include necessary local anesthesia, introduction of needles or catheter, injection of contrast media with or without automatic power injection, and/or necessary pre- and postinjection care specifically related to the injection procedure.

Selective vascular catheterization should be coded to include introduction and all lesser order selective catheterization used in the approach (eg, the description for a selective right middle cerebral artery catheterization includes the introduction and placement catheterization of the right common and internal carotid arteries).

Additional second and/or third order arterial catheterization within the same family of arteries or veins supplied by a single first order vessel should be expressed by 36012, 36218, or 36248.

Additional first order or higher catheterization in vascular families supplied by a first order vessel different from a previously selected and coded family should be separately coded using the conventions described above.

Surgical Procedures on Arteries and Veins

Primary vascular procedure listings include establishing both inflow and outflow by whatever procedures necessary. Also included is that portion of the operative arteriogram performed by the surgeon, as indicated. Sympathectomy, when done, is included in the listed aortic procedures. For unlisted vascular procedure, use 37799.

Please see the Surgery Guidelines section for the following guidelines:

- *Surgical Procedures on the Cardiovascular System*

AMA Coding Notes

Central Venous Access Procedures

(For refilling and maintenance of an implantable pump or reservoir for intravenous or intra-arterial drug delivery, use 96522)

Vascular Introduction and Injection Procedures

(For radiological supervision and interpretation, see Radiology)

(For injection procedures in conjunction with cardiac catheterization, see 93452-93461, 93563-93568)

(For chemotherapy of malignant disease, see 96401-96549)

AMA *CPT Assistant*

36589: Dec 04: 11, Jun 08: 8, Nov 15: 10
36590: Dec 04: 11, Jun 08: 8, Jul 10: 10

Plain English Description

A tunneled central venous catheter (CVC) is removed. A local anesthetic is injected. In 36589, a tunneled CVC without a subcutaneous port or pump is removed. The skin over the venous access site is incised and sutures removed. The CVC is dissected free of the tunnel and removed. Bleeding is controlled with manual pressure over the venous access site. The incision is closed and a dressing applied. In 36590, a tunneled CVC with a subcutaneous port or pump is removed. The subcutaneous pocket is incised and the port of pump dissected free. The CVC is dissected free of the tunnel and the port or pump and catheter are removed. Bleeding is controlled with manual pressure over the venous access site. The incision is closed and a dressing applied.

Removal of tunneled central venous catheter or access device

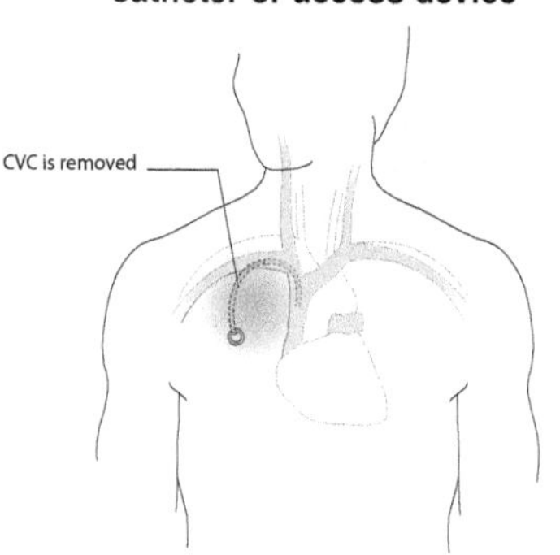

Without subcutaneous port or pump (36589); with subcutaneous port or pump, central or peripheral insertion (36590)

ICD-10-CM Diagnostic Codes

⑦	T80.211	Bloodstream infection due to central venous catheter
⑦	T80.212	Local infection due to central venous catheter
⑦	T80.218	Other infection due to central venous catheter
⑦	T82.518	Breakdown (mechanical) of other cardiac and vascular devices and implants
⑦	T82.538	Leakage of other cardiac and vascular devices and implants
⑦	T82.598	Other mechanical complication of other cardiac and vascular devices and implants
⑦	T82.818	Embolism due to vascular prosthetic devices, implants and grafts
⑦	T82.828	Fibrosis due to vascular prosthetic devices, implants and grafts
⑦	T82.838	Hemorrhage due to vascular prosthetic devices, implants and grafts
⑦	T82.848	Pain due to vascular prosthetic devices, implants and grafts
⑦	T82.868	Thrombosis due to vascular prosthetic devices, implants and grafts
⑦	T82.898	Other specified complication of vascular prosthetic devices, implants and grafts

CPT © 2018 American Medical Association. All Rights Reserved.

Z45.2	Encounter for adjustment and management of vascular access device

ICD-10-CM Coding Notes

For codes requiring a 7th character extension, refer to your ICD-10-CM book. Review the character descriptions and coding guidelines for proper selection. For some procedures, only certain characters will apply.

CCI Edits

Refer to Appendix A for CCI edits.

Facility RVUs

Code	Work	PE Facility	MP	Total Facility
36589	2.28	1.36	0.32	3.96
36590	3.10	1.86	0.53	5.49

Non-facility RVUs

Code	Work	PE Non-Facility	MP	Total Non-Facility
36589	2.28	2.11	0.32	4.71
36590	3.10	2.71	0.53	6.34

Modifiers (PAR)

Code	Mod 50	Mod 51	Mod 62	Mod 66	Mod 80
36589	0	2	0	0	0
36590	0	2	0	0	0

Global Period

Code	Days
36589	010
36590	010

CPT © 2018 American Medical Association. All Rights Reserved.

36591

36591 Collection of blood specimen from a completely implantable venous access device

(Do not report 36591 in conjunction with other services except a laboratory service)

(For collection of venous blood specimen by venipuncture, use 36415)

(For collection of capillary blood specimen, use 36416)

AMA Coding Guideline

Central Venous Access Procedures

To qualify as a central venous access catheter or device, the tip of the catheter/device must terminate in the subclavian, brachiocephalic (innominate) or iliac veins, the superior or inferior vena cava, or the right atrium. The venous access device may be either centrally inserted (jugular, subclavian, femoral vein or inferior vena cava catheter entry site) or peripherally inserted (eg, basilic, cephalic, or saphenous vein entry site). The device may be accessed for use either via exposed catheter (external to the skin), via a subcutaneous port or via a subcutaneous pump.

The procedures involving these types of devices fall into five categories:

1. Insertion (placement of catheter through a newly established venous access)
2. Repair (fixing device without replacement of either catheter or port/pump, other than pharmacologic or mechanical correction of intracatheter or pericatheter occlusion [see 36595 or 36596])
3. Partial replacement of only the catheter component associated with a port/pump device, but not entire device
4. Complete replacement of entire device via same venous access site (complete exchange)
5. Removal of entire device.

There is no coding distinction between venous access achieved percutaneously versus by cutdown or based on catheter size.

For the repair, partial (catheter only) replacement, complete replacement, or removal of both catheters (placed from separate venous access sites) of a multi-catheter device, with or without subcutaneous ports/pumps, use the appropriate code describing the service with a frequency of two.

If an existing central venous access device is removed and a new one placed via a separate venous access site, appropriate codes for both procedures (removal of old, if code exists, and insertion of new device) should be reported.

When imaging guidance is used for centrally inserted central venous catheters, for gaining access to the venous entry site and/or for manipulating the catheter into final central position, imaging guidance codes (eg, 76937, 77001) may be reported separately. Do not use 76937, 77001 in conjunction with 36568, 36569, 36572, 36573, 36584.

Please see the Surgical Guidelines section for the following table: The Central Venous Access Procedures Table

Vascular Introduction and Injection Procedures

Listed services for injection procedures include necessary local anesthesia, introduction of needles or catheter, injection of contrast media with or without automatic power injection, and/or necessary pre- and postinjection care specifically related to the injection procedure.

Selective vascular catheterization should be coded to include introduction and all lesser order selective catheterization used in the approach (eg, the description for a selective right middle cerebral artery catheterization includes the introduction and placement catheterization of the right common and internal carotid arteries).

Additional second and/or third order arterial catheterization within the same family of arteries or veins supplied by a single first order vessel should be expressed by 36012, 36218, or 36248.

Additional first order or higher catheterization in vascular families supplied by a first order vessel different from a previously selected and coded family should be separately coded using the conventions described above.

Surgical Procedures on Arteries and Veins

Primary vascular procedure listings include establishing both inflow and outflow by whatever procedures necessary. Also included is that portion of the operative arteriogram performed by the surgeon, as indicated. Sympathectomy, when done, is included in the listed aortic procedures. For unlisted vascular procedure, use 37799.

Please see the Surgery Guidelines section for the following guidelines:

- *Surgical Procedures on the Cardiovascular System*

AMA Coding Notes

Central Venous Access Procedures

(For refilling and maintenance of an implantable pump or reservoir for intravenous or intra-arterial drug delivery, use 96522)

Vascular Introduction and Injection Procedures

(For radiological supervision and interpretation, see Radiology)

(For injection procedures in conjunction with cardiac catheterization, see 93452-93461, 93563-93568)

(For chemotherapy of malignant disease, see 96401-96549)

AMA *CPT Assistant* ☐

36591: Apr 08: 9, Jul 11: 16, May 14: 4

Plain English Description

The septum of the IVAD is located by palpating the skin over the IVAD. The skin over the IVAD is cleansed and a Huber needle (special side-holed needle) with attached syringe and extension tubing primed with normal saline is inserted into the IVAD at a 90 degree angle. A small amount of blood is aspirated into the syringe and the IVAD is flushed with normal saline. The extension tubing is clamped. The syringe is then disconnected and an intermittent injection cap is attached. A Vacutainer is inserted into the injection cap. A discard tube is inserted onto the Vacutainer needle. The tubing is unclamped and the discard tube is filled. The extension tubing is clamped and the discard tube is removed and discarded. A blood specimen tube is then inserted onto the Vacutainer needle, the extension tubing is again unclamped, and the blood specimen is collected. One or more blood specimen tubes may be filled in this manner, then the Vacutainer is removed, and the line is flushed with 20 ml of normal saline. If no other procedures are to be performed, such as infusion of medications, the syringe is disconnected and the extension tubing is flushed with heparin. The Huber needle is then removed.

Collection of blood specimen from a completely implantable venous access device

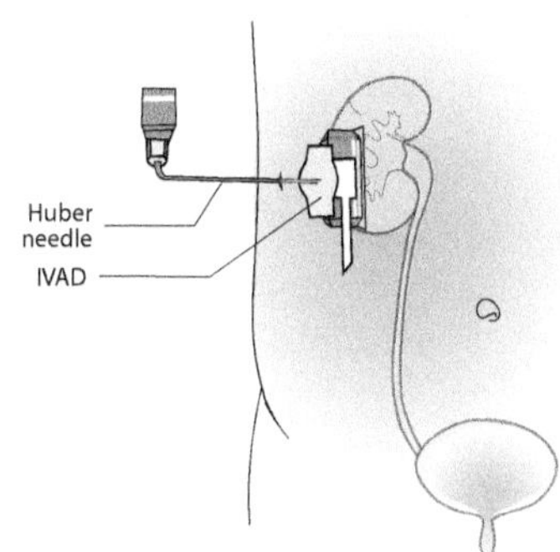

ICD-10-CM Diagnostic Codes

There are too many ICD-10-CM codes to list. Refer to ICD-10-CM code book for associated diagnostic codes.

CCI Edits

Refer to Appendix A for CCI edits.

Pub 100

36591: Pub 100-04, 12, 30.6.12

CPT © 2018 American Medical Association. All Rights Reserved.

Facility RVUs □

Code	Work	PE Facility	MP	Total Facility
36591	0.00	0.68	0.01	0.69

Non-facility RVUs □

Code	Work	PE Non-Facility	MP	Total Non-Facility
36591	0.00	0.68	0.01	0.69

Modifiers (PAR) □

Code	Mod 50	Mod 51	Mod 62	Mod 66	Mod 80
36591	0	0	0	0	0

Global Period

Code	Days
36591	XXX

CPT © 2018 American Medical Association. All Rights Reserved.

36592

36592 Collection of blood specimen using established central or peripheral catheter, venous, not otherwise specified

(For blood collection from an established arterial catheter, use 37799)

(Do not report 36592 in conjunction with other services except a laboratory service)

AMA Coding Guideline

Central Venous Access Procedures

To qualify as a central venous access catheter or device, the tip of the catheter/device must terminate in the subclavian, brachiocephalic (innominate) or iliac veins, the superior or inferior vena cava, or the right atrium. The venous access device may be either centrally inserted (jugular, subclavian, femoral vein or inferior vena cava catheter entry site) or peripherally inserted (eg, basilic, cephalic, or saphenous vein entry site). The device may be accessed for use either via exposed catheter (external to the skin), via a subcutaneous port or via a subcutaneous pump.

The procedures involving these types of devices fall into five categories:

1. Insertion (placement of catheter through a newly established venous access)
2. Repair (fixing device without replacement of either catheter or port/pump, other than pharmacologic or mechanical correction of intracatheter or pericatheter occlusion [see 36595 or 36596])
3. Partial replacement of only the catheter component associated with a port/pump device, but not entire device
4. Complete replacement of entire device via same venous access site (complete exchange)
5. Removal of entire device.

There is no coding distinction between venous access achieved percutaneously versus by cutdown or based on catheter size.

For the repair, partial (catheter only) replacement, complete replacement, or removal of both catheters (placed from separate venous access sites) of a multi-catheter device, with or without subcutaneous ports/pumps, use the appropriate code describing the service with a frequency of two.

If an existing central venous access device is removed and a new one placed via a separate venous access site, appropriate codes for both procedures (removal of old, if code exists, and insertion of new device) should be reported.

When imaging guidance is used for centrally inserted central venous catheters, for gaining access to the venous entry site and/or for manipulating the catheter into final central position, imaging guidance codes (eg, 76937, 77001) may be reported separately. Do not use 76937, 77001 in conjunction with 36568, 36569, 36572, 36573, 36584.

Please see the Surgical Guidelines section for the following table: The Central Venous Access Procedures Table

Vascular Introduction and Injection Procedures

Listed services for injection procedures include necessary local anesthesia, introduction of needles or catheter, injection of contrast media with or without automatic power injection, and/or necessary pre- and postinjection care specifically related to the injection procedure.

Selective vascular catheterization should be coded to include introduction and all lesser order selective catheterization used in the approach (eg, the description for a selective right middle cerebral artery catheterization includes the introduction and placement catheterization of the right common and internal carotid arteries).

Additional second and/or third order arterial catheterization within the same family of arteries or veins supplied by a single first order vessel should be expressed by 36012, 36218, or 36248.

Additional first order or higher catheterization in vascular families supplied by a first order vessel different from a previously selected and coded family should be separately coded using the conventions described above.

Surgical Procedures on Arteries and Veins

Primary vascular procedure listings include establishing both inflow and outflow by whatever procedures necessary. Also included is that portion of the operative arteriogram performed by the surgeon, as indicated. Sympathectomy, when done, is included in the listed aortic procedures. For unlisted vascular procedure, use 37799.

Please see the Surgery Guidelines section for the following guidelines:

- *Surgical Procedures on the Cardiovascular System*

AMA Coding Notes

Central Venous Access Procedures

(For refilling and maintenance of an implantable pump or reservoir for intravenous or intra-arterial drug delivery, use 96522)

Vascular Introduction and Injection Procedures

(For radiological supervision and interpretation, see Radiology)

(For injection procedures in conjunction with cardiac catheterization, see 93452-93461, 93563-93568)

(For chemotherapy of malignant disease, see 96401-96549)

AMA *CPT Assistant* □

36592: Apr 08: 9, Jul 11: 16

Plain English Description

The catheter hub is cleansed and a syringe is attached. The catheter is flushed with normal saline. Blood is then allowed to fill the central line and five ml of blood is aspirated into the syringe and discarded. If a Vacutainer system is used, it is attached. Labeled blood tubes are attached to the Vacutainer and filled. The Vacutainer system is removed and the central line is flushed with normal saline if an infusion procedure is to follow the blood collection. The line is flushed with heparin, otherwise. Alternatively, a syringe without a Vacutainer system can also be used to collect a blood specimen.

Collection of blood specimen from established central catheter

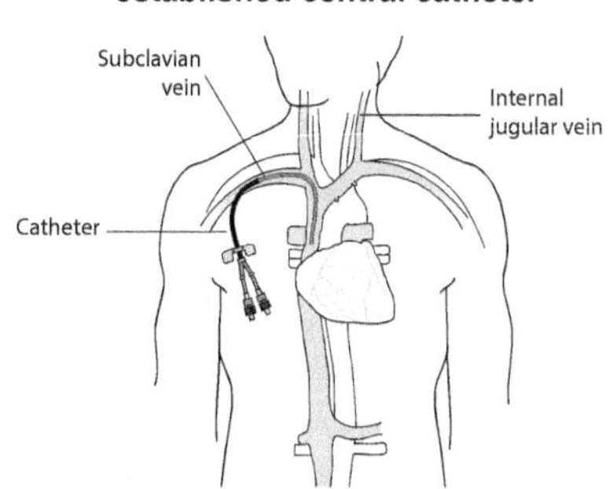

Blood is removed through an existing central or peripheral venous catheter.

ICD-10-CM Diagnostic Codes

There are too many ICD-10-CM codes to list. Refer to ICD-10-CM code book for associated diagnostic codes.

CCI Edits

Refer to Appendix A for CCI edits.

Facility RVUs □

Code	Work	PE Facility	MP	Total Facility
36592	0.00	0.76	0.01	0.77

Non-facility RVUs □

Code	Work	PE Non-Facility	MP	Total Non-Facility
36592	0.00	0.76	0.01	0.77

Modifiers (PAR) □

Code	Mod 50	Mod 51	Mod 62	Mod 66	Mod 80
36592	0	0	0	0	0

Global Period

Code	Days
36592	XXX

CPT © 2018 American Medical Association. All Rights Reserved.

36593

36593 Declotting by thrombolytic agent of implanted vascular access device or catheter

AMA Coding Guideline

Central Venous Access Procedures

To qualify as a central venous access catheter or device, the tip of the catheter/device must terminate in the subclavian, brachiocephalic (innominate) or iliac veins, the superior or inferior vena cava, or the right atrium. The venous access device may be either centrally inserted (jugular, subclavian, femoral vein or inferior vena cava catheter entry site) or peripherally inserted (eg, basilic, cephalic, or saphenous vein entry site). The device may be accessed for use either via exposed catheter (external to the skin), via a subcutaneous port or via a subcutaneous pump.

The procedures involving these types of devices fall into five categories:

1. Insertion (placement of catheter through a newly established venous access)
2. Repair (fixing device without replacement of either catheter or port/pump, other than pharmacologic or mechanical correction of intracatheter or pericatheter occlusion [see 36595 or 36596])
3. Partial replacement of only the catheter component associated with a port/pump device, but not entire device
4. Complete replacement of entire device via same venous access site (complete exchange)
5. Removal of entire device.

There is no coding distinction between venous access achieved percutaneously versus by cutdown or based on catheter size.

For the repair, partial (catheter only) replacement, complete replacement, or removal of both catheters (placed from separate venous access sites) of a multi-catheter device, with or without subcutaneous ports/pumps, use the appropriate code describing the service with a frequency of two.

If an existing central venous access device is removed and a new one placed via a separate venous access site, appropriate codes for both procedures (removal of old, if code exists, and insertion of new device) should be reported.

When imaging guidance is used for centrally inserted central venous catheters, for gaining access to the venous entry site and/or for manipulating the catheter into final central position, imaging guidance codes (eg, 76937, 77001) may be reported separately. Do not use 76937, 77001 in conjunction with 36568, 36569, 36572, 36573, 36584.

Please see the Surgical Guidelines section for the following table: The Central Venous Access Procedures Table

Vascular Introduction and Injection Procedures

Listed services for injection procedures include necessary local anesthesia, introduction of needles or catheter, injection of contrast media with or without automatic power injection, and/or necessary pre- and postinjection care specifically related to the injection procedure.

Selective vascular catheterization should be coded to include introduction and all lesser order selective catheterization used in the approach (eg, the description for a selective right middle cerebral artery catheterization includes the introduction and placement catheterization of the right common and internal carotid arteries).

Additional second and/or third order arterial catheterization within the same family of arteries or veins supplied by a single first order vessel should be expressed by 36012, 36218, or 36248.

Additional first order or higher catheterization in vascular families supplied by a first order vessel different from a previously selected and coded family should be separately coded using the conventions described above.

Surgical Procedures on Arteries and Veins

Primary vascular procedure listings include establishing both inflow and outflow by whatever procedures necessary. Also included is that portion of the operative arteriogram performed by the surgeon, as indicated. Sympathectomy, when done, is included in the listed aortic procedures. For unlisted vascular procedure, use 37799.

Please see the Surgery Guidelines section for the following guidelines:

- *Surgical Procedures on the Cardiovascular System*

AMA Coding Notes

Central Venous Access Procedures

(For refilling and maintenance of an implantable pump or reservoir for intravenous or intra-arterial drug delivery, use 96522)

Vascular Introduction and Injection Procedures

(For radiological supervision and interpretation, see Radiology)

(For injection procedures in conjunction with cardiac catheterization, see 93452-93461, 93563-93568)

(For chemotherapy of malignant disease, see 96401-96549)

AMA *CPT Assistant* □

36593: Apr 08: 9, Dec 09: 11, Aug 11: 9, Feb 13: 3

Plain English Description

A thrombolytic agent, such as streptokinase, tissue-type plasminogen activator (t-PA), urokinase, or heparin, is instilled into an implanted vascular access device (IVAD) or central venous catheter (CVC) to dissolve a thrombus (blood clot) obstructing the IVAD or catheter. The thrombolytic agent is prepared using the drug manufacturer's protocol. The skin over the IVAD or the catheter hub is cleansed. The thrombolytic agent is instilled into the IVAD or into each lumen of the CVC. The thrombolytic agent is left in the catheter for the required dwell time as indicated by the drug manufacturer. Dwell time may be from 30 to 60 minutes. Patency is checked by attempting to draw blood or infuse fluids. If the IVAD or catheter is still obstructed, a second instillation of the thrombolytic agent may be attempted.

Declotting by thrombolytic agent of implanted vascular access device or catheter

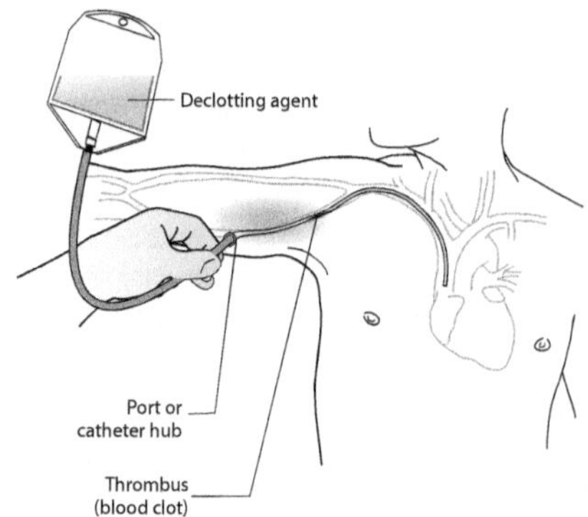

ICD-10-CM Diagnostic Codes

➐	T82.598	Other mechanical complication of other cardiac and vascular devices and implants
➐	T82.7	Infection and inflammatory reaction due to other cardiac and vascular devices, implants and grafts
➐	T82.818	Embolism due to vascular prosthetic devices, implants and grafts
➐	T82.868	Thrombosis due to vascular prosthetic devices, implants and grafts
➐	T82.898	Other specified complication of vascular prosthetic devices, implants and grafts
	Z45.2	Encounter for adjustment and management of vascular access device

ICD-10-CM Coding Notes

For codes requiring a 7th character extension, refer to your ICD-10-CM book. Review the character descriptions and coding guidelines for proper selection. For some procedures, only certain characters will apply.

CCI Edits

Refer to Appendix A for CCI edits.

CPT © 2018 American Medical Association. All Rights Reserved.

Facility RVUs

Code	Work	PE Facility	MP	Total Facility
36593	0.00	0.87	0.02	0.89

Non-facility RVUs

Code	Work	PE Non-Facility	MP	Total Non-Facility
36593	0.00	0.87	0.02	0.89

Modifiers (PAR)

Code	Mod 50	Mod 51	Mod 62	Mod 66	Mod 80
36593	0	0	0	0	0

Global Period

Code	Days
36593	XXX

CPT © 2018 American Medical Association. All Rights Reserved.

36595

36595 Mechanical removal of pericatheter obstructive material (eg, fibrin sheath) from central venous device via separate venous access

(Do not report 36595 in conjunction with 36593)

(For venous catheterization, see 36010-36012)

(For radiological supervision and interpretation, use 75901)

AMA Coding Guideline

Central Venous Access Procedures

To qualify as a central venous access catheter or device, the tip of the catheter/device must terminate in the subclavian, brachiocephalic (innominate) or iliac veins, the superior or inferior vena cava, or the right atrium. The venous access device may be either centrally inserted (jugular, subclavian, femoral vein or inferior vena cava catheter entry site) or peripherally inserted (eg, basilic, cephalic, or saphenous vein entry site). The device may be accessed for use either via exposed catheter (external to the skin), via a subcutaneous port or via a subcutaneous pump.

The procedures involving these types of devices fall into five categories:

1. Insertion (placement of catheter through a newly established venous access)
2. Repair (fixing device without replacement of either catheter or port/pump, other than pharmacologic or mechanical correction of intracatheter or pericatheter occlusion [see 36595 or 36596])
3. Partial replacement of only the catheter component associated with a port/pump device, but not entire device
4. Complete replacement of entire device via same venous access site (complete exchange)
5. Removal of entire device.

There is no coding distinction between venous access achieved percutaneously versus by cutdown or based on catheter size.

For the repair, partial (catheter only) replacement, complete replacement, or removal of both catheters (placed from separate venous access sites) of a multi-catheter device, with or without subcutaneous ports/pumps, use the appropriate code describing the service with a frequency of two.

If an existing central venous access device is removed and a new one placed via a separate venous access site, appropriate codes for both procedures (removal of old, if code exists, and insertion of new device) should be reported.

When imaging guidance is used for centrally inserted central venous catheters, for gaining access to the venous entry site and/or for manipulating the catheter into final central position, imaging guidance codes (eg, 76937, 77001) may be reported separately. Do not use 76937, 77001 in conjunction with 36568, 36569, 36572, 36573, 36584.

Please see the Surgical Guidelines section for the following table: The Central Venous Access Procedures Table

Vascular Introduction and Injection Procedures

Listed services for injection procedures include necessary local anesthesia, introduction of needles or catheter, injection of contrast media with or without automatic power injection, and/or necessary pre- and postinjection care specifically related to the injection procedure.

Selective vascular catheterization should be coded to include introduction and all lesser order selective catheterization used in the approach (eg, the description for a selective right middle cerebral artery catheterization includes the introduction and placement catheterization of the right common and internal carotid arteries).

Additional second and/or third order arterial catheterization within the same family of arteries or veins supplied by a single first order vessel should be expressed by 36012, 36218, or 36248.

Additional first order or higher catheterization in vascular families supplied by a first order vessel different from a previously selected and coded family should be separately coded using the conventions described above.

Surgical Procedures on Arteries and Veins

Primary vascular procedure listings include establishing both inflow and outflow by whatever procedures necessary. Also included is that portion of the operative arteriogram performed by the surgeon, as indicated. Sympathectomy, when done, is included in the listed aortic procedures. For unlisted vascular procedure, use 37799.

Please see the Surgery Guidelines section for the following guidelines:

- *Surgical Procedures on the Cardiovascular System*

AMA Coding Notes

Central Venous Access Procedures

(For refilling and maintenance of an implantable pump or reservoir for intravenous or intra-arterial drug delivery, use 96522)

Vascular Introduction and Injection Procedures

(For radiological supervision and interpretation, see Radiology)

(For injection procedures in conjunction with cardiac catheterization, see 93452-93461, 93563-93568)

(For chemotherapy of malignant disease, see 96401-96549)

AMA *CPT Assistant* □

36595: Dec 04: 9, 12

Plain English Description

One common complication of a semi-permanent CVC is the formation of a fibrin sheath at the tip of the catheter that causes obstruction or reduced flow through the CVC. A separately reportable venogram is performed and the existence of a fibrin sheath or other pericatheter obstructive material confirmed. A separate venous access site is prepped. The vein is incised and a sheath placed. A guidewire is placed and a snare guiding catheter introduced over the guidewire using separately reportable radiological guidance. The snare guiding catheter is advanced to the site of the pericatheter obstruction at the tip of the existing CVC. The guidewire is removed and a snare advanced to the site of the obstruction. The fibrin sheath or other obstructive material is mechanically removed by stripping it away with the snare. Patency of the CVC is evaluated by injecting intravenous fluid. The snare and snare guiding catheter are removed. The separate venous access site is closed with sutures.

Removal of pericatheter obstructive material from central venous device

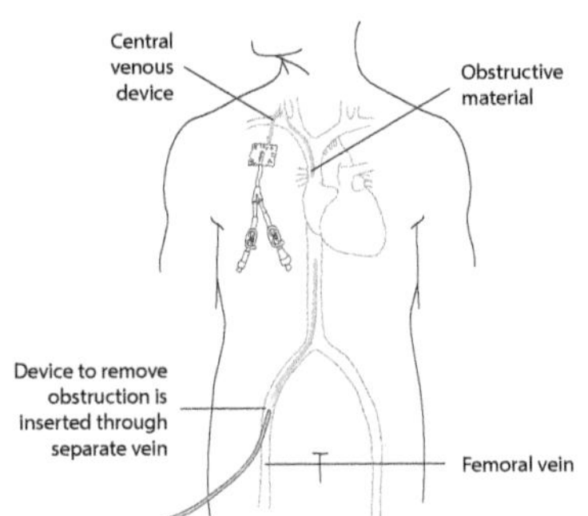

ICD-10-CM Diagnostic Codes

➐	T82.598	Other mechanical complication of other cardiac and vascular devices and implants
➐	T82.818	Embolism due to vascular prosthetic devices, implants and grafts
➐	T82.828	Fibrosis due to vascular prosthetic devices, implants and grafts
➐	T82.848	Pain due to vascular prosthetic devices, implants and grafts
➐	T82.868	Thrombosis due to vascular prosthetic devices, implants and grafts
➐	T82.898	Other specified complication of vascular prosthetic devices, implants and grafts
	Z45.2	Encounter for adjustment and management of vascular access device

ICD-10-CM Coding Notes

For codes requiring a 7th character extension, refer to your ICD-10-CM book. Review the character descriptions and coding guidelines for proper selection. For some procedures, only certain characters will apply.

CPT © 2018 American Medical Association. All Rights Reserved.

CCI Edits

Refer to Appendix A for CCI edits.

Facility RVUs

Code	Work	PE Facility	MP	Total Facility
36595	3.59	1.32	0.39	5.30

Non-facility RVUs

Code	Work	PE Non-Facility	MP	Total Non-Facility
36595	3.59	13.32	0.39	17.30

Modifiers (PAR)

Code	Mod 50	Mod 51	Mod 62	Mod 66	Mod 80
36595	0	2	0	0	1

Global Period

Code	Days
36595	000

CPT © 2018 American Medical Association. All Rights Reserved.

36596

36596 Mechanical removal of intraluminal (intracatheter) obstructive material from central venous device through device lumen

(Do not report 36596 in conjunction with 36593)

(For venous catheterization, see 36010-36012)

(For radiological supervision and interpretation, use 75902)

AMA Coding Guideline

Central Venous Access Procedures

To qualify as a central venous access catheter or device, the tip of the catheter/device must terminate in the subclavian, brachiocephalic (innominate) or iliac veins, the superior or inferior vena cava, or the right atrium. The venous access device may be either centrally inserted (jugular, subclavian, femoral vein or inferior vena cava catheter entry site) or peripherally inserted (eg, basilic, cephalic, or saphenous vein entry site). The device may be accessed for use either via exposed catheter (external to the skin), via a subcutaneous port or via a subcutaneous pump.

The procedures involving these types of devices fall into five categories:

1. Insertion (placement of catheter through a newly established venous access)
2. Repair (fixing device without replacement of either catheter or port/pump, other than pharmacologic or mechanical correction of intracatheter or pericatheter occlusion [see 36595 or 36596])
3. Partial replacement of only the catheter component associated with a port/pump device, but not entire device
4. Complete replacement of entire device via same venous access site (complete exchange)
5. Removal of entire device.

There is no coding distinction between venous access achieved percutaneously versus by cutdown or based on catheter size.

For the repair, partial (catheter only) replacement, complete replacement, or removal of both catheters (placed from separate venous access sites) of a multi-catheter device, with or without subcutaneous ports/pumps, use the appropriate code describing the service with a frequency of two.

If an existing central venous access device is removed and a new one placed via a separate venous access site, appropriate codes for both procedures (removal of old, if code exists, and insertion of new device) should be reported.

When imaging guidance is used for centrally inserted central venous catheters, for gaining access to the venous entry site and/or for manipulating the catheter into final central position, imaging guidance codes (eg, 76937, 77001) may be reported separately. Do not use 76937, 77001 in conjunction with 36568, 36569, 36572, 36573, 36584.

Please see the Surgical Guidelines section for the following table: The Central Venous Access Procedures Table

Vascular Introduction and Injection Procedures

Listed services for injection procedures include necessary local anesthesia, introduction of needles or catheter, injection of contrast media with or without automatic power injection, and/or necessary pre- and postinjection care specifically related to the injection procedure.

Selective vascular catheterization should be coded to include introduction and all lesser order selective catheterization used in the approach (eg, the description for a selective right middle cerebral artery catheterization includes the introduction and placement catheterization of the right common and internal carotid arteries).

Additional second and/or third order arterial catheterization within the same family of arteries or veins supplied by a single first order vessel should be expressed by 36012, 36218, or 36248.

Additional first order or higher catheterization in vascular families supplied by a first order vessel different from a previously selected and coded family should be separately coded using the conventions described above.

Surgical Procedures on Arteries and Veins

Primary vascular procedure listings include establishing both inflow and outflow by whatever procedures necessary. Also included is that portion of the operative arteriogram performed by the surgeon, as indicated. Sympathectomy, when done, is included in the listed aortic procedures. For unlisted vascular procedure, use 37799.

Please see the Surgery Guidelines section for the following guidelines:

- *Surgical Procedures on the Cardiovascular System*

AMA Coding Notes

Central Venous Access Procedures

(For refilling and maintenance of an implantable pump or reservoir for intravenous or intra-arterial drug delivery, use 96522)

Vascular Introduction and Injection Procedures

(For radiological supervision and interpretation, see Radiology)

(For injection procedures in conjunction with cardiac catheterization, see 93452-93461, 93563-93568)

(For chemotherapy of malignant disease, see 96401-96549)

AMA *CPT Assistant*

36596: Dec 04: 9, 12

Plain English Description

One common complication of a semi-permanent CVC is the accumulation of intraluminal obstructive material that causes complete occlusion or reduced flow through the CVC. A CVC without a subcutaneous port is accessed using a guidewire. A CVC with a port or pump is accessed using a Huber needle. A guidewire is then advanced into the port or pump reservoir. A snare guiding catheter or balloon catheter is advanced over the guidewire through the existing catheter lumen or the port or pump. The guidewire is removed. A snare is then used to strip away the obstructive material or the balloon catheter is inflated to open the obstruction. The snare and snare guiding catheter or the balloon catheter are removed. Patency of the CVC is evaluated by injecting intravenous fluid.

Mechanical removal of intracatheter obstructive material; CVD, device lumen

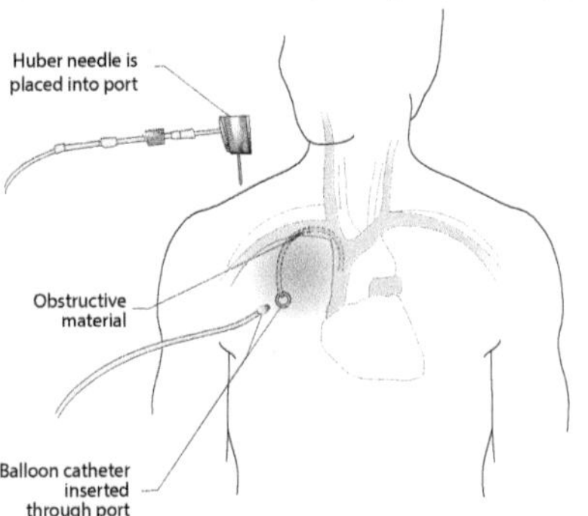

ICD-10-CM Diagnostic Codes

➐	T82.598	Other mechanical complication of other cardiac and vascular devices and implants
➐	T82.818	Embolism due to vascular prosthetic devices, implants and grafts
➐	T82.828	Fibrosis due to vascular prosthetic devices, implants and grafts
➐	T82.848	Pain due to vascular prosthetic devices, implants and grafts
➐	T82.868	Thrombosis due to vascular prosthetic devices, implants and grafts
➐	T82.898	Other specified complication of vascular prosthetic devices, implants and grafts
	Z45.2	Encounter for adjustment and management of vascular access device

ICD-10-CM Coding Notes

For codes requiring a 7th character extension, refer to your ICD-10-CM book. Review the character descriptions and coding guidelines for proper selection. For some procedures, only certain characters will apply.

CCI Edits

Refer to Appendix A for CCI edits.

CPT © 2018 American Medical Association. All Rights Reserved.

Facility RVUs

Code	Work	PE Facility	MP	Total Facility
36596	0.75	0.43	0.10	1.28

Non-facility RVUs

Code	Work	PE Non-Facility	MP	Total Non-Facility
36596	0.75	2.72	0.10	3.57

Modifiers (PAR)

Code	Mod 50	Mod 51	Mod 62	Mod 66	Mod 80
36596	0	2	0	0	1

Global Period

Code	Days
36596	000

CPT © 2018 American Medical Association. All Rights Reserved.

36597

36597 Repositioning of previously placed central venous catheter under fluoroscopic guidance

(For fluoroscopic guidance, use 76000)

AMA Coding Guideline

Central Venous Access Procedures

To qualify as a central venous access catheter or device, the tip of the catheter/device must terminate in the subclavian, brachiocephalic (innominate) or iliac veins, the superior or inferior vena cava, or the right atrium. The venous access device may be either centrally inserted (jugular, subclavian, femoral vein or inferior vena cava catheter entry site) or peripherally inserted (eg, basilic, cephalic, or saphenous vein entry site). The device may be accessed for use either via exposed catheter (external to the skin), via a subcutaneous port or via a subcutaneous pump.

The procedures involving these types of devices fall into five categories:

1. Insertion (placement of catheter through a newly established venous access)
2. Repair (fixing device without replacement of either catheter or port/pump, other than pharmacologic or mechanical correction of intracatheter or pericatheter occlusion [see 36595 or 36596])
3. Partial replacement of only the catheter component associated with a port/pump device, but not entire device
4. Complete replacement of entire device via same venous access site (complete exchange)
5. Removal of entire device.

There is no coding distinction between venous access achieved percutaneously versus by cutdown or based on catheter size.

For the repair, partial (catheter only) replacement, complete replacement, or removal of both catheters (placed from separate venous access sites) of a multi-catheter device, with or without subcutaneous ports/pumps, use the appropriate code describing the service with a frequency of two.

If an existing central venous access device is removed and a new one placed via a separate venous access site, appropriate codes for both procedures (removal of old, if code exists, and insertion of new device) should be reported.

When imaging guidance is used for centrally inserted central venous catheters, for gaining access to the venous entry site and/or for manipulating the catheter into final central position, imaging guidance codes (eg, 76937, 77001) may be reported separately. Do not use 76937, 77001 in conjunction with 36568, 36569, 36572, 36573, 36584.

Please see the Surgical Guidelines section for the following table: The Central Venous Access Procedures Table

Vascular Introduction and Injection Procedures

Listed services for injection procedures include necessary local anesthesia, introduction of needles or catheter, injection of contrast media with or without automatic power injection, and/or necessary pre- and postinjection care specifically related to the injection procedure.

Selective vascular catheterization should be coded to include introduction and all lesser order selective catheterization used in the approach (eg, the description for a selective right middle cerebral artery catheterization includes the introduction and placement catheterization of the right common and internal carotid arteries).

Additional second and/or third order arterial catheterization within the same family of arteries or veins supplied by a single first order vessel should be expressed by 36012, 36218, or 36248.

Additional first order or higher catheterization in vascular families supplied by a first order vessel different from a previously selected and coded family should be separately coded using the conventions described above.

Surgical Procedures on Arteries and Veins

Primary vascular procedure listings include establishing both inflow and outflow by whatever procedures necessary. Also included is that portion of the operative arteriogram performed by the surgeon, as indicated. Sympathectomy, when done, is included in the listed aortic procedures. For unlisted vascular procedure, use 37799.

Please see the Surgery Guidelines section for the following guidelines:

- *Surgical Procedures on the Cardiovascular System*

AMA Coding Notes

Central Venous Access Procedures

(For refilling and maintenance of an implantable pump or reservoir for intravenous or intra-arterial drug delivery, use 96522)

Vascular Introduction and Injection Procedures

(For radiological supervision and interpretation, see Radiology)

(For injection procedures in conjunction with cardiac catheterization, see 93452-93461, 93563-93568)

(For chemotherapy of malignant disease, see 96401-96549)

AMA *CPT Assistant* ▢

36597: Dec 04: 12, Sep 14: 5

Plain English Description

A separately reportable chest radiograph is obtained and the CVC tip is determined to be improperly positioned. Any sutures anchoring the CVC to the skin are removed. The physician then manipulates the catheter tip into the desired location under separately reportable fluoroscopic guidance. The catheter is secured with sutures and a dressing applied.

Repositioning of previously placed central venous catheter; fluoroscopic guidance

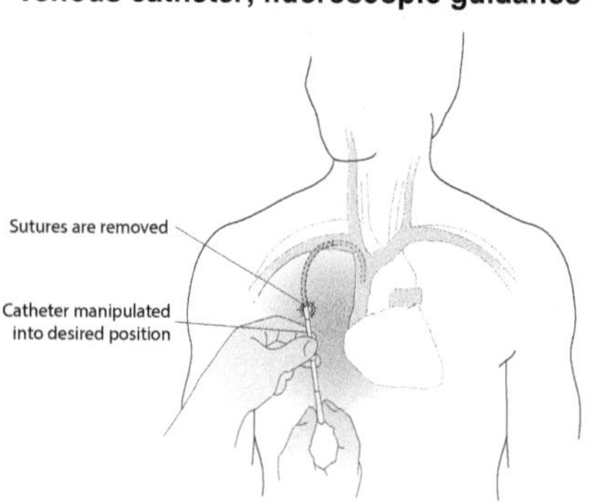

ICD-10-CM Diagnostic Codes

⑦	T80.212	Local infection due to central venous catheter
⑦	T82.528	Displacement of other cardiac and vascular devices and implants
⑦	T82.598	Other mechanical complication of other cardiac and vascular devices and implants
⑦	T82.828	Fibrosis due to vascular prosthetic devices, implants and grafts
⑦	T82.898	Other specified complication of vascular prosthetic devices, implants and grafts
	Z45.2	Encounter for adjustment and management of vascular access device

ICD-10-CM Coding Notes

For codes requiring a 7th character extension, refer to your ICD-10-CM book. Review the character descriptions and coding guidelines for proper selection. For some procedures, only certain characters will apply.

CCI Edits

Refer to Appendix A for CCI edits.

Facility RVUs ▢

Code	Work	PE Facility	MP	Total Facility
36597	1.21	0.43	0.13	1.77

Non-facility RVUs ▢

Code	Work	PE Non-Facility	MP	Total Non-Facility
36597	1.21	2.35	0.13	3.69

Modifiers (PAR) ▢

Code	Mod 50	Mod 51	Mod 62	Mod 66	Mod 80
36597	0	2	0	0	1

Global Period

Code	Days
36597	000

● New ▲ Revised ✚ Add On ⊘Modifier 51 Exempt ★Telemedicine ▢ CPT QuickRef ⁄FDA Pending ⇄ Laterality ⑦Seventh Character ♂Male ♀Female

CPT © 2018 American Medical Association. All Rights Reserved.

36598

36598 Contrast injection(s) for radiologic evaluation of existing central venous access device, including fluoroscopy, image documentation and report

(Do not report 36598 in conjunction with 76000)

(Do not report 36598 in conjunction with 36595, 36596)

(For complete diagnostic studies, see 75820, 75825, 75827)

AMA Coding Guideline

Central Venous Access Procedures

To qualify as a central venous access catheter or device, the tip of the catheter/device must terminate in the subclavian, brachiocephalic (innominate) or iliac veins, the superior or inferior vena cava, or the right atrium. The venous access device may be either centrally inserted (jugular, subclavian, femoral vein or inferior vena cava catheter entry site) or peripherally inserted (eg, basilic, cephalic, or saphenous vein entry site). The device may be accessed for use either via exposed catheter (external to the skin), via a subcutaneous port or via a subcutaneous pump.

The procedures involving these types of devices fall into five categories:

1. Insertion (placement of catheter through a newly established venous access)
2. Repair (fixing device without replacement of either catheter or port/pump, other than pharmacologic or mechanical correction of intracatheter or pericatheter occlusion [see 36595 or 36596])
3. Partial replacement of only the catheter component associated with a port/pump device, but not entire device
4. Complete replacement of entire device via same venous access site (complete exchange)
5. Removal of entire device.

There is no coding distinction between venous access achieved percutaneously versus by cutdown or based on catheter size.

For the repair, partial (catheter only) replacement, complete replacement, or removal of both catheters (placed from separate venous access sites) of a multi-catheter device, with or without subcutaneous ports/pumps, use the appropriate code describing the service with a frequency of two.

If an existing central venous access device is removed and a new one placed via a separate venous access site, appropriate codes for both procedures (removal of old, if code exists, and insertion of new device) should be reported.

When imaging guidance is used for centrally inserted central venous catheters, for gaining access to the venous entry site and/or for manipulating the catheter into final central position, imaging guidance codes (eg, 76937, 77001) may be reported separately. Do not use 76937, 77001 in conjunction with 36568, 36569, 36572, 36573, 36584.

Please see the Surgical Guidelines section for the following table: The Central Venous Access Procedures Table

Vascular Introduction and Injection Procedures

Listed services for injection procedures include necessary local anesthesia, introduction of needles or catheter, injection of contrast media with or without automatic power injection, and/or necessary pre- and postinjection care specifically related to the injection procedure.

Selective vascular catheterization should be coded to include introduction and all lesser order selective catheterization used in the approach (eg, the description for a selective right middle cerebral artery catheterization includes the introduction and placement catheterization of the right common and internal carotid arteries).

Additional second and/or third order arterial catheterization within the same family of arteries or veins supplied by a single first order vessel should be expressed by 36012, 36218, or 36248.

Additional first order or higher catheterization in vascular families supplied by a first order vessel different from a previously selected and coded family should be separately coded using the conventions described above.

Surgical Procedures on Arteries and Veins

Primary vascular procedure listings include establishing both inflow and outflow by whatever procedures necessary. Also included is that portion of the operative arteriogram performed by the surgeon, as indicated. Sympathectomy, when done, is included in the listed aortic procedures. For unlisted vascular procedure, use 37799.

Please see the Surgery Guidelines section for the following guidelines:

- *Surgical Procedures on the Cardiovascular System*

AMA Coding Notes

Central Venous Access Procedures

(For refilling and maintenance of an implantable pump or reservoir for intravenous or intra-arterial drug delivery, use 96522)

Vascular Introduction and Injection Procedures

(For radiological supervision and interpretation, see Radiology)

(For injection procedures in conjunction with cardiac catheterization, see 93452-93461, 93563-93568)

(For chemotherapy of malignant disease, see 96401-96549)

Plain English Description

Fluoroscopic evaluation is performed to confirm that the tip is properly positioned and that the catheter has not fractured or kinked. A CVC without a subcutaneous port is accessed by inserting a needle through the catheter hub. A CVC with a port or pump is accessed using a Huber needle. Contrast is injected. Fluoroscopic images are obtained of the catheter tip and along the course of the catheter to evaluate patency of the catheter and determine if there are any leaks. Upon completion of the contrast evaluation, the catheter is flushed with saline followed by an anticoagulant solution.

Contrast injection for radiologic evaluation of existing central venous access device

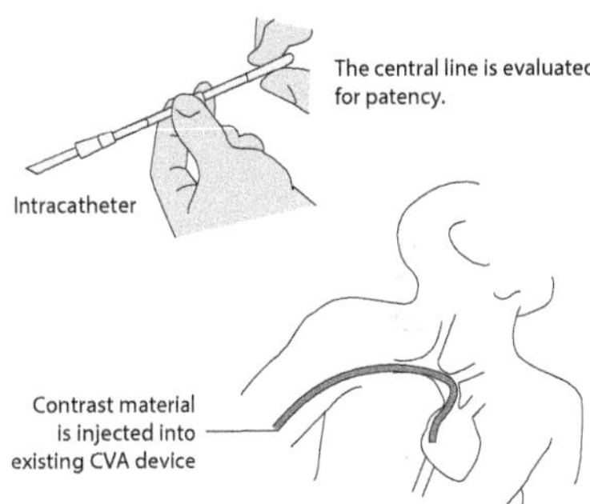

ICD-10-CM Diagnostic Codes

❼	T80.212	Local infection due to central venous catheter
❼	T80.218	Other infection due to central venous catheter
❼	T82.528	Displacement of other cardiac and vascular devices and implants
❼	T82.538	Leakage of other cardiac and vascular devices and implants
❼	T82.598	Other mechanical complication of other cardiac and vascular devices and implants
❼	T82.828	Fibrosis due to vascular prosthetic devices, implants and grafts
❼	T82.898	Other specified complication of vascular prosthetic devices, implants and grafts
	Z45.2	Encounter for adjustment and management of vascular access device

ICD-10-CM Coding Notes

For codes requiring a 7th character extension, refer to your ICD-10-CM book. Review the character descriptions and coding guidelines for proper selection. For some procedures, only certain characters will apply.

CCI Edits

Refer to Appendix A for CCI edits.

Pub 100

36598: Pub 100-04, 6, 20.6

CPT © 2018 American Medical Association. All Rights Reserved.

Facility RVUs

Code	Work	PE Facility	MP	Total Facility
36598	0.74	0.25	0.07	1.06

Non-facility RVUs

Code	Work	PE Non-Facility	MP	Total Non-Facility
36598	0.74	2.49	0.07	3.30

Modifiers (PAR)

Code	Mod 50	Mod 51	Mod 62	Mod 66	Mod 80
36598	1	2	0	0	0

Global Period

Code	Days
36598	000

CPT © 2018 American Medical Association. All Rights Reserved.

36600

36600 Arterial puncture, withdrawal of blood for diagnosis

AMA Coding Guideline

Surgical Procedures on Arteries and Veins

Primary vascular procedure listings include establishing both inflow and outflow by whatever procedures necessary. Also included is that portion of the operative arteriogram performed by the surgeon, as indicated. Sympathectomy, when done, is included in the listed aortic procedures. For unlisted vascular procedure, use 37799.

Please see the Surgery Guidelines section for the following guidelines:

- *Surgical Procedures on the Cardiovascular System*

AMA *CPT Assistant* ▢

36600: Fall 95: 7, Aug 00: 2, Oct 03: 2, Jul 05: 11, Jul 06: 4, Feb 07: 10, Jul 07: 1, May 14: 4

Plain English Description

The radial artery is the most common site for arterial puncture with alternative sites being the axillary and femoral arteries. The arterial puncture site is selected. The skin is prepped for sterile entry. The selected artery is punctured and the necessary blood samples obtained for separately reportable laboratory studies. The needle is withdrawn and pressure applied to the puncture site.

Arterial puncture, for blood sampling

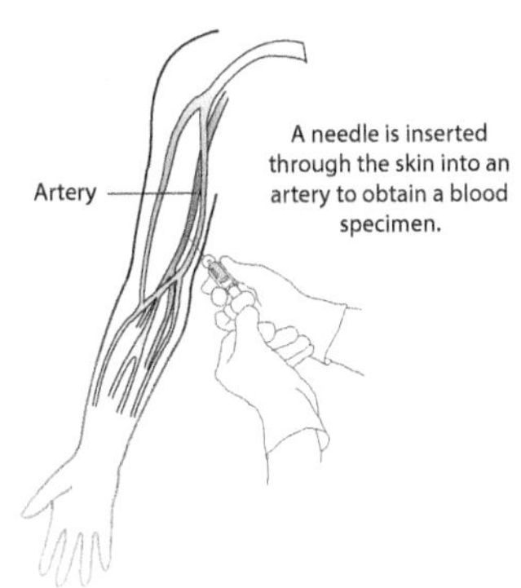
A needle is inserted through the skin into an artery to obtain a blood specimen.
Artery

ICD-10-CM Diagnostic Codes

There are too many ICD-10-CM codes to list. Refer to ICD-10-CM code book for associated diagnostic codes.

CCI Edits

Refer to Appendix A for CCI edits.

Pub 100

36600: Pub 100-04, 12, 30.6.12

Facility RVUs ▢

Code	Work	PE Facility	MP	Total Facility
36600	0.32	0.10	0.03	0.45

Non-facility RVUs ▢

Code	Work	PE Non-Facility	MP	Total Non-Facility
36600	0.32	0.52	0.03	0.87

Modifiers (PAR) ▢

Code	Mod 50	Mod 51	Mod 62	Mod 66	Mod 80
36600	0	2	0	0	1

Global Period

Code	Days
36600	XXX

CPT © 2018 American Medical Association. All Rights Reserved.

36620-36625

⊘ **36620 Arterial catheterization or cannulation for sampling, monitoring or transfusion (separate procedure); percutaneous**

36625 Arterial catheterization or cannulation for sampling, monitoring or transfusion (separate procedure); cutdown

AMA Coding Guideline

Surgical Procedures on Arteries and Veins

Primary vascular procedure listings include establishing both inflow and outflow by whatever procedures necessary. Also included is that portion of the operative arteriogram performed by the surgeon, as indicated. Sympathectomy, when done, is included in the listed aortic procedures. For unlisted vascular procedure, use 37799.

Please see the Surgery Guidelines section for the following guidelines:

- *Surgical Procedures on the Cardiovascular System*

AMA *CPT Assistant* ▢

36620: Fall 95: 7, Apr 98: 3, Nov 99: 32-33, Aug 00: 2, Oct 03: 2, Jul 06: 4, Jul 07: 1
36625: Fall 95: 7

Plain English Description

Arterial catheterization or cannulation is performed for sampling, monitoring or transfusion. This procedure may be performed to obtain arterial blood samples for blood gas monitoring, to monitor blood pressure, or for blood transfusion. The radial artery is the most common site for arterial catheterization or cannulation with alternative sites being the axillary and femoral arteries. The insertion site is selected, the skin is prepped for sterile entry, and a local anesthetic injected. Using a Seldinger technique, the skin and artery are punctured with a needle or a cutdown is performed to expose the artery followed by needle puncture. A guidewire is inserted through the needle and advanced several centimeters. An introducer sheath and dilator are advanced over the guidewire and the guidewire and dilator removed. The arterial line is then advanced through the introducer sheath and into the artery. Placement is checked as needed by separately reportable radiographs. The catheter or cannula is secured with tape and a dressing applied over the insertion site. Use 36620 for percutaneous insertion by puncturing the skin and artery. Use 36625 for cutdown, which involves incising the skin over the artery and then dissecting the artery free of surrounding tissue prior to needle puncture.

Arterial catheterization/cannulation

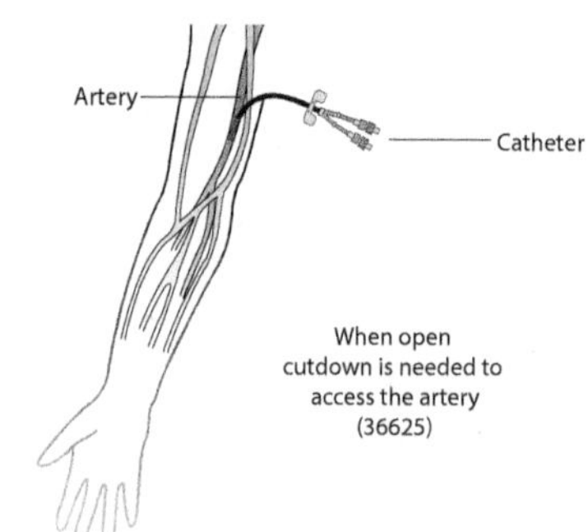
Artery
Catheter
When open cutdown is needed to access the artery (36625)

A needle is inserted through the skin to introduce a catheter or cannula into an artery for blood sampling, monitoring, or transfusion (36620).

ICD-10-CM Diagnostic Codes

There are too many ICD-10-CM codes to list. Refer to ICD-10-CM code book for associated diagnostic codes.

CCI Edits

Refer to Appendix A for CCI edits.

Facility RVUs ▢

Code	Work	PE Facility	MP	Total Facility
36620	1.00	0.20	0.08	1.28
36625	2.11	0.61	0.33	3.05

Non-facility RVUs ▢

Code	Work	PE Non-Facility	MP	Total Non-Facility
36620	1.00	0.20	0.08	1.28
36625	2.11	0.61	0.33	3.05

Modifiers (PAR) ▢

Code	Mod 50	Mod 51	Mod 62	Mod 66	Mod 80
36620	0	0	0	0	1
36625	0	0	0	0	1

Global Period

Code	Days
36620	000
36625	000

CPT © 2018 American Medical Association. All Rights Reserved.

61050-61055

61050 Cisternal or lateral cervical (C1-C2) puncture; without injection (separate procedure)

61055 Cisternal or lateral cervical (C1-C2) puncture; with injection of medication or other substance for diagnosis or treatment

(Do not report 61055 in conjunction with 62302, 62303, 62304, 62305)

(For radiological supervision and interpretation by a different physician or qualified health care professional, see Radiology)

AMA Coding Notes

Surgical Procedures on the Skull, Meninges, and Brain

(For injection procedure for cerebral angiography, see 36100-36218)

(For injection procedure for ventriculography, see 61026, 61120)

(For injection procedure for pneumoencephalography, use 61055)

Plain English Description

A cisternal or lateral cervical (C1-2) puncture is performed with or without injection. A cisternal puncture uses a spinal needle placed below the occipital bone at the back of the skull. Alternatively, the subarachnoid space in the posterior aspect of the spinal canal can be approached from a lateral direction. The needle shaft is held in place by the muscles in the lateral neck. After insertion of the needle, the stylet is removed and cerebrospinal fluid and blood is drained. The stylet is then replaced and a dressing is applied. Use code 61055 for a cisternal or lateral cervical (C1-2) punctured performed with injection of medication or other substance for diagnosis or treatment. The puncture procedure is performed as described above. As cerebrospinal fluid is withdrawn from the subarachnoid space, an equal amount of medication or other substance, such as gas, contrast media, dye, or radioactive material, is instilled. If the injection is performed for gas myelography or other radiologic procedure, separately reportable radiographs are obtained.

Cisternal or lateral cervical puncture (C1-C2)

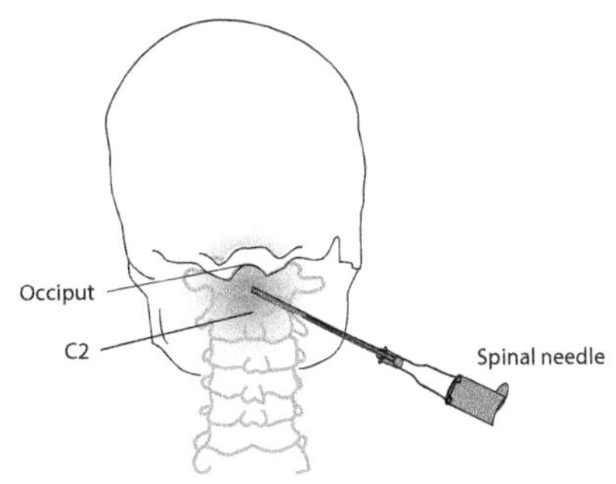

Without injection (61050); with injection of medication or other substance for diagnosis or treatment (61055)

ICD-10-CM Diagnostic Codes

G95.89	Other specified diseases of spinal cord
G95.9	Disease of spinal cord, unspecified
G96.12	Meningeal adhesions (cerebral) (spinal)
G96.19	Other disorders of meninges, not elsewhere classified

CCI Edits

Refer to Appendix A for CCI edits.

Facility RVUs ☐

Code	Work	PE Facility	MP	Total Facility
61050	1.51	0.80	0.14	2.45
61055	2.10	1.08	0.44	3.62

Non-facility RVUs ☐

Code	Work	PE Non-Facility	MP	Total Non-Facility
61050	1.51	0.80	0.14	2.45
61055	2.10	1.08	0.44	3.62

Modifiers (PAR) ☐

Code	Mod 50	Mod 51	Mod 62	Mod 66	Mod 80
61050	0	2	0	0	0
61055	0	0	0	0	1

Global Period

Code	Days
61050	000
61055	000

CPT © 2018 American Medical Association. All Rights Reserved.

62270-62272

62270 Spinal puncture, lumbar, diagnostic

62272 Spinal puncture, therapeutic, for drainage of cerebrospinal fluid (by needle or catheter)

AMA Coding Guideline

Injection, Drainage, or Aspiration Procedures on the Spine and Spinal Cord

Injection of contrast during fluoroscopic guidance and localization is an inclusive component of 62263, 62264, 62267, 62270, 62272, 62273, 62280, 62281, 62282, 62302, 62303, 62304, 62305, 62321, 62323, 62325, 62327. Fluoroscopic guidance and localization is reported with 77003, unless a formal contrast study (myelography, epidurography, or arthrography) is performed, in which case the use of fluoroscopy is included in the supervision and interpretation codes or the myelography via lumbar injection code. Image guidance and the injection of contrast are inclusive components and are required for the performance of myelography, as described by codes 62302, 62303, 62304, 62305.

For radiologic supervision and interpretation of epidurography, use 72275. Code 72275 is only to be used when an epidurogram is performed, images documented, and a formal radiologic report is issued.

Code 62263 describes a catheter-based treatment involving targeted injection of various substances (eg, hypertonic saline, steroid, anesthetic) via an indwelling epidural catheter. Code 62263 includes percutaneous insertion and removal of an epidural catheter (remaining in place over a several-day period), for the administration of multiple injections of a neurolytic agent(s) performed during serial treatment sessions (ie, spanning two or more treatment days). If required, adhesions or scarring may also be lysed by mechanical means. Code 62263 is not reported for each adhesiolysis treatment, but should be reported once to describe the entire series of injections/infusions spanning two or more treatment days.

Code 62264 describes multiple adhesiolysis treatment sessions performed on the same day. Adhesions or scarring may be lysed by injections of neurolytic agent(s). If required, adhesions or scarring may also be lysed mechanically using a percutaneously-deployed catheter.

Codes 62263 and 62264 include the procedure of injections of contrast for epidurography (72275) and fluoroscopic guidance and localization (77003) during initial or subsequent sessions.

Fluoroscopy or CT and any injection of contrast are inclusive components of 62321, 62323, 62325, 62327. For epidurography, use 72275.

The placement and use of a catheter to administer one or more epidural or subarachnoid injections on a single calendar day should be reported in the same manner as if a needle had been used, ie, as a single injection using either 62320, 62321, 62322, or 62323. Such injections should not be reported with 62324, 62325, 62326, or 62327. Threading a catheter into the epidural space, injecting substances at one or more levels and then removing the catheter should be treated as a single injection (62320, 62321, 62322, 62323). If the catheter is left in place to deliver substance(s) over a prolonged period (ie, more than a single calendar day) either continuously or via intermittent bolus, use 62324, 62325, 62326, 62327 as appropriate.

When reporting 62320, 62321, 62322, 62323, 62324, 62325, 62326, 62327 code choice is based on the region at which the needle or catheter entered the body (eg, lumbar). Codes 62320, 62321, 62322, 62323, 62324, 62325, 62326, 62327 should be reported only once, when the substance injected spreads or catheter tip insertion moves into another spinal region (eg, 62322 is reported only once for injection or catheter insertion at L3-4 with spread of the substance or placement of the catheter tip to the thoracic region).

Percutaneous spinal procedures are done with indirect visualization (eg, image guidance) (eg, 62287). Endoscopic assistance during an open procedure with continuous and direct visualization (light-based) is reported using excision codes (eg, 63020-63035).

Definitions

For purposes of CPT coding, the following definitions of approach and visualization apply. The primary approach and visualization define the service, whether another method is incidentally applied. Surgical services are presumed open, unless otherwise specified.

Percutaneous: Image-guided procedures (eg, computer tomography [CT] or fluoroscopy) performed with indirect visualization of the spine without the use of any device that allows visualization through a surgical incision.

Endoscopic: Spinal procedures performed with continuous direct visualization of the spine through an endoscope.

Open: Spinal procedures performed with continuous direct visualization of the spine through a surgical opening.

Indirect visualization: Image-guided (eg, CT or fluoroscopy), not light-based visualization.

Direct visualization: Light-based visualization; can be performed by eye, or with surgical loupes, microscope, or endoscope.

AMA Coding Notes

Injection, Drainage, or Aspiration Procedures on the Spine and Spinal Cord

(For transforaminal epidural injection, see 64479-64484)

(Report 01996 for daily hospital management of continuous epidural or subarachnoid drug administration performed in conjunction with 62324, 62325, 62326, 62327)

(For the techniques of microsurgery and/or use of microscope, use 69990)

Surgical Procedures on the Spine and Spinal Cord

(For application of caliper or tongs, use 20660)

(For treatment of fracture or dislocation of spine, see 22310-22327)

AMA *CPT Assistant* □

62270: Nov 99: 32-33, Oct 03: 2, Jul 06: 4, Jul 07: 1, Oct 09: 12, Nov 10: 3, Jan 11: 8, Mar 12: 3

62272: Nov 99: 32-33, Nov 10: 3, Dec 13: 14

Plain English Description

A lumbar spinal puncture is performed for diagnostic or therapeutic purposes. In 62270, a diagnostic lumbar puncture is performed for symptoms that may be indicative of an infection, such as meningitis; a malignant neoplasm; bleeding, such as subarachnoid hemorrhage; multiple sclerosis; Guillain-Barre syndrome. It may also be performed to measure cerebrospinal fluid (CSF) pressure. The skin over the lumbar spine is disinfected and a local anesthetic administered. A lumbar puncture needle is then inserted into the spinal canal and CSF specimens collected. The CSF specimens are sent to the laboratory for separately reportable evaluation. In 62272, a therapeutic spinal puncture is performed for elevated CSF pressure and CSF is drained using a needle or catheter placed as described above. CSF pressure is monitored during the drainage procedure and when the desired pressure is reached, the needle or catheter is removed.

Spinal puncture

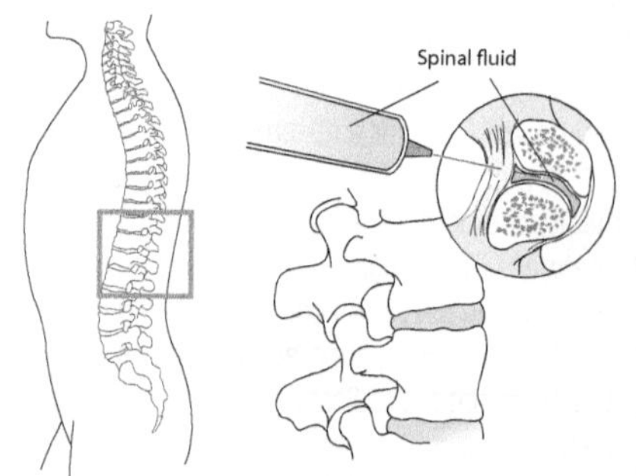

A small amount of spinal fluid is removed through a needle/catheter. Lumbar, diagnostic (62270); therapeutic drainage (62272)

ICD-10-CM Diagnostic Codes

A39.0	Meningococcal meningitis
A39.81	Meningococcal encephalitis
C91.00	Acute lymphoblastic leukemia not having achieved remission
C91.02	Acute lymphoblastic leukemia, in relapse
C92.00	Acute myeloblastic leukemia, not having achieved remission
C92.02	Acute myeloblastic leukemia, in relapse
G00.0	Hemophilus meningitis
G00.1	Pneumococcal meningitis
G00.2	Streptococcal meningitis
G00.3	Staphylococcal meningitis

CPT © 2018 American Medical Association. All Rights Reserved.

G00.8	Other bacterial meningitis
G00.9	Bacterial meningitis, unspecified
G01	Meningitis in bacterial diseases classified elsewhere
G02	Meningitis in other infectious and parasitic diseases classified elsewhere
G03.9	Meningitis, unspecified
G44.52	New daily persistent headache (NDPH)
G93.2	Benign intracranial hypertension
I60.8	Other nontraumatic subarachnoid hemorrhage
I60.9	Nontraumatic subarachnoid hemorrhage, unspecified
P10.3	Subarachnoid hemorrhage due to birth injury
P52.5	Subarachnoid (nontraumatic) hemorrhage of newborn
R51	Headache

CCI Edits

Refer to Appendix A for CCI edits.

Facility RVUs ☐

Code	Work	PE Facility	MP	Total Facility
62270	1.37	0.68	0.18	2.23
62272	1.35	0.76	0.30	2.41

Non-facility RVUs ☐

Code	Work	PE Non-Facility	MP	Total Non-Facility
62270	1.37	2.67	0.18	4.22
62272	1.35	3.92	0.30	5.57

Modifiers (PAR) ☐

Code	Mod 50	Mod 51	Mod 62	Mod 66	Mod 80
62270	0	2	0	0	1
62272	0	2	0	0	1

Global Period

Code	Days
62270	000
62272	000

CPT © 2018 American Medical Association. All Rights Reserved.

62273

62273 Injection, epidural, of blood or clot patch

(For injection of diagnostic or therapeutic substance[s], see 62320, 62321, 62322, 62323, 62324, 62325, 62326, 62327)

AMA Coding Guideline

Injection, Drainage, or Aspiration Procedures on the Spine and Spinal Cord

Injection of contrast during fluoroscopic guidance and localization is an inclusive component of 62263, 62264, 62267, 62270, 62272, 62273, 62280, 62281, 62282, 62302, 62303, 62304, 62305, 62321, 62323, 62325, 62327. Fluoroscopic guidance and localization is reported with 77003, unless a formal contrast study (myelography, epidurography, or arthrography) is performed, in which case the use of fluoroscopy is included in the supervision and interpretation codes or the myelography via lumbar injection code. Image guidance and the injection of contrast are inclusive components and are required for the performance of myelography, as described by codes 62302, 62303, 62304, 62305.

For radiologic supervision and interpretation of epidurography, use 72275. Code 72275 is only to be used when an epidurogram is performed, images documented, and a formal radiologic report is issued.

Code 62263 describes a catheter-based treatment involving targeted injection of various substances (eg, hypertonic saline, steroid, anesthetic) via an indwelling epidural catheter. Code 62263 includes percutaneous insertion and removal of an epidural catheter (remaining in place over a several-day period), for the administration of multiple injections of a neurolytic agent(s) performed during serial treatment sessions (ie, spanning two or more treatment days). If required, adhesions or scarring may also be lysed by mechanical means. Code 62263 is not reported for each adhesiolysis treatment, but should be reported once to describe the entire series of injections/infusions spanning two or more treatment days.

Code 62264 describes multiple adhesiolysis treatment sessions performed on the same day. Adhesions or scarring may be lysed by injections of neurolytic agent(s). If required, adhesions or scarring may also be lysed mechanically using a percutaneously-deployed catheter.

Codes 62263 and 62264 include the procedure of injections of contrast for epidurography (72275) and fluoroscopic guidance and localization (77003) during initial or subsequent sessions.

Fluoroscopy or CT and any injection of contrast are inclusive components of 62321, 62323, 62325, 62327. For epidurography, use 72275.

The placement and use of a catheter to administer one or more epidural or subarachnoid injections on a single calendar day should be reported in the same manner as if a needle had been used, ie, as a single injection using either 62320, 62321, 62322, or 62323. Such injections should not be reported with 62324, 62325, 62326, or 62327.

Threading a catheter into the epidural space, injecting substances at one or more levels and then removing the catheter should be treated as a single injection (62320, 62321, 62322, 62323). If the catheter is left in place to deliver substance(s) over a prolonged period (ie, more than a single calendar day) either continuously or via intermittent bolus, use 62324, 62325, 62326, 62327 as appropriate.

When reporting 62320, 62321, 62322, 62323, 62324, 62325, 62326, 62327 code choice is based on the region at which the needle or catheter entered the body (eg, lumbar). Codes 62320, 62321, 62322, 62323, 62324, 62325, 62326, 62327 should be reported only once, when the substance injected spreads or catheter tip insertion moves into another spinal region (eg, 62322 is reported only once for injection or catheter insertion at L3-4 with spread of the substance or placement of the catheter tip to the thoracic region).

Percutaneous spinal procedures are done with indirect visualization (eg, image guidance) (eg, 62287). Endoscopic assistance during an open procedure with continuous and direct visualization (light-based) is reported using excision codes (eg, 63020-63035).

Definitions

For purposes of CPT coding, the following definitions of approach and visualization apply. The primary approach and visualization define the service, whether another method is incidentally applied. Surgical services are presumed open, unless otherwise specified.

Percutaneous: Image-guided procedures (eg, computer tomography [CT] or fluoroscopy) performed with indirect visualization of the spine without the use of any device that allows visualization through a surgical incision.

Endoscopic: Spinal procedures performed with continuous direct visualization of the spine through an endoscope.

Open: Spinal procedures performed with continuous direct visualization of the spine through a surgical opening.

Indirect visualization: Image-guided (eg, CT or fluoroscopy), not light-based visualization.

Direct visualization: Light-based visualization; can be performed by eye, or with surgical loupes, microscope, or endoscope.

AMA Coding Notes

Injection, Drainage, or Aspiration Procedures on the Spine and Spinal Cord

(For transforaminal epidural injection, see 64479-64484)

(Report 01996 for daily hospital management of continuous epidural or subarachnoid drug administration performed in conjunction with 62324, 62325, 62326, 62327)

(For the techniques of microsurgery and/or use of microscope, use 69990)

Surgical Procedures on the Spine and Spinal Cord

(For application of caliper or tongs, use 20660)

(For treatment of fracture or dislocation of spine, see 22310-22327)

AMA *CPT Assistant* □

62273: Nov 99: 32-34, Oct 09: 12, Nov 10: 3

Plain English Description

The physician injects a blood or clot patch into the epidural space. Epidural blood patches are used to treat the complication of severe headache caused by a leak of spinal fluid into the epidural space following epidural anesthesia or diagnostic or therapeutic spinal punctures. The skin over the lower back is disinfected and local anesthetic injected. A separate site is prepped for a venipuncture and an intravenous catheter is placed in the vein. The epidural needle is placed in the epidural space near the site of the previous puncture site. Blood is withdrawn from the venous catheter and the blood is then injected into the epidural space. The patient rests for approximately 30 minutes while the blood forms a patch over the CSF leak.

Blood or clot patch injection

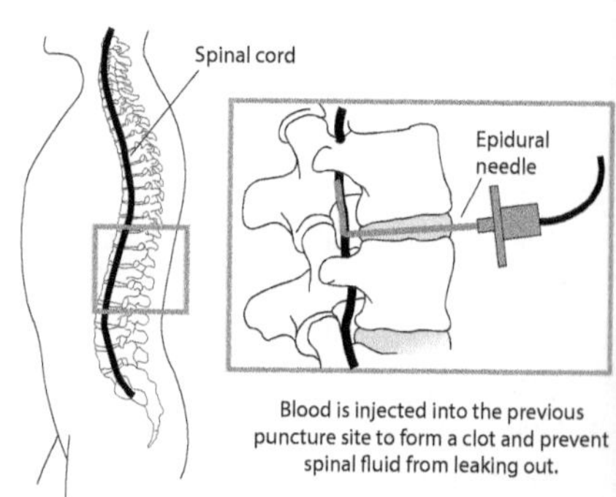

Blood is injected into the previous puncture site to form a clot and prevent spinal fluid from leaking out.

ICD-10-CM Diagnostic Codes

G97.0	Cerebrospinal fluid leak from spinal puncture
G97.1	Other reaction to spinal and lumbar puncture

CCI Edits

Refer to Appendix A for CCI edits.

CPT © 2018 American Medical Association. All Rights Reserved.

Facility RVUs

Code	Work	PE Facility	MP	Total Facility
62273	2.15	0.92	0.19	3.26

Non-facility RVUs

Code	Work	PE Non-Facility	MP	Total Non-Facility
62273	2.15	2.59	0.19	4.93

Modifiers (PAR)

Code	Mod 50	Mod 51	Mod 62	Mod 66	Mod 80
62273	0	2	0	0	1

Global Period

Code	Days
62273	000

CPT © 2018 American Medical Association. All Rights Reserved.

62280-62282

62280 Injection/infusion of neurolytic substance (eg, alcohol, phenol, iced saline solutions), with or without other therapeutic substance; subarachnoid

62281 Injection/infusion of neurolytic substance (eg, alcohol, phenol, iced saline solutions), with or without other therapeutic substance; epidural, cervical or thoracic

62282 Injection/infusion of neurolytic substance (eg, alcohol, phenol, iced saline solutions), with or without other therapeutic substance; epidural, lumbar, sacral (caudal)

AMA Coding Guideline

Injection, Drainage, or Aspiration Procedures on the Spine and Spinal Cord

Injection of contrast during fluoroscopic guidance and localization is an inclusive component of 62263, 62264, 62267, 62270, 62272, 62273, 62280, 62281, 62282, 62302, 62303, 62304, 62305, 62321, 62323, 62325, 62327. Fluoroscopic guidance and localization is reported with 77003, unless a formal contrast study (myelography, epidurography, or arthrography) is performed, in which case the use of fluoroscopy is included in the supervision and interpretation codes or the myelography via lumbar injection code. Image guidance and the injection of contrast are inclusive components and are required for the performance of myelography, as described by codes 62302, 62303, 62304, 62305.

For radiologic supervision and interpretation of epidurography, use 72275. Code 72275 is only to be used when an epidurogram is performed, images documented, and a formal radiologic report is issued.

Code 62263 describes a catheter-based treatment involving targeted injection of various substances (eg, hypertonic saline, steroid, anesthetic) via an indwelling epidural catheter. Code 62263 includes percutaneous insertion and removal of an epidural catheter (remaining in place over a several-day period), for the administration of multiple injections of a neurolytic agent(s) performed during serial treatment sessions (ie, spanning two or more treatment days). If required, adhesions or scarring may also be lysed by mechanical means. Code 62263 is not reported for each adhesiolysis treatment, but should be reported once to describe the entire series of injections/infusions spanning two or more treatment days.

Code 62264 describes multiple adhesiolysis treatment sessions performed on the same day. Adhesions or scarring may be lysed by injections of neurolytic agent(s). If required, adhesions or scarring may also be lysed mechanically using a percutaneously-deployed catheter.

Codes 62263 and 62264 include the procedure of injections of contrast for epidurography (72275) and fluoroscopic guidance and localization (77003) during initial or subsequent sessions.

Fluoroscopy or CT and any injection of contrast are inclusive components of 62321, 62323, 62325, 62327. For epidurography, use 72275.

The placement and use of a catheter to administer one or more epidural or subarachnoid injections on a single calendar day should be reported in the same manner as if a needle had been used, ie, as a single injection using either 62320, 62321, 62322, or 62323. Such injections should not be reported with 62324, 62325, 62326, or 62327.

Threading a catheter into the epidural space, injecting substances at one or more levels and then removing the catheter should be treated as a single injection (62320, 62321, 62322, 62323). If the catheter is left in place to deliver substance(s) over a prolonged period (ie, more than a single calendar day) either continuously or via intermittent bolus, use 62324, 62325, 62326, 62327 as appropriate.

When reporting 62320, 62321, 62322, 62323, 62324, 62325, 62326, 62327 code choice is based on the region at which the needle or catheter entered the body (eg, lumbar). Codes 62320, 62321, 62322, 62323, 62324, 62325, 62326, 62327 should be reported only once, when the substance injected spreads or catheter tip insertion moves into another spinal region (eg, 62322 is reported only once for injection or catheter insertion at L3-4 with spread of the substance or placement of the catheter tip to the thoracic region).

Percutaneous spinal procedures are done with indirect visualization (eg, image guidance) (eg, 62287). Endoscopic assistance during an open procedure with continuous and direct visualization (light-based) is reported using excision codes (eg, 63020-63035).

Definitions

For purposes of CPT coding, the following definitions of approach and visualization apply. The primary approach and visualization define the service, whether another method is incidentally applied. Surgical services are presumed open, unless otherwise specified.

Percutaneous: Image-guided procedures (eg, computer tomography [CT] or fluoroscopy) performed with indirect visualization of the spine without the use of any device that allows visualization through a surgical incision.

Endoscopic: Spinal procedures performed with continuous direct visualization of the spine through an endoscope.

Open: Spinal procedures performed with continuous direct visualization of the spine through a surgical opening.

Indirect visualization: Image-guided (eg, CT or fluoroscopy), not light-based visualization.

Direct visualization: Light-based visualization; can be performed by eye, or with surgical loupes, microscope, or endoscope.

AMA Coding Notes

Injection, Drainage, or Aspiration Procedures on the Spine and Spinal Cord

(For transforaminal epidural injection, see 64479-64484)

(Report 01996 for daily hospital management of continuous epidural or subarachnoid drug administration performed in conjunction with 62324, 62325, 62326, 62327)

(For the techniques of microsurgery and/or use of microscope, use 69990)

Surgical Procedures on the Spine and Spinal Cord

(For application of caliper or tongs, use 20660)

(For treatment of fracture or dislocation of spine, see 22310-22327)

AMA *CPT Assistant* □

62280: Nov 99: 32-34, Jan 00: 2, Jul 08: 9, Oct 09: 12, Feb 10: 11, Nov 10: 3, Jan 11: 8, Jun 12: 12

62281: Apr 96: 11, Nov 99: 32-34, Jan 00: 2, Jul 08: 9, Oct 09: 12, Feb 10: 11, May 10: 10, Nov 10: 3, Jan 11: 8, Jun 12: 12

62282: Apr 96: 11, Nov 99: 32-34, Jan 00: 2, Jul 08: 9, Oct 09: 12, Feb 10: 11, Nov 10: 3, Jan 11: 8, Jun 12: 12

Plain English Description

This procedure may also be referred to as a neurolytic block. Neurolytic substances such as alcohol, phenol, or iced saline destroy neural structures involved in pain perception and provide long-lasting pain relief. Types of conditions treated include chronic, intractable, non-terminal pain that is not responsive to other pain management modalities or cancer pain. Neurolytic blocks can be performed by injection or infusion of a neurolytic substance into the subarachnoid space which lies between the arachnoid mater and pia mater, or into the epidural space which lies between the bone and the outermost membrane covering the spinal cord or dura mater. The patient is positioned on an x-ray table with the back exposed. The site where the injection is to be performed is cleansed and a local anesthetic administered. Using separately reportable fluoroscopic guidance, a spinal needle or cannula is inserted into the subarachnoid or epidural space. A small amount of contrast is injected to ensure that the needle or cannula is properly positioned. The neurolytic substance is then injected or infused. Use 62280 for a subarachnoid injection or infusion at any level of the spine; use 62281 for an epidural injection or infusion in the cervical or thoracic region; and use 62282 for an epidural injection or infusion in the lumbar or sacral (caudal) region.

CPT © 2018 American Medical Association. All Rights Reserved.

Injection/infusion of neurolytic substance

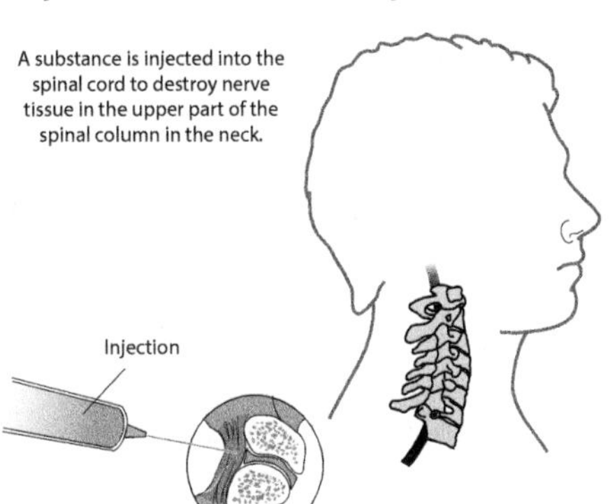

A substance is injected into the spinal cord to destroy nerve tissue in the upper part of the spinal column in the neck.
Injection

ICD-10-CM Diagnostic Codes

C76.0 Malignant neoplasm of head, face and neck
C76.1 Malignant neoplasm of thorax
C76.2 Malignant neoplasm of abdomen
C76.3 Malignant neoplasm of pelvis
C79.51 Secondary malignant neoplasm of bone
C79.89 Secondary malignant neoplasm of other specified sites
G89.11 Acute pain due to trauma
G89.12 Acute post-thoracotomy pain
G89.18 Other acute postprocedural pain
G89.21 Chronic pain due to trauma
G89.22 Chronic post-thoracotomy pain
G89.28 Other chronic postprocedural pain
G89.29 Other chronic pain
G89.3 Neoplasm related pain (acute) (chronic)
G89.4 Chronic pain syndrome
M54.11 Radiculopathy, occipito-atlanto-axial region
M54.12 Radiculopathy, cervical region
M54.13 Radiculopathy, cervicothoracic region
M54.14 Radiculopathy, thoracic region
M54.15 Radiculopathy, thoracolumbar region
M54.16 Radiculopathy, lumbar region
M54.17 Radiculopathy, lumbosacral region
M54.18 Radiculopathy, sacral and sacrococcygeal region
M54.2 Cervicalgia
⇄ M54.31 Sciatica, right side
⇄ M54.32 Sciatica, left side
⇄ M54.41 Lumbago with sciatica, right side
⇄ M54.42 Lumbago with sciatica, left side
M54.5 Low back pain
M54.6 Pain in thoracic spine
M54.81 Occipital neuralgia
M54.89 Other dorsalgia
M54.9 Dorsalgia, unspecified

CCI Edits

Refer to Appendix A for CCI edits.

Facility RVUs 🗆

Code	Work	PE Facility	MP	Total Facility
62280	2.63	1.66	0.47	4.76
62281	2.66	1.68	0.24	4.58
62282	2.33	1.60	0.23	4.16

Non-facility RVUs 🗆

Code	Work	PE Non-Facility	MP	Total Non-Facility
62280	2.63	6.35	0.47	9.45
62281	2.66	4.04	0.24	6.94
62282	2.33	6.07	0.23	8.63

Modifiers (PAR) 🗆

Code	Mod 50	Mod 51	Mod 62	Mod 66	Mod 80
62280	0	2	0	0	1
62281	0	2	0	0	1
62282	0	2	0	0	1

Global Period

Code	Days
62280	010
62281	010
62282	010

CPT © 2018 American Medical Association. All Rights Reserved.

62284

62284 Injection procedure for myelography and/or computed tomography, lumbar

(Do not report 62284 in conjunction with 62302, 62303, 62304, 62305, 72240, 72255, 72265, 72270)

(When both 62284 and 72240, 72255, 72265, 72270 are performed by the same physician or other qualified health care professional for myelography, see 62302, 62303, 62304, 62305)

(For injection procedure at C1-C2, use 61055)

(For radiological supervision and interpretation, see Radiology)

AMA Coding Guideline

Injection, Drainage, or Aspiration Procedures on the Spine and Spinal Cord

Injection of contrast during fluoroscopic guidance and localization is an inclusive component of 62263, 62264, 62267, 62270, 62272, 62273, 62280, 62281, 62282, 62302, 62303, 62304, 62305, 62321, 62323, 62325, 62327. Fluoroscopic guidance and localization is reported with 77003, unless a formal contrast study (myelography, epidurography, or arthrography) is performed, in which case the use of fluoroscopy is included in the supervision and interpretation codes or the myelography via lumbar injection code. Image guidance and the injection of contrast are inclusive components and are required for the performance of myelography, as described by codes 62302, 62303, 62304, 62305.

For radiologic supervision and interpretation of epidurography, use 72275. Code 72275 is only to be used when an epidurogram is performed, images documented, and a formal radiologic report is issued.

Code 62263 describes a catheter-based treatment involving targeted injection of various substances (eg, hypertonic saline, steroid, anesthetic) via an indwelling epidural catheter. Code 62263 includes percutaneous insertion and removal of an epidural catheter (remaining in place over a several-day period), for the administration of multiple injections of a neurolytic agent(s) performed during serial treatment sessions (ie, spanning two or more treatment days). If required, adhesions or scarring may also be lysed by mechanical means. Code 62263 is not reported for each adhesiolysis treatment, but should be reported once to describe the entire series of injections/infusions spanning two or more treatment days.

Code 62264 describes multiple adhesiolysis treatment sessions performed on the same day. Adhesions or scarring may be lysed by injections of neurolytic agent(s). If required, adhesions or scarring may also be lysed mechanically using a percutaneously-deployed catheter.

Codes 62263 and 62264 include the procedure of injections of contrast for epidurography (72275) and fluoroscopic guidance and localization (77003) during initial or subsequent sessions.

Fluoroscopy or CT and any injection of contrast are inclusive components of 62321, 62323, 62325, 62327. For epidurography, use 72275.

The placement and use of a catheter to administer one or more epidural or subarachnoid injections on a single calendar day should be reported in the same manner as if a needle had been used, ie, as a single injection using either 62320, 62321, 62322, or 62323. Such injections should not be reported with 62324, 62325, 62326, or 62327. Threading a catheter into the epidural space, injecting substances at one or more levels and then removing the catheter should be treated as a single injection (62320, 62321, 62322, 62323). If the catheter is left in place to deliver substance(s) over a prolonged period (ie, more than a single calendar day) either continuously or via intermittent bolus, use 62324, 62325, 62326, 62327 as appropriate.

When reporting 62320, 62321, 62322, 62323, 62324, 62325, 62326, 62327 code choice is based on the region at which the needle or catheter entered the body (eg, lumbar). Codes 62320, 62321, 62322, 62323, 62324, 62325, 62326, 62327 should be reported only once, when the substance injected spreads or catheter tip insertion moves into another spinal region (eg, 62322 is reported only once for injection or catheter insertion at L3-4 with spread of the substance or placement of the catheter tip to the thoracic region).

Percutaneous spinal procedures are done with indirect visualization (eg, image guidance) (eg, 62287). Endoscopic assistance during an open procedure with continuous and direct visualization (light-based) is reported using excision codes (eg, 63020-63035).

Definitions

For purposes of CPT coding, the following definitions of approach and visualization apply. The primary approach and visualization define the service, whether another method is incidentally applied. Surgical services are presumed open, unless otherwise specified.

Percutaneous: Image-guided procedures (eg, computer tomography [CT] or fluoroscopy) performed with indirect visualization of the spine without the use of any device that allows visualization through a surgical incision.

Endoscopic: Spinal procedures performed with continuous direct visualization of the spine through an endoscope.

Open: Spinal procedures performed with continuous direct visualization of the spine through a surgical opening.

Indirect visualization: Image-guided (eg, CT or fluoroscopy), not light-based visualization.

Direct visualization: Light-based visualization; can be performed by eye, or with surgical loupes, microscope, or endoscope.

AMA Coding Notes

Injection, Drainage, or Aspiration Procedures on the Spine and Spinal Cord

(For transforaminal epidural injection, see 64479-64484)

(Report 01996 for daily hospital management of continuous epidural or subarachnoid drug administration performed in conjunction with 62324, 62325, 62326, 62327)

(For the techniques of microsurgery and/or use of microscope, use 69990)

Surgical Procedures on the Spine and Spinal Cord

(For application of caliper or tongs, use 20660)

(For treatment of fracture or dislocation of spine, see 22310-22327)

AMA *CPT Assistant* ☐

62284: Fall 93: 13, Sep 04: 13

Plain English Description

The spinal canal (subarachnoid space) is injected with contrast material to visualize structures including the spinal cord and spinal nerve roots for separately reportable myelography and/or computed tomography (CT). This code is used to report injection procedures of the lumbar region of the spine. The patient is placed face-down on the examination table. The spine is visualized using separately reportable fluoroscopy. The skin over the planned injection site, usually the lower lumbar spine, is cleansed and a local anesthetic is injected. The patient may be repositioned if needed on the side or in a sitting position. A needle is then inserted into the subarachnoid space and contrast material is then injected and observed as it moves through the subarachnoid space enhancing visualization of the spinal cord, nerve roots, and surrounding soft tissues.

Injection procedure for myelography/CT

The spinal canal (subarachnoid space) is injected with contrast material to visualize the spinal cord and nerve roots.

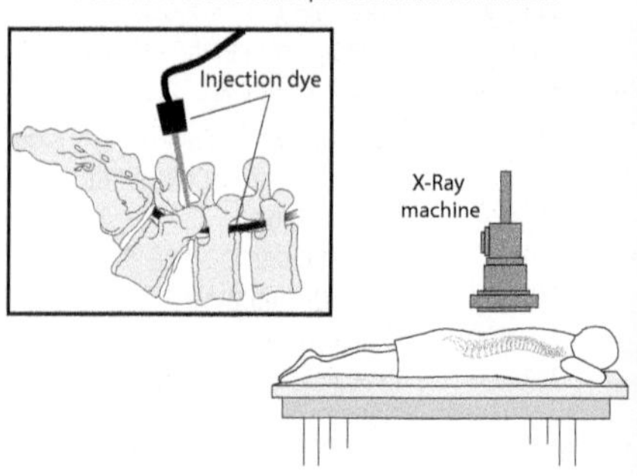

CPT © 2018 American Medical Association. All Rights Reserved.

ICD-10-CM Diagnostic Codes

M43.05 Spondylolysis, thoracolumbar region
M43.06 Spondylolysis, lumbar region
M43.07 Spondylolysis, lumbosacral region
M43.15 Spondylolisthesis, thoracolumbar region
M43.16 Spondylolisthesis, lumbar region
M43.17 Spondylolisthesis, lumbosacral region
M47.15 Other spondylosis with myelopathy, thoracolumbar region
M47.16 Other spondylosis with myelopathy, lumbar region
M47.25 Other spondylosis with radiculopathy, thoracolumbar region
M47.26 Other spondylosis with radiculopathy, lumbar region
M47.27 Other spondylosis with radiculopathy, lumbosacral region
M47.815 Spondylosis without myelopathy or radiculopathy, thoracolumbar region
M47.816 Spondylosis without myelopathy or radiculopathy, lumbar region
M47.817 Spondylosis without myelopathy or radiculopathy, lumbosacral region
M48.15 Ankylosing hyperostosis [Forestier], thoracolumbar region
M48.16 Ankylosing hyperostosis [Forestier], lumbar region
M48.17 Ankylosing hyperostosis [Forestier], lumbosacral region
M51.05 Intervertebral disc disorders with myelopathy, thoracolumbar region
M51.06 Intervertebral disc disorders with myelopathy, lumbar region
M51.15 Intervertebral disc disorders with radiculopathy, thoracolumbar region
M51.16 Intervertebral disc disorders with radiculopathy, lumbar region
M51.17 Intervertebral disc disorders with radiculopathy, lumbosacral region
M51.25 Other intervertebral disc displacement, thoracolumbar region
M51.26 Other intervertebral disc displacement, lumbar region
M51.27 Other intervertebral disc displacement, lumbosacral region
M51.35 Other intervertebral disc degeneration, thoracolumbar region
M51.36 Other intervertebral disc degeneration, lumbar region
M51.37 Other intervertebral disc degeneration, lumbosacral region
M51.45 Schmorl's nodes, thoracolumbar region
M51.46 Schmorl's nodes, lumbar region
M51.47 Schmorl's nodes, lumbosacral region
M51.85 Other intervertebral disc disorders, thoracolumbar region
M51.86 Other intervertebral disc disorders, lumbar region
M51.87 Other intervertebral disc disorders, lumbosacral region
M54.15 Radiculopathy, thoracolumbar region
M54.16 Radiculopathy, lumbar region
M54.17 Radiculopathy, lumbosacral region
⇄ M54.31 Sciatica, right side
⇄ M54.32 Sciatica, left side
⇄ M54.41 Lumbago with sciatica, right side
⇄ M54.42 Lumbago with sciatica, left side
M54.5 Low back pain
M54.89 Other dorsalgia
M96.1 Postlaminectomy syndrome, not elsewhere classified

CCI Edits

Refer to Appendix A for CCI edits.

Facility RVUs ☐

Code	Work	PE Facility	MP	Total Facility
62284	1.54	0.79	0.21	2.54

Non-facility RVUs ☐

Code	Work	PE Non-Facility	MP	Total Non-Facility
62284	1.54	3.86	0.21	5.61

Modifiers (PAR) ☐

Code	Mod 50	Mod 51	Mod 62	Mod 66	Mod 80
62284	0	2	0	0	1

Global Period

Code	Days
62284	000

CPT © 2018 American Medical Association. All Rights Reserved.

62290-62291

62290 Injection procedure for discography, each level; lumbar

62291 Injection procedure for discography, each level; cervical or thoracic

(For radiological supervision and interpretation, see 72285, 72295)

AMA Coding Guideline

Injection, Drainage, or Aspiration Procedures on the Spine and Spinal Cord

Injection of contrast during fluoroscopic guidance and localization is an inclusive component of 62263, 62264, 62267, 62270, 62272, 62273, 62280, 62281, 62282, 62302, 62303, 62304, 62305, 62321, 62323, 62325, 62327. Fluoroscopic guidance and localization is reported with 77003, unless a formal contrast study (myelography, epidurography, or arthrography) is performed, in which case the use of fluoroscopy is included in the supervision and interpretation codes or the myelography via lumbar injection code. Image guidance and the injection of contrast are inclusive components and are required for the performance of myelography, as described by codes 62302, 62303, 62304, 62305.

For radiologic supervision and interpretation of epidurography, use 72275. Code 72275 is only to be used when an epidurogram is performed, images documented, and a formal radiologic report is issued.

Code 62263 describes a catheter-based treatment involving targeted injection of various substances (eg, hypertonic saline, steroid, anesthetic) via an indwelling epidural catheter. Code 62263 includes percutaneous insertion and removal of an epidural catheter (remaining in place over a several-day period), for the administration of multiple injections of a neurolytic agent(s) performed during serial treatment sessions (ie, spanning two or more treatment days). If required, adhesions or scarring may also be lysed by mechanical means. Code 62263 is not reported for each adhesiolysis treatment, but should be reported once to describe the entire series of injections/infusions spanning two or more treatment days.

Code 62264 describes multiple adhesiolysis treatment sessions performed on the same day. Adhesions or scarring may be lysed by injections of neurolytic agent(s). If required, adhesions or scarring may also be lysed mechanically using a percutaneously-deployed catheter.

Codes 62263 and 62264 include the procedure of injections of contrast for epidurography (72275) and fluoroscopic guidance and localization (77003) during initial or subsequent sessions.

Fluoroscopy or CT and any injection of contrast are inclusive components of 62321, 62323, 62325, 62327. For epidurography, use 72275.

The placement and use of a catheter to administer one or more epidural or subarachnoid injections on a single calendar day should be reported in the same manner as if a needle had been used, ie, as a single injection using either 62320, 62321, 62322, or 62323. Such injections should not be reported with 62324, 62325, 62326, or 62327.

Threading a catheter into the epidural space, injecting substances at one or more levels and then removing the catheter should be treated as a single injection (62320, 62321, 62322, 62323). If the catheter is left in place to deliver substance(s) over a prolonged period (ie, more than a single calendar day) either continuously or via intermittent bolus, use 62324, 62325, 62326, 62327 as appropriate.

When reporting 62320, 62321, 62322, 62323, 62324, 62325, 62326, 62327 code choice is based on the region at which the needle or catheter entered the body (eg, lumbar). Codes 62320, 62321, 62322, 62323, 62324, 62325, 62326, 62327 should be reported only once, when the substance injected spreads or catheter tip insertion moves into another spinal region (eg, 62322 is reported only once for injection or catheter insertion at L3-4 with spread of the substance or placement of the catheter tip to the thoracic region).

Percutaneous spinal procedures are done with indirect visualization (eg, image guidance) (eg, 62287). Endoscopic assistance during an open procedure with continuous and direct visualization (light-based) is reported using excision codes (eg, 63020-63035).

Definitions

For purposes of CPT coding, the following definitions of approach and visualization apply. The primary approach and visualization define the service, whether another method is incidentally applied. Surgical services are presumed open, unless otherwise specified.

Percutaneous: Image-guided procedures (eg, computer tomography [CT] or fluoroscopy) performed with indirect visualization of the spine without the use of any device that allows visualization through a surgical incision.

Endoscopic: Spinal procedures performed with continuous direct visualization of the spine through an endoscope.

Open: Spinal procedures performed with continuous direct visualization of the spine through a surgical opening.

Indirect visualization: Image-guided (eg, CT or fluoroscopy), not light-based visualization.

Direct visualization: Light-based visualization; can be performed by eye, or with surgical loupes, microscope, or endoscope.

AMA Coding Notes

Injection, Drainage, or Aspiration Procedures on the Spine and Spinal Cord

(For transforaminal epidural injection, see 64479-64484)

(Report 01996 for daily hospital management of continuous epidural or subarachnoid drug administration performed in conjunction with 62324, 62325, 62326, 62327)

(For the techniques of microsurgery and/or use of microscope, use 69990)

Surgical Procedures on the Spine and Spinal Cord

(For application of caliper or tongs, use 20660)

(For treatment of fracture or dislocation of spine, see 22310-22327)

AMA *CPT Assistant* □

62290: Nov 99: 35, Apr 03: 27, Mar 11: 7, Jul 12: 3

62291: Nov 99: 35, Mar 11: 7

Plain English Description

Discography is performed to determine if an intervertebral disc abnormality is the cause of back pain. The patient is positioned on the side and the site of the injection is cleansed with an antiseptic solution. A local anesthetic is injected. Using separately reportable fluoroscopic supervision, a large bore needle is advanced through the skin to the disc. A discography needle is advanced through the first needle and into the center of the disc. Contrast is injected and separately reportable radiographs obtained. The procedure may be repeated on multiple discs and is reported for each level injected. Use 62290 for each lumbar disc injected; use 62291 for each cervical or thoracic disc injected.

Injection procedure for discography, each level

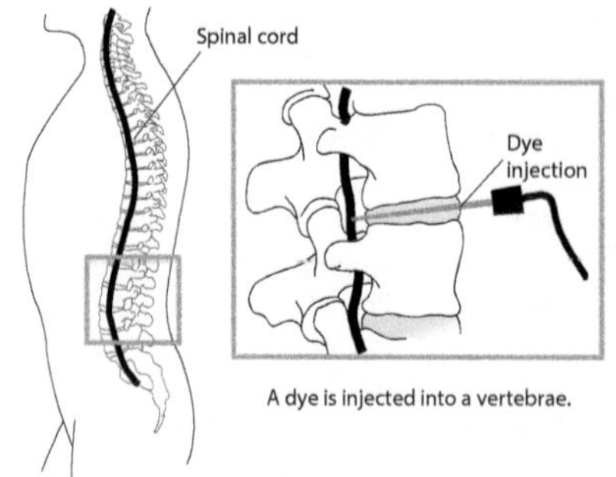

Lumbar (62290), cervical or thoracic (62291)

ICD-10-CM Diagnostic Codes

M46.31	Infection of intervertebral disc (pyogenic), occipito-atlanto-axial region
M46.32	Infection of intervertebral disc (pyogenic), cervical region
M46.33	Infection of intervertebral disc (pyogenic), cervicothoracic region
M46.34	Infection of intervertebral disc (pyogenic), thoracic region
M46.45	Discitis, unspecified, thoracolumbar region
M46.46	Discitis, unspecified, lumbar region
M46.47	Discitis, unspecified, lumbosacral region

CPT © 2018 American Medical Association. All Rights Reserved.

M50.01 Cervical disc disorder with myelopathy, high cervical region
M50.021 Cervical disc disorder at C4-C5 level with myelopathy
M50.022 Cervical disc disorder at C5-C6 level with myelopathy
M50.023 Cervical disc disorder at C6-C7 level with myelopathy
M50.03 Cervical disc disorder with myelopathy, cervicothoracic region
M50.11 Cervical disc disorder with radiculopathy, high cervical region
M50.121 Cervical disc disorder at C4-C5 level with radiculopathy
M50.122 Cervical disc disorder at C5-C6 level with radiculopathy
M50.123 Cervical disc disorder at C6-C7 level with radiculopathy
M50.13 Cervical disc disorder with radiculopathy, cervicothoracic region
M50.21 Other cervical disc displacement, high cervical region
M50.221 Other cervical disc displacement at C4-C5 level
M50.222 Other cervical disc displacement at C5-C6 level
M50.223 Other cervical disc displacement at C6-C7 level
M50.321 Other cervical disc degeneration at C4-C5 level
M50.322 Other cervical disc degeneration at C5-C6 level
M50.323 Other cervical disc degeneration at C6-C7 level
M50.83 Other cervical disc disorders, cervicothoracic region
M51.04 Intervertebral disc disorders with myelopathy, thoracic region
M51.05 Intervertebral disc disorders with myelopathy, thoracolumbar region
M51.06 Intervertebral disc disorders with myelopathy, lumbar region
M51.14 Intervertebral disc disorders with radiculopathy, thoracic region
M51.15 Intervertebral disc disorders with radiculopathy, thoracolumbar region
M51.16 Intervertebral disc disorders with radiculopathy, lumbar region
M51.17 Intervertebral disc disorders with radiculopathy, lumbosacral region
M51.24 Other intervertebral disc displacement, thoracic region
M51.25 Other intervertebral disc displacement, thoracolumbar region
M51.36 Other intervertebral disc degeneration, lumbar region
M51.37 Other intervertebral disc degeneration, lumbosacral region
M51.44 Schmorl's nodes, thoracic region
M51.45 Schmorl's nodes, thoracolumbar region
M51.46 Schmorl's nodes, lumbar region
M51.47 Schmorl's nodes, lumbosacral region
M51.84 Other intervertebral disc disorders, thoracic region
M51.85 Other intervertebral disc disorders, thoracolumbar region
M51.86 Other intervertebral disc disorders, lumbar region
M51.87 Other intervertebral disc disorders, lumbosacral region
M54.12 Radiculopathy, cervical region
M54.13 Radiculopathy, cervicothoracic region
M54.14 Radiculopathy, thoracic region
M54.15 Radiculopathy, thoracolumbar region
M54.16 Radiculopathy, lumbar region
M54.17 Radiculopathy, lumbosacral region
M54.2 Cervicalgia
⇄ M54.31 Sciatica, right side
⇄ M54.32 Sciatica, left side
⇄ M54.41 Lumbago with sciatica, right side
⇄ M54.42 Lumbago with sciatica, left side
M54.5 Low back pain
M54.6 Pain in thoracic spine
M96.1 Postlaminectomy syndrome, not elsewhere classified

CCI Edits

Refer to Appendix A for CCI edits.

Facility RVUs ☐

Code	Work	PE Facility	MP	Total Facility
62290	3.00	1.55	0.26	4.81
62291	2.91	1.49	0.25	4.65

Non-facility RVUs ☐

Code	Work	PE Non-Facility	MP	Total Non-Facility
62290	3.00	6.36	0.26	9.62
62291	2.91	6.12	0.25	9.28

Modifiers (PAR) ☐

Code	Mod 50	Mod 51	Mod 62	Mod 66	Mod 80
62290	0	2	0	0	1
62291	0	2	0	0	1

Global Period

Code	Days
62290	000
62291	000

CPT © 2018 American Medical Association. All Rights Reserved.

62302-62305

62302 Myelography via lumbar injection, including radiological supervision and interpretation; cervical

(Do not report 62302 in conjunction with 62284, 62303, 62304, 62305, 72240, 72255, 72265, 72270)

62303 Myelography via lumbar injection, including radiological supervision and interpretation; thoracic

(Do not report 62303 in conjunction with 62284, 62302, 62304, 62305, 72240, 72255, 72265, 72270)

62304 Myelography via lumbar injection, including radiological supervision and interpretation; lumbosacral

(Do not report 62304 in conjunction with 62284, 62302, 62303, 62305, 72240, 72255, 72265, 72270)

62305 Myelography via lumbar injection, including radiological supervision and interpretation; 2 or more regions (eg, lumbar/thoracic, cervical/thoracic, lumbar/cervical, lumbar/thoracic/cervical)

(Do not report 62305 in conjunction with 62284, 62302, 62303, 62304, 72240, 72255, 72265, 72270)

(For myelography lumbar injection and imaging performed by different physicians or other qualified health care professionals, see 62284 or 72240, 72255, 72265, 72270)

(For injection procedure at C1-C2, use 61055)

AMA Coding Guideline

Injection, Drainage, or Aspiration Procedures on the Spine and Spinal Cord

Injection of contrast during fluoroscopic guidance and localization is an inclusive component of 62263, 62264, 62267, 62270, 62272, 62273, 62280, 62281, 62282, 62302, 62303, 62304, 62305, 62321, 62323, 62325, 62327. Fluoroscopic guidance and localization is reported with 77003, unless a formal contrast study (myelography, epidurography, or arthrography) is performed, in which case the use of fluoroscopy is included in the supervision and interpretation codes or the myelography via lumbar injection code. Image guidance and the injection of contrast are inclusive components and are required for the performance of myelography, as described by codes 62302, 62303, 62304, 62305.

For radiologic supervision and interpretation of epidurography, use 72275. Code 72275 is only to be used when an epidurogram is performed, images documented, and a formal radiologic report is issued.

Code 62263 describes a catheter-based treatment involving targeted injection of various substances (eg, hypertonic saline, steroid, anesthetic) via an indwelling epidural catheter. Code 62263 includes percutaneous insertion and removal of an epidural catheter (remaining in place over a several-day period), for the administration of multiple injections of a neurolytic agent(s) performed during serial treatment sessions (ie, spanning two or more treatment days). If required, adhesions or scarring may also be lysed by mechanical means. Code 62263 is not reported for each adhesiolysis treatment, but should be reported once to describe the entire series of injections/infusions spanning two or more treatment days.

Code 62264 describes multiple adhesiolysis treatment sessions performed on the same day. Adhesions or scarring may be lysed by injections of neurolytic agent(s). If required, adhesions or scarring may also be lysed mechanically using a percutaneously-deployed catheter.

Codes 62263 and 62264 include the procedure of injections of contrast for epidurography (72275) and fluoroscopic guidance and localization (77003) during initial or subsequent sessions.

Fluoroscopy or CT and any injection of contrast are inclusive components of 62321, 62323, 62325, 62327. For epidurography, use 72275.

The placement and use of a catheter to administer one or more epidural or subarachnoid injections on a single calendar day should be reported in the same manner as if a needle had been used, ie, as a single injection using either 62320, 62321, 62322, or 62323. Such injections should not be reported with 62324, 62325, 62326, or 62327.

Threading a catheter into the epidural space, injecting substances at one or more levels and then removing the catheter should be treated as a single injection (62320, 62321, 62322, 62323). If the catheter is left in place to deliver substance(s) over a prolonged period (ie, more than a single calendar day) either continuously or via intermittent bolus, use 62324, 62325, 62326, 62327 as appropriate.

When reporting 62320, 62321, 62322, 62323, 62324, 62325, 62326, 62327 code choice is based on the region at which the needle or catheter entered the body (eg, lumbar). Codes 62320, 62321, 62322, 62323, 62324, 62325, 62326, 62327 should be reported only once, when the substance injected spreads or catheter tip insertion moves into another spinal region (eg, 62322 is reported only once for injection or catheter insertion at L3-4 with spread of the substance or placement of the catheter tip to the thoracic region).

Percutaneous spinal procedures are done with indirect visualization (eg, image guidance) (eg, 62287). Endoscopic assistance during an open procedure with continuous and direct visualization (light-based) is reported using excision codes (eg, 63020-63035).

Definitions

For purposes of CPT coding, the following definitions of approach and visualization apply. The primary approach and visualization define the service, whether another method is incidentally applied. Surgical services are presumed open, unless otherwise specified.

Percutaneous: Image-guided procedures (eg, computer tomography [CT] or fluoroscopy) performed with indirect visualization of the spine without the use of any device that allows visualization through a surgical incision.

Endoscopic: Spinal procedures performed with continuous direct visualization of the spine through an endoscope.

Open: Spinal procedures performed with continuous direct visualization of the spine through a surgical opening.

Indirect visualization: Image-guided (eg, CT or fluoroscopy), not light-based visualization.

Direct visualization: Light-based visualization; can be performed by eye, or with surgical loupes, microscope, or endoscope.

AMA Coding Notes

Injection, Drainage, or Aspiration Procedures on the Spine and Spinal Cord

(For transforaminal epidural injection, see 64479-64484)

(Report 01996 for daily hospital management of continuous epidural or subarachnoid drug administration performed in conjunction with 62324, 62325, 62326, 62327)

(For the techniques of microsurgery and/or use of microscope, use 69990)

Surgical Procedures on the Spine and Spinal Cord

(For application of caliper or tongs, use 20660)

(For treatment of fracture or dislocation of spine, see 22310-22327)

Plain English Description

Myelography is an imaging technique that provides a detailed picture of the spinal canal, spinal cord, and spinal nerve roots using real time fluoroscopy and x-rays. The procedure is done under the direct supervision of a radiologist and may be used to diagnose intervertebral disc herniation, spinal stenosis, tumors, infection, inflammation, and other lesions caused by disease or trauma. The patient is positioned lying on the abdomen or side. Under fluoroscopy, a spinal needle is advanced into the spinal canal at the lumbar region until a free flow of cerebrospinal fluid (CSF) is observed. A contrast material (non-ionic dye) is injected through the needle into the subarachnoid space and the needle is withdrawn. The procedure table is slowly tilted up or down to allow the contrast dye to flow within the subarachnoid space. The flow of dye is monitored using fluoroscopy and x-rays may then be obtained to document abnormalities. When the procedure is complete, the table is returned to a horizontal position and the patient is allowed to assume a comfortable position. Code 62302 is used for examination of the cervical region of the spine; code 62303 for the thoracic region; code

CPT © 2018 American Medical Association. All Rights Reserved.

62304 for the lumbosacral area; and code 62305 is reported when 2 or more areas of the spine are examined.

ICD-10-CM Diagnostic Codes

M43.01	Spondylolysis, occipito-atlanto-axial region
M43.02	Spondylolysis, cervical region
M43.03	Spondylolysis, cervicothoracic region
M43.04	Spondylolysis, thoracic region
M43.15	Spondylolisthesis, thoracolumbar region
M43.16	Spondylolisthesis, lumbar region
M43.17	Spondylolisthesis, lumbosacral region
M43.19	Spondylolisthesis, multiple sites in spine
M47.11	Other spondylosis with myelopathy, occipito-atlanto-axial region
M47.12	Other spondylosis with myelopathy, cervical region
M47.13	Other spondylosis with myelopathy, cervicothoracic region
M47.14	Other spondylosis with myelopathy, thoracic region
M47.15	Other spondylosis with myelopathy, thoracolumbar region
M47.16	Other spondylosis with myelopathy, lumbar region
M47.21	Other spondylosis with radiculopathy, occipito-atlanto-axial region
M47.22	Other spondylosis with radiculopathy, cervical region
M47.23	Other spondylosis with radiculopathy, cervicothoracic region
M47.24	Other spondylosis with radiculopathy, thoracic region
M47.25	Other spondylosis with radiculopathy, thoracolumbar region
M47.26	Other spondylosis with radiculopathy, lumbar region
M47.27	Other spondylosis with radiculopathy, lumbosacral region
M48.02	Spinal stenosis, cervical region
M48.04	Spinal stenosis, thoracic region
M48.06	Spinal stenosis, lumbar region
M50.01	Cervical disc disorder with myelopathy, high cervical region
M50.021	Cervical disc disorder at C4-C5 level with myelopathy
M50.022	Cervical disc disorder at C5-C6 level with myelopathy
M50.023	Cervical disc disorder at C6-C7 level with myelopathy
M50.03	Cervical disc disorder with myelopathy, cervicothoracic region
M51.04	Intervertebral disc disorders with myelopathy, thoracic region
M51.05	Intervertebral disc disorders with myelopathy, thoracolumbar region
M51.06	Intervertebral disc disorders with myelopathy, lumbar region
M51.14	Intervertebral disc disorders with radiculopathy, thoracic region
M51.15	Intervertebral disc disorders with radiculopathy, thoracolumbar region
M51.16	Intervertebral disc disorders with radiculopathy, lumbar region
M53.0	Cervicocranial syndrome
M53.1	Cervicobrachial syndrome
M54.12	Radiculopathy, cervical region
M54.14	Radiculopathy, thoracic region
M54.16	Radiculopathy, lumbar region
M54.2	Cervicalgia
⇄ M54.41	Lumbago with sciatica, right side
⇄ M54.42	Lumbago with sciatica, left side

CCI Edits

Refer to Appendix A for CCI edits.

Facility RVUs ▢

Code	Work	PE Facility	MP	Total Facility
62302	2.29	1.02	0.20	3.51
62303	2.29	1.02	0.20	3.51
62304	2.25	1.00	0.20	3.45
62305	2.35	1.04	0.21	3.60

Non-facility RVUs ▢

Code	Work	PE Non-Facility	MP	Total Non-Facility
62302	2.29	4.64	0.20	7.13
62303	2.29	4.80	0.20	7.29
62304	2.25	4.59	0.20	7.04
62305	2.35	5.09	0.21	7.65

Modifiers (PAR) ▢

Code	Mod 50	Mod 51	Mod 62	Mod 66	Mod 80
62302	0	2	0	0	1
62303	0	2	0	0	1
62304	0	2	0	0	1
62305	0	2	0	0	1

Global Period

Code	Days
62302	000
62303	000
62304	000
62305	000

CPT © 2018 American Medical Association. All Rights Reserved.

62320-62321

62320 Injection(s), of diagnostic or therapeutic substance(s) (eg, anesthetic, antispasmodic, opioid, steroid, other solution), not including neurolytic substances, including needle or catheter placement, interlaminar epidural or subarachnoid, cervical or thoracic; without imaging guidance

62321 Injection(s), of diagnostic or therapeutic substance(s) (eg, anesthetic, antispasmodic, opioid, steroid, other solution), not including neurolytic substances, including needle or catheter placement, interlaminar epidural or subarachnoid, cervical or thoracic; with imaging guidance (ie, fluoroscopy or CT)

(Do not report 62321 in conjunction with 77003, 77012, 76942)

AMA Coding Guideline

Injection, Drainage, or Aspiration Procedures on the Spine and Spinal Cord

Injection of contrast during fluoroscopic guidance and localization is an inclusive component of 62263, 62264, 62267, 62270, 62272, 62273, 62280, 62281, 62282, 62302, 62303, 62304, 62305, 62321, 62323, 62325, 62327. Fluoroscopic guidance and localization is reported with 77003, unless a formal contrast study (myelography, epidurography, or arthrography) is performed, in which case the use of fluoroscopy is included in the supervision and interpretation codes or the myelography via lumbar injection code. Image guidance and the injection of contrast are inclusive components and are required for the performance of myelography, as described by codes 62302, 62303, 62304, 62305.

For radiologic supervision and interpretation of epidurography, use 72275. Code 72275 is only to be used when an epidurogram is performed, images documented, and a formal radiologic report is issued.

Code 62263 describes a catheter-based treatment involving targeted injection of various substances (eg, hypertonic saline, steroid, anesthetic) via an indwelling epidural catheter. Code 62263 includes percutaneous insertion and removal of an epidural catheter (remaining in place over a several-day period), for the administration of multiple injections of a neurolytic agent(s) performed during serial treatment sessions (ie, spanning two or more treatment days). If required, adhesions or scarring may also be lysed by mechanical means. Code 62263 is not reported for each adhesiolysis treatment, but should be reported once to describe the entire series of injections/infusions spanning two or more treatment days.

Code 62264 describes multiple adhesiolysis treatment sessions performed on the same day. Adhesions or scarring may be lysed by injections of neurolytic agent(s). If required, adhesions or scarring may also be lysed mechanically using a percutaneously-deployed catheter.

Codes 62263 and 62264 include the procedure of injections of contrast for epidurography (72275) and fluoroscopic guidance and localization (77003) during initial or subsequent sessions.

Fluoroscopy or CT and any injection of contrast are inclusive components of 62321, 62323, 62325, 62327. For epidurography, use 72275.

The placement and use of a catheter to administer one or more epidural or subarachnoid injections on a single calendar day should be reported in the same manner as if a needle had been used, ie, as a single injection using either 62320, 62321, 62322, or 62323. Such injections should not be reported with 62324, 62325, 62326, or 62327.

Threading a catheter into the epidural space, injecting substances at one or more levels and then removing the catheter should be treated as a single injection (62320, 62321, 62322, 62323). If the catheter is left in place to deliver substance(s) over a prolonged period (ie, more than a single calendar day) either continuously or via intermittent bolus, use 62324, 62325, 62326, 62327 as appropriate.

When reporting 62320, 62321, 62322, 62323, 62324, 62325, 62326, 62327 code choice is based on the region at which the needle or catheter entered the body (eg, lumbar). Codes 62320, 62321, 62322, 62323, 62324, 62325, 62326, 62327 should be reported only once, when the substance injected spreads or catheter tip insertion moves into another spinal region (eg, 62322 is reported only once for injection or catheter insertion at L3-4 with spread of the substance or placement of the catheter tip to the thoracic region).

Percutaneous spinal procedures are done with indirect visualization (eg, image guidance) (eg, 62287). Endoscopic assistance during an open procedure with continuous and direct visualization (light-based) is reported using excision codes (eg, 63020-63035).

Definitions

For purposes of CPT coding, the following definitions of approach and visualization apply. The primary approach and visualization define the service, whether another method is incidentally applied. Surgical services are presumed open, unless otherwise specified.

Percutaneous: Image-guided procedures (eg, computer tomography [CT] or fluoroscopy) performed with indirect visualization of the spine without the use of any device that allows visualization through a surgical incision.

Endoscopic: Spinal procedures performed with continuous direct visualization of the spine through an endoscope.

Open: Spinal procedures performed with continuous direct visualization of the spine through a surgical opening.

Indirect visualization: Image-guided (eg, CT or fluoroscopy), not light-based visualization.

Direct visualization: Light-based visualization; can be performed by eye, or with surgical loupes, microscope, or endoscope.

AMA Coding Notes

Injection, Drainage, or Aspiration Procedures on the Spine and Spinal Cord

(For transforaminal epidural injection, see 64479-64484)

(Report 01996 for daily hospital management of continuous epidural or subarachnoid drug administration performed in conjunction with 62324, 62325, 62326, 62327)

(For the techniques of microsurgery and/or use of microscope, use 69990)

Surgical Procedures on the Spine and Spinal Cord

(For application of caliper or tongs, use 20660)

(For treatment of fracture or dislocation of spine, see 22310-22327)

AMA *CPT Assistant*

62320: Sep 17: 6

62321: Sep 17: 6

Plain English Description

The skin over the spinal region to be injected is cleansed with an antiseptic solution and a local anesthetic is injected. A thin spinal needle or catheter is inserted into the back of the epidural or subarachnoid space through a paramedian or midline interlaminar approach, usually under fluoroscopic guidance. The epidural space is the outermost area of the spinal canal filled with cerebrospinal fluid that lies between the outermost protective membrane (dura mater) surrounding the nerve roots and the vertebral wall. The subarachnoid space lies closer to the spinal cord and is located between the middle protective membrane, the arachnoid, and the innermost delicate membrane surrounding the spinal cord, the pia mater. Contrast dye may be injected first to confirm proper needle placement, to perform an epidurography, and to see that the medication is traveling into the desired area. A diagnostic or therapeutic substance, such as an anesthetic, antispasmodic, opioid, steroid, or other solution, such as a steroid and local anesthetic mix, excluding a neurolytic substance, is injected into the epidural or subarachnoid space. Following injection, the patient is monitored for any adverse effects. Use 62320 for interlaminar epidural or subarachnoid injection(s) in the cervical or thoracic region without imaging guidance; use 62321 for similar injection(s) done with imaging guidance, such as fluoroscopy or CT.

CPT © 2018 American Medical Association. All Rights Reserved.

ICD-10-CM Diagnostic Codes

G89.11 Acute pain due to trauma
G89.12 Acute post-thoracotomy pain
G89.18 Other acute postprocedural pain
G89.21 Chronic pain due to trauma
G89.22 Chronic post-thoracotomy pain
G89.28 Other chronic postprocedural pain
G89.29 Other chronic pain
G89.3 Neoplasm related pain (acute) (chronic)
M43.02 Spondylolysis, cervical region
M43.03 Spondylolysis, cervicothoracic region
M43.04 Spondylolysis, thoracic region
M43.05 Spondylolysis, thoracolumbar region
M43.12 Spondylolisthesis, cervical region
M43.13 Spondylolisthesis, cervicothoracic region
M43.14 Spondylolisthesis, thoracic region
M47.12 Other spondylosis with myelopathy, cervical region
M47.13 Other spondylosis with myelopathy, cervicothoracic region
M47.14 Other spondylosis with myelopathy, thoracic region
M47.15 Other spondylosis with myelopathy, thoracolumbar region
M47.23 Other spondylosis with radiculopathy, cervicothoracic region
M47.24 Other spondylosis with radiculopathy, thoracic region
M47.25 Other spondylosis with radiculopathy, thoracolumbar region
M47.812 Spondylosis without myelopathy or radiculopathy, cervical region
M47.813 Spondylosis without myelopathy or radiculopathy, cervicothoracic region
M47.814 Spondylosis without myelopathy or radiculopathy, thoracic region
M47.815 Spondylosis without myelopathy or radiculopathy, thoracolumbar region
M47.892 Other spondylosis, cervical region
M47.893 Other spondylosis, cervicothoracic region
M47.894 Other spondylosis, thoracic region
M47.895 Other spondylosis, thoracolumbar region
M48.02 Spinal stenosis, cervical region
M48.03 Spinal stenosis, cervicothoracic region
M48.04 Spinal stenosis, thoracic region
M50.021 Cervical disc disorder at C4-C5 level with myelopathy
M50.022 Cervical disc disorder at C5-C6 level with myelopathy
M50.023 Cervical disc disorder at C6-C7 level with myelopathy
M50.03 Cervical disc disorder with myelopathy, cervicothoracic region
M50.121 Cervical disc disorder at C4-C5 level with radiculopathy
M50.122 Cervical disc disorder at C5-C6 level with radiculopathy
M50.123 Cervical disc disorder at C6-C7 level with radiculopathy
M50.13 Cervical disc disorder with radiculopathy, cervicothoracic region
M50.221 Other cervical disc displacement at C4-C5 level
M50.222 Other cervical disc displacement at C5-C6 level
M50.223 Other cervical disc displacement at C6-C7 level
M50.23 Other cervical disc displacement, cervicothoracic region
M50.321 Other cervical disc degeneration at C4-C5 level
M50.322 Other cervical disc degeneration at C5-C6 level
M50.323 Other cervical disc degeneration at C6-C7 level
M50.33 Other cervical disc degeneration, cervicothoracic region
M50.821 Other cervical disc disorders at C4-C5 level
M50.822 Other cervical disc disorders at C5-C6 level
M50.823 Other cervical disc disorders at C6-C7 level
M50.83 Other cervical disc disorders, cervicothoracic region
M50.921 Unspecified cervical disc disorder at C4-C5 level
M50.922 Unspecified cervical disc disorder at C5-C6 level
M50.923 Unspecified cervical disc disorder at C6-C7 level
M50.93 Cervical disc disorder, unspecified, cervicothoracic region
M51.04 Intervertebral disc disorders with myelopathy, thoracic region
M51.05 Intervertebral disc disorders with myelopathy, thoracolumbar region
M51.24 Other intervertebral disc displacement, thoracic region
M51.25 Other intervertebral disc displacement, thoracolumbar region
M51.34 Other intervertebral disc degeneration, thoracic region
M51.35 Other intervertebral disc degeneration, thoracolumbar region
M54.11 Radiculopathy, occipito-atlanto-axial region
M54.12 Radiculopathy, cervical region
M54.13 Radiculopathy, cervicothoracic region
M54.14 Radiculopathy, thoracic region
M54.15 Radiculopathy, thoracolumbar region
M54.6 Pain in thoracic spine
M54.81 Occipital neuralgia

CCI Edits

Refer to Appendix A for CCI edits.

Facility RVUs ☐

Code	Work	PE Facility	MP	Total Facility
62320	1.80	0.89	0.16	2.85
62321	1.95	0.96	0.16	3.07

Non-facility RVUs ☐

Code	Work	PE Non-Facility	MP	Total Non-Facility
62320	1.80	2.72	0.16	4.68
62321	1.95	5.08	0.16	7.19

Modifiers (PAR) ☐

Code	Mod 50	Mod 51	Mod 62	Mod 66	Mod 80
62320	9	2	0	0	1
62321	9	2	0	0	1

Global Period

Code	Days
62320	000
62321	000

CPT © 2018 American Medical Association. All Rights Reserved.

62322-62323

62322 Injection(s), of diagnostic or therapeutic substance(s) (eg, anesthetic, antispasmodic, opioid, steroid, other solution), not including neurolytic substances, including needle or catheter placement, interlaminar epidural or subarachnoid, lumbar or sacral (caudal); without imaging guidance

62323 Injection(s), of diagnostic or therapeutic substance(s) (eg, anesthetic, antispasmodic, opioid, steroid, other solution), not including neurolytic substances, including needle or catheter placement, interlaminar epidural or subarachnoid, lumbar or sacral (caudal); with imaging guidance (ie, fluoroscopy or CT)

(Do not report 62323 in conjunction with 77003, 77012, 76942)

AMA Coding Guideline

Injection, Drainage, or Aspiration Procedures on the Spine and Spinal Cord

Injection of contrast during fluoroscopic guidance and localization is an inclusive component of 62263, 62264, 62267, 62270, 62272, 62273, 62280, 62281, 62282, 62302, 62303, 62304, 62305, 62321, 62323, 62325, 62327. Fluoroscopic guidance and localization is reported with 77003, unless a formal contrast study (myelography, epidurography, or arthrography) is performed, in which case the use of fluoroscopy is included in the supervision and interpretation codes or the myelography via lumbar injection code. Image guidance and the injection of contrast are inclusive components and are required for the performance of myelography, as described by codes 62302, 62303, 62304, 62305.

For radiologic supervision and interpretation of epidurography, use 72275. Code 72275 is only to be used when an epidurogram is performed, images documented, and a formal radiologic report is issued.

Code 62263 describes a catheter-based treatment involving targeted injection of various substances (eg, hypertonic saline, steroid, anesthetic) via an indwelling epidural catheter. Code 62263 includes percutaneous insertion and removal of an epidural catheter (remaining in place over a several-day period), for the administration of multiple injections of a neurolytic agent(s) performed during serial treatment sessions (ie, spanning two or more treatment days). If required, adhesions or scarring may also be lysed by mechanical means. Code 62263 is not reported for each adhesiolysis treatment, but should be reported once to describe the entire series of injections/infusions spanning two or more treatment days.

Code 62264 describes multiple adhesiolysis treatment sessions performed on the same day. Adhesions or scarring may be lysed by injections of neurolytic agent(s). If required, adhesions or scarring may also be lysed mechanically using a percutaneously-deployed catheter.

Codes 62263 and 62264 include the procedure of injections of contrast for epidurography (72275) and fluoroscopic guidance and localization (77003) during initial or subsequent sessions.

Fluoroscopy or CT and any injection of contrast are inclusive components of 62321, 62323, 62325, 62327. For epidurography, use 72275.

The placement and use of a catheter to administer one or more epidural or subarachnoid injections on a single calendar day should be reported in the same manner as if a needle had been used, ie, as a single injection using either 62320, 62321, 62322, or 62323. Such injections should not be reported with 62324, 62325, 62326, or 62327.

Threading a catheter into the epidural space, injecting substances at one or more levels and then removing the catheter should be treated as a single injection (62320, 62321, 62322, 62323). If the catheter is left in place to deliver substance(s) over a prolonged period (ie, more than a single calendar day) either continuously or via intermittent bolus, use 62324, 62325, 62326, 62327 as appropriate.

When reporting 62320, 62321, 62322, 62323, 62324, 62325, 62326, 62327 code choice is based on the region at which the needle or catheter entered the body (eg, lumbar). Codes 62320, 62321, 62322, 62323, 62324, 62325, 62326, 62327 should be reported only once, when the substance injected spreads or catheter tip insertion moves into another spinal region (eg, 62322 is reported only once for injection or catheter insertion at L3-4 with spread of the substance or placement of the catheter tip to the thoracic region).

Percutaneous spinal procedures are done with indirect visualization (eg, image guidance) (eg, 62287). Endoscopic assistance during an open procedure with continuous and direct visualization (light-based) is reported using excision codes (eg, 63020-63035).

Definitions

For purposes of CPT coding, the following definitions of approach and visualization apply. The primary approach and visualization define the service, whether another method is incidentally applied. Surgical services are presumed open, unless otherwise specified.

Percutaneous: Image-guided procedures (eg, computer tomography [CT] or fluoroscopy) performed with indirect visualization of the spine without the use of any device that allows visualization through a surgical incision.

Endoscopic: Spinal procedures performed with continuous direct visualization of the spine through an endoscope.

Open: Spinal procedures performed with continuous direct visualization of the spine through a surgical opening.

Indirect visualization: Image-guided (eg, CT or fluoroscopy), not light-based visualization.

Direct visualization: Light-based visualization; can be performed by eye, or with surgical loupes, microscope, or endoscope.

AMA Coding Notes

Injection, Drainage, or Aspiration Procedures on the Spine and Spinal Cord

(For transforaminal epidural injection, see 64479-64484)

(Report 01996 for daily hospital management of continuous epidural or subarachnoid drug administration performed in conjunction with 62324, 62325, 62326, 62327)

(For the techniques of microsurgery and/or use of microscope, use 69990)

Surgical Procedures on the Spine and Spinal Cord

(For application of caliper or tongs, use 20660)

(For treatment of fracture or dislocation of spine, see 22310-22327)

AMA *CPT Assistant*

62322: Sep 17: 6

62323: Sep 17: 6

Plain English Description

The skin over the spinal region to be injected is cleansed with an antiseptic solution and a local anesthetic is injected. A thin spinal needle or catheter is inserted into the skin and advanced into the back of the epidural or subarachnoid space through a paramedian or midline interlaminar approach, usually under fluoroscopic guidance. The epidural space is the outermost area of the spinal canal filled with cerebrospinal fluid that lies between the outermost protective membrane (dura mater) surrounding the nerve roots and the vertebral wall. The subarachnoid space lies closer to the spinal cord and is located between the middle protective membrane, the arachnoid, and the innermost delicate membrane surrounding the spinal cord, the pia mater. Contrast dye may be injected first to confirm proper needle placement, to perform an epidurography, and to see that the medication is traveling into the desired area. A diagnostic or therapeutic substance, such as an anesthetic, antispasmodic, opioid, steroid, or other solution, such as a steroid and local anesthetic mix, excluding a neurolytic substance, is injected into the epidural or subarachnoid space. Following injection, the patient is monitored for any adverse effects. Use 62322 for interlaminar epidural or subarachnoid injection(s) in the lumbar or sacral (caudal) region without imaging guidance; use 62323 for similar injection(s) done with imaging guidance, such as fluoroscopy or CT.

CPT © 2018 American Medical Association. All Rights Reserved.

ICD-10-CM Diagnostic Codes

	B02.23	Postherpetic polyneuropathy
	B02.7	Disseminated zoster
	B02.8	Zoster with other complications
	B02.9	Zoster without complications
	G89.11	Acute pain due to trauma
	G89.12	Acute post-thoracotomy pain
	G89.18	Other acute postprocedural pain
	G89.21	Chronic pain due to trauma
	G89.22	Chronic post-thoracotomy pain
	G89.28	Other chronic postprocedural pain
	G89.29	Other chronic pain
	G89.3	Neoplasm related pain (acute) (chronic)
	G97.1	Other reaction to spinal and lumbar puncture
	M43.05	Spondylolysis, thoracolumbar region
	M43.06	Spondylolysis, lumbar region
	M43.07	Spondylolysis, lumbosacral region
	M43.08	Spondylolysis, sacral and sacrococcygeal region
	M43.15	Spondylolisthesis, thoracolumbar region
	M43.16	Spondylolisthesis, lumbar region
	M43.17	Spondylolisthesis, lumbosacral region
	M43.18	Spondylolisthesis, sacral and sacrococcygeal region
	M47.26	Other spondylosis with radiculopathy, lumbar region
	M47.816	Spondylosis without myelopathy or radiculopathy, lumbar region
	M47.817	Spondylosis without myelopathy or radiculopathy, lumbosacral region
	M47.818	Spondylosis without myelopathy or radiculopathy, sacral and sacrococcygeal region
	M48.07	Spinal stenosis, lumbosacral region
	M51.05	Intervertebral disc disorders with myelopathy, thoracolumbar region
	M51.06	Intervertebral disc disorders with myelopathy, lumbar region
	M51.15	Intervertebral disc disorders with radiculopathy, thoracolumbar region
	M51.16	Intervertebral disc disorders with radiculopathy, lumbar region
	M51.17	Intervertebral disc disorders with radiculopathy, lumbosacral region
	M51.25	Other intervertebral disc displacement, thoracolumbar region
	M51.26	Other intervertebral disc displacement, lumbar region
	M51.27	Other intervertebral disc displacement, lumbosacral region
	M51.35	Other intervertebral disc degeneration, thoracolumbar region
	M51.36	Other intervertebral disc degeneration, lumbar region
	M51.37	Other intervertebral disc degeneration, lumbosacral region
	M51.85	Other intervertebral disc disorders, thoracolumbar region
	M51.86	Other intervertebral disc disorders, lumbar region
	M51.87	Other intervertebral disc disorders, lumbosacral region
	M54.15	Radiculopathy, thoracolumbar region
	M54.16	Radiculopathy, lumbar region
	M54.17	Radiculopathy, lumbosacral region
	M54.18	Radiculopathy, sacral and sacrococcygeal region
⇄	M54.31	Sciatica, right side
⇄	M54.32	Sciatica, left side
⇄	M54.41	Lumbago with sciatica, right side
⇄	M54.42	Lumbago with sciatica, left side
	M54.89	Other dorsalgia
	M96.1	Postlaminectomy syndrome, not elsewhere classified
	M99.23	Subluxation stenosis of neural canal of lumbar region
	M99.33	Osseous stenosis of neural canal of lumbar region
	M99.43	Connective tissue stenosis of neural canal of lumbar region
	M99.53	Intervertebral disc stenosis of neural canal of lumbar region
	M99.63	Osseous and subluxation stenosis of intervertebral foramina of lumbar region
	M99.73	Connective tissue and disc stenosis of intervertebral foramina of lumbar region

CCI Edits

Refer to Appendix A for CCI edits.

Facility RVUs ▢

Code	Work	PE Facility	MP	Total Facility
62322	1.55	0.77	0.14	2.46
62323	1.80	0.88	0.16	2.84

Non-facility RVUs ▢

Code	Work	PE Non-Facility	MP	Total Non-Facility
62322	1.55	2.67	0.14	4.36
62323	1.80	5.15	0.16	7.11

Modifiers (PAR) ▢

Code	Mod 50	Mod 51	Mod 62	Mod 66	Mod 80
62322	9	2	0	0	1
62323	9	2	0	0	1

Global Period

Code	Days
62322	000
62323	000

CPT © 2018 American Medical Association. All Rights Reserved.

62324-62325

62324 Injection(s), including indwelling catheter placement, continuous infusion or intermittent bolus, of diagnostic or therapeutic substance(s) (eg, anesthetic, antispasmodic, opioid, steroid, other solution), not including neurolytic substances, interlaminar epidural or subarachnoid, cervical or thoracic; without imaging guidance

62325 Injection(s), including indwelling catheter placement, continuous infusion or intermittent bolus, of diagnostic or therapeutic substance(s) (eg, anesthetic, antispasmodic, opioid, steroid, other solution), not including neurolytic substances, interlaminar epidural or subarachnoid, cervical or thoracic; with imaging guidance (ie, fluoroscopy or CT)

(Do not report 62325 in conjunction with 77003, 77012, 76942)

AMA Coding Guideline

Injection, Drainage, or Aspiration Procedures on the Spine and Spinal Cord

Injection of contrast during fluoroscopic guidance and localization is an inclusive component of 62263, 62264, 62267, 62270, 62272, 62273, 62280, 62281, 62282, 62302, 62303, 62304, 62305, 62321, 62323, 62325, 62327. Fluoroscopic guidance and localization is reported with 77003, unless a formal contrast study (myelography, epidurography, or arthrography) is performed, in which case the use of fluoroscopy is included in the supervision and interpretation codes or the myelography via lumbar injection code. Image guidance and the injection of contrast are inclusive components and are required for the performance of myelography, as described by codes 62302, 62303, 62304, 62305.

For radiologic supervision and interpretation of epidurography, use 72275. Code 72275 is only to be used when an epidurogram is performed, images documented, and a formal radiologic report is issued.

Code 62263 describes a catheter-based treatment involving targeted injection of various substances (eg, hypertonic saline, steroid, anesthetic) via an indwelling epidural catheter. Code 62263 includes percutaneous insertion and removal of an epidural catheter (remaining in place over a several-day period), for the administration of multiple injections of a neurolytic agent(s) performed during serial treatment sessions (ie, spanning two or more treatment days). If required, adhesions or scarring may also be lysed by mechanical means. Code 62263 is not reported for each adhesiolysis treatment, but should be reported once to describe the entire series of injections/infusions spanning two or more treatment days.

Code 62264 describes multiple adhesiolysis treatment sessions performed on the same day. Adhesions or scarring may be lysed by injections of neurolytic agent(s). If required, adhesions or scarring may also be lysed mechanically using a percutaneously-deployed catheter.

Codes 62263 and 62264 include the procedure of injections of contrast for epidurography (72275) and fluoroscopic guidance and localization (77003) during initial or subsequent sessions.

Fluoroscopy or CT and any injection of contrast are inclusive components of 62321, 62323, 62325, 62327. For epidurography, use 72275.

The placement and use of a catheter to administer one or more epidural or subarachnoid injections on a single calendar day should be reported in the same manner as if a needle had been used, ie, as a single injection using either 62320, 62321, 62322, or 62323. Such injections should not be reported with 62324, 62325, 62326, or 62327.

Threading a catheter into the epidural space, injecting substances at one or more levels and then removing the catheter should be treated as a single injection (62320, 62321, 62322, 62323). If the catheter is left in place to deliver substance(s) over a prolonged period (ie, more than a single calendar day) either continuously or via intermittent bolus, use 62324, 62325, 62326, 62327 as appropriate.

When reporting 62320, 62321, 62322, 62323, 62324, 62325, 62326, 62327 code choice is based on the region at which the needle or catheter entered the body (eg, lumbar). Codes 62320, 62321, 62322, 62323, 62324, 62325, 62326, 62327 should be reported only once, when the substance injected spreads or catheter tip insertion moves into another spinal region (eg, 62322 is reported only once for injection or catheter insertion at L3-4 with spread of the substance or placement of the catheter tip to the thoracic region).

Percutaneous spinal procedures are done with indirect visualization (eg, image guidance) (eg, 62287). Endoscopic assistance during an open procedure with continuous and direct visualization (light-based) is reported using excision codes (eg, 63020-63035).

Definitions

For purposes of CPT coding, the following definitions of approach and visualization apply. The primary approach and visualization define the service, whether another method is incidentally applied. Surgical services are presumed open, unless otherwise specified.

Percutaneous: Image-guided procedures (eg, computer tomography [CT] or fluoroscopy) performed with indirect visualization of the spine without the use of any device that allows visualization through a surgical incision.

Endoscopic: Spinal procedures performed with continuous direct visualization of the spine through an endoscope.

Open: Spinal procedures performed with continuous direct visualization of the spine through a surgical opening.

Indirect visualization: Image-guided (eg, CT or fluoroscopy), not light-based visualization.

Direct visualization: Light-based visualization; can be performed by eye, or with surgical loupes, microscope, or endoscope.

AMA Coding Notes

Injection, Drainage, or Aspiration Procedures on the Spine and Spinal Cord

(For transforaminal epidural injection, see 64479-64484)

(Report 01996 for daily hospital management of continuous epidural or subarachnoid drug administration performed in conjunction with 62324, 62325, 62326, 62327)

(For the techniques of microsurgery and/or use of microscope, use 69990)

Surgical Procedures on the Spine and Spinal Cord

(For application of caliper or tongs, use 20660)

(For treatment of fracture or dislocation of spine, see 22310-22327)

AMA *CPT Assistant* □

62324: May 17: 10, Sep 17: 6
62325: May 17: 10, Sep 17: 6

Plain English Description

The skin over the spinal region to be catheterized is cleansed with an antiseptic solution and a local anesthetic is injected. A spinal needle is inserted into the back of the epidural or subarachnoid space through a paramedian or midline interlaminar approach, usually under fluoroscopic guidance. The epidural space is the outermost area of the spinal canal filled with cerebrospinal fluid that lies between the outermost protective membrane (dura mater) surrounding the nerve roots and the vertebral wall. The subarachnoid space lies closer to the spinal cord and is located between the middle protective membrane, the arachnoid, and the innermost delicate membrane surrounding the spinal cord, the pia mater. Contrast dye may be injected first to confirm proper needle placement or perform an epidurography. A catheter is then threaded through the needle and advanced within the target space to ensure secure placement. A diagnostic or therapeutic substance, such as an anesthetic, antispasmodic, opioid, steroid, or other solution, such as a steroid and local anesthetic mix, excluding a neurolytic substance, is then continuously infused or injected as an intermittent bolus into the epidural or subarachnoid space. Following infusion, the patient is monitored for any adverse effects. Use 62324 for interlaminar epidural or subarachnoid infusion or intermittent

CPT © 2018 American Medical Association. All Rights Reserved.

bolus injection(s) in the cervical or thoracic region without imaging guidance and 62325 with imaging guidance.

ICD-10-CM Diagnostic Codes

G89.11 Acute pain due to trauma
G89.12 Acute post-thoracotomy pain
G89.18 Other acute postprocedural pain
G89.21 Chronic pain due to trauma
G89.22 Chronic post-thoracotomy pain
G89.28 Other chronic postprocedural pain
G89.29 Other chronic pain
G89.3 Neoplasm related pain (acute) (chronic)
G89.4 Chronic pain syndrome
M43.02 Spondylolysis, cervical region
M43.03 Spondylolysis, cervicothoracic region
M43.04 Spondylolysis, thoracic region
M43.12 Spondylolisthesis, cervical region
M43.13 Spondylolisthesis, cervicothoracic region
M43.14 Spondylolisthesis, thoracic region
M47.21 Other spondylosis with radiculopathy, occipito-atlanto-axial region
M47.22 Other spondylosis with radiculopathy, cervical region
M47.23 Other spondylosis with radiculopathy, cervicothoracic region
M47.24 Other spondylosis with radiculopathy, thoracic region
M47.812 Spondylosis without myelopathy or radiculopathy, cervical region
M47.813 Spondylosis without myelopathy or radiculopathy, cervicothoracic region
M47.814 Spondylosis without myelopathy or radiculopathy, thoracic region
M47.815 Spondylosis without myelopathy or radiculopathy, thoracolumbar region
M48.01 Spinal stenosis, occipito-atlanto-axial region
M48.02 Spinal stenosis, cervical region
M48.03 Spinal stenosis, cervicothoracic region
M48.04 Spinal stenosis, thoracic region
M50.01 Cervical disc disorder with myelopathy, high cervical region
M50.11 Cervical disc disorder with radiculopathy, high cervical region
M50.121 Cervical disc disorder at C4-C5 level with radiculopathy
M50.122 Cervical disc disorder at C5-C6 level with radiculopathy
M50.123 Cervical disc disorder at C6-C7 level with radiculopathy
M50.13 Cervical disc disorder with radiculopathy, cervicothoracic region
M50.21 Other cervical disc displacement, high cervical region
M50.23 Other cervical disc displacement, cervicothoracic region
M50.31 Other cervical disc degeneration, high cervical region
M50.32 Other cervical disc degeneration, mid-cervical region
M50.321 Other cervical disc degeneration at C4-C5 level
M50.322 Other cervical disc degeneration at C5-C6 level
M50.323 Other cervical disc degeneration at C6-C7 level
M50.33 Other cervical disc degeneration, cervicothoracic region
M50.81 Other cervical disc disorders, high cervical region
M50.821 Other cervical disc disorders at C4-C5 level
M50.822 Other cervical disc disorders at C5-C6 level
M50.823 Other cervical disc disorders at C6-C7 level
M50.83 Other cervical disc disorders, cervicothoracic region
M50.91 Cervical disc disorder, unspecified, high cervical region
M50.921 Unspecified cervical disc disorder at C4-C5 level
M50.922 Unspecified cervical disc disorder at C5-C6 level
M50.923 Unspecified cervical disc disorder at C6-C7 level
M50.93 Cervical disc disorder, unspecified, cervicothoracic region
M51.04 Intervertebral disc disorders with myelopathy, thoracic region
M51.05 Intervertebral disc disorders with myelopathy, thoracolumbar region
M51.14 Intervertebral disc disorders with radiculopathy, thoracic region
M51.24 Other intervertebral disc displacement, thoracic region
M51.34 Other intervertebral disc degeneration, thoracic region
M54.11 Radiculopathy, occipito-atlanto-axial region
M54.12 Radiculopathy, cervical region
M54.13 Radiculopathy, cervicothoracic region

CCI Edits

Refer to Appendix A for CCI edits.

Facility RVUs ☐

Code	Work	PE Facility	MP	Total Facility
62324	1.89	0.56	0.15	2.60
62325	2.20	0.70	0.18	3.08

Non-facility RVUs ☐

Code	Work	PE Non-Facility	MP	Total Non-Facility
62324	1.89	2.08	0.15	4.12
62325	2.20	4.29	0.18	6.67

Modifiers (PAR) ☐

Code	Mod 50	Mod 51	Mod 62	Mod 66	Mod 80
62324	9	2	0	0	1
62325	9	2	0	0	1

Global Period

Code	Days
62324	000
62325	000

CPT © 2018 American Medical Association. All Rights Reserved.

62326-62327

62326 Injection(s), including indwelling catheter placement, continuous infusion or intermittent bolus, of diagnostic or therapeutic substance(s) (eg, anesthetic, antispasmodic, opioid, steroid, other solution), not including neurolytic substances, interlaminar epidural or subarachnoid, lumbar or sacral (caudal); without imaging guidance

62327 Injection(s), including indwelling catheter placement, continuous infusion or intermittent bolus, of diagnostic or therapeutic substance(s) (eg, anesthetic, antispasmodic, opioid, steroid, other solution), not including neurolytic substances, interlaminar epidural or subarachnoid, lumbar or sacral (caudal); with imaging guidance (ie, fluoroscopy or CT)

(Do not report 62327 in conjunction with 77003, 77012, 76942)

(Report 01996 for daily hospital management of continuous epidural or subarachnoid drug administration performed in conjunction with 62324, 62325, 62326, 62327)

AMA Coding Guideline

Injection, Drainage, or Aspiration Procedures on the Spine and Spinal Cord

Injection of contrast during fluoroscopic guidance and localization is an inclusive component of 62263, 62264, 62267, 62270, 62272, 62273, 62280, 62281, 62282, 62302, 62303, 62304, 62305, 62321, 62323, 62325, 62327. Fluoroscopic guidance and localization is reported with 77003, unless a formal contrast study (myelography, epidurography, or arthrography) is performed, in which case the use of fluoroscopy is included in the supervision and interpretation codes or the myelography via lumbar injection code. Image guidance and the injection of contrast are inclusive components and are required for the performance of myelography, as described by codes 62302, 62303, 62304, 62305.

For radiologic supervision and interpretation of epidurography, use 72275. Code 72275 is only to be used when an epidurogram is performed, images documented, and a formal radiologic report is issued.

Code 62263 describes a catheter-based treatment involving targeted injection of various substances (eg, hypertonic saline, steroid, anesthetic) via an indwelling epidural catheter. Code 62263 includes percutaneous insertion and removal of an epidural catheter (remaining in place over a several-day period), for the administration of multiple injections of a neurolytic agent(s) performed during serial treatment sessions (ie, spanning two or more treatment days). If required, adhesions or scarring may also be lysed by mechanical means. Code 62263 is not reported for each adhesiolysis treatment, but should be reported once to describe the entire series of injections/infusions spanning two or more treatment days.

Code 62264 describes multiple adhesiolysis treatment sessions performed on the same day. Adhesions or scarring may be lysed by injections of neurolytic agent(s). If required, adhesions or scarring may also be lysed mechanically using a percutaneously-deployed catheter.

Codes 62263 and 62264 include the procedure of injections of contrast for epidurography (72275) and fluoroscopic guidance and localization (77003) during initial or subsequent sessions.

Fluoroscopy or CT and any injection of contrast are inclusive components of 62321, 62323, 62325, 62327. For epidurography, use 72275.

The placement and use of a catheter to administer one or more epidural or subarachnoid injections on a single calendar day should be reported in the same manner as if a needle had been used, ie, as a single injection using either 62320, 62321, 62322, or 62323. Such injections should not be reported with 62324, 62325, 62326, or 62327.

Threading a catheter into the epidural space, injecting substances at one or more levels and then removing the catheter should be treated as a single injection (62320, 62321, 62322, 62323). If the catheter is left in place to deliver substance(s) over a prolonged period (ie, more than a single calendar day) either continuously or via intermittent bolus, use 62324, 62325, 62326, 62327 as appropriate.

When reporting 62320, 62321, 62322, 62323, 62324, 62325, 62326, 62327 code choice is based on the region at which the needle or catheter entered the body (eg, lumbar). Codes 62320, 62321, 62322, 62323, 62324, 62325, 62326, 62327 should be reported only once, when the substance injected spreads or catheter tip insertion moves into another spinal region (eg, 62322 is reported only once for injection or catheter insertion at L3-4 with spread of the substance or placement of the catheter tip to the thoracic region).

Percutaneous spinal procedures are done with indirect visualization (eg, image guidance) (eg, 62287). Endoscopic assistance during an open procedure with continuous and direct visualization (light-based) is reported using excision codes (eg, 63020-63035).

Definitions

For purposes of CPT coding, the following definitions of approach and visualization apply. The primary approach and visualization define the service, whether another method is incidentally applied. Surgical services are presumed open, unless otherwise specified.

Percutaneous: Image-guided procedures (eg, computer tomography [CT] or fluoroscopy) performed with indirect visualization of the spine without the use of any device that allows visualization through a surgical incision.

Endoscopic: Spinal procedures performed with continuous direct visualization of the spine through an endoscope.

Open: Spinal procedures performed with continuous direct visualization of the spine through a surgical opening.

Indirect visualization: Image-guided (eg, CT or fluoroscopy), not light-based visualization.

Direct visualization: Light-based visualization; can be performed by eye, or with surgical loupes, microscope, or endoscope.

AMA Coding Notes

Injection, Drainage, or Aspiration Procedures on the Spine and Spinal Cord

(For transforaminal epidural injection, see 64479-64484)

(Report 01996 for daily hospital management of continuous epidural or subarachnoid drug administration performed in conjunction with 62324, 62325, 62326, 62327)

(For the techniques of microsurgery and/or use of microscope, use 69990)

Surgical Procedures on the Spine and Spinal Cord

(For application of caliper or tongs, use 20660)

(For treatment of fracture or dislocation of spine, see 22310-22327)

AMA *CPT Assistant*

62326: May 17: 10, Sep 17: 7

62327: May 17: 10, Sep 17: 7

Plain English Description

The skin over the spinal region to be catheterized is cleansed with an antiseptic solution and a local anesthetic is injected. A spinal needle is inserted into the back of the epidural or subarachnoid space through a paramedian or midline interlaminar approach, usually under fluoroscopic guidance. The epidural space is the outermost area of the spinal canal filled with cerebrospinal fluid that lies between the outermost protective membrane (dura mater) surrounding the nerve roots and the vertebral wall. The subarachnoid space lies closer to the spinal cord and is located between the middle protective membrane, the arachnoid, and the innermost delicate membrane surrounding the spinal cord, the pia mater. Contrast dye may be injected first to confirm proper needle placement or perform an epidurography. A catheter is then threaded through the needle and advanced within the target space to ensure secure placement. A diagnostic or therapeutic substance, such as an anesthetic, antispasmodic, opioid, steroid, or other solution, such as a steroid and local anesthetic mix, excluding a neurolytic substance, is then continuously infused or injected as an intermittent

CPT © 2018 American Medical Association. All Rights Reserved.

bolus into the epidural or subarachnoid space. Following infusion, the patient is monitored for any adverse effects. Use 62326 for interlaminar epidural or subarachnoid infusion or bolus injection(s) in the lumbar or sacral (caudal) region without imaging guidance and 62327 with imaging guidance.

ICD-10-CM Diagnostic Codes

B02.23 Postherpetic polyneuropathy
B02.7 Disseminated zoster
B02.8 Zoster with other complications
B02.9 Zoster without complications
G89.11 Acute pain due to trauma
G89.12 Acute post-thoracotomy pain
G89.18 Other acute postprocedural pain
G89.21 Chronic pain due to trauma
G89.22 Chronic post-thoracotomy pain
G89.28 Other chronic postprocedural pain
G89.29 Other chronic pain
G97.1 Other reaction to spinal and lumbar puncture
M43.05 Spondylolysis, thoracolumbar region
M43.06 Spondylolysis, lumbar region
M43.07 Spondylolysis, lumbosacral region
M43.08 Spondylolysis, sacral and sacrococcygeal region
M43.15 Spondylolisthesis, thoracolumbar region
M43.16 Spondylolisthesis, lumbar region
M43.17 Spondylolisthesis, lumbosacral region
M43.18 Spondylolisthesis, sacral and sacrococcygeal region
M47.26 Other spondylosis with radiculopathy, lumbar region
M47.816 Spondylosis without myelopathy or radiculopathy, lumbar region
M47.817 Spondylosis without myelopathy or radiculopathy, lumbosacral region
M47.818 Spondylosis without myelopathy or radiculopathy, sacral and sacrococcygeal region
M48.062 Spinal stenosis, lumbar region with neurogenic claudication
M48.07 Spinal stenosis, lumbosacral region
M51.05 Intervertebral disc disorders with myelopathy, thoracolumbar region
M51.06 Intervertebral disc disorders with myelopathy, lumbar region
M51.15 Intervertebral disc disorders with radiculopathy, thoracolumbar region
M51.16 Intervertebral disc disorders with radiculopathy, lumbar region
M51.17 Intervertebral disc disorders with radiculopathy, lumbosacral region
M51.25 Other intervertebral disc displacement, thoracolumbar region
M51.26 Other intervertebral disc displacement, lumbar region
M51.27 Other intervertebral disc displacement, lumbosacral region
M51.35 Other intervertebral disc degeneration, thoracolumbar region
M51.36 Other intervertebral disc degeneration, lumbar region
M51.37 Other intervertebral disc degeneration, lumbosacral region
M54.15 Radiculopathy, thoracolumbar region
M54.16 Radiculopathy, lumbar region
M54.17 Radiculopathy, lumbosacral region
M54.18 Radiculopathy, sacral and sacrococcygeal region
⇄ M54.31 Sciatica, right side
⇄ M54.32 Sciatica, left side
⇄ M54.41 Lumbago with sciatica, right side
⇄ M54.42 Lumbago with sciatica, left side
M54.5 Low back pain
M96.1 Postlaminectomy syndrome, not elsewhere classified
M99.23 Subluxation stenosis of neural canal of lumbar region
M99.33 Osseous stenosis of neural canal of lumbar region
M99.43 Connective tissue stenosis of neural canal of lumbar region
M99.53 Intervertebral disc stenosis of neural canal of lumbar region
M99.63 Osseous and subluxation stenosis of intervertebral foramina of lumbar region
M99.73 Connective tissue and disc stenosis of intervertebral foramina of lumbar region

CCI Edits

Refer to Appendix A for CCI edits.

Facility RVUs ☐

Code	Work	PE Facility	MP	Total Facility
62326	1.78	0.63	0.15	2.56
62327	1.90	0.72	0.16	2.78

Non-facility RVUs ☐

Code	Work	PE Non-Facility	MP	Total Non-Facility
62326	1.78	2.35	0.15	4.28
62327	1.90	4.63	0.16	6.69

Modifiers (PAR) ☐

Code	Mod 50	Mod 51	Mod 62	Mod 66	Mod 80
62326	9	2	0	0	1
62327	9	2	0	0	1

Global Period

Code	Days
62326	000
62327	000

CPT © 2018 American Medical Association. All Rights Reserved.

62350-62351

62350 Implantation, revision or repositioning of tunneled intrathecal or epidural catheter, for long-term medication administration via an external pump or implantable reservoir/infusion pump; without laminectomy

62351 Implantation, revision or repositioning of tunneled intrathecal or epidural catheter, for long-term medication administration via an external pump or implantable reservoir/infusion pump; with laminectomy

(For refilling and maintenance of an implantable infusion pump for spinal or brain drug therapy, see 95990, 95991)

AMA Coding Notes

Catheter Implantation Procedures on the Spine and Spinal Cord

(For percutaneous placement of intrathecal or epidural catheter, see 62270, 62272, 62273, 62280, 62281, 62282, 62284, 62320, 62321, 62322, 62323, 62324, 62325, 62326, 62327)

Surgical Procedures on the Spine and Spinal Cord

(For application of caliper or tongs, use 20660)

(For treatment of fracture or dislocation of spine, see 22310-22327)

AMA *CPT Assistant* □

62350: Nov 99: 36
62351: Nov 99: 36

Plain English Description

Implantation, revision, or repositioning of an intrathecal or epidural catheter may be performed with or without a laminectomy. In 62350, the procedure is performed without a laminectomy. For initial implantation, the overlying skin is cleansed with an antiseptic solution and a local anesthetic injected. A spinal needle is inserted into the skin and advanced into the intrathecal or epidural space. A catheter is then threaded through the needle and the catheter tip advanced cephalad to the selected level for pain control or other medication administration. The catheter is then tunneled subcutaneously approximately 5-10 cm away from the insertion site. The catheter is secured with sutures. The catheter is then connected to an external pump or an implantable reservoir or infusion pump. If revision of the catheter is performed the catheter is exposed and the connection site at the reservoir or pump is inspected. The catheter may be disconnected and trimmed and reconnected or other revisions made. If repositioning is performed, the catheter is disconnected from the internal or external pump or reservoir. The catheter is manipulated into a different site within the intrathecal or epidural space. The revised or repositioned catheter is secured with sutures and reconnected to the pump or reservoir. In 62351, the procedure is performed with a laminectomy. The skin is incised over the catheter placement site and extended down to the spinous processes. Muscle is retracted off the lamina and facet joint. A bone drill is used to remove part or all of the lamina. The intrathecal or epidural catheter is implanted, revised, or repositioned as described above. The catheter is tunneled through the subcutaneous tissue and connected to the pump or reservoir. The surgical wound is closed.

Implantation, revision or repositioning of tunneled intrathecal or epidural catheter

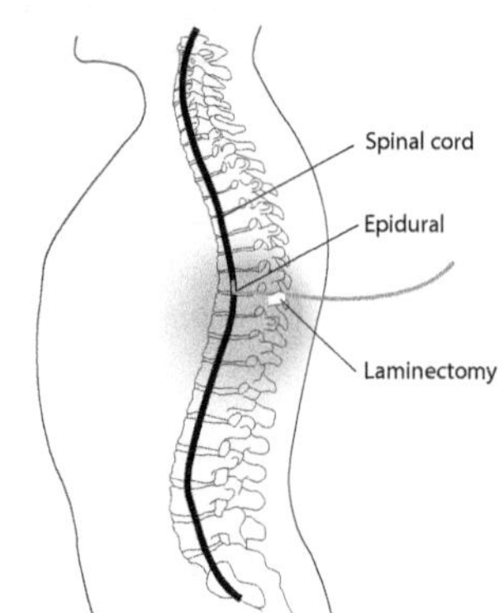

Without laminectomy (62350); with laminectomy (62351)

ICD-10-CM Diagnostic Codes

	C16.8	Malignant neoplasm of overlapping sites of stomach
	C16.9	Malignant neoplasm of stomach, unspecified
	C17.8	Malignant neoplasm of overlapping sites of small intestine
	C17.9	Malignant neoplasm of small intestine, unspecified
	C18.8	Malignant neoplasm of overlapping sites of colon
	C18.9	Malignant neoplasm of colon, unspecified
	C22.0	Liver cell carcinoma
	C22.1	Intrahepatic bile duct carcinoma
	C22.2	Hepatoblastoma
	C22.3	Angiosarcoma of liver
	C22.4	Other sarcomas of liver
	C22.7	Other specified carcinomas of liver
	C22.8	Malignant neoplasm of liver, primary, unspecified as to type
	C22.9	Malignant neoplasm of liver, not specified as primary or secondary
	C25.0	Malignant neoplasm of head of pancreas
	C25.1	Malignant neoplasm of body of pancreas
	C25.2	Malignant neoplasm of tail of pancreas
	C25.3	Malignant neoplasm of pancreatic duct
	C25.4	Malignant neoplasm of endocrine pancreas
	C25.7	Malignant neoplasm of other parts of pancreas
	C25.8	Malignant neoplasm of overlapping sites of pancreas
	C25.9	Malignant neoplasm of pancreas, unspecified
	C26.0	Malignant neoplasm of intestinal tract, part unspecified
	C26.9	Malignant neoplasm of ill-defined sites within the digestive system
⇄	C34.81	Malignant neoplasm of overlapping sites of right bronchus and lung
⇄	C34.82	Malignant neoplasm of overlapping sites of left bronchus and lung
	C39.9	Malignant neoplasm of lower respiratory tract, part unspecified
	C41.2	Malignant neoplasm of vertebral column
	C41.3	Malignant neoplasm of ribs, sternum and clavicle
	C41.4	Malignant neoplasm of pelvic bones, sacrum and coccyx
	C48.0	Malignant neoplasm of retroperitoneum
	C48.1	Malignant neoplasm of specified parts of peritoneum
	C48.8	Malignant neoplasm of overlapping sites of retroperitoneum and peritoneum
	C76.0	Malignant neoplasm of head, face and neck
	C76.1	Malignant neoplasm of thorax
	C76.2	Malignant neoplasm of abdomen
	C76.3	Malignant neoplasm of pelvis
	C79.9	Secondary malignant neoplasm of unspecified site
	G89.11	Acute pain due to trauma
	G89.12	Acute post-thoracotomy pain
	G89.18	Other acute postprocedural pain
	G89.21	Chronic pain due to trauma
	G89.22	Chronic post-thoracotomy pain
	G89.28	Other chronic postprocedural pain
	G89.29	Other chronic pain
	G89.3	Neoplasm related pain (acute) (chronic)
	M96.1	Postlaminectomy syndrome, not elsewhere classified

CCI Edits

Refer to Appendix A for CCI edits.

CPT © 2018 American Medical Association. All Rights Reserved.

Facility RVUs

Code	Work	PE Facility	MP	Total Facility
62350	6.05	4.30	1.15	11.50
62351	11.66	9.87	3.36	24.89

Non-facility RVUs

Code	Work	PE Non-Facility	MP	Total Non-Facility
62350	6.05	4.30	1.15	11.50
62351	11.66	9.87	3.36	24.89

Modifiers (PAR)

Code	Mod 50	Mod 51	Mod 62	Mod 66	Mod 80
62350	0	2	1	0	1
62351	0	2	2	0	2

Global Period

Code	Days
62350	010
62351	090

CPT © 2018 American Medical Association. All Rights Reserved.

62355

62355 Removal of previously implanted intrathecal or epidural catheter

AMA Coding Notes

Catheter Implantation Procedures on the Spine and Spinal Cord

(For percutaneous placement of intrathecal or epidural catheter, see 62270, 62272, 62273, 62280, 62281, 62282, 62284, 62320, 62321, 62322, 62323, 62324, 62325, 62326, 62327)

Surgical Procedures on the Spine and Spinal Cord

(For application of caliper or tongs, use 20660)

(For treatment of fracture or dislocation of spine, see 22310-22327)

Plain English Description

The previously placed intrathecal or epidural catheter is exposed at the distal aspect of the tunnel and disconnected from the pump or reservoir. Distal sutures are removed. The tunneled portion of the catheter is then palpated from the pump or reservoir site to the site where it enters the spinal canal. A small incision is made over the site where the catheter enters the spinal canal. The subcutaneous tunneled portion of the catheter is removed. Proximal sutures are removed. The catheter is then removed from the intrathecal or epidural space. The skin is closed with a suture or steristrips.

Removal of previously implanted intrathecal or epidural catheter

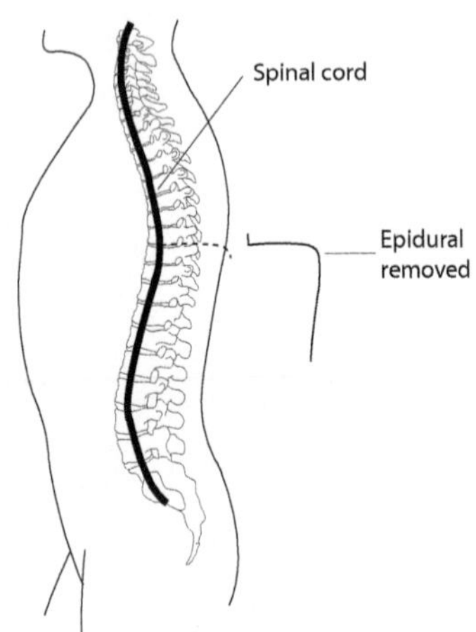

ICD-10-CM Diagnostic Codes

➐	T85.610	Breakdown (mechanical) of cranial or spinal infusion catheter
➐	T85.620	Displacement of cranial or spinal infusion catheter
➐	T85.630	Leakage of cranial or spinal infusion catheter
➐	T85.690	Other mechanical complication of cranial or spinal infusion catheter
➐	T85.735	Infection and inflammatory reaction due to cranial or spinal infusion catheter
➐	T85.810	Embolism due to nervous system prosthetic devices, implants and grafts
➐	T85.820	Fibrosis due to nervous system prosthetic devices, implants and grafts
➐	T85.830	Hemorrhage due to nervous system prosthetic devices, implants and grafts
➐	T85.840	Pain due to nervous system prosthetic devices, implants and grafts
➐	T85.850	Stenosis due to nervous system prosthetic devices, implants and grafts
➐	T85.860	Thrombosis due to nervous system prosthetic devices, implants and grafts
➐	T85.890	Other specified complication of nervous system prosthetic devices, implants and grafts
	Z45.1	Encounter for adjustment and management of infusion pump
	Z45.49	Encounter for adjustment and management of other implanted nervous system device

ICD-10-CM Coding Notes

For codes requiring a 7th character extension, refer to your ICD-10-CM book. Review the character descriptions and coding guidelines for proper selection. For some procedures, only certain characters will apply.

CCI Edits

Refer to Appendix A for CCI edits.

Facility RVUs ☐

Code	Work	PE Facility	MP	Total Facility
62355	3.55	3.43	0.75	7.73

Non-facility RVUs ☐

Code	Work	PE Non-Facility	MP	Total Non-Facility
62355	3.55	3.43	0.75	7.73

Modifiers (PAR) ☐

Code	Mod 50	Mod 51	Mod 62	Mod 66	Mod 80
62355	0	2	0	0	0

Global Period

Code	Days
62355	010

CPT © 2018 American Medical Association. All Rights Reserved.

62360-62362

62360 Implantation or replacement of device for intrathecal or epidural drug infusion; subcutaneous reservoir

62361 Implantation or replacement of device for intrathecal or epidural drug infusion; nonprogrammable pump

62362 Implantation or replacement of device for intrathecal or epidural drug infusion; programmable pump, including preparation of pump, with or without programming

AMA Coding Notes

Surgical Procedures on the Spine and Spinal Cord

(For application of caliper or tongs, use 20660)

(For treatment of fracture or dislocation of spine, see 22310-22327)

AMA *CPT Assistant* ☐

62362: Mar 97: 11

Plain English Description

For initial implantation of a subcutaneous reservoir or pump, the skin is incised, typically in the lateral aspect of the lower abdomen. A subcutaneous pocket is fashioned. The subcutaneous reservoir or pump is connected to the catheter and placed in the pocket. The skin is closed over the device. For replacement of a subcutaneous reservoir or pump, the old device is first removed in a separately reportable procedure. The new device is then inserted. Use 62360 for placement of a subcutaneous reservoir. Use 62361 for placement of a nonprogrammable pump. Use 62362 for placement of a programmable pump. Placement of a programmable pump requires preparation of the pump. The reservoir and alarm status are checked to ensure that the pump will function properly once implanted. Dosing, continuous infusion rate and/or time intervals for bolus infusion may be programmed at this time.

Implantation or replacement of device for intrathecal or epidural drug infusion; programmable pump

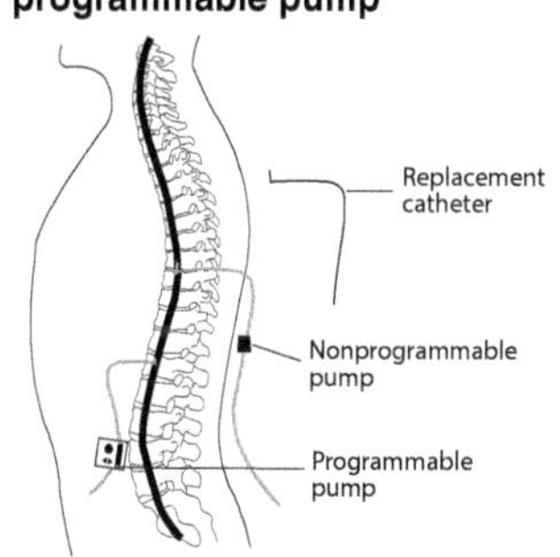

Subcutaneous reservoir (62360); nonprogrammable pump (62361); programmable pump (62362)

ICD-10-CM Diagnostic Codes

	C76.0	Malignant neoplasm of head, face and neck
	C76.1	Malignant neoplasm of thorax
	C76.2	Malignant neoplasm of abdomen
	C76.3	Malignant neoplasm of pelvis
	C79.9	Secondary malignant neoplasm of unspecified site
	G89.21	Chronic pain due to trauma
	G89.22	Chronic post-thoracotomy pain
	G89.28	Other chronic postprocedural pain
	G89.29	Other chronic pain
	G89.3	Neoplasm related pain (acute) (chronic)
	M96.1	Postlaminectomy syndrome, not elsewhere classified
⓿	T85.610	Breakdown (mechanical) of cranial or spinal infusion catheter
⓿	T85.620	Displacement of cranial or spinal infusion catheter
⓿	T85.630	Leakage of cranial or spinal infusion catheter
⓿	T85.690	Other mechanical complication of cranial or spinal infusion catheter
⓿	T85.735	Infection and inflammatory reaction due to cranial or spinal infusion catheter
⓿	T85.810	Embolism due to nervous system prosthetic devices, implants and grafts
⓿	T85.820	Fibrosis due to nervous system prosthetic devices, implants and grafts
⓿	T85.830	Hemorrhage due to nervous system prosthetic devices, implants and grafts
⓿	T85.840	Pain due to nervous system prosthetic devices, implants and grafts
⓿	T85.850	Stenosis due to nervous system prosthetic devices, implants and grafts
⓿	T85.860	Thrombosis due to nervous system prosthetic devices, implants and grafts
⓿	T85.890	Other specified complication of nervous system prosthetic devices, implants and grafts
	Z45.1	Encounter for adjustment and management of infusion pump
	Z45.49	Encounter for adjustment and management of other implanted nervous system device

ICD-10-CM Coding Notes

For codes requiring a 7th character extension, refer to your ICD-10-CM book. Review the character descriptions and coding guidelines for proper selection. For some procedures, only certain characters will apply.

CCI Edits

Refer to Appendix A for CCI edits.

Facility RVUs ☐

Code	Work	PE Facility	MP	Total Facility
62360	4.33	3.81	0.99	9.13
62361	5.00	5.42	2.04	12.46
62362	5.60	4.25	1.19	11.04

Non-facility RVUs ☐

Code	Work	PE Non-Facility	MP	Total Non-Facility
62360	4.33	3.81	0.99	9.13
62361	5.00	5.42	2.04	12.46
62362	5.60	4.25	1.19	11.04

Modifiers (PAR) ☐

Code	Mod 50	Mod 51	Mod 62	Mod 66	Mod 80
62360	0	2	1	0	0
62361	0	2	1	0	0
62362	0	2	1	0	0

Global Period

Code	Days
62360	010
62361	010
62362	010

CPT © 2018 American Medical Association. All Rights Reserved.

62367-62368

62367 Electronic analysis of programmable, implanted pump for intrathecal or epidural drug infusion (includes evaluation of reservoir status, alarm status, drug prescription status); without reprogramming or refill

62368 Electronic analysis of programmable, implanted pump for intrathecal or epidural drug infusion (includes evaluation of reservoir status, alarm status, drug prescription status); with reprogramming

(For refilling and maintenance of an implantable infusion pump for spinal or brain drug therapy, see 95990-95991)

AMA Coding Notes

Surgical Procedures on the Spine and Spinal Cord

(For application of caliper or tongs, use 20660)

(For treatment of fracture or dislocation of spine, see 22310-22327)

AMA *CPT Assistant* ▢

62367: Jul 12: 5, 6, Aug 12: 10, 11, 12, 15

62368: Nov 02: 10, Jul 06: 1, Jul 12: 5, 6, Aug 12: 10, 11, 12, 15

Plain English Description

A previously placed programmable implanted intrathecal or epidural drug infusion pump is evaluated using electronic analysis. A connection is established between the programmable pump and the interrogation device. The interrogation device provides information on reservoir status, alarm status and drug flow rates, which are evaluated to ensure that these are within normal parameters. The physician reviews the data obtained by the interrogation device and provides a written report of findings. In 62367, the pump is not reprogrammed or refilled. In 62368, the physician reprograms the pump using a telemetry device. Reprogramming may include adjusting alarm parameters and drug flow rates. The new settings are verified with the interrogation device. The pump is not refilled

Electronic analysis of programmable, implanted pump for intrathecal or epidural drug infusion

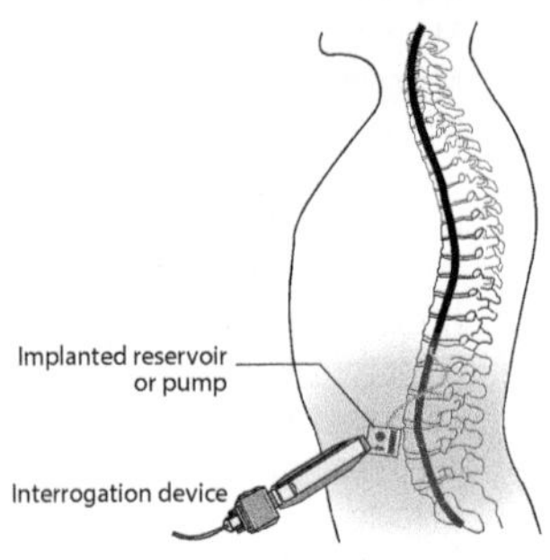

Without reprogramming (62367); with reprogramming 62368

ICD-10-CM Diagnostic Codes

Z45.1	Encounter for adjustment and management of infusion pump
Z45.49	Encounter for adjustment and management of other implanted nervous system device

CCI Edits

Refer to Appendix A for CCI edits.

Facility RVUs ▢

Code	Work	PE Facility	MP	Total Facility
62367	0.48	0.19	0.05	0.72
62368	0.67	0.27	0.07	1.01

Non-facility RVUs ▢

Code	Work	PE Non-Facility	MP	Total Non-Facility
62367	0.48	0.61	0.05	1.14
62368	0.67	0.83	0.07	1.57

Modifiers (PAR) ▢

Code	Mod 50	Mod 51	Mod 62	Mod 66	Mod 80
62367	0	0	0	0	1
62368	0	0	0	0	1

Global Period

Code	Days
62367	XXX
62368	XXX

CPT © 2018 American Medical Association. All Rights Reserved.

62369-62370

62369 Electronic analysis of programmable, implanted pump for intrathecal or epidural drug infusion (includes evaluation of reservoir status, alarm status, drug prescription status); with reprogramming and refill

62370 Electronic analysis of programmable, implanted pump for intrathecal or epidural drug infusion (includes evaluation of reservoir status, alarm status, drug prescription status); with reprogramming and refill (requiring skill of a physician or other qualified health care professional)

(Do not report 62367-62370 in conjunction with 95990, 95991. For refilling and maintenance of a reservoir or an implantable infusion pump for spinal or brain drug delivery without reprogramming, see 95990, 95991)

AMA Coding Notes

Surgical Procedures on the Spine and Spinal Cord

(For application of caliper or tongs, use 20660)

(For treatment of fracture or dislocation of spine, see 22310-22327)

AMA *CPT Assistant*

62369: Jul 12: 5, 6, Aug 12: 10, 11, 12, 15
62370: Jul 12: 5, 6, Aug 12: 10, 11, 12, 15

Plain English Description

A previously placed programmable, implanted intrathecal or epidural drug infusion pump is evaluated using electronic analysis. A connection is established between the programmable pump and the interrogation device. The interrogation device provides information on reservoir status, alarm status, and drug flow rates, which are evaluated to ensure that these are within normal parameters. The technician or physician reviews the data obtained by the interrogation device and determines that reprogramming is needed. Reprogramming is performed using a telemetry device and may include adjusting alarm parameters and drug flow rates. The new settings are verified with the interrogation device. The pump is also refilled. A written report of findings is provided. Use 62369 when the evaluation, reprogramming, and refilling of the pump is performed by a technician. Use 62370 when the skill of a physician or other qualified health care professional is required.

Electronic analysis of programmable, implanted pump for intrathecal or epidural drug infusion

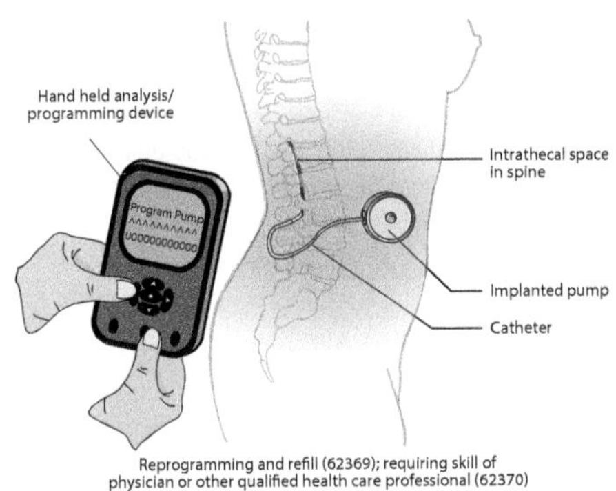

Reprogramming and refill (62369); requiring skill of physician or other qualified health care professional (62370)

ICD-10-CM Diagnostic Codes

Z45.1	Encounter for adjustment and management of infusion pump
Z45.49	Encounter for adjustment and management of other implanted nervous system device

CCI Edits

Refer to Appendix A for CCI edits.

Facility RVUs

Code	Work	PE Facility	MP	Total Facility
62369	0.67	0.27	0.07	1.01
62370	0.90	0.35	0.08	1.33

Non-facility RVUs

Code	Work	PE Non-Facility	MP	Total Non-Facility
62369	0.67	2.60	0.07	3.34
62370	0.90	2.49	0.08	3.47

Modifiers (PAR)

Code	Mod 50	Mod 51	Mod 62	Mod 66	Mod 80
62369	0	0	0	0	1
62370	0	0	0	0	1

Global Period

Code	Days
62369	XXX
62370	XXX

CPT © 2018 American Medical Association. All Rights Reserved.

62380

62380 Endoscopic decompression of spinal cord, nerve root(s), including laminotomy, partial facetectomy, foraminotomy, discectomy and/or excision of herniated intervertebral disc, 1 interspace, lumbar

(For open procedures, see 63030, 63056)

(For bilateral procedure, report 62380 with modifier 50)

AMA Coding Guideline

Endoscopic Decompression of Neural Elements and/or Excision of Herniated Intervertebral Discs

Definitions

For purposes of CPT coding, the following definitions of approach and visualization apply. The primary approach and visualization define the service, whether another method is incidentally applied. Surgical services are presumed open, unless otherwise specified.

Percutaneous: Image-guided procedures (eg, computer tomography [CT] or fluoroscopy) performed with indirect visualization of the spine without the use of any device that allows visualization through a surgical incision.

Endoscopic: Spinal procedures performed with continuous direct visualization of the spine through an endoscope.

Open: Spinal procedures performed with continuous direct visualization of the spine through a surgical opening.

Indirect visualization: Image-guided (eg, CT or fluoroscopy), not light-based visualization.

Direct visualization: Light-based visualization; can be performed by eye, or with surgical loupes, microscope, or endoscope.

AMA Coding Notes

Endoscopic Decompression of Neural Elements and/or Excision of Herniated Intervertebral Discs

(For the techniques of microsurgery and/or use of microscope, use 69990)

(For percutaneous decompression, see 62287, 0274T, 0275T)

Surgical Procedures on the Spine and Spinal Cord

(For application of caliper or tongs, use 20660)

(For treatment of fracture or dislocation of spine, see 22310-22327)

AMA *CPT Assistant* ▯

62380: Feb 17: 12

Plain English Description

Spinal cord and/or nerve root(s) decompression is done endoscopically. Compression symptoms include local or radiating pain, reduced mobility, and neurologic compromise. A needle/guidewire is inserted through the skin on one side of the midline and advanced to the involved level using fluoroscopic guidance. Small incisions are made around the needle/guidewire. Metal dilating tubes in graduating sizes are passed over the guidewire, gently spreading soft tissue and muscles away from the vertebrae. The needle/guidewire is removed. A hollow metal cylinder is passed over the metal dilator and the dilator is removed. The endoscope is inserted through the metal cylinder and the surgeon visualizes the targeted area on a projection screen. A nerve retractor is passed down a working channel of the endoscope and the spinal nerve is gently moved aside. Surgical instruments are then passed down another working channel of the endoscope and bony lamina is removed (laminotomy) ,as well as facet joints (partial facetectomy) and bone from around the neural foramen (foraminotomy). Herniated intervertebral disc may be partially or totally removed (discectomy). The retracted nerve is allowed to move back into place. The endoscope is removed. The metal cylinder is removed allowing soft tissue to close the incision. Skin may be closed with suture or staple or covered with a dressing.

ICD-10-CM Diagnostic Codes

	M51.05	Intervertebral disc disorders with myelopathy, thoracolumbar region
	M51.06	Intervertebral disc disorders with myelopathy, lumbar region
	M51.15	Intervertebral disc disorders with radiculopathy, thoracolumbar region
	M51.16	Intervertebral disc disorders with radiculopathy, lumbar region
	M51.17	Intervertebral disc disorders with radiculopathy, lumbosacral region
	M51.25	Other intervertebral disc displacement, thoracolumbar region
	M51.26	Other intervertebral disc displacement, lumbar region
	M51.27	Other intervertebral disc displacement, lumbosacral region
	M51.35	Other intervertebral disc degeneration, thoracolumbar region
	M51.36	Other intervertebral disc degeneration, lumbar region
	M51.37	Other intervertebral disc degeneration, lumbosacral region
	M51.46	Schmorl's nodes, lumbar region
	M51.47	Schmorl's nodes, lumbosacral region
	M51.85	Other intervertebral disc disorders, thoracolumbar region
	M51.86	Other intervertebral disc disorders, lumbar region
	M51.87	Other intervertebral disc disorders, lumbosacral region
	M53.85	Other specified dorsopathies, thoracolumbar region
	M53.86	Other specified dorsopathies, lumbar region
	M53.87	Other specified dorsopathies, lumbosacral region
	M54.15	Radiculopathy, thoracolumbar region
	M54.16	Radiculopathy, lumbar region
	M54.17	Radiculopathy, lumbosacral region
⇄	M54.31	Sciatica, right side
⇄	M54.32	Sciatica, left side
	M54.89	Other dorsalgia
	M99.53	Intervertebral disc stenosis of neural canal of lumbar region
	M99.73	Connective tissue and disc stenosis of intervertebral foramina of lumbar region

CCI Edits

Refer to Appendix A for CCI edits.

Facility RVUs ▯

Code	Work	PE Facility	MP	Total Facility
62380	0.00	0.00	0.00	0.00

Non-facility RVUs ▯

Code	Work	PE Non-Facility	MP	Total Non-Facility
62380	0.00	0.00	0.00	0.00

Modifiers (PAR) ▯

Code	Mod 50	Mod 51	Mod 62	Mod 66	Mod 80
62380	1	2	2	0	2

Global Period

Code	Days
62380	090

● New ▲ Revised ✚ Add On ⊘Modifier 51 Exempt ★Telemedicine ▯ CPT QuickRef ✗FDA Pending ⇄ Laterality ❼Seventh Character ♂Male ♀Female

CPT © 2018 American Medical Association. All Rights Reserved.

63650-63655

63650 Percutaneous implantation of neurostimulator electrode array, epidural

63655 Laminectomy for implantation of neurostimulator electrodes, plate/paddle, epidural

AMA Coding Guideline

Neurostimulators (Spinal) Procedures

For electronic analysis with programming, when performed, of spinal cord neurostimulator pulse generator/transmitters, see codes 95970, 95971, 95972. Test stimulation to confirm correct target site placement of the electrode array(s) and/or to confirm the functional status of the system is inherent to placement, and is not separately reported as electronic analysis or programming of the neurostimulator system. Electronic analysis (95970) at the time of implantation is not separately reported.

Codes 63650, 63655, and 63661-63664 describe the operative placement, revision, replacement, or removal of the spinal neurostimulator system components to provide spinal electrical stimulation. A neurostimulator system includes an implanted neurostimulator, external controller, extension, and collection of contacts. Multiple contacts or electrodes (4 or more) provide the actual electrical stimulation in the epidural space.

For percutaneously placed neurostimulator systems (63650, 63661, 63663), the contacts are on a catheter-like lead. An array defines the collection of contacts that are on one catheter.

For systems placed via an open surgical exposure (63655, 63662, 63664), the contacts are on a plate or paddle-shaped surface.

Do not report 63661 or 63663 when removing or replacing a temporary percutaneously placed array for an external generator.

AMA Coding Notes

Surgical Procedures on the Spine and Spinal Cord

(For application of caliper or tongs, use 20660)

(For treatment of fracture or dislocation of spine, see 22310-22327)

AMA *CPT Assistant* □

63650: Jun 98: 3-4, Nov 98: 18, Mar 99: 11, Apr 99: 10, Sep 99: 3, Dec 08: 8, Feb 10: 9, Aug 10: 8, Dec 10: 14, Apr 11: 10, Oct 13: 19, Dec 15: 17, Jan 16: 12, Dec 17: 16

63655: Jun 98: 3-4, Nov 98: 18, Sep 99: 3-4, Dec 08: 8, Aug 10: 8, Dec 10: 14, Apr 11: 10

Plain English Description

Placement of an implantable spinal cord stimulation system is performed to treat chronic back and/or leg pain. Electrical stimulation of the spinal cord alleviates pain by activating pain-inhibiting neurons and inducing a tingling sensation that masks pain sensations. In 63650, percutaneous placement of an electrode array in the epidural space is performed. Using separately reportable fluoroscopic guidance, a small incision is made in the skin over the planned insertion site. The vertebra is exposed and a small portion of the lamina removed (laminotomy). The electrode array, also referred to as leads, are advanced into the epidural space and secured with sutures. The patient is then awakened and the array tested to ensure that the neurostimulator is properly placed and that there is no pain from the electrode array implant itself. The neurostimulator will be tested at various settings and once the optimal settings are determined they will be used to program the pulse generator or receiver that will be implanted in a separately reportable procedure. The lead wires are then tunneled to the pulse generator/receiver pocket where they are attached to the generator/receiver. In 63655, an electrode plate or paddle is placed in the epidural space using an open technique requiring a laminectomy. An incision between 2-5 inches in length is made over the spine. Overlying soft tissue is dissected and the lamina exposed. Part or all of the lamina is excised to allow access to the epidural space. The plate or paddle is positioned in the epidural space and secured to the spine. Once the plate or paddle is in place, the patient is awakened and the device is tested. Tunneling of the leads to the pulse generator/receiver pocket and connection of the leads is performed as described above.

Implantation of neurostimulator electrode array, epidural

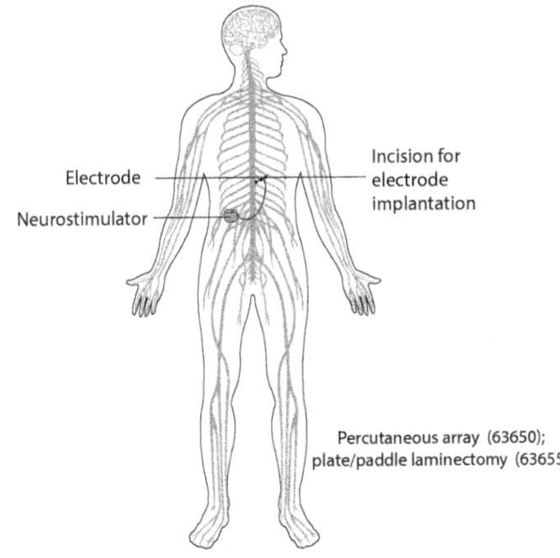

ICD-10-CM Diagnostic Codes

	G03.1	Chronic meningitis
	G03.9	Meningitis, unspecified
⇄	G56.41	Causalgia of right upper limb
⇄	G56.42	Causalgia of left upper limb
⇄	G56.43	Causalgia of bilateral upper limbs
⇄	G57.71	Causalgia of right lower limb
⇄	G57.72	Causalgia of left lower limb
⇄	G57.73	Causalgia of bilateral lower limbs
	G89.21	Chronic pain due to trauma
	G89.22	Chronic post-thoracotomy pain
	G89.28	Other chronic postprocedural pain
	G89.29	Other chronic pain
⇄	G90.511	Complex regional pain syndrome I of right upper limb
⇄	G90.512	Complex regional pain syndrome I of left upper limb
⇄	G90.513	Complex regional pain syndrome I of upper limb, bilateral
⇄	G90.521	Complex regional pain syndrome I of right lower limb
⇄	G90.522	Complex regional pain syndrome I of left lower limb
⇄	G90.523	Complex regional pain syndrome I of lower limb, bilateral
	G96.12	Meningeal adhesions (cerebral) (spinal)
	M47.21	Other spondylosis with radiculopathy, occipito-atlanto-axial region
	M47.22	Other spondylosis with radiculopathy, cervical region
	M47.23	Other spondylosis with radiculopathy, cervicothoracic region
	M47.24	Other spondylosis with radiculopathy, thoracic region
	M47.25	Other spondylosis with radiculopathy, thoracolumbar region
	M47.26	Other spondylosis with radiculopathy, lumbar region
	M47.27	Other spondylosis with radiculopathy, lumbosacral region
	M47.28	Other spondylosis with radiculopathy, sacral and sacrococcygeal region
	M50.11	Cervical disc disorder with radiculopathy, high cervical region
	M50.121	Cervical disc disorder at C4-C5 level with radiculopathy
	M50.122	Cervical disc disorder at C5-C6 level with radiculopathy
	M50.123	Cervical disc disorder at C6-C7 level with radiculopathy
	M50.13	Cervical disc disorder with radiculopathy, cervicothoracic region
	M51.14	Intervertebral disc disorders with radiculopathy, thoracic region
	M51.15	Intervertebral disc disorders with radiculopathy, thoracolumbar region
	M51.16	Intervertebral disc disorders with radiculopathy, lumbar region
	M51.17	Intervertebral disc disorders with radiculopathy, lumbosacral region
	M54.11	Radiculopathy, occipito-atlanto-axial region
	M54.12	Radiculopathy, cervical region
	M54.13	Radiculopathy, cervicothoracic region
	M54.14	Radiculopathy, thoracic region
	M54.15	Radiculopathy, thoracolumbar region
	M54.16	Radiculopathy, lumbar region
	M54.17	Radiculopathy, lumbosacral region
	M54.18	Radiculopathy, sacral and sacrococcygeal region
	M54.2	Cervicalgia
⇄	M54.31	Sciatica, right side
⇄	M54.32	Sciatica, left side

CPT © 2018 American Medical Association. All Rights Reserved.

⇄	M54.41	Lumbago with sciatica, right side
⇄	M54.42	Lumbago with sciatica, left side
	M54.5	Low back pain
	M54.6	Pain in thoracic spine
	M54.89	Other dorsalgia
	M96.1	Postlaminectomy syndrome, not elsewhere classified

CCI Edits

Refer to Appendix A for CCI edits.

Pub 100

63650: Pub 100-03, 1, 160.19, Pub 100-03, 1, 160.26, Pub 100-03, 1, 160.7-160.7.1

63655: Pub 100-03, 1, 160.26, Pub 100-03, 1, 160.7-160.7.1

Facility RVUs ▯

Code	Work	PE Facility	MP	Total Facility
63650	7.15	3.99	0.68	11.82
63655	10.92	9.53	3.65	24.10

Non-facility RVUs ▯

Code	Work	PE Non-Facility	MP	Total Non-Facility
63650	7.15	38.15	0.68	45.98
63655	10.92	9.53	3.65	24.10

Modifiers (PAR) ▯

Code	Mod 50	Mod 51	Mod 62	Mod 66	Mod 80
63650	0	2	0	0	1
63655	0	2	1	0	2

Global Period

Code	Days
63650	010
63655	090

CPT © 2018 American Medical Association. All Rights Reserved.

63661-63662

63661 Removal of spinal neurostimulator electrode percutaneous array(s), including fluoroscopy, when performed

63662 Removal of spinal neurostimulator electrode plate/paddle(s) placed via laminotomy or laminectomy, including fluoroscopy, when performed

AMA Coding Guideline
Neurostimulators (Spinal) Procedures

For electronic analysis with programming, when performed, of spinal cord neurostimulator pulse generator/transmitters, see codes 95970, 95971, 95972. Test stimulation to confirm correct target site placement of the electrode array(s) and/or to confirm the functional status of the system is inherent to placement, and is not separately reported as electronic analysis or programming of the neurostimulator system. Electronic analysis (95970) at the time of implantation is not separately reported.

Codes 63650, 63655, and 63661-63664 describe the operative placement, revision, replacement, or removal of the spinal neurostimulator system components to provide spinal electrical stimulation. A neurostimulator system includes an implanted neurostimulator, external controller, extension, and collection of contacts. Multiple contacts or electrodes (4 or more) provide the actual electrical stimulation in the epidural space.

For percutaneously placed neurostimulator systems (63650, 63661, 63663), the contacts are on a catheter-like lead. An array defines the collection of contacts that are on one catheter.

For systems placed via an open surgical exposure (63655, 63662, 63664), the contacts are on a plate or paddle-shaped surface.

Do not report 63661 or 63663 when removing or replacing a temporary percutaneously placed array for an external generator.

AMA Coding Notes
Surgical Procedures on the Spine and Spinal Cord

(For application of caliper or tongs, use 20660)

(For treatment of fracture or dislocation of spine, see 22310-22327)

AMA *CPT Assistant* ▯

63661: Feb 10: 9, Aug 10: 8, Jan 11: 8, Apr 11: 10

63662: Feb 10: 9, Aug 10: 8, Apr 11: 10

Plain English Description

An implantable spinal cord stimulation system used to treat chronic back and/or leg pain. Electrical stimulation of the spinal cord alleviates pain by activating pain-inhibiting neurons and inducing a tingling sensation that masks pain sensations. Typically, a temporary electrode array, plate, or paddle is placed to determine the effectiveness of the device in alleviating pain. The temporary device is eventually removed and if effective replaced with a permanent device or if ineffective it is removed without replacement. In 63661, percutaneous removal of an electrode array in the epidural space is performed. The subcutaneous pocket containing the generator/receiver is opened and the leads are disconnected. Using fluoroscopic guidance as needed, a small incision is made in the skin over the insertion site. The vertebra is exposed and the electrode array, also referred to as leads, are located and removed from the epidural space. The leads are dissected free of the subcutaneous tunnel and removed. If a permanent electrode array is to be placed this is performed in a separately reportable procedure. If the electrode array is not being replaced, the incisions are closed. In 63662, an electrode plate or paddle that has been placed via a laminotomy or laminectomy is removed from the epidural space. The subcutaneous pocket containing the generator/receiver is opened and the leads are disconnected. Using fluoroscopic guidance as needed, an incision is made over the spine. Overlying soft tissue is dissected and the lamina exposed. The plate or paddle is located in the epidural space and removed. The leads are dissected free of the subcutaneous tunnel and removed. If a permanent electrode plate or paddle is to be placed this is performed in a separately reportable procedure. If the electrode plate or paddle is not being replaced, the incisions are closed.

Removal of spinal neurostimulator electrode percutaneous array(s) including fluoroscopy

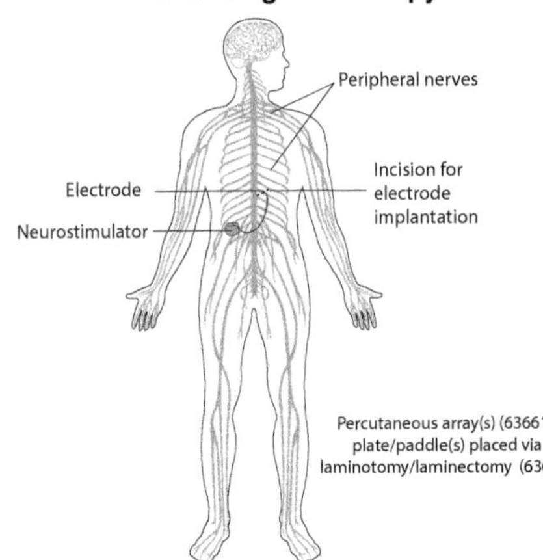

ICD-10-CM Diagnostic Codes

➐	T85.112	Breakdown (mechanical) of implanted electronic neurostimulator of spinal cord electrode (lead)
➐	T85.122	Displacement of implanted electronic neurostimulator of spinal cord electrode (lead)
➐	T85.192	Other mechanical complication of implanted electronic neurostimulator of spinal cord electrode (lead)
➐	T85.733	Infection and inflammatory reaction due to implanted electronic neurostimulator of spinal cord, electrode (lead)
➐	T85.810	Embolism due to nervous system prosthetic devices, implants and grafts
➐	T85.820	Fibrosis due to nervous system prosthetic devices, implants and grafts
➐	T85.830	Hemorrhage due to nervous system prosthetic devices, implants and grafts
➐	T85.840	Pain due to nervous system prosthetic devices, implants and grafts
➐	T85.850	Stenosis due to nervous system prosthetic devices, implants and grafts
➐	T85.860	Thrombosis due to nervous system prosthetic devices, implants and grafts
➐	T85.890	Other specified complication of nervous system prosthetic devices, implants and grafts
	Z45.42	Encounter for adjustment and management of neuropacemaker (brain) (peripheral nerve) (spinal cord)

ICD-10-CM Coding Notes

For codes requiring a 7th character extension, refer to your ICD-10-CM book. Review the character descriptions and coding guidelines for proper selection. For some procedures, only certain characters will apply.

CCI Edits

Refer to Appendix A for CCI edits.

Pub 100

63661: Pub 100-03, 1, 160.19, Pub 100-03, 1, 160.26, Pub 100-03, 1, 160.7-160.7.1

63662: Pub 100-03, 1, 160.19, Pub 100-03, 1, 160.26, Pub 100-03, 1, 160.7-160.7.1

CPT © 2018 American Medical Association. All Rights Reserved.

Facility RVUs

Code	Work	PE Facility	MP	Total Facility
63661	5.08	3.41	0.83	9.32
63662	11.00	9.68	3.72	24.40

Non-facility RVUs

Code	Work	PE Non-Facility	MP	Total Non-Facility
63661	5.08	11.60	0.83	17.51
63662	11.00	9.68	3.72	24.40

Modifiers (PAR)

Code	Mod 50	Mod 51	Mod 62	Mod 66	Mod 80
63661	0	2	1	0	2
63662	0	2	1	0	2

Global Period

Code	Days
63661	010
63662	090

CPT © 2018 American Medical Association. All Rights Reserved.

63663-63664

63663 Revision including replacement, when performed, of spinal neurostimulator electrode percutaneous array(s), including fluoroscopy, when performed

(Do not report 63663 in conjunction with 63661, 63662 for the same spinal level)

63664 Revision including replacement, when performed, of spinal neurostimulator electrode plate/ paddle(s) placed via laminotomy or laminectomy, including fluoroscopy, when performed

(Do not report 63664 in conjunction with 63661, 63662 for the same spinal level)

AMA Coding Guideline

Neurostimulators (Spinal) Procedures

For electronic analysis with programming, when performed, of spinal cord neurostimulator pulse generator/transmitters, see codes 95970, 95971, 95972. Test stimulation to confirm correct target site placement of the electrode array(s) and/ or to confirm the functional status of the system is inherent to placement, and is not separately reported as electronic analysis or programming of the neurostimulator system. Electronic analysis (95970) at the time of implantation is not separately reported.

Codes 63650, 63655, and 63661-63664 describe the operative placement, revision, replacement, or removal of the spinal neurostimulator system components to provide spinal electrical stimulation. A neurostimulator system includes an implanted neurostimulator, external controller, extension, and collection of contacts. Multiple contacts or electrodes (4 or more) provide the actual electrical stimulation in the epidural space.

For percutaneously placed neurostimulator systems (63650, 63661, 63663), the contacts are on a catheter-like lead. An array defines the collection of contacts that are on one catheter.

For systems placed via an open surgical exposure (63655, 63662, 63664), the contacts are on a plate or paddle-shaped surface.

Do not report 63661 or 63663 when removing or replacing a temporary percutaneously placed array for an external generator.

AMA Coding Notes

Surgical Procedures on the Spine and Spinal Cord

(For application of caliper or tongs, use 20660)

(For treatment of fracture or dislocation of spine, see 22310-22327)

AMA *CPT Assistant* □

63663: Feb 10: 9, Aug 10: 8, Apr 11: 10

63664: Feb 10: 9, Aug 10: 8, Apr 11: 10

Plain English Description

An implantable spinal cord stimulation system is used to treat chronic back and/or leg pain. Electrical stimulation of the spinal cord alleviates pain by activating pain-inhibiting neurons and inducing a tingling sensation that masks pain sensations. In 63663, revision including replacement of an electrode array in the epidural space is performed. Using separately reportable fluoroscopic guidance, a small incision is made in the skin over the insertion site. The electrode array is located and explored to determine whether it needs to be repositioned or removed and replaced. If it needs to be repositioned, any sutures are removed and the array is then moved as needed to obtain optimal pain control. If the array needs to be replaced it is removed in a separately reportable procedure. The new array is then advanced into the epidural space and secured with sutures. The patient is awakened and the revised or new array tested to ensure that the neurostimulator is properly placed and that there is no pain from the electrode array implant itself. The neurostimulator will be tested at various settings and once the optimal settings are determined they will be used to program the pulse generator or receiver that will be implanted in a separately reportable procedure. The lead wires are then tunneled to the pulse generator/receiver pocket where they are attached to the generator/receiver. In 63664, an electrode plate or paddle that has been placed via a laminotomy or laminectomy in the epidural space is revised and replaced as needed. An incision between 2-5 inches in length is made over the spine. Overlying soft tissue is dissected and the plate or paddle exposed and freed from the spine. If revision is performed, the plate or paddle is repositioned in the epidural space and secured to the spine. If the plate or paddle must be replaced it is removed in a separately reportable procedure. A new plate or paddle is then placed in the epidural space and secured to the spine. Once the plate or paddle is in place, the patient is awakened and testing of the device, tunneling of the leads to the pulse generator/receiver pocket, and connection of the leads is performed as described above.

Revision including replacement, when performed, of spinal neurostimulator electrode percutaneous array(s)

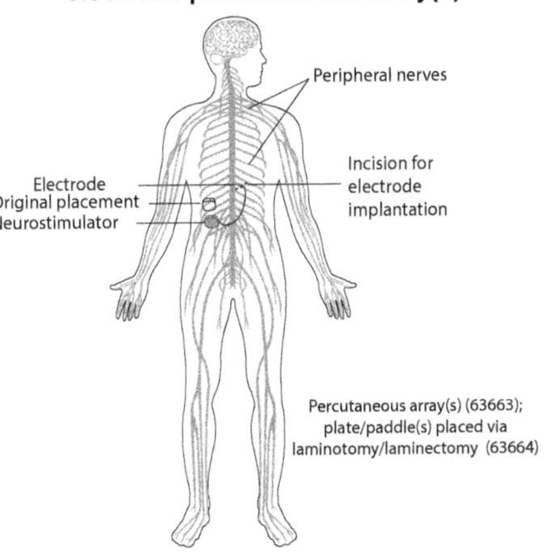

ICD-10-CM Diagnostic Codes

❼	T85.112	Breakdown (mechanical) of implanted electronic neurostimulator of spinal cord electrode (lead)
❼	T85.122	Displacement of implanted electronic neurostimulator of spinal cord electrode (lead)
❼	T85.192	Other mechanical complication of implanted electronic neurostimulator of spinal cord electrode (lead)
❼	T85.733	Infection and inflammatory reaction due to implanted electronic neurostimulator of spinal cord, electrode (lead)
❼	T85.810	Embolism due to nervous system prosthetic devices, implants and grafts
❼	T85.820	Fibrosis due to nervous system prosthetic devices, implants and grafts
❼	T85.830	Hemorrhage due to nervous system prosthetic devices, implants and grafts
❼	T85.840	Pain due to nervous system prosthetic devices, implants and grafts
❼	T85.850	Stenosis due to nervous system prosthetic devices, implants and grafts
❼	T85.860	Thrombosis due to nervous system prosthetic devices, implants and grafts
❼	T85.890	Other specified complication of nervous system prosthetic devices, implants and grafts
	Z45.42	Encounter for adjustment and management of neuropacemaker (brain) (peripheral nerve) (spinal cord)

ICD-10-CM Coding Notes

For codes requiring a 7th character extension, refer to your ICD-10-CM book. Review the character descriptions and coding guidelines for proper selection. For some procedures, only certain characters will apply.

CPT © 2018 American Medical Association. All Rights Reserved.

CCI Edits

Refer to Appendix A for CCI edits.

Pub 100

63663: Pub 100-03, 1, 160.19, Pub 100-03, 1, 160.26, Pub 100-03, 1, 160.7-160.7.1

63664: Pub 100-03, 1, 160.19, Pub 100-03, 1, 160.26, Pub 100-03, 1, 160.7-160.7.1

Facility RVUs

Code	Work	PE Facility	MP	Total Facility
63663	7.75	4.24	0.96	12.95
63664	11.52	9.87	3.90	25.29

Non-facility RVUs

Code	Work	PE Non-Facility	MP	Total Non-Facility
63663	7.75	14.73	0.96	23.44
63664	11.52	9.87	3.90	25.29

Modifiers (PAR)

Code	Mod 50	Mod 51	Mod 62	Mod 66	Mod 80
63663	0	2	1	0	2
63664	0	2	1	0	2

Global Period

Code	Days
63663	010
63664	090

CPT © 2018 American Medical Association. All Rights Reserved.

63685-63688

63685 Insertion or replacement of spinal neurostimulator pulse generator or receiver, direct or inductive coupling

(Do not report 63685 in conjunction with 63688 for the same pulse generator or receiver)

63688 Revision or removal of implanted spinal neurostimulator pulse generator or receiver

(For electronic analysis with programming, when performed, of implanted spinal cord neurostimulator pulse generator/transmitter, see 95970, 95971, 95972)

AMA Coding Guideline

Neurostimulators (Spinal) Procedures

For electronic analysis with programming, when performed, of spinal cord neurostimulator pulse generator/transmitters, see codes 95970, 95971, 95972. Test stimulation to confirm correct target site placement of the electrode array(s) and/or to confirm the functional status of the system is inherent to placement, and is not separately reported as electronic analysis or programming of the neurostimulator system. Electronic analysis (95970) at the time of implantation is not separately reported.

Codes 63650, 63655, and 63661-63664 describe the operative placement, revision, replacement, or removal of the spinal neurostimulator system components to provide spinal electrical stimulation. A neurostimulator system includes an implanted neurostimulator, external controller, extension, and collection of contacts. Multiple contacts or electrodes (4 or more) provide the actual electrical stimulation in the epidural space.

For percutaneously placed neurostimulator systems (63650, 63661, 63663), the contacts are on a catheter-like lead. An array defines the collection of contacts that are on one catheter.

For systems placed via an open surgical exposure (63655, 63662, 63664), the contacts are on a plate or paddle-shaped surface.

Do not report 63661 or 63663 when removing or replacing a temporary percutaneously placed array for an external generator.

AMA Coding Notes

Surgical Procedures on the Spine and Spinal Cord

(For application of caliper or tongs, use 20660)

(For treatment of fracture or dislocation of spine, see 22310-22327)

AMA *CPT Assistant* ☐

63685: Jun 98: 3-4, Sep 99: 5, Feb 10: 9, Oct 10: 14, Dec 10: 14, Apr 11: 10, Dec 17: 16

63688: Jun 98: 3-4, Sep 99: 5, Feb 10: 9, Apr 11: 11

Plain English Description

An implantable generator for spinal cord stimulation (SCS) generates electrical impulses to implanted electrodes in the spine. An implantable receiver receives electrical impulses from an external generator and then transmits those signals to the electrodes. In 63685, a pulse generator or receiver is inserted or replaced. For initial insertion, an incision is made in the skin overlying the planned insertion site for the neurostimulator pulse generator or receiver. A subcutaneous pocket is fashioned. The electrodes, which have been implanted and tunneled to the pocket in the separately reportable procedure, are connected to the generator or receiver and tested. Stimulation parameters are set and the device is placed in the skin pocket, which is closed with sutures. Replacement is performed in the same manner except that the existing generator or receiver is removed first by incising the skin over the existing generator or receiver. The skin pocket is opened and the existing device exposed. The electrodes are disconnected. The generator or receiver is dissected free of surrounding tissue and removed. The new generator or receiver is connected to the electrodes and tested. In 63688, an existing generator or receiver is revised or removed. Revision involves opening the skin pocket and removing the generator or receiver. The device is then evaluated and adjustments made as needed to ensure proper functioning. Removal is accomplished by exposing the device, disconnecting the electrodes (which are removed in a separate procedure) and closing the skin pocket.

Insertion or replacement of spinal neurostimulator pulse generator or receiver

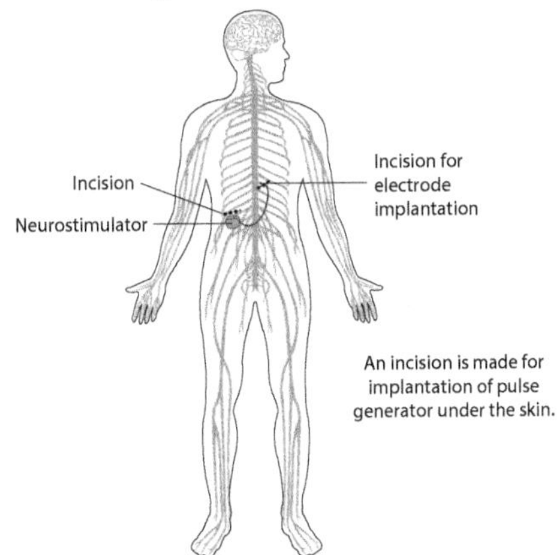

ICD-10-CM Diagnostic Codes

⇄	G56.41	Causalgia of right upper limb
⇄	G56.42	Causalgia of left upper limb
⇄	G56.43	Causalgia of bilateral upper limbs
⇄	G57.71	Causalgia of right lower limb
⇄	G57.72	Causalgia of left lower limb
⇄	G57.73	Causalgia of bilateral lower limbs
	G89.21	Chronic pain due to trauma
	G89.22	Chronic post-thoracotomy pain
	G89.28	Other chronic postprocedural pain
	G89.29	Other chronic pain
⇄	G90.511	Complex regional pain syndrome I of right upper limb
⇄	G90.512	Complex regional pain syndrome I of left upper limb
⇄	G90.513	Complex regional pain syndrome I of upper limb, bilateral
⇄	G90.521	Complex regional pain syndrome I of right lower limb
⇄	G90.522	Complex regional pain syndrome I of left lower limb
⇄	G90.523	Complex regional pain syndrome I of lower limb, bilateral
	M54.2	Cervicalgia
⇄	M54.31	Sciatica, right side
⇄	M54.32	Sciatica, left side
⇄	M54.41	Lumbago with sciatica, right side
⇄	M54.42	Lumbago with sciatica, left side
	M54.5	Low back pain
	M54.6	Pain in thoracic spine
	M54.89	Other dorsalgia
	M96.1	Postlaminectomy syndrome, not elsewhere classified
❼	T85.113	Breakdown (mechanical) of implanted electronic neurostimulator, generator
❼	T85.123	Displacement of implanted electronic neurostimulator, generator
❼	T85.193	Other mechanical complication of implanted electronic neurostimulator, generator
❼	T85.734	Infection and inflammatory reaction due to implanted electronic neurostimulator, generator
❼	T85.810	Embolism due to nervous system prosthetic devices, implants and grafts
❼	T85.820	Fibrosis due to nervous system prosthetic devices, implants and grafts
❼	T85.830	Hemorrhage due to nervous system prosthetic devices, implants and grafts
❼	T85.840	Pain due to nervous system prosthetic devices, implants and grafts
❼	T85.850	Stenosis due to nervous system prosthetic devices, implants and grafts
❼	T85.860	Thrombosis due to nervous system prosthetic devices, implants and grafts
❼	T85.890	Other specified complication of nervous system prosthetic devices, implants and grafts
	Z45.42	Encounter for adjustment and management of neuropacemaker (brain) (peripheral nerve) (spinal cord)

ICD-10-CM Coding Notes

For codes requiring a 7th character extension, refer to your ICD-10-CM book. Review the character descriptions and coding guidelines for proper selection. For some procedures, only certain characters will apply.

CCI Edits

Refer to Appendix A for CCI edits.

CPT © 2018 American Medical Association. All Rights Reserved.

Pub 100

63685: Pub 100-03, 1, 160.19, Pub 100-03, 1, 160.26, Pub 100-03, 1, 160.7-160.7.1

63688: Pub 100-03, 1, 160.19, Pub 100-03, 1, 160.26, Pub 100-03, 1, 160.7-160.7.1

Facility RVUs

Code	Work	PE Facility	MP	Total Facility
63685	5.19	4.15	1.06	10.40
63688	5.30	4.27	1.16	10.73

Non-facility RVUs

Code	Work	PE Non-Facility	MP	Total Non-Facility
63685	5.19	4.15	1.06	10.40
63688	5.30	4.27	1.16	10.73

Modifiers (PAR)

Code	Mod 50	Mod 51	Mod 62	Mod 66	Mod 80
63685	0	2	1	0	2
63688	0	2	0	0	1

Global Period

Code	Days
63685	010
63688	010

CPT © 2018 American Medical Association. All Rights Reserved.

64400-64405

64400 Injection, anesthetic agent; trigeminal nerve, any division or branch

64402 Injection, anesthetic agent; facial nerve

64405 Injection, anesthetic agent; greater occipital nerve

AMA Coding Notes

Introduction/Injection of Anesthetic Agent (Nerve Block), Diagnostic or Therapeutic Procedures on the Extracranial Nerves, Peripheral Nerves, and Autonomic Nervous System

(For destruction by neurolytic agent or chemodenervation, see 62280-62282, 64600-64681)

(For epidural or subarachnoid injection, see 62320, 62321, 62322, 62323, 62324, 62325, 62326, 62327)

(64479-64487, 64490-64495 are unilateral procedures. For bilateral procedures, use modifier 50)

Surgical Procedures on the Extracranial Nerves, Peripheral Nerves, and Autonomic Nervous System

(For intracranial surgery on cranial nerves, see 61450, 61460, 61790)

AMA *CPT Assistant*

64400: Jul 98: 10, May 99: 8, Nov 99: 36, Apr 05: 13, Feb 10: 9, Jan 13: 13

64402: Jul 98: 10, Apr 05: 13, Jan 13: 13

64405: Jul 98: 10, Apr 05: 13, Jan 13: 13, Oct 16: 11

Plain English Description

Injection of an anesthetic agent, also referred to as a nerve block, may be performed as either a diagnostic or therapeutic measure. In 64400, any division or branch of the trigeminal nerve is injected. The most common indication for injection of the trigeminal nerve is trigeminal neuralgia, which is characterized by shock-like stabbing pain, also referred to as lancinating pain. The trigeminal nerve divisions or branches may be injected using an intraoral or transcutaneous approach depending on the division or branch being injected. A needle is introduced into the trigeminal nerve at the base of the skull or along any of the divisions or branches. An anesthetic agent such as glycol is injected. The patient is asked to assess the degree of pain relief. In 64402, the facial nerve is injected. The facial nerve, also referred to as cranial nerve VII (CN VII), is a mixed nerve with both motor and sensory components and assists with facial expression. The nerve may be injected to treat muscle spasms or to interrupt transmission of sensory stimuli. The skin is cleansed over the facial nerve and an anesthetic is injected. In 64405, the greater occipital nerve is injected. The greater occipital nerves originate between the second and third vertebrae of the spine and supply the top of the scalp and the region above the ears and over the salivary glands. Injecting the nerve near the base of the skull treats occipital neuralgia.

Injection, anesthetic agent

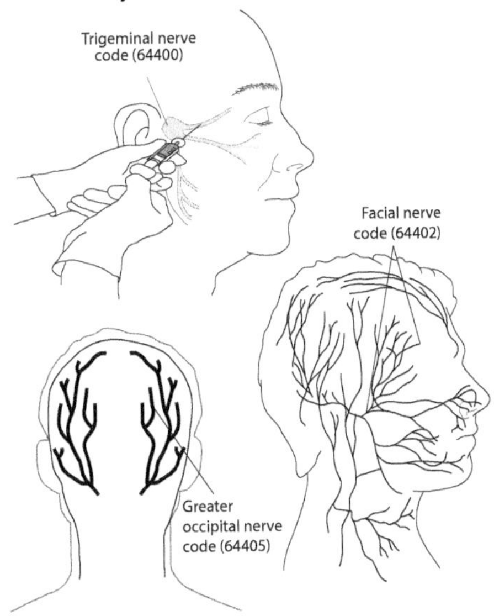

ICD-10-CM Diagnostic Codes

B02.22	Postherpetic trigeminal neuralgia
G44.001	Cluster headache syndrome, unspecified, intractable
G44.009	Cluster headache syndrome, unspecified, not intractable
G44.011	Episodic cluster headache, intractable
G44.019	Episodic cluster headache, not intractable
G44.021	Chronic cluster headache, intractable
G44.029	Chronic cluster headache, not intractable
G44.031	Episodic paroxysmal hemicrania, intractable
G44.039	Episodic paroxysmal hemicrania, not intractable
G44.041	Chronic paroxysmal hemicrania, intractable
G44.049	Chronic paroxysmal hemicrania, not intractable
G44.091	Other trigeminal autonomic cephalgias (TAC), intractable
G44.099	Other trigeminal autonomic cephalgias (TAC), not intractable
G44.89	Other headache syndrome
G50.0	Trigeminal neuralgia
G50.1	Atypical facial pain
G50.8	Other disorders of trigeminal nerve
G50.9	Disorder of trigeminal nerve, unspecified
G51.8	Other disorders of facial nerve
G51.9	Disorder of facial nerve, unspecified
G52.9	Cranial nerve disorder, unspecified
G58.8	Other specified mononeuropathies
G89.11	Acute pain due to trauma
G89.18	Other acute postprocedural pain
G89.21	Chronic pain due to trauma
G89.28	Other chronic postprocedural pain
G89.29	Other chronic pain
G89.3	Neoplasm related pain (acute) (chronic)
G89.4	Chronic pain syndrome
M53.0	Cervicocranial syndrome
M54.11	Radiculopathy, occipito-atlanto-axial region
M54.12	Radiculopathy, cervical region
M54.81	Occipital neuralgia
M62.838	Other muscle spasm
M79.2	Neuralgia and neuritis, unspecified
➐⇄ S04.30	Injury of trigeminal nerve, unspecified side
➐⇄ S04.31	Injury of trigeminal nerve, right side
➐⇄ S04.32	Injury of trigeminal nerve, left side
➐⇄ S04.50	Injury of facial nerve, unspecified side
➐⇄ S04.51	Injury of facial nerve, right side
➐⇄ S04.52	Injury of facial nerve, left side
➐ S13.4	Sprain of ligaments of cervical spine
➐ S14.2	Injury of nerve root of cervical spine
➐ S14.8	Injury of other specified nerves of neck
➐ S16.1	Strain of muscle, fascia and tendon at neck level

ICD-10-CM Coding Notes

For codes requiring a 7th character extension, refer to your ICD-10-CM book. Review the character descriptions and coding guidelines for proper selection. For some procedures, only certain characters will apply.

CCI Edits

Refer to Appendix A for CCI edits.

CPT © 2018 American Medical Association. All Rights Reserved.

Facility RVUs

Code	Work	PE Facility	MP	Total Facility
64400	1.11	0.72	0.25	2.08
64402	1.25	0.84	0.36	2.45
64405	0.94	0.40	0.20	1.54

Non-facility RVUs

Code	Work	PE Non-Facility	MP	Total Non-Facility
64400	1.11	2.52	0.25	3.88
64402	1.25	2.68	0.36	4.29
64405	0.94	1.23	0.20	2.37

Modifiers (PAR)

Code	Mod 50	Mod 51	Mod 62	Mod 66	Mod 80
64400	1	2	0	0	1
64402	1	2	0	0	1
64405	1	2	0	0	1

Global Period

Code	Days
64400	000
64402	000
64405	000

CPT © 2018 American Medical Association. All Rights Reserved.

64408

64408 Injection, anesthetic agent; vagus nerve

AMA Coding Notes

Introduction/Injection of Anesthetic Agent (Nerve Block), Diagnostic or Therapeutic Procedures on the Extracranial Nerves, Peripheral Nerves, and Autonomic Nervous System

(For destruction by neurolytic agent or chemodenervation, see 62280-62282, 64600-64681)

(For epidural or subarachnoid injection, see 62320, 62321, 62322, 62323, 62324, 62325, 62326, 62327)

(64479-64487, 64490-64495 are unilateral procedures. For bilateral procedures, use modifier 50)

Surgical Procedures on the Extracranial Nerves, Peripheral Nerves, and Autonomic Nervous System

(For intracranial surgery on cranial nerves, see 61450, 61460, 61790)

AMA *CPT Assistant* ▢

64408: Jul 98: 10, Apr 05: 13, Jan 13: 13

Plain English Description

Injection of an anesthetic agent, also referred to as a nerve block, may be performed as either a diagnostic or therapeutic measure. The vagus nerve, also referred to as cranial nerve X (CN X), is a mixed nerve that originates in the medulla and exits the skull at the jugular foramen. The motor portion innervates muscles of the pharynx, larynx, respiratory tract, heart, stomach, small intestine, most of large intestine and gallbladder. The sensory portion transmits sensation from the same structures that the motor portion innervates. The skin over the styloid process of the temporal bone is cleansed. A needle is advanced perpendicular to the skin until the styloid process is encountered. The needle is then retracted slightly and repositioned in a slightly inferior trajectory. The needle is advanced in this position until it is approximately 0.5 cm deeper than the point at which the styloid process was encountered. Positioning is checked by aspiration. If no blood or cerebral spinal fluid is aspirated, the anesthetic agent is injected.

Injection, anesthetic agent vagus nerve

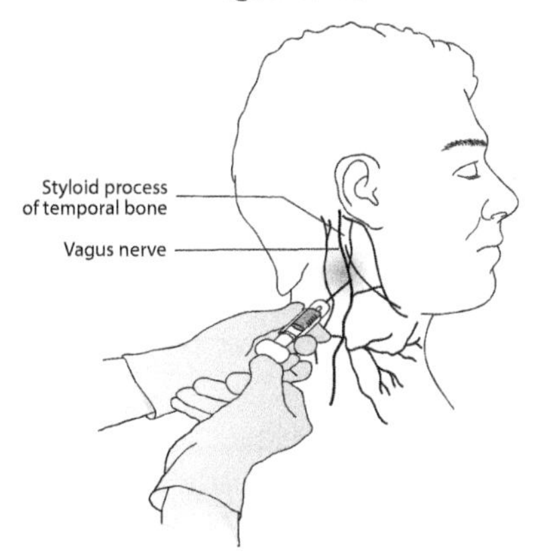

ICD-10-CM Diagnostic Codes

	C12	Malignant neoplasm of pyriform sinus
	C13.0	Malignant neoplasm of postcricoid region
	C13.1	Malignant neoplasm of aryepiglottic fold, hypopharyngeal aspect
	C13.2	Malignant neoplasm of posterior wall of hypopharynx
	C13.8	Malignant neoplasm of overlapping sites of hypopharynx
	C13.9	Malignant neoplasm of hypopharynx, unspecified
	C32.0	Malignant neoplasm of glottis
	C32.1	Malignant neoplasm of supraglottis
	C32.2	Malignant neoplasm of subglottis
	C32.3	Malignant neoplasm of laryngeal cartilage
	C32.8	Malignant neoplasm of overlapping sites of larynx
	C32.9	Malignant neoplasm of larynx, unspecified
	G24.1	Genetic torsion dystonia
	G24.2	Idiopathic nonfamilial dystonia
	G24.8	Other dystonia
	G24.9	Dystonia, unspecified
	G52.2	Disorders of vagus nerve
	G53	Cranial nerve disorders in diseases classified elsewhere
	G89.11	Acute pain due to trauma
	G89.18	Other acute postprocedural pain
	G89.21	Chronic pain due to trauma
	G89.28	Other chronic postprocedural pain
	G89.29	Other chronic pain
	G89.3	Neoplasm related pain (acute) (chronic)
	G89.4	Chronic pain syndrome
	J38.5	Laryngeal spasm
	J38.7	Other diseases of larynx
❼⇄	S04.891	Injury of other cranial nerves, right side
❼⇄	S04.892	Injury of other cranial nerves, left side
❼⇄	S04.899	Injury of other cranial nerves, unspecified side
❼	S12.8	Fracture of other parts of neck
❼	T27.0	Burn of larynx and trachea
❼	T27.1	Burn involving larynx and trachea with lung
❼	T27.4	Corrosion of larynx and trachea
❼	T27.5	Corrosion involving larynx and trachea with lung

ICD-10-CM Coding Notes

For codes requiring a 7th character extension, refer to your ICD-10-CM book. Review the character descriptions and coding guidelines for proper selection. For some procedures, only certain characters will apply.

CCI Edits

Refer to Appendix A for CCI edits.

Facility RVUs ▢

Code	Work	PE Facility	MP	Total Facility
64408	1.41	0.92	0.11	2.44

Non-facility RVUs ▢

Code	Work	PE Non-Facility	MP	Total Non-Facility
64408	1.41	1.83	0.11	3.35

Modifiers (PAR) ▢

Code	Mod 50	Mod 51	Mod 62	Mod 66	Mod 80
64408	1	2	0	0	0

Global Period

Code	Days
64408	000

CPT® Procedural Coding

CPT © 2018 American Medical Association. All Rights Reserved.

64410

64410 Injection, anesthetic agent; phrenic nerve

AMA Coding Notes

Introduction/Injection of Anesthetic Agent (Nerve Block), Diagnostic or Therapeutic Procedures on the Extracranial Nerves, Peripheral Nerves, and Autonomic Nervous System

(For destruction by neurolytic agent or chemodenervation, see 62280-62282, 64600-64681)

(For epidural or subarachnoid injection, see 62320, 62321, 62322, 62323, 62324, 62325, 62326, 62327)

(64479-64487, 64490-64495 are unilateral procedures. For bilateral procedures, use modifier 50)

Surgical Procedures on the Extracranial Nerves, Peripheral Nerves, and Autonomic Nervous System

(For intracranial surgery on cranial nerves, see 61450, 61460, 61790)

AMA *CPT Assistant* ☐

64410: Jul 98: 10, Apr 05: 13, Jan 13: 13

Plain English Description

Injection of an anesthetic agent, also referred to as a nerve block, may be performed as either a diagnostic or therapeutic measure. The phrenic nerve is a mixed spinal nerve originating from C4. It innervates muscles of the diaphragm and carries sensory information from the pleura, lungs, and pericardium. The skin over the C4 region of the spine is cleansed. A needle is inserted into the phrenic nerve, aspirated to ensure that it is not in a blood vessel, and an anesthetic agent is then injected.

Injection, anesthetic agent; phrenic nerve

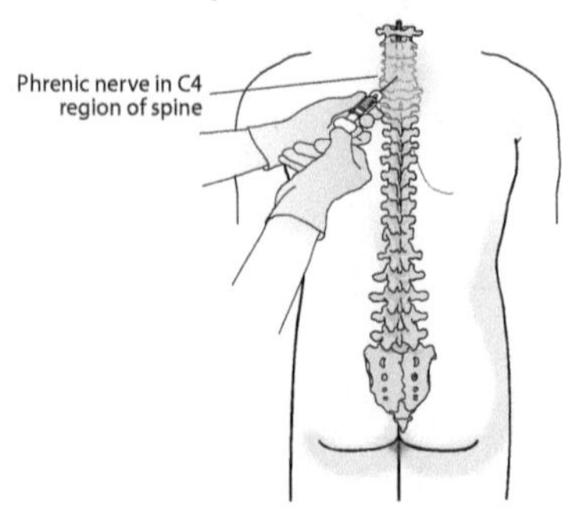

ICD-10-CM Diagnostic Codes

C49.3	Malignant neoplasm of connective and soft tissue of thorax
C76.1	Malignant neoplasm of thorax
C76.2	Malignant neoplasm of abdomen
C80.0	Disseminated malignant neoplasm, unspecified
G89.11	Acute pain due to trauma
G89.12	Acute post-thoracotomy pain
G89.18	Other acute postprocedural pain
G89.21	Chronic pain due to trauma
G89.22	Chronic post-thoracotomy pain
G89.28	Other chronic postprocedural pain
G89.29	Other chronic pain
G89.3	Neoplasm related pain (acute) (chronic)
G89.4	Chronic pain syndrome
R06.6	Hiccough
❼ S14.2	Injury of nerve root of cervical spine
❼ S14.8	Injury of other specified nerves of neck

ICD-10-CM Coding Notes

For codes requiring a 7th character extension, refer to your ICD-10-CM book. Review the character descriptions and coding guidelines for proper selection. For some procedures, only certain characters will apply.

CCI Edits

Refer to Appendix A for CCI edits.

Facility RVUs ☐

Code	Work	PE Facility	MP	Total Facility
64410	1.43	0.65	0.34	2.42

Non-facility RVUs ☐

Code	Work	PE Non-Facility	MP	Total Non-Facility
64410	1.43	2.66	0.34	4.43

Modifiers (PAR) ☐

Code	Mod 50	Mod 51	Mod 62	Mod 66	Mod 80
64410	1	2	0	0	0

Global Period

Code	Days
64410	000

CPT © 2018 American Medical Association. All Rights Reserved.

64413

64413 Injection, anesthetic agent; cervical plexus

AMA Coding Notes

Introduction/Injection of Anesthetic Agent (Nerve Block), Diagnostic or Therapeutic Procedures on the Extracranial Nerves, Peripheral Nerves, and Autonomic Nervous System

(For destruction by neurolytic agent or chemodenervation, see 62280-62282, 64600-64681)

(For epidural or subarachnoid injection, see 62320, 62321, 62322, 62323, 62324, 62325, 62326, 62327)

(64479-64487, 64490-64495 are unilateral procedures. For bilateral procedures, use modifier 50)

Surgical Procedures on the Extracranial Nerves, Peripheral Nerves, and Autonomic Nervous System

(For intracranial surgery on cranial nerves, see 61450, 61460, 61790)

AMA *CPT Assistant* ☐

64413: Jul 98: 10, Apr 05: 13, Jan 13: 13

Plain English Description

The cervical plexus is formed by then anterior rami of the C1-C4 nerve roots. It is located anterior to the cervical spine and posterior to the sternocleidomastoid muscle. The posterior border sternocleidomastoid is identified in the neck and marked. The planned injection site(s) is also marked. For a superficial cervical plexus block, a single injection is typically given at the midpoint of the sternocleidomastoid muscle. For a deep cervical plexus block, multiple injections between C2 and C6 may be given. The needle is inserted and aspirated to ensure that the needle is not in a blood vessel or for a deep block to ensure that it has not penetrated the subarachnoid space. The anesthetic is then injected. If multiple injections are performed, this is repeated until the desired level of anesthesia or analgesia has been attained.

Injection, anesthetic agent; cervical plexus

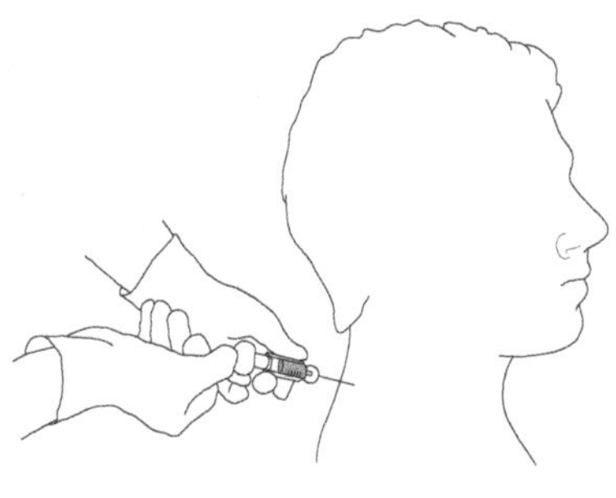

The physician injects a drug to numb the back of the neck and head.

ICD-10-CM Diagnostic Codes

	C41.2	Malignant neoplasm of vertebral column
	C49.0	Malignant neoplasm of connective and soft tissue of head, face and neck
	C79.89	Secondary malignant neoplasm of other specified sites
	G44.031	Episodic paroxysmal hemicrania, intractable
	G44.039	Episodic paroxysmal hemicrania, not intractable
	G44.041	Chronic paroxysmal hemicrania, intractable
	G44.049	Chronic paroxysmal hemicrania, not intractable
	G50.1	Atypical facial pain
	G54.2	Cervical root disorders, not elsewhere classified
	G54.8	Other nerve root and plexus disorders
	G54.9	Nerve root and plexus disorder, unspecified
	G55	Nerve root and plexus compressions in diseases classified elsewhere
	G89.11	Acute pain due to trauma
	G89.18	Other acute postprocedural pain
	G89.21	Chronic pain due to trauma
	G89.28	Other chronic postprocedural pain
	G89.29	Other chronic pain
	G89.3	Neoplasm related pain (acute) (chronic)
	G89.4	Chronic pain syndrome
	M46.02	Spinal enthesopathy, cervical region
	M47.12	Other spondylosis with myelopathy, cervical region
	M47.22	Other spondylosis with radiculopathy, cervical region
	M48.02	Spinal stenosis, cervical region
	M48.32	Traumatic spondylopathy, cervical region
❼	M48.42	Fatigue fracture of vertebra, cervical region
❼	M48.52	Collapsed vertebra, not elsewhere classified, cervical region
	M48.8X2	Other specified spondylopathies, cervical region
	M50.021	Cervical disc disorder at C4-C5 level with myelopathy
	M50.022	Cervical disc disorder at C5-C6 level with myelopathy
	M50.023	Cervical disc disorder at C6-C7 level with myelopathy
	M50.121	Cervical disc disorder at C4-C5 level with radiculopathy
	M50.122	Cervical disc disorder at C5-C6 level with radiculopathy
	M50.123	Cervical disc disorder at C6-C7 level with radiculopathy
	M50.221	Other cervical disc displacement at C4-C5 level
	M50.222	Other cervical disc displacement at C5-C6 level
	M50.223	Other cervical disc displacement at C6-C7 level
	M50.321	Other cervical disc degeneration at C4-C5 level
	M50.322	Other cervical disc degeneration at C5-C6 level
	M50.323	Other cervical disc degeneration at C6-C7 level
	M50.821	Other cervical disc disorders at C4-C5 level
	M50.822	Other cervical disc disorders at C5-C6 level
	M50.823	Other cervical disc disorders at C6-C7 level
	M53.82	Other specified dorsopathies, cervical region
	M54.12	Radiculopathy, cervical region
	M54.2	Cervicalgia
❼	M84.58	Pathological fracture in neoplastic disease, other specified site
	M96.1	Postlaminectomy syndrome, not elsewhere classified
	M99.01	Segmental and somatic dysfunction of cervical region
	M99.11	Subluxation complex (vertebral) of cervical region
	M99.21	Subluxation stenosis of neural canal of cervical region
	M99.31	Osseous stenosis of neural canal of cervical region
	M99.41	Connective tissue stenosis of neural canal of cervical region
	M99.51	Intervertebral disc stenosis of neural canal of cervical region
	M99.61	Osseous and subluxation stenosis of intervertebral foramina of cervical region
	M99.71	Connective tissue and disc stenosis of intervertebral foramina of cervical region
	M99.81	Other biomechanical lesions of cervical region
❼	S14.2	Injury of nerve root of cervical spine

ICD-10-CM Coding Notes

For codes requiring a 7th character extension, refer to your ICD-10-CM book. Review the character descriptions and coding guidelines for proper selection. For some procedures, only certain characters will apply.

CCI Edits

Refer to Appendix A for CCI edits.

CPT © 2018 American Medical Association. All Rights Reserved.

Facility RVUs

Code	Work	PE Facility	MP	Total Facility
64413	1.40	0.72	0.22	2.34

Non-facility RVUs

Code	Work	PE Non-Facility	MP	Total Non-Facility
64413	1.40	1.98	0.22	3.60

Modifiers (PAR)

Code	Mod 50	Mod 51	Mod 62	Mod 66	Mod 80
64413	1	2	0	0	1

Global Period

Code	Days
64413	000

CPT © 2018 American Medical Association. All Rights Reserved.

64415-64416

64415 Injection, anesthetic agent; brachial plexus, single

64416 Injection, anesthetic agent; brachial plexus, continuous infusion by catheter (including catheter placement)

(Do not report 64416 in conjunction with 01996)

AMA Coding Notes

Introduction/Injection of Anesthetic Agent (Nerve Block), Diagnostic or Therapeutic Procedures on the Extracranial Nerves, Peripheral Nerves, and Autonomic Nervous System

(For destruction by neurolytic agent or chemodenervation, see 62280-62282, 64600-64681)

(For epidural or subarachnoid injection, see 62320, 62321, 62322, 62323, 62324, 62325, 62326, 62327)

(64479-64487, 64490-64495 are unilateral procedures. For bilateral procedures, use modifier 50)

Surgical Procedures on the Extracranial Nerves, Peripheral Nerves, and Autonomic Nervous System

(For intracranial surgery on cranial nerves, see 61450, 61460, 61790)

AMA *CPT Assistant* ▢

64415: Fall 92: 17, Jul 98: 10, May 99: 8, Oct 01: 9, Feb 04: 7, Apr 05: 13, Nov 06: 23, Jan 13: 13

64416: Feb 04: 7, Apr 05: 13, Jan 13: 13

Plain English Description

The physician makes a single injection of a drug to numb the nerves in the arm. For code 64416, an anesthetic is injected into the brachial plexus by continuous infusion. The arm is abducted with the elbow flexed and the hand above the shoulder. The skin is cleansed and anesthetized before a needle is placed in the infraclavicular or supraclavicular region and advanced into position in the brachial plexus sheath. Proper placement of the needle is verified with electrical nerve stimulation and/or with the onset of numbness, tingling, or prickling sensations, or through separately reportable ultrasound imaging. The cannula for the nerve block is then threaded over the needle through the brachial plexus sheath. The needle is removed when the cannula is in position. Next, the epidural-type catheter for administering the anesthetic is threaded through the cannula into position in the brachial plexus sheath. The nerve block into the brachial plexus is then injected using a local anesthetic medication like lidocaine or bupivacaine. The function of the nerve block is determined, and the continuous infusion is started.

Brachial plexus injection, anesthetic agent

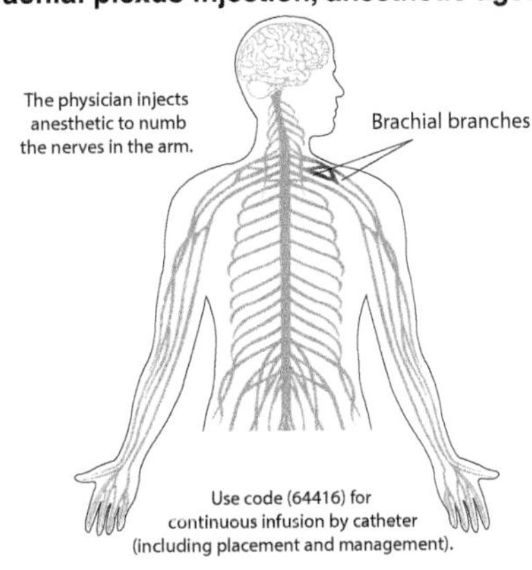
The physician injects anesthetic to numb the nerves in the arm.
Brachial branches
Use code (64416) for continuous infusion by catheter (including placement and management).

ICD-10-CM Diagnostic Codes

	Code	Description
	B02.29	Other postherpetic nervous system involvement
⇄	C40.01	Malignant neoplasm of scapula and long bones of right upper limb
⇄	C40.02	Malignant neoplasm of scapula and long bones of left upper limb
⇄	C47.11	Malignant neoplasm of peripheral nerves of right upper limb, including shoulder
⇄	C47.12	Malignant neoplasm of peripheral nerves of left upper limb, including shoulder
⇄	C49.11	Malignant neoplasm of connective and soft tissue of right upper limb, including shoulder
⇄	C49.12	Malignant neoplasm of connective and soft tissue of left upper limb, including shoulder
	C79.89	Secondary malignant neoplasm of other specified sites
	G54.0	Brachial plexus disorders
	G54.5	Neuralgic amyotrophy
	G54.6	Phantom limb syndrome with pain
⇄	G56.41	Causalgia of right upper limb
⇄	G56.42	Causalgia of left upper limb
	G89.11	Acute pain due to trauma
	G89.18	Other acute postprocedural pain
	G89.21	Chronic pain due to trauma
	G89.28	Other chronic postprocedural pain
	G89.29	Other chronic pain
	G89.3	Neoplasm related pain (acute) (chronic)
	G89.4	Chronic pain syndrome
⇄	G90.511	Complex regional pain syndrome I of right upper limb
⇄	G90.512	Complex regional pain syndrome I of left upper limb
⇄	G90.513	Complex regional pain syndrome I of upper limb, bilateral
⇄	M25.511	Pain in right shoulder
⇄	M25.512	Pain in left shoulder
	M54.13	Radiculopathy, cervicothoracic region
❼	S14.3	Injury of brachial plexus

ICD-10-CM Coding Notes

For codes requiring a 7th character extension, refer to your ICD-10-CM book. Review the character descriptions and coding guidelines for proper selection. For some procedures, only certain characters will apply.

CCI Edits

Refer to Appendix A for CCI edits.

Facility RVUs ▢

Code	Work	PE Facility	MP	Total Facility
64415	1.48	0.27	0.12	1.87
64416	1.81	0.33	0.14	2.28

Non-facility RVUs ▢

Code	Work	PE Non-Facility	MP	Total Non-Facility
64415	1.48	1.78	0.12	3.38
64416	1.81	0.33	0.14	2.28

Modifiers (PAR) ▢

Code	Mod 50	Mod 51	Mod 62	Mod 66	Mod 80
64415	1	2	0	0	1
64416	1	2	0	0	1

Global Period

Code	Days
64415	000
64416	000

CPT © 2018 American Medical Association. All Rights Reserved.

64417-64418

64417 Injection, anesthetic agent; axillary nerve

64418 Injection, anesthetic agent; suprascapular nerve

AMA Coding Notes

Introduction/Injection of Anesthetic Agent (Nerve Block), Diagnostic or Therapeutic Procedures on the Extracranial Nerves, Peripheral Nerves, and Autonomic Nervous System

(For destruction by neurolytic agent or chemodenervation, see 62280-62282, 64600-64681)

(For epidural or subarachnoid injection, see 62320, 62321, 62322, 62323, 62324, 62325, 62326, 62327)

(64479-64487, 64490-64495 are unilateral procedures. For bilateral procedures, use modifier 50)

Surgical Procedures on the Extracranial Nerves, Peripheral Nerves, and Autonomic Nervous System

(For intracranial surgery on cranial nerves, see 61450, 61460, 61790)

AMA *CPT Assistant* ▯

64417: Jul 98: 10, Apr 05: 13, Jan 13: 13

64418: Jul 98: 10, Apr 05: 13, Aug 07: 15, Jan 13: 13

Plain English Description

Injection of an anesthetic agent, also referred to as a nerve block, may be performed as either a diagnostic or therapeutic measure. In 64417, an axillary nerve block is performed. The axillary nerve originates from the brachial plexus at the level of the axilla. It divides into anterior and posterior trunks. The anterior trunk branches and supplies the middle and anterior surface of the deltoid. The posterior trunk branches supply the teres minor and posterior deltoid muscle. In 64418, a subscapular nerve block is performed. The subscapular nerve arises from the brachial plexus and divides into upper and lower branches. The upper branch supplies the upper part of the subscapularis muscle and the lower part branches and one branch supplies the lower part of the subscapularis and another the teres major. The skin over the planned injection site is cleansed. A needle is inserted into the axillary or subscapular nerve, aspirated to ensure that it is not in a blood vessel, and an anesthetic is injected.

Injection, anesthetic agent

Axillary nerve

Suprascapular nerve

Axillary nerve (64417); suprascapular nerve (64418)

ICD-10-CM Diagnostic Codes

	B02.29	Other postherpetic nervous system involvement
⇄	C40.01	Malignant neoplasm of scapula and long bones of right upper limb
⇄	C40.02	Malignant neoplasm of scapula and long bones of left upper limb
⇄	C47.11	Malignant neoplasm of peripheral nerves of right upper limb, including shoulder
⇄	C47.12	Malignant neoplasm of peripheral nerves of left upper limb, including shoulder
⇄	C49.11	Malignant neoplasm of connective and soft tissue of right upper limb, including shoulder
⇄	C49.12	Malignant neoplasm of connective and soft tissue of left upper limb, including shoulder
	C79.89	Secondary malignant neoplasm of other specified sites
	G54.0	Brachial plexus disorders
	G54.6	Phantom limb syndrome with pain
⇄	G56.40	Causalgia of unspecified upper limb
⇄	G56.41	Causalgia of right upper limb
⇄	G56.42	Causalgia of left upper limb
⇄	G56.43	Causalgia of bilateral upper limbs
⇄	G56.81	Other specified mononeuropathies of right upper limb
⇄	G56.82	Other specified mononeuropathies of left upper limb
⇄	G56.83	Other specified mononeuropathies of bilateral upper limbs
	G89.11	Acute pain due to trauma
	G89.18	Other acute postprocedural pain
	G89.21	Chronic pain due to trauma
	G89.28	Other chronic postprocedural pain
	G89.29	Other chronic pain
	G89.3	Neoplasm related pain (acute) (chronic)
	G89.4	Chronic pain syndrome
⇄	G90.511	Complex regional pain syndrome I of right upper limb
⇄	G90.512	Complex regional pain syndrome I of left upper limb
⇄	G90.513	Complex regional pain syndrome I of upper limb, bilateral
⇄	M25.51	Pain in shoulder
⇄	M25.52	Pain in elbow
⇄	M75.01	Adhesive capsulitis of right shoulder
⇄	M75.02	Adhesive capsulitis of left shoulder
⇄	M75.11	Incomplete rotator cuff tear or rupture not specified as traumatic
⇄	M75.111	Incomplete rotator cuff tear or rupture of right shoulder, not specified as traumatic
⇄	M75.112	Incomplete rotator cuff tear or rupture of left shoulder, not specified as traumatic
⇄	M75.12	Complete rotator cuff tear or rupture not specified as traumatic
⇄	M75.121	Complete rotator cuff tear or rupture of right shoulder, not specified as traumatic
⇄	M75.122	Complete rotator cuff tear or rupture of left shoulder, not specified as traumatic
⇄	M75.31	Calcific tendinitis of right shoulder
⇄	M75.32	Calcific tendinitis of left shoulder
⇄	M75.41	Impingement syndrome of right shoulder
⇄	M75.42	Impingement syndrome of left shoulder
⇄	M75.81	Other shoulder lesions, right shoulder
⇄	M75.82	Other shoulder lesions, left shoulder
⇄	M79.601	Pain in right arm
⇄	M79.602	Pain in left arm
⇄	M79.621	Pain in right upper arm
⇄	M79.622	Pain in left upper arm
❼⇄	S43.011	Anterior subluxation of right humerus
❼⇄	S43.012	Anterior subluxation of left humerus
❼⇄	S43.014	Anterior dislocation of right humerus
❼⇄	S43.015	Anterior dislocation of left humerus
❼⇄	S43.021	Posterior subluxation of right humerus
❼⇄	S43.022	Posterior subluxation of left humerus
❼⇄	S43.024	Posterior dislocation of right humerus
❼⇄	S43.025	Posterior dislocation of left humerus
❼⇄	S43.031	Inferior subluxation of right humerus
❼⇄	S43.032	Inferior subluxation of left humerus
❼⇄	S43.034	Inferior dislocation of right humerus
❼⇄	S43.035	Inferior dislocation of left humerus
❼⇄	S43.081	Other subluxation of right shoulder joint
❼⇄	S43.082	Other subluxation of left shoulder joint
❼⇄	S43.084	Other dislocation of right shoulder joint
❼⇄	S43.085	Other dislocation of left shoulder joint
❼⇄	S44.31	Injury of axillary nerve, right arm
❼⇄	S44.32	Injury of axillary nerve, left arm
❼⇄	S44.8X1	Injury of other nerves at shoulder and upper arm level, right arm
❼⇄	S44.8X2	Injury of other nerves at shoulder and upper arm level, left arm

CPT © 2018 American Medical Association. All Rights Reserved.

⑦⇄	S44.8X9	Injury of other nerves at shoulder and upper arm level, unspecified arm
⑦⇄	S46.011	Strain of muscle(s) and tendon(s) of the rotator cuff of right shoulder
⑦⇄	S46.012	Strain of muscle(s) and tendon(s) of the rotator cuff of left shoulder

ICD-10-CM Coding Notes

For codes requiring a 7th character extension, refer to your ICD-10-CM book. Review the character descriptions and coding guidelines for proper selection. For some procedures, only certain characters will apply.

CCI Edits

Refer to Appendix A for CCI edits.

Facility RVUs ▯

Code	Work	PE Facility	MP	Total Facility
64417	1.44	0.46	0.12	2.02
64418	1.10	0.42	0.12	1.64

Non-facility RVUs ▯

Code	Work	PE Non-Facility	MP	Total Non-Facility
64417	1.44	2.20	0.12	3.76
64418	1.10	1.49	0.12	2.71

Modifiers (PAR) ▯

Code	Mod 50	Mod 51	Mod 62	Mod 66	Mod 80
64417	1	2	0	0	1
64418	1	2	0	0	1

Global Period

Code	Days
64417	000
64418	000

CPT © 2018 American Medical Association. All Rights Reserved.

64420-64421

64420 Injection, anesthetic agent; intercostal nerve, single

64421 Injection, anesthetic agent; intercostal nerves, multiple, regional block

AMA Coding Notes

Introduction/Injection of Anesthetic Agent (Nerve Block), Diagnostic or Therapeutic Procedures on the Extracranial Nerves, Peripheral Nerves, and Autonomic Nervous System

(For destruction by neurolytic agent or chemodenervation, see 62280-62282, 64600-64681)

(For epidural or subarachnoid injection, see 62320, 62321, 62322, 62323, 62324, 62325, 62326, 62327)

(64479-64487, 64490-64495 are unilateral procedures. For bilateral procedures, use modifier 50)

Surgical Procedures on the Extracranial Nerves, Peripheral Nerves, and Autonomic Nervous System

(For intracranial surgery on cranial nerves, see 61450, 61460, 61790)

AMA *CPT Assistant* ☐

64420: Jul 98: 10, Apr 05: 13, Aug 10: 12, Nov 10: 9, Jan 13: 13, Jun 15: 3

64421: Jul 98: 10, Apr 05: 13, Aug 10: 12, Nov 10: 9, Jan 13: 13, Jun 15: 3, May 18: 10

Plain English Description

The intercostal nerves are mixed nerves that supply the skin and muscles of the upper extremities, thorax, and abdominal wall. The intercostal nerves exit the posterior aspect of the intercostal membrane just distal to the intervertebral foramen and then enter the intercostal groove running parallel to the rib. Branches of the intercostal nerves may be found between the ribs. Intercostal nerves are most often blocked along the posterior axillary line or just lateral to the paraspinal muscles at the angle of the rib. The planned injection site(s) is identified and marked along the inferior border of the rib(s). The needle is introduced underneath the inferior border of the rib and advanced until it reaches the subcostal groove. The anesthetic agent is then injected. Use 64420 for injection of a single intercostal nerve. Use 64421 if multiple intercostal nerves are injected.

Injection, anesthetic agent; intercostal nerve(s), regional block

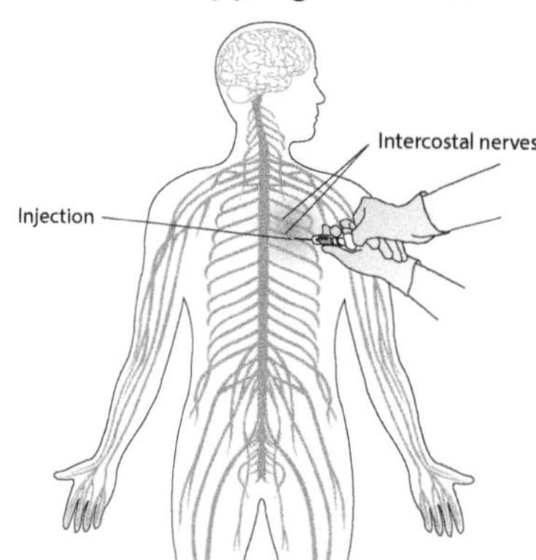

Single (64420); multiple, regional block (64421)

ICD-10-CM Diagnostic Codes

	B02.29	Other postherpetic nervous system involvement
	C41.3	Malignant neoplasm of ribs, sternum and clavicle
	C47.3	Malignant neoplasm of peripheral nerves of thorax
	C76.1	Malignant neoplasm of thorax
	C79.51	Secondary malignant neoplasm of bone
	C79.89	Secondary malignant neoplasm of other specified sites
	G58.0	Intercostal neuropathy
	G89.11	Acute pain due to trauma
	G89.12	Acute post-thoracotomy pain
	G89.18	Other acute postprocedural pain
	G89.21	Chronic pain due to trauma
	G89.22	Chronic post-thoracotomy pain
	G89.28	Other chronic postprocedural pain
	G89.29	Other chronic pain
	G89.3	Neoplasm related pain (acute) (chronic)
	G89.4	Chronic pain syndrome
	M54.14	Radiculopathy, thoracic region
	M54.6	Pain in thoracic spine
	M54.9	Dorsalgia, unspecified
	M79.2	Neuralgia and neuritis, unspecified
	R07.82	Intercostal pain
	R10.10	Upper abdominal pain, unspecified
⇄	R10.11	Right upper quadrant pain
⇄	R10.12	Left upper quadrant pain
❼	S22.21	Fracture of manubrium
❼	S22.22	Fracture of body of sternum
❼	S22.23	Sternal manubrial dissociation
❼	S22.24	Fracture of xiphoid process
❼⇄	S22.31	Fracture of one rib, right side
❼⇄	S22.32	Fracture of one rib, left side
❼⇄	S22.41	Multiple fractures of ribs, right side
❼⇄	S22.42	Multiple fractures of ribs, left side
❼⇄	S22.43	Multiple fractures of ribs, bilateral
❼	S22.5	Flail chest
❼	S23.41	Sprain of ribs
❼	S23.421	Sprain of chondrosternal joint
❼	S23.428	Other sprain of sternum
❼	S23.8	Sprain of other specified parts of thorax
❼	S29.011	Strain of muscle and tendon of front wall of thorax
❼	S29.012	Strain of muscle and tendon of back wall of thorax

ICD-10-CM Coding Notes

For codes requiring a 7th character extension, refer to your ICD-10-CM book. Review the character descriptions and coding guidelines for proper selection. For some procedures, only certain characters will apply.

CCI Edits

Refer to Appendix A for CCI edits.

Facility RVUs ☐

Code	Work	PE Facility	MP	Total Facility
64420	1.18	0.63	0.11	1.92
64421	1.68	0.82	0.14	2.64

Non-facility RVUs ☐

Code	Work	PE Non-Facility	MP	Total Non-Facility
64420	1.18	1.86	0.11	3.15
64421	1.68	2.64	0.14	4.46

Modifiers (PAR) ☐

Code	Mod 50	Mod 51	Mod 62	Mod 66	Mod 80
64420	0	2	0	0	1
64421	1	2	0	0	1

Global Period

Code	Days
64420	000
64421	000

CPT © 2018 American Medical Association. All Rights Reserved.

64425

64425 Injection, anesthetic agent; ilioinguinal, iliohypogastric nerves

AMA Coding Notes

Introduction/Injection of Anesthetic Agent (Nerve Block), Diagnostic or Therapeutic Procedures on the Extracranial Nerves, Peripheral Nerves, and Autonomic Nervous System

(For destruction by neurolytic agent or chemodenervation, see 62280-62282, 64600-64681)

(For epidural or subarachnoid injection, see 62320, 62321, 62322, 62323, 62324, 62325, 62326, 62327)

(64479-64487, 64490-64495 are unilateral procedures. For bilateral procedures, use modifier 50)

Surgical Procedures on the Extracranial Nerves, Peripheral Nerves, and Autonomic Nervous System

(For intracranial surgery on cranial nerves, see 61450, 61460, 61790)

AMA *CPT Assistant* ▫

64425: Jul 98: 10, Apr 05: 13, Jan 13: 13, Jun 15: 3

Plain English Description

The ilioinguinal and iliohypogastric nerves arise from L1. Both nerves emerge from the upper part of the lateral border of the psoas major muscle and then penetrate the transversus abdominus muscle just above and medial to the anterior superior iliac spine. The nerves run between the transversus abdominus and the internal oblique muscles for a short distance then penetrate the internal oblique. They run between the internal and external oblique muscles before branching and penetrating the external oblique muscle where branches provide skin sensation. The anterior superior iliac spine is located and the planned injection site medial and superior to it is marked. A needle is positioned perpendicular to the skin and the skin is punctured. The needle is advanced through the external oblique muscle and into the space between the internal and external oblique. The needle is aspirated to ensure that the needle is not in a blood vessel and the anesthetic agent is injected between the oblique muscles. The needle is then advanced through the internal oblique muscle into the space between the internal oblique and transversus abdominus. The space is aspirated and injected as described above. The needle is withdrawn and inserted at a 45-degree angle laterally and the procedure repeated.

Injection, anesthetic agent; ilioinguinal, iliohypogastric nerves

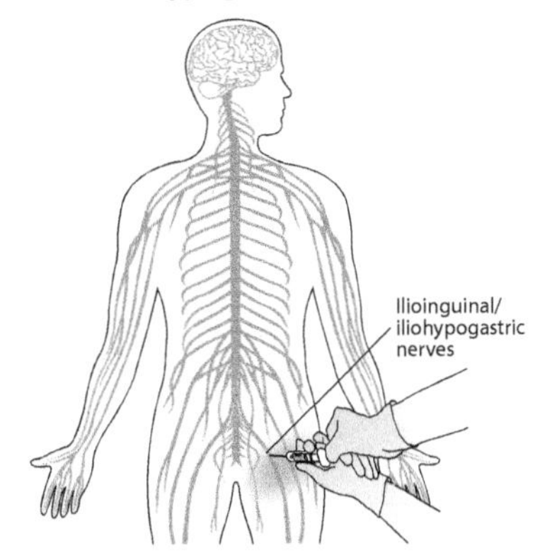

ICD-10-CM Diagnostic Codes

	C76.3	Malignant neoplasm of pelvis
	C79.89	Secondary malignant neoplasm of other specified sites
⇄	G57.80	Other specified mononeuropathies of unspecified lower limb
⇄	G57.81	Other specified mononeuropathies of right lower limb
⇄	G57.82	Other specified mononeuropathies of left lower limb
	G89.11	Acute pain due to trauma
	G89.18	Other acute postprocedural pain
	G89.21	Chronic pain due to trauma
	G89.28	Other chronic postprocedural pain
	G89.29	Other chronic pain
	G89.3	Neoplasm related pain (acute) (chronic)
	G89.4	Chronic pain syndrome
⇄	M79.651	Pain in right thigh
⇄	M79.652	Pain in left thigh
⇄	M79.659	Pain in unspecified thigh
	R10.2	Pelvic and perineal pain
	R10.30	Lower abdominal pain, unspecified
⇄	R10.31	Right lower quadrant pain
⇄	R10.32	Left lower quadrant pain
❼	S34.6	Injury of peripheral nerve(s) at abdomen, lower back and pelvis level
❼	S34.8	Injury of other nerves at abdomen, lower back and pelvis level
❼	S34.9	Injury of unspecified nerves at abdomen, lower back and pelvis level
❼	S38.01	Crushing injury of penis
❼	S38.02	Crushing injury of scrotum and testis
❼	S38.03	Crushing injury of vulva
❼	S39.013	Strain of muscle, fascia and tendon of pelvis
❼	S39.093	Other injury of muscle, fascia and tendon of pelvis
❼	S39.83	Other specified injuries of pelvis
❼	S39.840	Fracture of corpus cavernosum penis
❼	S39.848	Other specified injuries of external genitals
❼⇄	S74.8X1	Injury of other nerves at hip and thigh level, right leg
❼⇄	S74.8X2	Injury of other nerves at hip and thigh level, left leg

ICD-10-CM Coding Notes

For codes requiring a 7th character extension, refer to your ICD-10-CM book. Review the character descriptions and coding guidelines for proper selection. For some procedures, only certain characters will apply.

CCI Edits

Refer to Appendix A for CCI edits.

Facility RVUs ▫

Code	Work	PE Facility	MP	Total Facility
64425	1.75	0.80	0.17	2.72

Non-facility RVUs ▫

Code	Work	PE Non-Facility	MP	Total Non-Facility
64425	1.75	2.01	0.17	3.93

Modifiers (PAR) ▫

Code	Mod 50	Mod 51	Mod 62	Mod 66	Mod 80
64425	1	2	0	0	1

Global Period

Code	Days
64425	000

● New ▲ Revised ✚ Add On ⊘Modifier 51 Exempt ★Telemedicine ▫ CPT QuickRef ✗FDA Pending ⇄ Laterality ❼ Seventh Character ♂Male ♀Female

CPT © 2018 American Medical Association. All Rights Reserved.

64430

64430 Injection, anesthetic agent; pudendal nerve

AMA Coding Notes

Introduction/Injection of Anesthetic Agent (Nerve Block), Diagnostic or Therapeutic Procedures on the Extracranial Nerves, Peripheral Nerves, and Autonomic Nervous System

(For destruction by neurolytic agent or chemodenervation, see 62280-62282, 64600-64681)

(For epidural or subarachnoid injection, see 62320, 62321, 62322, 62323, 62324, 62325, 62326, 62327)

(64479-64487, 64490-64495 are unilateral procedures. For bilateral procedures, use modifier 50)

Surgical Procedures on the Extracranial Nerves, Peripheral Nerves, and Autonomic Nervous System

(For intracranial surgery on cranial nerves, see 61450, 61460, 61790)

AMA *CPT Assistant* ▯

64430: Jul 98: 10, Apr 05: 13, Jan 13: 13

Plain English Description

The physician performs a pudendal nerve block by injecting an anesthetic agent into the nerve. Pudendal nerve block is used during the second stage of labor to provide pain relief, for pelvic floor relaxation when forceps delivery is needed, and to provide anesthesia of the perineum for creation or repair of an episiotomy. The block may be administered via a transvaginal or transcutaneous perineal approach. Using a transvaginal approach, the ischial spine on the first side to be injected is palpated. A Huber needle is used to limit the depth of submucosal penetration. The needle is passed through the sacrospinous ligament and advanced about 1 cm. The physician ensures that the needle is in the proper location and that it has not penetrated the pudendal vessels by pulling back on the syringe. If blood is aspirated the needle is reposited. Aspiration is again performed and if no blood is present, the anesthetic is injected. The procedure is repeated on the opposite side. Using a transcutaneous perineal approach, the ischial tuberosity is palpated and the needle introduced slightly medial to the tuberosity. The needle is advanced approximately 2.5 cm. Aspiration is performed to ensure that the needle is not in a blood vessel and then the anesthetic is injected. The needle is withdrawn and directed into the deep superficial tissue of the vulva and anesthetic is again injected to block the ilioinguinal and genitofemoral components of the pudendal nerve. This is repeated on the opposite side.

Injection, anesthetic agent; pudendal nerve

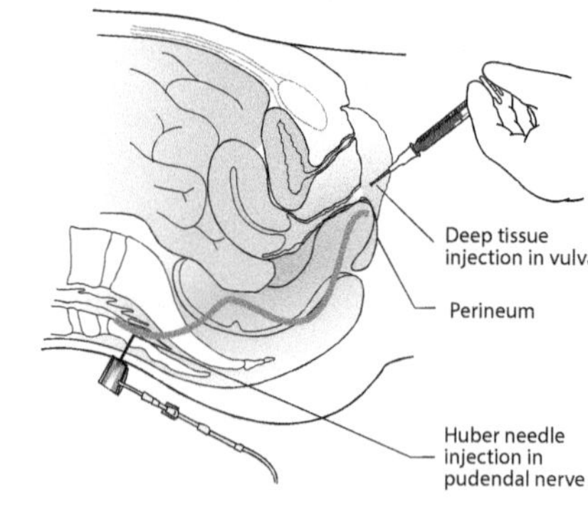

ICD-10-CM Diagnostic Codes

	C76.3	Malignant neoplasm of pelvis
	C79.89	Secondary malignant neoplasm of other specified sites
	G58.8	Other specified mononeuropathies
	G89.11	Acute pain due to trauma
	G89.18	Other acute postprocedural pain
	G89.21	Chronic pain due to trauma
	G89.28	Other chronic postprocedural pain
	G89.29	Other chronic pain
	G89.3	Neoplasm related pain (acute) (chronic)
	G89.4	Chronic pain syndrome
	N80.3	Endometriosis of pelvic peritoneum ♀
	N80.4	Endometriosis of rectovaginal septum and vagina ♀
	N94.810	Vulvar vestibulitis ♀
	N94.818	Other vulvodynia ♀
	N94.819	Vulvodynia, unspecified ♀
	N94.89	Other specified conditions associated with female genital organs and menstrual cycle ♀
	O71.89	Other specified obstetric trauma ♀
	R10.2	Pelvic and perineal pain
❼	S34.6	Injury of peripheral nerve(s) at abdomen, lower back and pelvis level
❼	S34.8	Injury of other nerves at abdomen, lower back and pelvis level
❼	S34.9	Injury of unspecified nerves at abdomen, lower back and pelvis level
❼	S38.03	Crushing injury of vulva
❼	S39.848	Other specified injuries of external genitals
❼	S39.94	Unspecified injury of external genitals

ICD-10-CM Coding Notes

For codes requiring a 7th character extension, refer to your ICD-10-CM book. Review the character descriptions and coding guidelines for proper selection. For some procedures, only certain characters will apply.

CCI Edits

Refer to Appendix A for CCI edits.

Facility RVUs ▯

Code	Work	PE Facility	MP	Total Facility
64430	1.46	0.70	0.14	2.30

Non-facility RVUs ▯

Code	Work	PE Non-Facility	MP	Total Non-Facility
64430	1.46	2.54	0.14	4.14

Modifiers (PAR) ▯

Code	Mod 50	Mod 51	Mod 62	Mod 66	Mod 80
64430	1	2	0	0	1

Global Period

Code	Days
64430	000

● New ▲ Revised ✚ Add On ⊘Modifier 51 Exempt ★Telemedicine ▯ CPT QuickRef ✗FDA Pending ⇄ Laterality ❼ Seventh Character ♂Male ♀Female

CPT © 2018 American Medical Association. All Rights Reserved.

64435

64435 Injection, anesthetic agent; paracervical (uterine) nerve

AMA Coding Notes

Introduction/Injection of Anesthetic Agent (Nerve Block), Diagnostic or Therapeutic Procedures on the Extracranial Nerves, Peripheral Nerves, and Autonomic Nervous System

(For destruction by neurolytic agent or chemodenervation, see 62280-62282, 64600-64681)

(For epidural or subarachnoid injection, see 62320, 62321, 62322, 62323, 62324, 62325, 62326, 62327)

(64479-64487, 64490-64495 are unilateral procedures. For bilateral procedures, use modifier 50)

Surgical Procedures on the Extracranial Nerves, Peripheral Nerves, and Autonomic Nervous System

(For intracranial surgery on cranial nerves, see 61450, 61460, 61790)

AMA *CPT Assistant* ▯

64435: Jul 98: 10, Mar 03: 22, Jul 03: 15, Apr 05: 13, Feb 12: 11, Jan 13: 13

Plain English Description

Paracervical nerve block is used to reduce pain during the first stage of labor. An 18.5 cm needle with a security tip is used to administer the injection. The needle is advanced transvaginally just deep to the lateral fornices of the vagina and into the broad ligament. The needle is aspirated to ensure that it is not in a blood vessel. The anesthetic agent is injected at various sites along the broad ligament. The procedure is repeated on the opposite side.

Injection, anesthetic agent; paracervical (uterine) nerve

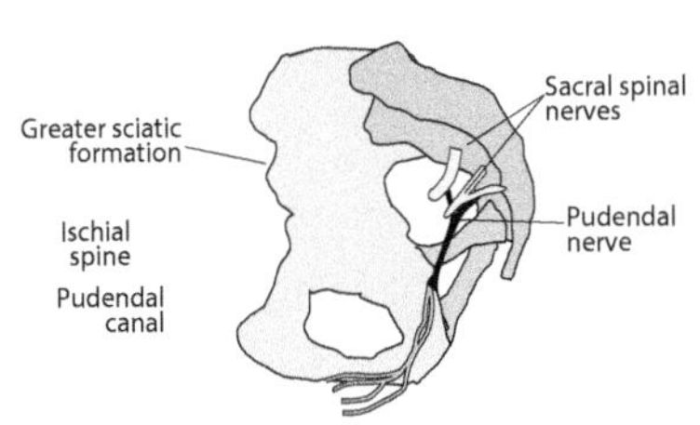

The physician injects a drug to numb the nerve around the cervix and relieve pain during childbirth.

ICD-10-CM Diagnostic Codes

❼	O32.1	Maternal care for breech presentation
❼	O32.2	Maternal care for transverse and oblique lie
❼	O32.3	Maternal care for face, brow and chin presentation
❼	O32.8	Maternal care for other malpresentation of fetus
❼	O33.5	Maternal care for disproportion due to unusually large fetus
❼	O64.0	Obstructed labor due to incomplete rotation of fetal head
❼	O64.1	Obstructed labor due to breech presentation
❼	O64.2	Obstructed labor due to face presentation
❼	O64.3	Obstructed labor due to brow presentation
❼	O64.4	Obstructed labor due to shoulder presentation
	O66.0	Obstructed labor due to shoulder dystocia ♀
	O66.2	Obstructed labor due to unusually large fetus ♀
	O66.5	Attempted application of vacuum extractor and forceps ♀

ICD-10-CM Coding Notes

For codes requiring a 7th character extension, refer to your ICD-10-CM book. Review the character descriptions and coding guidelines for proper selection. For some procedures, only certain characters will apply.

CCI Edits

Refer to Appendix A for CCI edits.

Facility RVUs ▯

Code	Work	PE Facility	MP	Total Facility
64435	1.45	0.73	0.17	2.35

Non-facility RVUs ▯

Code	Work	PE Non-Facility	MP	Total Non-Facility
64435	1.45	2.38	0.17	4.00

Modifiers (PAR) ▯

Code	Mod 50	Mod 51	Mod 62	Mod 66	Mod 80
64435	1	2	0	0	1

Global Period

Code	Days
64435	000

CPT © 2018 American Medical Association. All Rights Reserved.

64445

64445 Injection, anesthetic agent; sciatic nerve, single

AMA Coding Notes

Introduction/Injection of Anesthetic Agent (Nerve Block), Diagnostic or Therapeutic Procedures on the Extracranial Nerves, Peripheral Nerves, and Autonomic Nervous System

(For destruction by neurolytic agent or chemodenervation, see 62280-62282, 64600-64681)

(For epidural or subarachnoid injection, see 62320, 62321, 62322, 62323, 62324, 62325, 62326, 62327)

(64479-64487, 64490-64495 are unilateral procedures. For bilateral procedures, use modifier 50)

Surgical Procedures on the Extracranial Nerves, Peripheral Nerves, and Autonomic Nervous System

(For intracranial surgery on cranial nerves, see 61450, 61460, 61790)

AMA *CPT Assistant* ▢

64445: Jul 98: 10, May 99: 8, Feb 04: 8, Apr 05: 13, Dec 11: 8, Apr 12: 19, Jan 13: 13

Plain English Description

The thigh is flexed at the hip. A line is marked from the back of the knee to a point between the greater trochanter and the ischial tuberosity. The skin is cleansed. A needle is introduced just above the marked line to test the sciatic nerve using electrical nerve stimulation. After a motor response in the ankle, foot, or toes has been elicited, a sciatic nerve block is performed using a single injection of an anesthetic agent.

Injection, anesthetic agent; sciatic nerve

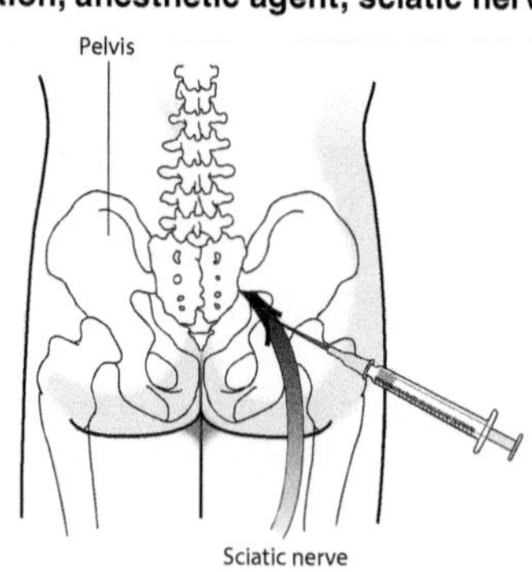

ICD-10-CM Diagnostic Codes

⇄	C47.21	Malignant neoplasm of peripheral nerves of right lower limb, including hip
⇄	C47.22	Malignant neoplasm of peripheral nerves of left lower limb, including hip
⇄	C49.21	Malignant neoplasm of connective and soft tissue of right lower limb, including hip
⇄	C49.22	Malignant neoplasm of connective and soft tissue of left lower limb, including hip
⇄	C76.51	Malignant neoplasm of right lower limb
⇄	C76.52	Malignant neoplasm of left lower limb
	C79.89	Secondary malignant neoplasm of other specified sites
⇄	G57.00	Lesion of sciatic nerve, unspecified lower limb
⇄	G57.01	Lesion of sciatic nerve, right lower limb
⇄	G57.02	Lesion of sciatic nerve, left lower limb
	G58.8	Other specified mononeuropathies
	G89.11	Acute pain due to trauma
	G89.18	Other acute postprocedural pain
	G89.21	Chronic pain due to trauma
	G89.28	Other chronic postprocedural pain
	G89.29	Other chronic pain
	G89.3	Neoplasm related pain (acute) (chronic)
⇄	M79.661	Pain in right lower leg
⇄	M79.662	Pain in left lower leg
⇄	M79.671	Pain in right foot
⇄	M79.672	Pain in left foot
⇄	M79.674	Pain in right toe(s)
⇄	M79.675	Pain in left toe(s)
❼⇄	S74.01	Injury of sciatic nerve at hip and thigh level, right leg
❼⇄	S74.02	Injury of sciatic nerve at hip and thigh level, left leg

ICD-10-CM Coding Notes

For codes requiring a 7th character extension, refer to your ICD-10-CM book. Review the character descriptions and coding guidelines for proper selection. For some procedures, only certain characters will apply.

CCI Edits

Refer to Appendix A for CCI edits.

Facility RVUs ▢

Code	Work	PE Facility	MP	Total Facility
64445	1.48	0.46	0.15	2.09

Non-facility RVUs ▢

Code	Work	PE Non-Facility	MP	Total Non-Facility
64445	1.48	2.26	0.15	3.89

Modifiers (PAR) ▢

Code	Mod 50	Mod 51	Mod 62	Mod 66	Mod 80
64445	1	2	0	0	1

Global Period

Code	Days
64445	000

CPT © 2018 American Medical Association. All Rights Reserved.

64446

64446 Injection, anesthetic agent; sciatic nerve, continuous infusion by catheter (including catheter placement)

(Do not report 64446 in conjunction with 01996)

AMA Coding Notes

Introduction/Injection of Anesthetic Agent (Nerve Block), Diagnostic or Therapeutic Procedures on the Extracranial Nerves, Peripheral Nerves, and Autonomic Nervous System

(For destruction by neurolytic agent or chemodenervation, see 62280-62282, 64600-64681)

(For epidural or subarachnoid injection, see 62320, 62321, 62322, 62323, 62324, 62325, 62326, 62327)

(64479-64487, 64490-64495 are unilateral procedures. For bilateral procedures, use modifier 50)

Surgical Procedures on the Extracranial Nerves, Peripheral Nerves, and Autonomic Nervous System

(For intracranial surgery on cranial nerves, see 61450, 61460, 61790)

AMA *CPT Assistant* ☐

64446: Feb 04: 9, Apr 05: 13, Jan 13: 13

Plain English Description

The thigh is flexed at the hip. A line is marked from the back of the knee to a point between the greater trochanter and the ischial tuberosity. The skin is cleansed and anesthetized before a needle is introduced just above the marked line to test the sciatic nerve and elicit a motor response in the ankle, foot, or toes. Next, an insulated, epidural-type needle is inserted to intersect with the tip of the first. A catheter is then threaded through the epidural needle and out the tip. Electrical nerve stimulation is tested again through the catheter. The epidural needle is removed when the cannula is secured in position. The nerve block is then injected into the sciatic nerve using a local anesthetic medication like lidocaine or bupivacaine. The function of the nerve block is determined, and continuous infusion is started.

Injection, anesthetic agent; sciatic nerve, continuous infusion by

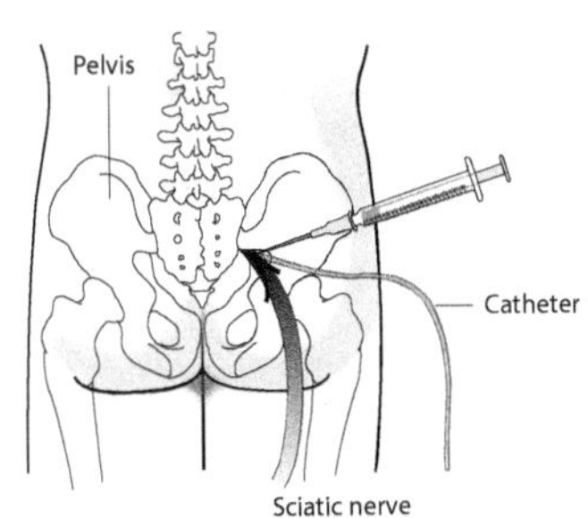

After the injection a catheter is inserted for continuous infusion.

ICD-10-CM Diagnostic Codes

⇄	C47.21	Malignant neoplasm of peripheral nerves of right lower limb, including hip
⇄	C47.22	Malignant neoplasm of peripheral nerves of left lower limb, including hip
⇄	C49.21	Malignant neoplasm of connective and soft tissue of right lower limb, including hip
⇄	C49.22	Malignant neoplasm of connective and soft tissue of left lower limb, including hip
⇄	C76.51	Malignant neoplasm of right lower limb
⇄	C76.52	Malignant neoplasm of left lower limb
	C79.89	Secondary malignant neoplasm of other specified sites
⇄	G57.00	Lesion of sciatic nerve, unspecified lower limb
⇄	G57.01	Lesion of sciatic nerve, right lower limb
⇄	G57.02	Lesion of sciatic nerve, left lower limb
	G58.8	Other specified mononeuropathies
	G89.11	Acute pain due to trauma
	G89.18	Other acute postprocedural pain
	G89.21	Chronic pain due to trauma
	G89.28	Other chronic postprocedural pain
	G89.29	Other chronic pain
	G89.3	Neoplasm related pain (acute) (chronic)
	M54.18	Radiculopathy, sacral and sacrococcygeal region
⇄	M54.30	Sciatica, unspecified side
⇄	M54.31	Sciatica, right side
⇄	M54.32	Sciatica, left side
⇄	M54.40	Lumbago with sciatica, unspecified side
⇄	M54.41	Lumbago with sciatica, right side
⇄	M54.42	Lumbago with sciatica, left side
⇄	M79.661	Pain in right lower leg
⇄	M79.662	Pain in left lower leg
⇄	M79.671	Pain in right foot
⇄	M79.672	Pain in left foot
⇄	M79.674	Pain in right toe(s)
⇄	M79.675	Pain in left toe(s)
❼⇄	S74.01	Injury of sciatic nerve at hip and thigh level, right leg
❼⇄	S74.02	Injury of sciatic nerve at hip and thigh level, left leg

ICD-10-CM Coding Notes

For codes requiring a 7th character extension, refer to your ICD-10-CM book. Review the character descriptions and coding guidelines for proper selection. For some procedures, only certain characters will apply.

CCI Edits

Refer to Appendix A for CCI edits.

Facility RVUs ☐

Code	Work	PE Facility	MP	Total Facility
64446	1.81	0.33	0.14	2.28

Non-facility RVUs ☐

Code	Work	PE Non-Facility	MP	Total Non-Facility
64446	1.81	0.33	0.14	2.28

Modifiers (PAR) ☐

Code	Mod 50	Mod 51	Mod 62	Mod 66	Mod 80
64446	1	2	0	0	1

Global Period

Code	Days
64446	000

CPT © 2018 American Medical Association. All Rights Reserved.

64447

64447 Injection, anesthetic agent; femoral nerve, single

(Do not report 64447 in conjunction with 01996)

AMA Coding Notes

Introduction/Injection of Anesthetic Agent (Nerve Block), Diagnostic or Therapeutic Procedures on the Extracranial Nerves, Peripheral Nerves, and Autonomic Nervous System

(For destruction by neurolytic agent or chemodenervation, see 62280-62282, 64600-64681)

(For epidural or subarachnoid injection, see 62320, 62321, 62322, 62323, 62324, 62325, 62326, 62327)

(64479-64487, 64490-64495 are unilateral procedures. For bilateral procedures, use modifier 50)

Surgical Procedures on the Extracranial Nerves, Peripheral Nerves, and Autonomic Nervous System

(For intracranial surgery on cranial nerves, see 61450, 61460, 61790)

AMA *CPT Assistant* ▯

64447: Feb 04: 9, Apr 05: 13, Jan 13: 13, Nov 14: 14, Dec 14: 16, Sep 15: 12

Plain English Description

The groin is cleansed and prepped with a small amount of local anesthetic on the affected side. The planned injection site is marked. A needle is introduced and electrical nerve stimulation performed to ensure that the needle is properly positioned. A femoral nerve block is performed using a single injection of an anesthetic agent.

Injection, anesthetic agent, femoral nerve

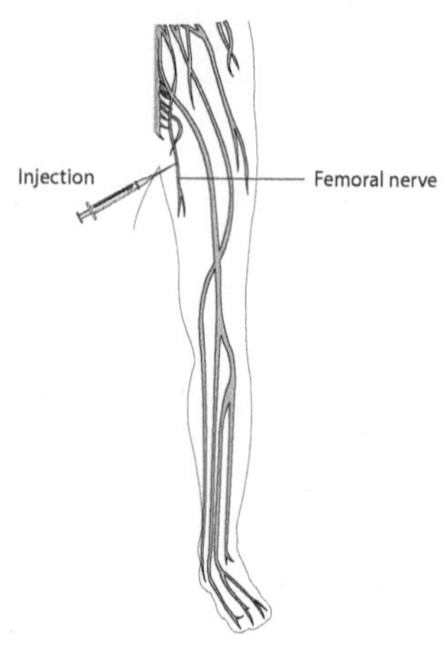

ICD-10-CM Diagnostic Codes

⇄	C47.21	Malignant neoplasm of peripheral nerves of right lower limb, including hip
⇄	C47.22	Malignant neoplasm of peripheral nerves of left lower limb, including hip
⇄	C49.21	Malignant neoplasm of connective and soft tissue of right lower limb, including hip
⇄	C49.22	Malignant neoplasm of connective and soft tissue of left lower limb, including hip
⇄	C76.51	Malignant neoplasm of right lower limb
⇄	C76.52	Malignant neoplasm of left lower limb
	C79.89	Secondary malignant neoplasm of other specified sites
	E08.41	Diabetes mellitus due to underlying condition with diabetic mononeuropathy
	E09.41	Drug or chemical induced diabetes mellitus with neurological complications with diabetic mononeuropathy
	E10.41	Type 1 diabetes mellitus with diabetic mononeuropathy
	E11.41	Type 2 diabetes mellitus with diabetic mononeuropathy
	E13.41	Other specified diabetes mellitus with diabetic mononeuropathy
⇄	G57.20	Lesion of femoral nerve, unspecified lower limb
⇄	G57.21	Lesion of femoral nerve, right lower limb
⇄	G57.22	Lesion of femoral nerve, left lower limb
	G89.11	Acute pain due to trauma
	G89.18	Other acute postprocedural pain
	G89.21	Chronic pain due to trauma
	G89.28	Other chronic postprocedural pain
	G89.29	Other chronic pain
	G89.3	Neoplasm related pain (acute) (chronic)
⇄	M79.604	Pain in right leg
⇄	M79.605	Pain in left leg
⇄	M79.651	Pain in right thigh
⇄	M79.652	Pain in left thigh
⇄	M79.661	Pain in right lower leg
⇄	M79.662	Pain in left lower leg
❼⇄	S74.11	Injury of femoral nerve at hip and thigh level, right leg
❼⇄	S74.12	Injury of femoral nerve at hip and thigh level, left leg

ICD-10-CM Coding Notes

For codes requiring a 7th character extension, refer to your ICD-10-CM book. Review the character descriptions and coding guidelines for proper selection. For some procedures, only certain characters will apply.

CCI Edits

Refer to Appendix A for CCI edits.

Facility RVUs ▯

Code	Work	PE Facility	MP	Total Facility
64447	1.50	0.29	0.12	1.91

Non-facility RVUs ▯

Code	Work	PE Non-Facility	MP	Total Non-Facility
64447	1.50	1.84	0.12	3.46

Modifiers (PAR) ▯

Code	Mod 50	Mod 51	Mod 62	Mod 66	Mod 80
64447	1	2	0	0	1

Global Period

Code	Days
64447	000

CPT © 2018 American Medical Association. All Rights Reserved.

64448

64448 Injection, anesthetic agent; femoral nerve, continuous infusion by catheter (including catheter placement)

(Do not report 64448 in conjunction with 01996)

AMA Coding Notes

Introduction/Injection of Anesthetic Agent (Nerve Block), Diagnostic or Therapeutic Procedures on the Extracranial Nerves, Peripheral Nerves, and Autonomic Nervous System

(For destruction by neurolytic agent or chemodenervation, see 62280-62282, 64600-64681)

(For epidural or subarachnoid injection, see 62320, 62321, 62322, 62323, 62324, 62325, 62326, 62327)

(64479-64487, 64490-64495 are unilateral procedures. For bilateral procedures, use modifier 50)

Surgical Procedures on the Extracranial Nerves, Peripheral Nerves, and Autonomic Nervous System

(For intracranial surgery on cranial nerves, see 61450, 61460, 61790)

AMA *CPT Assistant* □

64448: Feb 04: 10, Apr 05: 13, Jan 13: 13, Nov 14: 14, Dec 14: 16, Sep 15: 12

Plain English Description

An anesthetic is injected into the femoral nerve by continuous infusion. The patient's groin is cleansed and prepped with a small amount of local anesthetic on the affected side. An insulated needle is inserted within a long cannula, and the needle is placed through the anesthetized area of skin near the femoral artery and the inguinal ligament into the femoral nerve sheath. Proper placement of the needle is verified with electrical nerve stimulation and/or with the onset of numbness, tingling, or prickling sensations, or through separately reportable ultrasound imaging. The cannula is then advanced over the needle into the femoral nerve sheath. A long-acting local anesthetic like bupivacaine with epinephrine is carefully injected through the cannula and monitored for nerve block function. Periodic aspiration is performed to ensure that there is no possibility of intravascular injection. An epidural catheter is then threaded through the cannula and secured in position. The cannula is removed. Continuous infusion is started.

Injection, anesthetic agent, femoral nerve, continuous infusion by catheter

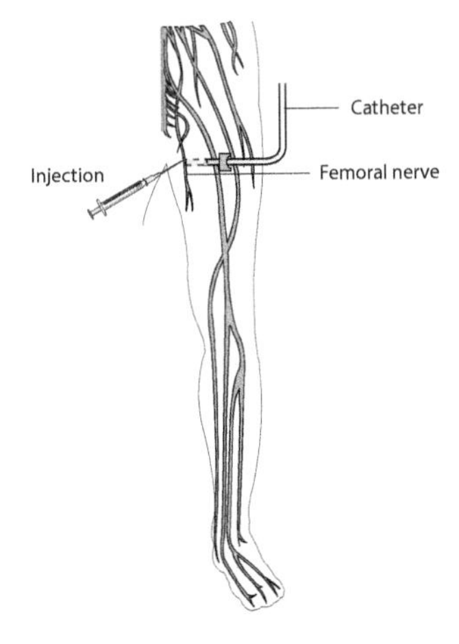

ICD-10-CM Diagnostic Codes

⇄	C40.21	Malignant neoplasm of long bones of right lower limb
⇄	C40.22	Malignant neoplasm of long bones of left lower limb
⇄	C47.21	Malignant neoplasm of peripheral nerves of right lower limb, including hip
⇄	C47.22	Malignant neoplasm of peripheral nerves of left lower limb, including hip
⇄	C49.21	Malignant neoplasm of connective and soft tissue of right lower limb, including hip
⇄	C49.22	Malignant neoplasm of connective and soft tissue of left lower limb, including hip
⇄	C76.51	Malignant neoplasm of right lower limb
⇄	C76.52	Malignant neoplasm of left lower limb
	C79.89	Secondary malignant neoplasm of other specified sites
	G89.11	Acute pain due to trauma
	G89.18	Other acute postprocedural pain
	G89.21	Chronic pain due to trauma
	G89.28	Other chronic postprocedural pain
	G89.29	Other chronic pain
	G89.3	Neoplasm related pain (acute) (chronic)
❼⇄	S72.031	Displaced midcervical fracture of right femur
❼⇄	S72.032	Displaced midcervical fracture of left femur
❼⇄	S72.041	Displaced fracture of base of neck of right femur
❼⇄	S72.042	Displaced fracture of base of neck of left femur
❼⇄	S72.111	Displaced fracture of greater trochanter of right femur
❼⇄	S72.112	Displaced fracture of greater trochanter of left femur
❼⇄	S72.121	Displaced fracture of lesser trochanter of right femur
❼⇄	S72.122	Displaced fracture of lesser trochanter of left femur
❼⇄	S72.131	Displaced apophyseal fracture of right femur
❼⇄	S72.132	Displaced apophyseal fracture of left femur
❼⇄	S72.141	Displaced intertrochanteric fracture of right femur
❼⇄	S72.142	Displaced intertrochanteric fracture of left femur
❼⇄	S72.21	Displaced subtrochanteric fracture of right femur
❼⇄	S72.22	Displaced subtrochanteric fracture of left femur
❼⇄	S72.321	Displaced transverse fracture of shaft of right femur
❼⇄	S72.322	Displaced transverse fracture of shaft of left femur
❼⇄	S72.331	Displaced oblique fracture of shaft of right femur
❼⇄	S72.332	Displaced oblique fracture of shaft of left femur
❼⇄	S72.341	Displaced spiral fracture of shaft of right femur
❼⇄	S72.342	Displaced spiral fracture of shaft of left femur
❼⇄	S72.351	Displaced comminuted fracture of shaft of right femur
❼⇄	S72.352	Displaced comminuted fracture of shaft of left femur
❼⇄	S72.361	Displaced segmental fracture of shaft of right femur
❼⇄	S72.362	Displaced segmental fracture of shaft of left femur

ICD-10-CM Coding Notes

For codes requiring a 7th character extension, refer to your ICD-10-CM book. Review the character descriptions and coding guidelines for proper selection. For some procedures, only certain characters will apply.

CCI Edits

Refer to Appendix A for CCI edits.

Facility RVUs □

Code	Work	PE Facility	MP	Total Facility
64448	1.63	0.29	0.13	2.05

Non-facility RVUs □

Code	Work	PE Non-Facility	MP	Total Non-Facility
64448	1.63	0.29	0.13	2.05

Modifiers (PAR) □

Code	Mod 50	Mod 51	Mod 62	Mod 66	Mod 80
64448	1	2	0	0	1

Global Period

Code	Days
64448	000

CPT © 2018 American Medical Association. All Rights Reserved.

64449

64449 Injection, anesthetic agent; lumbar plexus, posterior approach, continuous infusion by catheter (including catheter placement)

(Do not report 64449 in conjunction with 01996)

AMA Coding Notes

Introduction/Injection of Anesthetic Agent (Nerve Block), Diagnostic or Therapeutic Procedures on the Extracranial Nerves, Peripheral Nerves, and Autonomic Nervous System

(For destruction by neurolytic agent or chemodenervation, see 62280-62282, 64600-64681)

(For epidural or subarachnoid injection, see 62320, 62321, 62322, 62323, 62324, 62325, 62326, 62327)

(64479-64487, 64490-64495 are unilateral procedures. For bilateral procedures, use modifier 50)

Surgical Procedures on the Extracranial Nerves, Peripheral Nerves, and Autonomic Nervous System

(For intracranial surgery on cranial nerves, see 61450, 61460, 61790)

AMA *CPT Assistant* □

64449: Apr 05: 13, Jan 13: 13

Plain English Description

The needle insertion site is marked near the area between the iliac crests. The skin of the lower back is cleansed and prepped with a small amount of local anesthetic placed into deeper tissues. A special needle connected to a peripheral nerve stimulator is advanced into the psoas compartment. Proper positioning of the needle is verified by stimulating the lumbar plexus, which results in elevation of the patella and contraction of the quadriceps and sartorius. Aspiration is done to test for blood and cerebrospinal fluid, and a test dose of anesthesia is given to rule out intravenous or intrathecal injection. An infusion catheter is inserted through the needle after a small amount of local anesthetic is injected for the block. The function of the block is checked for analgesia of the left leg and hip. The correct catheter position is also verified for intravenous or intrathecal placement and secured in place. Continuous infusion of a dilute local anesthetic is started.

Injection, anesthetic agent; lumbar plexus, posterior approach, continuous infusion by catheter

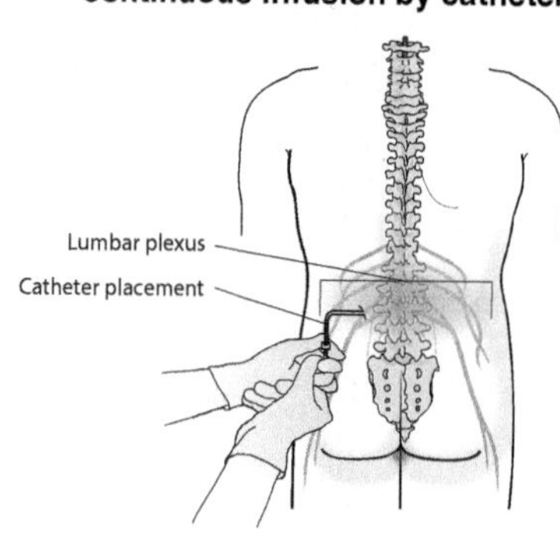

ICD-10-CM Diagnostic Codes

	B02.29	Other postherpetic nervous system involvement
⇄	C47.21	Malignant neoplasm of peripheral nerves of right lower limb, including hip
⇄	C47.22	Malignant neoplasm of peripheral nerves of left lower limb, including hip
⇄	C49.21	Malignant neoplasm of connective and soft tissue of right lower limb, including hip
⇄	C49.22	Malignant neoplasm of connective and soft tissue of left lower limb, including hip
	C76.3	Malignant neoplasm of pelvis
⇄	C76.51	Malignant neoplasm of right lower limb
⇄	C76.52	Malignant neoplasm of left lower limb
	C79.49	Secondary malignant neoplasm of other parts of nervous system
	C79.89	Secondary malignant neoplasm of other specified sites
	G89.11	Acute pain due to trauma
	G89.18	Other acute postprocedural pain
	G89.21	Chronic pain due to trauma
	G89.28	Other chronic postprocedural pain
	G89.29	Other chronic pain
	G89.3	Neoplasm related pain (acute) (chronic)
⇄	M79.604	Pain in right leg
⇄	M79.605	Pain in left leg
⇄	M79.651	Pain in right thigh
⇄	M79.652	Pain in left thigh
⇄	M79.661	Pain in right lower leg
⇄	M79.662	Pain in left lower leg
	R10.30	Lower abdominal pain, unspecified
⇄	R10.31	Right lower quadrant pain
⇄	R10.32	Left lower quadrant pain
❼⇄	S32.411	Displaced fracture of anterior wall of right acetabulum
❼⇄	S32.412	Displaced fracture of anterior wall of left acetabulum
❼⇄	S32.421	Displaced fracture of posterior wall of right acetabulum
❼⇄	S32.422	Displaced fracture of posterior wall of left acetabulum
❼⇄	S32.431	Displaced fracture of anterior column [iliopubic] of right acetabulum
❼⇄	S32.432	Displaced fracture of anterior column [iliopubic] of left acetabulum
❼⇄	S32.441	Displaced fracture of posterior column [ilioischial] of right acetabulum
❼⇄	S32.442	Displaced fracture of posterior column [ilioischial] of left acetabulum
❼⇄	S32.451	Displaced transverse fracture of right acetabulum
❼⇄	S32.452	Displaced transverse fracture of left acetabulum
❼⇄	S32.461	Displaced associated transverse-posterior fracture of right acetabulum
❼⇄	S32.462	Displaced associated transverse-posterior fracture of left acetabulum
❼⇄	S32.471	Displaced fracture of medial wall of right acetabulum
❼⇄	S32.472	Displaced fracture of medial wall of left acetabulum
❼⇄	S32.481	Displaced dome fracture of right acetabulum
❼⇄	S32.482	Displaced dome fracture of left acetabulum

ICD-10-CM Coding Notes

For codes requiring a 7th character extension, refer to your ICD-10-CM book. Review the character descriptions and coding guidelines for proper selection. For some procedures, only certain characters will apply.

CCI Edits

Refer to Appendix A for CCI edits.

Facility RVUs □

Code	Work	PE Facility	MP	Total Facility
64449	1.81	0.45	0.18	2.44

Non-facility RVUs □

Code	Work	PE Non-Facility	MP	Total Non-Facility
64449	1.81	0.45	0.18	2.44

Modifiers (PAR) □

Code	Mod 50	Mod 51	Mod 62	Mod 66	Mod 80
64449	1	2	0	0	1

Global Period

Code	Days
64449	000

CPT © 2018 American Medical Association. All Rights Reserved.

64450

64450 Injection, anesthetic agent; other peripheral nerve or branch

AMA Coding Notes

Introduction/Injection of Anesthetic Agent (Nerve Block), Diagnostic or Therapeutic Procedures on the Extracranial Nerves, Peripheral Nerves, and Autonomic Nervous System

(For destruction by neurolytic agent or chemodenervation, see 62280-62282, 64600-64681)

(For epidural or subarachnoid injection, see 62320, 62321, 62322, 62323, 62324, 62325, 62326, 62327)

(64479-64487, 64490-64495 are unilateral procedures. For bilateral procedures, use modifier 50)

Surgical Procedures on the Extracranial Nerves, Peripheral Nerves, and Autonomic Nervous System

(For intracranial surgery on cranial nerves, see 61450, 61460, 61790)

AMA *CPT Assistant* ▢

64450: Jul 98: 10, Nov 99: 37, Dec 99: 7, Oct 01: 9, Aug 03: 6, Apr 05: 13, Jan 09: 6, Jan 13: 13, Sep 15: 12, Nov 15: 11, Oct 16: 11, May 18: 10

Plain English Description

An anesthetic agent is injected into a peripheral nerve or branch not specifically described by another code. This procedure may also be referred to as a peripheral nerve block. Generally, this is performed on peripheral nerves or branches in the arm or leg. The specific nerve or branch is identified. The skin over the planned puncture site is disinfected. The needle is inserted, aspirated to ensure it is not in a blood vessel, and the anesthetic is injected.

Injection, anesthetic agent; other peripheral nerve or branch

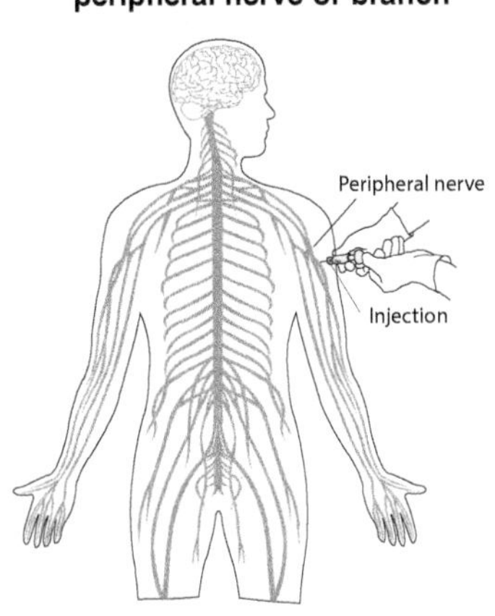

ICD-10-CM Diagnostic Codes

⇄	G56.81	Other specified mononeuropathies of right upper limb
⇄	G56.82	Other specified mononeuropathies of left upper limb
⇄	G56.83	Other specified mononeuropathies of bilateral upper limbs
⇄	G57.51	Tarsal tunnel syndrome, right lower limb
⇄	G57.52	Tarsal tunnel syndrome, left lower limb
⇄	G57.53	Tarsal tunnel syndrome, bilateral lower limbs
⇄	G57.81	Other specified mononeuropathies of right lower limb
⇄	G57.82	Other specified mononeuropathies of left lower limb
⇄	G57.83	Other specified mononeuropathies of bilateral lower limbs
	G58.9	Mononeuropathy, unspecified
	G89.11	Acute pain due to trauma
	G89.18	Other acute postprocedural pain
	G89.21	Chronic pain due to trauma
	G89.28	Other chronic postprocedural pain
	G89.29	Other chronic pain
	G89.3	Neoplasm related pain (acute) (chronic)
	M79.2	Neuralgia and neuritis, unspecified

CCI Edits

Refer to Appendix A for CCI edits.

Facility RVUs ▢

Code	Work	PE Facility	MP	Total Facility
64450	0.75	0.46	0.07	1.28

Non-facility RVUs ▢

Code	Work	PE Non-Facility	MP	Total Non-Facility
64450	0.75	1.37	0.07	2.19

Modifiers (PAR) ▢

Code	Mod 50	Mod 51	Mod 62	Mod 66	Mod 80
64450	1	2	0	0	1

Global Period

Code	Days
64450	000

CPT © 2018 American Medical Association. All Rights Reserved.

64455

64455 Injection(s), anesthetic agent and/or steroid, plantar common digital nerve(s) (eg, Morton's neuroma)

(Do not report 64455 in conjunction with 64632)

(Imaging guidance [fluoroscopy or CT] and any injection of contrast are inclusive components of 64479-64484. Imaging guidance and localization are required for the performance of 64479-64484)

Injection(s), anesthetic agent and/or steroid, plantar common digital nerve(s)

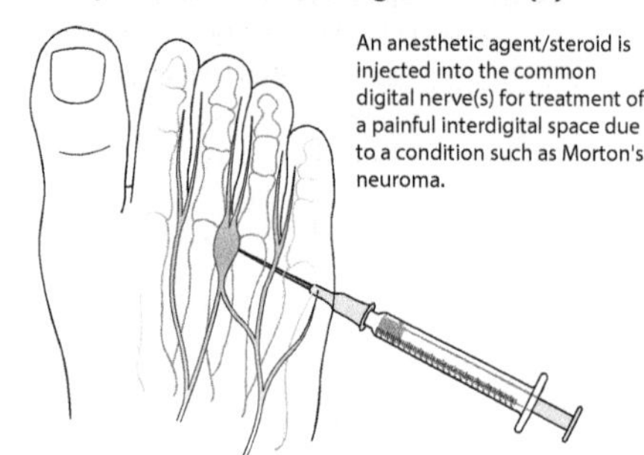

An anesthetic agent/steroid is injected into the common digital nerve(s) for treatment of a painful interdigital space due to a condition such as Morton's neuroma.

AMA Coding Notes

Introduction/Injection of Anesthetic Agent (Nerve Block), Diagnostic or Therapeutic Procedures on the Extracranial Nerves, Peripheral Nerves, and Autonomic Nervous System

(For destruction by neurolytic agent or chemodenervation, see 62280-62282, 64600-64681)

(For epidural or subarachnoid injection, see 62320, 62321, 62322, 62323, 62324, 62325, 62326, 62327)

(64479-64487, 64490-64495 are unilateral procedures. For bilateral procedures, use modifier 50)

Surgical Procedures on the Extracranial Nerves, Peripheral Nerves, and Autonomic Nervous System

(For intracranial surgery on cranial nerves, see 61450, 61460, 61790)

AMA *CPT Assistant* ▯

64455: Jan 13: 13

Plain English Description

With the patient in a supine position, the knee is flexed and supported with a pillow and the foot is maintained in a relaxed neutral position. The interdigital spaces are palpated and any tenderness or fullness is noted. The needle is inserted on the dorsal foot surface in a distal to proximal direction at a point 1-2 cm proximal to the web space and in line with the metatarsophalangeal joints. The needle is held at an angle of approximately 45 degrees and advanced through the mid-web space into the area of fullness at the plantar aspect of the foot. The needle is advanced until it tents the skin and then withdrawn to the tip of the neuroma. Taking care to avoid the plantar fat pad, an anesthetic agent is injected first to confirm the diagnosis, followed by steroid injection. A steroid/anesthetic mix may be used. One or more common digital nerves may be injected.

ICD-10-CM Diagnostic Codes

⇄	G57.61	Lesion of plantar nerve, right lower limb
⇄	G57.62	Lesion of plantar nerve, left lower limb
⇄	G57.63	Lesion of plantar nerve, bilateral lower limbs
⇄	G57.71	Causalgia of right lower limb
⇄	G57.72	Causalgia of left lower limb
⇄	G57.73	Causalgia of bilateral lower limbs
⇄	G90.521	Complex regional pain syndrome I of right lower limb
⇄	G90.522	Complex regional pain syndrome I of left lower limb
⇄	G90.523	Complex regional pain syndrome I of lower limb, bilateral

CCI Edits

Refer to Appendix A for CCI edits.

Facility RVUs ▯

Code	Work	PE Facility	MP	Total Facility
64455	0.75	0.19	0.06	1.00

Non-facility RVUs ▯

Code	Work	PE Non-Facility	MP	Total Non-Facility
64455	0.75	0.55	0.06	1.36

Modifiers (PAR) ▯

Code	Mod 50	Mod 51	Mod 62	Mod 66	Mod 80
64455	1	2	0	0	0

Global Period

Code	Days
64455	000

CPT © 2018 American Medical Association. All Rights Reserved.

64461-64463

64461 Paravertebral block (PVB) (paraspinous block), thoracic; single injection site (includes imaging guidance, when performed)

+ **64462 Paravertebral block (PVB) (paraspinous block), thoracic; second and any additional injection site(s) (includes imaging guidance, when performed) (List separately in addition to code for primary procedure)**

(Use 64462 in conjunction with 64461)

(Do not report 64462 more than once per day)

64463 Paravertebral block (PVB) (paraspinous block), thoracic; continuous infusion by catheter (includes imaging guidance, when performed)

(Do not report 64461, 64462, 64463 in conjunction with 62320, 62324, 64420, 64421, 64479, 64480, 64490, 64491, 64492, 76942, 77002, 77003)

AMA Coding Notes

Introduction/Injection of Anesthetic Agent (Nerve Block), Diagnostic or Therapeutic Procedures on the Extracranial Nerves, Peripheral Nerves, and Autonomic Nervous System

(For destruction by neurolytic agent or chemodenervation, see 62280-62282, 64600-64681)

(For epidural or subarachnoid injection, see 62320, 62321, 62322, 62323, 62324, 62325, 62326, 62327)

(64479-64487, 64490-64495 are unilateral procedures. For bilateral procedures, use modifier 50)

Surgical Procedures on the Extracranial Nerves, Peripheral Nerves, and Autonomic Nervous System

(For intracranial surgery on cranial nerves, see 61450, 61460, 61790)

AMA *CPT Assistant* ▯

64461: Jan 16: 9
64462: Jan 16: 9
64463: Jan 16: 9

Plain English Description

A thoracic paravertebral block (PVB) or paraspinous block is performed to provide unilateral anesthesia in patients undergoing thoracic or breast surgery or those with chest trauma and rib fractures. The paravertebral space is a wedge-shaped compartment adjacent to the vertebral bodies communicating superiorly and inferiorly across the ribs. The spinal nerves emerge from the intervertebral foramina into the paravertebral space and with the intercostal nerves branch laterally and extend medially into the epidural spaces. A thoracic PVB produces ipsilateral somatic and sympathetic nerve blockage with minimal cardiovascular or respiratory compromise. With the patient in a supported sitting position or resting lateral decubitus with the side to be blocked in the uppermost position, the spinous processes are marked on the skin, and a parasagittal line is measured and drawn lateral to the midline. The subcutaneous tissue and paravertebral muscles are infiltrated with local anesthetic along the parasagittal line. Using visual and tactile landmarking and ultrasound imaging as indicated, a spinal needle with extension tubing attached to the syringe containing local anesthetic is inserted into the paravertebral space and the anesthetic is injected. Code 64461 reports a single thoracic injection site with imaging, when performed. Code 64462 reports PVB at a second and any additional thoracic injection site. Code 64463 reports PVB via continuous anesthetic infusion though an indwelling catheter. A thin, flexible, epidural catheter is threaded through the spinal needle inserted into the paravertebral space; the spinal needle is removed; the catheter is secured in place and connected to an infusion pump. The anesthetic is then delivered continuously.

ICD-10-CM Diagnostic Codes

	G89.11	Acute pain due to trauma
	G89.12	Acute post-thoracotomy pain
	G89.18	Other acute postprocedural pain
	G89.21	Chronic pain due to trauma
	G89.22	Chronic post-thoracotomy pain
	G89.28	Other chronic postprocedural pain
	G89.29	Other chronic pain
	O63.0	Prolonged first stage (of labor) ♀
	R07.2	Precordial pain
	R07.81	Pleurodynia
	R07.82	Intercostal pain
	R07.89	Other chest pain
	R07.9	Chest pain, unspecified
❼⇄	S22.31	Fracture of one rib, right side
❼⇄	S22.32	Fracture of one rib, left side
❼⇄	S22.41	Multiple fractures of ribs, right side
❼⇄	S22.42	Multiple fractures of ribs, left side
❼⇄	S22.43	Multiple fractures of ribs, bilateral

ICD-10-CM Coding Notes

For codes requiring a 7th character extension, refer to your ICD-10-CM book. Review the character descriptions and coding guidelines for proper selection. For some procedures, only certain characters will apply.

CCI Edits

Refer to Appendix A for CCI edits.

Facility RVUs ▯

Code	Work	PE Facility	MP	Total Facility
64461	1.75	0.44	0.14	2.33
64462	1.10	0.28	0.09	1.47
64463	1.90	0.37	0.15	2.42

Non-facility RVUs ▯

Code	Work	PE Non-Facility	MP	Total Non-Facility
64461	1.75	2.07	0.14	3.96
64462	1.10	1.01	0.09	2.20
64463	1.90	3.08	0.15	5.13

Modifiers (PAR) ▯

Code	Mod 50	Mod 51	Mod 62	Mod 66	Mod 80
64461	1	2	0	0	1
64462	1	0	0	0	1
64463	1	2	0	0	1

Global Period

Code	Days
64461	000
64462	ZZZ
64463	000

CPT © 2018 American Medical Association. All Rights Reserved.

64479-64480

64479 Injection(s), anesthetic agent and/or steroid, transforaminal epidural, with imaging guidance (fluoroscopy or CT); cervical or thoracic, single level

(For transforaminal epidural injection under ultrasound guidance, use 0228T)

+ 64480 Injection(s), anesthetic agent and/or steroid, transforaminal epidural, with imaging guidance (fluoroscopy or CT); cervical or thoracic, each additional level (List separately in addition to code for primary procedure)

(Use 64480 in conjunction with 64479)

(For transforaminal epidural injection under ultrasound guidance, use 0229T)

(For transforaminal epidural injection at the T12-L1 level, use 64479)

AMA Coding Notes

Introduction/Injection of Anesthetic Agent (Nerve Block), Diagnostic or Therapeutic Procedures on the Extracranial Nerves, Peripheral Nerves, and Autonomic Nervous System

(For destruction by neurolytic agent or chemodenervation, see 62280-62282, 64600-64681)

(For epidural or subarachnoid injection, see 62320, 62321, 62322, 62323, 62324, 62325, 62326, 62327)

(64479-64487, 64490-64495 are unilateral procedures. For bilateral procedures, use modifier 50)

Surgical Procedures on the Extracranial Nerves, Peripheral Nerves, and Autonomic Nervous System

(For intracranial surgery on cranial nerves, see 61450, 61460, 61790)

AMA *CPT Assistant* ☐

64479: Nov 99: 33, 37, Feb 00: 4, Jul 08: 9, Nov 08: 11, Feb 10: 9, Jan 11: 8, Feb 11: 4, Jul 11: 16, Jul 12: 5, Jan 16: 9

64480: Nov 99: 33, 37, Feb 00: 4, Feb 05: 14, Jul 08: 9, Feb 10: 9, Jan 11: 8, Feb 11: 4, Jul 11: 16, Jul 12: 5

Plain English Description

A transforaminal epidural injection allows for a very selective injection around a specific nerve root. Nerve roots exit the spinal canal through the foramina, which are small openings between the vertebrae. The skin is cleansed and prepped over the affected cervical or thoracic vertebra. Using CT or fluoroscopic imaging, a needle is advanced through the skin and into the foramen. A small amount of radiopaque contrast material may be injected to enhance fluoroscopic images and to confirm proper placement of the spinal needle. The anesthetic and/or steroid is then injected around the nerve root. Use 64479 for transforaminal epidural injection at a single cervical or thoracic level. Use 64480 for each additional level injected.

Injection, anesthetic agent/steroid, transforaminal epidural; cervical/thoracic

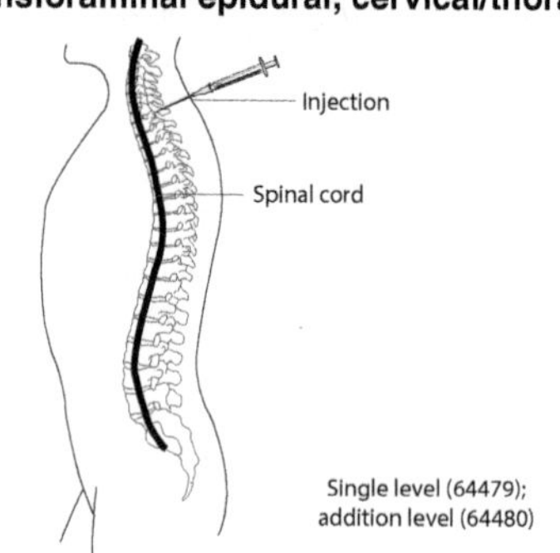

ICD-10-CM Diagnostic Codes

G54.2	Cervical root disorders, not elsewhere classified
G54.3	Thoracic root disorders, not elsewhere classified
G89.29	Other chronic pain
M47.21	Other spondylosis with radiculopathy, occipito-atlanto-axial region
M47.22	Other spondylosis with radiculopathy, cervical region
M47.23	Other spondylosis with radiculopathy, cervicothoracic region
M47.24	Other spondylosis with radiculopathy, thoracic region
M47.25	Other spondylosis with radiculopathy, thoracolumbar region
M50.10	Cervical disc disorder with radiculopathy, unspecified cervical region
M50.11	Cervical disc disorder with radiculopathy, high cervical region
M50.120	Mid-cervical disc disorder, unspecified
M50.121	Cervical disc disorder at C4-C5 level with radiculopathy
M50.122	Cervical disc disorder at C5-C6 level with radiculopathy
M50.123	Cervical disc disorder at C6-C7 level with radiculopathy
M50.13	Cervical disc disorder with radiculopathy, cervicothoracic region
M54.11	Radiculopathy, occipito-atlanto-axial region
M54.12	Radiculopathy, cervical region
M54.13	Radiculopathy, cervicothoracic region
M54.14	Radiculopathy, thoracic region
M54.15	Radiculopathy, thoracolumbar region
M54.2	Cervicalgia
M54.6	Pain in thoracic spine
❼ S14.2	Injury of nerve root of cervical spine
❼ S24.2	Injury of nerve root of thoracic spine

ICD-10-CM Coding Notes

For codes requiring a 7th character extension, refer to your ICD-10-CM book. Review the character descriptions and coding guidelines for proper selection. For some procedures, only certain characters will apply.

CCI Edits

Refer to Appendix A for CCI edits.

Facility RVUs ☐

Code	Work	PE Facility	MP	Total Facility
64479	2.29	1.27	0.20	3.76
64480	1.20	0.48	0.12	1.80

Non-facility RVUs ☐

Code	Work	PE Non-Facility	MP	Total Non-Facility
64479	2.29	4.46	0.20	6.95
64480	1.20	2.10	0.12	3.42

Modifiers (PAR) ☐

Code	Mod 50	Mod 51	Mod 62	Mod 66	Mod 80
64479	1	2	0	0	1
64480	1	0	0	0	1

Global Period

Code	Days
64479	000
64480	ZZZ

CPT © 2018 American Medical Association. All Rights Reserved.

64483-64484

64483 Injection(s), anesthetic agent and/or steroid, transforaminal epidural, with imaging guidance (fluoroscopy or CT); lumbar or sacral, single level

(For transforaminal epidural injection under ultrasound guidance, use 0230T)

+ 64484 Injection(s), anesthetic agent and/or steroid, transforaminal epidural, with imaging guidance (fluoroscopy or CT); lumbar or sacral, each additional level (List separately in addition to code for primary procedure)

(Use 64484 in conjunction with 64483)

(For transforaminal epidural injection under ultrasound guidance, use 0231T)

(64479-64484 are unilateral procedures. For bilateral procedures, use modifier 50)

AMA Coding Notes

Introduction/Injection of Anesthetic Agent (Nerve Block), Diagnostic or Therapeutic Procedures on the Extracranial Nerves, Peripheral Nerves, and Autonomic Nervous System

(For destruction by neurolytic agent or chemodenervation, see 62280-62282, 64600-64681)

(For epidural or subarachnoid injection, see 62320, 62321, 62322, 62323, 62324, 62325, 62326, 62327)

(64479-64487, 64490-64495 are unilateral procedures. For bilateral procedures, use modifier 50)

Surgical Procedures on the Extracranial Nerves, Peripheral Nerves, and Autonomic Nervous System

(For intracranial surgery on cranial nerves, see 61450, 61460, 61790)

AMA *CPT Assistant*

64483: Nov 99: 33, 37, Feb 00: 4, Jul 08: 9, Feb 10: 9, Jan 11: 8, Feb 11: 4, Jul 11: 16, May 12: 14, Jul 12: 5, Oct 16: 11

64484: Nov 99: 33, 37, Feb 00: 4, Feb 05: 14, Jul 08: 9, Nov 08: 11, Feb 10: 9, Feb 11: 4, Jul 11: 16, Jul 12: 5, Jan 16: 9

Plain English Description

A transforaminal epidural injection allows very selective injection around a specific nerve root. Nerve roots exit the spinal canal through the foramina, which are small openings between the vertebrae. The skin is cleansed and prepped over the affected lumbar or sacral vertebra. Using CT or fluoroscopic imaging, a needle is advanced through the skin and into the foramen. A small amount of radiopaque contrast material may be injected to enhance fluoroscopic images and to confirm proper placement of the spinal needle. The anesthetic and/or steroid is then injected around the nerve root. Use 64483 for transforaminal epidural injection at a single lumbar or sacral level. Use 64484 for each additional level injected.

Injection, anesthetic agent/steroid, transforaminal epidural; lumbar/sacral

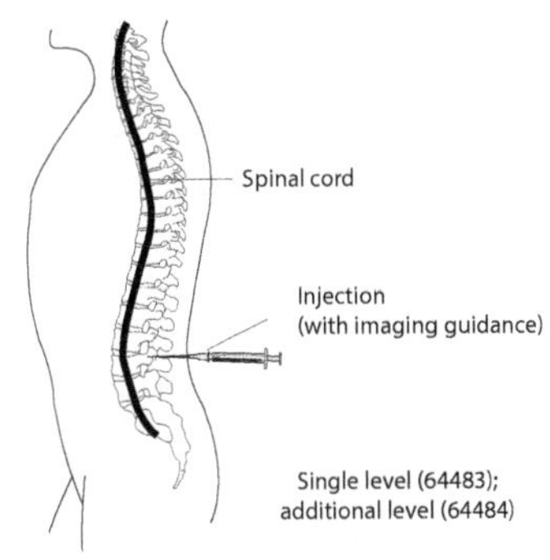

ICD-10-CM Diagnostic Codes

	G54.1	Lumbosacral plexus disorders
	G54.4	Lumbosacral root disorders, not elsewhere classified
	G89.29	Other chronic pain
	M47.25	Other spondylosis with radiculopathy, thoracolumbar region
	M47.26	Other spondylosis with radiculopathy, lumbar region
	M47.27	Other spondylosis with radiculopathy, lumbosacral region
	M47.28	Other spondylosis with radiculopathy, sacral and sacrococcygeal region
	M51.15	Intervertebral disc disorders with radiculopathy, thoracolumbar region
	M51.16	Intervertebral disc disorders with radiculopathy, lumbar region
	M51.17	Intervertebral disc disorders with radiculopathy, lumbosacral region
	M54.15	Radiculopathy, thoracolumbar region
	M54.16	Radiculopathy, lumbar region
	M54.17	Radiculopathy, lumbosacral region
	M54.18	Radiculopathy, sacral and sacrococcygeal region
	M54.5	Low back pain
	M54.89	Other dorsalgia
❼	S34.21	Injury of nerve root of lumbar spine
❼	S34.22	Injury of nerve root of sacral spine

ICD-10-CM Coding Notes

For codes requiring a 7th character extension, refer to your ICD-10-CM book. Review the character descriptions and coding guidelines for proper selection. For some procedures, only certain characters will apply.

CCI Edits

Refer to Appendix A for CCI edits.

Facility RVUs

Code	Work	PE Facility	MP	Total Facility
64483	1.90	1.14	0.15	3.19
64484	1.00	0.41	0.08	1.49

Non-facility RVUs

Code	Work	PE Non-Facility	MP	Total Non-Facility
64483	1.90	4.39	0.15	6.44
64484	1.00	1.71	0.08	2.79

Modifiers (PAR)

Code	Mod 50	Mod 51	Mod 62	Mod 66	Mod 80
64483	1	2	0	0	1
64484	1	0	0	0	1

Global Period

Code	Days
64483	000
64484	ZZZ

CPT © 2018 American Medical Association. All Rights Reserved.

64486-64489

64486 Transversus abdominis plane (TAP) block (abdominal plane block, rectus sheath block) unilateral; by injection(s) (includes imaging guidance, when performed)

64487 Transversus abdominis plane (TAP) block (abdominal plane block, rectus sheath block) unilateral; by continuous infusion(s) (includes imaging guidance, when performed)

64488 Transversus abdominis plane (TAP) block (abdominal plane block, rectus sheath block) bilateral; by injections (includes imaging guidance, when performed)

64489 Transversus abdominis plane (TAP) block (abdominal plane block, rectus sheath block) bilateral; by continuous infusions (includes imaging guidance, when performed)

AMA Coding Notes

Introduction/Injection of Anesthetic Agent (Nerve Block), Diagnostic or Therapeutic Procedures on the Extracranial Nerves, Peripheral Nerves, and Autonomic Nervous System

(For destruction by neurolytic agent or chemodenervation, see 62280-62282, 64600-64681)

(For epidural or subarachnoid injection, see 62320, 62321, 62322, 62323, 62324, 62325, 62326, 62327)

(64479-64487, 64490-64495 are unilateral procedures. For bilateral procedures, use modifier 50)

Surgical Procedures on the Extracranial Nerves, Peripheral Nerves, and Autonomic Nervous System

(For intracranial surgery on cranial nerves, see 61450, 61460, 61790)

AMA *CPT Assistant* ☐

64486: Jun 15: 3
64487: Jun 15: 3
64488: Jun 15: 3
64489: Jun 15: 3

Plain English Description

A transversus abdominis plane (TAP) block provides anesthesia to nerves in the anterior abdominal wall at the level of T6-L1 and is used as an adjunct therapy in abdominal surgery for postoperative pain control. The TAP block can be performed preoperatively, intraoperatively, or postoperatively. A unilateral TAP block is most effective when the surgical incision is located to the right or left of the midline. A bilateral block may be used when the incision is in the midline of the abdomen. A single injection of a long acting local anesthetic such as bupivacaine can provide pain relief up to 36 hours. Continuous infusion can provide pain relief for 36-72 hours. For a unilateral TAP block injection (64486), when using a blind approach, the triangle of Petit is identified and a needle is inserted perpendicular to the skin, cephalad to the iliac crest, and near the midaxillary line. The needle is then advanced through the external and internal abdominal oblique muscles into the fascia above the transversus abdominis muscle. Local anesthetic is injected at measured intervals following aspiration to ensure that the needle is not within a blood vessel. The procedure is repeated on the opposite side in 64488 for bilateral injection. For TAP block by continuous infusion(s), ultrasound guidance is normally used which allows the physician to visualize the layers of muscle and fascia and the hypoechoic spread of fluid when the anesthetic is given. A Touhy needle is inserted into the skin and advanced into the fascia directly above the transversus abdominis muscle. This layer of fascia, the transversus abdominis plane (TAP), is hydrodissected with 10 ml of isotonic saline. An epidural catheter is introduced through the Touhy needle and advanced 10-20 cm into the TAP. The Touhy needle is removed and the epidural catheter is connected to tubing. A bolus injection of local anesthetic is given and monitored by ultrasound. Once placement has been confirmed, the epidural catheter is secured to the skin. This is repeated on the opposite side for a bilateral block (64489). Once the catheter(s) are in place, continuous infusion(s) or intermittent bolus injections of anesthetic are administered.

ICD-10-CM Diagnostic Codes

	C18.0	Malignant neoplasm of cecum
	C18.1	Malignant neoplasm of appendix
	C18.2	Malignant neoplasm of ascending colon
	C18.3	Malignant neoplasm of hepatic flexure
	C18.4	Malignant neoplasm of transverse colon
	C18.5	Malignant neoplasm of splenic flexure
	C18.6	Malignant neoplasm of descending colon
	C18.7	Malignant neoplasm of sigmoid colon
	C18.8	Malignant neoplasm of overlapping sites of colon
	C22.0	Liver cell carcinoma
	C22.1	Intrahepatic bile duct carcinoma
	C22.2	Hepatoblastoma
	C22.3	Angiosarcoma of liver
	C22.4	Other sarcomas of liver
	C22.7	Other specified carcinomas of liver
	C22.8	Malignant neoplasm of liver, primary, unspecified as to type
	C25.0	Malignant neoplasm of head of pancreas
	C25.1	Malignant neoplasm of body of pancreas
	C25.2	Malignant neoplasm of tail of pancreas
	C25.3	Malignant neoplasm of pancreatic duct
	C25.4	Malignant neoplasm of endocrine pancreas
	C25.7	Malignant neoplasm of other parts of pancreas
	C25.8	Malignant neoplasm of overlapping sites of pancreas
⇄	C56.1	Malignant neoplasm of right ovary ♀
⇄	C56.2	Malignant neoplasm of left ovary ♀
⇄	C57.01	Malignant neoplasm of right fallopian tube ♀
⇄	C57.02	Malignant neoplasm of left fallopian tube ♀
	C78.7	Secondary malignant neoplasm of liver and intrahepatic bile duct
	C7A.020	Malignant carcinoid tumor of the appendix
	C7A.021	Malignant carcinoid tumor of the cecum
	C7A.022	Malignant carcinoid tumor of the ascending colon
	C7A.023	Malignant carcinoid tumor of the transverse colon
	C7A.024	Malignant carcinoid tumor of the descending colon
	C7A.025	Malignant carcinoid tumor of the sigmoid colon
	C7A.026	Malignant carcinoid tumor of the rectum
	D01.0	Carcinoma in situ of colon
	K35.20	Acute appendicitis with generalized peritonitis, without abscess
	K35.21	Acute appendicitis with generalized peritonitis, with abscess
	K35.30	Acute appendicitis with localized peritonitis, without perforation or gangrene
	K35.31	Acute appendicitis with localized peritonitis and gangrene, without perforation
	K35.32	Acute appendicitis with perforation and localized peritonitis, without abscess
	K35.33	Acute appendicitis with perforation and localized peritonitis, with abscess
	K35.80	Unspecified acute appendicitis
	K35.89	Other acute appendicitis
	K40.30	Unilateral inguinal hernia, with obstruction, without gangrene, not specified as recurrent
	K40.31	Unilateral inguinal hernia, with obstruction, without gangrene, recurrent
	K40.90	Unilateral inguinal hernia, without obstruction or gangrene, not specified as recurrent
	K40.91	Unilateral inguinal hernia, without obstruction or gangrene, recurrent
	K50.112	Crohn's disease of large intestine with intestinal obstruction

CPT © 2018 American Medical Association. All Rights Reserved.

K50.113	Crohn's disease of large intestine with fistula
K50.114	Crohn's disease of large intestine with abscess
K50.118	Crohn's disease of large intestine with other complication
K51.012	Ulcerative (chronic) pancolitis with intestinal obstruction
K51.013	Ulcerative (chronic) pancolitis with fistula
K51.014	Ulcerative (chronic) pancolitis with abscess
K51.018	Ulcerative (chronic) pancolitis with other complication
K51.512	Left sided colitis with intestinal obstruction
K51.513	Left sided colitis with fistula
K51.514	Left sided colitis with abscess
K51.518	Left sided colitis with other complication
K51.812	Other ulcerative colitis with intestinal obstruction
K51.813	Other ulcerative colitis with fistula
K51.814	Other ulcerative colitis with abscess
K51.818	Other ulcerative colitis with other complication
K55.041	Focal (segmental) acute infarction of large intestine
K55.042	Diffuse acute infarction of large intestine
K55.049	Acute infarction of large intestine, extent unspecified
K55.1	Chronic vascular disorders of intestine
K55.33	Stage 3 necrotizing enterocolitis
K55.9	Vascular disorder of intestine, unspecified
K56.1	Intussusception
K56.2	Volvulus
K56.3	Gallstone ileus
K56.52	Intestinal adhesions [bands] with complete obstruction
K56.601	Complete intestinal obstruction, unspecified as to cause
K56.691	Other complete intestinal obstruction
K57.20	Diverticulitis of large intestine with perforation and abscess without bleeding
K57.21	Diverticulitis of large intestine with perforation and abscess with bleeding
K57.31	Diverticulosis of large intestine without perforation or abscess with bleeding
K57.33	Diverticulitis of large intestine without perforation or abscess with bleeding
K75.0	Abscess of liver
K85.00	Idiopathic acute pancreatitis without necrosis or infection
K85.01	Idiopathic acute pancreatitis with uninfected necrosis
K85.02	Idiopathic acute pancreatitis with infected necrosis
K85.10	Biliary acute pancreatitis without necrosis or infection
K85.11	Biliary acute pancreatitis with uninfected necrosis
K85.12	Biliary acute pancreatitis with infected necrosis
K85.90	Acute pancreatitis without necrosis or infection, unspecified
K85.91	Acute pancreatitis with uninfected necrosis, unspecified
K85.92	Acute pancreatitis with infected necrosis, unspecified
K86.1	Other chronic pancreatitis
K86.89	Other specified diseases of pancreas
N73.0	Acute parametritis and pelvic cellulitis ♀
N73.3	Female acute pelvic peritonitis ♀
N73.6	Female pelvic peritoneal adhesions (postinfective) ♀
N80.0	Endometriosis of uterus ♀
N80.1	Endometriosis of ovary ♀
N80.2	Endometriosis of fallopian tube ♀
N80.3	Endometriosis of pelvic peritoneum ♀
N80.4	Endometriosis of rectovaginal septum and vagina ♀
N80.5	Endometriosis of intestine ♀
N99.4	Postprocedural pelvic peritoneal adhesions
O00.00	Abdominal pregnancy without intrauterine pregnancy ♀
O00.01	Abdominal pregnancy with intrauterine pregnancy ♀
⇄ O00.101	Right tubal pregnancy without intrauterine pregnancy ♀
⇄ O00.102	Left tubal pregnancy without intrauterine pregnancy ♀
⇄ O00.201	Right ovarian pregnancy without intrauterine pregnancy ♀
⇄ O00.202	Left ovarian pregnancy without intrauterine pregnancy ♀
⇄ O00.211	Right ovarian pregnancy with intrauterine pregnancy ♀
⇄ O00.212	Left ovarian pregnancy with intrauterine pregnancy ♀

CCI Edits

Refer to Appendix A for CCI edits.

Facility RVUs □

Code	Work	PE Facility	MP	Total Facility
64486	1.27	0.24	0.10	1.61
64487	1.48	0.27	0.12	1.87
64488	1.60	0.29	0.13	2.02
64489	1.80	0.33	0.14	2.27

Non-facility RVUs □

Code	Work	PE Non-Facility	MP	Total Non-Facility
64486	1.27	1.75	0.10	3.12
64487	1.48	2.89	0.12	4.49
64488	1.60	2.10	0.13	3.83
64489	1.80	4.71	0.14	6.65

Modifiers (PAR) □

Code	Mod 50	Mod 51	Mod 62	Mod 66	Mod 80
64486	1	2	0	0	1
64487	1	2	0	0	1
64488	2	2	0	0	1
64489	2	2	0	0	1

Global Period

Code	Days
64486	000
64487	000
64488	000
64489	000

CPT® Procedural Coding

CPT © 2018 American Medical Association. All Rights Reserved.

64490-64492

64490 Injection(s), diagnostic or therapeutic agent, paravertebral facet (zygapophyseal) joint (or nerves innervating that joint) with image guidance (fluoroscopy or CT), cervical or thoracic; single level

✚ **64491 Injection(s), diagnostic or therapeutic agent, paravertebral facet (zygapophyseal) joint (or nerves innervating that joint) with image guidance (fluoroscopy or CT), cervical or thoracic; second level (List separately in addition to code for primary procedure)**

(Use 64491 in conjunction with 64490)

✚ **64492 Injection(s), diagnostic or therapeutic agent, paravertebral facet (zygapophyseal) joint (or nerves innervating that joint) with image guidance (fluoroscopy or CT), cervical or thoracic; third and any additional level(s) (List separately in addition to code for primary procedure)**

(Do not report 64492 more than once per day)

(Use 64492 in conjunction with 64490, 64491)

AMA Coding Notes

Introduction/Injection of Anesthetic Agent (Nerve Block), Diagnostic or Therapeutic Procedures on the Paravertebral Spinal Nerves and Branches

(Image guidance [fluoroscopy or CT] and any injection of contrast are inclusive components of 64490-64495. Imaging guidance and localization are required for the performance of paravertebral facet joint injections described by codes 64490-64495. If imaging is not used, report 20552-20553. If ultrasound guidance is used, report 0213T-0218T)

(For bilateral paravertebral facet injection procedures, use modifier 50)

(For paravertebral facet injection of the T12-L1 joint, or nerves innervating that joint, use 64490)

Introduction/Injection of Anesthetic Agent (Nerve Block), Diagnostic or Therapeutic Procedures on the Extracranial Nerves, Peripheral Nerves, and Autonomic Nervous System

(For destruction by neurolytic agent or chemodenervation, see 62280-62282, 64600-64681)

(For epidural or subarachnoid injection, see 62320, 62321, 62322, 62323, 62324, 62325, 62326, 62327)

(64479-64487, 64490-64495 are unilateral procedures. For bilateral procedures, use modifier 50)

Surgical Procedures on the Extracranial Nerves, Peripheral Nerves, and Autonomic Nervous System

(For intracranial surgery on cranial nerves, see 61450, 61460, 61790)

AMA *CPT Assistant*

64490: Feb 10: 9, Aug 10: 12, Dec 10: 13, Jan 11: 8, Feb 11: 4, Jun 12: 10, Oct 12: 15

64491: Aug 10: 12, Jun 12: 10, Oct 12: 15

64492: Feb 10: 9, Aug 10: 12, Jan 11: 8, Feb 11: 4, Jun 12: 10, Oct 12: 15

Plain English Description

Paravertebral facet joints, also called zygapophyseal joints, are located on the back (posterior) of the spine on each side of the vertebra at the point where one vertebra overlaps the next. Facet joint pain may be associated with post laminectomy syndrome or other spine surgery due to destabilization of the spinal joints, scar tissue formation, or recurrent disc herniation. Other causes include spondylosis, spondylolisthesis, and arthritis. Using fluoroscopic or CT guidance, a diagnostic or therapeutic facet joint injection or injection of nerves innervating the joint is performed. The skin overlying the facet joint is prepped and a local anesthetic injected. A spinal needle is directed into the facet joint space until bone or cartilage is encountered. A small amount of contrast material is injected to verify that the needle is correctly positioned. This is followed by injection of a local anesthetic and/or steroid. Diagnostic facet joint injection uses a local anesthetic to identify the specific area generating the pain. If the patient experiences pain relief for a significant period of time following a diagnostic injection, the physician will perform a therapeutic injection on a subsequent date of service using a long acting local anesthetic in conjunction with a steroid. Use 64490 for a single cervical or thoracic facet joint injection; use 64491 for the second level; use 64492 for the third and any additional cervical or thoracic levels injected.

Paravertebral facet joint injection

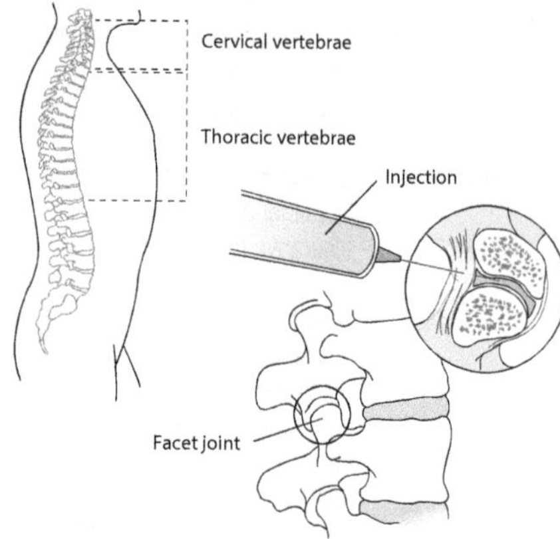

Single cervical or thoracic facet joint injection (64490); second level (64491); third and any additional cervical or thoracic levels (64492)

ICD-10-CM Diagnostic Codes

M46.81	Other specified inflammatory spondylopathies, occipito-atlanto-axial region
M46.82	Other specified inflammatory spondylopathies, cervical region
M46.83	Other specified inflammatory spondylopathies, cervicothoracic region
M46.84	Other specified inflammatory spondylopathies, thoracic region
M46.85	Other specified inflammatory spondylopathies, thoracolumbar region
M46.91	Unspecified inflammatory spondylopathy, occipito-atlanto-axial region
M46.92	Unspecified inflammatory spondylopathy, cervical region
M46.93	Unspecified inflammatory spondylopathy, cervicothoracic region
M46.94	Unspecified inflammatory spondylopathy, thoracic region
M46.95	Unspecified inflammatory spondylopathy, thoracolumbar region
M47.11	Other spondylosis with myelopathy, occipito-atlanto-axial region
M47.12	Other spondylosis with myelopathy, cervical region
M47.13	Other spondylosis with myelopathy, cervicothoracic region
M47.14	Other spondylosis with myelopathy, thoracic region
M47.15	Other spondylosis with myelopathy, thoracolumbar region
M47.21	Other spondylosis with radiculopathy, occipito-atlanto-axial region
M47.22	Other spondylosis with radiculopathy, cervical region
M47.23	Other spondylosis with radiculopathy, cervicothoracic region
M47.24	Other spondylosis with radiculopathy, thoracic region

CPT © 2018 American Medical Association. All Rights Reserved.

M47.25	Other spondylosis with radiculopathy, thoracolumbar region
M47.811	Spondylosis without myelopathy or radiculopathy, occipito-atlanto-axial region
M47.812	Spondylosis without myelopathy or radiculopathy, cervical region
M47.813	Spondylosis without myelopathy or radiculopathy, cervicothoracic region
M47.814	Spondylosis without myelopathy or radiculopathy, thoracic region
M54.11	Radiculopathy, occipito-atlanto-axial region
M54.12	Radiculopathy, cervical region
M54.13	Radiculopathy, cervicothoracic region
M54.14	Radiculopathy, thoracic region
M54.15	Radiculopathy, thoracolumbar region
M54.2	Cervicalgia
M54.6	Pain in thoracic spine

CCI Edits

Refer to Appendix A for CCI edits.

Facility RVUs ▢

Code	Work	PE Facility	MP	Total Facility
64490	1.82	1.05	0.16	3.03
64491	1.16	0.46	0.10	1.72
64492	1.16	0.48	0.10	1.74

Non-facility RVUs ▢

Code	Work	PE Non-Facility	MP	Total Non-Facility
64490	1.82	3.41	0.16	5.39
64491	1.16	1.42	0.10	2.68
64492	1.16	1.44	0.10	2.70

Modifiers (PAR) ▢

Code	Mod 50	Mod 51	Mod 62	Mod 66	Mod 80
64490	1	2	0	0	2
64491	1	0	0	0	2
64492	1	0	0	0	2

Global Period

Code	Days
64490	000
64491	ZZZ
64492	ZZZ

CPT © 2018 American Medical Association. All Rights Reserved.

64493-64495

64493 Injection(s), diagnostic or therapeutic agent, paravertebral facet (zygapophyseal) joint (or nerves innervating that joint) with image guidance (fluoroscopy or CT), lumbar or sacral; single level

+ 64494 Injection(s), diagnostic or therapeutic agent, paravertebral facet (zygapophyseal) joint (or nerves innervating that joint) with image guidance (fluoroscopy or CT), lumbar or sacral; second level (List separately in addition to code for primary procedure)

(Use 64494 in conjunction with 64493)

+ 64495 Injection(s), diagnostic or therapeutic agent, paravertebral facet (zygapophyseal) joint (or nerves innervating that joint) with image guidance (fluoroscopy or CT), lumbar or sacral; third and any additional level(s) (List separately in addition to code for primary procedure)

(Do not report 64495 more than once per day)

(Use 64495 in conjunction with 64493, 64494)

AMA Coding Notes

Introduction/Injection of Anesthetic Agent (Nerve Block), Diagnostic or Therapeutic Procedures on the Paravertebral Spinal Nerves and Branches

(Image guidance [fluoroscopy or CT] and any injection of contrast are inclusive components of 64490-64495. Imaging guidance and localization are required for the performance of paravertebral facet joint injections described by codes 64490-64495. If imaging is not used, report 20552-20553. If ultrasound guidance is used, report 0213T-0218T)

(For bilateral paravertebral facet injection procedures, use modifier 50)

(For paravertebral facet injection of the T12-L1 joint, or nerves innervating that joint, use 64490)

Introduction/Injection of Anesthetic Agent (Nerve Block), Diagnostic or Therapeutic Procedures on the Extracranial Nerves, Peripheral Nerves, and Autonomic Nervous System

(For destruction by neurolytic agent or chemodenervation, see 62280-62282, 64600-64681)

(For epidural or subarachnoid injection, see 62320, 62321, 62322, 62323, 62324, 62325, 62326, 62327)

(64479-64487, 64490-64495 are unilateral procedures. For bilateral procedures, use modifier 50)

Surgical Procedures on the Extracranial Nerves, Peripheral Nerves, and Autonomic Nervous System

(For intracranial surgery on cranial nerves, see 61450, 61460, 61790)

AMA *CPT Assistant*

64493: Feb 10: 9, Aug 10: 12, Jan 11: 8, Feb 11: 4, Jun 12: 10, Oct 12: 15, May 18: 10

64494: Feb 10: 9, Aug 10: 12, Jan 11: 8, Feb 11: 4, Jun 12: 10, May 18: 10

64495: Feb 10: 9, Aug 10: 12, Jan 11: 8, Feb 11: 4, Jun 12: 10, Oct 12: 15, May 18: 10

Plain English Description

Paravertebral facet joints, also called zygapophyseal joints, are located on the back (posterior) of the spine on each side of the vertebra at the point where one vertebra overlaps the next. Facet joint pain may is associated with post laminectomy syndrome or other spine surgery due to destabilization of the spinal joints, scar tissue formation, or recurrent disc herniation. Other causes include spondylosis, spondylolisthesis, and arthritis. Using fluoroscopic or CT guidance, a diagnostic or therapeutic facet joint injection or injection of nerves innervating the joint is performed. The skin overlying the facet joint is prepped and a local anesthetic injected. A spinal needle is directed into the facet joint space until bone or cartilage is encountered. A small amount of contrast material is injected to verify that the needle is correctly positioned. This is followed by injection of a local anesthetic and/or steroid. Diagnostic facet joint injection uses a local anesthetic to identify the specific area generating the pain. If the patient experiences pain relief for a significant period of time following a diagnostic injection, the physician will perform a therapeutic injection on a subsequent date of service using a long acting local anesthetic in conjunction with a steroid. Use 64493 for a single lumbar or sacral facet joint injection; use 64494 for the second level; use 64495 for the third and any additional lumbar or sacral levels injected.

Injection, diagnostic or therapeutic agent, paravertebral facet joint, lumbar or sacral

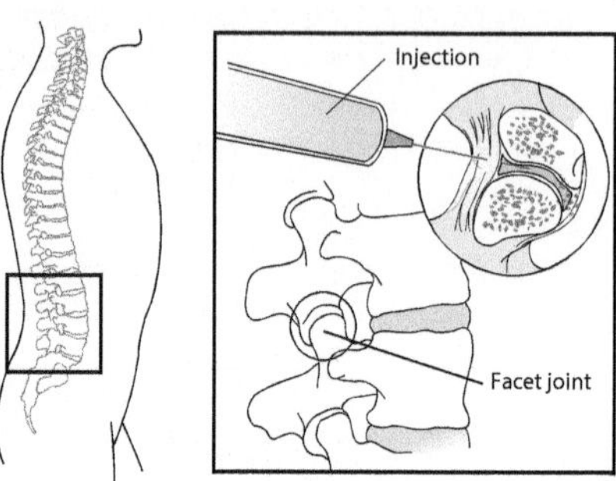

Single lumbar or sacral facet joint injection (64493); second level (64494); third and any additional levels (64495)

ICD-10-CM Diagnostic Codes

M46.86	Other specified inflammatory spondylopathies, lumbar region
M46.87	Other specified inflammatory spondylopathies, lumbosacral region
M46.96	Unspecified inflammatory spondylopathy, lumbar region
M46.97	Unspecified inflammatory spondylopathy, lumbosacral region
M47.16	Other spondylosis with myelopathy, lumbar region
M47.26	Other spondylosis with radiculopathy, lumbar region
M47.27	Other spondylosis with radiculopathy, lumbosacral region
M47.816	Spondylosis without myelopathy or radiculopathy, lumbar region
M54.16	Radiculopathy, lumbar region
M54.17	Radiculopathy, lumbosacral region
M54.5	Low back pain
M54.89	Other dorsalgia

CCI Edits

Refer to Appendix A for CCI edits.

Facility RVUs

Code	Work	PE Facility	MP	Total Facility
64493	1.52	0.93	0.13	2.58
64494	1.00	0.40	0.09	1.49
64495	1.00	0.42	0.09	1.51

Non-facility RVUs

Code	Work	PE Non-Facility	MP	Total Non-Facility
64493	1.52	3.26	0.13	4.91
64494	1.00	1.40	0.09	2.49
64495	1.00	1.40	0.09	2.49

Modifiers (PAR)

Code	Mod 50	Mod 51	Mod 62	Mod 66	Mod 80
64493	1	2	0	0	2
64494	1	0	0	0	2
64495	1	0	0	0	2

Global Period

Code	Days
64493	000
64494	ZZZ
64495	ZZZ

CPT © 2018 American Medical Association. All Rights Reserved.

64505

64505 Injection, anesthetic agent; sphenopalatine ganglion

AMA Coding Notes

Introduction/Injection of Anesthetic Agent (Nerve Block), Diagnostic or Therapeutic Procedures on the Extracranial Nerves, Peripheral Nerves, and Autonomic Nervous System

(For destruction by neurolytic agent or chemodenervation, see 62280-62282, 64600-64681)

(For epidural or subarachnoid injection, see 62320, 62321, 62322, 62323, 62324, 62325, 62326, 62327)

(64479-64487, 64490-64495 are unilateral procedures. For bilateral procedures, use modifier 50)

Surgical Procedures on the Extracranial Nerves, Peripheral Nerves, and Autonomic Nervous System

(For intracranial surgery on cranial nerves, see 61450, 61460, 61790)

AMA *CPT Assistant* ☐

64505: Jul 98: 10, Apr 05: 13, Jan 13: 13, Jun 13: 13, Jul 14: 8

Plain English Description

The sphenopalatine ganglion, also referred to as the pterygopalatine, nasal, Meckel's ganglion, or SPG, is a very small collection of nerves that includes sympathetic, parasympathetic and sensory nerves. Blocking this ganglion has been proven to relieve headaches of varying etiology and such ailments such as trigeminal neuralgia that cause facial pain. The ganglion is located behind the nose. In the procedure described by CPT code 64505, a needle is inserted through the cheek into the SPG and local anesthetic is injected. The coder should be cautioned that other techniques such as placing an anesthetic coated cotton swab intra-nasally or the use of a catheter (e.g. the SphenoCath) to apply anesthetic are not injections and therefore do not meet the description of code 64505. In the case of the cotton swab, this procedure would be inclusive of an E/M service, or if not performed in addition to a visit, would be reported with the unlisted code 64999. The SphenoCath technique would also be reported with unlisted code 64999.

Injection, anesthetic agent; spenopalatine ganglion

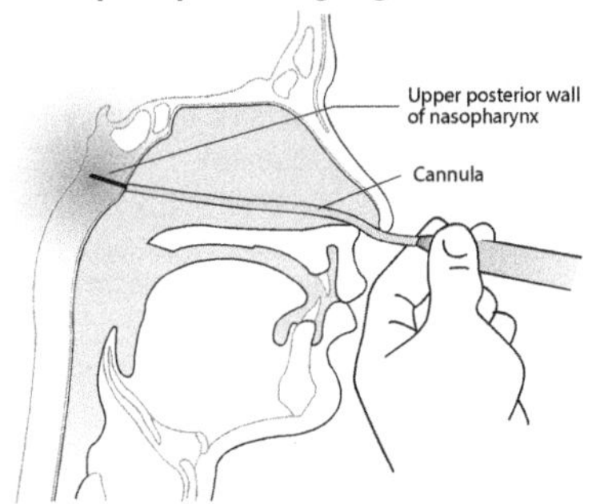

ICD-10-CM Diagnostic Codes

B02.29	Other postherpetic nervous system involvement
G43.001	Migraine without aura, not intractable, with status migrainosus
G43.009	Migraine without aura, not intractable, without status migrainosus
G43.011	Migraine without aura, intractable, with status migrainosus
G43.019	Migraine without aura, intractable, without status migrainosus
G43.101	Migraine with aura, not intractable, with status migrainosus
G43.109	Migraine with aura, not intractable, without status migrainosus
G43.111	Migraine with aura, intractable, with status migrainosus
G43.119	Migraine with aura, intractable, without status migrainosus
G43.401	Hemiplegic migraine, not intractable, with status migrainosus
G43.409	Hemiplegic migraine, not intractable, without status migrainosus
G43.411	Hemiplegic migraine, intractable, with status migrainosus
G43.419	Hemiplegic migraine, intractable, without status migrainosus
G43.501	Persistent migraine aura without cerebral infarction, not intractable, with status migrainosus
G43.509	Persistent migraine aura without cerebral infarction, not intractable, without status migrainosus
G43.511	Persistent migraine aura without cerebral infarction, intractable, with status migrainosus
G43.519	Persistent migraine aura without cerebral infarction, intractable, without status migrainosus
G43.701	Chronic migraine without aura, not intractable, with status migrainosus
G43.709	Chronic migraine without aura, not intractable, without status migrainosus
G43.711	Chronic migraine without aura, intractable, with status migrainosus
G43.719	Chronic migraine without aura, intractable, without status migrainosus
G43.801	Other migraine, not intractable, with status migrainosus
G43.809	Other migraine, not intractable, without status migrainosus
G43.811	Other migraine, intractable, with status migrainosus
G43.819	Other migraine, intractable, without status migrainosus
G43.901	Migraine, unspecified, not intractable, with status migrainosus
G43.909	Migraine, unspecified, not intractable, without status migrainosus
G43.911	Migraine, unspecified, intractable, with status migrainosus
G43.919	Migraine, unspecified, intractable, without status migrainosus
G44.001	Cluster headache syndrome, unspecified, intractable
G44.009	Cluster headache syndrome, unspecified, not intractable
G44.011	Episodic cluster headache, intractable
G44.019	Episodic cluster headache, not intractable
G44.021	Chronic cluster headache, intractable
G44.029	Chronic cluster headache, not intractable
G44.89	Other headache syndrome

CCI Edits

Refer to Appendix A for CCI edits.

Facility RVUs ☐

Code	Work	PE Facility	MP	Total Facility
64505	1.36	1.08	0.25	2.69

Non-facility RVUs ☐

Code	Work	PE Non-Facility	MP	Total Non-Facility
64505	1.36	1.75	0.25	3.36

Modifiers (PAR) ☐

Code	Mod 50	Mod 51	Mod 62	Mod 66	Mod 80
64505	1	2	0	0	1

Global Period

Code	Days
64505	000

CPT © 2018 American Medical Association. All Rights Reserved.

64510

64510 Injection, anesthetic agent; stellate ganglion (cervical sympathetic)

AMA Coding Notes

Introduction/Injection of Anesthetic Agent (Nerve Block), Diagnostic or Therapeutic Procedures on the Extracranial Nerves, Peripheral Nerves, and Autonomic Nervous System

(For destruction by neurolytic agent or chemodenervation, see 62280-62282, 64600-64681)

(For epidural or subarachnoid injection, see 62320, 62321, 62322, 62323, 62324, 62325, 62326, 62327)

(64479-64487, 64490-64495 are unilateral procedures. For bilateral procedures, use modifier 50)

Surgical Procedures on the Extracranial Nerves, Peripheral Nerves, and Autonomic Nervous System

(For intracranial surgery on cranial nerves, see 61450, 61460, 61790)

AMA *CPT Assistant* ☐

64510: Jul 98: 10, Apr 05: 13, Jan 13: 13

Plain English Description

A stellate ganglion block is performed to diagnose or treat sympathetic nerve mediated pain in the head, neck, chest or arm caused by conditions such as reflex sympathetic dystrophy, nerve injury, herpes zoster, or intractable angina. The front of the neck in the region of the voice box is palpated to identify the correct location for needle placement. The neck is prepped and the needle inserted into the skin and then advanced into the deeper tissues. When the needle is in the correct location, an anesthetic is injected. The patient is monitored for 10-20 minutes while the anesthetic takes effect.

Injection, anesthetic agent; stellate ganglion

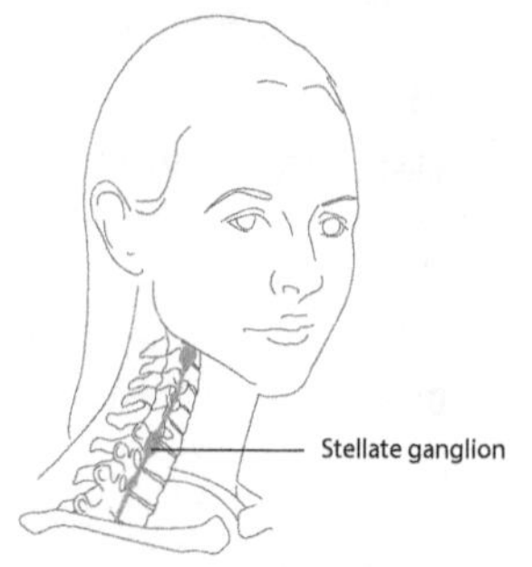

The physician injects a drug to numb the stellate ganglion, which lies at the base of the neck and provides sensation to parts of the face, neck, and arms.

ICD-10-CM Diagnostic Codes

	B02.22	Postherpetic trigeminal neuralgia
	B02.23	Postherpetic polyneuropathy
	B02.24	Postherpetic myelitis
	B02.29	Other postherpetic nervous system involvement
	C76.0	Malignant neoplasm of head, face and neck
	C76.1	Malignant neoplasm of thorax
⇄	G56.41	Causalgia of right upper limb
⇄	G56.42	Causalgia of left upper limb
⇄	G56.43	Causalgia of bilateral upper limbs
	G89.11	Acute pain due to trauma
	G89.12	Acute post-thoracotomy pain
	G89.18	Other acute postprocedural pain
	G89.21	Chronic pain due to trauma
	G89.22	Chronic post-thoracotomy pain
	G89.28	Other chronic postprocedural pain
	G89.29	Other chronic pain
	G89.3	Neoplasm related pain (acute) (chronic)
⇄	G90.511	Complex regional pain syndrome I of right upper limb
⇄	G90.512	Complex regional pain syndrome I of left upper limb
⇄	G90.513	Complex regional pain syndrome I of upper limb, bilateral
	I73.00	Raynaud's syndrome without gangrene
	I73.89	Other specified peripheral vascular diseases
	I73.9	Peripheral vascular disease, unspecified
❼	T33.09	Superficial frostbite of other part of head
❼	T33.1	Superficial frostbite of neck
❼	T33.2	Superficial frostbite of thorax
❼⇄	T33.41	Superficial frostbite of right arm
❼⇄	T33.42	Superficial frostbite of left arm
❼	T34.09	Frostbite with tissue necrosis of other part of head
❼	T34.1	Frostbite with tissue necrosis of neck
❼	T34.2	Frostbite with tissue necrosis of thorax
❼⇄	T34.41	Frostbite with tissue necrosis of right arm
❼⇄	T34.42	Frostbite with tissue necrosis of left arm

ICD-10-CM Coding Notes

For codes requiring a 7th character extension, refer to your ICD-10-CM book. Review the character descriptions and coding guidelines for proper selection. For some procedures, only certain characters will apply.

CCI Edits

Refer to Appendix A for CCI edits.

Facility RVUs ☐

Code	Work	PE Facility	MP	Total Facility
64510	1.22	0.81	0.10	2.13

Non-facility RVUs ☐

Code	Work	PE Non-Facility	MP	Total Non-Facility
64510	1.22	2.46	0.10	3.78

Modifiers (PAR) ☐

Code	Mod 50	Mod 51	Mod 62	Mod 66	Mod 80
64510	1	2	0	0	1

Global Period

Code	Days
64510	000

CPT © 2018 American Medical Association. All Rights Reserved.

64517

64517 Injection, anesthetic agent; superior hypogastric plexus

AMA Coding Notes

Introduction/Injection of Anesthetic Agent (Nerve Block), Diagnostic or Therapeutic Procedures on the Extracranial Nerves, Peripheral Nerves, and Autonomic Nervous System

(For destruction by neurolytic agent or chemodenervation, see 62280-62282, 64600-64681)

(For epidural or subarachnoid injection, see 62320, 62321, 62322, 62323, 62324, 62325, 62326, 62327)

(64479-64487, 64490-64495 are unilateral procedures. For bilateral procedures, use modifier 50)

Surgical Procedures on the Extracranial Nerves, Peripheral Nerves, and Autonomic Nervous System

(For intracranial surgery on cranial nerves, see 61450, 61460, 61790)

AMA *CPT Assistant* ▢

64517: Oct 04: 11, Apr 05: 13, Jan 13: 13

Plain English Description

A superior hypogastric plexus block is performed to relieve intractable pain in the pelvic region. This type of pain is often due to malignant primary and metastatic neoplasms in the pelvic region. The back is prepped over the L5-S1 interspace. Using separately reportable radiologic guidance, a spinal needle is inserted into the skin, passed through the L5-S1 interspace, and positioned anterolateral to the interspace. The needle is aspirated to ensure that the tip is located outside the ureters, spinal canal and blood vessels. Radiographic contrast is injected to ensure that the needle is properly placed in the pre-vertebral space anterior to the psoas muscle fascia. The needle is aspirated again and then a local anesthetic is injected.

Injection, anesthetic agent; superior hypogastric plexus

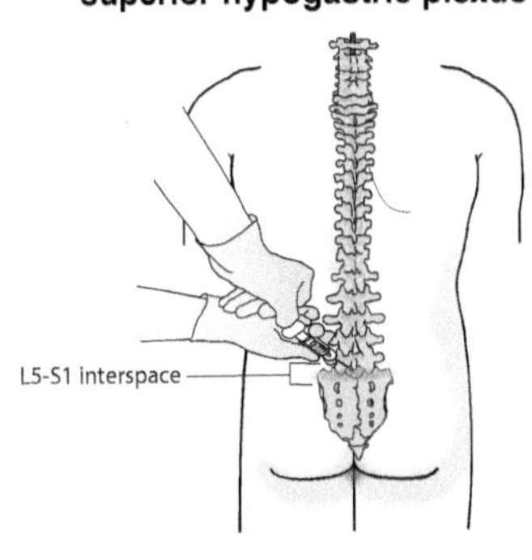

ICD-10-CM Diagnostic Codes

	B02.23	Postherpetic polyneuropathy
	B02.24	Postherpetic myelitis
	B02.29	Other postherpetic nervous system involvement
	C47.5	Malignant neoplasm of peripheral nerves of pelvis
	C48.0	Malignant neoplasm of retroperitoneum
	C48.1	Malignant neoplasm of specified parts of peritoneum
	C48.2	Malignant neoplasm of peritoneum, unspecified
	C48.8	Malignant neoplasm of overlapping sites of retroperitoneum and peritoneum
	C49.5	Malignant neoplasm of connective and soft tissue of pelvis
	C76.3	Malignant neoplasm of pelvis
	C78.6	Secondary malignant neoplasm of retroperitoneum and peritoneum
	C79.9	Secondary malignant neoplasm of unspecified site
	G58.8	Other specified mononeuropathies
	G89.11	Acute pain due to trauma
	G89.18	Other acute postprocedural pain
	G89.21	Chronic pain due to trauma
	G89.28	Other chronic postprocedural pain
	G89.29	Other chronic pain
	G89.3	Neoplasm related pain (acute) (chronic)
	G90.59	Complex regional pain syndrome I of other specified site
	K52.0	Gastroenteritis and colitis due to radiation
	K59.4	Anal spasm
	M54.16	Radiculopathy, lumbar region
	M54.17	Radiculopathy, lumbosacral region
	M54.18	Radiculopathy, sacral and sacrococcygeal region
	N80.3	Endometriosis of pelvic peritoneum ♀
	N80.5	Endometriosis of intestine ♀
	N80.8	Other endometriosis ♀
	N80.9	Endometriosis, unspecified ♀
	R10.2	Pelvic and perineal pain
	R10.30	Lower abdominal pain, unspecified
⇄	R10.31	Right lower quadrant pain
⇄	R10.32	Left lower quadrant pain
❼	S34.5	Injury of lumbar, sacral and pelvic sympathetic nerves

ICD-10-CM Coding Notes

For codes requiring a 7th character extension, refer to your ICD-10-CM book. Review the character descriptions and coding guidelines for proper selection. For some procedures, only certain characters will apply.

CCI Edits

Refer to Appendix A for CCI edits.

Facility RVUs ▢

Code	Work	PE Facility	MP	Total Facility
64517	2.20	1.23	0.17	3.60

Non-facility RVUs ▢

Code	Work	PE Non-Facility	MP	Total Non-Facility
64517	2.20	3.06	0.17	5.43

Modifiers (PAR) ▢

Code	Mod 50	Mod 51	Mod 62	Mod 66	Mod 80
64517	0	2	0	0	1

Global Period

Code	Days
64517	000

CPT © 2018 American Medical Association. All Rights Reserved.

64520

64520 Injection, anesthetic agent; lumbar or thoracic (paravertebral sympathetic)

AMA Coding Notes

Introduction/Injection of Anesthetic Agent (Nerve Block), Diagnostic or Therapeutic Procedures on the Extracranial Nerves, Peripheral Nerves, and Autonomic Nervous System

(For destruction by neurolytic agent or chemodenervation, see 62280-62282, 64600-64681)

(For epidural or subarachnoid injection, see 62320, 62321, 62322, 62323, 62324, 62325, 62326, 62327)

(64479-64487, 64490-64495 are unilateral procedures. For bilateral procedures, use modifier 50)

Surgical Procedures on the Extracranial Nerves, Peripheral Nerves, and Autonomic Nervous System

(For intracranial surgery on cranial nerves, see 61450, 61460, 61790)

AMA *CPT Assistant* □

64520: Jul 98: 10, Apr 05: 13, Dec 10: 14, Jan 13: 13

Plain English Description

Thoracic or lumbar paravertebral nerve block is used to treat acute or chronic pain in the thoracic or abdominal regions. The paravertebral space is a wedge-shaped area immediately adjacent to the vertebral bodies on either side of the spine where the spinal nerves emerge from the intervertebral foramen. Injection of a local anesthetic in this region produces unilateral motor, sensory, and sympathetic nerve blocks. The level of the blocks is determined, and the superior aspect of the spinous process is identified and marked. A needle entry site is marked approximately 2.5 cm lateral to the superior aspect of the spinous process. A local anesthetic is injected at the planned needle insertion site. A spinal epidural needle with tubing attached to a syringe is then inserted through the skin and advanced until contact is made with the transverse process. The needle is then withdrawn to the subcutaneous tissue and angled so that is can be walked off the lower (caudad) edge of the transverse process. The needle is reinserted and advanced into the paravertebral space. The needle is aspirated to ensure that it is not in the spinal canal or a blood vessel. The anesthetic is injected.

Injection, anesthetic agent; lumbar or thoracic

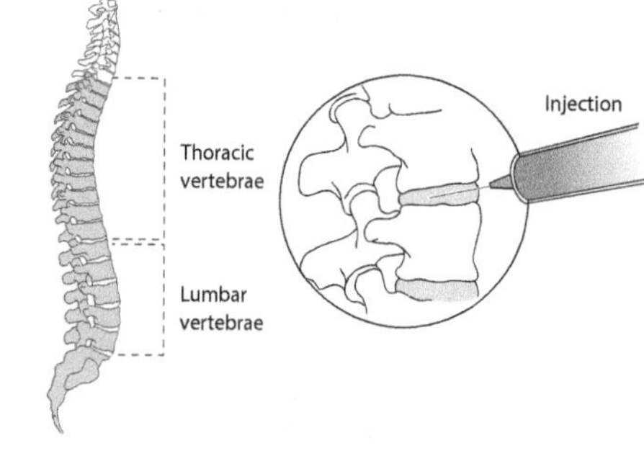

The physician injects a drug to numb the lumbar or thoracic sympathetic nerve to block pain to the pelvis, torso, and the legs.

ICD-10-CM Diagnostic Codes

	B02.29	Other postherpetic nervous system involvement
	C41.2	Malignant neoplasm of vertebral column
	G89.11	Acute pain due to trauma
	G89.12	Acute post-thoracotomy pain
	G89.18	Other acute postprocedural pain
	G89.21	Chronic pain due to trauma
	G89.22	Chronic post-thoracotomy pain
	G89.28	Other chronic postprocedural pain
	G89.29	Other chronic pain
	G89.3	Neoplasm related pain (acute) (chronic)
❼	M48.54	Collapsed vertebra, not elsewhere classified, thoracic region
❼	M48.55	Collapsed vertebra, not elsewhere classified, thoracolumbar region
❼	M48.56	Collapsed vertebra, not elsewhere classified, lumbar region
⇄	M54.40	Lumbago with sciatica, unspecified side
⇄	M54.41	Lumbago with sciatica, right side
⇄	M54.42	Lumbago with sciatica, left side
	M54.5	Low back pain
	M54.6	Pain in thoracic spine
⇄	M79.604	Pain in right leg
⇄	M79.605	Pain in left leg
❼	M80.88	Other osteoporosis with current pathological fracture, vertebra(e)
❼	M84.58	Pathological fracture in neoplastic disease, other specified site
	R10.10	Upper abdominal pain, unspecified
⇄	R10.11	Right upper quadrant pain
⇄	R10.12	Left upper quadrant pain
	R10.2	Pelvic and perineal pain
❼	S22.010	Wedge compression fracture of first thoracic vertebra
❼	S22.020	Wedge compression fracture of second thoracic vertebra
❼	S22.030	Wedge compression fracture of third thoracic vertebra
❼	S22.040	Wedge compression fracture of fourth thoracic vertebra
❼	S22.050	Wedge compression fracture of T5-T6 vertebra
❼	S22.060	Wedge compression fracture of T7-T8 vertebra
❼	S22.070	Wedge compression fracture of T9-T10 vertebra
❼	S22.080	Wedge compression fracture of T11-T12 vertebra
❼	S32.010	Wedge compression fracture of first lumbar vertebra
❼	S32.020	Wedge compression fracture of second lumbar vertebra
❼	S32.030	Wedge compression fracture of third lumbar vertebra
❼	S32.040	Wedge compression fracture of fourth lumbar vertebra
❼	S32.050	Wedge compression fracture of fifth lumbar vertebra

ICD-10-CM Coding Notes

For codes requiring a 7th character extension, refer to your ICD-10-CM book. Review the character descriptions and coding guidelines for proper selection. For some procedures, only certain characters will apply.

CCI Edits

Refer to Appendix A for CCI edits.

Facility RVUs □

Code	Work	PE Facility	MP	Total Facility
64520	1.35	0.86	0.13	2.34

Non-facility RVUs □

Code	Work	PE Non-Facility	MP	Total Non-Facility
64520	1.35	4.27	0.13	5.75

Modifiers (PAR) □

Code	Mod 50	Mod 51	Mod 62	Mod 66	Mod 80
64520	1	2	0	0	1

Global Period

Code	Days
64520	000

CPT © 2018 American Medical Association. All Rights Reserved.

64530

64530 Injection, anesthetic agent; celiac plexus, with or without radiologic monitoring

(For transendoscopic ultrasound-guided transmural injection, anesthetic, celiac plexus, use 43253)

AMA Coding Notes

Introduction/Injection of Anesthetic Agent (Nerve Block), Diagnostic or Therapeutic Procedures on the Extracranial Nerves, Peripheral Nerves, and Autonomic Nervous System

(For destruction by neurolytic agent or chemodenervation, see 62280-62282, 64600-64681)

(For epidural or subarachnoid injection, see 62320, 62321, 62322, 62323, 62324, 62325, 62326, 62327)

(64479-64487, 64490-64495 are unilateral procedures. For bilateral procedures, use modifier 50)

Surgical Procedures on the Extracranial Nerves, Peripheral Nerves, and Autonomic Nervous System

(For intracranial surgery on cranial nerves, see 61450, 61460, 61790)

AMA *CPT Assistant* ▯

64530: Jul 98: 10, Apr 05: 13, Jan 13: 13

Plain English Description

The celiac nerve plexus is a network of nerves located anterior to the aorta at the level of the T12 vertebra. The celiac plexus transmits nerve impulses from the pancreas, liver, gall bladder stomach and intestine to the brain. Celiac plexus block in performed to treat chronic pain due to disease or injury of these organs including malignant neoplasm, inflammation (pancreatitis), or other conditions. The skin of the back over the T12 vertebra is prepped. A local anesthetic is injected. Using radiological guidance, a needle is advanced into celiac plexus, which is the region immediately superior to the celiac artery. The needle is aspirated to ensure that the tip is not in a blood vessel. Contrast is injected to ensure that the needle is in the proper location. The needle is aspirated again and anesthetic is injected.

Injection, anesthetic agent; celiac plexus

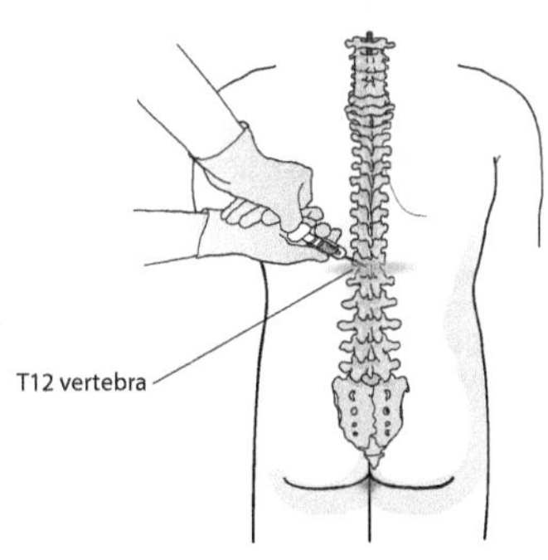

ICD-10-CM Diagnostic Codes

C22.0	Liver cell carcinoma
C22.1	Intrahepatic bile duct carcinoma
C22.2	Hepatoblastoma
C22.3	Angiosarcoma of liver
C22.4	Other sarcomas of liver
C22.7	Other specified carcinomas of liver
C22.8	Malignant neoplasm of liver, primary, unspecified as to type
C22.9	Malignant neoplasm of liver, not specified as primary or secondary
C25.0	Malignant neoplasm of head of pancreas
C25.1	Malignant neoplasm of body of pancreas
C25.2	Malignant neoplasm of tail of pancreas
C25.3	Malignant neoplasm of pancreatic duct
C25.4	Malignant neoplasm of endocrine pancreas
C25.7	Malignant neoplasm of other parts of pancreas
C25.8	Malignant neoplasm of overlapping sites of pancreas
C25.9	Malignant neoplasm of pancreas, unspecified
C48.0	Malignant neoplasm of retroperitoneum
C48.1	Malignant neoplasm of specified parts of peritoneum
C48.2	Malignant neoplasm of peritoneum, unspecified
C48.8	Malignant neoplasm of overlapping sites of retroperitoneum and peritoneum
C76.2	Malignant neoplasm of abdomen
C78.6	Secondary malignant neoplasm of retroperitoneum and peritoneum
C78.7	Secondary malignant neoplasm of liver and intrahepatic bile duct
G89.11	Acute pain due to trauma
G89.18	Other acute postprocedural pain
G89.21	Chronic pain due to trauma
G89.28	Other chronic postprocedural pain
G89.29	Other chronic pain
G89.3	Neoplasm related pain (acute) (chronic)
K55.1	Chronic vascular disorders of intestine
K55.8	Other vascular disorders of intestine
K85.00	Idiopathic acute pancreatitis without necrosis or infection
K85.01	Idiopathic acute pancreatitis with uninfected necrosis
K85.02	Idiopathic acute pancreatitis with infected necrosis
K85.10	Biliary acute pancreatitis without necrosis or infection
K85.11	Biliary acute pancreatitis with uninfected necrosis
K85.12	Biliary acute pancreatitis with infected necrosis
K85.20	Alcohol induced acute pancreatitis without necrosis or infection
K85.21	Alcohol induced acute pancreatitis with uninfected necrosis
K85.22	Alcohol induced acute pancreatitis with infected necrosis
K85.30	Drug induced acute pancreatitis without necrosis or infection
K85.31	Drug induced acute pancreatitis with uninfected necrosis
K85.32	Drug induced acute pancreatitis with infected necrosis
K85.80	Other acute pancreatitis without necrosis or infection
K85.81	Other acute pancreatitis with uninfected necrosis
K85.82	Other acute pancreatitis with infected necrosis
K86.0	Alcohol-induced chronic pancreatitis
K86.1	Other chronic pancreatitis
R10.10	Upper abdominal pain, unspecified
⇄ R10.11	Right upper quadrant pain
⇄ R10.12	Left upper quadrant pain

CCI Edits

Refer to Appendix A for CCI edits.

Facility RVUs ▯

Code	Work	PE Facility	MP	Total Facility
64530	1.58	0.92	0.13	2.63

Non-facility RVUs ▯

Code	Work	PE Non-Facility	MP	Total Non-Facility
64530	1.58	4.02	0.13	5.73

Modifiers (PAR) ▯

Code	Mod 50	Mod 51	Mod 62	Mod 66	Mod 80
64530	0	2	0	0	1

Global Period

Code	Days
64530	000

CPT © 2018 American Medical Association. All Rights Reserved.

64555

64555 Percutaneous implantation of neurostimulator electrode array; peripheral nerve (excludes sacral nerve)

(Do not report 64555 in conjunction with 64566)

(For percutaneous electrical stimulation of a peripheral nerve using needle[s] or needle electrode[s] [eg, PENS, PNT], use 64999)

AMA Coding Guideline

Neurostimulator Procedures on the Peripheral Nerves

For electronic analysis with programming, when performed, of peripheral nerve neurostimulator pulse generator/transmitters, see codes 95970, 95971, 95972. An electrode array is a catheter or other device with more than one contact. The function of each contact may be capable of being adjusted during programming services. Test stimulation to confirm correct target site placement of the electrode array(s) and/or to confirm the functional status of the system is inherent to placement, and is not separately reported as electronic analysis or programming of the neurostimulator system. Electronic analysis (95970) at the time of implantation is not separately reported.

Codes 64553, 64555, and 64561 may be used to report both temporary and permanent placement of percutaneous electrode arrays.

AMA Coding Notes

Neurostimulator Procedures on the Peripheral Nerves

(For transcutaneous nerve stimulation [TENS], use 97014 for electrical stimulation requiring supervision only or use 97032 for electrical stimulation requiring constant attendance)

Surgical Procedures on the Extracranial Nerves, Peripheral Nerves, and Autonomic Nervous System

(For intracranial surgery on cranial nerves, see 61450, 61460, 61790)

AMA *CPT Assistant* ▯

64555: Jan 15: 14, Feb 16: 13, Dec 17: 16, Aug 18: 10

Plain English Description

When implanting a neurostimulator electrode array, the exact procedure depends on which of the peripheral nerves is being stimulated. The planned insertion site is prepped. Anatomical landmarks are located and separately reportable ultrasound guidance is used as needed to facilitate correct placement of the electrodes. An electrically insulated needle is inserted into the skin and advanced parallel to the peripheral nerve. A power source is connected to the needle, stimulation is applied, and motor and sensory responses are evaluated as the position of the needle is changed until the desired response is achieved. The needle is disconnected from the power source. An electrode array is then passed through the lumen of the needle and positioned in the desired location next to the peripheral nerve. The needle is removed leaving the electrode array in place, which is then attached to an external generator/receiver.

Percutaneous implantation of neurostimulator electrode array; peripheral

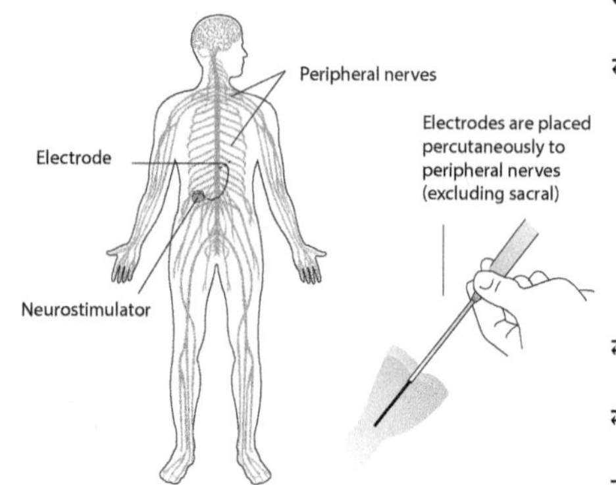

ICD-10-CM Diagnostic Codes

	B02.29	Other postherpetic nervous system involvement
⇄	G56.31	Lesion of radial nerve, right upper limb
⇄	G56.32	Lesion of radial nerve, left upper limb
⇄	G56.33	Lesion of radial nerve, bilateral upper limbs
⇄	G56.41	Causalgia of right upper limb
⇄	G56.42	Causalgia of left upper limb
⇄	G56.43	Causalgia of bilateral upper limbs
⇄	G56.81	Other specified mononeuropathies of right upper limb
⇄	G56.82	Other specified mononeuropathies of left upper limb
⇄	G56.83	Other specified mononeuropathies of bilateral upper limbs
⇄	G57.01	Lesion of sciatic nerve, right lower limb
⇄	G57.02	Lesion of sciatic nerve, left lower limb
⇄	G57.03	Lesion of sciatic nerve, bilateral lower limbs
⇄	G57.11	Meralgia paresthetica, right lower limb
⇄	G57.12	Meralgia paresthetica, left lower limb
⇄	G57.13	Meralgia paresthetica, bilateral lower limbs
⇄	G57.21	Lesion of femoral nerve, right lower limb
⇄	G57.22	Lesion of femoral nerve, left lower limb
⇄	G57.23	Lesion of femoral nerve, bilateral lower limbs
⇄	G57.31	Lesion of lateral popliteal nerve, right lower limb
⇄	G57.32	Lesion of lateral popliteal nerve, left lower limb
⇄	G57.33	Lesion of lateral popliteal nerve, bilateral lower limbs
⇄	G57.41	Lesion of medial popliteal nerve, right lower limb
⇄	G57.42	Lesion of medial popliteal nerve, left lower limb
⇄	G57.43	Lesion of medial popliteal nerve, bilateral lower limbs
⇄	G57.71	Causalgia of right lower limb
⇄	G57.72	Causalgia of left lower limb
⇄	G57.73	Causalgia of bilateral lower limbs
⇄	G57.81	Other specified mononeuropathies of right lower limb
⇄	G57.82	Other specified mononeuropathies of left lower limb
⇄	G57.83	Other specified mononeuropathies of bilateral lower limbs
	G58.0	Intercostal neuropathy
	G58.9	Mononeuropathy, unspecified
	G89.21	Chronic pain due to trauma
	G89.22	Chronic post-thoracotomy pain
	G89.28	Other chronic postprocedural pain
	G89.29	Other chronic pain
⇄	G90.511	Complex regional pain syndrome I of right upper limb
⇄	G90.512	Complex regional pain syndrome I of left upper limb
⇄	G90.513	Complex regional pain syndrome I of upper limb, bilateral
⇄	G90.521	Complex regional pain syndrome I of right lower limb
⇄	G90.522	Complex regional pain syndrome I of left lower limb
⇄	G90.523	Complex regional pain syndrome I of lower limb, bilateral
	M79.2	Neuralgia and neuritis, unspecified
⇄	M79.601	Pain in right arm
⇄	M79.602	Pain in left arm
⇄	M79.604	Pain in right leg
⇄	M79.605	Pain in left leg
❼⇄	S54.21	Injury of radial nerve at forearm level, right arm
❼⇄	S54.22	Injury of radial nerve at forearm level, left arm
❼⇄	S64.21	Injury of radial nerve at wrist and hand level of right arm
❼⇄	S64.22	Injury of radial nerve at wrist and hand level of left arm
❼⇄	S74.01	Injury of sciatic nerve at hip and thigh level, right leg
❼⇄	S74.02	Injury of sciatic nerve at hip and thigh level, left leg
❼⇄	S74.11	Injury of femoral nerve at hip and thigh level, right leg
❼⇄	S74.12	Injury of femoral nerve at hip and thigh level, left leg
❼⇄	S84.01	Injury of tibial nerve at lower leg level, right leg
❼⇄	S84.02	Injury of tibial nerve at lower leg level, left leg
❼⇄	S84.11	Injury of peroneal nerve at lower leg level, right leg
❼⇄	S84.12	Injury of peroneal nerve at lower leg level, left leg
❼⇄	S94.21	Injury of deep peroneal nerve at ankle and foot level, right leg
❼⇄	S94.22	Injury of deep peroneal nerve at ankle and foot level, left leg

CPT © 2018 American Medical Association. All Rights Reserved.

ICD-10-CM Coding Notes

For codes requiring a 7th character extension, refer to your ICD-10-CM book. Review the character descriptions and coding guidelines for proper selection. For some procedures, only certain characters will apply.

CCI Edits

Refer to Appendix A for CCI edits.

Pub 100

64555: Pub 100-03, 1, 160.7-160.7.1

Facility RVUs □

Code	Work	PE Facility	MP	Total Facility
64555	5.76	3.34	0.75	9.85

Non-facility RVUs □

Code	Work	PE Non-Facility	MP	Total Non-Facility
64555	5.76	37.80	0.75	44.31

Modifiers (PAR) □

Code	Mod 50	Mod 51	Mod 62	Mod 66	Mod 80
64555	0	2	0	0	1

Global Period

Code	Days
64555	010

CPT © 2018 American Medical Association. All Rights Reserved.

64561

64561 Percutaneous implantation of neurostimulator electrode array; sacral nerve (transforaminal placement) including image guidance, if performed

(For percutaneous electrical neuromuscular stimulation or neuromodulation using needle[s] or needle electrode[s] [eg, PENS, PNT], use 64999)

AMA Coding Guideline

Neurostimulator Procedures on the Peripheral Nerves

For electronic analysis with programming, when performed, of peripheral nerve neurostimulator pulse generator/transmitters, see codes 95970, 95971, 95972. An electrode array is a catheter or other device with more than one contact. The function of each contact may be capable of being adjusted during programming services. Test stimulation to confirm correct target site placement of the electrode array(s) and/or to confirm the functional status of the system is inherent to placement, and is not separately reported as electronic analysis or programming of the neurostimulator system. Electronic analysis (95970) at the time of implantation is not separately reported.

Codes 64553, 64555, and 64561 may be used to report both temporary and permanent placement of percutaneous electrode arrays.

AMA Coding Notes

Neurostimulator Procedures on the Peripheral Nerves

(For transcutaneous nerve stimulation [TENS], use 97014 for electrical stimulation requiring supervision only or use 97032 for electrical stimulation requiring constant attendance)

Surgical Procedures on the Extracranial Nerves, Peripheral Nerves, and Autonomic Nervous System

(For intracranial surgery on cranial nerves, see 61450, 61460, 61790)

AMA *CPT Assistant* ☐

64561: Dec 12: 14, Sep 14: 5

Plain English Description

A neurostimulator electrode array is placed for direct transforaminal sacral nerve stimulation, which is used to treat voiding dysfunction, including urge incontinence, urgency, frequency, and nonobstructive retention. The sacral foramen are located using bony landmarks or with imaging guidance such as fluoroscopy. The skin is prepped and a local anesthetic is injected into the skin and the periosteum of the sacrum. Percutaneous placement is accomplished using an electrically insulated spinal needle advanced through the skin and deeper tissues into the selected sacral foramen. A power source is connected to the needle, stimulation is applied, and motor and sensory responses are evaluated as the position of the needle is changed until the desired response is achieved. The needle is disconnected from the power source. An electrode array is then passed through the lumen of the needle and positioned in the desired location next to the sacral nerve. The needle is removed leaving the electrode array in place, which is then attached to an external generator/receiver.

Percutaneous implantation of neurostimulator electrode array; sacral nerve

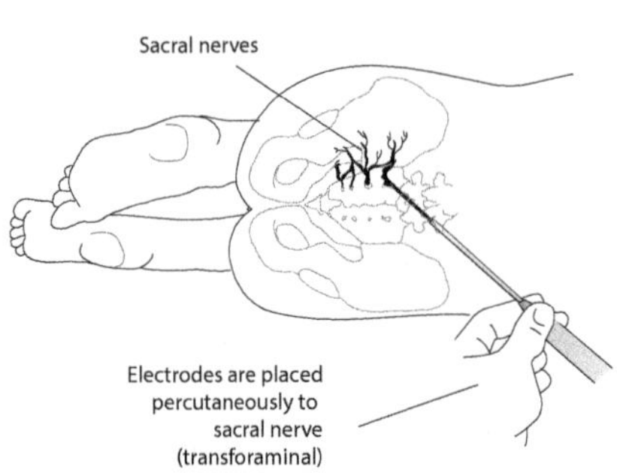

ICD-10-CM Diagnostic Codes

	G58.8	Other specified mononeuropathies
	G83.4	Cauda equina syndrome
	G95.89	Other specified diseases of spinal cord
	M79.2	Neuralgia and neuritis, unspecified
	N31.0	Uninhibited neuropathic bladder, not elsewhere classified
	N31.1	Reflex neuropathic bladder, not elsewhere classified
	N31.2	Flaccid neuropathic bladder, not elsewhere classified
	N31.8	Other neuromuscular dysfunction of bladder
	N31.9	Neuromuscular dysfunction of bladder, unspecified
	N39.41	Urge incontinence
	N39.42	Incontinence without sensory awareness
	N39.43	Post-void dribbling
	N39.44	Nocturnal enuresis
	N39.45	Continuous leakage
	N39.46	Mixed incontinence
	N39.490	Overflow incontinence
	N39.498	Other specified urinary incontinence
	N39.8	Other specified disorders of urinary system
	R10.2	Pelvic and perineal pain
	R32	Unspecified urinary incontinence
	R33.8	Other retention of urine
	R33.9	Retention of urine, unspecified
	R35.0	Frequency of micturition
	R35.1	Nocturia
	R35.8	Other polyuria
❼	S34.3	Injury of cauda equina

ICD-10-CM Coding Notes

For codes requiring a 7th character extension, refer to your ICD-10-CM book. Review the character descriptions and coding guidelines for proper selection. For some procedures, only certain characters will apply.

CCI Edits

Refer to Appendix A for CCI edits.

Pub 100

64561: Pub 100-03, 1, 230.18, Pub 100-04, 32, 40.2.1

Facility RVUs ☐

Code	Work	PE Facility	MP	Total Facility
64561	5.44	2.69	0.62	8.75

Non-facility RVUs ☐

Code	Work	PE Non-Facility	MP	Total Non-Facility
64561	5.44	14.86	0.62	20.92

Modifiers (PAR) ☐

Code	Mod 50	Mod 51	Mod 62	Mod 66	Mod 80
64561	1	2	0	0	1

Global Period

Code	Days
64561	010

CPT © 2018 American Medical Association. All Rights Reserved.

64575

64575 Incision for implantation of neurostimulator electrode array; peripheral nerve (excludes sacral nerve)

AMA Coding Guideline

Neurostimulator Procedures on the Peripheral Nerves

For electronic analysis with programming, when performed, of peripheral nerve neurostimulator pulse generator/transmitters, see codes 95970, 95971, 95972. An electrode array is a catheter or other device with more than one contact. The function of each contact may be capable of being adjusted during programming services. Test stimulation to confirm correct target site placement of the electrode array(s) and/or to confirm the functional status of the system is inherent to placement, and is not separately reported as electronic analysis or programming of the neurostimulator system. Electronic analysis (95970) at the time of implantation is not separately reported.

Codes 64553, 64555, and 64561 may be used to report both temporary and permanent placement of percutaneous electrode arrays.

AMA Coding Notes

Neurostimulator Procedures on the Peripheral Nerves

(For transcutaneous nerve stimulation [TENS], use 97014 for electrical stimulation requiring supervision only or use 97032 for electrical stimulation requiring constant attendance)

Surgical Procedures on the Extracranial Nerves, Peripheral Nerves, and Autonomic Nervous System

(For intracranial surgery on cranial nerves, see 61450, 61460, 61790)

Plain English Description

For placement of a neurostimulator electrode array, the exact procedure depends on which peripheral nerve is being stimulated. For open placement of a peripheral nerve neurostimulator electrode array, the planned insertion site is prepped and the skin is incised. Soft tissues are dissected to expose the targeted peripheral nerve. An electrode array is then positioned in the desired location next to the peripheral nerve and connected to a power source. Stimulation is applied and motor responses are evaluated. The electrode array is repositioned and retested until the desired responses are attained. The electrode array is then secured and tunneled to the generator/receiver which is implanted in a separately reportable procedure. Tissues are closed in layers over the electrode array.

Incision for implantation of peripheral nerve neurostimulator electrode array (excludes sacral nerve)

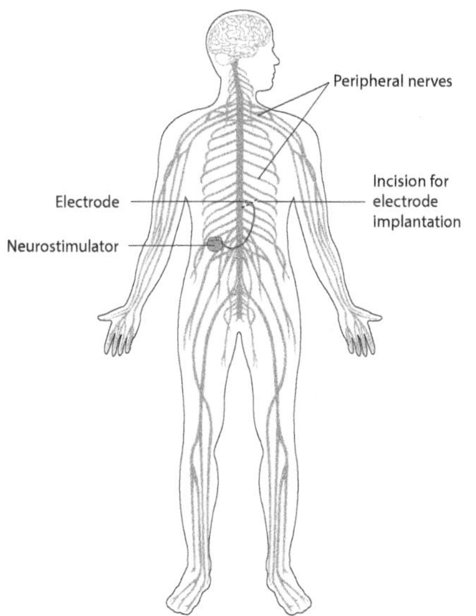

ICD-10-CM Diagnostic Codes

⇄	G56.03	Carpal tunnel syndrome, bilateral upper limbs
⇄	G56.11	Other lesions of median nerve, right upper limb
⇄	G56.12	Other lesions of median nerve, left upper limb
⇄	G56.13	Other lesions of median nerve, bilateral upper limbs
⇄	G56.21	Lesion of ulnar nerve, right upper limb
⇄	G56.22	Lesion of ulnar nerve, left upper limb
⇄	G56.23	Lesion of ulnar nerve, bilateral upper limbs
⇄	G56.31	Lesion of radial nerve, right upper limb
⇄	G56.32	Lesion of radial nerve, left upper limb
⇄	G56.33	Lesion of radial nerve, bilateral upper limbs
⇄	G56.41	Causalgia of right upper limb
⇄	G56.42	Causalgia of left upper limb
⇄	G56.43	Causalgia of bilateral upper limbs
⇄	G56.81	Other specified mononeuropathies of right upper limb
⇄	G56.82	Other specified mononeuropathies of left upper limb
⇄	G56.83	Other specified mononeuropathies of bilateral upper limbs
⇄	G57.01	Lesion of sciatic nerve, right lower limb
⇄	G57.02	Lesion of sciatic nerve, left lower limb
⇄	G57.03	Lesion of sciatic nerve, bilateral lower limbs
⇄	G57.11	Meralgia paresthetica, right lower limb
⇄	G57.12	Meralgia paresthetica, left lower limb
⇄	G57.13	Meralgia paresthetica, bilateral lower limbs
⇄	G57.21	Lesion of femoral nerve, right lower limb
⇄	G57.22	Lesion of femoral nerve, left lower limb
⇄	G57.23	Lesion of femoral nerve, bilateral lower limbs
⇄	G57.31	Lesion of lateral popliteal nerve, right lower limb
⇄	G57.32	Lesion of lateral popliteal nerve, left lower limb
⇄	G57.33	Lesion of lateral popliteal nerve, bilateral lower limbs
⇄	G57.41	Lesion of medial popliteal nerve, right lower limb
⇄	G57.42	Lesion of medial popliteal nerve, left lower limb
⇄	G57.43	Lesion of medial popliteal nerve, bilateral lower limbs
⇄	G57.71	Causalgia of right lower limb
⇄	G57.72	Causalgia of left lower limb
⇄	G57.73	Causalgia of bilateral lower limbs
⇄	G57.81	Other specified mononeuropathies of right lower limb
⇄	G57.82	Other specified mononeuropathies of left lower limb
⇄	G57.83	Other specified mononeuropathies of bilateral lower limbs
	G58.0	Intercostal neuropathy
	G58.9	Mononeuropathy, unspecified
	G89.21	Chronic pain due to trauma
	G89.22	Chronic post-thoracotomy pain
	G89.28	Other chronic postprocedural pain
	G89.29	Other chronic pain
⇄	G90.511	Complex regional pain syndrome I of right upper limb
⇄	G90.512	Complex regional pain syndrome I of left upper limb
⇄	G90.513	Complex regional pain syndrome I of upper limb, bilateral
⇄	G90.521	Complex regional pain syndrome I of right lower limb
⇄	G90.522	Complex regional pain syndrome I of left lower limb
⇄	G90.523	Complex regional pain syndrome I of lower limb, bilateral
	G90.8	Other disorders of autonomic nervous system
	M79.2	Neuralgia and neuritis, unspecified
⇄	M79.601	Pain in right arm
⇄	M79.602	Pain in left arm
⇄	M79.604	Pain in right leg
⇄	M79.605	Pain in left leg
➐⇄	S54.21	Injury of radial nerve at forearm level, right arm
➐⇄	S54.22	Injury of radial nerve at forearm level, left arm
➐⇄	S64.21	Injury of radial nerve at wrist and hand level of right arm
➐⇄	S64.22	Injury of radial nerve at wrist and hand level of left arm
➐⇄	S74.01	Injury of sciatic nerve at hip and thigh level, right leg
➐⇄	S74.02	Injury of sciatic nerve at hip and thigh level, left leg
➐⇄	S74.11	Injury of femoral nerve at hip and thigh level, right leg
➐⇄	S74.12	Injury of femoral nerve at hip and thigh level, left leg
➐⇄	S84.01	Injury of tibial nerve at lower leg level, right leg

CPT © 2018 American Medical Association. All Rights Reserved.

❼⇄	S84.02	Injury of tibial nerve at lower leg level, left leg
❼⇄	S84.11	Injury of peroneal nerve at lower leg level, right leg
❼⇄	S84.12	Injury of peroneal nerve at lower leg level, left leg

ICD-10-CM Coding Notes

For codes requiring a 7th character extension, refer to your ICD-10-CM book. Review the character descriptions and coding guidelines for proper selection. For some procedures, only certain characters will apply.

CCI Edits

Refer to Appendix A for CCI edits.

Pub 100

64575: Pub 100-03, 1, 160.19, Pub 100-03, 1, 160.26, Pub 100-03, 1, 160.7-160.7.1

Facility RVUs ☐

Code	Work	PE Facility	MP	Total Facility
64575	4.42	4.11	1.07	9.60

Non-facility RVUs ☐

Code	Work	PE Non-Facility	MP	Total Non-Facility
64575	4.42	4.11	1.07	9.60

Modifiers (PAR) ☐

Code	Mod 50	Mod 51	Mod 62	Mod 66	Mod 80
64575	0	2	0	0	1

Global Period

Code	Days
64575	090

CPT © 2018 American Medical Association. All Rights Reserved.

64580

64580 Incision for implantation of neurostimulator electrode array; neuromuscular

AMA Coding Guideline

Neurostimulator Procedures on the Peripheral Nerves

For electronic analysis with programming, when performed, of peripheral nerve neurostimulator pulse generator/transmitters, see codes 95970, 95971, 95972. An electrode array is a catheter or other device with more than one contact. The function of each contact may be capable of being adjusted during programming services. Test stimulation to confirm correct target site placement of the electrode array(s) and/or to confirm the functional status of the system is inherent to placement, and is not separately reported as electronic analysis or programming of the neurostimulator system. Electronic analysis (95970) at the time of implantation is not separately reported.

Codes 64553, 64555, and 64561 may be used to report both temporary and permanent placement of percutaneous electrode arrays.

AMA Coding Notes

Neurostimulator Procedures on the Peripheral Nerves

(For transcutaneous nerve stimulation [TENS], use 97014 for electrical stimulation requiring supervision only or use 97032 for electrical stimulation requiring constant attendance)

Surgical Procedures on the Extracranial Nerves, Peripheral Nerves, and Autonomic Nervous System

(For intracranial surgery on cranial nerves, see 61450, 61460, 61790)

Plain English Description

The exact procedure for implanting a neurostimulator electrode array depends on which neuromuscular site is being stimulated. For open neuromuscular neurostimulator electrode array placement, the planned insertion site is prepped and the skin is incised. Soft tissues are dissected. An electrode array is positioned in the desired location for neuromuscular stimulation and connected to a power source. Electrical stimulation is then applied and the targeted neuromuscular responses are evaluated. The electrode array is repositioned and retested until the desired responses are attained. The electrode array is then secured and tunneled to the generator/receiver which is implanted in a separately reportable procedure. Tissues are closed in layers over the electrode array.

Incision for implantation of neurostimulator electrode array; neuromuscular

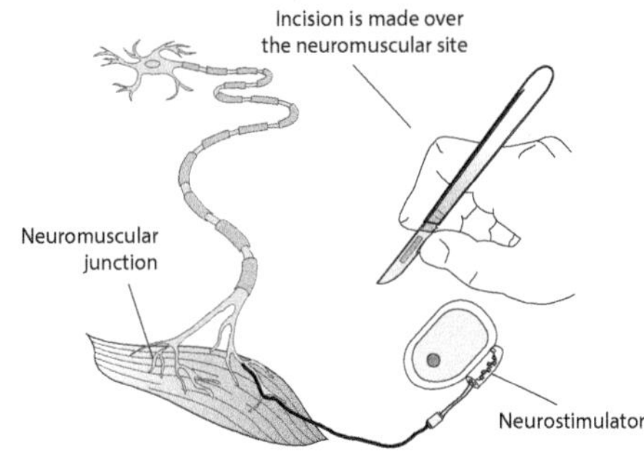

ICD-10-CM Diagnostic Codes

	G89.21	Chronic pain due to trauma
	G89.22	Chronic post-thoracotomy pain
	G89.28	Other chronic postprocedural pain
	G89.29	Other chronic pain
	M54.11	Radiculopathy, occipito-atlanto-axial region
	M54.12	Radiculopathy, cervical region
	M54.13	Radiculopathy, cervicothoracic region
	M54.14	Radiculopathy, thoracic region
	M54.15	Radiculopathy, thoracolumbar region
	M54.16	Radiculopathy, lumbar region
	M54.17	Radiculopathy, lumbosacral region
	M54.18	Radiculopathy, sacral and sacrococcygeal region
	M54.2	Cervicalgia
	M54.5	Low back pain
	M54.6	Pain in thoracic spine
	M54.81	Occipital neuralgia
	M54.89	Other dorsalgia
	M54.9	Dorsalgia, unspecified
	M79.2	Neuralgia and neuritis, unspecified
⇄	M79.601	Pain in right arm
⇄	M79.602	Pain in left arm
⇄	M79.604	Pain in right leg
⇄	M79.605	Pain in left leg
⇄	M79.621	Pain in right upper arm
⇄	M79.622	Pain in left upper arm
⇄	M79.631	Pain in right forearm
⇄	M79.632	Pain in left forearm
⇄	M79.651	Pain in right thigh
⇄	M79.652	Pain in left thigh
⇄	M79.661	Pain in right lower leg
⇄	M79.662	Pain in left lower leg
	M79.7	Fibromyalgia

CCI Edits

Refer to Appendix A for CCI edits.

Pub 100

64580: Pub 100-03, 1, 160.7-160.7.1

Facility RVUs ☐

Code	Work	PE Facility	MP	Total Facility
64580	4.19	3.67	1.00	8.86

Non-facility RVUs ☐

Code	Work	PE Non-Facility	MP	Total Non-Facility
64580	4.19	3.67	1.00	8.86

Modifiers (PAR) ☐

Code	Mod 50	Mod 51	Mod 62	Mod 66	Mod 80
64580	0	2	0	0	2

Global Period

Code	Days
64580	090

CPT © 2018 American Medical Association. All Rights Reserved.

64581

64581 Incision for implantation of neurostimulator electrode array; sacral nerve (transforaminal placement)

AMA Coding Guideline

Neurostimulator Procedures on the Peripheral Nerves

For electronic analysis with programming, when performed, of peripheral nerve neurostimulator pulse generator/transmitters, see codes 95970, 95971, 95972. An electrode array is a catheter or other device with more than one contact. The function of each contact may be capable of being adjusted during programming services. Test stimulation to confirm correct target site placement of the electrode array(s) and/or to confirm the functional status of the system is inherent to placement, and is not separately reported as electronic analysis or programming of the neurostimulator system. Electronic analysis (95970) at the time of implantation is not separately reported.

Codes 64553, 64555, and 64561 may be used to report both temporary and permanent placement of percutaneous electrode arrays.

AMA Coding Notes

Neurostimulator Procedures on the Peripheral Nerves

(For transcutaneous nerve stimulation [TENS], use 97014 for electrical stimulation requiring supervision only or use 97032 for electrical stimulation requiring constant attendance)

Surgical Procedures on the Extracranial Nerves, Peripheral Nerves, and Autonomic Nervous System

(For intracranial surgery on cranial nerves, see 61450, 61460, 61790)

AMA *CPT Assistant* □

64581: Dec 12: 14, Sep 14: 5

Plain English Description

Direct transforaminal sacral nerve stimulation is used to treat voiding dysfunction, including urge incontinence, urgency, frequency, and nonobstructive urinary retention. For open transforaminal implantation of a sacral nerve neurostimulator electrode array, the skin is prepped and a local anesthetic is injected into the skin and periosteum of the sacrum. The skin over the sacrum is incised in the midline. Overlying tissue is dissected and the sacrum is exposed. A foramen needle is inserted into the selected sacral foramen. A power source is connected to the needle; stimulation is applied; and the motor responses are evaluated as the position of the needle is changed until the desired response is achieved. The needle is disconnected from the power source and removed. An electrode array is then passed through the foramen and positioned in the desired location next to the sacral nerve. Correct placement is verified by testing motor response to stimulation. The electrode array is tunneled to the site of the generator/receiver which is implanted in a separately reportable procedure. The presacral fascia is closed over the electrode array, followed by closure of the subcutaneous tissue and skin.

Incision for implantation of neurostimulator electrode array; sacral nerve

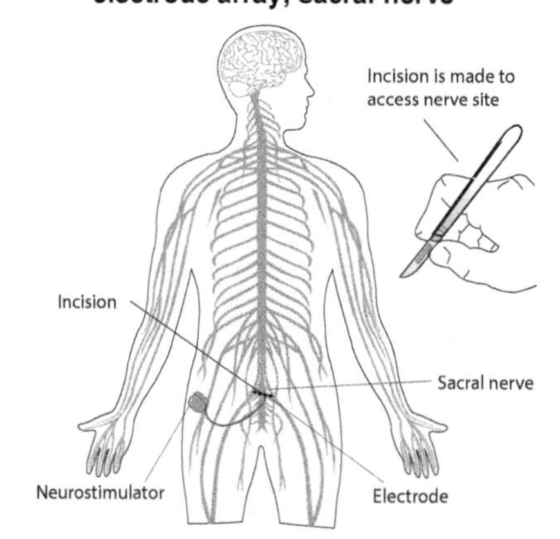

ICD-10-CM Diagnostic Codes

	G83.4	Cauda equina syndrome
	G95.89	Other specified diseases of spinal cord
	N31.0	Uninhibited neuropathic bladder, not elsewhere classified
	N31.1	Reflex neuropathic bladder, not elsewhere classified
	N31.2	Flaccid neuropathic bladder, not elsewhere classified
	N31.8	Other neuromuscular dysfunction of bladder
	N31.9	Neuromuscular dysfunction of bladder, unspecified
	N39.41	Urge incontinence
	N39.42	Incontinence without sensory awareness
	N39.43	Post-void dribbling
	N39.44	Nocturnal enuresis
	N39.45	Continuous leakage
	N39.46	Mixed incontinence
	N39.490	Overflow incontinence
	N39.498	Other specified urinary incontinence
	N39.8	Other specified disorders of urinary system
	R32	Unspecified urinary incontinence
	R33.8	Other retention of urine
	R33.9	Retention of urine, unspecified
	R35.0	Frequency of micturition
	R35.1	Nocturia
	R35.8	Other polyuria
❼	S34.3	Injury of cauda equina

ICD-10-CM Coding Notes

For codes requiring a 7th character extension, refer to your ICD-10-CM book. Review the character descriptions and coding guidelines for proper selection. For some procedures, only certain characters will apply.

CCI Edits

Refer to Appendix A for CCI edits.

Pub 100

64581: Pub 100-04, 32, 40.2.1

Facility RVUs □

Code	Work	PE Facility	MP	Total Facility
64581	12.20	5.47	1.42	19.09

Non-facility RVUs □

Code	Work	PE Non-Facility	MP	Total Non-Facility
64581	12.20	5.47	1.42	19.09

Modifiers (PAR) □

Code	Mod 50	Mod 51	Mod 62	Mod 66	Mod 80
64581	0	2	0	0	1

Global Period

Code	Days
64581	090

CPT © 2018 American Medical Association. All Rights Reserved.

64585

64585 Revision or removal of peripheral neurostimulator electrode array

AMA Coding Guideline

Neurostimulator Procedures on the Peripheral Nerves

For electronic analysis with programming, when performed, of peripheral nerve neurostimulator pulse generator/transmitters, see codes 95970, 95971, 95972. An electrode array is a catheter or other device with more than one contact. The function of each contact may be capable of being adjusted during programming services. Test stimulation to confirm correct target site placement of the electrode array(s) and/or to confirm the functional status of the system is inherent to placement, and is not separately reported as electronic analysis or programming of the neurostimulator system. Electronic analysis (95970) at the time of implantation is not separately reported.

Codes 64553, 64555, and 64561 may be used to report both temporary and permanent placement of percutaneous electrode arrays.

AMA Coding Notes

Neurostimulator Procedures on the Peripheral Nerves

(For transcutaneous nerve stimulation [TENS], use 97014 for electrical stimulation requiring supervision only or use 97032 for electrical stimulation requiring constant attendance)

Surgical Procedures on the Extracranial Nerves, Peripheral Nerves, and Autonomic Nervous System

(For intracranial surgery on cranial nerves, see 61450, 61460, 61790)

Plain English Description

The exact revision or removal procedure depends on the location of the existing peripheral neurostimulator electrode array. A skin incision is made over the existing array. Soft tissues are dissected and the electrode array is exposed. The device is inspected and detached from the generator/receiver. The array is tested and any malfunctioning components are replaced. The array is then positioned in the desired location next to the peripheral nerve. Correct placement is verified by testing motor response to stimulation. The electrode array is reconnected to the generator/receiver. Alternatively, the array may be removed and the surgical wound closed in layers.

Revision or removal of peripheral neurostimulator electrode array

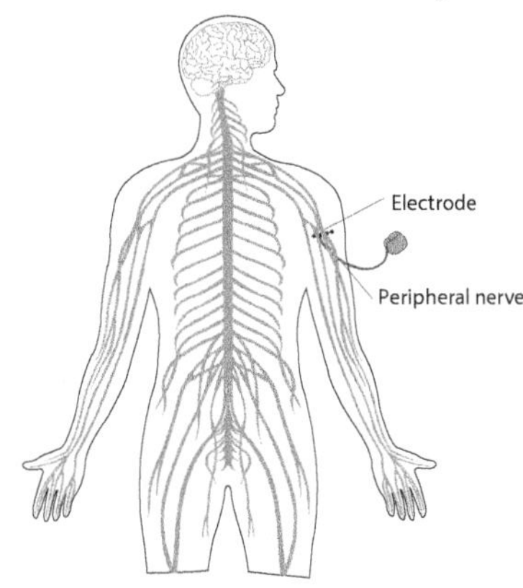

The electrodes used to stimulate the peripheral nervous tissues are removed or revised.

ICD-10-CM Diagnostic Codes

➐	T85.111	Breakdown (mechanical) of implanted electronic neurostimulator of peripheral nerve electrode (lead)
➐	T85.121	Displacement of implanted electronic neurostimulator of peripheral nerve electrode (lead)
➐	T85.191	Other mechanical complication of implanted electronic neurostimulator of peripheral nerve electrode (lead)
➐	T85.732	Infection and inflammatory reaction due to implanted electronic neurostimulator of peripheral nerve, electrode (lead)
➐	T85.810	Embolism due to nervous system prosthetic devices, implants and grafts
➐	T85.820	Fibrosis due to nervous system prosthetic devices, implants and grafts
➐	T85.830	Hemorrhage due to nervous system prosthetic devices, implants and grafts
➐	T85.840	Pain due to nervous system prosthetic devices, implants and grafts
➐	T85.850	Stenosis due to nervous system prosthetic devices, implants and grafts
➐	T85.860	Thrombosis due to nervous system prosthetic devices, implants and grafts
➐	T85.890	Other specified complication of nervous system prosthetic devices, implants and grafts
	Z45.42	Encounter for adjustment and management of neuropacemaker (brain) (peripheral nerve) (spinal cord)
	Z45.49	Encounter for adjustment and management of other implanted nervous system device
	Z46.2	Encounter for fitting and adjustment of other devices related to nervous system and special senses

ICD-10-CM Coding Notes

For codes requiring a 7th character extension, refer to your ICD-10-CM book. Review the character descriptions and coding guidelines for proper selection. For some procedures, only certain characters will apply.

CCI Edits

Refer to Appendix A for CCI edits.

Pub 100

64585: Pub 100-03, 1, 160.19, Pub 100-03, 1, 160.7-160.7.1, Pub 100-04, 32, 40.2.1

Facility RVUs ▯

Code	Work	PE Facility	MP	Total Facility
64585	2.11	1.76	0.27	4.14

Non-facility RVUs ▯

Code	Work	PE Non-Facility	MP	Total Non-Facility
64585	2.11	4.65	0.27	7.03

Modifiers (PAR) ▯

Code	Mod 50	Mod 51	Mod 62	Mod 66	Mod 80
64585	0	2	0	0	1

Global Period

Code	Days
64585	010

CPT © 2018 American Medical Association. All Rights Reserved.

64590

64590 Insertion or replacement of peripheral or gastric neurostimulator pulse generator or receiver, direct or inductive coupling

(Do not report 64590 in conjunction with 64595)

AMA Coding Guideline

Neurostimulator Procedures on the Peripheral Nerves

For electronic analysis with programming, when performed, of peripheral nerve neurostimulator pulse generator/transmitters, see codes 95970, 95971, 95972. An electrode array is a catheter or other device with more than one contact. The function of each contact may be capable of being adjusted during programming services. Test stimulation to confirm correct target site placement of the electrode array(s) and/or to confirm the functional status of the system is inherent to placement, and is not separately reported as electronic analysis or programming of the neurostimulator system. Electronic analysis (95970) at the time of implantation is not separately reported.

Codes 64553, 64555, and 64561 may be used to report both temporary and permanent placement of percutaneous electrode arrays.

AMA Coding Notes

Neurostimulator Procedures on the Peripheral Nerves

(For transcutaneous nerve stimulation [TENS], use 97014 for electrical stimulation requiring supervision only or use 97032 for electrical stimulation requiring constant attendance)

Surgical Procedures on the Extracranial Nerves, Peripheral Nerves, and Autonomic Nervous System

(For intracranial surgery on cranial nerves, see 61450, 61460, 61790)

AMA *CPT Assistant* ▢

64590: Sep 99: 4, Apr 01: 8, Mar 07: 4, Apr 07: 7, Sep 11: 9, Dec 12: 14, Jan 15: 14, Dec 17: 16, Aug 18: 10

Plain English Description

The physician inserts or replaces a pulse generator or receiver under the skin. The device is connected to an electrode(s) using direct or inductive coupling, and is used to stimulate peripheral nervous tissue, or gastric tissue.

Insertion or replacement of peripheral or gastric neurostimulator pulse generator or receiver

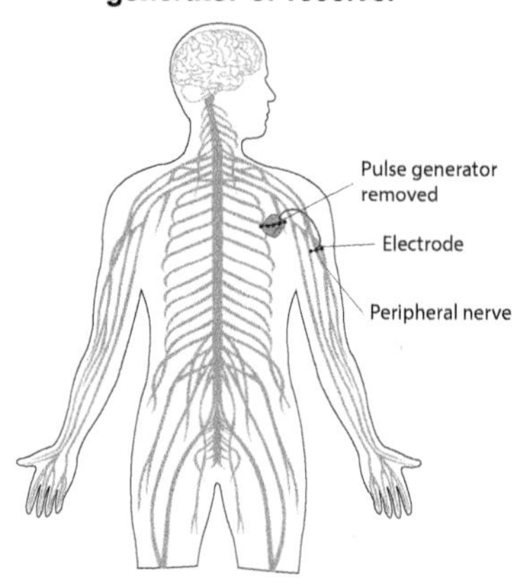

ICD-10-CM Diagnostic Codes

	B02.23	Postherpetic polyneuropathy
	B02.24	Postherpetic myelitis
	B02.29	Other postherpetic nervous system involvement
	G54.6	Phantom limb syndrome with pain
⇄	G56.01	Carpal tunnel syndrome, right upper limb
⇄	G56.02	Carpal tunnel syndrome, left upper limb
⇄	G56.03	Carpal tunnel syndrome, bilateral upper limbs
⇄	G56.11	Other lesions of median nerve, right upper limb
⇄	G56.12	Other lesions of median nerve, left upper limb
⇄	G56.13	Other lesions of median nerve, bilateral upper limbs
⇄	G56.21	Lesion of ulnar nerve, right upper limb
⇄	G56.22	Lesion of ulnar nerve, left upper limb
⇄	G56.23	Lesion of ulnar nerve, bilateral upper limbs
⇄	G56.31	Lesion of radial nerve, right upper limb
⇄	G56.32	Lesion of radial nerve, left upper limb
⇄	G56.33	Lesion of radial nerve, bilateral upper limbs
⇄	G56.41	Causalgia of right upper limb
⇄	G56.42	Causalgia of left upper limb
⇄	G56.43	Causalgia of bilateral upper limbs
⇄	G56.81	Other specified mononeuropathies of right upper limb
⇄	G56.82	Other specified mononeuropathies of left upper limb
⇄	G56.83	Other specified mononeuropathies of bilateral upper limbs
⇄	G57.01	Lesion of sciatic nerve, right lower limb
⇄	G57.02	Lesion of sciatic nerve, left lower limb
⇄	G57.11	Meralgia paresthetica, right lower limb
⇄	G57.12	Meralgia paresthetica, left lower limb
⇄	G57.21	Lesion of femoral nerve, right lower limb
⇄	G57.22	Lesion of femoral nerve, left lower limb
⇄	G57.31	Lesion of lateral popliteal nerve, right lower limb
⇄	G57.32	Lesion of lateral popliteal nerve, left lower limb
⇄	G57.41	Lesion of medial popliteal nerve, right lower limb
⇄	G57.42	Lesion of medial popliteal nerve, left lower limb
⇄	G57.71	Causalgia of right lower limb
⇄	G57.72	Causalgia of left lower limb
⇄	G57.81	Other specified mononeuropathies of right lower limb
⇄	G57.82	Other specified mononeuropathies of left lower limb
	G58.0	Intercostal neuropathy
	G58.9	Mononeuropathy, unspecified
	G89.21	Chronic pain due to trauma
	G89.22	Chronic post-thoracotomy pain
	G89.28	Other chronic postprocedural pain
	G89.29	Other chronic pain
	G89.4	Chronic pain syndrome
⇄	G90.511	Complex regional pain syndrome I of right upper limb
⇄	G90.512	Complex regional pain syndrome I of left upper limb
⇄	G90.513	Complex regional pain syndrome I of upper limb, bilateral
⇄	G90.521	Complex regional pain syndrome I of right lower limb
⇄	G90.522	Complex regional pain syndrome I of left lower limb
⇄	G90.523	Complex regional pain syndrome I of lower limb, bilateral
	M79.2	Neuralgia and neuritis, unspecified
⇄	M79.601	Pain in right arm
⇄	M79.602	Pain in left arm
⇄	M79.604	Pain in right leg
⇄	M79.605	Pain in left leg
⇄	M79.621	Pain in right upper arm
⇄	M79.622	Pain in left upper arm
⇄	M79.631	Pain in right forearm
⇄	M79.632	Pain in left forearm
⇄	M79.651	Pain in right thigh
⇄	M79.652	Pain in left thigh
⇄	M79.661	Pain in right lower leg
⇄	M79.662	Pain in left lower leg
❼	T85.113	Breakdown (mechanical) of implanted electronic neurostimulator, generator
❼	T85.123	Displacement of implanted electronic neurostimulator, generator
❼	T85.193	Other mechanical complication of implanted electronic neurostimulator, generator
❼	T85.734	Infection and inflammatory reaction due to implanted electronic neurostimulator, generator
❼	T85.830	Hemorrhage due to nervous system prosthetic devices, implants and grafts
❼	T85.840	Pain due to nervous system prosthetic devices, implants and grafts
❼	T85.850	Stenosis due to nervous system prosthetic devices, implants and grafts

CPT © 2018 American Medical Association. All Rights Reserved.

➐	T85.890	Other specified complication of nervous system prosthetic devices, implants and grafts
	Z45.42	Encounter for adjustment and management of neuropacemaker (brain) (peripheral nerve) (spinal cord)
	Z45.49	Encounter for adjustment and management of other implanted nervous system device
	Z46.2	Encounter for fitting and adjustment of other devices related to nervous system and special senses

ICD-10-CM Coding Notes

For codes requiring a 7th character extension, refer to your ICD-10-CM book. Review the character descriptions and coding guidelines for proper selection. For some procedures, only certain characters will apply.

CCI Edits

Refer to Appendix A for CCI edits.

Pub 100

64590: Pub 100-04, 32, 40.2.1

Facility RVUs ☐

Code	Work	PE Facility	MP	Total Facility
64590	2.45	1.87	0.32	4.64

Non-facility RVUs ☐

Code	Work	PE Non-Facility	MP	Total Non-Facility
64590	2.45	4.83	0.32	7.60

Modifiers (PAR) ☐

Code	Mod 50	Mod 51	Mod 62	Mod 66	Mod 80
64590	0	2	1	0	1

Global Period

Code	Days
64590	010

CPT © 2018 American Medical Association. All Rights Reserved.

CPT® Procedural Coding

64595

64595 Revision or removal of peripheral or gastric neurostimulator pulse generator or receiver

AMA Coding Guideline

Neurostimulator Procedures on the Peripheral Nerves

For electronic analysis with programming, when performed, of peripheral nerve neurostimulator pulse generator/transmitters, see codes 95970, 95971, 95972. An electrode array is a catheter or other device with more than one contact. The function of each contact may be capable of being adjusted during programming services. Test stimulation to confirm correct target site placement of the electrode array(s) and/or to confirm the functional status of the system is inherent to placement, and is not separately reported as electronic analysis or programming of the neurostimulator system. Electronic analysis (95970) at the time of implantation is not separately reported.

Codes 64553, 64555, and 64561 may be used to report both temporary and permanent placement of percutaneous electrode arrays.

AMA Coding Notes

Neurostimulator Procedures on the Peripheral Nerves

(For transcutaneous nerve stimulation [TENS], use 97014 for electrical stimulation requiring supervision only or use 97032 for electrical stimulation requiring constant attendance)

Surgical Procedures on the Extracranial Nerves, Peripheral Nerves, and Autonomic Nervous System

(For intracranial surgery on cranial nerves, see 61450, 61460, 61790)

AMA *CPT Assistant*

64595: Sep 99: 3, Mar 07: 4, Jan 08: 8

Plain English Description

The physician removes or revises a pulse generator or receiver which is located under the skin and connected to an electrode used to stimulate peripheral nervous tissue or gastric tissue.

Revision or removal of peripheral or gastric neurostimulator pulse generator or receiver

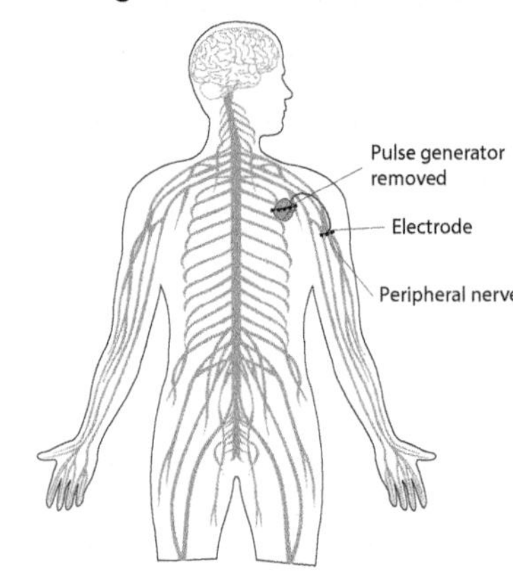

ICD-10-CM Diagnostic Codes

➐	T85.113	Breakdown (mechanical) of implanted electronic neurostimulator, generator
➐	T85.123	Displacement of implanted electronic neurostimulator, generator
➐	T85.193	Other mechanical complication of implanted electronic neurostimulator, generator
➐	T85.734	Infection and inflammatory reaction due to implanted electronic neurostimulator, generator
➐	T85.820	Fibrosis due to nervous system prosthetic devices, implants and grafts
➐	T85.830	Hemorrhage due to nervous system prosthetic devices, implants and grafts
➐	T85.840	Pain due to nervous system prosthetic devices, implants and grafts
➐	T85.890	Other specified complication of nervous system prosthetic devices, implants and grafts
	Z45.42	Encounter for adjustment and management of neuropacemaker (brain) (peripheral nerve) (spinal cord)
	Z45.49	Encounter for adjustment and management of other implanted nervous system device
	Z46.2	Encounter for fitting and adjustment of other devices related to nervous system and special senses

ICD-10-CM Coding Notes

For codes requiring a 7th character extension, refer to your ICD-10-CM book. Review the character descriptions and coding guidelines for proper selection. For some procedures, only certain characters will apply.

CCI Edits

Refer to Appendix A for CCI edits.

Pub 100

64595: Pub 100-04, 32, 40.2.1

Facility RVUs

Code	Work	PE Facility	MP	Total Facility
64595	1.78	1.62	0.23	3.63

Non-facility RVUs

Code	Work	PE Non-Facility	MP	Total Non-Facility
64595	1.78	4.88	0.23	6.89

Modifiers (PAR)

Code	Mod 50	Mod 51	Mod 62	Mod 66	Mod 80
64595	0	2	0	0	1

Global Period

Code	Days
64595	010

CPT © 2018 American Medical Association. All Rights Reserved.

64600-64610

64600 Destruction by neurolytic agent, trigeminal nerve; supraorbital, infraorbital, mental, or inferior alveolar branch

64605 Destruction by neurolytic agent, trigeminal nerve; second and third division branches at foramen ovale

64610 Destruction by neurolytic agent, trigeminal nerve; second and third division branches at foramen ovale under radiologic monitoring

AMA Coding Guideline

Destruction by Neurolytic Agent (eg, Chemical, Thermal, Electrical or Radiofrequency) and Chemodenervation Procedures on the Extracranial Nerves, Peripheral Nerves, and Autonomic Nervous System

Codes 64600-64681 include the injection of other therapeutic agents (eg, corticosteroids). Do not report diagnostic/therapeutic injections separately. Do not report a code labeled as destruction when using therapies that are not destructive of the target nerve (eg, pulsed radiofrequency), use 64999. For codes labeled as chemodenervation, the supply of the chemodenervation agent is reported separately.

AMA Coding Notes

Destruction by Neurolytic Agent (eg, Chemical, Thermal, Electrical or Radiofrequency) and Chemodenervation Procedures on the Extracranial Nerves, Peripheral Nerves, and Autonomic Nervous System

(For chemodenervation of internal anal sphincter, use 46505)

(For chemodenervation of the bladder, use 52287)

(For chemodenervation for strabismus involving the extraocular muscles, use 67345)

(For chemodenervation guided by needle electromyography or muscle electrical stimulation, see 95873, 95874)

Surgical Procedures on the Extracranial Nerves, Peripheral Nerves, and Autonomic Nervous System

(For intracranial surgery on cranial nerves, see 61450, 61460, 61790)

AMA *CPT Assistant* ▯

64600: Aug 05: 13, Feb 10: 9, Sep 12: 14

64605: Aug 05: 13, Feb 10: 9, Sep 12: 14

64610: Aug 05: 13, Feb 10: 9, Sep 12: 14, Apr 17: 10

Plain English Description

Destruction of a nerve is performed to treat chronic pain and may be performed by injection of a chemical neurolytic agent or using thermal, electrical or radiofrequency techniques. The most common technique used today is radiofrequency destruction, although the other techniques may also be used for certain pain syndromes. Prior to the destruction procedure, an electrode needle is introduced through the skin and advanced toward the targeted neural tissue. The needle is connected to a generator for motor and sensory testing performed to ensure that the needle is correctly positioned at the nerve responsible for the pain. Once the correct nerve pathway has been identified, the nerve is destroyed. If a chemical agent is used, the chemical agent is injected along the nerve pathway. Neurolytic chemical agents include: phenol, ethyl alcohol, glycerol, ammonium salt compounds and hypertonic or hypotonic solutions. Thermal or electrical modalities involve the use of a probe or needle that is inserted through the skin and activated to produce heat and destroy nerve tissue. To perform radiofrequency nerve destruction, an electrode needle is introduced through the skin and advanced toward the targeted neural tissue. The electrode is adjusted as needed until correct positioning is achieved. The radiofrequency device is then activated and an electric current generated that produces heat at the tip of the electrode and destroys the targeted nerve tissue. Use 64600 for destruction of the supraorbital, infraorbital, mental, or inferior alveolar branch of the trigeminal nerve. For second or third division branches of the trigeminal nerve at the foramen ovale use 64605 when the procedure is performed without the use of radiologic monitoring; use 64610 when the procedure is performed with radiologic monitoring.

Destruction by neurolytic agent, trigeminal nerve

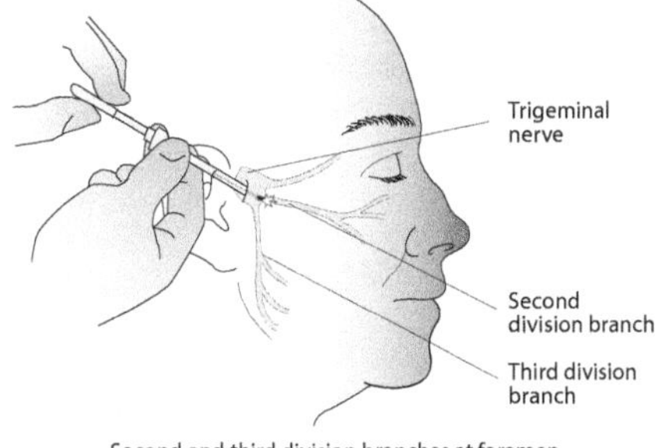

Second and third division branches at foramen ovale (64605); under radiologic monitoring (64610)

ICD-10-CM Diagnostic Codes

C03.0	Malignant neoplasm of upper gum
C03.1	Malignant neoplasm of lower gum
C04.0	Malignant neoplasm of anterior floor of mouth
C04.1	Malignant neoplasm of lateral floor of mouth
C04.8	Malignant neoplasm of overlapping sites of floor of mouth
C05.0	Malignant neoplasm of hard palate
C05.1	Malignant neoplasm of soft palate
C05.2	Malignant neoplasm of uvula
C05.8	Malignant neoplasm of overlapping sites of palate
C06.0	Malignant neoplasm of cheek mucosa
C06.1	Malignant neoplasm of vestibule of mouth
C06.2	Malignant neoplasm of retromolar area
C06.80	Malignant neoplasm of overlapping sites of unspecified parts of mouth
C07	Malignant neoplasm of parotid gland
C08.0	Malignant neoplasm of submandibular gland
C08.1	Malignant neoplasm of sublingual gland
C31.0	Malignant neoplasm of maxillary sinus
C41.0	Malignant neoplasm of bones of skull and face
C41.1	Malignant neoplasm of mandible
C76.0	Malignant neoplasm of head, face and neck
G89.3	Neoplasm related pain (acute) (chronic)

CCI Edits

Refer to Appendix A for CCI edits.

Facility RVUs ▯

Code	Work	PE Facility	MP	Total Facility
64600	3.49	2.43	0.74	6.66
64605	5.65	3.40	1.04	10.09
64610	7.20	4.63	2.44	14.27

Non-facility RVUs ▯

Code	Work	PE Non-Facility	MP	Total Non-Facility
64600	3.49	8.12	0.74	12.35
64605	5.65	10.20	1.04	16.89
64610	7.20	12.45	2.44	22.09

Modifiers (PAR) ▯

Code	Mod 50	Mod 51	Mod 62	Mod 66	Mod 80
64600	2	2	0	0	1
64605	1	2	0	0	0
64610	1	2	0	0	1

Global Period

Code	Days
64600	010
64605	010
64610	010

CPT © 2018 American Medical Association. All Rights Reserved.

64612

64612 Chemodenervation of muscle(s); muscle(s) innervated by facial nerve, unilateral (eg, for blepharospasm, hemifacial spasm)

(For bilateral procedure, report 64612 with modifier 50)

AMA Coding Guideline

Destruction by Neurolytic Agent (eg, Chemical, Thermal, Electrical or Radiofrequency) and Chemodenervation Procedures on the Extracranial Nerves, Peripheral Nerves, and Autonomic Nervous System

Codes 64600-64681 include the injection of other therapeutic agents (eg, corticosteroids). Do not report diagnostic/therapeutic injections separately. Do not report a code labeled as destruction when using therapies that are not destructive of the target nerve (eg, pulsed radiofrequency), use 64999. For codes labeled as chemodenervation, the supply of the chemodenervation agent is reported separately.

AMA Coding Notes

Destruction by Neurolytic Agent (eg, Chemical, Thermal, Electrical or Radiofrequency) and Chemodenervation Procedures on the Extracranial Nerves, Peripheral Nerves, and Autonomic Nervous System

(For chemodenervation of internal anal sphincter, use 46505)

(For chemodenervation of the bladder, use 52287)

(For chemodenervation for strabismus involving the extraocular muscles, use 67345)

(For chemodenervation guided by needle electromyography or muscle electrical stimulation, see 95873, 95874)

Surgical Procedures on the Extracranial Nerves, Peripheral Nerves, and Autonomic Nervous System

(For intracranial surgery on cranial nerves, see 61450, 61460, 61790)

AMA *CPT Assistant* ▢

64612: Oct 98: 10, Apr 01: 2, Aug 05: 13, Sep 06: 5, Dec 08: 9, Jan 09: 8, Feb 10: 9, 13, Dec 11: 19, Sep 12: 14, Apr 13: 5, Dec 13: 10, Jan 14: 6, May 14: 5

Plain English Description

Chemodenervation is performed on muscles innervated by the facial nerve unilaterally to treat involuntary muscle contractions or muscle spasms, such as blepharospasm or for treatment of hemifacial pain. Injection of botulinum toxin (type A or B) directly into a muscle produces temporary muscle paralysis by blocking the release of acetylcholine at the peripheral nerve endings which interrupts neuromuscular transmission of nerve impulses. The muscle and the specific muscle sites to be injected are determined either by use of electromyography or by examining and palpating the facial muscles and noting the location of the muscle spasm. The side of the face to be treated is prepped. The affected muscle or muscle group is then injected at carefully selected sites to accomplish the denervation.

Chemodenervation of muscle(s)

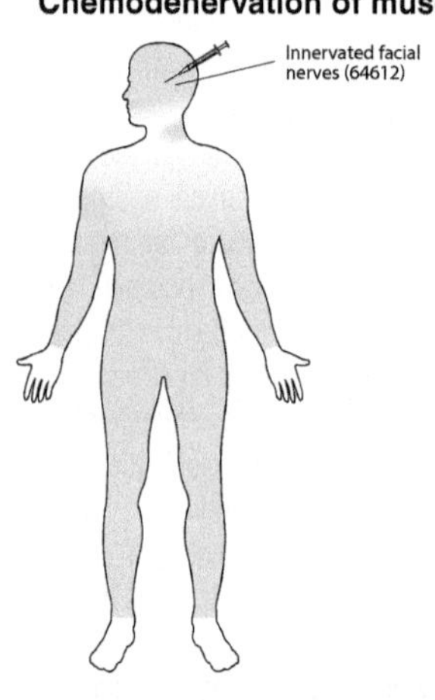

ICD-10-CM Diagnostic Codes

	G11.4	Hereditary spastic paraplegia
	G20	Parkinson's disease
	G24.1	Genetic torsion dystonia
	G24.4	Idiopathic orofacial dystonia
	G24.5	Blepharospasm
	G35	Multiple sclerosis
	G51.2	Melkersson's syndrome
⇄	G51.31	Clonic hemifacial spasm, right
⇄	G51.32	Clonic hemifacial spasm, left
⇄	G51.33	Clonic hemifacial spasm, bilateral
⇄	G51.39	Clonic hemifacial spasm, unspecified
	G51.4	Facial myokymia
	G51.8	Other disorders of facial nerve
	G51.9	Disorder of facial nerve, unspecified
	P11.3	Birth injury to facial nerve

CCI Edits

Refer to Appendix A for CCI edits.

Facility RVUs ▢

Code	Work	PE Facility	MP	Total Facility
64612	1.41	1.68	0.30	3.39

Non-facility RVUs ▢

Code	Work	PE Non-Facility	MP	Total Non-Facility
64612	1.41	2.12	0.30	3.83

Modifiers (PAR) ▢

Code	Mod 50	Mod 51	Mod 62	Mod 66	Mod 80
64612	1	2	0	0	1

Global Period

Code	Days
64612	010

● New ▲ Revised ✚ Add On ⊘Modifier 51 Exempt ★Telemedicine ▢ CPT QuickRef FDA Pending ⇄ Laterality Seventh Character ♂Male ♀Female

CPT © 2018 American Medical Association. All Rights Reserved.

64615

64615 Chemodenervation of muscle(s); muscle(s) innervated by facial, trigeminal, cervical spinal and accessory nerves, bilateral (eg, for chronic migraine)

(Report 64615 only once per session)

(Do not report 64615 in conjunction with 64612, 64616, 64617, 64642, 64643, 64644, 64645, 64646, 64647)

(For guidance see 95873, 95874. Do not report more than one guidance code for 64615)

AMA Coding Guideline

Destruction by Neurolytic Agent (eg, Chemical, Thermal, Electrical or Radiofrequency) and Chemodenervation Procedures on the Extracranial Nerves, Peripheral Nerves, and Autonomic Nervous System

Codes 64600-64681 include the injection of other therapeutic agents (eg, corticosteroids). Do not report diagnostic/therapeutic injections separately. Do not report a code labeled as destruction when using therapies that are not destructive of the target nerve (eg, pulsed radiofrequency), use 64999. For codes labeled as chemodenervation, the supply of the chemodenervation agent is reported separately.

AMA Coding Notes

Destruction by Neurolytic Agent (eg, Chemical, Thermal, Electrical or Radiofrequency) and Chemodenervation Procedures on the Extracranial Nerves, Peripheral Nerves, and Autonomic Nervous System

(For chemodenervation of internal anal sphincter, use 46505)

(For chemodenervation of the bladder, use 52287)

(For chemodenervation for strabismus involving the extraocular muscles, use 67345)

(For chemodenervation guided by needle electromyography or muscle electrical stimulation, see 95873, 95874)

Surgical Procedures on the Extracranial Nerves, Peripheral Nerves, and Autonomic Nervous System

(For intracranial surgery on cranial nerves, see 61450, 61460, 61790)

AMA *CPT Assistant* ☐

64615: Apr 13: 5, Jan 14: 6

Plain English Description

Chemical denervation involves the injection of a toxin (type A botulinum) directly into a muscle to produce temporary muscle paralysis by blocking the release of acetylcholine. Botulinum toxin injections have been shown to be effective in the prevention of migraines by blocking the neurotransmitter responsible for muscle contractions and pain. To perform chemical denervation of the muscles innervated by the facial, trigeminal, cervical spinal and accessory nerves small doses of Botox are injected bilaterally into muscles of the forehead, the side and back of the head, and the neck and shoulders.

ICD-10-CM Diagnostic Codes

G43.001	Migraine without aura, not intractable, with status migrainosus
G43.011	Migraine without aura, intractable, with status migrainosus
G43.019	Migraine without aura, intractable, without status migrainosus
G43.101	Migraine with aura, not intractable, with status migrainosus
G43.111	Migraine with aura, intractable, with status migrainosus
G43.119	Migraine with aura, intractable, without status migrainosus
G43.401	Hemiplegic migraine, not intractable, with status migrainosus
G43.411	Hemiplegic migraine, intractable, with status migrainosus
G43.419	Hemiplegic migraine, intractable, without status migrainosus
G43.501	Persistent migraine aura without cerebral infarction, not intractable, with status migrainosus
G43.511	Persistent migraine aura without cerebral infarction, intractable, with status migrainosus
G43.519	Persistent migraine aura without cerebral infarction, intractable, without status migrainosus
G43.701	Chronic migraine without aura, not intractable, with status migrainosus
G43.711	Chronic migraine without aura, intractable, with status migrainosus
G43.719	Chronic migraine without aura, intractable, without status migrainosus
G43.801	Other migraine, not intractable, with status migrainosus
G43.811	Other migraine, intractable, with status migrainosus
G43.819	Other migraine, intractable, without status migrainosus
G43.901	Migraine, unspecified, not intractable, with status migrainosus
G43.911	Migraine, unspecified, intractable, with status migrainosus
G43.919	Migraine, unspecified, intractable, without status migrainosus

CCI Edits

Refer to Appendix A for CCI edits.

Facility RVUs ☐

Code	Work	PE Facility	MP	Total Facility
64615	1.85	1.12	0.61	3.58

Non-facility RVUs ☐

Code	Work	PE Non-Facility	MP	Total Non-Facility
64615	1.85	1.81	0.61	4.27

Modifiers (PAR) ☐

Code	Mod 50	Mod 51	Mod 62	Mod 66	Mod 80
64615	2	2	0	0	1

Global Period

Code	Days
64615	010

CPT © 2018 American Medical Association. All Rights Reserved.

64616

64616 Chemodenervation of muscle(s); neck muscle(s), excluding muscles of the larynx, unilateral (eg, for cervical dystonia, spasmodic torticollis)

(For bilateral procedure, report 64616 with modifier 50)

(For chemodenervation guided by needle electromyography or muscle electrical stimulation, see 95873, 95874. Do not report more than one guidance code for any unit of 64616)

AMA Coding Guideline

Destruction by Neurolytic Agent (eg, Chemical, Thermal, Electrical or Radiofrequency) and Chemodenervation Procedures on the Extracranial Nerves, Peripheral Nerves, and Autonomic Nervous System

Codes 64600-64681 include the injection of other therapeutic agents (eg, corticosteroids). Do not report diagnostic/therapeutic injections separately. Do not report a code labeled as destruction when using therapies that are not destructive of the target nerve (eg, pulsed radiofrequency), use 64999. For codes labeled as chemodenervation, the supply of the chemodenervation agent is reported separately.

AMA Coding Notes

Destruction by Neurolytic Agent (eg, Chemical, Thermal, Electrical or Radiofrequency) and Chemodenervation Procedures on the Extracranial Nerves, Peripheral Nerves, and Autonomic Nervous System

(For chemodenervation of internal anal sphincter, use 46505)

(For chemodenervation of the bladder, use 52287)

(For chemodenervation for strabismus involving the extraocular muscles, use 67345)

(For chemodenervation guided by needle electromyography or muscle electrical stimulation, see 95873, 95874)

Surgical Procedures on the Extracranial Nerves, Peripheral Nerves, and Autonomic Nervous System

(For intracranial surgery on cranial nerves, see 61450, 61460, 61790)

AMA *CPT Assistant* □

64616: Jan 14: 6, May 14: 5

Plain English Description

Chemodenervation is performed on neck muscles unilaterally to treat involuntary muscle contractions or muscle spasms in the neck. This condition may be referred to as cervical dystonia or spasmodic torticollis. Injection of botulinum toxin (type A or B) directly into a muscle produces temporary muscle paralysis by blocking the release of acetylcholine at the peripheral nerve endings which interrupts neuromuscular transmission of nerve impulses. The muscle and the specific muscle sites to be injected are determined either by use of electromyography or by examining the position of the head, palpating the neck muscles, and noting the location of the muscle spasm. The side of the neck to be treated is prepped. The affected muscle or muscle group is then injected at carefully selected sites to accomplish the denervation.

ICD-10-CM Diagnostic Codes

G24.02	Drug induced acute dystonia
G24.1	Genetic torsion dystonia
G24.2	Idiopathic nonfamilial dystonia
G24.3	Spasmodic torticollis
G24.8	Other dystonia
G89.21	Chronic pain due to trauma
G89.28	Other chronic postprocedural pain
G89.29	Other chronic pain
G89.3	Neoplasm related pain (acute) (chronic)
M54.2	Cervicalgia

CCI Edits

Refer to Appendix A for CCI edits.

Facility RVUs □

Code	Work	PE Facility	MP	Total Facility
64616	1.53	1.13	0.52	3.18

Non-facility RVUs □

Code	Work	PE Non-Facility	MP	Total Non-Facility
64616	1.53	1.75	0.52	3.80

Modifiers (PAR) □

Code	Mod 50	Mod 51	Mod 62	Mod 66	Mod 80
64616	1	2	0	0	1

Global Period

Code	Days
64616	010

CPT © 2018 American Medical Association. All Rights Reserved.

64620

64620 Destruction by neurolytic agent, intercostal nerve

AMA Coding Guideline

Destruction by Neurolytic Agent (eg, Chemical, Thermal, Electrical or Radiofrequency) and Chemodenervation Procedures on the Extracranial Nerves, Peripheral Nerves, and Autonomic Nervous System

Codes 64600-64681 include the injection of other therapeutic agents (eg, corticosteroids). Do not report diagnostic/therapeutic injections separately. Do not report a code labeled as destruction when using therapies that are not destructive of the target nerve (eg, pulsed radiofrequency), use 64999. For codes labeled as chemodenervation, the supply of the chemodenervation agent is reported separately.

AMA Coding Notes

Destruction by Neurolytic Agent (eg, Chemical, Thermal, Electrical or Radiofrequency) and Chemodenervation Procedures on the Extracranial Nerves, Peripheral Nerves, and Autonomic Nervous System

(For chemodenervation of internal anal sphincter, use 46505)

(For chemodenervation of the bladder, use 52287)

(For chemodenervation for strabismus involving the extraocular muscles, use 67345)

(For chemodenervation guided by needle electromyography or muscle electrical stimulation, see 95873, 95874)

Surgical Procedures on the Extracranial Nerves, Peripheral Nerves, and Autonomic Nervous System

(For intracranial surgery on cranial nerves, see 61450, 61460, 61790)

AMA *CPT Assistant* ▢

64620: Nov 99: 38, Aug 05: 13, Sep 12: 14, Jan 14: 6

Plain English Description

Destruction of an intercostal nerve is performed to treat chronic pain and may be performed by injection of a chemical neurolytic agent or using thermal, electrical or radiofrequency techniques. The most common technique used today is radiofrequency destruction, although the other techniques may also be used for certain pain syndromes. Prior to the destruction procedure, an electrode needle is introduced through the skin and advanced toward the targeted neural tissue. The needle is connected to a generator for motor and sensory testing performed to ensure that the needle is correctly positioned at the nerve responsible for the pain. Once the correct nerve pathway has been identified, the nerve is destroyed. If a chemical agent is used, the chemical agent is injected along the nerve pathway. Neurolytic chemical agents include: phenol, ethyl alcohol, glycerol, ammonium salt compounds and hypertonic or hypotonic solutions. Thermal or electrical modalities involve the use of a probe or needle that is inserted through the skin and activated to produce heat and destroy nerve tissue. To perform radiofrequency nerve destruction, an electrode needle is introduced through the skin and advanced toward the targeted neural tissue. The electrode is adjusted as needed until correct positioning is achieved. The radiofrequency device is then activated and an electric current generated that produces heat at the tip of the electrode and destroys the targeted nerve tissue.

Destruction by neurolytic agent, intercostal nerve

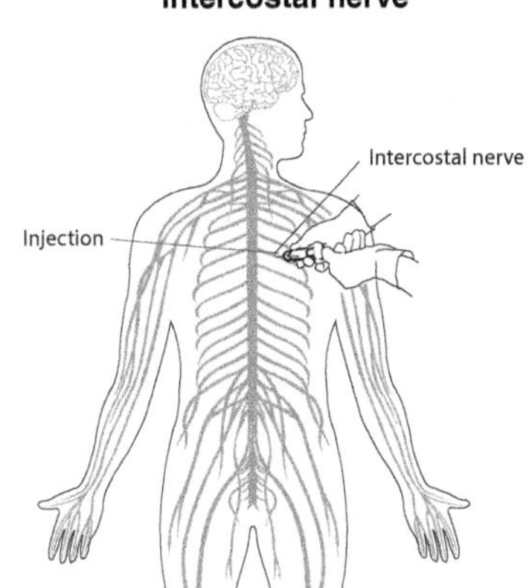

ICD-10-CM Diagnostic Codes

	B02.29	Other postherpetic nervous system involvement
	C41.3	Malignant neoplasm of ribs, sternum and clavicle
	C47.3	Malignant neoplasm of peripheral nerves of thorax
	C76.1	Malignant neoplasm of thorax
	C79.51	Secondary malignant neoplasm of bone
	C79.89	Secondary malignant neoplasm of other specified sites
	G58.0	Intercostal neuropathy
	G89.21	Chronic pain due to trauma
	G89.22	Chronic post-thoracotomy pain
	G89.28	Other chronic postprocedural pain
	G89.29	Other chronic pain
	G89.3	Neoplasm related pain (acute) (chronic)
	G89.4	Chronic pain syndrome
	M54.14	Radiculopathy, thoracic region
	M54.6	Pain in thoracic spine
	M54.9	Dorsalgia, unspecified
	M79.2	Neuralgia and neuritis, unspecified
	R07.89	Other chest pain
	R10.10	Upper abdominal pain, unspecified
⇄	R10.11	Right upper quadrant pain
⇄	R10.12	Left upper quadrant pain

CCI Edits

Refer to Appendix A for CCI edits.

Pub 100

64620: Pub 100-03, 1, 160.1

Facility RVUs ▢

Code	Work	PE Facility	MP	Total Facility
64620	2.89	1.86	0.25	5.00

Non-facility RVUs ▢

Code	Work	PE Non-Facility	MP	Total Non-Facility
64620	2.89	2.77	0.25	5.91

Modifiers (PAR) ▢

Code	Mod 50	Mod 51	Mod 62	Mod 66	Mod 80
64620	0	2	0	0	1

Global Period

Code	Days
64620	010

CPT © 2018 American Medical Association. All Rights Reserved.

64630

64630 Destruction by neurolytic agent; pudendal nerve

AMA Coding Guideline

Destruction by Neurolytic Agent (eg, Chemical, Thermal, Electrical or Radiofrequency) and Chemodenervation Procedures on the Extracranial Nerves, Peripheral Nerves, and Autonomic Nervous System

Codes 64600-64681 include the injection of other therapeutic agents (eg, corticosteroids). Do not report diagnostic/therapeutic injections separately. Do not report a code labeled as destruction when using therapies that are not destructive of the target nerve (eg, pulsed radiofrequency), use 64999. For codes labeled as chemodenervation, the supply of the chemodenervation agent is reported separately.

AMA Coding Notes

Destruction by Neurolytic Agent (eg, Chemical, Thermal, Electrical or Radiofrequency) and Chemodenervation Procedures on the Extracranial Nerves, Peripheral Nerves, and Autonomic Nervous System

(For chemodenervation of internal anal sphincter, use 46505)

(For chemodenervation of the bladder, use 52287)

(For chemodenervation for strabismus involving the extraocular muscles, use 67345)

(For chemodenervation guided by needle electromyography or muscle electrical stimulation, see 95873, 95874)

Surgical Procedures on the Extracranial Nerves, Peripheral Nerves, and Autonomic Nervous System

(For intracranial surgery on cranial nerves, see 61450, 61460, 61790)

AMA *CPT Assistant* ▢

64630: Aug 05: 13, Feb 10: 9, Sep 12: 14, Oct 17: 9

Plain English Description

The pudendal nerve controls sensation in the area between the genitals and the anus, the rectum, and the external genitalia. Destruction of the pudendal nerve is performed to treat chronic pain and may be performed by injection of a chemical neurolytic agent or using thermal, electrical or radiofrequency techniques. The most common technique used today is radiofrequency destruction, although the other techniques may also be used for certain pain syndromes. Prior to the destruction procedure, an electrode needle is introduced through the skin and advanced toward the targeted neural tissue. The needle is connected to a generator for motor and sensory testing performed to ensure that the needle is correctly positioned at the nerve responsible for the pain. Once the correct nerve pathway has been identified, the nerve is destroyed. If a chemical agent is used, the chemical agent is injected along the nerve pathway. Neurolytic chemical agents include: phenol, ethyl alcohol, glycerol, ammonium salt compounds and hypertonic or hypotonic solutions. Thermal or electrical modalities involve the use of a probe or needle that is inserted through the skin and activated to produce heat and destroy nerve tissue. To perform radiofrequency nerve destruction, an electrode needle is introduced through the skin and advanced toward the targeted neural tissue. The electrode is adjusted as needed until correct positioning is achieved. The radiofrequency device is then activated and an electric current generated that produces heat at the tip of the electrode and destroys the targeted nerve tissue.

ICD-10-CM Diagnostic Codes

	C76.3	Malignant neoplasm of pelvis
	C79.89	Secondary malignant neoplasm of other specified sites
	G58.8	Other specified mononeuropathies
	G89.21	Chronic pain due to trauma
	G89.28	Other chronic postprocedural pain
	G89.29	Other chronic pain
	G89.3	Neoplasm related pain (acute) (chronic)
	G89.4	Chronic pain syndrome
	N80.3	Endometriosis of pelvic peritoneum ♀
	N80.4	Endometriosis of rectovaginal septum and vagina ♀
	N94.810	Vulvar vestibulitis ♀
	N94.818	Other vulvodynia ♀
	N94.819	Vulvodynia, unspecified ♀
	N94.89	Other specified conditions associated with female genital organs and menstrual cycle ♀
	O71.89	Other specified obstetric trauma ♀
	R10.2	Pelvic and perineal pain
	R10.30	Lower abdominal pain, unspecified
⇄	R10.31	Right lower quadrant pain
⇄	R10.32	Left lower quadrant pain
	R10.9	Unspecified abdominal pain
❼	S34.6	Injury of peripheral nerve(s) at abdomen, lower back and pelvis level
❼	S34.8	Injury of other nerves at abdomen, lower back and pelvis level
❼	S34.9	Injury of unspecified nerves at abdomen, lower back and pelvis level
❼	S38.03	Crushing injury of vulva
❼	S39.848	Other specified injuries of external genitals
❼	S39.94	Unspecified injury of external genitals

ICD-10-CM Coding Notes

For codes requiring a 7th character extension, refer to your ICD-10-CM book. Review the character descriptions and coding guidelines for proper selection. For some procedures, only certain characters will apply.

CCI Edits

Refer to Appendix A for CCI edits.

Facility RVUs ▢

Code	Work	PE Facility	MP	Total Facility
64630	3.05	2.01	0.41	5.47

Non-facility RVUs ▢

Code	Work	PE Non-Facility	MP	Total Non-Facility
64630	3.05	3.31	0.41	6.77

Modifiers (PAR) ▢

Code	Mod 50	Mod 51	Mod 62	Mod 66	Mod 80
64630	0	2	0	0	0

Global Period

Code	Days
64630	010

CPT © 2018 American Medical Association. All Rights Reserved.

64632

64632 Destruction by neurolytic agent; plantar common digital nerve

(Do not report 64632 in conjunction with 64455)

AMA Coding Guideline

Destruction by Neurolytic Agent (eg, Chemical, Thermal, Electrical or Radiofrequency) and Chemodenervation Procedures on the Extracranial Nerves, Peripheral Nerves, and Autonomic Nervous System

Codes 64600-64681 include the injection of other therapeutic agents (eg, corticosteroids). Do not report diagnostic/therapeutic injections separately. Do not report a code labeled as destruction when using therapies that are not destructive of the target nerve (eg, pulsed radiofrequency), use 64999. For codes labeled as chemodenervation, the supply of the chemodenervation agent is reported separately.

AMA Coding Notes

Destruction by Neurolytic Agent (eg, Chemical, Thermal, Electrical or Radiofrequency) and Chemodenervation Procedures on the Extracranial Nerves, Peripheral Nerves, and Autonomic Nervous System

(For chemodenervation of internal anal sphincter, use 46505)

(For chemodenervation of the bladder, use 52287)

(For chemodenervation for strabismus involving the extraocular muscles, use 67345)

(For chemodenervation guided by needle electromyography or muscle electrical stimulation, see 95873, 95874)

Surgical Procedures on the Extracranial Nerves, Peripheral Nerves, and Autonomic Nervous System

(For intracranial surgery on cranial nerves, see 61450, 61460, 61790)

AMA *CPT Assistant* □

64632: Jan 09: 6, Sep 12: 14, Jan 13: 13, Jul 15: 11, Oct 17: 9

Plain English Description

This procedure is performed to treat pain in the interdigital space caused by conditions such as Morton's neuroma. With the patient in a supine position, the knee is flexed and supported with a pillow and the foot is maintained in a relaxed neutral position. The interdigital spaces are palpated and any tenderness or fullness is noted. The needle is inserted on the dorsal foot surface in a distal to proximal direction at a point 1-2 cm proximal to the web space and in line with the metatarsophalangeal joints. The needle is held at an angle of approximately 45 degrees and advanced through the mid web space at the plantar aspect of the foot. The needle is advanced until it tents the skin and then withdrawn approximately 1 cm. Taking care to avoid the plantar fat pad, a neurolytic agent such as ethyl alcohol is injected in an alcohol/anesthetic mix. Alcohol causes chemical neurolysis of the plantar common digital nerve due to dehydration, necrosis, and precipitation of protoplasm.

ICD-10-CM Diagnostic Codes

⇄	G57.61	Lesion of plantar nerve, right lower limb
⇄	G57.62	Lesion of plantar nerve, left lower limb
⇄	G57.63	Lesion of plantar nerve, bilateral lower limbs
⇄	G57.81	Other specified mononeuropathies of right lower limb
⇄	G57.82	Other specified mononeuropathies of left lower limb
⇄	G57.83	Other specified mononeuropathies of bilateral lower limbs
⇄	M79.671	Pain in right foot
⇄	M79.672	Pain in left foot
⇄	M79.674	Pain in right toe(s)
⇄	M79.675	Pain in left toe(s)

CCI Edits

Refer to Appendix A for CCI edits.

Facility RVUs □

Code	Work	PE Facility	MP	Total Facility
64632	1.23	0.65	0.08	1.96

Non-facility RVUs □

Code	Work	PE Non-Facility	MP	Total Non-Facility
64632	1.23	1.14	0.08	2.45

Modifiers (PAR) □

Code	Mod 50	Mod 51	Mod 62	Mod 66	Mod 80
64632	1	2	0	0	0

Global Period

Code	Days
64632	010

CPT © 2018 American Medical Association. All Rights Reserved.

64633-64636

64633 Destruction by neurolytic agent, paravertebral facet joint nerve(s), with imaging guidance (fluoroscopy or CT); cervical or thoracic, single facet joint

(For bilateral procedure, report 64633 with modifier 50)

+ 64634 Destruction by neurolytic agent, paravertebral facet joint nerve(s), with imaging guidance (fluoroscopy or CT); cervical or thoracic, each additional facet joint (List separately in addition to code for primary procedure)

(Use 64634 in conjunction with 64633)

(For bilateral procedure, report 64634 with modifier 50)

64635 Destruction by neurolytic agent, paravertebral facet joint nerve(s), with imaging guidance (fluoroscopy or CT); lumbar or sacral, single facet joint

(For bilateral procedure, report 64635 with modifier 50)

+ 64636 Destruction by neurolytic agent, paravertebral facet joint nerve(s), with imaging guidance (fluoroscopy or CT); lumbar or sacral, each additional facet joint (List separately in addition to code for primary procedure)

(Use 64636 in conjunction with 64635)

(For bilateral procedure, report 64636 with modifier 50)

(Do not report 64633-64636 in conjunction with 77003, 77012)

(For destruction by neurolytic agent, individual nerves, sacroiliac joint, use 64640)

AMA Coding Guideline

Destruction by Neurolytic Agent (eg, Chemical, Thermal, Electrical or Radiofrequency) and Chemodenervation Procedures on the Extracranial Nerves, Peripheral Nerves, and Autonomic Nervous System

Codes 64600-64681 include the injection of other therapeutic agents (eg, corticosteroids). Do not report diagnostic/therapeutic injections separately. Do not report a code labeled as destruction when using therapies that are not destructive of the target nerve (eg, pulsed radiofrequency), use 64999. For codes labeled as chemodenervation, the supply of the chemodenervation agent is reported separately.

AMA Coding Notes

Destruction by Neurolytic Agent (eg, Chemical, Thermal, Electrical or Radiofrequency) and Chemodenervation Procedures on the Extracranial Nerves, Peripheral Nerves, and Autonomic Nervous System

(For chemodenervation of internal anal sphincter, use 46505)

(For chemodenervation of the bladder, use 52287)

(For chemodenervation for strabismus involving the extraocular muscles, use 67345)

(For chemodenervation guided by needle electromyography or muscle electrical stimulation, see 95873, 95874)

Surgical Procedures on the Extracranial Nerves, Peripheral Nerves, and Autonomic Nervous System

(For intracranial surgery on cranial nerves, see 61450, 61460, 61790)

AMA *CPT Assistant* □

64633: Jun 12: 10, Jul 12: 6, Sep 12: 14, Apr 13: 10, Feb 15: 9

64634: Jun 12: 10, Jul 12: 6, Sep 12: 14, Apr 13: 10, Feb 15: 9

64635: Jun 12: 10, Jul 12: 6, 14, Sep 12: 14, Apr 13: 10, Feb 15: 9

64636: Jun 12: 10, Jul 12: 6, 14, Sep 12: 14, Apr 13: 10, Feb 15: 9

Plain English Description

Paravertebral facet joints, also called zygapophyseal joints, are located on the posterior aspect of the spine on each side of the vertebra at the point where one vertebra overlaps the next. Using fluoroscopic or CT guidance, the paravertebral facet joint nerve is destroyed using a neurolytic agent. The skin overlying the facet joint is prepped and a local anesthetic is injected. If a chemical neurolytic agent is used, a spinal needle is directed into the facet joint space until bone or cartilage is encountered. A small amount of contrast material is injected to verify that the needle is correctly positioned. This may be followed by injection of a local anesthetic and/or steroid. The selected chemical neurolytic agent is then injected along the nerve pathway. Neurolytic chemical agents include: phenol, ethyl alcohol, glycerol, ammonium salt compounds, and hypertonic or hypotonic solutions. Thermal or electrical modalities for neurolysis involve the use of a probe, needle, or electrode inserted through the skin and activated to produce heat and destroy nerve tissue. Using fluoroscopic or CT guidance, an electrode needle is introduced through the skin and advanced toward the targeted neural tissue. The needle is connected to a generator for performing motor and sensory testing to ensure that the needle is correctly positioned along the facet joint nerve. Once the correct nerve pathway has been identified, the nerve is destroyed. The probe, needle, or electrode is activated and an electric current is generated that produces heat at the tip of the device and destroys the targeted nerve tissue. Use 64633 for a single cervical or thoracic facet joint nerve; use 64634 for each additional cervical or thoracic level. Use 64635 for a single lumbar or sacral facet joint nerve; use 64636 for each additional lumbar or sacral level.

ICD-10-CM Diagnostic Codes

	C41.2	Malignant neoplasm of vertebral column
	C41.4	Malignant neoplasm of pelvic bones, sacrum and coccyx
	C76.0	Malignant neoplasm of head, face and neck
	C76.1	Malignant neoplasm of thorax
	C76.3	Malignant neoplasm of pelvis
	G89.29	Other chronic pain
	G89.3	Neoplasm related pain (acute) (chronic)
	M54.2	Cervicalgia
	M54.5	Low back pain
	M54.6	Pain in thoracic spine
	M54.9	Dorsalgia, unspecified
	R10.10	Upper abdominal pain, unspecified
⇄	R10.11	Right upper quadrant pain
⇄	R10.12	Left upper quadrant pain
	R10.2	Pelvic and perineal pain
⇄	R10.3	Pain localized to other parts of lower abdomen
⇄	R10.31	Right lower quadrant pain
⇄	R10.32	Left lower quadrant pain
	R10.9	Unspecified abdominal pain

CCI Edits

Refer to Appendix A for CCI edits.

Pub 100

64633: Pub 100-03, 1, 160.1

64634: Pub 100-03, 1, 160.1

64635: Pub 100-03, 1, 160.1

64636: Pub 100-03, 1, 160.1

CPT © 2018 American Medical Association. All Rights Reserved.

Facility RVUs

Code	Work	PE Facility	MP	Total Facility
64633	3.84	2.28	0.31	6.43
64634	1.32	0.52	0.11	1.95
64635	3.78	2.26	0.30	6.34
64636	1.16	0.46	0.09	1.71

Non-facility RVUs

Code	Work	PE Non-Facility	MP	Total Non-Facility
64633	3.84	7.74	0.31	11.89
64634	1.32	3.91	0.11	5.34
64635	3.78	7.68	0.30	11.76
64636	1.16	3.60	0.09	4.85

Modifiers (PAR)

Code	Mod 50	Mod 51	Mod 62	Mod 66	Mod 80
64633	1	2	0	0	1
64634	1	0	0	0	1
64635	1	2	0	0	1
64636	1	0	0	0	1

Global Period

Code	Days
64633	010
64634	ZZZ
64635	010
64636	ZZZ

CPT © 2018 American Medical Association. All Rights Reserved.

64640

64640 Destruction by neurolytic agent; other peripheral nerve or branch

AMA Coding Guideline

Destruction by Neurolytic Agent (eg, Chemical, Thermal, Electrical or Radiofrequency) and Chemodenervation Procedures on the Extracranial Nerves, Peripheral Nerves, and Autonomic Nervous System

Codes 64600-64681 include the injection of other therapeutic agents (eg, corticosteroids). Do not report diagnostic/therapeutic injections separately. Do not report a code labeled as destruction when using therapies that are not destructive of the target nerve (eg, pulsed radiofrequency), use 64999. For codes labeled as chemodenervation, the supply of the chemodenervation agent is reported separately.

AMA Coding Notes

Destruction by Neurolytic Agent (eg, Chemical, Thermal, Electrical or Radiofrequency) and Chemodenervation Procedures on the Extracranial Nerves, Peripheral Nerves, and Autonomic Nervous System

(For chemodenervation of internal anal sphincter, use 46505)

(For chemodenervation of the bladder, use 52287)

(For chemodenervation for strabismus involving the extraocular muscles, use 67345)

(For chemodenervation guided by needle electromyography or muscle electrical stimulation, see 95873, 95874)

Surgical Procedures on the Extracranial Nerves, Peripheral Nerves, and Autonomic Nervous System

(For intracranial surgery on cranial nerves, see 61450, 61460, 61790)

AMA *CPT Assistant* □

64640: Aug 05: 13, Dec 09: 11, Feb 10: 9, Jun 12: 15, Sep 12: 14, May 17: 10, Oct 17: 9, Jan 18: 7

Plain English Description

Destruction of a nerve is performed to treat chronic pain and may be performed by injection of a chemical neurolytic agent or using thermal, electrical or radiofrequency techniques. The most common technique used today is radiofrequency destruction, although the other techniques may also be used for certain pain syndromes. Prior to the destruction procedure, an electrode needle is introduced through the skin and advanced toward the targeted neural tissue. The needle is connected to a generator for motor and sensory testing performed to ensure that the needle is correctly positioned at the nerve responsible for the pain. Once the correct nerve pathway has been identified, the nerve is destroyed. If a chemical agent is used, the chemical agent is injected along the nerve pathway. Neurolytic chemical agents include: phenol, ethyl alcohol, glycerol, ammonium salt compounds and hypertonic or hypotonic solutions. Thermal or electrical modalities involve the use of a probe or needle that is inserted through the skin and activated to produce heat and destroy nerve tissue. To perform radiofrequency nerve destruction, an electrode needle is introduced through the skin and advanced toward the targeted neural tissue. The electrode is adjusted as needed until correct positioning is achieved. The radiofrequency device is then activated and an electric current generated that produces heat at the tip of the electrode and destroys the targeted nerve tissue. Use 64640 for destruction of a peripheral nerve or branch that does not have a more specific code listed.

Destruction by neurolytic agent; other peripheral nerve or branch

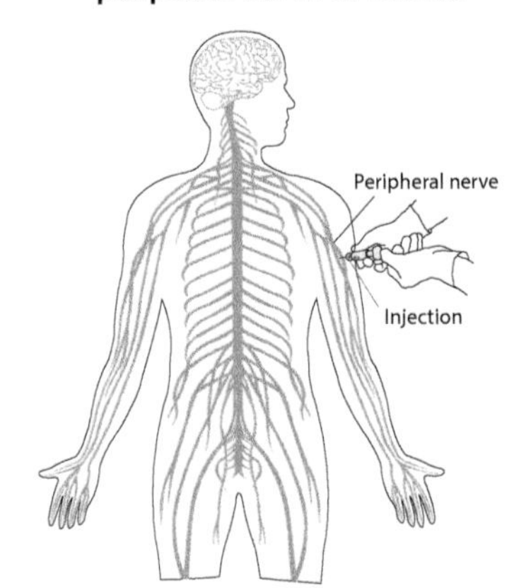

ICD-10-CM Diagnostic Codes

⇄	C76.51	Malignant neoplasm of right lower limb
⇄	C76.52	Malignant neoplasm of left lower limb
⇄	G57.11	Meralgia paresthetica, right lower limb
⇄	G57.12	Meralgia paresthetica, left lower limb
⇄	G57.21	Lesion of femoral nerve, right lower limb
⇄	G57.22	Lesion of femoral nerve, left lower limb
⇄	G57.31	Lesion of lateral popliteal nerve, right lower limb
⇄	G57.32	Lesion of lateral popliteal nerve, left lower limb
⇄	G57.33	Lesion of lateral popliteal nerve, bilateral lower limbs
⇄	G57.41	Lesion of medial popliteal nerve, right lower limb
⇄	G57.42	Lesion of medial popliteal nerve, left lower limb
⇄	G57.43	Lesion of medial popliteal nerve, bilateral lower limbs
⇄	G57.61	Lesion of plantar nerve, right lower limb
⇄	G57.62	Lesion of plantar nerve, left lower limb
⇄	G57.63	Lesion of plantar nerve, bilateral lower limbs
⇄	G57.71	Causalgia of right lower limb
⇄	G57.72	Causalgia of left lower limb
⇄	G57.73	Causalgia of bilateral lower limbs
⇄	G57.81	Other specified mononeuropathies of right lower limb
⇄	G57.82	Other specified mononeuropathies of left lower limb
⇄	G57.83	Other specified mononeuropathies of bilateral lower limbs
	G89.21	Chronic pain due to trauma
	G89.28	Other chronic postprocedural pain
	G89.29	Other chronic pain
	G89.3	Neoplasm related pain (acute) (chronic)
	G89.4	Chronic pain syndrome
⇄	G90.521	Complex regional pain syndrome I of right lower limb
⇄	G90.522	Complex regional pain syndrome I of left lower limb
⇄	G90.523	Complex regional pain syndrome I of lower limb, bilateral
⇄	M79.604	Pain in right leg
⇄	M79.605	Pain in left leg
⇄	M79.651	Pain in right thigh
⇄	M79.652	Pain in left thigh
⇄	M79.661	Pain in right lower leg
⇄	M79.662	Pain in left lower leg
➐⇄	S74.11	Injury of femoral nerve at hip and thigh level, right leg
➐⇄	S74.12	Injury of femoral nerve at hip and thigh level, left leg
➐⇄	S74.21	Injury of cutaneous sensory nerve at hip and high level, right leg
➐⇄	S74.22	Injury of cutaneous sensory nerve at hip and thigh level, left leg
➐⇄	S74.8X1	Injury of other nerves at hip and thigh level, right leg
➐⇄	S74.8X2	Injury of other nerves at hip and thigh level, left leg
➐⇄	S84.01	Injury of tibial nerve at lower leg level, right leg
➐⇄	S84.02	Injury of tibial nerve at lower leg level, left leg
➐⇄	S84.11	Injury of peroneal nerve at lower leg level, right leg
➐⇄	S84.12	Injury of peroneal nerve at lower leg level, left leg
➐⇄	S84.21	Injury of cutaneous sensory nerve at lower leg level, right leg
➐⇄	S84.22	Injury of cutaneous sensory nerve at lower leg level, left leg
➐⇄	S84.801	Injury of other nerves at lower leg level, right leg
➐⇄	S84.802	Injury of other nerves at lower leg level, left leg

ICD-10-CM Coding Notes

For codes requiring a 7th character extension, refer to your ICD-10-CM book. Review the character descriptions and coding guidelines for proper selection. For some procedures, only certain characters will apply.

CCI Edits

Refer to Appendix A for CCI edits.

CPT © 2018 American Medical Association. All Rights Reserved.

Facility RVUs □

Code	Work	PE Facility	MP	Total Facility
64640	1.23	1.36	0.10	2.69

Non-facility RVUs □

Code	Work	PE Non-Facility	MP	Total Non-Facility
64640	1.23	2.53	0.10	3.86

Modifiers (PAR) □

Code	Mod 50	Mod 51	Mod 62	Mod 66	Mod 80
64640	1	2	0	0	1

Global Period

Code	Days
64640	010

CPT © 2018 American Medical Association. All Rights Reserved.

64642-64643

64642 Chemodenervation of one extremity; 1-4 muscle(s)

+ 64643 Chemodenervation of one extremity; each additional extremity, 1-4 muscle(s) (List separately in addition to code for primary procedure)

(Use 64643 in conjunction with 64642, 64644)

AMA Coding Guideline

Destruction by Neurolytic Agent (eg, Chemical, Thermal, Electrical or Radiofrequency) and Chemodenervation Procedures on the Extracranial Nerves, Peripheral Nerves, and Autonomic Nervous System

Codes 64600-64681 include the injection of other therapeutic agents (eg, corticosteroids). Do not report diagnostic/therapeutic injections separately. Do not report a code labeled as destruction when using therapies that are not destructive of the target nerve (eg, pulsed radiofrequency), use 64999. For codes labeled as chemodenervation, the supply of the chemodenervation agent is reported separately.

AMA Coding Notes

Destruction by Neurolytic Agent (eg, Chemical, Thermal, Electrical or Radiofrequency) and Chemodenervation Procedures on the Extracranial Nerves, Peripheral Nerves, and Autonomic Nervous System

(For chemodenervation of internal anal sphincter, use 46505)

(For chemodenervation of the bladder, use 52287)

(For chemodenervation for strabismus involving the extraocular muscles, use 67345)

(For chemodenervation guided by needle electromyography or muscle electrical stimulation, see 95873, 95874)

Surgical Procedures on the Extracranial Nerves, Peripheral Nerves, and Autonomic Nervous System

(For intracranial surgery on cranial nerves, see 61450, 61460, 61790)

AMA *CPT Assistant* □

64642: Jan 14: 6, Oct 14: 15
64643: Jan 14: 6, Oct 14: 15

Plain English Description

Chemodenervation is performed on the muscles of one extremity to treat involuntary muscle contractions or muscle spasms such as those due to dystonia, cerebral palsy, or multiple sclerosis. Injection of botulinum toxin (type A or B) directly into a muscle produces temporary muscle paralysis by blocking the release of acetylcholine at the peripheral nerve endings which interrupts neuromuscular transmission of nerve impulses. The muscle and muscle sites to be injected are determined either by use of electromyography or by examining the affected extremity, palpating the muscles, and noting the location of the muscle spasm. The extremity to be treated is prepped. The affected muscle or muscle group is then injected at carefully selected sites to accomplish the denervation. Use 64642 for 1-4 muscles of one extremity and 64643 for 1-4 muscles in each additional extremity.

ICD-10-CM Diagnostic Codes

	G24.02	Drug induced acute dystonia
	G24.1	Genetic torsion dystonia
	G24.2	Idiopathic nonfamilial dystonia
	G24.9	Dystonia, unspecified
	G35	Multiple sclerosis
	G80.0	Spastic quadriplegic cerebral palsy
	G80.1	Spastic diplegic cerebral palsy
	G80.2	Spastic hemiplegic cerebral palsy
	G80.3	Athetoid cerebral palsy
	G80.4	Ataxic cerebral palsy
	G80.8	Other cerebral palsy
	G80.9	Cerebral palsy, unspecified
	G89.21	Chronic pain due to trauma
	G89.28	Other chronic postprocedural pain
	G89.29	Other chronic pain
	G89.3	Neoplasm related pain (acute) (chronic)
	M62.831	Muscle spasm of calf
	M62.838	Other muscle spasm
	M79.18	Myalgia, other site
⇄	M79.601	Pain in right arm
⇄	M79.602	Pain in left arm
⇄	M79.604	Pain in right leg
⇄	M79.605	Pain in left leg

CCI Edits

Refer to Appendix A for CCI edits.

Facility RVUs □

Code	Work	PE Facility	MP	Total Facility
64642	1.65	1.09	0.38	3.12
64643	1.22	0.62	0.24	2.08

Non-facility RVUs □

Code	Work	PE Non-Facility	MP	Total Non-Facility
64642	1.65	2.12	0.38	4.15
64643	1.22	1.19	0.24	2.65

Modifiers (PAR) □

Code	Mod 50	Mod 51	Mod 62	Mod 66	Mod 80
64642	0	2	0	0	1
64643	0	0	0	0	1

Global Period

Code	Days
64642	000
64643	ZZZ

CPT © 2018 American Medical Association. All Rights Reserved.

64644-64645

64644 Chemodenervation of one extremity; 5 or more muscles

+ **64645 Chemodenervation of one extremity; each additional extremity, 5 or more muscles (List separately in addition to code for primary procedure)**

(Use 64645 in conjunction with 64644)

AMA Coding Guideline

Destruction by Neurolytic Agent (eg, Chemical, Thermal, Electrical or Radiofrequency) and Chemodenervation Procedures on the Extracranial Nerves, Peripheral Nerves, and Autonomic Nervous System

Codes 64600-64681 include the injection of other therapeutic agents (eg, corticosteroids). Do not report diagnostic/therapeutic injections separately. Do not report a code labeled as destruction when using therapies that are not destructive of the target nerve (eg, pulsed radiofrequency), use 64999. For codes labeled as chemodenervation, the supply of the chemodenervation agent is reported separately.

AMA Coding Notes

Destruction by Neurolytic Agent (eg, Chemical, Thermal, Electrical or Radiofrequency) and Chemodenervation Procedures on the Extracranial Nerves, Peripheral Nerves, and Autonomic Nervous System

(For chemodenervation of internal anal sphincter, use 46505)

(For chemodenervation of the bladder, use 52287)

(For chemodenervation for strabismus involving the extraocular muscles, use 67345)

(For chemodenervation guided by needle electromyography or muscle electrical stimulation, see 95873, 95874)

Surgical Procedures on the Extracranial Nerves, Peripheral Nerves, and Autonomic Nervous System

(For intracranial surgery on cranial nerves, see 61450, 61460, 61790)

AMA *CPT Assistant* ▯

64644: Jan 14: 6, Oct 14: 15
64645: Jan 14: 6, Oct 14: 15

Plain English Description

Chemodenervation is performed on the muscles of one extremity to treat involuntary muscle contractions or muscle spasms such as those due to dystonia, cerebral palsy, or multiple sclerosis. Injection of botulinum toxin (type A or B) directly into a muscle produces temporary muscle paralysis by blocking the release of acetylcholine at the peripheral nerve endings which interrupts neuromuscular transmission of nerve impulses. The muscle and muscle sites to be injected are determined either by use of electromyography or by examining the affected extremity, palpating the muscles, and noting the location of the muscle spasm. The extremity to be treated is prepped. The affected muscles or muscle group(s) are then injected at carefully selected sites to accomplish the denervation. Use 64644 for 5 or more muscles of one extremity and 64645 for 5 or more muscles in each additional extremity.

ICD-10-CM Diagnostic Codes

	G24.02	Drug induced acute dystonia
	G24.1	Genetic torsion dystonia
	G24.2	Idiopathic nonfamilial dystonia
	G24.9	Dystonia, unspecified
	G35	Multiple sclerosis
	G80.0	Spastic quadriplegic cerebral palsy
	G80.1	Spastic diplegic cerebral palsy
	G80.2	Spastic hemiplegic cerebral palsy
	G80.3	Athetoid cerebral palsy
	G80.4	Ataxic cerebral palsy
	G80.8	Other cerebral palsy
	G80.9	Cerebral palsy, unspecified
	G89.21	Chronic pain due to trauma
	G89.28	Other chronic postprocedural pain
	G89.29	Other chronic pain
	G89.3	Neoplasm related pain (acute) (chronic)
	M62.831	Muscle spasm of calf
	M62.838	Other muscle spasm
	M79.18	Myalgia, other site
⇄	M79.601	Pain in right arm
⇄	M79.602	Pain in left arm
⇄	M79.604	Pain in right leg
⇄	M79.605	Pain in left leg

CCI Edits

Refer to Appendix A for CCI edits.

Facility RVUs ▯

Code	Work	PE Facility	MP	Total Facility
64644	1.82	1.19	0.41	3.42
64645	1.39	0.69	0.32	2.40

Non-facility RVUs ▯

Code	Work	PE Non-Facility	MP	Total Non-Facility
64644	1.82	2.59	0.41	4.82
64645	1.39	1.62	0.32	3.33

Modifiers (PAR) ▯

Code	Mod 50	Mod 51	Mod 62	Mod 66	Mod 80
64644	0	2	0	0	1
64645	0	0	0	0	1

Global Period

Code	Days
64644	000
64645	ZZZ

CPT © 2018 American Medical Association. All Rights Reserved.

64646-64647

64646 Chemodenervation of trunk muscle(s); 1-5 muscle(s)

64647 Chemodenervation of trunk muscle(s); 6 or more muscles

(Report either 64646 or 64647 only once per session)

AMA Coding Guideline

Destruction by Neurolytic Agent (eg, Chemical, Thermal, Electrical or Radiofrequency) and Chemodenervation Procedures on the Extracranial Nerves, Peripheral Nerves, and Autonomic Nervous System

Codes 64600-64681 include the injection of other therapeutic agents (eg, corticosteroids). Do not report diagnostic/therapeutic injections separately. Do not report a code labeled as destruction when using therapies that are not destructive of the target nerve (eg, pulsed radiofrequency), use 64999. For codes labeled as chemodenervation, the supply of the chemodenervation agent is reported separately.

AMA Coding Notes

Destruction by Neurolytic Agent (eg, Chemical, Thermal, Electrical or Radiofrequency) and Chemodenervation Procedures on the Extracranial Nerves, Peripheral Nerves, and Autonomic Nervous System

(For chemodenervation of internal anal sphincter, use 46505)

(For chemodenervation of the bladder, use 52287)

(For chemodenervation for strabismus involving the extraocular muscles, use 67345)

(For chemodenervation guided by needle electromyography or muscle electrical stimulation, see 95873, 95874)

Surgical Procedures on the Extracranial Nerves, Peripheral Nerves, and Autonomic Nervous System

(For intracranial surgery on cranial nerves, see 61450, 61460, 61790)

AMA *CPT Assistant*

64646: Jan 14: 6

64647: Jan 14: 6

Plain English Description

Chemodenervation is performed on the muscles of the trunk to treat involuntary muscle contractions or muscle spasms such as those due to dystonia, cerebral palsy, or multiple sclerosis. Injection of botulinum toxin (type A or B) directly into a muscle produces temporary muscle paralysis by blocking the release of acetylcholine at the peripheral nerve endings which interrupts neuromuscular transmission of nerve impulses. The muscle and muscle sites to be injected are determined either by use of electromyography or by examining the trunk, palpating the muscles, and noting the location of the muscle spasm. The trunk is prepped. The affected muscle(s) or muscle group is then injected at carefully selected sites to accomplish the denervation. Use 64646 for 1-5 muscles of the trunk and 64647 for 6 or more muscles in the trunk.

ICD-10-CM Diagnostic Codes

G24.02	Drug induced acute dystonia
G24.1	Genetic torsion dystonia
G24.2	Idiopathic nonfamilial dystonia
G24.9	Dystonia, unspecified
G35	Multiple sclerosis
G80.0	Spastic quadriplegic cerebral palsy
G80.1	Spastic diplegic cerebral palsy
G80.2	Spastic hemiplegic cerebral palsy
G80.3	Athetoid cerebral palsy
G80.4	Ataxic cerebral palsy
G80.8	Other cerebral palsy
G80.9	Cerebral palsy, unspecified
G89.21	Chronic pain due to trauma
G89.28	Other chronic postprocedural pain
G89.29	Other chronic pain
G89.3	Neoplasm related pain (acute) (chronic)
M54.5	Low back pain
M54.6	Pain in thoracic spine
M54.9	Dorsalgia, unspecified
M62.830	Muscle spasm of back
M62.838	Other muscle spasm

CCI Edits

Refer to Appendix A for CCI edits.

Facility RVUs

Code	Work	PE Facility	MP	Total Facility
64646	1.80	1.11	0.43	3.34
64647	2.11	1.23	0.62	3.96

Non-facility RVUs

Code	Work	PE Non-Facility	MP	Total Non-Facility
64646	1.80	2.12	0.43	4.35
64647	2.11	2.39	0.62	5.12

Modifiers (PAR)

Code	Mod 50	Mod 51	Mod 62	Mod 66	Mod 80
64646	0	2	0	0	1
64647	0	2	0	0	1

Global Period

Code	Days
64646	000
64647	000

CPT © 2018 American Medical Association. All Rights Reserved.

64680

64680 Destruction by neurolytic agent, with or without radiologic monitoring; celiac plexus

(For transendoscopic ultrasound-guided transmural injection, neurolytic agent, celiac plexus, use 43253)

AMA Coding Guideline

Destruction by Neurolytic Agent (eg, Chemical, Thermal, Electrical or Radiofrequency) and Chemodenervation Procedures on the Extracranial Nerves, Peripheral Nerves, and Autonomic Nervous System

Codes 64600-64681 include the injection of other therapeutic agents (eg, corticosteroids). Do not report diagnostic/therapeutic injections separately. Do not report a code labeled as destruction when using therapies that are not destructive of the target nerve (eg, pulsed radiofrequency), use 64999. For codes labeled as chemodenervation, the supply of the chemodenervation agent is reported separately.

AMA Coding Notes

Destruction by Neurolytic Agent (eg, Chemical, Thermal, Electrical or Radiofrequency) and Chemodenervation Procedures on the Extracranial Nerves, Peripheral Nerves, and Autonomic Nervous System

(For chemodenervation of internal anal sphincter, use 46505)

(For chemodenervation of the bladder, use 52287)

(For chemodenervation for strabismus involving the extraocular muscles, use 67345)

(For chemodenervation guided by needle electromyography or muscle electrical stimulation, see 95873, 95874)

Surgical Procedures on the Extracranial Nerves, Peripheral Nerves, and Autonomic Nervous System

(For intracranial surgery on cranial nerves, see 61450, 61460, 61790)

AMA *CPT Assistant* ☐

64680: Feb 99: 10, Aug 05: 13, Jun 08: 9, Sep 12: 14

Plain English Description

The celiac plexus is located in the retroperitoneum of the upper abdomen at the level of the T12-L1 vertebra lying anterior to the crura of the diaphragm. The celiac plexus surrounds the abdominal aorta, celiac and superior mesenteric arteries. Destruction of the celiac plexus is performed to treat pain due to metastatic cancer as well as nonmalignant pain, such as pain due to acute and chronic pancreatitis. Destruction may be performed by injection of a chemical neurolytic agent or using thermal, electrical or radiofrequency techniques. This procedure may be performed with or without radiologic monitoring. If radiologic monitoring is used, two needles are inserted on each side of the upper abdomen and directed toward the body of L1. Alternatively, the needles may be directed toward T12 if neurolysis is performed only on the splanchnic nerves. Contrast is then injected to confirm proper needle placement. If a chemical agent is used, the chemical agent is injected. Neurolytic chemical agents include: phenol, ethyl alcohol, glycerol, ammonium salt compounds and hypertonic or hypotonic solutions. Thermal or electrical modalities involve the use of a probe or needle that is inserted through the skin and activated to produce heat and destroy nerve tissue. To perform radiofrequency nerve destruction, an electrode needle is introduced through the skin and advanced toward the targeted neural tissue. The electrode is adjusted as needed until correct positioning is achieved. The radiofrequency device is then activated and an electric current generated that produces heat at the tip of the electrode and destroys the targeted nerve tissue.

ICD-10-CM Diagnostic Codes

	C22.0	Liver cell carcinoma
	C22.1	Intrahepatic bile duct carcinoma
	C22.2	Hepatoblastoma
	C22.3	Angiosarcoma of liver
	C22.4	Other sarcomas of liver
	C22.7	Other specified carcinomas of liver
	C22.8	Malignant neoplasm of liver, primary, unspecified as to type
	C22.9	Malignant neoplasm of liver, not specified as primary or secondary
	C25.0	Malignant neoplasm of head of pancreas
	C25.1	Malignant neoplasm of body of pancreas
	C25.2	Malignant neoplasm of tail of pancreas
	C25.3	Malignant neoplasm of pancreatic duct
	C25.4	Malignant neoplasm of endocrine pancreas
	C25.7	Malignant neoplasm of other parts of pancreas
	C25.8	Malignant neoplasm of overlapping sites of pancreas
	C25.9	Malignant neoplasm of pancreas, unspecified
	C48.0	Malignant neoplasm of retroperitoneum
	C48.1	Malignant neoplasm of specified parts of peritoneum
	C48.2	Malignant neoplasm of peritoneum, unspecified
	C48.8	Malignant neoplasm of overlapping sites of retroperitoneum and peritoneum
	C76.2	Malignant neoplasm of abdomen
	C78.6	Secondary malignant neoplasm of retroperitoneum and peritoneum
	C78.7	Secondary malignant neoplasm of liver and intrahepatic bile duct
	G89.21	Chronic pain due to trauma
	G89.28	Other chronic postprocedural pain
	G89.29	Other chronic pain
	G89.3	Neoplasm related pain (acute) (chronic)
	K86.0	Alcohol-induced chronic pancreatitis
	K86.1	Other chronic pancreatitis
	R10.10	Upper abdominal pain, unspecified
⇄	R10.11	Right upper quadrant pain
⇄	R10.12	Left upper quadrant pain

CCI Edits

Refer to Appendix A for CCI edits.

Facility RVUs ☐

Code	Work	PE Facility	MP	Total Facility
64680	2.67	1.75	0.24	4.66

Non-facility RVUs ☐

Code	Work	PE Non-Facility	MP	Total Non-Facility
64680	2.67	6.16	0.24	9.07

Modifiers (PAR) ☐

Code	Mod 50	Mod 51	Mod 62	Mod 66	Mod 80
64680	0	2	0	0	1

Global Period

Code	Days
64680	010

CPT © 2018 American Medical Association. All Rights Reserved.

64681

64681 Destruction by neurolytic agent, with or without radiologic monitoring; superior hypogastric plexus

AMA Coding Guideline

Destruction by Neurolytic Agent (eg, Chemical, Thermal, Electrical or Radiofrequency) and Chemodenervation Procedures on the Extracranial Nerves, Peripheral Nerves, and Autonomic Nervous System

Codes 64600-64681 include the injection of other therapeutic agents (eg, corticosteroids). Do not report diagnostic/therapeutic injections separately. Do not report a code labeled as destruction when using therapies that are not destructive of the target nerve (eg, pulsed radiofrequency), use 64999. For codes labeled as chemodenervation, the supply of the chemodenervation agent is reported separately.

AMA Coding Notes

Destruction by Neurolytic Agent (eg, Chemical, Thermal, Electrical or Radiofrequency) and Chemodenervation Procedures on the Extracranial Nerves, Peripheral Nerves, and Autonomic Nervous System

(For chemodenervation of internal anal sphincter, use 46505)

(For chemodenervation of the bladder, use 52287)

(For chemodenervation for strabismus involving the extraocular muscles, use 67345)

(For chemodenervation guided by needle electromyography or muscle electrical stimulation, see 95873, 95874)

Surgical Procedures on the Extracranial Nerves, Peripheral Nerves, and Autonomic Nervous System

(For intracranial surgery on cranial nerves, see 61450, 61460, 61790)

AMA *CPT Assistant* ▯

64681: Aug 05: 13, Dec 07: 13, Sep 12: 14

Plain English Description

The superior hypogastric plexus is a bilateral structure located in the retroperitoneum between the L5 and S1 vertebrae. Destruction of the superior hypogastric plexus is performed to treat pain due to a metastatic cancer in the pelvic region as well as nonmalignant chronic pain. Destruction may be performed by injection of a chemical neurolytic agent or using thermal, electrical or radiofrequency techniques. This procedure may be performed with or without radiologic monitoring. If radiologic monitoring is used, a needle is inserted into the ventral lateral surface of the spine at the L5-S1 interspace. Contrast is then injected to confirm proper needle placement in the prevertebral space just ventral to the psoas fascia. If a chemical agent is used, the chemical agent is injected. Neurolytic chemical agents include: phenol, ethyl alcohol, glycerol, ammonium salt compounds and hypertonic or hypotonic solutions. Thermal or electrical modalities involve the use of a probe or needle that is inserted through the skin and activated to produce heat and destroy nerve tissue. To perform radiofrequency nerve destruction, an electrode needle is introduced through the skin and advanced toward the targeted neural tissue. The electrode is adjusted as needed until correct positioning is achieved. The radiofrequency device is then activated and an electric current generated that produces heat at the tip of the electrode and destroys the targeted nerve tissue.

Destruction by neurolytic agent, with or without radiologic monitoring; superior hypogastric plexus

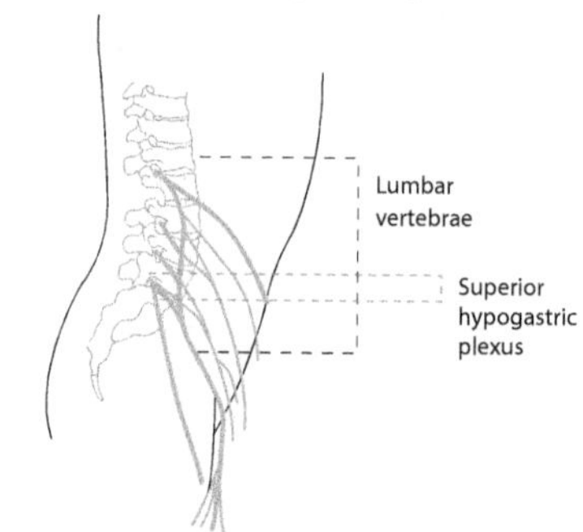

ICD-10-CM Diagnostic Codes

C47.5	Malignant neoplasm of peripheral nerves of pelvis
C48.0	Malignant neoplasm of retroperitoneum
C48.1	Malignant neoplasm of specified parts of peritoneum
C48.2	Malignant neoplasm of peritoneum, unspecified
C48.8	Malignant neoplasm of overlapping sites of retroperitoneum and peritoneum
C49.5	Malignant neoplasm of connective and soft tissue of pelvis
C76.3	Malignant neoplasm of pelvis
C78.6	Secondary malignant neoplasm of retroperitoneum and peritoneum
C79.9	Secondary malignant neoplasm of unspecified site
G89.21	Chronic pain due to trauma
G89.28	Other chronic postprocedural pain
G89.29	Other chronic pain
G89.3	Neoplasm related pain (acute) (chronic)
M54.16	Radiculopathy, lumbar region
M54.17	Radiculopathy, lumbosacral region
M54.18	Radiculopathy, sacral and sacrococcygeal region
R10.2	Pelvic and perineal pain
❼ S34.5	Injury of lumbar, sacral and pelvic sympathetic nerves

ICD-10-CM Coding Notes

For codes requiring a 7th character extension, refer to your ICD-10-CM book. Review the character descriptions and coding guidelines for proper selection. For some procedures, only certain characters will apply.

CCI Edits

Refer to Appendix A for CCI edits.

Facility RVUs ▯

Code	Work	PE Facility	MP	Total Facility
64681	3.78	2.97	1.12	7.87

Non-facility RVUs ▯

Code	Work	PE Non-Facility	MP	Total Non-Facility
64681	3.78	11.53	1.12	16.43

Modifiers (PAR) ▯

Code	Mod 50	Mod 51	Mod 62	Mod 66	Mod 80
64681	0	2	0	0	1

Global Period

Code	Days
64681	010

CPT © 2018 American Medical Association. All Rights Reserved.

71045-71048

71045 Radiologic examination, chest; single view

71046 Radiologic examination, chest; 2 views

71047 Radiologic examination, chest; 3 views

71048 Radiologic examination, chest; 4 or more views

(For acute abdomen series that includes a single view of the chest and one or more views of the abdomen, use 74022)

(For concurrent computer-aided detection [CAD] performed in addition to 71045, 71046, 71047, 71048, use 0174T)

(Do not report 71045, 71046, 71047, 71048 in conjunction with 0175T for computer-aided detection [CAD] performed remotely from the primary interpretation)

Plain English Description

A radiologic examination of the chest is performed. Chest radiographs (X-rays) provide images of the heart, lungs, bronchi, major blood vessels (aorta, vena cava, pulmonary vessels), and bones, (sternum, ribs, clavicle, scapula, spine). In 71045, a single view of the chest is obtained; 2 views in 71056; 3 views in 71047; and 4 views in 71048. The most common views are frontal (also referred to as anteroposterior or AP), posteroanterior (PA), and lateral. To obtain a frontal view, the patient is positioned facing the x-ray machine. A PA view is obtained with the patient's back toward the x-ray machine. For a lateral view, the patient is positioned with side of the chest toward the machine. Other views that may be obtained include apical lordotic, oblique, and lateral decubitus. An apical lordotic image provides better visualization of the apical (top) regions of the lungs. The patient is positioned with the back arched so that the tops of the lungs can be x-rayed. Oblique views may be obtained to evaluate a pulmonary or mediastinal mass or opacity or to provide additional images of the heart and great vessels. There are four positions used for oblique views including right and left anterior oblique, and right and left posterior oblique. Anterior oblique views are obtained with the patient standing and the chest rotated 45 degrees. The arm closest to the x-ray cassette is flexed with the hand resting on the hip. The opposite arm is raised as high as possible. The part of the chest farthest away from the x-ray cassette is the area being studied. Posterior oblique views are typically obtained only when the patient is too ill to stand or lay prone for anterior oblique views. A lateral decubitus view is obtained with the patient lying on the side; the patient's head rests on one arm, and the other arm is raised over the head with the elbow bent. Images are recorded on hard copy film or stored electronically as digital images. The physician reviews the images, notes any abnormalities, and provides a written interpretation of the findings.

RVUs

Code	Work	PE	PE Non-Facility	MP	Total Non-Facility	Total Facility	Global
71045	0.18	0.50	0.50	0.02	0.70	0.70	XXX
71046	0.22	0.65	0.65	0.02	0.89	0.89	XXX
71047	0.27	0.83	0.83	0.02	1.12	1.12	XXX
71048	0.31	0.88	0.88	0.02	1.21	1.21	XXX

72020

72020 Radiologic examination, spine, single view, specify level

(For a single view that includes the entire thoracic and lumbar spine, use 72081)

Plain English Description

A diagnostic x-ray is taken of one area of the spine. X-ray uses indirect ionizing radiation to take pictures inside the body. X-rays work on non-uniform material, such as human tissue, because of the different density and composition of the object, which allows some of the x-rays to be absorbed and some to pass through and be captured behind the object on a detector. This produces a 2D image of the structures. This code reports a single view of the spine to look for abnormalities or problems related to injury or pain and must be specified for the level.

RVUs

Code	Work	PE	PE Non-Facility	MP	Total Non-Facility	Total Facility	Global
72020	0.15	0.48	0.48	0.02	0.65	0.65	XXX

72040-72052

72040 Radiologic examination, spine, cervical; 2 or 3 views

72050 Radiologic examination, spine, cervical; 4 or 5 views

72052 Radiologic examination, spine, cervical; 6 or more views

Plain English Description

A radiologic exam is done of the cervical spine. Anteroposterior and lateral views are the most common projections taken. X-ray uses indirect ionizing radiation to take pictures inside the body. X-rays work on non-uniform material, such as human tissue, because of the different density and composition of the object, which allows some of the x-rays to be absorbed and some to pass through and be captured behind the object on a detector. This produces a 2D image of the structures. When 2-3 views or less are taken of the cervical spine, report 72040. If 4 or 5 views are taken, report 72050. A cervical spine x-ray examination with 6 or more views is reported with 72052.

RVUs

Code	Work	PE	PE Non-Facility	MP	Total Non-Facility	Total Facility	Global
72040	0.22	0.79	0.79	0.02	1.03	1.03	XXX
72050	0.31	1.08	1.08	0.03	1.42	1.42.	XXX
72052	0.36	1.30	1.30	0.03	1.69	1.69	XXX

72070-72074

72070 Radiologic examination, spine; thoracic, 2 views

72072 Radiologic examination, spine; thoracic, 3 views

72074 Radiologic examination, spine; thoracic, minimum of 4 views

Plain English Description

A radiologic exam is done of the thoracic spine. X-ray uses indirect ionizing radiation to take pictures inside the body. X-rays work on non-uniform material, such as human tissue, because of the different density and composition of the object, which allows some of the x-rays to be absorbed and some to pass through and be captured behind the object on a detector. This produces a 2D image of the structures. X-rays are taken of the thoracic spine to evaluate for back pain or suspected disease or injury. Films are taken from differing views that commonly include anteroposterior, lateral, posteroanterior, and a swimmer's view for the upper thoracic spine in which the patient reaches up with one arm and down with the other as if taking a swimming stroke. Report 72070 for 2 views of the thoracic spine; 72072 for 3 views; and 72074 for a minimum of 4 views of the thoracic spine.

RVUs

Code	Work	PE	PE Non-Facility	MP	Total Non-Facility	Total Facility	Global
72070	0.22	0.72	0.72	0.02	0.96	0.96	XXX
72072	0.22	0.78	0.78	0.02	1.02	1.02	XXX
72074	0.22	0.88	0.88	0.02	1.12	1.12	XXX

CPT © 2018 American Medical Association. All Rights Reserved.

72080

72080 Radiologic examination, spine; thoracolumbar junction, minimum of 2 views

(For a single view examination of the thoracolumbar junction, use 72020)

Plain English Description

A radiologic x-ray exam is done of the thoracolumbar junction of the spine. X-ray uses indirect ionizing radiation to take pictures inside the body. X-rays work on non-uniform material, such as human tissue, because of the different density and composition of the object, which allows some of the x-rays to be absorbed and some to pass through and be captured behind the object on a detector. This produces a 2D image of the structures. A minimum of two views are taken of the thoracolumbar junction of the spine to evaluate for back pain or suspected disease or injury. X-ray films are commonly taken from frontal and lateral views or posteroanterior and lateral views.

RVUs

Code	Work	PE	PE Non-Facility	MP	Total Non-Facility	Total Facility	Global
72080	0.22	0.71	0.71	0.02	0.95	0.95	XXX

72081-72084

72081 Radiologic examination, spine, entire thoracic and lumbar, including skull, cervical and sacral spine if performed (eg, scoliosis evaluation); one view

72082 Radiologic examination, spine, entire thoracic and lumbar, including skull, cervical and sacral spine if performed (eg, scoliosis evaluation); 2 or 3 views

72083 Radiologic examination, spine, entire thoracic and lumbar, including skull, cervical and sacral spine if performed (eg, scoliosis evaluation); 4 or 5 views

72084 Radiologic examination, spine, entire thoracic and lumbar, including skull, cervical and sacral spine if performed (eg, scoliosis evaluation); minimum of 6 views

Plain English Description

A diagnostic radiographic examination is done of the entire thoracic and lumbar spine for a scoliosis evaluation. This study is done to assess scoliosis, such as the type of scoliosis, and the location and degree of curvature. X-ray uses indirect ionizing radiation to take pictures inside the body. X-rays work on non-uniform material, such as human tissue, because of the different density and composition of the object, which allows some of the x-rays to be absorbed and some to pass through and be captured behind the object on a detector. This produces a 2D image of the structures. Code 72081 reports a single view x-ray of the entire thoracic and lumbar spine; code 72082 reports 2 or 3 views; code 72083 reports 4 or 5 views; and 72084 reports a spinal evaluation with a minimum of 6 views being taken. Posteroanterior, frontal, and lateral views are commonly taken of the spine while in an erect, standing, or upright position to help assess lateral curvature. The patient stands in front of a vertical grid with the knees together in full extension. The field of view includes the entire thoracic and lumbar spine and also the cervical and sacral spinal areas as well as the skull, whenever necessary. The vertebral bodies above and below the apex of the spinal curve that are the most tilted are measured by intersecting lines to give the degree of curvature. Lateral projections for viewing scoliosis may be taken with the patient's arms placed straight out in front for a better view of the curvature. Other views may also be taken of the spine while the patient is lying down face up.

RVUs

Code	Work	PE	PE Non-Facility	MP	Total Non-Facility	Total Facility	Global
72081	0.26	0.85	0.85	0.03	1.14	1.14	XXX
72082	0.31	1.49	1.49	0.03	1.83	1.83	XXX
72083	0.35	1.78	1.78	0.03	2.16	2.16	XXX
72084	0.41	2.07	2.07	0.04	2.52	2.52	XXX

72100-72114

72100 Radiologic examination, spine, lumbosacral; 2 or 3 views

72110 Radiologic examination, spine, lumbosacral; minimum of 4 views

72114 Radiologic examination, spine, lumbosacral; complete, including bending views, minimum of 6 views

Plain English Description

A radiologic exam is done of the lumbosacral spine. Frontal, posteroanterior, and lateral views are the most common projections taken. X-ray uses indirect ionizing radiation to take pictures inside the body. X-rays work on non-uniform material, such as human tissue, because of the different density and composition of the object, which allows some of the x-rays to be absorbed and some to pass through and be captured behind the object on a detector. This produces a 2D image of the structures. When 2 or 3 views are taken of the lumbosacral spine, report 72100. If at least 4 views are taken, report 72110. A complete lumbosacral spine exam (72114) includes a minimum of 6 views, which may include views taken from oblique angles as well as in bending positions, flexion and extension. Lateral bending positions may also be taken with the patient sitting on a stool with the back against a contact to avoid moving the torso forward. The patient flexes the back over to each side as far as possible without losing contact with the stool. The complete exam is often done by taking anteroposterior and lateral views first, particularly to 'clear' the spine before the technologist moves the patient into position for oblique angles and bending views if evaluating for trauma.

RVUs

Code	Work	PE	PE Non-Facility	MP	Total Non-Facility	Total Facility	Global
72100	0.22	0.79	0.79	0.02	1.03	1.03	XXX
72110	0.31	1.10	1.10	0.03	1.44	1.44	XXX
72114	0.32	1.29	1.29	0.03	1.64	1.64	XXX

72120

72120 Radiologic examination, spine, lumbosacral; bending views only, 2 or 3 views

(Contrast material in CT of spine is either by intrathecal or intravenous injection. For intrathecal injection, use also 61055 or 62284. IV injection of contrast material is part of the CT procedure)

Plain English Description

A radiologic exam of the lumbosacral spine is done taking 2 or 3 views with the patient in bending positions only. X-ray uses indirect ionizing radiation to take pictures inside the body. X-rays work on non-uniform material, such as human tissue, because of the different density and composition of the object, which allows some of the x-rays to be absorbed and some to pass through and be captured behind the object on a detector. This produces a 2D image of the structures. Biomechanical dysfunction of the lumbar spine is revealed with lateral bending views. The patient is placed sitting on a stool with the back against a contact to avoid moving the torso forward. The patient flexes the back over to each side as far as possible without losing contact with the stool. Sitting instead of standing helps block out effects of gross musculature. These

CPT © 2018 American Medical Association. All Rights Reserved.

views are helpful when plain films seem normal and symptoms of dysfunction are not explained. Flexion or extension bending views may also be taken with the patient standing, such as bending over forward with the knees straight and the arms dangling.

RVUs

Code	Work	PE	PE Non-Facility	MP	Total Non-Facility	Total Facility	Global
72120	0.22	0.97	0.97	0.02	1.21	1.21	XXX

72125-72127

72125 Computed tomography, cervical spine; without contrast material

72126 Computed tomography, cervical spine; with contrast material

72127 Computed tomography, cervical spine; without contrast material, followed by contrast material(s) and further sections

(For intrathecal injection procedure, see 61055, 62284)

Plain English Description

Diagnostic computed tomography (CT) is done on the cervical spine. CT uses multiple, narrow x-ray beams aimed around a single rotational axis, taking a series of 2D images of the target structure from multiple angles. Contrast material is used to enhance the images. Computer software processes the data and produces several images of thin, cross-sectional 2D slices of the targeted organ or area. Three-dimensional models of the spine can be created by stacking multiple, individual 2D slices together. The patient is placed inside the CT scanner on the table and images are obtained of the cervical spine. In 72125, no contrast medium is used. In 72126, an iodine contrast dye is injected either intrathecally into the C1-C2 or other cervical level, or administered intravenously to see the target area better before images are taken. If intrathecal injection is performed it is reported separately. In 72127, images are taken without contrast and again after the administration of the contrast. The physician reviews the images to look for suspected problems with the spine such as bone disease, fractures or other injuries, or birth defects of the spine in children.

RVUs

Code	Work	PE	PE Non-Facility	MP	Total Non-Facility	Total Facility	Global
72125	1.07	4.04	4.04	0.07	5.18	5.18	XXX
72126	1.22	5.10	5.10	0.08	6.40	6.40	XXX
72127	1.27	6.23	6.23	0.08	7.58	7.58	XXX

72128-72130

72128 Computed tomography, thoracic spine; without contrast material

72129 Computed tomography, thoracic spine; with contrast material

(For intrathecal injection procedure, see 61055, 62284)

72130 Computed tomography, thoracic spine; without contrast material, followed by contrast material(s) and further sections

(For intrathecal injection procedure, see 61055, 62284)

Plain English Description

Diagnostic computed tomography (CT) is done on the thoracic spine. CT uses multiple, narrow x-ray beams aimed around a single rotational axis, taking a series of 2D images of the target structure from multiple angles. Contrast material is used to enhance the images. Computer software processes the data and produces several images of thin, cross-sectional 2D slices of the targeted organ or area. Three-dimensional models of the spine can be created by stacking multiple, individual 2D slices together. The patient is placed inside the CT scanner on the table and images are obtained of the thoracic spine. In 72128, no contrast medium is used. In 72129, an iodine contrast dye is injected either intrathecally or administered intravenously to see the target area better before images are taken. If intrathecal injection is performed it is reported separately. In 72130, images are taken without contrast and again after the administration of the contrast. The physician reviews the images to look for suspected problems with the spine such as bone disease, and evaluate for fractures or other injuries as well as birth defects of the spine in children.

RVUs

Code	Work	PE	PE Non-Facility	MP	Total Non-Facility	Total Facility	Global
72128	1.00	4.01	4.01	0.07	5.08	5.08	XXX
72129	1.22	5.14	5.14	0.08	6.44	6.44	XXX
72130	1.27	6.24	6.24	0.08	7.59	7.59	XXX

72131-72133

72131 Computed tomography, lumbar spine; without contrast material

72132 Computed tomography, lumbar spine; with contrast material

72133 Computed tomography, lumbar spine; without contrast material, followed by contrast material(s) and further sections

(For intrathecal injection procedure, see 61055, 62284)

(To report 3D rendering, see 76376, 76377)

Plain English Description

Diagnostic computed tomography (CT) is done on the lumbar spine. CT uses multiple, narrow x-ray beams aimed around a single rotational axis, taking a series of 2D images of the target structure from multiple angles. Contrast material is used to enhance the images. Computer software processes the data and produces several images of thin, cross-sectional 2D slices of the targeted organ or area. Three-dimensional models of the spine can be created by stacking multiple, individual 2D slices together. The patient is placed inside the CT scanner on the table and images are obtained of the lumbar spine. In 72131, no contrast medium is used. In 72132, an iodine contrast dye is injected either intrathecally or administered intravenously to see the target area better before images are taken. If intrathecal injection is performed it is reported separately. In 72133, images are taken without contrast and again after the administration of the contrast. The physician reviews the images to look for suspected problems with the spine such as bone disease, and evaluate for fractures or other injuries as well as birth defects of the spine in children.

RVUs

Code	Work	PE	PE Non-Facility	MP	Total Non-Facility	Total Facility	Global
72131	1.00	3.99	3.99	0.07	5.06	5.06	XXX
72132	1.22	5.11	5.11	0.08	6.41	6.41	XXX
72133	1.27	6.20	6.20	0.09	7.56	7.56	XXX

CPT © 2018 American Medical Association. All Rights Reserved.

72141-72142

72141 Magnetic resonance (eg, proton) imaging, spinal canal and contents, cervical; without contrast material

72142 Magnetic resonance (eg, proton) imaging, spinal canal and contents, cervical; with contrast material(s)

(For cervical spinal canal imaging without contrast material followed by contrast material, use 72156)

Plain English Description

Magnetic resonance imaging (MRI) is done on the cervical spinal canal and contents. MRI is a noninvasive, non-radiating imaging technique that uses the magnetic properties of nuclei within hydrogen atoms of the body. The powerful magnetic field forces the hydrogen atoms to line up. Radiowaves are then transmitted within the strong magnetic field. Protons in the nuclei of different types of tissues emit a specific radiofrequency signal that bounces back to the computer, which records the images. The computer processes the signals and converts the data into tomographic, 3D, sectional images in slices with very high resolution. The patient is placed on a motorized table within a large MRI tunnel scanner that contains the magnet. MRI scans of the spine are often done when conservative treatment of back/neck pain is unsuccessful and more aggressive treatments are considered or following surgery. In 72141, no contrast medium is used. In 72142, a contrast dye is administered first to see the spinal area better before images are taken. The physician reviews the images to look for specific information that may correlate to the patient's symptoms, such as abnormal spinal alignment; disease or injury of vertebral bodies; intervertebral disc herniation, degeneration, or dehydration; the size of the spinal canal to accommodate the cord and nerve roots; pinched or inflamed nerves; or any changes since surgery.

RVUs

Code	Work	PE	PE Non-Facility	MP	Total Non-Facility	Total Facility	Global
72141	1.48	4.64	4.64	0.10	6.22	6.22	XXX
72142	1.78	7.12	7.12	0.13	9.03	9.03	XXX

72146-72147

72146 Magnetic resonance (eg, proton) imaging, spinal canal and contents, thoracic; without contrast material

72147 Magnetic resonance (eg, proton) imaging, spinal canal and contents, thoracic; with contrast material(s)

(For thoracic spinal canal imaging without contrast material followed by contrast material, use 72157)

Plain English Description

Magnetic resonance imaging (MRI) is done on the thoracic spinal canal and contents. MRI is a noninvasive, non-radiating imaging technique that uses the magnetic properties of nuclei within hydrogen atoms of the body. The powerful magnetic field forces the hydrogen atoms to line up. Radiowaves are then transmitted within the strong magnetic field. Protons in the nuclei of different types of tissues emit a specific radiofrequency signal that bounces back to the computer, which records the images. The computer processes the signals and converts the data into tomographic, 3D, sectional images in slices with very high resolution. The patient is placed on a motorized table within a large MRI tunnel scanner that contains the magnet. MRI scans of the spine are often done when conservative treatment of back/neck pain is unsuccessful and more aggressive treatments are considered or following surgery. In 72146, no contrast medium is used. In 72147, a contrast dye is administered first to see the spinal area better before images are taken. The physician reviews the images to look for specific information that may correlate to the patient's symptoms, such as abnormal spinal alignment; disease or injury of vertebral bodies; intervertebral disc herniation, degeneration, or dehydration; the size of the spinal canal to accommodate the cord and nerve roots; pinched or inflamed nerves; or any changes since surgery.

RVUs

Code	Work	PE	PE Non-Facility	MP	Total Non-Facility	Total Facility	Global
72146	1.48	4.65	4.65	0.10	6.23	6.23	XXX
72147	1.78	7.08	7.08	0.12	8.98	8.98	XXX

72148-72149

72148 Magnetic resonance (eg, proton) imaging, spinal canal and contents, lumbar; without contrast material

72149 Magnetic resonance (eg, proton) imaging, spinal canal and contents, lumbar; with contrast material(s)

(For lumbar spinal canal imaging without contrast material followed by contrast material, use 72158)

Plain English Description

Magnetic resonance imaging (MRI) is done on the lumbar spinal canal and contents. MRI is a noninvasive, non-radiating imaging technique that uses the magnetic properties of nuclei within hydrogen atoms of the body. The powerful magnetic field forces the hydrogen atoms to line up. Radiowaves are then transmitted within the strong magnetic field. Protons in the nuclei of different types of tissues emit a specific radiofrequency signal that bounces back to the computer, which records the images. The computer processes the signals and coverts the data into tomographic, 3D, sectional images in slices with very high resolution. The patient is placed on a motorized table within a large MRI tunnel scanner that contains the magnet. MRI scans of the spine are often done when conservative treatment of back pain is unsuccessful and more aggressive treatments are considered or following surgery. In 72148, no contrast medium is used. In 72149, a contrast dye is administered first to see the spinal area better before images are taken. The physician reviews the images to look for specific information that may correlate to the patient's symptoms, such as abnormal spinal alignment; disease or injury of vertebral bodies; intervertebral disc herniation, degeneration, or dehydration; the size of the spinal canal to accommodate the cord and nerve roots; pinched or inflamed nerves; or any changes since surgery.

RVUs

Code	Work	PE	PE Non-Facility	MP	Total Non-Facility	Total Facility	Global
72148	1.48	4.65	4.65	0.10	6.23	6.23	XXX
72149	1.78	7.01	7.01	0.13	8.92	8.92	XXX

72156-72158

72156 Magnetic resonance (eg, proton) imaging, spinal canal and contents, without contrast material, followed by contrast material(s) and further sequences; cervical

72157 Magnetic resonance (eg, proton) imaging, spinal canal and contents, without contrast material, followed by contrast material(s) and further sequences; thoracic

72158 Magnetic resonance (eg, proton) imaging, spinal canal and contents, without contrast material, followed by contrast material(s) and further sequences; lumbar

Plain English Description

Magnetic resonance imaging (MRI) is done on the cervical, thoracic, or lumbar spinal canal and contents. MRI is a noninvasive, non-radiating imaging technique that uses the magnetic properties of nuclei within hydrogen atoms of the body. The powerful magnetic field forces the hydrogen atoms to line

CPT © 2018 American Medical Association. All Rights Reserved.

up. Radiowaves are then transmitted within the strong magnetic field. Protons in the nuclei of different types of tissues emit a specific radiofrequency signal that bounces back to the computer, which records the images. The computer processes the signals and coverts the data into tomographic, 3D, sectional images in slices with very high resolution. The patient is placed on a motorized table within a large MRI tunnel scanner that contains the magnet. MRI scans of the spine are often done when conservative treatment of back/neck pain is unsuccessful and more aggressive treatments are considered or following surgery. Images are taken first without contrast and again after the administration of contrast to see the spinal area better. The physician reviews the images to look for specific information that may correlate to the patient's symptoms, such as abnormal spinal alignment; disease or injury of vertebral bodies; intervertebral disc herniation, degeneration, or dehydration; the size of the spinal canal to accommodate the cord and nerve roots; pinched or inflamed nerves; or any changes since surgery. Use 72156 for MRI of the cervical spine, 72157 for the thoracic spine, and 72158 for the lumbar spine.

RVUs

Code	Work	PE	PE Non-Facility	MP	Total Non-Facility	Total Facility	Global
72156	2.29	8.08	8.08	0.15	10.52	10.52	XXX
72157	2.29	8.11	8.11	0.15	10.55	10.55	XXX
72158	2.29	8.06	8.06	0.15	10.50	10.50	XXX

72200-72202

72200 Radiologic examination, sacroiliac joints; less than 3 views

72202 Radiologic examination, sacroiliac joints; 3 or more views

Plain English Description

A radiologic examination of the sacroiliac (SI) joints is performed. This is the area where the left and right winged pelvic bones join with the sacrum in the back to form the posterior portion of the pelvic ring. Because of its complex anatomy and irregular surfaces, the sacroiliac joint can be difficult to image. An anteroposterior (AP) view with the patient supine and knees or hips flexed, if possible, is typically done first for routine exam, along with left and right oblique views with the patient recumbent and rotated 25-30 degrees from the AP position. When imaging SI joints, the oblique views take the x-ray of the side that is up, although the patient is positioned for the opposite side down. Posteroanterior views may also be taken with the patient prone. X-rays are taken of the sacroiliac joints to help diagnose spondyloarthropathies in rheumatic disease, inflammatory lesions affecting the joint, sacroiliitis, ankylosing spondylitis, juvenile spondyloarthropathy, arthritis associated with inflammatory bowel disease, psoriatic arthritis, and reactive arthritis, as well as fractures or dislocations. X-ray imaging uses indirect ionizing radiation to take pictures inside the body. X-rays work on non-uniform material, such as human tissue, because of the different density and composition of the object, which allows some of the x-rays to be absorbed and some to pass through and be captured behind the object on a detector. This produces a 2D image of the structures. If less than 3 views are taken, report 72200. Use 72202 when 3 views or more are taken for a complete exam.

RVUs

Code	Work	PE	PE Non-Facility	MP	Total Non-Facility	Total Facility	Global
72200	0.17	0.68	0.68	0.02	0.87	0.87	XXX
72202	0.19	0.77	0.77	0.02	0.98	0.98	XXX

72240-72270

72240 Myelography, cervical, radiological supervision and interpretation

(Do not report 72240 in conjunction with 62284, 62302, 62303, 62304, 62305)

(When both 62284 and 72240 are performed by the same physician or other qualified health care professional for cervical myelography, use 62302)

(For complete cervical myelography via injection procedure at C1-C2, see 61055, 72240)

72255 Myelography, thoracic, radiological supervision and interpretation

(Do not report 72255 in conjunction with 62284, 62302, 62303, 62304, 62305)

(When both 62284 and 72255 are performed by the same physician or other qualified health care professional for thoracic myelography, use 62303)

(For complete thoracic myelography via injection procedure at C1-C2, see 61055, 72255)

72265 Myelography, lumbosacral, radiological supervision and interpretation

(Do not report 72265 in conjunction with 62284, 62302, 62303, 62304, 62305)

(When both 62284 and 72265 are performed by the same physician or other qualified health care professional for lumbosacral myelography, use 62304)

(For complete lumbosacral myelography via injection procedure at C1-C2, see 61055, 72265)

72270 Myelography, 2 or more regions (eg, lumbar/thoracic, cervical/thoracic, lumbar/cervical, lumbar/thoracic/cervical), radiological supervision and interpretation

(Do not report 72270 in conjunction with 62284, 62302, 62303, 62304, 62305)

(When both 62284 and 72270 are performed by the same physician or other qualified health care professional for myelography of 2 or more regions, use 62305)

(For complete myelography of 2 or more regions via injection procedure at C1-C2, see 61055, 72270)

Plain English Description

Myelography is a type of diagnostic imaging that uses contrast material injected into the subarachnoid space and real-time fluoroscopic x-ray imaging. After introducing a needle into the spinal canal and injecting contrast material into the subarachnoid space, the radiologist evaluates the spinal cord, spinal canal, nerve roots, meninges, and blood vessels in real time as contrast flows through the space around the spinal cord and nerve roots. Permanent x-ray images may also be taken. Spinal myelography is used to diagnose intervertebral disc herniation, meningeal inflammation, spinal stenosis, tumors, and other spinal lesions caused by infection or previous trauma. Report 72240 for myelography of the cervical spine, 72255 for thoracic myelography, 72265 for lumbosacral myelography, and 72270 when two or more regions of the spine are examined together.

CPT © 2018 American Medical Association. All Rights Reserved.

RVUs

Code	Work	PE	PE Non-Facility	MP	Total Non-Facility	Total Facility	Global
72240	0.91	1.97	1.97	0.06	2.94	2.94	XXX
72255	0.91	1.99	1.99	0.09	2.99	2.99	XXX
72265	0.83	1.86	1.86	0.06	2.75	2.75	XXX
72270	1.33	2.40	2.40	0.09	3.82	3.82	XXX

72275

72275 Epidurography, radiological supervision and interpretation

(72275 includes 77003)

(For injection procedure, see 62280, 62281, 62282, 62320, 62321, 62322, 62323, 62324, 62325, 62326, 62327, 64479, 64480, 64483, 64484)

(Use 72275 only when an epidurogram is performed, images documented, and a formal radiologic report is issued)

(Do not report 72275 in conjunction with 22586)

Plain English Description

Images of the epidural space surrounding the spinal cord are documented under radiological supervision while a therapeutic or diagnostic epidurography is performed. The radiologist also provides a formal radiologic report of the procedure after it is performed. The injection portion of the procedure to perform the epidurography is done by cleansing the skin over the targeted spinal region with an antiseptic solution and then injecting a local anesthetic. A spinal needle is inserted into the skin and advanced into the epidural space. Contrast may be injected to confirm proper needle placement or to perform the procedure itself. A diagnostic or therapeutic substance, such as an anesthetic, antispasmodic, opioid, steroid, or neurolytic substance is injected into the epidural space. Images are taken. Following injection, the patient is monitored for 15-20 minutes to ensure that there are no adverse effects. Report 72275 for radiological supervision during the procedure that includes documented imaging and provision of a formal interpretation of the procedure by the radiologist.

RVUs

Code	Work	PE	PE Non-Facility	MP	Total Non-Facility	Total Facility	Global
72275	0.76	2.67	2.67	0.05	3.48	3.48	XXX

72285

72285 Discography, cervical or thoracic, radiological supervision and interpretation

Plain English Description

Images of a cervical or thoracic intervertebral disc are documented under radiological supervision while a discography is performed. A formal interpretation of the procedure is also provided. Discography is done to determine if an intervertebral disc abnormality is the cause of back pain. To perform the injection portion of the discography, the patient is positioned on the side and the site of the injection is cleansed with an antiseptic solution. A local anesthetic is injected. A large bore needle is advanced through the skin to the targeted cervical or thoracic disc. A discography needle is advanced through the first needle and into the center of the disc. Contrast is injected and radiographs are obtained under supervision. Report 72285 for radiological supervision during the discography procedure and provision of a written interpretation after completion.

RVUs

Code	Work	PE	PE Non-Facility	MP	Total Non-Facility	Total Facility	Global
72285	1.16	2.09	2.09	0.07	3.32	3.32	XXX

72295

72295 Discography, lumbar, radiological supervision and interpretation

Plain English Description

Images of a lumbar intervertebral disc are documented under radiological supervision while a discography is performed. A formal interpretation of the procedure is also provided. Discography is done to determine if an intervertebral disc abnormality is the cause of back pain. To perform the injection portion of the discography, the patient is positioned on the side and the site of the injection is cleansed with an antiseptic solution. A local anesthetic is injected. A large bore needle is advanced through the skin to the targeted lumbar disc. A discography needle is advanced through the first needle and into the center of the disc. Contrast is injected and radiographs are obtained under supervision. Report 72295 for radiological supervision during the discography procedure and provision of a written interpretation after completion.

RVUs

Code	Work	PE	PE Non-Facility	MP	Total Non-Facility	Total Facility	Global
72295	0.83	2.00	2.00	0.07	2.90	2.90	XXX

75901

75901 Mechanical removal of pericatheter obstructive material (eg, fibrin sheath) from central venous device via separate venous access, radiologic supervision and interpretation

(For procedure, use 36595)

(For venous catheterization, see 36010-36012)

Plain English Description

The provider removes obstructive fibrous build-up from around a central venous catheter that was previously inserted. An accumulation of thrombotic or fibrous material can cause catheter failure. A special type of loop snare instrument is inserted through another access point, usually in the femoral vein, and advanced to the central venous catheter, where it is encircled snugly under radiologic supervision. The loop snare instrument is then pulled down along the length of the central venous catheter, stripping off the periobstructive material that has collected around it, and pulling it off the tip of the catheter.

RVUs

Code	Work	PE	PE Non-Facility	MP	Total Non-Facility	Total Facility	Global
75901	0.49	5.09	5.09	0.04	5.62	5.62	XXX

CPT © 2018 American Medical Association. All Rights Reserved.

75902

75902 Mechanical removal of intraluminal (intracatheter) obstructive material from central venous device through device lumen, radiologic supervision and interpretation

(For procedure, use 36596)

(For venous catheterization, see 36010-36012)

Plain English Description

The provider removes obstructive fibrous build-up from within the lumen of a central venous catheter that was previously inserted. An accumulation of thrombotic or fibrous material can cause catheter failure. Another catheter is inserted into the lumen of the central venous catheter through its entry port. The obstructing material is disrupted and removed and the central venous catheter lumen is flushed and checked for patency and unimpeded flow.

RVUs

Code	Work	PE	PE Non-Facility	MP	Total Non-Facility	Total Facility	Global
75902	0.39	1.79	1.79	0.04	2.22	2.22	XXX

76800

76800 Ultrasound, spinal canal and contents

Plain English Description

An ultrasound examination of the spinal canal and contents is performed. Ultrasound visualizes the body internally using sound waves far above human perception bounced off interior anatomical structures. As the sound waves pass through different densities of tissue, they are reflected back to the receiving unit at varying speeds and converted into pictures displayed on screen. Transdermal spinal ultrasound is used primarily in evaluation of newborns and infants because of the minimal ossification of the spine and the short distance between the skin and the spinal subarachnoid space. Spinal ultrasound may be used intraoperatively in adults and older children but is generally not considered an effective diagnostic tool in these patients. With the newborn or infant placed in a prone position, the neck is flexed. Acoustic coupling gel is applied to the skin along the spine. The spinal canal and contents are examined using a linear probe in both the sagittal and axial plane along the entire length of the spine. The physician reviews the images and provides a written interpretation.

RVUs

Code	Work	PE	PE Non-Facility	MP	Total Non-Facility	Total Facility	Global
76800	1.13	2.75	2.75	0.16	4.04	4.04	XXX

76942

76942 Ultrasonic guidance for needle placement (eg, biopsy, aspiration, injection, localization device), imaging supervision and interpretation

(Do not report 76942 in conjunction with 10004, 10005, 10006, 10021, 10030, 19083, 19285, 20604, 20606, 20611, 27096, 32554, 32555, 32556, 32557, 37760, 37761, 43232, 43237, 43242, 45341, 45342, 55874, 64479, 64480, 64483, 64484, 64490, 64491, 64493, 64494, 64495, 76975, 0213T, 0214T, 0215T, 0216T, 0217T, 0218T, 0228T, 0229T, 0230T, 0231T, 0232T, 0249T, 0481T)

(For harvesting, preparation, and injection[s] of platelet rich plasma, use 0232T)

Plain English Description

Ultrasound guidance including imaging supervision and interpretation is performed for needle placement during a separately reportable biopsy, aspiration, injection, or placement of a localization device. A local anesthetic is injected at the site of the planned needle or localization device placement. A transducer is then used to locate the lesion, site of the planned injection, or site of the planned placement of the localization device. The radiologist constantly monitors needle placement with the ultrasound probe to ensure the needle is properly placed. The radiologist also uses ultrasound imaging to monitor separately reportable biopsy, aspiration, injection, or device localization procedures. Upon completion of the procedure, the needle is withdrawn and pressure applied to control bleeding. A dressing is applied as needed. The radiologist then provides a written report of the ultrasound imaging component of the procedure.

RVUs

Code	Work	PE	PE Non-Facility	MP	Total Non-Facility	Total Facility	Global
76942	0.67	0.90	0.90	0.04	1.61	1.61	XXX

77001

+ 77001 Fluoroscopic guidance for central venous access device placement, replacement (catheter only or complete), or removal (includes fluoroscopic guidance for vascular access and catheter manipulation, any necessary contrast injections through access site or catheter with related venography radiologic supervision and interpretation, and radiographic documentation of final catheter position) (List separately in addition to code for primary procedure)

(Do not report 77001 in conjunction with 33957, 33958, 33959, 33962, 33963, 33964, 36568, 36569, 36572, 36573, 36584, 77002)

(If formal extremity venography is performed from separate venous access and separately interpreted, use 36005 and 75820, 75822, 75825, or 75827)

Plain English Description

This code reports the radiological portion of fluoroscopic guidance used throughout the procedure of placing, replacing, or removing a central venous access device, or CVAD. This includes contrast injections through the access site or catheter, related venography supervision and interpretation, and radiographic verification of the final catheter position. A CVAD is a catheter inserted with its tip in the superior or inferior vena cava or the right atrium for purposes of administering large amounts of blood, fluid, or repeated transfusions, such as antibiotics or cytotoxic therapy. Central veins are those in the thorax with direct continuity to the right atrium. The most commonly used access veins are the internal and external jugular and subclavian veins.

CPT © 2018 American Medical Association. All Rights Reserved.

A CVAD may be a peripherally inserted central catheter, or PICC line, which is placed through the antecubital veins in the arm and advanced to the central vein with the tip in the superior vena cava. CVADs may also be nontunneled, which are placed more directly into the central vein by access through the chest wall in the clavicular area. These have multiple lumen access within the catheter and are used mainly in intensive care settings for therapies under three weeks. A tunneled CVAD is placed through a subcutaneous tunnel created from the venous access site on the chest wall to a more distant exit site in the skin of the abdomen. CVADs may also be a totally implantable port with a silicone catheter and septum placed in a subcutaneous pocket and accessed across the skin by a needle into the port. This code is reported in addition to the primary procedure.

RVUs

Code	Work	PE	PE Non-Facility	MP	Total Non-Facility	Total Facility	Global
77001	0.38	2.13	2.13	0.04	2.55	2.55	ZZZ

77002

✚ **77002 Fluoroscopic guidance for needle placement (eg, biopsy, aspiration, injection, localization device) (List separately in addition to code for primary procedure)**

(See appropriate surgical code for procedure and anatomic location)

(Use 77002 in conjunction with 10160, 20206, 20220, 20225, 20520, 20525, 20526, 20550, 20551, 20552, 20553, 20555, 20600, 20605, 20610, 20612, 20615, 21116, 21550, 23350, 24220, 25246, 27093, 27095, 27369, 27648, 32400, 32405, 32553, 36002, 38220, 38221, 38222, 38505, 38794, 41019, 42400, 42405, 47000, 47001, 48102, 49180, 49411, 50200, 50390, 51100, 51101, 51102, 55700, 55876, 60100, 62268, 62269, 64505, 64600, 64605)

(77002 is included in all arthrography radiological supervision and interpretation codes. See Administration of Contrast Material[s] introductory guidelines for reporting of arthrography procedures)

Plain English Description

This code reports the radiological portion of fluoroscopic guidance used in needle placement for biopsy, aspiration, injection, or localization type procedures. Fluoroscopy is a continuous, x-ray beam passed through the body part being examined and projected onto a TV-like monitor to create a kind of x-ray movie. This uses more radiation than standard x-rays and can image many different body systems to study a specific structure or organ, localize a tumor or foreign body, and also study movement within the body. The area is identified with fluoroscopy and anesthetized. The appropriate type of needle is inserted under fluoroscopic guidance to perform the specified procedure such as removing aspirate or tissue samples for biopsy, injecting a therapeutic or diagnostic substance, or localizing a tumor or mass for further study. The primary procedural code reports the type of procedure and anatomic location.

RVUs

Code	Work	PE	PE Non-Facility	MP	Total Non-Facility	Total Facility	Global
77002	0.54	2.28	2.28	0.04	2.86	2.86	ZZZ

77003

✚ **77003 Fluoroscopic guidance and localization of needle or catheter tip for spine or paraspinous diagnostic or therapeutic injection procedures (epidural or subarachnoid) (List separately in addition to code for primary procedure)**

(Use 77003 in conjunction with 61050, 61055, 62267, 62270, 62272, 62273, 62280, 62281, 62282, 62284, 64510, 64517, 64520, 64610, 96450)

(Do not report 77003 in conjunction with 62320, 62321, 62322, 62323, 62324, 62325, 62326, 62327)

Plain English Description

Fluoroscopic guidance is used to locate the target site for inserting a needle or catheter tip for spinal or paraspinous diagnostic or therapeutic injection procedures. Fluoroscopy is a continuous, x-ray beam passed through the body part being examined and projected onto a TV-like monitor to create a kind of x-ray movie. This uses more radiation than standard x-rays and can image many different body systems to locate a specific structure or organ, as well as study movement within the body. The needle or catheter tip is inserted and a small amount of contrast material is injected and observed fluoroscopically to ensure correct positioning for an injection. The separately reportable primary injection procedure may be performed for diagnostic or therapeutic purposes, including injection of an anesthetic, a steroid, or destruction by neurolytic agent. Under fluoroscopic guidance, the physician monitors the injection procedure as it is carried out and provides a written report of the radiological component of the procedure.

RVUs

Code	Work	PE	PE Non-Facility	MP	Total Non-Facility	Total Facility	Global
77003	0.60	2.12	2.12	0.05	2.77	2.77	ZZZ

77021

▲ **77021 Magnetic resonance imaging guidance for needle placement (eg, for biopsy, needle aspiration, injection, or placement of localization device) radiological supervision and interpretation**

(For procedure, see appropriate organ or site)

(Do not report 77021 in conjunction with 10011, 10012, 10030, 19085, 19287, 32554, 32555, 32556, 32557, 0232T, 0481T)

(For harvesting, preparation, and injection[s] of platelet-rich plasma, use 0232T)

Plain English Description

This code reports the radiological supervision and interpretation portion of magnetic resonance imaging (MRI) guidance used in needle placement for biopsy, aspiration, injection, or localization procedures. The target area is localized using magnetic resonance imaging and then anesthetized. The appropriate type of needle is inserted under MRI guidance to perform the specified procedure such as removing aspirate or tissue samples for biopsy, injecting a therapeutic or diagnostic substance, or localizing a tumor or mass for further study. The surgical code reports the procedure and anatomic location. Magnetic resonance imaging is a noninvasive, non-radiating imaging technique that uses the magnetic properties of hydrogen atoms in the body. The nuclei of hydrogen atoms emit radiofrequency signals when the body is exposed to radiowaves transmitted within a strong magnetic field. The computer processes the signals and converts the data into tomographic, 3D images with very high resolution. The needle being used with MRI guidance may have special metallic ringlets around it, be coated with contrast material, or have a signal receiving coil in its tip.

CPT © 2018 American Medical Association. All Rights Reserved.

RVUs

Code	Work	PE	PE Non-Facility	MP	Total Non-Facility	Total Facility	Global
77021	1.50	11.85	11.85	0.09	13.44	13.44	XXX

80047-80048

80047 Basic metabolic panel (Calcium, ionized)

This panel must include the following:

Calcium, ionized (82330); Carbon dioxide (bicarbonate) (82374); Chloride (82435); Creatinine (82565); Glucose (82947); Potassium (84132); Sodium (84295); Urea Nitrogen (BUN) (84520)

80048 Basic metabolic panel (Calcium, total)

This panel must include the following:

Calcium, total (82310); Carbon dioxide (bicarbonate) (82374); Chloride (82435); Creatinine (82565); Glucose (82947); Potassium (84132); Sodium (84295); Urea nitrogen (BUN) (84520)

Plain English Description

A basic metabolic blood panel is obtained that includes ionized calcium levels along with carbon dioxide (bicarbonate) (CO2), chloride, creatinine, glucose, potassium, sodium, and urea nitrogen (BUN). A basic metabolic panel with measurement of ionized calcium may be used to screen for or monitor overall metabolic function or identify imbalances. Ionized or free calcium flows freely in the blood, is not attached to any proteins, and represents the amount of calcium available to support metabolic processes such as heart function, muscle contraction, nerve function, and blood clotting. Total carbon dioxide (bicarbonate) (CO2) level is composed of CO2, bicarbonate (HCO3-), and carbonic acid (H2CO3) with the primary constituent being bicarbonate, a negatively charged electrolyte that works in conjunction with other electrolytes, such as potassium, sodium, and chloride, to maintain proper acid-base balance and electrical neutrality at the cellular level. Chloride is also a negatively charged electrolyte that helps regulate body fluid and maintain proper acid-base balance. Creatinine is a waste product excreted by the kidneys that is produced in the muscles while breaking down creatine, a compound used by the muscles to create energy. Blood levels of creatinine provide a good measurement of renal function. Glucose is a simple sugar and the main source of energy for the body, regulated by insulin. When more glucose is available than is required, it is stored in the liver as glycogen or stored in adipose tissue as fat. Glucose measurement determines whether the glucose/insulin metabolic process is functioning properly. Both potassium and sodium are positively charged electrolytes that work in conjunction with other electrolytes to regulate body fluid, stimulate muscle contraction, and maintain proper acid-base balance and both are essential for maintaining normal metabolic processes. Urea is a waste product produced in the liver by the breakdown of protein from a sequence of chemical reactions referred to as the urea or Krebs-Henseleit cycle. Urea is taken up by the kidneys and excreted in the urine. Blood urea nitrogen, BUN, is a measure of renal function, and helps monitor renal disease and the effectiveness of dialysis. Report 80048 for the same basic metabolic panel, but with total calcium measured instead of ionized calcium. Total calcium is a measurement of the total amount of both ionized (free) calcium and calcium attached (bound) to proteins circulating in the blood. The measurement can screen for or monitor a number of conditions, including those affecting the bones, heart, nerves, kidneys, and teeth.

RVUs

Code	Work	PE	PE Non-Facility	MP	Total Non-Facility	Total Facility	Global
80047	0.00	0.00	0.00	0.00	0.00	0.00	XXX
80048	0.00	0.00	0.00	0.00	0.00	0.00	XXX

80050

80050 General health panel

This panel must include the following:

Comprehensive metabolic panel (80053); Blood count, complete (CBC), automated and automated differential WBC count (85025 or 85027 and 85004); OR Blood count, complete (CBC), automated (85027); and appropriate manual differential WBC count (85007 or 85009); Thyroid stimulating hormone (TSH) (84443)

Plain English Description

A general health panel is obtained that includes a comprehensive metabolic panel with albumin, bilirubin, total calcium, carbon dioxide, chloride, creatinine, glucose, alkaline phosphatase, potassium, total protein, sodium, alanine amino transferase (ALT) (SGPT), aspartate amino transferase (AST) (SGOT), urea nitrogen (BUN); a complete blood count with differential white count; and thyroid stimulating hormone (TSH). This test is used to evaluate electrolytes and fluid balance, liver and kidney function, and is used to help rule out conditions such as diabetes, thyroid disease, and anemia. Tests related to electrolytes and fluid balance include: carbon dioxide, chloride, potassium, and sodium. Tests specific to liver function include: albumin, bilirubin, alkaline phosphatase, ALT, AST, and total protein. Tests specific to kidney function: include BUN and creatinine. Calcium is needed to support metabolic processes such as heart function, muscle contraction, nerve function, and blood clotting. Glucose is the main source of energy for the body and is regulated by insulin. Glucose measurement determines whether the glucose/insulin metabolic process is functioning properly. A CBC is performed to test for anemia, infection, blood clotting disorders, as well as many other diseases. TSH is produced in the pituitary and helps to regulate two other thyroid hormones, T3 and T4, which in turn help regulate the body's metabolic processes.

RVUs

Code	Work	PE	PE Non-Facility	MP	Total Non-Facility	Total Facility	Global
80050	0.00	0.00	0.00	0.00	0.00	0.00	XXX

80051

80051 Electrolyte panel

This panel must include the following:

Carbon dioxide (bicarbonate) (82374); Chloride (82435); Potassium (84132); Sodium (84295)

Plain English Description

An electrolyte panel is obtained to detect problems with fluid and electrolyte balance and monitor the health status of persons with acute or chronic medical conditions including high blood pressure, heart failure, and kidney or liver disease. The test measures electrically charged minerals such as sodium, potassium, and chloride found in body tissues and blood. Sodium is primarily found outside cells and maintains water balance in the tissues, as well as nerve and muscle function. Potassium is primarily found inside cells and affects heart rhythm, cell metabolism, and muscle function. Chloride moves freely in and out of cells to regulate fluid levels and help maintain electrical neutrality. Carbon dioxide, or bicarbonate, maintains body pH and the acid/base balance of the blood. A test called an "anion gap" may be included in the electrolyte panel. Anion gap is a calculated value of the test components that measures the difference between the negatively charged ions (anions) and the positivity charged ions (cations). Anion gap values can be affected by many conditions such as metabolic disorders, starvation, and diabetes, or exposure to toxins. A blood sample is obtained by separately reportable venipuncture, heel or finger stick. Serum/plasma is tested using quantitative ion-selective electrode/enzymatic method.

CPT © 2018 American Medical Association. All Rights Reserved.

RVUs

Code	Work	PE	PE Non-Facility	MP	Total Non-Facility	Total Facility	Global
80051	0.00	0.00	0.00	0.00	0.00	0.00	XXX

80053

80053 Comprehensive metabolic panel
This panel must include the following:
Albumin (82040); Bilirubin, total (82247); Calcium, total (82310); Carbon dioxide (bicarbonate) (82374); Chloride (82435); Creatinine (82565); Glucose (82947); Phosphatase, alkaline (84075); Potassium (84132); Protein, total (84155); Sodium (84295); Transferase, alanine amino (ALT) (SGPT) (84460); Transferase, aspartate amino (AST) (SGOT) (84450); Urea nitrogen (BUN) (84520)

Plain English Description

A comprehensive metabolic panel is obtained that includes albumin, bilirubin, total calcium, carbon dioxide, chloride, creatinine, glucose, alkaline phosphatase, potassium, total protein, sodium, alanine amino transferase (ALT) (SGPT), aspartate amino transferase (AST) (SGOT), and urea nitrogen (BUN). This test is used to evaluate electrolytes and fluid balance as well as liver and kidney function. It is also used to help rule out conditions such as diabetes. Tests related to electrolytes and fluid balance include: carbon dioxide, chloride, potassium, and sodium. Tests specific to liver function include: albumin, bilirubin, alkaline phosphatase, ALT, AST, and total protein. Tests specific to kidney function include: BUN and creatinine. Calcium is needed to support metabolic processes such as heart function, muscle contraction, nerve function, and blood clotting. Glucose is the main source of energy for the body and is regulated by insulin. Glucose measurement determines whether the glucose/insulin metabolic process is functioning properly.

RVUs

Code	Work	PE	PE Non-Facility	MP	Total Non-Facility	Total Facility	Global
80053	0.00	0.00	0.00	0.00	0.00	0.00	XXX

80171

80171 Gabapentin, whole blood, serum, or plasma

Plain English Description

A blood test is performed to measure gabapentin levels. Gabapentin (Gabarone, Neurontin) is an analog of gamma-aminobutyric acid (GABA), a neurotransmitter produced by the brain, and is used to treat seizure disorders and chronic neuropathic pain. The drug may also be prescribed off label for migraine headaches and bipolar disorder. A blood sample is obtained by separately reportable venipuncture. Whole blood, serum, or plasma is tested using quantitative liquid chromatography-tandem mass spectrometry.

RVUs

Code	Work	PE	PE Non-Facility	MP	Total Non-Facility	Total Facility	Global
80171	0.00	0.00	0.00	0.00	0.00	0.00	XXX

80175

80175 Lamotrigine

Plain English Description

A blood test is performed to measure lamotrigine levels. Lamotrigine (Lamictal) is an anticonvulsant from the phenyltriazine class of medications and is used to treat seizure disorders and bipolar disorders. The drug may also be prescribed "off label" for peripheral neuropathy, migraine headaches and depression (without mania). A blood sample is obtained by separately reportable venipuncture. Serum/plasma is tested using quantitative enzyme immunoassay.

RVUs

Code	Work	PE	PE Non-Facility	MP	Total Non-Facility	Total Facility	Global
80175	0.00	0.00	0.00	0.00	0.00	0.00	XXX

80177

80177 Levetiracetam

Plain English Description

A blood test is performed to measure levetiracetam levels. Levetiracetam (Keppra) is an anticonvulsant medication used to treat seizure disorders. The drug may also be prescribed off label for neuropathic pain, Tourette's syndrome, autism, bipolar disorder, anxiety disorder and Alzheimer's disease. A blood sample is obtained by separately reportable venipuncture. Serum/plasma is tested using quantitative enzyme immunoassay.

RVUs

Code	Work	PE	PE Non-Facility	MP	Total Non-Facility	Total Facility	Global
80177	0.00	0.00	0.00	0.00	0.00	0.00	XXX

80199

80199 Tiagabine

Plain English Description

A blood test is performed to measure tiagabine levels. Tiagabine (Gabitril) is an anticonvulsant medication used as an adjunct treatment for partial seizure disorders in patients over the age of 12. The drug may also be prescribed off label for anxiety disorders and neuropathic pain. Tiagabine levels should be monitored by pre-dose (trough) blood draws. A blood sample is obtained by separately reportable venipuncture. Serum/plasma is tested using high performance liquid chromatography/tandem mass spectrometry.

RVUs

Code	Work	PE	PE Non-Facility	MP	Total Non-Facility	Total Facility	Global
80199	0.00	0.00	0.00	0.00	0.00	0.00	XXX

80203

80203 Zonisamide

Plain English Description

A blood test is performed to measure zonisamide levels. Zonisamide (Excegran, Zonegran) is a sulfonamide anticonvulsant medication used as an adjunct treatment for partial-onset seizures in adults. The drug may also be prescribed off label for migraine headaches, neuropathic pain and bipolar disorder. Zonisamide is currently in clinical trials for Parkinson's Disease under the trade name Tremode and for obesity under the trade name Empatic.

CPT © 2018 American Medical Association. All Rights Reserved.

Zonisamide levels should be monitored by pre-dose (trough) blood draws. A blood sample is obtained by separately reportable venipuncture. Serum/plasma is tested using quantitative enzyme multiplied immunoassay technique.

RVUs

Code	Work	PE	PE Non-Facility	MP	Total Non-Facility	Total Facility	Global
80203	0.00	0.00	0.00	0.00	0.00	0.00	XXX

80305-80307

80305 Drug test(s), presumptive, any number of drug classes, any number of devices or procedures; capable of being read by direct optical observation only (eg, utilizing immunoassay [eg, dipsticks, cups, cards, or cartridges]), includes sample validation when performed, per date of service

80306 Drug test(s), presumptive, any number of drug classes, any number of devices or procedures; read by instrument assisted direct optical observation (eg, utilizing immunoassay [eg, dipsticks, cups, cards, or cartridges]), includes sample validation when performed, per date of service

80307 Drug test(s), presumptive, any number of drug classes, any number of devices or procedures; by instrument chemistry analyzers (eg, utilizing immunoassay [eg, EIA, ELISA, EMIT, FPIA, IA, KIMS, RIA]), chromatography (eg, GC, HPLC), and mass spectrometry either with or without chromatography, (eg, DART, DESI, GC-MS, GC-MS/MS, LC-MS, LC-MS/MS, LDTD, MALDI, TOF) includes sample validation when performed, per date of service

Plain English Description

A laboratory test is performed to detect the presence or absence of drugs classes in a patient's system during a specific encounter. Presumptive screening is commonly done first, followed by test(s) for definitive drug identification as presumptive testing will not provide qualitative identification of individual drugs, nor quantitative levels present. A sample of blood or urine is obtained by separately reported procedure. Methods used include immunoassays, chromatography, and mass spectrometry. Code 80305 reports presumptive drug testing for any number of drug classes, any number of drug devices or procedures using CLIA waived methodologies for direct optical observation only, including dipsticks, cups, cards, or cartridges with sample validation, such as pH, nitrite, and specific gravity, when performed. Code 80306 reports presumptive drug testing using FDA specific equipment for moderate complexity testing methodologies with instrument assisted direct optical observation, including dipstick, cups, cards, and cartridges with sample validation, when performed. Code 80307 reports presumptive drug testing using FDA specific equipment for high complexity testing methodologies by instrument chemistry analyzers for immunoassay, chromatography, and mass spectrometry including sample validation when performed.

RVUs

Code	Work	PE	PE Non-Facility	MP	Total Non-Facility	Total Facility	Global
80305	0.00	0.00	0.00	0.00	0.00	0.00	XXX
80306	0.00	0.00	0.00	0.00	0.00	0.00	XXX
80307	0.00	0.00	0.00	0.00	0.00	0.00	XXX

80323

80323 Alkaloids, not otherwise specified

Plain English Description

A laboratory test is performed to measure alkaloids. Alkaloids are naturally occurring chemical compounds comprised of basic nitrogen atoms. The two most common forms are true alkaloids, which contain nitrogen in the heterocycle that originates from amino acids, and protoalkaloids that have nitrogen originating directly from the amino acids. Bacteria, fungi, plants, and animals can all produce alkaloid compounds that may be toxic to people, animals, and the environment. The pharmacological effects of alkaloids have been used for centuries in medications, for recreational drug use, and for entheogenic rituals. Alkaloid examples include local anesthetics, cocaine, caffeine, and nicotine (stimulants), morphine (analgesic), atropine (anti-cholinergic), quinidine (anti-arrhythmic), quinine (anti-malarial), berberine (antibacterial), vincristine (anti-neoplastic), reserpine (antihypertensive), ephedrine (bronchodilator), and the hallucinogens, psilocin and mescaline. Serum and urine may be tested using high performance liquid chromatography/tandem mass spectrometry.

RVUs

Code	Work	PE	PE Non-Facility	MP	Total Non-Facility	Total Facility	Global
80323	0.00	0.00	0.00	0.00	0.00	0.00	XXX

80329-80331

80329 Analgesics, non-opioid; 1 or 2

80330 Analgesics, non-opioid; 3-5

80331 Analgesics, non-opioid; 6 or more

Plain English Description

A laboratory test is performed to measure non-opioid analgesics in urine, serum, or plasma. Non-opioid analgesics include salicylates (aspirin), acetaminophen, the non-steroidal anti-inflammatory drugs (NSAIDS) ibuprofen and naproxen sodium, and selective cyclooxygenase-2 (COX-2) inhibitors (Celebrex). These drugs can be used to treat acute or chronic, mild to moderate pain and may be combined with opioids or other compounds to treat moderate to severe pain. In addition to relieving pain, many analgesics have anti-inflammatory and/or anti-pyretic properties. Salicylates in serum or plasma and acetaminophen in plasma are tested for using spectrophotometry. Ibuprofen in serum or plasma and naproxen sodium is tested for using high performance liquid chromatography. Code 80329 is used when testing for 1 or 2 non-opioid analgesic compounds. Code 80330 is used for 3-5 non-opioid analgesics, and code 80331 is used when identifying 6 or more.

RVUs

Code	Work	PE	PE Non-Facility	MP	Total Non-Facility	Total Facility	Global
80329	0.00	0.00	0.00	0.00	0.00	0.00	XXX
80330	0.00	0.00	0.00	0.00	0.00	0.00	XXX
80331	0.00	0.00	0.00	0.00	0.00	0.00	XXX

80332-80334

80332 Antidepressants, serotonergic class; 1 or 2

80333 Antidepressants, serotonergic class; 3-5

80334 Antidepressants, serotonergic class; 6 or more

Plain English Description

A laboratory test is performed to measure serotonergic antidepressants. Selective serotonin reuptake inhibitors (SSRIs) increase circulating levels of serotonin by inhibiting the reuptake of the neurotransmitter by the brain.

CPT © 2018 American Medical Association. All Rights Reserved.

They may be used to treat depression, anxiety disorders, chronic pain, and posttraumatic stress disorder (PTSD). Drugs in this class include citalopram (Celexa), escitalopram (Lexapro), fluvoxamine (Luvox), paroxetine (Paxil), fluoxetine (Prozac), and sertraline (Zoloft). A blood sample is obtained by separately reportable venipuncture. Serum or plasma is tested for citalopram, escitalopram, paroxetine, or sertraline using quantitative liquid chromatography-tandem mass spectrometry, for fluvoxamine using gas chromatography, and for fluoxetine using quantitative high performance liquid chromatography. Code 80332 is used when testing for 1 or 2 compounds; code 80333 is used for 3-5 compounds; and code 80334 is used when evaluating 6 or more serotonergic antidepressants.

RVUs

Code	Work	PE	PE Non-Facility	MP	Total Non-Facility	Total Facility	Global
80332	0.00	0.00	0.00	0.00	0.00	0.00	XXX
80333	0.00	0.00	0.00	0.00	0.00	0.00	XXX
80334	0.00	0.00	0.00	0.00	0.00	0.00	XXX

80335-80337

80335 Antidepressants, tricyclic and other cyclicals; 1 or 2
80336 Antidepressants, tricyclic and other cyclicals; 3-5
80337 Antidepressants, tricyclic and other cyclicals; 6 or more

Plain English Description

A laboratory test is performed to measure tricyclic and other cyclical antidepressants in urine, serum, or plasma. Tricyclic antidepressants (TCAs) and tetracyclic antidepressants (TeCAs) increase levels of the brain neurotransmitters, norepinephrine and serotonin while blocking acetylcholine. These drugs may be prescribed to treat depression, anxiety, fibromyalgia, chronic pain, and bedwetting. Tricyclic antidepressants include clomipramine (Anafranil), amitriptyline (Elavil), desipramine (Norpramin), nortriptyline (Pamelor), doxepin (Sinequan), and trimipramine (Surmontil). Tetracyclic antidepressants include amoxapine (Asendin), loxapine (Loxapac, Loxitan), mirtazapine (Remeron, Avinza), and maprotiline (Ludiomil). A blood sample is obtained by separately reportable venipuncture; urine sample by random void or catheterization. Urine, serum, or plasma is tested for all TCAs using quantitative liquid chromatography-tandem mass spectrometry. Serum or plasma is tested for the TeCA loxapine using high performance liquid chromatography. Urine, serum, or plasma is tested for amoxapine using quantitative high performance liquid chromatography. Serum or plasma is tested for maprotiline using quantitative gas chromatography and urine, serum, or plasma is tested for mirtazapine using quantitative gas chromatography/gas chromatography-mass spectrometry. Code 80335 is used when testing for 1 or 2 cyclical antidepressants; code 80336 is used for 3-5 compounds; and code 80337 is used when evaluating for 6 or more.

RVUs

Code	Work	PE	PE Non-Facility	MP	Total Non-Facility	Total Facility	Global
80335	0.00	0.00	0.00	0.00	0.00	0.00	XXX
80336	0.00	0.00	0.00	0.00	0.00	0.00	XXX
80337	0.00	0.00	0.00	0.00	0.00	0.00	XXX

80338

80338 Antidepressants, not otherwise specified

Plain English Description

A laboratory test is performed to measure antidepressants, not otherwise specified. The serotonin and norepinephrine reuptake inhibitor (SNRI) drugs venlafaxine (Effexor) and desvenlafaxine (Pristiq) may be prescribed to treat depression and can be tested for in serum or plasma using quantitative liquid chromatography-tandem mass spectrometry. The SNRI duloxetine (Cymbalta) is used to treat depression and chronic pain and can be tested for in serum or plasma using quantitative high performance liquid chromatography-tandem mass spectrometry. Atypical antidepressants include bupropion (Wellbutrin), used to treat depression and aid smoking cessation, and trazodone, a powerful sleep aid. Both can be tested for in serum or plasma using quantitative liquid chromatography-tandem mass spectrometry.

RVUs

Code	Work	PE	PE Non-Facility	MP	Total Non-Facility	Total Facility	Global
80338	0.00	0.00	0.00	0.00	0.00	0.00	XXX

80345

80345 Barbiturates

Plain English Description

A laboratory test is performed to measure barbiturates in stool, serum, plasma, or urine. Barbiturates are a class of drugs that cause central nervous system depression and may be prescribed to treat anxiety, insomnia, or seizures, and are used to produce mild sedation and general anesthesia. Barbiturates decrease tension and calm the brain. They can be highly addictive and produce withdrawal symptoms including rebound effects on REM sleep. The effects of barbiturates may vary and drugs are usually assigned to a class (very short, short, medium, or long acting) in relationship to their half-life. Very short acting barbiturates include methohexital (Brevital), thiamylal (Surital), and thiopental (pentobarbital) and are used primarily for anesthesia. Short acting barbiturates include pentobarbital (Nembutal), amobarbital (Amytal), butabarbital (Butisol, Soneryl), secobarbital (Seconal), aprobarbital (Alurate). Medium acting drugs are talbutal (Lotusate), cyclobarbital (Phanodorn), and butalbital (Fiorinal, Fioricet); the long acting drugs are mephobarbital (Mebaral), methylphenobarbital (Prominal), and phenobarbital (Luminal). A blood sample is obtained by separately reportable venipuncture, urine specimen by random void or catheterization, and meconium stool is collected from a diaper. Serum or plasma and urine are tested using quantitative gas chromatography-mass spectrometry. Stool may be tested using multiple chromatography and mass spectrometry procedures.

RVUs

Code	Work	PE	PE Non-Facility	MP	Total Non-Facility	Total Facility	Global
80345	0.00	0.00	0.00	0.00	0.00	0.00	XXX

80346-80347

80346 Benzodiazepines; 1-12
80347 Benzodiazepines; 13 or more

Plain English Description

A laboratory test is performed to measure benzodiazepines in stool, urine, serum, or plasma. Benzodiazepines are a class of drugs with sedative, hypnotic, anxiolytic, anti-convulsive, and muscle relaxant capabilities. Some short acting benzodiazepines have amnesic-dissociative actions. They may be prescribed to treat anxiety, panic disorders, insomnia, alcohol withdrawal, or seizures, and may be used as preoperative or intra-operative anesthesia. Common benzodiazepines and their uses include chlordiazepoxide (Librium) for alcohol withdrawal; diazepam (Valium) for anxiety, panic disorders, seizures, and insomnia; flurazepam (Dalmane) for insomnia and preoperative anesthesia; lorazepam (Ativan) for anxiety, insomnia, and seizures; temazepam (Restoril) for insomnia; clonazepam (Klonopin) for seizures and panic disorders; flunitrazepam (Rohypnol) for insomnia often implicated as a "date rape" drug; alprazolam (Xanax) for anxiety and panic disorders; triazolam (Halcion)

CPT © 2018 American Medical Association. All Rights Reserved.

for insomnia, and midazolam (Versed) for preoperative and intra-operative anesthesia. A blood sample is obtained by separately reportable venipuncture, urine specimen by random void or catheterization; and meconium stool is collected from a diaper. Serum, plasma, and meconium are tested using quantitative liquid chromatography-tandem mass spectrometry. Urine is tested using quantitative high performance liquid chromatography-tandem mass spectrometry. Code 80346 is used when testing for 1-12 benzodiazepines and code 80347 is reported when identifying 13 or more.

RVUs

Code	Work	PE	PE Non-Facility	MP	Total Non-Facility	Total Facility	Global
80346	0.00	0.00	0.00	0.00	0.00	0.00	XXX
80347	0.00	0.00	0.00	0.00	0.00	0.00	XXX

80348

80348 Buprenorphine

Plain English Description

A laboratory test is performed to measure buprenorphine and its metabolites in urine, serum, or plasma. Buprenorphine is a semi-synthetic opioid partial agonist used to treat opioid addiction and control acute or chronic pain in non-opioid tolerant persons. The drug is available in an oral form (Subutex, Suboxone, Zubsolv) to treat opioid addiction, or as a sublingual preparation (Temgesic) for moderate to severe pain. It may also be injected (Buprenex) for acute pain or administered via transdermal patch (Norspan, Butrans) to treat chronic pain. A blood sample is obtained by separately reportable venipuncture, urine by random void or catheterization. Serum or plasma is tested using quantitative high performance liquid chromatography-tandem mass spectrometry. Urine is tested using quantitative liquid chromatography-tandem mass spectrometry.

RVUs

Code	Work	PE	PE Non-Facility	MP	Total Non-Facility	Total Facility	Global
80348	0.00	0.00	0.00	0.00	0.00	0.00	XXX

80349

80349 Cannabinoids, natural

Plain English Description

A laboratory test is performed to measure natural cannabinoids in meconium stool, urine, serum, or plasma. Cannabinoids occur naturally in the marijuana plant (Cannabis sativa). Tetrahydrocannabinol, or THC, is the principal mind altering constituent of cannabis. When smoked or ingested, THC primarily affects the limbic system responsible for memory, cognition, and psychomotor performance, and the mesolimbic pathways responsible for the feeling of reward and pain perception. The chemical is fat soluble with a long elimination half-life. Cannabinoids may be detected in urine for several weeks and in serum or plasma for up to 12 hours. A blood sample is obtained by separately reportable venipuncture, urine sample by random void or catheterization, and meconium stool is collected from a diaper. Samples are tested for THC and its metabolite 9-carboxy-THC using quantitative liquid chromatography-tandem mass spectrometry.

RVUs

Code	Work	PE	PE Non-Facility	MP	Total Non-Facility	Total Facility	Global
80349	0.00	0.00	0.00	0.00	0.00	0.00	XXX

80353

80353 Cocaine

Plain English Description

A laboratory test is performed to measure cocaine in meconium stool, urine, serum, or plasma. Cocaine is a highly addictive, central nervous system stimulant and anesthetic derived from the leaves of the coca plant. It is a triple reuptake inhibitor (TRI) that affects serotonin, norepinephrine, and dopamine receptors in the brain. The drug can be inhaled, injected, or absorbed topically. A blood sample is obtained by separately reportable venipuncture. Urine is collected by random void or catheterization, and meconium stool is collected from a diaper. Serum, plasma, meconium stool, and a positive urine screen are tested using quantitative gas chromatography-mass spectrometry/quantitative liquid chromatography-tandem mass spectrometry.

RVUs

Code	Work	PE	PE Non-Facility	MP	Total Non-Facility	Total Facility	Global
80353	0.00	0.00	0.00	0.00	0.00	0.00	XXX

80354

80354 Fentanyl

Plain English Description

A laboratory test is performed to measure fentanyl in urine, serum, or plasma. Fentanyl is a potent synthetic opioid analgesic which has a rapid onset but short duration of action. It is often administered with benzodiazepines for conscious sedation. It may be used to treat acute postoperative pain, breakthrough pain associated with cancer or bone fractures, and chronic pain conditions. Fentanyl may be administered intravenously (Sublimaze), intrathecally with spinal or epidural anesthesia, via a transdermal patch (Duragesic), and orally in the form of a lollipop/lozenge (Actiq), buccal tablet (Fentora), or a sublingual spray. A blood sample is obtained by separately reportable venipuncture; urine specimen by random void or catheterization. Urine, serum, and plasma are tested using quantitative liquid chromatography-tandem mass spectrometry.

RVUs

Code	Work	PE	PE Non-Facility	MP	Total Non-Facility	Total Facility	Global
80354	0.00	0.00	0.00	0.00	0.00	0.00	XXX

80355

80355 Gabapentin, non-blood

(For therapeutic drug assay, use 80171)

Plain English Description

A laboratory test is performed to measure gabapentin in urine. Gabapentin (Neurontin) is an anticonvulsant, analgesic used to treat seizure disorders, neuropathic pain like diabetic neuropathy and post herpetic neuralgia, and restless leg syndrome. A urine sample is obtained by separately reportable random void or catheterization and tested using quantitative high performance liquid chromatography/tandem mass spectrometry.

RVUs

Code	Work	PE	PE Non-Facility	MP	Total Non-Facility	Total Facility	Global
80355	0.00	0.00	0.00	0.00	0.00	0.00	XXX

CPT © 2018 American Medical Association. All Rights Reserved.

80357

80357 Ketamine and norketamine

Plain English Description

A laboratory test is performed to measure ketamine and its metabolite, norketamine in serum or plasma. Ketamine is an N-methyl-D-aspartate receptor (NMDAR) antagonist that can be injected, ingested, or inhaled. It is a potent analgesic, sedative, amnesic that is used clinically for anesthesia, pain management, and to treat bronchospasm. Ketamine can provide stable cardiovascular function with protection of airway reflexes making it a safe anesthetic choice for many patients. However, the dissociative effects of the drug have made it attractive to individuals for recreational use and abuse. A blood sample is obtained by separately reportable venipuncture. Serum or plasma is tested using quantitative gas chromatography-mass spectrometry.

RVUs

Code	Work	PE	PE Non-Facility	MP	Total Non-Facility	Total Facility	Global
80357	0.00	0.00	0.00	0.00	0.00	0.00	XXX

80358

80358 Methadone

Plain English Description

A laboratory test is performed to measure methadone in meconium stool, urine, serum, or plasma. Methadone is a synthetic opioid with a long duration of action and strong analgesic effect. It is most commonly prescribed as part of a medically supervised drug addiction detoxification and maintenance program but may also be used to treat severe chronic pain. Methadone can decrease the symptoms of withdrawal in persons who are opioid addicted without producing the pleasurable symptoms associated with opioid abuse. A blood sample is obtained by separately reportable venipuncture. A urine sample is obtained by random void or catheterization, and meconium stool is collected from a diaper. Urine, serum, plasma, and stool may all be tested using quantitative liquid chromatography-tandem mass spectrometry.

RVUs

Code	Work	PE	PE Non-Facility	MP	Total Non-Facility	Total Facility	Global
80358	0.00	0.00	0.00	0.00	0.00	0.00	XXX

80361

80361 Opiates, 1 or more

Plain English Description

A laboratory test is performed to measure opiates in meconium stool, urine, serum, or plasma. Opiates are the naturally occurring opioid alkaloids found in the resin of the opium poppy plant (Papaver somniferum) and include morphine, codeine, and thebaine. Naturally occurring hydromorphone and hydrocodone may rarely be detected in opium. Dihydrocodeine, oxymorphol, oxycodone, oxymorphone, and metopon are also occasionally found in trace amounts. The semi-synthetic versions of these compounds are more appropriately defined as opioids or opiate analogs. Opiates fall into the class of narcotic analgesics and are prescribed clinically to treat moderate to severe pain. Opiates are central nervous system depressants but also affect areas of the brain that mediate pleasure to produce a euphoric state along with pain relief. These drugs may be consumed by individuals for recreational abuse. A blood sample is obtained by separately reportable venipuncture. A urine sample is obtained by random void or catheterization, and meconium stool is collected from a diaper. All samples are confirmed using quantitative liquid chromatography-tandem mass spectrometry.

RVUs

Code	Work	PE	PE Non-Facility	MP	Total Non-Facility	Total Facility	Global
80361	0.00	0.00	0.00	0.00	0.00	0.00	XXX

80362-80364

80362 Opioids and opiate analogs; 1 or 2

80363 Opioids and Opiate analogs; 3 or 4

80364 Opioids and Opiate analogs; 5 or more

Plain English Description

A laboratory test is performed to measure opioids and opiate analogs in meconium stool, urine, serum, or plasma. Opioids and opiate analogs are a class of drugs comprised of any naturally occurring opiate (codeine, morphine, thebaine) or semi-synthetic opioid (hydromorphone, hydrocodone, oxycodone, oxymorphone, buprenorphine, meperidine, methadone, propoxyphene, tapentadol, tramadol) that share a similar chemical structure and pharmacological effects. Opioids and opiate analogs are narcotic analgesic, central nervous system depressants prescribed clinically to treat moderate to severe, acute or chronic pain. These drugs also have an effect on areas of the brain that mediate pleasure and may produce a euphoric state along with pain relief. Opioids and opiate analogs may be abused by recreational drug users. A blood sample is obtained by separately reportable venipuncture. A urine sample is obtained by random void or catheterization, and meconium stool is collected from a diaper. Serum, plasma, urine, and stool are tested using quantitative liquid chromatography-tandem mass spectrometry. Code 80362 is used when testing for 1 or 2 opioids/opiate analogs; code 80363 is used for 3 or 4; and code 80364 is used when evaluating a sample for 5 or more opioids/opiate analogs.

RVUs

Code	Work	PE	PE Non-Facility	MP	Total Non-Facility	Total Facility	Global
80362	0.00	0.00	0.00	0.00	0.00	0.00	XXX
80363	0.00	0.00	0.00	0.00	0.00	0.00	XXX
80364	0.00	0.00	0.00	0.00	0.00	0.00	XXX

80365

80365 Oxycodone

Plain English Description

A laboratory test is performed to measure oxycodone (oxymorphone) in urine, serum, or plasma. Oxycodone is a semi-synthetic opioid, narcotic analgesic that is used to treat moderate to severe, acute or chronic pain. The drug can be used alone or in combination with aspirin or acetaminophen. Oxycodone may be injected or ingested orally. A blood sample is obtained by separately reportable venipuncture; urine by random void or catheterization. Urine is screened using qualitative enzyme immunoassay and urine, serum, and plasma are tested by quantitative liquid chromatography-tandem mass spectrometry.

RVUs

Code	Work	PE	PE Non-Facility	MP	Total Non-Facility	Total Facility	Global
80365	0.00	0.00	0.00	0.00	0.00	0.00	XXX

CPT © 2018 American Medical Association. All Rights Reserved.

80366

80366 Pregabalin

Plain English Description

A laboratory test is performed to measure pregabalin in urine, serum, or plasma. Pregabalin is marketed in the United States as Lyrica. It is an anticonvulsant prescribed to treat neuropathic pain like post herpetic neuralgia and diabetic peripheral neuropathy, chronic pain conditions such as fibromyalgia, and as an adjunct therapy in patients diagnosed with partial seizure disorder with or without secondary generalization. A blood sample is obtained by separately reportable venipuncture and urine by random void or catheterization. Urine, serum, and plasma are tested using quantitative high performance liquid chromatography/tandem mass spectrometry.

RVUs

Code	Work	PE	PE Non-Facility	MP	Total Non-Facility	Total Facility	Global
80366	0.00	0.00	0.00	0.00	0.00	0.00	XXX

80368

80368 Sedative hypnotics (non-benzodiazepines)

Plain English Description

A laboratory test is performed to measure non-benzodiazepine sedative hypnotics in urine, serum, or plasma. This class of psychoactive drugs provides the same benefits, side effects, and risks as benzodiazepines but has a very different chemical structure. Non-benzodiazepine drugs include eszopiclone (Lunesta), zaleplon (Sonata), Zolpidem (Ambien), Zolpidem tartrate (Intermezzo sublingual), ramelteon (Rozerem), chloral hydrate (Noctec), dexmedetomidine hydrochloride (Precedex). Most drugs in this class induce sleep by binding to a specific benzodiazepine brain receptor called omega-1 and are believed to be less disruptive to REM sleep cycles than benzodiazepines. Eszopiclone differs somewhat by increasing gamma-aminobutyric acid (GABA) at receptor sites in the brain and ramelteon is a melatonin receptor stimulator. Non-benzodiazepine sedative hypnotics are used as short term treatment for insomnia. Dexmedetomidine is used primarily for anesthesia. A blood sample is obtained by separately reportable venipuncture, and urine by random void or catheterization. Samples are tested for eszopiclone, zolpidem, and ramelteon using high performance liquid chromatography-tandem mass spectrometry. Zaleplon is tested for using high performance liquid chromatography alone. Serum and plasma are tested for chloral hydrate using gas chromatography and for dexmedetomidine using gas chromatography-mass spectrometry.

RVUs

Code	Work	PE	PE Non-Facility	MP	Total Non-Facility	Total Facility	Global
80368	0.00	0.00	0.00	0.00	0.00	0.00	XXX

80369-80370

80369 Skeletal muscle relaxants; 1 or 2
80370 Skeletal muscle relaxants; 3 or more

Plain English Description

A laboratory test is performed to measure skeletal muscle relaxants in urine, serum, or plasma. Skeletal muscle relaxants belong to several drug classes including neuromuscular blockers that prevent transmission of signals at the neuromuscular end plates causing paralysis (succinylcholine, pancuronium, botulinum toxins) and central nervous system spasmolytics that increase the inhibition of motor neurons, or decrease the level of excitation in the neocortex, brain stem, and/or spinal cord. Skeletal muscle relaxants may be used to treat conditions such as cerebral palsy, multiple sclerosis, spinal cord injury, low back pain, neck pain, fibromyalgia, myofascial pain syndrome, and tension headaches. Common antispasmodics include dantrolene (Dantrium), carisoprodol (Soma), baclofen (Lioresal), tizanidine (Zanaflex), cyclobenzaprine (Flexeril), metaxalone (Skelaxin), methocarbamol (Robaxin), and chlorzoxazone (Parafon Forte). A blood sample is obtained by separately reportable venipuncture, and a urine sample by random void or catheterization. Samples are tested for baclofen and cyclobenzaprine using quantitative high performance liquid chromatography/tandem mass spectrometry. Serum and plasma are tested for dantrolene using spectrofluorometry and for carisoprodol using quantitative gas chromatography-mass spectrometry. Code 80369 is reported for 1 or 2 relaxants, and 80370 for 3 or more.

RVUs

Code	Work	PE	PE Non-Facility	MP	Total Non-Facility	Total Facility	Global
80369	0.00	0.00	0.00	0.00	0.00	0.00	XXX
80370	0.00	0.00	0.00	0.00	0.00	0.00	XXX

80372

80372 Tapentadol

Plain English Description

A laboratory test is performed to measure tapentadol in urine, serum, or plasma. Tapentadol is marketed under the brand name Nucynta. It is a central acting opioid analgesic that works as an agonist of the ¦-opioid receptor to inhibit the reuptake of norepinephrine. Tapentadol is used to treat moderate to severe acute pain as an alternative to opiates. It may also be prescribed in an extend release formula to treat diabetic peripheral neuropathy. A blood sample is obtained by separately reportable venipuncture, and urine by random void or catheterization. Urine, serum, and plasma are tested using quantitative liquid chromatography-tandem mass spectrometry.

RVUs

Code	Work	PE	PE Non-Facility	MP	Total Non-Facility	Total Facility	Global
80372	0.00	0.00	0.00	0.00	0.00	0.00	XXX

80373

80373 Tramadol

Plain English Description

A laboratory test is performed to measure tramadol in urine, serum, or plasma. Tramadol may be marketed under the brand name Ultram. It is a central acting opioid analgesic that works as an agonist of the ¦-opioid receptor to inhibit the reuptake of norepinephrine and serotonin. Tramadol is used to treat moderate to moderate-severe acute or chronic pain as an alternative to opiates. It may also be prescribed in an extend release formula to treat fibromyalgia. A blood sample is obtained by separately reportable venipuncture, and urine by random void or catheterization. Urine, serum, and plasma are tested using quantitative liquid chromatography-tandem mass spectrometry.

RVUs

Code	Work	PE	PE Non-Facility	MP	Total Non-Facility	Total Facility	Global
80373	0.00	0.00	0.00	0.00	0.00	0.00	XXX

82286

82286 Bradykinin

Plain English Description

A laboratory test is performed to measure bradykinin. Bradykinin (BK) is a peptide molecule that causes vasodilation, contraction of non-vascular smooth muscle in the bronchus and gut, increases vascular permeability,

CPT © 2018 American Medical Association. All Rights Reserved.

and synthesizes prostaglandins. Bradykinin is broken down by angiotensin-converting enzyme (ACE), aminopeptidase P (APP) and carboxypeptidase N (CPN). Elevated levels of bradykinin may be present with hereditary angioedema and in patients who have tissue injury, chronic pain, or inflammatory disorders. A blood sample is obtained by separately reportable venipuncture. Serum/plasma is tested using enzyme-linked immunosorbent assay (ELISA).

RVUs

Code	Work	PE	PE Non-Facility	MP	Total Non-Facility	Total Facility	Global
82286	0.00	0.00	0.00	0.00	0.00	0.00	XXX

82310

82310 Calcium; total

Plain English Description

A blood sample is taken to measure the amount of total calcium. Calcium is one of the most important minerals in the body. About 99% of the calcium found the body is stored in the bones. The remaining 1% circulates in the blood. Calcium may be ionized (free) or attached (bound) to proteins. Free calcium is the calcium metabolically active in the body. Bound calcium is inactive. Total calcium is a measurement of the total amount of both free calcium and bound calcium circulating in the blood. Total calcium is measured to screen for or monitor a number of conditions, including those affecting the bones, heart, nerves, kidneys and teeth. Total calcium is measured using spectrophotometry.

RVUs

Code	Work	PE	PE Non-Facility	MP	Total Non-Facility	Total Facility	Global
82310	0.00	0.00	0.00	0.00	0.00	0.00	XXX

82330

82330 Calcium; ionized

Plain English Description

A blood sample is taken to measure the amount of ionized or free calcium. Ionized or free calcium is calcium that flows freely in the blood and is not attached to any proteins. Ionized calcium is metabolically active and available to support and regulate heart function, muscle contraction, central nervous system function, and blood clotting. Ionized calcium measurements may be obtained prior to major surgery, in critically ill patients, or when protein levels are abnormal. Ionized calcium is measured by ion selective electrode (ISE) or pH electrode methodology.

RVUs

Code	Work	PE	PE Non-Facility	MP	Total Non-Facility	Total Facility	Global
82330	0.00	0.00	0.00	0.00	0.00	0.00	XXX

82374

82374 Carbon dioxide (bicarbonate)

(See also 82803)

Plain English Description

A blood sample is taken to measure the total carbon dioxide (CO_2) level. The total CO_2 level is composed of CO_2, bicarbonate (HCO_3^-), and carbonic acid (H_2CO_3), with the primary constituent being bicarbonate. Bicarbonate is a negatively charged electrolyte that works in conjunction with other electrolytes, such as potassium, sodium, and chloride, to maintain proper acid-base balance and electrical neutrality at the cellular level. Bicarbonate is excreted and reabsorbed by the kidneys. Total CO_2 gives a rough estimate of bicarbonate concentration in the blood. CO_2 is measured by enzymatic methodology.

RVUs

Code	Work	PE	PE Non-Facility	MP	Total Non-Facility	Total Facility	Global
82374	0.00	0.00	0.00	0.00	0.00	0.00	XXX

82435

82435 Chloride; blood

Plain English Description

A blood sample is taken to measure chloride level. Chloride is a negatively charged electrolyte that works in conjunction with other electrolytes, such as potassium, sodium, and carbon dioxide (CO_2), to regulate fluid in the body and maintain proper acid-base balance. Chloride is found in all body fluids, but is concentrated in the blood. Chloride levels mirror sodium levels, increasing and decreasing in direct relationship to sodium, except when there is an acid-base imbalance. When an acid-base imbalance occurs, chloride acts as a buffer and chloride levels move independently of sodium. Chloride is measured to screen for or monitor electrolyte or acid-base balance. Chloride is measured by ion-selective electrode (ISE) methodology.

RVUs

Code	Work	PE	PE Non-Facility	MP	Total Non-Facility	Total Facility	Global
82435	0.00	0.00	0.00	0.00	0.00	0.00	XXX

82947-82948

82947 Glucose; quantitative, blood (except reagent strip)
82948 Glucose; blood, reagent strip

Plain English Description

A blood sample is obtained to measure total (quantitative) blood glucose level. Glucose is a simple sugar that is the main source of energy for the body. Carbohydrates are broken down into simple sugars, primarily glucose, absorbed by the intestine, and circulated in the blood. Insulin, a hormone produced by the pancreas, regulates glucose level in the blood and transports glucose to cells in other tissues and organs. When more glucose is available in the blood than is required, it is converted to glycogen and stored in the liver or converted to fat and stored in adipose (fat) tissue. If the glucose/insulin metabolic process is working properly, blood glucose will remain at a fairly constant, healthy level. Glucose is measured to determine whether the glucose/insulin metabolic process is functioning properly. It is used to monitor glucose levels and determine whether they are too low (hypoglycemia) or too high (hyperglycemia) as well as test for diabetes and monitor blood sugar control in diabetics. Use 82947 for quantitative blood glucose determination by enzymatic methodology or any method other than reagent strip. Use 82948 for blood glucose determination by reagent strip. A drop of blood is placed on a reagent strip, which is then compared to a calibrated color scale and a visual determination is made as to the amount of glucose present in the specimen.

RVUs

Code	Work	PE	PE Non-Facility	MP	Total Non-Facility	Total Facility	Global
82947	0.00	0.00	0.00	0.00	0.00	0.00	XXX
82948	0.00	0.00	0.00	0.00	0.00	0.00	XXX

CPT © 2018 American Medical Association. All Rights Reserved.

83873

83873 Myelin basic protein, cerebrospinal fluid

(For oligoclonal bands, use 83916)

Plain English Description

A test is performed on cerebral spinal fluid (CSF) to measure myelin basic protein (MBP) levels. MBP is a protective covering on nerve cells. When the protein breaks down, levels become elevated in cerebrospinal fluid. The most common cause of breakdown is multiple sclerosis (MS). Other causes include: central nervous system (CNS) trauma, infection or bleeding, encephalopathies and stroke. A sample of CSF is obtained by separately reportable lumbar puncture (spinal tap). Fluid is tested using quantitative enzyme-linked immunosorbent assay.

RVUs

Code	Work	PE	PE Non-Facility	MP	Total Non-Facility	Total Facility	Global
83873	0.00	0.00	0.00	0.00	0.00	0.00	XXX

84132

84132 Potassium; serum, plasma or whole blood

Plain English Description

A blood sample is obtained to measure potassium level. Potassium is a positively charged electrolyte that works in conjunction with other electrolytes, such as sodium, chloride, and carbon dioxide (CO2), to regulate body fluid, stimulate muscle contraction, and maintain proper acid-base balance. Potassium is found in all body fluids but mostly stored within cells, not in extracellular fluids, blood serum, or plasma. Small fluctuations in blood potassium, either too high (hyperkalemia) or too low (hypokalemia), can have serious, even life-threatening, consequences. Potassium level is used to screen for and monitor renal disease; monitor patients on certain medications, such as diuretics, as well as patients with acute and chronic conditions, such as dehydration or endocrine disorders. Because blood potassium affects heart rhythm and respiratory rate, it is routinely checked prior to major surgical procedures. Potassium is measured by ion-selective electrode (ISE) methodology.

RVUs

Code	Work	PE	PE Non-Facility	MP	Total Non-Facility	Total Facility	Global
84132	0.00	0.00	0.00	0.00	0.00	0.00	XXX

84260

84260 Serotonin

(For urine metabolites (HIAA), use 83497)

Plain English Description

A blood test is performed to measure serotonin levels. Serotonin is a monoamine neurotransmitter derived from tryptophan. Most serotonin is produced by the intestine where it regulates motility. It moves out of intestinal cells into the blood and is carried on platelets, helping to regulate hemostasis and blood clotting. The central nervous system (CNS) also produces a small amount of serotonin which helps to regulate mood, appetite, and sleep. Elevated levels may be found with intestinal obstruction, metastatic abdominal cancer, myocardial infarction, cystic fibrosis, dumping syndrome, and non-tropical sprue. Serotonin levels may be affected by certain medications if used within 72 hours of the blood test: lithium, MAO inhibitors, methyldopa, morphine, and reserpine. A blood sample is obtained by separately reportable venipuncture. Whole blood or serum is tested using quantitative high performance liquid chromatography.

RVUs

Code	Work	PE	PE Non-Facility	MP	Total Non-Facility	Total Facility	Global
84260	0.00	0.00	0.00	0.00	0.00	0.00	XXX

84295

84295 Sodium; serum, plasma or whole blood

Plain English Description

A blood sample is obtained to measure sodium level in 84295. A urine sample is obtained to measure sodium level in 84300. A sample other than urine, blood, plasma, or serum is obtained to measure sodium level in 84302. Sodium is a positively charged electrolyte that works in conjunction with other electrolytes, such as potassium, chloride, and carbon dioxide (CO2), to regulate fluid in the body and maintain proper acid-base balance. Sodium is an essential mineral in the body, necessary for maintaining normal metabolic processes, fluid levels, and vascular pressure. Sodium level is used to screen for and monitor elevated blood sodium (hypernatremia), low blood sodium (hyponatremia), and electrolyte imbalances. Sodium may be monitored in patients on certain medications, such as diuretics, that can cause electrolyte imbalance. Sodium is measured by ion-selective electrode (ISE) methodology.

RVUs

Code	Work	PE	PE Non-Facility	MP	Total Non-Facility	Total Facility	Global
84295	0.00	0.00	0.00	0.00	0.00	0.00	XXX

85002

85002 Bleeding time

Plain English Description

A test is performed to determine bleeding time. A laboratory test for platelet count may be ordered prior to the bleeding time test. A blood pressure cuff is placed on the upper arm and inflated to 20-40 mmHg. Two small cuts are made on the lower arm using a lancet or Surgicutt bleeding device. The time is noted and the blood pressure cuff is deflated. Blotting paper is touched to the cuts every 30 seconds until the bleeding stops completely. The time is again noted. Bleeding time is a coagulation test used to measure platelet function and the integrity of blood vessel walls.

RVUs

Code	Work	PE	PE Non-Facility	MP	Total Non-Facility	Total Facility	Global
85002	0.00	0.00	0.00	0.00	0.00	0.00	XXX

85004

85004 Blood count; automated differential WBC count

Plain English Description

A WBC is a count of the number of white blood cells (leukocytes) in a specific volume of blood. This test is performed to evaluate overall health and can help the physician evaluate conditions such as infection, allergy, systemic illness, inflammation, and leukemia. There are five types of WBCs, neutrophils, eosinophils, basophils, monocytes, and lymphocytes. In an automated WBC count each of the five types are counted separately using an electronic cell counter or an image analysis instrument.

RVUs

Code	Work	PE	PE Non-Facility	MP	Total Non-Facility	Total Facility	Global
85004	0.00	0.00	0.00	0.00	0.00	0.00	XXX

CPT © 2018 American Medical Association. All Rights Reserved.

85013-85014

85013 Blood count; spun microhematocrit
85014 Blood count; hematocrit (Hct)

Plain English Description

A blood test is performed to determine hematocrit (Hct). Hematocrit refers to the volume of red blood cells (erythrocytes) in a given volume of blood and is usually expressed as a percentage of total blood volume. A blood sample is obtained by separately reportable venipuncture or finger, heel, or ear stick. In 85013, the blood sample is collected in a microhematocrit tube which is centrifuged (spun) to separate the WBCs and plasma from the RBCs. The Hct (volume of RBCs) is then calculated and expressed as a percentage of total blood volume (RBCs + WBCs + plasma). In 85014, Hct is calculated using an electronic cell counter.

RVUs

Code	Work	PE	PE Non-Facility	MP	Total Non-Facility	Total Facility	Global
85013	0.00	0.00	0.00	0.00	0.00	0.00	XXX
85014	0.00	0.00	0.00	0.00	0.00	0.00	XXX

85018

85018 Blood count; hemoglobin (Hgb)

(For other hemoglobin determination, see 83020-83069)
(For immunoassay, hemoglobin, fecal, use 82274)
(For transcutaneous hemoglobin measurement, use 88738)

Plain English Description

A blood test is performed to determine hemoglobin (Hgb) which is a measurement of the amount of oxygen-carrying protein in the blood. Hgb is measured to determine the severity of anemia or polycythemia, monitor response to treatment for these conditions, or determine the need for blood transfusion. A blood sample is collected by separately reportable venipuncture or finger, heel, or ear stick. The sample may be sent to the lab or a rapid testing system may be used in the physician's office. Systems consist of a portable photometer and pipettes that contain reagent. The pipette is used to collect the blood sample from a capillary stick and the blood is automatically mixed with the reagent in the pipette. The photometer is then used to read the result which is displayed on the photometer device.

RVUs

Code	Work	PE	PE Non-Facility	MP	Total Non-Facility	Total Facility	Global
85018	0.00	0.00	0.00	0.00	0.00	0.00	XXX

85025-85027

85025 Blood count; complete (CBC), automated (Hgb, Hct, RBC, WBC and platelet count) and automated differential WBC count
85027 Blood count; complete (CBC), automated (Hgb, Hct, RBC, WBC and platelet count)

Plain English Description

An automated complete blood count (CBC) is performed with or without automated differential white blood cell (WBC) count. A CBC is used as a screening test to evaluate overall health and symptoms such as fatigue, bruising, bleeding, and inflammation, or to help diagnose infection. A CBC includes measurement of hemoglobin (Hgb) and hematocrit (Hct), red blood cell (RBC) count, white blood cell (WBC) count with or without differential, and platelet count. Hgb measures the amount of oxygen-carrying protein in the blood. Hct refers to the volume of red blood cells (erythrocytes) in a given volume of blood and is usually expressed as a percentage of total blood volume. RBC count is the number of red blood cells (erythrocytes) in a specific volume of blood. WBC count is the number of white blood cells (leukocytes) in a specific volume of blood. There are five types of WBCs: neutrophils, eosinophils, basophils, monocytes, and lymphocytes. If a differential is performed, each of the five types is counted separately. Platelet count is the number of platelets (thrombocytes) in the blood. Platelets are responsible for blood clotting. The CBC is performed with an automated blood cell counting instrument that can also be programmed to provide an automated WBC differential count. Use 85025 for CBC with automated differential WBC count or 85027 for CBC without differential WBC count.

RVUs

Code	Work	PE	PE Non-Facility	MP	Total Non-Facility	Total Facility	Global
85025	0.00	0.00	0.00	0.00	0.00	0.00	XXX
85027	0.00	0.00	0.00	0.00	0.00	0.00	XXX

85041

85041 Blood count; red blood cell (RBC), automated

(Do not report code 85041 in conjunction with 85025 or 85027)

Plain English Description

An automated red blood cell (RBC) count is performed to evaluate any decrease or increase in the number of RBCs in a specific volume of blood. RBC count may be performed as part of a general health screen or prior to a surgical procedure. It may also be performed to monitor patients undergoing chemotherapy or radiation therapy, or to monitor and evaluate response to treatment in patients with bleeding disorders, chronic anemia, or polycythemia. The RBC count is performed with an automated blood cell counting instrument.

RVUs

Code	Work	PE	PE Non-Facility	MP	Total Non-Facility	Total Facility	Global
85041	0.00	0.00	0.00	0.00	0.00	0.00	XXX

85045-85046

85045 Blood count; reticulocyte, automated
85046 Blood count; reticulocytes, automated, including 1 or more cellular parameters (eg, reticulocyte hemoglobin content [CHr], immature reticulocyte fraction [IRF], reticulocyte volume [MRV], RNA content), direct measurement

Plain English Description

An automated reticulocyte count is performed. Reticulocytes are new red blood cells (RBCs) that circulate in the peripheral blood for 1-2 days before losing sufficient RNA to become mature RBCs. A reticulocyte count may be performed when a blood test shows decreased RBCs and/or decreased hemoglobin or hematocrit measurements. The test can help determine if the bone marrow is responding to the body's need for RBCs. Indications for monitoring reticulocytes include vitamin B12 or folate deficiency, kidney disease, chemotherapy, bone marrow transplant, and treatment with erythropoietin or darbepoetin. A blood sample is obtained. A reticulocyte count is performed with an automated blood cell counting instrument. Automated reticulocyte count performed alone is reported with 85045. When automated reticulocyte count is performed with direct measurement of one or more cellular parameters, such as reticulocyte hemoglobin content (CHr), immature reticulocyte fraction (IRF), mean reticulocyte volume (MRV), or RNA content, 85046 is reported. CHr measures the amount of hemoglobin in reticulocytes, which is an indicator of iron utilization for RBC production, and is used to diagnosis iron deficiency. IRF is used to determine whether reticulocytes are being released prematurely and

CPT © 2018 American Medical Association. All Rights Reserved.

to quantify the proportion of immature reticulocytes. Premature release occurs during periods of high demand for RBCs in chronic kidney disease, following chemotherapy or bone marrow transplant, or in patients with AIDs or malignant disease, as well as other conditions. IRF is calculated as a ratio of immature reticulocytes to the total number of reticulocytes (both immature and mature). MRV looks at the total volume of reticulocytes compared to total red blood cells and is used to evaluate iron utilization. RNA content is evaluated to determine the maturity of circulating reticulocytes.

RVUs

Code	Work	PE	PE Non-Facility	MP	Total Non-Facility	Total Facility	Global
85045	0.00	0.00	0.00	0.00	0.00	0.00	XXX
85046	0.00	0.00	0.00	0.00	0.00	0.00	XXX

85048

85048 Blood count; leukocyte (WBC), automated

Plain English Description

An automated white blood cell (WBC/leukocyte) count is performed to evaluate any decrease or increase in the number of leukocytes in a specific volume of blood. Leukocyte count may be performed to monitor conditions such as HIV and AIDs, or to monitor medical therapies such as chemotherapy or radiation therapy that weaken the immune system and cause a decrease in WBCs. It may also be performed to screen for elevated levels found with bacterial infections, inflammation, leukemia, or trauma. The leukocyte count is performed with an automated blood cell counting instrument.

RVUs

Code	Work	PE	PE Non-Facility	MP	Total Non-Facility	Total Facility	Global
85048	0.00	0.00	0.00	0.00	0.00	0.00	XXX

85049

85049 Blood count; platelet, automated

Plain English Description

An automated platelet count is performed. Platelets, also referred to as thrombocytes, are responsible for blood clotting. A platelet count is performed to diagnose bleeding disorders such as Von Willebrand disease, or bone marrow diseases such as leukemia, or other blood cancers. Platelet levels may also be monitored in patients who have undergone bone marrow transplant, who are receiving chemotherapy, or who have chronic kidney disease or autoimmune disorders. Platelets are counted electronically using an automated device.

RVUs

Code	Work	PE	PE Non-Facility	MP	Total Non-Facility	Total Facility	Global
85049	0.00	0.00	0.00	0.00	0.00	0.00	XXX

85345

85345 Coagulation time; Lee and White

Plain English Description

A laboratory test is performed to measure coagulation time using Lee-White method. Coagulation time measures the number of minutes it takes a sample of blood to form a clot and may be used to assess platelet function. The Lee-White coagulation test requires human observation of 3 test tubes containing one patient's whole blood sample and timing with a stop watch the clot formation in each of the tubes. The number of minutes it takes each tube to form a clot is averaged to determine the coagulation time. This test is nonspecific and less accurate than other available coagulation time tests. It has largely been replaced with automated tests such as prothrombin time (PT) or activated partial thromboplastin time (PTT, aPTT).

RVUs

Code	Work	PE	PE Non-Facility	MP	Total Non-Facility	Total Facility	Global
85345	0.00	0.00	0.00	0.00	0.00	0.00	XXX

85610-85611

85610 Prothrombin time

85611 Prothrombin time; substitution, plasma fractions, each

Plain English Description

Prothrombin time (PT) measures how long it takes for blood to clot. Prothrombin, also called factor II, is one of the clotting factors made by the liver and adequate levels of vitamin K are needed for the liver to produce sufficient prothrombin. Prothrombin time is used to help identify the cause of abnormal bleeding or bruising; to check whether blood thinning medication, such as warfarin (Coumadin), is working; to check for low levels of blood clotting factors I, II, V, VII, and X; to check for low levels of vitamin K; to check liver function, to see how quickly the body is using up its clotting factors. The test is performed using electromagnetic mechanical clot detection. If prothrombin time is elevated and the patient is not on a blood thinning medication, a second prothrombin time using substitution plasma fractions (85611), also referred to as a prothrombin time mixing study, may be performed. This is performed by mixing patient plasma with normal plasma using a 1:1 mix. The mixture is incubated and the clotting time is again measured. If the result does not correct, it may be indicative that the patient has an inhibitor, such as lupus anticoagulant. If the result does correct, the patient may have a coagulation factor deficiency. Code 85611 is reported for each prothrombin time mixing study performed.

RVUs

Code	Work	PE	PE Non-Facility	MP	Total Non-Facility	Total Facility	Global
85610	0.00	0.00	0.00	0.00	0.00	0.00	XXX
85611	0.00	0.00	0.00	0.00	0.00	0.00	XXX

85651-85652

85651 Sedimentation rate, erythrocyte; non-automated

85652 Sedimentation rate, erythrocyte; automated

Plain English Description

A blood sample is obtained and a nonautomated erythrocyte sedimentation rate (ESR) performed. This test may also be referred to as a Westergren ESR. ESR is a non-specific test used to identify conditions associated with acute and chronic inflammation such as infection, cancer, and autoimmune diseases. ESR is typically used in conjunction with other tests that can more specifically identify the cause of the inflammatory process. The blood sample is anti-coagulated and placed in a tall thin tube. The distance erythrocytes (red blood cells) have fallen in one hour in a vertical column under the influence of gravity is then measured. In 85652, an automated ESR is performed. The blood sample is anti-coagulated, aspirated, and put into the automated system. An automated sedimentation rate reading is provided after the required sedimentation time has elapsed. There are a number of different automated systems available and the technique varies slightly depending on the automated system used.

CPT © 2018 American Medical Association. All Rights Reserved.

RVUs

Code	Work	PE	PE Non-Facility	MP	Total Non-Facility	Total Facility	Global
85651	0.00	0.00	0.00	0.00	0.00	0.00	XXX
85652	0.00	0.00	0.00	0.00	0.00	0.00	XXX

90791-90792

★ **90791 Psychiatric diagnostic evaluation**

★ **90792 Psychiatric diagnostic evaluation with medical services**

(Do not report 90791 or 90792 in conjunction with 99201-99337, 99341-99350, 99366-99368, 99401-99444, 97151, 97152, 97153, 97154, 97155, 97156, 97157, 97158, 0362T, 0373T)

(Use 90785 in conjunction with 90791, 90792 when the diagnostic evaluation includes interactive complexity services)

Plain English Description

Code 90791 reports a psychiatric diagnostic interview exam including a complete medical and psychiatric history, a mental status exam, ordering of laboratory and other diagnostic studies with interpretation, and communication with other sources or informants. The psychiatrist then establishes a tentative diagnosis and determines the patient's capacity to benefit from psychotherapy treatment. The patient's condition will determine the extent of the mental status exam needed during the diagnostic interview. In determining mental status, the doctor looks for symptoms of psychopathology in appearance, attitude, behavior, speech, stream of talk, emotional reactions, mood, and content of thoughts, perceptions, and sometimes cognition. The diagnostic interview exam is done when the provider first sees a patient, but may also be utilized again for a new episode of illness, or for re-admission as an inpatient due to underlying complications. When a psychiatric diagnostic evaluation is performed alone, report code 90791. When medical services are provided in conjunction with the psychiatric diagnostic evaluation, report code 90792.

RVUs

Code	Work	PE	PE Non-Facility	MP	Total Non-Facility	Total Facility	Global
90791	3.00	0.43	0.78	0.11	3.89	3.54	XXX
90792	3.25	0.60	0.96	0.16	4.37	4.01	XXX

90832-90838

★ **90832 Psychotherapy, 30 minutes with patient**

★✚ **90833 Psychotherapy, 30 minutes with patient when performed with an evaluation and management service (List separately in addition to the code for primary procedure)**

(Use 90833 in conjunction with 99201-99255, 99304-99337, 99341-99350)

★ **90834 Psychotherapy, 45 minutes with patient**

★✚ **90836 Psychotherapy, 45 minutes with patient when performed with an evaluation and management service (List separately in addition to the code for primary procedure)**

(Use 90836 in conjunction with 99201-99255, 99304-99337, 99341-99350)

★ **90837 Psychotherapy, 60 minutes with patient**

(Use the appropriate prolonged services code [99354, 99355, 99356, 99357] for psychotherapy services not performed with an E/M service of 90 minutes or longer face-to-face with the patient)

★✚ **90838 Psychotherapy, 60 minutes with patient when performed with an evaluation and management service (List separately in addition to the code for primary procedure)**

(Use 90838 in conjunction with 99201-99255, 99304-99337, 99341-99350)

(Use 90785 in conjunction with 90832, 90833, 90834, 90836, 90837, 90838 when psychotherapy includes interactive complexity services)

Plain English Description

Individual psychotherapy is provided to a patient utilizing reeducation, support and reassurance, insight discussions, and occasionally medication to affect behavior-modification through self-understanding, or to evaluate and improve family relationship dynamics as they relate to the patient's condition. If psychotherapy alone is provided, report 90832 for 30 minutes, 90834 for 45 minutes, and 90837 for 60 minutes. If medical evaluation and management services are performed with the psychotherapy, report code 90833 for 30 minutes, 90836 for 45 minutes, and 90838 for 60 minutes.

RVUs

Code	Work	PE	PE Non-Facility	MP	Total Non-Facility	Total Facility	Global
90832	1.50	0.21	0.35	0.05	1.90	1.76	XXX
90833	1.50	0.27	0.40	0.07	1.97	1.84	ZZZ
90834	2.00	0.28	0.46	0.07	2.53	2.35	XXX
90836	1.90	0.35	0.51	0.08	2.49	2.33	ZZZ
90837	3.00	0.42	0.69	0.11	3.80	3.53	XXX
90838	2.50	0.47	0.68	0.11	3.29	3.08	ZZZ

CPT © 2018 American Medical Association. All Rights Reserved.

90863

★✚ 90863 Pharmacologic management, including prescription and review of medication, when performed with psychotherapy services (List separately in addition to the code for primary procedure)

(Use 90863 in conjunction with 90832, 90834, 90837)

(For pharmacologic management with psychotherapy services performed by a physician or other qualified health care professional who may report evaluation and management codes, use the appropriate evaluation and management codes 99201-99255, 99281-99285, 99304-99337, 99341-99350 and the appropriate psychotherapy with evaluation and management service 90833, 90836, 90838)

(Do not count time spent on providing pharmacologic management services in the time used for selection of the psychotherapy service)

Plain English Description

Management of psychotropic medications is often required to ensure that the prescribed medication is achieving the desired results. In addition, many psychotropic drugs have side effects that must be monitored. In each psychotherapy session, the interval history and mental status examination of the patient focuses on response to medication and a review of side effects. The physician queries the patient about the perceived effectiveness of the medication and any side effects. Separately reportable laboratory tests may be performed to evaluate blood levels of the medication or to screen for adverse effects. The physician may then increase or decrease the dosage of a medication. The physician may discontinue the use of a drug which may require weaning the patient off the drug to avoid adverse effects. A new medication may be prescribed to replace an ineffective medication or one that is causing adverse effects. A new medication may be added to the treatment regimen in an effort to obtain better management of the mental health problem being treated. Code 90863 is an add-on code that is reported when pharmacologic management is provided with psychotherapy services.

RVUs

Code	Work	PE	PE Non-Facility	MP	Total Non-Facility	Total Facility	Global
90863	0.48	0.19	0.23	0.03	0.74	0.70	XXX

90865

90865 Narcosynthesis for psychiatric diagnostic and therapeutic purposes (eg, sodium amobarbital (Amytal) interview)

Plain English Description

Narcosynthesis involves intravenous administration of a sedative such as amobarbital (Amytal), thiopental (Pentothal), or pentobarbital (Nembutal) for psychiatric diagnostic and/or therapeutic purposes. An intravenous line is placed and a 5% solution of the selected sedative is administered at a rate of 25-50 mg per minute up to a total dose of 200-500 mg. The physician talks with the patient while administrating the sedative and halts the administration temporarily when the desired level of sedation is achieved as evidenced by physical signs such as lateral nystagmus for light sedation or slurred speech for deeper sedation. Intravenous administration of the drug is then resumed as a rate that will maintain the desired level of sedation. The patient experiences a relaxed, sleepy state. While in this state, patients with certain conditions may become more talkative, uninhibited, and spontaneous and this may be helpful in diagnosing the mental disorder. In addition, the calming effect of sedatives during narcosynthesis may also have therapeutic effects, such as assisting the patient in recalling and coping with traumatic images or memories.

RVUs

Code	Work	PE	PE Non-Facility	MP	Total Non-Facility	Total Facility	Global
90865	2.84	0.64	1.84	0.11	4.79	3.59	XXX

90867-90869

90867 Therapeutic repetitive transcranial magnetic stimulation (TMS) treatment; initial, including cortical mapping, motor threshold determination, delivery and management

(Report only once per course of treatment)

(Do not report 90867 in conjunction with 90868, 90869, 95860, 95870, 95928, 95929, 95939)

90868 Therapeutic repetitive transcranial magnetic stimulation (TMS) treatment; subsequent delivery and management, per session

90869 Therapeutic repetitive transcranial magnetic stimulation (TMS) treatment; subsequent motor threshold re-determination with delivery and management

(Do not report 90869 in conjunction with 90867, 90868, 95860-95870, 95928, 95929, 95939)

(If a significant, separately identifiable evaluation and management, medication management, or psychotherapy service is performed, the appropriate E/M or psychotherapy code may be reported in addition to 90867-90869. Evaluation and management activities directly related to cortical mapping, motor threshold determination, delivery and management of TMS are not separately reported)

Plain English Description

Repetitive transcranial magnetic stimulation (rTMS) is used primarily to treat depression in individuals who have not responded to other treatment modalities. rTMS may also be used as a treatment for anxiety, obsessive compulsive disorder, auditory hallucinations, and migraines. In these disorders, one part of the brain is overactive or sluggish. For example, the left prefrontal cortex is less active in people with depression. The procedure involves the use of magnetic fields to stimulate nerve cells in the region of the brain associated with the mood or other disorder. A large electromagnetic coil is placed against the scalp over the appropriate region of the brain. The electromagnetic coil delivers painless electric currents that stimulate the nerve cells. This therapy alters the brain's biochemistry, the firing patterns of neurons in the cortex, and the levels of neurotransmitters like serotonin. In 90867, in an initial planning, treatment, and management session, the physician determines the best sites on the forehead for placement of the magnets, the optimal rate of stimulating pulses, and the optimal dose of magnetic energy for treatment. The electromagnetic coil is placed against the forehead and switched on and off at a rate of up to 10 times per second. When the device is on, it delivers stimulating pulses that result in a tapping or clicking sound and a tapping sensation on the head. During the mapping process, the optimal site is identified by moving the electromagnetic coils and the optimal rate of the pulses is determined by varying the pulse rate. The physician then determines the optimal dose. The energy delivered is increased until the fingers or hands twitch to determine the motor threshold. Once the motor threshold has been determined, the physician calculates the optimal dose. During the course of treatment, the optimal dose may be adjusted depending on the response to treatment and side effects. Use 90868 for each subsequent delivery and management session when motor threshold does not require adjustment. During each subsequent treatment session, the magnets are placed on the head and the optimal level and duration of stimulation is delivered. Use 90869 for each subsequent delivery and management session requiring motor threshold re-determination. During each subsequent treatment session following re-determination of motor threshold, the magnets are placed on the head and the optimal level and duration of stimulation is delivered.

CPT © 2018 American Medical Association. All Rights Reserved.

RVUs

Code	Work	PE	PE Non-Facility	MP	Total Non-Facility	Total Facility	Global
90867	0.00	0.00	0.00	0.00	0.00	0.00	000
90868	0.00	0.00	0.00	0.00	0.00	0.00	000
90869	0.00	0.00	0.00	0.00	0.00	0.00	000

90870

90870 Electroconvulsive therapy (includes necessary monitoring)

Plain English Description

Electric currents are passed through the brain in electroconvulsive therapy (ECT) to deliberately trigger a brief seizure and cause chemical aspects of brain function to change. These chemical changes build on one another and help reduce the symptoms of severe depression and other mental illness such as schizophrenia, mania, and catatonia. ECT is done under general anesthesia. Electrode pads are placed on the patient's head, either unilaterally or bilaterally to receive the electric currents. Anesthesia and a muscle relaxant are given intravenously and a blood pressure cuff is placed around the ankle or forearm to prevent paralysis of those particular muscles. The physician sends a small amount of current through the electrodes to produce a seizure that lasts 30-60 seconds, and monitors the seizure by watching the movement in the cuffed hand or foot and the dramatic increase in brain activity on the EEG. Most people notice improvement after two or three treatments. ECT is more effective with multiple treatments.

RVUs

Code	Work	PE	PE Non-Facility	MP	Total Non-Facility	Total Facility	Global
90870	2.50	0.52	2.36	0.10	4.96	3.12	000

90875-90876

90875 Individual psychophysiological therapy incorporating biofeedback training by any modality (face-to-face with the patient), with psychotherapy (eg, insight oriented, behavior modifying or supportive psychotherapy); 30 minutes

90876 Individual psychophysiological therapy incorporating biofeedback training by any modality (face-to-face with the patient), with psychotherapy (eg, insight oriented, behavior modifying or supportive psychotherapy); 45 minutes

Plain English Description

Psychophysiological therapy using both biofeedback training and psychotherapy is provided in an individual, face-to-face setting. Psychophysiological therapy is designed to help individuals cope with stressors that cause anxiety disorders, chronic pain, and somatic symptoms. Biofeedback uses electronic sensory monitoring and feedback to help the patient achieve control over autonomic nervous system function. The biofeedback system monitors skin conductance (sweating), muscle tension, skin temperature and heart rate. Psychotherapy uses reeducation, support and reassurance, insight discussions, and occasionally medication to affect behavior-modification through self-understanding. Use code 90875 for a 30-minute session and 90876 for a 45-minute session.

RVUs

Code	Work	PE	PE Non-Facility	MP	Total Non-Facility	Total Facility	Global
90875	1.20	0.46	0.53	0.07	1.80	1.73	XXX
90876	1.90	0.73	1.04	0.11	3.05	2.74	XXX

90880

90880 Hypnotherapy

Plain English Description

Hypnotherapy is derived from the Greek term hypnos, meaning sleep. The aim of hypnotherapy is to reach an altered state of consciousness in which the conscious mind is relaxed, and the unconscious mind is more accessible. This state is used to explore memories, answer questions, and suggest specific goals, impressions, or new behaviors. Techniques for inducing an altered state of consciousness vary. There is no universally accepted standard. Sessions may vary from a single, brief encounter to longer, regularly scheduled appointments. Group sessions may also be done. Hypnotherapy is used in a multitude of applications to treat a wide variety of conditions and/or relieve symptoms. Examples for the use of hypnotherapy include anxiety, pain, psychosomatic disorders, headache, depression, bed-wetting, eating disorders, addictions, ulcers, erectile dysfunction, fibromyalgia, gastric disorders, insomnia, labor pain, and post-surgical recovery.

RVUs

Code	Work	PE	PE Non-Facility	MP	Total Non-Facility	Total Facility	Global
90880	2.19	0.31	0.71	0.08	2.98	2.58	XXX

90882

90882 Environmental intervention for medical management purposes on a psychiatric patient's behalf with agencies, employers, or institutions

Plain English Description

A psychiatrist or other mental health professional is called upon to intervene in a psychiatric patient's environment for any reason that helps manage the patient from a medical standpoint. This intervention takes place with the psychiatrist or mental health professional personally intervening with specific agencies, work places, or institutions with which the patient is engaged. For instance, the psychiatrist or mental health professional may appear in person at the patient's place of work to present information to the employer regarding the kind of work, or type of shift that may be inappropriate for that particular patient to attempt to perform. A psychiatrist or mental health professional may go to a child's school and be present in the classroom to aid in the management or treatment of a phobia-based condition.

RVUs

Code	Work	PE	PE Non-Facility	MP	Total Non-Facility	Total Facility	Global
90882	0.00	0.00	0.00	0.00	0.00	0.00	XXX

CPT © 2018 American Medical Association. All Rights Reserved.

90885

90885 Psychiatric evaluation of hospital records, other psychiatric reports, psychometric and/or projective tests, and other accumulated data for medical diagnostic purposes

Plain English Description

The psychiatrist or other mental health professional performs an evaluation of hospital records, other psychiatric reports, results of psychometric tests or other evaluations, and other types of accumulated data on the patient for the purpose of making a medical diagnosis. Records could be from inpatient or outpatient hospitalization, drug or alcohol rehabilitation programs or facilities, initial diagnostic interview examinations, group therapy sessions, or any other form or type of data collected on the patient for diagnostic purposes, or during treatment or medical management of specific condition(s).

RVUs

Code	Work	PE	PE Non-Facility	MP	Total Non-Facility	Total Facility	Global
90885	0.97	0.38	0.38	0.06	1.41	1.41	XXX

90887

90887 Interpretation or explanation of results of psychiatric, other medical examinations and procedures, or other accumulated data to family or other responsible persons, or advising them how to assist patient

(Do not report 90887 in conjunction with 97151, 97152, 97153, 97154, 97155, 97156, 97157, 97158, 0362T, 0373T)

Plain English Description

The physician meets with family members or other persons involved in the care of a patient with a mental or behavioral condition. The mental or behavioral condition is explained to the family, caregiver, and other individuals involved in the patient's care and their questions are answered. Any diagnostic tests that have been performed are explained. Treatment alternatives may be discussed and the current treatment plan will be described which may include the use of inpatient care, partial hospitalization, or outpatient care. Medications are discussed including dose, desired therapeutic effects, and side effects. Any planned procedures to help treat the condition are explained. The individuals involved in the patient's care may also be advised on what they can do to help the patient with their medical needs and activities of daily living.

RVUs

Code	Work	PE	PE Non-Facility	MP	Total Non-Facility	Total Facility	Global
90887	1.48	0.57	0.91	0.09	2.48	2.14	XXX

90889

90889 Preparation of report of patient's psychiatric status, history, treatment, or progress (other than for legal or consultative purposes) for other individuals, agencies, or insurance carriers

Plain English Description

A comprehensive report is prepared for a patient undergoing psychiatric treatment and is provided to other individual's, agencies or insurance carriers after appropriate written patient consent is obtained. The report provides information related to the patient's psychiatric status and includes pertinent historical and current information on the treatment provided and the patient's progress. Note that this code is not reported when the report is for legal purposes or is related to consultative services.

RVUs

Code	Work	PE	PE Non-Facility	MP	Total Non-Facility	Total Facility	Global
90889	0.00	0.00	0.00	0.00	0.00	0.00	XXX

90901

90901 Biofeedback training by any modality

Plain English Description

Biofeedback training is provided to help a patient learn to control automatic bodily responses. While biofeedback cannot cure disease, it can help patients learn to control physical responses that influence their health. Biofeedback is used by a variety of specialists to treat physical conditions, such as migraine headaches and other types of pain, digestive system disorders, high or low blood pressure, cardiac arrhythmias, Raynaud's disease, epilepsy, paralysis due to stroke, or cerebral palsy. Biofeedback includes identification of triggers that bring on symptoms and the use of relaxation techniques to help control symptoms. A clinician places electrical sensors on different parts of the body that monitor muscle tension, increased heart rate, temperature, or other physiologic signs. The sensors are attached to a biofeedback machine that provides cues such as a beeping sound or flashing light to indicate physiologic changes, such as increased muscle tension or heart rate, changes in temperature or other physiological responses. The patient then responds by concentrating on reducing muscle tension, slowing heart rate, modifying temperature, or providing another appropriate response to the biofeedback information. A typical biofeedback training session lasts from 30 to 60 minutes. The patient is also required to practice biofeedback methods at home on a day-to-day basis to help modify and control physiological responses.

RVUs

Code	Work	PE	PE Non-Facility	MP	Total Non-Facility	Total Facility	Global
90901	0.41	0.14	0.70	0.02	1.13	0.57	000

92960-92961

92960 Cardioversion, elective, electrical conversion of arrhythmia; external

92961 Cardioversion, elective, electrical conversion of arrhythmia; internal (separate procedure)

(Do not report 92961 in conjunction with 93282-93284, 93287, 93289, 93295, 93296, 93618-93624, 93631, 93640-93642, 93650, 93653-93657, 93662)

Plain English Description

Elective external cardioversion (92960) is performed to restore normal cardiac rhythm in patients who are experiencing an abnormally rapid heart rate (arrhythmia). Sedation is administered. Two defibrillator pads or paddles are used. One pad/paddle is placed on the patient's chest near the sternum and the second is placed either in the lower left chest or on the back under the left scapula. Electrical impulses (shocks) are delivered that restore normal cardiac rhythm. The strength of the electrical impulse depends on the type of arrhythmia and the patient's response. If the first attempt to restore the heart to normal rhythm is unsuccessful, a higher electrical impulse may be used and the procedure repeated. Internal cardioversion (92961) involves placing the defibrillator pads directly on the heart during open chest surgery. Electrical impulses (shocks) are delivered directly to the heart muscle.

CPT © 2018 American Medical Association. All Rights Reserved.

RVUs

Code	Work	PE	PE Non-Facility	MP	Total Non-Facility	Total Facility	Global
92960	2.00	0.99	2.37	0.14	4.51	3.13	000
92961	4.34	1.91	1.91	0.98	7.23	7.23	000

93000-93010

93000 Electrocardiogram, routine ECG with at least 12 leads; with interpretation and report

93005 Electrocardiogram, routine ECG with at least 12 leads; tracing only, without interpretation and report

93010 Electrocardiogram, routine ECG with at least 12 leads; interpretation and report only

(For ECG monitoring, see 99354-99360)

(Do not report 93000, 93005, 93010 in conjunction with, 0525T, 0526T, 0527T, 0528T, 0529T, 0530T, 0531T, 0532T)

Plain English Description

An ECG is used to evaluate the electrical activity of the heart. The test is performed with the patient lying prone on the exam table. Small plastic patches are attached at specific locations on the chest, abdomen, arms, and/or legs. Leads (wires) from the ECG tracing device are then attached to the patches. A tracing is obtained of the electrical signals from the heart. Electrical activity begins in the sinoatrial node which generates an electrical stimulus at regular intervals, usually 60 to 100 times per minute. This stimulus travels through the conduction pathways to the sinoatrial node causing the atria to contract. The stimulus then travels along the bundle of His which divides into right and left pathways providing electrical stimulation of the ventricles causing them to contract. Each contraction of the ventricles represents one heart beat. The ECG tracing includes the following elements: P wave, QRS complex, ST segment, and T wave. The P wave, a small upward notch in the tracing, indicates electrical stimulation of the atria. This is followed by the QRS complex which indicates the ventricles are electrically stimulated to contract. The short flat ST segment follows and indicates the time between the end of the ventricular contraction and the T wave. The T wave represents the recovery period of the ventricles. The physician reviews, interprets, and provides a written report of the ECG recording taking care to note any abnormalities. Use 93000 to report the complete procedure, including ECG tracing with physician review, interpretation, and report; use 93005 to report the tracing only; and use 93010 to report physician interpretation and written report only.

RVUs

Code	Work	PE	PE Non-Facility	MP	Total Non-Facility	Total Facility	Global
93000	0.17	0.29	0.29	0.02	0.48	0.48	XXX
93005	0.00	0.23	0.23	0.01	0.24	0.24	XXX
93010	0.17	0.06	0.06	0.01	0.24	0.24	XXX

93040-93042

93040 Rhythm ECG, 1-3 leads; with interpretation and report

93041 Rhythm ECG, 1-3 leads; tracing only without interpretation and report

93042 Rhythm ECG, 1-3 leads; interpretation and report only

Plain English Description

Electrocardiography (ECG or EKG) is an interpretation of the electrical activity of the heart over time captured and externally recorded by skin electrodes placed in the thoracic area. It is a noninvasive recording produced by an electrocardiographic device that transmits information, displayed on a report which indicates the overall rhythm of the heart and weaknesses in different parts of the heart muscle. It measures and diagnoses abnormal rhythms of the heart. In 93040, 1-3 leads are used and a report is generated. In 93041, only the procedure is reported. In 93042, only a physician report is generated without the procedure portion.

RVUs

Code	Work	PE	PE Non-Facility	MP	Total Non-Facility	Total Facility	Global
93040	0.15	0.19	0.19	0.02	0.36	0.36	XXX
93041	0.00	0.15	0.15	0.01	0.16	0.16	XXX
93042	0.15	0.04	0.04	0.01	0.20	0.20	XXX

93318

93318 Echocardiography, transesophageal (TEE) for monitoring purposes, including probe placement, real time 2-dimensional image acquisition and interpretation leading to ongoing (continuous) assessment of (dynamically changing) cardiac pumping function and to therapeutic measures on an immediate time basis

(Do not report 93318 in conjunction with 93355)

Plain English Description

Transesophageal echocardiography (TEE) is performed for monitoring purposes during surgery or other interventions that produce acute dynamic changes in cardiovascular function, such as procedures on the heart or aorta. The procedure includes probe placement, real time two-dimensional image acquisition, and interpretation with continuous assessment of cardiac pumping function and the effect of therapeutic measures as they are performed. A miniature high-frequency ultrasound transducer mounted on the tip of a tube is passed down through the mouth and advanced into the esophagus. The transducer directs ultrasound waves into the heart. The sound waves are then reflected back to the transducer and translated by a computer into an image of the heart that is displayed on a video screen. The images of the heart are continuously monitored as the surgical procedure or other intervention is performed. The monitoring physician reports changes to the physician performing the procedure or other intervention so that additional measures can be taken to minimize or counteract adverse changes in heart function.

RVUs

Code	Work	PE	PE Non-Facility	MP	Total Non-Facility	Total Facility	Global
93318	0.00	0.00	0.00	0.00	0.00	0.00	XXX

94002-94004

94002 Ventilation assist and management, initiation of pressure or volume preset ventilators for assisted or controlled breathing; hospital inpatient/observation, initial day

94003 Ventilation assist and management, initiation of pressure or volume preset ventilators for assisted or controlled breathing; hospital inpatient/observation, each subsequent day

94004 Ventilation assist and management, initiation of pressure or volume preset ventilators for assisted or controlled breathing; nursing facility, per day

(Do not report 94002-94004 in conjunction with Evaluation and Management services 99201-99499)

Plain English Description

Ventilation assist management is done for patients requiring breathing assistance. Ventilator use initiated by the therapist is either a pressure preset type (pressure support ventilator), or a volume preset type, (volume support

CPT © 2018 American Medical Association. All Rights Reserved.

ventilator). On a pressure preset ventilator, the therapist sets the inspiratory and expiratory positive airways pressure, the breath rate, and inspiratory time to match the patient's spontaneous respiratory effort, then sets the ventilator timing to allow the patient to trigger the breaths spontaneously and/or the machine to trigger breaths when apneic spells or slowed respiratory rate occur. Although a constant level of positive pressure is maintained with a pressure support ventilator, the tidal volume varies with the patient's effort and pulmonary mechanics, often resulting in ineffective respiratory efforts. The volume support machine uses the tidal volume as the feedback control. The therapist sets the tidal volume and respiratory frequency and the machine calculates a preset minute volume. The pressure support level is continuously adjusted to deliver the preset tidal volume, depending on the patient's respiratory efforts, breath by breath. Use 94002 for the initial day of ventilation assist and management for a hospital inpatient/observation stay, and 94003 for each subsequent day. Use 94004 for a nursing facility, per day.

RVUs

Code	Work	PE	PE Non-Facility	MP	Total Non-Facility	Total Facility	Global
94002	1.99	0.49	0.49	0.16	2.64	2.64	XXX
94003	1.37	0.41	0.41	0.11	1.89	1.89	XXX
94004	1.00	0.32	0.32	0.08	1.40	1.40	XXX

94760-94762

94760 Noninvasive ear or pulse oximetry for oxygen saturation; single determination

(For blood gases, see 82803-82810)

94761 Noninvasive ear or pulse oximetry for oxygen saturation; multiple determinations (eg, during exercise)

(Do not report 94760, 94761 in conjunction with 94617, 94618, 94621)

94762 Noninvasive ear or pulse oximetry for oxygen saturation; by continuous overnight monitoring (separate procedure)

(For other in vivo laboratory procedures, see 88720-88741)

Plain English Description

Ear or pulse oximetry measures the percentage of hemoglobin (Hb) that is saturated with oxygen and is used to monitor oxygen saturation of blood and detect lower than normal levels of oxygen in the blood. Oximeters also record pulse rate and provide a graphical display of blood flow past the probe. A probe is attached to the patient's ear lobe or finger. The probe is connected to a computerized unit. A light source from the probe is emitted at two wavelengths. The light is partially absorbed by Hb in amounts that differ based on whether the Hb is saturated or desaturated with oxygen. The absorption of the two wavelengths is then computed by the oximeter processer and the percentage of oxygenated Hb is displayed. The oximeter can be programmed to sound an audible alarm when the oxygen saturation of blood falls below a certain level. Use code 94760 for a single oxygen saturation determination, 94761 for multiple determinations, such as that obtained during exercise, or 94762 for continuous overnight monitoring.

RVUs

Code	Work	PE	PE Non-Facility	MP	Total Non-Facility	Total Facility	Global
94760	0.00	0.06	0.06	0.01	0.07	0.07	XXX
94761	0.00	0.11	0.11	0.01	0.12	0.12	XXX
94762	0.00	0.70	0.70	0.01	0.71	0.71	XXX

95812-95813

95812 Electroencephalogram (EEG) extended monitoring; 41-60 minutes

95813 Electroencephalogram (EEG) extended monitoring; greater than 1 hour

Plain English Description

An electroencephalogram (EEG) with extended monitoring is performed. An EEG may be performed to diagnose a seizure disorder, to determine the cause of confusion, to investigate periods of unconsciousness, to evaluate a head injury, or to identify other conditions affecting the brain such as a tumor, infection, degenerative disease, or metabolic disturbance. An EEG may also be used to evaluate a sleep disorder. An EEG technician applies sixteen or more electrodes in different positions on the scalp using a sticky paste. The electrodes are connected by wires to an amplifier and recording machine. The patient is instructed to lie still with the eyes closed. The machine is activated and the recording period begins. The machine converts electrical signals from the brain to wavy lines that are recorded on a moving piece of graph paper. During the recording the patient may be asked to hyperventilate or photic stimulation may be used in an attempt to trigger seizure activity. The physician reviews the EEG and provides a written interpretation of the test results. Use code 95812 for extended EEG monitoring lasting 41 to 60 minutes. Use code 95813 when the extended monitoring is for more than an hour.

RVUs

Code	Work	PE	PE Non-Facility	MP	Total Non-Facility	Total Facility	Global
95812	1.08	8.03	8.03	0.08	9.19	9.19	XXX
95813	1.63	9.67	9.67	0.12	11.42	11.42	XXX

95831-95834

95831 Muscle testing, manual (separate procedure) with report; extremity (excluding hand) or trunk

95832 Muscle testing, manual (separate procedure) with report; hand, with or without comparison with normal side

95833 Muscle testing, manual (separate procedure) with report; total evaluation of body, excluding hands

95834 Muscle testing, manual (separate procedure) with report; total evaluation of body, including hands

Plain English Description

Manual muscle testing is performed to evaluate function and strength of individual muscles and muscle groups. To perform manual muscle testing, a specific muscle or muscle group is isolated and then a movement such as flexion, extension, abduction, or adduction is performed while resistance is applied using either gravity or manual force. The patient is positioned for testing of the muscle or muscle group and stabilized as needed which may involve the use of a railing, bars, or external support belt. The patient is instructed on the movement, which may be demonstrated by the provider. Function is evaluated using passive range of motion as the provider moves the patient through the test movements, evaluating range of motion and any weakness or instability. The patient then performs the movements while resistance is applied to evaluate strength. The provider supplies a written report of findings and may quantify function and strength using a grading system such as the Medical Research Council's Manual Muscle Testing Grades. Use code 95831 for muscle testing of the trunk or an extremity excluding the hand. Use code 95832 for testing the hand with or without comparison to the hand on the normal side. Use code 95833 for a total evaluation of the body excluding the hands. Use code 95834 for total evaluation of the body including the hands.

CPT © 2018 American Medical Association. All Rights Reserved.

RVUs

Code	Work	PE	PE Non-Facility	MP	Total Non-Facility	Total Facility	Global
95831	0.28	0.11	0.61	0.03	0.92	0.42	XXX
95832	0.29	0.13	0.58	0.04	0.91	0.46	XXX
95833	0.47	0.14	0.71	0.02	1.20	0.63	XXX
95834	0.60	0.25	0.93	0.04	1.57	0.89	XXX

95851-95852

95851 Range of motion measurements and report (separate procedure); each extremity (excluding hand) or each trunk section (spine)

95852 Range of motion measurements and report (separate procedure); hand, with or without comparison with normal side

Plain English Description

Range of motion measurements are performed as a separate procedure to evaluate the function of specific joints and muscles or muscle groups. Passive range of motion is used. The provider moves the patient through the test movement while evaluating the patient's range of motion and noting any limitations to movement as well as any weakness or instability. Use code 95851 for range of motion testing of each extremity except the hand, or each section of the spine. Use code 95852 for range of motion testing of the hand with or without comparison to the hand on the normal side.

RVUs

Code	Work	PE	PE Non-Facility	MP	Total Non-Facility	Total Facility	Global
95851	0.16	0.05	0.42	0.01	0.59	0.22	XXX
95852	0.11	0.05	0.41	0.01	0.53	0.17	XXX

95857

95857 Cholinesterase inhibitor challenge test for myasthenia gravis

Plain English Description

Myasthenia gravis is a relatively rare autoimmune disorder in which antibodies form against acetylcholine nicotinic post-synaptic receptors at the myoneural junction. This results in progressively impaired muscle strength with continued use of the muscle and recovery of muscle strength following a period of rest. Myasthenia gravis may be generalized or limited to bulbar muscles causing facial muscle weakness, ptosis, double or blurred vision, difficulty swallowing, and speech disturbances. A cholinesterase challenge test is performed to diagnose myasthenia gravis or to determine treatment requirements. A cholinesterase inhibitor, such as edrophonium (generic for Tensilon) is administered intravenously. The patient is evaluated for improved muscle strength. If muscle strength does not improve with the initial dose, progressively higher doses may be administered in an attempt to elicit a positive response. If muscle strength improves, the test is positive for myasthenia gravis.

RVUs

Code	Work	PE	PE Non-Facility	MP	Total Non-Facility	Total Facility	Global
95857	0.53	0.28	0.97	0.04	1.54	0.85	XXX

95860-95864

95860 Needle electromyography; 1 extremity with or without related paraspinal areas

95861 Needle electromyography; 2 extremities with or without related paraspinal areas

(For dynamic electromyography performed during motion analysis studies, see 96002-96003)

95863 Needle electromyography; 3 extremities with or without related paraspinal areas

95864 Needle electromyography; 4 extremities with or without related paraspinal areas

Plain English Description

Needle electromyography (EMG) is a diagnostic test used to evaluate pain, weakness, numbness, or tingling in the upper or lower extremities. The test records the electrical activity of the muscles. Abnormal electrical activity of muscles can be caused by a number of diseases or conditions including inflammation of the muscles, pinched nerves, intervertebral disc herniation, peripheral nerve damage, muscular dystrophy, amyotrophic lateral sclerosis (ALS), myasthenia gravis, as well as other conditions. One or more pin electrodes are inserted through the skin and into the muscle. The electrode cable is attached to a recording device with a visual display. Electrical activity of the muscle is recorded. The patient may be asked to move the extremity so that electrical recordings can be obtained with the muscle flexed and extended. The ability of muscle fibers to respond to nervous stimulation, called the action potential, is displayed graphically as a wave form. The test includes any EMG recordings of related paraspinal areas. The physician reviews the EMG recordings and provides a written report of findings. Use 95860 for needle EMG of one extremity; 95861 for two extremities; 95863 for three extremities; and 95864 for four extremities.

RVUs

Code	Work	PE	PE Non-Facility	MP	Total Non-Facility	Total Facility	Global
95860	0.96	2.42	2.42	0.05	3.43	3.43	XXX
95861	1.54	3.26	3.26	0.10	4.90	4.90	XXX
95863	1.87	4.18	4.18	0.10	6.15	6.15	XXX
95864	1.99	4.96	4.96	0.12	7.07	7.07	XXX

95866

95866 Needle electromyography; hemidiaphragm

Plain English Description

Needle electromyography (EMG) is performed to evaluate muscle and nerve function of the right or left hemidiaphragm. It may also be used intraoperatively during procedures on the diaphragm. An EMG electrode is advanced through the skin, abdominal fascia, and abdominal wall muscles into the costal insertion of the diaphragm under the 8th, 9th, or 10th rib cartilage. Electrical responses are recorded with the patient breathing and holding the breath. The physician reviews the EMG recording and provides a written report of findings.

RVUs

Code	Work	PE	PE Non-Facility	MP	Total Non-Facility	Total Facility	Global
95866	1.25	2.56	2.56	0.09	3.90	3.90	XXX

CPT © 2018 American Medical Association. All Rights Reserved.

95867-95868

95867 Needle electromyography; cranial nerve supplied muscle(s), unilateral

95868 Needle electromyography; cranial nerve supplied muscles, bilateral

Plain English Description

Needle electromyography (EMG) is performed to evaluate muscle and nerve function of cranial nerve supplied muscles. Cranial nerves and their branches that can be tested by EMG include: CN III Oculomotor, CN IV Trochlear, CN V Trigeminal, CN VI Abducens, CN VII Facial, CN IX Glossopharyngeal, CN X Vagus, CN XI Spinal, and CN XII Hypoglossal. An EMG electrode needle is advanced through the skin and into the targeted muscle supplied by the cranial nerve. Electrical responses are recorded. The physician reviews the EMG recording and provides a written report of findings. Use code 95867 when the EMG is performed on one of the paired cranial nerves on only one side of the body. Use code 95868 when both of the paired cranial nerves are tested.

RVUs

Code	Work	PE	PE Non-Facility	MP	Total Non-Facility	Total Facility	Global
95867	0.79	2.15	2.15	0.06	3.00	3.00	XXX
95868	1.18	2.68	2.68	0.07	3.93	3.93	XXX

95869

95869 Needle electromyography; thoracic paraspinal muscles (excluding T1 or T12)

Plain English Description

Needle electromyography (EMG) is performed to evaluate muscle and nerve function of the thoracic paraspinal muscles, excluding those at levels T1 and T12. The paravertebral level where there is pain or other nerve or muscle symptoms is palpated. An EMG electrode needle is advanced through the skin and into the paravertebral gutter and positioned in the targeted thoracic paravertebral muscles. Electrical responses are recorded. The physician reviews the EMG recording and provides a written report of findings.

RVUs

Code	Work	PE	PE Non-Facility	MP	Total Non-Facility	Total Facility	Global
95869	0.37	2.27	2.27	0.03	2.67	2.67	XXX

95870

95870 Needle electromyography; limited study of muscles in 1 extremity or non-limb (axial) muscles (unilateral or bilateral), other than thoracic paraspinal, cranial nerve supplied muscles, or sphincters

(To report a complete study of the extremities, see 95860-95864)

(For anal or urethral sphincter, detrusor, urethra, perineum musculature, see 51785-51792)

(For eye muscles, use 92265)

Plain English Description

Needle electromyography (EMG) is a diagnostic test used to evaluate pain, weakness, numbness, or tingling in the muscles. In this procedure a limited study is performed on one extremity or the axial muscles excluding thoracic paraspinal muscles, cranial nerve supplied muscles or sphincters. The test records the electrical activity of the muscles. Abnormal electrical activity of muscles can be caused by a number of diseases or conditions including inflammation of the muscles, pinched nerves, intervertebral disc herniation, peripheral nerve damage, muscular dystrophy, amyotrophic lateral sclerosis (ALS), myasthenia gravis, as well as other conditions. One or more pin electrodes are inserted through the skin and into the muscle. The electrode cable is attached to a recording device with a visual display. Electrical activity of the muscle is recorded. The patient may be asked to move the extremity so that electrical recordings can be obtained with the muscle flexed and extended. The ability of muscle fibers to respond to nervous stimulation, called the action potential, is displayed graphically as a wave form. The physician reviews the EMG recordings and provides a written report of findings.

RVUs

Code	Work	PE	PE Non-Facility	MP	Total Non-Facility	Total Facility	Global
95870	0.37	2.18	2.18	0.03	2.58	2.58	XXX

95872

95872 Needle electromyography using single fiber electrode, with quantitative measurement of jitter, blocking and/or fiber density, any/all sites of each muscle studied

Plain English Description

Single-fiber electromyography (SFEMG) uses a specialized electrode with a 25 micrometer (μ) recording surface that is exposed at a port on the side of the electrode and a high pass filter of 500 hertz (Hz). The small recording surface allows the recording of action potentials from individual muscle fibers and also allows measurement of fiber density and evaluation of neuromuscular jitter and blocking. Neuromuscular jitter refers to abnormal transmission of nerve impulses and neuromuscular blocking refers to the failure of nerve transmission. One or more SFEMG electrode needles are positioned in the muscle fiber. The muscle is then activated by voluntary contraction by the patient or by electrical stimulation using a stimulating needle electrode. Recordings are then taken from 20 fibers of the same muscle. The recordings are then analyzed to identify jitter, blocking, and/or fiber density. The physician provides a written report of findings.

RVUs

Code	Work	PE	PE Non-Facility	MP	Total Non-Facility	Total Facility	Global
95872	2.88	2.55	2.55	0.21	5.64	5.64	XXX

95873

+ 95873 Electrical stimulation for guidance in conjunction with chemodenervation (List separately in addition to code for primary procedure)

(Do not report 95873 in conjunction with 64617, 95860-95870, 95874)

Plain English Description

Electrical stimulation is performed prior to chemodenervation to allow more precise localization of the chemodenervation injection site. A combination stimulation needle electrode and hypodermic containing the chemodenervation toxin is advanced through the skin and into the targeted injection site in the muscle. The stimulating device is activated and the stimulation needle is repositioned as needed until muscle contraction is observed or palpated by the physician. The position of the stimulation needle is manipulated until maximal contraction with a low level stimulus is achieved to ensure that the needle is in the most optimal position closest to the motor endplate of the nerve. The chemodenervation toxin is then injected in a separately reportable procedure. The stimulation and injection needle may be advanced along the muscle or may be withdrawn and reinserted at different sites in the muscle and the process repeated until the desired results are achieved.

CPT © 2018 American Medical Association. All Rights Reserved.

RVUs

Code	Work	PE	PE Non-Facility	MP	Total Non-Facility	Total Facility	Global
95873	0.37	1.75	1.75	0.01	2.13	2.13	ZZZ

95874

✚ **95874 Needle electromyography for guidance in conjunction with chemodenervation (List separately in addition to code for primary procedure)**

(Use 95873, 95874 in conjunction with 64612, 64615, 64616, 64642, 64643, 64644, 64645, 64646, 64647)

(Do not report more than one guidance code for each corresponding chemodenervation code)

(Do not report 95874 in conjunction with 64617, 95860-95870, 95873)

Plain English Description

Needle electromyography (EMG) is performed prior to chemodenervation to allow more precise localization of the chemodenervation injection site. A combination recording needle electrode and hypodermic containing the chemodenervation toxin is advanced through the skin and into the targeted injection site in the muscle. The recording device is activated to ensure that the needle is positioned in the spastic muscle and not in nearby blood vessels. The chemodenervation toxin is then injected in a separately reportable procedure. The recording and injection needle may be advanced along the muscle or may be withdrawn and reinserted at different sites in the muscle and additional injections performed until the desired results are achieved.

RVUs

Code	Work	PE	PE Non-Facility	MP	Total Non-Facility	Total Facility	Global
95874	0.37	1.79	1.79	0.02	2.18	2.18	ZZZ

95905

⊘ **95905 Motor and/or sensory nerve conduction, using preconfigured electrode array(s), amplitude and latency/velocity study, each limb, includes F-wave study when performed, with interpretation and report**

(Report 95905 only once per limb studied)

(Do not report 95905 in conjunction with 95885, 95886, 95907-95913)

Plain English Description

Nerve conduction studies are performed to diagnose and evaluate damage to nerves, nerve disorders such as carpal tunnel syndrome, and symptoms such as numbness, tingling, or other abnormal sensations. Automated systems are now available to perform tests on sensory and/or motor nerves. These automated systems are more commonly used on nerves of the wrist (median and ulnar nerves) and of the foot (peroneal, posterior tibia, and sural nerves). A preconfigured electrode array is attached to the skin of the limb being tested. Electrical pulses are sent through the array. The conduction time, which is the time it takes for the muscle to contract in response to the shock is recorded. The amplitude or strength of the response as well as the speed as reflected by latency or velocity of the response is also recorded. An F-wave study may also be performed. F-waves are small amplitude, long latency responses invoked by maximal stimulation of the motor nerve with the electrode directed away from the muscle being recorded. F-wave study provides information on the function of the proximal aspect of the nerve. Usually 10 or more F-wave recordings are made at each stimulus site. Recordings may be made on site or sent to a remote computer via a modem. The physician reviews the recordings and provides a written report of findings.

RVUs

Code	Work	PE	PE Non-Facility	MP	Total Non-Facility	Total Facility	Global
95905	0.05	1.73	1.73	0.02	1.80	1.80	XXX

95907-95913

95907 Nerve conduction studies; 1-2 studies
95908 Nerve conduction studies; 3-4 studies
95909 Nerve conduction studies; 5-6 studies
95910 Nerve conduction studies; 7-8 studies
95911 Nerve conduction studies; 9-10 studies
95912 Nerve conduction studies; 11-12 studies
95913 Nerve conduction studies; 13 or more studies

Plain English Description

Nerve conduction studies are performed to diagnose and evaluate damage to nerves, nerve disorders such as carpal tunnel syndrome, and symptoms such as numbness, tingling, or other abnormal sensations. Several flat metal disc electrodes are attached to the skin with paste or tape. A shock-emitting electrode is placed over the nerve to be studied and a recording electrode over the muscles innervated by the nerve. Electrical pulses are sent through the shock-emitting electrode. The conduction time, which is the time it takes for the muscle to contract in response to the shock, is recorded. The amplitude or strength of the response as well as the speed as reflected by latency or velocity of the response is also recorded. The physician reviews the recordings and provides a written report of findings. Use 95907 for 1-2 nerve conduction studies; 95908 for 3-4 nerve conduction studies; 95909 for 5-6 studies; 95910 for 7-8 studies; 95911 for 9-10 studies; 95912 for 11-12 studies; and 95913 for 13 studies or more.

RVUs

Code	Work	PE	PE Non-Facility	MP	Total Non-Facility	Total Facility	Global
95907	1.00	1.66	1.66	0.06	2.72	2.72	XXX
95908	1.25	2.20	2.20	0.07	3.52	3.52	XXX
95909	1.50	2.62	2.62	0.08	4.20	4.20	XXX
95910	2.00	3.40	3.40	0.11	5.51	5.51	XXX
95911	2.50	3.99	3.99	0.13	6.62	6.62	XXX
95912	3.00	4.28	4.28	0.16	7.44	7.44	XXX
95913	3.56	4.85	4.85	0.18	8.59	8.59	XXX

95921-95922

95921 Testing of autonomic nervous system function; cardiovagal innervation (parasympathetic function), including 2 or more of the following: heart rate response to deep breathing with recorded R-R interval, Valsalva ratio, and 30:15 ratio

95922 Testing of autonomic nervous system function; vasomotor adrenergic innervation (sympathetic adrenergic function), including beat-to-beat blood pressure and R-R interval changes during Valsalva maneuver and at least 5 minutes of passive tilt

(Do not report 95922 in conjunction with 95921)

Plain English Description

The autonomic nervous system (ANS) is divided into two parts, the sympathetic and parasympathetic nervous system. The sympathetic nervous system helps control blood pressure while the parasympathetic nervous system helps control heart rate. In 95921, cardiovagal innervation (parasympathetic

CPT © 2018 American Medical Association. All Rights Reserved.

function) is tested. An ECG rhythm strip is used to record heart rate, which varies in response to deep breathing, the Valsalva maneuver and moving from a lying to standing position if parasympathetic function is normal. The patient performs deep breathing and the recorded R-R interval on the ECG is evaluated. The Valsalva maneuver which involves attempting to forcibly exhale with the glottis closed so that no air escapes from the nose or mouth is also evaluated using the R-R interval on the ECG. The last test involves having the patient lie quietly on an exam table. The patient is then told to stand and the ratio of the longest R-R interval around 30th beat to the shortest R-R interval around the 15th beat is calculated (30:15 ratio). The physician reviews the tests and provides a written report of findings. In 95922, vasomotor adrenergic innervation (sympathetic adrenergic function) is tested. An ECG rhythm strip is used to record heart rate and R-R intervals and a blood pressure monitor is used to track changes in blood pressure. During the Valsalva maneuver beat-to-beat blood pressure and R-R intervals are recorded. The Valsalva maneuver increases intrathoracic pressure and reduces venous return which in turn should cause BP changes and reflex vasoconstriction if sympathetic adrenergic function is normal. A tilt test is also performed. The patient is placed on a tilt table in head down position for five minutes. The tilt table is then moved to a head-up position which causes blood to shift from the head to the extremities. If sympathetic adrenergic function is normal reflex responses occur in blood pressure.

RVUs

Code	Work	PE	PE Non-Facility	MP	Total Non-Facility	Total Facility	Global
95921	0.90	1.41	1.41	0.05	2.36	2.36	XXX
95922	0.96	1.68	1.68	0.06	2.70	2.70	XXX

95923

95923 Testing of autonomic nervous system function; sudomotor, including 1 or more of the following: quantitative sudomotor axon reflex test (QSART), silastic sweat imprint, thermoregulatory sweat test, and changes in sympathetic skin potential

Plain English Description

Sudomotor autonomic nervous system function is performed to evaluate small nerve fibers linked to sweat glands. There are a number of test methods available and the physician may use one or more of these methods. Quantitative sudomotor axon reflex test (QSART) begins by first measuring resting skin temperature and sweat output. Measurements are taken on the arms and/or legs. A plastic cup-shaped device is placed on the skin and the resting temperature and sweat output is measured. The patient is then given a chemical to stimulate sweat production which is delivered electrically through the skin to the sweat gland. Sweat production is measured. A computer is used to analyze the data to determine function of the portion of the autonomic nervous system that controls the sweat glands. Silastic sweat imprint uses silastic material placed on the skin a device that records the imprint of the sweat droplets on the silastic material. The thermoregulatory sweat test is performed by dusting the skin with an indicator powder. The patient is then placed in a heat cabinet to stimulate sweat production. The indicator powder changes color in response to sweat production. Changes in sympathetic peripheral autonomic skin potentials (PASP) are evoked using electrical stimulation of the skin. Electrical potential recordings are then made over the palms and soles of the feet to evaluate whether autonomic nerve fibers are functioning normally. The physician reviews the test results and provides a written report of findings.

RVUs

Code	Work	PE	PE Non-Facility	MP	Total Non-Facility	Total Facility	Global
95923	0.90	2.68	2.68	0.06	3.64	3.64	XXX

95925-95927

95925 Short-latency somatosensory evoked potential study, stimulation of any/all peripheral nerves or skin sites, recording from the central nervous system; in upper limbs

(Do not report 95925 in conjunction with 95926)

95926 Short-latency somatosensory evoked potential study, stimulation of any/all peripheral nerves or skin sites, recording from the central nervous system; in lower limbs

(Do not report 95926 in conjunction with 95925)

95927 Short-latency somatosensory evoked potential study, stimulation of any/all peripheral nerves or skin sites, recording from the central nervous system; in the trunk or head

(To report a unilateral study, use modifier 52)

(For auditory evoked potentials, use 92585)

Plain English Description

Somatosensory evoked potentials (SEPs) are electrical signals generated by afferent peripheral nerve fibers in response to sensory stimuli. SEPs are divided into three categories: short-latency, middle-latency, and long-latency. Short-latency SEPs refers to the portion of the SEP waveform that has the shortest delay (latency) time. The latency time varies depending on which nerve is being tested. Short-latency SEPs for the upper extremity nerves is the portion of the waveform occurring within 25 milliseconds of stimulation, while stimulation of the tibial nerve refers to the portion of the SEP waveform occurring within 50 milliseconds of stimulation. An abnormal SEP result indicates that there is dysfunction within the somatosensory pathways. Testing SEPs involves the use of electrical stimulation. Electrodes are placed on the skin over the selected peripheral nerve. A ground electrode is placed on the selected limb or other site to reduce stimulus artifact. Recording electrodes are placed over the scalp, spine, and peripheral nerves proximal to the stimulation site. Monophasic rectangular pulses are delivered using either constant voltage or a constant current stimulator. The stimulus causes the muscle to twitch and generates a SEP waveform. SEPs are recorded in a series of waves that reflect sequential activation of neural structures along the somatosensory pathways. The physician reviews the SEP recording and provides a written report of findings. Use 95925 for a short-latency SEP study of the upper limbs; use 95926 for the lower limbs; use 95927 for the trunk and head.

RVUs

Code	Work	PE	PE Non-Facility	MP	Total Non-Facility	Total Facility	Global
95925	0.54	3.14	3.14	0.05	3.73	3.73	XXX
95926	0.54	3.02	3.02	0.05	3.61	3.61	XXX
95927	0.54	3.14	3.14	0.06	3.74	3.74	XXX

CPT © 2018 American Medical Association. All Rights Reserved.

95928-95929

95928 Central motor evoked potential study (transcranial motor stimulation); upper limbs

(Do not report 95928 in conjunction with 95929)

95929 Central motor evoked potential study (transcranial motor stimulation); lower limbs

(Do not report 95929 in conjunction with 95928)

Plain English Description

A central motor evoked potential (MEP) study uses electrical stimulation of the motor area of the cerebral cortex with recording from peripheral muscles in the extremities to evaluate motor pathway function. In 95928, motor pathway function in the upper extremities is evaluated. Prior to MEP recording, baseline nerve conduction studies of the upper extremities are performed. Electrodes are placed on the skin over the appropriate muscles, usually the biceps, triceps, abductor pollicis brevis, and abductor digiti minimi muscles. Impedances are checked and the electrodes are adjusted as needed. Beginning with the abductor digiti minimi muscles, and for each additional muscle tested, the optimal scalp location for electrical stimulation is identified. The MEP threshold is then determined. The motor area of the cerebral cortex is stimulated and MEPs are recorded. Transcranial MEP amplitude or strength of response as well as the speed of response as reflected by onset latency is measured and compared to the baseline nerve conduction study. Next, compound muscle action potential (CMAP) is tested. For the abductor digiti minimi CMAP, the ulnar nerve is stimulated. The relative abductor digiti minimi MEP strength of response reflected as a percentage of CMAP strength of response is measured. The central motor conduction time (CMCT) is calculated. Stimulator output is reduced in 5% increments so that the dissociation between MEP threshold and the cortical stimulation silent period (CSSP) can be measured. Stimulator output is reduced until stimulation no longer alters the appearance of the average EMG for the muscle being tested. Dissociation between excitory and inhibitory effects of transcranial stimulation is defined as EMG inhibition without a preceding MEP at 2 or more stimulus intensities. The data is replicated and the signals are stored. The procedure is repeated on 3-4 muscles on the ipsilateral upper extremity and then the contralateral upper extremity is tested in the same manner. The physician reviews the recordings and provides a written report of findings. In 95929, motor pathway function of the lower extremities is evaluated. The procedure is performed as described above except that electrodes are placed over selected muscles in the legs.

RVUs

Code	Work	PE	PE Non-Facility	MP	Total Non-Facility	Total Facility	Global
95928	1.50	4.62	4.62	0.08	6.20	6.20	XXX
95929	1.50	4.77	4.77	0.08	6.35	6.35	XXX

95970-95972

▲ **95970 Electronic analysis of implanted neurostimulator pulse generator/transmitter (eg, contact group[s], interleaving, amplitude, pulse width, frequency [Hz], on/off cycling, burst, magnet mode, dose lockout, patient selectable parameters, responsive neurostimulation, detection algorithms, closed loop parameters, and passive parameters) by physician or other qualified health care professional; with brain, cranial nerve, spinal cord, peripheral nerve, or sacral nerve, neurostimulator pulse generator/transmitter, without programming**

(Do not report 95970 in conjunction with 43647, 43648, 43881, 43882, 61850, 61860, 61863, 61864, 61867, 61868, 61870, 61880, 61885, 61886, 61888, 63650, 63655, 63661, 63662, 63663, 63664, 63685, 63688, 64553, 64555, 64561, 64566, 64568, 64569, 64570, 64575, 64580, 64581, 64585, 64590, 64595, during the same operative session)

(Do not report 95970 in conjunction with 95971, 95972, 95976, 95977, 95983, 95984)

▲ **95971 Electronic analysis of implanted neurostimulator pulse generator/transmitter (eg, contact group[s], interleaving, amplitude, pulse width, frequency [Hz], on/off cycling, burst, magnet mode, dose lockout, patient selectable parameters, responsive neurostimulation, detection algorithms, closed loop parameters, and passive parameters) by physician or other qualified health care professional; with simple spinal cord or peripheral nerve (eg, sacral nerve) neurostimulator pulse generator/transmitter programming by physician or other qualified health care professional**

(Do not report 95971 in conjunction with 95972)

▲ **95972 Electronic analysis of implanted neurostimulator pulse generator/transmitter (eg, contact group[s], interleaving, amplitude, pulse width, frequency [Hz], on/off cycling, burst, magnet mode, dose lockout, patient selectable parameters, responsive neurostimulation, detection algorithms, closed loop parameters, and passive parameters) by physician or other qualified health care professional; with complex spinal cord or peripheral nerve (eg, sacral nerve) neurostimulator pulse generator/transmitter programming by physician or other qualified health care professional**

Plain English Description

An implanted neurostimulator pulse generator system consists of a generator/transmitter placed in a subcutaneous pocket and electrical leads connected from the nerve or area being stimulated to the transmitter. Electrical impulses from the generator/transmitter stimulate target regions of the brain, spinal cord, or fibers of a cranial nerve, peripheral nerve, or sacral nerve to treat a variety of conditions such as pain, epilepsy, and even depression. Neurostimulators are commonly used to treat chronic, intractable pain when other treatment modalities have failed or are contraindicated. The pulse generator/transmitter is analyzed and programmed at the time of implantation. Electronic analysis with or without reprogramming is then performed at regular intervals by the health care provider to ensure optimal functioning of the device. Electronic analysis involves documenting the values, settings, and impedances of the system's parameters prior to programming. Not all parameters are available in all systems. Stored data from the implanted device is downloaded to a computer software program. Some or all of the following parameters may be evaluated during routine electronic analysis: contact of the stimulator wires to target area(s) or group(s), interleaving, amplitude, pulse width, frequency (Hz), on/off cycling, burst, magnet mode, dose lockout, patient

CPT © 2018 American Medical Association. All Rights Reserved.

selectable parameters, responsive neurostimulation, detection algorithms, closed loop parameters, and passive parameters. Code 95970 is used to report electronic analysis only without reprogramming of the device. In 95971, the physician or other qualified professional performs simple programming of a spinal cord or peripheral nerve pulse generator/transmitter which involves adjusting 1-3 of the system parameters to improve therapy and address the patient's symptoms. Any parameter that needs to be adjusted at least two or more times during a session is counted. Report 95972 for complex programming of a spinal cord or peripheral nerve pulse generator/transmitter involving adjustment of more than three parameters.

RVUs

Code	Work	PE	PE Non-Facility	MP	Total Non-Facility	Total Facility	Global
95970	0.35	0.15	0.16	0.03	0.54	0.53	XXX
95971	0.78	0.32	0.59	0.07	1.44	1.17	XXX
95972	0.80	0.31	0.74	0.08	1.62	1.19	XXX

95990-95991

95990 Refilling and maintenance of implantable pump or reservoir for drug delivery, spinal (intrathecal, epidural) or brain (intraventricular), includes electronic analysis of pump, when performed

95991 Refilling and maintenance of implantable pump or reservoir for drug delivery, spinal (intrathecal, epidural) or brain (intraventricular), includes electronic analysis of pump, when performed; requiring skill of a physician or other qualified health care professional

(Do not report 95990, 95991 in conjunction with 62367-62370. For analysis and/or reprogramming of implantable infusion pump, see 62367-62370)

(For refill and maintenance of implanted infusion pump or reservoir for systemic drug therapy [eg, chemotherapy], use 96522)

Plain English Description

An implantable spinal or brain infusion pump provides long-term continuous or intermittent drug infusion. Because drugs are infused over an extended period of time, the pump or reservoir must be periodically refilled. When the pump is refilled, any pump or reservoir maintenance is performed and an electronic analysis may also be done. The drug is received from the pharmacy and the prescription and patient information are verified. An external needle is used to inject the drug into the pump or reservoir through a self-septum in the implantable infusion pump. Electronic analysis is performed as needed using an interrogation device. A connection is established between the programmable pump and the interrogation device, which provides information on reservoir status, alarm status, and drug flow rates, which are evaluated to ensure that they are all within normal parameters. Use 95991 when refilling and maintenance requires the skill of a physician or other qualified health care professional.

RVUs

Code	Work	PE	PE Non-Facility	MP	Total Non-Facility	Total Facility	Global
95990	0.00	2.59	2.59	0.03	2.62	2.62	XXX
95991	0.77	0.30	2.46	0.07	3.30	1.14	XXX

96150-96151

★ **96150 Health and behavior assessment (eg, health-focused clinical interview, behavioral observations, psychophysiological monitoring, health-oriented questionnaires), each 15 minutes face-to-face with the patient; initial assessment**

★ **96151 Health and behavior assessment (eg, health-focused clinical interview, behavioral observations, psychophysiological monitoring, health-oriented questionnaires), each 15 minutes face-to-face with the patient; re-assessment**

Plain English Description

A health and behavior assessment or reassessment may be performed by any health care professional with specialized training in health and behavior assessment including physicians, psychologists, advanced practice nurses, or clinical social workers. Health and behavioral assessment procedures are performed to identify biopsychosocial factors that may impact physical health problems and treatments in patients that have acute or chronic illnesses or disabilities. The patient is interviewed regarding medical, emotional, and social history. The patient's ability to manage problems related to the acute or chronic illness is assessed. Standardized questionnaires that evaluate anxiety, pain, coping strategies, and other contributing factors are used to obtain additional information. A treatment plan is developed that includes health and behavioral interventions including a plan for modifying any social factors that may be impacting the patient's health. Use 96150 for the initial face-to-face assessment and report once for each 15-minute time increment. Use 96151 for subsequent face-to-face reassessments and report once for each 15-minute time increment.

RVUs

Code	Work	PE	PE Non-Facility	MP	Total Non-Facility	Total Facility	Global
96150	0.50	0.08	0.13	0.02	0.65	0.60	XXX
96151	0.48	0.09	0.13	0.03	0.64	0.60	XXX

96152-96155

★ **96152 Health and behavior intervention, each 15 minutes, face-to-face; individual**

★ **96153 Health and behavior intervention, each 15 minutes, face-to-face; group (2 or more patients)**

★ **96154 Health and behavior intervention, each 15 minutes, face-to-face; family (with the patient present)**

96155 Health and behavior intervention, each 15 minutes, face-to-face; family (without the patient present)

Plain English Description

Health and behavior intervention services are performed that may include cognitive, behavioral, social, psychophysiological, or other procedures designed to improve health and treatment outcomes, reduce frequency and severity of disease-related problems, and improve overall well-being. The intervention services may be provided by any health care professional with specialized training in health and behavior interventions including physicians, psychologists, advanced practice nurses, or clinical social workers. Intervention services are specifically designed for the individual patient based on a separately reportable assessment. Techniques used might include education related to biopsychosocial factors influencing health, stress reduction techniques including relaxation and guided imagery, social support such as group discussions, social skills training. The family may be included in the intervention services if family dynamics are exacerbating the health issues of the patient. The provider may help improve communication,

CPT © 2018 American Medical Association. All Rights Reserved.

conflict resolution, and problem-solving skills within the family by providing instruction during the encounter and interpersonal communication exercises to be performed at home. Family members may also be instructed on how to manage biopsychosocial factors related to the care of children or terminally ill patients. For parents of young children, this may include behavior modification techniques such as praise and reward or distraction techniques to reduce fear and anxiety. In terminally ill patients, the caregiver may receive instruction and support related to improving communication, pain monitoring, and issues related to death and dying. Report the appropriate intervention code for each 15-minute time increment. Use 96152 for individual face-to-face encounters with the patient. Use 96153 for group face-to-face encounters. Use 96154 for family face-to-face encounters with the patient present and 96155 for family encounters without the patient present.

RVUs

Code	Work	PE	PE Non-Facility	MP	Total Non-Facility	Total Facility	Global
96152	0.46	0.07	0.11	0.02	0.59	0.55	XXX
96153	0.10	0.01	0.03	0.01	0.14	0.12	XXX
96154	0.45	0.06	0.11	0.02	0.58	0.53	XXX
96155	0.44	0.17	0.17	0.03	0.64	0.64	XXX

96360-96361

96360 Intravenous infusion, hydration; initial, 31 minutes to 1 hour

(Do not report 96360 if performed as a concurrent infusion service)

(Do not report intravenous infusion for hydration of 30 minutes or less)

+ **96361 Intravenous infusion, hydration; each additional hour (List separately in addition to code for primary procedure)**

(Use 96361 in conjunction with 96360)

(Report 96361 for hydration infusion intervals of greater than 30 minutes beyond 1 hour increments)

(Report 96361 to identify hydration if provided as a secondary or subsequent service after a different initial service [96360, 96365, 96374, 96409, 96413] is administered through the same IV access)

Plain English Description

An intravenous infusion is administered for hydration. An intravenous line is placed into a vein, usually in the arm, and fluid is administered to provide additional fluid levels and electrolytes to counteract the effects of dehydration or supplement deficient oral fluid intake. The physician provides direct supervision of the fluid administration and is immediately available to intervene should complications arise. The physician provides periodic assessments of the patient and documentation of the patient's response to treatment. Use 96360 for the initial 31 minutes to one hour of hydration. Use 96361 for each additional hour.

RVUs

Code	Work	PE	PE Non-Facility	MP	Total Non-Facility	Total Facility	Global
96360	0.17	0.88	0.88	0.02	1.07	1.07	XXX
96361	0.09	0.28	0.28	0.01	0.38	0.38	ZZZ

96365-96368

96365 Intravenous infusion, for therapy, prophylaxis, or diagnosis (specify substance or drug); initial, up to 1 hour

+ **96366 Intravenous infusion, for therapy, prophylaxis, or diagnosis (specify substance or drug); each additional hour (List separately in addition to code for primary procedure)**

(Report 96366 in conjunction with 96365, 96367)

(Report 96366 for additional hour[s] of sequential infusion)

(Report 96366 for infusion intervals of greater than 30 minutes beyond 1 hour increments)

(Report 96366 in conjunction with 96365 to identify each second and subsequent infusions of the same drug/substance)

+ **96367 Intravenous infusion, for therapy, prophylaxis, or diagnosis (specify substance or drug); additional sequential infusion of a new drug/substance, up to 1 hour (List separately in addition to code for primary procedure)**

(Report 96367 in conjunction with 96365, 96374, 96409, 96413 to identify the infusion of a new drug/substance provided as a secondary or subsequent service after a different initial service is administered through the same IV access. Report 96367 only once per sequential infusion of same infusate mix)

+ **96368 Intravenous infusion, for therapy, prophylaxis, or diagnosis (specify substance or drug); concurrent infusion (List separately in addition to code for primary procedure)**

(Report 96368 only once per date of service)

(Report 96368 in conjunction with 96365, 96366, 96413, 96415, 96416)

Plain English Description

An intravenous infusion of a specified substance or drug is administered for therapy, prophylaxis, or diagnosis. An intravenous line is placed into a vein, usually in the arm, and the specified substance or drug is administered. The physician provides direct supervision of the administration and is immediately available to intervene should complications arise. The physician provides periodic assessments of the patient and documentation of the patient's response to treatment. Use code 96365 for an intravenous infusion up to one hour. Use add-on code 96366 for each additional hour of the same infusion. Use add-on code 96367 for another, sequential infusion of a different substance or drug for up to one hour. Use add-on code 96368 when a different substance or drug is administered at the same time as another drug in a concurrent infusion.

RVUs

Code	Work	PE	PE Non-Facility	MP	Total Non-Facility	Total Facility	Global
96365	0.21	1.77	1.77	0.04	2.02	2.02	XXX
96366	0.18	0.42	0.42	0.01	0.61	0.61	ZZZ
96367	0.19	0.67	0.67	0.02	0.88	0.88	ZZZ
96368	0.17	0.41	0.41	0.01	0.59	0.59	ZZZ

CPT © 2018 American Medical Association. All Rights Reserved.

96369-96371

96369 Subcutaneous infusion for therapy or prophylaxis (specify substance or drug); initial, up to 1 hour, including pump set-up and establishment of subcutaneous infusion site(s)

(For infusions of 15 minutes or less, use 96372)

✚ **96370 Subcutaneous infusion for therapy or prophylaxis (specify substance or drug); each additional hour (List separately in addition to code for primary procedure)**

(Use 96370 in conjunction with 96369)

(Use 96370 for infusion intervals of greater than 30 minutes beyond 1 hour increments)

✚ **96371 Subcutaneous infusion for therapy or prophylaxis (specify substance or drug); additional pump set-up with establishment of new subcutaneous infusion site(s) (List separately in addition to code for primary procedure)**

(Use 96371 in conjunction with 96369)

(Use 96369, 96371 only once per encounter)

Plain English Description

A subcutaneous infusion for therapy or prophylaxis of up to one hour is performed (96369), including pump set-up and establishment of infusion site(s). Using aseptic technique, a sterile syringe and needle are used to withdraw the prescribed amount of the substance or drug to be infused. The pump reservoir is filled and the pump and tubing are prepared. The number and location of infusion sites are selected based on the total dosage of the prescribed medication. Common infusion sites include the abdomen, upper buttocks, lateral thigh or hip, and/or upper arm. The infusion sites are prepped with antiseptic solution and a needle is placed in the subcutaneous tissue at each site and tested to verify that it has not been placed in a blood vessel by pulling back on the syringe and checking for blood flow. As each needle is inserted and verified to be placed in subcutaneous tissue, it is secured with tape. When all sites are secured, the drug or medication is administered. Use 96370 for each additional hour of subcutaneous therapeutic or prophylactic infusion beyond the initial hour. Use 96371 for each additional pump set-up beyond the first with establishment of new subcutaneous infusion site(s).

RVUs

Code	Work	PE	PE Non-Facility	MP	Total Non-Facility	Total Facility	Global
96369	0.21	4.46	4.46	0.02	4.69	4.69	XXX
96370	0.18	0.25	0.25	0.01	0.44	0.44	ZZZ
96371	0.00	1.84	1.84	0.00	1.84	1.84	ZZZ

96372

96372 Therapeutic, prophylactic, or diagnostic injection (specify substance or drug); subcutaneous or intramuscular

(For administration of vaccines/toxoids, see 90460, 90461, 90471, 90472)

(Report 96372 for non-antineoplastic hormonal therapy injections)

(Report 96401 for anti-neoplastic nonhormonal injection therapy)

(Report 96402 for anti-neoplastic hormonal injection therapy)

(Do not report 96372 for injections given without direct physician or other qualified health care professional supervision. To report, use 99211. Hospitals may report 96372 when the physician or other qualified health care professional is not present)

(96372 does not include injections for allergen immunotherapy. For allergen immunotherapy injections, see 95115-95117)

Plain English Description

A subcutaneous or intramuscular injection of a therapeutic, prophylactic, or diagnostic substance or drug is given. A subcutaneous injection is administered just under the skin in the fatty tissue of the abdomen, upper arm, upper leg, or buttocks. The skin is cleansed. A two-inch fold of skin is pinched between the thumb and forefinger. The needle is inserted completely under the skin at a 45 to 90 degree angle using a quick, sharp thrust. The plunger is retracted to check for blood. If blood is present, a new site is selected. If no blood is present, the medication is injected slowly into the tissue. The needle is withdrawn and mild pressure is applied. An intramuscular injection is administered in a similar fashion deep into muscle tissue, differing only in the sites of administration and the angle of needle insertion. Common sites include the gluteal muscles of the buttocks, the vastus lateralis muscle of the thigh, or the deltoid muscle of the upper arm. The angle of insertion is 90 degrees. Intramuscular administration provides rapid systemic absorption and can be used for administration of relatively large doses of medication.

RVUs

Code	Work	PE	PE Non-Facility	MP	Total Non-Facility	Total Facility	Global
96372	0.17	0.29	0.29	0.01	0.47	0.47	XXX

96373

96373 Therapeutic, prophylactic, or diagnostic injection (specify substance or drug); intra-arterial

Plain English Description

An intra-arterial injection of a therapeutic, prophylactic, or diagnostic substance or drug is given. Intra-arterial injection delivers medication directly to an artery or organ. Very few medications are delivered into an artery. The arterial site is identified and the skin is cleansed. The artery is punctured and the specified substance or drug is injected.

RVUs

Code	Work	PE	PE Non-Facility	MP	Total Non-Facility	Total Facility	Global
96373	0.17	0.35	0.35	0.01	0.53	0.53	XXX

CPT © 2018 American Medical Association. All Rights Reserved.

96374-96376

96374 Therapeutic, prophylactic, or diagnostic injection (specify substance or drug); intravenous push, single or initial substance/drug

+ **96375 Therapeutic, prophylactic, or diagnostic injection (specify substance or drug); each additional sequential intravenous push of a new substance/drug (List separately in addition to code for primary procedure)**

(Use 96375 in conjunction with 96365, 96374, 96409, 96413)

(Report 96375 to identify intravenous push of a new substance/drug if provided as a secondary or subsequent service after a different initial service is administered through the same IV access)

+ **96376 Therapeutic, prophylactic, or diagnostic injection (specify substance or drug); each additional sequential intravenous push of the same substance/drug provided in a facility (List separately in addition to code for primary procedure)**

(Do not report 96376 for a push performed within 30 minutes of a reported push of the same substance or drug)

(96376 may be reported by facilities only)

(Report 96376 in conjunction with 96365, 96374, 96409, 96413)

Plain English Description

A therapeutic, prophylactic, or diagnostic injection is administered by intravenous push (IVP) technique. The specified substance or drug is injected using a syringe directly into an injection site of an existing intravenous line or intermittent infusion set (saline lock). The injection is given over a short period of time, usually less than 15 minutes. Use 96374 for a single or initial substance or drug. Use 96375 as an add-on code for each additional sequential push of a new substance or drug provided through the same venous access site. Use 96376 for the facility component for each additional sequential intravenous push of the same substance/drug when the interval between each administration is 30 minutes or more.

RVUs

Code	Work	PE	PE Non-Facility	MP	Total Non-Facility	Total Facility	Global
96374	0.18	0.90	0.90	0.02	1.10	1.10	XXX
96375	0.10	0.36	0.36	0.01	0.47	0.47	ZZZ
96376	0.00	0.00	0.00	0.00	0.00	0.00	ZZZ

97810-97814

97810 Acupuncture, 1 or more needles; without electrical stimulation, initial 15 minutes of personal one-on-one contact with the patient

(Do not report 97810 in conjunction with 97813)

+ **97811 Acupuncture, 1 or more needles; without electrical stimulation, each additional 15 minutes of personal one-on-one contact with the patient, with re-insertion of needle(s) (List separately in addition to code for primary procedure)**

(Use 97811 in conjunction with 97810, 97813)

97813 Acupuncture, 1 or more needles; with electrical stimulation, initial 15 minutes of personal one-on-one contact with the patient

(Do not report 97813 in conjunction with 97810)

+ **97814 Acupuncture, 1 or more needles; with electrical stimulation, each additional 15 minutes of personal one-on-one contact with the patient, with re-insertion of needle(s) (List separately in addition to code for primary procedure)**

(Use 97814 in conjunction with 97810, 97813)

Plain English Description

Acupuncture is a traditional Chinese medicine technique used most commonly for pain relief in which the practitioner stimulates specific acupuncture points on the body by inserting thin, sterile needles through the skin. Stimulation of the acupuncture points opens the flow of chi through the meridian pathways and corrects the imbalance of energy flow through the body. Traditional acupuncture may be used together with moxibustion or cupping therapy. Moxibustion is the burning of prepared cones of moxa, a dried, spongy herb known as mugwort, on or near the skin to facilitate healing. Cupping is the creation of local areas of suction to increase blood flow and facilitate healing. Acupuncture is done with or without electrical stimulation in which the needles that are inserted into the skin are then connected to a small generator device which sends continuous pulses of electrical stimulation through the needle into the tissue. Report 97810 for the first 15 minutes of acupuncture without electrical stimulation and 97811 for each additional 15 minutes without electrical stimulation including re-insertion of needles. Report 97813 for the first 15 minutes of acupuncture with electrical stimulation and 97814 for each additional 15 minutes with electrical stimulation including re-insertion of needles.

RVUs

Code	Work	PE	PE Non-Facility	MP	Total Non-Facility	Total Facility	Global
97810	0.60	0.23	0.39	0.04	1.03	0.87	XXX
97811	0.50	0.19	0.25	0.03	0.78	0.72	ZZZ
97813	0.65	0.25	0.44	0.04	1.13	0.94	XXX
97814	0.55	0.21	0.33	0.03	0.91	0.79	ZZZ

CPT © 2018 American Medical Association. All Rights Reserved.

99000-99001

99000 Handling and/or conveyance of specimen for transfer from the office to a laboratory

99001 Handling and/or conveyance of specimen for transfer from the patient in other than an office to a laboratory (distance may be indicated)

Plain English Description

A specimen is transported from the office (99000) or from another setting (99001) where it was obtained to the laboratory where the requested laboratory study will be performed. Prior to transport the specimen is stored in the office or other location where it was obtained following the specific protocol for handling of the specimen. The specimen is transported as required by the laboratory protocol designed for the specific specimen which may include keeping the specimen at a specific temperature (frozen or refrigerated). All safety precautions are adhered to when handling and transporting the specimen.

RVUs

Code	Work	PE	PE Non-Facility	MP	Total Non-Facility	Total Facility	Global
99000	0.00	0.00	0.00	0.00	0.00	0.00	XXX
99001	0.00	0.00	0.00	0.00	0.00	0.00	XXX

99024

99024 Postoperative follow-up visit, normally included in the surgical package, to indicate that an evaluation and management service was performed during a postoperative period for a reason(s) related to the original procedure

(As a component of a surgical "package," see Surgery Guidelines)

Plain English Description

Postoperative follow-up visit, normally included as a part of the surgical codes, reporting an evaluation and management service given for a reason(s) related to the surgical procedure provided as an adjunct to the basic services.

RVUs

Code	Work	PE	PE Non-Facility	MP	Total Non-Facility	Total Facility	Global
99024	0.00	0.00	0.00	0.00	0.00	0.00	XXX

99026-99027

99026 Hospital mandated on call service; in-hospital, each hour

99027 Hospital mandated on call service; out-of-hospital, each hour

(For standby services requiring prolonged attendance, use 99360, as appropriate. Time spent performing separately reportable procedure(s) or service(s) should not be included in the time reported as mandated on-call service)

Plain English Description

Code 99026 is reported for each hour the physician spends being on call while in the hospital. Code 99027 reports each hour a physician spends being on-call when he or she is not physically present within the hospital. Neither code includes physician time spent on other reportable services and/or procedures.

RVUs

Code	Work	PE	PE Non-Facility	MP	Total Non-Facility	Total Facility	Global
99026	0.00	0.00	0.00	0.00	0.00	0.00	XXX
99027	0.00	0.00	0.00	0.00	0.00	0.00	XXX

99050

99050 Services provided in the office at times other than regularly scheduled office hours, or days when the office is normally closed (eg, holidays, Saturday or Sunday), in addition to basic service

Plain English Description

Basic procedure or services provided to the patient in the office but under the special circumstances that the service is given outside of the times when office hours are regularly scheduled, or on days when the office is normally closed.

RVUs

Code	Work	PE	PE Non-Facility	MP	Total Non-Facility	Total Facility	Global
99050	0.00	0.00	0.00	0.00	0.00	0.00	XXX

99051

99051 Service(s) provided in the office during regularly scheduled evening, weekend, or holiday office hours, in addition to basic service

Plain English Description

Basic procedure or services provided to the patient in the office under the circumstances of regularly scheduled evening, weekend, or holiday office hours.

RVUs

Code	Work	PE	PE Non-Facility	MP	Total Non-Facility	Total Facility	Global
99051	0.00	0.00	0.00	0.00	0.00	0.00	XXX

99053

99053 Service(s) provided between 10:00 PM and 8:00 AM at 24-hour facility, in addition to basic service

Plain English Description

Services requested of the physician between 10:00 PM and 8:00 AM in addition to basic services, provided at a facility that remains open 24-hours/day.

RVUs

Code	Work	PE	PE Non-Facility	MP	Total Non-Facility	Total Facility	Global
99053	0.00	0.00	0.00	0.00	0.00	0.00	XXX

99056

99056 Service(s) typically provided in the office, provided out of the office at request of patient, in addition to basic service

Plain English Description

The physician or other qualified health care professional provides services to the patient at a location outside of the office setting that would normally be given inside the office at the patient's request.

CPT © 2018 American Medical Association. All Rights Reserved.

RVUs

Code	Work	PE	PE Non-Facility	MP	Total Non-Facility	Total Facility	Global
99056	0.00	0.00	0.00	0.00	0.00	0.00	XXX

99058-99060

99058 Service(s) provided on an emergency basis in the office, which disrupts other scheduled office services, in addition to basic service

99060 Service(s) provided on an emergency basis, out of the office, which disrupts other scheduled office services, in addition to basic service

Plain English Description

The physician or other qualified health care professional provides needed basic procedures or services in an emergency type situation either within the office (99058) or outside of the office (99060), which causes consequential disruption in the regularly scheduled office routine.

RVUs

Code	Work	PE	PE Non-Facility	MP	Total Non-Facility	Total Facility	Global
99058	0.00	0.00	0.00	0.00	0.00	0.00	XXX
99060	0.00	0.00	0.00	0.00	0.00	0.00	XXX

99070

99070 Supplies and materials (except spectacles), provided by the physician or other qualified health care professional over and above those usually included with the office visit or other services rendered (list drugs, trays, supplies, or materials provided)

(For supply of spectacles, use the appropriate supply codes)

Plain English Description

Supplies or other materials over and above those typically used in an office visit, such as drugs or surgical trays, are provided. This code should rarely be reported as most billable supplies and materials should be reported with a more specific HCPCS Level II code.

RVUs

Code	Work	PE	PE Non-Facility	MP	Total Non-Facility	Total Facility	Global
99070	0.00	0.00	0.00	0.00	0.00	0.00	XXX

99071

99071 Educational supplies, such as books, tapes, and pamphlets, for the patient's education at cost to physician or other qualified health care professional

Plain English Description

Educational supplies are provided at the expense of the physician or other qualified health care professional and the patient is then billed for those educational supplies. This code may be used to bill for books, tapes, pamphlets, or other educational material.

RVUs

Code	Work	PE	PE Non-Facility	MP	Total Non-Facility	Total Facility	Global
99071	0.00	0.00	0.00	0.00	0.00	0.00	XXX

99100

✚ **99100 Anesthesia for patient of extreme age, younger than 1 year and older than 70 (List separately in addition to code for primary anesthesia procedure)**

(For procedure performed on infants younger than 1 year of age at time of surgery, see 00326, 00561, 00834, 00836)

Plain English Description

This code reports an additional qualifying circumstance affecting the primary anesthesia service provided to the patient and cannot be reported alone. Use this code in conjunction with the codes for the primary anesthetic and surgical procedures when the patient is of extremely young or old age. Extreme age complicates the circumstances and character of the anesthesia service being provided and is defined as being under 1 year of age or over 70 years of age.

RVUs

Code	Work	PE	PE Non-Facility	MP	Total Non-Facility	Total Facility	Global
99100	0.00	0.00	0.00	0.00	0.00	0.00	ZZZ

99116

✚ **99116 Anesthesia complicated by utilization of total body hypothermia (List separately in addition to code for primary anesthesia procedure)**

Plain English Description

This code reports an additional qualifying circumstance affecting the primary anesthesia service provided to the patient and cannot be reported alone. Use this code in conjunction with the codes for the primary anesthetic and surgical procedures when total body hypothermia is utilized. Hypothermia complicates the circumstances and significantly affects the character of the anesthesia service being provided with additional operative condition risk factors. Hypothermia is the deliberate reduction in temperature of the whole body in order to slow the general metabolism of the tissues, i.e., lowering the metabolic rate for glucose and oxygen. It is often used in cardiac surgery and traumatic brain injury.

RVUs

Code	Work	PE	PE Non-Facility	MP	Total Non-Facility	Total Facility	Global
99116	0.00	0.00	0.00	0.00	0.00	0.00	ZZZ

99135

✚ **99135 Anesthesia complicated by utilization of controlled hypotension (List separately in addition to code for primary anesthesia procedure)**

Plain English Description

This code reports an additional qualifying circumstance affecting the primary anesthesia service provided to the patient and cannot be reported alone. Use this code in conjunction with the codes for the primary anesthetic and surgical procedures when controlled hypotension is utilized. Hypotension complicates the circumstances and significantly affects the character of the anesthesia service being provided with additional operative condition risk factors. Controlled hypotension has been used to reduce intraoperative blood loss and consequently the need for blood transfusions, as well as provide a bloodless operative field. Controlled hypotension is defined as a 30% reduction in the patient's baseline mean arterial pressure, a reduction in systolic blood pressure down to 80-90 mm Hg, or a reduction of mean arterial pressure to 50-65 mm Hg. Controlled hypotension is often used in spinal surgery, endoscopic microsurgery on the head, oromaxillofacial surgery, major orthopedic surgery, and cardiovascular surgery.

CPT © 2018 American Medical Association. All Rights Reserved.

RVUs

Code	Work	PE	PE Non-Facility	MP	Total Non-Facility	Total Facility	Global
99135	0.00	0.00	0.00	0.00	0.00	0.00	ZZZ

99140

✚ **99140 Anesthesia complicated by emergency conditions (specify) (List separately in addition to code for primary anesthesia procedure)**

(An emergency is defined as existing when delay in treatment of the patient would lead to a significant increase in the threat to life or body part)

Plain English Description

This code reports an additional qualifying circumstance affecting the primary anesthesia service provided to the patient and cannot be reported alone. Use this code in conjunction with the codes for the primary anesthetic and surgical procedures when emergency conditions exist. Emergency conditions complicate the circumstances and significantly affect the character of the anesthesia service being provided with additional, extraordinary risk factors. An emergency condition exists when any type of delay in patient treatment will significantly increase the threat to life and/or limb or other body part.

RVUs

Code	Work	PE	PE Non-Facility	MP	Total Non-Facility	Total Facility	Global
99140	0.00	0.00	0.00	0.00	0.00	0.00	ZZZ

99151-99153

⊘ **99151 Moderate sedation services provided by the same physician or other qualified health care professional performing the diagnostic or therapeutic service that the sedation supports, requiring the presence of an independent trained observer to assist in the monitoring of the patient's level of consciousness and physiological status; initial 15 minutes of intraservice time, patient younger than 5 years of age**

⊘ **99152 Moderate sedation services provided by the same physician or other qualified health care professional performing the diagnostic or therapeutic service that the sedation supports, requiring the presence of an independent trained observer to assist in the monitoring of the patient's level of consciousness and physiological status; initial 15 minutes of intraservice time, patient age 5 years or older**

✚ **99153 Moderate sedation services provided by the same physician or other qualified health care professional performing the diagnostic or therapeutic service that the sedation supports, requiring the presence of an independent trained observer to assist in the monitoring of the patient's level of consciousness and physiological status; each additional 15 minutes intraservice time (List separately in addition to code for primary service)**

(Use 99153 in conjunction with 99151, 99152)

(Do not report 99153 in conjunction with 99155, 99156)

Plain English Description

Moderate sedation services are provided by the same physician or other qualified health care professional who is performing the diagnostic or therapeutic service requiring the sedation with an independent trained observer to assist in monitoring the patient. A patient assessment is performed. An intravenous line is inserted and fluids are administered as needed. A sedative agent is then administered. The patient is maintained under moderate sedation, with monitoring of the patient's consciousness level and physiological status that includes oxygen saturation, heart rate, and blood pressure. Following completion of the procedure, the physician or other qualified health care professional continues to monitor the patient until he/she has recovered from the sedation and can be turned over to nursing staff for continued care. Use 99151 for the first 15 minutes of intraservice time for a patient younger than five years old; 99152 for the first 15 minutes of intraservice time for a patient age 5 years or older; and 99153 for each additional 15 minutes.

RVUs

Code	Work	PE	PE Non-Facility	MP	Total Non-Facility	Total Facility	Global
99151	0.50	0.17	1.57	0.05	2.12	0.72	XXX
99152	0.25	0.08	1.17	0.02	1.44	0.35	XXX
99153	0.00	0.29	0.29	0.01	0.30	0.30	ZZZ

99155-99157

99155 Moderate sedation services provided by a physician or other qualified health care professional other than the physician or other qualified health care professional performing the diagnostic or therapeutic service that the sedation supports; initial 15 minutes of intraservice time, patient younger than 5 years of age

99156 Moderate sedation services provided by a physician or other qualified health care professional other than the physician or other qualified health care professional performing the diagnostic or therapeutic service that the sedation supports; initial 15 minutes of intraservice time, patient age 5 years or older

✚ **99157 Moderate sedation services provided by a physician or other qualified health care professional other than the physician or other qualified health care professional performing the diagnostic or therapeutic service that the sedation supports; each additional 15 minutes intraservice time (List separately in addition to code for primary service)**

(Use 99157 in conjunction with 99155, 99156)

(Do not report 99157 in conjunction with 99151, 99152)

Plain English Description

Moderate sedation services are provided by a physician or other qualified health care professional other than the one performing the diagnostic or therapeutic service requiring the sedation. A patient assessment is performed. An intravenous line is inserted and fluids are administered as needed. A sedative agent is then administered. The patient is maintained under moderate sedation, with monitoring of the patient's consciousness level and physiological status that includes oxygen saturation, heart rate, and blood pressure. Following completion of the procedure, the physician or other qualified health care professional continues to monitor the patient until he/she has recovered from the sedation and can be turned over to nursing staff for continued care. Use 99155 for the first 15 minutes of intraservice time for a patient younger than five years old; 99156 for the first 15 minutes of intraservice time for a patient age 5 years or older; and 99157 for each additional 15 minutes.

CPT © 2018 American Medical Association. All Rights Reserved.

RVUs

Code	Work	PE	PE Non-Facility	MP	Total Non-Facility	Total Facility	Global
99155	1.90	0.46	0.46	0.18	2.54	2.54	XXX
99156	1.65	0.44	0.44	0.15	2.24	2.24	XXX
99157	1.25	0.47	0.47	0.10	1.82	1.82	ZZZ

99605-99607

99605 Medication therapy management service(s) provided by a pharmacist, individual, face-to-face with patient, with assessment and intervention if provided; initial 15 minutes, new patient

99606 Medication therapy management service(s) provided by a pharmacist, individual, face-to-face with patient, with assessment and intervention if provided; initial 15 minutes, established patient

+ **99607 Medication therapy management service(s) provided by a pharmacist, individual, face-to-face with patient, with assessment and intervention if provided; each additional 15 minutes (List separately in addition to code for primary service)**

(Use 99607 in conjunction with 99605, 99606)

Plain English Description

A pharmacist provides individual, face-to-face medication therapy management services to a patient, including assessment and intervention as needed. The pharmacist reviews the patient's pertinent history and medication profile, including both prescription and nonprescription medications, and identifies possible interactions and problems. The pharmacist then fine tunes the drug therapy for the best results, makes recommendations to improve health outcomes, and encourages compliance with the drug treatment regimen. Use 99605 for an initial new patient service of 15 minutes, 99606 for an established patient service of 15 minutes, and 99607 for each additional 15 minutes during the initial or established patient encounter.

RVUs

Code	Work	PE	PE Non-Facility	MP	Total Non-Facility	Total Facility	Global
99605	0.00	0.00	0.00	0.00	0.00	0.00	XXX
99606	0.00	0.00	0.00	0.00	0.00	0.00	XXX
99607	0.00	0.00	0.00	0.00	0.00	0.00	XXX

0106T-0110T

0106T Quantitative sensory testing (QST), testing and interpretation per extremity; using touch pressure stimuli to assess large diameter sensation

0107T Quantitative sensory testing (QST), testing and interpretation per extremity; using vibration stimuli to assess large diameter fiber sensation

0108T Quantitative sensory testing (QST), testing and interpretation per extremity; using cooling stimuli to assess small nerve fiber sensation and hyperalgesia

0109T Quantitative sensory testing (QST), testing and interpretation per extremity; using heat-pain stimuli to assess small nerve fiber sensation and hyperalgesia

0110T Quantitative sensory testing (QST), testing and interpretation per extremity; using other stimuli to assess sensation

Plain English Description

A device is used that provides specific sensory stimulation to test the sensory response of one of the patient's limbs. If the physician tests pressure stimulation, use 0106T. If vibration sensation is tested, use 0107T. If the patient's sensory response to cool temperatures is tested, use 0108T. For the testing of heat and/or pain stimuli, use 0109T. If other stimuli not found in codes 0106T-0109T are used to test sensation, use 0110T.

RVUs

Code	Work	PE	PE Non-Facility	MP	Total Non-Facility	Total Facility	Global
0106T	0.00	0.00	0.00	0.00	0.00	0.00	XXX
0107T	0.00	0.00	0.00	0.00	0.00	0.00	XXX
0108T	0.00	0.00	0.00	0.00	0.00	0.00	XXX
0109T	0.00	0.00	0.00	0.00	0.00	0.00	XXX
0110T	0.00	0.00	0.00	0.00	0.00	0.00	XXX

0213T-0215T

0213T Injection(s), diagnostic or therapeutic agent, paravertebral facet (zygapophyseal) joint (or nerves innervating that joint) with ultrasound guidance, cervical or thoracic; single level

(To report bilateral procedure, use 0213T with modifier 50)

+ **0214T Injection(s), diagnostic or therapeutic agent, paravertebral facet (zygapophyseal) joint (or nerves innervating that joint) with ultrasound guidance, cervical or thoracic; second level (List separately in addition to code for primary procedure)**

(Use 0214T in conjunction with 0213T)

(To report bilateral procedure, use 0214T with modifier 50)

+ **0215T Injection(s), diagnostic or therapeutic agent, paravertebral facet (zygapophyseal) joint (or nerves innervating that joint) with ultrasound guidance, cervical or thoracic; third and any additional level(s) (List separately in addition to code for primary procedure)**

(Do not report 0215T more than once per day)

(Use 0215T in conjunction with 0213T, 0214T)

(To report bilateral procedure, use 0215T with modifier 50)

Plain English Description

Paravertebral facet joints, also called zygapophyseal joints, are located on the back (posterior) of the spine on each side of the vertebra at the point where one vertebra overlaps the next. Facet joint pain may be associated with post-

CPT © 2018 American Medical Association. All Rights Reserved.

laminectomy syndrome or other spinal surgery with destabilization of the spinal joints, scar tissue formation, or recurrent disc herniation. Other causes include spondylosis, spondylolisthesis, and arthritis. Using ultrasound guidance, a diagnostic or therapeutic facet joint injection or injection of nerves innervating the joint is performed. The skin overlying the facet joint is prepped and a local anesthetic is injected. A spinal needle is directed into the facet joint space until bone or cartilage is encountered. A small amount of contrast material is injected to verify that the needle is correctly positioned. This is followed by injection of a local anesthetic and/or steroid. Diagnostic facet joint injection uses a local anesthetic to identify the specific area generating the pain. If the patient experiences pain relief for a significant period of time following a diagnostic injection, the physician will perform a therapeutic injection on a subsequent date of service using a long acting local anesthetic in conjunction with a steroid. Use 0213T for a single cervical or thoracic facet joint injection; use 0214T for the second level; use 0215T for the third and any additional cervical or thoracic levels injected.

RVUs

Code	Work	PE	PE Non-Facility	MP	Total Non-Facility	Total Facility	Global
0213T	0.00	0.00	0.00	0.00	0.00	0.00	XXX
0214T	0.00	0.00	0.00	0.00	0.00	0.00	ZZZ
0215T	0.00	0.00	0.00	0.00	0.00	0.00	ZZZ

0216T-0218T

0216T Injection(s), diagnostic or therapeutic agent, paravertebral facet (zygapophyseal) joint (or nerves innervating that joint) with ultrasound guidance, lumbar or sacral; single level

(To report bilateral procedure, use 0216T with modifier 50)

+ **0217T Injection(s), diagnostic or therapeutic agent, paravertebral facet (zygapophyseal) joint (or nerves innervating that joint) with ultrasound guidance, lumbar or sacral; second level (List separately in addition to code for primary procedure)**

(Use 0217T in conjunction with 0216T)

(To report bilateral procedure, use 0217T with modifier 50)

+ **0218T Injection(s), diagnostic or therapeutic agent, paravertebral facet (zygapophyseal) joint (or nerves innervating that joint) with ultrasound guidance, lumbar or sacral; third and any additional level(s) (List separately in addition to code for primary procedure)**

(Do not report 0218T more than once per day)

(Use 0218T in conjunction with 0216T, 0217T)

(If injection(s) are performed using fluoroscopy or CT, see 64490-64495)

(To report bilateral procedure, use 0218T with modifier 50)

Plain English Description

Paravertebral facet joints, also called zygapophyseal joints, are located on the back (posterior) of the spine on each side of the vertebra at the point where one vertebra overlaps the next. Facet joint pain may be associated with post laminectomy syndrome or other spinal surgery with destabilization of the spinal joints, scar tissue formation, or recurrent disc herniation. Other causes include spondylosis, spondylolisthesis, and arthritis. Using ultrasound guidance, a diagnostic or therapeutic facet joint injection or injection of nerves innervating the joint is performed. The skin overlying the facet joint is prepped and a local anesthetic is injected. A spinal needle is directed into the facet joint space until bone or cartilage is encountered. A small amount of contrast material is injected to verify that the needle is correctly positioned. This is followed by injection of a local anesthetic and/or steroid. Diagnostic facet joint injection uses a local anesthetic to identify the specific area generating the pain. If the patient experiences pain relief for a significant period of time following a diagnostic injection, the physician will perform a therapeutic injection on a subsequent date of service using a long acting local anesthetic in conjunction with a steroid. Use 0216T for a single lumbar or sacral facet joint injection; use 0217T for the second level; use 0218T for the third and any additional lumbar or sacral levels injected.

RVUs

Code	Work	PE	PE Non-Facility	MP	Total Non-Facility	Total Facility	Global
0216T	0.00	0.00	0.00	0.00	0.00	0.00	XXX
0217T	0.00	0.00	0.00	0.00	0.00	0.00	ZZZ
0218T	0.00	0.00	0.00	0.00	0.00	0.00	ZZZ

0228T-0229T

0228T Injection(s), anesthetic agent and/or steroid, transforaminal epidural, with ultrasound guidance, cervical or thoracic; single level

+ **0229T Injection(s), anesthetic agent and/or steroid, transforaminal epidural, with ultrasound guidance, cervical or thoracic; each additional level (List separately in addition to code for primary procedure)**

(Use 0229T in conjunction with 0228T)

Plain English Description

A transforaminal epidural injection is performed to treat foraminal stenosis and large or lateral disc herniations. The patient is positioned prone on the treatment table. Using fluoroscopic guidance, a needle is advanced through the skin and nerve root foramen of the affected vertebra and into the epidural space. Contrast is injected to ensure proper placement of the needle within the epidural space. An anesthetic agent and/or steroid is then injected. Use 0228T for the first injection of a cervical or thoracic vertebral level. Use 0229T for each additional cervical or thoracic level injected.

RVUs

Code	Work	PE	PE Non-Facility	MP	Total Non-Facility	Total Facility	Global
0228T	0.00	0.00	0.00	0.00	0.00	0.00	XXX
0229T	0.00	0.00	0.00	0.00	0.00	0.00	XXX

0230T-0231T

0230T Injection(s), anesthetic agent and/or steroid, transforaminal epidural, with ultrasound guidance, lumbar or sacral; single level

+ **0231T Injection(s), anesthetic agent and/or steroid, transforaminal epidural, with ultrasound guidance, lumbar or sacral; each additional level (List separately in addition to code for primary procedure)**

(Use 0231T in conjunction with 0230T)

(For transforaminal epidural injections performed under fluoroscopy or CT, see 64479-64484)

(Do not report 0228T-0231T in conjunction with 76942, 76998, 76999)

Plain English Description

A transforaminal epidural injection is performed to treat foraminal stenosis and large or lateral disc herniations. The patient is positioned prone on the treatment table. Using fluoroscopic guidance, a needle is advanced through the skin and nerve root foramen of the affected vertebra and into the epidural space. Contrast is injected to ensure proper placement of the needle within the

CPT © 2018 American Medical Association. All Rights Reserved.

epidural space. An anesthetic agent and/or steroid is then injected. Use 0230T for the first injection of a lumbar or sacral vertebral level. Use 0231T for each additional lumbar or sacral level injected.

RVUs

Code	Work	PE	PE Non-Facility	MP	Total Non-Facility	Total Facility	Global
0230T	0.00	0.00	0.00	0.00	0.00	0.00	XXX
0231T	0.00	0.00	0.00	0.00	0.00	0.00	XXX

0278T

0278T Transcutaneous electrical modulation pain reprocessing (eg, scrambler therapy), each treatment session (includes placement of electrodes)

(For implantation of trial or permanent electrode arrays or pulse generators for peripheral subcutaneous field stimulation, use 64999)

(For delivery of thermal energy to the muscle of the anal canal, use 46999)

Plain English Description

Transcutaneous electrical modulation pain reprocessing (TEMPR), also referred to as scrambler therapy, is used to treat intense, chronic pain, such as oncologic/cancer pain, pain due to failed back surgery, low back pain and sciatica, post-herpetic pain, trigeminal neuralgia, post-surgical nerve lesion neuropathy, pudendal neuropathy, brachial plexus neuropathy and other types of neuropathic pain. It works by interfering with pain signal transmission using transmission of non-pain impulses via surface electrodes that are picked up by the same nerve fibers transmitting the pain impulses. This mixes or scrambles the pain signal, modifying or overriding the pain signal received by the brain. Surface electrodes are applied to the skin at the sites of the pain. The electrodes are attached to a multiprocessor apparatus that stimulates the nerves with non-pain impulses during a treatment session which typically consists of 1-5 applications, each lasting approximately 30 minutes. Pain response is evaluated before and after each application. Patients may receive multiple treatment sessions over the course of several days or weeks. Report 0278T for each treatment session which may consist of 1 or more 30-minute applications.

RVUs

Code	Work	PE	PE Non-Facility	MP	Total Non-Facility	Total Facility	Global
0278T	0.00	0.00	0.00	0.00	0.00	0.00	XXX

0440T-0442T

0440T Ablation, percutaneous, cryoablation, includes imaging guidance; upper extremity distal/peripheral nerve

0441T Ablation, percutaneous, cryoablation, includes imaging guidance; lower extremity distal/peripheral nerve

0442T Ablation, percutaneous, cryoablation, includes imaging guidance; nerve plexus or other truncal nerve (eg, brachial plexus, pudendal nerve)

Plain English Description

A procedure is performed to relieve chronic nerve pain using cryoablation, a minimally invasive procedure performed under imaging guidance that utilizes a specialized needle, or cryoprobe, to deliver a cooling agent (helium, argon, liquid nitrogen) to the targeted nerve(s), destroying the myelin sheath and interrupting transmission of pain signals. The cryoprobe is comprised of a hollow cannula with a smaller inner lumen. Using image guidance, one or more probes are inserted through the skin to the targeted nerve(s). Correct placement may be confirmed by nerve stimulation test. The pressurized coolant is applied to the probe(s) and travels down the inner lumen in the form of an ice ball; expanding at the end of the probe to freeze the tissue. The gas formed from the coolant travels back up the probe and is expelled. The cryoprobe(s) are removed at the end of the procedure. Code 0440T reports percutaneous cryoablation of an upper extremity distal/peripheral nerve with imaging guidance, code 0441T is for a lower extremity distal/peripheral nerve and code 0442T is for a nerve plexus or other truncal nerve, such as the brachial plexus or pudendal nerve.

RVUs

Code	Work	PE	PE Non-Facility	MP	Total Non-Facility	Total Facility	Global
0440T	0.00	0.00	0.00	0.00	0.00	0.00	YYY
0441T	0.00	0.00	0.00	0.00	0.00	0.00	YYY
0442T	0.00	0.00	0.00	0.00	0.00	0.00	YYY

CPT © 2018 American Medical Association. All Rights Reserved.

J1100

J1100 Injection, dexamethasone sodium phosphate, 1 mg

RVUs Global: XXX

	Work	PE	MP	Total
Facility	0.00	0.00	0.00	0.00
Non-facility	0.00	0.00	0.00	0.00

Modifiers (PAR)

Mod 50	Mod 51	Mod 62	Mod 80
9	9	9	9

Pub 100

J1100: Pub 100-04, 17, 20

CCI Edits

Refer to Appendix A for CCI edits.

J1170

J1170 Injection, hydromorphone, up to 4 mg

RVUs Global: XXX

	Work	PE	MP	Total
Facility	0.00	0.00	0.00	0.00
Non-facility	0.00	0.00	0.00	0.00

Modifiers (PAR)

Mod 50	Mod 51	Mod 62	Mod 80
9	9	9	9

CCI Edits

Refer to Appendix A for CCI edits.

J2274

J2274 Injection, morphine sulfate, preservative-free for epidural or intrathecal use, 10 mg

RVUs Global: XXX

	Work	PE	MP	Total
Facility	0.00	0.00	0.00	0.00
Non-facility	0.00	0.00	0.00	0.00

Modifiers (PAR)

Mod 50	Mod 51	Mod 62	Mod 80
9	9	9	9

CCI Edits

Refer to Appendix A for CCI edits.

J2704

J2704 Injection, propofol, 10 mg

RVUs Global: XXX

	Work	PE	MP	Total
Facility	0.00	0.00	0.00	0.00
Non-facility	0.00	0.00	0.00	0.00

Modifiers (PAR)

Mod 50	Mod 51	Mod 62	Mod 80
9	9	9	9

CCI Edits

Refer to Appendix A for CCI edits.

J3010

ⓘJ3010 Injection, fentanyl citrate, 0.1 mg

RVUs Global: XXX

	Work	PE	MP	Total
Facility	0.00	0.00	0.00	0.00
Non-facility	0.00	0.00	0.00	0.00

Modifiers (PAR)

Mod 50	Mod 51	Mod 62	Mod 80
9	9	9	9

CCI Edits

Refer to Appendix A for CCI edits.

J3301

ⓘJ3301 Injection, triamcinolone acetonide, not otherwise specified, 10 mg

RVUs Global: XXX

	Work	PE	MP	Total
Facility	0.00	0.00	0.00	0.00
Non-facility	0.00	0.00	0.00	0.00

Modifiers (PAR)

Mod 50	Mod 51	Mod 62	Mod 80
9	9	9	9

AHA: 2Q 2013, 4

CCI Edits

Refer to Appendix A for CCI edits.

J7325

J7325 Hyaluronan or derivative, synvisc or synvisc-one, for intra-articular injection, 1 mg

RVUs Global: XXX

	Work	PE	MP	Total
Facility	0.00	0.00	0.00	0.00
Non-facility	0.00	0.00	0.00	0.00

Modifiers (PAR)

Mod 50	Mod 51	Mod 62	Mod 80
9	9	9	9

CCI Edits

Refer to Appendix A for CCI edits.

L8680

⊘L8680 Implantable neurostimulator electrode, each

RVUs Global:

	Work	PE	MP	Total
Facility	0.00	0.00	0.00	0.00
Non-facility	0.00	0.00	0.00	0.00

CCI Edits

Refer to Appendix A for CCI edits.

CPT © 2018 American Medical Association. All rights reserved.

Q9966

ⓘQ9966 Low osmolar contrast material, 200-299 mg/ml iodine concentration, per ml

RVUs

Global: XXX

	Work	PE	MP	Total
Facility	0.00	0.00	0.00	0.00
Non-facility	0.00	0.00	0.00	0.00

Modifiers (PAR)

Mod 50	Mod 51	Mod 62	Mod 80
9	9	9	9

CCI Edits

Refer to Appendix A for CCI edits.

CPT © 2018 American Medical Association. All rights reserved.

Modifiers

The CPT® code selected must be the one that most closely describes the service(s) and/or procedure(s) documented by the physician. However, sometimes certain services or procedures go above and beyond the definition of the assigned CPT code definition and require further clarification. For these and other reasons, modifiers were developed and implemented by the American Medical Association (AMA), the Centers for Medicare and Medicaid Services (CMS), and local Part B Medicare Administrative Contractors (MACs). These modifiers give health care providers a way to indicate that a service or procedure has been modified by some circumstance but still meets the code definition. Modifiers were designed to expand on the information already provided by the current CPT coding system and to assist in the prompt processing of claims. A CPT modifier is a two-digit numeric character reported with the appropriate CPT code, and is intended to transfer specific information regarding a certain procedure or service.

Modifiers are used to ensure payment accuracy, coding consistency, and editing under the outpatient prospective payment system (OPPS), and are also mandated for private practitioners (solo and multiple), ambulatory surgery centers (ASCs), and other outpatient hospital services.

Modifier Usage

Modifiers are indicated when:

- A service/procedure contains a professional and technical component but only one is applicable
- A service/procedure was performed by more than one physician and/or in more than one location
- The service reported was increased or decreased from that of the original definition
- Unusual events occurred during the service/procedure
- A service/procedure was performed more than once
- A bilateral procedure was performed
- Only part of a service was performed
- An adjunctive service was performed

If a modifier is to be utilized, the following must be documented in the patient's medical record:

- The special circumstances indicating the need to add that modifier
- All pertinent information and an adequate definition of the service/procedure performed supporting the use of the assigned modifier

CPT Modifiers

CPT modifiers are attached to the end of the appropriate CPT code. For professional services, modifiers will be reported as an attachment to the CPT code as reported on the CMS-1500 form, and for outpatient services, modifiers will be reported as an attachment to the CPT code as reported in the UB-04 form locator FL 44.

Some modifiers are strictly informational:

- Modifier 57, identifying a decision for surgery at the time of an evaluation and management service

Other modifiers are informational and indicate additional reimbursement may be warranted:

- Modifier 22, identifying an unusual service that is greater than what is typical for that code

Placement of a modifier after a CPT code does not always ensure additional reimbursement. A special report may be required if the service is rarely provided, unusual, variable, or new. The report should include pertinent information and an adequate definition or description of the nature, extent, and need for the service/procedure. It should also describe the complexity of the patient's symptoms, pertinent history and physical findings, diagnostic and therapeutic procedures, final diagnosis and associated conditions, and follow-up care.

Like CPT codes, the use of modifiers requires understanding of the purpose of each modifier. It is also important to identify when a modifier has been expanded or restricted by a payer prior to submission of a claim. There will also be times when the coding and modifier information issued by the CMS differs from that of the AMA's coding guidelines on the usage of modifiers.

Note: For the purposes of this Modifier chapter, payer-specific information is indicated with the symbol ⓘ. It is good to check with individual payers to determine modifier acceptance.

The following is a list of CPT modifiers:

22 Increased Procedural Services

When the work required to provide a service is substantially greater than typically required, it may be identified by adding modifier 22 to the usual procedure code. Documentation must support the substantial additional work and the reason for the additional work (i.e., increased intensity, time, technical difficulty of procedure, severity of patient's condition, physical and mental effort required).

Note: This modifier should not be appended to an E/M service.

ⓘ Claims submitted to Medicare, Medicaid, and other payers containing modifier 22 for unusual procedural services that do not have attached supporting documentation that illustrates the unusual distinction of the services will be processed as if the procedure codes were not appended

Modifiers

CPT © 2018 American Medical Association. All Rights Reserved.

with this modifier. Some payers might suspend the claims and request additional information from the provider, but this is the exception rather than the rule. For most payers, this modifier includes additional reimbursement to the provider for the additional work.

23 Unusual Anesthesia

Occasionally, a procedure which usually requires either no anesthesia or local anesthesia, because of unusual circumstances must be done under general anesthesia. This circumstance may be reported by adding modifier 23 to the procedure code of the basic service.

24 Unrelated Evaluation and Management Service by the Same Physician or Other Qualified Health Care Professional During a Postoperative Period

The physician or other qualified health care professional may need to indicate that an evaluation and management service was performed during a postoperative period for a reason(s) unrelated to the original procedure. This circumstance may be reported by adding modifier 24 to the appropriate level of E/M service.

ⓘ By payer definition, a postoperative period is one that has been determined to be included in the payment for the procedure that was performed. During this time, the provider offers treatment for the procedure in follow-up visits, which is not reimbursed. Medicare has postoperative periods for procedures of 0, 10, or 90 days (number of days applicable for each procedure can be found in the Federal Register or Physician Fee Schedule (RBRVS) put out by CMS.) Commercial payers may vary the postoperative days; check with each to determine the appropriate number of days for a given procedure.

25 Significant, Separately Identifiable Evaluation and Management Service by the Same Physician or Other Qualified Health Care Professional on the Same Day of the Procedure or Other Service

It may be necessary to indicate that on the day a procedure or service identified by a CPT code was performed, the patient's condition required a significant, separately identifiable E/M service above and beyond the other service provided or beyond the usual preoperative or postoperative care associated with the procedure that was performed. A significant, separately identifiable E/M service is defined or substantiated by documentation that satisfies the relevant criteria for the respective E/M service to be reported (see **Evaluation and Management Services Guidelines** for instructions on determining level of E/M service). The E/M service may be prompted by the symptom or condition for which the procedure and/or service was provided. As such, different diagnoses are not required for reporting of the E/M service on the same date. This circumstance may be reported by adding modifier 25 to the appropriate level of E/M service.

Note: This modifier is not used to report an E/M service that resulted in a decision to perform surgery. See modifier 57. For significant, separately identifiable non-E/M services, see modifier 59.

ⓘ Modifier 25 Guidelines

1. Modifier 25 should be used only when a visit is separately payable when billed in addition to a minor surgical procedure (any surgery with a 0- or 10-day postoperative period per Medicare). Payment for pre- and postoperative work in minor procedures is included in the payment for the procedure. Where the decision to perform the minor procedure is typically made immediately before the service (e.g., sutures are needed to close a wound), it is considered to be a routine preoperative service and an E/M service should not be billed in addition to the minor procedure. In circumstances in which the physician provides an E/M service that is beyond the usual pre- and postoperative work for the service, the visit may be billed with a modifier 25. A modifier is not needed if the visit was performed the day before a minor surgery because the global period for minor procedures does not include the day prior to the surgery.
2. The global surgery policy does not apply to services of other physicians who may be rendering services during the pre- or postoperative period unless the physician is a member of the same group as the operating physician.
3. The provider must determine if the E/M service for which they are billing is clearly distinct from the surgical service. When the decision to perform the minor procedure is typically done immediately before the procedure is rendered, the visit should not be billed separately.

26 Professional Component

Certain procedures are a combination of a physician or other qualified health care professional component and a technical component. When the physician or other qualified health care professional component is reported separately, the service may be identified by adding modifier 26 to the usual procedure number.

ⓘ To determine which codes have both a professional and technical component for CMS, review the Federal Register and/or the Physician Fee Schedule for a breakdown. Usually commercial payers go along with CMS determinations of professional and technical components. Some CPT codes are already broken down into professional and technical components. Examples of these are:

93005 Electrocardiography, routine ECG with at least 12 leads; tracing only, without interpretation and report (technical component)

93010 Electrocardiography, routine ECG with at least 12 leads; interpretation and report only

Modifier 26 should not be appended to either of the codes because the nomenclature itself has determined that they are already technical or professional components.

32 Mandated Services

Services related to *mandated* consultation and/or related services (e.g., third-party payer, governmental, legislative, or regulatory requirement) may be identified by adding modifier 32 to the basic procedure.

33 Preventive Services

When the primary purpose of the service is the delivery of an evidence based service in accordance with the US Preventive Services Task Force A or B rating in effect and other preventive services identified in preventive services mandates (legislative or regulatory), the service may be identified by adding 33 to the procedure. For separately reported services specifically identified as preventive, the modifier should not be used.

47 Anesthesia by Surgeon

Regional or general anesthesia provided by the surgeon may be reported by adding modifier 47 to the basic service. (This does not include local anesthesia.)

Note: Modifier 47 would not be used as a modifier for the anesthesia procedures.

ⓘ This service is not covered by Medicare and many state Medicaid programs. Commercial payers and managed care organizations may cover this additional service.

50 Bilateral Procedure

Unless otherwise identified in the listings, bilateral procedures that are performed at the same session should be identified by adding modifier 50 to the appropriate 5-digit code.

CPT © 2018 American Medical Association. All Rights Reserved.

ⓘ Reported as a one-line item for Medicare claims with the 50 modifier appended to the end of the code. Some carriers or payers may request that bilateral procedures be reported with the LT and RT HCPCS Level II modifiers as two-line items.

51 Multiple Procedures

When multiple procedures, other than E/M Services, Physical Medicine and Rehabilitation services, or provision of supplies (e.g., vaccines), are performed at the same session by the same individual, the primary procedure or service may be reported as listed. The additional procedure(s) or service(s) may be identified by appending modifier 51 to the additional procedure or service code(s).

Note: This modifier should not be appended to designated "add-on" codes (see Appendix D in the CPT codebook).

52 Reduced Services

Under certain circumstances a service or procedure is partially reduced or eliminated at the discretion of the physician or other qualified health care professional. Under these circumstances the service provided can be identified by its usual procedure number and the addition of the modifier 52, signifying that the service is reduced. This provides a means of reporting reduced services without disturbing the identification of the basic service.

Note: For hospital outpatient reporting of a previously scheduled procedure/ service that is partially reduced or cancelled as a result of extenuating circumstances or those that threaten the well-being of the patient prior to or after administration of anesthesia, see modifiers 73 and 74 (see modifiers approved for ASC hospital outpatient use in the CPT codebook).

ⓘ Procedures reported with modifier 52 are typically billed at a reduced amount. Most payers do not require documentation to support the use of modifier 52 and will reimburse the procedure at a reduced level.

53 Discontinued Procedure

Under certain circumstances, the physician or other qualified health care professional may elect to terminate a surgical or diagnostic procedure. Due to extenuating circumstances or those that threaten the well being of the patient, it may be necessary to indicate that a surgical or diagnostic procedure was started but discontinued. This circumstance may be reported by adding modifier 53 to the code reported by the individual for the discontinued procedure.

Note: This modifier is not used to report the elective cancellation of a procedure prior to the patient's anesthesia induction and/or surgical preparation in the operating suite.

Note: For outpatient hospital/ambulatory surgery center (ASC) reporting of a previously scheduled procedure/service that is partially reduced or cancelled as a result of extenuating circumstances or those that threaten the well being of the patient prior to or after administration of anesthesia, see modifiers 73 and 74 (see modifiers approved for ASC hospital outpatient use in the CPT codebook).

54 Surgical Care Only

When 1 physician or other qualified health care professional performs a surgical procedure and another provides preoperative and/or postoperative management, surgical services may be identified by adding modifier 54 to the usual procedure number.

ⓘ Both claims submitted by the surgeon and the other provider must report the date patient care was assumed and relinquished in block 19 of the CMS-1500 or electronic equivalent. Both the surgeon and the other provider must keep a copy of the written transfer agreement in the patient's medical record. Both providers will use the same CPT code, but they will use different modifiers that identify which portion of care they provided.

55 Postoperative Management Only

When 1 physician or other qualified health care professional performs the postoperative management and another physician has performed the surgical procedure, the postoperative component may be identified by adding modifier 55 to the usual procedure number.

ⓘ Both providers will use the same CPT code, but they will use different modifiers that identify which portion of care they provided.

56 Preoperative Management Only

When one physician or other qualified health care professional performs the preoperative care and evaluation and another physician performs the surgical procedure, the preoperative component may be identified by adding modifier 56 to the usual procedure number.

ⓘ Both providers will use the same CPT code, but will they will use different modifiers that identify which portion of care they provided. Some payers do not allow modifier 56 as by their definition the pre-operative care is included in the surgical component.

57 Decision for Surgery

An evaluation and management (E/M) service that resulted in the initial decision to perform the surgery may be identified by adding modifier 57 to the appropriate level of E/M service.

ⓘ **Major Surgical Procedures**

Major Surgery with a global period of 90 days (as defined by Medicare) include the day before and the day of surgery. For example, a visit the day before or the same day could be properly billed in addition to a cholecystotomy if the need for the surgery was found during the encounter. Modifier 57 should be added to the E/M code. Billing for a visit would not be appropriate if the physician was only discussing the upcoming surgical procedure.

Procedures with a 90 day global period are considered to be major surgery, as categorized by CMS. The RBRVS (Resource-Based Relative Value Scale) manual or Federal Register lists the global period for all procedure codes eligible for payment by Medicare.

ⓘ **Minor Surgical Procedures**

Procedures with a 0 or 10 day global period are considered to be minor or endoscopic surgeries, as categorized by CMS. E/M visits by the same physician on the same day as a minor surgery or endoscopy are included in the payment for the procedure, unless a significant, separately identifiable service is also performed.

58 Staged or Related Procedure or Service by the Same Physician or Other Qualified Health Care Professional During the Postoperative Period

It may be necessary to indicate that the performance of a procedure or service during the postoperative period was: (a) planned or anticipated (staged); (b) more extensive than the original procedure; or (c) for therapy following a diagnostic surgical procedure. This circumstance may be reported by adding modifier 58 to the staged or related procedure.

Note: For treatment of a problem that requires a return to the operating/ procedure room (eg, unanticipated clinical condition), see modifier 78.

ⓘ Modifier 58 must be used for purposes of identifying procedures performed by the original physician during the postoperative period of the original procedure, within the constraints of the modifier's definition. These procedures cannot be repeat operations (unless the procedures are more extensive than the original procedure) and cannot be for the treatment of complications requiring a return trip to the operating room.

Modifiers

CPT © 2018 American Medical Association. All Rights Reserved.

The existence of modifier 58 does not negate the global fee concept. Services that are included in CPT as multiple sessions or are defined as including multiple services or events may not be billed with this modifier. This modifier is designed to allow a method of reporting additional, related surgeries that are due to a progression of the disease and are not to be used to avoid global surgery edits applicable to staged procedures.

Modifier 58 should be used on surgical codes only and has no effect on the payment amount. It should not be used with the following codes because the codes are defined as "one or more sessions or stages":

65855	67031	67108	67145	67220
66762	67101	67110	67208	67227
66821	67105	67112	67210	67228
66840	67107	67141	67218	67229

59 Distinct Procedural Service

Under certain circumstances, the physician may need to indicate that a procedure or service was distinct or independent from other non-E/M services performed on the same day. Modifier 59 is used to identify procedures/services that are not normally reported together, but are appropriate under the circumstances. Documentation must support a different session, different procedure or surgery, different site or organ system, separate incision/excision, separate lesions, or separate injury (or area of injury in extensive injuries) not ordinarily encountered or performed on the same day by the same individual. However, when another already established modifier is more appropriate, it should be used rather than modifier 59. Only if no more descriptive modifier is available, and the use of modifier 59 best explains the circumstances, should modifier 59 be used.

Note: Modifier 59 should not be appended to an E/M service. To report a separate and distinct E/M service with a non-E/M service performed on the same date, see modifier 25.

ⓘ Modifier 59 was established to demonstrate that multiple, yet distinct, services were provided to a patient on the same date of service by the same provider. Because distinct procedures or services rendered on the same day by the same physician cannot be easily identified and properly adjudicated by simply listing the CPT procedure codes, modifier 59 assists the payer or Medicare carrier in applying the appropriate reimbursement protocol. If the modifier is not used in these circumstances, services may be denied, with the explanation of benefits stating that the payer does not reimburse for this service because it is part of another service that was performed at the same time.

62 Two Surgeons

When 2 surgeons work together as primary surgeons performing distinct part(s) of a procedure, each surgeon should report his/her distinct operative work by adding modifier 62 to the procedure code and any associated add-on code(s) for that procedure as long as both surgeons continue to work together as primary surgeons. Each surgeon should report the co-surgery once using the same procedure code. If additional procedure(s) (including add-on procedures(s)) are performed during the same surgical session, separate code(s) may also be reported with modifier 62 added.

Note: If a co-surgeon acts as an assistant in the performance of additional procedure(s), other than those reported with the modifier 62, during the same surgical session, those services may be reported using separate procedure code(s) with modifier 80 or modifier 82 added, as appropriate.

ⓘ According to Medicare, payment for the two physicians is based on the two physicians splitting 125% of the allowed charge(s). Check with other payers to determine payment based on this modifier. This modifier should not be confused with modifier 80 (assistant surgeon).

63 Procedure Performed on Infants Less Than 4 kg

Procedures performed on neonates and infants up to a present body weight of 4 kg may involve significantly increased complexity and physician or other qualified health care professional work commonly associated with these patients. This circumstance may be reported by adding modifier 63 to the procedure number.

Note: Unless otherwise designated, this modifier may only be appended to procedures/services listed in the 20100-69990 code series. Modifier 63 should not be appended to any CPT codes listed in the **Evaluation and Management Services, Anesthesia, Radiology, Pathology/Laboratory**, or **Medicine sections.**

66 Surgical Team

Under some circumstances, highly complex procedures (requiring the concomitant services of several physicians or other qualified health care professionals, often of different specialties, plus other highly skilled, specially trained personnel, various types of complex equipment) are carried out under the "surgical team "concept (e.g., organ transplants). Such circumstances may be identified by each participating individual with the addition of modifier 66 to the basic procedure code used for reporting services.

ⓘ Each surgeon that participates in the procedure would report the same CPT code with the 66 modifier. Only surgical CPT codes (10021-69990) should be used with modifier 66 unless otherwise stated by the payer.

76 Repeat Procedure or Service by Same Physician or Other Qualified Health Care Professional

It may be necessary to indicate that a procedure or service was repeated by the same physician or other qualified health care professional subsequent to the original procedure or service. This circumstance may be reported by adding modifier 76 to the repeated procedure or service.

Note: This modifier should not be appended to an E/M service.

77 Repeat Procedure or Service by Another Physician or Other Qualified Health Care Professional

It may be necessary to indicate that a basic procedure or service was repeated by another physician or other qualified health care professional subsequent to the original procedure or service. This circumstance may be reported by adding modifier 77 to the repeated procedure or service.

Note: This modifier should not be appended to an E/M service.

ⓘ Appending this modifier does not guarantee payment of the repeat procedure, but will assist in determining duplicate billings for the procedure.

78 Unplanned Return to the Operating/Procedure Room by the Same Physician or Other Qualified Health Care Professional Following Initial Procedure for a Related Procedure During the Postoperative Period

It may be necessary to indicate that another procedure was performed during the postoperative period of the initial procedure (unplanned procedure following initial procedure). When this procedure is related to the first, and requires the use of an operating/procedure room, it may be reported by adding modifier 78 to the related procedure. (For repeat procedures, see modifier 76.)

ⓘ Medicare includes specific medical and/or surgical care for postoperative complications within the global surgical package and does not allow additional payment. Included in the global surgical package are "additional medical and surgical services required of the surgeon during the postoperative period of the surgery because of complications which do not require additional trips to the operating room."

CPT © 2018 American Medical Association. All Rights Reserved.

79 Unrelated Procedure or Service by the Same Physician or Other Qualified Health Care Professional During the Postoperative Period

The individual may need to indicate that the performance of a procedure or service during the postoperative period was unrelated to the original procedure. This circumstance may be reported by using modifier 79. (For repeat procedures on the same day, see modifier 76.)

ⓘ When billing for an unrelated procedure by the same physician during the postoperative period of an original procedure, a new postoperative period will begin with the subsequent procedure. A different ICD-10-CM diagnosis should be indicated on the claim.

80 Assistant Surgeon

Surgical assistant services may be identified by adding modifier 80 to the usual procedure number(s).

ⓘ Some surgical procedures are not eligible for this modifier; check the Medicare physician fee schedule or with other payers to determine payment eligibility

81 Minimum Assistant Surgeon

Minimum surgical assistant services are identified by adding modifier 81 to the usual procedure number.

ⓘ Check with payers to determine if payment is allowed for this modifier.

82 Assistant Surgeon (When a Qualified Resident Is Not Available)

The unavailability of a qualified resident surgeon is a prerequisite for use of modifier 82 appended to the usual procedure code number(s).

ⓘ In some hospitals with residency programs, Medicare pays through the medical program or graduate medical education (GME) program. Because of this, they will not reimburse for a resident when they are used as an assistant surgeon. Although under special circumstances, payment may be made if there is a emergent situation that is life-threatening.

90 Reference (Outside) Laboratory

When laboratory procedures are performed by a party other than the treating or reporting physician or other qualified health care professional, the procedure may be identified by adding modifier 90 to the usual procedure number.

ⓘ Check with payers to determine if the provider may bill for the laboratory procedure if not performed by the provider.

91 Repeat Clinical Diagnostic Laboratory Test

In the course of treatment of the patient, it may be necessary to repeat the same laboratory test on the same day to obtain subsequent (multiple) test results. Under these circumstances, the laboratory test performed can be identified by its usual procedure number and the addition of the modifier 91.

Note: This modifier may not be used when tests are rerun to confirm initial results; due to testing problems with specimens or equipment; or for any other reason when a normal, one-time, reportable result is all that is required. This modifier may not be used when other code(s) describe a series of test results (eg, glucose tolerance tests, evocative/suppression testing). This modifier may only be used for laboratory test(s) performed more than once on the same day on the same patient.

92 Alternative Laboratory Platform Testing

When laboratory testing is performed using a kit or transportable instrument that wholly or in part consists of a single use, disposable analytical chamber, the service may be identified by adding modifier 92 to the usual laboratory procedure code (HIV testing 86701-86703 and 87389). The test does not require permanent dedicated space, hence by its design may be hand carried or transported to the vicinity of the patient for immediate testing at that site, although location of testing is not in itself determinative of the use of this modifier.

95 Synchronous Telemedicine Service Rendered Via a Real-Time Interactive Audio and Video Telecommunications System

Synchronous telemedicine service is defined as a real-time interaction between a physician or other qualified health care professional and a patient who is located at a distant site from the physician or other qualified health care professional. The totality of the communication of information exchanged between the physician or other qualified health care professional and the patient during the course of the synchronous telemedicine service must be of an amount and nature that would be sufficient to meet the key components and/or requirements of the same services when rendered via a face-to-face interaction. Modifier 95 may only be appended to the services listed in Appendix P. Appendix P is the list of the CPT codes for services that are typically performed face-to-face, but may be rendered via a real-time (synchronous) interactive audio and video telecommunications system.

96 Habilitative Services

When a service or procedure that may be either habilitative or rehabilitative in nature is provided for habilitative purposes, the physician or other qualified health care professional may add modifier 96 to the service or procedure code to indicate that the service or procedure provided was a habilitative service. Habilitative services help an individual learn skills and functioning for daily living that the individual has not yet developed, and then keep and/or improve those learned skills. Habilitative services also help an individual keep, learn, or improve skills and functioning for daily living.

97 Rehabilitative Services

When a service or procedure that may be either habilitative or rehabilitative in nature is provided for rehabilitative purposes, the physician or other qualified health care professional may add modifier 97 to the service or procedure code to indicate that the service or procedure provided was a rehabilitative service. Rehabilitative services help an individual keep, get back, or improve skills and functioning for daily living that have been lost or impaired because the individual was sick, hurt, or disabled.

99 Multiple Modifiers

Under certain circumstances 2 or more modifiers may be necessary to completely delineate a service. In such situations modifier 99 should be added to the basic procedure, and other applicable modifiers may be listed as part of the description of the service.

ⓘ Check with payers to determine if this modifier is necessary when reporting multiple modifiers.

Modifiers Approved for Ambulatory Surgery Center (ASC) Hospital Outpatient Use

There are some differences in modifiers for professional and ASC hospital use. The following list consists of the only approved modifiers that can be used in an ASC/hospital setting:

25 Significant, Separately Identifiable Evaluation and Management Service by the Same Physician or Other Qualified Health Care Professional on the Same Day of the Procedure or Other Service

It may be necessary to indicate that on the day a procedure or service identified by a CPT code was performed, the patient's condition required a significant,

Modifiers

CPT © 2018 American Medical Association. All Rights Reserved.

separately identifiable E/M service above and beyond the other service provided or beyond the usual preoperative and postoperative care associated with the procedure that was performed. A significant, separately identifiable E/M service is defined or substantiated by documentation that satisfies the relevant criteria for the respective E/M service to be reported (see **Evaluation and Management Services Guidelines** for instructions on determining level of E/M service). The E/M service may be prompted by the symptom or condition for which the procedure and/or service was provided. As such, different diagnoses are not required for reporting of the E/M services on the same date. This circumstance may be reported by adding modifier 25 to the appropriate level of E/M service.

Note: This modifier is not used to report an E/M service that resulted in a decision to perform surgery. See modifier 57. For significant, separately identifiable non-E/M services, see modifier 59.

ⓘ According to Medicare, modifier 25 may be appended to an Emergency Department Services E/M code (99281-99285) if provided on the same day as a diagnostic or therapeutic procedure.

27 Multiple Outpatient Hospital E/M Encounters on the Same Date

For hospital outpatient reporting purposes, utilization of hospital resources related to separate and distinct E/M encounters performed in multiple outpatient hospital settings on the same date may be reported by adding the modifier 27 to each appropriate level outpatient and/or emergency department E/M code(s). This modifier provides a means of reporting circumstances involving E/M services provided by physician(s) in more than one (multiple) outpatient hospital setting(s) (e.g., hospital emergency department, clinic).

Note: This modifier is not to be used for physician reporting of multiple E/M services performed by the same physician on the same date. For physician reporting of all outpatient E/M services provided by the same physician on the same date and performed in multiple outpatient setting(s) (eg, hospital emergency department, clinic), see **Evaluation and Management, Emergency Department**, or **Preventive Medicine Services** codes.

33 Preventive Services

When the primary purpose of the service is the delivery of evidence based service in accordance with a US Preventive Services Task Force A or B rating in effect and other preventive services identified in preventive services mandates (legislative or regulatory), the services may be identified by adding 33 to the procedure. For separately reported services specifically identified as preventive, the modifier should not be used.

50 Bilateral Procedure

Unless otherwise identified in the listings, bilateral procedures that are performed at the same operative session should be identified by adding modifier 50 to the appropriate 5-digit code.

ⓘ Reported on procedures performed at the same operative session, this modifier should be reported only once as a one-line item for Medicare, with the modifier appended to the end of the code.

ⓘ Some payers may accept the bilateral procedures as two-line items, with HCPCS Level II modifiers LT and RT appended to the end of the codes.

52 Reduced Services

Under certain circumstances a service or procedure is partially reduced or eliminated at the discretion of the physician or other qualified health care professional. Under these circumstances the service provided can be identified by its usual procedure number and the addition of modifier 52, signifying that the service is reduced. This provides a means of reporting reduced services without disturbing the identification of the basic service.

Note: For hospital outpatient reporting of a previously scheduled procedure/service that is partially reduced or cancelled as a result of extenuating circumstanced or those that threaten the well-being of the patient prior to or after administration of anesthesia, see modifiers 73 and 74.

ⓘ Procedures reported with modifier 52 are typically billed at a reduced amount. Most payers do not require documentation to support the use of modifier 52 and will reimburse the procedure at a reduced level.

58 Staged or Related Procedure or Service by the Same Physician or Other Qualified Health Care Professional During the Postoperative Period

It may be necessary to indicate that the performance of a procedure or service during the postoperative period was: (a) planned or anticipated (staged); (b) more extensive than the original procedure; or (c) for therapy following a diagnostic surgical procedure. This circumstance may be reported by adding modifier 58 to the staged or related procedure.

Note: For treatment of a problem that requires a return to the operating/procedure room (e.g., unanticipated clinical condition), see modifier 78.

ⓘ Modifier 58 must be used for purposes of identifying procedures performed by the original physician during the postoperative period of the original procedure, within the constraints of the modifier's definition. These procedures cannot be repeat operations (unless the procedures are more extensive than the original procedure) and cannot be for the treatment of complications requiring a return trip to the operating room.

The existence of modifier 58 does not negate the global fee concept. Services that are included in CPT as multiple sessions or are defined as including multiple services or events may not be billed with this modifier. This modifier is designed to allow a method of reporting additional, related surgeries that are due to a progression of the disease and are not to be used to avoid global surgery edits applicable to staged procedures.

Modifier 58 should be used on surgical codes only and has no effect on the payment amount.

Note: This modifier is not used to report the treatment of a problem that requires a return to the operating room. See modifier 78.

59 Distinct Procedural Service

Under certain circumstances, it may be necessary to indicate that a procedure or service was distinct or independent from other non-E/M services performed on the same day. Modifier 59 is used to identify procedures/services, other than E/M services, that are not normally reported together, but are appropriate under the circumstances. Documentation must support a different session, different procedure or surgery, different site or organ system, separate incision/excision, separate lesions, or separate injury (or area of injury in extensive injuries) not ordinarily encountered or performed on the same day by the same individual. However, when another already established modifier is appropriate, it should be used rather than modifier 59. Only if no more descriptive modifier is available, and the use of modifier 59 best explains the circumstances, should modifier 59 be used.

Note: Modifier 59 should not be appended to an E/M service. To report a separate and distinct E/M service with a non-E/M service performed on the same date, see modifier 25.

ⓘ Modifier 59 was established to demonstrate that multiple, yet distinct, services were provided to a patient on the same date of service by the same provider. Because distinct procedures or services rendered on the same day by the same physician cannot be easily identified and properly adjudicated by simply listing the CPT procedure codes, modifier 59 assists the payer or Medicare carrier in applying the appropriate reimbursement protocol. If the modifier is not used in

Modifiers

CPT © 2018 American Medical Association. All Rights Reserved.

these circumstances, services may be denied, with the explanation of benefits stating that the payer does not reimburse for this service because it is part of another service that was performed at the same time.

73 Discontinued Out-patient Hospital/Ambulatory Surgery Center (ASC) Procedure Prior to Administration of Anesthesia

Due to extenuating circumstances or those that threaten the well being of the patient, the physician may cancel a surgical or diagnostic procedure subsequent to the patient's surgical preparation (including sedation when provided, and being taken to the room where the procedure is to be performed), but prior to the administration of anesthesia (local, regional block(s), or general). Under these circumstances, the intended service that is prepared for but cancelled can be reported by its usual procedure number and the addition of modifier 73.

Note: The elective cancellation of a service prior to the administration of anesthesia and/or surgical preparation of the patient should not be reported. For physician reporting of a discontinued procedure, see modifier 53.

74 Discontinued Out-patient Hospital/Ambulatory Surgery Center (ASC) Procedure After Administration of Anesthesia

Due to extenuating circumstances or those that threaten the well being of the patient, the physician may terminate a surgical or diagnostic procedure after the administration of anesthesia (local, regional block(s), or general) or after the procedure was started (e.g., incision made, intubation started, scope inserted). Under these circumstances, the intended service that is prepared for but cancelled can be reported by its usual procedure number and the addition of modifier 74.

Note: The elective cancellation of a service prior to the administration of anesthesia and/or surgical preparation of the patient should not be reported. For physician reporting of a discontinued procedure, see modifier 53.

76 Repeat Procedure or Service by Same Physician or Other Qualified Health Care Professional

It may be necessary to indicate that a procedure or service was repeated subsequent to the original procedure or service. This circumstance may be reported by adding modifier 76 to the repeated procedure or service.

77 Repeat Procedure by Another Physician or Other Qualified Health Care Professional

It may be necessary to indicate that a basic procedure or service was repeated by another physician or other qualified health care professional subsequent to the original procedure or service. This circumstance may be reported by adding modifier 77 to the repeated procedure or service.

Note: This modifier should not be appended to an E/M service.

ⓘ Appending this modifier does not guarantee payment of the repeat procedure, but will assist in determining duplicate billings for the procedure.

78 Unplanned Return to the Operating/Procedure Room by the Same Physician or Other Qualified Health Care Professional Following Initial Procedure for a Related Procedure During the Postoperative Period

It may be necessary to indicate that another procedure was performed during the postoperative period of the initial procedure (unplanned procedure following initial procedure). When this procedure is related to the first, and requires the use of an operating/procedure room, it may be reported by adding modifier 78 to the related procedure. (For repeat procedures, see modifier 76.)

ⓘ Medicare includes specific medical and/or surgical care for postoperative complications within the global surgical package and does not allow additional payment. Included in the global surgical package are "additional medical and surgical services required of the surgeon during the postoperative period of the surgery because of complications which do not require additional trips to the operating room."

79 Unrelated Procedure or Service by the Same Physician or Other Qualified Health Care Professional During the Postoperative Period

The individual may need to indicate that the performance of a procedure or service during the postoperative period was unrelated to the original procedure. This circumstance may be reported by using modifier 79. (For repeat procedures on the same day, see modifier 76.)

ⓘ When billing for an unrelated procedure by the same physician during the postoperative period of an original procedure, a new postoperative period will begin with the subsequent procedure. A different diagnosis should be indicated on the claim to identify the unrelated procedure.

91 Repeat Clinical Diagnostic Laboratory Test

In the course of treatment of the patient, it may be necessary to repeat the same laboratory test on the same day to obtain subsequent (multiple) test results. Under these circumstances, the laboratory test performed can be identified by its usual procedure number and the addition of the modifier 91.

Note: This modifier may not be used when tests are rerun to confirm initial results due to testing problems with specimens or equipment; or for any other reason when a normal, one-time, reportable result is all that is required. This modifier may not be used when other code(s) describe a series of test results (e.g., glucose tolerance tests, evocative/suppression testing). This modifier may only be used for laboratory test(s) performed more than once on the same day on the same patient

Category II Modifiers

The following performance measurement modifiers may be used for Category II codes to indicate that a service specified in the associated measure(s) was considered but, due to either medical, patient, or system circumstance(s) documented in the medical record, the service was not provided. These modifiers serve as denominator exclusions from the performance measure. The user should note that not all listed measures provide for exclusions (see Alphabetical Clinical Topics Listing for more discussion regarding exclusion criteria).

Category II modifiers should only be reported with Category II codes—they should not be reported with Category I or Category III codes. In addition, the modifiers in the Category II section should only be used where specified in the guidelines, reporting instructions, parenthetic notes, or code descriptor language listed in the Category II section (code listing and the Alphabetical Clinical Topics Listing).

1P Performance Measure Exclusion Modifier due to Medical Reasons

Reasons include:

- Not indicated (absence of organ/limb, already received/performed, other)
- Contraindicated (patient allergic history, potential adverse drug interaction, other)
- Other medical reasons

Modifiers

CPT © 2018 American Medical Association. All Rights Reserved.

2P Performance Measure Exclusion Modifier due to Patient Reasons

Reasons include:

- Patient declined
- Economic, social, or religious reasons
- Other patient reasons

3P Performance Measure Exclusion Modifier due to System Reasons

Reasons include:

- Resources to perform the services not available
- Insurance coverage/payor-related limitations
- Other reasons attributable to health care delivery system

Modifier 8P is intended to be used as a "reporting modifier" to allow the reporting of circumstances when an action described in a measure's numerator is not performed and the reason is not otherwise specified.

8P Performance measure reporting modifier–action not performed, reason not otherwise specified

Level II (HCPCS/National) Modifiers

E1 Upper left, eyelid
E2 Lower left, eyelid
E3 Upper right, eyelid
E4 Lower right, eyelid
F1 Left hand, second digit
F2 Left hand, third digit
F3 Left hand, fourth digit
F4 Left hand, fifth digit
F5 Right hand, thumb
F6 Right hand, second digit
F7 Right hand, third digit
F8 Right hand, fourth digit
F9 Right hand, fifth digit
FA Left hand, thumb
GG Performance and payment of a screening mammogram and diagnostic mammogram on the same patient, same day
GH Diagnostic mammogram converted from screening mammogram on same day
LC Left circumflex coronary artery
LD Left anterior descending coronary artery
LM Left main coronary artery
LT Left side (used to identify procedures performed on the left side of the body)
QM Ambulance service provided under arrangement by a provider of services
QN Ambulance service furnished directly by a provider of services
RC Right coronary artery
RI Ramus intermedius coronary artery
RT Right side (used to identify procedures performed on the right side of the body)
T1 Left foot, second digit
T2 Left foot, third digit
T3 Left foot, fourth digit
T4 Left foot, fifth digit
T5 Right foot, great toe
T6 Right foot, second digit
T7 Right foot, third digit
T8 Right foot, fourth digit
T9 Right foot, fifth digit
TA Left foot, great toe
XE Separate Encounter *
XS Separate Structure *
XP Separate Practitioner *
XU Unusual Non-Overlapping Service *

(*HCPCS modifiers for selective identification of subsets of Distinct Procedural Services [59 modifier])

Modifier Rules

Mult Proc = Multiple Procedure (Modifier 51)

Indicates applicable payment adjustment rule for multiple procedures:

0 No payment adjustment rules for multiple procedures apply. If procedure is reported on the same day as another procedure, base the payment on the lower of (a) the actual charge, or (b) the fee schedule amount for the procedure.

1 Standard payment adjustment rules in effect before January 1, 1995 for multiple procedures apply. In the 1995 file, this indicator only applies to codes with a status code of "D." If procedure is reported on the same day as another procedure that has an indicator of 1, 2, or 3, rank the procedures by fee schedule amount and apply the appropriate reduction to this code (100%, 50%, 25%, 25%, 25%, and by report). Base the payment on the lower of (a) the actual charge, or (b) the fee schedule amount reduced by the appropriate percentage.

2 Standard payment adjustment rules for multiple procedures apply. If procedure is reported on the same day as another procedure with an indicator of 1, 2, or 3, rank the procedures by fee schedule amount and apply the appropriate reduction to this code (100%, 50%, 50%, 50%, 50% and by report). Base the payment on the lower of (a) the actual charge, or (b) the fee schedule amount reduced by the appropriate percentage.

3 Special rules for multiple endoscopic procedures apply if procedure is billed with another endoscopy in the same family (i.e., another endoscopy that has the same base procedure). The base procedure for each code with this indicator is identified in the ENDO BASE field of this file. Apply the multiple endoscopy rules to a family before ranking the family with the other procedures performed on the same day (for example, if multiple endoscopies in the same family are reported on the same day as endoscopies in another family or on the same day as a non-endoscopic procedure). If an endoscopic procedure is reported with only its base procedure, do not pay separately for the base procedure. Payment for the base procedure is included in the payment for the other endoscopy.

CPT © 2018 American Medical Association. All Rights Reserved.

5 Subject to 20% of the practice expense component for certain therapy services (25% reduction for services rendered in an institutional setting - effective for services January 1, 2012 and after).

9 Concept does not apply.

Bilat Surg = Bilateral Surgery (Modifier 50)

Indicates services subject to payment adjustment.

0 150% payment adjustment for bilateral procedures does not apply. If procedure is reported with modifier 50 or with modifiers RT and LT, base the payment for the two sides on the lower of: (a) the total actual charge for both sides or (b) 100% of the fee schedule amount for a single code. Example: The fee schedule amount for code XXXXX is $125. The physician reports code XXXXX-LT with an actual charge of $100 and XXXXX-RT with an actual charge of $100. Payment should be based on the fee schedule amount ($125) since it is lower than the total actual charges for the left and right sides ($200). The bilateral adjustment is inappropriate for codes in this category (a) because of physiology or anatomy, or (b) because the code description specifically states that it is a unilateral procedure and there is an existing code for the bilateral procedure.

1 150% payment adjustment for bilateral procedures applies. If the code is billed with the bilateral modifier or is reported twice on the same day by any other means (e.g., with RT and LT modifiers, or with a 2 in the units field), base the payment for these codes when reported as bilateral procedures on the lower of: (a) the total actual charge for both sides or (b) 150% of the fee schedule amount for a single code. If the code is reported as a bilateral procedure and is reported with other procedure codes on the same day, apply the bilateral adjustment before applying any multiple procedure rules.

2 150% payment adjustment does not apply. RVUs are already based on the procedure being performed as a bilateral procedure. If the procedure is reported with modifier 50 or is reported twice on the same day by any other means (e.g., with RT and LT modifiers or with a 2 in the units field), base the payment for both sides on the lower of (a) the total actual charge by the physician for both sides, or (b) 100% of the fee schedule for a single code. Example: The fee schedule amount for code YYYYY is $125. The physician reports code YYYYY-LT with an actual charge of $100 and YYYYY-RT with an actual charge of $100. Payment should be based on the fee schedule amount ($125) since it is lower than the total actual charges for the left and right sides ($200). The RVUs are based on a bilateral procedure because (a) the code descriptor specifically states that the procedure is bilateral,
(b) the code descriptor states that the procedure may be performed either unilaterally or bilaterally, or (c) the procedure is usually performed as a bilateral procedure.

3 The usual payment adjustment for bilateral procedures does not apply. If the procedure is reported with modifier 50 or is reported for both sides on the same day by any other means (e.g., with RT and LT modifiers or with a 2 in the units field), base the payment for each side or organ or site of a paired organ on the lower of (a) the actual charge for each side or (b) 100% of the fee schedule amount for each side. If the procedure is reported as a bilateral procedure and with other procedure codes on the same day, determine the fee schedule amount for a bilateral procedure before applying any multiple procedure rules. Services in this category are generally radiology procedures or other diagnostic tests which are not subject to the special payment rules for other bilateral surgeries.

9 Concept does not apply.

Asst Surg = Assistant at Surgery (Modifier 80)

Indicates services where an assistant at surgery is never paid for per Medicare Claims Manual.

0 Payment restriction for assistants at surgery applies to this procedure unless supporting documentation is submitted to establish medical necessity.

1 Statutory payment restriction for assistants at surgery applies to this procedure. Assistant at surgery may not be paid.

2 Payment restriction for assistants at surgery does not apply to this procedure. Assistant at surgery may be paid.

9 Concept does not apply.

Co Surg = Co-surgeons (Modifier 62)

Indicates services for which two surgeons, each in a different specialty, may be paid.

0 Co-surgeons not permitted for this procedure.

1 Co-surgeons could be paid, though supporting documentation is required to establish the medical necessity of two surgeons for the procedure.

2 Co-surgeons permitted and no documentation required if the two-specialty requirement is met.

9 Concept does not apply.

Team Surg = Team Surgery (Modifier 66)

Indicates services for which team surgeons may be paid.

0 Team surgeons not permitted for this procedure.

1 Team surgeons could be paid, though supporting documentation required to establish medical necessity of a team; pay by report.

2 Team surgeons permitted; pay by report.

9 Concept does not apply.

CPT © 2018 American Medical Association. All Rights Reserved.

National Correct Coding Initiative

A. Introduction

The principles of correct coding apply to the CPT codes in the range 00000-01999. Several general guidelines are repeated in this Chapter.

Physicians should report the HCPCS/CPT code that describes the procedure performed to the greatest specificity possible. A HCPCS/CPT code should be reported only if all services described by the code are performed. A physician should not report multiple HCPCS/CPT codes if a single HCPCS/CPT code exists that describes the services. This type of unbundling is incorrect coding.

HCPCS/CPT codes include all services usually performed as part of the procedure as a standard of medical/surgical practice. A physician should not separately report these services simply because HCPCS/CPT codes exist for them.

Specific issues unique to this section of CPT are clarified in this chapter.

Anesthesia care is provided by an anesthesia practitioner who may be a physician, a certified registered nurse anesthetist (CRNA) with or without medical direction, or an anesthesia assistant (AA) with medical direction. The anesthesia care package consists of preoperative evaluation, standard preparation and monitoring services, administration of anesthesia, and post- anesthesia recovery care.

Preoperative evaluation includes a sufficient history and physical examination so that the risk of adverse reactions can be minimized, alternative approaches to anesthesia planned, and all questions regarding the anesthesia procedure by the patient or family answered. Types of anesthesia include local, regional, epidural, general, moderate conscious sedation, or monitored anesthesia care (MAC). The anesthesia practitioner assumes responsibility for anesthesia and related care rendered in the post-anesthesia recovery period until the patient is released to the surgeon or another physician.

Anesthesiologists may personally perform anesthesia services or may supervise anesthesia services performed by a CRNA or AA. CRNAs may perform anesthesia services independently or under the supervision of an anesthesiologist or operating practitioner. An AA always performs anesthesia services under the direction of an anesthesiologist. Anesthesiologists personally performing anesthesia services and non-medically directed CRNAs bill in a standard fashion in accordance with CMS regulations as outlined in the Internet-Only Manuals (IOM), Medicare Claims Processing Manual, Publication 100-04, Chapter 12, Sections 50 and 140. CRNAs and AAs practicing under the medical direction of anesthesiologists follow instructions and regulations regarding this arrangement as outlined in the above sections of the Internet–Only Manual.

B. Standard Anesthesia Coding

The following policies reflect national Medicare correct coding guidelines for anesthesia services.

1. CPT codes 00100-01860 specify "Anesthesia for" followed by a description of a surgical intervention. CPT codes 01916-01933 describe anesthesia for diagnostic or interventional radiology procedures. Several CPT codes (01951-01999, excluding 01996) describe anesthesia services for burn excision/debridement, obstetrical, and other procedures. CPT codes *99151-99157* describe moderate (conscious) sedation services.

   Anesthesia services include, but are not limited to, preoperative evaluation of the patient, administration of anesthetic, other medications, blood, and fluids, monitoring of physiological parameters, and other supportive services.

   Anesthesia codes describe a general anatomic area or service which usually relates to a number of surgical procedures, often from multiple sections of the *CPT Manual*. For Medicare purposes, only one anesthesia code is reported unless the anesthesia code is an add-on code. In this case, both the code for the primary anesthesia service and the anesthesia add-on code are reported according to *CPT Manual* instructions.

2. A unique characteristic of anesthesia coding is the reporting of time units. Payment for anesthesia services increases with time. In addition to reporting a base unit value for an anesthesia service, the anesthesia practitioner reports anesthesia time. Anesthesia time is defined as the period during which an anesthesia practitioner is present with the patient. It starts when the anesthesia practitioner begins to prepare the patient for anesthesia services in the operating room or an equivalent area and ends when the anesthesia practitioner is no longer furnishing anesthesia services to the patient (i.e., when the patient may be placed safely under postoperative care). Anesthesia time is a continuous time period from the start of anesthesia to the end of an anesthesia service. In counting anesthesia time, the anesthesia practitioner can add blocks of time around an interruption in anesthesia time as long as the anesthesia practitioner is furnishing continuous anesthesia care within the time periods around the interruption.

   Example: A patient who undergoes a cataract extraction may require monitored anesthesia care (see below). This may require administration of a sedative in conjunction with a peri/retrobulbar injection for regional block anesthesia. Subsequently, an interval of 30 minutes or more may transpire during which time the patient does not require monitoring by an anesthesia practitioner. After this period, monitoring will commence again for the cataract extraction and ultimately the patient will be released to the surgeon's care or to recovery. The time that may be reported would include the time for the monitoring during the block and during the procedure. The interval time and the recovery time are not included in the anesthesia time calculation. Also, if unusual services not bundled into the anesthesia service are required, the time spent delivering these services before anesthesia time begins or after it ends may not be included as reportable anesthesia time.

However, if it is medically necessary for the anesthesia practitioner to continuously monitor the patient during the interval time and not perform any other service, the interval time may be included in the anesthesia time.

3. It is standard medical practice for an anesthesia practitioner to perform a patient examination and evaluation prior to surgery. This is considered part of the anesthesia service and is included in the base unit value of the anesthesia code. The evaluation and examination are not reported in the anesthesia time. If surgery is canceled, subsequent to the preoperative evaluation, payment may be allowed to the anesthesiologist for an evaluation and management service and the appropriate E/M code may be reported. (A non-medically directed CRNA may also report an E/M code under these circumstances if permitted by state law.)
Similarly, routine postoperative evaluation is included in the base unit for the anesthesia service. If this evaluation occurs after the anesthesia practitioner has safely placed the patient under postoperative care, neither additional anesthesia time units nor evaluation and management codes should be reported for this evaluation. Postoperative evaluation and management services related to the surgery are not separately reportable by the anesthesia practitioner except when an anesthesiologist provides significant, separately identifiable ongoing critical care services.

Anesthesia practitioners other than anesthesiologists and CRNAs cannot report evaluation and management codes except as described above when a surgical case is canceled.

If permitted by state law, anesthesia practitioners may separately report significant, separately identifiable postoperative management services after the anesthesia service time ends. These services include, but are not limited to, postoperative pain management and ventilator management unrelated to the anesthesia procedure.

Management of epidural or subarachnoid drug administration (CPT code 01996) is separately payable on dates of service subsequent to surgery but not on the date of surgery. If the only service provided is management of epidural/subarachnoid drug administration, then an evaluation and management service should not be reported in addition to CPT code 01996. Payment for management of epidural/subarachnoid drug administration is limited to one unit of service per postoperative day regardless of the number of visits necessary to manage the catheter per postoperative day (CPT definition). While an anesthesiologist or non-medically directed CRNA may be able to report this service, only one payment will be made per day.

Postoperative pain management services are generally provided by the surgeon who is reimbursed under a global payment policy related to the procedure and shall not be reported by the anesthesia practitioner unless separate, medically necessary services are required that cannot be rendered by the surgeon. The surgeon is responsible to document in the medical record the reason care is being referred to the anesthesia practitioner.

In certain circumstances critical care services are provided by the anesthesiologist. CRNAs may be paid for evaluation and management services in the critical care area if state law and/or regulation permits them to provide such services. In the case of anesthesiologists, the routine immediate postoperative care is not separately reported except as described above. Certain procedural services such as insertion of a Swan-Ganz catheter, insertion of a central venous pressure line, emergency intubation (outside of the operating suite), etc., are separately payable to anesthesiologists as well as non-medically directed CRNAs if these procedures are furnished within the parameters of state licensing laws.

4. Under certain circumstances an anesthesia practitioner may separately report an epidural or peripheral nerve block injection (bolus, intermittent bolus, or continuous infusion) for postoperative pain management when the surgeon requests assistance with postoperative pain management. An epidural injection (CPT code 623XX) for postoperative pain management may be reported separately with an anesthesia 0XXXX code only if the mode of intraoperative anesthesia is general anesthesia and the adequacy of the intraoperative anesthesia is not dependent on the epidural injection. A peripheral nerve block injection (CPT codes 64XXX) for postoperative pain management may be reported separately with an anesthesia 0XXXX code only if the mode of intraoperative anesthesia is general anesthesia, subarachnoid injection, or epidural injection, and the adequacy of the intraoperative anesthesia is not dependent on the peripheral nerve block injection. An epidural or peripheral nerve block injection (code numbers as identified above) administered preoperatively or intraoperatively is not separately reportable for postoperative pain management if the mode of anesthesia for the procedure is monitored anesthesia care (MAC), moderate conscious sedation, regional anesthesia by peripheral nerve block, or other type of anesthesia not identified above. If an epidural or peripheral nerve block injection (code numbers as identified above) for postoperative pain management is reported separately on the same date of service as an anesthesia 0XXXX code, modifier 59 may be appended to the epidural or peripheral nerve block injection code (code numbers as identified above) to indicate that it was administered for postoperative pain management. An epidural or peripheral nerve block injection (code numbers as identified above) for postoperative pain management in patients receiving general anesthesia, spinal (subarachnoid injection) anesthesia, or regional anesthesia by

epidural injection as described above may be administered preoperatively, intraoperatively, or postoperatively.

5. If an epidural or subarachnoid injection (bolus, intermittent bolus, or continuous) is utilized for intraoperative anesthesia and postoperative pain management, CPT code 01996 (daily hospital management of epidural or subarachnoid continuous drug administration) is not separately reportable on the day of insertion of the epidural or subarachnoid catheter. CPT code 01996 may only be reported for management for days subsequent to the date of insertion of the epidural or subarachnoid catheter.
6. Anesthesia HCPCS/CPT codes include all services integral to the anesthesia procedure such as preparation, monitoring, intra-operative care, and post-operative care until the patient is released by the anesthesia practitioner to the care of another physician. Examples of integral services include, but are not limited to, the following:
   - Transporting, positioning, prepping, draping of the patient for satisfactory anesthesia induction/surgical procedures.
   - Placement of external devices including, but not limited to, those for cardiac monitoring, oximetry, capnography, temperature monitoring, EEG, CNS evoked responses (e.g., BSER), Doppler flow.
   - Placement of peripheral intravenous lines for fluid and medication administration.
   - Placement of airway (e.g., endotracheal tube, orotracheal tube).
   - Laryngoscopy (direct or endoscopic) for placement of airway (e.g., endotracheal tube).
   - Placement of naso-gastric or oro-gastric tube.
   - Intra-operative interpretation of monitored functions (e.g., blood pressure, heart rate, respirations, oximetry, capnography, temperature, EEG, BSER, Doppler flow, CNS pressure).
   - Interpretation of laboratory determinations (e.g., arterial blood gases such as pH, pO2, pCO2, bicarbonate, CBC, blood chemistries, lactate) by the anesthesiologist/CRNA.
   - Nerve stimulation for determination of level of paralysis or localization of nerve(s). (Codes for EMG services are for diagnostic purposes for nerve dysfunction. To report these codes a complete diagnostic report must be present in the medical record.)
   - Insertion of urinary bladder catheter.
   - Blood sample procurement through existing lines or requiring venipuncture or arterial puncture.

   The NCCI contains many edits bundling standard preparation, monitoring, and procedural services into anesthesia CPT codes. Although some of these services may never be reported on the same date of service as an anesthesia service, many of these services could be provided at a separate patient encounter unrelated to the anesthesia service on the same date of service. Providers may utilize modifier 59 to bypass the edits under these circumstances.

   CPT codes describing services that are integral to an anesthesia service include, but are not limited to, the following:

   - 31505, 31515, 31527 (Laryngoscopy) (Laryngoscopy codes describe diagnostic or surgical services.)
   - 31622, 31645, 31646 (Bronchoscopy)
   - 36000, 36010-36015 (Introduction of needle or catheter)
   - 36400-36440 (Venipuncture and transfusion)
   - 62320-62327, 62318-62319 (Epidural or subarachnoid injections of diagnostic or therapeutic substance – bolus, intermittent bolus, or continuous infusion)

   CPT codes 62320-62327 and 62318-62319 (Epidural or subarachnoid injections of diagnostic or therapeutic substance - bolus, intermittent bolus, or continuous infusion) may be reported on the date of surgery if performed for postoperative pain management rather than as the means for providing the regional block for the surgical procedure. If a narcotic or other analgesic is injected postoperatively through the same catheter as the anesthetic agent, CPT codes 62320-62327 should not be reported for postoperative pain management. An epidural injection for postoperative pain management may be separately reportable with an anesthesia 0XXXX code only if the patient receives a general anesthetic and the adequacy of the intraoperative anesthesia is not dependent on the epidural injection. If an epidural injection is not utilized for operative anesthesia but is utilized for postoperative pain management, modifier 59 may be reported to indicate that the epidural injection was performed for postoperative pain management rather than intraoperative pain management.

   Pain management performed by an anesthesia practitioner after the postoperative anesthesia care period terminates may be separately reportable. However, postoperative pain management by the physician performing a surgical procedure is not separately reportable by that physician. Postoperative pain management is included in the global surgical package.

   Example: A patient has an epidural block with sedation and monitoring for arthroscopic knee surgery. The anesthesia practitioner reports CPT code 01382 (Anesthesia for diagnostic arthroscopic procedures of knee joint). The epidural catheter is left in place for postoperative pain management. The anesthesia practitioner should not also report CPT codes 62322/62323 or 62326/62327 (epidural/subarachnoid injection of diagnostic or therapeutic substance), or 01996 (daily management of epidural) on the date of surgery. CPT code 01996 may be reported with one unit of service per day on subsequent days until the catheter is removed. On the other hand, if the anesthesia practitioner performed general anesthesia reported as CPT code 01382 and at the request of the operating physician inserted an epidural catheter for treatment of anticipated postoperative pain, the anesthesia practitioner may report CPT code 62326-59 or 62327-59 indicating that this is a separate service from the anesthesia service. In this instance, the service is separately reportable whether the catheter is placed before, during, or after the surgery. Since treatment of postoperative pain is included in the global surgical package, the operating physician may request the assistance of the anesthesia practitioner if the degree of postoperative pain is expected to exceed the skills and experience of the operating physician to manage it. If the epidural catheter was placed on a different date than the surgery, modifier 59 would not be necessary. Effective January 1, 2004, daily hospital management of continuous epidural or subarachnoid drug administration performed on the day(s) subsequent to the placement of an epidural or subarachnoid catheter (CPT codes 62324-62327) may be reported as CPT code 01996.

- 64400-64530 (Peripheral nerve blocks – bolus injection or continuous infusion)
  CPT codes 64400-64530 (Peripheral nerve blocks – bolus injection or continuous infusion) may be reported on the date of surgery if performed for postoperative pain management only if the operative anesthesia is general anesthesia, subarachnoid injection, or epidural injection and the adequacy of the intraoperative anesthesia is not dependent on the peripheral nerve block. Peripheral nerve block codes should not be reported separately on the same date of service as a surgical procedure if used as the primary anesthetic technique or as a supplement to the primary anesthetic technique. Modifier 59 may be utilized to indicate that a peripheral nerve block injection was performed for postoperative pain management, rather than intraoperative anesthesia, and a procedure note should be included in the medical record.
- 67500 (Retrobulbar injection)
- 81000-81015, 82013, 82205, 82270, 82271(Performance and interpretation of laboratory tests)
- 43753, 43754, 43755 (Esophageal, gastric intubation)
- 92511-92520, 92543 (Special otorhinolaryngologic services)
- 92950 (Cardiopulmonary resuscitation)
- 92953 (Temporary transcutaneous pacemaker)
- 92960, 92961 (Cardioversion)
- 93000-93010 (Electrocardiography)
- 93040-93042 (Electrocardiography)
- 93303-93308 (Transthoracic echocardiography when utilized for monitoring purposes) However, when performed for diagnostic purposes with documentation including a formal report, this service may be considered a significant, separately identifiable, and separately reportable service.
- 93312-93317 (Transesophageal echocardiography when utilized for monitoring purposes) However, when performed for diagnostic purposes with documentation including a formal report, this service may be considered a significant, separately identifiable, and separately reportable service.
- 93318 (Transesophageal echocardiography for monitoring purposes)
- 93561-93562 (Indicator dilution studies)
- 93701 (Thoracic electrical bioimpedance)
- 93922-93981 (Extremity or visceral arterial or venous vascular studies) When performed diagnostically with a formal report, this service may be considered a significant, separately identifiable, and if medically necessary, a separately reportable service.
- 94640 (Inhalation/IPPB treatments)
- 94002-94004, 94660-94662 (Ventilation management/CPAP services) If these services are performed during a surgical procedure, they are included in the anesthesia service. These services may be separately reportable if performed by the anesthesia practitioner after post-operative care has been transferred to another physician by the anesthesia practitioner. Modifier 59 may be reported to indicate that these services are separately reportable. For example, if an anesthesia practitioner who provided anesthesia for a procedure initiates ventilation management in a post-operative recovery area prior to transfer of care to another physician, CPT codes 94002-94003 should not be reported for this service since it is included in the anesthesia procedure package. However, if the anesthesia practitioner transfers care to another physician and is called back to initiate ventilation because of a change in the patient's status, the initiation of ventilation may be separately reportable.
- 94664 (Inhalations)
- 94680-94690, 94770 (Expired gas analysis)
- 94760-94762 (Oximetry)
- 96360-96377 (Drug administration)
- 99201-99499 (Evaluation and management)

This list is not a comprehensive listing of all services included in anesthesia services.

7. Per Medicare Global Surgery rules the physician performing an operative procedure is responsible for treating postoperative pain. Treatment of postoperative pain by the operating physician is not separately reportable. However, the operating physician may request that an anesthesia practitioner assist in the treatment of postoperative pain management if it is medically reasonable and necessary. The actual or anticipated postoperative pain must be severe enough to require treatment by techniques beyond the experience of the operating physician. For example, the operating physician may request that the anesthesia practitioner administer an epidural or peripheral nerve block to treat actual or anticipated postoperative pain. The epidural or peripheral nerve block may be administered preoperatively, intraoperatively, or postoperatively. An epidural or peripheral nerve block that provides intraoperative pain management even if it also provides postoperative pain management is included in the 0XXXX anesthesia code and is not separately reportable. (See Chapter II (B) (#4) for guidelines regarding reporting anesthesia and postoperative pain management separately by an anesthesia practitioner on the same date of service.)

   If the operating physician requests that the anesthesia practitioner perform pain management services after the postoperative anesthesia care period terminates, the anesthesia practitioner may report it separately using modifier 59. Since postoperative pain management by the operating physician is included in the global surgical package, the operating physician may request the assistance of an anesthesia practitioner if it requires techniques beyond the experience of the operating physician.

8. Several nerve block CPT codes (e.g., 64416 (brachial plexus), 64446 (sciatic nerve), 64448 (femoral nerve), 64449 (lumbar plexus)) describe "continuous infusion by catheter (including catheter placement)." Two epidural/subarachnoid injection CPT codes 62324-62327 describe continuous infusion or intermittent bolus injection including placement of catheter. If an anesthesia practitioner places a catheter for continuous infusion epidural/subarachnoid or nerve block for intraoperative pain management, the service is included in the 0XXXX anesthesia procedure and is not separately reportable on the same date of service as the anesthesia 0XXXX code even if it is also utilized for postoperative pain management.
9. Per CMS Global Surgery rules postoperative pain management is a component of the global surgical package and is the responsibility of the physician performing the global surgical procedure. If the physician performing the global surgical procedure does not have the skills and experience to manage the postoperative pain and requests that an anesthesia practitioner assume the postoperative pain management, the anesthesia practitioner may report the additional services performed once this responsibility is transferred to the anesthesia practitioner. Pain management services subsequent to the date of insertion of the catheter for continuous infusion may be reported with CPT code 01996 for epidural/subarachnoid infusions and with evaluation and management codes for nerve block continuous infusions.

Radiologic Anesthesia Coding

Medicare's anesthesia billing guidelines allow only one anesthesia code to be reported for anesthesia services provided in conjunction with radiological procedures. Radiological Supervision and Interpretation (RS&I) codes may be applicable to radiological procedures being performed.

The appropriate RS&I code may be reported by the appropriate provider (e.g., radiologist, cardiologist, neurosurgeon, radiation oncologist). The RS&I codes are not included in anesthesia codes for these procedures.

Since Medicare anesthesia rules, with one exception, do not permit the physician performing a surgical or diagnostic procedure to separately report anesthesia for the procedure, the RS&I code(s) should not be reported by the same physician reporting the anesthesia service. Medicare rules allow physicians performing a surgical or diagnostic procedure to separately report medically reasonable and necessary moderate conscious sedation with a procedure unless the procedure is listed in Appendix G of the *CPT Manual.*

If a physician performing a radiologic procedure inserts a catheter as part of that procedure, and through the same site a catheter is utilized for monitoring purposes, it is inappropriate for either the anesthesia practitioner or the physician performing the radiologic procedure to separately report placement of the monitoring catheter (e.g., CPT codes 36500, 36555-36556, 36568-36569, 36580, 36584, 36597).

Monitored Anesthesia Care (MAC)

Monitored Anesthesia Care (MAC) may be performed by an anesthesia practitioner who administers sedatives, analgesics, hypnotics, or other anesthetic agents so that the patient remains responsive and breathes on his own. MAC provides anxiety relief, amnesia, pain relief, and comfort. MAC involves patient monitoring sufficient to anticipate the potential need to administer general anesthesia during a surgical or other procedure. MAC requires careful and continuous evaluation of various vital physiologic functions and the recognition and treatment of any adverse changes. CMS recognizes this type of anesthesia service as a payable service if medically reasonable and necessary.

Monitored anesthesia care includes the intraoperative monitoring by an anesthesia practitioner of the patient's vital physiological signs in anticipation of the need for administration of general anesthesia or of the development of adverse reaction to the surgical procedure. It also includes the performance of a pre-anesthesia evaluation and examination, prescription of the anesthesia care, administration of necessary oral or parenteral medications, and provision of indicated postoperative anesthesia care.

CPT code 01920 (Anesthesia for cardiac catheterization including coronary angiography and ventriculography (not to include Swan-Ganz catheter)) may be reported for monitored anesthesia care (MAC) in patients who are critically ill or critically unstable.

Issues of medical necessity are addressed by national CMS policy and local contractor coverage policies.

C. General Policy Statements

1. MUE and NCCI PTP edits are based on services provided by the same physician to the same beneficiary on the same date of service. Physicians should not inconvenience beneficiaries nor increase risks to beneficiaries by performing services on different dates of service to avoid MUE or NCCI PTP edits.
2. In this Manual many policies are described utilizing the term "physician." Unless indicated differently the usage of this term does not restrict the policies to physicians only but applies to all practitioners, hospitals, providers, or suppliers eligible to bill the relevant HCPCS/CPT codes pursuant to applicable portions of the Social Security Act (SSA) of 1965, the Code of Federal Regulations (CFR), and Medicare rules. In some sections of this Manual, the term "physician" would not include some of these entities because specific rules do not apply to them. For example, Anesthesia Rules [e.g., CMS Internet-Only Manual, Publication 100-04 (Medicare Claims Processing Manual), Chapter 12 (Physician/Nonphysician Practitioners), Section 50 (Payment for Anesthesiology Services)] and Global Surgery Rules [e.g., CMS Internet-Only Manual, Publication 100-04 (Medicare Claims Processing Manual), Chapter 12 (Physician/Nonphysician Practitioners), Section 40 (Surgeons and Global Surgery)] do not apply to hospitals.
3. Providers reporting services under Medicare's hospital outpatient prospective payment system (OPPS) should report all services in accordance with appropriate Medicare Internet- Only Manual (IOM) instructions.

4. In 2010 the CPT Manual modified the numbering of codes so that the sequence of codes as they appear in the *CPT Manual* does not necessarily correspond to a sequential numbering of codes. In the National Correct Coding Initiative Policy Manual for Medicare Services, use of a numerical range of codes reflects all codes that numerically fall within the range regardless of their sequential order in the *CPT Manual.*
5. Physicians should not report drug administration CPT codes 96360-96377 for anesthetic agents or other drugs administered between the patient's arrival at the operative center and discharge from the post-anesthesia care unit.
6. With limited exceptions Medicare Anesthesia Rules prevent separate payment for anesthesia for a medical or surgical procedure when provided by the physician performing the procedure. The physician should not report CPT codes 00100-01999, 62320-62327, or 64400-64530 for anesthesia for a procedure. Additionally, the physician should not unbundle the anesthesia procedure and report component codes individually. For example, introduction of a needle or intracatheter into a vein (CPT code 36000), venipuncture (CPT code 36410), drug administration (CPT codes 96360-96377) or cardiac assessment (e.g., CPT codes 93000-93010, 93040-93042) should not be reported when these procedures are related to the delivery of an anesthetic agent. Medicare allows separate reporting for moderate conscious sedation services (CPT codes 99151-99153) when provided by the same physician performing a medical or surgical procedure.
7. Intraoperative neurophysiology testing (HCPCS/CPT codes 95940, 95941/G0453) should not be reported by the physician/anesthesia practitioner performing an anesthesia procedure since it is included in the global package for the primary service code. The physician/anesthesia practitioner performing an anesthesia procedure should not report other 90000 neurophysiology testing codes for intraoperative neurophysiology testing (e.g., CPT codes 92585, 95822, 95860, 95861, 95867, 95868, 95870, 95907-95913, 95925-95937) since they are also included in the global package for the primary service code. However, when performed by a different physician during the procedure, intra-anesthesia neurophysiology testing may be separately reportable by the second physician.

CCI Table Information

The CCI Modification indicator is noted with superscript letters and is also located in the footer of each page for reference purposes. The codes are suffixed as **0** or **1**.

- **0** indicates there is no circumstance in which a modifier would be allowed or appropriate, meaning services represented by the code combination will not be paid separately.
- **1** signifies a modifier is allowed in order to differentiate between the services provided.

Note: The responsibility for the content of this product is the Centers for Medicare and Medicaid Services (CMS) and no endorsement by the American Medical Association (AMA) is intended or should be implied. The AMA disclaims responsibility for any consequences or liability attributable to or related to any uses, non-use, or interpretation of information contained or not contained in this product.

The NCCI edits on the following tables represent only the codes contained in this book. There are NCCI edits for CPT codes not found in this guide. The edits herein represent all active edits as of 1/1/2018. NCCI edits are updated quarterly. To view all NCCI edits, as well as quarterly updates, visit www.cms.gov/nationalcorrectcodeinited/.

Code 1	Code 2
00100	01996[1], 0213T[1], 0216T[1], 0228T[1], 0230T[1], 31505[1], 31515[1], 31527[1], 31622[1], 31634[1], 31645[1], 31647[1], 36000[1], 36010[0], 36011[1], 36012[1], 36013[1], 36014[1], 36015[1], 36400[1], 36405[1], 36406[1], 36410[1], 36420[1], 36425[1], 36430[1], 36440[1], 36591[0], 36592[0], 36600[1], 36640[1], 43752[1], 43753[1], 43754[1], 61026[1], 61055[1], 62280[1], 62281[1], 62282[1], 62284[1], 62320[1], 62321[1], 62322[1], 62323[1], 62324[1], 62325[1], 62326[1], 62327[1], 64400[1], 64402[1], 64405[1], 64408[1], 64410[1], 64413[1], 64415[1], 64416[1], 64417[1], 64418[1], 64420[1], 64421[1], 64425[1], 64430[1], 64435[1], 64445[1], 64446[1], 64447[1], 64448[1], 64449[1], 64450[1], 64461[1], 64463[1], 64479[1], 64483[1], 64486[1], 64487[1], 64488[1], 64489[1], 64490[1], 64493[1], 64505[1], 64510[1], 64517[1], 64520[1], 64530[1], 64553[1], 64555[1], 67500[1], 76000[1], 76970[1], 76998[0], 77002[0], 81000[1], 81002[1], 81003[1], 81005[1], 81015[1], 82013[1], 90865[1], 92511[1], 92512[1], 92516[1], 92520[1], 92537[1], 92538[1], 92950[1], 92953[1], 92960[1], 92961[1], 93000[1], 93005[1], 93010[1], 93040[1], 93041[1], 93042[1], 93050[0], 93303[0], 93304[0], 93306[1], 93307[1], 93308[1], 93312[1], 93313[1], 93314[1], 93315[1], 93316[1], 93317[1], 93318[0], 93351[1], 93355[0], 93451[1], 93456[1], 93457[1], 93561[0], 93562[0], 93701[0], 93922[1], 93923[1], 93924[1], 93925[1], 93926[1], 93930[1], 93931[1], 93970[1], 93971[1], 93975[1], 93976[1], 93978[1], 93979[1], 93980[1], 93981[1], 94002[1], 94004[1], 94200[1], 94250[0], 94640[1], 94644[1], 94660[1], 94662[1], 94680[1], 94681[1], 94690[1], 94760[0], 94761[0], 94762[1], 94770[1], 95812[0], 95813[0], 95816[0], 95819[0], 95822[0], 95829[0], 95955[0], 95956[0], 95957[0], 96360[0], 96365[0], 96372[0], 96373[0], 96374[0], 96375[0], 96376[0], 96377[0], 99151[0], 99152[0], 99153[0], 99155[0], 99156[0], 99157[0], 99201[0], 99202[0], 99203[0], 99204[0], 99205[0], 99211[0], 99212[0], 99213[0], 99214[0], 99215[0], 99217[0], 99218[0], 99219[0], 99220[0], 99221[0], 99222[0], 99223[0], 99224[0], 99225[0], 99226[0], 99231[0], 99232[0], 99233[0], 99234[0], 99235[0], 99236[0], 99238[0], 99239[0], 99281[0], 99282[0], 99283[0], 99284[0], 99285[0], 99304[0], 99305[0], 99306[0], 99307[0], 99308[0], 99309[0], 99310[0], 99315[0], 99318[0], 99324[0], 99325[0], 99326[0], 99327[0], 99328[0], 99334[0], 99335[0], 99336[0], 99337[0], 99341[0], 99342[0], 99343[0], 99347[0], 99348[0], 99349[0], 99354[0], 99355[0], 99356[0], 99357[0], 99358[0], 99359[0], 99415[0], 99416[0], 99446[0], 99447[0], 99448[0], 99449[0], 99451[0], 99452[0], 99466[0], 99468[0], 99469[0], 99471[0], 99472[0], 99475[0], 99476[0], 99477[0], 99478[0], 99479[0], 99480[0], 99483[0], 99485[0], 99497[0], C8921[1], C8922[1], C8923[1], C8924[1], C8925[1], C8926[1], C8927[0], C8929[1], C8930[1], G0380[1], G0381[1], G0382[1], G0383[1], G0384[1], G0406[0], G0407[0], G0408[0], G0425[0], G0426[0], G0427[0], G0463[0], G0500[0], G0508[0], G0509[0]
00102	01996[1], 0213T[1], 0216T[1], 0228T[1], 0230T[1], 31505[1], 31515[1], 31527[1], 31622[1], 31634[1], 31645[1], 31647[1], 36000[1], 36010[0], 36011[1], 36012[1], 36013[1], 36014[1], 36015[1], 36400[1], 36405[1], 36406[1], 36410[1], 36420[1], 36425[1], 36430[1], 36440[1], 36591[0], 36592[0], 36600[1], 36640[1], 43752[1], 43753[1], 43754[1], 61026[1], 61055[1], 62280[1], 62281[1], 62282[1], 62284[1], 62320[1], 62321[1], 62322[1], 62323[1], 62324[1], 62325[1], 62326[1], 62327[1], 64400[1], 64402[1], 64405[1], 64408[1], 64410[1], 64413[1], 64415[1], 64416[1], 64417[1], 64418[1], 64420[1], 64421[1], 64425[1], 64430[1], 64435[1], 64445[1], 64446[1], 64447[1], 64448[1], 64449[1], 64450[1], 64461[1], 64463[1], 64479[1], 64483[1], 64486[1], 64487[1], 64488[1], 64489[1], 64490[1], 64493[1], 64505[1], 64510[1], 64517[1], 64520[1], 64530[1], 64553[1], 64555[1], 67500[1], 76000[1], 76970[1], 76998[0], 77002[0], 81000[1], 81002[1], 81003[1], 81005[1], 81015[1], 82013[1], 90865[1], 92511[1], 92512[1], 92516[1], 92520[1], 92537[1], 92538[1], 92950[1], 92953[1], 92960[1], 92961[1], 93000[1], 93005[1], 93010[1], 93040[1], 93041[1], 93042[1], 93050[0], 93303[0], 93304[0], 93306[1], 93307[1], 93308[1], 93312[1], 93313[1], 93314[1], 93315[1], 93316[1], 93317[1], 93318[0], 93351[1], 93355[0], 93451[1], 93456[1], 93457[1], 93561[0], 93562[0], 93701[0], 93922[1], 93923[1], 93924[1], 93925[1], 93926[1], 93930[1], 93931[1], 93970[1], 93971[1], 93975[1], 93976[1], 93978[1], 93979[1], 93980[1], 93981[1], 94002[1], 94004[1], 94200[1], 94250[0], 94640[1], 94644[1], 94660[1], 94662[1], 94680[1], 94681[1], 94690[1], 94760[0], 94761[0], 94762[1], 94770[1], 95812[0], 95813[0], 95816[0], 95819[0], 95822[0], 95829[0], 95955[0], 95956[0], 95957[0], 96360[0], 96365[0], 96372[0], 96373[0], 96374[0], 96375[0], 96376[0], 96377[0], 99151[0], 99152[0], 99153[0], 99155[0], 99156[0], 99157[0], 99201[0], 99202[0], 99203[0], 99204[0], 99205[0], 99211[0], 99212[0], 99213[0], 99214[0], 99215[0], 99217[0], 99218[0], 99219[0], 99220[0], 99221[0], 99222[0], 99223[0], 99224[0], 99225[0], 99226[0], 99231[0], 99232[0], 99233[0], 99234[0], 99235[0], 99236[0], 99238[0], 99239[0], 99281[0], 99282[0], 99283[0], 99284[0], 99285[0], 99304[0], 99305[0], 99306[0], 99307[0], 99308[0], 99309[0], 99310[0], 99315[0], 99318[0], 99324[0], 99325[0], 99326[0], 99327[0], 99328[0], 99334[0], 99335[0], 99336[0], 99337[0], 99341[0], 99342[0], 99343[0], 99347[0], 99348[0], 99349[0], 99354[0], 99355[0], 99356[0], 99357[0], 99358[0], 99359[0], 99415[0], 99416[0], 99446[0], 99447[0], 99448[0], 99449[0], 99451[0], 99452[0], 99466[0], 99468[0], 99469[0], 99471[0], 99472[0], 99475[0], 99476[0], 99477[0], 99478[0], 99479[0], 99480[0], 99483[0], 99485[0], 99497[0], C8921[1], C8922[1], C8923[1], C8924[1], C8925[1], C8926[1], C8927[0], C8929[1], C8930[1], G0380[1], G0381[1], G0382[1], G0383[1], G0384[1], G0406[0], G0407[0], G0408[0], G0425[0], G0426[0], G0427[0], G0463[0], G0500[0], G0508[0], G0509[0]
00103	01996[1], 0213T[1], 0216T[1], 0228T[1], 0230T[1], 31505[1], 31515[1], 31527[1], 31622[1], 31634[1], 31645[1], 31647[1], 36000[1], 36010[0], 36011[1], 36012[1], 36013[1], 36014[1], 36015[1], 36400[1], 36405[1], 36406[1], 36410[1], 36420[1], 36425[1], 36430[1], 36440[1], 36591[0], 36592[0], 36600[1], 36640[1], 43752[1], 43753[1], 43754[1], 61026[1], 61055[1], 62280[1], 62281[1], 62282[1], 62284[1], 62320[1], 62321[1], 62322[1], 62323[1], 62324[1], 62325[1], 62326[1], 62327[1], 64400[1], 64402[1], 64405[1], 64408[1], 64410[1], 64413[1], 64415[1], 64416[1], 64417[1], 64418[1], 64420[1], 64421[1], 64425[1], 64430[1], 64435[1], 64445[1], 64446[1], 64447[1], 64448[1], 64449[1], 64450[1], 64461[1], 64463[1], 64479[1], 64483[1], 64486[1], 64487[1], 64488[1], 64489[1], 64490[1], 64493[1], 64505[1], 64510[1], 64517[1], 64520[1], 64530[1], 64553[1], 64555[1], 67500[1], 76000[1], 76970[1], 76998[0], 77002[0], 81000[1], 81002[1], 81003[1], 81005[1], 81015[1], 82013[1], 90865[1], 92511[1], 92512[1], 92516[1], 92520[1], 92537[1], 92538[1], 92950[1], 92953[1], 92960[1], 92961[1], 93000[1], 93005[1], 93010[1], 93040[1], 93041[1], 93042[1], 93050[0], 93303[0], 93304[0], 93306[1], 93307[1], 93308[1], 93312[1], 93313[1], 93314[1], 93315[1], 93316[1], 93317[1], 93318[0], 93351[1], 93355[0], 93451[1], 93456[1], 93457[1], 93561[0], 93562[0], 93701[0], 93922[1], 93923[1], 93924[1], 93925[1], 93926[1], 93930[1], 93931[1], 93970[1], 93971[1], 93975[1], 93976[1], 93978[1], 93979[1], 93980[1], 93981[1], 94002[1], 94004[1], 94200[1], 94250[0], 94640[1], 94644[1], 94660[1], 94662[1], 94680[1], 94681[1], 94690[1], 94760[0], 94761[0], 94762[1], 94770[1], 95812[0], 95813[0], 95816[0], 95819[0], 95822[0], 95829[0], 95955[0], 95956[0], 95957[0], 96360[0], 96365[0], 96372[0], 96373[0], 96374[0], 96375[0], 96376[0], 96377[0], 99151[0], 99152[0], 99153[0], 99155[0], 99156[0], 99157[0], 99201[0], 99202[0], 99203[0], 99204[0], 99205[0], 99211[0], 99212[0], 99213[0], 99214[0], 99215[0], 99217[0], 99218[0], 99219[0], 99220[0], 99221[0], 99222[0], 99223[0], 99224[0], 99225[0], 99226[0], 99231[0], 99232[0], 99233[0], 99234[0], 99235[0], 99236[0], 99238[0], 99239[0], 99281[0], 99282[0], 99283[0], 99284[0], 99285[0], 99304[0], 99305[0], 99306[0], 99307[0], 99308[0], 99309[0], 99310[0], 99315[0], 99318[0], 99324[0], 99325[0], 99326[0], 99327[0], 99328[0], 99334[0], 99335[0], 99336[0], 99337[0], 99341[0], 99342[0], 99343[0], 99347[0], 99348[0], 99349[0], 99354[0], 99355[0], 99356[0], 99357[0], 99358[0], 99359[0], 99415[0], 99416[0], 99446[0], 99447[0], 99448[0], 99449[0], 99451[0], 99452[0], 99466[0], 99468[0], 99469[0], 99471[0], 99472[0], 99475[0], 99476[0], 99477[0], 99478[0], 99479[0], 99480[0], 99483[0], 99485[0], 99497[0], C8921[1], C8922[1], C8923[1], C8924[1], C8925[1], C8926[1], C8927[0], C8929[1], C8930[1], G0380[1], G0381[1], G0382[1], G0383[1], G0384[1], G0406[0], G0407[0], G0408[0], G0425[0], G0426[0], G0427[0], G0463[0], G0500[0], G0508[0], G0509[0]
00104	01996[1], 0213T[1], 0216T[1], 0228T[1], 0230T[1], 0333T[0], 0464T[0], 31505[1], 31515[1], 31527[1], 31622[1], 31634[1], 31645[1], 31647[1], 36000[1], 36010[0], 36011[1], 36012[1], 36013[1], 36014[1], 36015[1], 36400[1], 36405[1], 36406[1], 36410[1], 36420[1], 36425[1], 36430[1], 36440[1], 36591[0], 36592[0], 36600[1], 36640[1], 43752[1], 43753[1], 43754[1], 61026[1], 61055[1], 62280[1], 62281[1], 62282[1], 62284[1], 62320[1], 62321[1], 62322[1], 62323[1], 62324[1], 62325[1], 62326[1], 62327[1], 64400[1], 64402[1], 64405[1], 64408[1], 64410[1], 64413[1], 64415[1], 64416[1], 64417[1], 64418[1], 64420[1], 64421[1], 64425[1], 64430[1], 64435[1], 64445[1], 64446[1], 64447[1], 64448[1], 64449[1], 64450[1], 64461[1], 64463[1], 64479[1], 64483[1], 64486[1], 64487[1], 64488[1], 64489[1], 64490[1], 64493[1], 64505[1], 64510[1], 64517[1], 64520[1], 64530[1], 64553[1], 64555[1], 67500[1], 76000[1], 76970[1], 76998[0], 77002[0], 81000[1], 81002[1], 81003[1], 81005[1], 81015[1], 82013[1], 90865[1], 92511[1], 92512[1], 92516[1], 92520[1], 92537[1], 92538[1], 92585[0], 92950[1], 92953[1], 92960[1], 92961[1], 93000[1], 93005[1], 93010[1], 93040[1], 93041[1], 93042[1], 93050[0], 93303[0], 93304[0], 93306[1], 93307[1], 93308[1], 93312[1], 93313[1], 93314[1], 93315[1], 93316[1], 93317[1], 93318[0], 93351[1], 93355[0], 93451[1], 93456[1], 93457[1], 93561[0], 93562[0], 93701[0], 93922[1], 93923[1], 93924[1], 93925[1], 93926[1], 93930[1], 93931[1], 93970[1], 93971[1], 93975[1], 93976[1], 93978[1], 93979[1], 93980[1], 93981[1], 94002[1], 94004[1], 94200[1], 94250[0], 94640[1], 94644[1], 94660[1], 94662[1], 94680[1], 94681[1], 94690[1], 94760[0], 94761[0], 94762[1], 94770[1], 95812[0], 95813[0], 95816[0], 95819[0], 95822[0], 95829[0], 95860[0], 95861[0], 95863[0], 95864[0], 95865[0], 95866[0], 95867[0], 95868[0], 95869[0], 95870[0], 95907[0], 95908[0], 95909[0], 95910[0], 95911[0], 95912[0], 95913[0], 95925[0], 95926[0], 95927[0], 95928[0], 95929[0], 95930[0], 95933[0], 95937[0], 95938[0], 95939[0], 95940[0], 95955[0], 95956[0], 95957[0], 96360[0], 96365[0], 96372[0], 96373[0], 96374[0], 96375[0], 96376[0], 96377[0], 99151[0], 99152[0], 99153[0], 99155[0], 99156[0], 99157[0], 99201[0], 99202[0], 99203[0], 99204[0], 99205[0], 99211[0], 99212[0], 99213[0], 99214[0], 99215[0], 99217[0], 99218[0], 99219[0], 99220[0], 99221[0], 99222[0], 99223[0], 99224[0], 99225[0], 99226[0], 99231[0], 99232[0], 99233[0], 99234[0], 99235[0], 99236[0], 99238[0], 99239[0], 99281[0], 99282[0], 99283[0], 99284[0], 99285[0], 99304[0], 99305[0], 99306[0], 99307[0], 99308[0], 99309[0], 99310[0], 99315[0], 99318[0], 99324[0], 99325[0], 99326[0], 99327[0], 99328[0], 99334[0], 99335[0], 99336[0], 99337[0], 99341[0], 99342[0], 99343[0], 99347[0], 99348[0], 99349[0], 99354[0], 99355[0], 99356[0], 99357[0], 99358[0], 99359[0], 99415[0], 99416[0], 99446[0], 99447[0], 99448[0], 99449[0], 99451[0], 99452[0], 99466[0], 99468[0], 99469[0], 99471[0], 99472[0], 99475[0], 99476[0], 99477[0], 99478[0], 99479[0], 99480[0], 99483[0], 99485[0], 99497[0], C8921[1], C8922[1], C8923[1], C8924[1], C8925[1], C8926[1], C8927[0], C8929[1], C8930[1], G0380[1], G0381[1], G0382[1], G0383[1], G0384[1], G0406[0], G0407[0], G0408[0], G0425[0], G0426[0], G0427[0], G0453[0], G0463[0], G0500[0], G0508[0], G0509[0]
00120	01996[1], 0213T[1], 0216T[1], 0228T[1], 0230T[1], 31505[1], 31515[1], 31527[1], 31622[1], 31634[1], 31645[1], 31647[1], 36000[1], 36010[0], 36011[1], 36012[1], 36013[1], 36014[1], 36015[1], 36400[1], 36405[1], 36406[1], 36410[1], 36420[1], 36425[1], 36430[1], 36440[1], 36591[0], 36592[0], 36600[1], 36640[1], 43752[1], 43753[1], 43754[1], 61026[1], 61055[1], 62280[1], 62281[1], 62282[1], 62284[1], 62320[1], 62321[1], 62322[1], 62323[1], 62324[1], 62325[1], 62326[1], 62327[1], 64400[1], 64402[1], 64405[1], 64408[1], 64410[1], 64413[1], 64415[1], 64416[1], 64417[1], 64418[1], 64420[1], 64421[1], 64425[1], 64430[1], 64435[1], 64445[1], 64446[1], 64447[1], 64448[1], 64449[1], 64450[1], 64461[1], 64463[1], 64479[1], 64483[1], 64486[1], 64487[1], 64488[1], 64489[1], 64490[1], 64493[1], 64505[1], 64510[1], 64517[1], 64520[1], 64530[1], 64553[1], 64555[1], 67500[1], 76000[1], 76970[1], 76998[0],

0 = Modifier usage not allowed or inappropriate 1 = Modifier usage allowed

CPT © 2018 American Medical Association. All Rights Reserved.

Code 1	Code 2
	77002[0], 81000[1], 81002[1], 81003[1], 81005[1], 81015[1], 82013[1], 90865[1], 92511[1], 92512[1], 92516[1], 92520[1], 92537[1], 92538[1], 92950[1], 92953[1], 92960[1], 92961[1], 93000[1], 93005[1], 93010[1], 93040[1], 93041[1], 93042[1], 93050[0], 93303[0], 93304[0], 93306[1], 93307[1], 93308[1], 93312[1], 93313[1], 93314[1], 93315[1], 93316[1], 93317[1], 93318[0], 93351[1], 93355[0], 93451[1], 93456[1], 93457[1], 93561[0], 93562[0], 93701[0], 93922[1], 93923[1], 93924[1], 93925[1], 93926[1], 93930[1], 93931[1], 93970[1], 93971[1], 93975[1], 93976[1], 93978[1], 93979[1], 93980[1], 93981[1], 94002[1], 94004[1], 94200[1], 94250[0], 94640[1], 94644[1], 94660[1], 94662[1], 94680[1], 94681[1], 94690[1], 94760[0], 94761[0], 94762[1], 94770[1], 95812[0], 95813[0], 95816[0], 95819[0], 95822[0], 95829[0], 95955[0], 95956[0], 95957[0], 96360[0], 96365[0], 96372[0], 96373[0], 96374[0], 96375[0], 96376[0], 96377[0], 99151[0], 99152[0], 99153[0], 99155[0], 99156[0], 99157[0], 99201[0], 99202[0], 99203[0], 99204[0], 99205[0], 99211[0], 99212[0], 99213[0], 99214[0], 99215[0], 99217[0], 99218[0], 99219[0], 99220[0], 99221[0], 99222[0], 99223[0], 99224[0], 99225[0], 99226[0], 99231[0], 99232[0], 99233[0], 99234[0], 99235[0], 99236[0], 99238[0], 99239[0], 99281[0], 99282[0], 99283[0], 99284[0], 99285[0], 99304[0], 99305[0], 99306[0], 99307[0], 99308[0], 99309[0], 99310[0], 99315[0], 99318[0], 99324[0], 99325[0], 99326[0], 99327[0], 99328[0], 99334[0], 99335[0], 99336[0], 99337[0], 99341[0], 99342[0], 99343[0], 99347[0], 99348[0], 99349[0], 99354[0], 99355[0], 99356[0], 99357[0], 99358[0], 99359[0], 99415[0], 99416[0], 99446[0], 99447[0], 99448[0], 99449[0], 99451[0], 99452[0], 99466[0], 99468[0], 99469[0], 99471[0], 99472[0], 99475[0], 99476[0], 99477[0], 99478[0], 99479[0], 99480[0], 99483[0], 99485[0], 99497[0], C8921[1], C8922[1], C8923[1], C8924[1], C8925[1], C8926[1], C8927[0], C8929[1], C8930[1], G0380[1], G0381[1], G0382[1], G0383[1], G0384[1], G0406[0], G0407[0], G0408[0], G0425[0], G0426[0], G0427[0], G0463[0], G0500[0], G0508[0], G0509[0]
00124	01996[1], 0213T[1], 0216T[1], 0228T[1], 0230T[1], 31505[1], 31515[1], 31527[1], 31622[1], 31634[1], 31645[1], 31647[1], 36000[1], 36010[0], 36011[1], 36012[1], 36013[1], 36014[1], 36015[1], 36400[1], 36405[1], 36406[1], 36410[1], 36420[1], 36425[1], 36430[1], 36440[1], 36591[0], 36592[0], 36600[1], 36640[1], 43752[1], 43753[1], 43754[1], 61026[1], 61055[1], 62280[1], 62281[1], 62282[1], 62284[1], 62320[1], 62321[1], 62322[1], 62323[1], 62324[1], 62325[1], 62326[1], 62327[1], 64400[1], 64402[1], 64405[1], 64408[1], 64410[1], 64413[1], 64415[1], 64416[1], 64417[1], 64418[1], 64420[1], 64421[1], 64425[1], 64430[1], 64435[1], 64445[1], 64446[1], 64447[1], 64448[1], 64449[1], 64450[1], 64461[1], 64463[1], 64479[1], 64483[1], 64486[1], 64487[1], 64488[1], 64489[1], 64490[1], 64493[1], 64505[1], 64510[1], 64517[1], 64520[1], 64530[1], 64553[1], 64555[1], 67500[1], 76000[1], 76100[1], 76970[1], 76998[0], 77002[0], 81000[1], 81002[1], 81003[1], 81005[1], 81015[1], 82013[1], 90865[1], 92511[1], 92512[1], 92516[1], 92520[1], 92537[1], 92538[1], 92950[1], 92953[1], 92960[1], 92961[1], 93000[1], 93005[1], 93010[1], 93040[1], 93041[1], 93042[1], 93050[0], 93303[0], 93304[0], 93306[1], 93307[1], 93308[1], 93312[1], 93313[1], 93314[1], 93315[1], 93316[1], 93317[1], 93318[0], 93351[1], 93355[0], 93451[1], 93456[1], 93457[1], 93561[0], 93562[0], 93701[0], 93922[1], 93923[1], 93924[1], 93925[1], 93926[1], 93930[1], 93931[1], 93970[1], 93971[1], 93975[1], 93976[1], 93978[1], 93979[1], 93980[1], 93981[1], 94002[1], 94004[1], 94200[1], 94250[0], 94640[1], 94644[1], 94660[1], 94662[1], 94680[1], 94681[1], 94690[1], 94760[0], 94761[0], 94762[1], 94770[1], 95812[0], 95813[0], 95816[0], 95819[0], 95822[0], 95829[0], 95955[0], 95956[0], 95957[0], 96360[0], 96365[0], 96372[0], 96373[0], 96374[0], 96375[0], 96376[0], 96377[0], 99151[0], 99152[0], 99153[0], 99155[0], 99156[0], 99157[0], 99201[0], 99202[0], 99203[0], 99204[0], 99205[0], 99211[0], 99212[0], 99213[0], 99214[0], 99215[0], 99217[0], 99218[0], 99219[0], 99220[0], 99221[0], 99222[0], 99223[0], 99224[0], 99225[0], 99226[0], 99231[0], 99232[0], 99233[0], 99234[0], 99235[0], 99236[0], 99238[0], 99239[0], 99281[0], 99282[0], 99283[0], 99284[0], 99285[0], 99304[0], 99305[0], 99306[0], 99307[0], 99308[0], 99309[0], 99310[0], 99315[0], 99318[0], 99324[0], 99325[0], 99326[0], 99327[0], 99328[0], 99334[0], 99335[0], 99336[0], 99337[0], 99341[0], 99342[0], 99343[0], 99347[0], 99348[0], 99349[0], 99354[0], 99355[0], 99356[0], 99357[0], 99358[0], 99359[0], 99415[0], 99416[0], 99446[0], 99447[0], 99448[0], 99449[0], 99451[0], 99452[0], 99466[0], 99468[0], 99469[0], 99471[0], 99472[0], 99475[0], 99476[0], 99477[0], 99478[0], 99479[0], 99480[0], 99483[0], 99485[0], 99497[0], C8921[1], C8922[1], C8923[1], C8924[1], C8925[1], C8926[1], C8927[0], C8929[1], C8930[1], G0380[1], G0381[1], G0382[1], G0383[1], G0384[1], G0406[0], G0407[0], G0408[0], G0425[0], G0426[0], G0427[0], G0463[0], G0500[0], G0508[0], G0509[0]
00126	01996[1], 0213T[1], 0216T[1], 0228T[1], 0230T[1], 31505[1], 31515[1], 31527[1], 31622[1], 31634[1], 31645[1], 31647[1], 36000[1], 36010[0], 36011[1], 36012[1], 36013[1], 36014[1], 36015[1], 36400[1], 36405[1], 36406[1], 36410[1], 36420[1], 36425[1], 36430[1], 36440[1], 36591[0], 36592[0], 36600[1], 36640[1], 43752[1], 43753[1], 43754[1], 61026[1], 61055[1], 62280[1], 62281[1], 62282[1], 62284[1], 62320[1], 62321[1], 62322[1], 62323[1], 62324[1], 62325[1], 62326[1], 62327[1], 64400[1], 64402[1], 64405[1], 64408[1], 64410[1], 64413[1], 64415[1], 64416[1], 64417[1], 64418[1], 64420[1], 64421[1], 64425[1], 64430[1], 64435[1], 64445[1], 64446[1], 64447[1], 64448[1], 64449[1], 64450[1], 64461[1], 64463[1], 64479[1], 64483[1], 64486[1], 64487[1], 64488[1], 64489[1], 64490[1], 64493[1], 64505[1], 64510[1], 64517[1], 64520[1], 64530[1], 64553[1], 64555[1], 67500[1], 76000[1], 76970[1], 76998[0], 77002[0], 81000[1], 81002[1], 81003[1], 81005[1], 81015[1], 82013[1], 90865[1], 92511[1], 92512[1], 92516[1], 92520[1], 92537[1], 92538[1], 92950[1], 92953[1], 92960[1], 92961[1], 93000[1], 93005[1], 93010[1], 93040[1], 93041[1], 93042[1], 93050[0], 93303[0], 93304[0], 93306[1], 93307[1], 93308[1], 93312[1], 93313[1], 93314[1], 93315[1], 93316[1], 93317[1], 93318[0], 93351[1], 93355[0], 93451[1], 93456[1], 93457[1], 93561[0], 93562[0], 93701[0], 93922[1], 93923[1], 93924[1], 93925[1], 93926[1], 93930[1], 93931[1], 93970[1], 93971[1], 93975[1], 93976[1], 93978[1], 93979[1], 93980[1], 93981[1], 94002[1], 94004[1], 94200[1], 94250[0], 94640[1], 94644[1], 94660[1], 94662[1], 94680[1], 94681[1], 94690[1], 94760[0], 94761[0], 94762[1], 94770[1], 95812[0], 95813[0], 95816[0], 95819[0], 95822[0], 95829[0], 95955[0], 95956[0], 95957[0], 96360[0], 96365[0], 96372[0], 96373[0], 96374[0], 96375[0], 96376[0], 96377[0], 99151[0], 99152[0], 99153[0], 99155[0], 99156[0], 99157[0], 99201[0], 99202[0], 99203[0], 99204[0], 99205[0], 99211[0], 99212[0], 99213[0], 99214[0], 99215[0], 99217[0], 99218[0], 99219[0], 99220[0], 99221[0], 99222[0], 99223[0], 99224[0], 99225[0], 99226[0], 99231[0], 99232[0], 99233[0], 99234[0], 99235[0], 99236[0], 99238[0], 99239[0], 99281[0], 99282[0], 99283[0], 99284[0], 99285[0], 99304[0], 99305[0], 99306[0], 99307[0], 99308[0], 99309[0], 99310[0], 99315[0], 99318[0], 99324[0], 99325[0], 99326[0], 99327[0], 99328[0], 99334[0], 99335[0], 99336[0], 99337[0], 99341[0], 99342[0], 99343[0], 99347[0], 99348[0], 99349[0], 99354[0], 99355[0], 99356[0], 99357[0], 99358[0], 99359[0], 99415[0], 99416[0], 99446[0], 99447[0], 99448[0], 99449[0], 99451[0], 99452[0], 99466[0], 99468[0], 99469[0], 99471[0], 99472[0], 99475[0], 99476[0], 99477[0], 99478[0], 99479[0], 99480[0], 99483[0], 99485[0], 99497[0], C8921[1], C8922[1], C8923[1], C8924[1], C8925[1], C8926[1], C8927[0], C8929[1], C8930[1], G0380[1], G0381[1], G0382[1], G0383[1], G0384[1], G0406[0], G0407[0], G0408[0], G0425[0], G0426[0], G0427[0], G0463[0], G0500[0], G0508[0], G0509[0]
00140	01996[1], 0213T[1], 0216T[1], 0228T[1], 0230T[1], 0329T[1], 31505[1], 31515[1], 31527[1], 31622[1], 31634[1], 31645[1], 31647[1], 36000[1], 36010[0], 36011[1], 36012[1], 36013[1], 36014[1], 36015[1], 36400[1], 36405[1], 36406[1], 36410[1], 36420[1], 36425[1], 36430[1], 36440[1], 36591[0], 36592[0], 36600[1], 36640[1], 43752[1], 43753[1], 43754[1], 61026[1], 61055[1], 62280[1], 62281[1], 62282[1], 62284[1], 62320[1], 62321[1], 62322[1], 62323[1], 62324[1], 62325[1], 62326[1], 62327[1], 64400[1], 64402[1], 64405[1], 64408[1], 64410[1], 64413[1], 64415[1], 64416[1], 64417[1], 64418[1], 64420[1], 64421[1], 64425[1], 64430[1], 64435[1], 64445[1], 64446[1], 64447[1], 64448[1], 64449[1], 64450[1], 64461[1], 64463[1], 64479[1], 64483[1], 64486[1], 64487[1], 64488[1], 64489[1], 64490[1], 64493[1], 64505[1], 64510[1], 64517[1], 64520[1], 64530[1], 64553[1], 64555[1], 67500[0], 76000[1], 76970[1], 76998[0], 77002[0], 81000[1], 81002[1], 81003[1], 81005[1], 81015[1], 82013[1], 90865[1], 92100[1], 92511[1], 92512[1], 92516[1], 92520[1], 92537[1], 92538[1], 92950[1], 92953[1], 92960[1], 92961[1], 93000[1], 93005[1], 93010[1], 93040[1], 93041[1], 93042[1], 93050[0], 93303[0], 93304[0], 93306[1], 93307[1], 93308[1], 93312[1], 93313[1], 93314[1], 93315[1], 93316[1], 93317[1], 93318[0], 93351[1], 93355[0], 93451[1], 93456[1], 93457[1], 93561[0], 93562[0], 93701[0], 93922[1], 93923[1], 93924[1], 93925[1], 93926[1], 93930[1], 93931[1], 93970[1], 93971[1], 93975[1], 93976[1], 93978[1], 93979[1], 93980[1], 93981[1], 94002[1], 94004[1], 94200[1], 94250[0], 94640[1], 94644[1], 94660[1], 94662[1], 94680[1], 94681[1], 94690[1], 94760[0], 94761[0], 94762[1], 94770[1], 95812[0], 95813[0], 95816[0], 95819[0], 95822[0], 95829[0], 95955[0], 95956[0], 95957[0], 96360[0], 96365[0], 96372[0], 96373[0], 96374[0], 96375[0], 96376[0], 96377[0], 99151[0], 99152[0], 99153[0], 99155[0], 99156[0], 99157[0], 99201[0], 99202[0], 99203[0], 99204[0], 99205[0], 99211[0], 99212[0], 99213[0], 99214[0], 99215[0], 99217[0], 99218[0], 99219[0], 99220[0], 99221[0], 99222[0], 99223[0], 99224[0], 99225[0], 99226[0], 99231[0], 99232[0], 99233[0], 99234[0], 99235[0], 99236[0], 99238[0], 99239[0], 99281[0], 99282[0], 99283[0], 99284[0], 99285[0], 99304[0], 99305[0], 99306[0], 99307[0], 99308[0], 99309[0], 99310[0], 99315[0], 99318[0], 99324[0], 99325[0], 99326[0], 99327[0], 99328[0], 99334[0], 99335[0], 99336[0], 99337[0], 99341[0], 99342[0], 99343[0], 99347[0], 99348[0], 99349[0], 99354[0], 99355[0], 99356[0], 99357[0], 99358[0], 99359[0], 99415[0], 99416[0], 99446[0], 99447[0], 99448[0], 99449[0], 99451[0], 99452[0], 99466[0], 99468[0], 99469[0], 99471[0], 99472[0], 99475[0], 99476[0], 99477[0], 99478[0], 99479[0], 99480[0], 99483[0], 99485[0], 99497[0], C8921[1], C8922[1], C8923[1], C8924[1], C8925[1], C8926[1], C8927[0], C8929[1], C8930[1], G0380[1], G0381[1], G0382[1], G0383[1], G0384[1], G0406[0], G0407[0], G0408[0], G0425[0], G0426[0], G0427[0], G0463[0], G0500[0], G0508[0], G0509[0]
00142	01996[1], 0213T[1], 0216T[1], 0228T[1], 0230T[1], 0329T[1], 31505[1], 31515[1], 31527[1], 31622[1], 31634[1], 31645[1], 31647[1], 36000[1], 36010[0], 36011[1], 36012[1], 36013[1], 36014[1], 36015[1], 36400[1], 36405[1], 36406[1], 36410[1], 36420[1], 36425[1], 36430[1], 36440[1], 36591[0], 36592[0], 36600[1], 36640[1], 43752[1], 43753[1], 43754[1], 61026[1], 61055[1], 62280[1], 62281[1], 62282[1], 62284[1], 62320[1], 62321[1], 62322[1], 62323[1], 62324[1], 62325[1], 62326[1], 62327[1], 64402[1], 64405[1], 64408[1], 64410[1], 64413[1], 64415[1], 64416[1], 64417[1], 64418[1], 64420[1], 64421[1], 64425[1], 64430[1], 64435[1], 64445[1], 64446[1], 64447[1], 64448[1], 64449[1], 64450[1], 64461[1], 64463[1], 64479[1], 64483[1], 64486[1], 64487[1], 64488[1], 64489[1], 64490[1], 64493[1], 64505[1], 64510[1], 64517[1], 64520[1], 64530[1], 64553[1], 64555[1], 67500[0], 76000[1], 76970[1], 76998[0], 77002[0], 81000[1], 81002[1], 81003[1], 81005[1], 81015[1], 82013[1], 90865[1], 92100[1], 92511[1], 92512[1], 92516[1], 92520[1], 92537[1], 92538[1], 92950[1], 92953[1], 92960[1], 92961[1], 93000[1], 93005[1], 93010[1], 93040[1], 93041[1], 93042[1], 93050[0], 93303[0], 93304[0], 93306[1], 93307[1], 93308[1], 93312[1], 93313[1], 93314[1], 93315[1], 93316[1], 93317[1], 93318[0], 93351[1], 93355[0], 93451[1], 93456[1], 93457[1], 93561[0], 93562[0], 93701[0], 93922[1], 93923[1], 93924[1], 93925[1], 93926[1], 93930[1], 93931[1], 93970[1], 93971[1], 93975[1], 93976[1], 93978[1], 93979[1], 93980[1], 93981[1], 94002[1], 94004[1], 94200[1], 94250[0], 94640[1], 94644[1], 94660[1], 94662[1], 94680[1], 94681[1], 94690[1], 94760[0], 94761[0], 94762[1], 94770[1], 95812[0], 95813[0], 95816[0], 95819[0], 95822[0], 95829[0], 95955[0], 95956[0], 95957[0], 96360[0], 96365[0], 96372[0], 96373[0], 96374[0], 96375[0], 96376[0], 96377[0], 99151[0], 99152[0], 99153[0], 99155[0], 99156[0], 99157[0], 99201[0], 99202[0], 99203[0], 99204[0], 99205[0], 99211[0], 99212[0], 99213[0], 99214[0], 99215[0], 99217[0], 99218[0], 99219[0], 99220[0], 99221[0], 99222[0], 99223[0], 99224[0], 99225[0], 99226[0], 99231[0],

0 = Modifier usage not allowed or inappropriate   1 = Modifier usage allowed

CPT © 2018 American Medical Association. All Rights Reserved.

Code 1	Code 2
	99232[0], 99233[0], 99234[0], 99235[0], 99236[0], 99238[0], 99239[0], 99281[0], 99282[0], 99283[0], 99284[0], 99285[0], 99304[0], 99305[0], 99306[0], 99307[0], 99308[0], 99309[0], 99310[0], 99315[0], 99318[0], 99324[0], 99325[0], 99326[0], 99327[0], 99328[0], 99334[0], 99335[0], 99336[0], 99337[0], 99341[0], 99342[0], 99343[0], 99347[0], 99348[0], 99349[0], 99354[0], 99355[0], 99356[0], 99357[0], 99358[0], 99359[0], 99415[0], 99416[0], 99446[0], 99447[0], 99448[0], 99449[0], 99451[0], 99452[0], 99466[0], 99468[0], 99469[0], 99471[0], 99472[0], 99475[0], 99476[0], 99477[0], 99478[0], 99479[0], 99480[0], 99483[0], 99485[0], 99497[0], C8921[1], C8922[1], C8923[1], C8924[1], C8925[1], C8926[1], C8927[0], C8929[1], C8930[1], G0380[1], G0381[1], G0382[1], G0383[1], G0384[1], G0406[0], G0407[0], G0408[0], G0425[0], G0426[0], G0427[0], G0463[0], G0500[0], G0508[0], G0509[0]
00144	01996[1], 0213T[1], 0216T[1], 0228T[1], 0230T[1], 31505[1], 31515[1], 31527[1], 31622[1], 31634[1], 31645[1], 31647[1], 36000[1], 36010[0], 36011[1], 36012[1], 36013[1], 36014[1], 36015[1], 36400[1], 36405[1], 36406[1], 36410[1], 36420[1], 36425[1], 36430[1], 36440[1], 36591[0], 36592[0], 36600[1], 36640[1], 43752[1], 43753[1], 43754[1], 61026[1], 61055[1], 62280[1], 62281[1], 62282[1], 62284[1], 62320[1], 62321[1], 62322[1], 62323[1], 62324[1], 62325[1], 62326[1], 62327[1], 64400[1], 64402[1], 64405[1], 64408[1], 64410[1], 64413[1], 64415[1], 64416[1], 64417[1], 64418[1], 64420[1], 64421[1], 64425[1], 64430[1], 64435[1], 64445[1], 64446[1], 64447[1], 64448[1], 64449[1], 64450[1], 64461[1], 64463[1], 64479[1], 64483[1], 64486[1], 64487[1], 64488[1], 64489[1], 64490[1], 64493[1], 64505[1], 64510[1], 64517[1], 64520[1], 64530[1], 64553[1], 64555[1], 67500[1], 76000[1], 76970[1], 76998[0], 77002[0], 81000[1], 81002[1], 81003[1], 81005[1], 81015[1], 82013[1], 90865[1], 92511[1], 92512[1], 92516[1], 92520[1], 92537[1], 92538[1], 92950[1], 92953[1], 92960[1], 92961[1], 93000[1], 93005[1], 93010[1], 93040[1], 93041[1], 93042[1], 93050[0], 93303[0], 93304[0], 93306[1], 93307[1], 93308[1], 93312[1], 93313[1], 93314[1], 93315[1], 93316[1], 93317[1], 93318[0], 93351[1], 93355[0], 93451[1], 93456[1], 93457[1], 93561[0], 93562[0], 93701[0], 93922[1], 93923[1], 93924[1], 93925[1], 93926[1], 93930[1], 93931[1], 93970[1], 93971[1], 93975[1], 93976[1], 93978[1], 93979[1], 93980[1], 93981[1], 94002[1], 94004[1], 94200[1], 94250[0], 94640[1], 94644[1], 94660[1], 94662[1], 94680[1], 94681[1], 94690[1], 94760[0], 94761[0], 94762[1], 94770[1], 95812[0], 95813[0], 95816[0], 95819[0], 95822[0], 95829[0], 95955[0], 95956[0], 95957[0], 96360[0], 96365[0], 96372[0], 96373[0], 96374[0], 96375[0], 96376[0], 96377[0], 99151[0], 99152[0], 99153[0], 99155[0], 99156[0], 99157[0], 99201[0], 99202[0], 99203[0], 99204[0], 99205[0], 99211[0], 99212[0], 99213[0], 99214[0], 99215[0], 99217[0], 99218[0], 99219[0], 99220[0], 99221[0], 99222[0], 99223[0], 99224[0], 99225[0], 99226[0], 99231[0], 99232[0], 99233[0], 99234[0], 99235[0], 99236[0], 99238[0], 99239[0], 99281[0], 99282[0], 99283[0], 99284[0], 99285[0], 99304[0], 99305[0], 99306[0], 99307[0], 99308[0], 99309[0], 99310[0], 99315[0], 99318[0], 99324[0], 99325[0], 99326[0], 99327[0], 99328[0], 99334[0], 99335[0], 99336[0], 99337[0], 99341[0], 99342[0], 99343[0], 99347[0], 99348[0], 99349[0], 99354[0], 99355[0], 99356[0], 99357[0], 99358[0], 99359[0], 99415[0], 99416[0], 99446[0], 99447[0], 99448[0], 99449[0], 99451[0], 99452[0], 99466[0], 99468[0], 99469[0], 99471[0], 99472[0], 99475[0], 99476[0], 99477[0], 99478[0], 99479[0], 99480[0], 99483[0], 99485[0], 99497[0], C8921[1], C8922[1], C8923[1], C8924[1], C8925[1], C8926[1], C8927[0], C8929[1], C8930[1], G0380[1], G0381[1], G0382[1], G0383[1], G0384[1], G0406[0], G0407[0], G0408[0], G0425[0], G0426[0], G0427[0], G0463[0], G0500[0], G0508[0], G0509[0]
00145	01996[1], 0213T[1], 0216T[1], 0228T[1], 0230T[1], 31505[1], 31515[1], 31527[1], 31622[1], 31634[1], 31645[1], 31647[1], 36000[1], 36010[0], 36011[1], 36012[1], 36013[1], 36014[1], 36015[1], 36400[1], 36405[1], 36406[1], 36410[1], 36420[1], 36425[1], 36430[1], 36440[1], 36591[0], 36592[0], 36600[1], 36640[1], 43752[1], 43753[1], 43754[1], 61026[1], 61055[1], 62280[1], 62281[1], 62282[1], 62284[1], 62320[1], 62321[1], 62322[1], 62323[1], 62324[1], 62325[1], 62326[1], 62327[1], 64400[1], 64402[1], 64405[1], 64408[1], 64410[1], 64413[1], 64415[1], 64416[1], 64417[1], 64418[1], 64420[1], 64421[1], 64425[1], 64430[1], 64435[1], 64445[1], 64446[1], 64447[1], 64448[1], 64449[1], 64450[1], 64461[1], 64463[1], 64479[1], 64483[1], 64486[1], 64487[1], 64488[1], 64489[1], 64490[1], 64493[1], 64505[1], 64510[1], 64517[1], 64520[1], 64530[1], 64553[1], 64555[1], 67500[0], 76000[1], 76970[1], 76998[0], 77002[0], 90865[1], 92511[1], 92512[1], 92516[1], 92520[1], 92537[1], 92538[1], 92950[1], 92953[1], 92960[1], 92961[1], 93000[1], 93005[1], 93010[1], 93040[1], 93041[1], 93042[1], 93050[0], 93303[0], 93304[0], 93306[1], 93307[1], 93308[1], 93312[1], 93313[1], 93314[1], 93315[1], 93316[1], 93317[1], 93318[0], 93351[1], 93355[0], 93451[1], 93456[1], 93457[1], 93561[0], 93562[0], 93701[0], 93922[1], 93923[1], 93924[1], 93925[1], 93926[1], 93930[1], 93931[1], 93970[1], 93971[1], 93975[1], 93976[1], 93978[1], 93979[1], 93980[1], 93981[1], 94002[1], 94004[1], 94200[1], 94250[0], 94640[1], 94644[1], 94660[1], 94662[1], 94680[1], 94681[1], 94690[1], 94760[0], 94761[0], 94762[1], 94770[1], 95812[0], 95813[0], 95816[0], 95819[0], 95822[0], 95829[0], 95955[0], 95956[0], 95957[0], 96360[0], 96365[0], 96372[0], 96373[0], 96374[0], 96375[0], 96376[0], 96377[0], 99151[0], 99152[0], 99153[0], 99155[0], 99156[0], 99157[0], 99201[0], 99202[0], 99203[0], 99204[0], 99205[0], 99211[0], 99212[0], 99213[0], 99214[0], 99215[0], 99217[0], 99218[0], 99219[0], 99220[0], 99221[0], 99222[0], 99223[0], 99224[0], 99225[0], 99226[0], 99231[0], 99232[0], 99233[0], 99234[0], 99235[0], 99236[0], 99238[0], 99239[0], 99281[0], 99282[0], 99283[0], 99284[0], 99285[0], 99304[0], 99305[0], 99306[0], 99307[0], 99308[0], 99309[0], 99310[0], 99315[0], 99318[0], 99324[0], 99325[0], 99326[0], 99327[0], 99328[0], 99334[0], 99335[0], 99336[0], 99337[0], 99341[0], 99342[0], 99343[0], 99347[0], 99348[0], 99349[0], 99354[0], 99355[0], 99356[0], 99357[0], 99358[0], 99359[0], 99415[0], 99416[0], 99446[0], 99447[0], 99448[0], 99449[0], 99451[0], 99452[0], 99466[0], 99468[0], 99469[0], 99471[0], 99472[0], 99475[0], 99476[0], 99477[0], 99478[0], 99479[0], 99480[0], 99483[0], 99485[0], 99497[0], C8921[1], C8922[1], C8923[1], C8924[1], C8925[1], C8926[1], C8927[0], C8929[1], C8930[1], G0380[1], G0381[1], G0382[1], G0383[1], G0384[1], G0406[0], G0407[0], G0408[0], G0425[0], G0426[0], G0427[0], G0463[0], G0500[0], G0508[0], G0509[0]
00147	01996[1], 0213T[1], 0216T[1], 0228T[1], 0230T[1], 31505[1], 31515[1], 31527[1], 31622[1], 31634[1], 31645[1], 31647[1], 36000[1], 36010[0], 36011[1], 36012[1], 36013[1], 36014[1], 36015[1], 36400[1], 36405[1], 36406[1], 36410[1], 36420[1], 36425[1], 36430[1], 36440[1], 36591[0], 36592[0], 36600[1], 36640[1], 43752[1], 43753[1], 43754[1], 61026[1], 61055[1], 62280[1], 62281[1], 62282[1], 62284[1], 62320[1], 62321[1], 62322[1], 62323[1], 62324[1], 62325[1], 62326[1], 62327[1], 64400[1], 64402[1], 64405[1], 64408[1], 64410[1], 64413[1], 64415[1], 64416[1], 64417[1], 64418[1], 64420[1], 64421[1], 64425[1], 64430[1], 64435[1], 64445[1], 64446[1], 64447[1], 64448[1], 64449[1], 64450[1], 64461[1], 64463[1], 64479[1], 64483[1], 64486[1], 64487[1], 64488[1], 64489[1], 64490[1], 64493[1], 64505[1], 64510[1], 64517[1], 64520[1], 64530[1], 64553[1], 64555[1], 67500[1], 76000[1], 76970[1], 76998[0], 77002[0], 90865[1], 92511[1], 92512[1], 92516[1], 92520[1], 92537[1], 92538[1], 92950[1], 92953[1], 92960[1], 92961[1], 93000[1], 93005[1], 93010[1], 93040[1], 93041[1], 93042[1], 93050[0], 93303[0], 93304[0], 93306[1], 93307[1], 93308[1], 93312[1], 93313[1], 93314[1], 93315[1], 93316[1], 93317[1], 93318[0], 93351[1], 93355[0], 93451[1], 93456[1], 93457[1], 93561[0], 93562[0], 93701[0], 93922[1], 93923[1], 93924[1], 93925[1], 93926[1], 93930[1], 93931[1], 93970[1], 93971[1], 93975[1], 93976[1], 93978[1], 93979[1], 93980[1], 93981[1], 94002[1], 94004[1], 94200[1], 94250[0], 94640[1], 94644[1], 94660[1], 94662[1], 94680[1], 94681[1], 94690[1], 94760[0], 94761[0], 94762[1], 94770[1], 95812[0], 95813[0], 95816[0], 95819[0], 95822[0], 95829[0], 95955[0], 95956[0], 95957[0], 96360[0], 96365[0], 96372[0], 96373[0], 96374[0], 96375[0], 96376[0], 96377[0], 99151[0], 99152[0], 99153[0], 99155[0], 99156[0], 99157[0], 99201[0], 99202[0], 99203[0], 99204[0], 99205[0], 99211[0], 99212[0], 99213[0], 99214[0], 99215[0], 99217[0], 99218[0], 99219[0], 99220[0], 99221[0], 99222[0], 99223[0], 99224[0], 99225[0], 99226[0], 99231[0], 99232[0], 99233[0], 99234[0], 99235[0], 99236[0], 99238[0], 99239[0], 99281[0], 99282[0], 99283[0], 99284[0], 99285[0], 99304[0], 99305[0], 99306[0], 99307[0], 99308[0], 99309[0], 99310[0], 99315[0], 99318[0], 99324[0], 99325[0], 99326[0], 99327[0], 99328[0], 99334[0], 99335[0], 99336[0], 99337[0], 99341[0], 99342[0], 99343[0], 99347[0], 99348[0], 99349[0], 99354[0], 99355[0], 99356[0], 99357[0], 99358[0], 99359[0], 99415[0], 99416[0], 99446[0], 99447[0], 99448[0], 99449[0], 99451[0], 99452[0], 99466[0], 99468[0], 99469[0], 99471[0], 99472[0], 99475[0], 99476[0], 99477[0], 99478[0], 99479[0], 99480[0], 99483[0], 99485[0], 99497[0], C8921[1], C8922[1], C8923[1], C8924[1], C8925[1], C8926[1], C8927[0], C8929[1], C8930[1], G0380[1], G0381[1], G0382[1], G0383[1], G0384[1], G0406[0], G0407[0], G0408[0], G0425[0], G0426[0], G0427[0], G0463[0], G0500[0], G0508[0], G0509[0]
00148	01996[1], 0213T[1], 0216T[1], 0228T[1], 0230T[1], 31505[1], 31515[1], 31527[1], 31622[1], 31634[1], 31645[1], 31647[1], 36000[1], 36010[0], 36011[1], 36012[1], 36013[1], 36014[1], 36015[1], 36400[1], 36405[1], 36406[1], 36410[1], 36420[1], 36425[1], 36430[1], 36440[1], 36591[0], 36592[0], 36600[1], 36640[1], 43752[1], 43753[1], 43754[1], 61026[1], 61055[1], 62280[1], 62281[1], 62282[1], 62284[1], 62320[1], 62321[1], 62322[1], 62323[1], 62324[1], 62325[1], 62326[1], 62327[1], 64400[1], 64402[1], 64405[1], 64408[1], 64410[1], 64413[1], 64415[1], 64416[1], 64417[1], 64418[1], 64420[1], 64421[1], 64425[1], 64430[1], 64435[1], 64445[1], 64446[1], 64447[1], 64448[1], 64449[1], 64450[1], 64461[1], 64463[1], 64479[1], 64483[1], 64486[1], 64487[1], 64488[1], 64489[1], 64490[1], 64493[1], 64505[1], 64510[1], 64517[1], 64520[1], 64530[1], 64553[1], 64555[1], 67500[1], 76000[1], 76970[1], 76998[0], 77002[0], 90865[1], 92511[1], 92512[1], 92516[1], 92520[1], 92537[1], 92538[1], 92950[1], 92953[1], 92960[1], 92961[1], 93000[1], 93005[1], 93010[1], 93040[1], 93041[1], 93042[1], 93050[0], 93303[0], 93304[0], 93306[1], 93307[1], 93308[1], 93312[1], 93313[1], 93314[1], 93315[1], 93316[1], 93317[1], 93318[0], 93351[1], 93355[0], 93451[1], 93456[1], 93457[1], 93561[0], 93562[0], 93701[0], 93922[1], 93923[1], 93924[1], 93925[1], 93926[1], 93930[1], 93931[1], 93970[1], 93971[1], 93975[1], 93976[1], 93978[1], 93979[1], 93980[1], 93981[1], 94002[1], 94004[1], 94200[1], 94250[0], 94640[1], 94644[1], 94660[1], 94662[1], 94680[1], 94681[1], 94690[1], 94760[0], 94761[0], 94762[1], 94770[1], 95812[0], 95813[0], 95816[0], 95819[0], 95822[0], 95829[0], 95955[0], 95956[0], 95957[0], 96360[0], 96365[0], 96372[0], 96373[0], 96374[0], 96375[0], 96376[0], 96377[0], 99151[0], 99152[0], 99153[0], 99155[0], 99156[0], 99157[0], 99201[0], 99202[0], 99203[0], 99204[0], 99205[0], 99211[0], 99212[0], 99213[0], 99214[0], 99215[0], 99217[0], 99218[0], 99219[0], 99220[0], 99221[0], 99222[0], 99223[0], 99224[0], 99225[0], 99226[0], 99231[0], 99232[0], 99233[0], 99234[0], 99235[0], 99236[0], 99238[0], 99239[0], 99281[0], 99282[0], 99283[0], 99284[0], 99285[0], 99304[0], 99305[0], 99306[0], 99307[0], 99308[0], 99309[0], 99310[0], 99315[0], 99318[0], 99324[0], 99325[0], 99326[0], 99327[0], 99328[0], 99334[0], 99335[0], 99336[0], 99337[0], 99341[0], 99342[0], 99343[0], 99347[0], 99348[0], 99349[0], 99354[0], 99355[0], 99356[0], 99357[0], 99358[0], 99359[0], 99415[0], 99416[0], 99446[0], 99447[0], 99448[0], 99449[0], 99451[0], 99452[0], 99466[0], 99468[0], 99469[0], 99471[0], 99472[0], 99475[0], 99476[0], 99477[0], 99478[0], 99479[0], 99480[0], 99483[0], 99485[0], 99497[0], C8921[1], C8922[1], C8923[1], C8924[1], C8925[1], C8926[1], C8927[0], C8929[1], C8930[1], G0380[1], G0381[1], G0382[1], G0383[1], G0384[1], G0406[0], G0407[0], G0408[0], G0425[0], G0426[0], G0427[0], G0463[0], G0500[0], G0508[0], G0509[0]
00160	01996[1], 0213T[1], 0216T[1], 0228T[1], 0230T[1], 31505[1], 31515[1], 31527[1], 31622[1], 31634[1], 31645[1], 31647[1], 36000[1], 36010[0], 36011[1], 36012[1], 36013[1], 36014[1], 36015[1], 36400[1],

0 = Modifier usage not allowed or inappropriate   1 = Modifier usage allowed

Appendix A: NCCI - CPT Codes

CPT © 2018 American Medical Association. All Rights Reserved.

Code 1	Code 2
	36405[1], 36406[1], 36410[1], 36420[1], 36425[1], 36430[1], 36440[1], 36591[0], 36592[0], 36600[1], 36640[1], 43752[1], 43753[1], 43754[1], 61026[1], 61055[1], 62280[1], 62281[1], 62282[1], 62284[1], 62320[1], 62321[1], 62322[1], 62323[1], 62324[1], 62325[1], 62326[1], 62327[1], 64400[1], 64402[1], 64405[1], 64408[1], 64410[1], 64413[1], 64415[1], 64416[1], 64417[1], 64418[1], 64420[1], 64421[1], 64425[1], 64430[1], 64435[1], 64445[1], 64446[1], 64447[1], 64448[1], 64449[1], 64450[1], 64461[1], 64463[1], 64479[1], 64483[1], 64486[1], 64487[1], 64488[1], 64489[1], 64490[1], 64493[1], 64505[1], 64510[1], 64517[1], 64520[1], 64530[1], 64553[1], 64555[1], 67500[1], 76000[1], 76970[1], 76998[0], 77002[0], 90865[1], 92511[1], 92512[1], 92516[1], 92520[1], 92537[1], 92538[1], 92950[1], 92953[1], 92960[1], 92961[1], 93000[1], 93005[1], 93010[1], 93040[1], 93041[1], 93042[1], 93050[0], 93303[0], 93304[0], 93306[1], 93307[1], 93308[1], 93312[1], 93313[1], 93314[1], 93315[1], 93316[1], 93317[1], 93318[0], 93351[1], 93355[0], 93451[1], 93456[1], 93457[1], 93561[0], 93562[0], 93701[0], 93922[1], 93923[1], 93924[1], 93925[1], 93926[1], 93930[1], 93931[1], 93970[1], 93971[1], 93975[1], 93976[1], 93978[1], 93979[1], 93980[1], 93981[1], 94002[1], 94004[1], 94200[1], 94250[0], 94640[1], 94644[1], 94660[1], 94662[1], 94680[1], 94681[1], 94690[1], 94760[0], 94761[0], 94762[1], 94770[1], 95812[0], 95813[0], 95816[0], 95819[0], 95822[0], 95829[0], 95955[0], 95956[0], 95957[0], 96360[0], 96365[0], 96372[0], 96373[0], 96374[0], 96375[0], 96376[0], 96377[0], 99151[0], 99152[0], 99153[0], 99155[0], 99156[0], 99157[0], 99201[0], 99202[0], 99203[0], 99204[0], 99205[0], 99211[0], 99212[0], 99213[0], 99214[0], 99215[0], 99217[0], 99218[0], 99219[0], 99220[0], 99221[0], 99222[0], 99223[0], 99224[0], 99225[0], 99226[0], 99231[0], 99232[0], 99233[0], 99234[0], 99235[0], 99236[0], 99238[0], 99239[0], 99281[0], 99282[0], 99283[0], 99284[0], 99285[0], 99304[0], 99305[0], 99306[0], 99307[0], 99308[0], 99309[0], 99310[0], 99315[0], 99318[0], 99324[0], 99325[0], 99326[0], 99327[0], 99328[0], 99334[0], 99335[0], 99336[0], 99337[0], 99341[0], 99342[0], 99343[0], 99347[0], 99348[0], 99349[0], 99354[0], 99355[0], 99356[0], 99357[0], 99358[0], 99359[0], 99415[0], 99416[0], 99446[0], 99447[0], 99448[0], 99449[0], 99451[0], 99452[0], 99466[0], 99468[0], 99469[0], 99471[0], 99472[0], 99475[0], 99476[0], 99477[0], 99478[0], 99479[0], 99480[0], 99483[0], 99485[0], 99497[0], C8921[1], C8922[1], C8923[1], C8924[1], C8925[1], C8926[1], C8927[0], C8929[1], C8930[1], G0380[1], G0381[1], G0382[1], G0383[1], G0384[1], G0406[0], G0407[0], G0408[0], G0425[0], G0426[0], G0427[0], G0463[0], G0500[0], G0508[0], G0509[0]
00162	01996[1], 0213T[1], 0216T[1], 0228T[1], 0230T[1], 31505[1], 31515[1], 31527[1], 31622[1], 31634[1], 31645[1], 31647[1], 36000[1], 36010[0], 36011[1], 36012[1], 36013[1], 36014[1], 36015[1], 36400[1], 36405[1], 36406[1], 36410[1], 36420[1], 36425[1], 36430[1], 36440[1], 36591[0], 36592[0], 36600[1], 36640[1], 43752[1], 43753[1], 43754[1], 61026[1], 61055[1], 62280[1], 62281[1], 62282[1], 62284[1], 62320[1], 62321[1], 62322[1], 62323[1], 62324[1], 62325[1], 62326[1], 62327[1], 64400[1], 64402[1], 64405[1], 64408[1], 64410[1], 64413[1], 64415[1], 64416[1], 64417[1], 64418[1], 64420[1], 64421[1], 64425[1], 64430[1], 64435[1], 64445[1], 64446[1], 64447[1], 64448[1], 64449[1], 64450[1], 64461[1], 64463[1], 64479[1], 64483[1], 64486[1], 64487[1], 64488[1], 64489[1], 64490[1], 64493[1], 64505[1], 64510[1], 64517[1], 64520[1], 64530[1], 64553[1], 64555[1], 67500[1], 76000[1], 76970[1], 76998[0], 77002[0], 90865[1], 92511[1], 92512[1], 92516[1], 92520[1], 92537[1], 92538[1], 92950[1], 92953[1], 92960[1], 92961[1], 93000[1], 93005[1], 93010[1], 93040[1], 93041[1], 93042[1], 93050[0], 93303[0], 93304[0], 93306[1], 93307[1], 93308[1], 93312[1], 93313[1], 93314[1], 93315[1], 93316[1], 93317[1], 93318[0], 93351[1], 93355[0], 93451[1], 93456[1], 93457[1], 93561[0], 93562[0], 93701[0], 93922[1], 93923[1], 93924[1], 93925[1], 93926[1], 93930[1], 93931[1], 93970[1], 93971[1], 93975[1], 93976[1], 93978[1], 93979[1], 93980[1], 93981[1], 94002[1], 94004[1], 94200[1], 94250[0], 94640[1], 94644[1], 94660[1], 94662[1], 94680[1], 94681[1], 94690[1], 94760[0], 94761[0], 94762[1], 94770[1], 95812[0], 95813[0], 95816[0], 95819[0], 95822[0], 95829[0], 95955[0], 95956[0], 95957[0], 96360[0], 96365[0], 96372[0], 96373[0], 96374[0], 96375[0], 96376[0], 96377[0], 99151[0], 99152[0], 99153[0], 99155[0], 99156[0], 99157[0], 99201[0], 99202[0], 99203[0], 99204[0], 99205[0], 99211[0], 99212[0], 99213[0], 99214[0], 99215[0], 99217[0], 99218[0], 99219[0], 99220[0], 99221[0], 99222[0], 99223[0], 99224[0], 99225[0], 99226[0], 99231[0], 99232[0], 99233[0], 99234[0], 99235[0], 99236[0], 99238[0], 99239[0], 99281[0], 99282[0], 99283[0], 99284[0], 99285[0], 99304[0], 99305[0], 99306[0], 99307[0], 99308[0], 99309[0], 99310[0], 99315[0], 99318[0], 99324[0], 99325[0], 99326[0], 99327[0], 99328[0], 99334[0], 99335[0], 99336[0], 99337[0], 99341[0], 99342[0], 99343[0], 99347[0], 99348[0], 99349[0], 99354[0], 99355[0], 99356[0], 99357[0], 99358[0], 99359[0], 99415[0], 99416[0], 99446[0], 99447[0], 99448[0], 99449[0], 99451[0], 99452[0], 99466[0], 99468[0], 99469[0], 99471[0], 99472[0], 99475[0], 99476[0], 99477[0], 99478[0], 99479[0], 99480[0], 99483[0], 99485[0], 99497[0], C8921[1], C8922[1], C8923[1], C8924[1], C8925[1], C8926[1], C8927[0], C8929[1], C8930[1], G0380[1], G0381[1], G0382[1], G0383[1], G0384[1], G0406[0], G0407[0], G0408[0], G0425[0], G0426[0], G0427[0], G0463[0], G0500[0], G0508[0], G0509[0]
00164	01996[1], 0213T[1], 0216T[1], 0228T[1], 0230T[1], 31505[1], 31515[1], 31527[1], 31622[1], 31634[1], 31645[1], 31647[1], 36000[1], 36010[0], 36011[1], 36012[1], 36013[1], 36014[1], 36015[1], 36400[1], 36405[1], 36406[1], 36410[1], 36420[1], 36425[1], 36430[1], 36440[1], 36591[0], 36592[0], 36600[1], 36640[1], 43752[1], 43753[1], 43754[1], 61026[1], 61055[1], 62280[1], 62281[1], 62282[1], 62284[1], 62320[1], 62321[1], 62322[1], 62323[1], 62324[1], 62325[1], 62326[1], 62327[1], 64400[1], 64402[1], 64405[1], 64408[1], 64410[1], 64413[1], 64415[1], 64416[1], 64417[1], 64418[1], 64420[1], 64421[1], 64425[1], 64430[1], 64435[1], 64445[1], 64446[1], 64447[1], 64448[1], 64449[1], 64450[1], 64461[1], 64463[1], 64479[1], 64483[1], 64486[1], 64487[1], 64488[1], 64489[1], 64490[1], 64493[1], 64505[1], 64510[1], 64517[1], 64520[1], 64530[1], 64553[1], 64555[1], 67500[1], 76000[1], 76970[1], 76998[0], 77002[0], 90865[1], 92511[1], 92512[1], 92516[1], 92520[1], 92537[1], 92538[1], 92950[1], 92953[1], 92960[1], 92961[1], 93000[1], 93005[1], 93010[1], 93040[1], 93041[1], 93042[1], 93050[0], 93303[0], 93304[0], 93306[1], 93307[1], 93308[1], 93312[1], 93313[1], 93314[1], 93315[1], 93316[1], 93317[1], 93318[0], 93351[1], 93355[0], 93451[1], 93456[1], 93457[1], 93561[0], 93562[0], 93701[0], 93922[1], 93923[1], 93924[1], 93925[1], 93926[1], 93930[1], 93931[1], 93970[1], 93971[1], 93975[1], 93976[1], 93978[1], 93979[1], 93980[1], 93981[1], 94002[1], 94004[1], 94200[1], 94250[0], 94640[1], 94644[1], 94660[1], 94662[1], 94680[1], 94681[1], 94690[1], 94760[0], 94761[0], 94762[1], 94770[1], 95812[0], 95813[0], 95816[0], 95819[0], 95822[0], 95829[0], 95955[0], 95956[0], 95957[0], 96360[0], 96365[0], 96372[0], 96373[0], 96374[0], 96375[0], 96376[0], 96377[0], 99151[0], 99152[0], 99153[0], 99155[0], 99156[0], 99157[0], 99201[0], 99202[0], 99203[0], 99204[0], 99205[0], 99211[0], 99212[0], 99213[0], 99214[0], 99215[0], 99217[0], 99218[0], 99219[0], 99220[0], 99221[0], 99222[0], 99223[0], 99224[0], 99225[0], 99226[0], 99231[0], 99232[0], 99233[0], 99234[0], 99235[0], 99236[0], 99238[0], 99239[0], 99281[0], 99282[0], 99283[0], 99284[0], 99285[0], 99304[0], 99305[0], 99306[0], 99307[0], 99308[0], 99309[0], 99310[0], 99315[0], 99318[0], 99324[0], 99325[0], 99326[0], 99327[0], 99328[0], 99334[0], 99335[0], 99336[0], 99337[0], 99341[0], 99342[0], 99343[0], 99347[0], 99348[0], 99349[0], 99354[0], 99355[0], 99356[0], 99357[0], 99358[0], 99359[0], 99415[0], 99416[0], 99446[0], 99447[0], 99448[0], 99449[0], 99451[0], 99452[0], 99466[0], 99468[0], 99469[0], 99471[0], 99472[0], 99475[0], 99476[0], 99477[0], 99478[0], 99479[0], 99480[0], 99483[0], 99485[0], 99497[0], C8921[1], C8922[1], C8923[1], C8924[1], C8925[1], C8926[1], C8927[0], C8929[1], C8930[1], G0380[1], G0381[1], G0382[1], G0383[1], G0384[1], G0406[0], G0407[0], G0408[0], G0425[0], G0426[0], G0427[0], G0463[0], G0500[0], G0508[0], G0509[0]
00170	01996[1], 0213T[1], 0216T[1], 0228T[1], 0230T[1], 31505[1], 31515[1], 31527[1], 31622[1], 31634[1], 31645[1], 31647[1], 36000[1], 36010[0], 36011[1], 36012[1], 36013[1], 36014[1], 36015[1], 36400[1], 36405[1], 36406[1], 36410[1], 36420[1], 36425[1], 36430[1], 36440[1], 36591[0], 36592[0], 36600[1], 36640[1], 43752[1], 43753[1], 43754[1], 61026[1], 61055[1], 62280[1], 62281[1], 62282[1], 62284[1], 62320[1], 62321[1], 62322[1], 62323[1], 62324[1], 62325[1], 62326[1], 62327[1], 64400[1], 64402[1], 64405[1], 64408[1], 64410[1], 64413[1], 64415[1], 64416[1], 64417[1], 64418[1], 64420[1], 64421[1], 64425[1], 64430[1], 64435[1], 64445[1], 64446[1], 64447[1], 64448[1], 64449[1], 64450[1], 64461[1], 64463[1], 64479[1], 64483[1], 64486[1], 64487[1], 64488[1], 64489[1], 64490[1], 64493[1], 64505[1], 64510[1], 64517[1], 64520[1], 64530[1], 64553[1], 64555[1], 67500[1], 76000[1], 76970[1], 76998[0], 77002[0], 90865[1], 92511[1], 92512[1], 92516[1], 92520[1], 92537[1], 92538[1], 92950[1], 92953[1], 92960[1], 92961[1], 93000[1], 93005[1], 93010[1], 93040[1], 93041[1], 93042[1], 93050[0], 93303[0], 93304[0], 93306[1], 93307[1], 93308[1], 93312[1], 93313[1], 93314[1], 93315[1], 93316[1], 93317[1], 93318[0], 93351[1], 93355[0], 93451[1], 93456[1], 93457[1], 93561[0], 93562[0], 93701[0], 93922[1], 93923[1], 93924[1], 93925[1], 93926[1], 93930[1], 93931[1], 93970[1], 93971[1], 93975[1], 93976[1], 93978[1], 93979[1], 93980[1], 93981[1], 94002[1], 94004[1], 94200[1], 94250[0], 94640[1], 94644[1], 94660[1], 94662[1], 94680[1], 94681[1], 94690[1], 94760[0], 94761[0], 94762[1], 94770[1], 95812[0], 95813[0], 95816[0], 95819[0], 95822[0], 95829[0], 95955[0], 95956[0], 95957[0], 96360[0], 96365[0], 96372[0], 96373[0], 96374[0], 96375[0], 96376[0], 96377[0], 99151[0], 99152[0], 99153[0], 99155[0], 99156[0], 99157[0], 99201[0], 99202[0], 99203[0], 99204[0], 99205[0], 99211[0], 99212[0], 99213[0], 99214[0], 99215[0], 99217[0], 99218[0], 99219[0], 99220[0], 99221[0], 99222[0], 99223[0], 99224[0], 99225[0], 99226[0], 99231[0], 99232[0], 99233[0], 99234[0], 99235[0], 99236[0], 99238[0], 99239[0], 99281[0], 99282[0], 99283[0], 99284[0], 99285[0], 99304[0], 99305[0], 99306[0], 99307[0], 99308[0], 99309[0], 99310[0], 99315[0], 99318[0], 99324[0], 99325[0], 99326[0], 99327[0], 99328[0], 99334[0], 99335[0], 99336[0], 99337[0], 99341[0], 99342[0], 99343[0], 99347[0], 99348[0], 99349[0], 99354[0], 99355[0], 99356[0], 99357[0], 99358[0], 99359[0], 99415[0], 99416[0], 99446[0], 99447[0], 99448[0], 99449[0], 99451[0], 99452[0], 99466[0], 99468[0], 99469[0], 99471[0], 99472[0], 99475[0], 99476[0], 99477[0], 99478[0], 99479[0], 99480[0], 99483[0], 99485[0], 99497[0], C8921[1], C8922[1], C8923[1], C8924[1], C8925[1], C8926[1], C8927[0], C8929[1], C8930[1], G0380[1], G0381[1], G0382[1], G0383[1], G0384[1], G0406[0], G0407[0], G0408[0], G0425[0], G0426[0], G0427[0], G0463[0], G0500[0], G0508[0], G0509[0]
00172	01996[1], 0213T[1], 0216T[1], 0228T[1], 0230T[1], 31505[1], 31515[1], 31527[1], 31622[1], 31634[1], 31645[1], 31647[1], 36000[1], 36010[0], 36011[1], 36012[1], 36013[1], 36014[1], 36015[1], 36400[1], 36405[1], 36406[1], 36410[1], 36420[1], 36425[1], 36430[1], 36440[1], 36591[0], 36592[0], 36600[1], 36640[1], 43752[1], 43753[1], 43754[1], 61026[1], 61055[1], 62280[1], 62281[1], 62282[1], 62284[1], 62320[1], 62321[1], 62322[1], 62323[1], 62324[1], 62325[1], 62326[1], 62327[1], 64400[1], 64402[1], 64405[1], 64408[1], 64410[1], 64413[1], 64415[1], 64416[1], 64417[1], 64418[1], 64420[1], 64421[1], 64425[1], 64430[1], 64435[1], 64445[1], 64446[1], 64447[1], 64448[1], 64449[1], 64450[1], 64461[1], 64463[1], 64479[1], 64483[1], 64486[1], 64487[1], 64488[1], 64489[1], 64490[1], 64493[1], 64505[1], 64510[1], 64517[1], 64520[1], 64530[1], 64553[1], 64555[1], 67500[1], 76000[1], 76970[1], 76998[0], 77002[0], 90865[1], 92511[1], 92512[1], 92516[1], 92520[1], 92537[1], 92538[1], 92950[1], 92953[1], 92960[1], 92961[1], 93000[1], 93005[1], 93010[1], 93040[1], 93041[1], 93042[1], 93050[0], 93303[0], 93304[0], 93306[1], 93307[1], 93308[1], 93312[1], 93313[1], 93314[1], 93315[1], 93316[1], 93317[1], 93318[0], 93351[1], 93355[0], 93451[1], 93456[1], 93457[1], 93561[0], 93562[0], 93701[0], 93922[1], 93923[1], 93924[1], 93925[1], 93926[1], 93930[1], 93931[1], 93970[1], 93971[1], 93975[1], 93976[1],

0 = Modifier usage not allowed or inappropriate 1 = Modifier usage allowed

CPT © 2018 American Medical Association. All Rights Reserved.

Code 1	Code 2
	93978[1], 93979[1], 93980[1], 93981[1], 94002[1], 94004[1], 94200[1], 94250[0], 94640[1], 94644[1], 94660[1], 94662[1], 94680[1], 94681[1], 94690[1], 94760[0], 94761[0], 94762[1], 94770[1], 95812[0], 95813[0], 95816[0], 95819[0], 95822[0], 95829[0], 95955[0], 95956[0], 95957[0], 96360[0], 96365[0], 96372[0], 96373[0], 96374[0], 96375[0], 96376[0], 96377[0], 99151[0], 99152[0], 99153[0], 99155[0], 99156[0], 99157[0], 99201[0], 99202[0], 99203[0], 99204[0], 99205[0], 99211[0], 99212[0], 99213[0], 99214[0], 99215[0], 99217[0], 99218[0], 99219[0], 99220[0], 99221[0], 99222[0], 99223[0], 99224[0], 99225[0], 99226[0], 99231[0], 99232[0], 99233[0], 99234[0], 99235[0], 99236[0], 99238[0], 99239[0], 99281[0], 99282[0], 99283[0], 99284[0], 99285[0], 99304[0], 99305[0], 99306[0], 99307[0], 99308[0], 99309[0], 99310[0], 99315[0], 99318[0], 99324[0], 99325[0], 99326[0], 99327[0], 99328[0], 99334[0], 99335[0], 99336[0], 99337[0], 99341[0], 99342[0], 99343[0], 99347[0], 99348[0], 99349[0], 99354[0], 99355[0], 99356[0], 99357[0], 99358[0], 99359[0], 99415[0], 99416[0], 99446[0], 99447[0], 99448[0], 99449[0], 99451[0], 99452[0], 99466[0], 99468[0], 99469[0], 99471[0], 99472[0], 99475[0], 99476[0], 99477[0], 99478[0], 99479[0], 99480[0], 99483[0], 99485[0], 99497[0], C8921[1], C8922[1], C8923[1], C8924[1], C8925[1], C8926[1], C8927[0], C8929[1], C8930[1], G0380[1], G0381[1], G0382[1], G0383[1], G0384[1], G0406[0], G0407[0], G0408[0], G0425[0], G0426[0], G0427[0], G0463[0], G0500[0], G0508[0], G0509[0]
00174	01996[1], 0213T[1], 0216T[1], 0228T[1], 0230T[1], 31505[1], 31515[1], 31527[1], 31622[1], 31634[1], 31645[1], 31647[1], 36000[1], 36010[0], 36011[1], 36012[1], 36013[1], 36014[1], 36015[1], 36400[1], 36405[1], 36406[1], 36410[1], 36420[1], 36425[1], 36430[1], 36440[1], 36591[0], 36592[0], 36600[1], 36640[1], 43752[1], 43753[1], 43754[1], 61026[1], 61055[1], 62280[1], 62281[1], 62282[1], 62284[1], 62320[1], 62321[1], 62322[1], 62323[1], 62324[1], 62325[1], 62326[1], 62327[1], 64400[1], 64402[1], 64405[1], 64408[1], 64410[1], 64413[1], 64415[1], 64416[1], 64417[1], 64418[1], 64420[1], 64421[1], 64425[1], 64430[1], 64435[1], 64445[1], 64446[1], 64447[1], 64448[1], 64449[1], 64450[1], 64461[1], 64463[1], 64479[1], 64483[1], 64486[1], 64487[1], 64488[1], 64489[1], 64490[1], 64493[1], 64505[1], 64510[1], 64517[1], 64520[1], 64530[1], 64553[1], 64555[1], 67500[1], 76000[1], 76970[1], 76998[0], 77002[0], 90865[1], 92511[1], 92512[1], 92516[1], 92520[1], 92537[1], 92538[1], 92950[1], 92953[1], 92960[1], 92961[1], 93000[1], 93005[1], 93010[1], 93040[1], 93041[1], 93042[1], 93050[0], 93303[0], 93304[0], 93306[1], 93307[1], 93308[1], 93312[1], 93313[1], 93314[1], 93315[1], 93316[1], 93317[1], 93318[0], 93351[1], 93355[0], 93451[1], 93456[1], 93457[1], 93561[0], 93562[0], 93701[0], 93922[1], 93923[1], 93924[1], 93925[1], 93926[1], 93930[1], 93931[1], 93970[1], 93971[1], 93975[1], 93976[1], 93978[1], 93979[1], 93980[1], 93981[1], 94002[1], 94004[1], 94200[1], 94250[0], 94640[1], 94644[1], 94660[1], 94662[1], 94680[1], 94681[1], 94690[1], 94760[0], 94761[0], 94762[1], 94770[1], 95812[0], 95813[0], 95816[0], 95819[0], 95822[0], 95829[0], 95955[0], 95956[0], 95957[0], 96360[0], 96365[0], 96372[0], 96373[0], 96374[0], 96375[0], 96376[0], 96377[0], 99151[0], 99152[0], 99153[0], 99155[0], 99156[0], 99157[0], 99201[0], 99202[0], 99203[0], 99204[0], 99205[0], 99211[0], 99212[0], 99213[0], 99214[0], 99215[0], 99217[0], 99218[0], 99219[0], 99220[0], 99221[0], 99222[0], 99223[0], 99224[0], 99225[0], 99226[0], 99231[0], 99232[0], 99233[0], 99234[0], 99235[0], 99236[0], 99238[0], 99239[0], 99281[0], 99282[0], 99283[0], 99284[0], 99285[0], 99304[0], 99305[0], 99306[0], 99307[0], 99308[0], 99309[0], 99310[0], 99315[0], 99318[0], 99324[0], 99325[0], 99326[0], 99327[0], 99328[0], 99334[0], 99335[0], 99336[0], 99337[0], 99341[0], 99342[0], 99343[0], 99347[0], 99348[0], 99349[0], 99354[0], 99355[0], 99356[0], 99357[0], 99358[0], 99359[0], 99415[0], 99416[0], 99446[0], 99447[0], 99448[0], 99449[0], 99451[0], 99452[0], 99466[0], 99468[0], 99469[0], 99471[0], 99472[0], 99475[0], 99476[0], 99477[0], 99478[0], 99479[0], 99480[0], 99483[0], 99485[0], 99497[0], C8921[1], C8922[1], C8923[1], C8924[1], C8925[1], C8926[1], C8927[0], C8929[1], C8930[1], G0380[1], G0381[1], G0382[1], G0383[1], G0384[1], G0406[0], G0407[0], G0408[0], G0425[0], G0426[0], G0427[0], G0463[0], G0500[0], G0508[0], G0509[0]
00176	01996[1], 0213T[1], 0216T[1], 0228T[1], 0230T[1], 31505[1], 31515[1], 31527[1], 31622[1], 31634[1], 31645[1], 31647[1], 36000[1], 36010[0], 36011[1], 36012[1], 36013[1], 36014[1], 36015[1], 36400[1], 36405[1], 36406[1], 36410[1], 36420[1], 36425[1], 36430[1], 36440[1], 36591[0], 36592[0], 36600[1], 36640[1], 43752[1], 43753[1], 43754[1], 61026[1], 61055[1], 62280[1], 62281[1], 62282[1], 62284[1], 62320[1], 62321[1], 62322[1], 62323[1], 62324[1], 62325[1], 62326[1], 62327[1], 64400[1], 64402[1], 64405[1], 64408[1], 64410[1], 64413[1], 64415[1], 64416[1], 64417[1], 64418[1], 64420[1], 64421[1], 64425[1], 64430[1], 64435[1], 64445[1], 64446[1], 64447[1], 64448[1], 64449[1], 64450[1], 64461[1], 64463[1], 64479[1], 64483[1], 64486[1], 64487[1], 64488[1], 64489[1], 64490[1], 64493[1], 64505[1], 64510[1], 64517[1], 64520[1], 64530[1], 64553[1], 64555[1], 67500[1], 76000[1], 76970[1], 76998[0], 77002[0], 90865[1], 92511[1], 92512[1], 92516[1], 92520[1], 92537[1], 92538[1], 92950[1], 92953[1], 92960[1], 92961[1], 93000[1], 93005[1], 93010[1], 93040[1], 93041[1], 93042[1], 93050[0], 93303[0], 93304[0], 93306[1], 93307[1], 93308[1], 93312[1], 93313[1], 93314[1], 93315[1], 93316[1], 93317[1], 93318[0], 93351[1], 93355[0], 93451[1], 93456[1], 93457[1], 93561[0], 93562[0], 93701[0], 93922[1], 93923[1], 93924[1], 93925[1], 93926[1], 93930[1], 93931[1], 93970[1], 93971[1], 93975[1], 93976[1], 93978[1], 93979[1], 93980[1], 93981[1], 94002[1], 94004[1], 94200[1], 94250[0], 94640[1], 94644[1], 94660[1], 94662[1], 94680[1], 94681[1], 94690[1], 94760[0], 94761[0], 94762[1], 94770[1], 95812[0], 95813[0], 95816[0], 95819[0], 95822[0], 95829[0], 95955[0], 95956[0], 95957[0], 96360[0], 96365[0], 96372[0], 96373[0], 96374[0], 96375[0], 96376[0], 96377[0], 99151[0], 99152[0], 99153[0], 99155[0], 99156[0], 99157[0], 99201[0], 99202[0], 99203[0], 99204[0], 99205[0], 99211[0], 99212[0], 99213[0], 99214[0], 99215[0], 99217[0], 99218[0], 99219[0], 99220[0], 99221[0], 99222[0], 99223[0], 99224[0], 99225[0], 99226[0], 99231[0], 99232[0], 99233[0], 99234[0], 99235[0], 99236[0], 99238[0], 99239[0], 99281[0], 99282[0], 99283[0], 99284[0], 99285[0], 99304[0], 99305[0], 99306[0], 99307[0], 99308[0], 99309[0], 99310[0], 99315[0], 99318[0], 99324[0], 99325[0], 99326[0], 99327[0], 99328[0], 99334[0], 99335[0], 99336[0], 99337[0], 99341[0], 99342[0], 99343[0], 99347[0], 99348[0], 99349[0], 99354[0], 99355[0], 99356[0], 99357[0], 99358[0], 99359[0], 99415[0], 99416[0], 99446[0], 99447[0], 99448[0], 99449[0], 99451[0], 99452[0], 99466[0], 99468[0], 99469[0], 99471[0], 99472[0], 99475[0], 99476[0], 99477[0], 99478[0], 99479[0], 99480[0], 99483[0], 99485[0], 99497[0], C8921[1], C8922[1], C8923[1], C8924[1], C8925[1], C8926[1], C8927[0], C8929[1], C8930[1], G0380[1], G0381[1], G0382[1], G0383[1], G0384[1], G0406[0], G0407[0], G0408[0], G0425[0], G0426[0], G0427[0], G0463[0], G0500[0], G0508[0], G0509[0]
00190	01996[1], 0213T[1], 0216T[1], 0228T[1], 0230T[1], 31505[1], 31515[1], 31527[1], 31622[1], 31634[1], 31645[1], 31647[1], 36000[1], 36010[0], 36011[1], 36012[1], 36013[1], 36014[1], 36015[1], 36400[1], 36405[1], 36406[1], 36410[1], 36420[1], 36425[1], 36430[1], 36440[1], 36591[0], 36592[0], 36600[1], 36640[1], 43752[1], 43753[1], 43754[1], 61026[1], 61055[1], 62280[1], 62281[1], 62282[1], 62284[1], 62320[1], 62321[1], 62322[1], 62323[1], 62324[1], 62325[1], 62326[1], 62327[1], 64400[1], 64402[1], 64405[1], 64408[1], 64410[1], 64413[1], 64415[1], 64416[1], 64417[1], 64418[1], 64420[1], 64421[1], 64425[1], 64430[1], 64435[1], 64445[1], 64446[1], 64447[1], 64448[1], 64449[1], 64450[1], 64461[1], 64463[1], 64479[1], 64483[1], 64486[1], 64487[1], 64488[1], 64489[1], 64490[1], 64493[1], 64505[1], 64510[1], 64517[1], 64520[1], 64530[1], 64553[1], 64555[1], 67500[1], 76000[1], 76970[1], 76998[0], 77002[0], 90865[1], 92511[1], 92512[1], 92516[1], 92520[1], 92537[1], 92538[1], 92950[1], 92953[1], 92960[1], 92961[1], 93000[1], 93005[1], 93010[1], 93040[1], 93041[1], 93042[1], 93050[0], 93303[0], 93304[0], 93306[1], 93307[1], 93308[1], 93312[1], 93313[1], 93314[1], 93315[1], 93316[1], 93317[1], 93318[0], 93351[1], 93355[0], 93451[1], 93456[1], 93457[1], 93561[0], 93562[0], 93701[0], 93922[1], 93923[1], 93924[1], 93925[1], 93926[1], 93930[1], 93931[1], 93970[1], 93971[1], 93975[1], 93976[1], 93978[1], 93979[1], 93980[1], 93981[1], 94002[1], 94004[1], 94200[1], 94250[0], 94640[1], 94644[1], 94660[1], 94662[1], 94680[1], 94681[1], 94690[1], 94760[0], 94761[0], 94762[1], 94770[1], 95812[0], 95813[0], 95816[0], 95819[0], 95822[0], 95829[0], 95955[0], 95956[0], 95957[0], 96360[0], 96365[0], 96372[0], 96373[0], 96374[0], 96375[0], 96376[0], 96377[0], 99151[0], 99152[0], 99153[0], 99155[0], 99156[0], 99157[0], 99201[0], 99202[0], 99203[0], 99204[0], 99205[0], 99211[0], 99212[0], 99213[0], 99214[0], 99215[0], 99217[0], 99218[0], 99219[0], 99220[0], 99221[0], 99222[0], 99223[0], 99224[0], 99225[0], 99226[0], 99231[0], 99232[0], 99233[0], 99234[0], 99235[0], 99236[0], 99238[0], 99239[0], 99281[0], 99282[0], 99283[0], 99284[0], 99285[0], 99304[0], 99305[0], 99306[0], 99307[0], 99308[0], 99309[0], 99310[0], 99315[0], 99318[0], 99324[0], 99325[0], 99326[0], 99327[0], 99328[0], 99334[0], 99335[0], 99336[0], 99337[0], 99341[0], 99342[0], 99343[0], 99347[0], 99348[0], 99349[0], 99354[0], 99355[0], 99356[0], 99357[0], 99358[0], 99359[0], 99415[0], 99416[0], 99446[0], 99447[0], 99448[0], 99449[0], 99451[0], 99452[0], 99466[0], 99468[0], 99469[0], 99471[0], 99472[0], 99475[0], 99476[0], 99477[0], 99478[0], 99479[0], 99480[0], 99483[0], 99485[0], 99497[0], C8921[1], C8922[1], C8923[1], C8924[1], C8925[1], C8926[1], C8927[0], C8929[1], C8930[1], G0380[1], G0381[1], G0382[1], G0383[1], G0384[1], G0406[0], G0407[0], G0408[0], G0425[0], G0426[0], G0427[0], G0463[0], G0500[0], G0508[0], G0509[0]
00192	01996[1], 0213T[1], 0216T[1], 0228T[1], 0230T[1], 31505[1], 31515[1], 31527[1], 31622[1], 31634[1], 31645[1], 31647[1], 36000[1], 36010[0], 36011[1], 36012[1], 36013[1], 36014[1], 36015[1], 36400[1], 36405[1], 36406[1], 36410[1], 36420[1], 36425[1], 36430[1], 36440[1], 36591[0], 36592[0], 36600[1], 36640[1], 43752[1], 43753[1], 43754[1], 61026[1], 61055[1], 62280[1], 62281[1], 62282[1], 62284[1], 62320[1], 62321[1], 62322[1], 62323[1], 62324[1], 62325[1], 62326[1], 62327[1], 64400[1], 64402[1], 64405[1], 64408[1], 64410[1], 64413[1], 64415[1], 64416[1], 64417[1], 64418[1], 64420[1], 64421[1], 64425[1], 64430[1], 64435[1], 64445[1], 64446[1], 64447[1], 64448[1], 64449[1], 64450[1], 64461[1], 64463[1], 64479[1], 64483[1], 64486[1], 64487[1], 64488[1], 64489[1], 64490[1], 64493[1], 64505[1], 64510[1], 64517[1], 64520[1], 64530[1], 64553[1], 64555[1], 67500[1], 76000[1], 76970[1], 76998[0], 77002[0], 90865[1], 92511[1], 92512[1], 92516[1], 92520[1], 92537[1], 92538[1], 92950[1], 92953[1], 92960[1], 92961[1], 93000[1], 93005[1], 93010[1], 93040[1], 93041[1], 93042[1], 93050[0], 93303[0], 93304[0], 93306[1], 93307[1], 93308[1], 93312[1], 93313[1], 93314[1], 93315[1], 93316[1], 93317[1], 93318[0], 93351[1], 93355[0], 93451[1], 93456[1], 93457[1], 93561[0], 93562[0], 93701[0], 93922[1], 93923[1], 93924[1], 93925[1], 93926[1], 93930[1], 93931[1], 93970[1], 93971[1], 93975[1], 93976[1], 93978[1], 93979[1], 93980[1], 93981[1], 94002[1], 94004[1], 94200[1], 94250[0], 94640[1], 94644[1], 94660[1], 94662[1], 94680[1], 94681[1], 94690[1], 94760[0], 94761[0], 94762[1], 94770[1], 95812[0], 95813[0], 95816[0], 95819[0], 95822[0], 95829[0], 95955[0], 95956[0], 95957[0], 96360[0], 96365[0], 96372[0], 96373[0], 96374[0], 96375[0], 96376[0], 96377[0], 99151[0], 99152[0], 99153[0], 99155[0], 99156[0], 99157[0], 99201[0], 99202[0], 99203[0], 99204[0], 99205[0], 99211[0], 99212[0], 99213[0], 99214[0], 99215[0], 99217[0], 99218[0], 99219[0], 99220[0], 99221[0], 99222[0], 99223[0], 99224[0], 99225[0], 99226[0], 99231[0], 99232[0], 99233[0], 99234[0], 99235[0], 99236[0], 99238[0], 99239[0], 99281[0], 99282[0], 99283[0], 99284[0], 99285[0], 99304[0], 99305[0], 99306[0], 99307[0], 99308[0], 99309[0], 99310[0], 99315[0], 99318[0], 99324[0], 99325[0], 99326[0], 99327[0], 99328[0], 99334[0], 99335[0], 99336[0], 99337[0], 99341[0], 99342[0], 99343[0], 99347[0], 99348[0], 99349[0], 99354[0], 99355[0], 99356[0], 99357[0], 99358[0], 99359[0], 99415[0], 99416[0], 99446[0], 99447[0], 99448[0], 99449[0], 99451[0], 99452[0], 99466[0], 99468[0], 99469[0], 99471[0], 99472[0], 99475[0], 99476[0],

Appendix A: NCCI - CPT Codes

0 = Modifier usage not allowed or inappropriate 1 = Modifier usage allowed

CPT © 2018 American Medical Association. All Rights Reserved.

Code 1	Code 2
	99477[0], 99478[0], 99479[0], 99480[0], 99483[0], 99485[0], 99497[0], C8921[1], C8922[1], C8923[1], C8924[1], C8925[1], C8926[1], C8927[0], C8929[1], C8930[1], G0380[1], G0381[1], G0382[1], G0383[1], G0384[1], G0406[0], G0407[0], G0408[0], G0425[0], G0426[0], G0427[0], G0463[0], G0500[0], G0508[0], G0509[0]
00210	01996[1], 0213T[1], 0216T[1], 0228T[1], 0230T[1], 0333T[0], 0464T[0], 31505[1], 31515[1], 31527[1], 31622[1], 31634[1], 31645[1], 31647[1], 36000[1], 36010[0], 36011[1], 36012[1], 36013[1], 36014[1], 36015[1], 36400[1], 36405[1], 36406[1], 36410[1], 36420[1], 36425[1], 36430[1], 36440[1], 36591[0], 36592[0], 36600[1], 36640[1], 43752[1], 43753[1], 43754[1], 61026[1], 61055[1], 62280[1], 62281[1], 62282[1], 62284[1], 62320[1], 62321[1], 62322[1], 62323[1], 62324[1], 62325[1], 62326[1], 62327[1], 64400[1], 64402[1], 64405[1], 64408[1], 64410[1], 64413[1], 64415[1], 64416[1], 64417[1], 64418[1], 64420[1], 64421[1], 64425[1], 64430[1], 64435[1], 64445[1], 64446[1], 64447[1], 64448[1], 64449[1], 64450[1], 64461[1], 64463[1], 64479[1], 64483[1], 64486[1], 64487[1], 64488[1], 64489[1], 64490[1], 64493[1], 64505[1], 64510[1], 64517[1], 64520[1], 64530[1], 64553[1], 64555[1], 67500[1], 76000[1], 76970[1], 76998[0], 77002[0], 90865[1], 92511[1], 92512[1], 92516[1], 92520[1], 92537[1], 92538[1], 92585[0], 92950[1], 92953[1], 92960[1], 92961[1], 93000[1], 93005[1], 93010[1], 93040[1], 93041[1], 93042[1], 93050[0], 93303[0], 93304[0], 93306[1], 93307[1], 93308[1], 93312[1], 93313[1], 93314[1], 93315[1], 93316[1], 93317[1], 93318[0], 93351[1], 93355[0], 93451[1], 93456[1], 93457[1], 93561[0], 93562[0], 93701[0], 93922[1], 93923[1], 93924[1], 93925[1], 93926[1], 93930[1], 93931[1], 93970[1], 93971[1], 93975[1], 93976[1], 93978[1], 93979[1], 93980[1], 93981[1], 94002[1], 94004[1], 94200[1], 94250[0], 94640[1], 94644[1], 94660[1], 94662[1], 94680[1], 94681[1], 94690[1], 94760[0], 94761[0], 94762[1], 94770[1], 95812[0], 95813[0], 95816[0], 95819[0], 95822[0], 95829[0], 95860[0], 95861[0], 95863[0], 95864[0], 95865[0], 95866[0], 95867[0], 95868[0], 95869[0], 95870[0], 95907[0], 95908[0], 95909[0], 95910[0], 95911[0], 95912[0], 95913[0], 95925[0], 95926[0], 95927[0], 95928[0], 95929[0], 95930[0], 95933[0], 95937[0], 95938[0], 95939[0], 95940[0], 95955[0], 95956[0], 95957[0], 96360[0], 96365[0], 96372[0], 96373[0], 96374[0], 96375[0], 96376[0], 96377[0], 99151[0], 99152[0], 99153[0], 99155[0], 99156[0], 99157[0], 99201[0], 99202[0], 99203[0], 99204[0], 99205[0], 99211[0], 99212[0], 99213[0], 99214[0], 99215[0], 99217[0], 99218[0], 99219[0], 99220[0], 99221[0], 99222[0], 99223[0], 99224[0], 99225[0], 99226[0], 99231[0], 99232[0], 99233[0], 99234[0], 99235[0], 99236[0], 99238[0], 99239[0], 99281[0], 99282[0], 99283[0], 99284[0], 99285[0], 99304[0], 99305[0], 99306[0], 99307[0], 99308[0], 99309[0], 99310[0], 99315[0], 99318[0], 99324[0], 99325[0], 99326[0], 99327[0], 99328[0], 99334[0], 99335[0], 99336[0], 99337[0], 99341[0], 99342[0], 99343[0], 99347[0], 99348[0], 99349[0], 99354[0], 99355[0], 99356[0], 99357[0], 99358[0], 99359[0], 99415[0], 99416[0], 99446[0], 99447[0], 99448[0], 99449[0], 99451[0], 99452[0], 99466[0], 99468[0], 99469[0], 99471[0], 99472[0], 99475[0], 99476[0], 99477[0], 99478[0], 99479[0], 99480[0], 99483[0], 99485[0], 99497[0], C8921[1], C8922[1], C8923[1], C8924[1], C8925[1], C8926[1], C8927[0], C8929[1], C8930[1], G0380[1], G0381[1], G0382[1], G0383[1], G0384[1], G0406[0], G0407[0], G0408[0], G0425[0], G0426[0], G0427[0], G0453[0], G0463[0], G0500[0], G0508[0], G0509[0]
00211	01996[1], 0213T[1], 0216T[1], 0228T[1], 0230T[1], 0333T[0], 0464T[0], 31505[1], 31515[1], 31527[1], 31622[1], 31634[1], 31645[1], 31647[1], 36000[1], 36010[0], 36011[1], 36012[1], 36013[1], 36014[1], 36015[1], 36400[1], 36405[1], 36406[1], 36410[1], 36420[1], 36425[1], 36430[1], 36440[1], 36591[0], 36592[0], 36600[1], 36640[1], 43752[1], 43753[1], 43754[1], 61026[1], 61055[1], 62280[1], 62281[1], 62282[1], 62284[1], 62320[1], 62321[1], 62322[1], 62323[1], 62324[1], 62325[1], 62326[1], 62327[1], 64400[1], 64402[1], 64405[1], 64408[1], 64410[1], 64413[1], 64415[1], 64416[1], 64417[1], 64418[1], 64420[1], 64421[1], 64425[1], 64430[1], 64435[1], 64445[1], 64446[1], 64447[1], 64448[1], 64449[1], 64450[1], 64461[1], 64463[1], 64479[1], 64483[1], 64486[1], 64487[1], 64488[1], 64489[1], 64490[1], 64493[1], 64505[1], 64510[1], 64517[1], 64520[1], 64530[1], 64553[1], 64555[1], 67500[1], 76000[1], 76970[1], 76998[0], 77002[0], 90865[1], 92511[1], 92512[1], 92516[1], 92520[1], 92537[1], 92538[1], 92585[0], 92950[1], 92953[1], 92960[1], 92961[1], 93000[1], 93005[1], 93010[1], 93040[1], 93041[1], 93042[1], 93050[0], 93303[0], 93304[0], 93307[1], 93308[1], 93312[1], 93313[1], 93314[1], 93315[1], 93316[1], 93317[1], 93318[0], 93355[0], 93451[1], 93456[1], 93457[1], 93561[0], 93562[0], 93701[0], 93922[1], 93923[1], 93924[1], 93925[1], 93926[1], 93930[1], 93931[1], 93970[1], 93971[1], 93975[1], 93976[1], 93978[1], 93979[1], 93980[1], 93981[1], 94002[1], 94004[1], 94200[1], 94250[0], 94640[1], 94660[1], 94662[1], 94680[1], 94681[1], 94690[1], 94760[0], 94761[0], 94762[1], 94770[1], 95812[0], 95813[0], 95816[0], 95819[0], 95822[0], 95829[0], 95860[0], 95861[0], 95863[0], 95864[0], 95865[0], 95866[0], 95867[0], 95868[0], 95869[0], 95870[0], 95907[0], 95908[0], 95909[0], 95910[0], 95911[0], 95912[0], 95913[0], 95925[0], 95926[0], 95927[0], 95928[0], 95929[0], 95930[0], 95933[0], 95937[0], 95938[0], 95939[0], 95940[0], 95955[0], 95956[0], 95957[0], 96360[0], 96365[0], 96372[0], 96373[0], 96374[0], 96375[0], 96376[0], 96377[0], 99151[0], 99152[0], 99153[0], 99155[0], 99156[0], 99157[0], 99201[0], 99202[0], 99203[0], 99204[0], 99205[0], 99211[0], 99212[0], 99213[0], 99214[0], 99215[0], 99217[0], 99218[0], 99219[0], 99220[0], 99221[0], 99222[0], 99223[0], 99224[0], 99225[0], 99226[0], 99231[0], 99232[0], 99233[0], 99234[0], 99235[0], 99236[0], 99238[0], 99239[0], 99281[0], 99282[0], 99283[0], 99284[0], 99285[0], 99304[0], 99305[0], 99306[0], 99307[0], 99308[0], 99309[0], 99310[0], 99315[0], 99318[0], 99324[0], 99325[0], 99326[0], 99327[0], 99328[0], 99334[0], 99335[0], 99336[0], 99337[0], 99341[0], 99342[0], 99343[0], 99347[0], 99348[0], 99349[0], 99354[0], 99355[0], 99356[0], 99357[0], 99358[0], 99359[0], 99415[0], 99416[0], 99446[0], 99447[0], 99448[0], 99449[0], 99451[0], 99452[0], 99466[0], 99468[0], 99469[0], 99471[0], 99472[0], 99475[0], 99476[0], 99477[0], 99478[0],
	99479[0], 99480[0], 99483[0], 99485[0], 99497[0], C8921[1], C8922[1], C8923[1], C8924[1], C8925[1], C8926[1], C8927[1], C8929[1], G0406[0], G0407[0], G0408[0], G0425[0], G0426[0], G0427[0], G0453[0], G0463[0], G0500[0], G0508[0], G0509[0]
00212	01996[1], 0213T[1], 0216T[1], 0228T[1], 0230T[1], 0333T[0], 0464T[0], 31505[1], 31515[1], 31527[1], 31622[1], 31634[1], 31645[1], 31647[1], 36000[1], 36010[0], 36011[1], 36012[1], 36013[1], 36014[1], 36015[1], 36400[1], 36405[1], 36406[1], 36410[1], 36420[1], 36425[1], 36430[1], 36440[1], 36591[0], 36592[0], 36600[1], 36640[1], 43752[1], 43753[1], 43754[1], 61026[1], 61055[1], 62280[1], 62281[1], 62282[1], 62284[1], 62320[1], 62321[1], 62322[1], 62323[1], 62324[1], 62325[1], 62326[1], 62327[1], 64400[1], 64402[1], 64405[1], 64408[1], 64410[1], 64413[1], 64415[1], 64416[1], 64417[1], 64418[1], 64420[1], 64421[1], 64425[1], 64430[1], 64435[1], 64445[1], 64446[1], 64447[1], 64448[1], 64449[1], 64450[1], 64461[1], 64463[1], 64479[1], 64483[1], 64486[1], 64487[1], 64488[1], 64489[1], 64490[1], 64493[1], 64505[1], 64510[1], 64517[1], 64520[1], 64530[1], 64553[1], 64555[1], 67500[1], 76000[1], 76970[1], 76998[0], 77002[0], 90865[1], 92511[1], 92512[1], 92516[1], 92520[1], 92537[1], 92538[1], 92585[0], 92950[1], 92953[1], 92960[1], 92961[1], 93000[1], 93005[1], 93010[1], 93040[1], 93041[1], 93042[1], 93050[0], 93303[0], 93304[0], 93306[1], 93307[1], 93308[1], 93312[1], 93313[1], 93314[1], 93315[1], 93316[1], 93317[1], 93318[0], 93351[1], 93355[0], 93451[1], 93456[1], 93457[1], 93561[0], 93562[0], 93701[0], 93922[1], 93923[1], 93924[1], 93925[1], 93926[1], 93930[1], 93931[1], 93970[1], 93971[1], 93975[1], 93976[1], 93978[1], 93979[1], 93980[1], 93981[1], 94002[1], 94004[1], 94200[1], 94250[0], 94640[1], 94644[1], 94660[1], 94662[1], 94680[1], 94681[1], 94690[1], 94760[0], 94761[0], 94762[1], 94770[1], 95812[0], 95813[0], 95816[0], 95819[0], 95822[0], 95829[0], 95860[0], 95861[0], 95863[0], 95864[0], 95865[0], 95866[0], 95867[0], 95868[0], 95869[0], 95870[0], 95907[0], 95908[0], 95909[0], 95910[0], 95911[0], 95912[0], 95913[0], 95925[0], 95926[0], 95927[0], 95928[0], 95929[0], 95930[0], 95933[0], 95937[0], 95938[0], 95939[0], 95940[0], 95955[0], 95956[0], 95957[0], 96360[0], 96365[0], 96372[0], 96373[0], 96374[0], 96375[0], 96376[0], 96377[0], 99151[0], 99152[0], 99153[0], 99155[0], 99156[0], 99157[0], 99201[0], 99202[0], 99203[0], 99204[0], 99205[0], 99211[0], 99212[0], 99213[0], 99214[0], 99215[0], 99217[0], 99218[0], 99219[0], 99220[0], 99221[0], 99222[0], 99223[0], 99224[0], 99225[0], 99226[0], 99231[0], 99232[0], 99233[0], 99234[0], 99235[0], 99236[0], 99238[0], 99239[0], 99281[0], 99282[0], 99283[0], 99284[0], 99285[0], 99304[0], 99305[0], 99306[0], 99307[0], 99308[0], 99309[0], 99310[0], 99315[0], 99318[0], 99324[0], 99325[0], 99326[0], 99327[0], 99328[0], 99334[0], 99335[0], 99336[0], 99337[0], 99341[0], 99342[0], 99343[0], 99347[0], 99348[0], 99349[0], 99354[0], 99355[0], 99356[0], 99357[0], 99358[0], 99359[0], 99415[0], 99416[0], 99446[0], 99447[0], 99448[0], 99449[0], 99451[0], 99452[0], 99466[0], 99468[0], 99469[0], 99471[0], 99472[0], 99475[0], 99476[0], 99477[0], 99478[0], 99479[0], 99480[0], 99483[0], 99485[0], 99497[0], C8921[1], C8922[1], C8923[1], C8924[1], C8925[1], C8926[1], C8927[0], C8929[1], C8930[1], G0380[1], G0381[1], G0382[1], G0383[1], G0384[1], G0406[0], G0407[0], G0408[0], G0425[0], G0426[0], G0427[0], G0453[0], G0463[0], G0500[0], G0508[0], G0509[0]
00214	01996[1], 0213T[1], 0216T[1], 0228T[1], 0230T[1], 0333T[0], 0464T[0], 31505[1], 31515[1], 31527[1], 31622[1], 31634[1], 31645[1], 31647[1], 36000[1], 36010[0], 36011[1], 36012[1], 36013[1], 36014[1], 36015[1], 36400[1], 36405[1], 36406[1], 36410[1], 36420[1], 36425[1], 36430[1], 36440[1], 36591[0], 36592[0], 36600[1], 36640[1], 43752[1], 43753[1], 43754[1], 61026[1], 61055[1], 62280[1], 62281[1], 62282[1], 62284[1], 62320[1], 62321[1], 62322[1], 62323[1], 62324[1], 62325[1], 62326[1], 62327[1], 64400[1], 64402[1], 64405[1], 64408[1], 64410[1], 64413[1], 64415[1], 64416[1], 64417[1], 64418[1], 64420[1], 64421[1], 64425[1], 64430[1], 64435[1], 64445[1], 64446[1], 64447[1], 64448[1], 64449[1], 64450[1], 64461[1], 64463[1], 64479[1], 64483[1], 64486[1], 64487[1], 64488[1], 64489[1], 64490[1], 64493[1], 64505[1], 64510[1], 64517[1], 64520[1], 64530[1], 64553[1], 64555[1], 67500[1], 76000[1], 76970[1], 76998[0], 77002[0], 90865[1], 92511[1], 92512[1], 92516[1], 92520[1], 92537[1], 92538[1], 92585[0], 92950[1], 92953[1], 92960[1], 92961[1], 93000[1], 93005[1], 93010[1], 93040[1], 93041[1], 93042[1], 93050[0], 93303[0], 93304[0], 93306[1], 93307[1], 93308[1], 93312[1], 93313[1], 93314[1], 93315[1], 93316[1], 93317[1], 93318[0], 93351[1], 93355[0], 93451[1], 93456[1], 93457[1], 93561[0], 93562[0], 93701[0], 93922[1], 93923[1], 93924[1], 93925[1], 93926[1], 93930[1], 93931[1], 93970[1], 93971[1], 93975[1], 93976[1], 93978[1], 93979[1], 93980[1], 93981[1], 94002[1], 94004[1], 94200[1], 94250[0], 94640[1], 94644[1], 94660[1], 94662[1], 94680[1], 94681[1], 94690[1], 94760[0], 94761[0], 94762[1], 94770[1], 95812[0], 95813[0], 95816[0], 95819[0], 95822[0], 95829[0], 95860[0], 95861[0], 95863[0], 95864[0], 95865[0], 95866[0], 95867[0], 95868[0], 95869[0], 95870[0], 95907[0], 95908[0], 95909[0], 95910[0], 95911[0], 95912[0], 95913[0], 95925[0], 95926[0], 95927[0], 95928[0], 95929[0], 95930[0], 95933[0], 95937[0], 95938[0], 95939[0], 95940[0], 95955[0], 95956[0], 95957[0], 96360[0], 96365[0], 96372[0], 96373[0], 96374[0], 96375[0], 96376[0], 96377[0], 99151[0], 99152[0], 99153[0], 99155[0], 99156[0], 99157[0], 99201[0], 99202[0], 99203[0], 99204[0], 99205[0], 99211[0], 99212[0], 99213[0], 99214[0], 99215[0], 99217[0], 99218[0], 99219[0], 99220[0], 99221[0], 99222[0], 99223[0], 99224[0], 99225[0], 99226[0], 99231[0], 99232[0], 99233[0], 99234[0], 99235[0], 99236[0], 99238[0], 99239[0], 99281[0], 99282[0], 99283[0], 99284[0], 99285[0], 99304[0], 99305[0], 99306[0], 99307[0], 99308[0], 99309[0], 99310[0], 99315[0], 99318[0], 99324[0], 99325[0], 99326[0], 99327[0], 99328[0], 99334[0], 99335[0], 99336[0], 99337[0], 99341[0], 99342[0], 99343[0], 99347[0], 99348[0], 99349[0], 99354[0], 99355[0], 99356[0], 99357[0], 99358[0], 99359[0], 99415[0], 99416[0], 99446[0], 99447[0], 99448[0], 99449[0], 99451[0], 99452[0], 99466[0], 99468[0], 99469[0], 99471[0], 99472[0], 99475[0], 99476[0], 99477[0], 99478[0], 99479[0], 99480[0], 99483[0], 99485[0], 99497[0], C8921[1], C8922[1],

0 = Modifier usage not allowed or inappropriate   1 = Modifier usage allowed

CPT © 2018 American Medical Association. All Rights Reserved.

Code 1	Code 2
	C8923[1], C8924[1], C8925[1], C8926[1], C8927[0], C8929[1], C8930[1], G0380[1], G0381[1], G0382[1], G0383[1], G0384[1], G0406[0], G0407[0], G0408[0], G0425[0], G0426[0], G0427[0], G0453[0], G0463[0], G0500[0], G0508[0], G0509[0]
00215	01996[1], 0213T[1], 0216T[1], 0228T[1], 0230T[1], 0333T[0], 0464T[0], 31505[1], 31515[1], 31527[1], 31622[1], 31634[1], 31645[1], 31647[1], 36000[1], 36010[0], 36011[1], 36012[1], 36013[1], 36014[1], 36015[1], 36400[1], 36405[1], 36406[1], 36410[1], 36420[1], 36425[1], 36430[1], 36440[1], 36591[0], 36592[0], 36600[1], 36640[1], 43752[1], 43753[1], 43754[1], 61026[1], 61055[1], 62280[1], 62281[1], 62282[1], 62284[1], 62320[1], 62321[1], 62322[1], 62323[1], 62324[1], 62325[1], 62326[1], 62327[1], 64400[1], 64402[1], 64405[1], 64408[1], 64410[1], 64413[1], 64415[1], 64416[1], 64417[1], 64418[1], 64420[1], 64421[1], 64425[1], 64430[1], 64435[1], 64445[1], 64446[1], 64447[1], 64448[1], 64449[1], 64450[1], 64461[1], 64463[1], 64479[1], 64483[1], 64486[1], 64487[1], 64488[1], 64489[1], 64490[1], 64493[1], 64505[1], 64510[1], 64517[1], 64520[1], 64530[1], 64553[1], 64555[1], 67500[1], 76000[1], 76970[1], 76998[0], 77002[0], 90865[1], 92511[1], 92512[1], 92516[1], 92520[1], 92537[1], 92538[1], 92585[0], 92950[1], 92953[1], 92960[1], 92961[1], 93000[1], 93005[1], 93010[1], 93040[1], 93041[1], 93042[1], 93050[0], 93303[0], 93304[0], 93306[1], 93307[1], 93308[1], 93312[1], 93313[1], 93314[1], 93315[1], 93316[1], 93317[1], 93318[0], 93351[1], 93355[0], 93451[1], 93456[1], 93457[1], 93561[0], 93562[0], 93701[0], 93922[1], 93923[1], 93924[1], 93925[1], 93926[1], 93930[1], 93931[1], 93970[1], 93971[1], 93975[1], 93976[1], 93978[1], 93979[1], 93980[1], 93981[1], 94002[1], 94004[1], 94200[1], 94250[0], 94640[1], 94644[1], 94660[1], 94662[1], 94680[1], 94681[1], 94690[1], 94760[0], 94761[0], 94762[1], 94770[1], 95812[0], 95813[0], 95816[0], 95819[0], 95822[0], 95829[0], 95860[0], 95861[0], 95863[0], 95864[0], 95865[0], 95866[0], 95867[0], 95868[0], 95869[0], 95870[0], 95907[0], 95908[0], 95909[0], 95910[0], 95911[0], 95912[0], 95913[0], 95925[0], 95926[0], 95927[0], 95928[0], 95929[0], 95930[0], 95933[0], 95937[0], 95938[0], 95939[0], 95940[0], 95955[0], 95956[0], 95957[0], 96360[0], 96365[0], 96372[0], 96373[0], 96374[0], 96375[0], 96376[0], 96377[0], 99151[0], 99152[0], 99153[0], 99155[0], 99156[0], 99157[0], 99201[0], 99202[0], 99203[0], 99204[0], 99205[0], 99211[0], 99212[0], 99213[0], 99214[0], 99215[0], 99217[0], 99218[0], 99219[0], 99220[0], 99221[0], 99222[0], 99223[0], 99224[0], 99225[0], 99226[0], 99231[0], 99232[0], 99233[0], 99234[0], 99235[0], 99236[0], 99238[0], 99239[0], 99281[0], 99282[0], 99283[0], 99284[0], 99285[0], 99304[0], 99305[0], 99306[0], 99307[0], 99308[0], 99309[0], 99310[0], 99315[0], 99318[0], 99324[0], 99325[0], 99326[0], 99327[0], 99328[0], 99334[0], 99335[0], 99336[0], 99337[0], 99341[0], 99342[0], 99343[0], 99347[0], 99348[0], 99349[0], 99354[0], 99355[0], 99356[0], 99357[0], 99358[0], 99359[0], 99415[0], 99416[0], 99446[0], 99447[0], 99448[0], 99449[0], 99451[0], 99452[0], 99466[0], 99468[0], 99469[0], 99471[0], 99472[0], 99475[0], 99476[0], 99477[0], 99478[0], 99479[0], 99480[0], 99483[0], 99485[0], 99497[0], C8921[1], C8922[1], C8923[1], C8924[1], C8925[1], C8926[1], C8927[0], C8929[1], C8930[1], G0380[1], G0381[1], G0382[1], G0383[1], G0384[1], G0406[0], G0407[0], G0408[0], G0425[0], G0426[0], G0427[0], G0453[0], G0463[0], G0500[0], G0508[0], G0509[0]
00216	01996[1], 0213T[1], 0216T[1], 0228T[1], 0230T[1], 0333T[0], 0464T[0], 31505[1], 31515[1], 31527[1], 31622[1], 31634[1], 31645[1], 31647[1], 36000[1], 36010[0], 36011[1], 36012[1], 36013[1], 36014[1], 36015[1], 36400[1], 36405[1], 36406[1], 36410[1], 36420[1], 36425[1], 36430[1], 36440[1], 36591[0], 36592[0], 36600[1], 36640[1], 43752[1], 43753[1], 43754[1], 61026[1], 61055[1], 62280[1], 62281[1], 62282[1], 62284[1], 62320[1], 62321[1], 62322[1], 62323[1], 62324[1], 62325[1], 62326[1], 62327[1], 64400[1], 64402[1], 64405[1], 64408[1], 64410[1], 64413[1], 64415[1], 64416[1], 64417[1], 64418[1], 64420[1], 64421[1], 64425[1], 64430[1], 64435[1], 64445[1], 64446[1], 64447[1], 64448[1], 64449[1], 64450[1], 64461[1], 64463[1], 64479[1], 64483[1], 64486[1], 64487[1], 64488[1], 64489[1], 64490[1], 64493[1], 64505[1], 64510[1], 64517[1], 64520[1], 64530[1], 64553[1], 64555[1], 67500[1], 76000[1], 76970[1], 76998[0], 77002[0], 90865[1], 92511[1], 92512[1], 92516[1], 92520[1], 92537[1], 92538[1], 92585[0], 92950[1], 92953[1], 92960[1], 92961[1], 93000[1], 93005[1], 93010[1], 93040[1], 93041[1], 93042[1], 93050[0], 93303[0], 93304[0], 93306[1], 93307[1], 93308[1], 93312[1], 93313[1], 93314[1], 93315[1], 93316[1], 93317[1], 93318[0], 93351[1], 93355[0], 93451[1], 93456[1], 93457[1], 93561[0], 93562[0], 93701[0], 93922[1], 93923[1], 93924[1], 93925[1], 93926[1], 93930[1], 93931[1], 93970[1], 93971[1], 93975[1], 93976[1], 93978[1], 93979[1], 93980[1], 93981[1], 94002[1], 94004[1], 94200[1], 94250[0], 94640[1], 94644[1], 94660[1], 94662[1], 94680[1], 94681[1], 94690[1], 94760[0], 94761[0], 94762[1], 94770[1], 95812[0], 95813[0], 95816[0], 95819[0], 95822[0], 95829[0], 95860[0], 95861[0], 95863[0], 95864[0], 95865[0], 95866[0], 95867[0], 95868[0], 95869[0], 95870[0], 95907[0], 95908[0], 95909[0], 95910[0], 95911[0], 95912[0], 95913[0], 95925[0], 95926[0], 95927[0], 95928[0], 95929[0], 95930[0], 95933[0], 95937[0], 95938[0], 95939[0], 95940[0], 95955[0], 95956[0], 95957[0], 96360[0], 96365[0], 96372[0], 96373[0], 96374[0], 96375[0], 96376[0], 96377[0], 99151[0], 99152[0], 99153[0], 99155[0], 99156[0], 99157[0], 99201[0], 99202[0], 99203[0], 99204[0], 99205[0], 99211[0], 99212[0], 99213[0], 99214[0], 99215[0], 99217[0], 99218[0], 99219[0], 99220[0], 99221[0], 99222[0], 99223[0], 99224[0], 99225[0], 99226[0], 99231[0], 99232[0], 99233[0], 99234[0], 99235[0], 99236[0], 99238[0], 99239[0], 99281[0], 99282[0], 99283[0], 99284[0], 99285[0], 99304[0], 99305[0], 99306[0], 99307[0], 99308[0], 99309[0], 99310[0], 99315[0], 99318[0], 99324[0], 99325[0], 99326[0], 99327[0], 99328[0], 99334[0], 99335[0], 99336[0], 99337[0], 99341[0], 99342[0], 99343[0], 99347[0], 99348[0], 99349[0], 99354[0], 99355[0], 99356[0], 99357[0], 99358[0], 99359[0], 99415[0], 99416[0], 99446[0], 99447[0], 99448[0], 99449[0], 99451[0], 99452[0], 99466[0], 99468[0], 99469[0], 99471[0], 99472[0], 99475[0], 99476[0], 99477[0], 99478[0], 99479[0], 99480[0], 99483[0], 99485[0], 99497[0], C8921[1], C8922[1],
	C8923[1], C8924[1], C8925[1], C8926[1], C8927[0], C8929[1], C8930[1], G0380[1], G0381[1], G0382[1], G0383[1], G0384[1], G0406[0], G0407[0], G0408[0], G0425[0], G0426[0], G0427[0], G0453[0], G0463[0], G0500[0], G0508[0], G0509[0]
00218	01996[1], 0213T[1], 0216T[1], 0228T[1], 0230T[1], 0333T[0], 0464T[0], 31505[1], 31515[1], 31527[1], 31622[1], 31634[1], 31645[1], 31647[1], 36000[1], 36010[0], 36011[1], 36012[1], 36013[1], 36014[1], 36015[1], 36400[1], 36405[1], 36406[1], 36410[1], 36420[1], 36425[1], 36430[1], 36440[1], 36591[0], 36592[0], 36600[1], 36640[1], 43752[1], 43753[1], 43754[1], 61026[1], 61055[1], 62280[1], 62281[1], 62282[1], 62284[1], 62320[1], 62321[1], 62322[1], 62323[1], 62324[1], 62325[1], 62326[1], 62327[1], 64400[1], 64402[1], 64405[1], 64408[1], 64410[1], 64413[1], 64415[1], 64416[1], 64417[1], 64418[1], 64420[1], 64421[1], 64425[1], 64430[1], 64435[1], 64445[1], 64446[1], 64447[1], 64448[1], 64449[1], 64450[1], 64461[1], 64463[1], 64479[1], 64483[1], 64486[1], 64487[1], 64488[1], 64489[1], 64490[1], 64493[1], 64505[1], 64510[1], 64517[1], 64520[1], 64530[1], 64553[1], 64555[1], 67500[1], 76000[1], 76970[1], 76998[0], 77002[0], 90865[1], 92511[1], 92512[1], 92516[1], 92520[1], 92537[1], 92538[1], 92585[0], 92950[1], 92953[1], 92960[1], 92961[1], 93000[1], 93005[1], 93010[1], 93040[1], 93041[1], 93042[1], 93050[0], 93303[0], 93304[0], 93306[1], 93307[1], 93308[1], 93312[1], 93313[1], 93314[1], 93315[1], 93316[1], 93317[1], 93318[0], 93351[1], 93355[0], 93451[1], 93456[1], 93457[1], 93561[0], 93562[0], 93701[0], 93922[1], 93923[1], 93924[1], 93925[1], 93926[1], 93930[1], 93931[1], 93970[1], 93971[1], 93975[1], 93976[1], 93978[1], 93979[1], 93980[1], 93981[1], 94002[1], 94004[1], 94200[1], 94250[0], 94640[1], 94644[1], 94660[1], 94662[1], 94680[1], 94681[1], 94690[1], 94760[0], 94761[0], 94762[1], 94770[1], 95812[0], 95813[0], 95816[0], 95819[0], 95822[0], 95829[0], 95860[0], 95861[0], 95863[0], 95864[0], 95865[0], 95866[0], 95867[0], 95868[0], 95869[0], 95870[0], 95907[0], 95908[0], 95909[0], 95910[0], 95911[0], 95912[0], 95913[0], 95925[0], 95926[0], 95927[0], 95928[0], 95929[0], 95930[0], 95933[0], 95937[0], 95938[0], 95939[0], 95940[0], 95955[0], 95956[0], 95957[0], 96360[0], 96365[0], 96372[0], 96373[0], 96374[0], 96375[0], 96376[0], 96377[0], 99151[0], 99152[0], 99153[0], 99155[0], 99156[0], 99157[0], 99201[0], 99202[0], 99203[0], 99204[0], 99205[0], 99211[0], 99212[0], 99213[0], 99214[0], 99215[0], 99217[0], 99218[0], 99219[0], 99220[0], 99221[0], 99222[0], 99223[0], 99224[0], 99225[0], 99226[0], 99231[0], 99232[0], 99233[0], 99234[0], 99235[0], 99236[0], 99238[0], 99239[0], 99281[0], 99282[0], 99283[0], 99284[0], 99285[0], 99304[0], 99305[0], 99306[0], 99307[0], 99308[0], 99309[0], 99310[0], 99315[0], 99318[0], 99324[0], 99325[0], 99326[0], 99327[0], 99328[0], 99334[0], 99335[0], 99336[0], 99337[0], 99341[0], 99342[0], 99343[0], 99347[0], 99348[0], 99349[0], 99354[0], 99355[0], 99356[0], 99357[0], 99358[0], 99359[0], 99415[0], 99416[0], 99446[0], 99447[0], 99448[0], 99449[0], 99451[0], 99452[0], 99466[0], 99468[0], 99469[0], 99471[0], 99472[0], 99475[0], 99476[0], 99477[0], 99478[0], 99479[0], 99480[0], 99483[0], 99485[0], 99497[0], C8921[1], C8922[1], C8923[1], C8924[1], C8925[1], C8926[1], C8927[0], C8929[1], C8930[1], G0380[1], G0381[1], G0382[1], G0383[1], G0384[1], G0406[0], G0407[0], G0408[0], G0425[0], G0426[0], G0427[0], G0453[0], G0463[0], G0500[0], G0508[0], G0509[0]
00220	01996[1], 0213T[1], 0216T[1], 0228T[1], 0230T[1], 0333T[0], 0464T[0], 31505[1], 31515[1], 31527[1], 31622[1], 31634[1], 31645[1], 31647[1], 36000[1], 36010[0], 36011[1], 36012[1], 36013[1], 36014[1], 36015[1], 36400[1], 36405[1], 36406[1], 36410[1], 36420[1], 36425[1], 36430[1], 36440[1], 36591[0], 36592[0], 36600[1], 36640[1], 43752[1], 43753[1], 43754[1], 61026[1], 61055[1], 62280[1], 62281[1], 62282[1], 62284[1], 62320[1], 62321[1], 62322[1], 62323[1], 62324[1], 62325[1], 62326[1], 62327[1], 64400[1], 64402[1], 64405[1], 64408[1], 64410[1], 64413[1], 64415[1], 64416[1], 64417[1], 64418[1], 64420[1], 64421[1], 64425[1], 64430[1], 64435[1], 64445[1], 64446[1], 64447[1], 64448[1], 64449[1], 64450[1], 64461[1], 64463[1], 64479[1], 64483[1], 64486[1], 64487[1], 64488[1], 64489[1], 64490[1], 64493[1], 64505[1], 64510[1], 64517[1], 64520[1], 64530[1], 64553[1], 64555[1], 67500[1], 76000[1], 76970[1], 76998[0], 77002[0], 90865[1], 92511[1], 92512[1], 92516[1], 92520[1], 92537[1], 92538[1], 92585[0], 92950[1], 92953[1], 92960[1], 92961[1], 93000[1], 93005[1], 93010[1], 93040[1], 93041[1], 93042[1], 93050[0], 93303[0], 93304[0], 93306[1], 93307[1], 93308[1], 93312[1], 93313[1], 93314[1], 93315[1], 93316[1], 93317[1], 93318[0], 93351[1], 93355[0], 93451[1], 93456[1], 93457[1], 93561[0], 93562[0], 93701[0], 93922[1], 93923[1], 93924[1], 93925[1], 93926[1], 93930[1], 93931[1], 93970[1], 93971[1], 93975[1], 93976[1], 93978[1], 93979[1], 93980[1], 93981[1], 94002[1], 94004[1], 94200[1], 94250[0], 94640[1], 94644[1], 94660[1], 94662[1], 94680[1], 94681[1], 94690[1], 94760[0], 94761[0], 94762[1], 94770[1], 95812[0], 95813[0], 95816[0], 95819[0], 95822[0], 95829[0], 95860[0], 95861[0], 95863[0], 95864[0], 95865[0], 95866[0], 95867[0], 95868[0], 95869[0], 95870[0], 95907[0], 95908[0], 95909[0], 95910[0], 95911[0], 95912[0], 95913[0], 95925[0], 95926[0], 95927[0], 95928[0], 95929[0], 95930[0], 95933[0], 95937[0], 95938[0], 95939[0], 95940[0], 95955[0], 95956[0], 95957[0], 96360[0], 96365[0], 96372[0], 96373[0], 96374[0], 96375[0], 96376[0], 96377[0], 99151[0], 99152[0], 99153[0], 99155[0], 99156[0], 99157[0], 99201[0], 99202[0], 99203[0], 99204[0], 99205[0], 99211[0], 99212[0], 99213[0], 99214[0], 99215[0], 99217[0], 99218[0], 99219[0], 99220[0], 99221[0], 99222[0], 99223[0], 99224[0], 99225[0], 99226[0], 99231[0], 99232[0], 99233[0], 99234[0], 99235[0], 99236[0], 99238[0], 99239[0], 99281[0], 99282[0], 99283[0], 99284[0], 99285[0], 99304[0], 99305[0], 99306[0], 99307[0], 99308[0], 99309[0], 99310[0], 99315[0], 99318[0], 99324[0], 99325[0], 99326[0], 99327[0], 99328[0], 99334[0], 99335[0], 99336[0], 99337[0], 99341[0], 99342[0], 99343[0], 99347[0], 99348[0], 99349[0], 99354[0], 99355[0], 99356[0], 99357[0], 99358[0], 99359[0], 99415[0], 99416[0], 99446[0], 99447[0], 99448[0], 99449[0], 99451[0], 99452[0], 99466[0], 99468[0], 99469[0], 99471[0], 99472[0], 99475[0], 99476[0], 99477[0], 99478[0], 99479[0], 99480[0], 99483[0], 99485[0], 99497[0], C8921[1], C8922[1],

Appendix A: NCCI - CPT Codes

0 = Modifier usage not allowed or inappropriate 1 = Modifier usage allowed

CPT © 2018 American Medical Association. All Rights Reserved.

Code 1	Code 2
	C8923[1], C8924[1], C8925[1], C8926[1], C8927[0], C8929[1], C8930[1], G0380[1], G0381[1], G0382[1], G0383[1], G0384[1], G0406[0], G0407[0], G0408[0], G0425[0], G0426[0], G0427[0], G0453[0], G0463[0], G0500[0], G0508[0], G0509[0]
00222	01996[1], 0213T[1], 0216T[1], 0228T[1], 0230T[1], 0333T[0], 0464T[0], 31505[1], 31515[1], 31527[1], 31622[1], 31634[1], 31645[1], 31647[1], 36000[1], 36010[0], 36011[1], 36012[1], 36013[1], 36014[1], 36015[1], 36400[1], 36405[1], 36406[1], 36410[1], 36420[1], 36425[1], 36430[1], 36440[1], 36591[0], 36592[0], 36600[1], 36640[1], 43752[1], 43753[1], 43754[1], 61026[1], 61055[1], 62280[1], 62281[1], 62282[1], 62284[1], 62320[1], 62321[1], 62322[1], 62323[1], 62324[1], 62325[1], 62326[1], 62327[1], 64400[1], 64402[1], 64405[1], 64408[1], 64410[1], 64413[1], 64415[1], 64416[1], 64417[1], 64418[1], 64420[1], 64421[1], 64425[1], 64430[1], 64435[1], 64445[1], 64446[1], 64447[1], 64448[1], 64449[1], 64450[1], 64461[1], 64463[1], 64479[1], 64483[1], 64486[1], 64487[1], 64488[1], 64489[1], 64490[1], 64493[1], 64505[1], 64510[1], 64517[1], 64520[1], 64530[1], 64553[1], 64555[1], 67500[1], 76000[1], 76970[1], 76998[0], 77002[0], 90865[1], 92511[1], 92512[1], 92516[1], 92520[1], 92537[1], 92538[1], 92585[0], 92950[1], 92953[1], 92960[1], 92961[1], 93000[1], 93005[1], 93010[1], 93040[1], 93041[1], 93042[1], 93050[0], 93303[0], 93304[0], 93306[1], 93307[1], 93308[1], 93312[1], 93313[1], 93314[1], 93315[1], 93316[1], 93317[1], 93318[0], 93351[1], 93355[0], 93451[1], 93456[1], 93457[1], 93561[0], 93562[0], 93701[0], 93922[1], 93923[1], 93924[1], 93925[1], 93926[1], 93930[1], 93931[1], 93970[1], 93971[1], 93975[1], 93976[1], 93978[1], 93979[1], 93980[1], 93981[1], 94002[1], 94004[1], 94200[1], 94250[0], 94640[1], 94644[1], 94660[1], 94662[1], 94680[1], 94681[1], 94690[1], 94760[0], 94761[0], 94762[1], 94770[1], 95812[0], 95813[0], 95816[0], 95819[0], 95822[0], 95829[0], 95860[0], 95861[0], 95863[0], 95864[0], 95865[0], 95866[0], 95867[0], 95868[0], 95869[0], 95870[0], 95907[0], 95908[0], 95909[0], 95910[0], 95911[0], 95912[0], 95913[0], 95925[0], 95926[0], 95927[0], 95928[0], 95929[0], 95930[0], 95933[0], 95937[0], 95938[0], 95939[0], 95940[0], 95955[0], 95956[0], 95957[0], 96360[0], 96365[0], 96372[0], 96373[0], 96374[0], 96375[0], 96376[0], 96377[0], 99151[0], 99152[0], 99153[0], 99155[0], 99156[0], 99157[0], 99201[0], 99202[0], 99203[0], 99204[0], 99205[0], 99211[0], 99212[0], 99213[0], 99214[0], 99215[0], 99217[0], 99218[0], 99219[0], 99220[0], 99221[0], 99222[0], 99223[0], 99224[0], 99225[0], 99226[0], 99231[0], 99232[0], 99233[0], 99234[0], 99235[0], 99236[0], 99238[0], 99239[0], 99281[0], 99282[0], 99283[0], 99284[0], 99285[0], 99304[0], 99305[0], 99306[0], 99307[0], 99308[0], 99309[0], 99310[0], 99315[0], 99318[0], 99324[0], 99325[0], 99326[0], 99327[0], 99328[0], 99334[0], 99335[0], 99336[0], 99337[0], 99341[0], 99342[0], 99343[0], 99347[0], 99348[0], 99349[0], 99354[0], 99355[0], 99356[0], 99357[0], 99358[0], 99359[0], 99415[0], 99416[0], 99446[0], 99447[0], 99448[0], 99449[0], 99451[0], 99452[0], 99466[0], 99468[0], 99469[0], 99471[0], 99472[0], 99475[0], 99476[0], 99477[0], 99478[0], 99479[0], 99480[0], 99483[0], 99485[0], 99497[0], C8921[1], C8922[1], C8923[1], C8924[1], C8925[1], C8926[1], C8927[0], C8929[1], C8930[1], G0380[1], G0381[1], G0382[1], G0383[1], G0384[1], G0406[0], G0407[0], G0408[0], G0425[0], G0426[0], G0427[0], G0453[0], G0463[0], G0500[0], G0508[0], G0509[0]
00300	01996[1], 0213T[1], 0216T[1], 0228T[1], 0230T[1], 0333T[0], 0464T[0], 31505[1], 31515[1], 31527[1], 31622[1], 31634[1], 31645[1], 31647[1], 36000[1], 36010[0], 36011[1], 36012[1], 36013[1], 36014[1], 36015[1], 36400[1], 36405[1], 36406[1], 36410[1], 36420[1], 36425[1], 36430[1], 36440[1], 36591[0], 36592[0], 36600[1], 36640[1], 43752[1], 43753[1], 43754[1], 61026[1], 61055[1], 62280[1], 62281[1], 62282[1], 62284[1], 62320[1], 62321[1], 62322[1], 62323[1], 62324[1], 62325[1], 62326[1], 62327[1], 64400[1], 64402[1], 64405[1], 64408[1], 64410[1], 64413[1], 64415[1], 64416[1], 64417[1], 64418[1], 64420[1], 64421[1], 64425[1], 64430[1], 64435[1], 64445[1], 64446[1], 64447[1], 64448[1], 64449[1], 64450[1], 64461[1], 64463[1], 64479[1], 64483[1], 64486[1], 64487[1], 64488[1], 64489[1], 64490[1], 64493[1], 64505[1], 64510[1], 64517[1], 64520[1], 64530[1], 64553[1], 64555[1], 67500[1], 76000[1], 76970[1], 76998[0], 77002[0], 90865[1], 92511[1], 92512[1], 92516[1], 92520[1], 92537[1], 92538[1], 92585[0], 92950[1], 92953[1], 92960[1], 92961[1], 93000[1], 93005[1], 93010[1], 93040[1], 93041[1], 93042[1], 93050[0], 93303[0], 93304[0], 93306[1], 93307[1], 93308[1], 93312[1], 93313[1], 93314[1], 93315[1], 93316[1], 93317[1], 93318[0], 93351[1], 93355[0], 93451[1], 93456[1], 93457[1], 93561[0], 93562[0], 93701[0], 93922[1], 93923[1], 93924[1], 93925[1], 93926[1], 93930[1], 93931[1], 93970[1], 93971[1], 93975[1], 93976[1], 93978[1], 93979[1], 93980[1], 93981[1], 94002[1], 94004[1], 94200[1], 94250[0], 94640[1], 94644[1], 94660[1], 94662[1], 94680[1], 94681[1], 94690[1], 94760[0], 94761[0], 94762[1], 94770[1], 95812[0], 95813[0], 95816[0], 95819[0], 95822[0], 95829[0], 95860[0], 95861[0], 95863[0], 95864[0], 95865[0], 95866[0], 95867[0], 95868[0], 95869[0], 95870[0], 95907[0], 95908[0], 95909[0], 95910[0], 95911[0], 95912[0], 95913[0], 95925[0], 95926[0], 95927[0], 95928[0], 95929[0], 95930[0], 95933[0], 95937[0], 95938[0], 95939[0], 95940[0], 95955[0], 95956[0], 95957[0], 96360[0], 96365[0], 96372[0], 96373[0], 96374[0], 96375[0], 96376[0], 96377[0], 99151[0], 99152[0], 99153[0], 99155[0], 99156[0], 99157[0], 99201[0], 99202[0], 99203[0], 99204[0], 99205[0], 99211[0], 99212[0], 99213[0], 99214[0], 99215[0], 99217[0], 99218[0], 99219[0], 99220[0], 99221[0], 99222[0], 99223[0], 99224[0], 99225[0], 99226[0], 99231[0], 99232[0], 99233[0], 99234[0], 99235[0], 99236[0], 99238[0], 99239[0], 99281[0], 99282[0], 99283[0], 99284[0], 99285[0], 99304[0], 99305[0], 99306[0], 99307[0], 99308[0], 99309[0], 99310[0], 99315[0], 99318[0], 99324[0], 99325[0], 99326[0], 99327[0], 99328[0], 99334[0], 99335[0], 99336[0], 99337[0], 99341[0], 99342[0], 99343[0], 99347[0], 99348[0], 99349[0], 99354[0], 99355[0], 99356[0], 99357[0], 99358[0], 99359[0], 99415[0], 99416[0], 99446[0], 99447[0], 99448[0], 99449[0], 99451[0], 99452[0], 99466[0], 99468[0], 99469[0], 99471[0], 99472[0], 99475[0], 99476[0], 99477[0], 99478[0], 99479[0], 99480[0], 99483[0], 99485[0], 99497[0], C8921[1], C8922[1],
	C8923[1], C8924[1], C8925[1], C8926[1], C8927[0], C8929[1], C8930[1], G0380[1], G0381[1], G0382[1], G0383[1], G0384[1], G0406[0], G0407[0], G0408[0], G0425[0], G0426[0], G0427[0], G0453[0], G0463[0], G0500[0], G0508[0], G0509[0]
00320	01996[1], 0213T[1], 0216T[1], 0228T[1], 0230T[1], 31505[1], 31515[1], 31527[1], 31622[1], 31634[1], 31645[1], 31647[1], 36000[1], 36010[0], 36011[1], 36012[1], 36013[1], 36014[1], 36015[1], 36400[1], 36405[1], 36406[1], 36410[1], 36420[1], 36425[1], 36430[1], 36440[1], 36591[0], 36592[0], 36600[1], 36640[1], 43752[1], 43753[1], 43754[1], 61026[1], 61055[1], 62280[1], 62281[1], 62282[1], 62284[1], 62320[1], 62321[1], 62322[1], 62323[1], 62324[1], 62325[1], 62326[1], 62327[1], 64400[1], 64402[1], 64405[1], 64408[1], 64410[1], 64413[1], 64415[1], 64416[1], 64417[1], 64418[1], 64420[1], 64421[1], 64425[1], 64430[1], 64435[1], 64445[1], 64446[1], 64447[1], 64448[1], 64449[1], 64450[1], 64461[1], 64463[1], 64479[1], 64483[1], 64486[1], 64487[1], 64488[1], 64489[1], 64490[1], 64493[1], 64505[1], 64510[1], 64517[1], 64520[1], 64530[1], 64553[1], 64555[1], 67500[1], 76000[1], 76970[1], 76998[0], 77002[0], 90865[1], 92511[1], 92512[1], 92516[1], 92520[1], 92537[1], 92538[1], 92950[1], 92953[1], 92960[1], 92961[1], 93000[1], 93005[1], 93010[1], 93040[1], 93041[1], 93042[1], 93050[0], 93303[0], 93304[0], 93306[1], 93307[1], 93308[1], 93312[1], 93313[1], 93314[1], 93315[1], 93316[1], 93317[1], 93318[0], 93351[1], 93355[0], 93451[1], 93456[1], 93457[1], 93561[0], 93562[0], 93701[0], 93922[1], 93923[1], 93924[1], 93925[1], 93926[1], 93930[1], 93931[1], 93970[1], 93971[1], 93975[1], 93976[1], 93978[1], 93979[1], 93980[1], 93981[1], 94002[1], 94004[1], 94200[1], 94250[0], 94640[1], 94644[1], 94660[1], 94662[1], 94680[1], 94681[1], 94690[1], 94760[0], 94761[0], 94762[1], 94770[1], 95812[0], 95813[0], 95816[0], 95819[0], 95822[0], 95829[0], 95955[0], 95956[0], 95957[0], 96360[0], 96365[0], 96372[0], 96373[0], 96374[0], 96375[0], 96376[0], 96377[0], 99151[0], 99152[0], 99153[0], 99155[0], 99156[0], 99157[0], 99201[0], 99202[0], 99203[0], 99204[0], 99205[0], 99211[0], 99212[0], 99213[0], 99214[0], 99215[0], 99217[0], 99218[0], 99219[0], 99220[0], 99221[0], 99222[0], 99223[0], 99224[0], 99225[0], 99226[0], 99231[0], 99232[0], 99233[0], 99234[0], 99235[0], 99236[0], 99238[0], 99239[0], 99281[0], 99282[0], 99283[0], 99284[0], 99285[0], 99304[0], 99305[0], 99306[0], 99307[0], 99308[0], 99309[0], 99310[0], 99315[0], 99318[0], 99324[0], 99325[0], 99326[0], 99327[0], 99328[0], 99334[0], 99335[0], 99336[0], 99337[0], 99341[0], 99342[0], 99343[0], 99347[0], 99348[0], 99349[0], 99354[0], 99355[0], 99356[0], 99357[0], 99358[0], 99359[0], 99415[0], 99416[0], 99446[0], 99447[0], 99448[0], 99449[0], 99451[0], 99452[0], 99466[0], 99468[0], 99469[0], 99471[0], 99472[0], 99475[0], 99476[0], 99477[0], 99478[0], 99479[0], 99480[0], 99483[0], 99485[0], 99497[0], C8921[1], C8922[1], C8923[1], C8924[1], C8925[1], C8926[1], C8927[0], C8929[1], C8930[1], G0380[1], G0381[1], G0382[1], G0383[1], G0384[1], G0406[0], G0407[0], G0408[0], G0425[0], G0426[0], G0427[0], G0463[0], G0500[0], G0508[0], G0509[0]
00322	01996[1], 0213T[1], 0216T[1], 0228T[1], 0230T[1], 31505[1], 31515[1], 31527[1], 31622[1], 31634[1], 31645[1], 31647[1], 36000[1], 36010[0], 36011[1], 36012[1], 36013[1], 36014[1], 36015[1], 36400[1], 36405[1], 36406[1], 36410[1], 36420[1], 36425[1], 36430[1], 36591[0], 36592[0], 36600[1], 36640[1], 43752[1], 43753[1], 43754[1], 61026[1], 61055[1], 62280[1], 62281[1], 62282[1], 62284[1], 62320[1], 62321[1], 62322[1], 62323[1], 62324[1], 62325[1], 62326[1], 62327[1], 64400[1], 64402[1], 64405[1], 64408[1], 64410[1], 64413[1], 64415[1], 64416[1], 64417[1], 64418[1], 64420[1], 64421[1], 64425[1], 64430[1], 64435[1], 64445[1], 64446[1], 64447[1], 64448[1], 64449[1], 64450[1], 64461[1], 64463[1], 64479[1], 64483[1], 64486[1], 64487[1], 64488[1], 64489[1], 64490[1], 64493[1], 64505[1], 64510[1], 64517[1], 64520[1], 64530[1], 64553[1], 64555[1], 67500[1], 76000[1], 76970[1], 76998[0], 77002[0], 90865[1], 92511[1], 92512[1], 92516[1], 92520[1], 92537[1], 92538[1], 92950[1], 92953[1], 92960[1], 92961[1], 93000[1], 93005[1], 93010[1], 93040[1], 93041[1], 93042[1], 93050[0], 93303[0], 93304[0], 93306[1], 93307[1], 93308[1], 93312[1], 93313[1], 93314[1], 93315[1], 93316[1], 93317[1], 93318[0], 93351[1], 93355[0], 93451[1], 93456[1], 93457[1], 93561[0], 93562[0], 93701[0], 93922[1], 93923[1], 93924[1], 93925[1], 93926[1], 93930[1], 93931[1], 93970[1], 93971[1], 93975[1], 93976[1], 93978[1], 93979[1], 93980[1], 93981[1], 94002[1], 94004[1], 94200[1], 94250[0], 94640[1], 94644[1], 94660[1], 94662[1], 94680[1], 94681[1], 94690[1], 94760[0], 94761[0], 94762[1], 94770[1], 95812[0], 95813[0], 95816[0], 95819[0], 95822[0], 95829[0], 95955[0], 95956[0], 95957[0], 96360[0], 96365[0], 96372[0], 96373[0], 96374[0], 96375[0], 96376[0], 96377[0], 99151[0], 99152[0], 99153[0], 99155[0], 99156[0], 99157[0], 99201[0], 99202[0], 99203[0], 99204[0], 99205[0], 99211[0], 99212[0], 99213[0], 99214[0], 99215[0], 99217[0], 99218[0], 99219[0], 99220[0], 99221[0], 99222[0], 99223[0], 99224[0], 99225[0], 99226[0], 99231[0], 99232[0], 99233[0], 99234[0], 99235[0], 99236[0], 99238[0], 99239[0], 99281[0], 99282[0], 99283[0], 99284[0], 99285[0], 99304[0], 99305[0], 99306[0], 99307[0], 99308[0], 99309[0], 99310[0], 99315[0], 99318[0], 99324[0], 99325[0], 99326[0], 99327[0], 99328[0], 99334[0], 99335[0], 99336[0], 99337[0], 99341[0], 99342[0], 99343[0], 99347[0], 99348[0], 99349[0], 99354[0], 99355[0], 99356[0], 99357[0], 99358[0], 99359[0], 99415[0], 99416[0], 99446[0], 99447[0], 99448[0], 99449[0], 99451[0], 99452[0], 99466[0], 99468[0], 99469[0], 99471[0], 99472[0], 99475[0], 99476[0], 99477[0], 99478[0], 99479[0], 99480[0], 99483[0], 99485[0], 99497[0], C8921[1], C8922[1], C8923[1], C8924[1], C8925[1], C8926[1], C8927[0], C8929[1], C8930[1], G0380[1], G0381[1], G0382[1], G0383[1], G0384[1], G0406[0], G0407[0], G0408[0], G0425[0], G0426[0], G0427[0], G0463[0], G0500[0], G0508[0], G0509[0]
00326	01996[1], 0213T[1], 0216T[1], 0228T[1], 0230T[1], 31622[1], 31634[1], 31645[1], 31647[1], 36000[1], 36010[0], 36011[1], 36012[1], 36013[1], 36014[1], 36015[1], 36400[1], 36405[1], 36406[1], 36410[1], 36420[1], 36425[1], 36430[1], 36440[1], 36591[0], 36592[0], 36600[1], 36640[1], 43752[1], 43753[1],

0 = Modifier usage not allowed or inappropriate   1 = Modifier usage allowed

CPT © 2018 American Medical Association. All Rights Reserved.

Code 1	Code 2
	43754[1], 61026[1], 61055[1], 62280[1], 62281[1], 62282[1], 62284[1], 62320[1], 62321[1], 62322[1], 62323[1], 62324[1], 62325[1], 62326[1], 62327[1], 64400[1], 64402[1], 64405[1], 64408[1], 64410[1], 64413[1], 64415[1], 64416[1], 64417[1], 64418[1], 64420[1], 64421[1], 64425[1], 64430[1], 64435[1], 64445[1], 64446[1], 64447[1], 64448[1], 64449[1], 64450[1], 64461[1], 64463[1], 64479[1], 64483[1], 64486[1], 64487[1], 64488[1], 64489[1], 64490[1], 64493[1], 64505[1], 64510[1], 64517[1], 64520[1], 64530[1], 64553[1], 64555[1], 67500[0], 76000[1], 76970[1], 76998[0], 77002[0], 90865[1], 92511[1], 92512[1], 92516[1], 92520[1], 92537[1], 92538[1], 92950[1], 92953[1], 92960[1], 92961[1], 93000[1], 93005[1], 93010[1], 93040[1], 93041[1], 93042[1], 93050[0], 93303[0], 93304[0], 93306[1], 93307[1], 93308[1], 93312[1], 93313[1], 93314[1], 93315[1], 93316[1], 93317[1], 93318[0], 93351[1], 93355[0], 93451[1], 93456[1], 93457[1], 93561[0], 93562[0], 93701[0], 93922[1], 93923[1], 93924[1], 93925[1], 93926[1], 93930[1], 93931[1], 93970[1], 93971[1], 93975[1], 93976[1], 93978[1], 93979[1], 93980[1], 93981[1], 94002[1], 94004[1], 94200[1], 94250[0], 94640[1], 94644[1], 94660[1], 94662[1], 94680[1], 94681[1], 94690[1], 94760[0], 94761[0], 94762[1], 94770[1], 95812[0], 95813[0], 95816[0], 95819[0], 95822[0], 95829[0], 95955[0], 95956[0], 95957[0], 96360[0], 96365[0], 96372[0], 96373[0], 96374[0], 96375[0], 96376[0], 96377[0], 99100[1], 99151[0], 99152[0], 99153[0], 99155[0], 99156[0], 99157[0], 99201[0], 99202[0], 99203[0], 99204[0], 99205[0], 99211[0], 99212[0], 99213[0], 99214[0], 99215[0], 99217[0], 99218[0], 99219[0], 99220[0], 99221[0], 99222[0], 99223[0], 99224[0], 99225[0], 99226[0], 99231[0], 99232[0], 99233[0], 99234[0], 99235[0], 99236[0], 99238[0], 99239[0], 99281[0], 99282[0], 99283[0], 99284[0], 99285[0], 99304[0], 99305[0], 99306[0], 99307[0], 99308[0], 99309[0], 99310[0], 99315[0], 99318[0], 99324[0], 99325[0], 99326[0], 99327[0], 99328[0], 99334[0], 99335[0], 99336[0], 99337[0], 99341[0], 99342[0], 99343[0], 99347[0], 99348[0], 99349[0], 99354[0], 99355[0], 99356[0], 99357[0], 99358[0], 99359[0], 99415[0], 99416[0], 99446[0], 99447[0], 99448[0], 99449[0], 99451[0], 99452[0], 99468[0], 99469[0], 99471[0], 99472[0], 99475[0], 99476[0], 99477[0], 99478[0], 99479[0], 99480[0], 99483[0], 99497[0], C8921[1], C8922[1], C8923[1], C8924[1], C8925[1], C8926[1], C8927[0], C8929[1], C8930[1], G0380[1], G0381[1], G0382[1], G0383[1], G0384[1], G0406[0], G0407[0], G0408[0], G0425[0], G0426[0], G0427[0], G0463[0], G0500[0], G0508[0], G0509[0]
00350	01996[1], 0213T[1], 0216T[1], 0228T[1], 0230T[1], 31505[1], 31515[1], 31527[1], 31622[1], 31634[1], 31645[1], 31647[1], 36000[1], 36010[0], 36011[1], 36012[1], 36013[1], 36014[1], 36015[1], 36400[1], 36405[1], 36406[1], 36410[1], 36420[1], 36425[1], 36430[1], 36440[1], 36591[0], 36592[0], 36600[1], 36640[1], 43752[1], 43753[1], 43754[1], 61026[1], 61055[1], 62280[1], 62281[1], 62282[1], 62284[1], 62320[1], 62321[1], 62322[1], 62323[1], 62324[1], 62325[1], 62326[1], 62327[1], 64400[1], 64402[1], 64405[1], 64408[1], 64410[1], 64413[1], 64415[1], 64416[1], 64417[1], 64418[1], 64420[1], 64421[1], 64425[1], 64430[1], 64435[1], 64445[1], 64446[1], 64447[1], 64448[1], 64449[1], 64450[1], 64461[1], 64463[1], 64479[1], 64483[1], 64486[1], 64487[1], 64488[1], 64489[1], 64490[1], 64493[1], 64505[1], 64510[1], 64517[1], 64520[1], 64530[1], 64553[1], 64555[1], 67500[1], 76000[1], 76970[1], 76998[0], 77002[0], 90865[1], 92511[1], 92512[1], 92516[1], 92520[1], 92537[1], 92538[1], 92950[1], 92953[1], 92960[1], 92961[1], 93000[1], 93005[1], 93010[1], 93040[1], 93041[1], 93042[1], 93050[0], 93303[0], 93304[0], 93306[1], 93307[1], 93308[1], 93312[1], 93313[1], 93314[1], 93315[1], 93316[1], 93317[1], 93318[0], 93351[1], 93355[0], 93451[1], 93456[1], 93457[1], 93561[0], 93562[0], 93701[0], 93922[1], 93923[1], 93924[1], 93925[1], 93926[1], 93930[1], 93931[1], 93970[1], 93971[1], 93975[1], 93976[1], 93978[1], 93979[1], 93980[1], 93981[1], 94002[1], 94004[1], 94200[1], 94250[0], 94640[1], 94644[1], 94660[1], 94662[1], 94680[1], 94681[1], 94690[1], 94760[0], 94761[0], 94762[1], 94770[1], 95812[0], 95813[0], 95816[0], 95819[0], 95822[0], 95829[0], 95955[0], 95956[0], 95957[0], 96360[0], 96365[0], 96372[0], 96373[0], 96374[0], 96375[0], 96376[0], 96377[0], 99151[0], 99152[0], 99153[0], 99155[0], 99156[0], 99157[0], 99201[0], 99202[0], 99203[0], 99204[0], 99205[0], 99211[0], 99212[0], 99213[0], 99214[0], 99215[0], 99217[0], 99218[0], 99219[0], 99220[0], 99221[0], 99222[0], 99223[0], 99224[0], 99225[0], 99226[0], 99231[0], 99232[0], 99233[0], 99234[0], 99235[0], 99236[0], 99238[0], 99239[0], 99281[0], 99282[0], 99283[0], 99284[0], 99285[0], 99304[0], 99305[0], 99306[0], 99307[0], 99308[0], 99309[0], 99310[0], 99315[0], 99318[0], 99324[0], 99325[0], 99326[0], 99327[0], 99328[0], 99334[0], 99335[0], 99336[0], 99337[0], 99341[0], 99342[0], 99343[0], 99347[0], 99348[0], 99349[0], 99354[0], 99355[0], 99356[0], 99357[0], 99358[0], 99359[0], 99415[0], 99416[0], 99446[0], 99447[0], 99448[0], 99449[0], 99451[0], 99452[0], 99466[0], 99468[0], 99469[0], 99471[0], 99472[0], 99475[0], 99476[0], 99477[0], 99478[0], 99479[0], 99480[0], 99483[0], 99485[0], 99497[0], C8921[1], C8922[1], C8923[1], C8924[1], C8925[1], C8926[1], C8927[0], C8929[1], C8930[1], G0380[1], G0381[1], G0382[1], G0383[1], G0384[1], G0406[0], G0407[0], G0408[0], G0425[0], G0426[0], G0427[0], G0463[0], G0500[0], G0508[0], G0509[0]
00352	01996[1], 0213T[1], 0216T[1], 0228T[1], 0230T[1], 31505[1], 31515[1], 31527[1], 31622[1], 31634[1], 31645[1], 31647[1], 36000[1], 36010[0], 36011[1], 36012[1], 36013[1], 36014[1], 36015[1], 36400[1], 36405[1], 36406[1], 36410[1], 36420[1], 36425[1], 36430[1], 36440[1], 36591[0], 36592[0], 36600[1], 36640[1], 43752[1], 43753[1], 43754[1], 61026[1], 61055[1], 62280[1], 62281[1], 62282[1], 62284[1], 62320[1], 62321[1], 62322[1], 62323[1], 62324[1], 62325[1], 62326[1], 62327[1], 64400[1], 64402[1], 64405[1], 64408[1], 64410[1], 64413[1], 64415[1], 64416[1], 64417[1], 64418[1], 64420[1], 64421[1], 64425[1], 64430[1], 64435[1], 64445[1], 64446[1], 64447[1], 64448[1], 64449[1], 64450[1], 64461[1], 64463[1], 64479[1], 64483[1], 64486[1], 64487[1], 64488[1], 64489[1], 64490[1], 64493[1], 64505[1], 64510[1], 64517[1], 64520[1], 64530[1], 64553[1], 64555[1], 67500[1], 76000[1], 76970[1], 76998[0], 77002[0], 90865[1], 92511[1], 92512[1], 92516[1], 92520[1], 92537[1], 92538[1], 92950[1], 92953[1], 92960[1], 92961[1], 93000[1], 93005[1], 93010[1], 93040[1], 93041[1], 93042[1], 93050[0], 93303[0], 93304[0], 93306[1], 93307[1], 93308[1], 93312[1], 93313[1], 93314[1], 93315[1], 93316[1], 93317[1], 93318[0], 93351[1], 93355[0], 93451[1], 93456[1], 93457[1], 93561[0], 93562[0], 93701[0], 93922[1], 93923[1], 93924[1], 93925[1], 93926[1], 93930[1], 93931[1], 93970[1], 93971[1], 93975[1], 93976[1], 93978[1], 93979[1], 93980[1], 93981[1], 94002[1], 94004[1], 94200[1], 94250[0], 94640[1], 94644[1], 94660[1], 94662[1], 94680[1], 94681[1], 94690[1], 94760[0], 94761[0], 94762[1], 94770[1], 95812[0], 95813[0], 95816[0], 95819[0], 95822[0], 95829[0], 95955[0], 95956[0], 95957[0], 96360[0], 96365[0], 96372[0], 96373[0], 96374[0], 96375[0], 96376[0], 96377[0], 99151[0], 99152[0], 99153[0], 99155[0], 99156[0], 99157[0], 99201[0], 99202[0], 99203[0], 99204[0], 99205[0], 99211[0], 99212[0], 99213[0], 99214[0], 99215[0], 99217[0], 99218[0], 99219[0], 99220[0], 99221[0], 99222[0], 99223[0], 99224[0], 99225[0], 99226[0], 99231[0], 99232[0], 99233[0], 99234[0], 99235[0], 99236[0], 99238[0], 99239[0], 99281[0], 99282[0], 99283[0], 99284[0], 99285[0], 99304[0], 99305[0], 99306[0], 99307[0], 99308[0], 99309[0], 99310[0], 99315[0], 99318[0], 99324[0], 99325[0], 99326[0], 99327[0], 99328[0], 99334[0], 99335[0], 99336[0], 99337[0], 99341[0], 99342[0], 99343[0], 99347[0], 99348[0], 99349[0], 99354[0], 99355[0], 99356[0], 99357[0], 99358[0], 99359[0], 99415[0], 99416[0], 99446[0], 99447[0], 99448[0], 99449[0], 99451[0], 99452[0], 99466[0], 99468[0], 99469[0], 99471[0], 99472[0], 99475[0], 99476[0], 99477[0], 99478[0], 99479[0], 99480[0], 99483[0], 99485[0], 99497[0], C8921[1], C8922[1], C8923[1], C8924[1], C8925[1], C8926[1], C8927[0], C8929[1], C8930[1], G0380[1], G0381[1], G0382[1], G0383[1], G0384[1], G0406[0], G0407[0], G0408[0], G0425[0], G0426[0], G0427[0], G0463[0], G0500[0], G0508[0], G0509[0]
00400	01996[1], 0213T[1], 0216T[1], 0228T[1], 0230T[1], 0333T[0], 0464T[0], 31505[1], 31515[1], 31527[1], 31622[1], 31634[1], 31645[1], 31647[1], 36000[1], 36010[0], 36011[1], 36012[1], 36013[1], 36014[1], 36015[1], 36400[1], 36405[1], 36406[1], 36410[1], 36420[1], 36425[1], 36430[1], 36440[1], 36591[0], 36592[0], 36600[1], 36640[1], 43752[1], 43753[1], 43754[1], 61026[1], 61055[1], 62280[1], 62281[1], 62282[1], 62284[1], 62320[1], 62321[1], 62322[1], 62323[1], 62324[1], 62325[1], 62326[1], 62327[1], 64400[1], 64402[1], 64405[1], 64408[1], 64410[1], 64413[1], 64415[1], 64416[1], 64417[1], 64418[1], 64420[1], 64421[1], 64425[1], 64430[1], 64435[1], 64445[1], 64446[1], 64447[1], 64448[1], 64449[1], 64450[1], 64461[1], 64463[1], 64479[1], 64483[1], 64486[1], 64487[1], 64488[1], 64489[1], 64490[1], 64493[1], 64505[1], 64510[1], 64517[1], 64520[1], 64530[1], 64553[1], 64555[1], 67500[1], 76000[1], 76970[1], 76998[0], 77002[0], 90865[1], 92511[1], 92512[1], 92516[1], 92520[1], 92537[1], 92538[1], 92585[0], 92950[1], 92953[1], 92960[1], 92961[1], 93000[1], 93005[1], 93010[1], 93040[1], 93041[1], 93042[1], 93050[0], 93303[0], 93304[0], 93306[1], 93307[1], 93308[1], 93312[1], 93313[1], 93314[1], 93315[1], 93316[1], 93317[1], 93318[0], 93351[1], 93355[0], 93451[1], 93456[1], 93457[1], 93561[0], 93562[0], 93701[0], 93922[1], 93923[1], 93924[1], 93925[1], 93926[1], 93930[1], 93931[1], 93970[1], 93971[1], 93975[1], 93976[1], 93978[1], 93979[1], 93980[1], 93981[1], 94002[1], 94004[1], 94200[1], 94250[0], 94640[1], 94644[1], 94660[1], 94662[1], 94680[1], 94681[1], 94690[1], 94760[0], 94761[0], 94762[1], 94770[1], 95812[0], 95813[0], 95816[0], 95819[0], 95822[0], 95829[0], 95860[0], 95861[0], 95863[0], 95864[0], 95865[0], 95866[0], 95867[0], 95868[0], 95869[0], 95870[0], 95907[0], 95908[0], 95909[0], 95910[0], 95911[0], 95912[0], 95913[0], 95925[0], 95926[0], 95927[0], 95928[0], 95929[0], 95930[0], 95933[0], 95937[0], 95938[0], 95939[0], 95940[0], 95955[0], 95956[0], 95957[0], 96360[0], 96365[0], 96372[0], 96373[0], 96374[0], 96375[0], 96376[0], 96377[0], 99151[0], 99152[0], 99153[0], 99155[0], 99156[0], 99157[0], 99201[0], 99202[0], 99203[0], 99204[0], 99205[0], 99211[0], 99212[0], 99213[0], 99214[0], 99215[0], 99217[0], 99218[0], 99219[0], 99220[0], 99221[0], 99222[0], 99223[0], 99224[0], 99225[0], 99226[0], 99231[0], 99232[0], 99233[0], 99234[0], 99235[0], 99236[0], 99238[0], 99239[0], 99281[0], 99282[0], 99283[0], 99284[0], 99285[0], 99304[0], 99305[0], 99306[0], 99307[0], 99308[0], 99309[0], 99310[0], 99315[0], 99318[0], 99324[0], 99325[0], 99326[0], 99327[0], 99328[0], 99334[0], 99335[0], 99336[0], 99337[0], 99341[0], 99342[0], 99343[0], 99347[0], 99348[0], 99349[0], 99354[0], 99355[0], 99356[0], 99357[0], 99358[0], 99359[0], 99415[0], 99416[0], 99446[0], 99447[0], 99448[0], 99449[0], 99451[0], 99452[0], 99466[0], 99468[0], 99469[0], 99471[0], 99472[0], 99475[0], 99476[0], 99477[0], 99478[0], 99479[0], 99480[0], 99483[0], 99485[0], 99497[0], C8921[1], C8922[1], C8923[1], C8924[1], C8925[1], C8926[1], C8927[0], C8929[1], C8930[1], G0380[1], G0381[1], G0382[1], G0383[1], G0384[1], G0406[0], G0407[0], G0408[0], G0425[0], G0426[0], G0427[0], G0453[0], G0463[0], G0500[0], G0508[0], G0509[0]
00402	01996[1], 0213T[1], 0216T[1], 0228T[1], 0230T[1], 31505[1], 31515[1], 31527[1], 31622[1], 31634[1], 31645[1], 31647[1], 36000[1], 36010[0], 36011[1], 36012[1], 36013[1], 36014[1], 36015[1], 36400[1], 36405[1], 36406[1], 36410[1], 36420[1], 36425[1], 36430[1], 36440[1], 36591[0], 36592[0], 36600[1], 36640[1], 43752[1], 43753[1], 43754[1], 61026[1], 61055[1], 62280[1], 62281[1], 62282[1], 62284[1], 62320[1], 62321[1], 62322[1], 62323[1], 62324[1], 62325[1], 62326[1], 62327[1], 64400[1], 64402[1], 64405[1], 64408[1], 64410[1], 64413[1], 64415[1], 64416[1], 64417[1], 64418[1], 64420[1], 64421[1], 64425[1], 64430[1], 64435[1], 64445[1], 64446[1], 64447[1], 64448[1], 64449[1], 64450[1], 64461[1], 64463[1], 64479[1], 64483[1], 64486[1], 64487[1], 64488[1], 64489[1], 64490[1], 64493[1], 64505[1], 64510[1], 64517[1], 64520[1], 64530[1], 64553[1], 64555[1], 67500[1], 76000[1], 76970[1], 76998[0], 77002[0], 90865[1], 92511[1], 92512[1], 92516[1], 92520[1], 92537[1], 92538[1], 92950[1], 92953[1], 92960[1], 92961[1], 93000[1], 93005[1], 93010[1], 93040[1], 93041[1], 93042[1], 93050[0], 93303[0], 93304[0], 93306[1], 93307[1], 93308[1], 93312[1], 93313[1], 93314[1], 93315[1], 93316[1], 93317[1], 93318[0], 93351[1], 93355[0], 93451[1], 93456[1], 93457[1], 93561[0], 93562[0], 93701[0], 93922[1],

0 = Modifier usage not allowed or inappropriate   1 = Modifier usage allowed

CPT © 2018 American Medical Association. All Rights Reserved.

Code 1	Code 2
	93923[1], 93924[1], 93925[1], 93926[1], 93930[1], 93931[1], 93970[1], 93971[1], 93975[1], 93976[1], 93978[1], 93979[1], 93980[1], 93981[1], 94002[1], 94004[1], 94200[1], 94250[0], 94640[1], 94644[1], 94660[1], 94662[1], 94680[1], 94681[1], 94690[1], 94760[0], 94761[0], 94762[1], 94770[1], 95812[0], 95813[0], 95816[0], 95819[0], 95822[0], 95829[0], 95955[0], 95956[0], 95957[0], 96360[0], 96365[0], 96372[0], 96373[0], 96374[0], 96375[0], 96376[0], 96377[0], 99151[0], 99152[0], 99153[0], 99155[0], 99156[0], 99157[0], 99201[0], 99202[0], 99203[0], 99204[0], 99205[0], 99211[0], 99212[0], 99213[0], 99214[0], 99215[0], 99217[0], 99218[0], 99219[0], 99220[0], 99221[0], 99222[0], 99223[0], 99224[0], 99225[0], 99226[0], 99231[0], 99232[0], 99233[0], 99234[0], 99235[0], 99236[0], 99238[0], 99239[0], 99281[0], 99282[0], 99283[0], 99284[0], 99285[0], 99304[0], 99305[0], 99306[0], 99307[0], 99308[0], 99309[0], 99310[0], 99315[0], 99318[0], 99324[0], 99325[0], 99326[0], 99327[0], 99328[0], 99334[0], 99335[0], 99336[0], 99337[0], 99341[0], 99342[0], 99343[0], 99347[0], 99348[0], 99349[0], 99354[0], 99355[0], 99356[0], 99357[0], 99358[0], 99359[0], 99415[0], 99416[0], 99446[0], 99447[0], 99448[0], 99449[0], 99451[0], 99452[0], 99466[0], 99468[0], 99469[0], 99471[0], 99472[0], 99475[0], 99476[0], 99477[0], 99478[0], 99479[0], 99480[0], 99483[0], 99485[0], 99497[0], C8921[1], C8922[1], C8923[1], C8924[1], C8925[1], C8926[1], C8927[0], C8929[1], C8930[1], G0380[1], G0381[1], G0382[1], G0383[1], G0384[1], G0406[0], G0407[0], G0408[0], G0425[0], G0426[0], G0427[0], G0463[0], G0500[0], G0508[0], G0509[0]
00404	01996[1], 0213T[1], 0216T[1], 0228T[1], 0230T[1], 31505[1], 31515[1], 31527[1], 31622[1], 31634[1], 31645[1], 31647[1], 36000[1], 36010[0], 36011[1], 36012[1], 36013[1], 36014[1], 36015[1], 36400[1], 36405[1], 36406[1], 36410[1], 36420[1], 36425[1], 36430[1], 36440[1], 36591[0], 36592[0], 36600[1], 36640[1], 43752[1], 43753[1], 43754[1], 61026[1], 61055[1], 62280[1], 62281[1], 62282[1], 62284[1], 62320[1], 62321[1], 62322[1], 62323[1], 62324[1], 62325[1], 62326[1], 62327[1], 64400[1], 64402[1], 64405[1], 64408[1], 64410[1], 64413[1], 64415[1], 64416[1], 64417[1], 64418[1], 64420[1], 64421[1], 64425[1], 64430[1], 64435[1], 64445[1], 64446[1], 64447[1], 64448[1], 64449[1], 64450[1], 64461[1], 64463[1], 64479[1], 64483[1], 64486[1], 64487[1], 64488[1], 64489[1], 64490[1], 64493[1], 64505[1], 64510[1], 64517[1], 64520[1], 64530[1], 64553[1], 64555[1], 67500[1], 76000[1], 76970[1], 76998[0], 77002[0], 90865[1], 92511[1], 92512[1], 92516[1], 92520[1], 92537[1], 92538[1], 92950[1], 92953[1], 92960[1], 92961[1], 93000[1], 93005[1], 93010[1], 93040[1], 93041[1], 93042[1], 93050[0], 93303[0], 93304[0], 93306[1], 93307[1], 93308[1], 93312[1], 93313[1], 93314[1], 93315[1], 93316[1], 93317[1], 93318[0], 93351[1], 93355[0], 93451[1], 93456[1], 93457[1], 93561[0], 93562[0], 93701[0], 93922[1], 93923[1], 93924[1], 93925[1], 93926[1], 93930[1], 93931[1], 93970[1], 93971[1], 93975[1], 93976[1], 93978[1], 93979[1], 93980[1], 93981[1], 94002[1], 94004[1], 94200[1], 94250[0], 94640[1], 94644[1], 94660[1], 94662[1], 94680[1], 94681[1], 94690[1], 94760[0], 94761[0], 94762[1], 94770[1], 95812[0], 95813[0], 95816[0], 95819[0], 95822[0], 95829[0], 95955[0], 95956[0], 95957[0], 96360[0], 96365[0], 96372[0], 96373[0], 96374[0], 96375[0], 96376[0], 96377[0], 99151[0], 99152[0], 99153[0], 99155[0], 99156[0], 99157[0], 99201[0], 99202[0], 99203[0], 99204[0], 99205[0], 99211[0], 99212[0], 99213[0], 99214[0], 99215[0], 99217[0], 99218[0], 99219[0], 99220[0], 99221[0], 99222[0], 99223[0], 99224[0], 99225[0], 99226[0], 99231[0], 99232[0], 99233[0], 99234[0], 99235[0], 99236[0], 99238[0], 99239[0], 99281[0], 99282[0], 99283[0], 99284[0], 99285[0], 99304[0], 99305[0], 99306[0], 99307[0], 99308[0], 99309[0], 99310[0], 99315[0], 99318[0], 99324[0], 99325[0], 99326[0], 99327[0], 99328[0], 99334[0], 99335[0], 99336[0], 99337[0], 99341[0], 99342[0], 99343[0], 99347[0], 99348[0], 99349[0], 99354[0], 99355[0], 99356[0], 99357[0], 99358[0], 99359[0], 99415[0], 99416[0], 99446[0], 99447[0], 99448[0], 99449[0], 99451[0], 99452[0], 99466[0], 99468[0], 99469[0], 99471[0], 99472[0], 99475[0], 99476[0], 99477[0], 99478[0], 99479[0], 99480[0], 99483[0], 99485[0], 99497[0], C8921[1], C8922[1], C8923[1], C8924[1], C8925[1], C8926[1], C8927[0], C8929[1], C8930[1], G0380[1], G0381[1], G0382[1], G0383[1], G0384[1], G0406[0], G0407[0], G0408[0], G0425[0], G0426[0], G0427[0], G0463[0], G0500[0], G0508[0], G0509[0]
00406	01996[1], 0213T[1], 0216T[1], 0228T[1], 0230T[1], 31505[1], 31515[1], 31527[1], 31622[1], 31634[1], 31645[1], 31647[1], 36000[1], 36010[0], 36011[1], 36012[1], 36013[1], 36014[1], 36015[1], 36400[1], 36405[1], 36406[1], 36410[1], 36420[1], 36425[1], 36430[1], 36440[1], 36591[0], 36592[0], 36600[1], 36640[1], 43752[1], 43753[1], 43754[1], 61026[1], 61055[1], 62280[1], 62281[1], 62282[1], 62284[1], 62320[1], 62321[1], 62322[1], 62323[1], 62324[1], 62325[1], 62326[1], 62327[1], 64400[1], 64402[1], 64405[1], 64408[1], 64410[1], 64413[1], 64415[1], 64416[1], 64417[1], 64418[1], 64420[1], 64421[1], 64425[1], 64430[1], 64435[1], 64445[1], 64446[1], 64447[1], 64448[1], 64449[1], 64450[1], 64461[1], 64463[1], 64479[1], 64483[1], 64486[1], 64487[1], 64488[1], 64489[1], 64490[1], 64493[1], 64505[1], 64510[1], 64517[1], 64520[1], 64530[1], 64553[1], 64555[1], 67500[1], 76000[1], 76970[1], 76998[0], 77002[0], 90865[1], 92511[1], 92512[1], 92516[1], 92520[1], 92537[1], 92538[1], 92950[1], 92953[1], 92960[1], 92961[1], 93000[1], 93005[1], 93010[1], 93040[1], 93041[1], 93042[1], 93050[0], 93303[0], 93304[0], 93306[1], 93307[1], 93308[1], 93312[1], 93313[1], 93314[1], 93315[1], 93316[1], 93317[1], 93318[0], 93351[1], 93355[0], 93451[1], 93456[1], 93457[1], 93561[0], 93562[0], 93701[0], 93922[1], 93923[1], 93924[1], 93925[1], 93926[1], 93930[1], 93931[1], 93970[1], 93971[1], 93975[1], 93976[1], 93978[1], 93979[1], 93980[1], 93981[1], 94002[1], 94004[1], 94200[1], 94250[0], 94640[1], 94644[1], 94660[1], 94662[1], 94680[1], 94681[1], 94690[1], 94760[0], 94761[0], 94762[1], 94770[1], 95812[0], 95813[0], 95816[0], 95819[0], 95822[0], 95829[0], 95955[0], 95956[0], 95957[0], 96360[0], 96365[0], 96372[0], 96373[0], 96374[0], 96375[0], 96376[0], 96377[0], 99151[0], 99152[0], 99153[0], 99155[0], 99156[0], 99157[0], 99201[0], 99202[0], 99203[0], 99204[0], 99205[0], 99211[0], 99212[0], 99213[0], 99214[0], 99215[0], 99217[0], 99218[0], 99219[0], 99220[0], 99221[0], 99222[0], 99223[0], 99224[0], 99225[0], 99226[0], 99231[0], 99232[0], 99233[0], 99234[0], 99235[0], 99236[0], 99238[0], 99239[0], 99281[0], 99282[0], 99283[0], 99284[0], 99285[0], 99304[0], 99305[0], 99306[0], 99307[0], 99308[0], 99309[0], 99310[0], 99315[0], 99318[0], 99324[0], 99325[0], 99326[0], 99327[0], 99328[0], 99334[0], 99335[0], 99336[0], 99337[0], 99341[0], 99342[0], 99343[0], 99347[0], 99348[0], 99349[0], 99354[0], 99355[0], 99356[0], 99357[0], 99358[0], 99359[0], 99415[0], 99416[0], 99446[0], 99447[0], 99448[0], 99449[0], 99451[0], 99452[0], 99466[0], 99468[0], 99469[0], 99471[0], 99472[0], 99475[0], 99476[0], 99477[0], 99478[0], 99479[0], 99480[0], 99483[0], 99485[0], 99497[0], C8921[1], C8922[1], C8923[1], C8924[1], C8925[1], C8926[1], C8927[0], C8929[1], C8930[1], G0380[1], G0381[1], G0382[1], G0383[1], G0384[1], G0406[0], G0407[0], G0408[0], G0425[0], G0426[0], G0427[0], G0463[0], G0500[0], G0508[0], G0509[0]
00410	01996[1], 0213T[1], 0216T[1], 0228T[1], 0230T[1], 31505[1], 31515[1], 31527[1], 31622[1], 31634[1], 31645[1], 31647[1], 36000[1], 36010[0], 36011[1], 36012[1], 36013[1], 36014[1], 36015[1], 36400[1], 36405[1], 36406[1], 36410[1], 36420[1], 36425[1], 36430[1], 36440[1], 36591[0], 36592[0], 36600[1], 36640[1], 43752[1], 43753[1], 43754[1], 61026[1], 61055[1], 62280[1], 62281[1], 62282[1], 62284[1], 62320[1], 62321[1], 62322[1], 62323[1], 62324[1], 62325[1], 62326[1], 62327[1], 64400[1], 64402[1], 64405[1], 64408[1], 64410[1], 64413[1], 64415[1], 64416[1], 64417[1], 64418[1], 64420[1], 64421[1], 64425[1], 64430[1], 64435[1], 64445[1], 64446[1], 64447[1], 64448[1], 64449[1], 64450[1], 64461[1], 64463[1], 64479[1], 64483[1], 64486[1], 64487[1], 64488[1], 64489[1], 64490[1], 64493[1], 64505[1], 64510[1], 64517[1], 64520[1], 64530[1], 64553[1], 64555[1], 67500[1], 76000[1], 76970[1], 76998[0], 77002[0], 90865[1], 92511[1], 92512[1], 92516[1], 92520[1], 92537[1], 92538[1], 92950[1], 92953[1], 92960[1], 92961[1], 93000[1], 93005[1], 93010[1], 93040[1], 93041[1], 93042[1], 93050[0], 93303[0], 93304[0], 93306[1], 93307[1], 93308[1], 93312[1], 93313[1], 93314[1], 93315[1], 93316[1], 93317[1], 93318[0], 93351[1], 93355[0], 93451[1], 93456[1], 93457[1], 93561[0], 93562[0], 93701[0], 93922[1], 93923[1], 93924[1], 93925[1], 93926[1], 93930[1], 93931[1], 93970[1], 93971[1], 93975[1], 93976[1], 93978[1], 93979[1], 93980[1], 93981[1], 94002[1], 94004[1], 94200[1], 94250[0], 94640[1], 94644[1], 94660[1], 94662[1], 94680[1], 94681[1], 94690[1], 94760[0], 94761[0], 94762[1], 94770[1], 95812[0], 95813[0], 95816[0], 95819[0], 95822[0], 95829[0], 95955[0], 95956[0], 95957[0], 96360[0], 96365[0], 96372[0], 96373[0], 96374[0], 96375[0], 96376[0], 96377[0], 99151[0], 99152[0], 99153[0], 99155[0], 99156[0], 99157[0], 99201[0], 99202[0], 99203[0], 99204[0], 99205[0], 99211[0], 99212[0], 99213[0], 99214[0], 99215[0], 99217[0], 99218[0], 99219[0], 99220[0], 99221[0], 99222[0], 99223[0], 99224[0], 99225[0], 99226[0], 99231[0], 99232[0], 99233[0], 99234[0], 99235[0], 99236[0], 99238[0], 99239[0], 99281[0], 99282[0], 99283[0], 99284[0], 99285[0], 99304[0], 99305[0], 99306[0], 99307[0], 99308[0], 99309[0], 99310[0], 99315[0], 99318[0], 99324[0], 99325[0], 99326[0], 99327[0], 99328[0], 99334[0], 99335[0], 99336[0], 99337[0], 99341[0], 99342[0], 99343[0], 99347[0], 99348[0], 99349[0], 99354[0], 99355[0], 99356[0], 99357[0], 99358[0], 99359[0], 99415[0], 99416[0], 99446[0], 99447[0], 99448[0], 99449[0], 99451[0], 99452[0], 99466[0], 99468[0], 99469[0], 99471[0], 99472[0], 99475[0], 99476[0], 99477[0], 99478[0], 99479[0], 99480[0], 99483[0], 99485[0], 99497[0], C8921[1], C8922[1], C8923[1], C8924[1], C8925[1], C8926[1], C8927[0], C8929[1], C8930[1], G0380[1], G0381[1], G0382[1], G0383[1], G0384[1], G0406[0], G0407[0], G0408[0], G0425[0], G0426[0], G0427[0], G0463[0], G0500[0], G0508[0], G0509[0]
00450	01996[1], 0213T[1], 0216T[1], 0228T[1], 0230T[1], 31505[1], 31515[1], 31527[1], 31622[1], 31634[1], 31645[1], 31647[1], 36000[1], 36010[0], 36011[1], 36012[1], 36013[1], 36014[1], 36015[1], 36400[1], 36405[1], 36406[1], 36410[1], 36420[1], 36425[1], 36430[1], 36440[1], 36591[0], 36592[0], 36600[1], 36640[1], 43752[1], 43753[1], 43754[1], 61026[1], 61055[1], 62280[1], 62281[1], 62282[1], 62284[1], 62320[1], 62321[1], 62322[1], 62323[1], 62324[1], 62325[1], 62326[1], 62327[1], 64400[1], 64402[1], 64405[1], 64408[1], 64410[1], 64413[1], 64415[1], 64416[1], 64417[1], 64418[1], 64420[1], 64421[1], 64425[1], 64430[1], 64435[1], 64445[1], 64446[1], 64447[1], 64448[1], 64449[1], 64450[1], 64461[1], 64463[1], 64479[1], 64483[1], 64486[1], 64487[1], 64488[1], 64489[1], 64490[1], 64493[1], 64505[1], 64510[1], 64517[1], 64520[1], 64530[1], 64553[1], 64555[1], 67500[1], 76000[1], 76970[1], 76998[0], 77002[0], 90865[1], 92511[1], 92512[1], 92516[1], 92520[1], 92537[1], 92538[1], 92950[1], 92953[1], 92960[1], 92961[1], 93000[1], 93005[1], 93010[1], 93040[1], 93041[1], 93042[1], 93050[0], 93303[0], 93304[0], 93306[1], 93307[1], 93308[1], 93312[1], 93313[1], 93314[1], 93315[1], 93316[1], 93317[1], 93318[0], 93351[1], 93355[0], 93451[1], 93456[1], 93457[1], 93561[0], 93562[0], 93701[0], 93922[1], 93923[1], 93924[1], 93925[1], 93926[1], 93930[1], 93931[1], 93970[1], 93971[1], 93975[1], 93976[1], 93978[1], 93979[1], 93980[1], 93981[1], 94002[1], 94004[1], 94200[1], 94250[0], 94640[1], 94644[1], 94660[1], 94662[1], 94680[1], 94681[1], 94690[1], 94760[0], 94761[0], 94762[1], 94770[1], 95812[0], 95813[0], 95816[0], 95819[0], 95822[0], 95829[0], 95955[0], 95956[0], 95957[0], 96360[0], 96365[0], 96372[0], 96373[0], 96374[0], 96375[0], 96376[0], 96377[0], 99151[0], 99152[0], 99153[0], 99155[0], 99156[0], 99157[0], 99201[0], 99202[0], 99203[0], 99204[0], 99205[0], 99211[0], 99212[0], 99213[0], 99214[0], 99215[0], 99217[0], 99218[0], 99219[0], 99220[0], 99221[0], 99222[0], 99223[0], 99224[0], 99225[0], 99226[0], 99231[0], 99232[0], 99233[0], 99234[0], 99235[0], 99236[0], 99238[0], 99239[0], 99281[0], 99282[0], 99283[0], 99284[0], 99285[0], 99304[0], 99305[0], 99306[0], 99307[0], 99308[0], 99309[0], 99310[0], 99315[0], 99318[0], 99324[0], 99325[0], 99326[0], 99327[0], 99328[0], 99334[0], 99335[0], 99336[0], 99337[0], 99341[0], 99342[0], 99343[0], 99347[0], 99348[0], 99349[0], 99354[0], 99355[0], 99356[0], 99357[0], 99358[0], 99359[0], 99415[0], 99416[0], 99446[0], 99447[0], 99448[0],

0 = Modifier usage not allowed or inappropriate 1 = Modifier usage allowed

CPT © 2018 American Medical Association. All Rights Reserved.

Code 1	Code 2
	99449[0], 99451[0], 99452[0], 99466[0], 99468[0], 99469[0], 99471[0], 99472[0], 99475[0], 99476[0], 99477[0], 99478[0], 99479[0], 99480[0], 99483[0], 99485[0], 99497[0], C8921[1], C8922[1], C8923[1], C8924[1], C8925[1], C8926[1], C8927[0], C8929[1], C8930[1], G0380[1], G0381[1], G0382[1], G0383[1], G0384[1], G0406[0], G0407[0], G0408[0], G0425[0], G0426[0], G0427[0], G0463[0], G0500[0], G0508[0], G0509[0]
00454	01996[1], 0213T[1], 0216T[1], 0228T[1], 0230T[1], 31505[1], 31515[1], 31527[1], 31622[1], 31634[1], 31645[1], 31647[1], 36000[1], 36010[0], 36011[1], 36012[1], 36013[1], 36014[1], 36015[1], 36400[1], 36405[1], 36406[1], 36410[1], 36420[1], 36425[1], 36430[1], 36440[1], 36591[0], 36592[0], 36600[1], 36640[1], 43752[1], 43753[1], 43754[1], 61026[1], 61055[1], 62280[1], 62281[1], 62282[1], 62284[1], 62320[1], 62321[1], 62322[1], 62323[1], 62324[1], 62325[1], 62326[1], 62327[1], 64400[1], 64402[1], 64405[1], 64408[1], 64410[1], 64413[1], 64415[1], 64416[1], 64417[1], 64418[1], 64420[1], 64421[1], 64425[1], 64430[1], 64435[1], 64445[1], 64446[1], 64447[1], 64448[1], 64449[1], 64450[1], 64461[1], 64463[1], 64479[1], 64483[1], 64486[1], 64487[1], 64488[1], 64489[1], 64490[1], 64493[1], 64505[1], 64510[1], 64517[1], 64520[1], 64530[1], 64553[1], 64555[1], 67500[1], 76000[1], 76970[1], 76998[0], 77002[0], 90865[1], 92511[1], 92512[1], 92516[1], 92520[1], 92537[1], 92538[1], 92950[1], 92953[1], 92960[1], 92961[1], 93000[1], 93005[1], 93010[1], 93040[1], 93041[1], 93042[1], 93050[0], 93303[0], 93304[0], 93306[1], 93307[1], 93308[1], 93312[1], 93313[1], 93314[1], 93315[1], 93316[1], 93317[1], 93318[0], 93351[1], 93355[0], 93451[1], 93456[1], 93457[1], 93561[0], 93562[0], 93701[0], 93922[1], 93923[1], 93924[1], 93925[1], 93926[1], 93930[1], 93931[1], 93970[1], 93971[1], 93975[1], 93976[1], 93978[1], 93979[1], 93980[1], 93981[1], 94002[1], 94004[1], 94200[1], 94250[0], 94640[1], 94644[1], 94660[1], 94662[1], 94680[1], 94681[1], 94690[1], 94760[0], 94761[0], 94762[1], 94770[1], 95812[0], 95813[0], 95816[0], 95819[0], 95822[0], 95829[0], 95955[0], 95956[0], 95957[0], 96360[0], 96365[0], 96372[0], 96373[0], 96374[0], 96375[0], 96376[0], 96377[0], 99151[0], 99152[0], 99153[0], 99155[0], 99156[0], 99157[0], 99201[0], 99202[0], 99203[0], 99204[0], 99205[0], 99211[0], 99212[0], 99213[0], 99214[0], 99215[0], 99217[0], 99218[0], 99219[0], 99220[0], 99221[0], 99222[0], 99223[0], 99224[0], 99225[0], 99226[0], 99231[0], 99232[0], 99233[0], 99234[0], 99235[0], 99236[0], 99238[0], 99239[0], 99281[0], 99282[0], 99283[0], 99284[0], 99285[0], 99304[0], 99305[0], 99306[0], 99307[0], 99308[0], 99309[0], 99310[0], 99315[0], 99318[0], 99324[0], 99325[0], 99326[0], 99327[0], 99328[0], 99334[0], 99335[0], 99336[0], 99337[0], 99341[0], 99342[0], 99343[0], 99347[0], 99348[0], 99349[0], 99354[0], 99355[0], 99356[0], 99357[0], 99358[0], 99359[0], 99415[0], 99416[0], 99446[0], 99447[0], 99448[0], 99449[0], 99451[0], 99452[0], 99466[0], 99468[0], 99469[0], 99471[0], 99472[0], 99475[0], 99476[0], 99477[0], 99478[0], 99479[0], 99480[0], 99483[0], 99485[0], 99497[0], C8921[1], C8922[1], C8923[1], C8924[1], C8925[1], C8926[1], C8927[0], C8929[1], C8930[1], G0380[1], G0381[1], G0382[1], G0383[1], G0384[1], G0406[0], G0407[0], G0408[0], G0425[0], G0426[0], G0427[0], G0463[0], G0500[0], G0508[0], G0509[0]
00470	01996[1], 0213T[1], 0216T[1], 0228T[1], 0230T[1], 31505[1], 31515[1], 31527[1], 31622[1], 31634[1], 31645[1], 31647[1], 36000[1], 36010[0], 36011[1], 36012[1], 36013[1], 36014[1], 36015[1], 36400[1], 36405[1], 36406[1], 36410[1], 36420[1], 36425[1], 36430[1], 36440[1], 36591[0], 36592[0], 36600[1], 36640[1], 43752[1], 43753[1], 43754[1], 61026[1], 61055[1], 62280[1], 62281[1], 62282[1], 62284[1], 62320[1], 62321[1], 62322[1], 62323[1], 62324[1], 62325[1], 62326[1], 62327[1], 64400[1], 64402[1], 64405[1], 64408[1], 64410[1], 64413[1], 64415[1], 64416[1], 64417[1], 64418[1], 64420[1], 64421[1], 64425[1], 64430[1], 64435[1], 64445[1], 64446[1], 64447[1], 64448[1], 64449[1], 64450[1], 64461[1], 64463[1], 64479[1], 64483[1], 64486[1], 64487[1], 64488[1], 64489[1], 64490[1], 64493[1], 64505[1], 64510[1], 64517[1], 64520[1], 64530[1], 64553[1], 64555[1], 67500[1], 76000[1], 76970[1], 76998[0], 77002[0], 90865[1], 92511[1], 92512[1], 92516[1], 92520[1], 92537[1], 92538[1], 92950[1], 92953[1], 92960[1], 92961[1], 93000[1], 93005[1], 93010[1], 93040[1], 93041[1], 93042[1], 93050[0], 93303[0], 93304[0], 93306[1], 93307[1], 93308[1], 93312[1], 93313[1], 93314[1], 93315[1], 93316[1], 93317[1], 93318[0], 93351[1], 93355[0], 93451[1], 93456[1], 93457[1], 93561[0], 93562[0], 93701[0], 93922[1], 93923[1], 93924[1], 93925[1], 93926[1], 93930[1], 93931[1], 93970[1], 93971[1], 93975[1], 93976[1], 93978[1], 93979[1], 93980[1], 93981[1], 94002[1], 94004[1], 94200[1], 94250[0], 94640[1], 94644[1], 94660[1], 94662[1], 94680[1], 94681[1], 94690[1], 94760[0], 94761[0], 94762[1], 94770[1], 95812[0], 95813[0], 95816[0], 95819[0], 95822[0], 95829[0], 95955[0], 95956[0], 95957[0], 96360[0], 96365[0], 96372[0], 96373[0], 96374[0], 96375[0], 96376[0], 96377[0], 99151[0], 99152[0], 99153[0], 99155[0], 99156[0], 99157[0], 99201[0], 99202[0], 99203[0], 99204[0], 99205[0], 99211[0], 99212[0], 99213[0], 99214[0], 99215[0], 99217[0], 99218[0], 99219[0], 99220[0], 99221[0], 99222[0], 99223[0], 99224[0], 99225[0], 99226[0], 99231[0], 99232[0], 99233[0], 99234[0], 99235[0], 99236[0], 99238[0], 99239[0], 99281[0], 99282[0], 99283[0], 99284[0], 99285[0], 99304[0], 99305[0], 99306[0], 99307[0], 99308[0], 99309[0], 99310[0], 99315[0], 99318[0], 99324[0], 99325[0], 99326[0], 99327[0], 99328[0], 99334[0], 99335[0], 99336[0], 99337[0], 99341[0], 99342[0], 99343[0], 99347[0], 99348[0], 99349[0], 99354[0], 99355[0], 99356[0], 99357[0], 99358[0], 99359[0], 99415[0], 99416[0], 99446[0], 99447[0], 99448[0], 99449[0], 99451[0], 99452[0], 99466[0], 99468[0], 99469[0], 99471[0], 99472[0], 99475[0], 99476[0], 99477[0], 99478[0], 99479[0], 99480[0], 99483[0], 99485[0], 99497[0], C8921[1], C8922[1], C8923[1], C8924[1], C8925[1], C8926[1], C8927[0], C8929[1], C8930[1], G0380[1], G0381[1], G0382[1], G0383[1], G0384[1], G0406[0], G0407[0], G0408[0], G0425[0], G0426[0], G0427[0], G0463[0], G0500[0], G0508[0], G0509[0]
00472	01996[1], 0213T[1], 0216T[1], 0228T[1], 0230T[1], 31505[1], 31515[1], 31527[1], 31622[1], 31634[1], 31645[1], 31647[1], 36000[1], 36010[0], 36011[1], 36012[1], 36013[1], 36014[1], 36015[1], 36400[1], 36405[1], 36406[1], 36410[1], 36420[1], 36425[1], 36430[1], 36440[1], 36591[0], 36592[0], 36600[1], 36640[1], 43752[1], 43753[1], 43754[1], 61026[1], 61055[1], 62280[1], 62281[1], 62282[1], 62284[1], 62320[1], 62321[1], 62322[1], 62323[1], 62324[1], 62325[1], 62326[1], 62327[1], 64400[1], 64402[1], 64405[1], 64408[1], 64410[1], 64413[1], 64415[1], 64416[1], 64417[1], 64418[1], 64420[1], 64421[1], 64425[1], 64430[1], 64435[1], 64445[1], 64446[1], 64447[1], 64448[1], 64449[1], 64450[1], 64461[1], 64463[1], 64479[1], 64483[1], 64486[1], 64487[1], 64488[1], 64489[1], 64490[1], 64493[1], 64505[1], 64510[1], 64517[1], 64520[1], 64530[1], 64553[1], 64555[1], 67500[1], 76000[1], 76970[1], 76998[0], 77002[0], 90865[1], 92511[1], 92512[1], 92516[1], 92520[1], 92537[1], 92538[1], 92950[1], 92953[1], 92960[1], 92961[1], 93000[1], 93005[1], 93010[1], 93040[1], 93041[1], 93042[1], 93050[0], 93303[0], 93304[0], 93306[1], 93307[1], 93308[1], 93312[1], 93313[1], 93314[1], 93315[1], 93316[1], 93317[1], 93318[0], 93351[1], 93355[0], 93451[1], 93456[1], 93457[1], 93561[0], 93562[0], 93701[0], 93922[1], 93923[1], 93924[1], 93925[1], 93926[1], 93930[1], 93931[1], 93970[1], 93971[1], 93975[1], 93976[1], 93978[1], 93979[1], 93980[1], 93981[1], 94002[1], 94004[1], 94200[1], 94250[0], 94640[1], 94644[1], 94660[1], 94662[1], 94680[1], 94681[1], 94690[1], 94760[0], 94761[0], 94762[1], 94770[1], 95812[0], 95813[0], 95816[0], 95819[0], 95822[0], 95829[0], 95955[0], 95956[0], 95957[0], 96360[0], 96365[0], 96372[0], 96373[0], 96374[0], 96375[0], 96376[0], 96377[0], 99151[0], 99152[0], 99153[0], 99155[0], 99156[0], 99157[0], 99201[0], 99202[0], 99203[0], 99204[0], 99205[0], 99211[0], 99212[0], 99213[0], 99214[0], 99215[0], 99217[0], 99218[0], 99219[0], 99220[0], 99221[0], 99222[0], 99223[0], 99224[0], 99225[0], 99226[0], 99231[0], 99232[0], 99233[0], 99234[0], 99235[0], 99236[0], 99238[0], 99239[0], 99281[0], 99282[0], 99283[0], 99284[0], 99285[0], 99304[0], 99305[0], 99306[0], 99307[0], 99308[0], 99309[0], 99310[0], 99315[0], 99318[0], 99324[0], 99325[0], 99326[0], 99327[0], 99328[0], 99334[0], 99335[0], 99336[0], 99337[0], 99341[0], 99342[0], 99343[0], 99347[0], 99348[0], 99349[0], 99354[0], 99355[0], 99356[0], 99357[0], 99358[0], 99359[0], 99415[0], 99416[0], 99446[0], 99447[0], 99448[0], 99449[0], 99451[0], 99452[0], 99466[0], 99468[0], 99469[0], 99471[0], 99472[0], 99475[0], 99476[0], 99477[0], 99478[0], 99479[0], 99480[0], 99483[0], 99485[0], 99497[0], C8921[1], C8922[1], C8923[1], C8924[1], C8925[1], C8926[1], C8927[0], C8929[1], C8930[1], G0380[1], G0381[1], G0382[1], G0383[1], G0384[1], G0406[0], G0407[0], G0408[0], G0425[0], G0426[0], G0427[0], G0463[0], G0500[0], G0508[0], G0509[0]
00474	01996[1], 0213T[1], 0216T[1], 0228T[1], 0230T[1], 31505[1], 31515[1], 31527[1], 31622[1], 31634[1], 31645[1], 31647[1], 36000[1], 36010[0], 36011[1], 36012[1], 36013[1], 36014[1], 36015[1], 36400[1], 36405[1], 36406[1], 36410[1], 36420[1], 36425[1], 36430[1], 36440[1], 36591[0], 36592[0], 36600[1], 36640[1], 43752[1], 43753[1], 43754[1], 61026[1], 61055[1], 62280[1], 62281[1], 62282[1], 62284[1], 62320[1], 62321[1], 62322[1], 62323[1], 62324[1], 62325[1], 62326[1], 62327[1], 64400[1], 64402[1], 64405[1], 64408[1], 64410[1], 64413[1], 64415[1], 64416[1], 64417[1], 64418[1], 64420[1], 64421[1], 64425[1], 64430[1], 64435[1], 64445[1], 64446[1], 64447[1], 64448[1], 64449[1], 64450[1], 64461[1], 64463[1], 64479[1], 64483[1], 64486[1], 64487[1], 64488[1], 64489[1], 64490[1], 64493[1], 64505[1], 64510[1], 64517[1], 64520[1], 64530[1], 64553[1], 64555[1], 67500[1], 76000[1], 76970[1], 76998[0], 77002[0], 90865[1], 92511[1], 92512[1], 92516[1], 92520[1], 92537[1], 92538[1], 92950[1], 92953[1], 92960[1], 92961[1], 93000[1], 93005[1], 93010[1], 93040[1], 93041[1], 93042[1], 93050[0], 93303[0], 93304[0], 93306[1], 93307[1], 93308[1], 93312[1], 93313[1], 93314[1], 93315[1], 93316[1], 93317[1], 93318[0], 93351[1], 93355[0], 93451[1], 93456[1], 93457[1], 93561[0], 93562[0], 93701[0], 93922[1], 93923[1], 93924[1], 93925[1], 93926[1], 93930[1], 93931[1], 93970[1], 93971[1], 93975[1], 93976[1], 93978[1], 93979[1], 93980[1], 93981[1], 94002[1], 94004[1], 94200[1], 94250[0], 94640[1], 94644[1], 94660[1], 94662[1], 94680[1], 94681[1], 94690[1], 94760[0], 94761[0], 94762[1], 94770[1], 95812[0], 95813[0], 95816[0], 95819[0], 95822[0], 95829[0], 95955[0], 95956[0], 95957[0], 96360[0], 96365[0], 96372[0], 96373[0], 96374[0], 96375[0], 96376[0], 96377[0], 99151[0], 99152[0], 99153[0], 99155[0], 99156[0], 99157[0], 99201[0], 99202[0], 99203[0], 99204[0], 99205[0], 99211[0], 99212[0], 99213[0], 99214[0], 99215[0], 99217[0], 99218[0], 99219[0], 99220[0], 99221[0], 99222[0], 99223[0], 99224[0], 99225[0], 99226[0], 99231[0], 99232[0], 99233[0], 99234[0], 99235[0], 99236[0], 99238[0], 99239[0], 99281[0], 99282[0], 99283[0], 99284[0], 99285[0], 99304[0], 99305[0], 99306[0], 99307[0], 99308[0], 99309[0], 99310[0], 99315[0], 99318[0], 99324[0], 99325[0], 99326[0], 99327[0], 99328[0], 99334[0], 99335[0], 99336[0], 99337[0], 99341[0], 99342[0], 99343[0], 99347[0], 99348[0], 99349[0], 99354[0], 99355[0], 99356[0], 99357[0], 99358[0], 99359[0], 99415[0], 99416[0], 99446[0], 99447[0], 99448[0], 99449[0], 99451[0], 99452[0], 99466[0], 99468[0], 99469[0], 99471[0], 99472[0], 99475[0], 99476[0], 99477[0], 99478[0], 99479[0], 99480[0], 99483[0], 99485[0], 99497[0], C8921[1], C8922[1], C8923[1], C8924[1], C8925[1], C8926[1], C8927[0], C8929[1], C8930[1], G0380[1], G0381[1], G0382[1], G0383[1], G0384[1], G0406[0], G0407[0], G0408[0], G0425[0], G0426[0], G0427[0], G0463[0], G0500[0], G0508[0], G0509[0]
00500	01996[1], 0213T[1], 0216T[1], 0228T[1], 0230T[1], 31505[1], 31515[1], 31527[1], 31622[1], 31634[1], 31645[1], 31647[1], 36000[1], 36010[0], 36011[1], 36012[1], 36013[1], 36014[1], 36015[1], 36400[1], 36405[1], 36406[1], 36410[1], 36420[1], 36425[1], 36430[1], 36440[1], 36591[0], 36592[0], 36600[1], 36640[1], 43752[1], 43753[1], 43754[1], 61026[1], 61055[1], 62280[1], 62281[1], 62282[1], 62284[1], 62320[1], 62321[1], 62322[1], 62323[1], 62324[1], 62325[1], 62326[1], 62327[1], 64400[1], 64402[1], 64405[1], 64408[1], 64410[1], 64413[1], 64415[1], 64416[1], 64417[1], 64418[1], 64420[1], 64421[1],

0 = Modifier usage not allowed or inappropriate 1 = Modifier usage allowed

CPT © 2018 American Medical Association. All Rights Reserved.

Code 1	Code 2
	64425[1], 64430[1], 64435[1], 64445[1], 64446[1], 64447[1], 64448[1], 64449[1], 64450[1], 64461[1], 64463[1], 64479[1], 64483[1], 64486[1], 64487[1], 64488[1], 64489[1], 64490[1], 64493[1], 64505[1], 64510[1], 64517[1], 64520[1], 64530[1], 64553[1], 64555[1], 67500[1], 76000[1], 76970[1], 76998[0], 77002[0], 90865[1], 92511[1], 92512[1], 92516[1], 92520[1], 92537[1], 92538[1], 92950[1], 92953[1], 92960[1], 92961[1], 93000[1], 93005[1], 93010[1], 93040[1], 93041[1], 93042[1], 93050[0], 93303[0], 93304[0], 93306[1], 93307[1], 93308[1], 93312[1], 93313[1], 93314[1], 93315[1], 93316[1], 93317[1], 93318[0], 93351[1], 93355[0], 93451[1], 93456[1], 93457[1], 93561[0], 93562[0], 93701[0], 93922[1], 93923[1], 93924[1], 93925[1], 93926[1], 93930[1], 93931[1], 93970[1], 93971[1], 93975[1], 93976[1], 93978[1], 93979[1], 93980[1], 93981[1], 94002[1], 94004[1], 94200[1], 94250[0], 94640[1], 94644[1], 94660[1], 94662[1], 94680[1], 94681[1], 94690[1], 94760[0], 94761[0], 94762[1], 94770[1], 95812[0], 95813[0], 95816[0], 95819[0], 95822[0], 95829[0], 95955[0], 95956[0], 95957[0], 96360[0], 96365[0], 96372[0], 96373[0], 96374[0], 96375[0], 96376[0], 96377[0], 99151[0], 99152[0], 99153[0], 99155[0], 99156[0], 99157[0], 99201[0], 99202[0], 99203[0], 99204[0], 99205[0], 99211[0], 99212[0], 99213[0], 99214[0], 99215[0], 99217[0], 99218[0], 99219[0], 99220[0], 99221[0], 99222[0], 99223[0], 99224[0], 99225[0], 99226[0], 99231[0], 99232[0], 99233[0], 99234[0], 99235[0], 99236[0], 99238[0], 99239[0], 99281[0], 99282[0], 99283[0], 99284[0], 99285[0], 99304[0], 99305[0], 99306[0], 99307[0], 99308[0], 99309[0], 99310[0], 99315[0], 99318[0], 99324[0], 99325[0], 99326[0], 99327[0], 99328[0], 99334[0], 99335[0], 99336[0], 99337[0], 99341[0], 99342[0], 99343[0], 99347[0], 99348[0], 99349[0], 99354[0], 99355[0], 99356[0], 99357[0], 99358[0], 99359[0], 99415[0], 99416[0], 99446[0], 99447[0], 99448[0], 99449[0], 99451[0], 99452[0], 99466[0], 99468[0], 99469[0], 99471[0], 99472[0], 99475[0], 99476[0], 99477[0], 99478[0], 99479[0], 99480[0], 99483[0], 99485[0], 99497[0], C8921[1], C8922[1], C8923[1], C8924[1], C8925[1], C8926[1], C8927[0], C8929[1], C8930[1], G0380[1], G0381[1], G0382[1], G0383[1], G0384[1], G0406[0], G0407[0], G0408[0], G0425[0], G0426[0], G0427[0], G0463[0], G0500[0], G0508[0], G0509[0]
00520	01996[1], 0213T[1], 0216T[1], 0228T[1], 0230T[1], 31505[1], 31515[1], 31527[1], 36000[1], 36010[0], 36011[1], 36012[1], 36013[1], 36014[1], 36015[1], 36400[1], 36405[1], 36406[1], 36410[1], 36420[1], 36425[1], 36430[1], 36440[1], 36591[0], 36592[0], 36600[1], 36640[1], 43752[1], 43753[1], 43754[1], 61026[1], 61055[1], 62280[1], 62281[1], 62282[1], 62284[1], 62320[1], 62321[1], 62322[1], 62323[1], 62324[1], 62325[1], 62326[1], 62327[1], 64400[1], 64402[1], 64405[1], 64408[1], 64410[1], 64413[1], 64415[1], 64416[1], 64417[1], 64418[1], 64420[1], 64421[1], 64425[1], 64430[1], 64435[1], 64445[1], 64446[1], 64447[1], 64448[1], 64449[1], 64450[1], 64461[1], 64463[1], 64479[1], 64483[1], 64486[1], 64487[1], 64488[1], 64489[1], 64490[1], 64493[1], 64505[1], 64510[1], 64517[1], 64520[1], 64530[1], 64553[1], 64555[1], 67500[1], 76000[1], 76970[1], 76998[0], 77002[0], 90865[1], 92511[1], 92512[1], 92516[1], 92520[1], 92537[1], 92538[1], 92950[1], 92953[1], 92960[1], 92961[1], 93000[1], 93005[1], 93010[1], 93040[1], 93041[1], 93042[1], 93050[0], 93303[0], 93304[0], 93306[1], 93307[1], 93308[1], 93312[1], 93313[1], 93314[1], 93315[1], 93316[1], 93317[1], 93318[0], 93351[1], 93355[0], 93451[1], 93456[1], 93457[1], 93561[0], 93562[0], 93701[0], 93922[1], 93923[1], 93924[1], 93925[1], 93926[1], 93930[1], 93931[1], 93970[1], 93971[1], 93975[1], 93976[1], 93978[1], 93979[1], 93980[1], 93981[1], 94002[1], 94004[1], 94200[1], 94250[0], 94640[1], 94644[1], 94660[1], 94662[1], 94680[1], 94681[1], 94690[1], 94760[0], 94761[0], 94762[1], 94770[1], 95812[0], 95813[0], 95816[0], 95819[0], 95822[0], 95829[0], 95955[0], 95956[0], 95957[0], 96360[0], 96365[0], 96372[0], 96373[0], 96374[0], 96375[0], 96376[0], 96377[0], 99151[0], 99152[0], 99153[0], 99155[0], 99156[0], 99157[0], 99201[0], 99202[0], 99203[0], 99204[0], 99205[0], 99211[0], 99212[0], 99213[0], 99214[0], 99215[0], 99217[0], 99218[0], 99219[0], 99220[0], 99221[0], 99222[0], 99223[0], 99224[0], 99225[0], 99226[0], 99231[0], 99232[0], 99233[0], 99234[0], 99235[0], 99236[0], 99238[0], 99239[0], 99281[0], 99282[0], 99283[0], 99284[0], 99285[0], 99304[0], 99305[0], 99306[0], 99307[0], 99308[0], 99309[0], 99310[0], 99315[0], 99318[0], 99324[0], 99325[0], 99326[0], 99327[0], 99328[0], 99334[0], 99335[0], 99336[0], 99337[0], 99341[0], 99342[0], 99343[0], 99347[0], 99348[0], 99349[0], 99354[0], 99355[0], 99356[0], 99357[0], 99358[0], 99359[0], 99415[0], 99416[0], 99446[0], 99447[0], 99448[0], 99449[0], 99451[0], 99452[0], 99466[0], 99468[0], 99469[0], 99471[0], 99472[0], 99475[0], 99476[0], 99477[0], 99478[0], 99479[0], 99480[0], 99483[0], 99485[0], 99497[0], C8921[1], C8922[1], C8923[1], C8924[1], C8925[1], C8926[1], C8927[0], C8929[1], C8930[1], G0380[1], G0381[1], G0382[1], G0383[1], G0384[1], G0406[0], G0407[0], G0408[0], G0425[0], G0426[0], G0427[0], G0463[0], G0500[0], G0508[0], G0509[0]
00522	01996[1], 0213T[1], 0216T[1], 0228T[1], 0230T[1], 31505[1], 31515[1], 31527[1], 31622[1], 31634[1], 31645[1], 31647[1], 36000[1], 36010[0], 36011[1], 36012[1], 36013[1], 36014[1], 36015[1], 36400[1], 36405[1], 36406[1], 36410[1], 36420[1], 36425[1], 36430[1], 36440[1], 36591[0], 36592[0], 36600[1], 36640[1], 43752[1], 43753[1], 43754[1], 61026[1], 61055[1], 62280[1], 62281[1], 62282[1], 62284[1], 62320[1], 62321[1], 62322[1], 62323[1], 62324[1], 62325[1], 62326[1], 62327[1], 64400[1], 64402[1], 64405[1], 64408[1], 64410[1], 64413[1], 64415[1], 64416[1], 64417[1], 64418[1], 64420[1], 64421[1], 64425[1], 64430[1], 64435[1], 64445[1], 64446[1], 64447[1], 64448[1], 64449[1], 64450[1], 64461[1], 64463[1], 64479[1], 64483[1], 64486[1], 64487[1], 64488[1], 64489[1], 64490[1], 64493[1], 64505[1], 64510[1], 64517[1], 64520[1], 64530[1], 64553[1], 64555[1], 67500[1], 76000[1], 76970[1], 76998[0], 77002[0], 90865[1], 92511[1], 92512[1], 92516[1], 92520[1], 92537[1], 92538[1], 92950[1], 92953[1], 92960[1], 92961[1], 93000[1], 93005[1], 93010[1], 93040[1], 93041[1], 93042[1], 93050[0], 93303[0], 93304[0], 93306[1], 93307[1], 93308[1], 93312[1], 93313[1], 93314[1], 93315[1], 93316[1], 93317[1], 93318[0], 93351[1], 93355[0], 93451[1], 93456[1], 93457[1], 93561[0], 93562[0], 93701[0], 93922[1], 93923[1], 93924[1], 93925[1], 93926[1], 93930[1], 93931[1], 93970[1], 93971[1], 93975[1], 93976[1], 93978[1], 93979[1], 93980[1], 93981[1], 94002[1], 94004[1], 94200[1], 94250[0], 94640[1], 94644[1], 94660[1], 94662[1], 94680[1], 94681[1], 94690[1], 94760[0], 94761[0], 94762[1], 94770[1], 95812[0], 95813[0], 95816[0], 95819[0], 95822[0], 95829[0], 95955[0], 95956[0], 95957[0], 96360[0], 96365[0], 96372[0], 96373[0], 96374[0], 96375[0], 96376[0], 96377[0], 99151[0], 99152[0], 99153[0], 99155[0], 99156[0], 99157[0], 99201[0], 99202[0], 99203[0], 99204[0], 99205[0], 99211[0], 99212[0], 99213[0], 99214[0], 99215[0], 99217[0], 99218[0], 99219[0], 99220[0], 99221[0], 99222[0], 99223[0], 99224[0], 99225[0], 99226[0], 99231[0], 99232[0], 99233[0], 99234[0], 99235[0], 99236[0], 99238[0], 99239[0], 99281[0], 99282[0], 99283[0], 99284[0], 99285[0], 99304[0], 99305[0], 99306[0], 99307[0], 99308[0], 99309[0], 99310[0], 99315[0], 99318[0], 99324[0], 99325[0], 99326[0], 99327[0], 99328[0], 99334[0], 99335[0], 99336[0], 99337[0], 99341[0], 99342[0], 99343[0], 99347[0], 99348[0], 99349[0], 99354[0], 99355[0], 99356[0], 99357[0], 99358[0], 99359[0], 99415[0], 99416[0], 99446[0], 99447[0], 99448[0], 99449[0], 99451[0], 99452[0], 99466[0], 99468[0], 99469[0], 99471[0], 99472[0], 99475[0], 99476[0], 99477[0], 99478[0], 99479[0], 99480[0], 99483[0], 99485[0], 99497[0], C8921[1], C8922[1], C8923[1], C8924[1], C8925[1], C8926[1], C8927[0], C8929[1], C8930[1], G0380[1], G0381[1], G0382[1], G0383[1], G0384[1], G0406[0], G0407[0], G0408[0], G0425[0], G0426[0], G0427[0], G0463[0], G0500[0], G0508[0], G0509[0]
00524	01996[1], 0213T[1], 0216T[1], 0228T[1], 0230T[1], 31505[1], 31515[1], 31527[1], 31622[1], 31634[1], 31645[1], 31647[1], 36000[1], 36010[0], 36011[1], 36012[1], 36013[1], 36014[1], 36015[1], 36400[1], 36405[1], 36406[1], 36410[1], 36420[1], 36425[1], 36430[1], 36440[1], 36591[0], 36592[0], 36600[1], 36640[1], 43752[1], 43753[1], 43754[1], 61026[1], 61055[1], 62280[1], 62281[1], 62282[1], 62284[1], 62320[1], 62321[1], 62322[1], 62323[1], 62324[1], 62325[1], 62326[1], 62327[1], 64400[1], 64402[1], 64405[1], 64408[1], 64410[1], 64413[1], 64415[1], 64416[1], 64417[1], 64418[1], 64420[1], 64421[1], 64425[1], 64430[1], 64435[1], 64445[1], 64446[1], 64447[1], 64448[1], 64449[1], 64450[1], 64461[1], 64463[1], 64479[1], 64483[1], 64486[1], 64487[1], 64488[1], 64489[1], 64490[1], 64493[1], 64505[1], 64510[1], 64517[1], 64520[1], 64530[1], 64553[1], 64555[1], 67500[1], 76000[1], 76970[1], 76998[0], 77002[0], 90865[1], 92511[1], 92512[1], 92516[1], 92520[1], 92537[1], 92538[1], 92950[1], 92953[1], 92960[1], 92961[1], 93000[1], 93005[1], 93010[1], 93040[1], 93041[1], 93042[1], 93050[0], 93303[0], 93304[0], 93306[1], 93307[1], 93308[1], 93312[1], 93313[1], 93314[1], 93315[1], 93316[1], 93317[1], 93318[0], 93351[1], 93355[0], 93451[1], 93456[1], 93457[1], 93561[0], 93562[0], 93701[0], 93922[1], 93923[1], 93924[1], 93925[1], 93926[1], 93930[1], 93931[1], 93970[1], 93971[1], 93975[1], 93976[1], 93978[1], 93979[1], 93980[1], 93981[1], 94002[1], 94004[1], 94200[1], 94250[0], 94640[1], 94644[1], 94660[1], 94662[1], 94680[1], 94681[1], 94690[1], 94760[0], 94761[0], 94762[1], 94770[1], 95812[0], 95813[0], 95816[0], 95819[0], 95822[0], 95829[0], 95955[0], 95956[0], 95957[0], 96360[0], 96365[0], 96372[0], 96373[0], 96374[0], 96375[0], 96376[0], 96377[0], 99151[0], 99152[0], 99153[0], 99155[0], 99156[0], 99157[0], 99201[0], 99202[0], 99203[0], 99204[0], 99205[0], 99211[0], 99212[0], 99213[0], 99214[0], 99215[0], 99217[0], 99218[0], 99219[0], 99220[0], 99221[0], 99222[0], 99223[0], 99224[0], 99225[0], 99226[0], 99231[0], 99232[0], 99233[0], 99234[0], 99235[0], 99236[0], 99238[0], 99239[0], 99281[0], 99282[0], 99283[0], 99284[0], 99285[0], 99304[0], 99305[0], 99306[0], 99307[0], 99308[0], 99309[0], 99310[0], 99315[0], 99318[0], 99324[0], 99325[0], 99326[0], 99327[0], 99328[0], 99334[0], 99335[0], 99336[0], 99337[0], 99341[0], 99342[0], 99343[0], 99347[0], 99348[0], 99349[0], 99354[0], 99355[0], 99356[0], 99357[0], 99358[0], 99359[0], 99415[0], 99416[0], 99446[0], 99447[0], 99448[0], 99449[0], 99451[0], 99452[0], 99466[0], 99468[0], 99469[0], 99471[0], 99472[0], 99475[0], 99476[0], 99477[0], 99478[0], 99479[0], 99480[0], 99483[0], 99485[0], 99497[0], C8921[1], C8922[1], C8923[1], C8924[1], C8925[1], C8926[1], C8927[0], C8929[1], C8930[1], G0380[1], G0381[1], G0382[1], G0383[1], G0384[1], G0406[0], G0407[0], G0408[0], G0425[0], G0426[0], G0427[0], G0463[0], G0500[0], G0508[0], G0509[0]
00528	01996[1], 0213T[1], 0216T[1], 0228T[1], 0230T[1], 31505[1], 31515[1], 31527[1], 31622[1], 31634[1], 31645[1], 31647[1], 36000[1], 36010[0], 36011[1], 36012[1], 36013[1], 36014[1], 36015[1], 36400[1], 36405[1], 36406[1], 36410[1], 36420[1], 36425[1], 36430[1], 36440[1], 36591[0], 36592[0], 36600[1], 36640[1], 43752[1], 43753[1], 43754[1], 61026[1], 61055[1], 62280[1], 62281[1], 62282[1], 62284[1], 62320[1], 62321[1], 62322[1], 62323[1], 62324[1], 62325[1], 62326[1], 62327[1], 64400[1], 64402[1], 64405[1], 64408[1], 64410[1], 64413[1], 64415[1], 64416[1], 64417[1], 64418[1], 64420[1], 64421[1], 64425[1], 64430[1], 64435[1], 64445[1], 64446[1], 64447[1], 64448[1], 64449[1], 64450[1], 64461[1], 64463[1], 64479[1], 64483[1], 64486[1], 64487[1], 64488[1], 64489[1], 64490[1], 64493[1], 64505[1], 64510[1], 64517[1], 64520[1], 64530[1], 64553[1], 64555[1], 67500[1], 76000[1], 76970[1], 76998[0], 77002[0], 90865[1], 92511[1], 92512[1], 92516[1], 92520[1], 92537[1], 92538[1], 92950[1], 92953[1], 92960[1], 92961[1], 93000[1], 93005[1], 93010[1], 93040[1], 93041[1], 93042[1], 93050[0], 93303[0], 93304[0], 93306[1], 93307[1], 93308[1], 93312[1], 93313[1], 93314[1], 93315[1], 93316[1], 93317[1], 93318[0], 93351[1], 93355[0], 93451[1], 93456[1], 93457[1], 93561[0], 93562[0], 93701[0], 93922[1], 93923[1], 93924[1], 93925[1], 93926[1], 93930[1], 93931[1], 93970[1], 93971[1], 93975[1], 93976[1], 93978[1], 93979[1], 93980[1], 93981[1], 94002[1], 94004[1], 94200[1], 94250[0], 94640[1], 94644[1], 94660[1], 94662[1], 94680[1], 94681[1], 94690[1], 94760[0], 94761[0], 94762[1], 94770[1], 95812[0], 95813[0], 95816[0], 95819[0], 95822[0], 95829[0], 95955[0], 95956[0], 95957[0], 96360[0], 96365[0], 96372[0], 96373[0], 96374[0], 96375[0], 96376[0], 96377[0], 99151[0], 99152[0], 99153[0], 99155[0], 99156[0], 99157[0], 99201[0], 99202[0], 99203[0], 99204[0], 99205[0], 99211[0], 99212[0], 99213[0],

0 = Modifier usage not allowed or inappropriate 1 = Modifier usage allowed

CPT © 2018 American Medical Association. All Rights Reserved.

Code 1	Code 2
	99214[0], 99215[0], 99217[0], 99218[0], 99219[0], 99220[0], 99221[0], 99222[0], 99223[0], 99224[0], 99225[0], 99226[0], 99231[0], 99232[0], 99233[0], 99234[0], 99235[0], 99236[0], 99238[0], 99239[0], 99281[0], 99282[0], 99283[0], 99284[0], 99285[0], 99304[0], 99305[0], 99306[0], 99307[0], 99308[0], 99309[0], 99310[0], 99315[0], 99318[0], 99324[0], 99325[0], 99326[0], 99327[0], 99328[0], 99334[0], 99335[0], 99336[0], 99337[0], 99341[0], 99342[0], 99343[0], 99347[0], 99348[0], 99349[0], 99354[0], 99355[0], 99356[0], 99357[0], 99358[0], 99359[0], 99415[0], 99416[0], 99446[0], 99447[0], 99448[0], 99449[0], 99451[0], 99452[0], 99466[0], 99468[0], 99469[0], 99471[0], 99472[0], 99475[0], 99476[0], 99477[0], 99478[0], 99479[0], 99480[0], 99483[0], 99485[0], 99497[0], C8921[1], C8922[1], C8923[1], C8924[1], C8925[1], C8926[1], C8927[0], C8929[1], C8930[1], G0380[1], G0381[1], G0382[1], G0383[1], G0384[1], G0406[0], G0407[0], G0408[0], G0425[0], G0426[0], G0427[0], G0463[0], G0500[0], G0508[0], G0509[0]
00529	01996[1], 0213T[1], 0216T[1], 0228T[1], 0230T[1], 31505[1], 31515[1], 31527[1], 31622[1], 31634[1], 31645[1], 31647[1], 36000[1], 36010[0], 36011[1], 36012[1], 36013[1], 36014[1], 36015[1], 36400[1], 36405[1], 36406[1], 36410[1], 36420[1], 36425[1], 36430[1], 36440[1], 36591[0], 36592[0], 36600[1], 36640[1], 43752[1], 43753[1], 43754[1], 61026[1], 61055[1], 62280[1], 62281[1], 62282[1], 62284[1], 62320[1], 62321[1], 62322[1], 62323[1], 62324[1], 62325[1], 62326[1], 62327[1], 64400[1], 64402[1], 64405[1], 64408[1], 64410[1], 64413[1], 64415[1], 64416[1], 64417[1], 64418[1], 64420[1], 64421[1], 64425[1], 64430[1], 64435[1], 64445[1], 64446[1], 64447[1], 64448[1], 64449[1], 64450[1], 64461[1], 64463[1], 64479[1], 64483[1], 64486[1], 64487[1], 64488[1], 64489[1], 64490[1], 64493[1], 64505[1], 64510[1], 64517[1], 64520[1], 64530[1], 64553[1], 64555[1], 67500[1], 76000[1], 76970[1], 76998[0], 77002[0], 90865[1], 92511[1], 92512[1], 92516[1], 92520[1], 92537[1], 92538[1], 92950[1], 92953[1], 92960[1], 92961[1], 93000[1], 93005[1], 93010[1], 93040[1], 93041[1], 93042[1], 93050[0], 93303[0], 93304[0], 93306[1], 93307[1], 93308[1], 93312[1], 93313[1], 93314[1], 93315[1], 93316[1], 93317[1], 93318[0], 93351[1], 93355[0], 93451[1], 93456[1], 93457[1], 93561[0], 93562[0], 93701[0], 93922[1], 93923[1], 93924[1], 93925[1], 93926[1], 93930[1], 93931[1], 93970[1], 93971[1], 93975[1], 93976[1], 93978[1], 93979[1], 93980[1], 93981[1], 94002[1], 94004[1], 94200[1], 94250[0], 94640[1], 94644[1], 94660[1], 94662[1], 94680[1], 94681[1], 94690[1], 94760[0], 94761[0], 94762[1], 94770[1], 95812[0], 95813[0], 95816[0], 95819[0], 95822[0], 95829[0], 95955[0], 95956[0], 95957[0], 96360[0], 96365[0], 96372[0], 96373[0], 96374[0], 96375[0], 96376[0], 96377[0], 99151[0], 99152[0], 99153[0], 99155[0], 99156[0], 99157[0], 99201[0], 99202[0], 99203[0], 99204[0], 99205[0], 99211[0], 99212[0], 99213[0], 99214[0], 99215[0], 99217[0], 99218[0], 99219[0], 99220[0], 99221[0], 99222[0], 99223[0], 99224[0], 99225[0], 99226[0], 99231[0], 99232[0], 99233[0], 99234[0], 99235[0], 99236[0], 99238[0], 99239[0], 99281[0], 99282[0], 99283[0], 99284[0], 99285[0], 99304[0], 99305[0], 99306[0], 99307[0], 99308[0], 99309[0], 99310[0], 99315[0], 99318[0], 99324[0], 99325[0], 99326[0], 99327[0], 99328[0], 99334[0], 99335[0], 99336[0], 99337[0], 99341[0], 99342[0], 99343[0], 99347[0], 99348[0], 99349[0], 99354[0], 99355[0], 99356[0], 99357[0], 99358[0], 99359[0], 99415[0], 99416[0], 99446[0], 99447[0], 99448[0], 99449[0], 99451[0], 99452[0], 99466[0], 99468[0], 99469[0], 99471[0], 99472[0], 99475[0], 99476[0], 99477[0], 99478[0], 99479[0], 99480[0], 99483[0], 99485[0], 99497[0], C8921[1], C8922[1], C8923[1], C8924[1], C8925[1], C8926[1], C8927[0], C8929[1], C8930[1], G0380[1], G0381[1], G0382[1], G0383[1], G0384[1], G0406[0], G0407[0], G0408[0], G0425[0], G0426[0], G0427[0], G0463[0], G0500[0], G0508[0], G0509[0]
00530	01996[1], 0213T[1], 0216T[1], 0228T[1], 0230T[1], 31505[1], 31515[1], 31527[1], 31622[1], 31634[1], 31645[1], 31647[1], 36000[1], 36010[0], 36011[1], 36012[1], 36013[1], 36014[1], 36015[1], 36400[1], 36405[1], 36406[1], 36410[1], 36420[1], 36425[1], 36430[1], 36440[1], 36591[0], 36592[0], 36600[1], 36640[1], 43752[1], 43753[1], 43754[1], 61026[1], 61055[1], 62280[1], 62281[1], 62282[1], 62284[1], 62320[1], 62321[1], 62322[1], 62323[1], 62324[1], 62325[1], 62326[1], 62327[1], 64400[1], 64402[1], 64405[1], 64408[1], 64410[1], 64413[1], 64415[1], 64416[1], 64417[1], 64418[1], 64420[1], 64421[1], 64425[1], 64430[1], 64435[1], 64445[1], 64446[1], 64447[1], 64448[1], 64449[1], 64450[1], 64461[1], 64463[1], 64479[1], 64483[1], 64486[1], 64487[1], 64488[1], 64489[1], 64490[1], 64493[1], 64505[1], 64510[1], 64517[1], 64520[1], 64530[1], 64553[1], 64555[1], 67500[1], 76000[1], 76970[1], 76998[0], 77002[0], 90865[1], 92511[1], 92512[1], 92516[1], 92520[1], 92537[1], 92538[1], 92950[1], 92953[1], 92960[1], 92961[1], 93000[1], 93005[1], 93010[1], 93040[1], 93041[1], 93042[1], 93050[0], 93303[0], 93304[0], 93306[1], 93307[1], 93308[1], 93312[1], 93313[1], 93314[1], 93315[1], 93316[1], 93317[1], 93318[0], 93351[1], 93355[0], 93451[1], 93456[1], 93457[1], 93561[0], 93562[0], 93701[0], 93922[1], 93923[1], 93924[1], 93925[1], 93926[1], 93930[1], 93931[1], 93970[1], 93971[1], 93975[1], 93976[1], 93978[1], 93979[1], 93980[1], 93981[1], 94002[1], 94004[1], 94200[1], 94250[0], 94640[1], 94644[1], 94660[1], 94662[1], 94680[1], 94681[1], 94690[1], 94760[0], 94761[0], 94762[1], 94770[1], 95812[0], 95813[0], 95816[0], 95819[0], 95822[0], 95829[0], 95955[0], 95956[0], 95957[0], 96360[0], 96365[0], 96372[0], 96373[0], 96374[0], 96375[0], 96376[0], 96377[0], 99151[0], 99152[0], 99153[0], 99155[0], 99156[0], 99157[0], 99201[0], 99202[0], 99203[0], 99204[0], 99205[0], 99211[0], 99212[0], 99213[0], 99214[0], 99215[0], 99217[0], 99218[0], 99219[0], 99220[0], 99221[0], 99222[0], 99223[0], 99224[0], 99225[0], 99226[0], 99231[0], 99232[0], 99233[0], 99234[0], 99235[0], 99236[0], 99238[0], 99239[0], 99281[0], 99282[0], 99283[0], 99284[0], 99285[0], 99304[0], 99305[0], 99306[0], 99307[0], 99308[0], 99309[0], 99310[0], 99315[0], 99318[0], 99324[0], 99325[0], 99326[0], 99327[0], 99328[0], 99334[0], 99335[0], 99336[0], 99337[0], 99341[0], 99342[0], 99343[0], 99347[0], 99348[0], 99349[0], 99354[0], 99355[0], 99356[0], 99357[0], 99358[0], 99359[0], 99415[0], 99416[0], 99446[0], 99447[0], 99448[0], 99449[0], 99451[0], 99452[0], 99466[0], 99468[0], 99469[0], 99471[0], 99472[0], 99475[0], 99476[0], 99477[0], 99478[0], 99479[0], 99480[0], 99483[0], 99485[0], 99497[0], C8921[1], C8922[1], C8923[1], C8924[1], C8925[1], C8926[1], C8927[0], C8929[1], C8930[1], G0380[1], G0381[1], G0382[1], G0383[1], G0384[1], G0406[0], G0407[0], G0408[0], G0425[0], G0426[0], G0427[0], G0463[0], G0500[0], G0508[0], G0509[0]
00532	01996[1], 0213T[1], 0216T[1], 0228T[1], 0230T[1], 31505[1], 31515[1], 31527[1], 31622[1], 31634[1], 31645[1], 31647[1], 36000[1], 36010[0], 36011[1], 36012[1], 36013[1], 36014[1], 36015[1], 36400[1], 36405[1], 36406[1], 36410[1], 36420[1], 36425[1], 36430[1], 36440[1], 36591[0], 36592[0], 36600[1], 36640[1], 43752[1], 43753[1], 43754[1], 61026[1], 61055[1], 62280[1], 62281[1], 62282[1], 62284[1], 62320[1], 62321[1], 62322[1], 62323[1], 62324[1], 62325[1], 62326[1], 62327[1], 64400[1], 64402[1], 64405[1], 64408[1], 64410[1], 64413[1], 64415[1], 64416[1], 64417[1], 64418[1], 64420[1], 64421[1], 64425[1], 64430[1], 64435[1], 64445[1], 64446[1], 64447[1], 64448[1], 64449[1], 64450[1], 64461[1], 64463[1], 64479[1], 64483[1], 64486[1], 64487[1], 64488[1], 64489[1], 64490[1], 64493[1], 64505[1], 64510[1], 64517[1], 64520[1], 64530[1], 64553[1], 64555[1], 67500[1], 76000[1], 76970[1], 76998[0], 77002[0], 90865[1], 92511[1], 92512[1], 92516[1], 92520[1], 92537[1], 92538[1], 92950[1], 92953[1], 92960[1], 92961[1], 93000[1], 93005[1], 93010[1], 93040[1], 93041[1], 93042[1], 93050[0], 93303[0], 93304[0], 93306[1], 93307[1], 93308[1], 93312[1], 93313[1], 93314[1], 93315[1], 93316[1], 93317[1], 93318[0], 93351[1], 93355[0], 93451[1], 93456[1], 93457[1], 93561[0], 93562[0], 93701[0], 93922[1], 93923[1], 93924[1], 93925[1], 93926[1], 93930[1], 93931[1], 93970[1], 93971[1], 93975[1], 93976[1], 93978[1], 93979[1], 93980[1], 93981[1], 94002[1], 94004[1], 94200[1], 94250[0], 94640[1], 94644[1], 94660[1], 94662[1], 94680[1], 94681[1], 94690[1], 94760[0], 94761[0], 94762[1], 94770[1], 95812[0], 95813[0], 95816[0], 95819[0], 95822[0], 95829[0], 95955[0], 95956[0], 95957[0], 96360[0], 96365[0], 96372[0], 96373[0], 96374[0], 96375[0], 96376[0], 96377[0], 99151[0], 99152[0], 99153[0], 99155[0], 99156[0], 99157[0], 99201[0], 99202[0], 99203[0], 99204[0], 99205[0], 99211[0], 99212[0], 99213[0], 99214[0], 99215[0], 99217[0], 99218[0], 99219[0], 99220[0], 99221[0], 99222[0], 99223[0], 99224[0], 99225[0], 99226[0], 99231[0], 99232[0], 99233[0], 99234[0], 99235[0], 99236[0], 99238[0], 99239[0], 99281[0], 99282[0], 99283[0], 99284[0], 99285[0], 99304[0], 99305[0], 99306[0], 99307[0], 99308[0], 99309[0], 99310[0], 99315[0], 99318[0], 99324[0], 99325[0], 99326[0], 99327[0], 99328[0], 99334[0], 99335[0], 99336[0], 99337[0], 99341[0], 99342[0], 99343[0], 99347[0], 99348[0], 99349[0], 99354[0], 99355[0], 99356[0], 99357[0], 99358[0], 99359[0], 99415[0], 99416[0], 99446[0], 99447[0], 99448[0], 99449[0], 99451[0], 99452[0], 99466[0], 99468[0], 99469[0], 99471[0], 99472[0], 99475[0], 99476[0], 99477[0], 99478[0], 99479[0], 99480[0], 99483[0], 99485[0], 99497[0], C8921[1], C8922[1], C8923[1], C8924[1], C8925[1], C8926[1], C8927[0], C8929[1], C8930[1], G0380[1], G0381[1], G0382[1], G0383[1], G0384[1], G0406[0], G0407[0], G0408[0], G0425[0], G0426[0], G0427[0], G0463[0], G0500[0], G0508[0], G0509[0]
00534	01996[1], 0213T[1], 0216T[1], 0228T[1], 0230T[1], 31505[1], 31515[1], 31527[1], 31622[1], 31634[1], 31645[1], 31647[1], 36000[1], 36010[0], 36011[1], 36012[1], 36013[1], 36014[1], 36015[1], 36400[1], 36405[1], 36406[1], 36410[1], 36420[1], 36425[1], 36430[1], 36440[1], 36591[0], 36592[0], 36600[1], 36640[1], 43752[1], 43753[1], 43754[1], 61026[1], 61055[1], 62280[1], 62281[1], 62282[1], 62284[1], 62320[1], 62321[1], 62322[1], 62323[1], 62324[1], 62325[1], 62326[1], 62327[1], 64400[1], 64402[1], 64405[1], 64408[1], 64410[1], 64413[1], 64415[1], 64416[1], 64417[1], 64418[1], 64420[1], 64421[1], 64425[1], 64430[1], 64435[1], 64445[1], 64446[1], 64447[1], 64448[1], 64449[1], 64450[1], 64461[1], 64463[1], 64479[1], 64483[1], 64486[1], 64487[1], 64488[1], 64489[1], 64490[1], 64493[1], 64505[1], 64510[1], 64517[1], 64520[1], 64530[1], 64553[1], 64555[1], 67500[1], 76000[1], 76970[1], 76998[0], 77002[0], 90865[1], 92511[1], 92512[1], 92516[1], 92520[1], 92537[1], 92538[1], 92950[1], 92953[1], 92960[1], 92961[1], 93000[1], 93005[1], 93010[1], 93040[1], 93041[1], 93042[1], 93050[0], 93303[0], 93304[0], 93306[1], 93307[1], 93308[1], 93312[1], 93313[1], 93314[1], 93315[1], 93316[1], 93317[1], 93318[0], 93351[1], 93355[0], 93451[1], 93456[1], 93457[1], 93561[0], 93562[0], 93701[0], 93922[1], 93923[1], 93924[1], 93925[1], 93926[1], 93930[1], 93931[1], 93970[1], 93971[1], 93975[1], 93976[1], 93978[1], 93979[1], 93980[1], 93981[1], 94002[1], 94004[1], 94200[1], 94250[0], 94640[1], 94644[1], 94660[1], 94662[1], 94680[1], 94681[1], 94690[1], 94760[0], 94761[0], 94762[1], 94770[1], 95812[0], 95813[0], 95816[0], 95819[0], 95822[0], 95829[0], 95955[0], 95956[0], 95957[0], 96360[0], 96365[0], 96372[0], 96373[0], 96374[0], 96375[0], 96376[0], 96377[0], 99151[0], 99152[0], 99153[0], 99155[0], 99156[0], 99157[0], 99201[0], 99202[0], 99203[0], 99204[0], 99205[0], 99211[0], 99212[0], 99213[0], 99214[0], 99215[0], 99217[0], 99218[0], 99219[0], 99220[0], 99221[0], 99222[0], 99223[0], 99224[0], 99225[0], 99226[0], 99231[0], 99232[0], 99233[0], 99234[0], 99235[0], 99236[0], 99238[0], 99239[0], 99281[0], 99282[0], 99283[0], 99284[0], 99285[0], 99304[0], 99305[0], 99306[0], 99307[0], 99308[0], 99309[0], 99310[0], 99315[0], 99318[0], 99324[0], 99325[0], 99326[0], 99327[0], 99328[0], 99334[0], 99335[0], 99336[0], 99337[0], 99341[0], 99342[0], 99343[0], 99347[0], 99348[0], 99349[0], 99354[0], 99355[0], 99356[0], 99357[0], 99358[0], 99359[0], 99415[0], 99416[0], 99446[0], 99447[0], 99448[0], 99449[0], 99451[0], 99452[0], 99466[0], 99468[0], 99469[0], 99471[0], 99472[0], 99475[0], 99476[0], 99477[0], 99478[0], 99479[0], 99480[0], 99483[0], 99485[0], 99497[0], C8921[1], C8922[1], C8923[1], C8924[1], C8925[1], C8926[1], C8927[0], C8929[1], C8930[1], G0380[1], G0381[1], G0382[1], G0383[1], G0384[1], G0406[0], G0407[0], G0408[0], G0425[0], G0426[0], G0427[0], G0463[0], G0500[0], G0508[0], G0509[0]

Appendix A: NCCI - CPT Codes

0 = Modifier usage not allowed or inappropriate 1 = Modifier usage allowed

CPT © 2018 American Medical Association. All Rights Reserved.

Code 1	Code 2
00537	01996[1], 0213T[1], 0216T[1], 0228T[1], 0230T[1], 31505[1], 31515[1], 31527[1], 31622[1], 31634[1], 31645[1], 31647[1], 36000[1], 36010[0], 36011[1], 36012[1], 36013[1], 36014[1], 36015[1], 36400[1], 36405[1], 36406[1], 36410[1], 36420[1], 36425[1], 36430[1], 36440[1], 36591[0], 36592[0], 36600[1], 36640[1], 43752[1], 43753[1], 43754[1], 61026[1], 61055[1], 62280[1], 62281[1], 62282[1], 62284[1], 62320[1], 62321[1], 62322[1], 62323[1], 62324[1], 62325[1], 62326[1], 62327[1], 64400[1], 64402[1], 64405[1], 64408[1], 64410[1], 64413[1], 64415[1], 64416[1], 64417[1], 64418[1], 64420[1], 64421[1], 64425[1], 64430[1], 64435[1], 64445[1], 64446[1], 64447[1], 64448[1], 64449[1], 64450[1], 64461[1], 64463[1], 64479[1], 64483[1], 64486[1], 64487[1], 64488[1], 64489[1], 64490[1], 64493[1], 64505[1], 64510[1], 64517[1], 64520[1], 64530[1], 64553[1], 64555[1], 67500[0], 76000[1], 76970[1], 76998[0], 77002[0], 90865[1], 92511[1], 92512[1], 92516[1], 92520[1], 92537[1], 92538[1], 92950[1], 92953[1], 92960[1], 92961[1], 93000[1], 93005[1], 93010[1], 93040[1], 93041[1], 93042[1], 93050[0], 93303[0], 93304[0], 93306[1], 93307[1], 93308[1], 93312[1], 93313[1], 93314[1], 93315[1], 93316[1], 93317[1], 93318[0], 93351[1], 93355[0], 93451[1], 93456[1], 93457[1], 93561[0], 93562[0], 93701[0], 93922[1], 93923[1], 93924[1], 93925[1], 93926[1], 93930[1], 93931[1], 93970[1], 93971[1], 93975[1], 93976[1], 93978[1], 93979[1], 93980[1], 93981[1], 94002[1], 94004[1], 94200[1], 94250[0], 94640[1], 94644[1], 94660[1], 94662[1], 94680[1], 94681[1], 94690[1], 94760[0], 94761[0], 94762[1], 94770[1], 95812[0], 95813[0], 95816[0], 95819[0], 95822[0], 95829[0], 95955[0], 95956[0], 95957[0], 96360[0], 96365[0], 96372[0], 96373[0], 96374[0], 96375[0], 96376[0], 96377[0], 99151[0], 99152[0], 99153[0], 99155[0], 99156[0], 99157[0], 99201[0], 99202[0], 99203[0], 99204[0], 99205[0], 99211[0], 99212[0], 99213[0], 99214[0], 99215[0], 99217[0], 99218[0], 99219[0], 99220[0], 99221[0], 99222[0], 99223[0], 99224[0], 99225[0], 99226[0], 99231[0], 99232[0], 99233[0], 99234[0], 99235[0], 99236[0], 99238[0], 99239[0], 99281[0], 99282[0], 99283[0], 99284[0], 99285[0], 99304[0], 99305[0], 99306[0], 99307[0], 99308[0], 99309[0], 99310[0], 99315[0], 99316[0], 99318[0], 99324[0], 99325[0], 99326[0], 99327[0], 99328[0], 99334[0], 99335[0], 99336[0], 99337[0], 99341[0], 99342[0], 99343[0], 99344[0], 99345[0], 99347[0], 99348[0], 99349[0], 99350[0], 99354[0], 99355[0], 99356[0], 99357[0], 99358[0], 99359[0], 99415[0], 99416[0], 99446[0], 99447[0], 99448[0], 99449[0], 99451[0], 99452[0], 99466[0], 99468[0], 99469[0], 99471[0], 99472[0], 99475[0], 99476[0], 99477[0], 99478[0], 99479[0], 99480[0], 99483[0], 99485[0], 99497[0], C8921[1], C8922[1], C8923[1], C8924[1], C8925[1], C8926[1], C8927[0], C8929[1], C8930[1], G0380[1], G0381[1], G0382[1], G0383[1], G0384[1], G0406[0], G0407[0], G0408[0], G0425[0], G0426[0], G0427[0], G0463[0], G0500[0], G0508[0], G0509[0]
00539	01996[1], 0213T[1], 0216T[1], 0228T[1], 0230T[1], 31505[1], 31515[1], 31527[1], 31622[1], 31634[1], 31645[1], 31647[1], 36000[1], 36010[0], 36011[1], 36012[1], 36013[1], 36014[1], 36015[1], 36400[1], 36405[1], 36406[1], 36410[1], 36420[1], 36425[1], 36430[1], 36440[1], 36591[0], 36592[0], 36600[1], 36640[1], 43752[1], 43753[1], 43754[1], 61026[1], 61055[1], 62280[1], 62281[1], 62282[1], 62284[1], 62320[1], 62321[1], 62322[1], 62323[1], 62324[1], 62325[1], 62326[1], 62327[1], 64400[1], 64402[1], 64405[1], 64408[1], 64410[1], 64413[1], 64415[1], 64416[1], 64417[1], 64418[1], 64420[1], 64421[1], 64425[1], 64430[1], 64435[1], 64445[1], 64446[1], 64447[1], 64448[1], 64449[1], 64450[1], 64461[1], 64463[1], 64479[1], 64483[1], 64486[1], 64487[1], 64488[1], 64489[1], 64490[1], 64493[1], 64505[1], 64510[1], 64517[1], 64520[1], 64530[1], 64553[1], 64555[1], 67500[0], 76000[1], 76970[1], 76998[0], 77002[0], 90865[1], 92511[1], 92512[1], 92516[1], 92520[1], 92537[1], 92538[1], 92950[1], 92953[1], 92960[1], 92961[1], 93000[1], 93005[1], 93010[1], 93040[1], 93041[1], 93042[1], 93050[0], 93303[0], 93304[0], 93306[1], 93307[1], 93308[1], 93312[1], 93313[1], 93314[1], 93315[1], 93316[1], 93317[1], 93318[0], 93351[1], 93355[0], 93451[1], 93456[1], 93457[1], 93561[0], 93562[0], 93701[0], 93922[1], 93923[1], 93924[1], 93925[1], 93926[1], 93930[1], 93931[1], 93970[1], 93971[1], 93975[1], 93976[1], 93978[1], 93979[1], 93980[1], 93981[1], 94002[1], 94004[1], 94200[1], 94250[0], 94640[1], 94644[1], 94660[1], 94662[1], 94680[1], 94681[1], 94690[1], 94760[0], 94761[0], 94762[1], 94770[1], 95812[0], 95813[0], 95816[0], 95819[0], 95822[0], 95829[0], 95955[0], 95956[0], 95957[0], 96360[0], 96365[0], 96372[0], 96373[0], 96374[0], 96375[0], 96376[0], 96377[0], 99151[0], 99152[0], 99153[0], 99155[0], 99156[0], 99157[0], 99201[0], 99202[0], 99203[0], 99204[0], 99205[0], 99211[0], 99212[0], 99213[0], 99214[0], 99215[0], 99217[0], 99218[0], 99219[0], 99220[0], 99221[0], 99222[0], 99223[0], 99224[0], 99225[0], 99226[0], 99231[0], 99232[0], 99233[0], 99234[0], 99235[0], 99236[0], 99238[0], 99239[0], 99281[0], 99282[0], 99283[0], 99284[0], 99285[0], 99304[0], 99305[0], 99306[0], 99307[0], 99308[0], 99309[0], 99310[0], 99315[0], 99318[0], 99324[0], 99325[0], 99326[0], 99327[0], 99328[0], 99334[0], 99335[0], 99336[0], 99337[0], 99341[0], 99342[0], 99343[0], 99347[0], 99348[0], 99349[0], 99354[0], 99355[0], 99356[0], 99357[0], 99358[0], 99359[0], 99415[0], 99416[0], 99446[0], 99447[0], 99448[0], 99449[0], 99451[0], 99452[0], 99468[0], 99469[0], 99471[0], 99472[0], 99475[0], 99476[0], 99477[0], 99478[0], 99479[0], 99480[0], 99483[0], 99497[0], C8921[1], C8922[1], C8923[1], C8924[1], C8925[1], C8926[1], C8927[0], C8929[1], C8930[1], G0380[1], G0381[1], G0382[1], G0383[1], G0384[1], G0406[0], G0407[0], G0408[0], G0425[0], G0426[0], G0427[0], G0463[0], G0500[0], G0508[0], G0509[0]
00540	01996[1], 0213T[1], 0216T[1], 0228T[1], 0230T[1], 31505[1], 31515[1], 31527[1], 31622[0], 31634[0], 31645[1], 31647[0], 36000[1], 36010[0], 36011[1], 36012[1], 36013[1], 36014[1], 36015[1], 36400[1], 36405[1], 36406[1], 36410[1], 36420[1], 36425[1], 36430[1], 36440[1], 36591[0], 36592[0], 36600[1], 36640[1], 43752[1], 43753[1], 43754[1], 61026[1], 61055[1], 62280[1], 62281[1], 62282[1], 62284[1], 62320[1], 62321[1], 62322[1], 62323[1], 62324[1], 62325[1], 62326[1], 62327[1], 64400[1], 64402[1], 64405[1], 64408[1], 64410[1], 64413[1], 64415[1], 64416[1], 64417[1], 64418[1], 64420[1], 64421[1], 64425[1], 64430[1], 64435[1], 64445[1], 64446[1], 64447[1], 64448[1], 64449[1], 64450[1], 64461[1], 64463[1], 64479[1], 64483[1], 64486[1], 64487[1], 64488[1], 64489[1], 64490[1], 64493[1], 64505[1], 64510[1], 64517[1], 64520[1], 64530[1], 64553[1], 64555[1], 67500[1], 76000[1], 76970[1], 76998[0], 77002[0], 90865[1], 92511[1], 92512[1], 92516[1], 92520[1], 92537[1], 92538[1], 92950[1], 92953[1], 92960[1], 92961[1], 93000[1], 93005[1], 93010[1], 93040[1], 93041[1], 93042[1], 93050[0], 93303[0], 93304[0], 93306[1], 93307[1], 93308[1], 93312[1], 93313[1], 93314[1], 93315[1], 93316[1], 93317[1], 93318[0], 93351[1], 93355[0], 93451[1], 93456[1], 93457[1], 93561[0], 93562[0], 93701[0], 93922[1], 93923[1], 93924[1], 93925[1], 93926[1], 93930[1], 93931[1], 93970[1], 93971[1], 93975[1], 93976[1], 93978[1], 93979[1], 93980[1], 93981[1], 94002[1], 94004[1], 94200[1], 94250[0], 94640[1], 94644[1], 94660[1], 94662[1], 94680[1], 94681[1], 94690[1], 94760[0], 94761[0], 94762[1], 94770[1], 95812[0], 95813[0], 95816[0], 95819[0], 95822[0], 95829[0], 95955[0], 95956[0], 95957[0], 96360[0], 96365[0], 96372[0], 96373[0], 96374[0], 96375[0], 96376[0], 96377[0], 99151[0], 99152[0], 99153[0], 99155[0], 99156[0], 99157[0], 99201[0], 99202[0], 99203[0], 99204[0], 99205[0], 99211[0], 99212[0], 99213[0], 99214[0], 99215[0], 99217[0], 99218[0], 99219[0], 99220[0], 99221[0], 99222[0], 99223[0], 99224[0], 99225[0], 99226[0], 99231[0], 99232[0], 99233[0], 99234[0], 99235[0], 99236[0], 99238[0], 99239[0], 99281[0], 99282[0], 99283[0], 99284[0], 99285[0], 99304[0], 99305[0], 99306[0], 99307[0], 99308[0], 99309[0], 99310[0], 99315[0], 99318[0], 99324[0], 99325[0], 99326[0], 99327[0], 99328[0], 99334[0], 99335[0], 99336[0], 99337[0], 99341[0], 99342[0], 99343[0], 99347[0], 99348[0], 99349[0], 99354[0], 99355[0], 99356[0], 99357[0], 99358[0], 99359[0], 99415[0], 99416[0], 99446[0], 99447[0], 99448[0], 99449[0], 99451[0], 99452[0], 99466[0], 99468[0], 99469[0], 99471[0], 99472[0], 99475[0], 99476[0], 99477[0], 99478[0], 99479[0], 99480[0], 99483[0], 99485[0], 99497[0], C8921[1], C8922[1], C8923[1], C8924[1], C8925[1], C8926[1], C8927[0], C8929[1], C8930[1], G0380[1], G0381[1], G0382[1], G0383[1], G0384[1], G0406[0], G0407[0], G0408[0], G0425[0], G0426[0], G0427[0], G0463[0], G0500[0], G0508[0], G0509[0]
00541	01996[1], 0213T[1], 0216T[1], 0228T[1], 0230T[1], 31505[1], 31515[1], 31527[1], 31622[1], 31634[1], 31645[1], 31647[1], 36000[1], 36010[0], 36011[1], 36012[1], 36013[1], 36014[1], 36015[1], 36400[1], 36405[1], 36406[1], 36410[1], 36420[1], 36425[1], 36430[1], 36440[1], 36591[0], 36592[0], 36600[1], 36640[1], 43752[1], 43753[1], 43754[1], 61026[1], 61055[1], 62280[1], 62281[1], 62282[1], 62284[1], 62320[1], 62321[1], 62322[1], 62323[1], 62324[1], 62325[1], 62326[1], 62327[1], 64400[1], 64402[1], 64405[1], 64408[1], 64410[1], 64413[1], 64415[1], 64416[1], 64417[1], 64418[1], 64420[1], 64421[1], 64425[1], 64430[1], 64435[1], 64445[1], 64446[1], 64447[1], 64448[1], 64449[1], 64450[1], 64461[1], 64463[1], 64479[1], 64483[1], 64486[1], 64487[1], 64488[1], 64489[1], 64490[1], 64493[1], 64505[1], 64510[1], 64517[1], 64520[1], 64530[1], 64553[1], 64555[1], 67500[0], 76000[1], 76970[1], 76998[0], 77002[0], 90865[1], 92511[1], 92512[1], 92516[1], 92520[1], 92537[1], 92538[1], 92950[1], 92953[1], 92960[1], 92961[1], 93000[1], 93005[1], 93010[1], 93040[1], 93041[1], 93042[1], 93050[0], 93303[0], 93304[0], 93306[1], 93307[1], 93308[1], 93312[1], 93313[1], 93314[1], 93315[1], 93316[1], 93317[1], 93318[0], 93351[1], 93355[0], 93451[1], 93456[1], 93457[1], 93561[0], 93562[0], 93701[0], 93922[1], 93923[1], 93924[1], 93925[1], 93926[1], 93930[1], 93931[1], 93970[1], 93971[1], 93975[1], 93976[1], 93978[1], 93979[1], 93980[1], 93981[1], 94002[1], 94004[1], 94200[1], 94250[0], 94640[1], 94644[1], 94660[1], 94662[1], 94680[1], 94681[1], 94690[1], 94760[0], 94761[0], 94762[1], 94770[1], 95812[0], 95813[0], 95816[0], 95819[0], 95822[0], 95829[0], 95955[0], 95956[0], 95957[0], 96360[0], 96365[0], 96372[0], 96373[0], 96374[0], 96375[0], 96376[0], 96377[0], 99151[0], 99152[0], 99153[0], 99155[0], 99156[0], 99157[0], 99201[0], 99202[0], 99203[0], 99204[0], 99205[0], 99211[0], 99212[0], 99213[0], 99214[0], 99215[0], 99217[0], 99218[0], 99219[0], 99220[0], 99221[0], 99222[0], 99223[0], 99224[0], 99225[0], 99226[0], 99231[0], 99232[0], 99233[0], 99234[0], 99235[0], 99236[0], 99238[0], 99239[0], 99281[0], 99282[0], 99283[0], 99284[0], 99285[0], 99304[0], 99305[0], 99306[0], 99307[0], 99308[0], 99309[0], 99310[0], 99315[0], 99318[0], 99324[0], 99325[0], 99326[0], 99327[0], 99328[0], 99334[0], 99335[0], 99336[0], 99337[0], 99341[0], 99342[0], 99343[0], 99347[0], 99348[0], 99349[0], 99354[0], 99355[0], 99356[0], 99357[0], 99358[0], 99359[0], 99415[0], 99416[0], 99446[0], 99447[0], 99448[0], 99449[0], 99451[0], 99452[0], 99468[0], 99469[0], 99471[0], 99472[0], 99475[0], 99476[0], 99477[0], 99478[0], 99479[0], 99480[0], 99483[0], 99497[0], C8921[1], C8922[1], C8923[1], C8924[1], C8925[1], C8926[1], C8927[0], C8929[1], C8930[1], G0380[1], G0381[1], G0382[1], G0383[1], G0384[1], G0406[0], G0407[0], G0408[0], G0425[0], G0426[0], G0427[0], G0463[0], G0500[0], G0508[0], G0509[0]
00542	01996[1], 0213T[1], 0216T[1], 0228T[1], 0230T[1], 31505[1], 31515[1], 31527[1], 31622[1], 31634[1], 31645[1], 31647[1], 36000[1], 36010[0], 36011[1], 36012[1], 36013[1], 36014[1], 36015[1], 36400[1], 36405[1], 36406[1], 36410[1], 36420[1], 36425[1], 36430[1], 36440[1], 36591[0], 36592[0], 36600[1], 36640[1], 43752[1], 43753[1], 43754[1], 61026[1], 61055[1], 62280[1], 62281[1], 62282[1], 62284[1], 62320[1], 62321[1], 62322[1], 62323[1], 62324[1], 62325[1], 62326[1], 62327[1], 64400[1], 64402[1], 64405[1], 64408[1], 64410[1], 64413[1], 64415[1], 64416[1], 64417[1], 64418[1], 64420[1], 64421[1], 64425[1], 64430[1], 64435[1], 64445[1], 64446[1], 64447[1], 64448[1], 64449[1], 64450[1], 64461[1], 64463[1], 64479[1], 64483[1], 64486[1], 64487[1], 64488[1], 64489[1], 64490[1], 64493[1], 64505[1], 64510[1], 64517[1], 64520[1], 64530[1], 64553[1], 64555[1], 67500[1], 76000[1], 76970[1], 76998[0], 77002[0], 90865[1], 92511[1], 92512[1], 92516[1], 92520[1], 92537[1], 92538[1], 92950[1], 92953[1], 92960[1], 92961[1], 93000[1], 93005[1], 93010[1], 93040[1], 93041[1], 93042[1], 93050[0], 93303[0], 93304[0], 93306[1], 93307[1], 93308[1], 93312[1], 93313[1], 93314[1], 93315[1], 93316[1], 93317[1], 93318[0], 93351[1], 93355[0], 93451[1], 93456[1], 93457[1], 93561[0], 93562[0], 93701[0], 93922[1], 93923[1], 93924[1], 93925[1], 93926[1], 93930[1], 93931[1], 93970[1], 93971[1], 93975[1], 93976[1],

CPT © 2018 American Medical Association. All Rights Reserved.

Code 1	Code 2
	93978[1], 93979[1], 93980[1], 93981[1], 94002[1], 94004[1], 94200[1], 94250[0], 94640[1], 94644[1], 94660[1], 94662[1], 94680[1], 94681[1], 94690[1], 94760[0], 94761[0], 94762[1], 94770[1], 95812[0], 95813[0], 95816[0], 95819[0], 95822[0], 95829[0], 95955[0], 95956[0], 95957[0], 96360[0], 96365[0], 96372[0], 96373[0], 96374[0], 96375[0], 96376[0], 96377[0], 99151[0], 99152[0], 99153[0], 99155[0], 99156[0], 99157[0], 99201[0], 99202[0], 99203[0], 99204[0], 99205[0], 99211[0], 99212[0], 99213[0], 99214[0], 99215[0], 99217[0], 99218[0], 99219[0], 99220[0], 99221[0], 99222[0], 99223[0], 99224[0], 99225[0], 99226[0], 99231[0], 99232[0], 99233[0], 99234[0], 99235[0], 99236[0], 99238[0], 99239[0], 99281[0], 99282[0], 99283[0], 99284[0], 99285[0], 99304[0], 99305[0], 99306[0], 99307[0], 99308[0], 99309[0], 99310[0], 99315[0], 99318[0], 99324[0], 99325[0], 99326[0], 99327[0], 99328[0], 99334[0], 99335[0], 99336[0], 99337[0], 99341[0], 99342[0], 99343[0], 99347[0], 99348[0], 99349[0], 99354[0], 99355[0], 99356[0], 99357[0], 99358[0], 99359[0], 99415[0], 99416[0], 99446[0], 99447[0], 99448[0], 99449[0], 99451[0], 99452[0], 99466[0], 99468[0], 99469[0], 99471[0], 99472[0], 99475[0], 99476[0], 99477[0], 99478[0], 99479[0], 99480[0], 99483[0], 99485[0], 99497[0], C8921[1], C8922[1], C8923[1], C8924[1], C8925[1], C8926[1], C8927[0], C8929[1], C8930[1], G0380[1], G0381[1], G0382[1], G0383[1], G0384[1], G0406[0], G0407[0], G0408[0], G0425[0], G0426[0], G0427[0], G0463[0], G0500[0], G0508[0], G0509[0]
00546	01996[1], 0213T[1], 0216T[1], 0228T[1], 0230T[1], 31505[1], 31515[1], 31527[1], 31622[1], 31634[1], 31645[1], 31647[1], 36000[1], 36010[0], 36011[1], 36012[1], 36013[1], 36014[1], 36015[1], 36400[1], 36405[1], 36406[1], 36410[1], 36420[1], 36425[1], 36430[1], 36440[1], 36591[0], 36592[0], 36600[1], 36640[1], 43752[1], 43753[1], 43754[1], 61026[1], 61055[1], 62280[1], 62281[1], 62282[1], 62284[1], 62320[1], 62321[1], 62322[1], 62323[1], 62324[1], 62325[1], 62326[1], 62327[1], 64400[1], 64402[1], 64405[1], 64408[1], 64410[1], 64413[1], 64415[1], 64416[1], 64417[1], 64418[1], 64420[1], 64421[1], 64425[1], 64430[1], 64435[1], 64445[1], 64446[1], 64447[1], 64448[1], 64449[1], 64450[1], 64461[1], 64463[1], 64479[1], 64483[1], 64486[1], 64487[1], 64488[1], 64489[1], 64490[1], 64493[1], 64505[1], 64510[1], 64517[1], 64520[1], 64530[1], 64553[1], 64555[1], 67500[1], 76000[1], 76970[1], 76998[0], 77002[0], 90865[1], 92511[1], 92512[1], 92516[1], 92520[1], 92537[1], 92538[1], 92950[1], 92953[1], 92960[1], 92961[1], 93000[1], 93005[1], 93010[1], 93040[1], 93041[1], 93042[1], 93050[0], 93303[0], 93304[0], 93306[1], 93307[1], 93308[1], 93312[1], 93313[1], 93314[1], 93315[1], 93316[1], 93317[1], 93318[0], 93351[1], 93355[0], 93451[1], 93456[1], 93457[1], 93561[0], 93562[0], 93701[0], 93922[1], 93923[1], 93924[1], 93925[1], 93926[1], 93930[1], 93931[1], 93970[1], 93971[1], 93975[1], 93976[1], 93978[1], 93979[1], 93980[1], 93981[1], 94002[1], 94004[1], 94200[1], 94250[0], 94640[1], 94644[1], 94660[1], 94662[1], 94680[1], 94681[1], 94690[1], 94760[0], 94761[0], 94762[1], 94770[1], 95812[0], 95813[0], 95816[0], 95819[0], 95822[0], 95829[0], 95955[0], 95956[0], 95957[0], 96360[0], 96365[0], 96372[0], 96373[0], 96374[0], 96375[0], 96376[0], 96377[0], 99151[0], 99152[0], 99153[0], 99155[0], 99156[0], 99157[0], 99201[0], 99202[0], 99203[0], 99204[0], 99205[0], 99211[0], 99212[0], 99213[0], 99214[0], 99215[0], 99217[0], 99218[0], 99219[0], 99220[0], 99221[0], 99222[0], 99223[0], 99224[0], 99225[0], 99226[0], 99231[0], 99232[0], 99233[0], 99234[0], 99235[0], 99236[0], 99238[0], 99239[0], 99281[0], 99282[0], 99283[0], 99284[0], 99285[0], 99304[0], 99305[0], 99306[0], 99307[0], 99308[0], 99309[0], 99310[0], 99315[0], 99318[0], 99324[0], 99325[0], 99326[0], 99327[0], 99328[0], 99334[0], 99335[0], 99336[0], 99337[0], 99341[0], 99342[0], 99343[0], 99347[0], 99348[0], 99349[0], 99354[0], 99355[0], 99356[0], 99357[0], 99358[0], 99359[0], 99415[0], 99416[0], 99446[0], 99447[0], 99448[0], 99449[0], 99451[0], 99452[0], 99466[0], 99468[0], 99469[0], 99471[0], 99472[0], 99475[0], 99476[0], 99477[0], 99478[0], 99479[0], 99480[0], 99483[0], 99485[0], 99497[0], C8921[1], C8922[1], C8923[1], C8924[1], C8925[1], C8926[1], C8927[0], C8929[1], C8930[1], G0380[1], G0381[1], G0382[1], G0383[1], G0384[1], G0406[0], G0407[0], G0408[0], G0425[0], G0426[0], G0427[0], G0463[0], G0500[0], G0508[0], G0509[0]
00548	01996[1], 0213T[1], 0216T[1], 0228T[1], 0230T[1], 31505[1], 31515[1], 31527[1], 31622[1], 31634[1], 31645[1], 31647[1], 36000[1], 36010[0], 36011[1], 36012[1], 36013[1], 36014[1], 36015[1], 36400[1], 36405[1], 36406[1], 36410[1], 36420[1], 36425[1], 36430[1], 36440[1], 36591[0], 36592[0], 36600[1], 36640[1], 43752[1], 43753[1], 43754[1], 61026[1], 61055[1], 62280[1], 62281[1], 62282[1], 62284[1], 62320[1], 62321[1], 62322[1], 62323[1], 62324[1], 62325[1], 62326[1], 62327[1], 64400[1], 64402[1], 64405[1], 64408[1], 64410[1], 64413[1], 64415[1], 64416[1], 64417[1], 64418[1], 64420[1], 64421[1], 64425[1], 64430[1], 64435[1], 64445[1], 64446[1], 64447[1], 64448[1], 64449[1], 64450[1], 64461[1], 64463[1], 64479[1], 64483[1], 64486[1], 64487[1], 64488[1], 64489[1], 64490[1], 64493[1], 64505[1], 64510[1], 64517[1], 64520[1], 64530[1], 64553[1], 64555[1], 67500[1], 76000[1], 76970[1], 76998[0], 77002[0], 90865[1], 92511[1], 92512[1], 92516[1], 92520[1], 92537[1], 92538[1], 92950[1], 92953[1], 92960[1], 92961[1], 93000[1], 93005[1], 93010[1], 93040[1], 93041[1], 93042[1], 93050[0], 93303[0], 93304[0], 93306[1], 93307[1], 93308[1], 93312[1], 93313[1], 93314[1], 93315[1], 93316[1], 93317[1], 93318[0], 93351[1], 93355[0], 93451[1], 93456[1], 93457[1], 93561[0], 93562[0], 93701[0], 93922[1], 93923[1], 93924[1], 93925[1], 93926[1], 93930[1], 93931[1], 93970[1], 93971[1], 93975[1], 93976[1], 93978[1], 93979[1], 93980[1], 93981[1], 94002[1], 94004[1], 94200[1], 94250[0], 94640[1], 94644[1], 94660[1], 94662[1], 94680[1], 94681[1], 94690[1], 94760[0], 94761[0], 94762[1], 94770[1], 95812[0], 95813[0], 95816[0], 95819[0], 95822[0], 95829[0], 95955[0], 95956[0], 95957[0], 96360[0], 96365[0], 96372[0], 96373[0], 96374[0], 96375[0], 96376[0], 96377[0], 99151[0], 99152[0], 99153[0], 99155[0], 99156[0], 99157[0], 99201[0], 99202[0], 99203[0], 99204[0], 99205[0], 99211[0], 99212[0], 99213[0], 99214[0], 99215[0], 99217[0], 99218[0], 99219[0], 99220[0], 99221[0], 99222[0], 99223[0], 99224[0], 99225[0], 99226[0], 99231[0], 99232[0], 99233[0], 99234[0], 99235[0], 99236[0], 99238[0], 99239[0], 99281[0], 99282[0], 99283[0], 99284[0], 99285[0], 99304[0], 99305[0], 99306[0], 99307[0], 99308[0], 99309[0], 99310[0], 99315[0], 99318[0], 99324[0], 99325[0], 99326[0], 99327[0], 99328[0], 99334[0], 99335[0], 99336[0], 99337[0], 99341[0], 99342[0], 99343[0], 99347[0], 99348[0], 99349[0], 99354[0], 99355[0], 99356[0], 99357[0], 99358[0], 99359[0], 99415[0], 99416[0], 99446[0], 99447[0], 99448[0], 99449[0], 99451[0], 99452[0], 99466[0], 99468[0], 99469[0], 99471[0], 99472[0], 99475[0], 99476[0], 99477[0], 99478[0], 99479[0], 99480[0], 99483[0], 99485[0], 99497[0], C8921[1], C8922[1], C8923[1], C8924[1], C8925[1], C8926[1], C8927[0], C8929[1], C8930[1], G0380[1], G0381[1], G0382[1], G0383[1], G0384[1], G0406[0], G0407[0], G0408[0], G0425[0], G0426[0], G0427[0], G0463[0], G0500[0], G0508[0], G0509[0]
00550	01996[1], 0213T[1], 0216T[1], 0228T[1], 0230T[1], 31505[1], 31515[1], 31527[1], 31622[1], 31634[1], 31645[1], 31647[1], 36000[1], 36010[0], 36011[1], 36012[1], 36013[1], 36014[1], 36015[1], 36400[1], 36405[1], 36406[1], 36410[1], 36420[1], 36425[1], 36430[1], 36440[1], 36591[0], 36592[0], 36600[1], 36640[1], 43752[1], 43753[1], 43754[1], 61026[1], 61055[1], 62280[1], 62281[1], 62282[1], 62284[1], 62320[1], 62321[1], 62322[1], 62323[1], 62324[1], 62325[1], 62326[1], 62327[1], 64400[1], 64402[1], 64405[1], 64408[1], 64410[1], 64413[1], 64415[1], 64416[1], 64417[1], 64418[1], 64420[1], 64421[1], 64425[1], 64430[1], 64435[1], 64445[1], 64446[1], 64447[1], 64448[1], 64449[1], 64450[1], 64461[1], 64463[1], 64479[1], 64483[1], 64486[1], 64487[1], 64488[1], 64489[1], 64490[1], 64493[1], 64505[1], 64510[1], 64517[1], 64520[1], 64530[1], 64553[1], 64555[1], 67500[0], 76000[1], 76970[1], 76998[0], 77002[0], 90865[1], 92511[1], 92512[1], 92516[1], 92520[1], 92537[1], 92538[1], 92950[1], 92953[1], 92960[1], 92961[1], 93000[1], 93005[1], 93010[1], 93040[1], 93041[1], 93042[1], 93050[0], 93303[0], 93304[0], 93306[1], 93307[1], 93308[1], 93312[1], 93313[1], 93314[1], 93315[1], 93316[1], 93317[1], 93318[0], 93351[1], 93355[0], 93451[1], 93456[1], 93457[1], 93561[0], 93562[0], 93701[0], 93922[1], 93923[1], 93924[1], 93925[1], 93926[1], 93930[1], 93931[1], 93970[1], 93971[1], 93975[1], 93976[1], 93978[1], 93979[1], 93980[1], 93981[1], 94002[1], 94004[1], 94200[1], 94250[0], 94640[1], 94644[1], 94660[1], 94662[1], 94680[1], 94681[1], 94690[1], 94760[0], 94761[0], 94762[1], 94770[1], 95812[0], 95813[0], 95816[0], 95819[0], 95822[0], 95829[0], 95955[0], 95956[0], 95957[0], 96360[0], 96365[0], 96372[0], 96373[0], 96374[0], 96375[0], 96376[0], 96377[0], 99151[0], 99152[0], 99153[0], 99155[0], 99156[0], 99157[0], 99201[0], 99202[0], 99203[0], 99204[0], 99205[0], 99211[0], 99212[0], 99213[0], 99214[0], 99215[0], 99217[0], 99218[0], 99219[0], 99220[0], 99221[0], 99222[0], 99223[0], 99224[0], 99225[0], 99226[0], 99231[0], 99232[0], 99233[0], 99234[0], 99235[0], 99236[0], 99238[0], 99239[0], 99281[0], 99282[0], 99283[0], 99284[0], 99285[0], 99304[0], 99305[0], 99306[0], 99307[0], 99308[0], 99309[0], 99310[0], 99315[0], 99316[0], 99318[0], 99324[0], 99325[0], 99326[0], 99327[0], 99328[0], 99334[0], 99335[0], 99336[0], 99337[0], 99341[0], 99342[0], 99343[0], 99344[0], 99345[0], 99347[0], 99348[0], 99349[0], 99350[0], 99354[0], 99355[0], 99356[0], 99357[0], 99358[0], 99359[0], 99415[0], 99416[0], 99446[0], 99447[0], 99448[0], 99449[0], 99451[0], 99452[0], 99466[0], 99468[0], 99469[0], 99471[0], 99472[0], 99475[0], 99476[0], 99477[0], 99478[0], 99479[0], 99480[0], 99483[0], 99485[0], 99497[0], C8921[1], C8922[1], C8923[1], C8924[1], C8925[1], C8926[1], C8927[0], C8929[1], C8930[1], G0380[1], G0381[1], G0382[1], G0383[1], G0384[1], G0406[0], G0407[0], G0408[0], G0425[0], G0426[0], G0427[0], G0463[0], G0500[0], G0508[0], G0509[0]
00560	00561[1], 00562[1], 00563[1], 00566[1], 01996[1], 0213T[1], 0216T[1], 0228T[1], 0230T[1], 31505[1], 31515[1], 31527[1], 31622[1], 31634[1], 31645[1], 31647[1], 36000[1], 36410[1], 36500[1], 36591[0], 36592[0], 36600[1], 36640[1], 43752[1], 43753[1], 43754[1], 61026[1], 61055[1], 62280[1], 62281[1], 62282[1], 62284[1], 62320[1], 62321[1], 62322[1], 62323[1], 62324[1], 62325[1], 62326[1], 62327[1], 64400[1], 64402[1], 64405[1], 64408[1], 64410[1], 64413[1], 64415[1], 64416[1], 64417[1], 64418[1], 64420[1], 64421[1], 64425[1], 64430[1], 64435[1], 64445[1], 64446[1], 64447[1], 64448[1], 64449[1], 64450[1], 64461[1], 64463[1], 64479[1], 64483[1], 64486[1], 64487[1], 64488[1], 64489[1], 64490[1], 64493[1], 64505[1], 64510[1], 64517[1], 64520[1], 64530[1], 64553[1], 64555[1], 67500[1], 76000[1], 76970[1], 76998[0], 77002[0], 90865[1], 92511[1], 92512[1], 92516[1], 92520[1], 92537[1], 92538[1], 92950[1], 92953[1], 92960[1], 92961[1], 93000[1], 93005[1], 93010[1], 93040[1], 93041[1], 93042[1], 93050[0], 93303[0], 93304[0], 93306[1], 93307[1], 93308[1], 93312[1], 93313[1], 93314[1], 93315[1], 93316[1], 93317[1], 93318[0], 93351[1], 93355[0], 93451[1], 93456[1], 93457[1], 93561[0], 93562[0], 93701[0], 93922[1], 93923[1], 93924[1], 93925[1], 93926[1], 93930[1], 93931[1], 93970[1], 93971[1], 93975[1], 93976[1], 93978[1], 93979[1], 93980[1], 93981[1], 94002[1], 94004[1], 94200[1], 94250[0], 94640[1], 94644[1], 94660[1], 94662[1], 94680[1], 94681[1], 94690[1], 94760[0], 94761[0], 94762[1], 94770[1], 95812[0], 95813[0], 95816[0], 95819[0], 95822[0], 95829[0], 95955[0], 95956[0], 95957[0], 96360[0], 96365[0], 96372[0], 96373[0], 96374[0], 96375[0], 96376[0], 96377[0], 99151[0], 99152[0], 99153[0], 99155[0], 99156[0], 99157[0], 99184[1], 99201[0], 99202[0], 99203[0], 99204[0], 99205[0], 99211[0], 99212[0], 99213[0], 99214[0], 99215[0], 99217[0], 99218[0], 99219[0], 99220[0], 99221[0], 99222[0], 99223[0], 99224[0], 99225[0], 99226[0], 99231[0], 99232[0], 99233[0], 99234[0], 99235[0], 99236[0], 99238[0], 99239[0], 99281[0], 99282[0], 99283[0], 99284[0], 99285[0], 99304[0], 99305[0], 99306[0], 99307[0], 99308[0], 99309[0], 99310[0], 99315[0], 99318[0], 99324[0], 99325[0], 99326[0], 99327[0], 99328[0], 99334[0], 99335[0], 99336[0], 99337[0], 99341[0], 99342[0], 99343[0], 99347[0], 99348[0], 99349[0], 99354[0], 99355[0], 99356[0], 99357[0], 99358[0], 99359[0], 99415[0], 99416[0], 99446[0], 99447[0], 99448[0], 99449[0], 99451[0], 99452[0], 99466[0], 99468[0], 99469[0], 99471[0], 99472[0], 99475[0], 99476[0], 99477[0], 99478[0], 99479[0], 99480[0], 99483[0], 99485[0], 99497[0],

0 = Modifier usage not allowed or inappropriate 1 = Modifier usage allowed

CPT © 2018 American Medical Association. All Rights Reserved.

Code 1	Code 2
	C8921[1], C8922[1], C8923[1], C8924[1], C8925[1], C8926[1], C8927[0], C8929[1], C8930[1], G0380[1], G0381[1], G0382[1], G0383[1], G0384[1], G0406[0], G0407[0], G0408[0], G0425[0], G0426[0], G0427[0], G0463[0], G0500[0], G0508[0], G0509[0]
00561	00567[1], 01996[1], 0213T[1], 0216T[1], 0228T[1], 0230T[1], 31505[1], 31515[1], 31527[1], 31622[1], 31634[1], 31645[1], 31647[1], 36000[1], 36010[0], 36011[1], 36012[1], 36013[1], 36014[1], 36015[1], 36400[1], 36405[1], 36406[1], 36410[1], 36420[1], 36425[1], 36430[1], 36440[1], 36500[1], 36591[0], 36592[0], 36600[1], 36640[1], 43752[1], 43753[1], 43754[1], 61026[1], 61055[1], 62280[1], 62281[1], 62282[1], 62284[1], 62320[1], 62321[1], 62322[1], 62323[1], 62324[1], 62325[1], 62326[1], 62327[1], 64400[1], 64402[1], 64405[1], 64408[1], 64410[1], 64413[1], 64415[1], 64416[1], 64417[1], 64418[1], 64420[1], 64421[1], 64425[1], 64430[1], 64435[1], 64445[1], 64446[1], 64447[1], 64448[1], 64449[1], 64450[1], 64461[1], 64463[1], 64479[1], 64483[1], 64486[1], 64487[1], 64488[1], 64489[1], 64490[1], 64493[1], 64505[1], 64510[1], 64517[1], 64520[1], 64530[1], 64553[1], 64555[1], 67500[1], 76000[1], 76970[1], 76998[0], 77002[0], 90865[1], 92511[1], 92512[1], 92516[1], 92520[1], 92537[1], 92538[1], 92950[1], 92953[1], 92960[1], 92961[1], 93000[1], 93005[1], 93010[1], 93040[1], 93041[1], 93042[1], 93050[0], 93303[0], 93304[0], 93306[1], 93307[1], 93308[1], 93312[1], 93313[1], 93314[1], 93315[1], 93316[1], 93317[1], 93318[0], 93351[1], 93355[0], 93451[1], 93456[1], 93457[1], 93561[0], 93562[0], 93701[0], 93922[1], 93923[1], 93924[1], 93925[1], 93926[1], 93930[1], 93931[1], 93970[1], 93971[1], 93975[1], 93976[1], 93978[1], 93979[1], 93980[1], 93981[1], 94002[1], 94004[1], 94200[1], 94250[0], 94640[1], 94644[1], 94660[1], 94662[1], 94680[1], 94681[1], 94690[1], 94760[0], 94761[0], 94762[1], 94770[1], 95812[0], 95813[0], 95816[0], 95819[0], 95822[0], 95829[0], 95955[0], 95956[0], 95957[0], 96360[0], 96365[0], 96372[0], 96373[0], 96374[0], 96375[0], 96376[0], 96377[0], 99100[1], 99116[1], 99135[1], 99151[0], 99152[0], 99153[0], 99155[0], 99156[0], 99157[0], 99184[1], 99201[0], 99202[0], 99203[0], 99204[0], 99205[0], 99211[0], 99212[0], 99213[0], 99214[0], 99215[0], 99217[0], 99218[0], 99219[0], 99220[0], 99221[0], 99222[0], 99223[0], 99224[0], 99225[0], 99226[0], 99231[0], 99232[0], 99233[0], 99234[0], 99235[0], 99236[0], 99238[0], 99239[0], 99281[0], 99282[0], 99283[0], 99284[0], 99285[0], 99304[0], 99305[0], 99306[0], 99307[0], 99308[0], 99309[0], 99310[0], 99315[0], 99318[0], 99324[0], 99325[0], 99326[0], 99327[0], 99328[0], 99334[0], 99335[0], 99336[0], 99337[0], 99341[0], 99342[0], 99343[0], 99347[0], 99348[0], 99349[0], 99354[0], 99355[0], 99356[0], 99357[0], 99358[0], 99359[0], 99415[0], 99416[0], 99446[0], 99447[0], 99448[0], 99449[0], 99451[0], 99452[0], 99466[0], 99468[0], 99469[0], 99471[0], 99472[0], 99475[0], 99476[0], 99477[0], 99478[0], 99479[0], 99480[0], 99483[0], 99485[0], 99497[0], C8921[1], C8922[1], C8923[1], C8924[1], C8925[1], C8926[1], C8927[0], C8929[1], C8930[1], G0380[1], G0381[1], G0382[1], G0383[1], G0384[1], G0406[0], G0407[0], G0408[0], G0425[0], G0426[0], G0427[0], G0463[0], G0500[0], G0508[0], G0509[0]
00562	00561[1], 00563[1], 00566[1], 00567[1], 01996[1], 0213T[1], 0216T[1], 0228T[1], 0230T[1], 31505[1], 31515[1], 31527[1], 31622[1], 31634[1], 31645[1], 31647[1], 36000[1], 36410[1], 36430[1], 36500[1], 36591[0], 36592[0], 36600[1], 36640[1], 43752[1], 43753[1], 43754[1], 61026[1], 61055[1], 62280[1], 62281[1], 62282[1], 62284[1], 62320[1], 62321[1], 62322[1], 62323[1], 62324[1], 62325[1], 62326[1], 62327[1], 64400[1], 64402[1], 64405[1], 64408[1], 64410[1], 64413[1], 64415[1], 64416[1], 64417[1], 64418[1], 64420[1], 64421[1], 64425[1], 64430[1], 64435[1], 64445[1], 64446[1], 64447[1], 64448[1], 64449[1], 64450[1], 64461[1], 64463[1], 64479[1], 64483[1], 64486[1], 64487[1], 64488[1], 64489[1], 64490[1], 64493[1], 64505[1], 64510[1], 64517[1], 64520[1], 64530[1], 64553[1], 64555[1], 67500[1], 76000[1], 76970[1], 76998[0], 77002[0], 90865[1], 92511[1], 92512[1], 92516[1], 92520[1], 92537[1], 92538[1], 92950[1], 92953[1], 92960[1], 92961[1], 93000[1], 93005[1], 93010[1], 93040[1], 93041[1], 93042[1], 93050[0], 93303[0], 93304[0], 93306[1], 93307[1], 93308[1], 93312[1], 93313[1], 93314[1], 93315[1], 93316[1], 93317[1], 93318[0], 93351[1], 93355[0], 93561[0], 93562[0], 93701[0], 93922[1], 93923[1], 93924[1], 93925[1], 93926[1], 93930[1], 93931[1], 93970[1], 93971[1], 93975[1], 93976[1], 93978[1], 93979[1], 93980[1], 93981[1], 94002[1], 94004[1], 94200[1], 94250[0], 94640[1], 94644[1], 94660[1], 94662[1], 94680[1], 94681[1], 94690[1], 94760[0], 94761[0], 94762[1], 94770[1], 95812[0], 95813[0], 95816[0], 95819[0], 95822[0], 95829[0], 95955[0], 95956[0], 95957[0], 96360[0], 96365[0], 96372[0], 96373[0], 96374[0], 96375[0], 96376[0], 96377[0], 99151[0], 99152[0], 99153[0], 99155[0], 99156[0], 99157[0], 99184[1], 99201[0], 99202[0], 99203[0], 99204[0], 99205[0], 99211[0], 99212[0], 99213[0], 99214[0], 99215[0], 99217[0], 99218[0], 99219[0], 99220[0], 99221[0], 99222[0], 99223[0], 99224[0], 99225[0], 99226[0], 99231[0], 99232[0], 99233[0], 99234[0], 99235[0], 99236[0], 99238[0], 99239[0], 99281[0], 99282[0], 99283[0], 99284[0], 99285[0], 99304[0], 99305[0], 99306[0], 99307[0], 99308[0], 99309[0], 99310[0], 99315[0], 99318[0], 99324[0], 99325[0], 99326[0], 99327[0], 99328[0], 99334[0], 99335[0], 99336[0], 99337[0], 99341[0], 99342[0], 99343[0], 99347[0], 99348[0], 99349[0], 99354[0], 99355[0], 99356[0], 99357[0], 99358[0], 99359[0], 99415[0], 99416[0], 99446[0], 99447[0], 99448[0], 99449[0], 99451[0], 99452[0], 99466[0], 99468[0], 99469[0], 99471[0], 99472[0], 99475[0], 99476[0], 99477[0], 99478[0], 99479[0], 99480[0], 99483[0], 99485[0], 99497[0], C8921[1], C8922[1], C8923[1], C8924[1], C8925[1], C8926[1], C8927[0], C8929[1], C8930[1], G0380[1], G0381[1], G0382[1], G0383[1], G0384[1], G0406[0], G0407[0], G0408[0], G0425[0], G0426[0], G0427[0], G0463[0], G0500[0], G0508[0], G0509[0]
00563	00561[1], 00566[1], 00567[1], 01996[1], 0213T[1], 0216T[1], 0228T[1], 0230T[1], 31505[1], 31515[1], 31527[1], 31622[1], 31634[1], 31645[1], 31647[1], 36000[1], 36010[0], 36011[1], 36012[1], 36013[1], 36014[1], 36015[1], 36400[1], 36405[1], 36406[1], 36410[1], 36420[1], 36425[1], 36430[1], 36440[1], 36591[0], 36592[0], 36600[1], 36640[1], 43752[1], 43753[1], 43754[1], 61026[1], 61055[1], 62280[1], 62281[1], 62282[1], 62284[1], 62320[1], 62321[1], 62322[1], 62323[1], 62324[1], 62325[1], 62326[1], 62327[1], 64400[1], 64402[1], 64405[1], 64408[1], 64410[1], 64413[1], 64415[1], 64416[1], 64417[1], 64418[1], 64420[1], 64421[1], 64425[1], 64430[1], 64435[1], 64445[1], 64446[1], 64447[1], 64448[1], 64449[1], 64450[1], 64461[1], 64463[1], 64479[1], 64483[1], 64486[1], 64487[1], 64488[1], 64489[1], 64490[1], 64493[1], 64505[1], 64510[1], 64517[1], 64520[1], 64530[1], 64553[1], 64555[1], 67500[0], 76000[1], 76970[1], 76998[0], 77002[0], 90865[1], 92511[1], 92512[1], 92516[1], 92520[1], 92537[1], 92538[1], 92950[1], 92953[1], 92960[1], 92961[1], 93000[1], 93005[1], 93010[1], 93040[1], 93041[1], 93042[1], 93050[0], 93303[0], 93304[0], 93306[1], 93307[1], 93308[1], 93312[1], 93313[1], 93314[1], 93315[1], 93316[1], 93317[1], 93318[0], 93351[1], 93355[0], 93451[1], 93456[1], 93457[1], 93561[0], 93562[0], 93701[0], 93922[1], 93923[1], 93924[1], 93925[1], 93926[1], 93930[1], 93931[1], 93970[1], 93971[1], 93975[1], 93976[1], 93978[1], 93979[1], 93980[1], 93981[1], 94002[1], 94004[1], 94200[1], 94250[0], 94640[1], 94644[1], 94660[1], 94662[1], 94680[1], 94681[1], 94690[1], 94760[0], 94761[0], 94762[1], 94770[1], 95812[0], 95813[0], 95816[0], 95819[0], 95822[0], 95829[0], 95955[0], 95956[0], 95957[0], 96360[0], 96365[0], 96372[0], 96373[0], 96374[0], 96375[0], 96376[0], 96377[0], 99151[0], 99152[0], 99153[0], 99155[0], 99156[0], 99157[0], 99184[1], 99201[0], 99202[0], 99203[0], 99204[0], 99205[0], 99211[0], 99212[0], 99213[0], 99214[0], 99215[0], 99217[0], 99218[0], 99219[0], 99220[0], 99221[0], 99222[0], 99223[0], 99224[0], 99225[0], 99226[0], 99231[0], 99232[0], 99233[0], 99234[0], 99235[0], 99236[0], 99238[0], 99239[0], 99281[0], 99282[0], 99283[0], 99284[0], 99285[0], 99304[0], 99305[0], 99306[0], 99307[0], 99308[0], 99309[0], 99310[0], 99315[0], 99316[0], 99318[0], 99324[0], 99325[0], 99326[0], 99327[0], 99328[0], 99334[0], 99335[0], 99336[0], 99337[0], 99341[0], 99342[0], 99343[0], 99344[0], 99345[0], 99347[0], 99348[0], 99349[0], 99350[0], 99354[0], 99355[0], 99356[0], 99357[0], 99358[0], 99359[0], 99415[0], 99416[0], 99446[0], 99447[0], 99448[0], 99449[0], 99451[0], 99452[0], 99466[0], 99468[0], 99469[0], 99471[0], 99472[0], 99475[0], 99476[0], 99477[0], 99478[0], 99479[0], 99480[0], 99483[0], 99485[0], 99497[0], C8921[1], C8922[1], C8923[1], C8924[1], C8925[1], C8926[1], C8927[0], C8929[1], C8930[1], G0380[1], G0381[1], G0382[1], G0383[1], G0384[1], G0406[0], G0407[0], G0408[0], G0425[0], G0426[0], G0427[0], G0463[0], G0500[0], G0508[0], G0509[0]
00566	00561[1], 00567[1], 01996[1], 0213T[1], 0216T[1], 0228T[1], 0230T[1], 31505[1], 31515[1], 31527[1], 31622[1], 31634[1], 31645[1], 31647[1], 36000[1], 36010[0], 36011[1], 36012[1], 36013[1], 36014[1], 36015[1], 36400[1], 36405[1], 36406[1], 36410[1], 36420[1], 36425[1], 36430[1], 36440[1], 36591[0], 36592[0], 36600[1], 36640[1], 43752[1], 43753[1], 43754[1], 61026[1], 61055[1], 62280[1], 62281[1], 62282[1], 62284[1], 62320[1], 62321[1], 62322[1], 62323[1], 62324[1], 62325[1], 62326[1], 62327[1], 64400[1], 64402[1], 64405[1], 64408[1], 64410[1], 64413[1], 64415[1], 64416[1], 64417[1], 64418[1], 64420[1], 64421[1], 64425[1], 64430[1], 64435[1], 64445[1], 64446[1], 64447[1], 64448[1], 64449[1], 64450[1], 64461[1], 64463[1], 64479[1], 64483[1], 64486[1], 64487[1], 64488[1], 64489[1], 64490[1], 64493[1], 64505[1], 64510[1], 64517[1], 64520[1], 64530[1], 64553[1], 64555[1], 67500[0], 76000[1], 76970[1], 76998[0], 77002[0], 90865[1], 92511[1], 92512[1], 92516[1], 92520[1], 92537[1], 92538[1], 92950[1], 92953[1], 92960[1], 92961[1], 93000[1], 93005[1], 93010[1], 93040[1], 93041[1], 93042[1], 93050[0], 93303[0], 93304[0], 93306[1], 93307[1], 93308[1], 93312[1], 93313[1], 93314[1], 93315[1], 93316[1], 93317[1], 93318[0], 93351[1], 93355[0], 93451[1], 93456[1], 93457[1], 93561[0], 93562[0], 93701[0], 93922[1], 93923[1], 93924[1], 93925[1], 93926[1], 93930[1], 93931[1], 93970[1], 93971[1], 93975[1], 93976[1], 93978[1], 93979[1], 93980[1], 93981[1], 94002[1], 94004[1], 94200[1], 94250[0], 94640[1], 94644[1], 94660[1], 94662[1], 94680[1], 94681[1], 94690[1], 94760[0], 94761[0], 94762[1], 94770[1], 95812[0], 95813[0], 95816[0], 95819[0], 95822[0], 95829[0], 95955[0], 95956[0], 95957[0], 96360[0], 96365[0], 96372[0], 96373[0], 96374[0], 96375[0], 96376[0], 96377[0], 99151[0], 99152[0], 99153[0], 99155[0], 99156[0], 99157[0], 99184[1], 99201[0], 99202[0], 99203[0], 99204[0], 99205[0], 99211[0], 99212[0], 99213[0], 99214[0], 99215[0], 99217[0], 99218[0], 99219[0], 99220[0], 99221[0], 99222[0], 99223[0], 99224[0], 99225[0], 99226[0], 99231[0], 99232[0], 99233[0], 99234[0], 99235[0], 99236[0], 99238[0], 99239[0], 99281[0], 99282[0], 99283[0], 99284[0], 99285[0], 99304[0], 99305[0], 99306[0], 99307[0], 99308[0], 99309[0], 99310[0], 99315[0], 99316[0], 99318[0], 99324[0], 99325[0], 99326[0], 99327[0], 99328[0], 99334[0], 99335[0], 99336[0], 99337[0], 99341[0], 99342[0], 99343[0], 99344[0], 99345[0], 99347[0], 99348[0], 99349[0], 99350[0], 99354[0], 99355[0], 99356[0], 99357[0], 99358[0], 99359[0], 99415[0], 99416[0], 99446[0], 99447[0], 99448[0], 99449[0], 99451[0], 99452[0], 99466[0], 99468[0], 99469[0], 99471[0], 99472[0], 99475[0], 99476[0], 99477[0], 99478[0], 99479[0], 99480[0], 99483[0], 99485[0], 99497[0], C8921[1], C8922[1], C8923[1], C8924[1], C8925[1], C8926[1], C8927[0], C8929[1], C8930[1], G0380[1], G0381[1], G0382[1], G0383[1], G0384[1], G0406[0], G0407[0], G0408[0], G0425[0], G0426[0], G0427[0], G0463[0], G0500[0], G0508[0], G0509[0]
00567	00560[1], 01996[1], 0213T[1], 0216T[1], 0228T[1], 0230T[1], 31505[1], 31515[1], 31527[1], 31622[1], 31634[1], 31645[1], 31647[1], 36000[1], 36010[0], 36011[1], 36012[1], 36013[1], 36014[1], 36015[1], 36400[1], 36405[1], 36406[1], 36410[1], 36420[1], 36425[1], 36430[1], 36440[1], 36591[0], 36592[0], 36600[1], 36640[1], 43752[1], 43753[1], 43754[1], 61026[1], 61055[1], 62280[1], 62281[1], 62282[1], 62284[1], 62320[1], 62321[1], 62322[1], 62323[1], 62324[1], 62325[1], 62326[1], 62327[1], 64400[1], 64402[1], 64405[1], 64408[1], 64410[1], 64413[1], 64415[1], 64416[1], 64417[1], 64418[1], 64420[1], 64421[1], 64425[1], 64430[1], 64435[1], 64445[1], 64446[1], 64447[1], 64448[1], 64449[1], 64450[1], 64461[1], 64463[1], 64479[1], 64483[1], 64486[1], 64487[1], 64488[1], 64489[1], 64490[1], 64493[1], 64505[1], 64510[1], 64517[1], 64520[1], 64530[1], 64553[1], 64555[1], 67500[1], 76000[1], 76970[1],

0 = Modifier usage not allowed or inappropriate 1 = Modifier usage allowed

CPT © 2018 American Medical Association. All Rights Reserved.

Code 1	Code 2
	76998[0], 77002[0], 90865[1], 92511[1], 92512[1], 92516[1], 92520[1], 92537[1], 92538[1], 92950[1], 92953[1], 92960[1], 92961[1], 93000[1], 93005[1], 93010[1], 93040[1], 93041[1], 93042[1], 93050[0], 93303[0], 93304[0], 93307[1], 93308[1], 93312[1], 93313[1], 93314[1], 93315[1], 93316[1], 93317[1], 93318[0], 93355[0], 93451[1], 93456[1], 93457[1], 93561[0], 93562[0], 93701[0], 93922[1], 93923[1], 93924[1], 93925[1], 93926[1], 93930[1], 93931[1], 93970[1], 93971[1], 93975[1], 93976[1], 93978[1], 93979[1], 93980[1], 93981[1], 94002[1], 94004[1], 94200[1], 94250[0], 94640[1], 94660[1], 94662[1], 94680[1], 94681[1], 94690[1], 94760[0], 94761[0], 94762[1], 94770[1], 95812[0], 95813[0], 95816[0], 95819[0], 95822[0], 95829[0], 95955[0], 95956[0], 95957[0], 96360[0], 96365[0], 96372[0], 96373[0], 96374[0], 96375[0], 96376[0], 96377[0], 99151[0], 99152[0], 99153[0], 99155[0], 99156[0], 99157[0], 99184[1], 99201[0], 99202[0], 99203[0], 99204[0], 99205[0], 99211[0], 99212[0], 99213[0], 99214[0], 99215[0], 99217[0], 99218[0], 99219[0], 99220[0], 99221[0], 99222[0], 99223[0], 99224[0], 99225[0], 99226[0], 99231[0], 99232[0], 99233[0], 99234[0], 99235[0], 99236[0], 99238[0], 99239[0], 99281[0], 99282[0], 99283[0], 99284[0], 99285[0], 99304[0], 99305[0], 99306[0], 99307[0], 99308[0], 99309[0], 99310[0], 99315[0], 99318[0], 99324[0], 99325[0], 99326[0], 99327[0], 99328[0], 99334[0], 99335[0], 99336[0], 99337[0], 99341[0], 99342[0], 99343[0], 99347[0], 99348[0], 99349[0], 99354[0], 99355[0], 99356[0], 99357[0], 99358[0], 99359[0], 99415[0], 99416[0], 99446[0], 99447[0], 99448[0], 99449[0], 99451[0], 99452[0], 99466[0], 99468[0], 99469[0], 99471[0], 99472[0], 99475[0], 99476[0], 99477[0], 99478[0], 99479[0], 99480[0], 99483[0], 99485[0], 99497[0], C8921[1], C8922[1], C8923[1], C8924[1], C8925[1], C8926[1], C8927[1], C8929[1], G0406[0], G0407[0], G0408[0], G0425[0], G0426[0], G0427[0], G0463[0], G0500[0], G0508[0], G0509[0]
00580	01996[1], 0213T[1], 0216T[1], 0228T[1], 0230T[1], 31505[1], 31515[1], 31527[1], 31622[1], 31634[1], 31645[1], 31647[1], 36000[1], 36410[1], 36500[1], 36591[0], 36592[0], 36600[1], 36640[1], 43752[1], 43753[1], 43754[1], 61026[1], 61055[1], 62280[1], 62281[1], 62282[1], 62284[1], 62320[1], 62321[1], 62322[1], 62323[1], 62324[1], 62325[1], 62326[1], 62327[1], 64400[1], 64402[1], 64405[1], 64408[1], 64410[1], 64413[1], 64415[1], 64416[1], 64417[1], 64418[1], 64420[1], 64421[1], 64425[1], 64430[1], 64435[1], 64445[1], 64446[1], 64447[1], 64448[1], 64449[1], 64450[1], 64461[1], 64463[1], 64479[1], 64483[1], 64486[1], 64487[1], 64488[1], 64489[1], 64490[1], 64493[1], 64505[1], 64510[1], 64517[1], 64520[1], 64530[1], 64553[1], 64555[1], 67500[1], 76000[1], 76970[1], 76998[0], 77002[0], 90865[1], 92511[1], 92512[1], 92516[1], 92520[1], 92537[1], 92538[1], 92950[1], 92953[1], 92960[1], 92961[1], 93000[1], 93005[1], 93010[1], 93040[1], 93041[1], 93042[1], 93050[0], 93303[0], 93304[0], 93306[1], 93307[1], 93308[1], 93312[1], 93313[1], 93314[1], 93315[1], 93316[1], 93317[1], 93318[0], 93351[1], 93355[0], 93451[1], 93456[1], 93457[1], 93561[0], 93562[0], 93701[0], 93922[1], 93923[1], 93924[1], 93925[1], 93926[1], 93930[1], 93931[1], 93970[1], 93971[1], 93975[1], 93976[1], 93978[1], 93979[1], 93980[1], 93981[1], 94002[1], 94004[1], 94200[1], 94250[0], 94640[1], 94644[1], 94660[1], 94662[1], 94680[1], 94681[1], 94690[1], 94760[0], 94761[0], 94762[1], 94770[1], 95812[0], 95813[0], 95816[0], 95819[0], 95822[0], 95829[0], 95955[0], 95956[0], 95957[0], 96360[0], 96365[0], 96372[0], 96373[0], 96374[0], 96375[0], 96376[0], 96377[0], 99151[0], 99152[0], 99153[0], 99155[0], 99156[0], 99157[0], 99184[1], 99201[0], 99202[0], 99203[0], 99204[0], 99205[0], 99211[0], 99212[0], 99213[0], 99214[0], 99215[0], 99217[0], 99218[0], 99219[0], 99220[0], 99221[0], 99222[0], 99223[0], 99224[0], 99225[0], 99226[0], 99231[0], 99232[0], 99233[0], 99234[0], 99235[0], 99236[0], 99238[0], 99239[0], 99281[0], 99282[0], 99283[0], 99284[0], 99285[0], 99304[0], 99305[0], 99306[0], 99307[0], 99308[0], 99309[0], 99310[0], 99315[0], 99318[0], 99324[0], 99325[0], 99326[0], 99327[0], 99328[0], 99334[0], 99335[0], 99336[0], 99337[0], 99341[0], 99342[0], 99343[0], 99347[0], 99348[0], 99349[0], 99354[0], 99355[0], 99356[0], 99357[0], 99358[0], 99359[0], 99415[0], 99416[0], 99446[0], 99447[0], 99448[0], 99449[0], 99451[0], 99452[0], 99466[0], 99468[0], 99469[0], 99471[0], 99472[0], 99475[0], 99476[0], 99477[0], 99478[0], 99479[0], 99480[0], 99483[0], 99485[0], 99497[0], C8921[1], C8922[1], C8923[1], C8924[1], C8925[1], C8926[1], C8927[0], C8929[1], C8930[1], G0380[1], G0381[1], G0382[1], G0383[1], G0384[1], G0406[0], G0407[0], G0408[0], G0425[0], G0426[0], G0427[0], G0463[0], G0500[0], G0508[0], G0509[0]
00600	01996[1], 0213T[1], 0216T[1], 0228T[1], 0230T[1], 0333T[0], 0464T[0], 31505[1], 31515[1], 31527[1], 31622[1], 31634[1], 31645[1], 31647[1], 36000[1], 36010[0], 36011[1], 36012[1], 36013[1], 36014[1], 36015[1], 36400[1], 36405[1], 36406[1], 36410[1], 36420[1], 36425[1], 36430[1], 36440[1], 36591[0], 36592[0], 36600[1], 36640[1], 43752[1], 43753[1], 43754[1], 61026[1], 61055[1], 62280[1], 62281[1], 62282[1], 62284[1], 62320[1], 62321[1], 62322[1], 62323[1], 62324[1], 62325[1], 62326[1], 62327[1], 64400[1], 64402[1], 64405[1], 64408[1], 64410[1], 64413[1], 64415[1], 64416[1], 64417[1], 64418[1], 64420[1], 64421[1], 64425[1], 64430[1], 64435[1], 64445[1], 64446[1], 64447[1], 64448[1], 64449[1], 64450[1], 64461[1], 64463[1], 64479[1], 64483[1], 64486[1], 64487[1], 64488[1], 64489[1], 64490[1], 64493[1], 64505[1], 64510[1], 64517[1], 64520[1], 64530[1], 64553[1], 64555[1], 67500[1], 76000[1], 76970[1], 76998[0], 77002[0], 90865[1], 92511[1], 92512[1], 92516[1], 92520[1], 92537[1], 92538[1], 92585[0], 92950[1], 92953[1], 92960[1], 92961[1], 93000[1], 93005[1], 93010[1], 93040[1], 93041[1], 93042[1], 93050[0], 93303[0], 93304[0], 93306[1], 93307[1], 93308[1], 93312[1], 93313[1], 93314[1], 93315[1], 93316[1], 93317[1], 93318[0], 93351[1], 93355[0], 93451[1], 93456[1], 93457[1], 93561[0], 93562[0], 93701[0], 93922[1], 93923[1], 93924[1], 93925[1], 93926[1], 93930[1], 93931[1], 93970[1], 93971[1], 93975[1], 93976[1], 93978[1], 93979[1], 93980[1], 93981[1], 94002[1], 94004[1], 94200[1], 94250[0], 94640[1], 94644[1], 94660[1], 94662[1], 94680[1], 94681[1], 94690[1], 94760[0], 94761[0], 94762[1], 94770[1], 95812[0], 95813[0], 95816[0], 95819[0], 95822[0], 95829[0], 95860[0], 95861[0], 95863[0], 95864[0], 95865[0], 95866[0], 95867[0], 95868[0], 95869[0], 95870[0], 95907[0], 95908[0], 95909[0], 95910[0], 95911[0], 95912[0], 95913[0], 95925[0], 95926[0], 95927[0], 95928[0], 95929[0], 95930[0], 95933[0], 95937[0], 95938[0], 95939[0], 95940[0], 95955[0], 95956[0], 95957[0], 96360[0], 96365[0], 96372[0], 96373[0], 96374[0], 96375[0], 96376[0], 96377[0], 99151[0], 99152[0], 99153[0], 99155[0], 99156[0], 99157[0], 99201[0], 99202[0], 99203[0], 99204[0], 99205[0], 99211[0], 99212[0], 99213[0], 99214[0], 99215[0], 99217[0], 99218[0], 99219[0], 99220[0], 99221[0], 99222[0], 99223[0], 99224[0], 99225[0], 99226[0], 99231[0], 99232[0], 99233[0], 99234[0], 99235[0], 99236[0], 99238[0], 99239[0], 99281[0], 99282[0], 99283[0], 99284[0], 99285[0], 99304[0], 99305[0], 99306[0], 99307[0], 99308[0], 99309[0], 99310[0], 99315[0], 99318[0], 99324[0], 99325[0], 99326[0], 99327[0], 99328[0], 99334[0], 99335[0], 99336[0], 99337[0], 99341[0], 99342[0], 99343[0], 99347[0], 99348[0], 99349[0], 99354[0], 99355[0], 99356[0], 99357[0], 99358[0], 99359[0], 99415[0], 99416[0], 99446[0], 99447[0], 99448[0], 99449[0], 99451[0], 99452[0], 99466[0], 99468[0], 99469[0], 99471[0], 99472[0], 99475[0], 99476[0], 99477[0], 99478[0], 99479[0], 99480[0], 99483[0], 99485[0], 99497[0], C8921[1], C8922[1], C8923[1], C8924[1], C8925[1], C8926[1], C8927[0], C8929[1], C8930[1], G0380[1], G0381[1], G0382[1], G0383[1], G0384[1], G0406[0], G0407[0], G0408[0], G0425[0], G0426[0], G0427[0], G0453[0], G0463[0], G0500[0], G0508[0], G0509[0]
00604	01996[1], 0213T[1], 0216T[1], 0228T[1], 0230T[1], 0333T[0], 0464T[0], 31505[1], 31515[1], 31527[1], 31622[1], 31634[1], 31645[1], 31647[1], 36000[1], 36010[0], 36011[1], 36012[1], 36013[1], 36014[1], 36015[1], 36400[1], 36405[1], 36406[1], 36410[1], 36420[1], 36425[1], 36430[1], 36440[1], 36591[0], 36592[0], 36600[1], 36640[1], 43752[1], 43753[1], 43754[1], 61026[1], 61055[1], 62280[1], 62281[1], 62282[1], 62284[1], 62320[1], 62321[1], 62322[1], 62323[1], 62324[1], 62325[1], 62326[1], 62327[1], 64400[1], 64402[1], 64405[1], 64408[1], 64410[1], 64413[1], 64415[1], 64416[1], 64417[1], 64418[1], 64420[1], 64421[1], 64425[1], 64430[1], 64435[1], 64445[1], 64446[1], 64447[1], 64448[1], 64449[1], 64450[1], 64461[1], 64463[1], 64479[1], 64483[1], 64486[1], 64487[1], 64488[1], 64489[1], 64490[1], 64493[1], 64505[1], 64510[1], 64517[1], 64520[1], 64530[1], 64553[1], 64555[1], 67500[1], 76000[1], 76970[1], 76998[0], 77002[0], 90865[1], 92511[1], 92512[1], 92516[1], 92520[1], 92537[1], 92538[1], 92585[0], 92950[1], 92953[1], 92960[1], 92961[1], 93000[1], 93005[1], 93010[1], 93040[1], 93041[1], 93042[1], 93050[0], 93303[0], 93304[0], 93306[1], 93307[1], 93308[1], 93312[1], 93313[1], 93314[1], 93315[1], 93316[1], 93317[1], 93318[0], 93351[1], 93355[0], 93451[1], 93456[1], 93457[1], 93561[0], 93562[0], 93701[0], 93922[1], 93923[1], 93924[1], 93925[1], 93926[1], 93930[1], 93931[1], 93970[1], 93971[1], 93975[1], 93976[1], 93978[1], 93979[1], 93980[1], 93981[1], 94002[1], 94004[1], 94200[1], 94250[0], 94640[1], 94644[1], 94660[1], 94662[1], 94680[1], 94681[1], 94690[1], 94760[0], 94761[0], 94762[1], 94770[1], 95812[0], 95813[0], 95816[0], 95819[0], 95822[0], 95829[0], 95860[0], 95861[0], 95863[0], 95864[0], 95865[0], 95866[0], 95867[0], 95868[0], 95869[0], 95870[0], 95907[0], 95908[0], 95909[0], 95910[0], 95911[0], 95912[0], 95913[0], 95925[0], 95926[0], 95927[0], 95928[0], 95929[0], 95930[0], 95933[0], 95937[0], 95938[0], 95939[0], 95940[0], 95955[0], 95956[0], 95957[0], 96360[0], 96365[0], 96372[0], 96373[0], 96374[0], 96375[0], 96376[0], 96377[0], 99151[0], 99152[0], 99153[0], 99155[0], 99156[0], 99157[0], 99201[0], 99202[0], 99203[0], 99204[0], 99205[0], 99211[0], 99212[0], 99213[0], 99214[0], 99215[0], 99217[0], 99218[0], 99219[0], 99220[0], 99221[0], 99222[0], 99223[0], 99224[0], 99225[0], 99226[0], 99231[0], 99232[0], 99233[0], 99234[0], 99235[0], 99236[0], 99238[0], 99239[0], 99281[0], 99282[0], 99283[0], 99284[0], 99285[0], 99304[0], 99305[0], 99306[0], 99307[0], 99308[0], 99309[0], 99310[0], 99315[0], 99318[0], 99324[0], 99325[0], 99326[0], 99327[0], 99328[0], 99334[0], 99335[0], 99336[0], 99337[0], 99341[0], 99342[0], 99343[0], 99347[0], 99348[0], 99349[0], 99354[0], 99355[0], 99356[0], 99357[0], 99358[0], 99359[0], 99415[0], 99416[0], 99446[0], 99447[0], 99448[0], 99449[0], 99451[0], 99452[0], 99466[0], 99468[0], 99469[0], 99471[0], 99472[0], 99475[0], 99476[0], 99477[0], 99478[0], 99479[0], 99480[0], 99483[0], 99485[0], 99497[0], C8921[1], C8922[1], C8923[1], C8924[1], C8925[1], C8926[1], C8927[0], C8929[1], C8930[1], G0380[1], G0381[1], G0382[1], G0383[1], G0384[1], G0406[0], G0407[0], G0408[0], G0425[0], G0426[0], G0427[0], G0453[0], G0463[0], G0500[0], G0508[0], G0509[0]
00625	01996[1], 0213T[1], 0216T[1], 0228T[1], 0230T[1], 0333T[0], 0464T[0], 31505[1], 31515[1], 31527[1], 31622[1], 31634[1], 31645[1], 31647[1], 36000[1], 36010[0], 36011[1], 36012[1], 36013[1], 36014[1], 36015[1], 36400[1], 36405[1], 36406[1], 36410[1], 36420[1], 36425[1], 36430[1], 36440[1], 36591[0], 36592[0], 36600[1], 36640[1], 43752[1], 43753[1], 43754[1], 61026[1], 61055[1], 62280[1], 62281[1], 62282[1], 62284[1], 62320[1], 62321[1], 62322[1], 62323[1], 62324[1], 62325[1], 62326[1], 62327[1], 64400[1], 64402[1], 64405[1], 64408[1], 64410[1], 64413[1], 64415[1], 64416[1], 64417[1], 64418[1], 64420[1], 64421[1], 64425[1], 64430[1], 64435[1], 64445[1], 64446[1], 64447[1], 64448[1], 64449[1], 64450[1], 64461[1], 64463[1], 64479[1], 64483[1], 64486[1], 64487[1], 64488[1], 64489[1], 64490[1], 64493[1], 64505[1], 64510[1], 64517[1], 64520[1], 64530[1], 64553[1], 64555[1], 67500[1], 76000[1], 76970[1], 76998[0], 77002[0], 90865[1], 92511[1], 92512[1], 92516[1], 92520[1], 92537[1], 92538[1], 92585[0], 92950[1], 92953[1], 92960[1], 92961[1], 93000[1], 93005[1], 93010[1], 93040[1], 93041[1], 93042[1], 93050[0], 93303[0], 93304[0], 93306[1], 93307[1], 93308[1], 93312[1], 93313[1], 93314[1], 93315[1], 93316[1], 93317[1], 93318[0], 93351[1], 93355[0], 93451[1], 93456[1], 93457[1], 93561[0], 93562[0], 93701[0], 93922[1], 93923[1], 93924[1], 93925[1], 93926[1], 93930[1], 93931[1], 93970[1], 93971[1], 93975[1], 93976[1], 93978[1], 93979[1], 93980[1], 93981[1], 94002[1], 94004[1], 94200[1], 94250[0], 94640[1], 94644[1], 94660[1], 94662[1], 94680[1], 94681[1], 94690[1], 94760[0], 94761[0], 94762[1], 94770[1], 95812[0], 95813[0], 95816[0], 95819[0], 95822[0], 95829[0], 95860[0], 95861[0], 95863[0], 95864[0], 95865[0], 95866[0], 95867[0], 95868[0], 95869[0], 95870[0], 95907[0], 95908[0],

0 = Modifier usage not allowed or inappropriate 1 = Modifier usage allowed

CPT © 2018 American Medical Association. All Rights Reserved.

Code 1	Code 2
	95909[0], 95910[0], 95911[0], 95912[0], 95913[0], 95925[0], 95926[0], 95927[0], 95928[0], 95929[0], 95930[0], 95933[0], 95937[0], 95938[0], 95939[0], 95940[0], 95955[0], 95956[0], 95957[0], 96360[0], 96365[0], 96372[0], 96373[0], 96374[0], 96375[0], 96376[0], 96377[0], 99151[0], 99152[0], 99153[0], 99155[0], 99156[0], 99157[0], 99201[0], 99202[0], 99203[0], 99204[0], 99205[0], 99211[0], 99212[0], 99213[0], 99214[0], 99215[0], 99217[0], 99218[0], 99219[0], 99220[0], 99221[0], 99222[0], 99223[0], 99224[0], 99225[0], 99226[0], 99231[0], 99232[0], 99233[0], 99234[0], 99235[0], 99236[0], 99238[0], 99239[0], 99281[0], 99282[0], 99283[0], 99284[0], 99285[0], 99304[0], 99305[0], 99306[0], 99307[0], 99308[0], 99309[0], 99310[0], 99315[0], 99316[0], 99318[0], 99324[0], 99325[0], 99326[0], 99327[0], 99328[0], 99334[0], 99335[0], 99336[0], 99337[0], 99341[0], 99342[0], 99343[0], 99344[0], 99345[0], 99347[0], 99348[0], 99349[0], 99350[0], 99354[0], 99355[0], 99356[0], 99357[0], 99358[0], 99359[0], 99415[0], 99416[0], 99446[0], 99447[0], 99448[0], 99449[0], 99451[0], 99452[0], 99466[0], 99467[0], 99468[0], 99469[0], 99471[0], 99472[0], 99475[0], 99476[0], 99477[0], 99478[0], 99479[0], 99480[0], 99483[0], 99485[0], 99497[0], C8921[1], C8922[1], C8923[1], C8924[1], C8925[1], C8926[1], C8927[0], C8929[1], C8930[1], G0380[1], G0381[1], G0382[1], G0383[1], G0384[1], G0406[0], G0407[0], G0408[0], G0425[0], G0426[0], G0427[0], G0453[0], G0463[0], G0500[0], G0508[0], G0509[0]
00626	00625[0], 01996[1], 0213T[1], 0216T[1], 0228T[1], 0230T[1], 0333T[0], 0464T[0], 31505[1], 31515[1], 31527[1], 31622[1], 31634[1], 31645[1], 31647[1], 36000[1], 36010[0], 36011[1], 36012[1], 36013[1], 36014[1], 36015[1], 36400[1], 36405[1], 36406[1], 36410[1], 36420[1], 36425[1], 36430[1], 36440[1], 36591[0], 36592[0], 36600[1], 36640[1], 43752[1], 43753[1], 43754[1], 61026[1], 61055[1], 62280[1], 62281[1], 62282[1], 62284[1], 62320[1], 62321[1], 62322[1], 62323[1], 62324[1], 62325[1], 62326[1], 62327[1], 64400[1], 64402[1], 64405[1], 64408[1], 64410[1], 64413[1], 64415[1], 64416[1], 64417[1], 64418[1], 64420[1], 64421[1], 64425[1], 64430[1], 64435[1], 64445[1], 64446[1], 64447[1], 64448[1], 64449[1], 64450[1], 64461[1], 64463[1], 64479[1], 64483[1], 64486[1], 64487[1], 64488[1], 64489[1], 64490[1], 64493[1], 64505[1], 64510[1], 64517[1], 64520[1], 64530[1], 64553[1], 64555[1], 67500[1], 76000[1], 76970[1], 76998[0], 77002[0], 90865[1], 92511[1], 92512[1], 92516[1], 92520[1], 92537[1], 92538[1], 92585[0], 92950[1], 92953[1], 92960[1], 92961[1], 93000[1], 93005[1], 93010[1], 93040[1], 93041[1], 93042[1], 93050[0], 93303[0], 93304[0], 93306[1], 93307[1], 93308[1], 93312[1], 93313[1], 93314[1], 93315[1], 93316[1], 93317[1], 93318[0], 93351[1], 93355[0], 93451[1], 93456[1], 93457[1], 93561[0], 93562[0], 93701[0], 93922[1], 93923[1], 93924[1], 93925[1], 93926[1], 93930[1], 93931[1], 93970[1], 93971[1], 93975[1], 93976[1], 93978[1], 93979[1], 93980[1], 93981[1], 94002[1], 94004[1], 94200[1], 94250[0], 94640[1], 94644[1], 94660[1], 94662[1], 94680[1], 94681[1], 94690[1], 94760[0], 94761[0], 94762[1], 94770[1], 95812[0], 95813[0], 95816[0], 95819[0], 95822[0], 95829[0], 95860[0], 95861[0], 95863[0], 95864[0], 95865[0], 95866[0], 95867[0], 95868[0], 95869[0], 95870[0], 95907[0], 95908[0], 95909[0], 95910[0], 95911[0], 95912[0], 95913[0], 95925[0], 95926[0], 95927[0], 95928[0], 95929[0], 95930[0], 95933[0], 95937[0], 95938[0], 95939[0], 95940[0], 95955[0], 95956[0], 95957[0], 96360[0], 96365[0], 96372[0], 96373[0], 96374[0], 96375[0], 96376[0], 96377[0], 99151[0], 99152[0], 99153[0], 99155[0], 99156[0], 99157[0], 99201[0], 99202[0], 99203[0], 99204[0], 99205[0], 99211[0], 99212[0], 99213[0], 99214[0], 99215[0], 99217[0], 99218[0], 99219[0], 99220[0], 99221[0], 99222[0], 99223[0], 99224[0], 99225[0], 99226[0], 99231[0], 99232[0], 99233[0], 99234[0], 99235[0], 99236[0], 99238[0], 99239[0], 99281[0], 99282[0], 99283[0], 99284[0], 99285[0], 99304[0], 99305[0], 99306[0], 99307[0], 99308[0], 99309[0], 99310[0], 99315[0], 99316[0], 99318[0], 99324[0], 99325[0], 99326[0], 99327[0], 99328[0], 99334[0], 99335[0], 99336[0], 99337[0], 99341[0], 99342[0], 99343[0], 99344[0], 99345[0], 99347[0], 99348[0], 99349[0], 99350[0], 99354[0], 99355[0], 99356[0], 99357[0], 99358[0], 99359[0], 99415[0], 99416[0], 99446[0], 99447[0], 99448[0], 99449[0], 99451[0], 99452[0], 99466[0], 99467[0], 99468[0], 99469[0], 99471[0], 99472[0], 99475[0], 99476[0], 99477[0], 99478[0], 99479[0], 99480[0], 99483[0], 99485[0], 99497[0], C8921[1], C8922[1], C8923[1], C8924[1], C8925[1], C8926[1], C8927[0], C8929[1], C8930[1], G0380[1], G0381[1], G0382[1], G0383[1], G0384[1], G0406[0], G0407[0], G0408[0], G0425[0], G0426[0], G0427[0], G0453[0], G0463[0], G0500[0], G0508[0], G0509[0]
00630	01996[1], 0213T[1], 0216T[1], 0228T[1], 0230T[1], 0333T[0], 0464T[0], 31505[1], 31515[1], 31527[1], 31622[1], 31634[1], 31645[1], 31647[1], 36000[1], 36010[0], 36011[1], 36012[1], 36013[1], 36014[1], 36015[1], 36400[1], 36405[1], 36406[1], 36410[1], 36420[1], 36425[1], 36430[1], 36440[1], 36591[0], 36592[0], 36600[1], 36640[1], 43752[1], 43753[1], 43754[1], 61026[1], 61055[1], 62280[1], 62281[1], 62282[1], 62284[1], 62320[1], 62321[1], 62322[1], 62323[1], 62324[1], 62325[1], 62326[1], 62327[1], 64400[1], 64402[1], 64405[1], 64408[1], 64410[1], 64413[1], 64415[1], 64416[1], 64417[1], 64418[1], 64420[1], 64421[1], 64425[1], 64430[1], 64435[1], 64445[1], 64446[1], 64447[1], 64448[1], 64449[1], 64450[1], 64461[1], 64463[1], 64479[1], 64483[1], 64486[1], 64487[1], 64488[1], 64489[1], 64490[1], 64493[1], 64505[1], 64510[1], 64517[1], 64520[1], 64530[1], 64553[1], 64555[1], 67500[1], 76000[1], 76970[1], 76998[0], 77002[0], 90865[1], 92511[1], 92512[1], 92516[1], 92520[1], 92537[1], 92538[1], 92585[0], 92950[1], 92953[1], 92960[1], 92961[1], 93000[1], 93005[1], 93010[1], 93040[1], 93041[1], 93042[1], 93050[0], 93303[0], 93304[0], 93306[1], 93307[1], 93308[1], 93312[1], 93313[1], 93314[1], 93315[1], 93316[1], 93317[1], 93318[0], 93351[1], 93355[0], 93451[1], 93456[1], 93457[1], 93561[0], 93562[0], 93701[0], 93922[1], 93923[1], 93924[1], 93925[1], 93926[1], 93930[1], 93931[1], 93970[1], 93971[1], 93975[1], 93976[1], 93978[1], 93979[1], 93980[1], 93981[1], 94002[1], 94004[1], 94200[1], 94250[0], 94640[1], 94644[1], 94660[1], 94662[1], 94680[1], 94681[1], 94690[1], 94760[0], 94761[0], 94762[1], 94770[1], 95812[0], 95813[0], 95816[0], 95819[0], 95822[0], 95829[0], 95860[0], 95861[0], 95863[0], 95864[0], 95865[0], 95866[0], 95867[0], 95868[0], 95869[0], 95870[0], 95907[0], 95908[0],
	95909[0], 95910[0], 95911[0], 95912[0], 95913[0], 95925[0], 95926[0], 95927[0], 95928[0], 95929[0], 95930[0], 95933[0], 95937[0], 95938[0], 95939[0], 95940[0], 95955[0], 95956[0], 95957[0], 96360[0], 96365[0], 96372[0], 96373[0], 96374[0], 96375[0], 96376[0], 96377[0], 99151[0], 99152[0], 99153[0], 99155[0], 99156[0], 99157[0], 99201[0], 99202[0], 99203[0], 99204[0], 99205[0], 99211[0], 99212[0], 99213[0], 99214[0], 99215[0], 99217[0], 99218[0], 99219[0], 99220[0], 99221[0], 99222[0], 99223[0], 99224[0], 99225[0], 99226[0], 99231[0], 99232[0], 99233[0], 99234[0], 99235[0], 99236[0], 99238[0], 99239[0], 99281[0], 99282[0], 99283[0], 99284[0], 99285[0], 99304[0], 99305[0], 99306[0], 99307[0], 99308[0], 99309[0], 99310[0], 99315[0], 99318[0], 99324[0], 99325[0], 99326[0], 99327[0], 99328[0], 99334[0], 99335[0], 99336[0], 99337[0], 99341[0], 99342[0], 99343[0], 99347[0], 99348[0], 99349[0], 99354[0], 99355[0], 99356[0], 99357[0], 99358[0], 99359[0], 99415[0], 99416[0], 99446[0], 99447[0], 99448[0], 99449[0], 99451[0], 99452[0], 99466[0], 99468[0], 99469[0], 99471[0], 99472[0], 99475[0], 99476[0], 99477[0], 99478[0], 99479[0], 99480[0], 99483[0], 99485[0], 99497[0], C8921[1], C8922[1], C8923[1], C8924[1], C8925[1], C8926[1], C8927[0], C8929[1], C8930[1], G0380[1], G0381[1], G0382[1], G0383[1], G0384[1], G0406[0], G0407[0], G0408[0], G0425[0], G0426[0], G0427[0], G0453[0], G0463[0], G0500[0], G0508[0], G0509[0]
00632	01996[1], 0213T[1], 0216T[1], 0228T[1], 0230T[1], 0333T[0], 0464T[0], 31505[1], 31515[1], 31527[1], 31622[1], 31634[1], 31645[1], 31647[1], 36000[1], 36010[0], 36011[1], 36012[1], 36013[1], 36014[1], 36015[1], 36400[1], 36405[1], 36406[1], 36410[1], 36420[1], 36425[1], 36430[1], 36440[1], 36591[0], 36592[0], 36600[1], 36640[1], 43752[1], 43753[1], 43754[1], 61026[1], 61055[1], 62280[1], 62281[1], 62282[1], 62284[1], 62320[1], 62321[1], 62322[1], 62323[1], 62324[1], 62325[1], 62326[1], 62327[1], 64400[1], 64402[1], 64405[1], 64408[1], 64410[1], 64413[1], 64415[1], 64416[1], 64417[1], 64418[1], 64420[1], 64421[1], 64425[1], 64430[1], 64435[1], 64445[1], 64446[1], 64447[1], 64448[1], 64449[1], 64450[1], 64461[1], 64463[1], 64479[1], 64483[1], 64486[1], 64487[1], 64488[1], 64489[1], 64490[1], 64493[1], 64505[1], 64510[1], 64517[1], 64520[1], 64530[1], 64553[1], 64555[1], 67500[1], 76000[1], 76970[1], 76998[0], 77002[0], 90865[1], 92511[1], 92512[1], 92516[1], 92520[1], 92537[1], 92538[1], 92585[0], 92950[1], 92953[1], 92960[1], 92961[1], 93000[1], 93005[1], 93010[1], 93040[1], 93041[1], 93042[1], 93050[0], 93303[0], 93304[0], 93306[1], 93307[1], 93308[1], 93312[1], 93313[1], 93314[1], 93315[1], 93316[1], 93317[1], 93318[0], 93351[1], 93355[0], 93451[1], 93456[1], 93457[1], 93561[0], 93562[0], 93701[0], 93922[1], 93923[1], 93924[1], 93925[1], 93926[1], 93930[1], 93931[1], 93970[1], 93971[1], 93975[1], 93976[1], 93978[1], 93979[1], 93980[1], 93981[1], 94002[1], 94004[1], 94200[1], 94250[0], 94640[1], 94644[1], 94660[1], 94662[1], 94680[1], 94681[1], 94690[1], 94760[0], 94761[0], 94762[1], 94770[1], 95812[0], 95813[0], 95816[0], 95819[0], 95822[0], 95829[0], 95860[0], 95861[0], 95863[0], 95864[0], 95865[0], 95866[0], 95867[0], 95868[0], 95869[0], 95870[0], 95907[0], 95908[0], 95909[0], 95910[0], 95911[0], 95912[0], 95913[0], 95925[0], 95926[0], 95927[0], 95928[0], 95929[0], 95930[0], 95933[0], 95937[0], 95938[0], 95939[0], 95940[0], 95955[0], 95956[0], 95957[0], 96360[0], 96365[0], 96372[0], 96373[0], 96374[0], 96375[0], 96376[0], 96377[0], 99151[0], 99152[0], 99153[0], 99155[0], 99156[0], 99157[0], 99201[0], 99202[0], 99203[0], 99204[0], 99205[0], 99211[0], 99212[0], 99213[0], 99214[0], 99215[0], 99217[0], 99218[0], 99219[0], 99220[0], 99221[0], 99222[0], 99223[0], 99224[0], 99225[0], 99226[0], 99231[0], 99232[0], 99233[0], 99234[0], 99235[0], 99236[0], 99238[0], 99239[0], 99281[0], 99282[0], 99283[0], 99284[0], 99285[0], 99304[0], 99305[0], 99306[0], 99307[0], 99308[0], 99309[0], 99310[0], 99315[0], 99318[0], 99324[0], 99325[0], 99326[0], 99327[0], 99328[0], 99334[0], 99335[0], 99336[0], 99337[0], 99341[0], 99342[0], 99343[0], 99347[0], 99348[0], 99349[0], 99354[0], 99355[0], 99356[0], 99357[0], 99358[0], 99359[0], 99415[0], 99416[0], 99446[0], 99447[0], 99448[0], 99449[0], 99451[0], 99452[0], 99466[0], 99468[0], 99469[0], 99471[0], 99472[0], 99475[0], 99476[0], 99477[0], 99478[0], 99479[0], 99480[0], 99483[0], 99485[0], 99497[0], C8921[1], C8922[1], C8923[1], C8924[1], C8925[1], C8926[1], C8927[0], C8929[1], C8930[1], G0380[1], G0381[1], G0382[1], G0383[1], G0384[1], G0406[0], G0407[0], G0408[0], G0425[0], G0426[0], G0427[0], G0453[0], G0463[0], G0500[0], G0508[0], G0509[0]
00635	01996[1], 0213T[1], 0216T[1], 0228T[1], 0230T[1], 0333T[0], 0464T[0], 31505[1], 31515[1], 31527[1], 31622[1], 31634[1], 31645[1], 31647[1], 36000[1], 36010[0], 36011[1], 36012[1], 36013[1], 36014[1], 36015[1], 36400[1], 36405[1], 36406[1], 36410[1], 36420[1], 36425[1], 36430[1], 36440[1], 36591[0], 36592[0], 36600[1], 36640[1], 43752[1], 43753[1], 43754[1], 61026[1], 61055[1], 62280[1], 62281[1], 62282[1], 62284[1], 62320[1], 62321[1], 62322[1], 62323[1], 62324[1], 62325[1], 62326[1], 62327[1], 64400[1], 64402[1], 64405[1], 64408[1], 64410[1], 64413[1], 64415[1], 64416[1], 64417[1], 64418[1], 64420[1], 64421[1], 64425[1], 64430[1], 64435[1], 64445[1], 64446[1], 64447[1], 64448[1], 64449[1], 64450[1], 64461[1], 64463[1], 64479[1], 64483[1], 64486[1], 64487[1], 64488[1], 64489[1], 64490[1], 64493[1], 64505[1], 64510[1], 64517[1], 64520[1], 64530[1], 64553[1], 64555[1], 67500[0], 76000[1], 76970[1], 76998[0], 77002[0], 90865[1], 92511[1], 92512[1], 92516[1], 92520[1], 92537[1], 92538[1], 92585[0], 92950[1], 92953[1], 92960[1], 92961[1], 93000[1], 93005[1], 93010[1], 93040[1], 93041[1], 93042[1], 93050[0], 93303[0], 93304[0], 93306[1], 93307[1], 93308[1], 93312[1], 93313[1], 93314[1], 93315[1], 93316[1], 93317[1], 93318[0], 93351[1], 93355[0], 93451[1], 93456[1], 93457[1], 93561[0], 93562[0], 93701[0], 93922[1], 93923[1], 93924[1], 93925[1], 93926[1], 93930[1], 93931[1], 93970[1], 93971[1], 93975[1], 93976[1], 93978[1], 93979[1], 93980[1], 93981[1], 94002[1], 94004[1], 94200[1], 94250[0], 94640[1], 94644[1], 94660[1], 94662[1], 94680[1], 94681[1], 94690[1], 94760[0], 94761[0], 94762[1], 94770[1], 95812[0], 95813[0], 95816[0], 95819[0], 95822[0], 95829[0], 95860[0], 95861[0], 95863[0], 95864[0], 95865[0], 95866[0], 95867[0], 95868[0], 95869[0], 95870[0], 95907[0], 95908[0],

0 = Modifier usage not allowed or inappropriate 1 = Modifier usage allowed

Appendix A: NCCI - CPT Codes

CPT © 2018 American Medical Association. All Rights Reserved.

Code 1	Code 2
	95909[0], 95910[0], 95911[0], 95912[0], 95913[0], 95925[0], 95926[0], 95927[0], 95928[0], 95929[0], 95930[0], 95933[0], 95937[0], 95938[0], 95939[0], 95940[0], 95955[0], 95956[0], 95957[0], 96360[0], 96365[0], 96372[0], 96373[0], 96374[0], 96375[0], 96376[0], 96377[0], 99151[0], 99152[0], 99153[0], 99155[0], 99156[0], 99157[0], 99201[0], 99202[0], 99203[0], 99204[0], 99205[0], 99211[0], 99212[0], 99213[0], 99214[0], 99215[0], 99217[0], 99218[0], 99219[0], 99220[0], 99221[0], 99222[0], 99223[0], 99224[0], 99225[0], 99226[0], 99231[0], 99232[0], 99233[0], 99234[0], 99235[0], 99236[0], 99238[0], 99239[0], 99281[0], 99282[0], 99283[0], 99284[0], 99285[0], 99304[0], 99305[0], 99306[0], 99307[0], 99308[0], 99309[0], 99310[0], 99315[0], 99316[0], 99318[0], 99324[0], 99325[0], 99326[0], 99327[0], 99328[0], 99334[0], 99335[0], 99336[0], 99337[0], 99341[0], 99342[0], 99343[0], 99344[0], 99345[0], 99347[0], 99348[0], 99349[0], 99350[0], 99354[0], 99355[0], 99356[0], 99357[0], 99358[0], 99359[0], 99415[0], 99416[0], 99446[0], 99447[0], 99448[0], 99449[0], 99451[0], 99452[0], 99466[0], 99468[0], 99469[0], 99471[0], 99472[0], 99475[0], 99476[0], 99477[0], 99478[0], 99479[0], 99480[0], 99483[0], 99485[0], 99497[0], C8921[1], C8922[1], C8923[1], C8924[1], C8925[1], C8926[1], C8927[0], C8929[1], C8930[1], G0380[1], G0381[1], G0382[1], G0383[1], G0384[1], G0406[0], G0407[0], G0408[0], G0425[0], G0426[0], G0427[0], G0453[0], G0463[0], G0500[0], G0508[0], G0509[0]
00640	01996[1], 0213T[1], 0216T[1], 0228T[1], 0230T[1], 0333T[0], 0464T[0], 31505[1], 31515[1], 31527[1], 31622[1], 31634[1], 31645[1], 31647[1], 36000[1], 36010[0], 36011[1], 36012[1], 36013[1], 36014[1], 36015[1], 36400[1], 36405[1], 36406[1], 36410[1], 36420[1], 36425[1], 36430[1], 36440[1], 36591[0], 36592[0], 36600[1], 36640[1], 43752[1], 43753[1], 43754[1], 61026[1], 61055[1], 62280[1], 62281[1], 62282[1], 62284[1], 62320[1], 62321[1], 62322[1], 62323[1], 62324[1], 62325[1], 62326[1], 62327[1], 64400[1], 64402[1], 64405[1], 64408[1], 64410[1], 64413[1], 64415[1], 64416[1], 64417[1], 64418[1], 64420[1], 64421[1], 64425[1], 64430[1], 64435[1], 64445[1], 64446[1], 64447[1], 64448[1], 64449[1], 64450[1], 64461[1], 64463[1], 64479[1], 64483[1], 64486[1], 64487[1], 64488[1], 64489[1], 64490[1], 64493[1], 64505[1], 64510[1], 64517[1], 64520[1], 64530[1], 64553[1], 64555[1], 67500[0], 76000[1], 76970[1], 76998[0], 77002[0], 90865[1], 92511[1], 92512[1], 92516[1], 92520[1], 92537[1], 92538[1], 92585[0], 92950[1], 92953[1], 92960[1], 92961[1], 93000[1], 93005[1], 93010[1], 93040[1], 93041[1], 93042[1], 93050[0], 93303[0], 93304[0], 93306[1], 93307[1], 93308[1], 93312[1], 93313[1], 93314[1], 93315[1], 93316[1], 93317[1], 93318[0], 93351[1], 93355[0], 93451[1], 93456[1], 93457[1], 93561[0], 93562[0], 93701[0], 93922[1], 93923[1], 93924[1], 93925[1], 93926[1], 93930[1], 93931[1], 93970[1], 93971[1], 93975[1], 93976[1], 93978[1], 93979[1], 93980[1], 93981[1], 94002[1], 94004[1], 94200[1], 94250[0], 94640[1], 94644[1], 94660[1], 94662[1], 94680[1], 94681[1], 94690[1], 94760[0], 94761[0], 94762[1], 94770[1], 95812[0], 95813[0], 95816[0], 95819[0], 95822[0], 95829[0], 95860[0], 95861[0], 95863[0], 95864[0], 95865[0], 95866[0], 95867[0], 95868[0], 95869[0], 95870[0], 95907[0], 95908[0], 95909[0], 95910[0], 95911[0], 95912[0], 95913[0], 95925[0], 95926[0], 95927[0], 95928[0], 95929[0], 95930[0], 95933[0], 95937[0], 95938[0], 95939[0], 95940[0], 95955[0], 95956[0], 95957[0], 96360[0], 96365[0], 96372[0], 96373[0], 96374[0], 96375[0], 96376[0], 96377[0], 99151[0], 99152[0], 99153[0], 99155[0], 99156[0], 99157[0], 99201[0], 99202[0], 99203[0], 99204[0], 99205[0], 99211[0], 99212[0], 99213[0], 99214[0], 99215[0], 99217[0], 99218[0], 99219[0], 99220[0], 99221[0], 99222[0], 99223[0], 99224[0], 99225[0], 99226[0], 99231[0], 99232[0], 99233[0], 99234[0], 99235[0], 99236[0], 99238[0], 99239[0], 99281[0], 99282[0], 99283[0], 99284[0], 99285[0], 99304[0], 99305[0], 99306[0], 99307[0], 99308[0], 99309[0], 99310[0], 99315[0], 99318[0], 99324[0], 99325[0], 99326[0], 99327[0], 99328[0], 99334[0], 99335[0], 99336[0], 99337[0], 99341[0], 99342[0], 99343[0], 99347[0], 99348[0], 99349[0], 99354[0], 99355[0], 99356[0], 99357[0], 99358[0], 99359[0], 99415[0], 99416[0], 99446[0], 99447[0], 99448[0], 99449[0], 99451[0], 99452[0], 99468[0], 99469[0], 99471[0], 99472[0], 99475[0], 99476[0], 99477[0], 99478[0], 99479[0], 99480[0], 99483[0], 99497[0], C8921[1], C8922[1], C8923[1], C8924[1], C8925[1], C8926[1], C8927[0], C8929[1], C8930[1], G0380[1], G0381[1], G0382[1], G0383[1], G0384[1], G0406[0], G0407[0], G0408[0], G0425[0], G0426[0], G0427[0], G0453[0], G0463[0], G0500[0], G0508[0], G0509[0]
00670	01996[1], 0213T[1], 0216T[1], 0228T[1], 0230T[1], 0333T[0], 0464T[0], 31505[1], 31515[1], 31527[1], 31622[1], 31634[1], 31645[1], 31647[1], 36000[1], 36010[0], 36011[1], 36012[1], 36013[1], 36014[1], 36015[1], 36400[1], 36405[1], 36406[1], 36410[1], 36420[1], 36425[1], 36430[1], 36440[1], 36591[0], 36592[0], 36600[1], 36640[1], 43752[1], 43753[1], 43754[1], 61026[1], 61055[1], 62280[1], 62281[1], 62282[1], 62284[1], 62320[1], 62321[1], 62322[1], 62323[1], 62324[1], 62325[1], 62326[1], 62327[1], 64400[1], 64402[1], 64405[1], 64408[1], 64410[1], 64413[1], 64415[1], 64416[1], 64417[1], 64418[1], 64420[1], 64421[1], 64425[1], 64430[1], 64435[1], 64445[1], 64446[1], 64447[1], 64448[1], 64449[1], 64450[1], 64461[1], 64463[1], 64479[1], 64483[1], 64486[1], 64487[1], 64488[1], 64489[1], 64490[1], 64493[1], 64505[1], 64510[1], 64517[1], 64520[1], 64530[1], 64553[1], 64555[1], 67500[1], 76000[1], 76970[1], 76998[0], 77002[0], 90865[1], 92511[1], 92512[1], 92516[1], 92520[1], 92537[1], 92538[1], 92585[0], 92950[1], 92953[1], 92960[1], 92961[1], 93000[1], 93005[1], 93010[1], 93040[1], 93041[1], 93042[1], 93050[0], 93303[0], 93304[0], 93306[1], 93307[1], 93308[1], 93312[1], 93313[1], 93314[1], 93315[1], 93316[1], 93317[1], 93318[0], 93351[1], 93355[0], 93451[1], 93456[1], 93457[1], 93561[0], 93562[0], 93701[0], 93922[1], 93923[1], 93924[1], 93925[1], 93926[1], 93930[1], 93931[1], 93970[1], 93971[1], 93975[1], 93976[1], 93978[1], 93979[1], 93980[1], 93981[1], 94002[1], 94004[1], 94200[1], 94250[0], 94640[1], 94644[1], 94660[1], 94662[1], 94680[1], 94681[1], 94690[1], 94760[0], 94761[0], 94762[1], 94770[1], 95812[0], 95813[0], 95816[0], 95819[0], 95822[0], 95829[0], 95860[0], 95861[0], 95863[0], 95864[0], 95865[0], 95866[0], 95867[0], 95868[0], 95869[0], 95870[0], 95907[0], 95908[0],
	95909[0], 95910[0], 95911[0], 95912[0], 95913[0], 95925[0], 95926[0], 95927[0], 95928[0], 95929[0], 95930[0], 95933[0], 95937[0], 95938[0], 95939[0], 95940[0], 95955[0], 95956[0], 95957[0], 96360[0], 96365[0], 96372[0], 96373[0], 96374[0], 96375[0], 96376[0], 96377[0], 99151[0], 99152[0], 99153[0], 99155[0], 99156[0], 99157[0], 99201[0], 99202[0], 99203[0], 99204[0], 99205[0], 99211[0], 99212[0], 99213[0], 99214[0], 99215[0], 99217[0], 99218[0], 99219[0], 99220[0], 99221[0], 99222[0], 99223[0], 99224[0], 99225[0], 99226[0], 99231[0], 99232[0], 99233[0], 99234[0], 99235[0], 99236[0], 99238[0], 99239[0], 99281[0], 99282[0], 99283[0], 99284[0], 99285[0], 99304[0], 99305[0], 99306[0], 99307[0], 99308[0], 99309[0], 99310[0], 99315[0], 99318[0], 99324[0], 99325[0], 99326[0], 99327[0], 99328[0], 99334[0], 99335[0], 99336[0], 99337[0], 99341[0], 99342[0], 99343[0], 99347[0], 99348[0], 99349[0], 99354[0], 99355[0], 99356[0], 99357[0], 99358[0], 99359[0], 99415[0], 99416[0], 99446[0], 99447[0], 99448[0], 99449[0], 99451[0], 99452[0], 99466[0], 99468[0], 99469[0], 99471[0], 99472[0], 99475[0], 99476[0], 99477[0], 99478[0], 99479[0], 99480[0], 99483[0], 99485[0], 99497[0], C8921[1], C8922[1], C8923[1], C8924[1], C8925[1], C8926[1], C8927[0], C8929[1], C8930[1], G0380[1], G0381[1], G0382[1], G0383[1], G0384[1], G0406[0], G0407[0], G0408[0], G0425[0], G0426[0], G0427[0], G0453[0], G0463[0], G0500[0], G0508[0], G0509[0]
00700	01996[1], 0213T[1], 0216T[1], 0228T[1], 0230T[1], 0333T[0], 0464T[0], 31505[1], 31515[1], 31527[1], 31622[1], 31634[1], 31645[1], 31647[1], 36000[1], 36010[0], 36011[1], 36012[1], 36013[1], 36014[1], 36015[1], 36400[1], 36405[1], 36406[1], 36410[1], 36420[1], 36425[1], 36430[1], 36440[1], 36591[0], 36592[0], 36600[1], 36640[1], 43752[1], 43753[1], 43754[1], 61026[1], 61055[1], 62280[1], 62281[1], 62282[1], 62284[1], 62320[1], 62321[1], 62322[1], 62323[1], 62324[1], 62325[1], 62326[1], 62327[1], 64400[1], 64402[1], 64405[1], 64408[1], 64410[1], 64413[1], 64415[1], 64416[1], 64417[1], 64418[1], 64420[1], 64421[1], 64425[1], 64430[1], 64435[1], 64445[1], 64446[1], 64447[1], 64448[1], 64449[1], 64450[1], 64461[1], 64463[1], 64479[1], 64483[1], 64486[1], 64487[1], 64488[1], 64489[1], 64490[1], 64493[1], 64505[1], 64510[1], 64517[1], 64520[1], 64530[1], 64553[1], 64555[1], 67500[1], 76000[1], 76970[1], 76998[0], 77002[0], 90865[1], 92511[1], 92512[1], 92516[1], 92520[1], 92537[1], 92538[1], 92585[0], 92950[1], 92953[1], 92960[1], 92961[1], 93000[1], 93005[1], 93010[1], 93040[1], 93041[1], 93042[1], 93050[0], 93303[0], 93304[0], 93306[1], 93307[1], 93308[1], 93312[1], 93313[1], 93314[1], 93315[1], 93316[1], 93317[1], 93318[0], 93351[1], 93355[0], 93451[1], 93456[1], 93457[1], 93561[0], 93562[0], 93701[0], 93922[1], 93923[1], 93924[1], 93925[1], 93926[1], 93930[1], 93931[1], 93970[1], 93971[1], 93975[1], 93976[1], 93978[1], 93979[1], 93980[1], 93981[1], 94002[1], 94004[1], 94200[1], 94250[0], 94640[1], 94644[1], 94660[1], 94662[1], 94680[1], 94681[1], 94690[1], 94760[0], 94761[0], 94762[1], 94770[1], 95812[0], 95813[0], 95816[0], 95819[0], 95822[0], 95829[0], 95860[0], 95861[0], 95863[0], 95864[0], 95865[0], 95866[0], 95867[0], 95868[0], 95869[0], 95870[0], 95907[0], 95908[0], 95909[0], 95910[0], 95911[0], 95912[0], 95913[0], 95925[0], 95926[0], 95927[0], 95928[0], 95929[0], 95930[0], 95933[0], 95937[0], 95938[0], 95939[0], 95940[0], 95955[0], 95956[0], 95957[0], 96360[0], 96365[0], 96372[0], 96373[0], 96374[0], 96375[0], 96376[0], 96377[0], 99151[0], 99152[0], 99153[0], 99155[0], 99156[0], 99157[0], 99201[0], 99202[0], 99203[0], 99204[0], 99205[0], 99211[0], 99212[0], 99213[0], 99214[0], 99215[0], 99217[0], 99218[0], 99219[0], 99220[0], 99221[0], 99222[0], 99223[0], 99224[0], 99225[0], 99226[0], 99231[0], 99232[0], 99233[0], 99234[0], 99235[0], 99236[0], 99238[0], 99239[0], 99281[0], 99282[0], 99283[0], 99284[0], 99285[0], 99304[0], 99305[0], 99306[0], 99307[0], 99308[0], 99309[0], 99310[0], 99315[0], 99318[0], 99324[0], 99325[0], 99326[0], 99327[0], 99328[0], 99334[0], 99335[0], 99336[0], 99337[0], 99341[0], 99342[0], 99343[0], 99347[0], 99348[0], 99349[0], 99354[0], 99355[0], 99356[0], 99357[0], 99358[0], 99359[0], 99415[0], 99416[0], 99446[0], 99447[0], 99448[0], 99449[0], 99451[0], 99452[0], 99466[0], 99468[0], 99469[0], 99471[0], 99472[0], 99475[0], 99476[0], 99477[0], 99478[0], 99479[0], 99480[0], 99483[0], 99485[0], 99497[0], C8921[1], C8922[1], C8923[1], C8924[1], C8925[1], C8926[1], C8927[0], C8929[1], C8930[1], G0380[1], G0381[1], G0382[1], G0383[1], G0384[1], G0406[0], G0407[0], G0408[0], G0425[0], G0426[0], G0427[0], G0453[0], G0463[0], G0500[0], G0508[0], G0509[0]
00702	01996[1], 0213T[1], 0216T[1], 0228T[1], 0230T[1], 31505[1], 31515[1], 31527[1], 31622[1], 31634[1], 31645[1], 31647[1], 36000[1], 36010[0], 36011[1], 36012[1], 36013[1], 36014[1], 36015[1], 36400[1], 36405[1], 36406[1], 36410[1], 36420[1], 36425[1], 36430[1], 36440[1], 36591[0], 36592[0], 36600[1], 36640[1], 43752[1], 43753[1], 43754[1], 61026[1], 61055[1], 62280[1], 62281[1], 62282[1], 62284[1], 62320[1], 62321[1], 62322[1], 62323[1], 62324[1], 62325[1], 62326[1], 62327[1], 64400[1], 64402[1], 64405[1], 64408[1], 64410[1], 64413[1], 64415[1], 64416[1], 64417[1], 64418[1], 64420[1], 64421[1], 64425[1], 64430[1], 64435[1], 64445[1], 64446[1], 64447[1], 64448[1], 64449[1], 64450[1], 64461[1], 64463[1], 64479[1], 64483[1], 64486[1], 64487[1], 64488[1], 64489[1], 64490[1], 64493[1], 64505[1], 64510[1], 64517[1], 64520[1], 64530[1], 64553[1], 64555[1], 67500[1], 76000[1], 76970[1], 76998[0], 77002[0], 90865[1], 92511[1], 92512[1], 92516[1], 92520[1], 92537[1], 92538[1], 92950[1], 92953[1], 92960[1], 92961[1], 93000[1], 93005[1], 93010[1], 93040[1], 93041[1], 93042[1], 93050[0], 93303[0], 93304[0], 93306[1], 93307[1], 93308[1], 93312[1], 93313[1], 93314[1], 93315[1], 93316[1], 93317[1], 93318[0], 93351[1], 93355[0], 93451[1], 93456[1], 93457[1], 93561[0], 93562[0], 93701[0], 93922[1], 93923[1], 93924[1], 93925[1], 93926[1], 93930[1], 93931[1], 93970[1], 93971[1], 93975[1], 93976[1], 93978[1], 93979[1], 93980[1], 93981[1], 94002[1], 94004[1], 94200[1], 94250[0], 94640[1], 94644[1], 94660[1], 94662[1], 94680[1], 94681[1], 94690[1], 94760[0], 94761[0], 94762[1], 94770[1], 95812[0], 95813[0], 95816[0], 95819[0], 95822[0], 95829[0], 95955[0], 95956[0], 95957[0], 96360[0], 96365[0], 96372[0], 96373[0], 96374[0], 96375[0], 96376[0], 96377[0], 99151[0], 99152[0], 99153[0], 99155[0],

0 = Modifier usage not allowed or inappropriate 1 = Modifier usage allowed

CPT © 2018 American Medical Association. All Rights Reserved.

Code 1	Code 2
	99156[0], 99157[0], 99201[0], 99202[0], 99203[0], 99204[0], 99205[0], 99211[0], 99212[0], 99213[0], 99214[0], 99215[0], 99217[0], 99218[0], 99219[0], 99220[0], 99221[0], 99222[0], 99223[0], 99224[0], 99225[0], 99226[0], 99231[0], 99232[0], 99233[0], 99234[0], 99235[0], 99236[0], 99238[0], 99239[0], 99281[0], 99282[0], 99283[0], 99284[0], 99285[0], 99304[0], 99305[0], 99306[0], 99307[0], 99308[0], 99309[0], 99310[0], 99315[0], 99318[0], 99324[0], 99325[0], 99326[0], 99327[0], 99328[0], 99334[0], 99335[0], 99336[0], 99337[0], 99341[0], 99342[0], 99343[0], 99347[0], 99348[0], 99349[0], 99354[0], 99355[0], 99356[0], 99357[0], 99358[0], 99359[0], 99415[0], 99416[0], 99446[0], 99447[0], 99448[0], 99449[0], 99451[0], 99452[0], 99466[0], 99468[0], 99469[0], 99471[0], 99472[0], 99475[0], 99476[0], 99477[0], 99478[0], 99479[0], 99480[0], 99483[0], 99485[0], 99497[0], C8921[1], C8922[1], C8923[1], C8924[1], C8925[1], C8926[1], C8927[0], C8929[1], C8930[1], G0380[1], G0381[1], G0382[1], G0383[1], G0384[1], G0406[0], G0407[0], G0408[0], G0425[0], G0426[0], G0427[0], G0463[0], G0500[0], G0508[0], G0509[0]
00730	01996[1], 0213T[1], 0216T[1], 0228T[1], 0230T[1], 0333T[0], 0464T[0], 31505[1], 31515[1], 31527[1], 31622[1], 31634[1], 31645[1], 31647[1], 36000[1], 36010[0], 36011[1], 36012[1], 36013[1], 36014[1], 36015[1], 36400[1], 36405[1], 36406[1], 36410[1], 36420[1], 36425[1], 36430[1], 36440[1], 36591[0], 36592[0], 36600[1], 36640[1], 43752[1], 43753[1], 43754[1], 61026[1], 61055[1], 62280[1], 62281[1], 62282[1], 62284[1], 62320[1], 62321[1], 62322[1], 62323[1], 62324[1], 62325[1], 62326[1], 62327[1], 64400[1], 64402[1], 64405[1], 64408[1], 64410[1], 64413[1], 64415[1], 64416[1], 64417[1], 64418[1], 64420[1], 64421[1], 64425[1], 64430[1], 64435[1], 64445[1], 64446[1], 64447[1], 64448[1], 64449[1], 64450[1], 64461[1], 64463[1], 64479[1], 64483[1], 64486[1], 64487[1], 64488[1], 64489[1], 64490[1], 64493[1], 64505[1], 64510[1], 64517[1], 64520[1], 64530[1], 64553[1], 64555[1], 67500[1], 76000[1], 76970[1], 76998[0], 77002[0], 90865[1], 92511[1], 92512[1], 92516[1], 92520[1], 92537[1], 92538[1], 92585[0], 92950[1], 92953[1], 92960[1], 92961[1], 93000[1], 93005[1], 93010[1], 93040[1], 93041[1], 93042[1], 93050[0], 93303[0], 93304[0], 93306[1], 93307[1], 93308[1], 93312[1], 93313[1], 93314[1], 93315[1], 93316[1], 93317[1], 93318[0], 93351[1], 93355[0], 93451[1], 93456[1], 93457[1], 93561[0], 93562[0], 93701[0], 93922[1], 93923[1], 93924[1], 93925[1], 93926[1], 93930[1], 93931[1], 93970[1], 93971[1], 93975[1], 93976[1], 93978[1], 93979[1], 93980[1], 93981[1], 94002[1], 94004[1], 94200[1], 94250[0], 94640[1], 94644[1], 94660[1], 94662[1], 94680[1], 94681[1], 94690[1], 94760[0], 94761[0], 94762[1], 94770[1], 95812[0], 95813[0], 95816[0], 95819[0], 95822[0], 95829[0], 95860[0], 95861[0], 95863[0], 95864[0], 95865[0], 95866[0], 95867[0], 95868[0], 95869[0], 95870[0], 95907[0], 95908[0], 95909[0], 95910[0], 95911[0], 95912[0], 95913[0], 95925[0], 95926[0], 95927[0], 95928[0], 95929[0], 95930[0], 95933[0], 95937[0], 95938[0], 95939[0], 95940[0], 95955[0], 95956[0], 95957[0], 96360[0], 96365[0], 96372[0], 96373[0], 96374[0], 96375[0], 96376[0], 96377[0], 99151[0], 99152[0], 99153[0], 99155[0], 99156[0], 99157[0], 99201[0], 99202[0], 99203[0], 99204[0], 99205[0], 99211[0], 99212[0], 99213[0], 99214[0], 99215[0], 99217[0], 99218[0], 99219[0], 99220[0], 99221[0], 99222[0], 99223[0], 99224[0], 99225[0], 99226[0], 99231[0], 99232[0], 99233[0], 99234[0], 99235[0], 99236[0], 99238[0], 99239[0], 99281[0], 99282[0], 99283[0], 99284[0], 99285[0], 99304[0], 99305[0], 99306[0], 99307[0], 99308[0], 99309[0], 99310[0], 99315[0], 99318[0], 99324[0], 99325[0], 99326[0], 99327[0], 99328[0], 99334[0], 99335[0], 99336[0], 99337[0], 99341[0], 99342[0], 99343[0], 99347[0], 99348[0], 99349[0], 99354[0], 99355[0], 99356[0], 99357[0], 99358[0], 99359[0], 99415[0], 99416[0], 99446[0], 99447[0], 99448[0], 99449[0], 99451[0], 99452[0], 99466[0], 99468[0], 99469[0], 99471[0], 99472[0], 99475[0], 99476[0], 99477[0], 99478[0], 99479[0], 99480[0], 99483[0], 99485[0], 99497[0], C8921[1], C8922[1], C8923[1], C8924[1], C8925[1], C8926[1], C8927[0], C8929[1], C8930[1], G0380[1], G0381[1], G0382[1], G0383[1], G0384[1], G0406[0], G0407[0], G0408[0], G0425[0], G0426[0], G0427[0], G0453[0], G0463[0], G0500[0], G0508[0], G0509[0]
00731	01996[1], 0213T[1], 0216T[1], 0228T[1], 0230T[1], 31505[1], 31515[1], 31527[1], 31622[1], 31634[1], 31645[1], 31647[1], 36000[1], 36010[0], 36011[1], 36012[1], 36013[1], 36014[1], 36015[1], 36400[1], 36405[1], 36406[1], 36410[1], 36420[1], 36425[1], 36430[1], 36440[1], 36591[0], 36592[0], 36600[1], 36640[1], 43752[1], 43753[1], 43754[1], 61026[1], 61055[1], 62280[1], 62281[1], 62282[1], 62284[1], 62320[1], 62321[1], 62322[1], 62323[1], 62324[1], 62325[1], 62326[1], 62327[1], 64400[1], 64402[1], 64405[1], 64408[1], 64410[1], 64413[1], 64415[1], 64416[1], 64417[1], 64418[1], 64420[1], 64421[1], 64425[1], 64430[1], 64435[1], 64445[1], 64446[1], 64447[1], 64448[1], 64449[1], 64450[1], 64461[1], 64463[1], 64479[1], 64483[1], 64486[1], 64487[1], 64488[1], 64489[1], 64490[1], 64493[1], 64505[1], 64510[1], 64517[1], 64520[1], 64530[1], 64553[1], 64555[1], 67500[1], 76000[1], 76970[1], 76998[0], 77002[0], 90865[1], 92511[1], 92512[1], 92516[1], 92520[1], 92537[1], 92538[1], 92950[1], 92953[1], 92960[1], 92961[1], 93000[1], 93005[1], 93010[1], 93040[1], 93041[1], 93042[1], 93050[0], 93303[0], 93304[0], 93306[1], 93307[1], 93308[1], 93312[1], 93313[1], 93314[1], 93315[1], 93316[1], 93317[1], 93318[0], 93351[1], 93355[0], 93451[1], 93456[1], 93457[1], 93561[0], 93562[0], 93701[0], 93922[1], 93923[1], 93924[1], 93925[1], 93926[1], 93930[1], 93931[1], 93970[1], 93971[1], 93975[1], 93976[1], 93978[1], 93979[1], 93980[1], 93981[1], 94002[1], 94004[1], 94200[1], 94250[0], 94640[1], 94644[1], 94660[1], 94662[1], 94680[1], 94681[1], 94690[1], 94760[0], 94761[0], 94762[1], 94770[1], 95812[0], 95813[0], 95816[0], 95819[0], 95822[0], 95829[0], 95955[0], 95956[0], 95957[0], 96360[0], 96365[0], 96372[0], 96373[0], 96374[0], 96375[0], 96376[0], 96377[0], 96523[0], 99151[0], 99152[0], 99153[0], 99155[0], 99156[0], 99157[0], 99201[0], 99202[0], 99203[0], 99204[0], 99205[0], 99211[0], 99212[0], 99213[0], 99214[0], 99215[0], 99217[0], 99218[0], 99219[0], 99220[0], 99221[0], 99222[0], 99223[0], 99224[0], 99225[0], 99226[0], 99231[0], 99232[0], 99233[0], 99234[0], 99235[0], 99236[0], 99238[0], 99239[0], 99281[0], 99282[0], 99283[0], 99284[0], 99285[0], 99304[0], 99305[0], 99306[0], 99307[0], 99308[0], 99309[0], 99310[0], 99315[0], 99318[0], 99324[0], 99325[0], 99326[0], 99327[0], 99328[0], 99334[0], 99335[0], 99336[0], 99337[0], 99341[0], 99342[0], 99343[0], 99347[0], 99348[0], 99349[0], 99354[0], 99355[0], 99356[0], 99357[0], 99358[0], 99359[0], 99415[0], 99416[0], 99446[0], 99447[0], 99448[0], 99449[0], 99451[0], 99452[0], 99466[0], 99468[0], 99469[0], 99471[0], 99472[0], 99475[0], 99476[0], 99477[0], 99478[0], 99479[0], 99480[0], 99483[0], 99485[0], 99497[0], C8921[1], C8922[1], C8923[1], C8924[1], C8925[1], C8926[1], C8927[0], C8929[1], C8930[1], G0380[1], G0381[1], G0382[1], G0383[1], G0384[1], G0406[0], G0407[0], G0408[0], G0425[0], G0426[0], G0427[0], G0463[0], G0500[0], G0508[0], G0509[0]
00732	01996[1], 0213T[1], 0216T[1], 0228T[1], 0230T[1], 31505[1], 31515[1], 31527[1], 31622[1], 31634[1], 31645[1], 31647[1], 36000[1], 36010[0], 36011[1], 36012[1], 36013[1], 36014[1], 36015[1], 36400[1], 36405[1], 36406[1], 36410[1], 36420[1], 36425[1], 36430[1], 36440[1], 36591[0], 36592[0], 36600[1], 36640[1], 43752[1], 43753[1], 43754[1], 61026[1], 61055[1], 62280[1], 62281[1], 62282[1], 62284[1], 62320[1], 62321[1], 62322[1], 62323[1], 62324[1], 62325[1], 62326[1], 62327[1], 64400[1], 64402[1], 64405[1], 64408[1], 64410[1], 64413[1], 64415[1], 64416[1], 64417[1], 64418[1], 64420[1], 64421[1], 64425[1], 64430[1], 64435[1], 64445[1], 64446[1], 64447[1], 64448[1], 64449[1], 64450[1], 64461[1], 64463[1], 64479[1], 64483[1], 64486[1], 64487[1], 64488[1], 64489[1], 64490[1], 64493[1], 64505[1], 64510[1], 64517[1], 64520[1], 64530[1], 64553[1], 64555[1], 67500[1], 76000[1], 76970[1], 76998[0], 77002[0], 90865[1], 92511[1], 92512[1], 92516[1], 92520[1], 92537[1], 92538[1], 92950[1], 92953[1], 92960[1], 92961[1], 93000[1], 93005[1], 93010[1], 93040[1], 93041[1], 93042[1], 93050[0], 93303[0], 93304[0], 93306[1], 93307[1], 93308[1], 93312[1], 93313[1], 93314[1], 93315[1], 93316[1], 93317[1], 93318[0], 93351[1], 93355[0], 93451[1], 93456[1], 93457[1], 93561[0], 93562[0], 93701[0], 93922[1], 93923[1], 93924[1], 93925[1], 93926[1], 93930[1], 93931[1], 93970[1], 93971[1], 93975[1], 93976[1], 93978[1], 93979[1], 93980[1], 93981[1], 94002[1], 94004[1], 94200[1], 94250[0], 94640[1], 94644[1], 94660[1], 94662[1], 94680[1], 94681[1], 94690[1], 94760[0], 94761[0], 94762[1], 94770[1], 95812[0], 95813[0], 95816[0], 95819[0], 95822[0], 95829[0], 95955[0], 95956[0], 95957[0], 96360[0], 96365[0], 96372[0], 96373[0], 96374[0], 96375[0], 96376[0], 96377[0], 96523[0], 99151[0], 99152[0], 99153[0], 99155[0], 99156[0], 99157[0], 99201[0], 99202[0], 99203[0], 99204[0], 99205[0], 99211[0], 99212[0], 99213[0], 99214[0], 99215[0], 99217[0], 99218[0], 99219[0], 99220[0], 99221[0], 99222[0], 99223[0], 99224[0], 99225[0], 99226[0], 99231[0], 99232[0], 99233[0], 99234[0], 99235[0], 99236[0], 99238[0], 99239[0], 99281[0], 99282[0], 99283[0], 99284[0], 99285[0], 99304[0], 99305[0], 99306[0], 99307[0], 99308[0], 99309[0], 99310[0], 99315[0], 99318[0], 99324[0], 99325[0], 99326[0], 99327[0], 99328[0], 99334[0], 99335[0], 99336[0], 99337[0], 99341[0], 99342[0], 99343[0], 99347[0], 99348[0], 99349[0], 99354[0], 99355[0], 99356[0], 99357[0], 99358[0], 99359[0], 99415[0], 99416[0], 99446[0], 99447[0], 99448[0], 99449[0], 99451[0], 99452[0], 99466[0], 99468[0], 99469[0], 99471[0], 99472[0], 99475[0], 99476[0], 99477[0], 99478[0], 99479[0], 99480[0], 99483[0], 99485[0], 99497[0], C8921[1], C8922[1], C8923[1], C8924[1], C8925[1], C8926[1], C8927[0], C8929[1], C8930[1], G0380[1], G0381[1], G0382[1], G0383[1], G0384[1], G0406[0], G0407[0], G0408[0], G0425[0], G0426[0], G0427[0], G0463[0], G0500[0], G0508[0], G0509[0]
00750	01996[1], 0213T[1], 0216T[1], 0228T[1], 0230T[1], 31505[1], 31515[1], 31527[1], 31622[1], 31634[1], 31645[1], 31647[1], 36000[1], 36010[0], 36011[1], 36012[1], 36013[1], 36014[1], 36015[1], 36400[1], 36405[1], 36406[1], 36410[1], 36420[1], 36425[1], 36430[1], 36440[1], 36591[0], 36592[0], 36600[1], 36640[1], 43752[1], 43753[1], 43754[1], 61026[1], 61055[1], 62280[1], 62281[1], 62282[1], 62284[1], 62320[1], 62321[1], 62322[1], 62323[1], 62324[1], 62325[1], 62326[1], 62327[1], 64400[1], 64402[1], 64405[1], 64408[1], 64410[1], 64413[1], 64415[1], 64416[1], 64417[1], 64418[1], 64420[1], 64421[1], 64425[1], 64430[1], 64435[1], 64445[1], 64446[1], 64447[1], 64448[1], 64449[1], 64450[1], 64461[1], 64463[1], 64479[1], 64483[1], 64486[1], 64487[1], 64488[1], 64489[1], 64490[1], 64493[1], 64505[1], 64510[1], 64517[1], 64520[1], 64530[1], 64553[1], 64555[1], 67500[1], 76000[1], 76970[1], 76998[0], 77002[0], 90865[1], 92511[1], 92512[1], 92516[1], 92520[1], 92537[1], 92538[1], 92950[1], 92953[1], 92960[1], 92961[1], 93000[1], 93005[1], 93010[1], 93040[1], 93041[1], 93042[1], 93050[0], 93303[0], 93304[0], 93306[1], 93307[1], 93308[1], 93312[1], 93313[1], 93314[1], 93315[1], 93316[1], 93317[1], 93318[0], 93351[1], 93355[0], 93451[1], 93456[1], 93457[1], 93561[0], 93562[0], 93701[0], 93922[1], 93923[1], 93924[1], 93925[1], 93926[1], 93930[1], 93931[1], 93970[1], 93971[1], 93975[1], 93976[1], 93978[1], 93979[1], 93980[1], 93981[1], 94002[1], 94004[1], 94200[1], 94250[0], 94640[1], 94644[1], 94660[1], 94662[1], 94680[1], 94681[1], 94690[1], 94760[0], 94761[0], 94762[1], 94770[1], 95812[0], 95813[0], 95816[0], 95819[0], 95822[0], 95829[0], 95955[0], 95956[0], 95957[0], 96360[0], 96365[0], 96372[0], 96373[0], 96374[0], 96375[0], 96376[0], 96377[0], 99151[0], 99152[0], 99153[0], 99155[0], 99156[0], 99157[0], 99201[0], 99202[0], 99203[0], 99204[0], 99205[0], 99211[0], 99212[0], 99213[0], 99214[0], 99215[0], 99217[0], 99218[0], 99219[0], 99220[0], 99221[0], 99222[0], 99223[0], 99224[0], 99225[0], 99226[0], 99231[0], 99232[0], 99233[0], 99234[0], 99235[0], 99236[0], 99238[0], 99239[0], 99281[0], 99282[0], 99283[0], 99284[0], 99285[0], 99304[0], 99305[0], 99306[0], 99307[0], 99308[0], 99309[0], 99310[0], 99315[0], 99318[0], 99324[0], 99325[0], 99326[0], 99327[0], 99328[0], 99334[0], 99335[0], 99336[0], 99337[0], 99341[0], 99342[0], 99343[0], 99347[0], 99348[0], 99349[0], 99354[0], 99355[0], 99356[0], 99357[0], 99358[0], 99359[0], 99415[0], 99416[0], 99446[0], 99447[0], 99448[0], 99449[0], 99451[0], 99452[0], 99466[0], 99468[0], 99469[0], 99471[0], 99472[0], 99475[0], 99476[0], 99477[0], 99478[0], 99479[0], 99480[0], 99483[0], 99485[0], 99497[0], C8921[1], C8922[1], C8923[1],

0 = Modifier usage not allowed or inappropriate 1 = Modifier usage allowed

CPT © 2018 American Medical Association. All Rights Reserved.

Code 1	Code 2
	C8924[1], C8925[1], C8926[1], C8927[0], C8929[1], C8930[1], G0380[1], G0381[1], G0382[1], G0383[1], G0384[1], G0406[0], G0407[0], G0408[0], G0425[0], G0426[0], G0427[0], G0463[0], G0500[0], G0508[0], G0509[0]
00752	01996[1], 0213T[1], 0216T[1], 0228T[1], 0230T[1], 31505[1], 31515[1], 31527[1], 31622[1], 31634[1], 31645[1], 31647[1], 36000[1], 36010[0], 36011[1], 36012[1], 36013[1], 36014[1], 36015[1], 36400[1], 36405[1], 36406[1], 36410[1], 36420[1], 36425[1], 36430[1], 36440[1], 36591[0], 36592[0], 36600[1], 36640[1], 43752[1], 43753[1], 43754[1], 61026[1], 61055[1], 62280[1], 62281[1], 62282[1], 62284[1], 62320[1], 62321[1], 62322[1], 62323[1], 62324[1], 62325[1], 62326[1], 62327[1], 64400[1], 64402[1], 64405[1], 64408[1], 64410[1], 64413[1], 64415[1], 64416[1], 64417[1], 64418[1], 64420[1], 64421[1], 64425[1], 64430[1], 64435[1], 64445[1], 64446[1], 64447[1], 64448[1], 64449[1], 64450[1], 64461[1], 64463[1], 64479[1], 64483[1], 64486[1], 64487[1], 64488[1], 64489[1], 64490[1], 64493[1], 64505[1], 64510[1], 64517[1], 64520[1], 64530[1], 64553[1], 64555[1], 67500[1], 76000[1], 76970[1], 76998[0], 77002[0], 90865[1], 92511[1], 92512[1], 92516[1], 92520[1], 92537[1], 92538[1], 92950[1], 92953[1], 92960[1], 92961[1], 93000[1], 93005[1], 93010[1], 93040[1], 93041[1], 93042[1], 93050[0], 93303[0], 93304[0], 93306[1], 93307[1], 93308[1], 93312[1], 93313[1], 93314[1], 93315[1], 93316[1], 93317[1], 93318[0], 93351[1], 93355[0], 93451[1], 93456[1], 93457[1], 93561[0], 93562[0], 93701[0], 93922[1], 93923[1], 93924[1], 93925[1], 93926[1], 93930[1], 93931[1], 93970[1], 93971[1], 93975[1], 93976[1], 93978[1], 93979[1], 93980[1], 93981[1], 94002[1], 94004[1], 94200[1], 94250[0], 94640[1], 94644[1], 94660[1], 94662[1], 94680[1], 94681[1], 94690[1], 94760[0], 94761[0], 94762[1], 94770[1], 95812[0], 95813[0], 95816[0], 95819[0], 95822[0], 95829[0], 95955[0], 95956[0], 95957[0], 96360[0], 96365[0], 96372[0], 96373[0], 96374[0], 96375[0], 96376[0], 96377[0], 99151[0], 99152[0], 99153[0], 99155[0], 99156[0], 99157[0], 99201[0], 99202[0], 99203[0], 99204[0], 99205[0], 99211[0], 99212[0], 99213[0], 99214[0], 99215[0], 99217[0], 99218[0], 99219[0], 99220[0], 99221[0], 99222[0], 99223[0], 99224[0], 99225[0], 99226[0], 99231[0], 99232[0], 99233[0], 99234[0], 99235[0], 99236[0], 99238[0], 99239[0], 99281[0], 99282[0], 99283[0], 99284[0], 99285[0], 99304[0], 99305[0], 99306[0], 99307[0], 99308[0], 99309[0], 99310[0], 99315[0], 99318[0], 99324[0], 99325[0], 99326[0], 99327[0], 99328[0], 99334[0], 99335[0], 99336[0], 99337[0], 99341[0], 99342[0], 99343[0], 99347[0], 99348[0], 99349[0], 99354[0], 99355[0], 99356[0], 99357[0], 99358[0], 99359[0], 99415[0], 99416[0], 99446[0], 99447[0], 99448[0], 99449[0], 99451[0], 99452[0], 99466[0], 99468[0], 99469[0], 99471[0], 99472[0], 99475[0], 99476[0], 99477[0], 99478[0], 99479[0], 99480[0], 99483[0], 99485[0], 99497[0], C8921[1], C8922[1], C8923[1], C8924[1], C8925[1], C8926[1], C8927[0], C8929[1], C8930[1], G0380[1], G0381[1], G0382[1], G0383[1], G0384[1], G0406[0], G0407[0], G0408[0], G0425[0], G0426[0], G0427[0], G0463[0], G0500[0], G0508[0], G0509[0]
00754	01996[1], 0213T[1], 0216T[1], 0228T[1], 0230T[1], 31505[1], 31515[1], 31527[1], 31622[1], 31634[1], 31645[1], 31647[1], 36000[1], 36010[0], 36011[1], 36012[1], 36013[1], 36014[1], 36015[1], 36400[1], 36405[1], 36406[1], 36410[1], 36420[1], 36425[1], 36430[1], 36440[1], 36591[0], 36592[0], 36600[1], 36640[1], 43752[1], 43753[1], 43754[1], 61026[1], 61055[1], 62280[1], 62281[1], 62282[1], 62284[1], 62320[1], 62321[1], 62322[1], 62323[1], 62324[1], 62325[1], 62326[1], 62327[1], 64400[1], 64402[1], 64405[1], 64408[1], 64410[1], 64413[1], 64415[1], 64416[1], 64417[1], 64418[1], 64420[1], 64421[1], 64425[1], 64430[1], 64435[1], 64445[1], 64446[1], 64447[1], 64448[1], 64449[1], 64450[1], 64461[1], 64463[1], 64479[1], 64483[1], 64486[1], 64487[1], 64488[1], 64489[1], 64490[1], 64493[1], 64505[1], 64510[1], 64517[1], 64520[1], 64530[1], 64553[1], 64555[1], 67500[1], 76000[1], 76970[1], 76998[0], 77002[0], 90865[1], 92511[1], 92512[1], 92516[1], 92520[1], 92537[1], 92538[1], 92950[1], 92953[1], 92960[1], 92961[1], 93000[1], 93005[1], 93010[1], 93040[1], 93041[1], 93042[1], 93050[0], 93303[0], 93304[0], 93306[1], 93307[1], 93308[1], 93312[1], 93313[1], 93314[1], 93315[1], 93316[1], 93317[1], 93318[0], 93351[1], 93355[0], 93451[1], 93456[1], 93457[1], 93561[0], 93562[0], 93701[0], 93922[1], 93923[1], 93924[1], 93925[1], 93926[1], 93930[1], 93931[1], 93970[1], 93971[1], 93975[1], 93976[1], 93978[1], 93979[1], 93980[1], 93981[1], 94002[1], 94004[1], 94200[1], 94250[0], 94640[1], 94644[1], 94660[1], 94662[1], 94680[1], 94681[1], 94690[1], 94760[0], 94761[0], 94762[1], 94770[1], 95812[0], 95813[0], 95816[0], 95819[0], 95822[0], 95829[0], 95955[0], 95956[0], 95957[0], 96360[0], 96365[0], 96372[0], 96373[0], 96374[0], 96375[0], 96376[0], 96377[0], 99151[0], 99152[0], 99153[0], 99155[0], 99156[0], 99157[0], 99201[0], 99202[0], 99203[0], 99204[0], 99205[0], 99211[0], 99212[0], 99213[0], 99214[0], 99215[0], 99217[0], 99218[0], 99219[0], 99220[0], 99221[0], 99222[0], 99223[0], 99224[0], 99225[0], 99226[0], 99231[0], 99232[0], 99233[0], 99234[0], 99235[0], 99236[0], 99238[0], 99239[0], 99281[0], 99282[0], 99283[0], 99284[0], 99285[0], 99304[0], 99305[0], 99306[0], 99307[0], 99308[0], 99309[0], 99310[0], 99315[0], 99318[0], 99324[0], 99325[0], 99326[0], 99327[0], 99328[0], 99334[0], 99335[0], 99336[0], 99337[0], 99341[0], 99342[0], 99343[0], 99347[0], 99348[0], 99349[0], 99354[0], 99355[0], 99356[0], 99357[0], 99358[0], 99359[0], 99415[0], 99416[0], 99446[0], 99447[0], 99448[0], 99449[0], 99451[0], 99452[0], 99466[0], 99468[0], 99469[0], 99471[0], 99472[0], 99475[0], 99476[0], 99477[0], 99478[0], 99479[0], 99480[0], 99483[0], 99485[0], 99497[0], C8921[1], C8922[1], C8923[1], C8924[1], C8925[1], C8926[1], C8927[0], C8929[1], C8930[1], G0380[1], G0381[1], G0382[1], G0383[1], G0384[1], G0406[0], G0407[0], G0408[0], G0425[0], G0426[0], G0427[0], G0463[0], G0500[0], G0508[0], G0509[0]
00756	01996[1], 0213T[1], 0216T[1], 0228T[1], 0230T[1], 31505[1], 31515[1], 31527[1], 31622[1], 31634[1], 31645[1], 31647[1], 36000[1], 36010[0], 36011[1], 36012[1], 36013[1], 36014[1], 36015[1], 36400[1], 36405[1], 36406[1], 36410[1], 36420[1], 36425[1], 36430[1], 36440[1], 36591[0], 36592[0], 36600[1], 36640[1], 43752[1], 43753[1], 43754[1], 61026[1], 61055[1], 62280[1], 62281[1], 62282[1], 62284[1], 62320[1], 62321[1], 62322[1], 62323[1], 62324[1], 62325[1], 62326[1], 62327[1], 64400[1], 64402[1], 64405[1], 64408[1], 64410[1], 64413[1], 64415[1], 64416[1], 64417[1], 64418[1], 64420[1], 64421[1], 64425[1], 64430[1], 64435[1], 64445[1], 64446[1], 64447[1], 64448[1], 64449[1], 64450[1], 64461[1], 64463[1], 64479[1], 64483[1], 64486[1], 64487[1], 64488[1], 64489[1], 64490[1], 64493[1], 64505[1], 64510[1], 64517[1], 64520[1], 64530[1], 64553[1], 64555[1], 67500[1], 76000[1], 76970[1], 76998[0], 77002[0], 90865[1], 92511[1], 92512[1], 92516[1], 92520[1], 92537[1], 92538[1], 92950[1], 92953[1], 92960[1], 92961[1], 93000[1], 93005[1], 93010[1], 93040[1], 93041[1], 93042[1], 93050[0], 93303[0], 93304[0], 93306[1], 93307[1], 93308[1], 93312[1], 93313[1], 93314[1], 93315[1], 93316[1], 93317[1], 93318[0], 93351[1], 93355[0], 93451[1], 93456[1], 93457[1], 93561[0], 93562[0], 93701[0], 93922[1], 93923[1], 93924[1], 93925[1], 93926[1], 93930[1], 93931[1], 93970[1], 93971[1], 93975[1], 93976[1], 93978[1], 93979[1], 93980[1], 93981[1], 94002[1], 94004[1], 94200[1], 94250[0], 94640[1], 94644[1], 94660[1], 94662[1], 94680[1], 94681[1], 94690[1], 94760[0], 94761[0], 94762[1], 94770[1], 95812[0], 95813[0], 95816[0], 95819[0], 95822[0], 95829[0], 95955[0], 95956[0], 95957[0], 96360[0], 96365[0], 96372[0], 96373[0], 96374[0], 96375[0], 96376[0], 96377[0], 99151[0], 99152[0], 99153[0], 99155[0], 99156[0], 99157[0], 99201[0], 99202[0], 99203[0], 99204[0], 99205[0], 99211[0], 99212[0], 99213[0], 99214[0], 99215[0], 99217[0], 99218[0], 99219[0], 99220[0], 99221[0], 99222[0], 99223[0], 99224[0], 99225[0], 99226[0], 99231[0], 99232[0], 99233[0], 99234[0], 99235[0], 99236[0], 99238[0], 99239[0], 99281[0], 99282[0], 99283[0], 99284[0], 99285[0], 99304[0], 99305[0], 99306[0], 99307[0], 99308[0], 99309[0], 99310[0], 99315[0], 99318[0], 99324[0], 99325[0], 99326[0], 99327[0], 99328[0], 99334[0], 99335[0], 99336[0], 99337[0], 99341[0], 99342[0], 99343[0], 99347[0], 99348[0], 99349[0], 99354[0], 99355[0], 99356[0], 99357[0], 99358[0], 99359[0], 99415[0], 99416[0], 99446[0], 99447[0], 99448[0], 99449[0], 99451[0], 99452[0], 99466[0], 99468[0], 99469[0], 99471[0], 99472[0], 99475[0], 99476[0], 99477[0], 99478[0], 99479[0], 99480[0], 99483[0], 99485[0], 99497[0], C8921[1], C8922[1], C8923[1], C8924[1], C8925[1], C8926[1], C8927[0], C8929[1], C8930[1], G0380[1], G0381[1], G0382[1], G0383[1], G0384[1], G0406[0], G0407[0], G0408[0], G0425[0], G0426[0], G0427[0], G0463[0], G0500[0], G0508[0], G0509[0]
00770	01996[1], 0213T[1], 0216T[1], 0228T[1], 0230T[1], 31505[1], 31515[1], 31527[1], 31622[1], 31634[1], 31645[1], 31647[1], 36000[1], 36010[0], 36011[1], 36012[1], 36013[1], 36014[1], 36015[1], 36400[1], 36405[1], 36406[1], 36410[1], 36420[1], 36425[1], 36430[1], 36440[1], 36591[0], 36592[0], 36600[1], 36640[1], 43752[1], 43753[1], 43754[1], 61026[1], 61055[1], 62280[1], 62281[1], 62282[1], 62284[1], 62320[1], 62321[1], 62322[1], 62323[1], 62324[1], 62325[1], 62326[1], 62327[1], 64400[1], 64402[1], 64405[1], 64408[1], 64410[1], 64413[1], 64415[1], 64416[1], 64417[1], 64418[1], 64420[1], 64421[1], 64425[1], 64430[1], 64435[1], 64445[1], 64446[1], 64447[1], 64448[1], 64449[1], 64450[1], 64461[1], 64463[1], 64479[1], 64483[1], 64486[1], 64487[1], 64488[1], 64489[1], 64490[1], 64493[1], 64505[1], 64510[1], 64517[1], 64520[1], 64530[1], 64553[1], 64555[1], 67500[1], 76000[1], 76970[1], 76998[0], 77002[0], 90865[1], 92511[1], 92512[1], 92516[1], 92520[1], 92537[1], 92538[1], 92950[1], 92953[1], 92960[1], 92961[1], 93000[1], 93005[1], 93010[1], 93040[1], 93041[1], 93042[1], 93050[0], 93303[0], 93304[0], 93306[1], 93307[1], 93308[1], 93312[1], 93313[1], 93314[1], 93315[1], 93316[1], 93317[1], 93318[0], 93351[1], 93355[0], 93561[0], 93562[0], 93701[0], 93922[1], 93923[1], 93924[1], 93925[1], 93926[1], 93930[1], 93931[1], 93970[1], 93971[1], 93975[1], 93976[1], 93978[1], 93979[1], 93980[1], 93981[1], 94002[1], 94004[1], 94200[1], 94250[0], 94640[1], 94644[1], 94660[1], 94662[1], 94680[1], 94681[1], 94690[1], 94760[0], 94761[0], 94762[1], 94770[1], 95812[0], 95813[0], 95816[0], 95819[0], 95822[0], 95829[0], 95955[0], 95956[0], 95957[0], 96360[0], 96365[0], 96372[0], 96373[0], 96374[0], 96375[0], 96376[0], 96377[0], 99151[0], 99152[0], 99153[0], 99155[0], 99156[0], 99157[0], 99201[0], 99202[0], 99203[0], 99204[0], 99205[0], 99211[0], 99212[0], 99213[0], 99214[0], 99215[0], 99217[0], 99218[0], 99219[0], 99220[0], 99221[0], 99222[0], 99223[0], 99224[0], 99225[0], 99226[0], 99231[0], 99232[0], 99233[0], 99234[0], 99235[0], 99236[0], 99238[0], 99239[0], 99281[0], 99282[0], 99283[0], 99284[0], 99285[0], 99304[0], 99305[0], 99306[0], 99307[0], 99308[0], 99309[0], 99310[0], 99315[0], 99318[0], 99324[0], 99325[0], 99326[0], 99327[0], 99328[0], 99334[0], 99335[0], 99336[0], 99337[0], 99341[0], 99342[0], 99343[0], 99347[0], 99348[0], 99349[0], 99354[0], 99355[0], 99356[0], 99357[0], 99358[0], 99359[0], 99415[0], 99416[0], 99446[0], 99447[0], 99448[0], 99449[0], 99451[0], 99452[0], 99466[0], 99468[0], 99469[0], 99471[0], 99472[0], 99475[0], 99476[0], 99477[0], 99478[0], 99479[0], 99480[0], 99483[0], 99485[0], 99497[0], C8921[1], C8922[1], C8923[1], C8924[1], C8925[1], C8926[1], C8927[0], C8929[1], C8930[1], G0380[1], G0381[1], G0382[1], G0383[1], G0384[1], G0406[0], G0407[0], G0408[0], G0425[0], G0426[0], G0427[0], G0463[0], G0500[0], G0508[0], G0509[0]
00790	01996[1], 0213T[1], 0216T[1], 0228T[1], 0230T[1], 31505[1], 31515[1], 31527[1], 31622[1], 31634[1], 31645[1], 31647[1], 36000[1], 36010[0], 36011[1], 36012[1], 36013[1], 36014[1], 36015[1], 36400[1], 36405[1], 36406[1], 36410[1], 36420[1], 36425[1], 36430[1], 36440[1], 36591[0], 36592[0], 36600[1], 36640[1], 43752[1], 43754[1], 61026[1], 61055[1], 62280[1], 62281[1], 62282[1], 62284[1], 62320[1], 62321[1], 62322[1], 62323[1], 62324[1], 62325[1], 62326[1], 62327[1], 64400[1], 64402[1], 64405[1], 64408[1], 64410[1], 64413[1], 64415[1], 64416[1], 64417[1], 64418[1], 64420[1], 64421[1], 64425[1], 64430[1], 64435[1], 64445[1], 64446[1], 64447[1], 64448[1], 64449[1], 64450[1], 64461[1], 64463[1], 64479[1], 64483[1], 64486[1], 64487[1], 64488[1], 64489[1], 64490[1], 64493[1], 64505[1], 64510[1], 64517[1], 64520[1], 64530[1], 64553[1], 64555[1], 67500[1], 76000[1], 76970[1], 76998[0], 77002[0],

0 = Modifier usage not allowed or inappropriate 1 = Modifier usage allowed

CPT © 2018 American Medical Association. All Rights Reserved.

Code 1	Code 2
	90865[1], 92511[1], 92512[1], 92516[1], 92520[1], 92537[1], 92538[1], 92950[1], 92953[1], 92960[1], 92961[1], 93000[1], 93005[1], 93010[1], 93040[1], 93041[1], 93042[1], 93050[0], 93303[0], 93304[0], 93306[1], 93307[1], 93308[1], 93312[1], 93313[1], 93314[1], 93315[1], 93316[1], 93317[1], 93318[0], 93351[1], 93355[0], 93451[1], 93456[1], 93457[1], 93561[0], 93562[0], 93701[0], 93922[1], 93923[1], 93924[1], 93925[1], 93926[1], 93930[1], 93931[1], 93970[1], 93971[1], 93975[1], 93976[1], 93978[1], 93979[1], 93980[1], 93981[1], 94002[1], 94004[1], 94200[1], 94250[0], 94640[1], 94644[1], 94660[1], 94662[1], 94680[1], 94681[1], 94690[1], 94760[0], 94761[0], 94762[1], 94770[1], 95812[0], 95813[0], 95816[0], 95819[0], 95822[0], 95829[0], 95955[0], 95956[0], 95957[0], 96360[0], 96365[0], 96372[0], 96373[0], 96374[0], 96375[0], 96376[0], 96377[0], 99151[0], 99152[0], 99153[0], 99155[0], 99156[0], 99157[0], 99201[0], 99202[0], 99203[0], 99204[0], 99205[0], 99211[0], 99212[0], 99213[0], 99214[0], 99215[0], 99217[0], 99218[0], 99219[0], 99220[0], 99221[0], 99222[0], 99223[0], 99224[0], 99225[0], 99226[0], 99231[0], 99232[0], 99233[0], 99234[0], 99235[0], 99236[0], 99238[0], 99239[0], 99281[0], 99282[0], 99283[0], 99284[0], 99285[0], 99304[0], 99305[0], 99306[0], 99307[0], 99308[0], 99309[0], 99310[0], 99315[0], 99318[0], 99324[0], 99325[0], 99326[0], 99327[0], 99328[0], 99334[0], 99335[0], 99336[0], 99337[0], 99341[0], 99342[0], 99343[0], 99347[0], 99348[0], 99349[0], 99354[0], 99355[0], 99356[0], 99357[0], 99358[0], 99359[0], 99415[0], 99416[0], 99446[0], 99447[0], 99448[0], 99449[0], 99451[0], 99452[0], 99466[0], 99468[0], 99469[0], 99471[0], 99472[0], 99475[0], 99476[0], 99477[0], 99478[0], 99479[0], 99480[0], 99483[0], 99485[0], 99497[0], C8921[1], C8922[1], C8923[1], C8924[1], C8925[1], C8926[1], C8927[0], C8929[1], C8930[1], G0380[1], G0381[1], G0382[1], G0383[1], G0384[1], G0406[0], G0407[0], G0408[0], G0425[0], G0426[0], G0427[0], G0463[0], G0500[0], G0508[0], G0509[0]
00792	01996[1], 0213T[1], 0216T[1], 0228T[1], 0230T[1], 31505[1], 31515[1], 31527[1], 31622[1], 31634[1], 31645[1], 31647[1], 36000[1], 36010[0], 36011[1], 36012[1], 36013[1], 36014[1], 36015[1], 36400[1], 36405[1], 36406[1], 36410[1], 36420[1], 36425[1], 36430[1], 36440[1], 36591[0], 36592[0], 36600[1], 36640[1], 43752[1], 43753[1], 43754[1], 61026[1], 61055[1], 62280[1], 62281[1], 62282[1], 62284[1], 62320[1], 62321[1], 62322[1], 62323[1], 62324[1], 62325[1], 62326[1], 62327[1], 64400[1], 64402[1], 64405[1], 64408[1], 64410[1], 64413[1], 64415[1], 64416[1], 64417[1], 64418[1], 64420[1], 64421[1], 64425[1], 64430[1], 64435[1], 64445[1], 64446[1], 64447[1], 64448[1], 64449[1], 64450[1], 64461[1], 64463[1], 64479[1], 64483[1], 64486[1], 64487[1], 64488[1], 64489[1], 64490[1], 64493[1], 64505[1], 64510[1], 64517[1], 64520[1], 64530[1], 64553[1], 64555[1], 67500[1], 76000[1], 76970[1], 76998[0], 77002[0], 90865[1], 92511[1], 92512[1], 92516[1], 92520[1], 92537[1], 92538[1], 92950[1], 92953[1], 92960[1], 92961[1], 93000[1], 93005[1], 93010[1], 93040[1], 93041[1], 93042[1], 93050[0], 93303[0], 93304[0], 93306[1], 93307[1], 93308[1], 93312[1], 93313[1], 93314[1], 93315[1], 93316[1], 93317[1], 93318[0], 93351[1], 93355[0], 93451[1], 93456[1], 93457[1], 93561[0], 93562[0], 93701[0], 93922[1], 93923[1], 93924[1], 93925[1], 93926[1], 93930[1], 93931[1], 93970[1], 93971[1], 93975[1], 93976[1], 93978[1], 93979[1], 93980[1], 93981[1], 94002[1], 94004[1], 94200[1], 94250[0], 94640[1], 94644[1], 94660[1], 94662[1], 94680[1], 94681[1], 94690[1], 94760[0], 94761[0], 94762[1], 94770[1], 95812[0], 95813[0], 95816[0], 95819[0], 95822[0], 95829[0], 95955[0], 95956[0], 95957[0], 96360[0], 96365[0], 96372[0], 96373[0], 96374[0], 96375[0], 96376[0], 96377[0], 99151[0], 99152[0], 99153[0], 99155[0], 99156[0], 99157[0], 99201[0], 99202[0], 99203[0], 99204[0], 99205[0], 99211[0], 99212[0], 99213[0], 99214[0], 99215[0], 99217[0], 99218[0], 99219[0], 99220[0], 99221[0], 99222[0], 99223[0], 99224[0], 99225[0], 99226[0], 99231[0], 99232[0], 99233[0], 99234[0], 99235[0], 99236[0], 99238[0], 99239[0], 99281[0], 99282[0], 99283[0], 99284[0], 99285[0], 99304[0], 99305[0], 99306[0], 99307[0], 99308[0], 99309[0], 99310[0], 99315[0], 99318[0], 99324[0], 99325[0], 99326[0], 99327[0], 99328[0], 99334[0], 99335[0], 99336[0], 99337[0], 99341[0], 99342[0], 99343[0], 99347[0], 99348[0], 99349[0], 99354[0], 99355[0], 99356[0], 99357[0], 99358[0], 99359[0], 99415[0], 99416[0], 99446[0], 99447[0], 99448[0], 99449[0], 99451[0], 99452[0], 99466[0], 99468[0], 99469[0], 99471[0], 99472[0], 99475[0], 99476[0], 99477[0], 99478[0], 99479[0], 99480[0], 99483[0], 99485[0], 99497[0], C8921[1], C8922[1], C8923[1], C8924[1], C8925[1], C8926[1], C8927[0], C8929[1], C8930[1], G0380[1], G0381[1], G0382[1], G0383[1], G0384[1], G0406[0], G0407[0], G0408[0], G0425[0], G0426[0], G0427[0], G0463[0], G0500[0], G0508[0], G0509[0]
00794	01996[1], 0213T[1], 0216T[1], 0228T[1], 0230T[1], 31505[1], 31515[1], 31527[1], 31622[1], 31634[1], 31645[1], 31647[1], 36000[1], 36010[0], 36011[1], 36012[1], 36013[1], 36014[1], 36015[1], 36400[1], 36405[1], 36406[1], 36410[1], 36420[1], 36425[1], 36430[1], 36440[1], 36591[0], 36592[0], 36600[1], 36640[1], 43752[1], 43753[1], 43754[1], 61026[1], 61055[1], 62280[1], 62281[1], 62282[1], 62284[1], 62320[1], 62321[1], 62322[1], 62323[1], 62324[1], 62325[1], 62326[1], 62327[1], 64400[1], 64402[1], 64405[1], 64408[1], 64410[1], 64413[1], 64415[1], 64416[1], 64417[1], 64418[1], 64420[1], 64421[1], 64425[1], 64430[1], 64435[1], 64445[1], 64446[1], 64447[1], 64448[1], 64449[1], 64450[1], 64461[1], 64463[1], 64479[1], 64483[1], 64486[1], 64487[1], 64488[1], 64489[1], 64490[1], 64493[1], 64505[1], 64510[1], 64517[1], 64520[1], 64530[1], 64553[1], 64555[1], 67500[1], 76000[1], 76970[1], 76998[0], 77002[0], 90865[1], 92511[1], 92512[1], 92516[1], 92520[1], 92537[1], 92538[1], 92950[1], 92953[1], 92960[1], 92961[1], 93000[1], 93005[1], 93010[1], 93040[1], 93041[1], 93042[1], 93050[0], 93303[0], 93304[0], 93306[1], 93307[1], 93308[1], 93312[1], 93313[1], 93314[1], 93315[1], 93316[1], 93317[1], 93318[0], 93351[1], 93355[0], 93451[1], 93456[1], 93457[1], 93561[0], 93562[0], 93701[0], 93922[1], 93923[1], 93924[1], 93925[1], 93926[1], 93930[1], 93931[1], 93970[1], 93971[1], 93975[1], 93976[1], 93978[1], 93979[1], 93980[1], 93981[1], 94002[1], 94004[1], 94200[1], 94250[0], 94640[1], 94644[1], 94660[1], 94662[1], 94680[1], 94681[1], 94690[1], 94760[0], 94761[0], 94762[1], 94770[1], 95812[0], 95813[0], 95816[0], 95819[0], 95822[0], 95829[0], 95955[0], 95956[0], 95957[0], 96360[0], 96365[0], 96372[0], 96373[0], 96374[0], 96375[0], 96376[0], 96377[0], 99151[0], 99152[0], 99153[0], 99155[0], 99156[0], 99157[0], 99201[0], 99202[0], 99203[0], 99204[0], 99205[0], 99211[0], 99212[0], 99213[0], 99214[0], 99215[0], 99217[0], 99218[0], 99219[0], 99220[0], 99221[0], 99222[0], 99223[0], 99224[0], 99225[0], 99226[0], 99231[0], 99232[0], 99233[0], 99234[0], 99235[0], 99236[0], 99238[0], 99239[0], 99281[0], 99282[0], 99283[0], 99284[0], 99285[0], 99304[0], 99305[0], 99306[0], 99307[0], 99308[0], 99309[0], 99310[0], 99315[0], 99318[0], 99324[0], 99325[0], 99326[0], 99327[0], 99328[0], 99334[0], 99335[0], 99336[0], 99337[0], 99341[0], 99342[0], 99343[0], 99347[0], 99348[0], 99349[0], 99354[0], 99355[0], 99356[0], 99357[0], 99358[0], 99359[0], 99415[0], 99416[0], 99446[0], 99447[0], 99448[0], 99449[0], 99451[0], 99452[0], 99466[0], 99468[0], 99469[0], 99471[0], 99472[0], 99475[0], 99476[0], 99477[0], 99478[0], 99479[0], 99480[0], 99483[0], 99485[0], 99497[0], C8921[1], C8922[1], C8923[1], C8924[1], C8925[1], C8926[1], C8927[0], C8929[1], C8930[1], G0380[1], G0381[1], G0382[1], G0383[1], G0384[1], G0406[0], G0407[0], G0408[0], G0425[0], G0426[0], G0427[0], G0463[0], G0500[0], G0508[0], G0509[0]
00796	01996[1], 0213T[1], 0216T[1], 0228T[1], 0230T[1], 31505[1], 31515[1], 31527[1], 31622[1], 31634[1], 31645[1], 31647[1], 36000[1], 36010[0], 36011[1], 36012[1], 36013[1], 36014[1], 36015[1], 36400[1], 36405[1], 36406[1], 36410[1], 36420[1], 36425[1], 36430[1], 36440[1], 36591[0], 36592[0], 36600[1], 36640[1], 43752[1], 43753[1], 43754[1], 61026[1], 61055[1], 62280[1], 62281[1], 62282[1], 62284[1], 62320[1], 62321[1], 62322[1], 62323[1], 62324[1], 62325[1], 62326[1], 62327[1], 64400[1], 64402[1], 64405[1], 64408[1], 64410[1], 64413[1], 64415[1], 64416[1], 64417[1], 64418[1], 64420[1], 64421[1], 64425[1], 64430[1], 64435[1], 64445[1], 64446[1], 64447[1], 64448[1], 64449[1], 64450[1], 64461[1], 64463[1], 64479[1], 64483[1], 64486[1], 64487[1], 64488[1], 64489[1], 64490[1], 64493[1], 64505[1], 64510[1], 64517[1], 64520[1], 64530[1], 64553[1], 64555[1], 67500[1], 76000[1], 76970[1], 76998[0], 77002[0], 90865[1], 92511[1], 92512[1], 92516[1], 92520[1], 92537[1], 92538[1], 92950[1], 92953[1], 92960[1], 92961[1], 93000[1], 93005[1], 93010[1], 93040[1], 93041[1], 93042[1], 93050[0], 93303[0], 93304[0], 93306[1], 93307[1], 93308[1], 93312[1], 93313[1], 93314[1], 93315[1], 93316[1], 93317[1], 93318[0], 93351[1], 93355[0], 93451[1], 93456[1], 93457[1], 93561[0], 93562[0], 93701[0], 93922[1], 93923[1], 93924[1], 93925[1], 93926[1], 93930[1], 93931[1], 93970[1], 93971[1], 93975[1], 93976[1], 93978[1], 93979[1], 93980[1], 93981[1], 94002[1], 94004[1], 94200[1], 94250[0], 94640[1], 94644[1], 94660[1], 94662[1], 94680[1], 94681[1], 94690[1], 94760[0], 94761[0], 94762[1], 94770[1], 95812[0], 95813[0], 95816[0], 95819[0], 95822[0], 95829[0], 95955[0], 95956[0], 95957[0], 96360[0], 96365[0], 96372[0], 96373[0], 96374[0], 96375[0], 96376[0], 96377[0], 99151[0], 99152[0], 99153[0], 99155[0], 99156[0], 99157[0], 99201[0], 99202[0], 99203[0], 99204[0], 99205[0], 99211[0], 99212[0], 99213[0], 99214[0], 99215[0], 99217[0], 99218[0], 99219[0], 99220[0], 99221[0], 99222[0], 99223[0], 99224[0], 99225[0], 99226[0], 99231[0], 99232[0], 99233[0], 99234[0], 99235[0], 99236[0], 99238[0], 99239[0], 99281[0], 99282[0], 99283[0], 99284[0], 99285[0], 99304[0], 99305[0], 99306[0], 99307[0], 99308[0], 99309[0], 99310[0], 99315[0], 99318[0], 99324[0], 99325[0], 99326[0], 99327[0], 99328[0], 99334[0], 99335[0], 99336[0], 99337[0], 99341[0], 99342[0], 99343[0], 99347[0], 99348[0], 99349[0], 99354[0], 99355[0], 99356[0], 99357[0], 99358[0], 99359[0], 99415[0], 99416[0], 99446[0], 99447[0], 99448[0], 99449[0], 99451[0], 99452[0], 99466[0], 99468[0], 99469[0], 99471[0], 99472[0], 99475[0], 99476[0], 99477[0], 99478[0], 99479[0], 99480[0], 99483[0], 99485[0], 99497[0], C8921[1], C8922[1], C8923[1], C8924[1], C8925[1], C8926[1], C8927[0], C8929[1], C8930[1], G0380[1], G0381[1], G0382[1], G0383[1], G0384[1], G0406[0], G0407[0], G0408[0], G0425[0], G0426[0], G0427[0], G0463[0], G0500[0], G0508[0], G0509[0]
00797	01996[1], 0213T[1], 0216T[1], 0228T[1], 0230T[1], 31505[1], 31515[1], 31527[1], 31622[1], 31634[1], 31645[1], 31647[1], 36000[1], 36010[0], 36011[1], 36012[1], 36013[1], 36014[1], 36015[1], 36400[1], 36405[1], 36406[1], 36410[1], 36420[1], 36425[1], 36430[1], 36440[1], 36591[0], 36592[0], 36600[1], 36640[1], 43752[1], 43753[1], 43754[1], 61026[1], 61055[1], 62280[1], 62281[1], 62282[1], 62284[1], 62320[1], 62321[1], 62322[1], 62323[1], 62324[1], 62325[1], 62326[1], 62327[1], 64400[1], 64402[1], 64405[1], 64408[1], 64410[1], 64413[1], 64415[1], 64416[1], 64417[1], 64418[1], 64420[1], 64421[1], 64425[1], 64430[1], 64435[1], 64445[1], 64446[1], 64447[1], 64448[1], 64449[1], 64450[1], 64461[1], 64463[1], 64479[1], 64483[1], 64486[1], 64487[1], 64488[1], 64489[1], 64490[1], 64493[1], 64505[1], 64510[1], 64517[1], 64520[1], 64530[1], 64553[1], 64555[1], 67500[0], 76000[1], 76970[1], 76998[0], 77002[0], 90865[1], 92511[1], 92512[1], 92516[1], 92520[1], 92537[1], 92538[1], 92950[1], 92953[1], 92960[1], 92961[1], 93000[1], 93005[1], 93010[1], 93040[1], 93041[1], 93042[1], 93050[0], 93303[0], 93304[0], 93306[1], 93307[1], 93308[1], 93312[1], 93313[1], 93314[1], 93315[1], 93316[1], 93317[1], 93318[0], 93351[1], 93355[0], 93451[1], 93456[1], 93457[1], 93561[0], 93562[0], 93701[0], 93922[1], 93923[1], 93924[1], 93925[1], 93926[1], 93930[1], 93931[1], 93970[1], 93971[1], 93975[1], 93976[1], 93978[1], 93979[1], 93980[1], 93981[1], 94002[1], 94004[1], 94200[1], 94250[0], 94640[1], 94644[1], 94660[1], 94662[1], 94680[1], 94681[1], 94690[1], 94760[0], 94761[0], 94762[1], 94770[1], 95812[0], 95813[0], 95816[0], 95819[0], 95822[0], 95829[0], 95955[0], 95956[0], 95957[0], 96360[0], 96365[0], 96372[0], 96373[0], 96374[0], 96375[0], 96376[0], 96377[0], 99151[0], 99152[0], 99153[0], 99155[0], 99156[0], 99157[0], 99201[0], 99202[0], 99203[0], 99204[0], 99205[0], 99211[0], 99212[0], 99213[0], 99214[0], 99215[0], 99217[0], 99218[0], 99219[0], 99220[0], 99221[0], 99222[0], 99223[0], 99224[0], 99225[0], 99226[0], 99231[0], 99232[0], 99233[0], 99234[0], 99235[0], 99236[0], 99238[0], 99239[0], 99281[0], 99282[0], 99283[0], 99284[0], 99285[0], 99304[0], 99305[0], 99306[0], 99307[0], 99308[0],

0 = Modifier usage not allowed or inappropriate 1 = Modifier usage allowed

CPT © 2018 American Medical Association. All Rights Reserved.

Code 1	Code 2
	99309[0], 99310[0], 99315[0], 99318[0], 99324[0], 99325[0], 99326[0], 99327[0], 99328[0], 99334[0], 99335[0], 99336[0], 99337[0], 99341[0], 99342[0], 99343[0], 99347[0], 99348[0], 99349[0], 99354[0], 99355[0], 99356[0], 99357[0], 99358[0], 99359[0], 99415[0], 99416[0], 99446[0], 99447[0], 99448[0], 99449[0], 99451[0], 99452[0], 99466[0], 99468[0], 99469[0], 99471[0], 99472[0], 99475[0], 99476[0], 99477[0], 99478[0], 99479[0], 99480[0], 99483[0], 99485[0], 99497[0], C8921[1], C8922[1], C8923[1], C8924[1], C8925[1], C8926[1], C8927[0], C8929[1], C8930[1], G0380[1], G0381[1], G0382[1], G0383[1], G0384[1], G0406[0], G0407[0], G0408[0], G0425[0], G0426[0], G0427[0], G0463[0], G0500[0], G0508[0], G0509[0]
00800	01996[1], 0213T[1], 0216T[1], 0228T[1], 0230T[1], 0333T[0], 0464T[0], 31505[1], 31515[1], 31527[1], 31622[1], 31634[1], 31645[1], 31647[1], 36000[1], 36010[0], 36011[1], 36012[1], 36013[1], 36014[1], 36015[1], 36400[1], 36405[1], 36406[1], 36410[1], 36420[1], 36425[1], 36430[1], 36440[1], 36591[0], 36592[0], 36600[1], 36640[1], 43752[1], 43753[1], 43754[1], 61026[1], 61055[1], 62280[1], 62281[1], 62282[1], 62284[1], 62320[1], 62321[1], 62322[1], 62323[1], 62324[1], 62325[1], 62326[1], 62327[1], 64400[1], 64402[1], 64405[1], 64408[1], 64410[1], 64413[1], 64415[1], 64416[1], 64417[1], 64418[1], 64420[1], 64421[1], 64425[1], 64430[1], 64435[1], 64445[1], 64446[1], 64447[1], 64448[1], 64449[1], 64450[1], 64461[1], 64463[1], 64479[1], 64483[1], 64486[1], 64487[1], 64488[1], 64489[1], 64490[1], 64493[1], 64505[1], 64510[1], 64517[1], 64520[1], 64530[1], 64553[1], 64555[1], 67500[1], 76000[1], 76970[1], 76998[0], 77002[0], 90865[1], 92511[1], 92512[1], 92516[1], 92520[1], 92537[1], 92538[1], 92585[0], 92950[1], 92953[1], 92960[1], 92961[1], 93000[1], 93005[1], 93010[1], 93040[1], 93041[1], 93042[1], 93050[0], 93303[0], 93304[0], 93306[1], 93307[1], 93308[1], 93312[1], 93313[1], 93314[1], 93315[1], 93316[1], 93317[1], 93318[0], 93351[1], 93355[0], 93451[1], 93456[1], 93457[1], 93561[0], 93562[0], 93701[0], 93922[1], 93923[1], 93924[1], 93925[1], 93926[1], 93930[1], 93931[1], 93970[1], 93971[1], 93975[1], 93976[1], 93978[1], 93979[1], 93980[1], 93981[1], 94002[1], 94004[1], 94200[1], 94250[0], 94640[1], 94644[1], 94660[1], 94662[1], 94680[1], 94681[1], 94690[1], 94760[0], 94761[0], 94762[1], 94770[1], 95812[0], 95813[0], 95816[0], 95819[0], 95822[0], 95829[0], 95860[0], 95861[0], 95863[0], 95864[0], 95865[0], 95866[0], 95867[0], 95868[0], 95869[0], 95870[0], 95907[0], 95908[0], 95909[0], 95910[0], 95911[0], 95912[0], 95913[0], 95925[0], 95926[0], 95927[0], 95928[0], 95929[0], 95930[0], 95933[0], 95937[0], 95938[0], 95939[0], 95940[0], 95955[0], 95956[0], 95957[0], 96360[0], 96365[0], 96372[0], 96373[0], 96374[0], 96375[0], 96376[0], 96377[0], 99151[0], 99152[0], 99153[0], 99155[0], 99156[0], 99157[0], 99201[0], 99202[0], 99203[0], 99204[0], 99205[0], 99211[0], 99212[0], 99213[0], 99214[0], 99215[0], 99217[0], 99218[0], 99219[0], 99220[0], 99221[0], 99222[0], 99223[0], 99224[0], 99225[0], 99226[0], 99231[0], 99232[0], 99233[0], 99234[0], 99235[0], 99236[0], 99238[0], 99239[0], 99281[0], 99282[0], 99283[0], 99284[0], 99285[0], 99304[0], 99305[0], 99306[0], 99307[0], 99308[0], 99309[0], 99310[0], 99315[0], 99318[0], 99324[0], 99325[0], 99326[0], 99327[0], 99328[0], 99334[0], 99335[0], 99336[0], 99337[0], 99341[0], 99342[0], 99343[0], 99347[0], 99348[0], 99349[0], 99354[0], 99355[0], 99356[0], 99357[0], 99358[0], 99359[0], 99415[0], 99416[0], 99446[0], 99447[0], 99448[0], 99449[0], 99451[0], 99452[0], 99466[0], 99468[0], 99469[0], 99471[0], 99472[0], 99475[0], 99476[0], 99477[0], 99478[0], 99479[0], 99480[0], 99483[0], 99485[0], 99497[0], C8921[1], C8922[1], C8923[1], C8924[1], C8925[1], C8926[1], C8927[0], C8929[1], C8930[1], G0380[1], G0381[1], G0382[1], G0383[1], G0384[1], G0406[0], G0407[0], G0408[0], G0425[0], G0426[0], G0427[0], G0453[0], G0463[0], G0500[0], G0508[0], G0509[0]
00802	01996[1], 0213T[1], 0216T[1], 0228T[1], 0230T[1], 31505[1], 31515[1], 31527[1], 31622[1], 31634[1], 31645[1], 31647[1], 36000[1], 36010[0], 36011[1], 36012[1], 36013[1], 36014[1], 36015[1], 36400[1], 36405[1], 36406[1], 36410[1], 36420[1], 36425[1], 36430[1], 36440[1], 36591[0], 36592[0], 36600[1], 36640[1], 43752[1], 43753[1], 43754[1], 61026[1], 61055[1], 62280[1], 62281[1], 62282[1], 62284[1], 62320[1], 62321[1], 62322[1], 62323[1], 62324[1], 62325[1], 62326[1], 62327[1], 64400[1], 64402[1], 64405[1], 64408[1], 64410[1], 64413[1], 64415[1], 64416[1], 64417[1], 64418[1], 64420[1], 64421[1], 64425[1], 64430[1], 64435[1], 64445[1], 64446[1], 64447[1], 64448[1], 64449[1], 64450[1], 64461[1], 64463[1], 64479[1], 64483[1], 64486[1], 64487[1], 64488[1], 64489[1], 64490[1], 64493[1], 64505[1], 64510[1], 64517[1], 64520[1], 64530[1], 64553[1], 64555[1], 67500[1], 76000[1], 76970[1], 76998[0], 77002[0], 90865[1], 92511[1], 92512[1], 92516[1], 92520[1], 92537[1], 92538[1], 92950[1], 92953[1], 92960[1], 92961[1], 93000[1], 93005[1], 93010[1], 93040[1], 93041[1], 93042[1], 93050[0], 93303[0], 93304[0], 93306[1], 93307[1], 93308[1], 93312[1], 93313[1], 93314[1], 93315[1], 93316[1], 93317[1], 93318[0], 93351[1], 93355[0], 93451[1], 93456[1], 93457[1], 93561[0], 93562[0], 93701[0], 93922[1], 93923[1], 93924[1], 93925[1], 93926[1], 93930[1], 93931[1], 93970[1], 93971[1], 93975[1], 93976[1], 93978[1], 93979[1], 93980[1], 93981[1], 94002[1], 94004[1], 94200[1], 94250[0], 94640[1], 94644[1], 94660[1], 94662[1], 94680[1], 94681[1], 94690[1], 94760[0], 94761[0], 94762[1], 94770[1], 95812[0], 95813[0], 95816[0], 95819[0], 95822[0], 95829[0], 95955[0], 95956[0], 95957[0], 96360[0], 96365[0], 96372[0], 96373[0], 96374[0], 96375[0], 96376[0], 96377[0], 99151[0], 99152[0], 99153[0], 99155[0], 99156[0], 99157[0], 99201[0], 99202[0], 99203[0], 99204[0], 99205[0], 99211[0], 99212[0], 99213[0], 99214[0], 99215[0], 99217[0], 99218[0], 99219[0], 99220[0], 99221[0], 99222[0], 99223[0], 99224[0], 99225[0], 99226[0], 99231[0], 99232[0], 99233[0], 99234[0], 99235[0], 99236[0], 99238[0], 99239[0], 99281[0], 99282[0], 99283[0], 99284[0], 99285[0], 99304[0], 99305[0], 99306[0], 99307[0], 99308[0], 99309[0], 99310[0], 99315[0], 99318[0], 99324[0], 99325[0], 99326[0], 99327[0], 99328[0], 99334[0], 99335[0], 99336[0], 99337[0], 99341[0], 99342[0], 99343[0], 99347[0], 99348[0], 99349[0], 99354[0], 99355[0], 99356[0], 99357[0], 99358[0], 99359[0], 99415[0], 99416[0], 99446[0], 99447[0], 99448[0], 99449[0], 99451[0], 99452[0], 99466[0], 99468[0], 99469[0], 99471[0], 99472[0], 99475[0], 99476[0], 99477[0], 99478[0], 99479[0], 99480[0], 99483[0], 99485[0], 99497[0], C8921[1], C8922[1], C8923[1], C8924[1], C8925[1], C8926[1], C8927[0], C8929[1], C8930[1], G0380[1], G0381[1], G0382[1], G0383[1], G0384[1], G0406[0], G0407[0], G0408[0], G0425[0], G0426[0], G0427[0], G0463[0], G0500[0], G0508[0], G0509[0]
00811	01996[1], 0213T[1], 0216T[1], 0228T[1], 0230T[1], 31505[1], 31515[1], 31527[1], 31622[1], 31634[1], 31645[1], 31647[1], 36000[1], 36010[0], 36011[1], 36012[1], 36013[1], 36014[1], 36015[1], 36400[1], 36405[1], 36406[1], 36410[1], 36420[1], 36425[1], 36430[1], 36440[1], 36591[0], 36592[0], 36600[1], 36640[1], 43752[1], 43754[1], 61026[1], 61055[1], 62280[1], 62281[1], 62282[1], 62284[1], 62320[1], 62321[1], 62322[1], 62323[1], 62324[1], 62325[1], 62326[1], 62327[1], 64400[1], 64402[1], 64405[1], 64408[1], 64410[1], 64413[1], 64415[1], 64416[1], 64417[1], 64418[1], 64420[1], 64421[1], 64425[1], 64430[1], 64435[1], 64445[1], 64446[1], 64447[1], 64448[1], 64449[1], 64450[1], 64461[1], 64463[1], 64479[1], 64483[1], 64486[1], 64487[1], 64488[1], 64489[1], 64490[1], 64493[1], 64505[1], 64510[1], 64517[1], 64520[1], 64530[1], 64553[1], 64555[1], 67500[1], 76000[1], 76970[1], 76998[0], 77002[0], 90865[1], 92511[1], 92512[1], 92516[1], 92520[1], 92537[1], 92538[1], 92950[1], 92953[1], 92960[1], 92961[1], 93000[1], 93005[1], 93010[1], 93040[1], 93041[1], 93042[1], 93050[0], 93303[0], 93304[0], 93306[1], 93307[1], 93308[1], 93312[1], 93313[1], 93314[1], 93315[1], 93316[1], 93317[1], 93318[0], 93351[1], 93355[0], 93451[1], 93456[1], 93457[1], 93561[0], 93562[0], 93701[0], 93922[1], 93923[1], 93924[1], 93925[1], 93926[1], 93930[1], 93931[1], 93970[1], 93971[1], 93975[1], 93976[1], 93978[1], 93979[1], 93980[1], 93981[1], 94002[1], 94004[1], 94200[1], 94250[0], 94640[1], 94644[1], 94660[1], 94662[1], 94680[1], 94681[1], 94690[1], 94760[0], 94761[0], 94762[1], 94770[1], 95812[0], 95813[0], 95816[0], 95819[0], 95822[0], 95829[0], 95955[0], 95956[0], 95957[0], 96360[0], 96365[0], 96372[0], 96373[0], 96374[0], 96375[0], 96376[0], 96377[0], 96523[0], 99151[0], 99152[0], 99153[0], 99155[0], 99156[0], 99157[0], 99201[0], 99202[0], 99203[0], 99204[0], 99205[0], 99211[0], 99212[0], 99213[0], 99214[0], 99215[0], 99217[0], 99218[0], 99219[0], 99220[0], 99221[0], 99222[0], 99223[0], 99224[0], 99225[0], 99226[0], 99231[0], 99232[0], 99233[0], 99234[0], 99235[0], 99236[0], 99238[0], 99239[0], 99281[0], 99282[0], 99283[0], 99284[0], 99285[0], 99304[0], 99305[0], 99306[0], 99307[0], 99308[0], 99309[0], 99310[0], 99315[0], 99318[0], 99324[0], 99325[0], 99326[0], 99327[0], 99328[0], 99334[0], 99335[0], 99336[0], 99337[0], 99341[0], 99342[0], 99343[0], 99347[0], 99348[0], 99349[0], 99354[0], 99355[0], 99356[0], 99357[0], 99358[0], 99359[0], 99415[0], 99416[0], 99446[0], 99447[0], 99448[0], 99449[0], 99451[0], 99452[0], 99466[0], 99468[0], 99469[0], 99471[0], 99472[0], 99475[0], 99476[0], 99477[0], 99478[0], 99479[0], 99480[0], 99483[0], 99485[0], 99497[0], C8921[1], C8922[1], C8923[1], C8924[1], C8925[1], C8926[1], C8927[0], C8929[1], C8930[1], G0380[1], G0381[1], G0382[1], G0383[1], G0384[1], G0406[0], G0407[0], G0408[0], G0425[0], G0426[0], G0427[0], G0463[0], G0500[0], G0508[0], G0509[0]
00812	01996[1], 0213T[1], 0216T[1], 0228T[1], 0230T[1], 31505[1], 31515[1], 31527[1], 31622[1], 31634[1], 31645[1], 31647[1], 36000[1], 36010[0], 36011[1], 36012[1], 36013[1], 36014[1], 36015[1], 36400[1], 36405[1], 36406[1], 36410[1], 36420[1], 36425[1], 36430[1], 36440[1], 36591[0], 36592[0], 36600[1], 36640[1], 43752[1], 43754[1], 61026[1], 61055[1], 62280[1], 62281[1], 62282[1], 62284[1], 62320[1], 62321[1], 62322[1], 62323[1], 62324[1], 62325[1], 62326[1], 62327[1], 64400[1], 64402[1], 64405[1], 64408[1], 64410[1], 64413[1], 64415[1], 64416[1], 64417[1], 64418[1], 64420[1], 64421[1], 64425[1], 64430[1], 64435[1], 64445[1], 64446[1], 64447[1], 64448[1], 64449[1], 64450[1], 64461[1], 64463[1], 64479[1], 64483[1], 64486[1], 64487[1], 64488[1], 64489[1], 64490[1], 64493[1], 64505[1], 64510[1], 64517[1], 64520[1], 64530[1], 64553[1], 64555[1], 67500[1], 76000[1], 76970[1], 76998[0], 77002[0], 90865[1], 92511[1], 92512[1], 92516[1], 92520[1], 92537[1], 92538[1], 92950[1], 92953[1], 92960[1], 92961[1], 93000[1], 93005[1], 93010[1], 93040[1], 93041[1], 93042[1], 93050[0], 93303[0], 93304[0], 93306[1], 93307[1], 93308[1], 93312[1], 93313[1], 93314[1], 93315[1], 93316[1], 93317[1], 93318[0], 93351[1], 93355[0], 93451[1], 93456[1], 93457[1], 93561[0], 93562[0], 93701[0], 93922[1], 93923[1], 93924[1], 93925[1], 93926[1], 93930[1], 93931[1], 93970[1], 93971[1], 93975[1], 93976[1], 93978[1], 93979[1], 93980[1], 93981[1], 94002[1], 94004[1], 94200[1], 94250[0], 94640[1], 94644[1], 94660[1], 94662[1], 94680[1], 94681[1], 94690[1], 94760[0], 94761[0], 94762[1], 94770[1], 95812[0], 95813[0], 95816[0], 95819[0], 95822[0], 95829[0], 95955[0], 95956[0], 95957[0], 96360[0], 96365[0], 96372[0], 96373[0], 96374[0], 96375[0], 96376[0], 96377[0], 96523[0], 99151[0], 99152[0], 99153[0], 99155[0], 99156[0], 99157[0], 99201[0], 99202[0], 99203[0], 99204[0], 99205[0], 99211[0], 99212[0], 99213[0], 99214[0], 99215[0], 99217[0], 99218[0], 99219[0], 99220[0], 99221[0], 99222[0], 99223[0], 99224[0], 99225[0], 99226[0], 99231[0], 99232[0], 99233[0], 99234[0], 99235[0], 99236[0], 99238[0], 99239[0], 99281[0], 99282[0], 99283[0], 99284[0], 99285[0], 99304[0], 99305[0], 99306[0], 99307[0], 99308[0], 99309[0], 99310[0], 99315[0], 99318[0], 99324[0], 99325[0], 99326[0], 99327[0], 99328[0], 99334[0], 99335[0], 99336[0], 99337[0], 99341[0], 99342[0], 99343[0], 99347[0], 99348[0], 99349[0], 99354[0], 99355[0], 99356[0], 99357[0], 99358[0], 99359[0], 99415[0], 99416[0], 99446[0], 99447[0], 99448[0], 99449[0], 99451[0], 99452[0], 99466[0], 99468[0], 99469[0], 99471[0], 99472[0], 99475[0], 99476[0], 99477[0], 99478[0], 99479[0], 99480[0], 99483[0], 99485[0], 99497[0], C8921[1], C8922[1], C8923[1], C8924[1], C8925[1], C8926[1], C8927[0], C8929[1], C8930[1], G0380[1], G0381[1], G0382[1], G0383[1], G0384[1], G0406[0], G0407[0], G0408[0], G0425[0], G0426[0], G0427[0], G0463[0], G0500[0], G0508[0], G0509[0]

0 = Modifier usage not allowed or inappropriate 1 = Modifier usage allowed

Appendix A: NCCI - CPT Codes

CPT © 2018 American Medical Association. All Rights Reserved.

Code 1	Code 2
00813	00731^1, 00732^1, 00811^1, 00812^1, 01996^1, 0213T^1, 0216T^1, 0228T^1, 0230T^1, 31505^1, 31515^1, 31527^1, 31622^1, 31634^1, 31645^1, 31647^1, 36000^1, 36010^0, 36011^1, 36012^1, 36013^1, 36014^1, 36015^1, 36400^1, 36405^1, 36406^1, 36410^1, 36420^1, 36425^1, 36430^1, 36440^1, 36591^0, 36592^0, 36600^1, 36640^1, 43752^1, 43753^1, 43754^1, 61026^1, 61055^1, 62280^1, 62281^1, 62282^1, 62284^1, 62320^1, 62321^1, 62322^1, 62323^1, 62324^1, 62325^1, 62326^1, 62327^1, 64400^1, 64402^1, 64405^1, 64408^1, 64410^1, 64413^1, 64415^1, 64416^1, 64417^1, 64418^1, 64420^1, 64421^1, 64425^1, 64430^1, 64435^1, 64445^1, 64446^1, 64447^1, 64448^1, 64449^1, 64450^1, 64461^1, 64463^1, 64479^1, 64483^1, 64486^1, 64487^1, 64488^1, 64489^1, 64490^1, 64493^1, 64505^1, 64510^1, 64517^1, 64520^1, 64530^1, 64553^1, 64555^1, 67500^1, 76000^1, 76970^1, 76998^0, 77002^0, 90865^1, 92511^1, 92512^1, 92516^1, 92520^1, 92537^1, 92538^1, 92950^1, 92953^1, 92960^1, 92961^1, 93000^1, 93005^1, 93010^1, 93040^1, 93041^1, 93042^1, 93050^0, 93303^0, 93304^0, 93306^1, 93307^1, 93308^1, 93312^1, 93313^1, 93314^1, 93315^1, 93316^1, 93317^1, 93318^0, 93351^1, 93355^0, 93451^1, 93456^1, 93457^1, 93561^0, 93562^0, 93701^0, 93922^1, 93923^1, 93924^1, 93925^1, 93926^1, 93930^1, 93931^1, 93970^1, 93971^1, 93975^1, 93976^1, 93978^1, 93979^1, 93980^1, 93981^1, 94002^1, 94004^1, 94200^1, 94250^0, 94640^1, 94644^1, 94660^1, 94662^1, 94680^1, 94681^1, 94690^1, 94760^0, 94761^0, 94762^1, 94770^1, 95812^0, 95813^0, 95816^0, 95819^0, 95822^0, 95829^0, 95955^0, 95956^0, 95957^0, 96360^0, 96365^0, 96372^0, 96373^0, 96374^0, 96375^0, 96376^0, 96377^0, 96523^0, 99151^0, 99152^0, 99153^0, 99155^0, 99156^0, 99157^0, 99201^0, 99202^0, 99203^0, 99204^0, 99205^0, 99211^0, 99212^0, 99213^0, 99214^0, 99215^0, 99217^0, 99218^0, 99219^0, 99220^0, 99221^0, 99222^0, 99223^0, 99224^0, 99225^0, 99226^0, 99231^0, 99232^0, 99233^0, 99234^0, 99235^0, 99236^0, 99238^0, 99239^0, 99281^0, 99282^0, 99283^0, 99284^0, 99285^0, 99304^0, 99305^0, 99306^0, 99307^0, 99308^0, 99309^0, 99310^0, 99315^0, 99318^0, 99324^0, 99325^0, 99326^0, 99327^0, 99328^0, 99334^0, 99335^0, 99336^0, 99337^0, 99341^0, 99342^0, 99343^0, 99347^0, 99348^0, 99349^0, 99354^0, 99355^0, 99356^0, 99357^0, 99358^0, 99359^0, 99415^0, 99416^0, 99446^0, 99447^0, 99448^0, 99449^0, 99451^0, 99452^0, 99466^0, 99468^0, 99469^0, 99471^0, 99472^0, 99475^0, 99476^0, 99477^0, 99478^0, 99479^0, 99480^0, 99483^0, 99485^0, 99497^0, C8921^1, C8922^1, C8923^1, C8924^1, C8925^1, C8926^1, C8927^0, C8929^1, C8930^1, G0380^1, G0381^1, G0382^1, G0383^1, G0384^1, G0406^0, G0407^0, G0408^0, G0425^0, G0426^0, G0427^0, G0463^0, G0500^0, G0508^0, G0509^0
00820	01996^1, 0213T^1, 0216T^1, 0228T^1, 0230T^1, 31505^1, 31515^1, 31527^1, 31622^1, 31634^1, 31645^1, 31647^1, 36000^1, 36010^0, 36011^1, 36012^1, 36013^1, 36014^1, 36015^1, 36400^1, 36405^1, 36406^1, 36410^1, 36420^1, 36425^1, 36430^1, 36440^1, 36591^0, 36592^0, 36600^1, 36640^1, 43752^1, 43753^1, 43754^1, 61026^1, 61055^1, 62280^1, 62281^1, 62282^1, 62284^1, 62320^1, 62321^1, 62322^1, 62323^1, 62324^1, 62325^1, 62326^1, 62327^1, 64400^1, 64402^1, 64405^1, 64408^1, 64410^1, 64413^1, 64415^1, 64416^1, 64417^1, 64418^1, 64420^1, 64421^1, 64425^1, 64430^1, 64435^1, 64445^1, 64446^1, 64447^1, 64448^1, 64449^1, 64450^1, 64461^1, 64463^1, 64479^1, 64483^1, 64486^1, 64487^1, 64488^1, 64489^1, 64490^1, 64493^1, 64505^1, 64510^1, 64517^1, 64520^1, 64530^1, 64553^1, 64555^1, 67500^1, 76000^1, 76970^1, 76998^0, 77002^0, 90865^1, 92511^1, 92512^1, 92516^1, 92520^1, 92537^1, 92538^1, 92950^1, 92953^1, 92960^1, 92961^1, 93000^1, 93005^1, 93010^1, 93040^1, 93041^1, 93042^1, 93050^0, 93303^0, 93304^0, 93306^1, 93307^1, 93308^1, 93312^1, 93313^1, 93314^1, 93315^1, 93316^1, 93317^1, 93318^0, 93351^1, 93355^0, 93451^1, 93456^1, 93457^1, 93561^0, 93562^0, 93701^0, 93922^1, 93923^1, 93924^1, 93925^1, 93926^1, 93930^1, 93931^1, 93970^1, 93971^1, 93975^1, 93976^1, 93978^1, 93979^1, 93980^1, 93981^1, 94002^1, 94004^1, 94200^1, 94250^0, 94640^1, 94644^1, 94660^1, 94662^1, 94680^1, 94681^1, 94690^1, 94760^0, 94761^0, 94762^1, 94770^1, 95812^0, 95813^0, 95816^0, 95819^0, 95822^0, 95829^0, 95955^0, 95956^0, 95957^0, 96360^0, 96365^0, 96372^0, 96373^0, 96374^0, 96375^0, 96376^0, 96377^0, 99151^0, 99152^0, 99153^0, 99155^0, 99156^0, 99157^0, 99201^0, 99202^0, 99203^0, 99204^0, 99205^0, 99211^0, 99212^0, 99213^0, 99214^0, 99215^0, 99217^0, 99218^0, 99219^0, 99220^0, 99221^0, 99222^0, 99223^0, 99224^0, 99225^0, 99226^0, 99231^0, 99232^0, 99233^0, 99234^0, 99235^0, 99236^0, 99238^0, 99239^0, 99281^0, 99282^0, 99283^0, 99284^0, 99285^0, 99304^0, 99305^0, 99306^0, 99307^0, 99308^0, 99309^0, 99310^0, 99315^0, 99318^0, 99324^0, 99325^0, 99326^0, 99327^0, 99328^0, 99334^0, 99335^0, 99336^0, 99337^0, 99341^0, 99342^0, 99343^0, 99347^0, 99348^0, 99349^0, 99354^0, 99355^0, 99356^0, 99357^0, 99358^0, 99359^0, 99415^0, 99416^0, 99446^0, 99447^0, 99448^0, 99449^0, 99451^0, 99452^0, 99466^0, 99468^0, 99469^0, 99471^0, 99472^0, 99475^0, 99476^0, 99477^0, 99478^0, 99479^0, 99480^0, 99483^0, 99485^0, 99497^0, C8921^1, C8922^1, C8923^1, C8924^1, C8925^1, C8926^1, C8927^0, C8929^1, C8930^1, G0380^1, G0381^1, G0382^1, G0383^1, G0384^1, G0406^0, G0407^0, G0408^0, G0425^0, G0426^0, G0427^0, G0463^0, G0500^0, G0508^0, G0509^0
00830	00834^1, 00836^1, 01996^1, 0213T^1, 0216T^1, 0228T^1, 0230T^1, 31505^1, 31515^1, 31527^1, 31622^1, 31634^1, 31645^1, 31647^1, 36000^1, 36010^0, 36011^1, 36012^1, 36013^1, 36014^1, 36015^1, 36400^1, 36405^1, 36406^1, 36410^1, 36420^1, 36425^1, 36430^1, 36440^1, 36591^0, 36592^0, 36600^1, 36640^1, 43752^1, 43753^1, 43754^1, 61026^1, 61055^1, 62280^1, 62281^1, 62282^1, 62284^1, 62320^1, 62321^1, 62322^1, 62323^1, 62324^1, 62325^1, 62326^1, 62327^1, 64400^1, 64402^1, 64405^1, 64408^1, 64410^1, 64413^1, 64415^1, 64416^1, 64417^1, 64418^1, 64420^1, 64421^1, 64425^1, 64430^1, 64435^1, 64445^1, 64446^1, 64447^1, 64448^1, 64449^1, 64450^1, 64461^1, 64463^1, 64479^1, 64483^1, 64486^1, 64487^1, 64488^1, 64489^1, 64490^1, 64493^1, 64505^1, 64510^1, 64517^1, 64520^1, 64530^1, 64553^1, 64555^1, 67500^1, 76000^1, 76970^1, 76998^0, 77002^0, 90865^1, 92511^1, 92512^1, 92516^1, 92520^1, 92537^1, 92538^1, 92950^1, 92953^1, 92960^1, 92961^1, 93000^1, 93005^1, 93010^1, 93040^1, 93041^1, 93042^1, 93050^0, 93303^0, 93304^0, 93306^1, 93307^1, 93308^1, 93312^1, 93313^1, 93314^1, 93315^1, 93316^1, 93317^1, 93318^0, 93351^1, 93355^0, 93451^1, 93456^1, 93457^1, 93561^0, 93562^0, 93701^0, 93922^1, 93923^1, 93924^1, 93925^1, 93926^1, 93930^1, 93931^1, 93970^1, 93971^1, 93975^1, 93976^1, 93978^1, 93979^1, 93980^1, 93981^1, 94002^1, 94004^1, 94200^1, 94250^0, 94640^1, 94644^1, 94660^1, 94662^1, 94680^1, 94681^1, 94690^1, 94760^0, 94761^0, 94762^1, 94770^1, 95812^0, 95813^0, 95816^0, 95819^0, 95822^0, 95829^0, 95955^0, 95956^0, 95957^0, 96360^0, 96365^0, 96372^0, 96373^0, 96374^0, 96375^0, 96376^0, 96377^0, 99151^0, 99152^0, 99153^0, 99155^0, 99156^0, 99157^0, 99201^0, 99202^0, 99203^0, 99204^0, 99205^0, 99211^0, 99212^0, 99213^0, 99214^0, 99215^0, 99217^0, 99218^0, 99219^0, 99220^0, 99221^0, 99222^0, 99223^0, 99224^0, 99225^0, 99226^0, 99231^0, 99232^0, 99233^0, 99234^0, 99235^0, 99236^0, 99238^0, 99239^0, 99281^0, 99282^0, 99283^0, 99284^0, 99285^0, 99304^0, 99305^0, 99306^0, 99307^0, 99308^0, 99309^0, 99310^0, 99315^0, 99318^0, 99324^0, 99325^0, 99326^0, 99327^0, 99328^0, 99334^0, 99335^0, 99336^0, 99337^0, 99341^0, 99342^0, 99343^0, 99347^0, 99348^0, 99349^0, 99354^0, 99355^0, 99356^0, 99357^0, 99358^0, 99359^0, 99415^0, 99416^0, 99446^0, 99447^0, 99448^0, 99449^0, 99451^0, 99452^0, 99466^0, 99468^0, 99469^0, 99471^0, 99472^0, 99475^0, 99476^0, 99477^0, 99478^0, 99479^0, 99480^0, 99483^0, 99485^0, 99497^0, C8921^1, C8922^1, C8923^1, C8924^1, C8925^1, C8926^1, C8927^0, C8929^1, C8930^1, G0380^1, G0381^1, G0382^1, G0383^1, G0384^1, G0406^0, G0407^0, G0408^0, G0425^0, G0426^0, G0427^0, G0463^0, G0500^0, G0508^0, G0509^0
00832	00834^1, 00836^1, 01996^1, 0213T^1, 0216T^1, 0228T^1, 0230T^1, 31505^1, 31515^1, 31527^1, 31622^1, 31634^1, 31645^1, 31647^1, 36000^1, 36010^0, 36011^1, 36012^1, 36013^1, 36014^1, 36015^1, 36400^1, 36405^1, 36406^1, 36410^1, 36420^1, 36425^1, 36430^1, 36440^1, 36591^0, 36592^0, 36600^1, 36640^1, 43752^1, 43753^1, 43754^1, 61026^1, 61055^1, 62280^1, 62281^1, 62282^1, 62284^1, 62320^1, 62321^1, 62322^1, 62323^1, 62324^1, 62325^1, 62326^1, 62327^1, 64400^1, 64402^1, 64405^1, 64408^1, 64410^1, 64413^1, 64415^1, 64416^1, 64417^1, 64418^1, 64420^1, 64421^1, 64425^1, 64430^1, 64435^1, 64445^1, 64446^1, 64447^1, 64448^1, 64449^1, 64450^1, 64461^1, 64463^1, 64479^1, 64483^1, 64486^1, 64487^1, 64488^1, 64489^1, 64490^1, 64493^1, 64505^1, 64510^1, 64517^1, 64520^1, 64530^1, 64553^1, 64555^1, 67500^1, 76000^1, 76970^1, 76998^0, 77002^0, 90865^1, 92511^1, 92512^1, 92516^1, 92520^1, 92537^1, 92538^1, 92950^1, 92953^1, 92960^1, 92961^1, 93000^1, 93005^1, 93010^1, 93040^1, 93041^1, 93042^1, 93050^0, 93303^0, 93304^0, 93306^1, 93307^1, 93308^1, 93312^1, 93313^1, 93314^1, 93315^1, 93316^1, 93317^1, 93318^0, 93351^1, 93355^0, 93451^1, 93456^1, 93457^1, 93561^0, 93562^0, 93701^0, 93922^1, 93923^1, 93924^1, 93925^1, 93926^1, 93930^1, 93931^1, 93970^1, 93971^1, 93975^1, 93976^1, 93978^1, 93979^1, 93980^1, 93981^1, 94002^1, 94004^1, 94200^1, 94250^0, 94640^1, 94644^1, 94660^1, 94662^1, 94680^1, 94681^1, 94690^1, 94760^0, 94761^0, 94762^1, 94770^1, 95812^0, 95813^0, 95816^0, 95819^0, 95822^0, 95829^0, 95955^0, 95956^0, 95957^0, 96360^0, 96365^0, 96372^0, 96373^0, 96374^0, 96375^0, 96376^0, 96377^0, 99151^0, 99152^0, 99153^0, 99155^0, 99156^0, 99157^0, 99201^0, 99202^0, 99203^0, 99204^0, 99205^0, 99211^0, 99212^0, 99213^0, 99214^0, 99215^0, 99217^0, 99218^0, 99219^0, 99220^0, 99221^0, 99222^0, 99223^0, 99224^0, 99225^0, 99226^0, 99231^0, 99232^0, 99233^0, 99234^0, 99235^0, 99236^0, 99238^0, 99239^0, 99281^0, 99282^0, 99283^0, 99284^0, 99285^0, 99304^0, 99305^0, 99306^0, 99307^0, 99308^0, 99309^0, 99310^0, 99315^0, 99318^0, 99324^0, 99325^0, 99326^0, 99327^0, 99328^0, 99334^0, 99335^0, 99336^0, 99337^0, 99341^0, 99342^0, 99343^0, 99347^0, 99348^0, 99349^0, 99354^0, 99355^0, 99356^0, 99357^0, 99358^0, 99359^0, 99415^0, 99416^0, 99446^0, 99447^0, 99448^0, 99449^0, 99451^0, 99452^0, 99466^0, 99468^0, 99469^0, 99471^0, 99472^0, 99475^0, 99476^0, 99477^0, 99478^0, 99479^0, 99480^0, 99483^0, 99485^0, 99497^0, C8921^1, C8922^1, C8923^1, C8924^1, C8925^1, C8926^1, C8927^0, C8929^1, C8930^1, G0380^1, G0381^1, G0382^1, G0383^1, G0384^1, G0406^0, G0407^0, G0408^0, G0425^0, G0426^0, G0427^0, G0463^0, G0500^0, G0508^0, G0509^0
00834	00836^1, 01996^1, 0213T^1, 0216T^1, 0228T^1, 0230T^1, 31505^1, 31515^1, 31527^1, 31622^1, 31634^1, 31645^1, 31647^1, 36000^1, 36010^0, 36011^1, 36012^1, 36013^1, 36014^1, 36015^1, 36400^1, 36405^1, 36406^1, 36410^1, 36420^1, 36425^1, 36430^1, 36440^1, 36591^0, 36592^0, 36600^1, 36640^1, 43752^1, 43753^1, 43754^1, 61026^1, 61055^1, 62280^1, 62281^1, 62282^1, 62284^1, 62320^1, 62321^1, 62322^1, 62323^1, 62324^1, 62325^1, 62326^1, 62327^1, 64400^1, 64402^1, 64405^1, 64408^1, 64410^1, 64413^1, 64415^1, 64416^1, 64417^1, 64418^1, 64420^1, 64421^1, 64425^1, 64430^1, 64435^1, 64445^1, 64446^1, 64447^1, 64448^1, 64449^1, 64450^1, 64461^1, 64463^1, 64479^1, 64483^1, 64486^1, 64487^1, 64488^1, 64489^1, 64490^1, 64493^1, 64505^1, 64510^1, 64517^1, 64520^1, 64530^1, 64553^1, 64555^1, 67500^0, 76000^1, 76970^1, 76998^0, 77002^0, 90865^1, 92511^1, 92512^1, 92516^1, 92520^1, 92537^1, 92538^1, 92950^1, 92953^1, 92960^1, 92961^1, 93000^1, 93005^1, 93010^1, 93040^1, 93041^1, 93042^1, 93050^0, 93303^0, 93304^0, 93306^1, 93307^1, 93308^1, 93312^1, 93313^1, 93314^1, 93315^1, 93316^1,

0 = Modifier usage not allowed or inappropriate 1 = Modifier usage allowed

CPT © 2018 American Medical Association. All Rights Reserved.

Code 1	Code 2
	93317[1], 93318[0], 93351[1], 93355[0], 93451[1], 93456[1], 93457[1], 93561[0], 93562[0], 93701[0], 93922[1], 93923[1], 93924[1], 93925[1], 93926[1], 93930[1], 93931[1], 93970[1], 93971[1], 93975[1], 93976[1], 93978[1], 93979[1], 93980[1], 93981[1], 94002[1], 94004[1], 94200[1], 94250[0], 94640[1], 94644[1], 94660[1], 94662[1], 94680[1], 94681[1], 94690[1], 94760[0], 94761[0], 94762[1], 94770[1], 95812[0], 95813[0], 95816[0], 95819[0], 95822[0], 95829[0], 95955[0], 95956[0], 95957[0], 96360[0], 96365[0], 96372[0], 96373[0], 96374[0], 96375[0], 96376[0], 96377[0], 99100[1], 99151[0], 99152[0], 99153[0], 99155[0], 99156[0], 99157[0], 99201[0], 99202[0], 99203[0], 99204[0], 99205[0], 99211[0], 99212[0], 99213[0], 99214[0], 99215[0], 99217[0], 99218[0], 99219[0], 99220[0], 99221[0], 99222[0], 99223[0], 99224[0], 99225[0], 99226[0], 99231[0], 99232[0], 99233[0], 99234[0], 99235[0], 99236[0], 99238[0], 99239[0], 99281[0], 99282[0], 99283[0], 99284[0], 99285[0], 99304[0], 99305[0], 99306[0], 99307[0], 99308[0], 99309[0], 99310[0], 99315[0], 99318[0], 99324[0], 99325[0], 99326[0], 99327[0], 99328[0], 99334[0], 99335[0], 99336[0], 99337[0], 99341[0], 99342[0], 99343[0], 99347[0], 99348[0], 99349[0], 99354[0], 99355[0], 99356[0], 99357[0], 99358[0], 99359[0], 99415[0], 99416[0], 99446[0], 99447[0], 99448[0], 99449[0], 99451[0], 99452[0], 99468[0], 99469[0], 99471[0], 99472[0], 99475[0], 99476[0], 99477[0], 99478[0], 99479[0], 99480[0], 99483[0], 99497[0], C8921[1], C8922[1], C8923[1], C8924[1], C8925[1], C8926[1], C8927[0], C8929[1], C8930[1], G0380[1], G0381[1], G0382[1], G0383[1], G0384[1], G0406[0], G0407[0], G0408[0], G0425[0], G0426[0], G0427[0], G0463[0], G0500[0], G0508[0], G0509[0]
00836	01996[1], 0213T[1], 0216T[1], 0228T[1], 0230T[1], 31505[1], 31515[1], 31527[1], 31622[1], 31634[1], 31645[1], 31647[1], 36000[1], 36010[0], 36011[1], 36012[1], 36013[1], 36014[1], 36015[1], 36400[1], 36405[1], 36406[1], 36410[1], 36420[1], 36425[1], 36430[1], 36440[1], 36591[0], 36592[0], 36600[1], 36640[1], 43752[1], 43753[1], 43754[1], 61026[1], 61055[1], 62280[1], 62281[1], 62282[1], 62284[1], 62320[1], 62321[1], 62322[1], 62323[1], 62324[1], 62325[1], 62326[1], 62327[1], 64400[1], 64402[1], 64405[1], 64408[1], 64410[1], 64413[1], 64415[1], 64416[1], 64417[1], 64418[1], 64420[1], 64421[1], 64425[1], 64430[1], 64435[1], 64445[1], 64446[1], 64447[1], 64448[1], 64449[1], 64450[1], 64461[1], 64463[1], 64479[1], 64483[1], 64486[1], 64487[1], 64488[1], 64489[1], 64490[1], 64493[1], 64505[1], 64510[1], 64517[1], 64520[1], 64530[1], 64553[1], 64555[1], 67500[0], 76000[1], 76970[1], 76998[0], 77002[0], 90865[1], 92511[1], 92512[1], 92516[1], 92520[1], 92537[1], 92538[1], 92950[1], 92953[1], 92960[1], 92961[1], 93000[1], 93005[1], 93010[1], 93040[1], 93041[1], 93042[1], 93050[0], 93303[0], 93304[0], 93306[1], 93307[1], 93308[1], 93312[1], 93313[1], 93314[1], 93315[1], 93316[1], 93317[1], 93318[0], 93351[1], 93355[0], 93451[1], 93456[1], 93457[1], 93561[0], 93562[0], 93701[0], 93922[1], 93923[1], 93924[1], 93925[1], 93926[1], 93930[1], 93931[1], 93970[1], 93971[1], 93975[1], 93976[1], 93978[1], 93979[1], 93980[1], 93981[1], 94002[1], 94004[1], 94200[1], 94250[0], 94640[1], 94644[1], 94660[1], 94662[1], 94680[1], 94681[1], 94690[1], 94760[0], 94761[0], 94762[1], 94770[1], 95812[0], 95813[0], 95816[0], 95819[0], 95822[0], 95829[0], 95955[0], 95956[0], 95957[0], 96360[0], 96365[0], 96372[0], 96373[0], 96374[0], 96375[0], 96376[0], 96377[0], 99100[1], 99151[0], 99152[0], 99153[0], 99155[0], 99156[0], 99157[0], 99201[0], 99202[0], 99203[0], 99204[0], 99205[0], 99211[0], 99212[0], 99213[0], 99214[0], 99215[0], 99217[0], 99218[0], 99219[0], 99220[0], 99221[0], 99222[0], 99223[0], 99224[0], 99225[0], 99226[0], 99231[0], 99232[0], 99233[0], 99234[0], 99235[0], 99236[0], 99238[0], 99239[0], 99281[0], 99282[0], 99283[0], 99284[0], 99285[0], 99304[0], 99305[0], 99306[0], 99307[0], 99308[0], 99309[0], 99310[0], 99315[0], 99318[0], 99324[0], 99325[0], 99326[0], 99327[0], 99328[0], 99334[0], 99335[0], 99336[0], 99337[0], 99341[0], 99342[0], 99343[0], 99347[0], 99348[0], 99349[0], 99354[0], 99355[0], 99356[0], 99357[0], 99358[0], 99359[0], 99415[0], 99416[0], 99446[0], 99447[0], 99448[0], 99449[0], 99451[0], 99452[0], 99468[0], 99469[0], 99471[0], 99472[0], 99475[0], 99476[0], 99477[0], 99478[0], 99479[0], 99480[0], 99483[0], 99497[0], C8921[1], C8922[1], C8923[1], C8924[1], C8925[1], C8926[1], C8927[0], C8929[1], C8930[1], G0380[1], G0381[1], G0382[1], G0383[1], G0384[1], G0406[0], G0407[0], G0408[0], G0425[0], G0426[0], G0427[0], G0463[0], G0500[0], G0508[0], G0509[0]
00840	01996[1], 0213T[1], 0216T[1], 0228T[1], 0230T[1], 31505[1], 31515[1], 31527[1], 31622[1], 31634[1], 31645[1], 31647[1], 36000[1], 36010[0], 36011[1], 36012[1], 36013[1], 36014[1], 36015[1], 36400[1], 36405[1], 36406[1], 36410[1], 36420[1], 36425[1], 36430[1], 36440[1], 36591[0], 36592[0], 36600[1], 36640[1], 43752[1], 43754[1], 61026[1], 61055[1], 62280[1], 62281[1], 62282[1], 62284[1], 62320[1], 62321[1], 62322[1], 62323[1], 62324[1], 62325[1], 62326[1], 62327[1], 64400[1], 64402[1], 64405[1], 64408[1], 64410[1], 64413[1], 64415[1], 64416[1], 64417[1], 64418[1], 64420[1], 64421[1], 64425[1], 64430[1], 64435[1], 64445[1], 64446[1], 64447[1], 64448[1], 64449[1], 64450[1], 64461[1], 64463[1], 64479[1], 64483[1], 64486[1], 64487[1], 64488[1], 64489[1], 64490[1], 64493[1], 64505[1], 64510[1], 64517[1], 64520[1], 64530[1], 64553[1], 64555[1], 67500[1], 76000[1], 76970[1], 76998[0], 77002[0], 90865[1], 92511[1], 92512[1], 92516[1], 92520[1], 92537[1], 92538[1], 92950[1], 92953[1], 92960[1], 92961[1], 93000[1], 93005[1], 93010[1], 93040[1], 93041[1], 93042[1], 93050[0], 93303[0], 93304[0], 93306[1], 93307[1], 93308[1], 93312[1], 93313[1], 93314[1], 93315[1], 93316[1], 93317[1], 93318[0], 93351[1], 93355[0], 93451[1], 93456[1], 93457[1], 93561[0], 93562[0], 93701[0], 93922[1], 93923[1], 93924[1], 93925[1], 93926[1], 93930[1], 93931[1], 93970[1], 93971[1], 93975[1], 93976[1], 93978[1], 93979[1], 93980[1], 93981[1], 94002[1], 94004[1], 94200[1], 94250[0], 94640[1], 94644[1], 94660[1], 94662[1], 94680[1], 94681[1], 94690[1], 94760[0], 94761[0], 94762[1], 94770[1], 95812[0], 95813[0], 95816[0], 95819[0], 95822[0], 95829[0], 95955[0], 95956[0], 95957[0], 96360[0], 96365[0], 96372[0], 96373[0], 96374[0], 96375[0], 96376[0], 96377[0], 99151[0], 99152[0], 99153[0], 99155[0], 99156[0], 99157[0], 99201[0], 99202[0], 99203[0], 99204[0], 99205[0], 99211[0], 99212[0], 99213[0], 99214[0], 99215[0], 99217[0], 99218[0], 99219[0], 99220[0], 99221[0], 99222[0], 99223[0], 99224[0], 99225[0], 99226[0], 99231[0], 99232[0], 99233[0], 99234[0], 99235[0], 99236[0], 99238[0], 99239[0], 99281[0], 99282[0], 99283[0], 99284[0], 99285[0], 99304[0], 99305[0], 99306[0], 99307[0], 99308[0], 99309[0], 99310[0], 99315[0], 99318[0], 99324[0], 99325[0], 99326[0], 99327[0], 99328[0], 99334[0], 99335[0], 99336[0], 99337[0], 99341[0], 99342[0], 99343[0], 99347[0], 99348[0], 99349[0], 99354[0], 99355[0], 99356[0], 99357[0], 99358[0], 99359[0], 99415[0], 99416[0], 99446[0], 99447[0], 99448[0], 99449[0], 99451[0], 99452[0], 99466[0], 99468[0], 99469[0], 99471[0], 99472[0], 99475[0], 99476[0], 99477[0], 99478[0], 99479[0], 99480[0], 99483[0], 99485[0], 99497[0], C8921[1], C8922[1], C8923[1], C8924[1], C8925[1], C8926[1], C8927[0], C8929[1], C8930[1], G0380[1], G0381[1], G0382[1], G0383[1], G0384[1], G0406[0], G0407[0], G0408[0], G0425[0], G0426[0], G0427[0], G0463[0], G0500[0], G0508[0], G0509[0]
00842	01996[1], 0213T[1], 0216T[1], 0228T[1], 0230T[1], 31505[1], 31515[1], 31527[1], 31622[1], 31634[1], 31645[1], 31647[1], 36000[1], 36010[0], 36011[1], 36012[1], 36013[1], 36014[1], 36015[1], 36400[1], 36405[1], 36406[1], 36410[1], 36420[1], 36425[1], 36430[1], 36440[1], 36591[0], 36592[0], 36600[1], 36640[1], 43752[1], 43753[1], 43754[1], 61026[1], 61055[1], 62280[1], 62281[1], 62282[1], 62284[1], 62320[1], 62321[1], 62322[1], 62323[1], 62324[1], 62325[1], 62326[1], 62327[1], 64400[1], 64402[1], 64405[1], 64408[1], 64410[1], 64413[1], 64415[1], 64416[1], 64417[1], 64418[1], 64420[1], 64421[1], 64425[1], 64430[1], 64435[1], 64445[1], 64446[1], 64447[1], 64448[1], 64449[1], 64450[1], 64461[1], 64463[1], 64479[1], 64483[1], 64486[1], 64487[1], 64488[1], 64489[1], 64490[1], 64493[1], 64505[1], 64510[1], 64517[1], 64520[1], 64530[1], 64553[1], 64555[1], 67500[1], 76000[1], 76970[1], 76998[0], 77002[0], 90865[1], 92511[1], 92512[1], 92516[1], 92520[1], 92537[1], 92538[1], 92950[1], 92953[1], 92960[1], 92961[1], 93000[1], 93005[1], 93010[1], 93040[1], 93041[1], 93042[1], 93050[0], 93303[0], 93304[0], 93306[1], 93307[1], 93308[1], 93312[1], 93313[1], 93314[1], 93315[1], 93316[1], 93317[1], 93318[0], 93351[1], 93355[0], 93451[1], 93456[1], 93457[1], 93561[0], 93562[0], 93701[0], 93922[1], 93923[1], 93924[1], 93925[1], 93926[1], 93930[1], 93931[1], 93970[1], 93971[1], 93975[1], 93976[1], 93978[1], 93979[1], 93980[1], 93981[1], 94002[1], 94004[1], 94200[1], 94250[0], 94640[1], 94644[1], 94660[1], 94662[1], 94680[1], 94681[1], 94690[1], 94760[0], 94761[0], 94762[1], 94770[1], 95812[0], 95813[0], 95816[0], 95819[0], 95822[0], 95829[0], 95955[0], 95956[0], 95957[0], 96360[0], 96365[0], 96372[0], 96373[0], 96374[0], 96375[0], 96376[0], 96377[0], 99151[0], 99152[0], 99153[0], 99155[0], 99156[0], 99157[0], 99201[0], 99202[0], 99203[0], 99204[0], 99205[0], 99211[0], 99212[0], 99213[0], 99214[0], 99215[0], 99217[0], 99218[0], 99219[0], 99220[0], 99221[0], 99222[0], 99223[0], 99224[0], 99225[0], 99226[0], 99231[0], 99232[0], 99233[0], 99234[0], 99235[0], 99236[0], 99238[0], 99239[0], 99281[0], 99282[0], 99283[0], 99284[0], 99285[0], 99304[0], 99305[0], 99306[0], 99307[0], 99308[0], 99309[0], 99310[0], 99315[0], 99318[0], 99324[0], 99325[0], 99326[0], 99327[0], 99328[0], 99334[0], 99335[0], 99336[0], 99337[0], 99341[0], 99342[0], 99343[0], 99347[0], 99348[0], 99349[0], 99354[0], 99355[0], 99356[0], 99357[0], 99358[0], 99359[0], 99415[0], 99416[0], 99446[0], 99447[0], 99448[0], 99449[0], 99451[0], 99452[0], 99466[0], 99468[0], 99469[0], 99471[0], 99472[0], 99475[0], 99476[0], 99477[0], 99478[0], 99479[0], 99480[0], 99483[0], 99485[0], 99497[0], C8921[1], C8922[1], C8923[1], C8924[1], C8925[1], C8926[1], C8927[0], C8929[1], C8930[1], G0380[1], G0381[1], G0382[1], G0383[1], G0384[1], G0406[0], G0407[0], G0408[0], G0425[0], G0426[0], G0427[0], G0463[0], G0500[0], G0508[0], G0509[0]
00844	01996[1], 0213T[1], 0216T[1], 0228T[1], 0230T[1], 31505[1], 31515[1], 31527[1], 31622[1], 31634[1], 31645[1], 31647[1], 36000[1], 36010[0], 36011[1], 36012[1], 36013[1], 36014[1], 36015[1], 36400[1], 36405[1], 36406[1], 36410[1], 36420[1], 36425[1], 36430[1], 36440[1], 36591[0], 36592[0], 36600[1], 36640[1], 43752[1], 43753[1], 43754[1], 61026[1], 61055[1], 62280[1], 62281[1], 62282[1], 62284[1], 62320[1], 62321[1], 62322[1], 62323[1], 62324[1], 62325[1], 62326[1], 62327[1], 64400[1], 64402[1], 64405[1], 64408[1], 64410[1], 64413[1], 64415[1], 64416[1], 64417[1], 64418[1], 64420[1], 64421[1], 64425[1], 64430[1], 64435[1], 64445[1], 64446[1], 64447[1], 64448[1], 64449[1], 64450[1], 64461[1], 64463[1], 64479[1], 64483[1], 64486[1], 64487[1], 64488[1], 64489[1], 64490[1], 64493[1], 64505[1], 64510[1], 64517[1], 64520[1], 64530[1], 64553[1], 64555[1], 67500[1], 76000[1], 76970[1], 76998[0], 77002[0], 90865[1], 92511[1], 92512[1], 92516[1], 92520[1], 92537[1], 92538[1], 92950[1], 92953[1], 92960[1], 92961[1], 93000[1], 93005[1], 93010[1], 93040[1], 93041[1], 93042[1], 93050[0], 93303[0], 93304[0], 93306[1], 93307[1], 93308[1], 93312[1], 93313[1], 93314[1], 93315[1], 93316[1], 93317[1], 93318[0], 93351[1], 93355[0], 93451[1], 93456[1], 93457[1], 93561[0], 93562[0], 93701[0], 93922[1], 93923[1], 93924[1], 93925[1], 93926[1], 93930[1], 93931[1], 93970[1], 93971[1], 93975[1], 93976[1], 93978[1], 93979[1], 93980[1], 93981[1], 94002[1], 94004[1], 94200[1], 94250[0], 94640[1], 94644[1], 94660[1], 94662[1], 94680[1], 94681[1], 94690[1], 94760[0], 94761[0], 94762[1], 94770[1], 95812[0], 95813[0], 95816[0], 95819[0], 95822[0], 95829[0], 95955[0], 95956[0], 95957[0], 96360[0], 96365[0], 96372[0], 96373[0], 96374[0], 96375[0], 96376[0], 96377[0], 99151[0], 99152[0], 99153[0], 99155[0], 99156[0], 99157[0], 99201[0], 99202[0], 99203[0], 99204[0], 99205[0], 99211[0], 99212[0], 99213[0], 99214[0], 99215[0], 99217[0], 99218[0], 99219[0], 99220[0], 99221[0], 99222[0], 99223[0], 99224[0], 99225[0], 99226[0], 99231[0], 99232[0], 99233[0], 99234[0], 99235[0], 99236[0], 99238[0], 99239[0], 99281[0], 99282[0], 99283[0], 99284[0], 99285[0], 99304[0], 99305[0], 99306[0], 99307[0], 99308[0], 99309[0], 99310[0], 99315[0], 99318[0], 99324[0], 99325[0], 99326[0], 99327[0], 99328[0], 99334[0], 99335[0], 99336[0], 99337[0], 99341[0], 99342[0], 99343[0], 99347[0], 99348[0], 99349[0], 99354[0], 99355[0], 99356[0], 99357[0], 99358[0], 99359[0], 99415[0], 99416[0], 99446[0], 99447[0], 99448[0], 99449[0], 99451[0], 99452[0], 99466[0], 99468[0], 99469[0], 99471[0], 99472[0], 99475[0], 99476[0],

Appendix A: NCCI - CPT Codes

0 = Modifier usage not allowed or inappropriate 1 = Modifier usage allowed

CPT © 2018 American Medical Association. All Rights Reserved.

Code 1	Code 2
	99477[0], 99478[0], 99479[0], 99480[0], 99483[0], 99485[0], 99497[0], C8921[1], C8922[1], C8923[1], C8924[1], C8925[1], C8926[1], C8927[0], C8929[1], C8930[1], G0380[1], G0381[1], G0382[1], G0383[1], G0384[1], G0406[0], G0407[0], G0408[0], G0425[0], G0426[0], G0427[0], G0463[0], G0500[0], G0508[0], G0509[0]
00846	01996[1], 0213T[1], 0216T[1], 0228T[1], 0230T[1], 31505[1], 31515[1], 31527[1], 31622[1], 31634[1], 31645[1], 31647[1], 36000[1], 36010[0], 36011[1], 36012[1], 36013[1], 36014[1], 36015[1], 36400[1], 36405[1], 36406[1], 36410[1], 36420[1], 36425[1], 36430[1], 36440[1], 36591[0], 36592[0], 36600[1], 36640[1], 43752[1], 43753[1], 43754[1], 61026[1], 61055[1], 62280[1], 62281[1], 62282[1], 62284[1], 62320[1], 62321[1], 62322[1], 62323[1], 62324[1], 62325[1], 62326[1], 62327[1], 64400[1], 64402[1], 64405[1], 64408[1], 64410[1], 64413[1], 64415[1], 64416[1], 64417[1], 64418[1], 64420[1], 64421[1], 64425[1], 64430[1], 64435[1], 64445[1], 64446[1], 64447[1], 64448[1], 64449[1], 64450[1], 64461[1], 64463[1], 64479[1], 64483[1], 64486[1], 64487[1], 64488[1], 64489[1], 64490[1], 64493[1], 64505[1], 64510[1], 64517[1], 64520[1], 64530[1], 64553[1], 64555[1], 67500[1], 76000[1], 76970[1], 76998[0], 77002[0], 90865[1], 92511[1], 92512[1], 92516[1], 92520[1], 92537[1], 92538[1], 92950[1], 92953[1], 92960[1], 92961[1], 93000[1], 93005[1], 93010[1], 93040[1], 93041[1], 93042[1], 93050[0], 93303[0], 93304[0], 93306[1], 93307[1], 93308[1], 93312[1], 93313[1], 93314[1], 93315[1], 93316[1], 93317[1], 93318[0], 93351[1], 93355[0], 93451[1], 93456[1], 93457[1], 93561[0], 93562[0], 93701[0], 93922[1], 93923[1], 93924[1], 93925[1], 93926[1], 93930[1], 93931[1], 93970[1], 93971[1], 93975[1], 93976[1], 93978[1], 93979[1], 93980[1], 93981[1], 94002[1], 94004[1], 94200[1], 94250[0], 94640[1], 94644[1], 94660[1], 94662[1], 94680[1], 94681[1], 94690[1], 94760[0], 94761[0], 94762[1], 94770[1], 95812[0], 95813[0], 95816[0], 95819[0], 95822[0], 95829[0], 95955[0], 95956[0], 95957[0], 96360[0], 96365[0], 96372[0], 96373[0], 96374[0], 96375[0], 96376[0], 96377[0], 99151[0], 99152[0], 99153[0], 99155[0], 99156[0], 99157[0], 99201[0], 99202[0], 99203[0], 99204[0], 99205[0], 99211[0], 99212[0], 99213[0], 99214[0], 99215[0], 99217[0], 99218[0], 99219[0], 99220[0], 99221[0], 99222[0], 99223[0], 99224[0], 99225[0], 99226[0], 99231[0], 99232[0], 99233[0], 99234[0], 99235[0], 99236[0], 99238[0], 99239[0], 99281[0], 99282[0], 99283[0], 99284[0], 99285[0], 99304[0], 99305[0], 99306[0], 99307[0], 99308[0], 99309[0], 99310[0], 99315[0], 99318[0], 99324[0], 99325[0], 99326[0], 99327[0], 99328[0], 99334[0], 99335[0], 99336[0], 99337[0], 99341[0], 99342[0], 99343[0], 99347[0], 99348[0], 99349[0], 99354[0], 99355[0], 99356[0], 99357[0], 99358[0], 99359[0], 99415[0], 99416[0], 99446[0], 99447[0], 99448[0], 99449[0], 99451[0], 99452[0], 99466[0], 99468[0], 99469[0], 99471[0], 99472[0], 99475[0], 99476[0], 99477[0], 99478[0], 99479[0], 99480[0], 99483[0], 99485[0], 99497[0], C8921[1], C8922[1], C8923[1], C8924[1], C8925[1], C8926[1], C8927[0], C8929[1], C8930[1], G0380[1], G0381[1], G0382[1], G0383[1], G0384[1], G0406[0], G0407[0], G0408[0], G0425[0], G0426[0], G0427[0], G0463[0], G0500[0], G0508[0], G0509[0]
00848	01996[1], 0213T[1], 0216T[1], 0228T[1], 0230T[1], 31505[1], 31515[1], 31527[1], 31622[1], 31634[1], 31645[1], 31647[1], 36000[1], 36010[0], 36011[1], 36012[1], 36013[1], 36014[1], 36015[1], 36400[1], 36405[1], 36406[1], 36410[1], 36420[1], 36425[1], 36430[1], 36440[1], 36591[0], 36592[0], 36600[1], 36640[1], 43752[1], 43753[1], 43754[1], 61026[1], 61055[1], 62280[1], 62281[1], 62282[1], 62284[1], 62320[1], 62321[1], 62322[1], 62323[1], 62324[1], 62325[1], 62326[1], 62327[1], 64400[1], 64402[1], 64405[1], 64408[1], 64410[1], 64413[1], 64415[1], 64416[1], 64417[1], 64418[1], 64420[1], 64421[1], 64425[1], 64430[1], 64435[1], 64445[1], 64446[1], 64447[1], 64448[1], 64449[1], 64450[1], 64461[1], 64463[1], 64479[1], 64483[1], 64486[1], 64487[1], 64488[1], 64489[1], 64490[1], 64493[1], 64505[1], 64510[1], 64517[1], 64520[1], 64530[1], 64553[1], 64555[1], 67500[1], 76000[1], 76970[1], 76998[0], 77002[0], 90865[1], 92511[1], 92512[1], 92516[1], 92520[1], 92537[1], 92538[1], 92950[1], 92953[1], 92960[1], 92961[1], 93000[1], 93005[1], 93010[1], 93040[1], 93041[1], 93042[1], 93050[0], 93303[0], 93304[0], 93306[1], 93307[1], 93308[1], 93312[1], 93313[1], 93314[1], 93315[1], 93316[1], 93317[1], 93318[0], 93351[1], 93355[0], 93451[1], 93456[1], 93457[1], 93561[0], 93562[0], 93701[0], 93922[1], 93923[1], 93924[1], 93925[1], 93926[1], 93930[1], 93931[1], 93970[1], 93971[1], 93975[1], 93976[1], 93978[1], 93979[1], 93980[1], 93981[1], 94002[1], 94004[1], 94200[1], 94250[0], 94640[1], 94644[1], 94660[1], 94662[1], 94680[1], 94681[1], 94690[1], 94760[0], 94761[0], 94762[1], 94770[1], 95812[0], 95813[0], 95816[0], 95819[0], 95822[0], 95829[0], 95955[0], 95956[0], 95957[0], 96360[0], 96365[0], 96372[0], 96373[0], 96374[0], 96375[0], 96376[0], 96377[0], 99151[0], 99152[0], 99153[0], 99155[0], 99156[0], 99157[0], 99201[0], 99202[0], 99203[0], 99204[0], 99205[0], 99211[0], 99212[0], 99213[0], 99214[0], 99215[0], 99217[0], 99218[0], 99219[0], 99220[0], 99221[0], 99222[0], 99223[0], 99224[0], 99225[0], 99226[0], 99231[0], 99232[0], 99233[0], 99234[0], 99235[0], 99236[0], 99238[0], 99239[0], 99281[0], 99282[0], 99283[0], 99284[0], 99285[0], 99304[0], 99305[0], 99306[0], 99307[0], 99308[0], 99309[0], 99310[0], 99315[0], 99318[0], 99324[0], 99325[0], 99326[0], 99327[0], 99328[0], 99334[0], 99335[0], 99336[0], 99337[0], 99341[0], 99342[0], 99343[0], 99347[0], 99348[0], 99349[0], 99354[0], 99355[0], 99356[0], 99357[0], 99358[0], 99359[0], 99415[0], 99416[0], 99446[0], 99447[0], 99448[0], 99449[0], 99451[0], 99452[0], 99466[0], 99468[0], 99469[0], 99471[0], 99472[0], 99475[0], 99476[0], 99477[0], 99478[0], 99479[0], 99480[0], 99483[0], 99485[0], 99497[0], C8921[1], C8922[1], C8923[1], C8924[1], C8925[1], C8926[1], C8927[0], C8929[1], C8930[1], G0380[1], G0381[1], G0382[1], G0383[1], G0384[1], G0406[0], G0407[0], G0408[0], G0425[0], G0426[0], G0427[0], G0463[0], G0500[0], G0508[0], G0509[0]
00851	01996[1], 0213T[1], 0216T[1], 0228T[1], 0230T[1], 31505[1], 31515[1], 31527[1], 31622[1], 31634[1], 31645[1], 31647[1], 36000[1], 36010[0], 36011[1], 36012[1], 36013[1], 36014[1], 36015[1], 36400[1], 36405[1], 36406[1], 36410[1], 36420[1], 36425[1], 36430[1], 36440[1], 36591[0], 36592[0], 36600[1], 36640[1], 43752[1], 43753[1], 43754[1], 61026[1], 61055[1], 62280[1], 62281[1], 62282[1], 62284[1], 62320[1], 62321[1], 62322[1], 62323[1], 62324[1], 62325[1], 62326[1], 62327[1], 64400[1], 64402[1], 64405[1], 64408[1], 64410[1], 64413[1], 64415[1], 64416[1], 64417[1], 64418[1], 64420[1], 64421[1], 64425[1], 64430[1], 64435[1], 64445[1], 64446[1], 64447[1], 64448[1], 64449[1], 64450[1], 64461[1], 64463[1], 64479[1], 64483[1], 64486[1], 64487[1], 64488[1], 64489[1], 64490[1], 64493[1], 64505[1], 64510[1], 64517[1], 64520[1], 64530[1], 64553[1], 64555[1], 67500[0], 76000[1], 76970[1], 76998[0], 77002[0], 90865[1], 92511[1], 92512[1], 92516[1], 92520[1], 92537[1], 92538[1], 92950[1], 92953[1], 92960[1], 92961[1], 93000[1], 93005[1], 93010[1], 93040[1], 93041[1], 93042[1], 93050[0], 93303[0], 93304[0], 93306[1], 93307[1], 93308[1], 93312[1], 93313[1], 93314[1], 93315[1], 93316[1], 93317[1], 93318[0], 93351[1], 93355[0], 93451[1], 93456[1], 93457[1], 93561[0], 93562[0], 93701[0], 93922[1], 93923[1], 93924[1], 93925[1], 93926[1], 93930[1], 93931[1], 93970[1], 93971[1], 93975[1], 93976[1], 93978[1], 93979[1], 93980[1], 93981[1], 94002[1], 94004[1], 94200[1], 94250[0], 94640[1], 94644[1], 94660[1], 94662[1], 94680[1], 94681[1], 94690[1], 94760[0], 94761[0], 94762[1], 94770[1], 95812[0], 95813[0], 95816[0], 95819[0], 95822[0], 95829[0], 95955[0], 95956[0], 95957[0], 96360[0], 96365[0], 96372[0], 96373[0], 96374[0], 96375[0], 96376[0], 96377[0], 99151[0], 99152[0], 99153[0], 99155[0], 99156[0], 99157[0], 99201[0], 99202[0], 99203[0], 99204[0], 99205[0], 99211[0], 99212[0], 99213[0], 99214[0], 99215[0], 99217[0], 99218[0], 99219[0], 99220[0], 99221[0], 99222[0], 99223[0], 99224[0], 99225[0], 99226[0], 99231[0], 99232[0], 99233[0], 99234[0], 99235[0], 99236[0], 99238[0], 99239[0], 99281[0], 99282[0], 99283[0], 99284[0], 99285[0], 99304[0], 99305[0], 99306[0], 99307[0], 99308[0], 99309[0], 99310[0], 99315[0], 99318[0], 99324[0], 99325[0], 99326[0], 99327[0], 99328[0], 99334[0], 99335[0], 99336[0], 99337[0], 99341[0], 99342[0], 99343[0], 99347[0], 99348[0], 99349[0], 99354[0], 99355[0], 99356[0], 99357[0], 99358[0], 99359[0], 99415[0], 99416[0], 99446[0], 99447[0], 99448[0], 99449[0], 99451[0], 99452[0], 99466[0], 99468[0], 99469[0], 99471[0], 99472[0], 99475[0], 99476[0], 99477[0], 99478[0], 99479[0], 99480[0], 99483[0], 99485[0], 99497[0], C8921[1], C8922[1], C8923[1], C8924[1], C8925[1], C8926[1], C8927[0], C8929[1], C8930[1], G0380[1], G0381[1], G0382[1], G0383[1], G0384[1], G0406[0], G0407[0], G0408[0], G0425[0], G0426[0], G0427[0], G0463[0], G0500[0], G0508[0], G0509[0]
00860	01996[1], 0213T[1], 0216T[1], 0228T[1], 0230T[1], 31505[1], 31515[1], 31527[1], 31622[1], 31634[1], 31645[1], 31647[1], 36000[1], 36010[0], 36011[1], 36012[1], 36013[1], 36014[1], 36015[1], 36400[1], 36405[1], 36406[1], 36410[1], 36420[1], 36425[1], 36430[1], 36440[1], 36591[0], 36592[0], 36600[1], 36640[1], 43752[1], 43753[1], 43754[1], 61026[1], 61055[1], 62280[1], 62281[1], 62282[1], 62284[1], 62320[1], 62321[1], 62322[1], 62323[1], 62324[1], 62325[1], 62326[1], 62327[1], 64400[1], 64402[1], 64405[1], 64408[1], 64410[1], 64413[1], 64415[1], 64416[1], 64417[1], 64418[1], 64420[1], 64421[1], 64425[1], 64430[1], 64435[1], 64445[1], 64446[1], 64447[1], 64448[1], 64449[1], 64450[1], 64461[1], 64463[1], 64479[1], 64483[1], 64486[1], 64487[1], 64488[1], 64489[1], 64490[1], 64493[1], 64505[1], 64510[1], 64517[1], 64520[1], 64530[1], 64553[1], 64555[1], 67500[1], 76000[1], 76970[1], 76998[0], 77002[0], 90865[1], 92511[1], 92512[1], 92516[1], 92520[1], 92537[1], 92538[1], 92950[1], 92953[1], 92960[1], 92961[1], 93000[1], 93005[1], 93010[1], 93040[1], 93041[1], 93042[1], 93050[0], 93303[0], 93304[0], 93306[1], 93307[1], 93308[1], 93312[1], 93313[1], 93314[1], 93315[1], 93316[1], 93317[1], 93318[0], 93351[1], 93355[0], 93451[1], 93456[1], 93457[1], 93561[0], 93562[0], 93701[0], 93922[1], 93923[1], 93924[1], 93925[1], 93926[1], 93930[1], 93931[1], 93970[1], 93971[1], 93975[1], 93976[1], 93978[1], 93979[1], 93980[1], 93981[1], 94002[1], 94004[1], 94200[1], 94250[0], 94640[1], 94644[1], 94660[1], 94662[1], 94680[1], 94681[1], 94690[1], 94760[0], 94761[0], 94762[1], 94770[1], 95812[0], 95813[0], 95816[0], 95819[0], 95822[0], 95829[0], 95955[0], 95956[0], 95957[0], 96360[0], 96365[0], 96372[0], 96373[0], 96374[0], 96375[0], 96376[0], 96377[0], 99151[0], 99152[0], 99153[0], 99155[0], 99156[0], 99157[0], 99201[0], 99202[0], 99203[0], 99204[0], 99205[0], 99211[0], 99212[0], 99213[0], 99214[0], 99215[0], 99217[0], 99218[0], 99219[0], 99220[0], 99221[0], 99222[0], 99223[0], 99224[0], 99225[0], 99226[0], 99231[0], 99232[0], 99233[0], 99234[0], 99235[0], 99236[0], 99238[0], 99239[0], 99281[0], 99282[0], 99283[0], 99284[0], 99285[0], 99304[0], 99305[0], 99306[0], 99307[0], 99308[0], 99309[0], 99310[0], 99315[0], 99318[0], 99324[0], 99325[0], 99326[0], 99327[0], 99328[0], 99334[0], 99335[0], 99336[0], 99337[0], 99341[0], 99342[0], 99343[0], 99347[0], 99348[0], 99349[0], 99354[0], 99355[0], 99356[0], 99357[0], 99358[0], 99359[0], 99415[0], 99416[0], 99446[0], 99447[0], 99448[0], 99449[0], 99451[0], 99452[0], 99466[0], 99468[0], 99469[0], 99471[0], 99472[0], 99475[0], 99476[0], 99477[0], 99478[0], 99479[0], 99480[0], 99483[0], 99485[0], 99497[0], C8921[1], C8922[1], C8923[1], C8924[1], C8925[1], C8926[1], C8927[0], C8929[1], C8930[1], G0380[1], G0381[1], G0382[1], G0383[1], G0384[1], G0406[0], G0407[0], G0408[0], G0425[0], G0426[0], G0427[0], G0463[0], G0500[0], G0508[0], G0509[0]
00862	01996[1], 0213T[1], 0216T[1], 0228T[1], 0230T[1], 31505[1], 31515[1], 31527[1], 31622[1], 31634[1], 31645[1], 31647[1], 36000[1], 36010[0], 36011[1], 36012[1], 36013[1], 36014[1], 36015[1], 36400[1], 36405[1], 36406[1], 36410[1], 36420[1], 36425[1], 36430[1], 36440[1], 36591[0], 36592[0], 36600[1], 36640[1], 43752[1], 43753[1], 43754[1], 61026[1], 61055[1], 62280[1], 62281[1], 62282[1], 62284[1], 62320[1], 62321[1], 62322[1], 62323[1], 62324[1], 62325[1], 62326[1], 62327[1], 64400[1], 64402[1], 64405[1], 64408[1], 64410[1], 64413[1], 64415[1], 64416[1], 64417[1], 64418[1], 64420[1], 64421[1],

0 = Modifier usage not allowed or inappropriate 1 = Modifier usage allowed

CPT © 2018 American Medical Association. All Rights Reserved.

Code 1	Code 2
	64425[1], 64430[1], 64435[1], 64445[1], 64446[1], 64447[1], 64448[1], 64449[1], 64450[1], 64461[1], 64463[1], 64479[1], 64483[1], 64486[1], 64487[1], 64488[1], 64489[1], 64490[1], 64493[1], 64505[1], 64510[1], 64517[1], 64520[1], 64530[1], 64553[1], 64555[1], 67500[1], 76000[1], 76970[1], 76998[0], 77002[0], 90865[1], 92511[1], 92512[1], 92516[1], 92520[1], 92537[1], 92538[1], 92950[1], 92953[1], 92960[1], 92961[1], 93000[1], 93005[1], 93010[1], 93040[1], 93041[1], 93042[1], 93050[0], 93303[0], 93304[0], 93306[1], 93307[1], 93308[1], 93312[1], 93313[1], 93314[1], 93315[1], 93316[1], 93317[1], 93318[0], 93351[1], 93355[0], 93451[1], 93456[1], 93457[1], 93561[0], 93562[0], 93701[0], 93922[1], 93923[1], 93924[1], 93925[1], 93926[1], 93930[1], 93931[1], 93970[1], 93971[1], 93975[1], 93976[1], 93978[1], 93979[1], 93980[1], 93981[1], 94002[1], 94004[1], 94200[1], 94250[0], 94640[1], 94644[1], 94660[1], 94662[1], 94680[1], 94681[1], 94690[1], 94760[0], 94761[0], 94762[1], 94770[1], 95812[0], 95813[0], 95816[0], 95819[0], 95822[0], 95829[0], 95955[0], 95956[0], 95957[0], 96360[0], 96365[0], 96372[0], 96373[0], 96374[0], 96375[0], 96376[0], 96377[0], 99151[0], 99152[0], 99153[0], 99155[0], 99156[0], 99157[0], 99201[0], 99202[0], 99203[0], 99204[0], 99205[0], 99211[0], 99212[0], 99213[0], 99214[0], 99215[0], 99217[0], 99218[0], 99219[0], 99220[0], 99221[0], 99222[0], 99223[0], 99224[0], 99225[0], 99226[0], 99231[0], 99232[0], 99233[0], 99234[0], 99235[0], 99236[0], 99238[0], 99239[0], 99281[0], 99282[0], 99283[0], 99284[0], 99285[0], 99304[0], 99305[0], 99306[0], 99307[0], 99308[0], 99309[0], 99310[0], 99315[0], 99318[0], 99324[0], 99325[0], 99326[0], 99327[0], 99328[0], 99334[0], 99335[0], 99336[0], 99337[0], 99341[0], 99342[0], 99343[0], 99347[0], 99348[0], 99349[0], 99354[0], 99355[0], 99356[0], 99357[0], 99358[0], 99359[0], 99415[0], 99416[0], 99446[0], 99447[0], 99448[0], 99449[0], 99451[0], 99452[0], 99466[0], 99468[0], 99469[0], 99471[0], 99472[0], 99475[0], 99476[0], 99477[0], 99478[0], 99479[0], 99480[0], 99483[0], 99485[0], 99497[0], C8921[1], C8922[1], C8923[1], C8924[1], C8925[1], C8926[1], C8927[0], C8929[1], C8930[1], G0380[1], G0381[1], G0382[1], G0383[1], G0384[1], G0406[0], G0407[0], G0408[0], G0425[0], G0426[0], G0427[0], G0463[0], G0500[0], G0508[0], G0509[0]
00864	01996[1], 0213T[1], 0216T[1], 0228T[1], 0230T[1], 31505[1], 31515[1], 31527[1], 31622[1], 31634[1], 31645[1], 31647[1], 36000[1], 36010[0], 36011[1], 36012[1], 36013[1], 36014[1], 36015[1], 36400[1], 36405[1], 36406[1], 36410[1], 36420[1], 36425[1], 36430[1], 36440[1], 36591[0], 36592[0], 36600[1], 36640[1], 43752[1], 43753[1], 43754[1], 61026[1], 61055[1], 62280[1], 62281[1], 62282[1], 62284[1], 62320[1], 62321[1], 62322[1], 62323[1], 62324[1], 62325[1], 62326[1], 62327[1], 64400[1], 64402[1], 64405[1], 64408[1], 64410[1], 64413[1], 64415[1], 64416[1], 64417[1], 64418[1], 64420[1], 64421[1], 64425[1], 64430[1], 64435[1], 64445[1], 64446[1], 64447[1], 64448[1], 64449[1], 64450[1], 64461[1], 64463[1], 64479[1], 64483[1], 64486[1], 64487[1], 64488[1], 64489[1], 64490[1], 64493[1], 64505[1], 64510[1], 64517[1], 64520[1], 64530[1], 64553[1], 64555[1], 67500[1], 76000[1], 76970[1], 76998[0], 77002[0], 90865[1], 92511[1], 92512[1], 92516[1], 92520[1], 92537[1], 92538[1], 92950[1], 92953[1], 92960[1], 92961[1], 93000[1], 93005[1], 93010[1], 93040[1], 93041[1], 93042[1], 93050[0], 93303[0], 93304[0], 93306[1], 93307[1], 93308[1], 93312[1], 93313[1], 93314[1], 93315[1], 93316[1], 93317[1], 93318[0], 93351[1], 93355[0], 93451[1], 93456[1], 93457[1], 93561[0], 93562[0], 93701[0], 93922[1], 93923[1], 93924[1], 93925[1], 93926[1], 93930[1], 93931[1], 93970[1], 93971[1], 93975[1], 93976[1], 93978[1], 93979[1], 93980[1], 93981[1], 94002[1], 94004[1], 94200[1], 94250[0], 94640[1], 94644[1], 94660[1], 94662[1], 94680[1], 94681[1], 94690[1], 94760[0], 94761[0], 94762[1], 94770[1], 95812[0], 95813[0], 95816[0], 95819[0], 95822[0], 95829[0], 95955[0], 95956[0], 95957[0], 96360[0], 96365[0], 96372[0], 96373[0], 96374[0], 96375[0], 96376[0], 96377[0], 99151[0], 99152[0], 99153[0], 99155[0], 99156[0], 99157[0], 99201[0], 99202[0], 99203[0], 99204[0], 99205[0], 99211[0], 99212[0], 99213[0], 99214[0], 99215[0], 99217[0], 99218[0], 99219[0], 99220[0], 99221[0], 99222[0], 99223[0], 99224[0], 99225[0], 99226[0], 99231[0], 99232[0], 99233[0], 99234[0], 99235[0], 99236[0], 99238[0], 99239[0], 99281[0], 99282[0], 99283[0], 99284[0], 99285[0], 99304[0], 99305[0], 99306[0], 99307[0], 99308[0], 99309[0], 99310[0], 99315[0], 99318[0], 99324[0], 99325[0], 99326[0], 99327[0], 99328[0], 99334[0], 99335[0], 99336[0], 99337[0], 99341[0], 99342[0], 99343[0], 99347[0], 99348[0], 99349[0], 99354[0], 99355[0], 99356[0], 99357[0], 99358[0], 99359[0], 99415[0], 99416[0], 99446[0], 99447[0], 99448[0], 99449[0], 99451[0], 99452[0], 99466[0], 99468[0], 99469[0], 99471[0], 99472[0], 99475[0], 99476[0], 99477[0], 99478[0], 99479[0], 99480[0], 99483[0], 99485[0], 99497[0], C8921[1], C8922[1], C8923[1], C8924[1], C8925[1], C8926[1], C8927[0], C8929[1], C8930[1], G0380[1], G0381[1], G0382[1], G0383[1], G0384[1], G0406[0], G0407[0], G0408[0], G0425[0], G0426[0], G0427[0], G0463[0], G0500[0], G0508[0], G0509[0]
00865	01996[1], 0213T[1], 0216T[1], 0228T[1], 0230T[1], 31505[1], 31515[1], 31527[1], 31622[1], 31634[1], 31645[1], 31647[1], 36000[1], 36010[1], 36011[1], 36012[1], 36013[1], 36014[1], 36015[1], 36400[1], 36405[1], 36406[1], 36410[1], 36420[1], 36425[1], 36430[1], 36440[1], 36591[0], 36592[0], 36600[1], 36640[1], 43752[1], 43753[1], 43754[1], 61026[1], 61055[1], 62280[1], 62281[1], 62282[1], 62284[1], 62320[1], 62321[1], 62322[1], 62323[1], 62324[1], 62325[1], 62326[1], 62327[1], 64400[1], 64402[1], 64405[1], 64408[1], 64410[1], 64413[1], 64415[1], 64416[1], 64417[1], 64418[1], 64420[1], 64421[1], 64425[1], 64430[1], 64435[1], 64445[1], 64446[1], 64447[1], 64448[1], 64449[1], 64450[1], 64461[1], 64463[1], 64479[1], 64483[1], 64486[1], 64487[1], 64488[1], 64489[1], 64490[1], 64493[1], 64505[1], 64510[1], 64517[1], 64520[1], 64530[1], 64553[1], 64555[1], 67500[1], 76000[1], 76970[1], 76998[0], 77002[0], 90865[1], 92511[1], 92512[1], 92516[1], 92520[1], 92537[1], 92538[1], 92950[1], 92953[1], 92960[1], 92961[1], 93000[1], 93005[1], 93010[1], 93040[1], 93041[1], 93042[1], 93050[0], 93303[1], 93304[1], 93306[1], 93307[1], 93308[1], 93312[1], 93313[1], 93314[1], 93315[1], 93316[1], 93317[1], 93318[0], 93351[1], 93355[0], 93451[1], 93456[1], 93457[1], 93561[0], 93562[0], 93701[0], 93922[1], 93923[1], 93924[1], 93925[1], 93926[1], 93930[1], 93931[1], 93970[1], 93971[1], 93975[1], 93976[1], 93978[1], 93979[1], 93980[1], 93981[1], 94002[1], 94004[1], 94200[1], 94250[0], 94640[1], 94644[1], 94660[1], 94662[1], 94680[1], 94681[1], 94690[1], 94760[0], 94761[0], 94762[1], 94770[1], 95812[0], 95813[0], 95816[0], 95819[0], 95822[0], 95829[0], 95955[0], 95956[0], 95957[0], 96360[0], 96365[0], 96372[0], 96373[0], 96374[0], 96375[0], 96376[0], 96377[0], 99151[0], 99152[0], 99153[0], 99155[0], 99156[0], 99157[0], 99201[0], 99202[0], 99203[0], 99204[0], 99205[0], 99211[0], 99212[0], 99213[0], 99214[0], 99215[0], 99217[0], 99218[0], 99219[0], 99220[0], 99221[0], 99222[0], 99223[0], 99224[0], 99225[0], 99226[0], 99231[0], 99232[0], 99233[0], 99234[0], 99235[0], 99236[0], 99238[0], 99239[0], 99281[0], 99282[0], 99283[0], 99284[0], 99285[0], 99304[0], 99305[0], 99306[0], 99307[0], 99308[0], 99309[0], 99310[0], 99315[0], 99318[0], 99324[0], 99325[0], 99326[0], 99327[0], 99328[0], 99334[0], 99335[0], 99336[0], 99337[0], 99341[0], 99342[0], 99343[0], 99347[0], 99348[0], 99349[0], 99354[0], 99355[0], 99356[0], 99357[0], 99358[0], 99359[0], 99415[0], 99416[0], 99446[0], 99447[0], 99448[0], 99449[0], 99451[0], 99452[0], 99466[0], 99468[0], 99469[0], 99471[0], 99472[0], 99475[0], 99476[0], 99477[0], 99478[0], 99479[0], 99480[0], 99483[0], 99485[0], 99497[0], C8921[1], C8922[1], C8923[1], C8924[1], C8925[1], C8926[1], C8927[0], C8929[1], C8930[1], G0380[1], G0381[1], G0382[1], G0383[1], G0384[1], G0406[0], G0407[0], G0408[0], G0425[0], G0426[0], G0427[0], G0463[0], G0500[0], G0508[0], G0509[0]
00866	01996[1], 0213T[1], 0216T[1], 0228T[1], 0230T[1], 31505[1], 31515[1], 31527[1], 31622[1], 31634[1], 31645[1], 31647[1], 36000[1], 36010[0], 36011[1], 36012[1], 36013[1], 36014[1], 36015[1], 36400[1], 36405[1], 36406[1], 36410[1], 36420[1], 36425[1], 36430[1], 36440[1], 36591[0], 36592[0], 36600[1], 36640[1], 43752[1], 43753[1], 43754[1], 61026[1], 61055[1], 62280[1], 62281[1], 62282[1], 62284[1], 62320[1], 62321[1], 62322[1], 62323[1], 62324[1], 62325[1], 62326[1], 62327[1], 64400[1], 64402[1], 64405[1], 64408[1], 64410[1], 64413[1], 64415[1], 64416[1], 64417[1], 64418[1], 64420[1], 64421[1], 64425[1], 64430[1], 64435[1], 64445[1], 64446[1], 64447[1], 64448[1], 64449[1], 64450[1], 64461[1], 64463[1], 64479[1], 64483[1], 64486[1], 64487[1], 64488[1], 64489[1], 64490[1], 64493[1], 64505[1], 64510[1], 64517[1], 64520[1], 64530[1], 64553[1], 64555[1], 67500[1], 76000[1], 76970[1], 76998[0], 77002[0], 90865[1], 92511[1], 92512[1], 92516[1], 92520[1], 92537[1], 92538[1], 92950[1], 92953[1], 92960[1], 92961[1], 93000[1], 93005[1], 93010[1], 93040[1], 93041[1], 93042[1], 93050[0], 93303[0], 93304[0], 93306[1], 93307[1], 93308[1], 93312[1], 93313[1], 93314[1], 93315[1], 93316[1], 93317[1], 93318[0], 93351[1], 93355[0], 93451[1], 93456[1], 93457[1], 93561[0], 93562[0], 93701[0], 93922[1], 93923[1], 93924[1], 93925[1], 93926[1], 93930[1], 93931[1], 93970[1], 93971[1], 93975[1], 93976[1], 93978[1], 93979[1], 93980[1], 93981[1], 94002[1], 94004[1], 94200[1], 94250[0], 94640[1], 94644[1], 94660[1], 94662[1], 94680[1], 94681[1], 94690[1], 94760[0], 94761[0], 94762[1], 94770[1], 95812[0], 95813[0], 95816[0], 95819[0], 95822[0], 95829[0], 95955[0], 95956[0], 95957[0], 96360[0], 96365[0], 96372[0], 96373[0], 96374[0], 96375[0], 96376[0], 96377[0], 99151[0], 99152[0], 99153[0], 99155[0], 99156[0], 99157[0], 99201[0], 99202[0], 99203[0], 99204[0], 99205[0], 99211[0], 99212[0], 99213[0], 99214[0], 99215[0], 99217[0], 99218[0], 99219[0], 99220[0], 99221[0], 99222[0], 99223[0], 99224[0], 99225[0], 99226[0], 99231[0], 99232[0], 99233[0], 99234[0], 99235[0], 99236[0], 99238[0], 99239[0], 99281[0], 99282[0], 99283[0], 99284[0], 99285[0], 99304[0], 99305[0], 99306[0], 99307[0], 99308[0], 99309[0], 99310[0], 99315[0], 99318[0], 99324[0], 99325[0], 99326[0], 99327[0], 99328[0], 99334[0], 99335[0], 99336[0], 99337[0], 99341[0], 99342[0], 99343[0], 99347[0], 99348[0], 99349[0], 99354[0], 99355[0], 99356[0], 99357[0], 99358[0], 99359[0], 99415[0], 99416[0], 99446[0], 99447[0], 99448[0], 99449[0], 99451[0], 99452[0], 99466[0], 99468[0], 99469[0], 99471[0], 99472[0], 99475[0], 99476[0], 99477[0], 99478[0], 99479[0], 99480[0], 99483[0], 99485[0], 99497[0], C8921[1], C8922[1], C8923[1], C8924[1], C8925[1], C8926[1], C8927[0], C8929[1], C8930[1], G0380[1], G0381[1], G0382[1], G0383[1], G0384[1], G0406[0], G0407[0], G0408[0], G0425[0], G0426[0], G0427[0], G0463[0], G0500[0], G0508[0], G0509[0]
00868	01996[1], 0213T[1], 0216T[1], 0228T[1], 0230T[1], 31505[1], 31515[1], 31527[1], 31622[1], 31634[1], 31645[1], 31647[1], 36000[1], 36010[0], 36011[1], 36012[1], 36013[1], 36014[1], 36015[1], 36400[1], 36405[1], 36406[1], 36410[1], 36420[1], 36425[1], 36430[1], 36440[1], 36591[0], 36592[0], 36600[1], 36640[1], 43752[1], 43753[1], 43754[1], 61026[1], 61055[1], 62280[1], 62281[1], 62282[1], 62284[1], 62320[1], 62321[1], 62322[1], 62323[1], 62324[1], 62325[1], 62326[1], 62327[1], 64400[1], 64402[1], 64405[1], 64408[1], 64410[1], 64413[1], 64415[1], 64416[1], 64417[1], 64418[1], 64420[1], 64421[1], 64425[1], 64430[1], 64435[1], 64445[1], 64446[1], 64447[1], 64448[1], 64449[1], 64450[1], 64461[1], 64463[1], 64479[1], 64483[1], 64486[1], 64487[1], 64488[1], 64489[1], 64490[1], 64493[1], 64505[1], 64510[1], 64517[1], 64520[1], 64530[1], 64553[1], 64555[1], 67500[1], 76000[1], 76970[1], 76998[0], 77002[0], 90865[1], 92511[1], 92512[1], 92516[1], 92520[1], 92537[1], 92538[1], 92950[1], 92953[1], 92960[1], 92961[1], 93000[1], 93005[1], 93010[1], 93040[1], 93041[1], 93042[1], 93050[0], 93303[0], 93304[0], 93306[1], 93307[1], 93308[1], 93312[1], 93313[1], 93314[1], 93315[1], 93316[1], 93317[1], 93318[0], 93351[1], 93355[0], 93451[1], 93456[1], 93457[1], 93561[0], 93562[0], 93701[0], 93922[1], 93923[1], 93924[1], 93925[1], 93926[1], 93930[1], 93931[1], 93970[1], 93971[1], 93975[1], 93976[1], 93978[1], 93979[1], 93980[1], 93981[1], 94002[1], 94004[1], 94200[1], 94250[0], 94640[1], 94644[1], 94660[1], 94662[1], 94680[1], 94681[1], 94690[1], 94760[0], 94761[0], 94762[1], 94770[1], 95812[0], 95813[0], 95816[0], 95819[0], 95822[0], 95829[0], 95955[0], 95956[0], 95957[0], 96360[0], 96365[0], 96372[0], 96373[0], 96374[0], 96375[0], 96376[0], 96377[0], 99151[0], 99152[0], 99153[0], 99155[0],

0 = Modifier usage not allowed or inappropriate 1 = Modifier usage allowed

CPT © 2018 American Medical Association. All Rights Reserved.

Code 1	Code 2
	99156^0, 99157^0, 99201^0, 99202^0, 99203^0, 99204^0, 99205^0, 99211^0, 99212^0, 99213^0, 99214^0, 99215^0, 99217^0, 99218^0, 99219^0, 99220^0, 99221^0, 99222^0, 99223^0, 99224^0, 99225^0, 99226^0, 99231^0, 99232^0, 99233^0, 99234^0, 99235^0, 99236^0, 99238^0, 99239^0, 99281^0, 99282^0, 99283^0, 99284^0, 99285^0, 99304^0, 99305^0, 99306^0, 99307^0, 99308^0, 99309^0, 99310^0, 99315^0, 99318^0, 99324^0, 99325^0, 99326^0, 99327^0, 99328^0, 99334^0, 99335^0, 99336^0, 99337^0, 99341^0, 99342^0, 99343^0, 99347^0, 99348^0, 99349^0, 99354^0, 99355^0, 99356^0, 99357^0, 99358^0, 99359^0, 99415^0, 99416^0, 99446^0, 99447^0, 99448^0, 99449^0, 99451^0, 99452^0, 99466^0, 99468^0, 99469^0, 99471^0, 99472^0, 99475^0, 99476^0, 99477^0, 99478^0, 99479^0, 99480^0, 99483^0, 99485^0, 99497^0, C8921^1, C8922^1, C8923^1, C8924^1, C8925^1, C8926^1, C8927^0, C8929^1, C8930^1, G0380^1, G0381^1, G0382^1, G0383^1, G0384^1, G0406^0, G0407^0, G0408^0, G0425^0, G0426^0, G0427^0, G0463^0, G0500^0, G0508^0, G0509^0
00870	01996^1, 0213T^1, 0216T^1, 0228T^1, 0230T^1, 31505^1, 31515^1, 31527^1, 31622^1, 31634^1, 31645^1, 31647^1, 36000^1, 36010^0, 36011^1, 36012^1, 36013^1, 36014^1, 36015^1, 36400^1, 36405^1, 36406^1, 36410^1, 36420^1, 36425^1, 36430^1, 36440^1, 36591^0, 36592^0, 36600^1, 36640^1, 43752^1, 43753^1, 43754^1, 61026^1, 61055^1, 62280^1, 62281^1, 62282^1, 62284^1, 62320^1, 62321^1, 62322^1, 62323^1, 62324^1, 62325^1, 62326^1, 62327^1, 64400^1, 64402^1, 64405^1, 64408^1, 64410^1, 64413^1, 64415^1, 64416^1, 64417^1, 64418^1, 64420^1, 64421^1, 64425^1, 64430^1, 64435^1, 64445^1, 64446^1, 64447^1, 64448^1, 64449^1, 64450^1, 64461^1, 64463^1, 64479^1, 64483^1, 64486^1, 64487^1, 64488^1, 64489^1, 64490^1, 64493^1, 64505^1, 64510^1, 64517^1, 64520^1, 64530^1, 64553^1, 64555^1, 67500^1, 76000^1, 76970^1, 76998^0, 77002^0, 90865^1, 92511^1, 92512^1, 92516^1, 92520^1, 92537^1, 92538^1, 92950^1, 92953^1, 92960^1, 92961^1, 93000^1, 93005^1, 93010^1, 93040^1, 93041^1, 93042^1, 93050^0, 93303^0, 93304^0, 93306^1, 93307^1, 93308^1, 93312^1, 93313^1, 93314^1, 93315^1, 93316^1, 93317^1, 93318^0, 93351^1, 93355^0, 93451^1, 93456^1, 93457^1, 93561^0, 93562^0, 93701^0, 93922^1, 93923^1, 93924^1, 93925^1, 93926^1, 93930^1, 93931^1, 93970^1, 93971^1, 93975^1, 93976^1, 93978^1, 93979^1, 93980^1, 93981^1, 94002^1, 94004^1, 94200^1, 94250^0, 94640^1, 94644^1, 94660^1, 94662^1, 94680^1, 94681^1, 94690^1, 94760^0, 94761^0, 94762^1, 94770^1, 95812^0, 95813^0, 95816^0, 95819^0, 95822^0, 95829^0, 95955^0, 95956^0, 95957^0, 96360^0, 96365^0, 96372^0, 96373^0, 96374^0, 96375^0, 96376^0, 96377^0, 99151^0, 99152^0, 99153^0, 99155^0, 99156^0, 99157^0, 99201^0, 99202^0, 99203^0, 99204^0, 99205^0, 99211^0, 99212^0, 99213^0, 99214^0, 99215^0, 99217^0, 99218^0, 99219^0, 99220^0, 99221^0, 99222^0, 99223^0, 99224^0, 99225^0, 99226^0, 99231^0, 99232^0, 99233^0, 99234^0, 99235^0, 99236^0, 99238^0, 99239^0, 99281^0, 99282^0, 99283^0, 99284^0, 99285^0, 99304^0, 99305^0, 99306^0, 99307^0, 99308^0, 99309^0, 99310^0, 99315^0, 99318^0, 99324^0, 99325^0, 99326^0, 99327^0, 99328^0, 99334^0, 99335^0, 99336^0, 99337^0, 99341^0, 99342^0, 99343^0, 99347^0, 99348^0, 99349^0, 99354^0, 99355^0, 99356^0, 99357^0, 99358^0, 99359^0, 99415^0, 99416^0, 99446^0, 99447^0, 99448^0, 99449^0, 99451^0, 99452^0, 99466^0, 99468^0, 99469^0, 99471^0, 99472^0, 99475^0, 99476^0, 99477^0, 99478^0, 99479^0, 99480^0, 99483^0, 99485^0, 99497^0, C8921^1, C8922^1, C8923^1, C8924^1, C8925^1, C8926^1, C8927^0, C8929^1, C8930^1, G0380^1, G0381^1, G0382^1, G0383^1, G0384^1, G0406^0, G0407^0, G0408^0, G0425^0, G0426^0, G0427^0, G0463^0, G0500^0, G0508^0, G0509^0
00872	01996^1, 0213T^1, 0216T^1, 0228T^1, 0230T^1, 31505^1, 31515^1, 31527^1, 31622^1, 31634^1, 31645^1, 31647^1, 36000^1, 36010^0, 36011^1, 36012^1, 36013^1, 36014^1, 36015^1, 36400^1, 36405^1, 36406^1, 36410^1, 36420^1, 36425^1, 36430^1, 36440^1, 36591^0, 36592^0, 36600^1, 36640^1, 43752^1, 43753^1, 43754^1, 61026^1, 61055^1, 62280^1, 62281^1, 62282^1, 62284^1, 62320^1, 62321^1, 62322^1, 62323^1, 62324^1, 62325^1, 62326^1, 62327^1, 64400^1, 64402^1, 64405^1, 64408^1, 64410^1, 64413^1, 64415^1, 64416^1, 64417^1, 64418^1, 64420^1, 64421^1, 64425^1, 64430^1, 64435^1, 64445^1, 64446^1, 64447^1, 64448^1, 64449^1, 64450^1, 64461^1, 64463^1, 64479^1, 64483^1, 64486^1, 64487^1, 64488^1, 64489^1, 64490^1, 64493^1, 64505^1, 64510^1, 64517^1, 64520^1, 64530^1, 64553^1, 64555^1, 67500^1, 76000^1, 76970^1, 76998^0, 77002^0, 90865^1, 92511^1, 92512^1, 92516^1, 92520^1, 92537^1, 92538^1, 92950^1, 92953^1, 92960^1, 92961^1, 93000^1, 93005^1, 93010^1, 93040^1, 93041^1, 93042^1, 93050^0, 93303^0, 93304^0, 93306^1, 93307^1, 93308^1, 93312^1, 93313^1, 93314^1, 93315^1, 93316^1, 93317^1, 93318^0, 93351^1, 93355^0, 93451^1, 93456^1, 93457^1, 93561^0, 93562^0, 93701^0, 93922^1, 93923^1, 93924^1, 93925^1, 93926^1, 93930^1, 93931^1, 93970^1, 93971^1, 93975^1, 93976^1, 93978^1, 93979^1, 93980^1, 93981^1, 94002^1, 94004^1, 94200^1, 94250^0, 94640^1, 94644^1, 94660^1, 94662^1, 94680^1, 94681^1, 94690^1, 94760^0, 94761^0, 94762^1, 94770^1, 95812^0, 95813^0, 95816^0, 95819^0, 95822^0, 95829^0, 95955^0, 95956^0, 95957^0, 96360^0, 96365^0, 96372^0, 96373^0, 96374^0, 96375^0, 96376^0, 96377^0, 99151^0, 99152^0, 99153^0, 99155^0, 99156^0, 99157^0, 99201^0, 99202^0, 99203^0, 99204^0, 99205^0, 99211^0, 99212^0, 99213^0, 99214^0, 99215^0, 99217^0, 99218^0, 99219^0, 99220^0, 99221^0, 99222^0, 99223^0, 99224^0, 99225^0, 99226^0, 99231^0, 99232^0, 99233^0, 99234^0, 99235^0, 99236^0, 99238^0, 99239^0, 99281^0, 99282^0, 99283^0, 99284^0, 99285^0, 99304^0, 99305^0, 99306^0, 99307^0, 99308^0, 99309^0, 99310^0, 99315^0, 99318^0, 99324^0, 99325^0, 99326^0, 99327^0, 99328^0, 99334^0, 99335^0, 99336^0, 99337^0, 99341^0, 99342^0, 99343^0, 99347^0, 99348^0, 99349^0, 99354^0,
	99355^0, 99356^0, 99357^0, 99358^0, 99359^0, 99415^0, 99416^0, 99446^0, 99447^0, 99448^0, 99449^0, 99451^0, 99452^0, 99466^0, 99468^0, 99469^0, 99471^0, 99472^0, 99475^0, 99476^0, 99477^0, 99478^0, 99479^0, 99480^0, 99483^0, 99485^0, 99497^0, C8921^1, C8922^1, C8923^1, C8924^1, C8925^1, C8926^1, C8927^0, C8929^1, C8930^1, G0380^1, G0381^1, G0382^1, G0383^1, G0384^1, G0406^0, G0407^0, G0408^0, G0425^0, G0426^0, G0427^0, G0463^0, G0500^0, G0508^0, G0509^0
00873	01996^1, 0213T^1, 0216T^1, 0228T^1, 0230T^1, 31505^1, 31515^1, 31527^1, 31622^1, 31634^1, 31645^1, 31647^1, 36000^1, 36010^0, 36011^1, 36012^1, 36013^1, 36014^1, 36015^1, 36400^1, 36405^1, 36406^1, 36410^1, 36420^1, 36425^1, 36430^1, 36440^1, 36591^0, 36592^0, 36600^1, 36640^1, 43752^1, 43753^1, 43754^1, 61026^1, 61055^1, 62280^1, 62281^1, 62282^1, 62284^1, 62320^1, 62321^1, 62322^1, 62323^1, 62324^1, 62325^1, 62326^1, 62327^1, 64400^1, 64402^1, 64405^1, 64408^1, 64410^1, 64413^1, 64415^1, 64416^1, 64417^1, 64418^1, 64420^1, 64421^1, 64425^1, 64430^1, 64435^1, 64445^1, 64446^1, 64447^1, 64448^1, 64449^1, 64450^1, 64461^1, 64463^1, 64479^1, 64483^1, 64486^1, 64487^1, 64488^1, 64489^1, 64490^1, 64493^1, 64505^1, 64510^1, 64517^1, 64520^1, 64530^1, 64553^1, 64555^1, 67500^1, 76000^1, 76970^1, 76998^0, 77002^0, 90865^1, 92511^1, 92512^1, 92516^1, 92520^1, 92537^1, 92538^1, 92950^1, 92953^1, 92960^1, 92961^1, 93000^1, 93005^1, 93010^1, 93040^1, 93041^1, 93042^1, 93050^0, 93303^0, 93304^0, 93306^1, 93307^1, 93308^1, 93312^1, 93313^1, 93314^1, 93315^1, 93316^1, 93317^1, 93318^0, 93351^1, 93355^0, 93451^1, 93456^1, 93457^1, 93561^0, 93562^0, 93701^0, 93922^1, 93923^1, 93924^1, 93925^1, 93926^1, 93930^1, 93931^1, 93970^1, 93971^1, 93975^1, 93976^1, 93978^1, 93979^1, 93980^1, 93981^1, 94002^1, 94004^1, 94200^1, 94250^0, 94640^1, 94644^1, 94660^1, 94662^1, 94680^1, 94681^1, 94690^1, 94760^0, 94761^0, 94762^1, 94770^1, 95812^0, 95813^0, 95816^0, 95819^0, 95822^0, 95829^0, 95955^0, 95956^0, 95957^0, 96360^0, 96365^0, 96372^0, 96373^0, 96374^0, 96375^0, 96376^0, 96377^0, 99151^0, 99152^0, 99153^0, 99155^0, 99156^0, 99157^0, 99201^0, 99202^0, 99203^0, 99204^0, 99205^0, 99211^0, 99212^0, 99213^0, 99214^0, 99215^0, 99217^0, 99218^0, 99219^0, 99220^0, 99221^0, 99222^0, 99223^0, 99224^0, 99225^0, 99226^0, 99231^0, 99232^0, 99233^0, 99234^0, 99235^0, 99236^0, 99238^0, 99239^0, 99281^0, 99282^0, 99283^0, 99284^0, 99285^0, 99304^0, 99305^0, 99306^0, 99307^0, 99308^0, 99309^0, 99310^0, 99315^0, 99318^0, 99324^0, 99325^0, 99326^0, 99327^0, 99328^0, 99334^0, 99335^0, 99336^0, 99337^0, 99341^0, 99342^0, 99343^0, 99347^0, 99348^0, 99349^0, 99354^0, 99355^0, 99356^0, 99357^0, 99358^0, 99359^0, 99415^0, 99416^0, 99446^0, 99447^0, 99448^0, 99449^0, 99451^0, 99452^0, 99466^0, 99468^0, 99469^0, 99471^0, 99472^0, 99475^0, 99476^0, 99477^0, 99478^0, 99479^0, 99480^0, 99483^0, 99485^0, 99497^0, C8921^1, C8922^1, C8923^1, C8924^1, C8925^1, C8926^1, C8927^0, C8929^1, C8930^1, G0380^1, G0381^1, G0382^1, G0383^1, G0384^1, G0406^0, G0407^0, G0408^0, G0425^0, G0426^0, G0427^0, G0463^0, G0500^0, G0508^0, G0509^0
00880	01996^1, 0213T^1, 0216T^1, 0228T^1, 0230T^1, 31505^1, 31515^1, 31527^1, 31622^1, 31634^1, 31645^1, 31647^1, 36000^1, 36010^0, 36011^1, 36012^1, 36013^1, 36014^1, 36015^1, 36400^1, 36405^1, 36406^1, 36410^1, 36420^1, 36425^1, 36430^1, 36440^1, 36591^0, 36592^0, 36600^1, 36640^1, 43752^1, 43753^1, 43754^1, 61026^1, 61055^1, 62280^1, 62281^1, 62282^1, 62284^1, 62320^1, 62321^1, 62322^1, 62323^1, 62324^1, 62325^1, 62326^1, 62327^1, 64400^1, 64402^1, 64405^1, 64408^1, 64410^1, 64413^1, 64415^1, 64416^1, 64417^1, 64418^1, 64420^1, 64421^1, 64425^1, 64430^1, 64435^1, 64445^1, 64446^1, 64447^1, 64448^1, 64449^1, 64450^1, 64461^1, 64463^1, 64479^1, 64483^1, 64486^1, 64487^1, 64488^1, 64489^1, 64490^1, 64493^1, 64505^1, 64510^1, 64517^1, 64520^1, 64530^1, 64553^1, 64555^1, 67500^1, 76000^1, 76970^1, 76998^0, 77002^0, 90865^1, 92511^1, 92512^1, 92516^1, 92520^1, 92537^1, 92538^1, 92950^1, 92953^1, 92960^1, 92961^1, 93000^1, 93005^1, 93010^1, 93040^1, 93041^1, 93042^1, 93050^0, 93303^0, 93304^0, 93306^1, 93307^1, 93308^1, 93312^1, 93313^1, 93314^1, 93315^1, 93316^1, 93317^1, 93318^0, 93351^1, 93355^0, 93451^1, 93456^1, 93457^1, 93561^0, 93562^0, 93701^0, 93922^1, 93923^1, 93924^1, 93925^1, 93926^1, 93930^1, 93931^1, 93970^1, 93971^1, 93975^1, 93976^1, 93978^1, 93979^1, 93980^1, 93981^1, 94002^1, 94004^1, 94200^1, 94250^0, 94640^1, 94644^1, 94660^1, 94662^1, 94680^1, 94681^1, 94690^1, 94760^0, 94761^0, 94762^1, 94770^1, 95812^0, 95813^0, 95816^0, 95819^0, 95822^0, 95829^0, 95955^0, 95956^0, 95957^0, 96360^0, 96365^0, 96372^0, 96373^0, 96374^0, 96375^0, 96376^0, 96377^0, 99151^0, 99152^0, 99153^0, 99155^0, 99156^0, 99157^0, 99201^0, 99202^0, 99203^0, 99204^0, 99205^0, 99211^0, 99212^0, 99213^0, 99214^0, 99215^0, 99217^0, 99218^0, 99219^0, 99220^0, 99221^0, 99222^0, 99223^0, 99224^0, 99225^0, 99226^0, 99231^0, 99232^0, 99233^0, 99234^0, 99235^0, 99236^0, 99238^0, 99239^0, 99281^0, 99282^0, 99283^0, 99284^0, 99285^0, 99304^0, 99305^0, 99306^0, 99307^0, 99308^0, 99309^0, 99310^0, 99315^0, 99318^0, 99324^0, 99325^0, 99326^0, 99327^0, 99328^0, 99334^0, 99335^0, 99336^0, 99337^0, 99341^0, 99342^0, 99343^0, 99347^0, 99348^0, 99349^0, 99354^0, 99355^0, 99356^0, 99357^0, 99358^0, 99359^0, 99415^0, 99416^0, 99446^0, 99447^0, 99448^0, 99449^0, 99451^0, 99452^0, 99466^0, 99468^0, 99469^0, 99471^0, 99472^0, 99475^0, 99476^0, 99477^0, 99478^0, 99479^0, 99480^0, 99483^0, 99485^0, 99497^0, C8921^1, C8922^1, C8923^1, C8924^1, C8925^1, C8926^1, C8927^0, C8929^1, C8930^1, G0380^1, G0381^1, G0382^1, G0383^1, G0384^1, G0406^0, G0407^0, G0408^0, G0425^0, G0426^0, G0427^0, G0463^0, G0500^0, G0508^0, G0509^0

0 = Modifier usage not allowed or inappropriate 1 = Modifier usage allowed

CPT © 2018 American Medical Association. All Rights Reserved.

Code 1	Code 2
00882	01996[1], 0213T[1], 0216T[1], 0228T[1], 0230T[1], 31505[1], 31515[1], 31527[1], 31622[1], 31634[1], 31645[1], 31647[1], 36000[1], 36010[0], 36011[1], 36012[1], 36013[1], 36014[1], 36015[1], 36400[1], 36405[1], 36406[1], 36410[1], 36420[1], 36425[1], 36430[1], 36440[1], 36591[0], 36592[0], 36600[1], 36640[1], 43752[1], 43753[1], 43754[1], 61026[1], 61055[1], 62280[1], 62281[1], 62282[1], 62284[1], 62320[1], 62321[1], 62322[1], 62323[1], 62324[1], 62325[1], 62326[1], 62327[1], 64400[1], 64402[1], 64405[1], 64408[1], 64410[1], 64413[1], 64415[1], 64416[1], 64417[1], 64418[1], 64420[1], 64421[1], 64425[1], 64430[1], 64435[1], 64445[1], 64446[1], 64447[1], 64448[1], 64449[1], 64450[1], 64461[1], 64463[1], 64479[1], 64483[1], 64486[1], 64487[1], 64488[1], 64489[1], 64490[1], 64493[1], 64505[1], 64510[1], 64517[1], 64520[1], 64530[1], 64553[1], 64555[1], 67500[1], 76000[1], 76970[1], 76998[0], 77002[0], 90865[1], 92511[1], 92512[1], 92516[1], 92520[1], 92537[1], 92538[1], 92950[1], 92953[1], 92960[1], 92961[1], 93000[1], 93005[1], 93010[1], 93040[1], 93041[1], 93042[1], 93050[0], 93303[0], 93304[0], 93306[1], 93307[1], 93308[1], 93312[1], 93313[1], 93314[1], 93315[1], 93316[1], 93317[1], 93318[0], 93351[1], 93355[0], 93451[1], 93456[1], 93457[1], 93561[0], 93562[0], 93701[0], 93922[1], 93923[1], 93924[1], 93925[1], 93926[1], 93930[1], 93931[1], 93970[1], 93971[1], 93975[1], 93976[1], 93978[1], 93979[1], 93980[1], 93981[1], 94002[1], 94004[1], 94200[1], 94250[0], 94640[1], 94644[1], 94660[1], 94662[1], 94680[1], 94681[1], 94690[1], 94760[0], 94761[0], 94762[1], 94770[1], 95812[0], 95813[0], 95816[0], 95819[0], 95822[0], 95829[0], 95955[0], 95956[0], 95957[0], 96360[0], 96365[0], 96372[0], 96373[0], 96374[0], 96375[0], 96376[0], 96377[0], 99151[0], 99152[0], 99153[0], 99155[0], 99156[0], 99157[0], 99201[0], 99202[0], 99203[0], 99204[0], 99205[0], 99211[0], 99212[0], 99213[0], 99214[0], 99215[0], 99217[0], 99218[0], 99219[0], 99220[0], 99221[0], 99222[0], 99223[0], 99224[0], 99225[0], 99226[0], 99231[0], 99232[0], 99233[0], 99234[0], 99235[0], 99236[0], 99238[0], 99239[0], 99281[0], 99282[0], 99283[0], 99284[0], 99285[0], 99304[0], 99305[0], 99306[0], 99307[0], 99308[0], 99309[0], 99310[0], 99315[0], 99318[0], 99324[0], 99325[0], 99326[0], 99327[0], 99328[0], 99334[0], 99335[0], 99336[0], 99337[0], 99341[0], 99342[0], 99343[0], 99347[0], 99348[0], 99349[0], 99354[0], 99355[0], 99356[0], 99357[0], 99358[0], 99359[0], 99415[0], 99416[0], 99446[0], 99447[0], 99448[0], 99449[0], 99451[0], 99452[0], 99466[0], 99468[0], 99469[0], 99471[0], 99472[0], 99475[0], 99476[0], 99477[0], 99478[0], 99479[0], 99480[0], 99483[0], 99485[0], 99497[0], C8921[1], C8922[1], C8923[1], C8924[1], C8925[1], C8926[1], C8927[0], C8929[1], C8930[1], G0380[1], G0381[1], G0382[1], G0383[1], G0384[1], G0406[0], G0407[0], G0408[0], G0425[0], G0426[0], G0427[0], G0463[0], G0500[0], G0508[0], G0509[0]
00902	01996[1], 0213T[1], 0216T[1], 0228T[1], 0230T[1], 31505[1], 31515[1], 31527[1], 31622[1], 31634[1], 31645[1], 31647[1], 36000[1], 36010[0], 36011[1], 36012[1], 36013[1], 36014[1], 36015[1], 36400[1], 36405[1], 36406[1], 36410[1], 36420[1], 36425[1], 36430[1], 36440[1], 36591[0], 36592[0], 36600[1], 36640[1], 43752[1], 43753[1], 43754[1], 61026[1], 61055[1], 62280[1], 62281[1], 62282[1], 62284[1], 62320[1], 62321[1], 62322[1], 62323[1], 62324[1], 62325[1], 62326[1], 62327[1], 64400[1], 64402[1], 64405[1], 64408[1], 64410[1], 64413[1], 64415[1], 64416[1], 64417[1], 64418[1], 64420[1], 64421[1], 64425[1], 64430[1], 64435[1], 64445[1], 64446[1], 64447[1], 64448[1], 64449[1], 64450[1], 64461[1], 64463[1], 64479[1], 64483[1], 64486[1], 64487[1], 64488[1], 64489[1], 64490[1], 64493[1], 64505[1], 64510[1], 64517[1], 64520[1], 64530[1], 64553[1], 64555[1], 67500[1], 76000[1], 76970[1], 76998[0], 77002[0], 90865[1], 92511[1], 92512[1], 92516[1], 92520[1], 92537[1], 92538[1], 92950[1], 92953[1], 92960[1], 92961[1], 93000[1], 93005[1], 93010[1], 93040[1], 93041[1], 93042[1], 93050[0], 93303[0], 93304[0], 93306[1], 93307[1], 93308[1], 93312[1], 93313[1], 93314[1], 93315[1], 93316[1], 93317[1], 93318[0], 93351[1], 93355[0], 93451[1], 93456[1], 93457[1], 93561[0], 93562[0], 93701[0], 93922[1], 93923[1], 93924[1], 93925[1], 93926[1], 93930[1], 93931[1], 93970[1], 93971[1], 93975[1], 93976[1], 93978[1], 93979[1], 93980[1], 93981[1], 94002[1], 94004[1], 94200[1], 94250[0], 94640[1], 94644[1], 94660[1], 94662[1], 94680[1], 94681[1], 94690[1], 94760[0], 94761[0], 94762[1], 94770[1], 95812[0], 95813[0], 95816[0], 95819[0], 95822[0], 95829[0], 95955[0], 95956[0], 95957[0], 96360[0], 96365[0], 96372[0], 96373[0], 96374[0], 96375[0], 96376[0], 96377[0], 99151[0], 99152[0], 99153[0], 99155[0], 99156[0], 99157[0], 99201[0], 99202[0], 99203[0], 99204[0], 99205[0], 99211[0], 99212[0], 99213[0], 99214[0], 99215[0], 99217[0], 99218[0], 99219[0], 99220[0], 99221[0], 99222[0], 99223[0], 99224[0], 99225[0], 99226[0], 99231[0], 99232[0], 99233[0], 99234[0], 99235[0], 99236[0], 99238[0], 99239[0], 99281[0], 99282[0], 99283[0], 99284[0], 99285[0], 99304[0], 99305[0], 99306[0], 99307[0], 99308[0], 99309[0], 99310[0], 99315[0], 99318[0], 99324[0], 99325[0], 99326[0], 99327[0], 99328[0], 99334[0], 99335[0], 99336[0], 99337[0], 99341[0], 99342[0], 99343[0], 99347[0], 99348[0], 99349[0], 99354[0], 99355[0], 99356[0], 99357[0], 99358[0], 99359[0], 99415[0], 99416[0], 99446[0], 99447[0], 99448[0], 99449[0], 99451[0], 99452[0], 99466[0], 99468[0], 99469[0], 99471[0], 99472[0], 99475[0], 99476[0], 99477[0], 99478[0], 99479[0], 99480[0], 99483[0], 99485[0], 99497[0], C8921[1], C8922[1], C8923[1], C8924[1], C8925[1], C8926[1], C8927[0], C8929[1], C8930[1], G0380[1], G0381[1], G0382[1], G0383[1], G0384[1], G0406[0], G0407[0], G0408[0], G0425[0], G0426[0], G0427[0], G0463[0], G0500[0], G0508[0], G0509[0]
00904	01996[1], 0213T[1], 0216T[1], 0228T[1], 0230T[1], 31505[1], 31515[1], 31527[1], 31622[1], 31634[1], 31645[1], 31647[1], 36000[1], 36010[0], 36011[1], 36012[1], 36013[1], 36014[1], 36015[1], 36400[1], 36405[1], 36406[1], 36410[1], 36420[1], 36425[1], 36430[1], 36440[1], 36591[0], 36592[0], 36600[1], 36640[1], 43752[1], 43753[1], 43754[1], 61026[1], 61055[1], 62280[1], 62281[1], 62282[1], 62284[1], 62320[1], 62321[1], 62322[1], 62323[1], 62324[1], 62325[1], 62326[1], 62327[1], 64400[1], 64402[1], 64405[1], 64408[1], 64410[1], 64413[1], 64415[1], 64416[1], 64417[1], 64418[1], 64420[1], 64421[1], 64425[1], 64430[1], 64435[1], 64445[1], 64446[1], 64447[1], 64448[1], 64449[1], 64450[1], 64461[1], 64463[1], 64479[1], 64483[1], 64486[1], 64487[1], 64488[1], 64489[1], 64490[1], 64493[1], 64505[1], 64510[1], 64517[1], 64520[1], 64530[1], 64553[1], 64555[1], 67500[1], 76000[1], 76970[1], 76998[0], 77002[0], 90865[1], 92511[1], 92512[1], 92516[1], 92520[1], 92537[1], 92538[1], 92950[1], 92953[1], 92960[1], 92961[1], 93000[1], 93005[1], 93010[1], 93040[1], 93041[1], 93042[1], 93050[0], 93303[0], 93304[0], 93306[1], 93307[1], 93308[1], 93312[1], 93313[1], 93314[1], 93315[1], 93316[1], 93317[1], 93318[0], 93351[1], 93355[0], 93451[1], 93456[1], 93457[1], 93561[0], 93562[0], 93701[0], 93922[1], 93923[1], 93924[1], 93925[1], 93926[1], 93930[1], 93931[1], 93970[1], 93971[1], 93975[1], 93976[1], 93978[1], 93979[1], 93980[1], 93981[1], 94002[1], 94004[1], 94200[1], 94250[0], 94640[1], 94644[1], 94660[1], 94662[1], 94680[1], 94681[1], 94690[1], 94760[0], 94761[0], 94762[1], 94770[1], 95812[0], 95813[0], 95816[0], 95819[0], 95822[0], 95829[0], 95955[0], 95956[0], 95957[0], 96360[0], 96365[0], 96372[0], 96373[0], 96374[0], 96375[0], 96376[0], 96377[0], 99151[0], 99152[0], 99153[0], 99155[0], 99156[0], 99157[0], 99201[0], 99202[0], 99203[0], 99204[0], 99205[0], 99211[0], 99212[0], 99213[0], 99214[0], 99215[0], 99217[0], 99218[0], 99219[0], 99220[0], 99221[0], 99222[0], 99223[0], 99224[0], 99225[0], 99226[0], 99231[0], 99232[0], 99233[0], 99234[0], 99235[0], 99236[0], 99238[0], 99239[0], 99281[0], 99282[0], 99283[0], 99284[0], 99285[0], 99304[0], 99305[0], 99306[0], 99307[0], 99308[0], 99309[0], 99310[0], 99315[0], 99318[0], 99324[0], 99325[0], 99326[0], 99327[0], 99328[0], 99334[0], 99335[0], 99336[0], 99337[0], 99341[0], 99342[0], 99343[0], 99347[0], 99348[0], 99349[0], 99354[0], 99355[0], 99356[0], 99357[0], 99358[0], 99359[0], 99415[0], 99416[0], 99446[0], 99447[0], 99448[0], 99449[0], 99451[0], 99452[0], 99466[0], 99468[0], 99469[0], 99471[0], 99472[0], 99475[0], 99476[0], 99477[0], 99478[0], 99479[0], 99480[0], 99483[0], 99485[0], 99497[0], C8921[1], C8922[1], C8923[1], C8924[1], C8925[1], C8926[1], C8927[0], C8929[1], C8930[1], G0380[1], G0381[1], G0382[1], G0383[1], G0384[1], G0406[0], G0407[0], G0408[0], G0425[0], G0426[0], G0427[0], G0463[0], G0500[0], G0508[0], G0509[0]
00906	01996[1], 0213T[1], 0216T[1], 0228T[1], 0230T[1], 31505[1], 31515[1], 31527[1], 31622[1], 31634[1], 31645[1], 31647[1], 36000[1], 36010[0], 36011[1], 36012[1], 36013[1], 36014[1], 36015[1], 36400[1], 36405[1], 36406[1], 36410[1], 36420[1], 36425[1], 36430[1], 36440[1], 36591[0], 36592[0], 36600[1], 36640[1], 43752[1], 43753[1], 43754[1], 61026[1], 61055[1], 62280[1], 62281[1], 62282[1], 62284[1], 62320[1], 62321[1], 62322[1], 62323[1], 62324[1], 62325[1], 62326[1], 62327[1], 64400[1], 64402[1], 64405[1], 64408[1], 64410[1], 64413[1], 64415[1], 64416[1], 64417[1], 64418[1], 64420[1], 64421[1], 64425[1], 64430[1], 64435[1], 64445[1], 64446[1], 64447[1], 64448[1], 64449[1], 64450[1], 64461[1], 64463[1], 64479[1], 64483[1], 64486[1], 64487[1], 64488[1], 64489[1], 64490[1], 64493[1], 64505[1], 64510[1], 64517[1], 64520[1], 64530[1], 64553[1], 64555[1], 67500[1], 76000[1], 76970[1], 76998[0], 77002[0], 90865[1], 92511[1], 92512[1], 92516[1], 92520[1], 92537[1], 92538[1], 92950[1], 92953[1], 92960[1], 92961[1], 93000[1], 93005[1], 93010[1], 93040[1], 93041[1], 93042[1], 93050[0], 93303[0], 93304[0], 93306[1], 93307[1], 93308[1], 93312[1], 93313[1], 93314[1], 93315[1], 93316[1], 93317[1], 93318[0], 93351[1], 93355[0], 93451[1], 93456[1], 93457[1], 93561[0], 93562[0], 93701[0], 93922[1], 93923[1], 93924[1], 93925[1], 93926[1], 93930[1], 93931[1], 93970[1], 93971[1], 93975[1], 93976[1], 93978[1], 93979[1], 93980[1], 93981[1], 94002[1], 94004[1], 94200[1], 94250[0], 94640[1], 94644[1], 94660[1], 94662[1], 94680[1], 94681[1], 94690[1], 94760[0], 94761[0], 94762[1], 94770[1], 95812[0], 95813[0], 95816[0], 95819[0], 95822[0], 95829[0], 95955[0], 95956[0], 95957[0], 96360[0], 96365[0], 96372[0], 96373[0], 96374[0], 96375[0], 96376[0], 96377[0], 99151[0], 99152[0], 99153[0], 99155[0], 99156[0], 99157[0], 99201[0], 99202[0], 99203[0], 99204[0], 99205[0], 99211[0], 99212[0], 99213[0], 99214[0], 99215[0], 99217[0], 99218[0], 99219[0], 99220[0], 99221[0], 99222[0], 99223[0], 99224[0], 99225[0], 99226[0], 99231[0], 99232[0], 99233[0], 99234[0], 99235[0], 99236[0], 99238[0], 99239[0], 99281[0], 99282[0], 99283[0], 99284[0], 99285[0], 99304[0], 99305[0], 99306[0], 99307[0], 99308[0], 99309[0], 99310[0], 99315[0], 99318[0], 99324[0], 99325[0], 99326[0], 99327[0], 99328[0], 99334[0], 99335[0], 99336[0], 99337[0], 99341[0], 99342[0], 99343[0], 99347[0], 99348[0], 99349[0], 99354[0], 99355[0], 99356[0], 99357[0], 99358[0], 99359[0], 99415[0], 99416[0], 99446[0], 99447[0], 99448[0], 99449[0], 99451[0], 99452[0], 99466[0], 99468[0], 99469[0], 99471[0], 99472[0], 99475[0], 99476[0], 99477[0], 99478[0], 99479[0], 99480[0], 99483[0], 99485[0], 99497[0], C8921[1], C8922[1], C8923[1], C8924[1], C8925[1], C8926[1], C8927[0], C8929[1], C8930[1], G0380[1], G0381[1], G0382[1], G0383[1], G0384[1], G0406[0], G0407[0], G0408[0], G0425[0], G0426[0], G0427[0], G0463[0], G0500[0], G0508[0], G0509[0]
00908	01996[1], 0213T[1], 0216T[1], 0228T[1], 0230T[1], 31505[1], 31515[1], 31527[1], 31622[1], 31634[1], 31645[1], 31647[1], 36000[1], 36010[0], 36011[1], 36012[1], 36013[1], 36014[1], 36015[1], 36400[1], 36405[1], 36406[1], 36410[1], 36420[1], 36425[1], 36430[1], 36440[1], 36591[0], 36592[0], 36600[1], 36640[1], 43752[1], 43753[1], 43754[1], 61026[1], 61055[1], 62280[1], 62281[1], 62282[1], 62284[1], 62320[1], 62321[1], 62322[1], 62323[1], 62324[1], 62325[1], 62326[1], 62327[1], 64400[1], 64402[1], 64405[1], 64408[1], 64410[1], 64413[1], 64415[1], 64416[1], 64417[1], 64418[1], 64420[1], 64421[1], 64425[1], 64430[1], 64435[1], 64445[1], 64446[1], 64447[1], 64448[1], 64449[1], 64450[1], 64461[1], 64463[1], 64479[1], 64483[1], 64486[1], 64487[1], 64488[1], 64489[1], 64490[1], 64493[1], 64505[1], 64510[1], 64517[1], 64520[1], 64530[1], 64553[1], 64555[1], 67500[1], 76000[1], 76970[1], 76998[0], 77002[0], 90865[1], 92511[1], 92512[1], 92516[1], 92520[1], 92537[1], 92538[1], 92950[1], 92953[1], 92960[1], 92961[1], 93000[1], 93005[1], 93010[1], 93040[1], 93041[1], 93042[1], 93050[0], 93303[0], 93304[0], 93306[1], 93307[1], 93308[1], 93312[1], 93313[1], 93314[1], 93315[1], 93316[1], 93317[1],

0 = Modifier usage not allowed or inappropriate 1 = Modifier usage allowed

CPT © 2018 American Medical Association. All Rights Reserved.

Code 1	Code 2
	93318[0], 93351[1], 93355[0], 93451[1], 93456[1], 93457[1], 93561[0], 93562[0], 93701[0], 93922[1], 93923[1], 93924[1], 93925[1], 93926[1], 93930[1], 93931[1], 93970[1], 93971[1], 93975[1], 93976[1], 93978[1], 93979[1], 93980[1], 93981[1], 94002[1], 94004[1], 94200[1], 94250[0], 94640[1], 94644[1], 94660[1], 94662[1], 94680[1], 94681[1], 94690[1], 94760[0], 94761[0], 94762[1], 94770[1], 95812[0], 95813[0], 95816[0], 95819[0], 95822[0], 95829[0], 95955[0], 95956[0], 95957[0], 96360[0], 96365[0], 96372[0], 96373[0], 96374[0], 96375[0], 96376[0], 96377[0], 99151[0], 99152[0], 99153[0], 99155[0], 99156[0], 99157[0], 99201[0], 99202[0], 99203[0], 99204[0], 99205[0], 99211[0], 99212[0], 99213[0], 99214[0], 99215[0], 99217[0], 99218[0], 99219[0], 99220[0], 99221[0], 99222[0], 99223[0], 99224[0], 99225[0], 99226[0], 99231[0], 99232[0], 99233[0], 99234[0], 99235[0], 99236[0], 99238[0], 99239[0], 99281[0], 99282[0], 99283[0], 99284[0], 99285[0], 99304[0], 99305[0], 99306[0], 99307[0], 99308[0], 99309[0], 99310[0], 99315[0], 99318[0], 99324[0], 99325[0], 99326[0], 99327[0], 99328[0], 99334[0], 99335[0], 99336[0], 99337[0], 99341[0], 99342[0], 99343[0], 99347[0], 99348[0], 99349[0], 99354[0], 99355[0], 99356[0], 99357[0], 99358[0], 99359[0], 99415[0], 99416[0], 99446[0], 99447[0], 99448[0], 99449[0], 99451[0], 99452[0], 99466[0], 99468[0], 99469[0], 99471[0], 99472[0], 99475[0], 99476[0], 99477[0], 99478[0], 99479[0], 99480[0], 99483[0], 99485[0], 99497[0], C8921[1], C8922[1], C8923[1], C8924[1], C8925[1], C8926[1], C8927[0], C8929[1], C8930[1], G0380[1], G0381[1], G0382[1], G0383[1], G0384[1], G0406[0], G0407[0], G0408[0], G0425[0], G0426[0], G0427[0], G0463[0], G0500[0], G0508[0], G0509[0]
00910	01996[1], 0213T[1], 0216T[1], 0228T[1], 0230T[1], 31505[1], 31515[1], 31527[1], 31622[1], 31634[1], 31645[1], 31647[1], 36000[1], 36010[0], 36011[1], 36012[1], 36013[1], 36014[1], 36015[1], 36400[1], 36405[1], 36406[1], 36410[1], 36420[1], 36425[1], 36430[1], 36440[1], 36591[0], 36592[0], 36600[1], 36640[1], 43752[1], 43753[1], 43754[1], 61026[1], 61055[1], 62280[1], 62281[1], 62282[1], 62284[1], 62320[1], 62321[1], 62322[1], 62323[1], 62324[1], 62325[1], 62326[1], 62327[1], 64400[1], 64402[1], 64405[1], 64408[1], 64410[1], 64413[1], 64415[1], 64416[1], 64417[1], 64418[1], 64420[1], 64421[1], 64425[1], 64430[1], 64435[1], 64445[1], 64446[1], 64447[1], 64448[1], 64449[1], 64450[1], 64461[1], 64463[1], 64479[1], 64483[1], 64486[1], 64487[1], 64488[1], 64489[1], 64490[1], 64493[1], 64505[1], 64510[1], 64517[1], 64520[1], 64530[1], 64553[1], 64555[1], 67500[1], 76000[1], 76970[1], 76998[0], 77002[0], 90865[1], 92511[1], 92512[1], 92516[1], 92520[1], 92537[1], 92538[1], 92950[1], 92953[1], 92960[1], 92961[1], 93000[1], 93005[1], 93010[1], 93040[1], 93041[1], 93042[1], 93050[0], 93303[0], 93304[0], 93306[1], 93307[1], 93308[1], 93312[1], 93313[1], 93314[1], 93315[1], 93316[1], 93317[1], 93318[0], 93351[1], 93355[0], 93451[1], 93456[1], 93457[1], 93561[0], 93562[0], 93701[0], 93922[1], 93923[1], 93924[1], 93925[1], 93926[1], 93930[1], 93931[1], 93970[1], 93971[1], 93975[1], 93976[1], 93978[1], 93979[1], 93980[1], 93981[1], 94002[1], 94004[1], 94200[1], 94250[0], 94640[1], 94644[1], 94660[1], 94662[1], 94680[1], 94681[1], 94690[1], 94760[0], 94761[0], 94762[1], 94770[1], 95812[0], 95813[0], 95816[0], 95819[0], 95822[0], 95829[0], 95955[0], 95956[0], 95957[0], 96360[0], 96365[0], 96372[0], 96373[0], 96374[0], 96375[0], 96376[0], 96377[0], 99151[0], 99152[0], 99153[0], 99155[0], 99156[0], 99157[0], 99201[0], 99202[0], 99203[0], 99204[0], 99205[0], 99211[0], 99212[0], 99213[0], 99214[0], 99215[0], 99217[0], 99218[0], 99219[0], 99220[0], 99221[0], 99222[0], 99223[0], 99224[0], 99225[0], 99226[0], 99231[0], 99232[0], 99233[0], 99234[0], 99235[0], 99236[0], 99238[0], 99239[0], 99281[0], 99282[0], 99283[0], 99284[0], 99285[0], 99304[0], 99305[0], 99306[0], 99307[0], 99308[0], 99309[0], 99310[0], 99315[0], 99318[0], 99324[0], 99325[0], 99326[0], 99327[0], 99328[0], 99334[0], 99335[0], 99336[0], 99337[0], 99341[0], 99342[0], 99343[0], 99347[0], 99348[0], 99349[0], 99354[0], 99355[0], 99356[0], 99357[0], 99358[0], 99359[0], 99415[0], 99416[0], 99446[0], 99447[0], 99448[0], 99449[0], 99451[0], 99452[0], 99466[0], 99468[0], 99469[0], 99471[0], 99472[0], 99475[0], 99476[0], 99477[0], 99478[0], 99479[0], 99480[0], 99483[0], 99485[0], 99497[0], C8921[1], C8922[1], C8923[1], C8924[1], C8925[1], C8926[1], C8927[0], C8929[1], C8930[1], G0380[1], G0381[1], G0382[1], G0383[1], G0384[1], G0406[0], G0407[0], G0408[0], G0425[0], G0426[0], G0427[0], G0463[0], G0500[0], G0508[0], G0509[0]
00912	01996[1], 0213T[1], 0216T[1], 0228T[1], 0230T[1], 31505[1], 31515[1], 31527[1], 31622[1], 31634[1], 31645[1], 31647[1], 36000[1], 36010[0], 36011[1], 36012[1], 36013[1], 36014[1], 36015[1], 36400[1], 36405[1], 36406[1], 36410[1], 36420[1], 36425[1], 36430[1], 36440[1], 36591[0], 36592[0], 36600[1], 36640[1], 43752[1], 43753[1], 43754[1], 61026[1], 61055[1], 62280[1], 62281[1], 62282[1], 62284[1], 62320[1], 62321[1], 62322[1], 62323[1], 62324[1], 62325[1], 62326[1], 62327[1], 64400[1], 64402[1], 64405[1], 64408[1], 64410[1], 64413[1], 64415[1], 64416[1], 64417[1], 64418[1], 64420[1], 64421[1], 64425[1], 64430[1], 64435[1], 64445[1], 64446[1], 64447[1], 64448[1], 64449[1], 64450[1], 64461[1], 64463[1], 64479[1], 64483[1], 64486[1], 64487[1], 64488[1], 64489[1], 64490[1], 64493[1], 64505[1], 64510[1], 64517[1], 64520[1], 64530[1], 64553[1], 64555[1], 67500[1], 76000[1], 76970[1], 76998[0], 77002[0], 90865[1], 92511[1], 92512[1], 92516[1], 92520[1], 92537[1], 92538[1], 92950[1], 92953[1], 92960[1], 92961[1], 93000[1], 93005[1], 93010[1], 93040[1], 93041[1], 93042[1], 93050[0], 93303[0], 93304[0], 93306[1], 93307[1], 93308[1], 93312[1], 93313[1], 93314[1], 93315[1], 93316[1], 93317[1], 93318[0], 93351[1], 93355[0], 93451[1], 93456[1], 93457[1], 93561[0], 93562[0], 93701[0], 93922[1], 93923[1], 93924[1], 93925[1], 93926[1], 93930[1], 93931[1], 93970[1], 93971[1], 93975[1], 93976[1], 93978[1], 93979[1], 93980[1], 93981[1], 94002[1], 94004[1], 94200[1], 94250[0], 94640[1], 94644[1], 94660[1], 94662[1], 94680[1], 94681[1], 94690[1], 94760[0], 94761[0], 94762[1], 94770[1], 95812[0], 95813[0], 95816[0], 95819[0], 95822[0], 95829[0], 95955[0], 95956[0], 95957[0], 96360[0], 96365[0], 96372[0], 96373[0], 96374[0], 96375[0], 96376[0], 96377[0], 99151[0], 99152[0], 99153[0], 99155[0], 99156[0], 99157[0], 99201[0], 99202[0], 99203[0], 99204[0], 99205[0], 99211[0], 99212[0], 99213[0], 99214[0], 99215[0], 99217[0], 99218[0], 99219[0], 99220[0], 99221[0], 99222[0], 99223[0], 99224[0], 99225[0], 99226[0], 99231[0], 99232[0], 99233[0], 99234[0], 99235[0], 99236[0], 99238[0], 99239[0], 99281[0], 99282[0], 99283[0], 99284[0], 99285[0], 99304[0], 99305[0], 99306[0], 99307[0], 99308[0], 99309[0], 99310[0], 99315[0], 99318[0], 99324[0], 99325[0], 99326[0], 99327[0], 99328[0], 99334[0], 99335[0], 99336[0], 99337[0], 99341[0], 99342[0], 99343[0], 99347[0], 99348[0], 99349[0], 99354[0], 99355[0], 99356[0], 99357[0], 99358[0], 99359[0], 99415[0], 99416[0], 99446[0], 99447[0], 99448[0], 99449[0], 99451[0], 99452[0], 99466[0], 99468[0], 99469[0], 99471[0], 99472[0], 99475[0], 99476[0], 99477[0], 99478[0], 99479[0], 99480[0], 99483[0], 99485[0], 99497[0], C8921[1], C8922[1], C8923[1], C8924[1], C8925[1], C8926[1], C8927[0], C8929[1], C8930[1], G0380[1], G0381[1], G0382[1], G0383[1], G0384[1], G0406[0], G0407[0], G0408[0], G0425[0], G0426[0], G0427[0], G0463[0], G0500[0], G0508[0], G0509[0]
00914	01996[1], 0213T[1], 0216T[1], 0228T[1], 0230T[1], 31505[1], 31515[1], 31527[1], 31622[1], 31634[1], 31645[1], 31647[1], 36000[1], 36010[0], 36011[1], 36012[1], 36013[1], 36014[1], 36015[1], 36400[1], 36405[1], 36406[1], 36410[1], 36420[1], 36425[1], 36430[1], 36440[1], 36591[0], 36592[0], 36600[1], 36640[1], 43752[1], 43753[1], 43754[1], 61026[1], 61055[1], 62280[1], 62281[1], 62282[1], 62284[1], 62320[1], 62321[1], 62322[1], 62323[1], 62324[1], 62325[1], 62326[1], 62327[1], 64400[1], 64402[1], 64405[1], 64408[1], 64410[1], 64413[1], 64415[1], 64416[1], 64417[1], 64418[1], 64420[1], 64421[1], 64425[1], 64430[1], 64435[1], 64445[1], 64446[1], 64447[1], 64448[1], 64449[1], 64450[1], 64461[1], 64463[1], 64479[1], 64483[1], 64486[1], 64487[1], 64488[1], 64489[1], 64490[1], 64493[1], 64505[1], 64510[1], 64517[1], 64520[1], 64530[1], 64553[1], 64555[1], 67500[1], 76000[1], 76970[1], 76998[0], 77002[0], 90865[1], 92511[1], 92512[1], 92516[1], 92520[1], 92537[1], 92538[1], 92950[1], 92953[1], 92960[1], 92961[1], 93000[1], 93005[1], 93010[1], 93040[1], 93041[1], 93042[1], 93050[0], 93303[0], 93304[0], 93306[1], 93307[1], 93308[1], 93312[1], 93313[1], 93314[1], 93315[1], 93316[1], 93317[1], 93318[0], 93351[1], 93355[0], 93451[1], 93456[1], 93457[1], 93561[0], 93562[0], 93701[0], 93922[1], 93923[1], 93924[1], 93925[1], 93926[1], 93930[1], 93931[1], 93970[1], 93971[1], 93975[1], 93976[1], 93978[1], 93979[1], 93980[1], 93981[1], 94002[1], 94004[1], 94200[1], 94250[0], 94640[1], 94644[1], 94660[1], 94662[1], 94680[1], 94681[1], 94690[1], 94760[0], 94761[0], 94762[1], 94770[1], 95812[0], 95813[0], 95816[0], 95819[0], 95822[0], 95829[0], 95955[0], 95956[0], 95957[0], 96360[0], 96365[0], 96372[0], 96373[0], 96374[0], 96375[0], 96376[0], 96377[0], 99151[0], 99152[0], 99153[0], 99155[0], 99156[0], 99157[0], 99201[0], 99202[0], 99203[0], 99204[0], 99205[0], 99211[0], 99212[0], 99213[0], 99214[0], 99215[0], 99217[0], 99218[0], 99219[0], 99220[0], 99221[0], 99222[0], 99223[0], 99224[0], 99225[0], 99226[0], 99231[0], 99232[0], 99233[0], 99234[0], 99235[0], 99236[0], 99238[0], 99239[0], 99281[0], 99282[0], 99283[0], 99284[0], 99285[0], 99304[0], 99305[0], 99306[0], 99307[0], 99308[0], 99309[0], 99310[0], 99315[0], 99318[0], 99324[0], 99325[0], 99326[0], 99327[0], 99328[0], 99334[0], 99335[0], 99336[0], 99337[0], 99341[0], 99342[0], 99343[0], 99347[0], 99348[0], 99349[0], 99354[0], 99355[0], 99356[0], 99357[0], 99358[0], 99359[0], 99415[0], 99416[0], 99446[0], 99447[0], 99448[0], 99449[0], 99451[0], 99452[0], 99466[0], 99468[0], 99469[0], 99471[0], 99472[0], 99475[0], 99476[0], 99477[0], 99478[0], 99479[0], 99480[0], 99483[0], 99485[0], 99497[0], C8921[1], C8922[1], C8923[1], C8924[1], C8925[1], C8926[1], C8927[0], C8929[1], C8930[1], G0380[1], G0381[1], G0382[1], G0383[1], G0384[1], G0406[0], G0407[0], G0408[0], G0425[0], G0426[0], G0427[0], G0463[0], G0500[0], G0508[0], G0509[0]
00916	01996[1], 0213T[1], 0216T[1], 0228T[1], 0230T[1], 31505[1], 31515[1], 31527[1], 31622[1], 31634[1], 31645[1], 31647[1], 36000[1], 36010[0], 36011[1], 36012[1], 36013[1], 36014[1], 36015[1], 36400[1], 36405[1], 36406[1], 36410[1], 36420[1], 36425[1], 36430[1], 36440[1], 36591[0], 36592[0], 36600[1], 36640[1], 43752[1], 43753[1], 43754[1], 61026[1], 61055[1], 62280[1], 62281[1], 62282[1], 62284[1], 62320[1], 62321[1], 62322[1], 62323[1], 62324[1], 62325[1], 62326[1], 62327[1], 64400[1], 64402[1], 64405[1], 64408[1], 64410[1], 64413[1], 64415[1], 64416[1], 64417[1], 64418[1], 64420[1], 64421[1], 64425[1], 64430[1], 64435[1], 64445[1], 64446[1], 64447[1], 64448[1], 64449[1], 64450[1], 64461[1], 64463[1], 64479[1], 64483[1], 64486[1], 64487[1], 64488[1], 64489[1], 64490[1], 64493[1], 64505[1], 64510[1], 64517[1], 64520[1], 64530[1], 64553[1], 64555[1], 67500[1], 76000[1], 76970[1], 76998[0], 77002[0], 90865[1], 92511[1], 92512[1], 92516[1], 92520[1], 92537[1], 92538[1], 92950[1], 92953[1], 92960[1], 92961[1], 93000[1], 93005[1], 93010[1], 93040[1], 93041[1], 93042[1], 93050[0], 93303[0], 93304[0], 93306[1], 93307[1], 93308[1], 93312[1], 93313[1], 93314[1], 93315[1], 93316[1], 93317[1], 93318[0], 93351[1], 93355[0], 93451[1], 93456[1], 93457[1], 93561[0], 93562[0], 93701[0], 93922[1], 93923[1], 93924[1], 93925[1], 93926[1], 93930[1], 93931[1], 93970[1], 93971[1], 93975[1], 93976[1], 93978[1], 93979[1], 93980[1], 93981[1], 94002[1], 94004[1], 94200[1], 94250[0], 94640[1], 94644[1], 94660[1], 94662[1], 94680[1], 94681[1], 94690[1], 94760[0], 94761[0], 94762[1], 94770[1], 95812[0], 95813[0], 95816[0], 95819[0], 95822[0], 95829[0], 95955[0], 95956[0], 95957[0], 96360[0], 96365[0], 96372[0], 96373[0], 96374[0], 96375[0], 96376[0], 96377[0], 99151[0], 99152[0], 99153[0], 99155[0], 99156[0], 99157[0], 99201[0], 99202[0], 99203[0], 99204[0], 99205[0], 99211[0], 99212[0], 99213[0], 99214[0], 99215[0], 99217[0], 99218[0], 99219[0], 99220[0], 99221[0], 99222[0], 99223[0], 99224[0], 99225[0], 99226[0], 99231[0], 99232[0], 99233[0], 99234[0], 99235[0], 99236[0], 99238[0], 99239[0], 99281[0], 99282[0], 99283[0], 99284[0], 99285[0], 99304[0], 99305[0], 99306[0], 99307[0], 99308[0], 99309[0], 99310[0], 99315[0], 99318[0], 99324[0], 99325[0], 99326[0], 99327[0], 99328[0], 99334[0], 99335[0], 99336[0], 99337[0], 99341[0], 99342[0], 99343[0], 99347[0], 99348[0], 99349[0], 99354[0],

0 = Modifier usage not allowed or inappropriate 1 = Modifier usage allowed

Appendix A: NCCI - CPT Codes

CPT © 2018 American Medical Association. All Rights Reserved.

Code 1	Code 2
	99355[0], 99356[0], 99357[0], 99358[0], 99359[0], 99415[0], 99416[0], 99446[0], 99447[0], 99448[0], 99449[0], 99451[0], 99452[0], 99466[0], 99468[0], 99469[0], 99471[0], 99472[0], 99475[0], 99476[0], 99477[0], 99478[0], 99479[0], 99480[0], 99483[0], 99485[0], 99497[0], C8921[1], C8922[1], C8923[1], C8924[1], C8925[1], C8926[1], C8927[0], C8929[1], C8930[1], G0380[1], G0381[1], G0382[1], G0383[1], G0384[1], G0406[0], G0407[0], G0408[0], G0425[0], G0426[0], G0427[0], G0463[0], G0500[0], G0508[0], G0509[0]
00918	01996[1], 0213T[1], 0216T[1], 0228T[1], 0230T[1], 31505[1], 31515[1], 31527[1], 31622[1], 31634[1], 31645[1], 31647[1], 36000[1], 36010[0], 36011[1], 36012[1], 36013[1], 36014[1], 36015[1], 36400[1], 36405[1], 36406[1], 36410[1], 36420[1], 36425[1], 36430[1], 36440[1], 36591[0], 36592[0], 36600[1], 36640[1], 43752[1], 43753[1], 43754[1], 61026[1], 61055[1], 62280[1], 62281[1], 62282[1], 62284[1], 62320[1], 62321[1], 62322[1], 62323[1], 62324[1], 62325[1], 62326[1], 62327[1], 64400[1], 64402[1], 64405[1], 64408[1], 64410[1], 64413[1], 64415[1], 64416[1], 64417[1], 64418[1], 64420[1], 64421[1], 64425[1], 64430[1], 64435[1], 64445[1], 64446[1], 64447[1], 64448[1], 64449[1], 64450[1], 64461[1], 64463[1], 64479[1], 64483[1], 64486[1], 64487[1], 64488[1], 64489[1], 64490[1], 64493[1], 64505[1], 64510[1], 64517[1], 64520[1], 64530[1], 64553[1], 64555[1], 67500[1], 76000[1], 76970[1], 76998[0], 77002[0], 90865[1], 92511[1], 92512[1], 92516[1], 92520[1], 92537[1], 92538[1], 92950[1], 92953[1], 92960[1], 92961[1], 93000[1], 93005[1], 93010[1], 93040[1], 93041[1], 93042[1], 93050[0], 93303[0], 93304[0], 93306[1], 93307[1], 93308[1], 93312[1], 93313[1], 93314[1], 93315[1], 93316[1], 93317[1], 93318[0], 93351[1], 93355[0], 93451[1], 93456[1], 93457[1], 93561[0], 93562[0], 93701[0], 93922[1], 93923[1], 93924[1], 93925[1], 93926[1], 93930[1], 93931[1], 93970[1], 93971[1], 93975[1], 93976[1], 93978[1], 93979[1], 93980[1], 93981[1], 94002[1], 94004[1], 94200[1], 94250[0], 94640[1], 94644[1], 94660[1], 94662[1], 94680[1], 94681[1], 94690[1], 94760[0], 94761[0], 94762[1], 94770[1], 95812[0], 95813[0], 95816[0], 95819[0], 95822[0], 95829[0], 95955[0], 95956[0], 95957[0], 96360[0], 96365[0], 96372[0], 96373[0], 96374[0], 96375[0], 96376[0], 96377[0], 99151[0], 99152[0], 99153[0], 99155[0], 99156[0], 99157[0], 99201[0], 99202[0], 99203[0], 99204[0], 99205[0], 99211[0], 99212[0], 99213[0], 99214[0], 99215[0], 99217[0], 99218[0], 99219[0], 99220[0], 99221[0], 99222[0], 99223[0], 99224[0], 99225[0], 99226[0], 99231[0], 99232[0], 99233[0], 99234[0], 99235[0], 99236[0], 99238[0], 99239[0], 99281[0], 99282[0], 99283[0], 99284[0], 99285[0], 99304[0], 99305[0], 99306[0], 99307[0], 99308[0], 99309[0], 99310[0], 99315[0], 99318[0], 99324[0], 99325[0], 99326[0], 99327[0], 99328[0], 99334[0], 99335[0], 99336[0], 99337[0], 99341[0], 99342[0], 99343[0], 99347[0], 99348[0], 99349[0], 99354[0], 99355[0], 99356[0], 99357[0], 99358[0], 99359[0], 99415[0], 99416[0], 99446[0], 99447[0], 99448[0], 99449[0], 99451[0], 99452[0], 99466[0], 99468[0], 99469[0], 99471[0], 99472[0], 99475[0], 99476[0], 99477[0], 99478[0], 99479[0], 99480[0], 99483[0], 99485[0], 99497[0], C8921[1], C8922[1], C8923[1], C8924[1], C8925[1], C8926[1], C8927[0], C8929[1], C8930[1], G0380[1], G0381[1], G0382[1], G0383[1], G0384[1], G0406[0], G0407[0], G0408[0], G0425[0], G0426[0], G0427[0], G0463[0], G0500[0], G0508[0], G0509[0]
00920	00942[0], 01996[1], 0213T[1], 0216T[1], 0228T[1], 0230T[1], 31505[1], 31515[1], 31527[1], 31622[1], 31634[1], 31645[1], 31647[1], 36000[1], 36010[0], 36011[1], 36012[1], 36013[1], 36014[1], 36015[1], 36400[1], 36405[1], 36406[1], 36410[1], 36420[1], 36425[1], 36430[1], 36440[1], 36591[0], 36592[0], 36600[1], 36640[1], 43752[1], 43753[1], 43754[1], 61026[1], 61055[1], 62280[1], 62281[1], 62282[1], 62284[1], 62320[1], 62321[1], 62322[1], 62323[1], 62324[1], 62325[1], 62326[1], 62327[1], 64400[1], 64402[1], 64405[1], 64408[1], 64410[1], 64413[1], 64415[1], 64416[1], 64417[1], 64418[1], 64420[1], 64421[1], 64425[1], 64430[1], 64435[1], 64445[1], 64446[1], 64447[1], 64448[1], 64449[1], 64450[1], 64461[1], 64463[1], 64479[1], 64483[1], 64486[1], 64487[1], 64488[1], 64489[1], 64490[1], 64493[1], 64505[1], 64510[1], 64517[1], 64520[1], 64530[1], 64553[1], 64555[1], 67500[1], 76000[1], 76970[1], 76998[0], 77002[0], 90865[1], 92511[1], 92512[1], 92516[1], 92520[1], 92537[1], 92538[1], 92950[1], 92953[1], 92960[1], 92961[1], 93000[1], 93005[1], 93010[1], 93040[1], 93041[1], 93042[1], 93050[0], 93303[0], 93304[0], 93306[1], 93307[1], 93308[1], 93312[1], 93313[1], 93314[1], 93315[1], 93316[1], 93317[1], 93318[0], 93351[1], 93355[0], 93451[1], 93456[1], 93457[1], 93561[0], 93562[0], 93701[0], 93922[1], 93923[1], 93924[1], 93925[1], 93926[1], 93930[1], 93931[1], 93970[1], 93971[1], 93975[1], 93976[1], 93978[1], 93979[1], 93980[1], 93981[1], 94002[1], 94004[1], 94200[1], 94250[0], 94640[1], 94644[1], 94660[1], 94662[1], 94680[1], 94681[1], 94690[1], 94760[0], 94761[0], 94762[1], 94770[1], 95812[0], 95813[0], 95816[0], 95819[0], 95822[0], 95829[0], 95955[0], 95956[0], 95957[0], 96360[0], 96365[0], 96372[0], 96373[0], 96374[0], 96375[0], 96376[0], 96377[0], 99151[0], 99152[0], 99153[0], 99155[0], 99156[0], 99157[0], 99201[0], 99202[0], 99203[0], 99204[0], 99205[0], 99211[0], 99212[0], 99213[0], 99214[0], 99215[0], 99217[0], 99218[0], 99219[0], 99220[0], 99221[0], 99222[0], 99223[0], 99224[0], 99225[0], 99226[0], 99231[0], 99232[0], 99233[0], 99234[0], 99235[0], 99236[0], 99238[0], 99239[0], 99281[0], 99282[0], 99283[0], 99284[0], 99285[0], 99304[0], 99305[0], 99306[0], 99307[0], 99308[0], 99309[0], 99310[0], 99315[0], 99318[0], 99324[0], 99325[0], 99326[0], 99327[0], 99328[0], 99334[0], 99335[0], 99336[0], 99337[0], 99341[0], 99342[0], 99343[0], 99347[0], 99348[0], 99349[0], 99354[0], 99355[0], 99356[0], 99357[0], 99358[0], 99359[0], 99415[0], 99416[0], 99446[0], 99447[0], 99448[0], 99449[0], 99451[0], 99452[0], 99466[0], 99468[0], 99469[0], 99471[0], 99472[0], 99475[0], 99476[0], 99477[0], 99478[0], 99479[0], 99480[0], 99483[0], 99485[0], 99497[0], C8921[1], C8922[1], C8923[1], C8924[1], C8925[1], C8926[1], C8927[0], C8929[1], C8930[1], G0380[1], G0381[1], G0382[1], G0383[1], G0384[1], G0406[0], G0407[0], G0408[0], G0425[0], G0426[0], G0427[0], G0463[0], G0500[0], G0508[0], G0509[0]
00921	01996[1], 0213T[1], 0216T[1], 0228T[1], 0230T[1], 31505[1], 31515[1], 31527[1], 31622[1], 31634[1], 31645[1], 31647[1], 36000[1], 36010[0], 36011[1], 36012[1], 36013[1], 36014[1], 36015[1], 36400[1], 36405[1], 36406[1], 36410[1], 36420[1], 36425[1], 36430[1], 36440[1], 36591[0], 36592[0], 36600[1], 36640[1], 43752[1], 43753[1], 43754[1], 61026[1], 61055[1], 62280[1], 62281[1], 62282[1], 62284[1], 62320[1], 62321[1], 62322[1], 62323[1], 62324[1], 62325[1], 62326[1], 62327[1], 64400[1], 64402[1], 64405[1], 64408[1], 64410[1], 64413[1], 64415[1], 64416[1], 64417[1], 64418[1], 64420[1], 64421[1], 64425[1], 64430[1], 64435[1], 64445[1], 64446[1], 64447[1], 64448[1], 64449[1], 64450[1], 64461[1], 64463[1], 64479[1], 64483[1], 64486[1], 64487[1], 64488[1], 64489[1], 64490[1], 64493[1], 64505[1], 64510[1], 64517[1], 64520[1], 64530[1], 64553[1], 64555[1], 67500[0], 76000[1], 76970[1], 76998[0], 77002[0], 90865[1], 92511[1], 92512[1], 92516[1], 92520[1], 92537[1], 92538[1], 92950[1], 92953[1], 92960[1], 92961[1], 93000[1], 93005[1], 93010[1], 93040[1], 93041[1], 93042[1], 93050[0], 93303[0], 93304[0], 93306[1], 93307[1], 93308[1], 93312[1], 93313[1], 93314[1], 93315[1], 93316[1], 93317[1], 93318[0], 93351[1], 93355[0], 93451[1], 93456[1], 93457[1], 93561[0], 93562[0], 93701[0], 93922[1], 93923[1], 93924[1], 93925[1], 93926[1], 93930[1], 93931[1], 93970[1], 93971[1], 93975[1], 93976[1], 93978[1], 93979[1], 93980[1], 93981[1], 94002[1], 94004[1], 94200[1], 94250[0], 94640[1], 94644[1], 94660[1], 94662[1], 94680[1], 94681[1], 94690[1], 94760[0], 94761[0], 94762[1], 94770[1], 95812[0], 95813[0], 95816[0], 95819[0], 95822[0], 95829[0], 95955[0], 95956[0], 95957[0], 96360[0], 96365[0], 96372[0], 96373[0], 96374[0], 96375[0], 96376[0], 96377[0], 99151[0], 99152[0], 99153[0], 99155[0], 99156[0], 99157[0], 99201[0], 99202[0], 99203[0], 99204[0], 99205[0], 99211[0], 99212[0], 99213[0], 99214[0], 99215[0], 99217[0], 99218[0], 99219[0], 99220[0], 99221[0], 99222[0], 99223[0], 99224[0], 99225[0], 99226[0], 99231[0], 99232[0], 99233[0], 99234[0], 99235[0], 99236[0], 99238[0], 99239[0], 99281[0], 99282[0], 99283[0], 99284[0], 99285[0], 99304[0], 99305[0], 99306[0], 99307[0], 99308[0], 99309[0], 99310[0], 99315[0], 99318[0], 99324[0], 99325[0], 99326[0], 99327[0], 99328[0], 99334[0], 99335[0], 99336[0], 99337[0], 99341[0], 99342[0], 99343[0], 99347[0], 99348[0], 99349[0], 99354[0], 99355[0], 99356[0], 99357[0], 99358[0], 99359[0], 99415[0], 99416[0], 99446[0], 99447[0], 99448[0], 99449[0], 99451[0], 99452[0], 99468[0], 99469[0], 99471[0], 99472[0], 99475[0], 99476[0], 99477[0], 99478[0], 99479[0], 99480[0], 99483[0], 99497[0], C8921[1], C8922[1], C8923[1], C8924[1], C8925[1], C8926[1], C8927[0], C8929[1], C8930[1], G0380[1], G0381[1], G0382[1], G0383[1], G0384[1], G0406[0], G0407[0], G0408[0], G0425[0], G0426[0], G0427[0], G0463[0], G0500[0], G0508[0], G0509[0]
00922	01996[1], 0213T[1], 0216T[1], 0228T[1], 0230T[1], 31505[1], 31515[1], 31527[1], 31622[1], 31634[1], 31645[1], 31647[1], 36000[1], 36010[0], 36011[1], 36012[1], 36013[1], 36014[1], 36015[1], 36400[1], 36405[1], 36406[1], 36410[1], 36420[1], 36425[1], 36430[1], 36440[1], 36591[0], 36592[0], 36600[1], 36640[1], 43752[1], 43753[1], 43754[1], 61026[1], 61055[1], 62280[1], 62281[1], 62282[1], 62284[1], 62320[1], 62321[1], 62322[1], 62323[1], 62324[1], 62325[1], 62326[1], 62327[1], 64400[1], 64402[1], 64405[1], 64408[1], 64410[1], 64413[1], 64415[1], 64416[1], 64417[1], 64418[1], 64420[1], 64421[1], 64425[1], 64430[1], 64435[1], 64445[1], 64446[1], 64447[1], 64448[1], 64449[1], 64450[1], 64461[1], 64463[1], 64479[1], 64483[1], 64486[1], 64487[1], 64488[1], 64489[1], 64490[1], 64493[1], 64505[1], 64510[1], 64517[1], 64520[1], 64530[1], 64553[1], 64555[1], 67500[1], 76000[1], 76970[1], 76998[0], 77002[0], 90865[1], 92511[1], 92512[1], 92516[1], 92520[1], 92537[1], 92538[1], 92950[1], 92953[1], 92960[1], 92961[1], 93000[1], 93005[1], 93010[1], 93040[1], 93041[1], 93042[1], 93050[0], 93303[0], 93304[0], 93306[1], 93307[1], 93308[1], 93312[1], 93313[1], 93314[1], 93315[1], 93316[1], 93317[1], 93318[0], 93351[1], 93355[0], 93451[1], 93456[1], 93457[1], 93561[0], 93562[0], 93701[0], 93922[1], 93923[1], 93924[1], 93925[1], 93926[1], 93930[1], 93931[1], 93970[1], 93971[1], 93975[1], 93976[1], 93978[1], 93979[1], 93980[1], 93981[1], 94002[1], 94004[1], 94200[1], 94250[0], 94640[1], 94644[1], 94660[1], 94662[1], 94680[1], 94681[1], 94690[1], 94760[0], 94761[0], 94762[1], 94770[1], 95812[0], 95813[0], 95816[0], 95819[0], 95822[0], 95829[0], 95955[0], 95956[0], 95957[0], 96360[0], 96365[0], 96372[0], 96373[0], 96374[0], 96375[0], 96376[0], 96377[0], 99151[0], 99152[0], 99153[0], 99155[0], 99156[0], 99157[0], 99201[0], 99202[0], 99203[0], 99204[0], 99205[0], 99211[0], 99212[0], 99213[0], 99214[0], 99215[0], 99217[0], 99218[0], 99219[0], 99220[0], 99221[0], 99222[0], 99223[0], 99224[0], 99225[0], 99226[0], 99231[0], 99232[0], 99233[0], 99234[0], 99235[0], 99236[0], 99238[0], 99239[0], 99281[0], 99282[0], 99283[0], 99284[0], 99285[0], 99304[0], 99305[0], 99306[0], 99307[0], 99308[0], 99309[0], 99310[0], 99315[0], 99318[0], 99324[0], 99325[0], 99326[0], 99327[0], 99328[0], 99334[0], 99335[0], 99336[0], 99337[0], 99341[0], 99342[0], 99343[0], 99347[0], 99348[0], 99349[0], 99354[0], 99355[0], 99356[0], 99357[0], 99358[0], 99359[0], 99415[0], 99416[0], 99446[0], 99447[0], 99448[0], 99449[0], 99451[0], 99452[0], 99466[0], 99468[0], 99469[0], 99471[0], 99472[0], 99475[0], 99476[0], 99477[0], 99478[0], 99479[0], 99480[0], 99483[0], 99485[0], 99497[0], C8921[1], C8922[1], C8923[1], C8924[1], C8925[1], C8926[1], C8927[0], C8929[1], C8930[1], G0380[1], G0381[1], G0382[1], G0383[1], G0384[1], G0406[0], G0407[0], G0408[0], G0425[0], G0426[0], G0427[0], G0463[0], G0500[0], G0508[0], G0509[0]
00924	01996[1], 0213T[1], 0216T[1], 0228T[1], 0230T[1], 31505[1], 31515[1], 31527[1], 31622[1], 31634[1], 31645[1], 31647[1], 36000[1], 36010[0], 36011[1], 36012[1], 36013[1], 36014[1], 36015[1], 36400[1], 36405[1], 36406[1], 36410[1], 36420[1], 36425[1], 36430[1], 36440[1], 36591[0], 36592[0], 36600[1], 36640[1], 43752[1], 43753[1], 43754[1], 61026[1], 61055[1], 62280[1], 62281[1], 62282[1], 62284[1], 62320[1], 62321[1], 62322[1], 62323[1], 62324[1], 62325[1], 62326[1], 62327[1], 64400[1], 64402[1], 64405[1], 64408[1], 64410[1], 64413[1], 64415[1], 64416[1], 64417[1], 64418[1], 64420[1], 64421[1], 64425[1], 64430[1], 64435[1], 64445[1], 64446[1], 64447[1], 64448[1], 64449[1], 64450[1], 64461[1],

0 = Modifier usage not allowed or inappropriate 1 = Modifier usage allowed

CPT © 2018 American Medical Association. All Rights Reserved.

Code 1	Code 2
	64463[1], 64479[1], 64483[1], 64486[1], 64487[1], 64488[1], 64489[1], 64490[1], 64493[1], 64505[1], 64510[1], 64517[1], 64520[1], 64530[1], 64553[1], 64555[1], 67500[1], 76000[1], 76970[1], 76998[0], 77002[0], 90865[1], 92511[1], 92512[1], 92516[1], 92520[1], 92537[1], 92538[1], 92950[1], 92953[1], 92960[1], 92961[1], 93000[1], 93005[1], 93010[1], 93040[1], 93041[1], 93042[1], 93050[0], 93303[0], 93304[0], 93306[1], 93307[1], 93308[1], 93312[1], 93313[1], 93314[1], 93315[1], 93316[1], 93317[1], 93318[0], 93351[1], 93355[0], 93451[1], 93456[1], 93457[1], 93561[0], 93562[0], 93701[0], 93922[1], 93923[1], 93924[1], 93925[1], 93926[1], 93930[1], 93931[1], 93970[1], 93971[1], 93975[1], 93976[1], 93978[1], 93979[1], 93980[1], 93981[1], 94002[1], 94004[1], 94200[1], 94250[0], 94640[1], 94644[1], 94660[1], 94662[1], 94680[1], 94681[1], 94690[1], 94760[0], 94761[0], 94762[1], 94770[1], 95812[0], 95813[0], 95816[0], 95819[0], 95822[0], 95829[0], 95955[0], 95956[0], 95957[0], 96360[0], 96365[0], 96372[0], 96373[0], 96374[0], 96375[0], 96376[0], 96377[0], 99151[0], 99152[0], 99153[0], 99155[0], 99156[0], 99157[0], 99201[0], 99202[0], 99203[0], 99204[0], 99205[0], 99211[0], 99212[0], 99213[0], 99214[0], 99215[0], 99217[0], 99218[0], 99219[0], 99220[0], 99221[0], 99222[0], 99223[0], 99224[0], 99225[0], 99226[0], 99231[0], 99232[0], 99233[0], 99234[0], 99235[0], 99236[0], 99238[0], 99239[0], 99281[0], 99282[0], 99283[0], 99284[0], 99285[0], 99304[0], 99305[0], 99306[0], 99307[0], 99308[0], 99309[0], 99310[0], 99315[0], 99318[0], 99324[0], 99325[0], 99326[0], 99327[0], 99328[0], 99334[0], 99335[0], 99336[0], 99337[0], 99341[0], 99342[0], 99343[0], 99347[0], 99348[0], 99349[0], 99354[0], 99355[0], 99356[0], 99357[0], 99358[0], 99359[0], 99415[0], 99416[0], 99446[0], 99447[0], 99448[0], 99449[0], 99451[0], 99452[0], 99466[0], 99468[0], 99469[0], 99471[0], 99472[0], 99475[0], 99476[0], 99477[0], 99478[0], 99479[0], 99480[0], 99483[0], 99485[0], 99497[0], C8921[1], C8922[1], C8923[1], C8924[1], C8925[1], C8926[1], C8927[0], C8929[1], C8930[1], G0380[1], G0381[1], G0382[1], G0383[1], G0384[1], G0406[0], G0407[0], G0408[0], G0425[0], G0426[0], G0427[0], G0463[0], G0500[0], G0508[0], G0509[0]
00926	01996[1], 0213T[1], 0216T[1], 0228T[1], 0230T[1], 31505[1], 31515[1], 31527[1], 31622[1], 31634[1], 31645[1], 31647[1], 36000[1], 36010[0], 36011[1], 36012[1], 36013[1], 36014[1], 36015[1], 36400[1], 36405[1], 36406[1], 36410[1], 36420[1], 36425[1], 36430[1], 36440[1], 36591[0], 36592[0], 36600[1], 36640[1], 43752[1], 43753[1], 43754[1], 61026[1], 61055[1], 62280[1], 62281[1], 62282[1], 62284[1], 62320[1], 62321[1], 62322[1], 62323[1], 62324[1], 62325[1], 62326[1], 62327[1], 64400[1], 64402[1], 64405[1], 64408[1], 64410[1], 64413[1], 64415[1], 64416[1], 64417[1], 64418[1], 64420[1], 64421[1], 64425[1], 64430[1], 64435[1], 64445[1], 64446[1], 64447[1], 64448[1], 64449[1], 64450[1], 64461[1], 64463[1], 64479[1], 64483[1], 64486[1], 64487[1], 64488[1], 64489[1], 64490[1], 64493[1], 64505[1], 64510[1], 64517[1], 64520[1], 64530[1], 64553[1], 64555[1], 67500[1], 76000[1], 76970[1], 76998[0], 77002[0], 90865[1], 92511[1], 92512[1], 92516[1], 92520[1], 92537[1], 92538[1], 92950[1], 92953[1], 92960[1], 92961[1], 93000[1], 93005[1], 93010[1], 93040[1], 93041[1], 93042[1], 93050[0], 93303[0], 93304[0], 93306[1], 93307[1], 93308[1], 93312[1], 93313[1], 93314[1], 93315[1], 93316[1], 93317[1], 93318[0], 93351[1], 93355[0], 93451[1], 93456[1], 93457[1], 93561[0], 93562[0], 93701[0], 93922[1], 93923[1], 93924[1], 93925[1], 93926[1], 93930[1], 93931[1], 93970[1], 93971[1], 93975[1], 93976[1], 93978[1], 93979[1], 93980[1], 93981[1], 94002[1], 94004[1], 94200[1], 94250[0], 94640[1], 94644[1], 94660[1], 94662[1], 94680[1], 94681[1], 94690[1], 94760[0], 94761[0], 94762[1], 94770[1], 95812[0], 95813[0], 95816[0], 95819[0], 95822[0], 95829[0], 95955[0], 95956[0], 95957[0], 96360[0], 96365[0], 96372[0], 96373[0], 96374[0], 96375[0], 96376[0], 96377[0], 99151[0], 99152[0], 99153[0], 99155[0], 99156[0], 99157[0], 99201[0], 99202[0], 99203[0], 99204[0], 99205[0], 99211[0], 99212[0], 99213[0], 99214[0], 99215[0], 99217[0], 99218[0], 99219[0], 99220[0], 99221[0], 99222[0], 99223[0], 99224[0], 99225[0], 99226[0], 99231[0], 99232[0], 99233[0], 99234[0], 99235[0], 99236[0], 99238[0], 99239[0], 99281[0], 99282[0], 99283[0], 99284[0], 99285[0], 99304[0], 99305[0], 99306[0], 99307[0], 99308[0], 99309[0], 99310[0], 99315[0], 99318[0], 99324[0], 99325[0], 99326[0], 99327[0], 99328[0], 99334[0], 99335[0], 99336[0], 99337[0], 99341[0], 99342[0], 99343[0], 99347[0], 99348[0], 99349[0], 99354[0], 99355[0], 99356[0], 99357[0], 99358[0], 99359[0], 99415[0], 99416[0], 99446[0], 99447[0], 99448[0], 99449[0], 99451[0], 99452[0], 99466[0], 99468[0], 99469[0], 99471[0], 99472[0], 99475[0], 99476[0], 99477[0], 99478[0], 99479[0], 99480[0], 99483[0], 99485[0], 99497[0], C8921[1], C8922[1], C8923[1], C8924[1], C8925[1], C8926[1], C8927[0], C8929[1], C8930[1], G0380[1], G0381[1], G0382[1], G0383[1], G0384[1], G0406[0], G0407[0], G0408[0], G0425[0], G0426[0], G0427[0], G0463[0], G0500[0], G0508[0], G0509[0]
00928	01996[1], 0213T[1], 0216T[1], 0228T[1], 0230T[1], 31505[1], 31515[1], 31527[1], 31622[1], 31634[1], 31645[1], 31647[1], 36000[1], 36010[0], 36011[1], 36012[1], 36013[1], 36014[1], 36015[1], 36400[1], 36405[1], 36406[1], 36410[1], 36420[1], 36425[1], 36430[1], 36440[1], 36591[0], 36592[0], 36600[1], 36640[1], 43752[1], 43753[1], 43754[1], 61026[1], 61055[1], 62280[1], 62281[1], 62282[1], 62284[1], 62320[1], 62321[1], 62322[1], 62323[1], 62324[1], 62325[1], 62326[1], 62327[1], 64400[1], 64402[1], 64405[1], 64408[1], 64410[1], 64413[1], 64415[1], 64416[1], 64417[1], 64418[1], 64420[1], 64421[1], 64425[1], 64430[1], 64435[1], 64445[1], 64446[1], 64447[1], 64448[1], 64449[1], 64450[1], 64461[1], 64463[1], 64479[1], 64483[1], 64486[1], 64487[1], 64488[1], 64489[1], 64490[1], 64493[1], 64505[1], 64510[1], 64517[1], 64520[1], 64530[1], 64553[1], 64555[1], 67500[1], 76000[1], 76970[1], 76998[0], 77002[0], 90865[1], 92511[1], 92512[1], 92516[1], 92520[1], 92537[1], 92538[1], 92950[1], 92953[1], 92960[1], 92961[1], 93000[1], 93005[1], 93010[1], 93040[1], 93041[1], 93042[1], 93050[0], 93303[0], 93304[0], 93306[1], 93307[1], 93308[1], 93312[1], 93313[1], 93314[1], 93315[1], 93316[1], 93317[1], 93318[0], 93351[1], 93355[0], 93451[1], 93456[1], 93457[1], 93561[0], 93562[0], 93701[0], 93922[1], 93923[1], 93924[1], 93925[1], 93926[1], 93930[1], 93931[1], 93970[1], 93971[1], 93975[1], 93976[1], 93978[1], 93979[1], 93980[1], 93981[1], 94002[1], 94004[1], 94200[1], 94250[0], 94640[1], 94644[1], 94660[1], 94662[1], 94680[1], 94681[1], 94690[1], 94760[0], 94761[0], 94762[1], 94770[1], 95812[0], 95813[0], 95816[0], 95819[0], 95822[0], 95829[0], 95955[0], 95956[0], 95957[0], 96360[0], 96365[0], 96372[0], 96373[0], 96374[0], 96375[0], 96376[0], 96377[0], 99151[0], 99152[0], 99153[0], 99155[0], 99156[0], 99157[0], 99201[0], 99202[0], 99203[0], 99204[0], 99205[0], 99211[0], 99212[0], 99213[0], 99214[0], 99215[0], 99217[0], 99218[0], 99219[0], 99220[0], 99221[0], 99222[0], 99223[0], 99224[0], 99225[0], 99226[0], 99231[0], 99232[0], 99233[0], 99234[0], 99235[0], 99236[0], 99238[0], 99239[0], 99281[0], 99282[0], 99283[0], 99284[0], 99285[0], 99304[0], 99305[0], 99306[0], 99307[0], 99308[0], 99309[0], 99310[0], 99315[0], 99318[0], 99324[0], 99325[0], 99326[0], 99327[0], 99328[0], 99334[0], 99335[0], 99336[0], 99337[0], 99341[0], 99342[0], 99343[0], 99347[0], 99348[0], 99349[0], 99354[0], 99355[0], 99356[0], 99357[0], 99358[0], 99359[0], 99415[0], 99416[0], 99446[0], 99447[0], 99448[0], 99449[0], 99451[0], 99452[0], 99466[0], 99468[0], 99469[0], 99471[0], 99472[0], 99475[0], 99476[0], 99477[0], 99478[0], 99479[0], 99480[0], 99483[0], 99485[0], 99497[0], C8921[1], C8922[1], C8923[1], C8924[1], C8925[1], C8926[1], C8927[0], C8929[1], C8930[1], G0380[1], G0381[1], G0382[1], G0383[1], G0384[1], G0406[0], G0407[0], G0408[0], G0425[0], G0426[0], G0427[0], G0463[0], G0500[0], G0508[0], G0509[0]
00930	01996[1], 0213T[1], 0216T[1], 0228T[1], 0230T[1], 31505[1], 31515[1], 31527[1], 31622[1], 31634[1], 31645[1], 31647[1], 36000[1], 36010[0], 36011[1], 36012[1], 36013[1], 36014[1], 36015[1], 36400[1], 36405[1], 36406[1], 36410[1], 36420[1], 36425[1], 36430[1], 36440[1], 36591[0], 36592[0], 36600[1], 36640[1], 43752[1], 43753[1], 43754[1], 61026[1], 61055[1], 62280[1], 62281[1], 62282[1], 62284[1], 62320[1], 62321[1], 62322[1], 62323[1], 62324[1], 62325[1], 62326[1], 62327[1], 64400[1], 64402[1], 64405[1], 64408[1], 64410[1], 64413[1], 64415[1], 64416[1], 64417[1], 64418[1], 64420[1], 64421[1], 64425[1], 64430[1], 64435[1], 64445[1], 64446[1], 64447[1], 64448[1], 64449[1], 64450[1], 64461[1], 64463[1], 64479[1], 64483[1], 64486[1], 64487[1], 64488[1], 64489[1], 64490[1], 64493[1], 64505[1], 64510[1], 64517[1], 64520[1], 64530[1], 64553[1], 64555[1], 67500[1], 76000[1], 76970[1], 76998[0], 77002[0], 90865[1], 92511[1], 92512[1], 92516[1], 92520[1], 92537[1], 92538[1], 92950[1], 92953[1], 92960[1], 92961[1], 93000[1], 93005[1], 93010[1], 93040[1], 93041[1], 93042[1], 93050[0], 93303[0], 93304[0], 93306[1], 93307[1], 93308[1], 93312[1], 93313[1], 93314[1], 93315[1], 93316[1], 93317[1], 93318[0], 93351[1], 93355[0], 93451[1], 93456[1], 93457[1], 93561[0], 93562[0], 93701[0], 93922[1], 93923[1], 93924[1], 93925[1], 93926[1], 93930[1], 93931[1], 93970[1], 93971[1], 93975[1], 93976[1], 93978[1], 93979[1], 93980[1], 93981[1], 94002[1], 94004[1], 94200[1], 94250[0], 94640[1], 94644[1], 94660[1], 94662[1], 94680[1], 94681[1], 94690[1], 94760[0], 94761[0], 94762[1], 94770[1], 95812[0], 95813[0], 95816[0], 95819[0], 95822[0], 95829[0], 95955[0], 95956[0], 95957[0], 96360[0], 96365[0], 96372[0], 96373[0], 96374[0], 96375[0], 96376[0], 96377[0], 99151[0], 99152[0], 99153[0], 99155[0], 99156[0], 99157[0], 99201[0], 99202[0], 99203[0], 99204[0], 99205[0], 99211[0], 99212[0], 99213[0], 99214[0], 99215[0], 99217[0], 99218[0], 99219[0], 99220[0], 99221[0], 99222[0], 99223[0], 99224[0], 99225[0], 99226[0], 99231[0], 99232[0], 99233[0], 99234[0], 99235[0], 99236[0], 99238[0], 99239[0], 99281[0], 99282[0], 99283[0], 99284[0], 99285[0], 99304[0], 99305[0], 99306[0], 99307[0], 99308[0], 99309[0], 99310[0], 99315[0], 99318[0], 99324[0], 99325[0], 99326[0], 99327[0], 99328[0], 99334[0], 99335[0], 99336[0], 99337[0], 99341[0], 99342[0], 99343[0], 99347[0], 99348[0], 99349[0], 99354[0], 99355[0], 99356[0], 99357[0], 99358[0], 99359[0], 99415[0], 99416[0], 99446[0], 99447[0], 99448[0], 99449[0], 99451[0], 99452[0], 99466[0], 99468[0], 99469[0], 99471[0], 99472[0], 99475[0], 99476[0], 99477[0], 99478[0], 99479[0], 99480[0], 99483[0], 99485[0], 99497[0], C8921[1], C8922[1], C8923[1], C8924[1], C8925[1], C8926[1], C8927[0], C8929[1], C8930[1], G0380[1], G0381[1], G0382[1], G0383[1], G0384[1], G0406[0], G0407[0], G0408[0], G0425[0], G0426[0], G0427[0], G0463[0], G0500[0], G0508[0], G0509[0]
00932	01996[1], 0213T[1], 0216T[1], 0228T[1], 0230T[1], 31505[1], 31515[1], 31527[1], 31622[1], 31634[1], 31645[1], 31647[1], 36000[1], 36010[0], 36011[1], 36012[1], 36013[1], 36014[1], 36015[1], 36400[1], 36405[1], 36406[1], 36410[1], 36420[1], 36425[1], 36430[1], 36440[1], 36591[0], 36592[0], 36600[1], 36640[1], 43752[1], 43753[1], 43754[1], 61026[1], 61055[1], 62280[1], 62281[1], 62282[1], 62284[1], 62320[1], 62321[1], 62322[1], 62323[1], 62324[1], 62325[1], 62326[1], 62327[1], 64400[1], 64402[1], 64405[1], 64408[1], 64410[1], 64413[1], 64415[1], 64416[1], 64417[1], 64418[1], 64420[1], 64421[1], 64425[1], 64430[1], 64435[1], 64445[1], 64446[1], 64447[1], 64448[1], 64449[1], 64450[1], 64461[1], 64463[1], 64479[1], 64483[1], 64486[1], 64487[1], 64488[1], 64489[1], 64490[1], 64493[1], 64505[1], 64510[1], 64517[1], 64520[1], 64530[1], 64553[1], 64555[1], 67500[1], 76000[1], 76970[1], 76998[0], 77002[0], 90865[1], 92511[1], 92512[1], 92516[1], 92520[1], 92537[1], 92538[1], 92950[1], 92953[1], 92960[1], 92961[1], 93000[1], 93005[1], 93010[1], 93040[1], 93041[1], 93042[1], 93050[0], 93303[0], 93304[0], 93306[1], 93307[1], 93308[1], 93312[1], 93313[1], 93314[1], 93315[1], 93316[1], 93317[1], 93318[0], 93351[1], 93355[0], 93451[1], 93456[1], 93457[1], 93561[0], 93562[0], 93701[0], 93922[1], 93923[1], 93924[1], 93925[1], 93926[1], 93930[1], 93931[1], 93970[1], 93971[1], 93975[1], 93976[1], 93978[1], 93979[1], 93980[1], 93981[1], 94002[1], 94004[1], 94200[1], 94250[0], 94640[1], 94644[1], 94660[1], 94662[1], 94680[1], 94681[1], 94690[1], 94760[0], 94761[0], 94762[1], 94770[1], 95812[0], 95813[0], 95816[0], 95819[0], 95822[0], 95829[0], 95955[0], 95956[0], 95957[0], 96360[0], 96365[0], 96372[0], 96373[0], 96374[0], 96375[0], 96376[0], 96377[0], 99151[0], 99152[0], 99153[0], 99155[0], 99156[0], 99157[0], 99201[0], 99202[0], 99203[0], 99204[0], 99205[0], 99211[0], 99212[0], 99213[0],

0 = Modifier usage not allowed or inappropriate 1 = Modifier usage allowed

Appendix A: NCCI - CPT Codes

CPT © 2018 American Medical Association. All Rights Reserved.

Code 1	Code 2
	99214^0, 99215^0, 99217^0, 99218^0, 99219^0, 99220^0, 99221^0, 99222^0, 99223^0, 99224^0, 99225^0, 99226^0, 99231^0, 99232^0, 99233^0, 99234^0, 99235^0, 99236^0, 99238^0, 99239^0, 99281^0, 99282^0, 99283^0, 99284^0, 99285^0, 99304^0, 99305^0, 99306^0, 99307^0, 99308^0, 99309^0, 99310^0, 99315^0, 99318^0, 99324^0, 99325^0, 99326^0, 99327^0, 99328^0, 99334^0, 99335^0, 99336^0, 99337^0, 99341^0, 99342^0, 99343^0, 99347^0, 99348^0, 99349^0, 99354^0, 99355^0, 99356^0, 99357^0, 99358^0, 99359^0, 99415^0, 99416^0, 99446^0, 99447^0, 99448^0, 99449^0, 99451^0, 99452^0, 99466^0, 99468^0, 99469^0, 99471^0, 99472^0, 99475^0, 99476^0, 99477^0, 99478^0, 99479^0, 99480^0, 99483^0, 99485^0, 99497^0, C8921^1, C8922^1, C8923^1, C8924^1, C8925^1, C8926^1, C8927^0, C8929^1, C8930^1, G0380^1, G0381^1, G0382^1, G0383^1, G0384^1, G0406^0, G0407^0, G0408^0, G0425^0, G0426^0, G0427^0, G0463^0, G0500^0, G0508^0, G0509^0
00934	01996^1, 0213T^1, 0216T^1, 0228T^1, 0230T^1, 31505^1, 31515^1, 31527^1, 31622^1, 31634^1, 31645^1, 31647^1, 36000^1, 36010^0, 36011^1, 36012^1, 36013^1, 36014^1, 36015^1, 36400^1, 36405^1, 36406^1, 36410^1, 36420^1, 36425^1, 36430^1, 36440^1, 36591^0, 36592^0, 36600^1, 36640^1, 43752^1, 43753^1, 43754^1, 61026^1, 61055^1, 62280^1, 62281^1, 62282^1, 62284^1, 62320^1, 62321^1, 62322^1, 62323^1, 62324^1, 62325^1, 62326^1, 62327^1, 64400^1, 64402^1, 64405^1, 64408^1, 64410^1, 64413^1, 64415^1, 64416^1, 64417^1, 64418^1, 64420^1, 64421^1, 64425^1, 64430^1, 64435^1, 64445^1, 64446^1, 64447^1, 64448^1, 64449^1, 64450^1, 64461^1, 64463^1, 64479^1, 64483^1, 64486^1, 64487^1, 64488^1, 64489^1, 64490^1, 64493^1, 64505^1, 64510^1, 64517^1, 64520^1, 64530^1, 64553^1, 64555^1, 67500^1, 76000^1, 76970^1, 76998^0, 77002^0, 90865^1, 92511^1, 92512^1, 92516^1, 92520^1, 92537^1, 92538^1, 92950^1, 92953^1, 92960^1, 92961^1, 93000^1, 93005^1, 93010^1, 93040^1, 93041^1, 93042^1, 93050^0, 93303^0, 93304^0, 93306^1, 93307^1, 93308^1, 93312^1, 93313^1, 93314^1, 93315^1, 93316^1, 93317^1, 93318^0, 93351^1, 93355^0, 93451^1, 93456^1, 93457^1, 93561^0, 93562^0, 93701^0, 93922^1, 93923^1, 93924^1, 93925^1, 93926^1, 93930^1, 93931^1, 93970^1, 93971^1, 93975^1, 93976^1, 93978^1, 93979^1, 93980^1, 93981^1, 94002^1, 94004^1, 94200^1, 94250^0, 94640^1, 94644^1, 94660^1, 94662^1, 94680^1, 94681^1, 94690^1, 94760^0, 94761^0, 94762^1, 94770^1, 95812^0, 95813^0, 95816^0, 95819^0, 95822^0, 95829^0, 95955^0, 95956^0, 95957^0, 96360^0, 96365^0, 96372^0, 96373^0, 96374^0, 96375^0, 96376^0, 96377^0, 99151^0, 99152^0, 99153^0, 99155^0, 99156^0, 99157^0, 99201^0, 99202^0, 99203^0, 99204^0, 99205^0, 99211^0, 99212^0, 99213^0, 99214^0, 99215^0, 99217^0, 99218^0, 99219^0, 99220^0, 99221^0, 99222^0, 99223^0, 99224^0, 99225^0, 99226^0, 99231^0, 99232^0, 99233^0, 99234^0, 99235^0, 99236^0, 99238^0, 99239^0, 99281^0, 99282^0, 99283^0, 99284^0, 99285^0, 99304^0, 99305^0, 99306^0, 99307^0, 99308^0, 99309^0, 99310^0, 99315^0, 99318^0, 99324^0, 99325^0, 99326^0, 99327^0, 99328^0, 99334^0, 99335^0, 99336^0, 99337^0, 99341^0, 99342^0, 99343^0, 99347^0, 99348^0, 99349^0, 99354^0, 99355^0, 99356^0, 99357^0, 99358^0, 99359^0, 99415^0, 99416^0, 99446^0, 99447^0, 99448^0, 99449^0, 99451^0, 99452^0, 99466^0, 99468^0, 99469^0, 99471^0, 99472^0, 99475^0, 99476^0, 99477^0, 99478^0, 99479^0, 99480^0, 99483^0, 99485^0, 99497^0, C8921^1, C8922^1, C8923^1, C8924^1, C8925^1, C8926^1, C8927^0, C8929^1, C8930^1, G0380^1, G0381^1, G0382^1, G0383^1, G0384^1, G0406^0, G0407^0, G0408^0, G0425^0, G0426^0, G0427^0, G0463^0, G0500^0, G0508^0, G0509^0
00936	01996^1, 0213T^1, 0216T^1, 0228T^1, 0230T^1, 31505^1, 31515^1, 31527^1, 31622^1, 31634^1, 31645^1, 31647^1, 36000^1, 36010^0, 36011^1, 36012^1, 36013^1, 36014^1, 36015^1, 36400^1, 36405^1, 36406^1, 36410^1, 36420^1, 36425^1, 36430^1, 36440^1, 36591^0, 36592^0, 36600^1, 36640^1, 43752^1, 43753^1, 43754^1, 61026^1, 61055^1, 62280^1, 62281^1, 62282^1, 62284^1, 62320^1, 62321^1, 62322^1, 62323^1, 62324^1, 62325^1, 62326^1, 62327^1, 64400^1, 64402^1, 64405^1, 64408^1, 64410^1, 64413^1, 64415^1, 64416^1, 64417^1, 64418^1, 64420^1, 64421^1, 64425^1, 64430^1, 64435^1, 64445^1, 64446^1, 64447^1, 64448^1, 64449^1, 64450^1, 64461^1, 64463^1, 64479^1, 64483^1, 64486^1, 64487^1, 64488^1, 64489^1, 64490^1, 64493^1, 64505^1, 64510^1, 64517^1, 64520^1, 64530^1, 64553^1, 64555^1, 67500^1, 76000^1, 76970^1, 76998^0, 77002^0, 90865^1, 92511^1, 92512^1, 92516^1, 92520^1, 92537^1, 92538^1, 92950^1, 92953^1, 92960^1, 92961^1, 93000^1, 93005^1, 93010^1, 93040^1, 93041^1, 93042^1, 93050^0, 93303^0, 93304^0, 93306^1, 93307^1, 93308^1, 93312^1, 93313^1, 93314^1, 93315^1, 93316^1, 93317^1, 93318^0, 93351^1, 93355^0, 93451^1, 93456^1, 93457^1, 93561^0, 93562^0, 93701^0, 93922^1, 93923^1, 93924^1, 93925^1, 93926^1, 93930^1, 93931^1, 93970^1, 93971^1, 93975^1, 93976^1, 93978^1, 93979^1, 93980^1, 93981^1, 94002^1, 94004^1, 94200^1, 94250^0, 94640^1, 94644^1, 94660^1, 94662^1, 94680^1, 94681^1, 94690^1, 94760^0, 94761^0, 94762^1, 94770^1, 95812^0, 95813^0, 95816^0, 95819^0, 95822^0, 95829^0, 95955^0, 95956^0, 95957^0, 96360^0, 96365^0, 96372^0, 96373^0, 96374^0, 96375^0, 96376^0, 96377^0, 99151^0, 99152^0, 99153^0, 99155^0, 99156^0, 99157^0, 99201^0, 99202^0, 99203^0, 99204^0, 99205^0, 99211^0, 99212^0, 99213^0, 99214^0, 99215^0, 99217^0, 99218^0, 99219^0, 99220^0, 99221^0, 99222^0, 99223^0, 99224^0, 99225^0, 99226^0, 99231^0, 99232^0, 99233^0, 99234^0, 99235^0, 99236^0, 99238^0, 99239^0, 99281^0, 99282^0, 99283^0, 99284^0, 99285^0, 99304^0, 99305^0, 99306^0, 99307^0, 99308^0, 99309^0, 99310^0, 99315^0, 99318^0, 99324^0, 99325^0, 99326^0, 99327^0, 99328^0, 99334^0, 99335^0, 99336^0, 99337^0, 99341^0, 99342^0, 99343^0, 99347^0, 99348^0, 99349^0, 99354^0, 99355^0, 99356^0, 99357^0, 99358^0, 99359^0, 99415^0, 99416^0, 99446^0, 99447^0, 99448^0, 99449^0, 99451^0, 99452^0, 99466^0, 99468^0, 99469^0, 99471^0, 99472^0, 99475^0, 99476^0, 99477^0, 99478^0, 99479^0, 99480^0, 99483^0, 99485^0, 99497^0, C8921^1, C8922^1, C8923^1, C8924^1, C8925^1, C8926^1, C8927^0, C8929^1, C8930^1, G0380^1, G0381^1, G0382^1, G0383^1, G0384^1, G0406^0, G0407^0, G0408^0, G0425^0, G0426^0, G0427^0, G0463^0, G0500^0, G0508^0, G0509^0
00938	01996^1, 0213T^1, 0216T^1, 0228T^1, 0230T^1, 31505^1, 31515^1, 31527^1, 31622^1, 31634^1, 31645^1, 31647^1, 36000^1, 36010^0, 36011^1, 36012^1, 36013^1, 36014^1, 36015^1, 36400^1, 36405^1, 36406^1, 36410^1, 36420^1, 36425^1, 36430^1, 36440^1, 36591^0, 36592^0, 36600^1, 36640^1, 43752^1, 43753^1, 43754^1, 61026^1, 61055^1, 62280^1, 62281^1, 62282^1, 62284^1, 62320^1, 62321^1, 62322^1, 62323^1, 62324^1, 62325^1, 62326^1, 62327^1, 64400^1, 64402^1, 64405^1, 64408^1, 64410^1, 64413^1, 64415^1, 64416^1, 64417^1, 64418^1, 64420^1, 64421^1, 64425^1, 64430^1, 64435^1, 64445^1, 64446^1, 64447^1, 64448^1, 64449^1, 64450^1, 64461^1, 64463^1, 64479^1, 64483^1, 64486^1, 64487^1, 64488^1, 64489^1, 64490^1, 64493^1, 64505^1, 64510^1, 64517^1, 64520^1, 64530^1, 64553^1, 64555^1, 67500^1, 76000^1, 76970^1, 76998^0, 77002^0, 90865^1, 92511^1, 92512^1, 92516^1, 92520^1, 92537^1, 92538^1, 92950^1, 92953^1, 92960^1, 92961^1, 93000^1, 93005^1, 93010^1, 93040^1, 93041^1, 93042^1, 93050^0, 93303^0, 93304^0, 93306^1, 93307^1, 93308^1, 93312^1, 93313^1, 93314^1, 93315^1, 93316^1, 93317^1, 93318^0, 93351^1, 93355^0, 93451^1, 93456^1, 93457^1, 93561^0, 93562^0, 93701^0, 93922^1, 93923^1, 93924^1, 93925^1, 93926^1, 93930^1, 93931^1, 93970^1, 93971^1, 93975^1, 93976^1, 93978^1, 93979^1, 93980^1, 93981^1, 94002^1, 94004^1, 94200^1, 94250^0, 94640^1, 94644^1, 94660^1, 94662^1, 94680^1, 94681^1, 94690^1, 94760^0, 94761^0, 94762^1, 94770^1, 95812^0, 95813^0, 95816^0, 95819^0, 95822^0, 95829^0, 95955^0, 95956^0, 95957^0, 96360^0, 96365^0, 96372^0, 96373^0, 96374^0, 96375^0, 96376^0, 96377^0, 99151^0, 99152^0, 99153^0, 99155^0, 99156^0, 99157^0, 99201^0, 99202^0, 99203^0, 99204^0, 99205^0, 99211^0, 99212^0, 99213^0, 99214^0, 99215^0, 99217^0, 99218^0, 99219^0, 99220^0, 99221^0, 99222^0, 99223^0, 99224^0, 99225^0, 99226^0, 99231^0, 99232^0, 99233^0, 99234^0, 99235^0, 99236^0, 99238^0, 99239^0, 99281^0, 99282^0, 99283^0, 99284^0, 99285^0, 99304^0, 99305^0, 99306^0, 99307^0, 99308^0, 99309^0, 99310^0, 99315^0, 99318^0, 99324^0, 99325^0, 99326^0, 99327^0, 99328^0, 99334^0, 99335^0, 99336^0, 99337^0, 99341^0, 99342^0, 99343^0, 99347^0, 99348^0, 99349^0, 99354^0, 99355^0, 99356^0, 99357^0, 99358^0, 99359^0, 99415^0, 99416^0, 99446^0, 99447^0, 99448^0, 99449^0, 99451^0, 99452^0, 99466^0, 99468^0, 99469^0, 99471^0, 99472^0, 99475^0, 99476^0, 99477^0, 99478^0, 99479^0, 99480^0, 99483^0, 99485^0, 99497^0, C8921^1, C8922^1, C8923^1, C8924^1, C8925^1, C8926^1, C8927^0, C8929^1, C8930^1, G0380^1, G0381^1, G0382^1, G0383^1, G0384^1, G0406^0, G0407^0, G0408^0, G0425^0, G0426^0, G0427^0, G0463^0, G0500^0, G0508^0, G0509^0
00940	01996^1, 0213T^1, 0216T^1, 0228T^1, 0230T^1, 31505^1, 31515^1, 31527^1, 31622^1, 31634^1, 31645^1, 31647^1, 36000^1, 36010^0, 36011^1, 36012^1, 36013^1, 36014^1, 36015^1, 36400^1, 36405^1, 36406^1, 36410^1, 36420^1, 36425^1, 36430^1, 36440^1, 36591^0, 36592^0, 36600^1, 36640^1, 43752^1, 43753^1, 43754^1, 61026^1, 61055^1, 62280^1, 62281^1, 62282^1, 62284^1, 62320^1, 62321^1, 62322^1, 62323^1, 62324^1, 62325^1, 62326^1, 62327^1, 64400^1, 64402^1, 64405^1, 64408^1, 64410^1, 64413^1, 64415^1, 64416^1, 64417^1, 64418^1, 64420^1, 64421^1, 64425^1, 64430^1, 64435^1, 64445^1, 64446^1, 64447^1, 64448^1, 64449^1, 64450^1, 64461^1, 64463^1, 64479^1, 64483^1, 64486^1, 64487^1, 64488^1, 64489^1, 64490^1, 64493^1, 64505^1, 64510^1, 64517^1, 64520^1, 64530^1, 64553^1, 64555^1, 67500^1, 76000^1, 76970^1, 76998^0, 77002^0, 90865^1, 92511^1, 92512^1, 92516^1, 92520^1, 92537^1, 92538^1, 92950^1, 92953^1, 92960^1, 92961^1, 93000^1, 93005^1, 93010^1, 93040^1, 93041^1, 93042^1, 93050^0, 93303^0, 93304^0, 93306^1, 93307^1, 93308^1, 93312^1, 93313^1, 93314^1, 93315^1, 93316^1, 93317^1, 93318^0, 93351^1, 93355^0, 93451^1, 93456^1, 93457^1, 93561^0, 93562^0, 93701^0, 93922^1, 93923^1, 93924^1, 93925^1, 93926^1, 93930^1, 93931^1, 93970^1, 93971^1, 93975^1, 93976^1, 93978^1, 93979^1, 93980^1, 93981^1, 94002^1, 94004^1, 94200^1, 94250^0, 94640^1, 94644^1, 94660^1, 94662^1, 94680^1, 94681^1, 94690^1, 94760^0, 94761^0, 94762^1, 94770^1, 95812^0, 95813^0, 95816^0, 95819^0, 95822^0, 95829^0, 95955^0, 95956^0, 95957^0, 96360^0, 96365^0, 96372^0, 96373^0, 96374^0, 96375^0, 96376^0, 96377^0, 99151^0, 99152^0, 99153^0, 99155^0, 99156^0, 99157^0, 99201^0, 99202^0, 99203^0, 99204^0, 99205^0, 99211^0, 99212^0, 99213^0, 99214^0, 99215^0, 99217^0, 99218^0, 99219^0, 99220^0, 99221^0, 99222^0, 99223^0, 99224^0, 99225^0, 99226^0, 99231^0, 99232^0, 99233^0, 99234^0, 99235^0, 99236^0, 99238^0, 99239^0, 99281^0, 99282^0, 99283^0, 99284^0, 99285^0, 99304^0, 99305^0, 99306^0, 99307^0, 99308^0, 99309^0, 99310^0, 99315^0, 99318^0, 99324^0, 99325^0, 99326^0, 99327^0, 99328^0, 99334^0, 99335^0, 99336^0, 99337^0, 99341^0, 99342^0, 99343^0, 99347^0, 99348^0, 99349^0, 99354^0, 99355^0, 99356^0, 99357^0, 99358^0, 99359^0, 99415^0, 99416^0, 99446^0, 99447^0, 99448^0, 99449^0, 99451^0, 99452^0, 99466^0, 99468^0, 99469^0, 99471^0, 99472^0, 99475^0, 99476^0, 99477^0, 99478^0, 99479^0, 99480^0, 99483^0, 99485^0, 99497^0, C8921^1, C8922^1, C8923^1, C8924^1, C8925^1, C8926^1, C8927^0, C8929^1, C8930^1, G0380^1, G0381^1, G0382^1, G0383^1, G0384^1, G0406^0, G0407^0, G0408^0, G0425^0, G0426^0, G0427^0, G0463^0, G0500^0, G0508^0, G0509^0

0 = Modifier usage not allowed or inappropriate 1 = Modifier usage allowed

CPT © 2018 American Medical Association. All Rights Reserved.

Code 1	Code 2
00942	01996[1], 0213T[1], 0216T[1], 0228T[1], 0230T[1], 31505[1], 31515[1], 31527[1], 31622[1], 31634[1], 31645[1], 31647[1], 36000[1], 36010[0], 36011[1], 36012[1], 36013[1], 36014[1], 36015[1], 36400[1], 36405[1], 36406[1], 36410[1], 36420[1], 36425[1], 36430[1], 36440[1], 36591[0], 36592[0], 36600[1], 36640[1], 43752[1], 43753[1], 43754[1], 61026[1], 61055[1], 62280[1], 62281[1], 62282[1], 62284[1], 62320[1], 62321[1], 62322[1], 62323[1], 62324[1], 62325[1], 62326[1], 62327[1], 64400[1], 64402[1], 64405[1], 64408[1], 64410[1], 64413[1], 64415[1], 64416[1], 64417[1], 64418[1], 64420[1], 64421[1], 64425[1], 64430[1], 64435[1], 64445[1], 64446[1], 64447[1], 64448[1], 64449[1], 64450[1], 64461[1], 64463[1], 64479[1], 64483[1], 64486[1], 64487[1], 64488[1], 64489[1], 64490[1], 64493[1], 64505[1], 64510[1], 64517[1], 64520[1], 64530[1], 64553[1], 64555[1], 67500[1], 76000[1], 76970[1], 76998[0], 77002[0], 90865[1], 92511[1], 92512[1], 92516[1], 92520[1], 92537[1], 92538[1], 92950[1], 92953[1], 92960[1], 92961[1], 93000[1], 93005[1], 93010[1], 93040[1], 93041[1], 93042[1], 93050[0], 93303[0], 93304[0], 93306[1], 93307[1], 93308[1], 93312[1], 93313[1], 93314[1], 93315[1], 93316[1], 93317[1], 93318[0], 93351[1], 93355[0], 93451[1], 93456[1], 93457[1], 93561[0], 93562[0], 93701[0], 93922[1], 93923[1], 93924[1], 93925[1], 93926[1], 93930[1], 93931[1], 93970[1], 93971[1], 93975[1], 93976[1], 93978[1], 93979[1], 93980[1], 93981[1], 94002[1], 94004[1], 94200[1], 94250[0], 94640[1], 94644[1], 94660[1], 94662[1], 94680[1], 94681[1], 94690[1], 94760[0], 94761[0], 94762[1], 94770[1], 95812[0], 95813[0], 95816[0], 95819[0], 95822[0], 95829[0], 95955[0], 95956[0], 95957[0], 96360[0], 96365[0], 96372[0], 96373[0], 96374[0], 96375[0], 96376[0], 96377[0], 99151[0], 99152[0], 99153[0], 99155[0], 99156[0], 99157[0], 99201[0], 99202[0], 99203[0], 99204[0], 99205[0], 99211[0], 99212[0], 99213[0], 99214[0], 99215[0], 99217[0], 99218[0], 99219[0], 99220[0], 99221[0], 99222[0], 99223[0], 99224[0], 99225[0], 99226[0], 99231[0], 99232[0], 99233[0], 99234[0], 99235[0], 99236[0], 99238[0], 99239[0], 99281[0], 99282[0], 99283[0], 99284[0], 99285[0], 99304[0], 99305[0], 99306[0], 99307[0], 99308[0], 99309[0], 99310[0], 99315[0], 99318[0], 99324[0], 99325[0], 99326[0], 99327[0], 99328[0], 99334[0], 99335[0], 99336[0], 99337[0], 99341[0], 99342[0], 99343[0], 99347[0], 99348[0], 99349[0], 99354[0], 99355[0], 99356[0], 99357[0], 99358[0], 99359[0], 99415[0], 99416[0], 99446[0], 99447[0], 99448[0], 99449[0], 99451[0], 99452[0], 99466[0], 99468[0], 99469[0], 99471[0], 99472[0], 99475[0], 99476[0], 99477[0], 99478[0], 99479[0], 99480[0], 99483[0], 99485[0], 99497[0], C8921[1], C8922[1], C8923[1], C8924[1], C8925[1], C8926[1], C8927[0], C8929[1], C8930[1], G0380[1], G0381[1], G0382[1], G0383[1], G0384[1], G0406[0], G0407[0], G0408[0], G0425[0], G0426[0], G0427[0], G0463[0], G0500[0], G0508[0], G0509[0]
00944	01996[1], 0213T[1], 0216T[1], 0228T[1], 0230T[1], 31505[1], 31515[1], 31527[1], 31622[1], 31634[1], 31645[1], 31647[1], 36000[1], 36010[0], 36011[1], 36012[1], 36013[1], 36014[1], 36015[1], 36400[1], 36405[1], 36406[1], 36410[1], 36420[1], 36425[1], 36430[1], 36440[1], 36591[0], 36592[0], 36600[1], 36640[1], 43752[1], 43753[1], 43754[1], 61026[1], 61055[1], 62280[1], 62281[1], 62282[1], 62284[1], 62320[1], 62321[1], 62322[1], 62323[1], 62324[1], 62325[1], 62326[1], 62327[1], 64400[1], 64402[1], 64405[1], 64408[1], 64410[1], 64413[1], 64415[1], 64416[1], 64417[1], 64418[1], 64420[1], 64421[1], 64425[1], 64430[1], 64435[1], 64445[1], 64446[1], 64447[1], 64448[1], 64449[1], 64450[1], 64461[1], 64463[1], 64479[1], 64483[1], 64486[1], 64487[1], 64488[1], 64489[1], 64490[1], 64493[1], 64505[1], 64510[1], 64517[1], 64520[1], 64530[1], 64553[1], 64555[1], 67500[1], 76000[1], 76970[1], 76998[0], 77002[0], 90865[1], 92511[1], 92512[1], 92516[1], 92520[1], 92537[1], 92538[1], 92950[1], 92953[1], 92960[1], 92961[1], 93000[1], 93005[1], 93010[1], 93040[1], 93041[1], 93042[1], 93050[0], 93303[0], 93304[0], 93306[1], 93307[1], 93308[1], 93312[1], 93313[1], 93314[1], 93315[1], 93316[1], 93317[1], 93318[0], 93351[1], 93355[0], 93451[1], 93456[1], 93457[1], 93561[0], 93562[0], 93701[0], 93922[1], 93923[1], 93924[1], 93925[1], 93926[1], 93930[1], 93931[1], 93970[1], 93971[1], 93975[1], 93976[1], 93978[1], 93979[1], 93980[1], 93981[1], 94002[1], 94004[1], 94200[1], 94250[0], 94640[1], 94644[1], 94660[1], 94662[1], 94680[1], 94681[1], 94690[1], 94760[0], 94761[0], 94762[1], 94770[1], 95812[0], 95813[0], 95816[0], 95819[0], 95822[0], 95829[0], 95955[0], 95956[0], 95957[0], 96360[0], 96365[0], 96372[0], 96373[0], 96374[0], 96375[0], 96376[0], 96377[0], 99151[0], 99152[0], 99153[0], 99155[0], 99156[0], 99157[0], 99201[0], 99202[0], 99203[0], 99204[0], 99205[0], 99211[0], 99212[0], 99213[0], 99214[0], 99215[0], 99217[0], 99218[0], 99219[0], 99220[0], 99221[0], 99222[0], 99223[0], 99224[0], 99225[0], 99226[0], 99231[0], 99232[0], 99233[0], 99234[0], 99235[0], 99236[0], 99238[0], 99239[0], 99281[0], 99282[0], 99283[0], 99284[0], 99285[0], 99304[0], 99305[0], 99306[0], 99307[0], 99308[0], 99309[0], 99310[0], 99315[0], 99318[0], 99324[0], 99325[0], 99326[0], 99327[0], 99328[0], 99334[0], 99335[0], 99336[0], 99337[0], 99341[0], 99342[0], 99343[0], 99347[0], 99348[0], 99349[0], 99354[0], 99355[0], 99356[0], 99357[0], 99358[0], 99359[0], 99415[0], 99416[0], 99446[0], 99447[0], 99448[0], 99449[0], 99451[0], 99452[0], 99466[0], 99468[0], 99469[0], 99471[0], 99472[0], 99475[0], 99476[0], 99477[0], 99478[0], 99479[0], 99480[0], 99483[0], 99485[0], 99497[0], C8921[1], C8922[1], C8923[1], C8924[1], C8925[1], C8926[1], C8927[0], C8929[1], C8930[1], G0380[1], G0381[1], G0382[1], G0383[1], G0384[1], G0406[0], G0407[0], G0408[0], G0425[0], G0426[0], G0427[0], G0463[0], G0500[0], G0508[0], G0509[0]
00948	01996[1], 0213T[1], 0216T[1], 0228T[1], 0230T[1], 31505[1], 31515[1], 31527[1], 31622[1], 31634[1], 31645[1], 31647[1], 36000[1], 36010[0], 36011[1], 36012[1], 36013[1], 36014[1], 36015[1], 36400[1], 36405[1], 36406[1], 36410[1], 36420[1], 36425[1], 36430[1], 36440[1], 36591[0], 36592[0], 36600[1], 36640[1], 43752[1], 43753[1], 43754[1], 61026[1], 61055[1], 62280[1], 62281[1], 62282[1], 62284[1], 62320[1], 62321[1], 62322[1], 62323[1], 62324[1], 62325[1], 62326[1], 62327[1], 64400[1], 64402[1], 64405[1], 64408[1], 64410[1], 64413[1], 64415[1], 64416[1], 64417[1], 64418[1], 64420[1], 64421[1], 64425[1], 64430[1], 64435[1], 64445[1], 64446[1], 64447[1], 64448[1], 64449[1], 64450[1], 64461[1], 64463[1], 64479[1], 64483[1], 64486[1], 64487[1], 64488[1], 64489[1], 64490[1], 64493[1], 64505[1], 64510[1], 64517[1], 64520[1], 64530[1], 64553[1], 64555[1], 67500[1], 76000[1], 76970[1], 76998[0], 77002[0], 90865[1], 92511[1], 92512[1], 92516[1], 92520[1], 92537[1], 92538[1], 92950[1], 92953[1], 92960[1], 92961[1], 93000[1], 93005[1], 93010[1], 93040[1], 93041[1], 93042[1], 93050[0], 93303[0], 93304[0], 93306[1], 93307[1], 93308[1], 93312[1], 93313[1], 93314[1], 93315[1], 93316[1], 93317[1], 93318[0], 93351[1], 93355[0], 93451[1], 93456[1], 93457[1], 93561[0], 93562[0], 93701[0], 93922[1], 93923[1], 93924[1], 93925[1], 93926[1], 93930[1], 93931[1], 93970[1], 93971[1], 93975[1], 93976[1], 93978[1], 93979[1], 93980[1], 93981[1], 94002[1], 94004[1], 94200[1], 94250[0], 94640[1], 94644[1], 94660[1], 94662[1], 94680[1], 94681[1], 94690[1], 94760[0], 94761[0], 94762[1], 94770[1], 95812[0], 95813[0], 95816[0], 95819[0], 95822[0], 95829[0], 95955[0], 95956[0], 95957[0], 96360[0], 96365[0], 96372[0], 96373[0], 96374[0], 96375[0], 96376[0], 96377[0], 99151[0], 99152[0], 99153[0], 99155[0], 99156[0], 99157[0], 99201[0], 99202[0], 99203[0], 99204[0], 99205[0], 99211[0], 99212[0], 99213[0], 99214[0], 99215[0], 99217[0], 99218[0], 99219[0], 99220[0], 99221[0], 99222[0], 99223[0], 99224[0], 99225[0], 99226[0], 99231[0], 99232[0], 99233[0], 99234[0], 99235[0], 99236[0], 99238[0], 99239[0], 99281[0], 99282[0], 99283[0], 99284[0], 99285[0], 99304[0], 99305[0], 99306[0], 99307[0], 99308[0], 99309[0], 99310[0], 99315[0], 99318[0], 99324[0], 99325[0], 99326[0], 99327[0], 99328[0], 99334[0], 99335[0], 99336[0], 99337[0], 99341[0], 99342[0], 99343[0], 99347[0], 99348[0], 99349[0], 99354[0], 99355[0], 99356[0], 99357[0], 99358[0], 99359[0], 99415[0], 99416[0], 99446[0], 99447[0], 99448[0], 99449[0], 99451[0], 99452[0], 99466[0], 99468[0], 99469[0], 99471[0], 99472[0], 99475[0], 99476[0], 99477[0], 99478[0], 99479[0], 99480[0], 99483[0], 99485[0], 99497[0], C8921[1], C8922[1], C8923[1], C8924[1], C8925[1], C8926[1], C8927[0], C8929[1], C8930[1], G0380[1], G0381[1], G0382[1], G0383[1], G0384[1], G0406[0], G0407[0], G0408[0], G0425[0], G0426[0], G0427[0], G0463[0], G0500[0], G0508[0], G0509[0]
00950	01996[1], 0213T[1], 0216T[1], 0228T[1], 0230T[1], 31505[1], 31515[1], 31527[1], 31622[1], 31634[1], 31645[1], 31647[1], 36000[1], 36010[0], 36011[1], 36012[1], 36013[1], 36014[1], 36015[1], 36400[1], 36405[1], 36406[1], 36410[1], 36420[1], 36425[1], 36430[1], 36440[1], 36591[0], 36592[0], 36600[1], 36640[1], 43752[1], 43753[1], 43754[1], 61026[1], 61055[1], 62280[1], 62281[1], 62282[1], 62284[1], 62320[1], 62321[1], 62322[1], 62323[1], 62324[1], 62325[1], 62326[1], 62327[1], 64400[1], 64402[1], 64405[1], 64408[1], 64410[1], 64413[1], 64415[1], 64416[1], 64417[1], 64418[1], 64420[1], 64421[1], 64425[1], 64430[1], 64435[1], 64445[1], 64446[1], 64447[1], 64448[1], 64449[1], 64450[1], 64461[1], 64463[1], 64479[1], 64483[1], 64486[1], 64487[1], 64488[1], 64489[1], 64490[1], 64493[1], 64505[1], 64510[1], 64517[1], 64520[1], 64530[1], 64553[1], 64555[1], 67500[1], 76000[1], 76970[1], 76998[0], 77002[0], 90865[1], 92511[1], 92512[1], 92516[1], 92520[1], 92537[1], 92538[1], 92950[1], 92953[1], 92960[1], 92961[1], 93000[1], 93005[1], 93010[1], 93040[1], 93041[1], 93042[1], 93050[0], 93303[0], 93304[0], 93306[1], 93307[1], 93308[1], 93312[1], 93313[1], 93314[1], 93315[1], 93316[1], 93317[1], 93318[0], 93351[1], 93355[0], 93451[1], 93456[1], 93457[1], 93561[0], 93562[0], 93701[0], 93922[1], 93923[1], 93924[1], 93925[1], 93926[1], 93930[1], 93931[1], 93970[1], 93971[1], 93975[1], 93976[1], 93978[1], 93979[1], 93980[1], 93981[1], 94002[1], 94004[1], 94200[1], 94250[0], 94640[1], 94644[1], 94660[1], 94662[1], 94680[1], 94681[1], 94690[1], 94760[0], 94761[0], 94762[1], 94770[1], 95812[0], 95813[0], 95816[0], 95819[0], 95822[0], 95829[0], 95955[0], 95956[0], 95957[0], 96360[0], 96365[0], 96372[0], 96373[0], 96374[0], 96375[0], 96376[0], 96377[0], 99151[0], 99152[0], 99153[0], 99155[0], 99156[0], 99157[0], 99201[0], 99202[0], 99203[0], 99204[0], 99205[0], 99211[0], 99212[0], 99213[0], 99214[0], 99215[0], 99217[0], 99218[0], 99219[0], 99220[0], 99221[0], 99222[0], 99223[0], 99224[0], 99225[0], 99226[0], 99231[0], 99232[0], 99233[0], 99234[0], 99235[0], 99236[0], 99238[0], 99239[0], 99281[0], 99282[0], 99283[0], 99284[0], 99285[0], 99304[0], 99305[0], 99306[0], 99307[0], 99308[0], 99309[0], 99310[0], 99315[0], 99318[0], 99324[0], 99325[0], 99326[0], 99327[0], 99328[0], 99334[0], 99335[0], 99336[0], 99337[0], 99341[0], 99342[0], 99343[0], 99347[0], 99348[0], 99349[0], 99354[0], 99355[0], 99356[0], 99357[0], 99358[0], 99359[0], 99415[0], 99416[0], 99446[0], 99447[0], 99448[0], 99449[0], 99451[0], 99452[0], 99466[0], 99468[0], 99469[0], 99471[0], 99472[0], 99475[0], 99476[0], 99477[0], 99478[0], 99479[0], 99480[0], 99483[0], 99485[0], 99497[0], C8921[1], C8922[1], C8923[1], C8924[1], C8925[1], C8926[1], C8927[0], C8929[1], C8930[1], G0380[1], G0381[1], G0382[1], G0383[1], G0384[1], G0406[0], G0407[0], G0408[0], G0425[0], G0426[0], G0427[0], G0463[0], G0500[0], G0508[0], G0509[0]
00952	01996[1], 0213T[1], 0216T[1], 0228T[1], 0230T[1], 31505[1], 31515[1], 31527[1], 31622[1], 31634[1], 31645[1], 31647[1], 36000[1], 36010[0], 36011[1], 36012[1], 36013[1], 36014[1], 36015[1], 36400[1], 36405[1], 36406[1], 36410[1], 36420[1], 36425[1], 36430[1], 36440[1], 36591[0], 36592[0], 36600[1], 36640[1], 43752[1], 43753[1], 43754[1], 61026[1], 61055[1], 62280[1], 62281[1], 62282[1], 62284[1], 62320[1], 62321[1], 62322[1], 62323[1], 62324[1], 62325[1], 62326[1], 62327[1], 64400[1], 64402[1], 64405[1], 64408[1], 64410[1], 64413[1], 64415[1], 64416[1], 64417[1], 64418[1], 64420[1], 64421[1], 64425[1], 64430[1], 64435[1], 64445[1], 64446[1], 64447[1], 64448[1], 64449[1], 64450[1], 64461[1], 64463[1], 64479[1], 64483[1], 64486[1], 64487[1], 64488[1], 64489[1], 64490[1], 64493[1], 64505[1], 64510[1], 64517[1], 64520[1], 64530[1], 64553[1], 64555[1], 67500[1], 76000[1], 76970[1], 76998[0], 77002[0], 90865[1], 92511[1], 92512[1], 92516[1], 92520[1], 92537[1], 92538[1], 92950[1], 92953[1], 92960[1], 92961[1], 93000[1], 93005[1], 93010[1], 93040[1], 93041[1], 93042[1], 93050[0], 93303[0], 93304[0], 93306[1], 93307[1], 93308[1], 93312[1], 93313[1], 93314[1], 93315[1], 93316[1], 93317[1],

Appendix A: NCCI - CPT Codes

0 = Modifier usage not allowed or inappropriate 1 = Modifier usage allowed

CPT © 2018 American Medical Association. All Rights Reserved.

Code 1	Code 2
	93318[0], 93351[1], 93355[0], 93451[1], 93456[1], 93457[1], 93561[0], 93562[0], 93701[0], 93922[1], 93923[1], 93924[1], 93925[1], 93926[1], 93930[1], 93931[1], 93970[1], 93971[1], 93975[1], 93976[1], 93978[1], 93979[1], 93980[1], 93981[1], 94002[1], 94004[1], 94200[1], 94250[0], 94640[1], 94644[1], 94660[1], 94662[1], 94680[1], 94681[1], 94690[1], 94760[0], 94761[0], 94762[1], 94770[1], 95812[0], 95813[0], 95816[0], 95819[0], 95822[0], 95829[0], 95955[0], 95956[0], 95957[0], 96360[0], 96365[0], 96372[0], 96373[0], 96374[0], 96375[0], 96376[0], 96377[0], 99151[0], 99152[0], 99153[0], 99155[0], 99156[0], 99157[0], 99201[0], 99202[0], 99203[0], 99204[0], 99205[0], 99211[0], 99212[0], 99213[0], 99214[0], 99215[0], 99217[0], 99218[0], 99219[0], 99220[0], 99221[0], 99222[0], 99223[0], 99224[0], 99225[0], 99226[0], 99231[0], 99232[0], 99233[0], 99234[0], 99235[0], 99236[0], 99238[0], 99239[0], 99281[0], 99282[0], 99283[0], 99284[0], 99285[0], 99304[0], 99305[0], 99306[0], 99307[0], 99308[0], 99309[0], 99310[0], 99315[0], 99318[0], 99324[0], 99325[0], 99326[0], 99327[0], 99328[0], 99334[0], 99335[0], 99336[0], 99337[0], 99341[0], 99342[0], 99343[0], 99347[0], 99348[0], 99349[0], 99354[0], 99355[0], 99356[0], 99357[0], 99358[0], 99359[0], 99415[0], 99416[0], 99446[0], 99447[0], 99448[0], 99449[0], 99451[0], 99452[0], 99466[0], 99468[0], 99469[0], 99471[0], 99472[0], 99475[0], 99476[0], 99477[0], 99478[0], 99479[0], 99480[0], 99483[0], 99485[0], 99497[0], C8921[1], C8922[1], C8923[1], C8924[1], C8925[1], C8926[1], C8927[0], C8929[1], C8930[1], G0380[1], G0381[1], G0382[1], G0383[1], G0384[1], G0406[0], G0407[0], G0408[0], G0425[0], G0426[0], G0427[0], G0463[0], G0500[0], G0508[0], G0509[0]
01112	01996[1], 0213T[1], 0216T[1], 0228T[1], 0230T[1], 31505[1], 31515[1], 31527[1], 31622[1], 31634[1], 31645[1], 31647[1], 36000[1], 36010[0], 36011[1], 36012[1], 36013[1], 36014[1], 36015[1], 36400[1], 36405[1], 36406[1], 36410[1], 36420[1], 36425[1], 36430[1], 36440[1], 36591[0], 36592[0], 36600[1], 36640[1], 43752[1], 43753[1], 43754[1], 61026[1], 61055[1], 62280[1], 62281[1], 62282[1], 62284[1], 62320[1], 62321[1], 62322[1], 62323[1], 62324[1], 62325[1], 62326[1], 62327[1], 64400[1], 64402[1], 64405[1], 64408[1], 64410[1], 64413[1], 64415[1], 64416[1], 64417[1], 64418[1], 64420[1], 64421[1], 64425[1], 64430[1], 64435[1], 64445[1], 64446[1], 64447[1], 64448[1], 64449[1], 64450[1], 64461[1], 64463[1], 64479[1], 64483[1], 64486[1], 64487[1], 64488[1], 64489[1], 64490[1], 64493[1], 64505[1], 64510[1], 64517[1], 64520[1], 64530[1], 64553[1], 64555[1], 67500[0], 76000[1], 76970[1], 76998[0], 77002[0], 90865[1], 92511[1], 92512[1], 92516[1], 92520[1], 92537[1], 92538[1], 92950[1], 92953[1], 92960[1], 92961[1], 93000[1], 93005[1], 93010[1], 93040[1], 93041[1], 93042[1], 93050[0], 93303[0], 93304[0], 93306[1], 93307[1], 93308[1], 93312[1], 93313[1], 93314[1], 93315[1], 93316[1], 93317[1], 93318[0], 93351[1], 93355[0], 93451[1], 93456[1], 93457[1], 93561[0], 93562[0], 93701[0], 93922[1], 93923[1], 93924[1], 93925[1], 93926[1], 93930[1], 93931[1], 93970[1], 93971[1], 93975[1], 93976[1], 93978[1], 93979[1], 93980[1], 93981[1], 94002[1], 94004[1], 94200[1], 94250[0], 94640[1], 94644[1], 94660[1], 94662[1], 94680[1], 94681[1], 94690[1], 94760[0], 94761[0], 94762[1], 94770[1], 95812[0], 95813[0], 95816[0], 95819[0], 95822[0], 95829[0], 95955[0], 95956[0], 95957[0], 96360[0], 96365[0], 96372[0], 96373[0], 96374[0], 96375[0], 96376[0], 96377[0], 99151[0], 99152[0], 99153[0], 99155[0], 99156[0], 99157[0], 99201[0], 99202[0], 99203[0], 99204[0], 99205[0], 99211[0], 99212[0], 99213[0], 99214[0], 99215[0], 99217[0], 99218[0], 99219[0], 99220[0], 99221[0], 99222[0], 99223[0], 99224[0], 99225[0], 99226[0], 99231[0], 99232[0], 99233[0], 99234[0], 99235[0], 99236[0], 99238[0], 99239[0], 99281[0], 99282[0], 99283[0], 99284[0], 99285[0], 99304[0], 99305[0], 99306[0], 99307[0], 99308[0], 99309[0], 99310[0], 99315[0], 99316[0], 99318[0], 99324[0], 99325[0], 99326[0], 99327[0], 99328[0], 99334[0], 99335[0], 99336[0], 99337[0], 99341[0], 99342[0], 99343[0], 99344[0], 99345[0], 99347[0], 99348[0], 99349[0], 99350[0], 99354[0], 99355[0], 99356[0], 99357[0], 99358[0], 99359[0], 99415[0], 99416[0], 99446[0], 99447[0], 99448[0], 99449[0], 99451[0], 99452[0], 99466[0], 99468[0], 99469[0], 99471[0], 99472[0], 99475[0], 99476[0], 99477[0], 99478[0], 99479[0], 99480[0], 99483[0], 99485[0], 99497[0], C8921[1], C8922[1], C8923[1], C8924[1], C8925[1], C8926[1], C8927[0], C8929[1], C8930[1], G0380[1], G0381[1], G0382[1], G0383[1], G0384[1], G0406[0], G0407[0], G0408[0], G0425[0], G0426[0], G0427[0], G0463[0], G0500[0], G0508[0], G0509[0]
01120	01996[1], 0213T[1], 0216T[1], 0228T[1], 0230T[1], 31505[1], 31515[1], 31527[1], 31622[1], 31634[1], 31645[1], 31647[1], 36000[1], 36010[0], 36011[1], 36012[1], 36013[1], 36014[1], 36015[1], 36400[1], 36405[1], 36406[1], 36410[1], 36420[1], 36425[1], 36430[1], 36440[1], 36591[0], 36592[0], 36600[1], 36640[1], 43752[1], 43753[1], 43754[1], 61026[1], 61055[1], 62280[1], 62281[1], 62282[1], 62284[1], 62320[1], 62321[1], 62322[1], 62323[1], 62324[1], 62325[1], 62326[1], 62327[1], 64400[1], 64402[1], 64405[1], 64408[1], 64410[1], 64413[1], 64415[1], 64416[1], 64417[1], 64418[1], 64420[1], 64421[1], 64425[1], 64430[1], 64435[1], 64445[1], 64446[1], 64447[1], 64448[1], 64449[1], 64450[1], 64461[1], 64463[1], 64479[1], 64483[1], 64486[1], 64487[1], 64488[1], 64489[1], 64490[1], 64493[1], 64505[1], 64510[1], 64517[1], 64520[1], 64530[1], 64553[1], 64555[1], 67500[1], 76000[1], 76970[1], 76998[0], 77002[0], 90865[1], 92511[1], 92512[1], 92516[1], 92520[1], 92537[1], 92538[1], 92950[1], 92953[1], 92960[1], 92961[1], 93000[1], 93005[1], 93010[1], 93040[1], 93041[1], 93042[1], 93050[0], 93303[0], 93304[0], 93306[1], 93307[1], 93308[1], 93312[1], 93313[1], 93314[1], 93315[1], 93316[1], 93317[1], 93318[0], 93351[1], 93355[0], 93451[1], 93456[1], 93457[1], 93561[0], 93562[0], 93701[0], 93922[1], 93923[1], 93924[1], 93925[1], 93926[1], 93930[1], 93931[1], 93970[1], 93971[1], 93975[1], 93976[1], 93978[1], 93979[1], 93980[1], 93981[1], 94002[1], 94004[1], 94200[1], 94250[0], 94640[1], 94644[1], 94660[1], 94662[1], 94680[1], 94681[1], 94690[1], 94760[0], 94761[0], 94762[1], 94770[1], 95812[0], 95813[0], 95816[0], 95819[0], 95822[0], 95829[0], 95955[0], 95956[0], 95957[0], 96360[0], 96365[0], 96372[0], 96373[0], 96374[0], 96375[0], 96376[0], 96377[0], 99151[0], 99152[0], 99153[0], 99155[0], 99156[0], 99157[0], 99201[0], 99202[0], 99203[0], 99204[0], 99205[0], 99211[0], 99212[0], 99213[0], 99214[0], 99215[0], 99217[0], 99218[0], 99219[0], 99220[0], 99221[0], 99222[0], 99223[0], 99224[0], 99225[0], 99226[0], 99231[0], 99232[0], 99233[0], 99234[0], 99235[0], 99236[0], 99238[0], 99239[0], 99281[0], 99282[0], 99283[0], 99284[0], 99285[0], 99304[0], 99305[0], 99306[0], 99307[0], 99308[0], 99309[0], 99310[0], 99315[0], 99318[0], 99324[0], 99325[0], 99326[0], 99327[0], 99328[0], 99334[0], 99335[0], 99336[0], 99337[0], 99341[0], 99342[0], 99343[0], 99347[0], 99348[0], 99349[0], 99354[0], 99355[0], 99356[0], 99357[0], 99358[0], 99359[0], 99415[0], 99416[0], 99446[0], 99447[0], 99448[0], 99449[0], 99451[0], 99452[0], 99466[0], 99468[0], 99469[0], 99471[0], 99472[0], 99475[0], 99476[0], 99477[0], 99478[0], 99479[0], 99480[0], 99483[0], 99485[0], 99497[0], C8921[1], C8922[1], C8923[1], C8924[1], C8925[1], C8926[1], C8927[0], C8929[1], C8930[1], G0380[1], G0381[1], G0382[1], G0383[1], G0384[1], G0406[0], G0407[0], G0408[0], G0425[0], G0426[0], G0427[0], G0463[0], G0500[0], G0508[0], G0509[0]
01130	01996[1], 0213T[1], 0216T[1], 0228T[1], 0230T[1], 31505[1], 31515[1], 31527[1], 31622[1], 31634[1], 31645[1], 31647[1], 36000[1], 36010[0], 36011[1], 36012[1], 36013[1], 36014[1], 36015[1], 36400[1], 36405[1], 36406[1], 36410[1], 36420[1], 36425[1], 36430[1], 36440[1], 36591[0], 36592[0], 36600[1], 36640[1], 43752[1], 43753[1], 43754[1], 61026[1], 61055[1], 62280[1], 62281[1], 62282[1], 62284[1], 62320[1], 62321[1], 62322[1], 62323[1], 62324[1], 62325[1], 62326[1], 62327[1], 64400[1], 64402[1], 64405[1], 64408[1], 64410[1], 64413[1], 64415[1], 64416[1], 64417[1], 64418[1], 64420[1], 64421[1], 64425[1], 64430[1], 64435[1], 64445[1], 64446[1], 64447[1], 64448[1], 64449[1], 64450[1], 64461[1], 64463[1], 64479[1], 64483[1], 64486[1], 64487[1], 64488[1], 64489[1], 64490[1], 64493[1], 64505[1], 64510[1], 64517[1], 64520[1], 64530[1], 64553[1], 64555[1], 67500[1], 76000[1], 76970[1], 76998[0], 77002[0], 90865[1], 92511[1], 92512[1], 92516[1], 92520[1], 92537[1], 92538[1], 92950[1], 92953[1], 92960[1], 92961[1], 93000[1], 93005[1], 93010[1], 93040[1], 93041[1], 93042[1], 93050[0], 93303[0], 93304[0], 93306[1], 93307[1], 93308[1], 93312[1], 93313[1], 93314[1], 93315[1], 93316[1], 93317[1], 93318[0], 93351[1], 93355[0], 93451[1], 93456[1], 93457[1], 93561[0], 93562[0], 93701[0], 93922[1], 93923[1], 93924[1], 93925[1], 93926[1], 93930[1], 93931[1], 93970[1], 93971[1], 93975[1], 93976[1], 93978[1], 93979[1], 93980[1], 93981[1], 94002[1], 94004[1], 94200[1], 94250[0], 94640[1], 94644[1], 94660[1], 94662[1], 94680[1], 94681[1], 94690[1], 94760[0], 94761[0], 94762[1], 94770[1], 95812[0], 95813[0], 95816[0], 95819[0], 95822[0], 95829[0], 95955[0], 95956[0], 95957[0], 96360[0], 96365[0], 96372[0], 96373[0], 96374[0], 96375[0], 96376[0], 96377[0], 99151[0], 99152[0], 99153[0], 99155[0], 99156[0], 99157[0], 99201[0], 99202[0], 99203[0], 99204[0], 99205[0], 99211[0], 99212[0], 99213[0], 99214[0], 99215[0], 99217[0], 99218[0], 99219[0], 99220[0], 99221[0], 99222[0], 99223[0], 99224[0], 99225[0], 99226[0], 99231[0], 99232[0], 99233[0], 99234[0], 99235[0], 99236[0], 99238[0], 99239[0], 99281[0], 99282[0], 99283[0], 99284[0], 99285[0], 99304[0], 99305[0], 99306[0], 99307[0], 99308[0], 99309[0], 99310[0], 99315[0], 99318[0], 99324[0], 99325[0], 99326[0], 99327[0], 99328[0], 99334[0], 99335[0], 99336[0], 99337[0], 99341[0], 99342[0], 99343[0], 99347[0], 99348[0], 99349[0], 99354[0], 99355[0], 99356[0], 99357[0], 99358[0], 99359[0], 99415[0], 99416[0], 99446[0], 99447[0], 99448[0], 99449[0], 99451[0], 99452[0], 99466[0], 99468[0], 99469[0], 99471[0], 99472[0], 99475[0], 99476[0], 99477[0], 99478[0], 99479[0], 99480[0], 99483[0], 99485[0], 99497[0], C8921[1], C8922[1], C8923[1], C8924[1], C8925[1], C8926[1], C8927[0], C8929[1], C8930[1], G0380[1], G0381[1], G0382[1], G0383[1], G0384[1], G0406[0], G0407[0], G0408[0], G0425[0], G0426[0], G0427[0], G0463[0], G0500[0], G0508[0], G0509[0]
01140	01996[1], 0213T[1], 0216T[1], 0228T[1], 0230T[1], 31505[1], 31515[1], 31527[1], 31622[1], 31634[1], 31645[1], 31647[1], 36000[1], 36010[0], 36011[1], 36012[1], 36013[1], 36014[1], 36015[1], 36400[1], 36405[1], 36406[1], 36410[1], 36420[1], 36425[1], 36430[1], 36440[1], 36591[0], 36592[0], 36600[1], 36640[1], 43752[1], 43753[1], 43754[1], 61026[1], 61055[1], 62280[1], 62281[1], 62282[1], 62284[1], 62320[1], 62321[1], 62322[1], 62323[1], 62324[1], 62325[1], 62326[1], 62327[1], 64400[1], 64402[1], 64405[1], 64408[1], 64410[1], 64413[1], 64415[1], 64416[1], 64417[1], 64418[1], 64420[1], 64421[1], 64425[1], 64430[1], 64435[1], 64445[1], 64446[1], 64447[1], 64448[1], 64449[1], 64450[1], 64461[1], 64463[1], 64479[1], 64483[1], 64486[1], 64487[1], 64488[1], 64489[1], 64490[1], 64493[1], 64505[1], 64510[1], 64517[1], 64520[1], 64530[1], 64553[1], 64555[1], 67500[1], 76000[1], 76970[1], 76998[0], 77002[0], 90865[1], 92511[1], 92512[1], 92516[1], 92520[1], 92537[1], 92538[1], 92950[1], 92953[1], 92960[1], 92961[1], 93000[1], 93005[1], 93010[1], 93040[1], 93041[1], 93042[1], 93050[0], 93303[0], 93304[0], 93306[1], 93307[1], 93308[1], 93312[1], 93313[1], 93314[1], 93315[1], 93316[1], 93317[1], 93318[0], 93351[1], 93355[0], 93451[1], 93456[1], 93457[1], 93561[0], 93562[0], 93701[0], 93922[1], 93923[1], 93924[1], 93925[1], 93926[1], 93930[1], 93931[1], 93970[1], 93971[1], 93975[1], 93976[1], 93978[1], 93979[1], 93980[1], 93981[1], 94002[1], 94004[1], 94200[1], 94250[0], 94640[1], 94644[1], 94660[1], 94662[1], 94680[1], 94681[1], 94690[1], 94760[0], 94761[0], 94762[1], 94770[1], 95812[0], 95813[0], 95816[0], 95819[0], 95822[0], 95829[0], 95955[0], 95956[0], 95957[0], 96360[0], 96365[0], 96372[0], 96373[0], 96374[0], 96375[0], 96376[0], 96377[0], 99151[0], 99152[0], 99153[0], 99155[0], 99156[0], 99157[0], 99201[0], 99202[0], 99203[0], 99204[0], 99205[0], 99211[0], 99212[0], 99213[0], 99214[0], 99215[0], 99217[0], 99218[0], 99219[0], 99220[0], 99221[0], 99222[0], 99223[0], 99224[0], 99225[0], 99226[0], 99231[0], 99232[0], 99233[0], 99234[0], 99235[0], 99236[0], 99238[0], 99239[0], 99281[0], 99282[0], 99283[0], 99284[0], 99285[0], 99304[0], 99305[0], 99306[0], 99307[0], 99308[0], 99309[0], 99310[0], 99315[0], 99318[0], 99324[0], 99325[0], 99326[0], 99327[0], 99328[0], 99334[0], 99335[0], 99336[0], 99337[0], 99341[0], 99342[0], 99343[0], 99347[0], 99348[0], 99349[0], 99354[0],

0 = Modifier usage not allowed or inappropriate 1 = Modifier usage allowed

CPT © 2018 American Medical Association. All Rights Reserved.

Code 1	Code 2
	99355[0], 99356[0], 99357[0], 99358[0], 99359[0], 99415[0], 99416[0], 99446[0], 99447[0], 99448[0], 99449[0], 99451[0], 99452[0], 99466[0], 99468[0], 99469[0], 99471[0], 99472[0], 99475[0], 99476[0], 99477[0], 99478[0], 99479[0], 99480[0], 99483[0], 99485[0], 99497[0], C8921[1], C8922[1], C8923[1], C8924[1], C8925[1], C8926[1], C8927[0], C8929[1], C8930[1], G0380[1], G0381[1], G0382[1], G0383[1], G0384[1], G0406[0], G0407[0], G0408[0], G0425[0], G0426[0], G0427[0], G0463[0], G0500[0], G0508[0], G0509[0]
01150	01996[1], 0213T[1], 0216T[1], 0228T[1], 0230T[1], 31505[1], 31515[1], 31527[1], 31622[1], 31634[1], 31645[1], 31647[1], 36000[1], 36010[0], 36011[1], 36012[1], 36013[1], 36014[1], 36015[1], 36400[1], 36405[1], 36406[1], 36410[1], 36420[1], 36425[1], 36430[1], 36440[1], 36591[0], 36592[0], 36600[1], 36640[1], 43752[1], 43753[1], 43754[1], 61026[1], 61055[1], 62280[1], 62281[1], 62282[1], 62284[1], 62320[1], 62321[1], 62322[1], 62323[1], 62324[1], 62325[1], 62326[1], 62327[1], 64400[1], 64402[1], 64405[1], 64408[1], 64410[1], 64413[1], 64415[1], 64416[1], 64417[1], 64418[1], 64420[1], 64421[1], 64425[1], 64430[1], 64435[1], 64445[1], 64446[1], 64447[1], 64448[1], 64449[1], 64450[1], 64461[1], 64463[1], 64479[1], 64483[1], 64486[1], 64487[1], 64488[1], 64489[1], 64490[1], 64493[1], 64505[1], 64510[1], 64517[1], 64520[1], 64530[1], 64553[1], 64555[1], 67500[1], 76000[1], 76970[1], 76998[0], 77002[0], 90865[1], 92511[1], 92512[1], 92516[1], 92520[1], 92537[1], 92538[1], 92950[1], 92953[1], 92960[1], 92961[1], 93000[1], 93005[1], 93010[1], 93040[1], 93041[1], 93042[1], 93050[0], 93303[0], 93304[0], 93306[1], 93307[1], 93308[1], 93312[1], 93313[1], 93314[1], 93315[1], 93316[1], 93317[1], 93318[0], 93351[1], 93355[0], 93451[1], 93456[1], 93457[1], 93561[0], 93562[0], 93701[0], 93922[1], 93923[1], 93924[1], 93925[1], 93926[1], 93930[1], 93931[1], 93970[1], 93971[1], 93975[1], 93976[1], 93978[1], 93979[1], 93980[1], 93981[1], 94002[1], 94004[1], 94200[1], 94250[0], 94640[1], 94644[1], 94660[1], 94662[1], 94680[1], 94681[1], 94690[1], 94760[0], 94761[0], 94762[1], 94770[1], 95812[0], 95813[0], 95816[0], 95819[0], 95822[0], 95829[0], 95955[0], 95956[0], 95957[0], 96360[0], 96365[0], 96372[0], 96373[0], 96374[0], 96375[0], 96376[0], 96377[0], 99151[0], 99152[0], 99153[0], 99155[0], 99156[0], 99157[0], 99201[0], 99202[0], 99203[0], 99204[0], 99205[0], 99211[0], 99212[0], 99213[0], 99214[0], 99215[0], 99217[0], 99218[0], 99219[0], 99220[0], 99221[0], 99222[0], 99223[0], 99224[0], 99225[0], 99226[0], 99231[0], 99232[0], 99233[0], 99234[0], 99235[0], 99236[0], 99238[0], 99239[0], 99281[0], 99282[0], 99283[0], 99284[0], 99285[0], 99304[0], 99305[0], 99306[0], 99307[0], 99308[0], 99309[0], 99310[0], 99315[0], 99318[0], 99324[0], 99325[0], 99326[0], 99327[0], 99328[0], 99334[0], 99335[0], 99336[0], 99337[0], 99341[0], 99342[0], 99343[0], 99347[0], 99348[0], 99349[0], 99354[0], 99355[0], 99356[0], 99357[0], 99358[0], 99359[0], 99415[0], 99416[0], 99446[0], 99447[0], 99448[0], 99449[0], 99451[0], 99452[0], 99466[0], 99468[0], 99469[0], 99471[0], 99472[0], 99475[0], 99476[0], 99477[0], 99478[0], 99479[0], 99480[0], 99483[0], 99485[0], 99497[0], C8921[1], C8922[1], C8923[1], C8924[1], C8925[1], C8926[1], C8927[0], C8929[1], C8930[1], G0380[1], G0381[1], G0382[1], G0383[1], G0384[1], G0406[0], G0407[0], G0408[0], G0425[0], G0426[0], G0427[0], G0463[0], G0500[0], G0508[0], G0509[0]
01160	01996[1], 0213T[1], 0216T[1], 0228T[1], 0230T[1], 31505[1], 31515[1], 31527[1], 31622[1], 31634[1], 31645[1], 31647[1], 36000[1], 36010[0], 36011[1], 36012[1], 36013[1], 36014[1], 36015[1], 36400[1], 36405[1], 36406[1], 36410[1], 36420[1], 36425[1], 36430[1], 36440[1], 36591[0], 36592[0], 36600[1], 36640[1], 43752[1], 43753[1], 43754[1], 61026[1], 61055[1], 62280[1], 62281[1], 62282[1], 62284[1], 62320[1], 62321[1], 62322[1], 62323[1], 62324[1], 62325[1], 62326[1], 62327[1], 64400[1], 64402[1], 64405[1], 64408[1], 64410[1], 64413[1], 64415[1], 64416[1], 64417[1], 64418[1], 64420[1], 64421[1], 64425[1], 64430[1], 64435[1], 64445[1], 64446[1], 64447[1], 64448[1], 64449[1], 64450[1], 64461[1], 64463[1], 64479[1], 64483[1], 64486[1], 64487[1], 64488[1], 64489[1], 64490[1], 64493[1], 64505[1], 64510[1], 64517[1], 64520[1], 64530[1], 64553[1], 64555[1], 67500[1], 76000[1], 76970[1], 76998[0], 77002[0], 90865[1], 92511[1], 92512[1], 92516[1], 92520[1], 92537[1], 92538[1], 92950[1], 92953[1], 92960[1], 92961[1], 93000[1], 93005[1], 93010[1], 93040[1], 93041[1], 93042[1], 93050[0], 93303[0], 93304[0], 93306[1], 93307[1], 93308[1], 93312[1], 93313[1], 93314[1], 93315[1], 93316[1], 93317[1], 93318[0], 93351[1], 93355[0], 93451[1], 93456[1], 93457[1], 93561[0], 93562[0], 93701[0], 93922[1], 93923[1], 93924[1], 93925[1], 93926[1], 93930[1], 93931[1], 93970[1], 93971[1], 93975[1], 93976[1], 93978[1], 93979[1], 93980[1], 93981[1], 94002[1], 94004[1], 94200[1], 94250[0], 94640[1], 94644[1], 94660[1], 94662[1], 94680[1], 94681[1], 94690[1], 94760[0], 94761[0], 94762[1], 94770[1], 95812[0], 95813[0], 95816[0], 95819[0], 95822[0], 95829[0], 95955[0], 95956[0], 95957[0], 96360[0], 96365[0], 96372[0], 96373[0], 96374[0], 96375[0], 96376[0], 96377[0], 99151[0], 99152[0], 99153[0], 99155[0], 99156[0], 99157[0], 99201[0], 99202[0], 99203[0], 99204[0], 99205[0], 99211[0], 99212[0], 99213[0], 99214[0], 99215[0], 99217[0], 99218[0], 99219[0], 99220[0], 99221[0], 99222[0], 99223[0], 99224[0], 99225[0], 99226[0], 99231[0], 99232[0], 99233[0], 99234[0], 99235[0], 99236[0], 99238[0], 99239[0], 99281[0], 99282[0], 99283[0], 99284[0], 99285[0], 99304[0], 99305[0], 99306[0], 99307[0], 99308[0], 99309[0], 99310[0], 99315[0], 99318[0], 99324[0], 99325[0], 99326[0], 99327[0], 99328[0], 99334[0], 99335[0], 99336[0], 99337[0], 99341[0], 99342[0], 99343[0], 99347[0], 99348[0], 99349[0], 99354[0], 99355[0], 99356[0], 99357[0], 99358[0], 99359[0], 99415[0], 99416[0], 99446[0], 99447[0], 99448[0], 99449[0], 99451[0], 99452[0], 99466[0], 99468[0], 99469[0], 99471[0], 99472[0], 99475[0], 99476[0], 99477[0], 99478[0], 99479[0], 99480[0], 99483[0], 99485[0], 99497[0], C8921[1], C8922[1], C8923[1], C8924[1], C8925[1], C8926[1], C8927[0], C8929[1], C8930[1], G0380[1], G0381[1], G0382[1], G0383[1], G0384[1], G0406[0], G0407[0], G0408[0], G0425[0], G0426[0], G0427[0], G0463[0], G0500[0], G0508[0], G0509[0]
01170	01996[1], 0213T[1], 0216T[1], 0228T[1], 0230T[1], 31505[1], 31515[1], 31527[1], 31622[1], 31634[1], 31645[1], 31647[1], 36000[1], 36010[0], 36011[1], 36012[1], 36013[1], 36014[1], 36015[1], 36400[1], 36405[1], 36406[1], 36410[1], 36420[1], 36425[1], 36430[1], 36440[1], 36591[0], 36592[0], 36600[1], 36640[1], 43752[1], 43753[1], 43754[1], 61026[1], 61055[1], 62280[1], 62281[1], 62282[1], 62284[1], 62320[1], 62321[1], 62322[1], 62323[1], 62324[1], 62325[1], 62326[1], 62327[1], 64400[1], 64402[1], 64405[1], 64408[1], 64410[1], 64413[1], 64415[1], 64416[1], 64417[1], 64418[1], 64420[1], 64421[1], 64425[1], 64430[1], 64435[1], 64445[1], 64446[1], 64447[1], 64448[1], 64449[1], 64450[1], 64461[1], 64463[1], 64479[1], 64483[1], 64486[1], 64487[1], 64488[1], 64489[1], 64490[1], 64493[1], 64505[1], 64510[1], 64517[1], 64520[1], 64530[1], 64553[1], 64555[1], 67500[1], 76000[1], 76970[1], 76998[0], 77002[0], 90865[1], 92511[1], 92512[1], 92516[1], 92520[1], 92537[1], 92538[1], 92950[1], 92953[1], 92960[1], 92961[1], 93000[1], 93005[1], 93010[1], 93040[1], 93041[1], 93042[1], 93050[0], 93303[0], 93304[0], 93306[1], 93307[1], 93308[1], 93312[1], 93313[1], 93314[1], 93315[1], 93316[1], 93317[1], 93318[0], 93351[1], 93355[0], 93451[1], 93456[1], 93457[1], 93561[0], 93562[0], 93701[0], 93922[1], 93923[1], 93924[1], 93925[1], 93926[1], 93930[1], 93931[1], 93970[1], 93971[1], 93975[1], 93976[1], 93978[1], 93979[1], 93980[1], 93981[1], 94002[1], 94004[1], 94200[1], 94250[0], 94640[1], 94644[1], 94660[1], 94662[1], 94680[1], 94681[1], 94690[1], 94760[0], 94761[0], 94762[1], 94770[1], 95812[0], 95813[0], 95816[0], 95819[0], 95822[0], 95829[0], 95955[0], 95956[0], 95957[0], 96360[0], 96365[0], 96372[0], 96373[0], 96374[0], 96375[0], 96376[0], 96377[0], 99151[0], 99152[0], 99153[0], 99155[0], 99156[0], 99157[0], 99201[0], 99202[0], 99203[0], 99204[0], 99205[0], 99211[0], 99212[0], 99213[0], 99214[0], 99215[0], 99217[0], 99218[0], 99219[0], 99220[0], 99221[0], 99222[0], 99223[0], 99224[0], 99225[0], 99226[0], 99231[0], 99232[0], 99233[0], 99234[0], 99235[0], 99236[0], 99238[0], 99239[0], 99281[0], 99282[0], 99283[0], 99284[0], 99285[0], 99304[0], 99305[0], 99306[0], 99307[0], 99308[0], 99309[0], 99310[0], 99315[0], 99318[0], 99324[0], 99325[0], 99326[0], 99327[0], 99328[0], 99334[0], 99335[0], 99336[0], 99337[0], 99341[0], 99342[0], 99343[0], 99347[0], 99348[0], 99349[0], 99354[0], 99355[0], 99356[0], 99357[0], 99358[0], 99359[0], 99415[0], 99416[0], 99446[0], 99447[0], 99448[0], 99449[0], 99451[0], 99452[0], 99466[0], 99468[0], 99469[0], 99471[0], 99472[0], 99475[0], 99476[0], 99477[0], 99478[0], 99479[0], 99480[0], 99483[0], 99485[0], 99497[0], C8921[1], C8922[1], C8923[1], C8924[1], C8925[1], C8926[1], C8927[0], C8929[1], C8930[1], G0380[1], G0381[1], G0382[1], G0383[1], G0384[1], G0406[0], G0407[0], G0408[0], G0425[0], G0426[0], G0427[0], G0463[0], G0500[0], G0508[0], G0509[0]
01173	01996[1], 0213T[1], 0216T[1], 0228T[1], 0229T[1], 0230T[1], 0231T[1], 31505[1], 31515[1], 31527[1], 31622[1], 31634[1], 31645[1], 31647[1], 36000[1], 36010[0], 36011[1], 36012[1], 36013[1], 36014[1], 36015[1], 36400[1], 36405[1], 36406[1], 36410[1], 36420[1], 36425[1], 36430[1], 36440[1], 36591[0], 36592[0], 36600[1], 36640[1], 43752[1], 43753[1], 43754[1], 61026[1], 61055[1], 62280[1], 62281[1], 62282[1], 62284[1], 62320[1], 62321[1], 62322[1], 62323[1], 62324[1], 62325[1], 62326[1], 62327[1], 64400[1], 64402[1], 64405[1], 64408[1], 64410[1], 64413[1], 64415[1], 64416[1], 64417[1], 64418[1], 64420[1], 64421[1], 64425[1], 64430[1], 64435[1], 64445[1], 64446[1], 64447[1], 64448[1], 64449[1], 64450[1], 64461[1], 64463[1], 64479[1], 64480[1], 64483[1], 64484[1], 64486[1], 64487[1], 64488[1], 64489[1], 64490[1], 64493[1], 64505[1], 64510[1], 64517[1], 64520[1], 64530[1], 64553[1], 64555[1], 67500[0], 76000[1], 76970[1], 76998[0], 77002[0], 90865[1], 92511[1], 92512[1], 92516[1], 92520[1], 92537[1], 92538[1], 92950[1], 92953[1], 92960[1], 92961[1], 93000[1], 93005[1], 93010[1], 93040[1], 93041[1], 93042[1], 93050[0], 93303[0], 93304[0], 93306[1], 93307[1], 93308[1], 93312[1], 93313[1], 93314[1], 93315[1], 93316[1], 93317[1], 93318[0], 93351[1], 93355[0], 93451[1], 93456[1], 93457[1], 93561[0], 93562[0], 93701[0], 93922[1], 93923[1], 93924[1], 93925[1], 93926[1], 93930[1], 93931[1], 93970[1], 93971[1], 93975[1], 93976[1], 93978[1], 93979[1], 93980[1], 93981[1], 94002[1], 94004[1], 94200[1], 94250[0], 94640[1], 94644[1], 94660[1], 94662[1], 94680[1], 94681[1], 94690[1], 94760[0], 94761[0], 94762[1], 94770[1], 95812[0], 95813[0], 95816[0], 95819[0], 95822[0], 95829[0], 95955[0], 95956[0], 95957[0], 96360[0], 96365[0], 96372[0], 96373[0], 96374[0], 96375[0], 96376[0], 96377[0], 99151[0], 99152[0], 99153[0], 99155[0], 99156[0], 99157[0], 99201[0], 99202[0], 99203[0], 99204[0], 99205[0], 99211[0], 99212[0], 99213[0], 99214[0], 99215[0], 99217[0], 99218[0], 99219[0], 99220[0], 99221[0], 99222[0], 99223[0], 99224[0], 99225[0], 99226[0], 99231[0], 99232[0], 99233[0], 99234[0], 99235[0], 99236[0], 99238[0], 99239[0], 99281[0], 99282[0], 99283[0], 99284[0], 99285[0], 99304[0], 99305[0], 99306[0], 99307[0], 99308[0], 99309[0], 99310[0], 99315[0], 99316[0], 99318[0], 99324[0], 99325[0], 99326[0], 99327[0], 99328[0], 99334[0], 99335[0], 99336[0], 99337[0], 99341[0], 99342[0], 99343[0], 99344[0], 99345[0], 99347[0], 99348[0], 99349[0], 99350[0], 99354[0], 99355[0], 99356[0], 99357[0], 99358[0], 99359[0], 99415[0], 99416[0], 99446[0], 99447[0], 99448[0], 99449[0], 99451[0], 99452[0], 99466[0], 99468[0], 99469[0], 99471[0], 99472[0], 99475[0], 99476[0], 99477[0], 99478[0], 99479[0], 99480[0], 99483[0], 99485[0], 99497[0], C8921[1], C8922[1], C8923[1], C8924[1], C8925[1], C8926[1], C8927[0], C8929[1], C8930[1], G0380[1], G0381[1], G0382[1], G0383[1], G0384[1], G0406[0], G0407[0], G0408[0], G0425[0], G0426[0], G0427[0], G0463[0], G0500[0], G0508[0], G0509[0]
01200	01996[1], 0213T[1], 0216T[1], 0228T[1], 0230T[1], 31505[1], 31515[1], 31527[1], 31622[1], 31634[1], 31645[1], 31647[1], 36000[1], 36010[0], 36011[1], 36012[1], 36013[1], 36014[1], 36015[1], 36400[1], 36405[1], 36406[1], 36410[1], 36420[1], 36425[1], 36430[1], 36440[1], 36591[0], 36592[0], 36600[1], 36640[1], 43752[1], 43753[1], 43754[1], 61026[1], 61055[1], 62280[1], 62281[1], 62282[1], 62284[1], 62320[1], 62321[1], 62322[1], 62323[1], 62324[1], 62325[1], 62326[1], 62327[1], 64400[1], 64402[1], 64405[1], 64408[1], 64410[1], 64413[1], 64415[1], 64416[1], 64417[1], 64418[1], 64420[1], 64421[1],

0 = Modifier usage not allowed or inappropriate   1 = Modifier usage allowed

CPT © 2018 American Medical Association. All Rights Reserved.

Code 1	Code 2
	64425[1], 64430[1], 64435[1], 64445[1], 64446[1], 64447[1], 64448[1], 64449[1], 64450[1], 64461[1], 64463[1], 64479[1], 64483[1], 64486[1], 64487[1], 64488[1], 64489[1], 64490[1], 64493[1], 64505[1], 64510[1], 64517[1], 64520[1], 64530[1], 64553[1], 64555[1], 67500[1], 76000[1], 76970[1], 76998[0], 77002[0], 90865[1], 92511[1], 92512[1], 92516[1], 92520[1], 92537[1], 92538[1], 92950[1], 92953[1], 92960[1], 92961[1], 93000[1], 93005[1], 93010[1], 93040[1], 93041[1], 93042[1], 93050[0], 93303[0], 93304[0], 93306[1], 93307[1], 93308[1], 93312[1], 93313[1], 93314[1], 93315[1], 93316[1], 93317[1], 93318[0], 93351[1], 93355[0], 93451[1], 93456[1], 93457[1], 93561[0], 93562[0], 93701[0], 93922[1], 93923[1], 93924[1], 93925[1], 93926[1], 93930[1], 93931[1], 93970[1], 93971[1], 93975[1], 93976[1], 93978[1], 93979[1], 93980[1], 93981[1], 94002[1], 94004[1], 94200[1], 94250[0], 94640[1], 94644[1], 94660[1], 94662[1], 94680[1], 94681[1], 94690[1], 94760[0], 94761[0], 94762[1], 94770[1], 95812[0], 95813[0], 95816[0], 95819[0], 95822[0], 95829[0], 95955[0], 95956[0], 95957[0], 96360[0], 96365[0], 96372[0], 96373[0], 96374[0], 96375[0], 96376[0], 96377[0], 99151[0], 99152[0], 99153[0], 99155[0], 99156[0], 99157[0], 99201[0], 99202[0], 99203[0], 99204[0], 99205[0], 99211[0], 99212[0], 99213[0], 99214[0], 99215[0], 99217[0], 99218[0], 99219[0], 99220[0], 99221[0], 99222[0], 99223[0], 99224[0], 99225[0], 99226[0], 99231[0], 99232[0], 99233[0], 99234[0], 99235[0], 99236[0], 99238[0], 99239[0], 99281[0], 99282[0], 99283[0], 99284[0], 99285[0], 99304[0], 99305[0], 99306[0], 99307[0], 99308[0], 99309[0], 99310[0], 99315[0], 99318[0], 99324[0], 99325[0], 99326[0], 99327[0], 99328[0], 99334[0], 99335[0], 99336[0], 99337[0], 99341[0], 99342[0], 99343[0], 99347[0], 99348[0], 99349[0], 99354[0], 99355[0], 99356[0], 99357[0], 99358[0], 99359[0], 99415[0], 99416[0], 99446[0], 99447[0], 99448[0], 99449[0], 99451[0], 99452[0], 99466[0], 99468[0], 99469[0], 99471[0], 99472[0], 99475[0], 99476[0], 99477[0], 99478[0], 99479[0], 99480[0], 99483[0], 99485[0], 99497[0], C8921[1], C8922[1], C8923[1], C8924[1], C8925[1], C8926[1], C8927[0], C8929[1], C8930[1], G0380[1], G0381[1], G0382[1], G0383[1], G0384[1], G0406[0], G0407[0], G0408[0], G0425[0], G0426[0], G0427[0], G0463[0], G0500[0], G0508[0], G0509[0]
01202	01996[1], 0213T[1], 0216T[1], 0228T[1], 0230T[1], 31505[1], 31515[1], 31527[1], 31622[1], 31634[1], 31645[1], 31647[1], 36000[1], 36010[0], 36011[1], 36012[1], 36013[1], 36014[1], 36015[1], 36400[1], 36405[1], 36406[1], 36410[1], 36420[1], 36425[1], 36430[1], 36440[1], 36591[0], 36592[0], 36600[1], 36640[1], 43752[1], 43753[1], 43754[1], 61026[1], 61055[1], 62280[1], 62281[1], 62282[1], 62284[1], 62320[1], 62321[1], 62322[1], 62323[1], 62324[1], 62325[1], 62326[1], 62327[1], 64400[1], 64402[1], 64405[1], 64408[1], 64410[1], 64413[1], 64415[1], 64416[1], 64417[1], 64418[1], 64420[1], 64421[1], 64425[1], 64430[1], 64435[1], 64445[1], 64446[1], 64447[1], 64448[1], 64449[1], 64450[1], 64461[1], 64463[1], 64479[1], 64483[1], 64486[1], 64487[1], 64488[1], 64489[1], 64490[1], 64493[1], 64505[1], 64510[1], 64517[1], 64520[1], 64530[1], 64553[1], 64555[1], 67500[1], 76000[1], 76970[1], 76998[0], 77002[0], 90865[1], 92511[1], 92512[1], 92516[1], 92520[1], 92537[1], 92538[1], 92950[1], 92953[1], 92960[1], 92961[1], 93000[1], 93005[1], 93010[1], 93040[1], 93041[1], 93042[1], 93050[0], 93303[0], 93304[0], 93306[1], 93307[1], 93308[1], 93312[1], 93313[1], 93314[1], 93315[1], 93316[1], 93317[1], 93318[0], 93351[1], 93355[0], 93451[1], 93456[1], 93457[1], 93561[0], 93562[0], 93701[0], 93922[1], 93923[1], 93924[1], 93925[1], 93926[1], 93930[1], 93931[1], 93970[1], 93971[1], 93975[1], 93976[1], 93978[1], 93979[1], 93980[1], 93981[1], 94002[1], 94004[1], 94200[1], 94250[0], 94640[1], 94644[1], 94660[1], 94662[1], 94680[1], 94681[1], 94690[1], 94760[0], 94761[0], 94762[1], 94770[1], 95812[0], 95813[0], 95816[0], 95819[0], 95822[0], 95829[0], 95955[0], 95956[0], 95957[0], 96360[0], 96365[0], 96372[0], 96373[0], 96374[0], 96375[0], 96376[0], 96377[0], 99151[0], 99152[0], 99153[0], 99155[0], 99156[0], 99157[0], 99201[0], 99202[0], 99203[0], 99204[0], 99205[0], 99211[0], 99212[0], 99213[0], 99214[0], 99215[0], 99217[0], 99218[0], 99219[0], 99220[0], 99221[0], 99222[0], 99223[0], 99224[0], 99225[0], 99226[0], 99231[0], 99232[0], 99233[0], 99234[0], 99235[0], 99236[0], 99238[0], 99239[0], 99281[0], 99282[0], 99283[0], 99284[0], 99285[0], 99304[0], 99305[0], 99306[0], 99307[0], 99308[0], 99309[0], 99310[0], 99315[0], 99318[0], 99324[0], 99325[0], 99326[0], 99327[0], 99328[0], 99334[0], 99335[0], 99336[0], 99337[0], 99341[0], 99342[0], 99343[0], 99347[0], 99348[0], 99349[0], 99354[0], 99355[0], 99356[0], 99357[0], 99358[0], 99359[0], 99415[0], 99416[0], 99446[0], 99447[0], 99448[0], 99449[0], 99451[0], 99452[0], 99466[0], 99468[0], 99469[0], 99471[0], 99472[0], 99475[0], 99476[0], 99477[0], 99478[0], 99479[0], 99480[0], 99483[0], 99485[0], 99497[0], C8921[1], C8922[1], C8923[1], C8924[1], C8925[1], C8926[1], C8927[0], C8929[1], C8930[1], G0380[1], G0381[1], G0382[1], G0383[1], G0384[1], G0406[0], G0407[0], G0408[0], G0425[0], G0426[0], G0427[0], G0463[0], G0500[0], G0508[0], G0509[0]
01210	01996[1], 0213T[1], 0216T[1], 0228T[1], 0230T[1], 31505[1], 31515[1], 31527[1], 31622[1], 31634[1], 31645[1], 31647[1], 36000[1], 36010[0], 36011[1], 36012[1], 36013[1], 36014[1], 36015[1], 36400[1], 36405[1], 36406[1], 36410[1], 36420[1], 36425[1], 36430[1], 36440[1], 36591[0], 36592[0], 36600[1], 36640[1], 43752[1], 43753[1], 43754[1], 61026[1], 61055[1], 62280[1], 62281[1], 62282[1], 62284[1], 62320[1], 62321[1], 62322[1], 62323[1], 62324[1], 62325[1], 62326[1], 62327[1], 64400[1], 64402[1], 64405[1], 64408[1], 64410[1], 64413[1], 64415[1], 64416[1], 64417[1], 64418[1], 64420[1], 64421[1], 64425[1], 64430[1], 64435[1], 64445[1], 64446[1], 64447[1], 64448[1], 64449[1], 64450[1], 64461[1], 64463[1], 64479[1], 64483[1], 64486[1], 64487[1], 64488[1], 64489[1], 64490[1], 64493[1], 64505[1], 64510[1], 64517[1], 64520[1], 64530[1], 64553[1], 64555[1], 67500[1], 76000[1], 76970[1], 76998[0], 77002[0], 90865[1], 92511[1], 92512[1], 92516[1], 92520[1], 92537[1], 92538[1], 92950[1], 92953[1], 92960[1], 92961[1], 93000[1], 93005[1], 93010[1], 93040[1], 93041[1], 93042[1], 93050[0], 93303[0], 93304[0], 93306[1], 93307[1], 93308[1], 93312[1], 93313[1], 93314[1], 93315[1], 93316[1], 93317[1], 93318[0], 93351[1], 93355[0], 93451[1], 93456[1], 93457[1], 93561[0], 93562[0], 93701[0], 93922[1], 93923[1], 93924[1], 93925[1], 93926[1], 93930[1], 93931[1], 93970[1], 93971[1], 93975[1], 93976[1], 93978[1], 93979[1], 93980[1], 93981[1], 94002[1], 94004[1], 94200[1], 94250[0], 94640[1], 94644[1], 94660[1], 94662[1], 94680[1], 94681[1], 94690[1], 94760[0], 94761[0], 94762[1], 94770[1], 95812[0], 95813[0], 95816[0], 95819[0], 95822[0], 95829[0], 95955[0], 95956[0], 95957[0], 96360[0], 96365[0], 96372[0], 96373[0], 96374[0], 96375[0], 96376[0], 96377[0], 99151[0], 99152[0], 99153[0], 99155[0], 99156[0], 99157[0], 99201[0], 99202[0], 99203[0], 99204[0], 99205[0], 99211[0], 99212[0], 99213[0], 99214[0], 99215[0], 99217[0], 99218[0], 99219[0], 99220[0], 99221[0], 99222[0], 99223[0], 99224[0], 99225[0], 99226[0], 99231[0], 99232[0], 99233[0], 99234[0], 99235[0], 99236[0], 99238[0], 99239[0], 99281[0], 99282[0], 99283[0], 99284[0], 99285[0], 99304[0], 99305[0], 99306[0], 99307[0], 99308[0], 99309[0], 99310[0], 99315[0], 99318[0], 99324[0], 99325[0], 99326[0], 99327[0], 99328[0], 99334[0], 99335[0], 99336[0], 99337[0], 99341[0], 99342[0], 99343[0], 99347[0], 99348[0], 99349[0], 99354[0], 99355[0], 99356[0], 99357[0], 99358[0], 99359[0], 99415[0], 99416[0], 99446[0], 99447[0], 99448[0], 99449[0], 99451[0], 99452[0], 99466[0], 99468[0], 99469[0], 99471[0], 99472[0], 99475[0], 99476[0], 99477[0], 99478[0], 99479[0], 99480[0], 99483[0], 99485[0], 99497[0], C8921[1], C8922[1], C8923[1], C8924[1], C8925[1], C8926[1], C8927[0], C8929[1], C8930[1], G0380[1], G0381[1], G0382[1], G0383[1], G0384[1], G0406[0], G0407[0], G0408[0], G0425[0], G0426[0], G0427[0], G0463[0], G0500[0], G0508[0], G0509[0]
01212	01996[1], 0213T[1], 0216T[1], 0228T[1], 0230T[1], 31505[1], 31515[1], 31527[1], 31622[1], 31634[1], 31645[1], 31647[1], 36000[1], 36010[0], 36011[1], 36012[1], 36013[1], 36014[1], 36015[1], 36400[1], 36405[1], 36406[1], 36410[1], 36420[1], 36425[1], 36430[1], 36440[1], 36591[0], 36592[0], 36600[1], 36640[1], 43752[1], 43753[1], 43754[1], 61026[1], 61055[1], 62280[1], 62281[1], 62282[1], 62284[1], 62320[1], 62321[1], 62322[1], 62323[1], 62324[1], 62325[1], 62326[1], 62327[1], 64400[1], 64402[1], 64405[1], 64408[1], 64410[1], 64413[1], 64415[1], 64416[1], 64417[1], 64418[1], 64420[1], 64421[1], 64425[1], 64430[1], 64435[1], 64445[1], 64446[1], 64447[1], 64448[1], 64449[1], 64450[1], 64461[1], 64463[1], 64479[1], 64483[1], 64486[1], 64487[1], 64488[1], 64489[1], 64490[1], 64493[1], 64505[1], 64510[1], 64517[1], 64520[1], 64530[1], 64553[1], 64555[1], 67500[1], 76000[1], 76970[1], 76998[0], 77002[0], 90865[1], 92511[1], 92512[1], 92516[1], 92520[1], 92537[1], 92538[1], 92950[1], 92953[1], 92960[1], 92961[1], 93000[1], 93005[1], 93010[1], 93040[1], 93041[1], 93042[1], 93050[0], 93303[0], 93304[0], 93306[1], 93307[1], 93308[1], 93312[1], 93313[1], 93314[1], 93315[1], 93316[1], 93317[1], 93318[0], 93351[1], 93355[0], 93451[1], 93456[1], 93457[1], 93561[0], 93562[0], 93701[0], 93922[1], 93923[1], 93924[1], 93925[1], 93926[1], 93930[1], 93931[1], 93970[1], 93971[1], 93975[1], 93976[1], 93978[1], 93979[1], 93980[1], 93981[1], 94002[1], 94004[1], 94200[1], 94250[0], 94640[1], 94644[1], 94660[1], 94662[1], 94680[1], 94681[1], 94690[1], 94760[0], 94761[0], 94762[1], 94770[1], 95812[0], 95813[0], 95816[0], 95819[0], 95822[0], 95829[0], 95955[0], 95956[0], 95957[0], 96360[0], 96365[0], 96372[0], 96373[0], 96374[0], 96375[0], 96376[0], 96377[0], 99151[0], 99152[0], 99153[0], 99155[0], 99156[0], 99157[0], 99201[0], 99202[0], 99203[0], 99204[0], 99205[0], 99211[0], 99212[0], 99213[0], 99214[0], 99215[0], 99217[0], 99218[0], 99219[0], 99220[0], 99221[0], 99222[0], 99223[0], 99224[0], 99225[0], 99226[0], 99231[0], 99232[0], 99233[0], 99234[0], 99235[0], 99236[0], 99238[0], 99239[0], 99281[0], 99282[0], 99283[0], 99284[0], 99285[0], 99304[0], 99305[0], 99306[0], 99307[0], 99308[0], 99309[0], 99310[0], 99315[0], 99318[0], 99324[0], 99325[0], 99326[0], 99327[0], 99328[0], 99334[0], 99335[0], 99336[0], 99337[0], 99341[0], 99342[0], 99343[0], 99347[0], 99348[0], 99349[0], 99354[0], 99355[0], 99356[0], 99357[0], 99358[0], 99359[0], 99415[0], 99416[0], 99446[0], 99447[0], 99448[0], 99449[0], 99451[0], 99452[0], 99466[0], 99468[0], 99469[0], 99471[0], 99472[0], 99475[0], 99476[0], 99477[0], 99478[0], 99479[0], 99480[0], 99483[0], 99485[0], 99497[0], C8921[1], C8922[1], C8923[1], C8924[1], C8925[1], C8926[1], C8927[0], C8929[1], C8930[1], G0380[1], G0381[1], G0382[1], G0383[1], G0384[1], G0406[0], G0407[0], G0408[0], G0425[0], G0426[0], G0427[0], G0463[0], G0500[0], G0508[0], G0509[0]
01214	01215[0], 01996[1], 0213T[1], 0216T[1], 0228T[1], 0230T[1], 31505[1], 31515[1], 31527[1], 31622[1], 31634[1], 31645[1], 31647[1], 36000[1], 36010[0], 36011[1], 36012[1], 36013[1], 36014[1], 36015[1], 36400[1], 36405[1], 36406[1], 36410[1], 36420[1], 36425[1], 36430[1], 36440[1], 36591[0], 36592[0], 36600[1], 36640[1], 43752[1], 43753[1], 43754[1], 61026[1], 61055[1], 62280[1], 62281[1], 62282[1], 62284[1], 62320[1], 62321[1], 62322[1], 62323[1], 62324[1], 62325[1], 62326[1], 62327[1], 64400[1], 64402[1], 64405[1], 64408[1], 64410[1], 64413[1], 64415[1], 64416[1], 64417[1], 64418[1], 64420[1], 64421[1], 64425[1], 64430[1], 64435[1], 64445[1], 64446[1], 64447[1], 64448[1], 64449[1], 64450[1], 64461[1], 64463[1], 64479[1], 64483[1], 64486[1], 64487[1], 64488[1], 64489[1], 64490[1], 64493[1], 64505[1], 64510[1], 64517[1], 64520[1], 64530[1], 64553[1], 64555[1], 67500[1], 76000[1], 76970[1], 76998[0], 77002[0], 90865[1], 92511[1], 92512[1], 92516[1], 92520[1], 92537[1], 92538[1], 92950[1], 92953[1], 92960[1], 92961[1], 93000[1], 93005[1], 93010[1], 93040[1], 93041[1], 93042[1], 93050[0], 93303[0], 93304[0], 93306[1], 93307[1], 93308[1], 93312[1], 93313[1], 93314[1], 93315[1], 93316[1], 93317[1], 93318[0], 93351[1], 93355[0], 93451[1], 93456[1], 93457[1], 93561[0], 93562[0], 93701[0], 93922[1], 93923[1], 93924[1], 93925[1], 93926[1], 93930[1], 93931[1], 93970[1], 93971[1], 93975[1], 93976[1], 93978[1], 93979[1], 93980[1], 93981[1], 94002[1], 94004[1], 94200[1], 94250[0], 94640[1], 94644[1], 94660[1], 94662[1], 94680[1], 94681[1], 94690[1], 94760[0], 94761[0], 94762[1], 94770[1], 95812[0], 95813[0], 95816[0], 95819[0], 95822[0], 95829[0], 95955[0], 95956[0], 95957[0], 96360[0], 96365[0], 96372[0], 96373[0], 96374[0], 96375[0], 96376[0], 96377[0], 99151[0], 99152[0], 99153[0],

0 = Modifier usage not allowed or inappropriate 1 = Modifier usage allowed

CPT © 2018 American Medical Association. All Rights Reserved.

Code 1	Code 2
	99155[0], 99156[0], 99157[0], 99201[0], 99202[0], 99203[0], 99204[0], 99205[0], 99211[0], 99212[0], 99213[0], 99214[0], 99215[0], 99217[0], 99218[0], 99219[0], 99220[0], 99221[0], 99222[0], 99223[0], 99224[0], 99225[0], 99226[0], 99231[0], 99232[0], 99233[0], 99234[0], 99235[0], 99236[0], 99238[0], 99239[0], 99281[0], 99282[0], 99283[0], 99284[0], 99285[0], 99304[0], 99305[0], 99306[0], 99307[0], 99308[0], 99309[0], 99310[0], 99315[0], 99318[0], 99324[0], 99325[0], 99326[0], 99327[0], 99328[0], 99334[0], 99335[0], 99336[0], 99337[0], 99341[0], 99342[0], 99343[0], 99347[0], 99348[0], 99349[0], 99354[0], 99355[0], 99356[0], 99357[0], 99358[0], 99359[0], 99415[0], 99416[0], 99446[0], 99447[0], 99448[0], 99449[0], 99451[0], 99452[0], 99466[0], 99468[0], 99469[0], 99471[0], 99472[0], 99475[0], 99476[0], 99477[0], 99478[0], 99479[0], 99480[0], 99483[0], 99485[0], 99497[0], C8921[1], C8922[1], C8923[1], C8924[1], C8925[1], C8926[1], C8927[0], C8929[1], C8930[1], G0380[1], G0381[1], G0382[1], G0383[1], G0384[1], G0406[0], G0407[0], G0408[0], G0425[0], G0426[0], G0427[0], G0463[0], G0500[0], G0508[0], G0509[0]
01215	01996[1], 0213T[1], 0216T[1], 0228T[1], 0230T[1], 31505[1], 31515[1], 31527[1], 31622[1], 31634[1], 31645[1], 31647[1], 36000[1], 36010[0], 36011[1], 36012[1], 36013[1], 36014[1], 36015[1], 36400[1], 36405[1], 36406[1], 36410[1], 36420[1], 36425[1], 36430[1], 36440[1], 36591[0], 36592[0], 36600[1], 36640[1], 43752[1], 43753[1], 43754[1], 61026[1], 61055[1], 62280[1], 62281[1], 62282[1], 62284[1], 62320[1], 62321[1], 62322[1], 62323[1], 62324[1], 62325[1], 62326[1], 62327[1], 64400[1], 64402[1], 64405[1], 64408[1], 64410[1], 64413[1], 64415[1], 64416[1], 64417[1], 64418[1], 64420[1], 64421[1], 64425[1], 64430[1], 64435[1], 64445[1], 64446[1], 64447[1], 64448[1], 64449[1], 64450[1], 64461[1], 64463[1], 64479[1], 64483[1], 64486[1], 64487[1], 64488[1], 64489[1], 64490[1], 64493[1], 64505[1], 64510[1], 64517[1], 64520[1], 64530[1], 64553[1], 64555[1], 67500[0], 76000[1], 76970[1], 76998[0], 77002[0], 90865[1], 92511[1], 92512[1], 92516[1], 92520[1], 92537[1], 92538[1], 92950[1], 92953[1], 92960[1], 92961[1], 93000[1], 93005[1], 93010[1], 93040[1], 93041[1], 93042[1], 93050[0], 93303[0], 93304[0], 93306[1], 93307[1], 93308[1], 93312[1], 93313[1], 93314[1], 93315[1], 93316[1], 93317[1], 93318[0], 93351[1], 93355[0], 93451[1], 93456[1], 93457[1], 93561[0], 93562[0], 93701[0], 93922[1], 93923[1], 93924[1], 93925[1], 93926[1], 93930[1], 93931[1], 93970[1], 93971[1], 93975[1], 93976[1], 93978[1], 93979[1], 93980[1], 93981[1], 94002[1], 94004[1], 94200[1], 94250[0], 94640[1], 94644[1], 94660[1], 94662[1], 94680[1], 94681[1], 94690[1], 94760[0], 94761[0], 94762[1], 94770[1], 95812[0], 95813[0], 95816[0], 95819[0], 95822[0], 95829[0], 95955[0], 95956[0], 95957[0], 96360[0], 96365[0], 96372[0], 96373[0], 96374[0], 96375[0], 96376[0], 96377[0], 99151[0], 99152[0], 99153[0], 99155[0], 99156[0], 99157[0], 99201[0], 99202[0], 99203[0], 99204[0], 99205[0], 99211[0], 99212[0], 99213[0], 99214[0], 99215[0], 99217[0], 99218[0], 99219[0], 99220[0], 99221[0], 99222[0], 99223[0], 99224[0], 99225[0], 99226[0], 99231[0], 99232[0], 99233[0], 99234[0], 99235[0], 99236[0], 99238[0], 99239[0], 99281[0], 99282[0], 99283[0], 99284[0], 99285[0], 99304[0], 99305[0], 99306[0], 99307[0], 99308[0], 99309[0], 99310[0], 99315[0], 99316[0], 99318[0], 99324[0], 99325[0], 99326[0], 99327[0], 99328[0], 99334[0], 99335[0], 99336[0], 99337[0], 99341[0], 99342[0], 99343[0], 99344[0], 99345[0], 99347[0], 99348[0], 99349[0], 99350[0], 99354[0], 99355[0], 99356[0], 99357[0], 99358[0], 99359[0], 99415[0], 99416[0], 99446[0], 99447[0], 99448[0], 99449[0], 99451[0], 99452[0], 99466[0], 99468[0], 99469[0], 99471[0], 99472[0], 99475[0], 99476[0], 99477[0], 99478[0], 99479[0], 99480[0], 99483[0], 99485[0], 99497[0], C8921[1], C8922[1], C8923[1], C8924[1], C8925[1], C8926[1], C8927[0], C8929[1], C8930[1], G0380[1], G0381[1], G0382[1], G0383[1], G0384[1], G0406[0], G0407[0], G0408[0], G0425[0], G0426[0], G0427[0], G0463[0], G0500[0], G0508[0], G0509[0]
01220	01996[1], 0213T[1], 0216T[1], 0228T[1], 0230T[1], 31505[1], 31515[1], 31527[1], 31622[1], 31634[1], 31645[1], 31647[1], 36000[1], 36010[0], 36011[1], 36012[1], 36013[1], 36014[1], 36015[1], 36400[1], 36405[1], 36406[1], 36410[1], 36420[1], 36425[1], 36430[1], 36440[1], 36591[0], 36592[0], 36600[1], 36640[1], 43752[1], 43753[1], 43754[1], 61026[1], 61055[1], 62280[1], 62281[1], 62282[1], 62284[1], 62320[1], 62321[1], 62322[1], 62323[1], 62324[1], 62325[1], 62326[1], 62327[1], 64400[1], 64402[1], 64405[1], 64408[1], 64410[1], 64413[1], 64415[1], 64416[1], 64417[1], 64418[1], 64420[1], 64421[1], 64425[1], 64430[1], 64435[1], 64445[1], 64446[1], 64447[1], 64448[1], 64449[1], 64450[1], 64461[1], 64463[1], 64479[1], 64483[1], 64486[1], 64487[1], 64488[1], 64489[1], 64490[1], 64493[1], 64505[1], 64510[1], 64517[1], 64520[1], 64530[1], 64553[1], 64555[1], 67500[1], 76000[1], 76970[1], 76998[0], 77002[0], 90865[1], 92511[1], 92512[1], 92516[1], 92520[1], 92537[1], 92538[1], 92950[1], 92953[1], 92960[1], 92961[1], 93000[1], 93005[1], 93010[1], 93040[1], 93041[1], 93042[1], 93050[0], 93303[0], 93304[0], 93306[1], 93307[1], 93308[1], 93312[1], 93313[1], 93314[1], 93315[1], 93316[1], 93317[1], 93318[0], 93351[1], 93355[0], 93451[1], 93456[1], 93457[1], 93561[0], 93562[0], 93701[0], 93922[1], 93923[1], 93924[1], 93925[1], 93926[1], 93930[1], 93931[1], 93970[1], 93971[1], 93975[1], 93976[1], 93978[1], 93979[1], 93980[1], 93981[1], 94002[1], 94004[1], 94200[1], 94250[0], 94640[1], 94644[1], 94660[1], 94662[1], 94680[1], 94681[1], 94690[1], 94760[0], 94761[0], 94762[1], 94770[1], 95812[0], 95813[0], 95816[0], 95819[0], 95822[0], 95829[0], 95955[0], 95956[0], 95957[0], 96360[0], 96365[0], 96372[0], 96373[0], 96374[0], 96375[0], 96376[0], 96377[0], 99151[0], 99152[0], 99153[0], 99155[0], 99156[0], 99157[0], 99201[0], 99202[0], 99203[0], 99204[0], 99205[0], 99211[0], 99212[0], 99213[0], 99214[0], 99215[0], 99217[0], 99218[0], 99219[0], 99220[0], 99221[0], 99222[0], 99223[0], 99224[0], 99225[0], 99226[0], 99231[0], 99232[0], 99233[0], 99234[0], 99235[0], 99236[0], 99238[0], 99239[0], 99281[0], 99282[0], 99283[0], 99284[0], 99285[0], 99304[0], 99305[0], 99306[0], 99307[0], 99308[0], 99309[0], 99310[0], 99315[0], 99318[0], 99324[0], 99325[0], 99326[0], 99327[0], 99328[0], 99334[0], 99335[0], 99336[0], 99337[0], 99341[0], 99342[0], 99343[0], 99347[0], 99348[0], 99349[0], 99354[0], 99355[0], 99356[0], 99357[0], 99358[0], 99359[0], 99415[0], 99416[0], 99446[0], 99447[0], 99448[0], 99449[0], 99451[0], 99452[0], 99466[0], 99468[0], 99469[0], 99471[0], 99472[0], 99475[0], 99476[0], 99477[0], 99478[0], 99479[0], 99480[0], 99483[0], 99485[0], 99497[0], C8921[1], C8922[1], C8923[1], C8924[1], C8925[1], C8926[1], C8927[0], C8929[1], C8930[1], G0380[1], G0381[1], G0382[1], G0383[1], G0384[1], G0406[0], G0407[0], G0408[0], G0425[0], G0426[0], G0427[0], G0463[0], G0500[0], G0508[0], G0509[0]
01230	01996[1], 0213T[1], 0216T[1], 0228T[1], 0230T[1], 31505[1], 31515[1], 31527[1], 31622[1], 31634[1], 31645[1], 31647[1], 36000[1], 36010[0], 36011[1], 36012[1], 36013[1], 36014[1], 36015[1], 36400[1], 36405[1], 36406[1], 36410[1], 36420[1], 36425[1], 36430[1], 36440[1], 36591[0], 36592[0], 36600[1], 36640[1], 43752[1], 43753[1], 43754[1], 61026[1], 61055[1], 62280[1], 62281[1], 62282[1], 62284[1], 62320[1], 62321[1], 62322[1], 62323[1], 62324[1], 62325[1], 62326[1], 62327[1], 64400[1], 64402[1], 64405[1], 64408[1], 64410[1], 64413[1], 64415[1], 64416[1], 64417[1], 64418[1], 64420[1], 64421[1], 64425[1], 64430[1], 64435[1], 64445[1], 64446[1], 64447[1], 64448[1], 64449[1], 64450[1], 64461[1], 64463[1], 64479[1], 64483[1], 64486[1], 64487[1], 64488[1], 64489[1], 64490[1], 64493[1], 64505[1], 64510[1], 64517[1], 64520[1], 64530[1], 64553[1], 64555[1], 67500[1], 76000[1], 76970[1], 76998[0], 77002[0], 90865[1], 92511[1], 92512[1], 92516[1], 92520[1], 92537[1], 92538[1], 92950[1], 92953[1], 92960[1], 92961[1], 93000[1], 93005[1], 93010[1], 93040[1], 93041[1], 93042[1], 93050[0], 93303[0], 93304[0], 93306[1], 93307[1], 93308[1], 93312[1], 93313[1], 93314[1], 93315[1], 93316[1], 93317[1], 93318[0], 93351[1], 93355[0], 93451[1], 93456[1], 93457[1], 93561[0], 93562[0], 93701[0], 93922[1], 93923[1], 93924[1], 93925[1], 93926[1], 93930[1], 93931[1], 93970[1], 93971[1], 93975[1], 93976[1], 93978[1], 93979[1], 93980[1], 93981[1], 94002[1], 94004[1], 94200[1], 94250[0], 94640[1], 94644[1], 94660[1], 94662[1], 94680[1], 94681[1], 94690[1], 94760[0], 94761[0], 94762[1], 94770[1], 95812[0], 95813[0], 95816[0], 95819[0], 95822[0], 95829[0], 95955[0], 95956[0], 95957[0], 96360[0], 96365[0], 96372[0], 96373[0], 96374[0], 96375[0], 96376[0], 96377[0], 99151[0], 99152[0], 99153[0], 99155[0], 99156[0], 99157[0], 99201[0], 99202[0], 99203[0], 99204[0], 99205[0], 99211[0], 99212[0], 99213[0], 99214[0], 99215[0], 99217[0], 99218[0], 99219[0], 99220[0], 99221[0], 99222[0], 99223[0], 99224[0], 99225[0], 99226[0], 99231[0], 99232[0], 99233[0], 99234[0], 99235[0], 99236[0], 99238[0], 99239[0], 99281[0], 99282[0], 99283[0], 99284[0], 99285[0], 99304[0], 99305[0], 99306[0], 99307[0], 99308[0], 99309[0], 99310[0], 99315[0], 99318[0], 99324[0], 99325[0], 99326[0], 99327[0], 99328[0], 99334[0], 99335[0], 99336[0], 99337[0], 99341[0], 99342[0], 99343[0], 99347[0], 99348[0], 99349[0], 99354[0], 99355[0], 99356[0], 99357[0], 99358[0], 99359[0], 99415[0], 99416[0], 99446[0], 99447[0], 99448[0], 99449[0], 99451[0], 99452[0], 99466[0], 99468[0], 99469[0], 99471[0], 99472[0], 99475[0], 99476[0], 99477[0], 99478[0], 99479[0], 99480[0], 99483[0], 99485[0], 99497[0], C8921[1], C8922[1], C8923[1], C8924[1], C8925[1], C8926[1], C8927[0], C8929[1], C8930[1], G0380[1], G0381[1], G0382[1], G0383[1], G0384[1], G0406[0], G0407[0], G0408[0], G0425[0], G0426[0], G0427[0], G0463[0], G0500[0], G0508[0], G0509[0]
01232	01996[1], 0213T[1], 0216T[1], 0228T[1], 0230T[1], 31505[1], 31515[1], 31527[1], 31622[1], 31634[1], 31645[1], 31647[1], 36000[1], 36010[0], 36011[1], 36012[1], 36013[1], 36014[1], 36015[1], 36400[1], 36405[1], 36406[1], 36410[1], 36420[1], 36425[1], 36430[1], 36440[1], 36591[0], 36592[0], 36600[1], 36640[1], 43752[1], 43753[1], 43754[1], 61026[1], 61055[1], 62280[1], 62281[1], 62282[1], 62284[1], 62320[1], 62321[1], 62322[1], 62323[1], 62324[1], 62325[1], 62326[1], 62327[1], 64400[1], 64402[1], 64405[1], 64408[1], 64410[1], 64413[1], 64415[1], 64416[1], 64417[1], 64418[1], 64420[1], 64421[1], 64425[1], 64430[1], 64435[1], 64445[1], 64446[1], 64447[1], 64448[1], 64449[1], 64450[1], 64461[1], 64463[1], 64479[1], 64483[1], 64486[1], 64487[1], 64488[1], 64489[1], 64490[1], 64493[1], 64505[1], 64510[1], 64517[1], 64520[1], 64530[1], 64553[1], 64555[1], 67500[1], 76000[1], 76970[1], 76998[0], 77002[0], 90865[1], 92511[1], 92512[1], 92516[1], 92520[1], 92537[1], 92538[1], 92950[1], 92953[1], 92960[1], 92961[1], 93000[1], 93005[1], 93010[1], 93040[1], 93041[1], 93042[1], 93050[0], 93303[0], 93304[0], 93306[1], 93307[1], 93308[1], 93312[1], 93313[1], 93314[1], 93315[1], 93316[1], 93317[1], 93318[0], 93351[1], 93355[0], 93451[1], 93456[1], 93457[1], 93561[0], 93562[0], 93701[0], 93922[1], 93923[1], 93924[1], 93925[1], 93926[1], 93930[1], 93931[1], 93970[1], 93971[1], 93975[1], 93976[1], 93978[1], 93979[1], 93980[1], 93981[1], 94002[1], 94004[1], 94200[1], 94250[0], 94640[1], 94644[1], 94660[1], 94662[1], 94680[1], 94681[1], 94690[1], 94760[0], 94761[0], 94762[1], 94770[1], 95812[0], 95813[0], 95816[0], 95819[0], 95822[0], 95829[0], 95955[0], 95956[0], 95957[0], 96360[0], 96365[0], 96372[0], 96373[0], 96374[0], 96375[0], 96376[0], 96377[0], 99151[0], 99152[0], 99153[0], 99155[0], 99156[0], 99157[0], 99201[0], 99202[0], 99203[0], 99204[0], 99205[0], 99211[0], 99212[0], 99213[0], 99214[0], 99215[0], 99217[0], 99218[0], 99219[0], 99220[0], 99221[0], 99222[0], 99223[0], 99224[0], 99225[0], 99226[0], 99231[0], 99232[0], 99233[0], 99234[0], 99235[0], 99236[0], 99238[0], 99239[0], 99281[0], 99282[0], 99283[0], 99284[0], 99285[0], 99304[0], 99305[0], 99306[0], 99307[0], 99308[0], 99309[0], 99310[0], 99315[0], 99318[0], 99324[0], 99325[0], 99326[0], 99327[0], 99328[0], 99334[0], 99335[0], 99336[0], 99337[0], 99341[0], 99342[0], 99343[0], 99347[0], 99348[0], 99349[0], 99354[0], 99355[0], 99356[0], 99357[0], 99358[0], 99359[0], 99415[0], 99416[0], 99446[0], 99447[0], 99448[0], 99449[0], 99451[0], 99452[0], 99466[0], 99468[0], 99469[0], 99471[0], 99472[0], 99475[0], 99476[0], 99477[0], 99478[0], 99479[0], 99480[0], 99483[0], 99485[0], 99497[0], C8921[1], C8922[1], C8923[1], C8924[1], C8925[1], C8926[1], C8927[0], C8929[1], C8930[1], G0380[1], G0381[1], G0382[1], G0383[1], G0384[1], G0406[0], G0407[0], G0408[0], G0425[0], G0426[0], G0427[0], G0463[0], G0500[0], G0508[0], G0509[0]

0 = Modifier usage not allowed or inappropriate 1 = Modifier usage allowed

Appendix A: NCCI - CPT Codes

CPT © 2018 American Medical Association. All Rights Reserved.

Code 1	Code 2
01234	01996[1], 0213T[1], 0216T[1], 0228T[1], 0230T[1], 31505[1], 31515[1], 31527[1], 31622[1], 31634[1], 31645[1], 31647[1], 36000[1], 36010[0], 36011[1], 36012[1], 36013[1], 36014[1], 36015[1], 36400[1], 36405[1], 36406[1], 36410[1], 36420[1], 36425[1], 36430[1], 36440[1], 36591[0], 36592[0], 36600[1], 36640[1], 43752[1], 43753[1], 43754[1], 61026[1], 61055[1], 62280[1], 62281[1], 62282[1], 62284[1], 62320[1], 62321[1], 62322[1], 62323[1], 62324[1], 62325[1], 62326[1], 62327[1], 64400[1], 64402[1], 64405[1], 64408[1], 64410[1], 64413[1], 64415[1], 64416[1], 64417[1], 64418[1], 64420[1], 64421[1], 64425[1], 64430[1], 64435[1], 64445[1], 64446[1], 64447[1], 64448[1], 64449[1], 64450[1], 64461[1], 64463[1], 64479[1], 64483[1], 64486[1], 64487[1], 64488[1], 64489[1], 64490[1], 64493[1], 64505[1], 64510[1], 64517[1], 64520[1], 64530[1], 64553[1], 64555[1], 67500[1], 76000[1], 76970[1], 76998[0], 77002[0], 90865[1], 92511[1], 92512[1], 92516[1], 92520[1], 92537[1], 92538[1], 92950[1], 92953[1], 92960[1], 92961[1], 93000[1], 93005[1], 93010[1], 93040[1], 93041[1], 93042[1], 93050[0], 93303[0], 93304[0], 93306[1], 93307[1], 93308[1], 93312[1], 93313[1], 93314[1], 93315[1], 93316[1], 93317[1], 93318[0], 93351[1], 93355[0], 93451[1], 93456[1], 93457[1], 93561[0], 93562[0], 93701[0], 93922[1], 93923[1], 93924[1], 93925[1], 93926[1], 93930[1], 93931[1], 93970[1], 93971[1], 93975[1], 93976[1], 93978[1], 93979[1], 93980[1], 93981[1], 94002[1], 94004[1], 94200[1], 94250[0], 94640[1], 94644[1], 94660[1], 94662[1], 94680[1], 94681[1], 94690[1], 94760[0], 94761[0], 94762[1], 94770[1], 95812[0], 95813[0], 95816[0], 95819[0], 95822[0], 95829[0], 95955[0], 95956[0], 95957[0], 96360[0], 96365[0], 96372[0], 96373[0], 96374[0], 96375[0], 96376[0], 96377[0], 99151[0], 99152[0], 99153[0], 99155[0], 99156[0], 99157[0], 99201[0], 99202[0], 99203[0], 99204[0], 99205[0], 99211[0], 99212[0], 99213[0], 99214[0], 99215[0], 99217[0], 99218[0], 99219[0], 99220[0], 99221[0], 99222[0], 99223[0], 99224[0], 99225[0], 99226[0], 99231[0], 99232[0], 99233[0], 99234[0], 99235[0], 99236[0], 99238[0], 99239[0], 99281[0], 99282[0], 99283[0], 99284[0], 99285[0], 99304[0], 99305[0], 99306[0], 99307[0], 99308[0], 99309[0], 99310[0], 99315[0], 99318[0], 99324[0], 99325[0], 99326[0], 99327[0], 99328[0], 99334[0], 99335[0], 99336[0], 99337[0], 99341[0], 99342[0], 99343[0], 99347[0], 99348[0], 99349[0], 99354[0], 99355[0], 99356[0], 99357[0], 99358[0], 99359[0], 99415[0], 99416[0], 99446[0], 99447[0], 99448[0], 99449[0], 99451[0], 99452[0], 99466[0], 99468[0], 99469[0], 99471[0], 99472[0], 99475[0], 99476[0], 99477[0], 99478[0], 99479[0], 99480[0], 99483[0], 99485[0], 99497[0], C8921[1], C8922[1], C8923[1], C8924[1], C8925[1], C8926[1], C8927[0], C8929[1], C8930[1], G0380[1], G0381[1], G0382[1], G0383[1], G0384[1], G0406[0], G0407[0], G0408[0], G0425[0], G0426[0], G0427[0], G0463[0], G0500[0], G0508[0], G0509[0]
01250	01996[1], 0213T[1], 0216T[1], 0228T[1], 0230T[1], 0333T[0], 0464T[0], 31505[1], 31515[1], 31527[1], 31622[1], 31634[1], 31645[1], 31647[1], 36000[1], 36010[0], 36011[1], 36012[1], 36013[1], 36014[1], 36015[1], 36400[1], 36405[1], 36406[1], 36410[1], 36420[1], 36425[1], 36430[1], 36440[1], 36591[0], 36592[0], 36600[1], 36640[1], 43752[1], 43753[1], 43754[1], 61026[1], 61055[1], 62280[1], 62281[1], 62282[1], 62284[1], 62320[1], 62321[1], 62322[1], 62323[1], 62324[1], 62325[1], 62326[1], 62327[1], 64400[1], 64402[1], 64405[1], 64408[1], 64410[1], 64413[1], 64415[1], 64416[1], 64417[1], 64418[1], 64420[1], 64421[1], 64425[1], 64430[1], 64435[1], 64445[1], 64446[1], 64447[1], 64448[1], 64449[1], 64450[1], 64461[1], 64463[1], 64479[1], 64483[1], 64486[1], 64487[1], 64488[1], 64489[1], 64490[1], 64493[1], 64505[1], 64510[1], 64517[1], 64520[1], 64530[1], 64553[1], 64555[1], 67500[1], 76000[1], 76970[1], 76998[0], 77002[0], 90865[1], 92511[1], 92512[1], 92516[1], 92520[1], 92537[1], 92538[1], 92585[0], 92950[1], 92953[1], 92960[1], 92961[1], 93000[1], 93005[1], 93010[1], 93040[1], 93041[1], 93042[1], 93050[0], 93303[0], 93304[0], 93306[1], 93307[1], 93308[1], 93312[1], 93313[1], 93314[1], 93315[1], 93316[1], 93317[1], 93318[0], 93351[1], 93355[0], 93451[1], 93456[1], 93457[1], 93561[0], 93562[0], 93701[0], 93922[1], 93923[1], 93924[1], 93925[1], 93926[1], 93930[1], 93931[1], 93970[1], 93971[1], 93975[1], 93976[1], 93978[1], 93979[1], 93980[1], 93981[1], 94002[1], 94004[1], 94200[1], 94250[0], 94640[1], 94644[1], 94660[1], 94662[1], 94680[1], 94681[1], 94690[1], 94760[0], 94761[0], 94762[1], 94770[1], 95812[0], 95813[0], 95816[0], 95819[0], 95822[0], 95829[0], 95860[0], 95861[0], 95863[0], 95864[0], 95865[0], 95866[0], 95867[0], 95868[0], 95869[0], 95870[0], 95907[0], 95908[0], 95909[0], 95910[0], 95911[0], 95912[0], 95913[0], 95925[0], 95926[0], 95927[0], 95928[0], 95929[0], 95930[0], 95933[0], 95937[0], 95938[0], 95939[0], 95940[0], 95955[0], 95956[0], 95957[0], 96360[0], 96365[0], 96372[0], 96373[0], 96374[0], 96375[0], 96376[0], 96377[0], 99151[0], 99152[0], 99153[0], 99155[0], 99156[0], 99157[0], 99201[0], 99202[0], 99203[0], 99204[0], 99205[0], 99211[0], 99212[0], 99213[0], 99214[0], 99215[0], 99217[0], 99218[0], 99219[0], 99220[0], 99221[0], 99222[0], 99223[0], 99224[0], 99225[0], 99226[0], 99231[0], 99232[0], 99233[0], 99234[0], 99235[0], 99236[0], 99238[0], 99239[0], 99281[0], 99282[0], 99283[0], 99284[0], 99285[0], 99304[0], 99305[0], 99306[0], 99307[0], 99308[0], 99309[0], 99310[0], 99315[0], 99318[0], 99324[0], 99325[0], 99326[0], 99327[0], 99328[0], 99334[0], 99335[0], 99336[0], 99337[0], 99341[0], 99342[0], 99343[0], 99347[0], 99348[0], 99349[0], 99354[0], 99355[0], 99356[0], 99357[0], 99358[0], 99359[0], 99415[0], 99416[0], 99446[0], 99447[0], 99448[0], 99449[0], 99451[0], 99452[0], 99466[0], 99468[0], 99469[0], 99471[0], 99472[0], 99475[0], 99476[0], 99477[0], 99478[0], 99479[0], 99480[0], 99483[0], 99485[0], 99497[0], C8921[1], C8922[1], C8923[1], C8924[1], C8925[1], C8926[1], C8927[0], C8929[1], C8930[1], G0380[1], G0381[1], G0382[1], G0383[1], G0384[1], G0406[0], G0407[0], G0408[0], G0425[0], G0426[0], G0427[0], G0453[0], G0463[0], G0500[0], G0508[0], G0509[0]
01260	01996[1], 0213T[1], 0216T[1], 0228T[1], 0230T[1], 31505[1], 31515[1], 31527[1], 31622[1], 31634[1], 31645[1], 31647[1], 36000[1], 36010[0], 36011[1], 36012[1], 36013[1], 36014[1], 36015[1], 36400[1], 36405[1], 36406[1], 36410[1], 36420[1], 36425[1], 36430[1], 36440[1], 36591[0], 36592[0], 36600[1], 36640[1], 43752[1], 43753[1], 43754[1], 61026[1], 61055[1], 62280[1], 62281[1], 62282[1], 62284[1], 62320[1], 62321[1], 62322[1], 62323[1], 62324[1], 62325[1], 62326[1], 62327[1], 64400[1], 64402[1], 64405[1], 64408[1], 64410[1], 64413[1], 64415[1], 64416[1], 64417[1], 64418[1], 64420[1], 64421[1], 64425[1], 64430[1], 64435[1], 64445[1], 64446[1], 64447[1], 64448[1], 64449[1], 64450[1], 64461[1], 64463[1], 64479[1], 64483[1], 64486[1], 64487[1], 64488[1], 64489[1], 64490[1], 64493[1], 64505[1], 64510[1], 64517[1], 64520[1], 64530[1], 64553[1], 64555[1], 67500[1], 76000[1], 76970[1], 76998[0], 77002[0], 90865[1], 92511[1], 92512[1], 92516[1], 92520[1], 92537[1], 92538[1], 92950[1], 92953[1], 92960[1], 92961[1], 93000[1], 93005[1], 93010[1], 93040[1], 93041[1], 93042[1], 93050[0], 93303[0], 93304[0], 93306[1], 93307[1], 93308[1], 93312[1], 93313[1], 93314[1], 93315[1], 93316[1], 93317[1], 93318[0], 93351[1], 93355[0], 93451[1], 93456[1], 93457[1], 93561[0], 93562[0], 93701[0], 93922[1], 93923[1], 93924[1], 93925[1], 93926[1], 93930[1], 93931[1], 93970[1], 93971[1], 93975[1], 93976[1], 93978[1], 93979[1], 93980[1], 93981[1], 94002[1], 94004[1], 94200[1], 94250[0], 94640[1], 94644[1], 94660[1], 94662[1], 94680[1], 94681[1], 94690[1], 94760[0], 94761[0], 94762[1], 94770[1], 95812[0], 95813[0], 95816[0], 95819[0], 95822[0], 95829[0], 95955[0], 95956[0], 95957[0], 96360[0], 96365[0], 96372[0], 96373[0], 96374[0], 96375[0], 96376[0], 96377[0], 99151[0], 99152[0], 99153[0], 99155[0], 99156[0], 99157[0], 99201[0], 99202[0], 99203[0], 99204[0], 99205[0], 99211[0], 99212[0], 99213[0], 99214[0], 99215[0], 99217[0], 99218[0], 99219[0], 99220[0], 99221[0], 99222[0], 99223[0], 99224[0], 99225[0], 99226[0], 99231[0], 99232[0], 99233[0], 99234[0], 99235[0], 99236[0], 99238[0], 99239[0], 99281[0], 99282[0], 99283[0], 99284[0], 99285[0], 99304[0], 99305[0], 99306[0], 99307[0], 99308[0], 99309[0], 99310[0], 99315[0], 99318[0], 99324[0], 99325[0], 99326[0], 99327[0], 99328[0], 99334[0], 99335[0], 99336[0], 99337[0], 99341[0], 99342[0], 99343[0], 99347[0], 99348[0], 99349[0], 99354[0], 99355[0], 99356[0], 99357[0], 99358[0], 99359[0], 99415[0], 99416[0], 99446[0], 99447[0], 99448[0], 99449[0], 99451[0], 99452[0], 99466[0], 99468[0], 99469[0], 99471[0], 99472[0], 99475[0], 99476[0], 99477[0], 99478[0], 99479[0], 99480[0], 99483[0], 99485[0], 99497[0], C8921[1], C8922[1], C8923[1], C8924[1], C8925[1], C8926[1], C8927[0], C8929[1], C8930[1], G0380[1], G0381[1], G0382[1], G0383[1], G0384[1], G0406[0], G0407[0], G0408[0], G0425[0], G0426[0], G0427[0], G0463[0], G0500[0], G0508[0], G0509[0]
01270	01996[1], 0213T[1], 0216T[1], 0228T[1], 0230T[1], 31505[1], 31515[1], 31527[1], 31622[1], 31634[1], 31645[1], 31647[1], 36000[1], 36010[0], 36011[1], 36012[1], 36013[1], 36014[1], 36015[1], 36400[1], 36405[1], 36406[1], 36410[1], 36420[1], 36425[1], 36430[1], 36440[1], 36591[0], 36592[0], 36600[1], 36640[1], 43752[1], 43753[1], 43754[1], 61026[1], 61055[1], 62280[1], 62281[1], 62282[1], 62284[1], 62320[1], 62321[1], 62322[1], 62323[1], 62324[1], 62325[1], 62326[1], 62327[1], 64400[1], 64402[1], 64405[1], 64408[1], 64410[1], 64413[1], 64415[1], 64416[1], 64417[1], 64418[1], 64420[1], 64421[1], 64425[1], 64430[1], 64435[1], 64445[1], 64446[1], 64447[1], 64448[1], 64449[1], 64450[1], 64461[1], 64463[1], 64479[1], 64483[1], 64486[1], 64487[1], 64488[1], 64489[1], 64490[1], 64493[1], 64505[1], 64510[1], 64517[1], 64520[1], 64530[1], 64553[1], 64555[1], 67500[1], 76000[1], 76970[1], 76998[0], 77002[0], 90865[1], 92511[1], 92512[1], 92516[1], 92520[1], 92537[1], 92538[1], 92950[1], 92953[1], 92960[1], 92961[1], 93000[1], 93005[1], 93010[1], 93040[1], 93041[1], 93042[1], 93050[0], 93303[0], 93304[0], 93306[1], 93307[1], 93308[1], 93312[1], 93313[1], 93314[1], 93315[1], 93316[1], 93317[1], 93318[0], 93351[1], 93355[0], 93451[1], 93456[1], 93457[1], 93561[0], 93562[0], 93701[0], 93922[1], 93923[1], 93924[1], 93925[1], 93926[1], 93930[1], 93931[1], 93970[1], 93971[1], 93975[1], 93976[1], 93978[1], 93979[1], 93980[1], 93981[1], 94002[1], 94004[1], 94200[1], 94250[0], 94640[1], 94644[1], 94660[1], 94662[1], 94680[1], 94681[1], 94690[1], 94760[0], 94761[0], 94762[1], 94770[1], 95812[0], 95813[0], 95816[0], 95819[0], 95822[0], 95829[0], 95955[0], 95956[0], 95957[0], 96360[0], 96365[0], 96372[0], 96373[0], 96374[0], 96375[0], 96376[0], 96377[0], 99151[0], 99152[0], 99153[0], 99155[0], 99156[0], 99157[0], 99201[0], 99202[0], 99203[0], 99204[0], 99205[0], 99211[0], 99212[0], 99213[0], 99214[0], 99215[0], 99217[0], 99218[0], 99219[0], 99220[0], 99221[0], 99222[0], 99223[0], 99224[0], 99225[0], 99226[0], 99231[0], 99232[0], 99233[0], 99234[0], 99235[0], 99236[0], 99238[0], 99239[0], 99281[0], 99282[0], 99283[0], 99284[0], 99285[0], 99304[0], 99305[0], 99306[0], 99307[0], 99308[0], 99309[0], 99310[0], 99315[0], 99318[0], 99324[0], 99325[0], 99326[0], 99327[0], 99328[0], 99334[0], 99335[0], 99336[0], 99337[0], 99341[0], 99342[0], 99343[0], 99347[0], 99348[0], 99349[0], 99354[0], 99355[0], 99356[0], 99357[0], 99358[0], 99359[0], 99415[0], 99416[0], 99446[0], 99447[0], 99448[0], 99449[0], 99451[0], 99452[0], 99466[0], 99468[0], 99469[0], 99471[0], 99472[0], 99475[0], 99476[0], 99477[0], 99478[0], 99479[0], 99480[0], 99483[0], 99485[0], 99497[0], C8921[1], C8922[1], C8923[1], C8924[1], C8925[1], C8926[1], C8927[0], C8929[1], C8930[1], G0380[1], G0381[1], G0382[1], G0383[1], G0384[1], G0406[0], G0407[0], G0408[0], G0425[0], G0426[0], G0427[0], G0463[0], G0500[0], G0508[0], G0509[0]
01272	01996[1], 0213T[1], 0216T[1], 0228T[1], 0230T[1], 31505[1], 31515[1], 31527[1], 31622[1], 31634[1], 31645[1], 31647[1], 36000[1], 36010[0], 36011[1], 36012[1], 36013[1], 36014[1], 36015[1], 36400[1], 36405[1], 36406[1], 36410[1], 36420[1], 36425[1], 36430[1], 36440[1], 36591[0], 36592[0], 36600[1], 36640[1], 43752[1], 43753[1], 43754[1], 61026[1], 61055[1], 62280[1], 62281[1], 62282[1], 62284[1], 62320[1], 62321[1], 62322[1], 62323[1], 62324[1], 62325[1], 62326[1], 62327[1], 64400[1], 64402[1], 64405[1], 64408[1], 64410[1], 64413[1], 64415[1], 64416[1], 64417[1], 64418[1], 64420[1], 64421[1], 64425[1], 64430[1], 64435[1], 64445[1], 64446[1], 64447[1], 64448[1], 64449[1], 64450[1], 64461[1], 64463[1], 64479[1], 64483[1], 64486[1], 64487[1], 64488[1], 64489[1], 64490[1], 64493[1], 64505[1], 64510[1], 64517[1], 64520[1], 64530[1], 64553[1], 64555[1], 67500[1], 76000[1], 76970[1], 76998[0],

Appendix A: NCCI - CPT Codes

0 = Modifier usage not allowed or inappropriate 1 = Modifier usage allowed

CPT © 2018 American Medical Association. All Rights Reserved.

Code 1	Code 2
	77002[0], 90865[1], 92511[1], 92512[1], 92516[1], 92520[1], 92537[1], 92538[1], 92950[1], 92953[1], 92960[1], 92961[1], 93000[1], 93005[1], 93010[1], 93040[1], 93041[1], 93042[1], 93050[0], 93303[0], 93304[0], 93306[1], 93307[1], 93308[1], 93312[1], 93313[1], 93314[1], 93315[1], 93316[1], 93317[1], 93318[0], 93351[1], 93355[0], 93451[1], 93456[1], 93457[1], 93561[0], 93562[0], 93701[0], 93922[1], 93923[1], 93924[1], 93925[1], 93926[1], 93930[1], 93931[1], 93970[1], 93971[1], 93975[1], 93976[1], 93978[1], 93979[1], 93980[1], 93981[1], 94002[1], 94004[1], 94200[1], 94250[0], 94640[1], 94644[1], 94660[1], 94662[1], 94680[1], 94681[1], 94690[1], 94760[0], 94761[0], 94762[1], 94770[1], 95812[0], 95813[0], 95816[0], 95819[0], 95822[0], 95829[0], 95955[0], 95956[0], 95957[0], 96360[0], 96365[0], 96372[0], 96373[0], 96374[0], 96375[0], 96376[0], 96377[0], 99151[0], 99152[0], 99153[0], 99155[0], 99156[0], 99157[0], 99201[0], 99202[0], 99203[0], 99204[0], 99205[0], 99211[0], 99212[0], 99213[0], 99214[0], 99215[0], 99217[0], 99218[0], 99219[0], 99220[0], 99221[0], 99222[0], 99223[0], 99224[0], 99225[0], 99226[0], 99231[0], 99232[0], 99233[0], 99234[0], 99235[0], 99236[0], 99238[0], 99239[0], 99281[0], 99282[0], 99283[0], 99284[0], 99285[0], 99304[0], 99305[0], 99306[0], 99307[0], 99308[0], 99309[0], 99310[0], 99315[0], 99318[0], 99324[0], 99325[0], 99326[0], 99327[0], 99328[0], 99334[0], 99335[0], 99336[0], 99337[0], 99341[0], 99342[0], 99343[0], 99347[0], 99348[0], 99349[0], 99354[0], 99355[0], 99356[0], 99357[0], 99358[0], 99359[0], 99415[0], 99416[0], 99446[0], 99447[0], 99448[0], 99449[0], 99451[0], 99452[0], 99466[0], 99468[0], 99469[0], 99471[0], 99472[0], 99475[0], 99476[0], 99477[0], 99478[0], 99479[0], 99480[0], 99483[0], 99485[0], 99497[0], C8921[1], C8922[1], C8923[1], C8924[1], C8925[1], C8926[1], C8927[0], C8929[1], C8930[1], G0380[1], G0381[1], G0382[1], G0383[1], G0384[1], G0406[0], G0407[0], G0408[0], G0425[0], G0426[0], G0427[0], G0463[0], G0500[0], G0508[0], G0509[0]
01274	01996[1], 0213T[1], 0216T[1], 0228T[1], 0230T[1], 31505[1], 31515[1], 31527[1], 31622[1], 31634[1], 31645[1], 31647[1], 36000[1], 36010[0], 36011[1], 36012[1], 36013[1], 36014[1], 36015[1], 36400[1], 36405[1], 36406[1], 36410[1], 36420[1], 36425[1], 36430[1], 36440[1], 36591[0], 36592[0], 36600[1], 36640[1], 43752[1], 43753[1], 43754[1], 61026[1], 61055[1], 62280[1], 62281[1], 62282[1], 62284[1], 62320[1], 62321[1], 62322[1], 62323[1], 62324[1], 62325[1], 62326[1], 62327[1], 64400[1], 64402[1], 64405[1], 64408[1], 64410[1], 64413[1], 64415[1], 64416[1], 64417[1], 64418[1], 64420[1], 64421[1], 64425[1], 64430[1], 64435[1], 64445[1], 64446[1], 64447[1], 64448[1], 64449[1], 64450[1], 64461[1], 64463[1], 64479[1], 64483[1], 64486[1], 64487[1], 64488[1], 64489[1], 64490[1], 64493[1], 64505[1], 64510[1], 64517[1], 64520[1], 64530[1], 64553[1], 64555[1], 67500[1], 76000[1], 76970[1], 76998[0], 77002[0], 90865[1], 92511[1], 92512[1], 92516[1], 92520[1], 92537[1], 92538[1], 92950[1], 92953[1], 92960[1], 92961[1], 93000[1], 93005[1], 93010[1], 93040[1], 93041[1], 93042[1], 93050[0], 93303[0], 93304[0], 93306[1], 93307[1], 93308[1], 93312[1], 93313[1], 93314[1], 93315[1], 93316[1], 93317[1], 93318[0], 93351[1], 93355[0], 93451[1], 93456[1], 93457[1], 93561[0], 93562[0], 93701[0], 93922[1], 93923[1], 93924[1], 93925[1], 93926[1], 93930[1], 93931[1], 93970[1], 93971[1], 93975[1], 93976[1], 93978[1], 93979[1], 93980[1], 93981[1], 94002[1], 94004[1], 94200[1], 94250[0], 94640[1], 94644[1], 94660[1], 94662[1], 94680[1], 94681[1], 94690[1], 94760[0], 94761[0], 94762[1], 94770[1], 95812[0], 95813[0], 95816[0], 95819[0], 95822[0], 95829[0], 95955[0], 95956[0], 95957[0], 96360[0], 96365[0], 96372[0], 96373[0], 96374[0], 96375[0], 96376[0], 96377[0], 99151[0], 99152[0], 99153[0], 99155[0], 99156[0], 99157[0], 99201[0], 99202[0], 99203[0], 99204[0], 99205[0], 99211[0], 99212[0], 99213[0], 99214[0], 99215[0], 99217[0], 99218[0], 99219[0], 99220[0], 99221[0], 99222[0], 99223[0], 99224[0], 99225[0], 99226[0], 99231[0], 99232[0], 99233[0], 99234[0], 99235[0], 99236[0], 99238[0], 99239[0], 99281[0], 99282[0], 99283[0], 99284[0], 99285[0], 99304[0], 99305[0], 99306[0], 99307[0], 99308[0], 99309[0], 99310[0], 99315[0], 99318[0], 99324[0], 99325[0], 99326[0], 99327[0], 99328[0], 99334[0], 99335[0], 99336[0], 99337[0], 99341[0], 99342[0], 99343[0], 99347[0], 99348[0], 99349[0], 99354[0], 99355[0], 99356[0], 99357[0], 99358[0], 99359[0], 99415[0], 99416[0], 99446[0], 99447[0], 99448[0], 99449[0], 99451[0], 99452[0], 99466[0], 99468[0], 99469[0], 99471[0], 99472[0], 99475[0], 99476[0], 99477[0], 99478[0], 99479[0], 99480[0], 99483[0], 99485[0], 99497[0], C8921[1], C8922[1], C8923[1], C8924[1], C8925[1], C8926[1], C8927[0], C8929[1], C8930[1], G0380[1], G0381[1], G0382[1], G0383[1], G0384[1], G0406[0], G0407[0], G0408[0], G0425[0], G0426[0], G0427[0], G0463[0], G0500[0], G0508[0], G0509[0]
01320	01996[1], 0213T[1], 0216T[1], 0228T[1], 0230T[1], 0333T[0], 0464T[0], 31505[1], 31515[1], 31527[1], 31622[1], 31634[1], 31645[1], 31647[1], 36000[1], 36010[0], 36011[1], 36012[1], 36013[1], 36014[1], 36015[1], 36400[1], 36405[1], 36406[1], 36410[1], 36420[1], 36425[1], 36430[1], 36440[1], 36591[0], 36592[0], 36600[1], 36640[1], 43752[1], 43753[1], 43754[1], 61026[1], 61055[1], 62280[1], 62281[1], 62282[1], 62284[1], 62320[1], 62321[1], 62322[1], 62323[1], 62324[1], 62325[1], 62326[1], 62327[1], 64400[1], 64402[1], 64405[1], 64408[1], 64410[1], 64413[1], 64415[1], 64416[1], 64417[1], 64418[1], 64420[1], 64421[1], 64425[1], 64430[1], 64435[1], 64445[1], 64446[1], 64447[1], 64448[1], 64449[1], 64450[1], 64461[1], 64463[1], 64479[1], 64483[1], 64486[1], 64487[1], 64488[1], 64489[1], 64490[1], 64493[1], 64505[1], 64510[1], 64517[1], 64520[1], 64530[1], 64553[1], 64555[1], 67500[1], 76000[1], 76970[1], 76998[0], 77002[0], 90865[1], 92511[1], 92512[1], 92516[1], 92520[1], 92537[1], 92538[1], 92585[0], 92950[1], 92953[1], 92960[1], 92961[1], 93000[1], 93005[1], 93010[1], 93040[1], 93041[1], 93042[1], 93050[0], 93303[0], 93304[0], 93306[1], 93307[1], 93308[1], 93312[1], 93313[1], 93314[1], 93315[1], 93316[1], 93317[1], 93318[0], 93351[1], 93355[0], 93451[1], 93456[1], 93457[1], 93561[0], 93562[0], 93701[0], 93922[1], 93923[1], 93924[1], 93925[1], 93926[1], 93930[1], 93931[1], 93970[1], 93971[1], 93975[1], 93976[1], 93978[1], 93979[1], 93980[1], 93981[1], 94002[1], 94004[1], 94200[1], 94250[0], 94640[1], 94644[1], 94660[1], 94662[1], 94680[1], 94681[1], 94690[1], 94760[0], 94761[0], 94762[1], 94770[1], 95812[0], 95813[0], 95816[0], 95819[0], 95822[0], 95829[0], 95860[0], 95861[0], 95863[0], 95864[0], 95865[0], 95866[0], 95867[0], 95868[0], 95869[0], 95870[0], 95907[0], 95908[0], 95909[0], 95910[0], 95911[0], 95912[0], 95913[0], 95925[0], 95926[0], 95927[0], 95928[0], 95929[0], 95930[0], 95933[0], 95937[0], 95938[0], 95939[0], 95940[0], 95955[0], 95956[0], 95957[0], 96360[0], 96365[0], 96372[0], 96373[0], 96374[0], 96375[0], 96376[0], 96377[0], 99151[0], 99152[0], 99153[0], 99155[0], 99156[0], 99157[0], 99201[0], 99202[0], 99203[0], 99204[0], 99205[0], 99211[0], 99212[0], 99213[0], 99214[0], 99215[0], 99217[0], 99218[0], 99219[0], 99220[0], 99221[0], 99222[0], 99223[0], 99224[0], 99225[0], 99226[0], 99231[0], 99232[0], 99233[0], 99234[0], 99235[0], 99236[0], 99238[0], 99239[0], 99281[0], 99282[0], 99283[0], 99284[0], 99285[0], 99304[0], 99305[0], 99306[0], 99307[0], 99308[0], 99309[0], 99310[0], 99315[0], 99318[0], 99324[0], 99325[0], 99326[0], 99327[0], 99328[0], 99334[0], 99335[0], 99336[0], 99337[0], 99341[0], 99342[0], 99343[0], 99347[0], 99348[0], 99349[0], 99354[0], 99355[0], 99356[0], 99357[0], 99358[0], 99359[0], 99415[0], 99416[0], 99446[0], 99447[0], 99448[0], 99449[0], 99451[0], 99452[0], 99466[0], 99468[0], 99469[0], 99471[0], 99472[0], 99475[0], 99476[0], 99477[0], 99478[0], 99479[0], 99480[0], 99483[0], 99485[0], 99497[0], C8921[1], C8922[1], C8923[1], C8924[1], C8925[1], C8926[1], C8927[0], C8929[1], C8930[1], G0380[1], G0381[1], G0382[1], G0383[1], G0384[1], G0406[0], G0407[0], G0408[0], G0425[0], G0426[0], G0427[0], G0453[0], G0463[0], G0500[0], G0508[0], G0509[0]
01340	01996[1], 0213T[1], 0216T[1], 0228T[1], 0230T[1], 31505[1], 31515[1], 31527[1], 31622[1], 31634[1], 31645[1], 31647[1], 36000[1], 36010[0], 36011[1], 36012[1], 36013[1], 36014[1], 36015[1], 36400[1], 36405[1], 36406[1], 36410[1], 36420[1], 36425[1], 36430[1], 36440[1], 36591[0], 36592[0], 36600[1], 36640[1], 43752[1], 43753[1], 43754[1], 61026[1], 61055[1], 62280[1], 62281[1], 62282[1], 62284[1], 62320[1], 62321[1], 62322[1], 62323[1], 62324[1], 62325[1], 62326[1], 62327[1], 64400[1], 64402[1], 64405[1], 64408[1], 64410[1], 64413[1], 64415[1], 64416[1], 64417[1], 64418[1], 64420[1], 64421[1], 64425[1], 64430[1], 64435[1], 64445[1], 64446[1], 64447[1], 64448[1], 64449[1], 64450[1], 64461[1], 64463[1], 64479[1], 64483[1], 64486[1], 64487[1], 64488[1], 64489[1], 64490[1], 64493[1], 64505[1], 64510[1], 64517[1], 64520[1], 64530[1], 64553[1], 64555[1], 67500[1], 76000[1], 76970[1], 76998[0], 77002[0], 90865[1], 92511[1], 92512[1], 92516[1], 92520[1], 92537[1], 92538[1], 92950[1], 92953[1], 92960[1], 92961[1], 93000[1], 93005[1], 93010[1], 93040[1], 93041[1], 93042[1], 93050[0], 93303[0], 93304[0], 93306[1], 93307[1], 93308[1], 93312[1], 93313[1], 93314[1], 93315[1], 93316[1], 93317[1], 93318[0], 93351[1], 93355[0], 93451[1], 93456[1], 93457[1], 93561[0], 93562[0], 93701[0], 93922[1], 93923[1], 93924[1], 93925[1], 93926[1], 93930[1], 93931[1], 93970[1], 93971[1], 93975[1], 93976[1], 93978[1], 93979[1], 93980[1], 93981[1], 94002[1], 94004[1], 94200[1], 94250[0], 94640[1], 94644[1], 94660[1], 94662[1], 94680[1], 94681[1], 94690[1], 94760[0], 94761[0], 94762[1], 94770[1], 95812[0], 95813[0], 95816[0], 95819[0], 95822[0], 95829[0], 95955[0], 95956[0], 95957[0], 96360[0], 96365[0], 96372[0], 96373[0], 96374[0], 96375[0], 96376[0], 96377[0], 99151[0], 99152[0], 99153[0], 99155[0], 99156[0], 99157[0], 99201[0], 99202[0], 99203[0], 99204[0], 99205[0], 99211[0], 99212[0], 99213[0], 99214[0], 99215[0], 99217[0], 99218[0], 99219[0], 99220[0], 99221[0], 99222[0], 99223[0], 99224[0], 99225[0], 99226[0], 99231[0], 99232[0], 99233[0], 99234[0], 99235[0], 99236[0], 99238[0], 99239[0], 99281[0], 99282[0], 99283[0], 99284[0], 99285[0], 99304[0], 99305[0], 99306[0], 99307[0], 99308[0], 99309[0], 99310[0], 99315[0], 99318[0], 99324[0], 99325[0], 99326[0], 99327[0], 99328[0], 99334[0], 99335[0], 99336[0], 99337[0], 99341[0], 99342[0], 99343[0], 99347[0], 99348[0], 99349[0], 99354[0], 99355[0], 99356[0], 99357[0], 99358[0], 99359[0], 99415[0], 99416[0], 99446[0], 99447[0], 99448[0], 99449[0], 99451[0], 99452[0], 99466[0], 99468[0], 99469[0], 99471[0], 99472[0], 99475[0], 99476[0], 99477[0], 99478[0], 99479[0], 99480[0], 99483[0], 99485[0], 99497[0], C8921[1], C8922[1], C8923[1], C8924[1], C8925[1], C8926[1], C8927[0], C8929[1], C8930[1], G0380[1], G0381[1], G0382[1], G0383[1], G0384[1], G0406[0], G0407[0], G0408[0], G0425[0], G0426[0], G0427[0], G0463[0], G0500[0], G0508[0], G0509[0]
01360	01996[1], 0213T[1], 0216T[1], 0228T[1], 0230T[1], 31505[1], 31515[1], 31527[1], 31622[1], 31634[1], 31645[1], 31647[1], 36000[1], 36010[0], 36011[1], 36012[1], 36013[1], 36014[1], 36015[1], 36400[1], 36405[1], 36406[1], 36410[1], 36420[1], 36425[1], 36430[1], 36440[1], 36591[0], 36592[0], 36600[1], 36640[1], 43752[1], 43753[1], 43754[1], 61026[1], 61055[1], 62280[1], 62281[1], 62282[1], 62284[1], 62320[1], 62321[1], 62322[1], 62323[1], 62324[1], 62325[1], 62326[1], 62327[1], 64400[1], 64402[1], 64405[1], 64408[1], 64410[1], 64413[1], 64415[1], 64416[1], 64417[1], 64418[1], 64420[1], 64421[1], 64425[1], 64430[1], 64435[1], 64445[1], 64446[1], 64447[1], 64448[1], 64449[1], 64450[1], 64461[1], 64463[1], 64479[1], 64483[1], 64486[1], 64487[1], 64488[1], 64489[1], 64490[1], 64493[1], 64505[1], 64510[1], 64517[1], 64520[1], 64530[1], 64553[1], 64555[1], 67500[1], 76000[1], 76970[1], 76998[0], 77002[0], 90865[1], 92511[1], 92512[1], 92516[1], 92520[1], 92537[1], 92538[1], 92950[1], 92953[1], 92960[1], 92961[1], 93000[1], 93005[1], 93010[1], 93040[1], 93041[1], 93042[1], 93050[0], 93303[0], 93304[0], 93306[1], 93307[1], 93308[1], 93312[1], 93313[1], 93314[1], 93315[1], 93316[1], 93317[1], 93318[0], 93351[1], 93355[0], 93451[1], 93456[1], 93457[1], 93561[0], 93562[0], 93701[0], 93922[1], 93923[1], 93924[1], 93925[1], 93926[1], 93930[1], 93931[1], 93970[1], 93971[1], 93975[1], 93976[1], 93978[1], 93979[1], 93980[1], 93981[1], 94002[1], 94004[1], 94200[1], 94250[0], 94640[1], 94644[1], 94660[1], 94662[1], 94680[1], 94681[1], 94690[1], 94760[0], 94761[0], 94762[1], 94770[1], 95812[0], 95813[0], 95816[0], 95819[0], 95822[0], 95829[0], 95955[0], 95956[0], 95957[0], 96360[0], 96365[0], 96372[0], 96373[0], 96374[0], 96375[0], 96376[0], 96377[0], 99151[0], 99152[0], 99153[0], 99155[0],

0 = Modifier usage not allowed or inappropriate 1 = Modifier usage allowed

CPT © 2018 American Medical Association. All Rights Reserved.

Code 1	Code 2
	99156^0, 99157^0, 99201^0, 99202^0, 99203^0, 99204^0, 99205^0, 99211^0, 99212^0, 99213^0, 99214^0, 99215^0, 99217^0, 99218^0, 99219^0, 99220^0, 99221^0, 99222^0, 99223^0, 99224^0, 99225^0, 99226^0, 99231^0, 99232^0, 99233^0, 99234^0, 99235^0, 99236^0, 99238^0, 99239^0, 99281^0, 99282^0, 99283^0, 99284^0, 99285^0, 99304^0, 99305^0, 99306^0, 99307^0, 99308^0, 99309^0, 99310^0, 99315^0, 99318^0, 99324^0, 99325^0, 99326^0, 99327^0, 99328^0, 99334^0, 99335^0, 99336^0, 99337^0, 99341^0, 99342^0, 99343^0, 99347^0, 99348^0, 99349^0, 99354^0, 99355^0, 99356^0, 99357^0, 99358^0, 99359^0, 99415^0, 99416^0, 99446^0, 99447^0, 99448^0, 99449^0, 99451^0, 99452^0, 99466^0, 99468^0, 99469^0, 99471^0, 99472^0, 99475^0, 99476^0, 99477^0, 99478^0, 99479^0, 99480^0, 99483^0, 99485^0, 99497^0, C8921^1, C8922^1, C8923^1, C8924^1, C8925^1, C8926^1, C8927^0, C8929^1, C8930^1, G0380^1, G0381^1, G0382^1, G0383^1, G0384^1, G0406^0, G0407^0, G0408^0, G0425^0, G0426^0, G0427^0, G0463^0, G0500^0, G0508^0, G0509^0
01380	01996^1, 0213T^1, 0216T^1, 0228T^1, 0230T^1, 31505^1, 31515^1, 31527^1, 31622^1, 31634^1, 31645^1, 31647^1, 36000^1, 36010^0, 36011^1, 36012^1, 36013^1, 36014^1, 36015^1, 36400^1, 36405^1, 36406^1, 36410^1, 36420^1, 36425^1, 36430^1, 36440^1, 36591^0, 36592^0, 36600^1, 36640^1, 43752^1, 43753^1, 43754^1, 61026^1, 61055^1, 62280^1, 62281^1, 62282^1, 62284^1, 62320^1, 62321^1, 62322^1, 62323^1, 62324^1, 62325^1, 62326^1, 62327^1, 64400^1, 64402^1, 64405^1, 64408^1, 64410^1, 64413^1, 64415^1, 64416^1, 64417^1, 64418^1, 64420^1, 64421^1, 64425^1, 64430^1, 64435^1, 64445^1, 64446^1, 64447^1, 64448^1, 64449^1, 64450^1, 64461^1, 64463^1, 64479^1, 64483^1, 64486^1, 64487^1, 64488^1, 64489^1, 64490^1, 64493^1, 64505^1, 64510^1, 64517^1, 64520^1, 64530^1, 64553^1, 64555^1, 67500^1, 76000^1, 76970^1, 76998^0, 77002^0, 90865^1, 92511^1, 92512^1, 92516^1, 92520^1, 92537^1, 92538^1, 92950^1, 92953^1, 92960^1, 92961^1, 93000^1, 93005^1, 93010^1, 93040^1, 93041^1, 93042^1, 93050^0, 93303^0, 93304^0, 93306^1, 93307^1, 93308^1, 93312^1, 93313^1, 93314^1, 93315^1, 93316^1, 93317^1, 93318^0, 93351^1, 93355^0, 93451^1, 93456^1, 93457^1, 93561^0, 93562^0, 93701^0, 93922^1, 93923^1, 93924^1, 93925^1, 93926^1, 93930^1, 93931^1, 93970^1, 93971^1, 93975^1, 93976^1, 93978^1, 93979^1, 93980^1, 93981^1, 94002^1, 94004^1, 94200^1, 94250^0, 94640^1, 94644^1, 94660^1, 94662^1, 94680^1, 94681^1, 94690^1, 94760^0, 94761^0, 94762^1, 94770^1, 95812^0, 95813^0, 95816^0, 95819^0, 95822^0, 95829^0, 95955^0, 95956^0, 95957^0, 96360^0, 96365^0, 96372^0, 96373^0, 96374^0, 96375^0, 96376^0, 96377^0, 99151^0, 99152^0, 99153^0, 99155^0, 99156^0, 99157^0, 99201^0, 99202^0, 99203^0, 99204^0, 99205^0, 99211^0, 99212^0, 99213^0, 99214^0, 99215^0, 99217^0, 99218^0, 99219^0, 99220^0, 99221^0, 99222^0, 99223^0, 99224^0, 99225^0, 99226^0, 99231^0, 99232^0, 99233^0, 99234^0, 99235^0, 99236^0, 99238^0, 99239^0, 99281^0, 99282^0, 99283^0, 99284^0, 99285^0, 99304^0, 99305^0, 99306^0, 99307^0, 99308^0, 99309^0, 99310^0, 99315^0, 99318^0, 99324^0, 99325^0, 99326^0, 99327^0, 99328^0, 99334^0, 99335^0, 99336^0, 99337^0, 99341^0, 99342^0, 99343^0, 99347^0, 99348^0, 99349^0, 99354^0, 99355^0, 99356^0, 99357^0, 99358^0, 99359^0, 99415^0, 99416^0, 99446^0, 99447^0, 99448^0, 99449^0, 99451^0, 99452^0, 99466^0, 99468^0, 99469^0, 99471^0, 99472^0, 99475^0, 99476^0, 99477^0, 99478^0, 99479^0, 99480^0, 99483^0, 99485^0, 99497^0, C8921^1, C8922^1, C8923^1, C8924^1, C8925^1, C8926^1, C8927^0, C8929^1, C8930^1, G0380^1, G0381^1, G0382^1, G0383^1, G0384^1, G0406^0, G0407^0, G0408^0, G0425^0, G0426^0, G0427^0, G0463^0, G0500^0, G0508^0, G0509^0
01382	01996^1, 0213T^1, 0216T^1, 0228T^1, 0230T^1, 31505^1, 31515^1, 31527^1, 31622^1, 31634^1, 31645^1, 31647^1, 36000^1, 36010^0, 36011^1, 36012^1, 36013^1, 36014^1, 36015^1, 36400^1, 36405^1, 36406^1, 36410^1, 36420^1, 36425^1, 36430^1, 36440^1, 36591^0, 36592^0, 36600^1, 36640^1, 43752^1, 43753^1, 43754^1, 61026^1, 61055^1, 62280^1, 62281^1, 62282^1, 62284^1, 62320^1, 62321^1, 62322^1, 62323^1, 62324^1, 62325^1, 62326^1, 62327^1, 64400^1, 64402^1, 64405^1, 64408^1, 64410^1, 64413^1, 64415^1, 64416^1, 64417^1, 64418^1, 64420^1, 64421^1, 64425^1, 64430^1, 64435^1, 64445^1, 64446^1, 64447^1, 64448^1, 64449^1, 64450^1, 64461^1, 64463^1, 64479^1, 64483^1, 64486^1, 64487^1, 64488^1, 64489^1, 64490^1, 64493^1, 64505^1, 64510^1, 64517^1, 64520^1, 64530^1, 64553^1, 64555^1, 67500^1, 76000^1, 76970^1, 76998^0, 77002^0, 90865^1, 92511^1, 92512^1, 92516^1, 92520^1, 92537^1, 92538^1, 92950^1, 92953^1, 92960^1, 92961^1, 93000^1, 93005^1, 93010^1, 93040^1, 93041^1, 93042^1, 93050^0, 93303^0, 93304^0, 93306^1, 93307^1, 93308^1, 93312^1, 93313^1, 93314^1, 93315^1, 93316^1, 93317^1, 93318^0, 93351^1, 93355^0, 93451^1, 93456^1, 93457^1, 93561^0, 93562^0, 93701^0, 93922^1, 93923^1, 93924^1, 93925^1, 93926^1, 93930^1, 93931^1, 93970^1, 93971^1, 93975^1, 93976^1, 93978^1, 93979^1, 93980^1, 93981^1, 94002^1, 94004^1, 94200^1, 94250^0, 94640^1, 94644^1, 94660^1, 94662^1, 94680^1, 94681^1, 94690^1, 94760^0, 94761^0, 94762^1, 94770^1, 95812^0, 95813^0, 95816^0, 95819^0, 95822^0, 95829^0, 95955^0, 95956^0, 95957^0, 96360^0, 96365^0, 96372^0, 96373^0, 96374^0, 96375^0, 96376^0, 96377^0, 99151^0, 99152^0, 99153^0, 99155^0, 99156^0, 99157^0, 99201^0, 99202^0, 99203^0, 99204^0, 99205^0, 99211^0, 99212^0, 99213^0, 99214^0, 99215^0, 99217^0, 99218^0, 99219^0, 99220^0, 99221^0, 99222^0, 99223^0, 99224^0, 99225^0, 99226^0, 99231^0, 99232^0, 99233^0, 99234^0, 99235^0, 99236^0, 99238^0, 99239^0, 99281^0, 99282^0, 99283^0, 99284^0, 99285^0, 99304^0, 99305^0, 99306^0, 99307^0, 99308^0, 99309^0, 99310^0, 99315^0, 99318^0, 99324^0, 99325^0, 99326^0, 99327^0, 99328^0, 99334^0, 99335^0, 99336^0, 99337^0, 99341^0, 99342^0, 99343^0, 99347^0, 99348^0, 99349^0, 99354^0, 99355^0, 99356^0, 99357^0, 99358^0, 99359^0, 99415^0, 99416^0, 99446^0, 99447^0, 99448^0, 99449^0, 99451^0, 99452^0, 99466^0, 99468^0, 99469^0, 99471^0, 99472^0, 99475^0, 99476^0, 99477^0, 99478^0, 99479^0, 99480^0, 99483^0, 99485^0, 99497^0, C8921^1, C8922^1, C8923^1, C8924^1, C8925^1, C8926^1, C8927^0, C8929^1, C8930^1, G0380^1, G0381^1, G0382^1, G0383^1, G0384^1, G0406^0, G0407^0, G0408^0, G0425^0, G0426^0, G0427^0, G0463^0, G0500^0, G0508^0, G0509^0
01390	01996^1, 0213T^1, 0216T^1, 0228T^1, 0230T^1, 31505^1, 31515^1, 31527^1, 31622^1, 31634^1, 31645^1, 31647^1, 36000^1, 36010^0, 36011^1, 36012^1, 36013^1, 36014^1, 36015^1, 36400^1, 36405^1, 36406^1, 36410^1, 36420^1, 36425^1, 36430^1, 36440^1, 36591^0, 36592^0, 36600^1, 36640^1, 43752^1, 43753^1, 43754^1, 61026^1, 61055^1, 62280^1, 62281^1, 62282^1, 62284^1, 62320^1, 62321^1, 62322^1, 62323^1, 62324^1, 62325^1, 62326^1, 62327^1, 64400^1, 64402^1, 64405^1, 64408^1, 64410^1, 64413^1, 64415^1, 64416^1, 64417^1, 64418^1, 64420^1, 64421^1, 64425^1, 64430^1, 64435^1, 64445^1, 64446^1, 64447^1, 64448^1, 64449^1, 64450^1, 64461^1, 64463^1, 64479^1, 64483^1, 64486^1, 64487^1, 64488^1, 64489^1, 64490^1, 64493^1, 64505^1, 64510^1, 64517^1, 64520^1, 64530^1, 64553^1, 64555^1, 67500^1, 76000^1, 76970^1, 76998^0, 77002^0, 90865^1, 92511^1, 92512^1, 92516^1, 92520^1, 92537^1, 92538^1, 92950^1, 92953^1, 92960^1, 92961^1, 93000^1, 93005^1, 93010^1, 93040^1, 93041^1, 93042^1, 93050^0, 93303^0, 93304^0, 93306^1, 93307^1, 93308^1, 93312^1, 93313^1, 93314^1, 93315^1, 93316^1, 93317^1, 93318^0, 93351^1, 93355^0, 93451^1, 93456^1, 93457^1, 93561^0, 93562^0, 93701^0, 93922^1, 93923^1, 93924^1, 93925^1, 93926^1, 93930^1, 93931^1, 93970^1, 93971^1, 93975^1, 93976^1, 93978^1, 93979^1, 93980^1, 93981^1, 94002^1, 94004^1, 94200^1, 94250^0, 94640^1, 94644^1, 94660^1, 94662^1, 94680^1, 94681^1, 94690^1, 94760^0, 94761^0, 94762^1, 94770^1, 95812^0, 95813^0, 95816^0, 95819^0, 95822^0, 95829^0, 95955^0, 95956^0, 95957^0, 96360^0, 96365^0, 96372^0, 96373^0, 96374^0, 96375^0, 96376^0, 96377^0, 99151^0, 99152^0, 99153^0, 99155^0, 99156^0, 99157^0, 99201^0, 99202^0, 99203^0, 99204^0, 99205^0, 99211^0, 99212^0, 99213^0, 99214^0, 99215^0, 99217^0, 99218^0, 99219^0, 99220^0, 99221^0, 99222^0, 99223^0, 99224^0, 99225^0, 99226^0, 99231^0, 99232^0, 99233^0, 99234^0, 99235^0, 99236^0, 99238^0, 99239^0, 99281^0, 99282^0, 99283^0, 99284^0, 99285^0, 99304^0, 99305^0, 99306^0, 99307^0, 99308^0, 99309^0, 99310^0, 99315^0, 99318^0, 99324^0, 99325^0, 99326^0, 99327^0, 99328^0, 99334^0, 99335^0, 99336^0, 99337^0, 99341^0, 99342^0, 99343^0, 99347^0, 99348^0, 99349^0, 99354^0, 99355^0, 99356^0, 99357^0, 99358^0, 99359^0, 99415^0, 99416^0, 99446^0, 99447^0, 99448^0, 99449^0, 99451^0, 99452^0, 99466^0, 99468^0, 99469^0, 99471^0, 99472^0, 99475^0, 99476^0, 99477^0, 99478^0, 99479^0, 99480^0, 99483^0, 99485^0, 99497^0, C8921^1, C8922^1, C8923^1, C8924^1, C8925^1, C8926^1, C8927^0, C8929^1, C8930^1, G0380^1, G0381^1, G0382^1, G0383^1, G0384^1, G0406^0, G0407^0, G0408^0, G0425^0, G0426^0, G0427^0, G0463^0, G0500^0, G0508^0, G0509^0
01392	01996^1, 0213T^1, 0216T^1, 0228T^1, 0230T^1, 31505^1, 31515^1, 31527^1, 31622^1, 31634^1, 31645^1, 31647^1, 36000^1, 36010^0, 36011^1, 36012^1, 36013^1, 36014^1, 36015^1, 36400^1, 36405^1, 36406^1, 36410^1, 36420^1, 36425^1, 36430^1, 36440^1, 36591^0, 36592^0, 36600^1, 36640^1, 43752^1, 43753^1, 43754^1, 61026^1, 61055^1, 62280^1, 62281^1, 62282^1, 62284^1, 62320^1, 62321^1, 62322^1, 62323^1, 62324^1, 62325^1, 62326^1, 62327^1, 64400^1, 64402^1, 64405^1, 64408^1, 64410^1, 64413^1, 64415^1, 64416^1, 64417^1, 64418^1, 64420^1, 64421^1, 64425^1, 64430^1, 64435^1, 64445^1, 64446^1, 64447^1, 64448^1, 64449^1, 64450^1, 64461^1, 64463^1, 64479^1, 64483^1, 64486^1, 64487^1, 64488^1, 64489^1, 64490^1, 64493^1, 64505^1, 64510^1, 64517^1, 64520^1, 64530^1, 64553^1, 64555^1, 67500^1, 76000^1, 76970^1, 76998^0, 77002^0, 90865^1, 92511^1, 92512^1, 92516^1, 92520^1, 92537^1, 92538^1, 92950^1, 92953^1, 92960^1, 92961^1, 93000^1, 93005^1, 93010^1, 93040^1, 93041^1, 93042^1, 93050^0, 93303^0, 93304^0, 93306^1, 93307^1, 93308^1, 93312^1, 93313^1, 93314^1, 93315^1, 93316^1, 93317^1, 93318^0, 93351^1, 93355^0, 93451^1, 93456^1, 93457^1, 93561^0, 93562^0, 93701^0, 93922^1, 93923^1, 93924^1, 93925^1, 93926^1, 93930^1, 93931^1, 93970^1, 93971^1, 93975^1, 93976^1, 93978^1, 93979^1, 93980^1, 93981^1, 94002^1, 94004^1, 94200^1, 94250^0, 94640^1, 94644^1, 94660^1, 94662^1, 94680^1, 94681^1, 94690^1, 94760^0, 94761^0, 94762^1, 94770^1, 95812^0, 95813^0, 95816^0, 95819^0, 95822^0, 95829^0, 95955^0, 95956^0, 95957^0, 96360^0, 96365^0, 96372^0, 96373^0, 96374^0, 96375^0, 96376^0, 96377^0, 99151^0, 99152^0, 99153^0, 99155^0, 99156^0, 99157^0, 99201^0, 99202^0, 99203^0, 99204^0, 99205^0, 99211^0, 99212^0, 99213^0, 99214^0, 99215^0, 99217^0, 99218^0, 99219^0, 99220^0, 99221^0, 99222^0, 99223^0, 99224^0, 99225^0, 99226^0, 99231^0, 99232^0, 99233^0, 99234^0, 99235^0, 99236^0, 99238^0, 99239^0, 99281^0, 99282^0, 99283^0, 99284^0, 99285^0, 99304^0, 99305^0, 99306^0, 99307^0, 99308^0, 99309^0, 99310^0, 99315^0, 99318^0, 99324^0, 99325^0, 99326^0, 99327^0, 99328^0, 99334^0, 99335^0, 99336^0, 99337^0, 99341^0, 99342^0, 99343^0, 99347^0, 99348^0, 99349^0, 99354^0, 99355^0, 99356^0, 99357^0, 99358^0, 99359^0, 99415^0, 99416^0, 99446^0, 99447^0, 99448^0, 99449^0, 99451^0, 99452^0, 99466^0, 99468^0, 99469^0, 99471^0, 99472^0, 99475^0, 99476^0, 99477^0, 99478^0, 99479^0, 99480^0, 99483^0, 99485^0, 99497^0, C8921^1, C8922^1, C8923^1, C8924^1, C8925^1, C8926^1, C8927^0, C8929^1, C8930^1, G0380^1, G0381^1, G0382^1, G0383^1, G0384^1, G0406^0, G0407^0, G0408^0, G0425^0, G0426^0, G0427^0, G0463^0, G0500^0, G0508^0, G0509^0

0 = Modifier usage not allowed or inappropriate   1 = Modifier usage allowed

CPT © 2018 American Medical Association. All Rights Reserved.

Code 1	Code 2
01400	01382[1], 01996[1], 0213T[1], 0216T[1], 0228T[1], 0230T[1], 31505[1], 31515[1], 31527[1], 31622[1], 31634[1], 31645[1], 31647[1], 36000[1], 36010[0], 36011[1], 36012[1], 36013[1], 36014[1], 36015[1], 36400[1], 36405[1], 36406[1], 36410[1], 36420[1], 36425[1], 36430[1], 36440[1], 36591[0], 36592[0], 36600[1], 36640[1], 43752[1], 43753[1], 43754[1], 61026[1], 61055[1], 62280[1], 62281[1], 62282[1], 62284[1], 62320[1], 62321[1], 62322[1], 62323[1], 62324[1], 62325[1], 62326[1], 62327[1], 64400[1], 64402[1], 64405[1], 64408[1], 64410[1], 64413[1], 64415[1], 64416[1], 64417[1], 64418[1], 64420[1], 64421[1], 64425[1], 64430[1], 64435[1], 64445[1], 64446[1], 64447[1], 64448[1], 64449[1], 64450[1], 64461[1], 64463[1], 64479[1], 64483[1], 64486[1], 64487[1], 64488[1], 64489[1], 64490[1], 64493[1], 64505[1], 64510[1], 64517[1], 64520[1], 64530[1], 64553[1], 64555[1], 67500[1], 76000[1], 76970[1], 76998[0], 77002[0], 90865[1], 92511[1], 92512[1], 92516[1], 92520[1], 92537[1], 92538[1], 92950[1], 92953[1], 92960[1], 92961[1], 93000[1], 93005[1], 93010[1], 93040[1], 93041[1], 93042[1], 93050[0], 93303[0], 93304[0], 93306[1], 93307[1], 93308[1], 93312[1], 93313[1], 93314[1], 93315[1], 93316[1], 93317[1], 93318[0], 93351[1], 93355[0], 93451[1], 93456[1], 93457[1], 93561[0], 93562[0], 93701[0], 93922[1], 93923[1], 93924[1], 93925[1], 93926[1], 93930[1], 93931[1], 93970[1], 93971[1], 93975[1], 93976[1], 93978[1], 93979[1], 93980[1], 93981[1], 94002[1], 94004[1], 94200[1], 94250[0], 94640[1], 94644[1], 94660[1], 94662[1], 94680[1], 94681[1], 94690[1], 94760[0], 94761[0], 94762[1], 94770[1], 95812[0], 95813[0], 95816[0], 95819[0], 95822[0], 95829[0], 95955[0], 95956[0], 95957[0], 96360[0], 96365[0], 96372[0], 96373[0], 96374[0], 96375[0], 96376[0], 96377[0], 99151[0], 99152[0], 99153[0], 99155[0], 99156[0], 99157[0], 99201[0], 99202[0], 99203[0], 99204[0], 99205[0], 99211[0], 99212[0], 99213[0], 99214[0], 99215[0], 99217[0], 99218[0], 99219[0], 99220[0], 99221[0], 99222[0], 99223[0], 99224[0], 99225[0], 99226[0], 99231[0], 99232[0], 99233[0], 99234[0], 99235[0], 99236[0], 99238[0], 99239[0], 99281[0], 99282[0], 99283[0], 99284[0], 99285[0], 99304[0], 99305[0], 99306[0], 99307[0], 99308[0], 99309[0], 99310[0], 99315[0], 99318[0], 99324[0], 99325[0], 99326[0], 99327[0], 99328[0], 99334[0], 99335[0], 99336[0], 99337[0], 99341[0], 99342[0], 99343[0], 99347[0], 99348[0], 99349[0], 99354[0], 99355[0], 99356[0], 99357[0], 99358[0], 99359[0], 99415[0], 99416[0], 99446[0], 99447[0], 99448[0], 99449[0], 99451[0], 99452[0], 99466[0], 99468[0], 99469[0], 99471[0], 99472[0], 99475[0], 99476[0], 99477[0], 99478[0], 99479[0], 99480[0], 99483[0], 99485[0], 99497[0], C8921[1], C8922[1], C8923[1], C8924[1], C8925[1], C8926[1], C8927[0], C8929[1], C8930[1], G0380[1], G0381[1], G0382[1], G0383[1], G0384[1], G0406[0], G0407[0], G0408[0], G0425[0], G0426[0], G0427[0], G0463[0], G0500[0], G0508[0], G0509[0]
01402	01996[1], 0213T[1], 0216T[1], 0228T[1], 0230T[1], 31505[1], 31515[1], 31527[1], 31622[1], 31634[1], 31645[1], 31647[1], 36000[1], 36010[0], 36011[1], 36012[1], 36013[1], 36014[1], 36015[1], 36400[1], 36405[1], 36406[1], 36410[1], 36420[1], 36425[1], 36430[1], 36440[1], 36591[0], 36592[0], 36600[1], 36640[1], 43752[1], 43753[1], 43754[1], 61026[1], 61055[1], 62280[1], 62281[1], 62282[1], 62284[1], 62320[1], 62321[1], 62322[1], 62323[1], 62324[1], 62325[1], 62326[1], 62327[1], 64400[1], 64402[1], 64405[1], 64408[1], 64410[1], 64413[1], 64415[1], 64416[1], 64417[1], 64418[1], 64420[1], 64421[1], 64425[1], 64430[1], 64435[1], 64445[1], 64446[1], 64447[1], 64448[1], 64449[1], 64450[1], 64461[1], 64463[1], 64479[1], 64483[1], 64486[1], 64487[1], 64488[1], 64489[1], 64490[1], 64493[1], 64505[1], 64510[1], 64517[1], 64520[1], 64530[1], 64553[1], 64555[1], 67500[1], 76000[1], 76970[1], 76998[0], 77002[0], 90865[1], 92511[1], 92512[1], 92516[1], 92520[1], 92537[1], 92538[1], 92950[1], 92953[1], 92960[1], 92961[1], 93000[1], 93005[1], 93010[1], 93040[1], 93041[1], 93042[1], 93050[0], 93303[0], 93304[0], 93306[1], 93307[1], 93308[1], 93312[1], 93313[1], 93314[1], 93315[1], 93316[1], 93317[1], 93318[0], 93351[1], 93355[0], 93451[1], 93456[1], 93457[1], 93561[0], 93562[0], 93701[0], 93922[1], 93923[1], 93924[1], 93925[1], 93926[1], 93930[1], 93931[1], 93970[1], 93971[1], 93975[1], 93976[1], 93978[1], 93979[1], 93980[1], 93981[1], 94002[1], 94004[1], 94200[1], 94250[0], 94640[1], 94644[1], 94660[1], 94662[1], 94680[1], 94681[1], 94690[1], 94760[0], 94761[0], 94762[1], 94770[1], 95812[0], 95813[0], 95816[0], 95819[0], 95822[0], 95829[0], 95955[0], 95956[0], 95957[0], 96360[0], 96365[0], 96372[0], 96373[0], 96374[0], 96375[0], 96376[0], 96377[0], 99151[0], 99152[0], 99153[0], 99155[0], 99156[0], 99157[0], 99201[0], 99202[0], 99203[0], 99204[0], 99205[0], 99211[0], 99212[0], 99213[0], 99214[0], 99215[0], 99217[0], 99218[0], 99219[0], 99220[0], 99221[0], 99222[0], 99223[0], 99224[0], 99225[0], 99226[0], 99231[0], 99232[0], 99233[0], 99234[0], 99235[0], 99236[0], 99238[0], 99239[0], 99281[0], 99282[0], 99283[0], 99284[0], 99285[0], 99304[0], 99305[0], 99306[0], 99307[0], 99308[0], 99309[0], 99310[0], 99315[0], 99318[0], 99324[0], 99325[0], 99326[0], 99327[0], 99328[0], 99334[0], 99335[0], 99336[0], 99337[0], 99341[0], 99342[0], 99343[0], 99347[0], 99348[0], 99349[0], 99354[0], 99355[0], 99356[0], 99357[0], 99358[0], 99359[0], 99415[0], 99416[0], 99446[0], 99447[0], 99448[0], 99449[0], 99451[0], 99452[0], 99466[0], 99468[0], 99469[0], 99471[0], 99472[0], 99475[0], 99476[0], 99477[0], 99478[0], 99479[0], 99480[0], 99483[0], 99485[0], 99497[0], C8921[1], C8922[1], C8923[1], C8924[1], C8925[1], C8926[1], C8927[0], C8929[1], C8930[1], G0380[1], G0381[1], G0382[1], G0383[1], G0384[1], G0406[0], G0407[0], G0408[0], G0425[0], G0426[0], G0427[0], G0463[0], G0500[0], G0508[0], G0509[0]
01404	01996[1], 0213T[1], 0216T[1], 0228T[1], 0230T[1], 31505[1], 31515[1], 31527[1], 31622[1], 31634[1], 31645[1], 31647[1], 36000[1], 36010[0], 36011[1], 36012[1], 36013[1], 36014[1], 36015[1], 36400[1], 36405[1], 36406[1], 36410[1], 36420[1], 36425[1], 36430[1], 36440[1], 36591[0], 36592[0], 36600[1], 36640[1], 43752[1], 43753[1], 43754[1], 61026[1], 61055[1], 62280[1], 62281[1], 62282[1], 62284[1], 62320[1], 62321[1], 62322[1], 62323[1], 62324[1], 62325[1], 62326[1], 62327[1], 64400[1], 64402[1], 64405[1], 64408[1], 64410[1], 64413[1], 64415[1], 64416[1], 64417[1], 64418[1], 64420[1], 64421[1], 64425[1], 64430[1], 64435[1], 64445[1], 64446[1], 64447[1], 64448[1], 64449[1], 64450[1], 64461[1], 64463[1], 64479[1], 64483[1], 64486[1], 64487[1], 64488[1], 64489[1], 64490[1], 64493[1], 64505[1], 64510[1], 64517[1], 64520[1], 64530[1], 64553[1], 64555[1], 67500[1], 76000[1], 76970[1], 76998[0], 77002[0], 90865[1], 92511[1], 92512[1], 92516[1], 92520[1], 92537[1], 92538[1], 92950[1], 92953[1], 92960[1], 92961[1], 93000[1], 93005[1], 93010[1], 93040[1], 93041[1], 93042[1], 93050[0], 93303[0], 93304[0], 93306[1], 93307[1], 93308[1], 93312[1], 93313[1], 93314[1], 93315[1], 93316[1], 93317[1], 93318[0], 93351[1], 93355[0], 93451[1], 93456[1], 93457[1], 93561[0], 93562[0], 93701[0], 93922[1], 93923[1], 93924[1], 93925[1], 93926[1], 93930[1], 93931[1], 93970[1], 93971[1], 93975[1], 93976[1], 93978[1], 93979[1], 93980[1], 93981[1], 94002[1], 94004[1], 94200[1], 94250[0], 94640[1], 94644[1], 94660[1], 94662[1], 94680[1], 94681[1], 94690[1], 94760[0], 94761[0], 94762[1], 94770[1], 95812[0], 95813[0], 95816[0], 95819[0], 95822[0], 95829[0], 95955[0], 95956[0], 95957[0], 96360[0], 96365[0], 96372[0], 96373[0], 96374[0], 96375[0], 96376[0], 96377[0], 99151[0], 99152[0], 99153[0], 99155[0], 99156[0], 99157[0], 99201[0], 99202[0], 99203[0], 99204[0], 99205[0], 99211[0], 99212[0], 99213[0], 99214[0], 99215[0], 99217[0], 99218[0], 99219[0], 99220[0], 99221[0], 99222[0], 99223[0], 99224[0], 99225[0], 99226[0], 99231[0], 99232[0], 99233[0], 99234[0], 99235[0], 99236[0], 99238[0], 99239[0], 99281[0], 99282[0], 99283[0], 99284[0], 99285[0], 99304[0], 99305[0], 99306[0], 99307[0], 99308[0], 99309[0], 99310[0], 99315[0], 99318[0], 99324[0], 99325[0], 99326[0], 99327[0], 99328[0], 99334[0], 99335[0], 99336[0], 99337[0], 99341[0], 99342[0], 99343[0], 99347[0], 99348[0], 99349[0], 99354[0], 99355[0], 99356[0], 99357[0], 99358[0], 99359[0], 99415[0], 99416[0], 99446[0], 99447[0], 99448[0], 99449[0], 99451[0], 99452[0], 99466[0], 99468[0], 99469[0], 99471[0], 99472[0], 99475[0], 99476[0], 99477[0], 99478[0], 99479[0], 99480[0], 99483[0], 99485[0], 99497[0], C8921[1], C8922[1], C8923[1], C8924[1], C8925[1], C8926[1], C8927[0], C8929[1], C8930[1], G0380[1], G0381[1], G0382[1], G0383[1], G0384[1], G0406[0], G0407[0], G0408[0], G0425[0], G0426[0], G0427[0], G0463[0], G0500[0], G0508[0], G0509[0]
01420	01996[1], 0213T[1], 0216T[1], 0228T[1], 0230T[1], 31505[1], 31515[1], 31527[1], 31622[1], 31634[1], 31645[1], 31647[1], 36000[1], 36010[0], 36011[1], 36012[1], 36013[1], 36014[1], 36015[1], 36400[1], 36405[1], 36406[1], 36410[1], 36420[1], 36425[1], 36430[1], 36440[1], 36591[0], 36592[0], 36600[1], 36640[1], 43752[1], 43753[1], 43754[1], 61026[1], 61055[1], 62280[1], 62281[1], 62282[1], 62284[1], 62320[1], 62321[1], 62322[1], 62323[1], 62324[1], 62325[1], 62326[1], 62327[1], 64400[1], 64402[1], 64405[1], 64408[1], 64410[1], 64413[1], 64415[1], 64416[1], 64417[1], 64418[1], 64420[1], 64421[1], 64425[1], 64430[1], 64435[1], 64445[1], 64446[1], 64447[1], 64448[1], 64449[1], 64450[1], 64461[1], 64463[1], 64479[1], 64483[1], 64486[1], 64487[1], 64488[1], 64489[1], 64490[1], 64493[1], 64505[1], 64510[1], 64517[1], 64520[1], 64530[1], 64553[1], 64555[1], 67500[1], 76000[1], 76970[1], 76998[0], 77002[0], 90865[1], 92511[1], 92512[1], 92516[1], 92520[1], 92537[1], 92538[1], 92950[1], 92953[1], 92960[1], 92961[1], 93000[1], 93005[1], 93010[1], 93040[1], 93041[1], 93042[1], 93050[0], 93303[0], 93304[0], 93306[1], 93307[1], 93308[1], 93312[1], 93313[1], 93314[1], 93315[1], 93316[1], 93317[1], 93318[0], 93351[1], 93355[0], 93451[1], 93456[1], 93457[1], 93561[0], 93562[0], 93701[0], 93922[1], 93923[1], 93924[1], 93925[1], 93926[1], 93930[1], 93931[1], 93970[1], 93971[1], 93975[1], 93976[1], 93978[1], 93979[1], 93980[1], 93981[1], 94002[1], 94004[1], 94200[1], 94250[0], 94640[1], 94644[1], 94660[1], 94662[1], 94680[1], 94681[1], 94690[1], 94760[0], 94761[0], 94762[1], 94770[1], 95812[0], 95813[0], 95816[0], 95819[0], 95822[0], 95829[0], 95955[0], 95956[0], 95957[0], 96360[0], 96365[0], 96372[0], 96373[0], 96374[0], 96375[0], 96376[0], 96377[0], 99151[0], 99152[0], 99153[0], 99155[0], 99156[0], 99157[0], 99201[0], 99202[0], 99203[0], 99204[0], 99205[0], 99211[0], 99212[0], 99213[0], 99214[0], 99215[0], 99217[0], 99218[0], 99219[0], 99220[0], 99221[0], 99222[0], 99223[0], 99224[0], 99225[0], 99226[0], 99231[0], 99232[0], 99233[0], 99234[0], 99235[0], 99236[0], 99238[0], 99239[0], 99281[0], 99282[0], 99283[0], 99284[0], 99285[0], 99304[0], 99305[0], 99306[0], 99307[0], 99308[0], 99309[0], 99310[0], 99315[0], 99318[0], 99324[0], 99325[0], 99326[0], 99327[0], 99328[0], 99334[0], 99335[0], 99336[0], 99337[0], 99341[0], 99342[0], 99343[0], 99347[0], 99348[0], 99349[0], 99354[0], 99355[0], 99356[0], 99357[0], 99358[0], 99359[0], 99415[0], 99416[0], 99446[0], 99447[0], 99448[0], 99449[0], 99451[0], 99452[0], 99466[0], 99468[0], 99469[0], 99471[0], 99472[0], 99475[0], 99476[0], 99477[0], 99478[0], 99479[0], 99480[0], 99483[0], 99485[0], 99497[0], C8921[1], C8922[1], C8923[1], C8924[1], C8925[1], C8926[1], C8927[0], C8929[1], C8930[1], G0380[1], G0381[1], G0382[1], G0383[1], G0384[1], G0406[0], G0407[0], G0408[0], G0425[0], G0426[0], G0427[0], G0463[0], G0500[0], G0508[0], G0509[0]
01430	01996[1], 0213T[1], 0216T[1], 0228T[1], 0230T[1], 31505[1], 31515[1], 31527[1], 31622[1], 31634[1], 31645[1], 31647[1], 36000[1], 36010[0], 36011[1], 36012[1], 36013[1], 36014[1], 36015[1], 36400[1], 36405[1], 36406[1], 36410[1], 36420[1], 36425[1], 36430[1], 36440[1], 36591[0], 36592[0], 36600[1], 36640[1], 43752[1], 43753[1], 43754[1], 61026[1], 61055[1], 62280[1], 62281[1], 62282[1], 62284[1], 62320[1], 62321[1], 62322[1], 62323[1], 62324[1], 62325[1], 62326[1], 62327[1], 64400[1], 64402[1], 64405[1], 64408[1], 64410[1], 64413[1], 64415[1], 64416[1], 64417[1], 64418[1], 64420[1], 64421[1], 64425[1], 64430[1], 64435[1], 64445[1], 64446[1], 64447[1], 64448[1], 64449[1], 64450[1], 64461[1], 64463[1], 64479[1], 64483[1], 64486[1], 64487[1], 64488[1], 64489[1], 64490[1], 64493[1], 64505[1], 64510[1], 64517[1], 64520[1], 64530[1], 64553[1], 64555[1], 67500[1], 76000[1], 76970[1], 76998[0], 77002[0], 90865[1], 92511[1], 92512[1], 92516[1], 92520[1], 92537[1], 92538[1], 92950[1], 92953[1], 92960[1], 92961[1], 93000[1], 93005[1], 93010[1], 93040[1], 93041[1], 93042[1], 93050[0], 93303[0], 93304[0], 93306[1], 93307[1], 93308[1], 93312[1], 93313[1], 93314[1], 93315[1], 93316[1], 93317[1],

0 = Modifier usage not allowed or inappropriate 1 = Modifier usage allowed

CPT © 2018 American Medical Association. All Rights Reserved.

Appendix A: NCCI - CPT Codes

Code 1	Code 2
	93318[0], 93351[1], 93355[0], 93451[1], 93456[1], 93457[1], 93561[0], 93562[0], 93701[0], 93922[1], 93923[1], 93924[1], 93925[1], 93926[1], 93930[1], 93931[1], 93970[1], 93971[1], 93975[1], 93976[1], 93978[1], 93979[1], 93980[1], 93981[1], 94002[1], 94004[1], 94200[1], 94250[0], 94640[1], 94644[1], 94660[1], 94662[1], 94680[1], 94681[1], 94690[1], 94760[0], 94761[0], 94762[1], 94770[1], 95812[0], 95813[0], 95816[0], 95819[0], 95822[0], 95829[0], 95955[0], 95956[0], 95957[0], 96360[0], 96365[0], 96372[0], 96373[0], 96374[0], 96375[0], 96376[0], 96377[0], 99151[0], 99152[0], 99153[0], 99155[0], 99156[0], 99157[0], 99201[0], 99202[0], 99203[0], 99204[0], 99205[0], 99211[0], 99212[0], 99213[0], 99214[0], 99215[0], 99217[0], 99218[0], 99219[0], 99220[0], 99221[0], 99222[0], 99223[0], 99224[0], 99225[0], 99226[0], 99231[0], 99232[0], 99233[0], 99234[0], 99235[0], 99236[0], 99238[0], 99239[0], 99281[0], 99282[0], 99283[0], 99284[0], 99285[0], 99304[0], 99305[0], 99306[0], 99307[0], 99308[0], 99309[0], 99310[0], 99315[0], 99318[0], 99324[0], 99325[0], 99326[0], 99327[0], 99328[0], 99334[0], 99335[0], 99336[0], 99337[0], 99341[0], 99342[0], 99343[0], 99347[0], 99348[0], 99349[0], 99354[0], 99355[0], 99356[0], 99357[0], 99358[0], 99359[0], 99415[0], 99416[0], 99446[0], 99447[0], 99448[0], 99449[0], 99451[0], 99452[0], 99466[0], 99468[0], 99469[0], 99471[0], 99472[0], 99475[0], 99476[0], 99477[0], 99478[0], 99479[0], 99480[0], 99483[0], 99485[0], 99497[0], C8921[1], C8922[1], C8923[1], C8924[1], C8925[1], C8926[1], C8927[0], C8929[1], C8930[1], G0380[1], G0381[1], G0382[1], G0383[1], G0384[1], G0406[0], G0407[0], G0408[0], G0425[0], G0426[0], G0427[0], G0463[0], G0500[0], G0508[0], G0509[0]
01432	01996[1], 0213T[1], 0216T[1], 0228T[1], 0230T[1], 31505[1], 31515[1], 31527[1], 31622[1], 31634[1], 31645[1], 31647[1], 36000[1], 36010[0], 36011[1], 36012[1], 36013[1], 36014[1], 36015[1], 36400[1], 36405[1], 36406[1], 36410[1], 36420[1], 36425[1], 36430[1], 36440[1], 36591[0], 36592[0], 36600[1], 36640[1], 43752[1], 43753[1], 43754[1], 61026[1], 61055[1], 62280[1], 62281[1], 62282[1], 62284[1], 62320[1], 62321[1], 62322[1], 62323[1], 62324[1], 62325[1], 62326[1], 62327[1], 64400[1], 64402[1], 64405[1], 64408[1], 64410[1], 64413[1], 64415[1], 64416[1], 64417[1], 64418[1], 64420[1], 64421[1], 64425[1], 64430[1], 64435[1], 64445[1], 64446[1], 64447[1], 64448[1], 64449[1], 64450[1], 64461[1], 64463[1], 64479[1], 64483[1], 64486[1], 64487[1], 64488[1], 64489[1], 64490[1], 64493[1], 64505[1], 64510[1], 64517[1], 64520[1], 64530[1], 64553[1], 64555[1], 67500[1], 76000[1], 76970[1], 76998[0], 77002[0], 90865[1], 92511[1], 92512[1], 92516[1], 92520[1], 92537[1], 92538[1], 92950[1], 92953[1], 92960[1], 92961[1], 93000[1], 93005[1], 93010[1], 93040[1], 93041[1], 93042[1], 93050[0], 93303[0], 93304[0], 93306[1], 93307[1], 93308[1], 93312[1], 93313[1], 93314[1], 93315[1], 93316[1], 93317[1], 93318[0], 93351[1], 93355[0], 93451[1], 93456[1], 93457[1], 93561[0], 93562[0], 93701[0], 93922[1], 93923[1], 93924[1], 93925[1], 93926[1], 93930[1], 93931[1], 93970[1], 93971[1], 93975[1], 93976[1], 93978[1], 93979[1], 93980[1], 93981[1], 94002[1], 94004[1], 94200[1], 94250[0], 94640[1], 94644[1], 94660[1], 94662[1], 94680[1], 94681[1], 94690[1], 94760[0], 94761[0], 94762[1], 94770[1], 95812[0], 95813[0], 95816[0], 95819[0], 95822[0], 95829[0], 95955[0], 95956[0], 95957[0], 96360[0], 96365[0], 96372[0], 96373[0], 96374[0], 96375[0], 96376[0], 96377[0], 99151[0], 99152[0], 99153[0], 99155[0], 99156[0], 99157[0], 99201[0], 99202[0], 99203[0], 99204[0], 99205[0], 99211[0], 99212[0], 99213[0], 99214[0], 99215[0], 99217[0], 99218[0], 99219[0], 99220[0], 99221[0], 99222[0], 99223[0], 99224[0], 99225[0], 99226[0], 99231[0], 99232[0], 99233[0], 99234[0], 99235[0], 99236[0], 99238[0], 99239[0], 99281[0], 99282[0], 99283[0], 99284[0], 99285[0], 99304[0], 99305[0], 99306[0], 99307[0], 99308[0], 99309[0], 99310[0], 99315[0], 99318[0], 99324[0], 99325[0], 99326[0], 99327[0], 99328[0], 99334[0], 99335[0], 99336[0], 99337[0], 99341[0], 99342[0], 99343[0], 99347[0], 99348[0], 99349[0], 99354[0], 99355[0], 99356[0], 99357[0], 99358[0], 99359[0], 99415[0], 99416[0], 99446[0], 99447[0], 99448[0], 99449[0], 99451[0], 99452[0], 99466[0], 99468[0], 99469[0], 99471[0], 99472[0], 99475[0], 99476[0], 99477[0], 99478[0], 99479[0], 99480[0], 99483[0], 99485[0], 99497[0], C8921[1], C8922[1], C8923[1], C8924[1], C8925[1], C8926[1], C8927[0], C8929[1], C8930[1], G0380[1], G0381[1], G0382[1], G0383[1], G0384[1], G0406[0], G0407[0], G0408[0], G0425[0], G0426[0], G0427[0], G0463[0], G0500[0], G0508[0], G0509[0]
01440	01996[1], 0213T[1], 0216T[1], 0228T[1], 0230T[1], 31505[1], 31515[1], 31527[1], 31622[1], 31634[1], 31645[1], 31647[1], 36000[1], 36010[0], 36011[1], 36012[1], 36013[1], 36014[1], 36015[1], 36400[1], 36405[1], 36406[1], 36410[1], 36420[1], 36425[1], 36430[1], 36440[1], 36591[0], 36592[0], 36600[1], 36640[1], 43752[1], 43753[1], 43754[1], 61026[1], 61055[1], 62280[1], 62281[1], 62282[1], 62284[1], 62320[1], 62321[1], 62322[1], 62323[1], 62324[1], 62325[1], 62326[1], 62327[1], 64400[1], 64402[1], 64405[1], 64408[1], 64410[1], 64413[1], 64415[1], 64416[1], 64417[1], 64418[1], 64420[1], 64421[1], 64425[1], 64430[1], 64435[1], 64445[1], 64446[1], 64447[1], 64448[1], 64449[1], 64450[1], 64461[1], 64463[1], 64479[1], 64483[1], 64486[1], 64487[1], 64488[1], 64489[1], 64490[1], 64493[1], 64505[1], 64510[1], 64517[1], 64520[1], 64530[1], 64553[1], 64555[1], 67500[1], 76000[1], 76970[1], 76998[0], 77002[0], 90865[1], 92511[1], 92512[1], 92516[1], 92520[1], 92537[1], 92538[1], 92950[1], 92953[1], 92960[1], 92961[1], 93000[1], 93005[1], 93010[1], 93040[1], 93041[1], 93042[1], 93050[0], 93303[0], 93304[0], 93306[1], 93307[1], 93308[1], 93312[1], 93313[1], 93314[1], 93315[1], 93316[1], 93317[1], 93318[0], 93351[1], 93355[0], 93451[1], 93456[1], 93457[1], 93561[0], 93562[0], 93701[0], 93922[1], 93923[1], 93924[1], 93925[1], 93926[1], 93930[1], 93931[1], 93970[1], 93971[1], 93975[1], 93976[1], 93978[1], 93979[1], 93980[1], 93981[1], 94002[1], 94004[1], 94200[1], 94250[0], 94640[1], 94644[1], 94660[1], 94662[1], 94680[1], 94681[1], 94690[1], 94760[0], 94761[0], 94762[1], 94770[1], 95812[0], 95813[0], 95816[0], 95819[0], 95822[0], 95829[0], 95955[0], 95956[0], 95957[0], 96360[0], 96365[0], 96372[0], 96373[0], 96374[0], 96375[0], 96376[0], 96377[0], 99151[0], 99152[0], 99153[0], 99155[0], 99156[0], 99157[0], 99201[0], 99202[0], 99203[0], 99204[0], 99205[0], 99211[0], 99212[0], 99213[0], 99214[0], 99215[0], 99217[0], 99218[0], 99219[0], 99220[0], 99221[0], 99222[0], 99223[0], 99224[0], 99225[0], 99226[0], 99231[0], 99232[0], 99233[0], 99234[0], 99235[0], 99236[0], 99238[0], 99239[0], 99281[0], 99282[0], 99283[0], 99284[0], 99285[0], 99304[0], 99305[0], 99306[0], 99307[0], 99308[0], 99309[0], 99310[0], 99315[0], 99318[0], 99324[0], 99325[0], 99326[0], 99327[0], 99328[0], 99334[0], 99335[0], 99336[0], 99337[0], 99341[0], 99342[0], 99343[0], 99347[0], 99348[0], 99349[0], 99354[0], 99355[0], 99356[0], 99357[0], 99358[0], 99359[0], 99415[0], 99416[0], 99446[0], 99447[0], 99448[0], 99449[0], 99451[0], 99452[0], 99466[0], 99468[0], 99469[0], 99471[0], 99472[0], 99475[0], 99476[0], 99477[0], 99478[0], 99479[0], 99480[0], 99483[0], 99485[0], 99497[0], C8921[1], C8922[1], C8923[1], C8924[1], C8925[1], C8926[1], C8927[0], C8929[1], C8930[1], G0380[1], G0381[1], G0382[1], G0383[1], G0384[1], G0406[0], G0407[0], G0408[0], G0425[0], G0426[0], G0427[0], G0463[0], G0500[0], G0508[0], G0509[0]
01442	01996[1], 0213T[1], 0216T[1], 0228T[1], 0230T[1], 31505[1], 31515[1], 31527[1], 31622[1], 31634[1], 31645[1], 31647[1], 36000[1], 36010[0], 36011[1], 36012[1], 36013[1], 36014[1], 36015[1], 36400[1], 36405[1], 36406[1], 36410[1], 36420[1], 36425[1], 36430[1], 36440[1], 36591[0], 36592[0], 36600[1], 36640[1], 43752[1], 43753[1], 43754[1], 61026[1], 61055[1], 62280[1], 62281[1], 62282[1], 62284[1], 62320[1], 62321[1], 62322[1], 62323[1], 62324[1], 62325[1], 62326[1], 62327[1], 64400[1], 64402[1], 64405[1], 64408[1], 64410[1], 64413[1], 64415[1], 64416[1], 64417[1], 64418[1], 64420[1], 64421[1], 64425[1], 64430[1], 64435[1], 64445[1], 64446[1], 64447[1], 64448[1], 64449[1], 64450[1], 64461[1], 64463[1], 64479[1], 64483[1], 64486[1], 64487[1], 64488[1], 64489[1], 64490[1], 64493[1], 64505[1], 64510[1], 64517[1], 64520[1], 64530[1], 64553[1], 64555[1], 67500[1], 76000[1], 76970[1], 76998[0], 77002[0], 90865[1], 92511[1], 92512[1], 92516[1], 92520[1], 92537[1], 92538[1], 92950[1], 92953[1], 92960[1], 92961[1], 93000[1], 93005[1], 93010[1], 93040[1], 93041[1], 93042[1], 93050[0], 93303[0], 93304[0], 93306[1], 93307[1], 93308[1], 93312[1], 93313[1], 93314[1], 93315[1], 93316[1], 93317[1], 93318[0], 93351[1], 93355[0], 93451[1], 93456[1], 93457[1], 93561[0], 93562[0], 93701[0], 93922[1], 93923[1], 93924[1], 93925[1], 93926[1], 93930[1], 93931[1], 93970[1], 93971[1], 93975[1], 93976[1], 93978[1], 93979[1], 93980[1], 93981[1], 94002[1], 94004[1], 94200[1], 94250[0], 94640[1], 94644[1], 94660[1], 94662[1], 94680[1], 94681[1], 94690[1], 94760[0], 94761[0], 94762[1], 94770[1], 95812[0], 95813[0], 95816[0], 95819[0], 95822[0], 95829[0], 95955[0], 95956[0], 95957[0], 96360[0], 96365[0], 96372[0], 96373[0], 96374[0], 96375[0], 96376[0], 96377[0], 99151[0], 99152[0], 99153[0], 99155[0], 99156[0], 99157[0], 99201[0], 99202[0], 99203[0], 99204[0], 99205[0], 99211[0], 99212[0], 99213[0], 99214[0], 99215[0], 99217[0], 99218[0], 99219[0], 99220[0], 99221[0], 99222[0], 99223[0], 99224[0], 99225[0], 99226[0], 99231[0], 99232[0], 99233[0], 99234[0], 99235[0], 99236[0], 99238[0], 99239[0], 99281[0], 99282[0], 99283[0], 99284[0], 99285[0], 99304[0], 99305[0], 99306[0], 99307[0], 99308[0], 99309[0], 99310[0], 99315[0], 99318[0], 99324[0], 99325[0], 99326[0], 99327[0], 99328[0], 99334[0], 99335[0], 99336[0], 99337[0], 99341[0], 99342[0], 99343[0], 99347[0], 99348[0], 99349[0], 99354[0], 99355[0], 99356[0], 99357[0], 99358[0], 99359[0], 99415[0], 99416[0], 99446[0], 99447[0], 99448[0], 99449[0], 99451[0], 99452[0], 99466[0], 99468[0], 99469[0], 99471[0], 99472[0], 99475[0], 99476[0], 99477[0], 99478[0], 99479[0], 99480[0], 99483[0], 99485[0], 99497[0], C8921[1], C8922[1], C8923[1], C8924[1], C8925[1], C8926[1], C8927[0], C8929[1], C8930[1], G0380[1], G0381[1], G0382[1], G0383[1], G0384[1], G0406[0], G0407[0], G0408[0], G0425[0], G0426[0], G0427[0], G0463[0], G0500[0], G0508[0], G0509[0]
01444	01996[1], 0213T[1], 0216T[1], 0228T[1], 0230T[1], 31505[1], 31515[1], 31527[1], 31622[1], 31634[1], 31645[1], 31647[1], 36000[1], 36010[0], 36011[1], 36012[1], 36013[1], 36014[1], 36015[1], 36400[1], 36405[1], 36406[1], 36410[1], 36420[1], 36425[1], 36430[1], 36440[1], 36591[0], 36592[0], 36600[1], 36640[1], 43752[1], 43753[1], 43754[1], 61026[1], 61055[1], 62280[1], 62281[1], 62282[1], 62284[1], 62320[1], 62321[1], 62322[1], 62323[1], 62324[1], 62325[1], 62326[1], 62327[1], 64400[1], 64402[1], 64405[1], 64408[1], 64410[1], 64413[1], 64415[1], 64416[1], 64417[1], 64418[1], 64420[1], 64421[1], 64425[1], 64430[1], 64435[1], 64445[1], 64446[1], 64447[1], 64448[1], 64449[1], 64450[1], 64461[1], 64463[1], 64479[1], 64483[1], 64486[1], 64487[1], 64488[1], 64489[1], 64490[1], 64493[1], 64505[1], 64510[1], 64517[1], 64520[1], 64530[1], 64553[1], 64555[1], 67500[1], 76000[1], 76970[1], 76998[0], 77002[0], 90865[1], 92511[1], 92512[1], 92516[1], 92520[1], 92537[1], 92538[1], 92950[1], 92953[1], 92960[1], 92961[1], 93000[1], 93005[1], 93010[1], 93040[1], 93041[1], 93042[1], 93050[0], 93303[0], 93304[0], 93306[1], 93307[1], 93308[1], 93312[1], 93313[1], 93314[1], 93315[1], 93316[1], 93317[1], 93318[0], 93351[1], 93355[0], 93451[1], 93456[1], 93457[1], 93561[0], 93562[0], 93701[0], 93922[1], 93923[1], 93924[1], 93925[1], 93926[1], 93930[1], 93931[1], 93970[1], 93971[1], 93975[1], 93976[1], 93978[1], 93979[1], 93980[1], 93981[1], 94002[1], 94004[1], 94200[1], 94250[0], 94640[1], 94644[1], 94660[1], 94662[1], 94680[1], 94681[1], 94690[1], 94760[0], 94761[0], 94762[1], 94770[1], 95812[0], 95813[0], 95816[0], 95819[0], 95822[0], 95829[0], 95955[0], 95956[0], 95957[0], 96360[0], 96365[0], 96372[0], 96373[0], 96374[0], 96375[0], 96376[0], 96377[0], 99151[0], 99152[0], 99153[0], 99155[0], 99156[0], 99157[0], 99201[0], 99202[0], 99203[0], 99204[0], 99205[0], 99211[0], 99212[0], 99213[0], 99214[0], 99215[0], 99217[0], 99218[0], 99219[0], 99220[0], 99221[0], 99222[0], 99223[0], 99224[0], 99225[0], 99226[0], 99231[0], 99232[0], 99233[0], 99234[0], 99235[0], 99236[0], 99238[0], 99239[0], 99281[0], 99282[0], 99283[0], 99284[0], 99285[0], 99304[0], 99305[0], 99306[0], 99307[0], 99308[0], 99309[0], 99310[0], 99315[0], 99318[0], 99324[0], 99325[0], 99326[0], 99327[0], 99328[0], 99334[0], 99335[0], 99336[0], 99337[0], 99341[0], 99342[0], 99343[0], 99347[0], 99348[0], 99349[0], 99354[0],

0 = Modifier usage not allowed or inappropriate 1 = Modifier usage allowed

CPT © 2018 American Medical Association. All Rights Reserved.

Code 1	Code 2
	99355[0], 99356[0], 99357[0], 99358[0], 99359[0], 99415[0], 99416[0], 99446[0], 99447[0], 99448[0], 99449[0], 99451[0], 99452[0], 99466[0], 99468[0], 99469[0], 99471[0], 99472[0], 99475[0], 99476[0], 99477[0], 99478[0], 99479[0], 99480[0], 99483[0], 99485[0], 99497[0], C8921[1], C8922[1], C8923[1], C8924[1], C8925[1], C8926[1], C8927[0], C8929[1], C8930[1], G0380[1], G0381[1], G0382[1], G0383[1], G0384[1], G0406[0], G0407[0], G0408[0], G0425[0], G0426[0], G0427[0], G0463[0], G0500[0], G0508[0], G0509[0]
01462	01996[1], 0213T[1], 0216T[1], 0228T[1], 0230T[1], 31505[1], 31515[1], 31527[1], 31622[1], 31634[1], 31645[1], 31647[1], 36000[1], 36010[0], 36011[1], 36012[1], 36013[1], 36014[1], 36015[1], 36400[1], 36405[1], 36406[1], 36410[1], 36420[1], 36425[1], 36430[1], 36440[1], 36591[0], 36592[0], 36600[1], 36640[1], 43752[1], 43753[1], 43754[1], 61026[1], 61055[1], 62280[1], 62281[1], 62282[1], 62284[1], 62320[1], 62321[1], 62322[1], 62323[1], 62324[1], 62325[1], 62326[1], 62327[1], 64400[1], 64402[1], 64405[1], 64408[1], 64410[1], 64413[1], 64415[1], 64416[1], 64417[1], 64418[1], 64420[1], 64421[1], 64425[1], 64430[1], 64435[1], 64445[1], 64446[1], 64447[1], 64448[1], 64449[1], 64450[1], 64461[1], 64463[1], 64479[1], 64483[1], 64486[1], 64487[1], 64488[1], 64489[1], 64490[1], 64493[1], 64505[1], 64510[1], 64517[1], 64520[1], 64530[1], 64553[1], 64555[1], 67500[1], 76000[1], 76970[1], 76998[0], 77002[0], 90865[1], 92511[1], 92512[1], 92516[1], 92520[1], 92537[1], 92538[1], 92950[1], 92953[1], 92960[1], 92961[1], 93000[1], 93005[1], 93010[1], 93040[1], 93041[1], 93042[1], 93050[0], 93303[0], 93304[0], 93306[1], 93307[1], 93308[1], 93312[1], 93313[1], 93314[1], 93315[1], 93316[1], 93317[1], 93318[0], 93351[1], 93355[0], 93451[1], 93456[1], 93457[1], 93561[0], 93562[0], 93701[0], 93922[1], 93923[1], 93924[1], 93925[1], 93926[1], 93930[1], 93931[1], 93970[1], 93971[1], 93975[1], 93976[1], 93978[1], 93979[1], 93980[1], 93981[1], 94002[1], 94004[1], 94200[1], 94250[0], 94640[1], 94644[1], 94660[1], 94662[1], 94680[1], 94681[1], 94690[1], 94760[0], 94761[0], 94762[1], 94770[1], 95812[0], 95813[0], 95816[0], 95819[0], 95822[0], 95829[0], 95955[0], 95956[0], 95957[0], 96360[0], 96365[0], 96372[0], 96373[0], 96374[0], 96375[0], 96376[0], 96377[0], 99151[0], 99152[0], 99153[0], 99155[0], 99156[0], 99157[0], 99201[0], 99202[0], 99203[0], 99204[0], 99205[0], 99211[0], 99212[0], 99213[0], 99214[0], 99215[0], 99217[0], 99218[0], 99219[0], 99220[0], 99221[0], 99222[0], 99223[0], 99224[0], 99225[0], 99226[0], 99231[0], 99232[0], 99233[0], 99234[0], 99235[0], 99236[0], 99238[0], 99239[0], 99281[0], 99282[0], 99283[0], 99284[0], 99285[0], 99304[0], 99305[0], 99306[0], 99307[0], 99308[0], 99309[0], 99310[0], 99315[0], 99318[0], 99324[0], 99325[0], 99326[0], 99327[0], 99328[0], 99334[0], 99335[0], 99336[0], 99337[0], 99341[0], 99342[0], 99343[0], 99347[0], 99348[0], 99349[0], 99354[0], 99355[0], 99356[0], 99357[0], 99358[0], 99359[0], 99415[0], 99416[0], 99446[0], 99447[0], 99448[0], 99449[0], 99451[0], 99452[0], 99466[0], 99468[0], 99469[0], 99471[0], 99472[0], 99475[0], 99476[0], 99477[0], 99478[0], 99479[0], 99480[0], 99483[0], 99485[0], 99497[0], C8921[1], C8922[1], C8923[1], C8924[1], C8925[1], C8926[1], C8927[0], C8929[1], C8930[1], G0380[1], G0381[1], G0382[1], G0383[1], G0384[1], G0406[0], G0407[0], G0408[0], G0425[0], G0426[0], G0427[0], G0463[0], G0500[0], G0508[0], G0509[0]
01464	01996[1], 0213T[1], 0216T[1], 0228T[1], 0230T[1], 31505[1], 31515[1], 31527[1], 31622[1], 31634[1], 31645[1], 31647[1], 36000[1], 36010[0], 36011[1], 36012[1], 36013[1], 36014[1], 36015[1], 36400[1], 36405[1], 36406[1], 36410[1], 36420[1], 36425[1], 36430[1], 36440[1], 36591[0], 36592[0], 36600[1], 36640[1], 43752[1], 43753[1], 43754[1], 61026[1], 61055[1], 62280[1], 62281[1], 62282[1], 62284[1], 62320[1], 62321[1], 62322[1], 62323[1], 62324[1], 62325[1], 62326[1], 62327[1], 64400[1], 64402[1], 64405[1], 64408[1], 64410[1], 64413[1], 64415[1], 64416[1], 64417[1], 64418[1], 64420[1], 64421[1], 64425[1], 64430[1], 64435[1], 64445[1], 64446[1], 64447[1], 64448[1], 64449[1], 64450[1], 64461[1], 64463[1], 64479[1], 64483[1], 64486[1], 64487[1], 64488[1], 64489[1], 64490[1], 64493[1], 64505[1], 64510[1], 64517[1], 64520[1], 64530[1], 64553[1], 64555[1], 67500[1], 76000[1], 76970[1], 76998[0], 77002[0], 90865[1], 92511[1], 92512[1], 92516[1], 92520[1], 92537[1], 92538[1], 92950[1], 92953[1], 92960[1], 92961[1], 93000[1], 93005[1], 93010[1], 93040[1], 93041[1], 93042[1], 93050[0], 93303[0], 93304[0], 93306[1], 93307[1], 93308[1], 93312[1], 93313[1], 93314[1], 93315[1], 93316[1], 93317[1], 93318[0], 93351[1], 93355[0], 93451[1], 93456[1], 93457[1], 93561[0], 93562[0], 93701[0], 93922[1], 93923[1], 93924[1], 93925[1], 93926[1], 93930[1], 93931[1], 93970[1], 93971[1], 93975[1], 93976[1], 93978[1], 93979[1], 93980[1], 93981[1], 94002[1], 94004[1], 94200[1], 94250[0], 94640[1], 94644[1], 94660[1], 94662[1], 94680[1], 94681[1], 94690[1], 94760[0], 94761[0], 94762[1], 94770[1], 95812[0], 95813[0], 95816[0], 95819[0], 95822[0], 95829[0], 95955[0], 95956[0], 95957[0], 96360[0], 96365[0], 96372[0], 96373[0], 96374[0], 96375[0], 96376[0], 96377[0], 99151[0], 99152[0], 99153[0], 99155[0], 99156[0], 99157[0], 99201[0], 99202[0], 99203[0], 99204[0], 99205[0], 99211[0], 99212[0], 99213[0], 99214[0], 99215[0], 99217[0], 99218[0], 99219[0], 99220[0], 99221[0], 99222[0], 99223[0], 99224[0], 99225[0], 99226[0], 99231[0], 99232[0], 99233[0], 99234[0], 99235[0], 99236[0], 99238[0], 99239[0], 99281[0], 99282[0], 99283[0], 99284[0], 99285[0], 99304[0], 99305[0], 99306[0], 99307[0], 99308[0], 99309[0], 99310[0], 99315[0], 99318[0], 99324[0], 99325[0], 99326[0], 99327[0], 99328[0], 99334[0], 99335[0], 99336[0], 99337[0], 99341[0], 99342[0], 99343[0], 99347[0], 99348[0], 99349[0], 99354[0], 99355[0], 99356[0], 99357[0], 99358[0], 99359[0], 99415[0], 99416[0], 99446[0], 99447[0], 99448[0], 99449[0], 99451[0], 99452[0], 99466[0], 99468[0], 99469[0], 99471[0], 99472[0], 99475[0], 99476[0], 99477[0], 99478[0], 99479[0], 99480[0], 99483[0], 99485[0], 99497[0], C8921[1], C8922[1], C8923[1], C8924[1], C8925[1], C8926[1], C8927[0], C8929[1], C8930[1], G0380[1], G0381[1], G0382[1], G0383[1], G0384[1], G0406[0], G0407[0], G0408[0], G0425[0], G0426[0], G0427[0], G0463[0], G0500[0], G0508[0], G0509[0]
01470	01996[1], 0213T[1], 0216T[1], 0228T[1], 0230T[1], 0333T[0], 0464T[0], 31505[1], 31515[1], 31527[1], 31622[1], 31634[1], 31645[1], 31647[1], 36000[1], 36010[0], 36011[1], 36012[1], 36013[1], 36014[1], 36015[1], 36400[1], 36405[1], 36406[1], 36410[1], 36420[1], 36425[1], 36430[1], 36440[1], 36591[0], 36592[0], 36600[1], 36640[1], 43752[1], 43753[1], 43754[1], 61026[1], 61055[1], 62280[1], 62281[1], 62282[1], 62284[1], 62320[1], 62321[1], 62322[1], 62323[1], 62324[1], 62325[1], 62326[1], 62327[1], 64400[1], 64402[1], 64405[1], 64408[1], 64410[1], 64413[1], 64415[1], 64416[1], 64417[1], 64418[1], 64420[1], 64421[1], 64425[1], 64430[1], 64435[1], 64445[1], 64446[1], 64447[1], 64448[1], 64449[1], 64450[1], 64461[1], 64463[1], 64479[1], 64483[1], 64486[1], 64487[1], 64488[1], 64489[1], 64490[1], 64493[1], 64505[1], 64510[1], 64517[1], 64520[1], 64530[1], 64553[1], 64555[1], 67500[1], 76000[1], 76970[1], 76998[0], 77002[0], 90865[1], 92511[1], 92512[1], 92516[1], 92520[1], 92537[1], 92538[1], 92585[0], 92950[1], 92953[1], 92960[1], 92961[1], 93000[1], 93005[1], 93010[1], 93040[1], 93041[1], 93042[1], 93050[0], 93303[0], 93304[0], 93306[1], 93307[1], 93308[1], 93312[1], 93313[1], 93314[1], 93315[1], 93316[1], 93317[1], 93318[0], 93351[1], 93355[0], 93451[1], 93456[1], 93457[1], 93561[0], 93562[0], 93701[0], 93922[1], 93923[1], 93924[1], 93925[1], 93926[1], 93930[1], 93931[1], 93970[1], 93971[1], 93975[1], 93976[1], 93978[1], 93979[1], 93980[1], 93981[1], 94002[1], 94004[1], 94200[1], 94250[0], 94640[1], 94644[1], 94660[1], 94662[1], 94680[1], 94681[1], 94690[1], 94760[0], 94761[0], 94762[1], 94770[1], 95812[0], 95813[0], 95816[0], 95819[0], 95822[0], 95829[0], 95860[0], 95861[0], 95863[0], 95864[0], 95865[0], 95866[0], 95867[0], 95868[0], 95869[0], 95870[0], 95907[0], 95908[0], 95909[0], 95910[0], 95911[0], 95912[0], 95913[0], 95925[0], 95926[0], 95927[0], 95928[0], 95929[0], 95930[0], 95933[0], 95937[0], 95938[0], 95939[0], 95940[0], 95955[0], 95956[0], 95957[0], 96360[0], 96365[0], 96372[0], 96373[0], 96374[0], 96375[0], 96376[0], 96377[0], 99151[0], 99152[0], 99153[0], 99155[0], 99156[0], 99157[0], 99201[0], 99202[0], 99203[0], 99204[0], 99205[0], 99211[0], 99212[0], 99213[0], 99214[0], 99215[0], 99217[0], 99218[0], 99219[0], 99220[0], 99221[0], 99222[0], 99223[0], 99224[0], 99225[0], 99226[0], 99231[0], 99232[0], 99233[0], 99234[0], 99235[0], 99236[0], 99238[0], 99239[0], 99281[0], 99282[0], 99283[0], 99284[0], 99285[0], 99304[0], 99305[0], 99306[0], 99307[0], 99308[0], 99309[0], 99310[0], 99315[0], 99318[0], 99324[0], 99325[0], 99326[0], 99327[0], 99328[0], 99334[0], 99335[0], 99336[0], 99337[0], 99341[0], 99342[0], 99343[0], 99347[0], 99348[0], 99349[0], 99354[0], 99355[0], 99356[0], 99357[0], 99358[0], 99359[0], 99415[0], 99416[0], 99446[0], 99447[0], 99448[0], 99449[0], 99451[0], 99452[0], 99466[0], 99468[0], 99469[0], 99471[0], 99472[0], 99475[0], 99476[0], 99477[0], 99478[0], 99479[0], 99480[0], 99483[0], 99485[0], 99497[0], C8921[1], C8922[1], C8923[1], C8924[1], C8925[1], C8926[1], C8927[0], C8929[1], C8930[1], G0380[1], G0381[1], G0382[1], G0383[1], G0384[1], G0406[0], G0407[0], G0408[0], G0425[0], G0426[0], G0427[0], G0453[0], G0463[0], G0500[0], G0508[0], G0509[0]
01472	01996[1], 0213T[1], 0216T[1], 0228T[1], 0230T[1], 31505[1], 31515[1], 31527[1], 31622[1], 31634[1], 31645[1], 31647[1], 36000[1], 36010[0], 36011[1], 36012[1], 36013[1], 36014[1], 36015[1], 36400[1], 36405[1], 36406[1], 36410[1], 36420[1], 36425[1], 36430[1], 36440[1], 36591[0], 36592[0], 36600[1], 36640[1], 43752[1], 43753[1], 43754[1], 61026[1], 61055[1], 62280[1], 62281[1], 62282[1], 62284[1], 62320[1], 62321[1], 62322[1], 62323[1], 62324[1], 62325[1], 62326[1], 62327[1], 64400[1], 64402[1], 64405[1], 64408[1], 64410[1], 64413[1], 64415[1], 64416[1], 64417[1], 64418[1], 64420[1], 64421[1], 64425[1], 64430[1], 64435[1], 64445[1], 64446[1], 64447[1], 64448[1], 64449[1], 64450[1], 64461[1], 64463[1], 64479[1], 64483[1], 64486[1], 64487[1], 64488[1], 64489[1], 64490[1], 64493[1], 64505[1], 64510[1], 64517[1], 64520[1], 64530[1], 64553[1], 64555[1], 67500[1], 76000[1], 76970[1], 76998[0], 77002[0], 90865[1], 92511[1], 92512[1], 92516[1], 92520[1], 92537[1], 92538[1], 92950[1], 92953[1], 92960[1], 92961[1], 93000[1], 93005[1], 93010[1], 93040[1], 93041[1], 93042[1], 93050[0], 93303[0], 93304[0], 93306[1], 93307[1], 93308[1], 93312[1], 93313[1], 93314[1], 93315[1], 93316[1], 93317[1], 93318[0], 93351[1], 93355[0], 93451[1], 93456[1], 93457[1], 93561[0], 93562[0], 93701[0], 93922[1], 93923[1], 93924[1], 93925[1], 93926[1], 93930[1], 93931[1], 93970[1], 93971[1], 93975[1], 93976[1], 93978[1], 93979[1], 93980[1], 93981[1], 94002[1], 94004[1], 94200[1], 94250[0], 94640[1], 94644[1], 94660[1], 94662[1], 94680[1], 94681[1], 94690[1], 94760[0], 94761[0], 94762[1], 94770[1], 95812[0], 95813[0], 95816[0], 95819[0], 95822[0], 95829[0], 95955[0], 95956[0], 95957[0], 96360[0], 96365[0], 96372[0], 96373[0], 96374[0], 96375[0], 96376[0], 96377[0], 99151[0], 99152[0], 99153[0], 99155[0], 99156[0], 99157[0], 99201[0], 99202[0], 99203[0], 99204[0], 99205[0], 99211[0], 99212[0], 99213[0], 99214[0], 99215[0], 99217[0], 99218[0], 99219[0], 99220[0], 99221[0], 99222[0], 99223[0], 99224[0], 99225[0], 99226[0], 99231[0], 99232[0], 99233[0], 99234[0], 99235[0], 99236[0], 99238[0], 99239[0], 99281[0], 99282[0], 99283[0], 99284[0], 99285[0], 99304[0], 99305[0], 99306[0], 99307[0], 99308[0], 99309[0], 99310[0], 99315[0], 99318[0], 99324[0], 99325[0], 99326[0], 99327[0], 99328[0], 99334[0], 99335[0], 99336[0], 99337[0], 99341[0], 99342[0], 99343[0], 99347[0], 99348[0], 99349[0], 99354[0], 99355[0], 99356[0], 99357[0], 99358[0], 99359[0], 99415[0], 99416[0], 99446[0], 99447[0], 99448[0], 99449[0], 99451[0], 99452[0], 99466[0], 99468[0], 99469[0], 99471[0], 99472[0], 99475[0], 99476[0], 99477[0], 99478[0], 99479[0], 99480[0], 99483[0], 99485[0], 99497[0], C8921[1], C8922[1], C8923[1], C8924[1], C8925[1], C8926[1], C8927[0], C8929[1], C8930[1], G0380[1], G0381[1], G0382[1], G0383[1], G0384[1], G0406[0], G0407[0], G0408[0], G0425[0], G0426[0], G0427[0], G0463[0], G0500[0], G0508[0], G0509[0]
01474	01996[1], 0213T[1], 0216T[1], 0228T[1], 0230T[1], 31505[1], 31515[1], 31527[1], 31622[1], 31634[1], 31645[1], 31647[1], 36000[1], 36010[0], 36011[1], 36012[1], 36013[1], 36014[1], 36015[1], 36400[1], 36405[1], 36406[1], 36410[1], 36420[1], 36425[1], 36430[1], 36440[1], 36591[0], 36592[0], 36600[1],

0 = Modifier usage not allowed or inappropriate 1 = Modifier usage allowed

CPT © 2018 American Medical Association. All Rights Reserved.

Code 1	Code 2
	36640[1], 43752[1], 43753[1], 43754[1], 61026[1], 61055[1], 62280[1], 62281[1], 62282[1], 62284[1], 62320[1], 62321[1], 62322[1], 62323[1], 62324[1], 62325[1], 62326[1], 62327[1], 64400[1], 64402[1], 64405[1], 64408[1], 64410[1], 64413[1], 64415[1], 64416[1], 64417[1], 64418[1], 64420[1], 64421[1], 64425[1], 64430[1], 64435[1], 64445[1], 64446[1], 64447[1], 64448[1], 64449[1], 64450[1], 64461[1], 64463[1], 64479[1], 64483[1], 64486[1], 64487[1], 64488[1], 64489[1], 64490[1], 64493[1], 64505[1], 64510[1], 64517[1], 64520[1], 64530[1], 64553[1], 64555[1], 67500[1], 76000[1], 76970[1], 76998[0], 77002[0], 90865[1], 92511[1], 92512[1], 92516[1], 92520[1], 92537[1], 92538[1], 92950[1], 92953[1], 92960[1], 92961[1], 93000[1], 93005[1], 93010[1], 93040[1], 93041[1], 93042[1], 93050[0], 93303[0], 93304[0], 93306[1], 93307[1], 93308[1], 93312[1], 93313[1], 93314[1], 93315[1], 93316[1], 93317[1], 93318[0], 93351[1], 93355[0], 93451[1], 93456[1], 93457[1], 93561[0], 93562[0], 93701[0], 93922[1], 93923[1], 93924[1], 93925[1], 93926[1], 93930[1], 93931[1], 93970[1], 93971[1], 93975[1], 93976[1], 93978[1], 93979[1], 93980[1], 93981[1], 94002[1], 94004[1], 94200[1], 94250[0], 94640[1], 94644[1], 94660[1], 94662[1], 94680[1], 94681[1], 94690[1], 94760[0], 94761[0], 94762[1], 94770[1], 95812[0], 95813[0], 95816[0], 95819[0], 95822[0], 95829[0], 95955[0], 95956[0], 95957[0], 96360[0], 96365[0], 96372[0], 96373[0], 96374[0], 96375[0], 96376[0], 96377[0], 99151[0], 99152[0], 99153[0], 99155[0], 99156[0], 99157[0], 99201[0], 99202[0], 99203[0], 99204[0], 99205[0], 99211[0], 99212[0], 99213[0], 99214[0], 99215[0], 99217[0], 99218[0], 99219[0], 99220[0], 99221[0], 99222[0], 99223[0], 99224[0], 99225[0], 99226[0], 99231[0], 99232[0], 99233[0], 99234[0], 99235[0], 99236[0], 99238[0], 99239[0], 99281[0], 99282[0], 99283[0], 99284[0], 99285[0], 99304[0], 99305[0], 99306[0], 99307[0], 99308[0], 99309[0], 99310[0], 99315[0], 99318[0], 99324[0], 99325[0], 99326[0], 99327[0], 99328[0], 99334[0], 99335[0], 99336[0], 99337[0], 99341[0], 99342[0], 99343[0], 99347[0], 99348[0], 99349[0], 99354[0], 99355[0], 99356[0], 99357[0], 99358[0], 99359[0], 99415[0], 99416[0], 99446[0], 99447[0], 99448[0], 99449[0], 99451[0], 99452[0], 99466[0], 99468[0], 99469[0], 99471[0], 99472[0], 99475[0], 99476[0], 99477[0], 99478[0], 99479[0], 99480[0], 99483[0], 99485[0], 99497[0], C8921[1], C8922[1], C8923[1], C8924[1], C8925[1], C8926[1], C8927[0], C8929[1], C8930[1], G0380[1], G0381[1], G0382[1], G0383[1], G0384[1], G0406[0], G0407[0], G0408[0], G0425[0], G0426[0], G0427[0], G0463[0], G0500[0], G0508[0], G0509[0]
01480	01996[1], 0213T[1], 0216T[1], 0228T[1], 0230T[1], 31505[1], 31515[1], 31527[1], 31622[1], 31634[1], 31645[1], 31647[1], 36000[1], 36010[0], 36011[1], 36012[1], 36013[1], 36014[1], 36015[1], 36400[1], 36405[1], 36406[1], 36410[1], 36420[1], 36425[1], 36430[1], 36440[1], 36591[0], 36592[0], 36600[1], 36640[1], 43752[1], 43753[1], 43754[1], 61026[1], 61055[1], 62280[1], 62281[1], 62282[1], 62284[1], 62320[1], 62321[1], 62322[1], 62323[1], 62324[1], 62325[1], 62326[1], 62327[1], 64400[1], 64402[1], 64405[1], 64408[1], 64410[1], 64413[1], 64415[1], 64416[1], 64417[1], 64418[1], 64420[1], 64421[1], 64425[1], 64430[1], 64435[1], 64445[1], 64446[1], 64447[1], 64448[1], 64449[1], 64450[1], 64461[1], 64463[1], 64479[1], 64483[1], 64486[1], 64487[1], 64488[1], 64489[1], 64490[1], 64493[1], 64505[1], 64510[1], 64517[1], 64520[1], 64530[1], 64553[1], 64555[1], 67500[1], 76000[1], 76970[1], 76998[0], 77002[0], 90865[1], 92511[1], 92512[1], 92516[1], 92520[1], 92537[1], 92538[1], 92950[1], 92953[1], 92960[1], 92961[1], 93000[1], 93005[1], 93010[1], 93040[1], 93041[1], 93042[1], 93050[0], 93303[0], 93304[0], 93306[1], 93307[1], 93308[1], 93312[1], 93313[1], 93314[1], 93315[1], 93316[1], 93317[1], 93318[0], 93351[1], 93355[0], 93451[1], 93456[1], 93457[1], 93561[0], 93562[0], 93701[0], 93922[1], 93923[1], 93924[1], 93925[1], 93926[1], 93930[1], 93931[1], 93970[1], 93971[1], 93975[1], 93976[1], 93978[1], 93979[1], 93980[1], 93981[1], 94002[1], 94004[1], 94200[1], 94250[0], 94640[1], 94644[1], 94660[1], 94662[1], 94680[1], 94681[1], 94690[1], 94760[0], 94761[0], 94762[1], 94770[1], 95812[0], 95813[0], 95816[0], 95819[0], 95822[0], 95829[0], 95955[0], 95956[0], 95957[0], 96360[0], 96365[0], 96372[0], 96373[0], 96374[0], 96375[0], 96376[0], 96377[0], 99151[0], 99152[0], 99153[0], 99155[0], 99156[0], 99157[0], 99201[0], 99202[0], 99203[0], 99204[0], 99205[0], 99211[0], 99212[0], 99213[0], 99214[0], 99215[0], 99217[0], 99218[0], 99219[0], 99220[0], 99221[0], 99222[0], 99223[0], 99224[0], 99225[0], 99226[0], 99231[0], 99232[0], 99233[0], 99234[0], 99235[0], 99236[0], 99238[0], 99239[0], 99281[0], 99282[0], 99283[0], 99284[0], 99285[0], 99304[0], 99305[0], 99306[0], 99307[0], 99308[0], 99309[0], 99310[0], 99315[0], 99318[0], 99324[0], 99325[0], 99326[0], 99327[0], 99328[0], 99334[0], 99335[0], 99336[0], 99337[0], 99341[0], 99342[0], 99343[0], 99347[0], 99348[0], 99349[0], 99354[0], 99355[0], 99356[0], 99357[0], 99358[0], 99359[0], 99415[0], 99416[0], 99446[0], 99447[0], 99448[0], 99449[0], 99451[0], 99452[0], 99466[0], 99468[0], 99469[0], 99471[0], 99472[0], 99475[0], 99476[0], 99477[0], 99478[0], 99479[0], 99480[0], 99483[0], 99485[0], 99497[0], C8921[1], C8922[1], C8923[1], C8924[1], C8925[1], C8926[1], C8927[0], C8929[1], C8930[1], G0380[1], G0381[1], G0382[1], G0383[1], G0384[1], G0406[0], G0407[0], G0408[0], G0425[0], G0426[0], G0427[0], G0463[0], G0500[0], G0508[0], G0509[0]
01482	01996[1], 0213T[1], 0216T[1], 0228T[1], 0230T[1], 31505[1], 31515[1], 31527[1], 31622[1], 31634[1], 31645[1], 31647[1], 36000[1], 36010[0], 36011[1], 36012[1], 36013[1], 36014[1], 36015[1], 36400[1], 36405[1], 36406[1], 36410[1], 36420[1], 36425[1], 36430[1], 36440[1], 36591[0], 36592[0], 36600[1], 36640[1], 43752[1], 43753[1], 43754[1], 61026[1], 61055[1], 62280[1], 62281[1], 62282[1], 62284[1], 62320[1], 62321[1], 62322[1], 62323[1], 62324[1], 62325[1], 62326[1], 62327[1], 64400[1], 64402[1], 64405[1], 64408[1], 64410[1], 64413[1], 64415[1], 64416[1], 64417[1], 64418[1], 64420[1], 64421[1], 64425[1], 64430[1], 64435[1], 64445[1], 64446[1], 64447[1], 64448[1], 64449[1], 64450[1], 64461[1], 64463[1], 64479[1], 64483[1], 64486[1], 64487[1], 64488[1], 64489[1], 64490[1], 64493[1], 64505[1], 64510[1], 64517[1], 64520[1], 64530[1], 64553[1], 64555[1], 67500[1], 76000[1], 76970[1], 76998[0], 77002[0], 90865[1], 92511[1], 92512[1], 92516[1], 92520[1], 92537[1], 92538[1], 92950[1], 92953[1], 92960[1], 92961[1], 93000[1], 93005[1], 93010[1], 93040[1], 93041[1], 93042[1], 93050[0], 93303[0], 93304[0], 93306[1], 93307[1], 93308[1], 93312[1], 93313[1], 93314[1], 93315[1], 93316[1], 93317[1], 93318[0], 93351[1], 93355[0], 93451[1], 93456[1], 93457[1], 93561[0], 93562[0], 93701[0], 93922[1], 93923[1], 93924[1], 93925[1], 93926[1], 93930[1], 93931[1], 93970[1], 93971[1], 93975[1], 93976[1], 93978[1], 93979[1], 93980[1], 93981[1], 94002[1], 94004[1], 94200[1], 94250[0], 94640[1], 94644[1], 94660[1], 94662[1], 94680[1], 94681[1], 94690[1], 94760[0], 94761[0], 94762[1], 94770[1], 95812[0], 95813[0], 95816[0], 95819[0], 95822[0], 95829[0], 95955[0], 95956[0], 95957[0], 96360[0], 96365[0], 96372[0], 96373[0], 96374[0], 96375[0], 96376[0], 96377[0], 99151[0], 99152[0], 99153[0], 99155[0], 99156[0], 99157[0], 99201[0], 99202[0], 99203[0], 99204[0], 99205[0], 99211[0], 99212[0], 99213[0], 99214[0], 99215[0], 99217[0], 99218[0], 99219[0], 99220[0], 99221[0], 99222[0], 99223[0], 99224[0], 99225[0], 99226[0], 99231[0], 99232[0], 99233[0], 99234[0], 99235[0], 99236[0], 99238[0], 99239[0], 99281[0], 99282[0], 99283[0], 99284[0], 99285[0], 99304[0], 99305[0], 99306[0], 99307[0], 99308[0], 99309[0], 99310[0], 99315[0], 99318[0], 99324[0], 99325[0], 99326[0], 99327[0], 99328[0], 99334[0], 99335[0], 99336[0], 99337[0], 99341[0], 99342[0], 99343[0], 99347[0], 99348[0], 99349[0], 99354[0], 99355[0], 99356[0], 99357[0], 99358[0], 99359[0], 99415[0], 99416[0], 99446[0], 99447[0], 99448[0], 99449[0], 99451[0], 99452[0], 99466[0], 99468[0], 99469[0], 99471[0], 99472[0], 99475[0], 99476[0], 99477[0], 99478[0], 99479[0], 99480[0], 99483[0], 99485[0], 99497[0], C8921[1], C8922[1], C8923[1], C8924[1], C8925[1], C8926[1], C8927[0], C8929[1], C8930[1], G0380[1], G0381[1], G0382[1], G0383[1], G0384[1], G0406[0], G0407[0], G0408[0], G0425[0], G0426[0], G0427[0], G0463[0], G0500[0], G0508[0], G0509[0]
01484	01996[1], 0213T[1], 0216T[1], 0228T[1], 0230T[1], 31505[1], 31515[1], 31527[1], 31622[1], 31634[1], 31645[1], 31647[1], 36000[1], 36010[0], 36011[1], 36012[1], 36013[1], 36014[1], 36015[1], 36400[1], 36405[1], 36406[1], 36410[1], 36420[1], 36425[1], 36430[1], 36440[1], 36591[0], 36592[0], 36600[1], 36640[1], 43752[1], 43753[1], 43754[1], 61026[1], 61055[1], 62280[1], 62281[1], 62282[1], 62284[1], 62320[1], 62321[1], 62322[1], 62323[1], 62324[1], 62325[1], 62326[1], 62327[1], 64400[1], 64402[1], 64405[1], 64408[1], 64410[1], 64413[1], 64415[1], 64416[1], 64417[1], 64418[1], 64420[1], 64421[1], 64425[1], 64430[1], 64435[1], 64445[1], 64446[1], 64447[1], 64448[1], 64449[1], 64450[1], 64461[1], 64463[1], 64479[1], 64483[1], 64486[1], 64487[1], 64488[1], 64489[1], 64490[1], 64493[1], 64505[1], 64510[1], 64517[1], 64520[1], 64530[1], 64553[1], 64555[1], 67500[1], 76000[1], 76970[1], 76998[0], 77002[0], 90865[1], 92511[1], 92512[1], 92516[1], 92520[1], 92537[1], 92538[1], 92950[1], 92953[1], 92960[1], 92961[1], 93000[1], 93005[1], 93010[1], 93040[1], 93041[1], 93042[1], 93050[0], 93303[0], 93304[0], 93306[1], 93307[1], 93308[1], 93312[1], 93313[1], 93314[1], 93315[1], 93316[1], 93317[1], 93318[0], 93351[1], 93355[0], 93451[1], 93456[1], 93457[1], 93561[0], 93562[0], 93701[0], 93922[1], 93923[1], 93924[1], 93925[1], 93926[1], 93930[1], 93931[1], 93970[1], 93971[1], 93975[1], 93976[1], 93978[1], 93979[1], 93980[1], 93981[1], 94002[1], 94004[1], 94200[1], 94250[0], 94640[1], 94644[1], 94660[1], 94662[1], 94680[1], 94681[1], 94690[1], 94760[0], 94761[0], 94762[1], 94770[1], 95812[0], 95813[0], 95816[0], 95819[0], 95822[0], 95829[0], 95955[0], 95956[0], 95957[0], 96360[0], 96365[0], 96372[0], 96373[0], 96374[0], 96375[0], 96376[0], 96377[0], 99151[0], 99152[0], 99153[0], 99155[0], 99156[0], 99157[0], 99201[0], 99202[0], 99203[0], 99204[0], 99205[0], 99211[0], 99212[0], 99213[0], 99214[0], 99215[0], 99217[0], 99218[0], 99219[0], 99220[0], 99221[0], 99222[0], 99223[0], 99224[0], 99225[0], 99226[0], 99231[0], 99232[0], 99233[0], 99234[0], 99235[0], 99236[0], 99238[0], 99239[0], 99281[0], 99282[0], 99283[0], 99284[0], 99285[0], 99304[0], 99305[0], 99306[0], 99307[0], 99308[0], 99309[0], 99310[0], 99315[0], 99318[0], 99324[0], 99325[0], 99326[0], 99327[0], 99328[0], 99334[0], 99335[0], 99336[0], 99337[0], 99341[0], 99342[0], 99343[0], 99347[0], 99348[0], 99349[0], 99354[0], 99355[0], 99356[0], 99357[0], 99358[0], 99359[0], 99415[0], 99416[0], 99446[0], 99447[0], 99448[0], 99449[0], 99451[0], 99452[0], 99466[0], 99468[0], 99469[0], 99471[0], 99472[0], 99475[0], 99476[0], 99477[0], 99478[0], 99479[0], 99480[0], 99483[0], 99485[0], 99497[0], C8921[1], C8922[1], C8923[1], C8924[1], C8925[1], C8926[1], C8927[0], C8929[1], C8930[1], G0380[1], G0381[1], G0382[1], G0383[1], G0384[1], G0406[0], G0407[0], G0408[0], G0425[0], G0426[0], G0427[0], G0463[0], G0500[0], G0508[0], G0509[0]
01486	01996[1], 0213T[1], 0216T[1], 0228T[1], 0230T[1], 31505[1], 31515[1], 31527[1], 31622[1], 31634[1], 31645[1], 31647[1], 36000[1], 36010[0], 36011[1], 36012[1], 36013[1], 36014[1], 36015[1], 36400[1], 36405[1], 36406[1], 36410[1], 36420[1], 36425[1], 36430[1], 36440[1], 36591[0], 36592[0], 36600[1], 36640[1], 43752[1], 43753[1], 43754[1], 61026[1], 61055[1], 62280[1], 62281[1], 62282[1], 62284[1], 62320[1], 62321[1], 62322[1], 62323[1], 62324[1], 62325[1], 62326[1], 62327[1], 64400[1], 64402[1], 64405[1], 64408[1], 64410[1], 64413[1], 64415[1], 64416[1], 64417[1], 64418[1], 64420[1], 64421[1], 64425[1], 64430[1], 64435[1], 64445[1], 64446[1], 64447[1], 64448[1], 64449[1], 64450[1], 64461[1], 64463[1], 64479[1], 64483[1], 64486[1], 64487[1], 64488[1], 64489[1], 64490[1], 64493[1], 64505[1], 64510[1], 64517[1], 64520[1], 64530[1], 64553[1], 64555[1], 67500[1], 76000[1], 76970[1], 76998[0], 77002[0], 90865[1], 92511[1], 92512[1], 92516[1], 92520[1], 92537[1], 92538[1], 92950[1], 92953[1], 92960[1], 92961[1], 93000[1], 93005[1], 93010[1], 93040[1], 93041[1], 93042[1], 93050[0], 93303[0], 93304[0], 93306[1], 93307[1], 93308[1], 93312[1], 93313[1], 93314[1], 93315[1], 93316[1], 93317[1], 93318[0], 93351[1], 93355[0], 93451[1], 93456[1], 93457[1], 93561[0], 93562[0], 93701[0], 93922[1], 93923[1], 93924[1], 93925[1], 93926[1], 93930[1], 93931[1], 93970[1], 93971[1], 93975[1], 93976[1], 93978[1], 93979[1], 93980[1], 93981[1], 94002[1], 94004[1], 94200[1], 94250[0], 94640[1], 94644[1],

0 = Modifier usage not allowed or inappropriate 1 = Modifier usage allowed

CPT © 2018 American Medical Association. All Rights Reserved.

Code 1	Code 2
	94660[1], 94662[1], 94680[1], 94681[1], 94690[1], 94760[0], 94761[0], 94762[1], 94770[1], 95812[0], 95813[0], 95816[0], 95819[0], 95822[0], 95829[0], 95955[0], 95956[0], 95957[0], 96360[0], 96365[0], 96372[0], 96373[0], 96374[0], 96375[0], 96376[0], 96377[0], 99151[0], 99152[0], 99153[0], 99155[0], 99156[0], 99157[0], 99201[0], 99202[0], 99203[0], 99204[0], 99205[0], 99211[0], 99212[0], 99213[0], 99214[0], 99215[0], 99217[0], 99218[0], 99219[0], 99220[0], 99221[0], 99222[0], 99223[0], 99224[0], 99225[0], 99226[0], 99231[0], 99232[0], 99233[0], 99234[0], 99235[0], 99236[0], 99238[0], 99239[0], 99281[0], 99282[0], 99283[0], 99284[0], 99285[0], 99304[0], 99305[0], 99306[0], 99307[0], 99308[0], 99309[0], 99310[0], 99315[0], 99318[0], 99324[0], 99325[0], 99326[0], 99327[0], 99328[0], 99334[0], 99335[0], 99336[0], 99337[0], 99341[0], 99342[0], 99343[0], 99347[0], 99348[0], 99349[0], 99354[0], 99355[0], 99356[0], 99357[0], 99358[0], 99359[0], 99415[0], 99416[0], 99446[0], 99447[0], 99448[0], 99449[0], 99451[0], 99452[0], 99466[0], 99468[0], 99469[0], 99471[0], 99472[0], 99475[0], 99476[0], 99477[0], 99478[0], 99479[0], 99480[0], 99483[0], 99485[0], 99497[0], C8921[1], C8922[1], C8923[1], C8924[1], C8925[1], C8926[1], C8927[0], C8929[1], C8930[1], G0380[1], G0381[1], G0382[1], G0383[1], G0384[1], G0406[0], G0407[0], G0408[0], G0425[0], G0426[0], G0427[0], G0463[0], G0500[0], G0508[0], G0509[0]
01490	01996[1], 0213T[1], 0216T[1], 0228T[1], 0230T[1], 31505[1], 31515[1], 31527[1], 31622[1], 31634[1], 31645[1], 31647[1], 36000[1], 36010[0], 36011[1], 36012[1], 36013[1], 36014[1], 36015[1], 36400[1], 36405[1], 36406[1], 36410[1], 36420[1], 36425[1], 36430[1], 36440[1], 36591[0], 36592[0], 36600[1], 36640[1], 43752[1], 43753[1], 43754[1], 61026[1], 61055[1], 62280[1], 62281[1], 62282[1], 62284[1], 62320[1], 62321[1], 62322[1], 62323[1], 62324[1], 62325[1], 62326[1], 62327[1], 64400[1], 64402[1], 64405[1], 64408[1], 64410[1], 64413[1], 64415[1], 64416[1], 64417[1], 64418[1], 64420[1], 64421[1], 64425[1], 64430[1], 64435[1], 64445[1], 64446[1], 64447[1], 64448[1], 64449[1], 64450[1], 64461[1], 64463[1], 64479[1], 64483[1], 64486[1], 64487[1], 64488[1], 64489[1], 64490[1], 64493[1], 64505[1], 64510[1], 64517[1], 64520[1], 64530[1], 64553[1], 64555[1], 67500[1], 76000[1], 76970[1], 76998[0], 77002[0], 90865[1], 92511[1], 92512[1], 92516[1], 92520[1], 92537[1], 92538[1], 92950[1], 92953[1], 92960[1], 92961[1], 93000[1], 93005[1], 93010[1], 93040[1], 93041[1], 93042[1], 93050[0], 93303[0], 93304[0], 93306[1], 93307[1], 93308[1], 93312[1], 93313[1], 93314[1], 93315[1], 93316[1], 93317[1], 93318[0], 93351[1], 93355[0], 93451[1], 93456[1], 93457[1], 93561[0], 93562[0], 93701[0], 93922[1], 93923[1], 93924[1], 93925[1], 93926[1], 93930[1], 93931[1], 93970[1], 93971[1], 93975[1], 93976[1], 93978[1], 93979[1], 93980[1], 93981[1], 94002[1], 94004[1], 94200[1], 94250[0], 94640[1], 94644[1], 94660[1], 94662[1], 94680[1], 94681[1], 94690[1], 94760[0], 94761[0], 94762[1], 94770[1], 95812[0], 95813[0], 95816[0], 95819[0], 95822[0], 95829[0], 95955[0], 95956[0], 95957[0], 96360[0], 96365[0], 96372[0], 96373[0], 96374[0], 96375[0], 96376[0], 96377[0], 99151[0], 99152[0], 99153[0], 99155[0], 99156[0], 99157[0], 99201[0], 99202[0], 99203[0], 99204[0], 99205[0], 99211[0], 99212[0], 99213[0], 99214[0], 99215[0], 99217[0], 99218[0], 99219[0], 99220[0], 99221[0], 99222[0], 99223[0], 99224[0], 99225[0], 99226[0], 99231[0], 99232[0], 99233[0], 99234[0], 99235[0], 99236[0], 99238[0], 99239[0], 99281[0], 99282[0], 99283[0], 99284[0], 99285[0], 99304[0], 99305[0], 99306[0], 99307[0], 99308[0], 99309[0], 99310[0], 99315[0], 99318[0], 99324[0], 99325[0], 99326[0], 99327[0], 99328[0], 99334[0], 99335[0], 99336[0], 99337[0], 99341[0], 99342[0], 99343[0], 99347[0], 99348[0], 99349[0], 99354[0], 99355[0], 99356[0], 99357[0], 99358[0], 99359[0], 99415[0], 99416[0], 99446[0], 99447[0], 99448[0], 99449[0], 99451[0], 99452[0], 99466[0], 99468[0], 99469[0], 99471[0], 99472[0], 99475[0], 99476[0], 99477[0], 99478[0], 99479[0], 99480[0], 99483[0], 99485[0], 99497[0], C8921[1], C8922[1], C8923[1], C8924[1], C8925[1], C8926[1], C8927[0], C8929[1], C8930[1], G0380[1], G0381[1], G0382[1], G0383[1], G0384[1], G0406[0], G0407[0], G0408[0], G0425[0], G0426[0], G0427[0], G0463[0], G0500[0], G0508[0], G0509[0]
01500	01996[1], 0213T[1], 0216T[1], 0228T[1], 0230T[1], 31505[1], 31515[1], 31527[1], 31622[1], 31634[1], 31645[1], 31647[1], 36000[1], 36010[0], 36011[1], 36012[1], 36013[1], 36014[1], 36015[1], 36400[1], 36405[1], 36406[1], 36410[1], 36420[1], 36425[1], 36430[1], 36440[1], 36591[0], 36592[0], 36600[1], 36640[1], 43752[1], 43753[1], 43754[1], 61026[1], 61055[1], 62280[1], 62281[1], 62282[1], 62284[1], 62320[1], 62321[1], 62322[1], 62323[1], 62324[1], 62325[1], 62326[1], 62327[1], 64400[1], 64402[1], 64405[1], 64408[1], 64410[1], 64413[1], 64415[1], 64416[1], 64417[1], 64418[1], 64420[1], 64421[1], 64425[1], 64430[1], 64435[1], 64445[1], 64446[1], 64447[1], 64448[1], 64449[1], 64450[1], 64461[1], 64463[1], 64479[1], 64483[1], 64486[1], 64487[1], 64488[1], 64489[1], 64490[1], 64493[1], 64505[1], 64510[1], 64517[1], 64520[1], 64530[1], 64553[1], 64555[1], 67500[1], 76000[1], 76970[1], 76998[0], 77002[0], 90865[1], 92511[1], 92512[1], 92516[1], 92520[1], 92537[1], 92538[1], 92950[1], 92953[1], 92960[1], 92961[1], 93000[1], 93005[1], 93010[1], 93040[1], 93041[1], 93042[1], 93050[0], 93303[0], 93304[0], 93306[1], 93307[1], 93308[1], 93312[1], 93313[1], 93314[1], 93315[1], 93316[1], 93317[1], 93318[0], 93351[1], 93355[0], 93451[1], 93456[1], 93457[1], 93561[0], 93562[0], 93701[0], 93922[1], 93923[1], 93924[1], 93925[1], 93926[1], 93930[1], 93931[1], 93970[1], 93971[1], 93975[1], 93976[1], 93978[1], 93979[1], 93980[1], 93981[1], 94002[1], 94004[1], 94200[1], 94250[0], 94640[1], 94644[1], 94660[1], 94662[1], 94680[1], 94681[1], 94690[1], 94760[0], 94761[0], 94762[1], 94770[1], 95812[0], 95813[0], 95816[0], 95819[0], 95822[0], 95829[0], 95955[0], 95956[0], 95957[0], 96360[0], 96365[0], 96372[0], 96373[0], 96374[0], 96375[0], 96376[0], 96377[0], 99151[0], 99152[0], 99153[0], 99155[0], 99156[0], 99157[0], 99201[0], 99202[0], 99203[0], 99204[0], 99205[0], 99211[0], 99212[0], 99213[0], 99214[0], 99215[0], 99217[0], 99218[0], 99219[0], 99220[0], 99221[0], 99222[0], 99223[0], 99224[0], 99225[0], 99226[0], 99231[0], 99232[0], 99233[0], 99234[0], 99235[0], 99236[0], 99238[0], 99239[0], 99281[0], 99282[0], 99283[0], 99284[0], 99285[0], 99304[0], 99305[0], 99306[0], 99307[0], 99308[0], 99309[0], 99310[0], 99315[0], 99318[0], 99324[0], 99325[0], 99326[0], 99327[0], 99328[0], 99334[0], 99335[0], 99336[0], 99337[0], 99341[0], 99342[0], 99343[0], 99347[0], 99348[0], 99349[0], 99354[0], 99355[0], 99356[0], 99357[0], 99358[0], 99359[0], 99415[0], 99416[0], 99446[0], 99447[0], 99448[0], 99449[0], 99451[0], 99452[0], 99466[0], 99468[0], 99469[0], 99471[0], 99472[0], 99475[0], 99476[0], 99477[0], 99478[0], 99479[0], 99480[0], 99483[0], 99485[0], 99497[0], C8921[1], C8922[1], C8923[1], C8924[1], C8925[1], C8926[1], C8927[0], C8929[1], C8930[1], G0380[1], G0381[1], G0382[1], G0383[1], G0384[1], G0406[0], G0407[0], G0408[0], G0425[0], G0426[0], G0427[0], G0463[0], G0500[0], G0508[0], G0509[0]
01502	01996[1], 0213T[1], 0216T[1], 0228T[1], 0230T[1], 31505[1], 31515[1], 31527[1], 31622[1], 31634[1], 31645[1], 31647[1], 36000[1], 36010[0], 36011[1], 36012[1], 36013[1], 36014[1], 36015[1], 36400[1], 36405[1], 36406[1], 36410[1], 36420[1], 36425[1], 36430[1], 36440[1], 36591[0], 36592[0], 36600[1], 36640[1], 43752[1], 43753[1], 43754[1], 61026[1], 61055[1], 62280[1], 62281[1], 62282[1], 62284[1], 62320[1], 62321[1], 62322[1], 62323[1], 62324[1], 62325[1], 62326[1], 62327[1], 64400[1], 64402[1], 64405[1], 64408[1], 64410[1], 64413[1], 64415[1], 64416[1], 64417[1], 64418[1], 64420[1], 64421[1], 64425[1], 64430[1], 64435[1], 64445[1], 64446[1], 64447[1], 64448[1], 64449[1], 64450[1], 64461[1], 64463[1], 64479[1], 64483[1], 64486[1], 64487[1], 64488[1], 64489[1], 64490[1], 64493[1], 64505[1], 64510[1], 64517[1], 64520[1], 64530[1], 64553[1], 64555[1], 67500[1], 76000[1], 76970[1], 76998[0], 77002[0], 90865[1], 92511[1], 92512[1], 92516[1], 92520[1], 92537[1], 92538[1], 92950[1], 92953[1], 92960[1], 92961[1], 93000[1], 93005[1], 93010[1], 93040[1], 93041[1], 93042[1], 93050[0], 93303[0], 93304[0], 93306[1], 93307[1], 93308[1], 93312[1], 93313[1], 93314[1], 93315[1], 93316[1], 93317[1], 93318[0], 93351[1], 93355[0], 93451[1], 93456[1], 93457[1], 93561[0], 93562[0], 93701[0], 93922[1], 93923[1], 93924[1], 93925[1], 93926[1], 93930[1], 93931[1], 93970[1], 93971[1], 93975[1], 93976[1], 93978[1], 93979[1], 93980[1], 93981[1], 94002[1], 94004[1], 94200[1], 94250[0], 94640[1], 94644[1], 94660[1], 94662[1], 94680[1], 94681[1], 94690[1], 94760[0], 94761[0], 94762[1], 94770[1], 95812[0], 95813[0], 95816[0], 95819[0], 95822[0], 95829[0], 95955[0], 95956[0], 95957[0], 96360[0], 96365[0], 96372[0], 96373[0], 96374[0], 96375[0], 96376[0], 96377[0], 99151[0], 99152[0], 99153[0], 99155[0], 99156[0], 99157[0], 99201[0], 99202[0], 99203[0], 99204[0], 99205[0], 99211[0], 99212[0], 99213[0], 99214[0], 99215[0], 99217[0], 99218[0], 99219[0], 99220[0], 99221[0], 99222[0], 99223[0], 99224[0], 99225[0], 99226[0], 99231[0], 99232[0], 99233[0], 99234[0], 99235[0], 99236[0], 99238[0], 99239[0], 99281[0], 99282[0], 99283[0], 99284[0], 99285[0], 99304[0], 99305[0], 99306[0], 99307[0], 99308[0], 99309[0], 99310[0], 99315[0], 99318[0], 99324[0], 99325[0], 99326[0], 99327[0], 99328[0], 99334[0], 99335[0], 99336[0], 99337[0], 99341[0], 99342[0], 99343[0], 99347[0], 99348[0], 99349[0], 99354[0], 99355[0], 99356[0], 99357[0], 99358[0], 99359[0], 99415[0], 99416[0], 99446[0], 99447[0], 99448[0], 99449[0], 99451[0], 99452[0], 99466[0], 99468[0], 99469[0], 99471[0], 99472[0], 99475[0], 99476[0], 99477[0], 99478[0], 99479[0], 99480[0], 99483[0], 99485[0], 99497[0], C8921[1], C8922[1], C8923[1], C8924[1], C8925[1], C8926[1], C8927[0], C8929[1], C8930[1], G0380[1], G0381[1], G0382[1], G0383[1], G0384[1], G0406[0], G0407[0], G0408[0], G0425[0], G0426[0], G0427[0], G0463[0], G0500[0], G0508[0], G0509[0]
01520	01996[1], 0213T[1], 0216T[1], 0228T[1], 0230T[1], 31505[1], 31515[1], 31527[1], 31622[1], 31634[1], 31645[1], 31647[1], 36000[1], 36010[0], 36011[1], 36012[1], 36013[1], 36014[1], 36015[1], 36400[1], 36405[1], 36406[1], 36410[1], 36420[1], 36425[1], 36430[1], 36440[1], 36591[0], 36592[0], 36600[1], 36640[1], 43752[1], 43753[1], 43754[1], 61026[1], 61055[1], 62280[1], 62281[1], 62282[1], 62284[1], 62320[1], 62321[1], 62322[1], 62323[1], 62324[1], 62325[1], 62326[1], 62327[1], 64400[1], 64402[1], 64405[1], 64408[1], 64410[1], 64413[1], 64415[1], 64416[1], 64417[1], 64418[1], 64420[1], 64421[1], 64425[1], 64430[1], 64435[1], 64445[1], 64446[1], 64447[1], 64448[1], 64449[1], 64450[1], 64461[1], 64463[1], 64479[1], 64483[1], 64486[1], 64487[1], 64488[1], 64489[1], 64490[1], 64493[1], 64505[1], 64510[1], 64517[1], 64520[1], 64530[1], 64553[1], 64555[1], 67500[1], 76000[1], 76970[1], 76998[0], 77002[0], 90865[1], 92511[1], 92512[1], 92516[1], 92520[1], 92537[1], 92538[1], 92950[1], 92953[1], 92960[1], 92961[1], 93000[1], 93005[1], 93010[1], 93040[1], 93041[1], 93042[1], 93050[0], 93303[0], 93304[0], 93306[1], 93307[1], 93308[1], 93312[1], 93313[1], 93314[1], 93315[1], 93316[1], 93317[1], 93318[0], 93351[1], 93355[0], 93451[1], 93456[1], 93457[1], 93561[0], 93562[0], 93701[0], 93922[1], 93923[1], 93924[1], 93925[1], 93926[1], 93930[1], 93931[1], 93970[1], 93971[1], 93975[1], 93976[1], 93978[1], 93979[1], 93980[1], 93981[1], 94002[1], 94004[1], 94200[1], 94250[0], 94640[1], 94644[1], 94660[1], 94662[1], 94680[1], 94681[1], 94690[1], 94760[0], 94761[0], 94762[1], 94770[1], 95812[0], 95813[0], 95816[0], 95819[0], 95822[0], 95829[0], 95955[0], 95956[0], 95957[0], 96360[0], 96365[0], 96372[0], 96373[0], 96374[0], 96375[0], 96376[0], 96377[0], 99151[0], 99152[0], 99153[0], 99155[0], 99156[0], 99157[0], 99201[0], 99202[0], 99203[0], 99204[0], 99205[0], 99211[0], 99212[0], 99213[0], 99214[0], 99215[0], 99217[0], 99218[0], 99219[0], 99220[0], 99221[0], 99222[0], 99223[0], 99224[0], 99225[0], 99226[0], 99231[0], 99232[0], 99233[0], 99234[0], 99235[0], 99236[0], 99238[0], 99239[0], 99281[0], 99282[0], 99283[0], 99284[0], 99285[0], 99304[0], 99305[0], 99306[0], 99307[0], 99308[0], 99309[0], 99310[0], 99315[0], 99318[0], 99324[0], 99325[0], 99326[0], 99327[0], 99328[0], 99334[0], 99335[0], 99336[0], 99337[0], 99341[0], 99342[0], 99343[0], 99347[0], 99348[0], 99349[0], 99354[0], 99355[0], 99356[0], 99357[0], 99358[0], 99359[0], 99415[0], 99416[0], 99446[0], 99447[0], 99448[0], 99449[0], 99451[0], 99452[0], 99466[0], 99468[0], 99469[0], 99471[0], 99472[0], 99475[0], 99476[0], 99477[0], 99478[0], 99479[0], 99480[0], 99483[0], 99485[0], 99497[0], C8921[1], C8922[1], C8923[1],

0 = Modifier usage not allowed or inappropriate 1 = Modifier usage allowed

CPT © 2018 American Medical Association. All Rights Reserved.

Code 1	Code 2
	C8924[1], C8925[1], C8926[1], C8927[0], C8929[1], C8930[1], G0380[1], G0381[1], G0382[1], G0383[1], G0384[1], G0406[0], G0407[0], G0408[0], G0425[0], G0426[0], G0427[0], G0463[0], G0500[0], G0508[0], G0509[0]
01522	01996[1], 0213T[1], 0216T[1], 0228T[1], 0230T[1], 31505[1], 31515[1], 31527[1], 31622[1], 31634[1], 31645[1], 31647[1], 36000[1], 36010[0], 36011[1], 36012[1], 36013[1], 36014[1], 36015[1], 36400[1], 36405[1], 36406[1], 36410[1], 36420[1], 36425[1], 36430[1], 36440[1], 36591[0], 36592[0], 36600[1], 36640[1], 43752[1], 43753[1], 43754[1], 61026[1], 61055[1], 62280[1], 62281[1], 62282[1], 62284[1], 62320[1], 62321[1], 62322[1], 62323[1], 62324[1], 62325[1], 62326[1], 62327[1], 64400[1], 64402[1], 64405[1], 64408[1], 64410[1], 64413[1], 64415[1], 64416[1], 64417[1], 64418[1], 64420[1], 64421[1], 64425[1], 64430[1], 64435[1], 64445[1], 64446[1], 64447[1], 64448[1], 64449[1], 64450[1], 64461[1], 64463[1], 64479[1], 64483[1], 64486[1], 64487[1], 64488[1], 64489[1], 64490[1], 64493[1], 64505[1], 64510[1], 64517[1], 64520[1], 64530[1], 64553[1], 64555[1], 67500[1], 76000[1], 76970[1], 76998[0], 77002[0], 90865[1], 92511[1], 92512[1], 92516[1], 92520[1], 92537[1], 92538[1], 92950[1], 92953[1], 92960[1], 92961[1], 93000[1], 93005[1], 93010[1], 93040[1], 93041[1], 93042[1], 93050[0], 93303[0], 93304[0], 93306[1], 93307[1], 93308[1], 93312[1], 93313[1], 93314[1], 93315[1], 93316[1], 93317[1], 93318[0], 93351[1], 93355[0], 93451[1], 93456[1], 93457[1], 93561[0], 93562[0], 93701[0], 93922[1], 93923[1], 93924[1], 93925[1], 93926[1], 93930[1], 93931[1], 93970[1], 93971[1], 93975[1], 93976[1], 93978[1], 93979[1], 93980[1], 93981[1], 94002[1], 94004[1], 94200[1], 94250[0], 94640[1], 94644[1], 94660[1], 94662[1], 94680[1], 94681[1], 94690[1], 94760[0], 94761[0], 94762[1], 94770[1], 95812[0], 95813[0], 95816[0], 95819[0], 95822[0], 95829[0], 95955[0], 95956[0], 95957[0], 96360[0], 96365[0], 96372[0], 96373[0], 96374[0], 96375[0], 96376[0], 96377[0], 99151[0], 99152[0], 99153[0], 99155[0], 99156[0], 99157[0], 99201[0], 99202[0], 99203[0], 99204[0], 99205[0], 99211[0], 99212[0], 99213[0], 99214[0], 99215[0], 99217[0], 99218[0], 99219[0], 99220[0], 99221[0], 99222[0], 99223[0], 99224[0], 99225[0], 99226[0], 99231[0], 99232[0], 99233[0], 99234[0], 99235[0], 99236[0], 99238[0], 99239[0], 99281[0], 99282[0], 99283[0], 99284[0], 99285[0], 99304[0], 99305[0], 99306[0], 99307[0], 99308[0], 99309[0], 99310[0], 99315[0], 99318[0], 99324[0], 99325[0], 99326[0], 99327[0], 99328[0], 99334[0], 99335[0], 99336[0], 99337[0], 99341[0], 99342[0], 99343[0], 99347[0], 99348[0], 99349[0], 99354[0], 99355[0], 99356[0], 99357[0], 99358[0], 99359[0], 99415[0], 99416[0], 99446[0], 99447[0], 99448[0], 99449[0], 99451[0], 99452[0], 99466[0], 99468[0], 99469[0], 99471[0], 99472[0], 99475[0], 99476[0], 99477[0], 99478[0], 99479[0], 99480[0], 99483[0], 99485[0], 99497[0], C8921[1], C8922[1], C8923[1], C8924[1], C8925[1], C8926[1], C8927[0], C8929[1], C8930[1], G0380[1], G0381[1], G0382[1], G0383[1], G0384[1], G0406[0], G0407[0], G0408[0], G0425[0], G0426[0], G0427[0], G0463[0], G0500[0], G0508[0], G0509[0]
01610	01996[1], 0213T[1], 0216T[1], 0228T[1], 0230T[1], 0333T[0], 0464T[0], 31505[1], 31515[1], 31527[1], 31622[1], 31634[1], 31645[1], 31647[1], 36000[1], 36010[0], 36011[1], 36012[1], 36013[1], 36014[1], 36015[1], 36400[1], 36405[1], 36406[1], 36410[1], 36420[1], 36425[1], 36430[1], 36440[1], 36591[0], 36592[0], 36600[1], 36640[1], 43752[1], 43753[1], 43754[1], 61026[1], 61055[1], 62280[1], 62281[1], 62282[1], 62284[1], 62320[1], 62321[1], 62322[1], 62323[1], 62324[1], 62325[1], 62326[1], 62327[1], 64400[1], 64402[1], 64405[1], 64408[1], 64410[1], 64413[1], 64415[1], 64416[1], 64417[1], 64418[1], 64420[1], 64421[1], 64425[1], 64430[1], 64435[1], 64445[1], 64446[1], 64447[1], 64448[1], 64449[1], 64450[1], 64461[1], 64463[1], 64479[1], 64483[1], 64486[1], 64487[1], 64488[1], 64489[1], 64490[1], 64493[1], 64505[1], 64510[1], 64517[1], 64520[1], 64530[1], 64553[1], 64555[1], 67500[1], 76000[1], 76970[1], 76998[0], 77002[0], 90865[1], 92511[1], 92512[1], 92516[1], 92520[1], 92537[1], 92538[1], 92585[0], 92950[1], 92953[1], 92960[1], 92961[1], 93000[1], 93005[1], 93010[1], 93040[1], 93041[1], 93042[1], 93050[0], 93303[0], 93304[0], 93306[1], 93307[1], 93308[1], 93312[1], 93313[1], 93314[1], 93315[1], 93316[1], 93317[1], 93318[0], 93351[1], 93355[0], 93451[1], 93456[1], 93457[1], 93561[0], 93562[0], 93701[0], 93922[1], 93923[1], 93924[1], 93925[1], 93926[1], 93930[1], 93931[1], 93970[1], 93971[1], 93975[1], 93976[1], 93978[1], 93979[1], 93980[1], 93981[1], 94002[1], 94004[1], 94200[1], 94250[0], 94640[1], 94644[1], 94660[1], 94662[1], 94680[1], 94681[1], 94690[1], 94760[0], 94761[0], 94762[1], 94770[1], 95812[0], 95813[0], 95816[0], 95819[0], 95822[0], 95829[0], 95860[0], 95861[0], 95863[0], 95864[0], 95865[0], 95866[0], 95867[0], 95868[0], 95869[0], 95870[0], 95907[0], 95908[0], 95909[0], 95910[0], 95911[0], 95912[0], 95913[0], 95925[0], 95926[0], 95927[0], 95928[0], 95929[0], 95930[0], 95933[0], 95937[0], 95938[0], 95939[0], 95940[0], 95955[0], 95956[0], 95957[0], 96360[0], 96365[0], 96372[0], 96373[0], 96374[0], 96375[0], 96376[0], 96377[0], 99151[0], 99152[0], 99153[0], 99155[0], 99156[0], 99157[0], 99201[0], 99202[0], 99203[0], 99204[0], 99205[0], 99211[0], 99212[0], 99213[0], 99214[0], 99215[0], 99217[0], 99218[0], 99219[0], 99220[0], 99221[0], 99222[0], 99223[0], 99224[0], 99225[0], 99226[0], 99231[0], 99232[0], 99233[0], 99234[0], 99235[0], 99236[0], 99238[0], 99239[0], 99281[0], 99282[0], 99283[0], 99284[0], 99285[0], 99304[0], 99305[0], 99306[0], 99307[0], 99308[0], 99309[0], 99310[0], 99315[0], 99318[0], 99324[0], 99325[0], 99326[0], 99327[0], 99328[0], 99334[0], 99335[0], 99336[0], 99337[0], 99341[0], 99342[0], 99343[0], 99347[0], 99348[0], 99349[0], 99354[0], 99355[0], 99356[0], 99357[0], 99358[0], 99359[0], 99415[0], 99416[0], 99446[0], 99447[0], 99448[0], 99449[0], 99451[0], 99452[0], 99466[0], 99468[0], 99469[0], 99471[0], 99472[0], 99475[0], 99476[0], 99477[0], 99478[0], 99479[0], 99480[0], 99483[0], 99485[0], 99497[0], C8921[1], C8922[1], C8923[1], C8924[1], C8925[1], C8926[1], C8927[0], C8929[1], C8930[1], G0380[1], G0381[1], G0382[1], G0383[1], G0384[1], G0406[0], G0407[0], G0408[0], G0425[0], G0426[0], G0427[0], G0453[0], G0463[0], G0500[0], G0508[0], G0509[0]
01620	01996[1], 0213T[1], 0216T[1], 0228T[1], 0230T[1], 31505[1], 31515[1], 31527[1], 31622[1], 31634[1], 31645[1], 31647[1], 36000[1], 36010[0], 36011[1], 36012[1], 36013[1], 36014[1], 36015[1], 36400[1], 36405[1], 36406[1], 36410[1], 36420[1], 36425[1], 36430[1], 36440[1], 36591[0], 36592[0], 36600[1], 36640[1], 43752[1], 43753[1], 43754[1], 61026[1], 61055[1], 62280[1], 62281[1], 62282[1], 62284[1], 62320[1], 62321[1], 62322[1], 62323[1], 62324[1], 62325[1], 62326[1], 62327[1], 64400[1], 64402[1], 64405[1], 64408[1], 64410[1], 64413[1], 64415[1], 64416[1], 64417[1], 64418[1], 64420[1], 64421[1], 64425[1], 64430[1], 64435[1], 64445[1], 64446[1], 64447[1], 64448[1], 64449[1], 64450[1], 64461[1], 64463[1], 64479[1], 64483[1], 64486[1], 64487[1], 64488[1], 64489[1], 64490[1], 64493[1], 64505[1], 64510[1], 64517[1], 64520[1], 64530[1], 64553[1], 64555[1], 67500[1], 76000[1], 76970[1], 76998[0], 77002[0], 90865[1], 92511[1], 92512[1], 92516[1], 92520[1], 92537[1], 92538[1], 92950[1], 92953[1], 92960[1], 92961[1], 93000[1], 93005[1], 93010[1], 93040[1], 93041[1], 93042[1], 93050[0], 93303[0], 93304[0], 93306[1], 93307[1], 93308[1], 93312[1], 93313[1], 93314[1], 93315[1], 93316[1], 93317[1], 93318[0], 93351[1], 93355[0], 93451[1], 93456[1], 93457[1], 93561[0], 93562[0], 93701[0], 93922[1], 93923[1], 93924[1], 93925[1], 93926[1], 93930[1], 93931[1], 93970[1], 93971[1], 93975[1], 93976[1], 93978[1], 93979[1], 93980[1], 93981[1], 94002[1], 94004[1], 94200[1], 94250[0], 94640[1], 94644[1], 94660[1], 94662[1], 94680[1], 94681[1], 94690[1], 94760[0], 94761[0], 94762[1], 94770[1], 95812[0], 95813[0], 95816[0], 95819[0], 95822[0], 95829[0], 95955[0], 95956[0], 95957[0], 96360[0], 96365[0], 96372[0], 96373[0], 96374[0], 96375[0], 96376[0], 96377[0], 99151[0], 99152[0], 99153[0], 99155[0], 99156[0], 99157[0], 99201[0], 99202[0], 99203[0], 99204[0], 99205[0], 99211[0], 99212[0], 99213[0], 99214[0], 99215[0], 99217[0], 99218[0], 99219[0], 99220[0], 99221[0], 99222[0], 99223[0], 99224[0], 99225[0], 99226[0], 99231[0], 99232[0], 99233[0], 99234[0], 99235[0], 99236[0], 99238[0], 99239[0], 99281[0], 99282[0], 99283[0], 99284[0], 99285[0], 99304[0], 99305[0], 99306[0], 99307[0], 99308[0], 99309[0], 99310[0], 99315[0], 99318[0], 99324[0], 99325[0], 99326[0], 99327[0], 99328[0], 99334[0], 99335[0], 99336[0], 99337[0], 99341[0], 99342[0], 99343[0], 99347[0], 99348[0], 99349[0], 99354[0], 99355[0], 99356[0], 99357[0], 99358[0], 99359[0], 99415[0], 99416[0], 99446[0], 99447[0], 99448[0], 99449[0], 99451[0], 99452[0], 99466[0], 99468[0], 99469[0], 99471[0], 99472[0], 99475[0], 99476[0], 99477[0], 99478[0], 99479[0], 99480[0], 99483[0], 99485[0], 99497[0], C8921[1], C8922[1], C8923[1], C8924[1], C8925[1], C8926[1], C8927[0], C8929[1], C8930[1], G0380[1], G0381[1], G0382[1], G0383[1], G0384[1], G0406[0], G0407[0], G0408[0], G0425[0], G0426[0], G0427[0], G0463[0], G0500[0], G0508[0], G0509[0]
01622	01996[1], 0213T[1], 0216T[1], 0228T[1], 0230T[1], 31505[1], 31515[1], 31527[1], 31622[1], 31634[1], 31645[1], 31647[1], 36000[1], 36010[0], 36011[1], 36012[1], 36013[1], 36014[1], 36015[1], 36400[1], 36405[1], 36406[1], 36410[1], 36420[1], 36425[1], 36430[1], 36440[1], 36591[0], 36592[0], 36600[1], 36640[1], 43752[1], 43753[1], 43754[1], 61026[1], 61055[1], 62280[1], 62281[1], 62282[1], 62284[1], 62320[1], 62321[1], 62322[1], 62323[1], 62324[1], 62325[1], 62326[1], 62327[1], 64400[1], 64402[1], 64405[1], 64408[1], 64410[1], 64413[1], 64415[1], 64416[1], 64417[1], 64418[1], 64420[1], 64421[1], 64425[1], 64430[1], 64435[1], 64445[1], 64446[1], 64447[1], 64448[1], 64449[1], 64450[1], 64461[1], 64463[1], 64479[1], 64483[1], 64486[1], 64487[1], 64488[1], 64489[1], 64490[1], 64493[1], 64505[1], 64510[1], 64517[1], 64520[1], 64530[1], 64553[1], 64555[1], 67500[1], 76000[1], 76970[1], 76998[0], 77002[0], 90865[1], 92511[1], 92512[1], 92516[1], 92520[1], 92537[1], 92538[1], 92950[1], 92953[1], 92960[1], 92961[1], 93000[1], 93005[1], 93010[1], 93040[1], 93041[1], 93042[1], 93050[0], 93303[0], 93304[0], 93306[1], 93307[1], 93308[1], 93312[1], 93313[1], 93314[1], 93315[1], 93316[1], 93317[1], 93318[0], 93351[1], 93355[0], 93451[1], 93456[1], 93457[1], 93561[0], 93562[0], 93701[0], 93922[1], 93923[1], 93924[1], 93925[1], 93926[1], 93930[1], 93931[1], 93970[1], 93971[1], 93975[1], 93976[1], 93978[1], 93979[1], 93980[1], 93981[1], 94002[1], 94004[1], 94200[1], 94250[0], 94640[1], 94644[1], 94660[1], 94662[1], 94680[1], 94681[1], 94690[1], 94760[0], 94761[0], 94762[1], 94770[1], 95812[0], 95813[0], 95816[0], 95819[0], 95822[0], 95829[0], 95955[0], 95956[0], 95957[0], 96360[0], 96365[0], 96372[0], 96373[0], 96374[0], 96375[0], 96376[0], 96377[0], 99151[0], 99152[0], 99153[0], 99155[0], 99156[0], 99157[0], 99201[0], 99202[0], 99203[0], 99204[0], 99205[0], 99211[0], 99212[0], 99213[0], 99214[0], 99215[0], 99217[0], 99218[0], 99219[0], 99220[0], 99221[0], 99222[0], 99223[0], 99224[0], 99225[0], 99226[0], 99231[0], 99232[0], 99233[0], 99234[0], 99235[0], 99236[0], 99238[0], 99239[0], 99281[0], 99282[0], 99283[0], 99284[0], 99285[0], 99304[0], 99305[0], 99306[0], 99307[0], 99308[0], 99309[0], 99310[0], 99315[0], 99318[0], 99324[0], 99325[0], 99326[0], 99327[0], 99328[0], 99334[0], 99335[0], 99336[0], 99337[0], 99341[0], 99342[0], 99343[0], 99347[0], 99348[0], 99349[0], 99354[0], 99355[0], 99356[0], 99357[0], 99358[0], 99359[0], 99415[0], 99416[0], 99446[0], 99447[0], 99448[0], 99449[0], 99451[0], 99452[0], 99466[0], 99468[0], 99469[0], 99471[0], 99472[0], 99475[0], 99476[0], 99477[0], 99478[0], 99479[0], 99480[0], 99483[0], 99485[0], 99497[0], C8921[1], C8922[1], C8923[1], C8924[1], C8925[1], C8926[1], C8927[0], C8929[1], C8930[1], G0380[1], G0381[1], G0382[1], G0383[1], G0384[1], G0406[0], G0407[0], G0408[0], G0425[0], G0426[0], G0427[0], G0463[0], G0500[0], G0508[0], G0509[0]
01630	01622[1], 01996[1], 0213T[1], 0216T[1], 0228T[1], 0230T[1], 31505[1], 31515[1], 31527[1], 31622[1], 31634[1], 31645[1], 31647[1], 36000[1], 36010[0], 36011[1], 36012[1], 36013[1], 36014[1], 36015[1], 36400[1], 36405[1], 36406[1], 36410[1], 36420[1], 36425[1], 36430[1], 36440[1], 36591[0], 36592[0], 36600[1], 36640[1], 43752[1], 43753[1], 43754[1], 61026[1], 61055[1], 62280[1], 62281[1], 62282[1], 62284[1], 62320[1], 62321[1], 62322[1], 62323[1], 62324[1], 62325[1], 62326[1], 62327[1], 64400[1], 64402[1], 64405[1], 64408[1], 64410[1], 64413[1], 64415[1], 64416[1], 64417[1], 64418[1], 64420[1],

0 = Modifier usage not allowed or inappropriate 1 = Modifier usage allowed

CPT © 2018 American Medical Association. All Rights Reserved.

Code 1	Code 2
	64421[1], 64425[1], 64430[1], 64435[1], 64445[1], 64446[1], 64447[1], 64448[1], 64449[1], 64450[1], 64461[1], 64463[1], 64479[1], 64483[1], 64486[1], 64487[1], 64488[1], 64489[1], 64490[1], 64493[1], 64505[1], 64510[1], 64517[1], 64520[1], 64530[1], 64553[1], 64555[1], 67500[1], 76000[1], 76970[1], 76998[0], 77002[0], 90865[1], 92511[1], 92512[1], 92516[1], 92520[1], 92537[1], 92538[1], 92950[1], 92953[1], 92960[1], 92961[1], 93000[1], 93005[1], 93010[1], 93040[1], 93041[1], 93042[1], 93050[0], 93303[0], 93304[0], 93306[1], 93307[1], 93308[1], 93312[1], 93313[1], 93314[1], 93315[1], 93316[1], 93317[1], 93318[0], 93351[1], 93355[0], 93451[1], 93456[1], 93457[1], 93561[0], 93562[0], 93701[0], 93922[1], 93923[1], 93924[1], 93925[1], 93926[1], 93930[1], 93931[1], 93970[1], 93971[1], 93975[1], 93976[1], 93978[1], 93979[1], 93980[1], 93981[1], 94002[1], 94004[1], 94200[1], 94250[0], 94640[1], 94644[1], 94660[1], 94662[1], 94680[1], 94681[1], 94690[1], 94760[0], 94761[0], 94762[1], 94770[1], 95812[0], 95813[0], 95816[0], 95819[0], 95822[0], 95829[0], 95955[0], 95956[0], 95957[0], 96360[0], 96365[0], 96372[0], 96373[0], 96374[0], 96375[0], 96376[0], 96377[0], 99151[0], 99152[0], 99153[0], 99155[0], 99156[0], 99157[0], 99201[0], 99202[0], 99203[0], 99204[0], 99205[0], 99211[0], 99212[0], 99213[0], 99214[0], 99215[0], 99217[0], 99218[0], 99219[0], 99220[0], 99221[0], 99222[0], 99223[0], 99224[0], 99225[0], 99226[0], 99231[0], 99232[0], 99233[0], 99234[0], 99235[0], 99236[0], 99238[0], 99239[0], 99281[0], 99282[0], 99283[0], 99284[0], 99285[0], 99304[0], 99305[0], 99306[0], 99307[0], 99308[0], 99309[0], 99310[0], 99315[0], 99318[0], 99324[0], 99325[0], 99326[0], 99327[0], 99328[0], 99334[0], 99335[0], 99336[0], 99337[0], 99341[0], 99342[0], 99343[0], 99347[0], 99348[0], 99349[0], 99354[0], 99355[0], 99356[0], 99357[0], 99358[0], 99359[0], 99415[0], 99416[0], 99446[0], 99447[0], 99448[0], 99449[0], 99451[0], 99452[0], 99466[0], 99468[0], 99469[0], 99471[0], 99472[0], 99475[0], 99476[0], 99477[0], 99478[0], 99479[0], 99480[0], 99483[0], 99485[0], 99497[0], C8921[1], C8922[1], C8923[1], C8924[1], C8925[1], C8926[1], C8927[0], C8929[1], C8930[1], G0380[1], G0381[1], G0382[1], G0383[1], G0384[1], G0406[0], G0407[0], G0408[0], G0425[0], G0426[0], G0427[0], G0463[0], G0500[0], G0508[0], G0509[0]
01634	01996[1], 0213T[1], 0216T[1], 0228T[1], 0230T[1], 31505[1], 31515[1], 31527[1], 31622[1], 31634[1], 31645[1], 31647[1], 36000[1], 36010[0], 36011[1], 36012[1], 36013[1], 36014[1], 36015[1], 36400[1], 36405[1], 36406[1], 36410[1], 36420[1], 36425[1], 36430[1], 36440[1], 36591[0], 36592[0], 36600[1], 36640[1], 43752[1], 43753[1], 43754[1], 61026[1], 61055[1], 62280[1], 62281[1], 62282[1], 62284[1], 62320[1], 62321[1], 62322[1], 62323[1], 62324[1], 62325[1], 62326[1], 62327[1], 64400[1], 64402[1], 64405[1], 64408[1], 64410[1], 64413[1], 64415[1], 64416[1], 64417[1], 64418[1], 64420[1], 64421[1], 64425[1], 64430[1], 64435[1], 64445[1], 64446[1], 64447[1], 64448[1], 64449[1], 64450[1], 64461[1], 64463[1], 64479[1], 64483[1], 64486[1], 64487[1], 64488[1], 64489[1], 64490[1], 64493[1], 64505[1], 64510[1], 64517[1], 64520[1], 64530[1], 64553[1], 64555[1], 67500[1], 76000[1], 76970[1], 76998[0], 77002[0], 90865[1], 92511[1], 92512[1], 92516[1], 92520[1], 92537[1], 92538[1], 92950[1], 92953[1], 92960[1], 92961[1], 93000[1], 93005[1], 93010[1], 93040[1], 93041[1], 93042[1], 93050[0], 93303[0], 93304[0], 93306[1], 93307[1], 93308[1], 93312[1], 93313[1], 93314[1], 93315[1], 93316[1], 93317[1], 93318[0], 93351[1], 93355[0], 93451[1], 93456[1], 93457[1], 93561[0], 93562[0], 93701[0], 93922[1], 93923[1], 93924[1], 93925[1], 93926[1], 93930[1], 93931[1], 93970[1], 93971[1], 93975[1], 93976[1], 93978[1], 93979[1], 93980[1], 93981[1], 94002[1], 94004[1], 94200[1], 94250[0], 94640[1], 94644[1], 94660[1], 94662[1], 94680[1], 94681[1], 94690[1], 94760[0], 94761[0], 94762[1], 94770[1], 95812[0], 95813[0], 95816[0], 95819[0], 95822[0], 95829[0], 95955[0], 95956[0], 95957[0], 96360[0], 96365[0], 96372[0], 96373[0], 96374[0], 96375[0], 96376[0], 96377[0], 99151[0], 99152[0], 99153[0], 99155[0], 99156[0], 99157[0], 99201[0], 99202[0], 99203[0], 99204[0], 99205[0], 99211[0], 99212[0], 99213[0], 99214[0], 99215[0], 99217[0], 99218[0], 99219[0], 99220[0], 99221[0], 99222[0], 99223[0], 99224[0], 99225[0], 99226[0], 99231[0], 99232[0], 99233[0], 99234[0], 99235[0], 99236[0], 99238[0], 99239[0], 99281[0], 99282[0], 99283[0], 99284[0], 99285[0], 99304[0], 99305[0], 99306[0], 99307[0], 99308[0], 99309[0], 99310[0], 99315[0], 99318[0], 99324[0], 99325[0], 99326[0], 99327[0], 99328[0], 99334[0], 99335[0], 99336[0], 99337[0], 99341[0], 99342[0], 99343[0], 99347[0], 99348[0], 99349[0], 99354[0], 99355[0], 99356[0], 99357[0], 99358[0], 99359[0], 99415[0], 99416[0], 99446[0], 99447[0], 99448[0], 99449[0], 99451[0], 99452[0], 99466[0], 99468[0], 99469[0], 99471[0], 99472[0], 99475[0], 99476[0], 99477[0], 99478[0], 99479[0], 99480[0], 99483[0], 99485[0], 99497[0], C8921[1], C8922[1], C8923[1], C8924[1], C8925[1], C8926[1], C8927[0], C8929[1], C8930[1], G0380[1], G0381[1], G0382[1], G0383[1], G0384[1], G0406[0], G0407[0], G0408[0], G0425[0], G0426[0], G0427[0], G0463[0], G0500[0], G0508[0], G0509[0]
01636	01996[1], 0213T[1], 0216T[1], 0228T[1], 0230T[1], 31505[1], 31515[1], 31527[1], 31622[1], 31634[1], 31645[1], 31647[1], 36000[1], 36010[0], 36011[1], 36012[1], 36013[1], 36014[1], 36015[1], 36400[1], 36405[1], 36406[1], 36410[1], 36420[1], 36425[1], 36430[1], 36440[1], 36591[0], 36592[0], 36600[1], 36640[1], 43752[1], 43753[1], 43754[1], 61026[1], 61055[1], 62280[1], 62281[1], 62282[1], 62284[1], 62320[1], 62321[1], 62322[1], 62323[1], 62324[1], 62325[1], 62326[1], 62327[1], 64400[1], 64402[1], 64405[1], 64408[1], 64410[1], 64413[1], 64415[1], 64416[1], 64417[1], 64418[1], 64420[1], 64421[1], 64425[1], 64430[1], 64435[1], 64445[1], 64446[1], 64447[1], 64448[1], 64449[1], 64450[1], 64461[1], 64463[1], 64479[1], 64483[1], 64486[1], 64487[1], 64488[1], 64489[1], 64490[1], 64493[1], 64505[1], 64510[1], 64517[1], 64520[1], 64530[1], 64553[1], 64555[1], 67500[1], 76000[1], 76970[1], 76998[0], 77002[0], 90865[1], 92511[1], 92512[1], 92516[1], 92520[1], 92537[1], 92538[1], 92950[1], 92953[1], 92960[1], 92961[1], 93000[1], 93005[1], 93010[1], 93040[1], 93041[1], 93042[1], 93050[0], 93303[0], 93304[0], 93306[1], 93307[1], 93308[1], 93312[1], 93313[1], 93314[1], 93315[1], 93316[1], 93317[1], 93318[0], 93351[1], 93355[0], 93451[1], 93456[1], 93457[1], 93561[0], 93562[0], 93701[0], 93922[1], 93923[1], 93924[1], 93925[1], 93926[1], 93930[1], 93931[1], 93970[1], 93971[1], 93975[1], 93976[1], 93978[1], 93979[1], 93980[1], 93981[1], 94002[1], 94004[1], 94200[1], 94250[0], 94640[1], 94644[1], 94660[1], 94662[1], 94680[1], 94681[1], 94690[1], 94760[0], 94761[0], 94762[1], 94770[1], 95812[0], 95813[0], 95816[0], 95819[0], 95822[0], 95829[0], 95955[0], 95956[0], 95957[0], 96360[0], 96365[0], 96372[0], 96373[0], 96374[0], 96375[0], 96376[0], 96377[0], 99151[0], 99152[0], 99153[0], 99155[0], 99156[0], 99157[0], 99201[0], 99202[0], 99203[0], 99204[0], 99205[0], 99211[0], 99212[0], 99213[0], 99214[0], 99215[0], 99217[0], 99218[0], 99219[0], 99220[0], 99221[0], 99222[0], 99223[0], 99224[0], 99225[0], 99226[0], 99231[0], 99232[0], 99233[0], 99234[0], 99235[0], 99236[0], 99238[0], 99239[0], 99281[0], 99282[0], 99283[0], 99284[0], 99285[0], 99304[0], 99305[0], 99306[0], 99307[0], 99308[0], 99309[0], 99310[0], 99315[0], 99318[0], 99324[0], 99325[0], 99326[0], 99327[0], 99328[0], 99334[0], 99335[0], 99336[0], 99337[0], 99341[0], 99342[0], 99343[0], 99347[0], 99348[0], 99349[0], 99354[0], 99355[0], 99356[0], 99357[0], 99358[0], 99359[0], 99415[0], 99416[0], 99446[0], 99447[0], 99448[0], 99449[0], 99451[0], 99452[0], 99466[0], 99468[0], 99469[0], 99471[0], 99472[0], 99475[0], 99476[0], 99477[0], 99478[0], 99479[0], 99480[0], 99483[0], 99485[0], 99497[0], C8921[1], C8922[1], C8923[1], C8924[1], C8925[1], C8926[1], C8927[0], C8929[1], C8930[1], G0380[1], G0381[1], G0382[1], G0383[1], G0384[1], G0406[0], G0407[0], G0408[0], G0425[0], G0426[0], G0427[0], G0463[0], G0500[0], G0508[0], G0509[0]
01638	01996[1], 0213T[1], 0216T[1], 0228T[1], 0230T[1], 31505[1], 31515[1], 31527[1], 31622[1], 31634[1], 31645[1], 31647[1], 36000[1], 36010[0], 36011[1], 36012[1], 36013[1], 36014[1], 36015[1], 36400[1], 36405[1], 36406[1], 36410[1], 36420[1], 36425[1], 36430[1], 36440[1], 36591[0], 36592[0], 36600[1], 36640[1], 43752[1], 43753[1], 43754[1], 61026[1], 61055[1], 62280[1], 62281[1], 62282[1], 62284[1], 62320[1], 62321[1], 62322[1], 62323[1], 62324[1], 62325[1], 62326[1], 62327[1], 64400[1], 64402[1], 64405[1], 64408[1], 64410[1], 64413[1], 64415[1], 64416[1], 64417[1], 64418[1], 64420[1], 64421[1], 64425[1], 64430[1], 64435[1], 64445[1], 64446[1], 64447[1], 64448[1], 64449[1], 64450[1], 64461[1], 64463[1], 64479[1], 64483[1], 64486[1], 64487[1], 64488[1], 64489[1], 64490[1], 64493[1], 64505[1], 64510[1], 64517[1], 64520[1], 64530[1], 64553[1], 64555[1], 67500[1], 76000[1], 76970[1], 76998[0], 77002[0], 90865[1], 92511[1], 92512[1], 92516[1], 92520[1], 92537[1], 92538[1], 92950[1], 92953[1], 92960[1], 92961[1], 93000[1], 93005[1], 93010[1], 93040[1], 93041[1], 93042[1], 93050[0], 93303[0], 93304[0], 93306[1], 93307[1], 93308[1], 93312[1], 93313[1], 93314[1], 93315[1], 93316[1], 93317[1], 93318[0], 93351[1], 93355[0], 93451[1], 93456[1], 93457[1], 93561[0], 93562[0], 93701[0], 93922[1], 93923[1], 93924[1], 93925[1], 93926[1], 93930[1], 93931[1], 93970[1], 93971[1], 93975[1], 93976[1], 93978[1], 93979[1], 93980[1], 93981[1], 94002[1], 94004[1], 94200[1], 94250[0], 94640[1], 94644[1], 94660[1], 94662[1], 94680[1], 94681[1], 94690[1], 94760[0], 94761[0], 94762[1], 94770[1], 95812[0], 95813[0], 95816[0], 95819[0], 95822[0], 95829[0], 95955[0], 95956[0], 95957[0], 96360[0], 96365[0], 96372[0], 96373[0], 96374[0], 96375[0], 96376[0], 96377[0], 99151[0], 99152[0], 99153[0], 99155[0], 99156[0], 99157[0], 99201[0], 99202[0], 99203[0], 99204[0], 99205[0], 99211[0], 99212[0], 99213[0], 99214[0], 99215[0], 99217[0], 99218[0], 99219[0], 99220[0], 99221[0], 99222[0], 99223[0], 99224[0], 99225[0], 99226[0], 99231[0], 99232[0], 99233[0], 99234[0], 99235[0], 99236[0], 99238[0], 99239[0], 99281[0], 99282[0], 99283[0], 99284[0], 99285[0], 99304[0], 99305[0], 99306[0], 99307[0], 99308[0], 99309[0], 99310[0], 99315[0], 99318[0], 99324[0], 99325[0], 99326[0], 99327[0], 99328[0], 99334[0], 99335[0], 99336[0], 99337[0], 99341[0], 99342[0], 99343[0], 99347[0], 99348[0], 99349[0], 99354[0], 99355[0], 99356[0], 99357[0], 99358[0], 99359[0], 99415[0], 99416[0], 99446[0], 99447[0], 99448[0], 99449[0], 99451[0], 99452[0], 99466[0], 99468[0], 99469[0], 99471[0], 99472[0], 99475[0], 99476[0], 99477[0], 99478[0], 99479[0], 99480[0], 99483[0], 99485[0], 99497[0], C8921[1], C8922[1], C8923[1], C8924[1], C8925[1], C8926[1], C8927[0], C8929[1], C8930[1], G0380[1], G0381[1], G0382[1], G0383[1], G0384[1], G0406[0], G0407[0], G0408[0], G0425[0], G0426[0], G0427[0], G0463[0], G0500[0], G0508[0], G0509[0]
01650	01996[1], 0213T[1], 0216T[1], 0228T[1], 0230T[1], 31505[1], 31515[1], 31527[1], 31622[1], 31634[1], 31645[1], 31647[1], 36000[1], 36010[0], 36011[1], 36012[1], 36013[1], 36014[1], 36015[1], 36400[1], 36405[1], 36406[1], 36410[1], 36420[1], 36425[1], 36430[1], 36440[1], 36591[0], 36592[0], 36600[1], 36640[1], 43752[1], 43753[1], 43754[1], 61026[1], 61055[1], 62280[1], 62281[1], 62282[1], 62284[1], 62320[1], 62321[1], 62322[1], 62323[1], 62324[1], 62325[1], 62326[1], 62327[1], 64400[1], 64402[1], 64405[1], 64408[1], 64410[1], 64413[1], 64415[1], 64416[1], 64417[1], 64418[1], 64420[1], 64421[1], 64425[1], 64430[1], 64435[1], 64445[1], 64446[1], 64447[1], 64448[1], 64449[1], 64450[1], 64461[1], 64463[1], 64479[1], 64483[1], 64486[1], 64487[1], 64488[1], 64489[1], 64490[1], 64493[1], 64505[1], 64510[1], 64517[1], 64520[1], 64530[1], 64553[1], 64555[1], 67500[1], 76000[1], 76970[1], 76998[0], 77002[0], 90865[1], 92511[1], 92512[1], 92516[1], 92520[1], 92537[1], 92538[1], 92950[1], 92953[1], 92960[1], 92961[1], 93000[1], 93005[1], 93010[1], 93040[1], 93041[1], 93042[1], 93050[0], 93303[0], 93304[0], 93306[1], 93307[1], 93308[1], 93312[1], 93313[1], 93314[1], 93315[1], 93316[1], 93317[1], 93318[0], 93351[1], 93355[0], 93451[1], 93456[1], 93457[1], 93561[0], 93562[0], 93701[0], 93922[1], 93923[1], 93924[1], 93925[1], 93926[1], 93930[1], 93931[1], 93970[1], 93971[1], 93975[1], 93976[1], 93978[1], 93979[1], 93980[1], 93981[1], 94002[1], 94004[1], 94200[1], 94250[0], 94640[1], 94644[1], 94660[1], 94662[1], 94680[1], 94681[1], 94690[1], 94760[0], 94761[0], 94762[1], 94770[1], 95812[0], 95813[0], 95816[0], 95819[0], 95822[0], 95829[0], 95955[0], 95956[0], 95957[0], 96360[0], 96365[0], 96372[0], 96373[0], 96374[0], 96375[0], 96376[0], 96377[0], 99151[0], 99152[0], 99153[0], 99155[0],

0 = Modifier usage not allowed or inappropriate 1 = Modifier usage allowed

CPT © 2018 American Medical Association. All Rights Reserved.

Appendix A: NCCI - CPT Codes

Code 1	Code 2
	99156[0], 99157[0], 99201[0], 99202[0], 99203[0], 99204[0], 99205[0], 99211[0], 99212[0], 99213[0], 99214[0], 99215[0], 99217[0], 99218[0], 99219[0], 99220[0], 99221[0], 99222[0], 99223[0], 99224[0], 99225[0], 99226[0], 99231[0], 99232[0], 99233[0], 99234[0], 99235[0], 99236[0], 99238[0], 99239[0], 99281[0], 99282[0], 99283[0], 99284[0], 99285[0], 99304[0], 99305[0], 99306[0], 99307[0], 99308[0], 99309[0], 99310[0], 99315[0], 99318[0], 99324[0], 99325[0], 99326[0], 99327[0], 99328[0], 99334[0], 99335[0], 99336[0], 99337[0], 99341[0], 99342[0], 99343[0], 99347[0], 99348[0], 99349[0], 99354[0], 99355[0], 99356[0], 99357[0], 99358[0], 99359[0], 99415[0], 99416[0], 99446[0], 99447[0], 99448[0], 99449[0], 99451[0], 99452[0], 99466[0], 99468[0], 99469[0], 99471[0], 99472[0], 99475[0], 99476[0], 99477[0], 99478[0], 99479[0], 99480[0], 99483[0], 99485[0], 99497[0], C8921[1], C8922[1], C8923[1], C8924[1], C8925[1], C8926[1], C8927[0], C8929[1], C8930[1], G0380[1], G0381[1], G0382[1], G0383[1], G0384[1], G0406[0], G0407[0], G0408[0], G0425[0], G0426[0], G0427[0], G0463[0], G0500[0], G0508[0], G0509[0]
01652	01996[1], 0213T[1], 0216T[1], 0228T[1], 0230T[1], 31505[1], 31515[1], 31527[1], 31622[1], 31634[1], 31645[1], 31647[1], 36000[1], 36010[0], 36011[1], 36012[1], 36013[1], 36014[1], 36015[1], 36400[1], 36405[1], 36406[1], 36410[1], 36420[1], 36425[1], 36430[1], 36440[1], 36591[0], 36592[0], 36600[1], 36640[1], 43752[1], 43753[1], 43754[1], 61026[1], 61055[1], 62280[1], 62281[1], 62282[1], 62284[1], 62320[1], 62321[1], 62322[1], 62323[1], 62324[1], 62325[1], 62326[1], 62327[1], 64400[1], 64402[1], 64405[1], 64408[1], 64410[1], 64413[1], 64415[1], 64416[1], 64417[1], 64418[1], 64420[1], 64421[1], 64425[1], 64430[1], 64435[1], 64445[1], 64446[1], 64447[1], 64448[1], 64449[1], 64450[1], 64461[1], 64463[1], 64479[1], 64483[1], 64486[1], 64487[1], 64488[1], 64489[1], 64490[1], 64493[1], 64505[1], 64510[1], 64517[1], 64520[1], 64530[1], 64553[1], 64555[1], 67500[1], 76000[1], 76970[1], 76998[0], 77002[0], 90865[1], 92511[1], 92512[1], 92516[1], 92520[1], 92537[1], 92538[1], 92950[1], 92953[1], 92960[1], 92961[1], 93000[1], 93005[1], 93010[1], 93040[1], 93041[1], 93042[1], 93050[0], 93303[0], 93304[0], 93306[1], 93307[1], 93308[1], 93312[1], 93313[1], 93314[1], 93315[1], 93316[1], 93317[1], 93318[0], 93351[1], 93355[0], 93451[1], 93456[1], 93457[1], 93561[0], 93562[0], 93701[0], 93922[1], 93923[1], 93924[1], 93925[1], 93926[1], 93930[1], 93931[1], 93970[1], 93971[1], 93975[1], 93976[1], 93978[1], 93979[1], 93980[1], 93981[1], 94002[1], 94004[1], 94200[1], 94250[0], 94640[1], 94644[1], 94660[1], 94662[1], 94680[1], 94681[1], 94690[1], 94760[0], 94761[0], 94762[1], 94770[1], 95812[0], 95813[0], 95816[0], 95819[0], 95822[0], 95829[0], 95955[0], 95956[0], 95957[0], 96360[0], 96365[0], 96372[0], 96373[0], 96374[0], 96375[0], 96376[0], 96377[0], 99151[0], 99152[0], 99153[0], 99155[0], 99156[0], 99157[0], 99201[0], 99202[0], 99203[0], 99204[0], 99205[0], 99211[0], 99212[0], 99213[0], 99214[0], 99215[0], 99217[0], 99218[0], 99219[0], 99220[0], 99221[0], 99222[0], 99223[0], 99224[0], 99225[0], 99226[0], 99231[0], 99232[0], 99233[0], 99234[0], 99235[0], 99236[0], 99238[0], 99239[0], 99281[0], 99282[0], 99283[0], 99284[0], 99285[0], 99304[0], 99305[0], 99306[0], 99307[0], 99308[0], 99309[0], 99310[0], 99315[0], 99318[0], 99324[0], 99325[0], 99326[0], 99327[0], 99328[0], 99334[0], 99335[0], 99336[0], 99337[0], 99341[0], 99342[0], 99343[0], 99347[0], 99348[0], 99349[0], 99354[0], 99355[0], 99356[0], 99357[0], 99358[0], 99359[0], 99415[0], 99416[0], 99446[0], 99447[0], 99448[0], 99449[0], 99451[0], 99452[0], 99466[0], 99468[0], 99469[0], 99471[0], 99472[0], 99475[0], 99476[0], 99477[0], 99478[0], 99479[0], 99480[0], 99483[0], 99485[0], 99497[0], C8921[1], C8922[1], C8923[1], C8924[1], C8925[1], C8926[1], C8927[0], C8929[1], C8930[1], G0380[1], G0381[1], G0382[1], G0383[1], G0384[1], G0406[0], G0407[0], G0408[0], G0425[0], G0426[0], G0427[0], G0463[0], G0500[0], G0508[0], G0509[0]
01654	01996[1], 0213T[1], 0216T[1], 0228T[1], 0230T[1], 31505[1], 31515[1], 31527[1], 31622[1], 31634[1], 31645[1], 31647[1], 36000[1], 36010[0], 36011[1], 36012[1], 36013[1], 36014[1], 36015[1], 36400[1], 36405[1], 36406[1], 36410[1], 36420[1], 36425[1], 36430[1], 36440[1], 36591[0], 36592[0], 36600[1], 36640[1], 43752[1], 43753[1], 43754[1], 61026[1], 61055[1], 62280[1], 62281[1], 62282[1], 62284[1], 62320[1], 62321[1], 62322[1], 62323[1], 62324[1], 62325[1], 62326[1], 62327[1], 64400[1], 64402[1], 64405[1], 64408[1], 64410[1], 64413[1], 64415[1], 64416[1], 64417[1], 64418[1], 64420[1], 64421[1], 64425[1], 64430[1], 64435[1], 64445[1], 64446[1], 64447[1], 64448[1], 64449[1], 64450[1], 64461[1], 64463[1], 64479[1], 64483[1], 64486[1], 64487[1], 64488[1], 64489[1], 64490[1], 64493[1], 64505[1], 64510[1], 64517[1], 64520[1], 64530[1], 64553[1], 64555[1], 67500[1], 76000[1], 76970[1], 76998[0], 77002[0], 90865[1], 92511[1], 92512[1], 92516[1], 92520[1], 92537[1], 92538[1], 92950[1], 92953[1], 92960[1], 92961[1], 93000[1], 93005[1], 93010[1], 93040[1], 93041[1], 93042[1], 93050[0], 93303[0], 93304[0], 93306[1], 93307[1], 93308[1], 93312[1], 93313[1], 93314[1], 93315[1], 93316[1], 93317[1], 93318[0], 93351[1], 93355[0], 93451[1], 93456[1], 93457[1], 93561[0], 93562[0], 93701[0], 93922[1], 93923[1], 93924[1], 93925[1], 93926[1], 93930[1], 93931[1], 93970[1], 93971[1], 93975[1], 93976[1], 93978[1], 93979[1], 93980[1], 93981[1], 94002[1], 94004[1], 94200[1], 94250[0], 94640[1], 94644[1], 94660[1], 94662[1], 94680[1], 94681[1], 94690[1], 94760[0], 94761[0], 94762[1], 94770[1], 95812[0], 95813[0], 95816[0], 95819[0], 95822[0], 95829[0], 95955[0], 95956[0], 95957[0], 96360[0], 96365[0], 96372[0], 96373[0], 96374[0], 96375[0], 96376[0], 96377[0], 99151[0], 99152[0], 99153[0], 99155[0], 99156[0], 99157[0], 99201[0], 99202[0], 99203[0], 99204[0], 99205[0], 99211[0], 99212[0], 99213[0], 99214[0], 99215[0], 99217[0], 99218[0], 99219[0], 99220[0], 99221[0], 99222[0], 99223[0], 99224[0], 99225[0], 99226[0], 99231[0], 99232[0], 99233[0], 99234[0], 99235[0], 99236[0], 99238[0], 99239[0], 99281[0], 99282[0], 99283[0], 99284[0], 99285[0], 99304[0], 99305[0], 99306[0], 99307[0], 99308[0], 99309[0], 99310[0], 99315[0], 99318[0], 99324[0], 99325[0], 99326[0], 99327[0], 99328[0], 99334[0], 99335[0], 99336[0], 99337[0], 99341[0], 99342[0], 99343[0], 99347[0], 99348[0], 99349[0], 99354[0], 99355[0], 99356[0], 99357[0], 99358[0], 99359[0], 99415[0], 99416[0], 99446[0], 99447[0], 99448[0], 99449[0], 99451[0], 99452[0], 99466[0], 99468[0], 99469[0], 99471[0], 99472[0], 99475[0], 99476[0], 99477[0], 99478[0], 99479[0], 99480[0], 99483[0], 99485[0], 99497[0], C8921[1], C8922[1], C8923[1], C8924[1], C8925[1], C8926[1], C8927[0], C8929[1], C8930[1], G0380[1], G0381[1], G0382[1], G0383[1], G0384[1], G0406[0], G0407[0], G0408[0], G0425[0], G0426[0], G0427[0], G0463[0], G0500[0], G0508[0], G0509[0]
01656	01996[1], 0213T[1], 0216T[1], 0228T[1], 0230T[1], 31505[1], 31515[1], 31527[1], 31622[1], 31634[1], 31645[1], 31647[1], 36000[1], 36010[0], 36011[1], 36012[1], 36013[1], 36014[1], 36015[1], 36400[1], 36405[1], 36406[1], 36410[1], 36420[1], 36425[1], 36430[1], 36440[1], 36591[0], 36592[0], 36600[1], 36640[1], 43752[1], 43753[1], 43754[1], 61026[1], 61055[1], 62280[1], 62281[1], 62282[1], 62284[1], 62320[1], 62321[1], 62322[1], 62323[1], 62324[1], 62325[1], 62326[1], 62327[1], 64400[1], 64402[1], 64405[1], 64408[1], 64410[1], 64413[1], 64415[1], 64416[1], 64417[1], 64418[1], 64420[1], 64421[1], 64425[1], 64430[1], 64435[1], 64445[1], 64446[1], 64447[1], 64448[1], 64449[1], 64450[1], 64461[1], 64463[1], 64479[1], 64483[1], 64486[1], 64487[1], 64488[1], 64489[1], 64490[1], 64493[1], 64505[1], 64510[1], 64517[1], 64520[1], 64530[1], 64553[1], 64555[1], 67500[1], 76000[1], 76970[1], 76998[0], 77002[0], 90865[1], 92511[1], 92512[1], 92516[1], 92520[1], 92537[1], 92538[1], 92950[1], 92953[1], 92960[1], 92961[1], 93000[1], 93005[1], 93010[1], 93040[1], 93041[1], 93042[1], 93050[0], 93303[0], 93304[0], 93306[1], 93307[1], 93308[1], 93312[1], 93313[1], 93314[1], 93315[1], 93316[1], 93317[1], 93318[0], 93351[1], 93355[0], 93451[1], 93456[1], 93457[1], 93561[0], 93562[0], 93701[0], 93922[1], 93923[1], 93924[1], 93925[1], 93926[1], 93930[1], 93931[1], 93970[1], 93971[1], 93975[1], 93976[1], 93978[1], 93979[1], 93980[1], 93981[1], 94002[1], 94004[1], 94200[1], 94250[0], 94640[1], 94644[1], 94660[1], 94662[1], 94680[1], 94681[1], 94690[1], 94760[0], 94761[0], 94762[1], 94770[1], 95812[0], 95813[0], 95816[0], 95819[0], 95822[0], 95829[0], 95955[0], 95956[0], 95957[0], 96360[0], 96365[0], 96372[0], 96373[0], 96374[0], 96375[0], 96376[0], 96377[0], 99151[0], 99152[0], 99153[0], 99155[0], 99156[0], 99157[0], 99201[0], 99202[0], 99203[0], 99204[0], 99205[0], 99211[0], 99212[0], 99213[0], 99214[0], 99215[0], 99217[0], 99218[0], 99219[0], 99220[0], 99221[0], 99222[0], 99223[0], 99224[0], 99225[0], 99226[0], 99231[0], 99232[0], 99233[0], 99234[0], 99235[0], 99236[0], 99238[0], 99239[0], 99281[0], 99282[0], 99283[0], 99284[0], 99285[0], 99304[0], 99305[0], 99306[0], 99307[0], 99308[0], 99309[0], 99310[0], 99315[0], 99318[0], 99324[0], 99325[0], 99326[0], 99327[0], 99328[0], 99334[0], 99335[0], 99336[0], 99337[0], 99341[0], 99342[0], 99343[0], 99347[0], 99348[0], 99349[0], 99354[0], 99355[0], 99356[0], 99357[0], 99358[0], 99359[0], 99415[0], 99416[0], 99446[0], 99447[0], 99448[0], 99449[0], 99451[0], 99452[0], 99466[0], 99468[0], 99469[0], 99471[0], 99472[0], 99475[0], 99476[0], 99477[0], 99478[0], 99479[0], 99480[0], 99483[0], 99485[0], 99497[0], C8921[1], C8922[1], C8923[1], C8924[1], C8925[1], C8926[1], C8927[0], C8929[1], C8930[1], G0380[1], G0381[1], G0382[1], G0383[1], G0384[1], G0406[0], G0407[0], G0408[0], G0425[0], G0426[0], G0427[0], G0463[0], G0500[0], G0508[0], G0509[0]
01670	01996[1], 0213T[1], 0216T[1], 0228T[1], 0230T[1], 31505[1], 31515[1], 31527[1], 31622[1], 31634[1], 31645[1], 31647[1], 36000[1], 36010[0], 36011[1], 36012[1], 36013[1], 36014[1], 36015[1], 36400[1], 36405[1], 36406[1], 36410[1], 36420[1], 36425[1], 36430[1], 36440[1], 36591[0], 36592[0], 36600[1], 36640[1], 43752[1], 43753[1], 43754[1], 61026[1], 61055[1], 62280[1], 62281[1], 62282[1], 62284[1], 62320[1], 62321[1], 62322[1], 62323[1], 62324[1], 62325[1], 62326[1], 62327[1], 64400[1], 64402[1], 64405[1], 64408[1], 64410[1], 64413[1], 64415[1], 64416[1], 64417[1], 64418[1], 64420[1], 64421[1], 64425[1], 64430[1], 64435[1], 64445[1], 64446[1], 64447[1], 64448[1], 64449[1], 64450[1], 64461[1], 64463[1], 64479[1], 64483[1], 64486[1], 64487[1], 64488[1], 64489[1], 64490[1], 64493[1], 64505[1], 64510[1], 64517[1], 64520[1], 64530[1], 64553[1], 64555[1], 67500[1], 76000[1], 76970[1], 76998[0], 77002[0], 90865[1], 92511[1], 92512[1], 92516[1], 92520[1], 92537[1], 92538[1], 92950[1], 92953[1], 92960[1], 92961[1], 93000[1], 93005[1], 93010[1], 93040[1], 93041[1], 93042[1], 93050[0], 93303[0], 93304[0], 93306[1], 93307[1], 93308[1], 93312[1], 93313[1], 93314[1], 93315[1], 93316[1], 93317[1], 93318[0], 93351[1], 93355[0], 93451[1], 93456[1], 93457[1], 93561[0], 93562[0], 93701[0], 93922[1], 93923[1], 93924[1], 93925[1], 93926[1], 93930[1], 93931[1], 93970[1], 93971[1], 93975[1], 93976[1], 93978[1], 93979[1], 93980[1], 93981[1], 94002[1], 94004[1], 94200[1], 94250[0], 94640[1], 94644[1], 94660[1], 94662[1], 94680[1], 94681[1], 94690[1], 94760[0], 94761[0], 94762[1], 94770[1], 95812[0], 95813[0], 95816[0], 95819[0], 95822[0], 95829[0], 95955[0], 95956[0], 95957[0], 96360[0], 96365[0], 96372[0], 96373[0], 96374[0], 96375[0], 96376[0], 96377[0], 99151[0], 99152[0], 99153[0], 99155[0], 99156[0], 99157[0], 99201[0], 99202[0], 99203[0], 99204[0], 99205[0], 99211[0], 99212[0], 99213[0], 99214[0], 99215[0], 99217[0], 99218[0], 99219[0], 99220[0], 99221[0], 99222[0], 99223[0], 99224[0], 99225[0], 99226[0], 99231[0], 99232[0], 99233[0], 99234[0], 99235[0], 99236[0], 99238[0], 99239[0], 99281[0], 99282[0], 99283[0], 99284[0], 99285[0], 99304[0], 99305[0], 99306[0], 99307[0], 99308[0], 99309[0], 99310[0], 99315[0], 99318[0], 99324[0], 99325[0], 99326[0], 99327[0], 99328[0], 99334[0], 99335[0], 99336[0], 99337[0], 99341[0], 99342[0], 99343[0], 99347[0], 99348[0], 99349[0], 99354[0], 99355[0], 99356[0], 99357[0], 99358[0], 99359[0], 99415[0], 99416[0], 99446[0], 99447[0], 99448[0], 99449[0], 99451[0], 99452[0], 99466[0], 99468[0], 99469[0], 99471[0], 99472[0], 99475[0], 99476[0], 99477[0], 99478[0], 99479[0], 99480[0], 99483[0], 99485[0], 99497[0], C8921[1], C8922[1], C8923[1], C8924[1], C8925[1], C8926[1], C8927[0], C8929[1], C8930[1], G0380[1], G0381[1], G0382[1], G0383[1], G0384[1], G0406[0], G0407[0], G0408[0], G0425[0], G0426[0], G0427[0], G0463[0], G0500[0], G0508[0], G0509[0]

0 = Modifier usage not allowed or inappropriate 1 = Modifier usage allowed

CPT © 2018 American Medical Association. All Rights Reserved.

Code 1	Code 2
01680	01996[1], 0213T[1], 0216T[1], 0228T[1], 0230T[1], 31505[1], 31515[1], 31527[1], 31622[1], 31634[1], 31645[1], 31647[1], 36000[1], 36010[0], 36011[1], 36012[1], 36013[1], 36014[1], 36015[1], 36400[1], 36405[1], 36406[1], 36410[1], 36420[1], 36425[1], 36430[1], 36440[1], 36591[0], 36592[0], 36600[1], 36640[1], 43752[1], 43753[1], 43754[1], 61026[1], 61055[1], 62280[1], 62281[1], 62282[1], 62284[1], 62320[1], 62321[1], 62322[1], 62323[1], 62324[1], 62325[1], 62326[1], 62327[1], 64400[1], 64402[1], 64405[1], 64408[1], 64410[1], 64413[1], 64415[1], 64416[1], 64417[1], 64418[1], 64420[1], 64421[1], 64425[1], 64430[1], 64435[1], 64445[1], 64446[1], 64447[1], 64448[1], 64449[1], 64450[1], 64461[1], 64463[1], 64479[1], 64483[1], 64486[1], 64487[1], 64488[1], 64489[1], 64490[1], 64493[1], 64505[1], 64510[1], 64517[1], 64520[1], 64530[1], 64553[1], 64555[1], 67500[1], 76000[1], 76970[1], 76998[0], 77002[0], 90865[1], 92511[1], 92512[1], 92516[1], 92520[1], 92537[1], 92538[1], 92950[1], 92953[1], 92960[1], 92961[1], 93000[1], 93005[1], 93010[1], 93040[1], 93041[1], 93042[1], 93050[0], 93303[0], 93304[0], 93306[1], 93307[1], 93308[1], 93312[1], 93313[1], 93314[1], 93315[1], 93316[1], 93317[1], 93318[0], 93351[1], 93355[0], 93451[1], 93456[1], 93457[1], 93561[0], 93562[0], 93701[0], 93922[1], 93923[1], 93924[1], 93925[1], 93926[1], 93930[1], 93931[1], 93970[1], 93971[1], 93975[1], 93976[1], 93978[1], 93979[1], 93980[1], 93981[1], 94002[1], 94004[1], 94200[1], 94250[0], 94640[1], 94644[1], 94660[1], 94662[1], 94680[1], 94681[1], 94690[1], 94760[0], 94761[0], 94762[1], 94770[1], 95812[0], 95813[0], 95816[0], 95819[0], 95822[0], 95829[0], 95955[0], 95956[0], 95957[0], 96360[0], 96365[0], 96372[0], 96373[0], 96374[0], 96375[0], 96376[0], 96377[0], 99151[0], 99152[0], 99153[0], 99155[0], 99156[0], 99157[0], 99201[0], 99202[0], 99203[0], 99204[0], 99205[0], 99211[0], 99212[0], 99213[0], 99214[0], 99215[0], 99217[0], 99218[0], 99219[0], 99220[0], 99221[0], 99222[0], 99223[0], 99224[0], 99225[0], 99226[0], 99231[0], 99232[0], 99233[0], 99234[0], 99235[0], 99236[0], 99238[0], 99239[0], 99281[0], 99282[0], 99283[0], 99284[0], 99285[0], 99304[0], 99305[0], 99306[0], 99307[0], 99308[0], 99309[0], 99310[0], 99315[0], 99318[0], 99324[0], 99325[0], 99326[0], 99327[0], 99328[0], 99334[0], 99335[0], 99336[0], 99337[0], 99341[0], 99342[0], 99343[0], 99347[0], 99348[0], 99349[0], 99354[0], 99355[0], 99356[0], 99357[0], 99358[0], 99359[0], 99415[0], 99416[0], 99446[0], 99447[0], 99448[0], 99449[0], 99451[0], 99452[0], 99466[0], 99468[0], 99469[0], 99471[0], 99472[0], 99475[0], 99476[0], 99477[0], 99478[0], 99479[0], 99480[0], 99483[0], 99485[0], 99497[0], C8921[1], C8922[1], C8923[1], C8924[1], C8925[1], C8926[1], C8927[0], C8929[1], C8930[1], G0380[1], G0381[1], G0382[1], G0383[1], G0384[1], G0406[0], G0407[0], G0408[0], G0425[0], G0426[0], G0427[0], G0463[0], G0500[0], G0508[0], G0509[0]
01710	01996[1], 0213T[1], 0216T[1], 0228T[1], 0230T[1], 0333T[0], 0464T[0], 31505[1], 31515[1], 31527[1], 31622[1], 31634[1], 31645[1], 31647[1], 36000[1], 36010[0], 36011[1], 36012[1], 36013[1], 36014[1], 36015[1], 36400[1], 36405[1], 36406[1], 36410[1], 36420[1], 36425[1], 36430[1], 36440[1], 36591[0], 36592[0], 36600[1], 36640[1], 43752[1], 43753[1], 43754[1], 61026[1], 61055[1], 62280[1], 62281[1], 62282[1], 62284[1], 62320[1], 62321[1], 62322[1], 62323[1], 62324[1], 62325[1], 62326[1], 62327[1], 64400[1], 64402[1], 64405[1], 64408[1], 64410[1], 64413[1], 64415[1], 64416[1], 64417[1], 64418[1], 64420[1], 64421[1], 64425[1], 64430[1], 64435[1], 64445[1], 64446[1], 64447[1], 64448[1], 64449[1], 64450[1], 64461[1], 64463[1], 64479[1], 64483[1], 64486[1], 64487[1], 64488[1], 64489[1], 64490[1], 64493[1], 64505[1], 64510[1], 64517[1], 64520[1], 64530[1], 64553[1], 64555[1], 67500[1], 76000[1], 76970[1], 76998[0], 77002[0], 90865[1], 92511[1], 92512[1], 92516[1], 92520[1], 92537[1], 92538[1], 92585[0], 92950[1], 92953[1], 92960[1], 92961[1], 93000[1], 93005[1], 93010[1], 93040[1], 93041[1], 93042[1], 93050[0], 93303[0], 93304[0], 93306[1], 93307[1], 93308[1], 93312[1], 93313[1], 93314[1], 93315[1], 93316[1], 93317[1], 93318[0], 93351[1], 93355[0], 93451[1], 93456[1], 93457[1], 93561[0], 93562[0], 93701[0], 93922[1], 93923[1], 93924[1], 93925[1], 93926[1], 93930[1], 93931[1], 93970[1], 93971[1], 93975[1], 93976[1], 93978[1], 93979[1], 93980[1], 93981[1], 94002[1], 94004[1], 94200[1], 94250[0], 94640[1], 94644[1], 94660[1], 94662[1], 94680[1], 94681[1], 94690[1], 94760[0], 94761[0], 94762[1], 94770[1], 95812[0], 95813[0], 95816[0], 95819[0], 95822[0], 95829[0], 95860[0], 95861[0], 95863[0], 95864[0], 95865[0], 95866[0], 95867[0], 95868[0], 95869[0], 95870[0], 95907[0], 95908[0], 95909[0], 95910[0], 95911[0], 95912[0], 95913[0], 95925[0], 95926[0], 95927[0], 95928[0], 95929[0], 95930[0], 95933[0], 95937[0], 95938[0], 95939[0], 95940[0], 95955[0], 95956[0], 95957[0], 96360[0], 96365[0], 96372[0], 96373[0], 96374[0], 96375[0], 96376[0], 96377[0], 99151[0], 99152[0], 99153[0], 99155[0], 99156[0], 99157[0], 99201[0], 99202[0], 99203[0], 99204[0], 99205[0], 99211[0], 99212[0], 99213[0], 99214[0], 99215[0], 99217[0], 99218[0], 99219[0], 99220[0], 99221[0], 99222[0], 99223[0], 99224[0], 99225[0], 99226[0], 99231[0], 99232[0], 99233[0], 99234[0], 99235[0], 99236[0], 99238[0], 99239[0], 99281[0], 99282[0], 99283[0], 99284[0], 99285[0], 99304[0], 99305[0], 99306[0], 99307[0], 99308[0], 99309[0], 99310[0], 99315[0], 99318[0], 99324[0], 99325[0], 99326[0], 99327[0], 99328[0], 99334[0], 99335[0], 99336[0], 99337[0], 99341[0], 99342[0], 99343[0], 99347[0], 99348[0], 99349[0], 99354[0], 99355[0], 99356[0], 99357[0], 99358[0], 99359[0], 99415[0], 99416[0], 99446[0], 99447[0], 99448[0], 99449[0], 99451[0], 99452[0], 99466[0], 99468[0], 99469[0], 99471[0], 99472[0], 99475[0], 99476[0], 99477[0], 99478[0], 99479[0], 99480[0], 99483[0], 99485[0], 99497[0], C8921[1], C8922[1], C8923[1], C8924[1], C8925[1], C8926[1], C8927[0], C8929[1], C8930[1], G0380[1], G0381[1], G0382[1], G0383[1], G0384[1], G0406[0], G0407[0], G0408[0], G0425[0], G0426[0], G0427[0], G0453[0], G0463[0], G0500[0], G0508[0], G0509[0]
01712	01996[1], 0213T[1], 0216T[1], 0228T[1], 0230T[1], 31505[1], 31515[1], 31527[1], 31622[1], 31634[1], 31645[1], 31647[1], 36000[1], 36010[0], 36011[1], 36012[1], 36013[1], 36014[1], 36015[1], 36400[1], 36405[1], 36406[1], 36410[1], 36420[1], 36425[1], 36430[1], 36440[1], 36591[0], 36592[0], 36600[1], 36640[1], 43752[1], 43753[1], 43754[1], 61026[1], 61055[1], 62280[1], 62281[1], 62282[1], 62284[1], 62320[1], 62321[1], 62322[1], 62323[1], 62324[1], 62325[1], 62326[1], 62327[1], 64400[1], 64402[1], 64405[1], 64408[1], 64410[1], 64413[1], 64415[1], 64416[1], 64417[1], 64418[1], 64420[1], 64421[1], 64425[1], 64430[1], 64435[1], 64445[1], 64446[1], 64447[1], 64448[1], 64449[1], 64450[1], 64461[1], 64463[1], 64479[1], 64483[1], 64486[1], 64487[1], 64488[1], 64489[1], 64490[1], 64493[1], 64505[1], 64510[1], 64517[1], 64520[1], 64530[1], 64553[1], 64555[1], 67500[1], 76000[1], 76970[1], 76998[0], 77002[0], 90865[1], 92511[1], 92512[1], 92516[1], 92520[1], 92537[1], 92538[1], 92950[1], 92953[1], 92960[1], 92961[1], 93000[1], 93005[1], 93010[1], 93040[1], 93041[1], 93042[1], 93050[0], 93303[0], 93304[0], 93306[1], 93307[1], 93308[1], 93312[1], 93313[1], 93314[1], 93315[1], 93316[1], 93317[1], 93318[0], 93351[1], 93355[0], 93451[1], 93456[1], 93457[1], 93561[0], 93562[0], 93701[0], 93922[1], 93923[1], 93924[1], 93925[1], 93926[1], 93930[1], 93931[1], 93970[1], 93971[1], 93975[1], 93976[1], 93978[1], 93979[1], 93980[1], 93981[1], 94002[1], 94004[1], 94200[1], 94250[0], 94640[1], 94644[1], 94660[1], 94662[1], 94680[1], 94681[1], 94690[1], 94760[0], 94761[0], 94762[1], 94770[1], 95812[0], 95813[0], 95816[0], 95819[0], 95822[0], 95829[0], 95955[0], 95956[0], 95957[0], 96360[0], 96365[0], 96372[0], 96373[0], 96374[0], 96375[0], 96376[0], 96377[0], 99151[0], 99152[0], 99153[0], 99155[0], 99156[0], 99157[0], 99201[0], 99202[0], 99203[0], 99204[0], 99205[0], 99211[0], 99212[0], 99213[0], 99214[0], 99215[0], 99217[0], 99218[0], 99219[0], 99220[0], 99221[0], 99222[0], 99223[0], 99224[0], 99225[0], 99226[0], 99231[0], 99232[0], 99233[0], 99234[0], 99235[0], 99236[0], 99238[0], 99239[0], 99281[0], 99282[0], 99283[0], 99284[0], 99285[0], 99304[0], 99305[0], 99306[0], 99307[0], 99308[0], 99309[0], 99310[0], 99315[0], 99318[0], 99324[0], 99325[0], 99326[0], 99327[0], 99328[0], 99334[0], 99335[0], 99336[0], 99337[0], 99341[0], 99342[0], 99343[0], 99347[0], 99348[0], 99349[0], 99354[0], 99355[0], 99356[0], 99357[0], 99358[0], 99359[0], 99415[0], 99416[0], 99446[0], 99447[0], 99448[0], 99449[0], 99451[0], 99452[0], 99466[0], 99468[0], 99469[0], 99471[0], 99472[0], 99475[0], 99476[0], 99477[0], 99478[0], 99479[0], 99480[0], 99483[0], 99485[0], 99497[0], C8921[1], C8922[1], C8923[1], C8924[1], C8925[1], C8926[1], C8927[0], C8929[1], C8930[1], G0380[1], G0381[1], G0382[1], G0383[1], G0384[1], G0406[0], G0407[0], G0408[0], G0425[0], G0426[0], G0427[0], G0463[0], G0500[0], G0508[0], G0509[0]
01714	01996[1], 0213T[1], 0216T[1], 0228T[1], 0230T[1], 31505[1], 31515[1], 31527[1], 31622[1], 31634[1], 31645[1], 31647[1], 36000[1], 36010[0], 36011[1], 36012[1], 36013[1], 36014[1], 36015[1], 36400[1], 36405[1], 36406[1], 36410[1], 36420[1], 36425[1], 36430[1], 36440[1], 36591[0], 36592[0], 36600[1], 36640[1], 43752[1], 43753[1], 43754[1], 61026[1], 61055[1], 62280[1], 62281[1], 62282[1], 62284[1], 62320[1], 62321[1], 62322[1], 62323[1], 62324[1], 62325[1], 62326[1], 62327[1], 64400[1], 64402[1], 64405[1], 64408[1], 64410[1], 64413[1], 64415[1], 64416[1], 64417[1], 64418[1], 64420[1], 64421[1], 64425[1], 64430[1], 64435[1], 64445[1], 64446[1], 64447[1], 64448[1], 64449[1], 64450[1], 64461[1], 64463[1], 64479[1], 64483[1], 64486[1], 64487[1], 64488[1], 64489[1], 64490[1], 64493[1], 64505[1], 64510[1], 64517[1], 64520[1], 64530[1], 64553[1], 64555[1], 67500[1], 76000[1], 76970[1], 76998[0], 77002[0], 90865[1], 92511[1], 92512[1], 92516[1], 92520[1], 92537[1], 92538[1], 92950[1], 92953[1], 92960[1], 92961[1], 93000[1], 93005[1], 93010[1], 93040[1], 93041[1], 93042[1], 93050[0], 93303[0], 93304[0], 93306[1], 93307[1], 93308[1], 93312[1], 93313[1], 93314[1], 93315[1], 93316[1], 93317[1], 93318[0], 93351[1], 93355[0], 93451[1], 93456[1], 93457[1], 93561[0], 93562[0], 93701[0], 93922[1], 93923[1], 93924[1], 93925[1], 93926[1], 93930[1], 93931[1], 93970[1], 93971[1], 93975[1], 93976[1], 93978[1], 93979[1], 93980[1], 93981[1], 94002[1], 94004[1], 94200[1], 94250[0], 94640[1], 94644[1], 94660[1], 94662[1], 94680[1], 94681[1], 94690[1], 94760[0], 94761[0], 94762[1], 94770[1], 95812[0], 95813[0], 95816[0], 95819[0], 95822[0], 95829[0], 95955[0], 95956[0], 95957[0], 96360[0], 96365[0], 96372[0], 96373[0], 96374[0], 96375[0], 96376[0], 96377[0], 99151[0], 99152[0], 99153[0], 99155[0], 99156[0], 99157[0], 99201[0], 99202[0], 99203[0], 99204[0], 99205[0], 99211[0], 99212[0], 99213[0], 99214[0], 99215[0], 99217[0], 99218[0], 99219[0], 99220[0], 99221[0], 99222[0], 99223[0], 99224[0], 99225[0], 99226[0], 99231[0], 99232[0], 99233[0], 99234[0], 99235[0], 99236[0], 99238[0], 99239[0], 99281[0], 99282[0], 99283[0], 99284[0], 99285[0], 99304[0], 99305[0], 99306[0], 99307[0], 99308[0], 99309[0], 99310[0], 99315[0], 99318[0], 99324[0], 99325[0], 99326[0], 99327[0], 99328[0], 99334[0], 99335[0], 99336[0], 99337[0], 99341[0], 99342[0], 99343[0], 99347[0], 99348[0], 99349[0], 99354[0], 99355[0], 99356[0], 99357[0], 99358[0], 99359[0], 99415[0], 99416[0], 99446[0], 99447[0], 99448[0], 99449[0], 99451[0], 99452[0], 99466[0], 99468[0], 99469[0], 99471[0], 99472[0], 99475[0], 99476[0], 99477[0], 99478[0], 99479[0], 99480[0], 99483[0], 99485[0], 99497[0], C8921[1], C8922[1], C8923[1], C8924[1], C8925[1], C8926[1], C8927[0], C8929[1], C8930[1], G0380[1], G0381[1], G0382[1], G0383[1], G0384[1], G0406[0], G0407[0], G0408[0], G0425[0], G0426[0], G0427[0], G0463[0], G0500[0], G0508[0], G0509[0]
01716	01996[1], 0213T[1], 0216T[1], 0228T[1], 0230T[1], 31505[1], 31515[1], 31527[1], 31622[1], 31634[1], 31645[1], 31647[1], 36000[1], 36010[0], 36011[1], 36012[1], 36013[1], 36014[1], 36015[1], 36400[1], 36405[1], 36406[1], 36410[1], 36420[1], 36425[1], 36430[1], 36440[1], 36591[0], 36592[0], 36600[1], 36640[1], 43752[1], 43753[1], 43754[1], 61026[1], 61055[1], 62280[1], 62281[1], 62282[1], 62284[1], 62320[1], 62321[1], 62322[1], 62323[1], 62324[1], 62325[1], 62326[1], 62327[1], 64400[1], 64402[1], 64405[1], 64408[1], 64410[1], 64413[1], 64415[1], 64416[1], 64417[1], 64418[1], 64420[1], 64421[1], 64425[1], 64430[1], 64435[1], 64445[1], 64446[1], 64447[1], 64448[1], 64449[1], 64450[1], 64461[1], 64463[1], 64479[1], 64483[1], 64486[1], 64487[1], 64488[1], 64489[1], 64490[1], 64493[1], 64505[1], 64510[1], 64517[1], 64520[1], 64530[1], 64553[1], 64555[1], 67500[1], 76000[1], 76970[1], 76998[0],

0 = Modifier usage not allowed or inappropriate 1 = Modifier usage allowed

CPT © 2018 American Medical Association. All Rights Reserved.

Code 1	Code 2
	77002[0], 90865[1], 92511[1], 92512[1], 92516[1], 92520[1], 92537[1], 92538[1], 92950[1], 92953[1], 92960[1], 92961[1], 93000[1], 93005[1], 93010[1], 93040[1], 93041[1], 93042[1], 93050[0], 93303[0], 93304[0], 93306[1], 93307[1], 93308[1], 93312[1], 93313[1], 93314[1], 93315[1], 93316[1], 93317[1], 93318[0], 93351[1], 93355[0], 93451[1], 93456[1], 93457[1], 93561[0], 93562[0], 93701[0], 93922[1], 93923[1], 93924[1], 93925[1], 93926[1], 93930[1], 93931[1], 93970[1], 93971[1], 93975[1], 93976[1], 93978[1], 93979[1], 93980[1], 93981[1], 94002[1], 94004[1], 94200[1], 94250[0], 94640[1], 94644[1], 94660[1], 94662[1], 94680[1], 94681[1], 94690[1], 94760[0], 94761[0], 94762[1], 94770[1], 95812[0], 95813[0], 95816[0], 95819[0], 95822[0], 95829[0], 95955[0], 95956[0], 95957[0], 96360[0], 96365[0], 96372[0], 96373[0], 96374[0], 96375[0], 96376[0], 96377[0], 99151[0], 99152[0], 99153[0], 99155[0], 99156[0], 99157[0], 99201[0], 99202[0], 99203[0], 99204[0], 99205[0], 99211[0], 99212[0], 99213[0], 99214[0], 99215[0], 99217[0], 99218[0], 99219[0], 99220[0], 99221[0], 99222[0], 99223[0], 99224[0], 99225[0], 99226[0], 99231[0], 99232[0], 99233[0], 99234[0], 99235[0], 99236[0], 99238[0], 99239[0], 99281[0], 99282[0], 99283[0], 99284[0], 99285[0], 99304[0], 99305[0], 99306[0], 99307[0], 99308[0], 99309[0], 99310[0], 99315[0], 99318[0], 99324[0], 99325[0], 99326[0], 99327[0], 99328[0], 99334[0], 99335[0], 99336[0], 99337[0], 99341[0], 99342[0], 99343[0], 99347[0], 99348[0], 99349[0], 99354[0], 99355[0], 99356[0], 99357[0], 99358[0], 99359[0], 99415[0], 99416[0], 99446[0], 99447[0], 99448[0], 99449[0], 99451[0], 99452[0], 99466[0], 99468[0], 99469[0], 99471[0], 99472[0], 99475[0], 99476[0], 99477[0], 99478[0], 99479[0], 99480[0], 99483[0], 99485[0], 99497[0], C8921[1], C8922[1], C8923[1], C8924[1], C8925[1], C8926[1], C8927[0], C8929[1], C8930[1], G0380[1], G0381[1], G0382[1], G0383[1], G0384[1], G0406[0], G0407[0], G0408[0], G0425[0], G0426[0], G0427[0], G0463[0], G0500[0], G0508[0], G0509[0]
01730	01996[1], 0213T[1], 0216T[1], 0228T[1], 0230T[1], 31505[1], 31515[1], 31527[1], 31622[1], 31634[1], 31645[1], 31647[1], 36000[1], 36010[0], 36011[1], 36012[1], 36013[1], 36014[1], 36015[1], 36400[1], 36405[1], 36406[1], 36410[1], 36420[1], 36425[1], 36430[1], 36440[1], 36591[0], 36592[0], 36600[1], 36640[1], 43752[1], 43753[1], 43754[1], 61026[1], 61055[1], 62280[1], 62281[1], 62282[1], 62284[1], 62320[1], 62321[1], 62322[1], 62323[1], 62324[1], 62325[1], 62326[1], 62327[1], 64400[1], 64402[1], 64405[1], 64408[1], 64410[1], 64413[1], 64415[1], 64416[1], 64417[1], 64418[1], 64420[1], 64421[1], 64425[1], 64430[1], 64435[1], 64445[1], 64446[1], 64447[1], 64448[1], 64449[1], 64450[1], 64461[1], 64463[1], 64479[1], 64483[1], 64486[1], 64487[1], 64488[1], 64489[1], 64490[1], 64493[1], 64505[1], 64510[1], 64517[1], 64520[1], 64530[1], 64553[1], 64555[1], 67500[1], 76000[1], 76970[1], 76998[0], 77002[0], 90865[1], 92511[1], 92512[1], 92516[1], 92520[1], 92537[1], 92538[1], 92950[1], 92953[1], 92960[1], 92961[1], 93000[1], 93005[1], 93010[1], 93040[1], 93041[1], 93042[1], 93050[0], 93303[0], 93304[0], 93306[1], 93307[1], 93308[1], 93312[1], 93313[1], 93314[1], 93315[1], 93316[1], 93317[1], 93318[0], 93351[1], 93355[0], 93451[1], 93456[1], 93457[1], 93561[0], 93562[0], 93701[0], 93922[1], 93923[1], 93924[1], 93925[1], 93926[1], 93930[1], 93931[1], 93970[1], 93971[1], 93975[1], 93976[1], 93978[1], 93979[1], 93980[1], 93981[1], 94002[1], 94004[1], 94200[1], 94250[0], 94640[1], 94644[1], 94660[1], 94662[1], 94680[1], 94681[1], 94690[1], 94760[0], 94761[0], 94762[1], 94770[1], 95812[0], 95813[0], 95816[0], 95819[0], 95822[0], 95829[0], 95955[0], 95956[0], 95957[0], 96360[0], 96365[0], 96372[0], 96373[0], 96374[0], 96375[0], 96376[0], 96377[0], 99151[0], 99152[0], 99153[0], 99155[0], 99156[0], 99157[0], 99201[0], 99202[0], 99203[0], 99204[0], 99205[0], 99211[0], 99212[0], 99213[0], 99214[0], 99215[0], 99217[0], 99218[0], 99219[0], 99220[0], 99221[0], 99222[0], 99223[0], 99224[0], 99225[0], 99226[0], 99231[0], 99232[0], 99233[0], 99234[0], 99235[0], 99236[0], 99238[0], 99239[0], 99281[0], 99282[0], 99283[0], 99284[0], 99285[0], 99304[0], 99305[0], 99306[0], 99307[0], 99308[0], 99309[0], 99310[0], 99315[0], 99318[0], 99324[0], 99325[0], 99326[0], 99327[0], 99328[0], 99334[0], 99335[0], 99336[0], 99337[0], 99341[0], 99342[0], 99343[0], 99347[0], 99348[0], 99349[0], 99354[0], 99355[0], 99356[0], 99357[0], 99358[0], 99359[0], 99415[0], 99416[0], 99446[0], 99447[0], 99448[0], 99449[0], 99451[0], 99452[0], 99466[0], 99468[0], 99469[0], 99471[0], 99472[0], 99475[0], 99476[0], 99477[0], 99478[0], 99479[0], 99480[0], 99483[0], 99485[0], 99497[0], C8921[1], C8922[1], C8923[1], C8924[1], C8925[1], C8926[1], C8927[0], C8929[1], C8930[1], G0380[1], G0381[1], G0382[1], G0383[1], G0384[1], G0406[0], G0407[0], G0408[0], G0425[0], G0426[0], G0427[0], G0463[0], G0500[0], G0508[0], G0509[0]
01732	01996[1], 0213T[1], 0216T[1], 0228T[1], 0230T[1], 31505[1], 31515[1], 31527[1], 31622[1], 31634[1], 31645[1], 31647[1], 36000[1], 36010[0], 36011[1], 36012[1], 36013[1], 36014[1], 36015[1], 36400[1], 36405[1], 36406[1], 36410[1], 36420[1], 36425[1], 36430[1], 36440[1], 36591[0], 36592[0], 36600[1], 36640[1], 43752[1], 43753[1], 43754[1], 61026[1], 61055[1], 62280[1], 62281[1], 62282[1], 62284[1], 62320[1], 62321[1], 62322[1], 62323[1], 62324[1], 62325[1], 62326[1], 62327[1], 64400[1], 64402[1], 64405[1], 64408[1], 64410[1], 64413[1], 64415[1], 64416[1], 64417[1], 64418[1], 64420[1], 64421[1], 64425[1], 64430[1], 64435[1], 64445[1], 64446[1], 64447[1], 64448[1], 64449[1], 64450[1], 64461[1], 64463[1], 64479[1], 64483[1], 64486[1], 64487[1], 64488[1], 64489[1], 64490[1], 64493[1], 64505[1], 64510[1], 64517[1], 64520[1], 64530[1], 64553[1], 64555[1], 67500[1], 76000[1], 76970[1], 76998[0], 77002[0], 90865[1], 92511[1], 92512[1], 92516[1], 92520[1], 92537[1], 92538[1], 92950[1], 92953[1], 92960[1], 92961[1], 93000[1], 93005[1], 93010[1], 93040[1], 93041[1], 93042[1], 93050[0], 93303[0], 93304[0], 93306[1], 93307[1], 93308[1], 93312[1], 93313[1], 93314[1], 93315[1], 93316[1], 93317[1], 93318[0], 93351[1], 93355[0], 93451[1], 93456[1], 93457[1], 93561[0], 93562[0], 93701[0], 93922[1], 93923[1], 93924[1], 93925[1], 93926[1], 93930[1], 93931[1], 93970[1], 93971[1], 93975[1], 93976[1], 93978[1], 93979[1], 93980[1], 93981[1], 94002[1], 94004[1], 94200[1], 94250[0], 94640[1], 94644[1], 94660[1], 94662[1], 94680[1], 94681[1], 94690[1], 94760[0], 94761[0], 94762[1], 94770[1], 95812[0], 95813[0], 95816[0], 95819[0], 95822[0], 95829[0], 95955[0], 95956[0], 95957[0], 96360[0], 96365[0], 96372[0], 96373[0], 96374[0], 96375[0], 96376[0], 96377[0], 99151[0], 99152[0], 99153[0], 99155[0], 99156[0], 99157[0], 99201[0], 99202[0], 99203[0], 99204[0], 99205[0], 99211[0], 99212[0], 99213[0], 99214[0], 99215[0], 99217[0], 99218[0], 99219[0], 99220[0], 99221[0], 99222[0], 99223[0], 99224[0], 99225[0], 99226[0], 99231[0], 99232[0], 99233[0], 99234[0], 99235[0], 99236[0], 99238[0], 99239[0], 99281[0], 99282[0], 99283[0], 99284[0], 99285[0], 99304[0], 99305[0], 99306[0], 99307[0], 99308[0], 99309[0], 99310[0], 99315[0], 99318[0], 99324[0], 99325[0], 99326[0], 99327[0], 99328[0], 99334[0], 99335[0], 99336[0], 99337[0], 99341[0], 99342[0], 99343[0], 99347[0], 99348[0], 99349[0], 99354[0], 99355[0], 99356[0], 99357[0], 99358[0], 99359[0], 99415[0], 99416[0], 99446[0], 99447[0], 99448[0], 99449[0], 99451[0], 99452[0], 99466[0], 99468[0], 99469[0], 99471[0], 99472[0], 99475[0], 99476[0], 99477[0], 99478[0], 99479[0], 99480[0], 99483[0], 99485[0], 99497[0], C8921[1], C8922[1], C8923[1], C8924[1], C8925[1], C8926[1], C8927[0], C8929[1], C8930[1], G0380[1], G0381[1], G0382[1], G0383[1], G0384[1], G0406[0], G0407[0], G0408[0], G0425[0], G0426[0], G0427[0], G0463[0], G0500[0], G0508[0], G0509[0]
01740	01732[1], 01996[1], 0213T[1], 0216T[1], 0228T[1], 0230T[1], 31505[1], 31515[1], 31527[1], 31622[1], 31634[1], 31645[1], 31647[1], 36000[1], 36010[0], 36011[1], 36012[1], 36013[1], 36014[1], 36015[1], 36400[1], 36405[1], 36406[1], 36410[1], 36420[1], 36425[1], 36430[1], 36440[1], 36591[0], 36592[0], 36600[1], 36640[1], 43752[1], 43753[1], 43754[1], 61026[1], 61055[1], 62280[1], 62281[1], 62282[1], 62284[1], 62320[1], 62321[1], 62322[1], 62323[1], 62324[1], 62325[1], 62326[1], 62327[1], 64400[1], 64402[1], 64405[1], 64408[1], 64410[1], 64413[1], 64415[1], 64416[1], 64417[1], 64418[1], 64420[1], 64421[1], 64425[1], 64430[1], 64435[1], 64445[1], 64446[1], 64447[1], 64448[1], 64449[1], 64450[1], 64461[1], 64463[1], 64479[1], 64483[1], 64486[1], 64487[1], 64488[1], 64489[1], 64490[1], 64493[1], 64505[1], 64510[1], 64517[1], 64520[1], 64530[1], 64553[1], 64555[1], 67500[1], 76000[1], 76970[1], 76998[0], 77002[0], 90865[1], 92511[1], 92512[1], 92516[1], 92520[1], 92537[1], 92538[1], 92950[1], 92953[1], 92960[1], 92961[1], 93000[1], 93005[1], 93010[1], 93040[1], 93041[1], 93042[1], 93050[0], 93303[0], 93304[0], 93306[1], 93307[1], 93308[1], 93312[1], 93313[1], 93314[1], 93315[1], 93316[1], 93317[1], 93318[0], 93351[1], 93355[0], 93451[1], 93456[1], 93457[1], 93561[0], 93562[0], 93701[0], 93922[1], 93923[1], 93924[1], 93925[1], 93926[1], 93930[1], 93931[1], 93970[1], 93971[1], 93975[1], 93976[1], 93978[1], 93979[1], 93980[1], 93981[1], 94002[1], 94004[1], 94200[1], 94250[0], 94640[1], 94644[1], 94660[1], 94662[1], 94680[1], 94681[1], 94690[1], 94760[0], 94761[0], 94762[1], 94770[1], 95812[0], 95813[0], 95816[0], 95819[0], 95822[0], 95829[0], 95955[0], 95956[0], 95957[0], 96360[0], 96365[0], 96372[0], 96373[0], 96374[0], 96375[0], 96376[0], 96377[0], 99151[0], 99152[0], 99153[0], 99155[0], 99156[0], 99157[0], 99201[0], 99202[0], 99203[0], 99204[0], 99205[0], 99211[0], 99212[0], 99213[0], 99214[0], 99215[0], 99217[0], 99218[0], 99219[0], 99220[0], 99221[0], 99222[0], 99223[0], 99224[0], 99225[0], 99226[0], 99231[0], 99232[0], 99233[0], 99234[0], 99235[0], 99236[0], 99238[0], 99239[0], 99281[0], 99282[0], 99283[0], 99284[0], 99285[0], 99304[0], 99305[0], 99306[0], 99307[0], 99308[0], 99309[0], 99310[0], 99315[0], 99318[0], 99324[0], 99325[0], 99326[0], 99327[0], 99328[0], 99334[0], 99335[0], 99336[0], 99337[0], 99341[0], 99342[0], 99343[0], 99347[0], 99348[0], 99349[0], 99354[0], 99355[0], 99356[0], 99357[0], 99358[0], 99359[0], 99415[0], 99416[0], 99446[0], 99447[0], 99448[0], 99449[0], 99451[0], 99452[0], 99466[0], 99468[0], 99469[0], 99471[0], 99472[0], 99475[0], 99476[0], 99477[0], 99478[0], 99479[0], 99480[0], 99483[0], 99485[0], 99497[0], C8921[1], C8922[1], C8923[1], C8924[1], C8925[1], C8926[1], C8927[0], C8929[1], C8930[1], G0380[1], G0381[1], G0382[1], G0383[1], G0384[1], G0406[0], G0407[0], G0408[0], G0425[0], G0426[0], G0427[0], G0463[0], G0500[0], G0508[0], G0509[0]
01742	01996[1], 0213T[1], 0216T[1], 0228T[1], 0230T[1], 31505[1], 31515[1], 31527[1], 31622[1], 31634[1], 31645[1], 31647[1], 36000[1], 36010[0], 36011[1], 36012[1], 36013[1], 36014[1], 36015[1], 36400[1], 36405[1], 36406[1], 36410[1], 36420[1], 36425[1], 36430[1], 36440[1], 36591[0], 36592[0], 36600[1], 36640[1], 43752[1], 43753[1], 43754[1], 61026[1], 61055[1], 62280[1], 62281[1], 62282[1], 62284[1], 62320[1], 62321[1], 62322[1], 62323[1], 62324[1], 62325[1], 62326[1], 62327[1], 64400[1], 64402[1], 64405[1], 64408[1], 64410[1], 64413[1], 64415[1], 64416[1], 64417[1], 64418[1], 64420[1], 64421[1], 64425[1], 64430[1], 64435[1], 64445[1], 64446[1], 64447[1], 64448[1], 64449[1], 64450[1], 64461[1], 64463[1], 64479[1], 64483[1], 64486[1], 64487[1], 64488[1], 64489[1], 64490[1], 64493[1], 64505[1], 64510[1], 64517[1], 64520[1], 64530[1], 64553[1], 64555[1], 67500[1], 76000[1], 76970[1], 76998[0], 77002[0], 90865[1], 92511[1], 92512[1], 92516[1], 92520[1], 92537[1], 92538[1], 92950[1], 92953[1], 92960[1], 92961[1], 93000[1], 93005[1], 93010[1], 93040[1], 93041[1], 93042[1], 93050[0], 93303[0], 93304[0], 93306[1], 93307[1], 93308[1], 93312[1], 93313[1], 93314[1], 93315[1], 93316[1], 93317[1], 93318[0], 93351[1], 93355[0], 93451[1], 93456[1], 93457[1], 93561[0], 93562[0], 93701[0], 93922[1], 93923[1], 93924[1], 93925[1], 93926[1], 93930[1], 93931[1], 93970[1], 93971[1], 93975[1], 93976[1], 93978[1], 93979[1], 93980[1], 93981[1], 94002[1], 94004[1], 94200[1], 94250[0], 94640[1], 94644[1], 94660[1], 94662[1], 94680[1], 94681[1], 94690[1], 94760[0], 94761[0], 94762[1], 94770[1], 95812[0], 95813[0], 95816[0], 95819[0], 95822[0], 95829[0], 95955[0], 95956[0], 95957[0], 96360[0], 96365[0], 96372[0], 96373[0], 96374[0], 96375[0], 96376[0], 96377[0], 99151[0], 99152[0], 99153[0], 99155[0], 99156[0], 99157[0], 99201[0], 99202[0], 99203[0], 99204[0], 99205[0], 99211[0], 99212[0], 99213[0], 99214[0], 99215[0], 99217[0], 99218[0], 99219[0], 99220[0], 99221[0], 99222[0], 99223[0], 99224[0], 99225[0], 99226[0], 99231[0], 99232[0], 99233[0], 99234[0], 99235[0], 99236[0], 99238[0], 99239[0],

CPT © 2018 American Medical Association. All Rights Reserved.

Code 1	Code 2
	99281[0], 99282[0], 99283[0], 99284[0], 99285[0], 99304[0], 99305[0], 99306[0], 99307[0], 99308[0], 99309[0], 99310[0], 99315[0], 99318[0], 99324[0], 99325[0], 99326[0], 99327[0], 99328[0], 99334[0], 99335[0], 99336[0], 99337[0], 99341[0], 99342[0], 99343[0], 99347[0], 99348[0], 99349[0], 99354[0], 99355[0], 99356[0], 99357[0], 99358[0], 99359[0], 99415[0], 99416[0], 99446[0], 99447[0], 99448[0], 99449[0], 99451[0], 99452[0], 99466[0], 99468[0], 99469[0], 99471[0], 99472[0], 99475[0], 99476[0], 99477[0], 99478[0], 99479[0], 99480[0], 99483[0], 99485[0], 99497[0], C8921[1], C8922[1], C8923[1], C8924[1], C8925[1], C8926[1], C8927[0], C8929[1], C8930[1], G0380[1], G0381[1], G0382[1], G0383[1], G0384[1], G0406[0], G0407[0], G0408[0], G0425[0], G0426[0], G0427[0], G0463[0], G0500[0], G0508[0], G0509[0]
01744	01996[1], 0213T[1], 0216T[1], 0228T[1], 0230T[1], 31505[1], 31515[1], 31527[1], 31622[1], 31634[1], 31645[1], 31647[1], 36000[1], 36010[0], 36011[1], 36012[1], 36013[1], 36014[1], 36015[1], 36400[1], 36405[1], 36406[1], 36410[1], 36420[1], 36425[1], 36430[1], 36440[1], 36591[0], 36592[0], 36600[1], 36640[1], 43752[1], 43753[1], 43754[1], 61026[1], 61055[1], 62280[1], 62281[1], 62282[1], 62284[1], 62320[1], 62321[1], 62322[1], 62323[1], 62324[1], 62325[1], 62326[1], 62327[1], 64400[1], 64402[1], 64405[1], 64408[1], 64410[1], 64413[1], 64415[1], 64416[1], 64417[1], 64418[1], 64420[1], 64421[1], 64425[1], 64430[1], 64435[1], 64445[1], 64446[1], 64447[1], 64448[1], 64449[1], 64450[1], 64461[1], 64463[1], 64479[1], 64483[1], 64486[1], 64487[1], 64488[1], 64489[1], 64490[1], 64493[1], 64505[1], 64510[1], 64517[1], 64520[1], 64530[1], 64553[1], 64555[1], 67500[1], 76000[1], 76970[1], 76998[0], 77002[0], 90865[1], 92511[1], 92512[1], 92516[1], 92520[1], 92537[1], 92538[1], 92950[1], 92953[1], 92960[1], 92961[1], 93000[1], 93005[1], 93010[1], 93040[1], 93041[1], 93042[1], 93050[0], 93303[0], 93304[0], 93306[1], 93307[1], 93308[1], 93312[1], 93313[1], 93314[1], 93315[1], 93316[1], 93317[1], 93318[0], 93351[1], 93355[0], 93451[1], 93456[1], 93457[1], 93561[0], 93562[0], 93701[0], 93922[1], 93923[1], 93924[1], 93925[1], 93926[1], 93930[1], 93931[1], 93970[1], 93971[1], 93975[1], 93976[1], 93978[1], 93979[1], 93980[1], 93981[1], 94002[1], 94004[1], 94200[1], 94250[0], 94640[1], 94644[1], 94660[1], 94662[1], 94680[1], 94681[1], 94690[1], 94760[0], 94761[0], 94762[1], 94770[1], 95812[0], 95813[0], 95816[0], 95819[0], 95822[0], 95829[0], 95955[0], 95956[0], 95957[0], 96360[0], 96365[0], 96372[0], 96373[0], 96374[0], 96375[0], 96376[0], 96377[0], 99151[0], 99152[0], 99153[0], 99155[0], 99156[0], 99157[0], 99201[0], 99202[0], 99203[0], 99204[0], 99205[0], 99211[0], 99212[0], 99213[0], 99214[0], 99215[0], 99217[0], 99218[0], 99219[0], 99220[0], 99221[0], 99222[0], 99223[0], 99224[0], 99225[0], 99226[0], 99231[0], 99232[0], 99233[0], 99234[0], 99235[0], 99236[0], 99238[0], 99239[0], 99281[0], 99282[0], 99283[0], 99284[0], 99285[0], 99304[0], 99305[0], 99306[0], 99307[0], 99308[0], 99309[0], 99310[0], 99315[0], 99318[0], 99324[0], 99325[0], 99326[0], 99327[0], 99328[0], 99334[0], 99335[0], 99336[0], 99337[0], 99341[0], 99342[0], 99343[0], 99347[0], 99348[0], 99349[0], 99354[0], 99355[0], 99356[0], 99357[0], 99358[0], 99359[0], 99415[0], 99416[0], 99446[0], 99447[0], 99448[0], 99449[0], 99451[0], 99452[0], 99466[0], 99468[0], 99469[0], 99471[0], 99472[0], 99475[0], 99476[0], 99477[0], 99478[0], 99479[0], 99480[0], 99483[0], 99485[0], 99497[0], C8921[1], C8922[1], C8923[1], C8924[1], C8925[1], C8926[1], C8927[0], C8929[1], C8930[1], G0380[1], G0381[1], G0382[1], G0383[1], G0384[1], G0406[0], G0407[0], G0408[0], G0425[0], G0426[0], G0427[0], G0463[0], G0500[0], G0508[0], G0509[0]
01756	01996[1], 0213T[1], 0216T[1], 0228T[1], 0230T[1], 31505[1], 31515[1], 31527[1], 31622[1], 31634[1], 31645[1], 31647[1], 36000[1], 36010[0], 36011[1], 36012[1], 36013[1], 36014[1], 36015[1], 36400[1], 36405[1], 36406[1], 36410[1], 36420[1], 36425[1], 36430[1], 36440[1], 36591[0], 36592[0], 36600[1], 36640[1], 43752[1], 43753[1], 43754[1], 61026[1], 61055[1], 62280[1], 62281[1], 62282[1], 62284[1], 62320[1], 62321[1], 62322[1], 62323[1], 62324[1], 62325[1], 62326[1], 62327[1], 64400[1], 64402[1], 64405[1], 64408[1], 64410[1], 64413[1], 64415[1], 64416[1], 64417[1], 64418[1], 64420[1], 64421[1], 64425[1], 64430[1], 64435[1], 64445[1], 64446[1], 64447[1], 64448[1], 64449[1], 64450[1], 64461[1], 64463[1], 64479[1], 64483[1], 64486[1], 64487[1], 64488[1], 64489[1], 64490[1], 64493[1], 64505[1], 64510[1], 64517[1], 64520[1], 64530[1], 64553[1], 64555[1], 67500[1], 76000[1], 76970[1], 76998[0], 77002[0], 90865[1], 92511[1], 92512[1], 92516[1], 92520[1], 92537[1], 92538[1], 92950[1], 92953[1], 92960[1], 92961[1], 93000[1], 93005[1], 93010[1], 93040[1], 93041[1], 93042[1], 93050[0], 93303[0], 93304[0], 93306[1], 93307[1], 93308[1], 93312[1], 93313[1], 93314[1], 93315[1], 93316[1], 93317[1], 93318[0], 93351[1], 93355[0], 93451[1], 93456[1], 93457[1], 93561[0], 93562[0], 93701[0], 93922[1], 93923[1], 93924[1], 93925[1], 93926[1], 93930[1], 93931[1], 93970[1], 93971[1], 93975[1], 93976[1], 93978[1], 93979[1], 93980[1], 93981[1], 94002[1], 94004[1], 94200[1], 94250[0], 94640[1], 94644[1], 94660[1], 94662[1], 94680[1], 94681[1], 94690[1], 94760[0], 94761[0], 94762[1], 94770[1], 95812[0], 95813[0], 95816[0], 95819[0], 95822[0], 95829[0], 95955[0], 95956[0], 95957[0], 96360[0], 96365[0], 96372[0], 96373[0], 96374[0], 96375[0], 96376[0], 96377[0], 99151[0], 99152[0], 99153[0], 99155[0], 99156[0], 99157[0], 99201[0], 99202[0], 99203[0], 99204[0], 99205[0], 99211[0], 99212[0], 99213[0], 99214[0], 99215[0], 99217[0], 99218[0], 99219[0], 99220[0], 99221[0], 99222[0], 99223[0], 99224[0], 99225[0], 99226[0], 99231[0], 99232[0], 99233[0], 99234[0], 99235[0], 99236[0], 99238[0], 99239[0], 99281[0], 99282[0], 99283[0], 99284[0], 99285[0], 99304[0], 99305[0], 99306[0], 99307[0], 99308[0], 99309[0], 99310[0], 99315[0], 99318[0], 99324[0], 99325[0], 99326[0], 99327[0], 99328[0], 99334[0], 99335[0], 99336[0], 99337[0], 99341[0], 99342[0], 99343[0], 99347[0], 99348[0], 99349[0], 99354[0], 99355[0], 99356[0], 99357[0], 99358[0], 99359[0], 99415[0], 99416[0], 99446[0], 99447[0], 99448[0], 99449[0], 99451[0], 99452[0], 99466[0], 99468[0], 99469[0], 99471[0], 99472[0], 99475[0], 99476[0], 99477[0], 99478[0], 99479[0], 99480[0], 99483[0], 99485[0], 99497[0], C8921[1], C8922[1], C8923[1], C8924[1], C8925[1], C8926[1], C8927[0], C8929[1], C8930[1], G0380[1], G0381[1], G0382[1], G0383[1], G0384[1], G0406[0], G0407[0], G0408[0], G0425[0], G0426[0], G0427[0], G0463[0], G0500[0], G0508[0], G0509[0]
01758	01996[1], 0213T[1], 0216T[1], 0228T[1], 0230T[1], 31505[1], 31515[1], 31527[1], 31622[1], 31634[1], 31645[1], 31647[1], 36000[1], 36010[0], 36011[1], 36012[1], 36013[1], 36014[1], 36015[1], 36400[1], 36405[1], 36406[1], 36410[1], 36420[1], 36425[1], 36430[1], 36440[1], 36591[0], 36592[0], 36600[1], 36640[1], 43752[1], 43753[1], 43754[1], 61026[1], 61055[1], 62280[1], 62281[1], 62282[1], 62284[1], 62320[1], 62321[1], 62322[1], 62323[1], 62324[1], 62325[1], 62326[1], 62327[1], 64400[1], 64402[1], 64405[1], 64408[1], 64410[1], 64413[1], 64415[1], 64416[1], 64417[1], 64418[1], 64420[1], 64421[1], 64425[1], 64430[1], 64435[1], 64445[1], 64446[1], 64447[1], 64448[1], 64449[1], 64450[1], 64461[1], 64463[1], 64479[1], 64483[1], 64486[1], 64487[1], 64488[1], 64489[1], 64490[1], 64493[1], 64505[1], 64510[1], 64517[1], 64520[1], 64530[1], 64553[1], 64555[1], 67500[1], 76000[1], 76970[1], 76998[0], 77002[0], 90865[1], 92511[1], 92512[1], 92516[1], 92520[1], 92537[1], 92538[1], 92950[1], 92953[1], 92960[1], 92961[1], 93000[1], 93005[1], 93010[1], 93040[1], 93041[1], 93042[1], 93050[0], 93303[0], 93304[0], 93306[1], 93307[1], 93308[1], 93312[1], 93313[1], 93314[1], 93315[1], 93316[1], 93317[1], 93318[0], 93351[1], 93355[0], 93451[1], 93456[1], 93457[1], 93561[0], 93562[0], 93701[0], 93922[1], 93923[1], 93924[1], 93925[1], 93926[1], 93930[1], 93931[1], 93970[1], 93971[1], 93975[1], 93976[1], 93978[1], 93979[1], 93980[1], 93981[1], 94002[1], 94004[1], 94200[1], 94250[0], 94640[1], 94644[1], 94660[1], 94662[1], 94680[1], 94681[1], 94690[1], 94760[0], 94761[0], 94762[1], 94770[1], 95812[0], 95813[0], 95816[0], 95819[0], 95822[0], 95829[0], 95955[0], 95956[0], 95957[0], 96360[0], 96365[0], 96372[0], 96373[0], 96374[0], 96375[0], 96376[0], 96377[0], 99151[0], 99152[0], 99153[0], 99155[0], 99156[0], 99157[0], 99201[0], 99202[0], 99203[0], 99204[0], 99205[0], 99211[0], 99212[0], 99213[0], 99214[0], 99215[0], 99217[0], 99218[0], 99219[0], 99220[0], 99221[0], 99222[0], 99223[0], 99224[0], 99225[0], 99226[0], 99231[0], 99232[0], 99233[0], 99234[0], 99235[0], 99236[0], 99238[0], 99239[0], 99281[0], 99282[0], 99283[0], 99284[0], 99285[0], 99304[0], 99305[0], 99306[0], 99307[0], 99308[0], 99309[0], 99310[0], 99315[0], 99318[0], 99324[0], 99325[0], 99326[0], 99327[0], 99328[0], 99334[0], 99335[0], 99336[0], 99337[0], 99341[0], 99342[0], 99343[0], 99347[0], 99348[0], 99349[0], 99354[0], 99355[0], 99356[0], 99357[0], 99358[0], 99359[0], 99415[0], 99416[0], 99446[0], 99447[0], 99448[0], 99449[0], 99451[0], 99452[0], 99466[0], 99468[0], 99469[0], 99471[0], 99472[0], 99475[0], 99476[0], 99477[0], 99478[0], 99479[0], 99480[0], 99483[0], 99485[0], 99497[0], C8921[1], C8922[1], C8923[1], C8924[1], C8925[1], C8926[1], C8927[0], C8929[1], C8930[1], G0380[1], G0381[1], G0382[1], G0383[1], G0384[1], G0406[0], G0407[0], G0408[0], G0425[0], G0426[0], G0427[0], G0463[0], G0500[0], G0508[0], G0509[0]
01760	01996[1], 0213T[1], 0216T[1], 0228T[1], 0230T[1], 31505[1], 31515[1], 31527[1], 31622[1], 31634[1], 31645[1], 31647[1], 36000[1], 36010[0], 36011[1], 36012[1], 36013[1], 36014[1], 36015[1], 36400[1], 36405[1], 36406[1], 36410[1], 36420[1], 36425[1], 36430[1], 36440[1], 36591[0], 36592[0], 36600[1], 36640[1], 43752[1], 43753[1], 43754[1], 61026[1], 61055[1], 62280[1], 62281[1], 62282[1], 62284[1], 62320[1], 62321[1], 62322[1], 62323[1], 62324[1], 62325[1], 62326[1], 62327[1], 64400[1], 64402[1], 64405[1], 64408[1], 64410[1], 64413[1], 64415[1], 64416[1], 64417[1], 64418[1], 64420[1], 64421[1], 64425[1], 64430[1], 64435[1], 64445[1], 64446[1], 64447[1], 64448[1], 64449[1], 64450[1], 64461[1], 64463[1], 64479[1], 64483[1], 64486[1], 64487[1], 64488[1], 64489[1], 64490[1], 64493[1], 64505[1], 64510[1], 64517[1], 64520[1], 64530[1], 64553[1], 64555[1], 67500[1], 76000[1], 76970[1], 76998[0], 77002[0], 90865[1], 92511[1], 92512[1], 92516[1], 92520[1], 92537[1], 92538[1], 92950[1], 92953[1], 92960[1], 92961[1], 93000[1], 93005[1], 93010[1], 93040[1], 93041[1], 93042[1], 93050[0], 93303[0], 93304[0], 93306[1], 93307[1], 93308[1], 93312[1], 93313[1], 93314[1], 93315[1], 93316[1], 93317[1], 93318[0], 93351[1], 93355[0], 93451[1], 93456[1], 93457[1], 93561[0], 93562[0], 93701[0], 93922[1], 93923[1], 93924[1], 93925[1], 93926[1], 93930[1], 93931[1], 93970[1], 93971[1], 93975[1], 93976[1], 93978[1], 93979[1], 93980[1], 93981[1], 94002[1], 94004[1], 94200[1], 94250[0], 94640[1], 94644[1], 94660[1], 94662[1], 94680[1], 94681[1], 94690[1], 94760[0], 94761[0], 94762[1], 94770[1], 95812[0], 95813[0], 95816[0], 95819[0], 95822[0], 95829[0], 95955[0], 95956[0], 95957[0], 96360[0], 96365[0], 96372[0], 96373[0], 96374[0], 96375[0], 96376[0], 96377[0], 99151[0], 99152[0], 99153[0], 99155[0], 99156[0], 99157[0], 99201[0], 99202[0], 99203[0], 99204[0], 99205[0], 99211[0], 99212[0], 99213[0], 99214[0], 99215[0], 99217[0], 99218[0], 99219[0], 99220[0], 99221[0], 99222[0], 99223[0], 99224[0], 99225[0], 99226[0], 99231[0], 99232[0], 99233[0], 99234[0], 99235[0], 99236[0], 99238[0], 99239[0], 99281[0], 99282[0], 99283[0], 99284[0], 99285[0], 99304[0], 99305[0], 99306[0], 99307[0], 99308[0], 99309[0], 99310[0], 99315[0], 99318[0], 99324[0], 99325[0], 99326[0], 99327[0], 99328[0], 99334[0], 99335[0], 99336[0], 99337[0], 99341[0], 99342[0], 99343[0], 99347[0], 99348[0], 99349[0], 99354[0], 99355[0], 99356[0], 99357[0], 99358[0], 99359[0], 99415[0], 99416[0], 99446[0], 99447[0], 99448[0], 99449[0], 99451[0], 99452[0], 99466[0], 99468[0], 99469[0], 99471[0], 99472[0], 99475[0], 99476[0], 99477[0], 99478[0], 99479[0], 99480[0], 99483[0], 99485[0], 99497[0], C8921[1], C8922[1], C8923[1], C8924[1], C8925[1], C8926[1], C8927[0], C8929[1], C8930[1], G0380[1], G0381[1], G0382[1], G0383[1], G0384[1], G0406[0], G0407[0], G0408[0], G0425[0], G0426[0], G0427[0], G0463[0], G0500[0], G0508[0], G0509[0]
01770	01996[1], 0213T[1], 0216T[1], 0228T[1], 0230T[1], 31505[1], 31515[1], 31527[1], 31622[1], 31634[1], 31645[1], 31647[1], 36000[1], 36010[0], 36011[1], 36012[1], 36013[1], 36014[1], 36015[1], 36400[1],

0 = Modifier usage not allowed or inappropriate 1 = Modifier usage allowed

Appendix A: NCCI - CPT Codes

CPT © 2018 American Medical Association. All Rights Reserved.

Code 1	Code 2
	36405[1], 36406[1], 36410[1], 36420[1], 36425[1], 36430[1], 36440[1], 36591[0], 36592[0], 36600[1], 36640[1], 43752[1], 43753[1], 43754[1], 61026[1], 61055[1], 62280[1], 62281[1], 62282[1], 62284[1], 62320[1], 62321[1], 62322[1], 62323[1], 62324[1], 62325[1], 62326[1], 62327[1], 64400[1], 64402[1], 64405[1], 64408[1], 64410[1], 64413[1], 64415[1], 64416[1], 64417[1], 64418[1], 64420[1], 64421[1], 64425[1], 64430[1], 64435[1], 64445[1], 64446[1], 64447[1], 64448[1], 64449[1], 64450[1], 64461[1], 64463[1], 64479[1], 64483[1], 64486[1], 64487[1], 64488[1], 64489[1], 64490[1], 64493[1], 64505[1], 64510[1], 64517[1], 64520[1], 64530[1], 64553[1], 64555[1], 67500[1], 76000[1], 76970[1], 76998[0], 77002[0], 90865[1], 92511[1], 92512[1], 92516[1], 92520[1], 92537[1], 92538[1], 92950[1], 92953[1], 92960[1], 92961[1], 93000[1], 93005[1], 93010[1], 93040[1], 93041[1], 93042[1], 93050[0], 93303[0], 93304[0], 93306[1], 93307[1], 93308[1], 93312[1], 93313[1], 93314[1], 93315[1], 93316[1], 93317[1], 93318[0], 93351[1], 93355[0], 93451[1], 93456[1], 93457[1], 93561[0], 93562[0], 93701[0], 93922[1], 93923[1], 93924[1], 93925[1], 93926[1], 93930[1], 93931[1], 93970[1], 93971[1], 93975[1], 93976[1], 93978[1], 93979[1], 93980[1], 93981[1], 94002[1], 94004[1], 94200[1], 94250[0], 94640[1], 94644[1], 94660[1], 94662[1], 94680[1], 94681[1], 94690[1], 94760[0], 94761[0], 94762[1], 94770[1], 95812[0], 95813[0], 95816[0], 95819[0], 95822[0], 95829[0], 95955[0], 95956[0], 95957[0], 96360[0], 96365[0], 96372[0], 96373[0], 96374[0], 96375[0], 96376[0], 96377[0], 99151[0], 99152[0], 99153[0], 99155[0], 99156[0], 99157[0], 99201[0], 99202[0], 99203[0], 99204[0], 99205[0], 99211[0], 99212[0], 99213[0], 99214[0], 99215[0], 99217[0], 99218[0], 99219[0], 99220[0], 99221[0], 99222[0], 99223[0], 99224[0], 99225[0], 99226[0], 99231[0], 99232[0], 99233[0], 99234[0], 99235[0], 99236[0], 99238[0], 99239[0], 99281[0], 99282[0], 99283[0], 99284[0], 99285[0], 99304[0], 99305[0], 99306[0], 99307[0], 99308[0], 99309[0], 99310[0], 99315[0], 99318[0], 99324[0], 99325[0], 99326[0], 99327[0], 99328[0], 99334[0], 99335[0], 99336[0], 99337[0], 99341[0], 99342[0], 99343[0], 99347[0], 99348[0], 99349[0], 99354[0], 99355[0], 99356[0], 99357[0], 99358[0], 99359[0], 99415[0], 99416[0], 99446[0], 99447[0], 99448[0], 99449[0], 99451[0], 99452[0], 99466[0], 99468[0], 99469[0], 99471[0], 99472[0], 99475[0], 99476[0], 99477[0], 99478[0], 99479[0], 99480[0], 99483[0], 99485[0], 99497[0], C8921[1], C8922[1], C8923[1], C8924[1], C8925[1], C8926[1], C8927[0], C8929[1], C8930[1], G0380[1], G0381[1], G0382[1], G0383[1], G0384[1], G0406[0], G0407[0], G0408[0], G0425[0], G0426[0], G0427[0], G0463[0], G0500[0], G0508[0], G0509[0]
01772	01996[1], 0213T[1], 0216T[1], 0228T[1], 0230T[1], 31505[1], 31515[1], 31527[1], 31622[1], 31634[1], 31645[1], 31647[1], 36000[1], 36010[0], 36011[1], 36012[1], 36013[1], 36014[1], 36015[1], 36400[1], 36405[1], 36406[1], 36410[1], 36420[1], 36425[1], 36430[1], 36440[1], 36591[0], 36592[0], 36600[1], 36640[1], 43752[1], 43753[1], 43754[1], 61026[1], 61055[1], 62280[1], 62281[1], 62282[1], 62284[1], 62320[1], 62321[1], 62322[1], 62323[1], 62324[1], 62325[1], 62326[1], 62327[1], 64400[1], 64402[1], 64405[1], 64408[1], 64410[1], 64413[1], 64415[1], 64416[1], 64417[1], 64418[1], 64420[1], 64421[1], 64425[1], 64430[1], 64435[1], 64445[1], 64446[1], 64447[1], 64448[1], 64449[1], 64450[1], 64461[1], 64463[1], 64479[1], 64483[1], 64486[1], 64487[1], 64488[1], 64489[1], 64490[1], 64493[1], 64505[1], 64510[1], 64517[1], 64520[1], 64530[1], 64553[1], 64555[1], 67500[1], 76000[1], 76970[1], 76998[0], 77002[0], 90865[1], 92511[1], 92512[1], 92516[1], 92520[1], 92537[1], 92538[1], 92950[1], 92953[1], 92960[1], 92961[1], 93000[1], 93005[1], 93010[1], 93040[1], 93041[1], 93042[1], 93050[0], 93303[0], 93304[0], 93306[1], 93307[1], 93308[1], 93312[1], 93313[1], 93314[1], 93315[1], 93316[1], 93317[1], 93318[0], 93351[1], 93355[0], 93451[1], 93456[1], 93457[1], 93561[0], 93562[0], 93701[0], 93922[1], 93923[1], 93924[1], 93925[1], 93926[1], 93930[1], 93931[1], 93970[1], 93971[1], 93975[1], 93976[1], 93978[1], 93979[1], 93980[1], 93981[1], 94002[1], 94004[1], 94200[1], 94250[0], 94640[1], 94644[1], 94660[1], 94662[1], 94680[1], 94681[1], 94690[1], 94760[0], 94761[0], 94762[1], 94770[1], 95812[0], 95813[0], 95816[0], 95819[0], 95822[0], 95829[0], 95955[0], 95956[0], 95957[0], 96360[0], 96365[0], 96372[0], 96373[0], 96374[0], 96375[0], 96376[0], 96377[0], 99151[0], 99152[0], 99153[0], 99155[0], 99156[0], 99157[0], 99201[0], 99202[0], 99203[0], 99204[0], 99205[0], 99211[0], 99212[0], 99213[0], 99214[0], 99215[0], 99217[0], 99218[0], 99219[0], 99220[0], 99221[0], 99222[0], 99223[0], 99224[0], 99225[0], 99226[0], 99231[0], 99232[0], 99233[0], 99234[0], 99235[0], 99236[0], 99238[0], 99239[0], 99281[0], 99282[0], 99283[0], 99284[0], 99285[0], 99304[0], 99305[0], 99306[0], 99307[0], 99308[0], 99309[0], 99310[0], 99315[0], 99318[0], 99324[0], 99325[0], 99326[0], 99327[0], 99328[0], 99334[0], 99335[0], 99336[0], 99337[0], 99341[0], 99342[0], 99343[0], 99347[0], 99348[0], 99349[0], 99354[0], 99355[0], 99356[0], 99357[0], 99358[0], 99359[0], 99415[0], 99416[0], 99446[0], 99447[0], 99448[0], 99449[0], 99451[0], 99452[0], 99466[0], 99468[0], 99469[0], 99471[0], 99472[0], 99475[0], 99476[0], 99477[0], 99478[0], 99479[0], 99480[0], 99483[0], 99485[0], 99497[0], C8921[1], C8922[1], C8923[1], C8924[1], C8925[1], C8926[1], C8927[0], C8929[1], C8930[1], G0380[1], G0381[1], G0382[1], G0383[1], G0384[1], G0406[0], G0407[0], G0408[0], G0425[0], G0426[0], G0427[0], G0463[0], G0500[0], G0508[0], G0509[0]
01780	01996[1], 0213T[1], 0216T[1], 0228T[1], 0230T[1], 31505[1], 31515[1], 31527[1], 31622[1], 31634[1], 31645[1], 31647[1], 36000[1], 36010[0], 36011[1], 36012[1], 36013[1], 36014[1], 36015[1], 36400[1], 36405[1], 36406[1], 36410[1], 36420[1], 36425[1], 36430[1], 36440[1], 36591[0], 36592[0], 36600[1], 36640[1], 43752[1], 43753[1], 43754[1], 61026[1], 61055[1], 62280[1], 62281[1], 62282[1], 62284[1], 62320[1], 62321[1], 62322[1], 62323[1], 62324[1], 62325[1], 62326[1], 62327[1], 64400[1], 64402[1], 64405[1], 64408[1], 64410[1], 64413[1], 64415[1], 64416[1], 64417[1], 64418[1], 64420[1], 64421[1], 64425[1], 64430[1], 64435[1], 64445[1], 64446[1], 64447[1], 64448[1], 64449[1], 64450[1], 64461[1], 64463[1], 64479[1], 64483[1], 64486[1], 64487[1], 64488[1], 64489[1], 64490[1], 64493[1], 64505[1], 64510[1], 64517[1], 64520[1], 64530[1], 64553[1], 64555[1], 67500[1], 76000[1], 76970[1], 76998[0], 77002[0], 90865[1], 92511[1], 92512[1], 92516[1], 92520[1], 92537[1], 92538[1], 92950[1], 92953[1], 92960[1], 92961[1], 93000[1], 93005[1], 93010[1], 93040[1], 93041[1], 93042[1], 93050[0], 93303[0], 93304[0], 93306[1], 93307[1], 93308[1], 93312[1], 93313[1], 93314[1], 93315[1], 93316[1], 93317[1], 93318[0], 93351[1], 93355[0], 93451[1], 93456[1], 93457[1], 93561[0], 93562[0], 93701[0], 93922[1], 93923[1], 93924[1], 93925[1], 93926[1], 93930[1], 93931[1], 93970[1], 93971[1], 93975[1], 93976[1], 93978[1], 93979[1], 93980[1], 93981[1], 94002[1], 94004[1], 94200[1], 94250[0], 94640[1], 94644[1], 94660[1], 94662[1], 94680[1], 94681[1], 94690[1], 94760[0], 94761[0], 94762[1], 94770[1], 95812[0], 95813[0], 95816[0], 95819[0], 95822[0], 95829[0], 95955[0], 95956[0], 95957[0], 96360[0], 96365[0], 96372[0], 96373[0], 96374[0], 96375[0], 96376[0], 96377[0], 99151[0], 99152[0], 99153[0], 99155[0], 99156[0], 99157[0], 99201[0], 99202[0], 99203[0], 99204[0], 99205[0], 99211[0], 99212[0], 99213[0], 99214[0], 99215[0], 99217[0], 99218[0], 99219[0], 99220[0], 99221[0], 99222[0], 99223[0], 99224[0], 99225[0], 99226[0], 99231[0], 99232[0], 99233[0], 99234[0], 99235[0], 99236[0], 99238[0], 99239[0], 99281[0], 99282[0], 99283[0], 99284[0], 99285[0], 99304[0], 99305[0], 99306[0], 99307[0], 99308[0], 99309[0], 99310[0], 99315[0], 99318[0], 99324[0], 99325[0], 99326[0], 99327[0], 99328[0], 99334[0], 99335[0], 99336[0], 99337[0], 99341[0], 99342[0], 99343[0], 99347[0], 99348[0], 99349[0], 99354[0], 99355[0], 99356[0], 99357[0], 99358[0], 99359[0], 99415[0], 99416[0], 99446[0], 99447[0], 99448[0], 99449[0], 99451[0], 99452[0], 99466[0], 99468[0], 99469[0], 99471[0], 99472[0], 99475[0], 99476[0], 99477[0], 99478[0], 99479[0], 99480[0], 99483[0], 99485[0], 99497[0], C8921[1], C8922[1], C8923[1], C8924[1], C8925[1], C8926[1], C8927[0], C8929[1], C8930[1], G0380[1], G0381[1], G0382[1], G0383[1], G0384[1], G0406[0], G0407[0], G0408[0], G0425[0], G0426[0], G0427[0], G0463[0], G0500[0], G0508[0], G0509[0]
01782	01996[1], 0213T[1], 0216T[1], 0228T[1], 0230T[1], 31505[1], 31515[1], 31527[1], 31622[1], 31634[1], 31645[1], 31647[1], 36000[1], 36010[0], 36011[1], 36012[1], 36013[1], 36014[1], 36015[1], 36400[1], 36405[1], 36406[1], 36410[1], 36420[1], 36425[1], 36430[1], 36440[1], 36591[0], 36592[0], 36600[1], 36640[1], 43752[1], 43753[1], 43754[1], 61026[1], 61055[1], 62280[1], 62281[1], 62282[1], 62284[1], 62320[1], 62321[1], 62322[1], 62323[1], 62324[1], 62325[1], 62326[1], 62327[1], 64400[1], 64402[1], 64405[1], 64408[1], 64410[1], 64413[1], 64415[1], 64416[1], 64417[1], 64418[1], 64420[1], 64421[1], 64425[1], 64430[1], 64435[1], 64445[1], 64446[1], 64447[1], 64448[1], 64449[1], 64450[1], 64461[1], 64463[1], 64479[1], 64483[1], 64486[1], 64487[1], 64488[1], 64489[1], 64490[1], 64493[1], 64505[1], 64510[1], 64517[1], 64520[1], 64530[1], 64553[1], 64555[1], 67500[1], 76000[1], 76970[1], 76998[0], 77002[0], 90865[1], 92511[1], 92512[1], 92516[1], 92520[1], 92537[1], 92538[1], 92950[1], 92953[1], 92960[1], 92961[1], 93000[1], 93005[1], 93010[1], 93040[1], 93041[1], 93042[1], 93050[0], 93303[0], 93304[0], 93306[1], 93307[1], 93308[1], 93312[1], 93313[1], 93314[1], 93315[1], 93316[1], 93317[1], 93318[0], 93351[1], 93355[0], 93451[1], 93456[1], 93457[1], 93561[0], 93562[0], 93701[0], 93922[1], 93923[1], 93924[1], 93925[1], 93926[1], 93930[1], 93931[1], 93970[1], 93971[1], 93975[1], 93976[1], 93978[1], 93979[1], 93980[1], 93981[1], 94002[1], 94004[1], 94200[1], 94250[0], 94640[1], 94644[1], 94660[1], 94662[1], 94680[1], 94681[1], 94690[1], 94760[0], 94761[0], 94762[1], 94770[1], 95812[0], 95813[0], 95816[0], 95819[0], 95822[0], 95829[0], 95955[0], 95956[0], 95957[0], 96360[0], 96365[0], 96372[0], 96373[0], 96374[0], 96375[0], 96376[0], 96377[0], 99151[0], 99152[0], 99153[0], 99155[0], 99156[0], 99157[0], 99201[0], 99202[0], 99203[0], 99204[0], 99205[0], 99211[0], 99212[0], 99213[0], 99214[0], 99215[0], 99217[0], 99218[0], 99219[0], 99220[0], 99221[0], 99222[0], 99223[0], 99224[0], 99225[0], 99226[0], 99231[0], 99232[0], 99233[0], 99234[0], 99235[0], 99236[0], 99238[0], 99239[0], 99281[0], 99282[0], 99283[0], 99284[0], 99285[0], 99304[0], 99305[0], 99306[0], 99307[0], 99308[0], 99309[0], 99310[0], 99315[0], 99318[0], 99324[0], 99325[0], 99326[0], 99327[0], 99328[0], 99334[0], 99335[0], 99336[0], 99337[0], 99341[0], 99342[0], 99343[0], 99347[0], 99348[0], 99349[0], 99354[0], 99355[0], 99356[0], 99357[0], 99358[0], 99359[0], 99415[0], 99416[0], 99446[0], 99447[0], 99448[0], 99449[0], 99451[0], 99452[0], 99466[0], 99468[0], 99469[0], 99471[0], 99472[0], 99475[0], 99476[0], 99477[0], 99478[0], 99479[0], 99480[0], 99483[0], 99485[0], 99497[0], C8921[1], C8922[1], C8923[1], C8924[1], C8925[1], C8926[1], C8927[0], C8929[1], C8930[1], G0380[1], G0381[1], G0382[1], G0383[1], G0384[1], G0406[0], G0407[0], G0408[0], G0425[0], G0426[0], G0427[0], G0463[0], G0500[0], G0508[0], G0509[0]
01810	01996[1], 0213T[1], 0216T[1], 0228T[1], 0230T[1], 0333T[0], 0464T[0], 31505[1], 31515[1], 31527[1], 31622[1], 31634[1], 31645[1], 31647[1], 36000[1], 36010[0], 36011[1], 36012[1], 36013[1], 36014[1], 36015[1], 36400[1], 36405[1], 36406[1], 36410[1], 36420[1], 36425[1], 36430[1], 36440[1], 36591[0], 36592[0], 36600[1], 36640[1], 43752[1], 43753[1], 43754[1], 61026[1], 61055[1], 62280[1], 62281[1], 62282[1], 62284[1], 62320[1], 62321[1], 62322[1], 62323[1], 62324[1], 62325[1], 62326[1], 62327[1], 64400[1], 64402[1], 64405[1], 64408[1], 64410[1], 64413[1], 64415[1], 64416[1], 64417[1], 64418[1], 64420[1], 64421[1], 64425[1], 64430[1], 64435[1], 64445[1], 64446[1], 64447[1], 64448[1], 64449[1], 64450[1], 64461[1], 64463[1], 64479[1], 64483[1], 64486[1], 64487[1], 64488[1], 64489[1], 64490[1], 64493[1], 64505[1], 64510[1], 64517[1], 64520[1], 64530[1], 64553[1], 64555[1], 67500[1], 76000[1], 76970[1], 76998[0], 77002[0], 90865[1], 92511[1], 92512[1], 92516[1], 92520[1], 92537[1], 92538[1], 92585[0], 92950[1], 92953[1], 92960[1], 92961[1], 93000[1], 93005[1], 93010[1], 93040[1], 93041[1], 93042[1], 93050[0], 93303[0], 93304[0], 93306[1], 93307[1], 93308[1], 93312[1], 93313[1], 93314[1], 93315[1], 93316[1], 93317[1], 93318[0], 93351[1], 93355[0], 93451[1], 93456[1], 93457[1], 93561[0], 93562[0], 93701[0], 93922[1], 93923[1], 93924[1], 93925[1], 93926[1], 93930[1], 93931[1], 93970[1],

Appendix A: NCCI - CPT Codes

0 = Modifier usage not allowed or inappropriate 1 = Modifier usage allowed

CPT © 2018 American Medical Association. All Rights Reserved.

Code 1	Code 2
	93971[1], 93975[1], 93976[1], 93978[1], 93979[1], 93980[1], 93981[1], 94002[1], 94004[1], 94200[1], 94250[0], 94640[1], 94644[1], 94660[1], 94662[1], 94680[1], 94681[1], 94690[1], 94760[0], 94761[0], 94762[1], 94770[1], 95812[0], 95813[0], 95816[0], 95819[0], 95822[0], 95829[0], 95860[0], 95861[0], 95863[0], 95864[0], 95865[0], 95866[0], 95867[0], 95868[0], 95869[0], 95870[0], 95907[0], 95908[0], 95909[0], 95910[0], 95911[0], 95912[0], 95913[0], 95925[0], 95926[0], 95927[0], 95928[0], 95929[0], 95930[0], 95933[0], 95937[0], 95938[0], 95939[0], 95940[0], 95955[0], 95956[0], 95957[0], 96360[0], 96365[0], 96372[0], 96373[0], 96374[0], 96375[0], 96376[0], 96377[0], 99151[0], 99152[0], 99153[0], 99155[0], 99156[0], 99157[0], 99201[0], 99202[0], 99203[0], 99204[0], 99205[0], 99211[0], 99212[0], 99213[0], 99214[0], 99215[0], 99217[0], 99218[0], 99219[0], 99220[0], 99221[0], 99222[0], 99223[0], 99224[0], 99225[0], 99226[0], 99231[0], 99232[0], 99233[0], 99234[0], 99235[0], 99236[0], 99238[0], 99239[0], 99281[0], 99282[0], 99283[0], 99284[0], 99285[0], 99304[0], 99305[0], 99306[0], 99307[0], 99308[0], 99309[0], 99310[0], 99315[0], 99318[0], 99324[0], 99325[0], 99326[0], 99327[0], 99328[0], 99334[0], 99335[0], 99336[0], 99337[0], 99341[0], 99342[0], 99343[0], 99347[0], 99348[0], 99349[0], 99354[0], 99355[0], 99356[0], 99357[0], 99358[0], 99359[0], 99415[0], 99416[0], 99446[0], 99447[0], 99448[0], 99449[0], 99451[0], 99452[0], 99466[0], 99468[0], 99469[0], 99471[0], 99472[0], 99475[0], 99476[0], 99477[0], 99478[0], 99479[0], 99480[0], 99483[0], 99485[0], 99497[0], C8921[1], C8922[1], C8923[1], C8924[1], C8925[1], C8926[1], C8927[0], C8929[1], C8930[1], G0380[1], G0381[1], G0382[1], G0383[1], G0384[1], G0406[0], G0407[0], G0408[0], G0425[0], G0426[0], G0427[0], G0453[0], G0463[0], G0500[0], G0508[0], G0509[0]
01820	01996[1], 0213T[1], 0216T[1], 0228T[1], 0230T[1], 31505[1], 31515[1], 31527[1], 31622[1], 31634[1], 31645[1], 31647[1], 36000[1], 36010[0], 36011[1], 36012[1], 36013[1], 36014[1], 36015[1], 36400[1], 36405[1], 36406[1], 36410[1], 36420[1], 36425[1], 36430[1], 36440[1], 36591[0], 36592[0], 36600[1], 36640[1], 43752[1], 43753[1], 43754[1], 61026[1], 61055[1], 62280[1], 62281[1], 62282[1], 62284[1], 62320[1], 62321[1], 62322[1], 62323[1], 62324[1], 62325[1], 62326[1], 62327[1], 64400[1], 64402[1], 64405[1], 64408[1], 64410[1], 64413[1], 64415[1], 64416[1], 64417[1], 64418[1], 64420[1], 64421[1], 64425[1], 64430[1], 64435[1], 64445[1], 64446[1], 64447[1], 64448[1], 64449[1], 64450[1], 64461[1], 64463[1], 64479[1], 64483[1], 64486[1], 64487[1], 64488[1], 64489[1], 64490[1], 64493[1], 64505[1], 64510[1], 64517[1], 64520[1], 64530[1], 64553[1], 64555[1], 67500[1], 76000[1], 76970[1], 76998[0], 77002[0], 90865[1], 92511[1], 92512[1], 92516[1], 92520[1], 92537[1], 92538[1], 92950[1], 92953[1], 92960[1], 92961[1], 93000[1], 93005[1], 93010[1], 93040[1], 93041[1], 93042[1], 93050[0], 93303[0], 93304[0], 93306[1], 93307[1], 93308[1], 93312[1], 93313[1], 93314[1], 93315[1], 93316[1], 93317[1], 93318[0], 93351[1], 93355[0], 93451[1], 93456[1], 93457[1], 93561[0], 93562[0], 93701[0], 93922[1], 93923[1], 93924[1], 93925[1], 93926[1], 93930[1], 93931[1], 93970[1], 93971[1], 93975[1], 93976[1], 93978[1], 93979[1], 93980[1], 93981[1], 94002[1], 94004[1], 94200[1], 94250[0], 94640[1], 94644[1], 94660[1], 94662[1], 94680[1], 94681[1], 94690[1], 94760[0], 94761[0], 94762[1], 94770[1], 95812[0], 95813[0], 95816[0], 95819[0], 95822[0], 95829[0], 95955[0], 95956[0], 95957[0], 96360[0], 96365[0], 96372[0], 96373[0], 96374[0], 96375[0], 96376[0], 96377[0], 99151[0], 99152[0], 99153[0], 99155[0], 99156[0], 99157[0], 99201[0], 99202[0], 99203[0], 99204[0], 99205[0], 99211[0], 99212[0], 99213[0], 99214[0], 99215[0], 99217[0], 99218[0], 99219[0], 99220[0], 99221[0], 99222[0], 99223[0], 99224[0], 99225[0], 99226[0], 99231[0], 99232[0], 99233[0], 99234[0], 99235[0], 99236[0], 99238[0], 99239[0], 99281[0], 99282[0], 99283[0], 99284[0], 99285[0], 99304[0], 99305[0], 99306[0], 99307[0], 99308[0], 99309[0], 99310[0], 99315[0], 99318[0], 99324[0], 99325[0], 99326[0], 99327[0], 99328[0], 99334[0], 99335[0], 99336[0], 99337[0], 99341[0], 99342[0], 99343[0], 99347[0], 99348[0], 99349[0], 99354[0], 99355[0], 99356[0], 99357[0], 99358[0], 99359[0], 99415[0], 99416[0], 99446[0], 99447[0], 99448[0], 99449[0], 99451[0], 99452[0], 99466[0], 99468[0], 99469[0], 99471[0], 99472[0], 99475[0], 99476[0], 99477[0], 99478[0], 99479[0], 99480[0], 99483[0], 99485[0], 99497[0], C8921[1], C8922[1], C8923[1], C8924[1], C8925[1], C8926[1], C8927[0], C8929[1], C8930[1], G0380[1], G0381[1], G0382[1], G0383[1], G0384[1], G0406[0], G0407[0], G0408[0], G0425[0], G0426[0], G0427[0], G0463[0], G0500[0], G0508[0], G0509[0]
01829	01996[1], 0213T[1], 0216T[1], 0228T[1], 0230T[1], 31505[1], 31515[1], 31527[1], 31622[1], 31634[1], 31645[1], 31647[1], 36000[1], 36010[0], 36011[1], 36012[1], 36013[1], 36014[1], 36015[1], 36400[1], 36405[1], 36406[1], 36410[1], 36420[1], 36425[1], 36430[1], 36440[1], 36591[0], 36592[0], 36600[1], 36640[1], 43752[1], 43753[1], 43754[1], 61026[1], 61055[1], 62280[1], 62281[1], 62282[1], 62284[1], 62320[1], 62321[1], 62322[1], 62323[1], 62324[1], 62325[1], 62326[1], 62327[1], 64400[1], 64402[1], 64405[1], 64408[1], 64410[1], 64413[1], 64415[1], 64416[1], 64417[1], 64418[1], 64420[1], 64421[1], 64425[1], 64430[1], 64435[1], 64445[1], 64446[1], 64447[1], 64448[1], 64449[1], 64450[1], 64461[1], 64463[1], 64479[1], 64483[1], 64486[1], 64487[1], 64488[1], 64489[1], 64490[1], 64493[1], 64505[1], 64510[1], 64517[1], 64520[1], 64530[1], 64553[1], 64555[1], 67500[0], 76000[1], 76970[1], 76998[0], 77002[0], 90865[1], 92511[1], 92512[1], 92516[1], 92520[1], 92537[1], 92538[1], 92950[1], 92953[1], 92960[1], 92961[1], 93000[1], 93005[1], 93010[1], 93040[1], 93041[1], 93042[1], 93050[0], 93303[0], 93304[0], 93306[1], 93307[1], 93308[1], 93312[1], 93313[1], 93314[1], 93315[1], 93316[1], 93317[1], 93318[0], 93351[1], 93355[0], 93451[1], 93456[1], 93457[1], 93561[0], 93562[0], 93701[0], 93922[1], 93923[1], 93924[1], 93925[1], 93926[1], 93930[1], 93931[1], 93970[1], 93971[1], 93975[1], 93976[1], 93978[1], 93979[1], 93980[1], 93981[1], 94002[1], 94004[1], 94200[1], 94250[0], 94640[1], 94644[1], 94660[1], 94662[1], 94680[1], 94681[1], 94690[1], 94760[0], 94761[0], 94762[1], 94770[1], 95812[0], 95813[0], 95816[0], 95819[0], 95822[0], 95829[0], 95955[0], 95956[0], 95957[0], 96360[0], 96365[0], 96372[0], 96373[0], 96374[0], 96375[0], 96376[0], 96377[0], 99151[0], 99152[0], 99153[0], 99155[0], 99156[0], 99157[0], 99201[0], 99202[0], 99203[0], 99204[0], 99205[0], 99211[0], 99212[0], 99213[0], 99214[0], 99215[0], 99217[0], 99218[0], 99219[0], 99220[0], 99221[0], 99222[0], 99223[0], 99224[0], 99225[0], 99226[0], 99231[0], 99232[0], 99233[0], 99234[0], 99235[0], 99236[0], 99238[0], 99239[0], 99281[0], 99282[0], 99283[0], 99284[0], 99285[0], 99304[0], 99305[0], 99306[0], 99307[0], 99308[0], 99309[0], 99310[0], 99315[0], 99318[0], 99324[0], 99325[0], 99326[0], 99327[0], 99328[0], 99334[0], 99335[0], 99336[0], 99337[0], 99341[0], 99342[0], 99343[0], 99347[0], 99348[0], 99349[0], 99354[0], 99355[0], 99356[0], 99357[0], 99358[0], 99359[0], 99415[0], 99416[0], 99446[0], 99447[0], 99448[0], 99449[0], 99451[0], 99452[0], 99468[0], 99469[0], 99471[0], 99472[0], 99475[0], 99476[0], 99477[0], 99478[0], 99479[0], 99480[0], 99483[0], 99497[0], C8921[1], C8922[1], C8923[1], C8924[1], C8925[1], C8926[1], C8927[0], C8929[1], C8930[1], G0380[1], G0381[1], G0382[1], G0383[1], G0384[1], G0406[0], G0407[0], G0408[0], G0425[0], G0426[0], G0427[0], G0463[0], G0500[0], G0508[0], G0509[0]
01830	01829[1], 01996[1], 0213T[1], 0216T[1], 0228T[1], 0230T[1], 31505[1], 31515[1], 31527[1], 31622[1], 31634[1], 31645[1], 31647[1], 36000[1], 36010[0], 36011[1], 36012[1], 36013[1], 36014[1], 36015[1], 36400[1], 36405[1], 36406[1], 36410[1], 36420[1], 36425[1], 36430[1], 36440[1], 36591[0], 36592[0], 36600[1], 36640[1], 43752[1], 43753[1], 43754[1], 61026[1], 61055[1], 62280[1], 62281[1], 62282[1], 62284[1], 62320[1], 62321[1], 62322[1], 62323[1], 62324[1], 62325[1], 62326[1], 62327[1], 64400[1], 64402[1], 64405[1], 64408[1], 64410[1], 64413[1], 64415[1], 64416[1], 64417[1], 64418[1], 64420[1], 64421[1], 64425[1], 64430[1], 64435[1], 64445[1], 64446[1], 64447[1], 64448[1], 64449[1], 64450[1], 64461[1], 64463[1], 64479[1], 64483[1], 64486[1], 64487[1], 64488[1], 64489[1], 64490[1], 64493[1], 64505[1], 64510[1], 64517[1], 64520[1], 64530[1], 64553[1], 64555[1], 67500[1], 76000[1], 76970[1], 76998[0], 77002[0], 90865[1], 92511[1], 92512[1], 92516[1], 92520[1], 92537[1], 92538[1], 92950[1], 92953[1], 92960[1], 92961[1], 93000[1], 93005[1], 93010[1], 93040[1], 93041[1], 93042[1], 93050[0], 93303[0], 93304[0], 93306[1], 93307[1], 93308[1], 93312[1], 93313[1], 93314[1], 93315[1], 93316[1], 93317[1], 93318[0], 93351[1], 93355[0], 93451[1], 93456[1], 93457[1], 93561[0], 93562[0], 93701[0], 93922[1], 93923[1], 93924[1], 93925[1], 93926[1], 93930[1], 93931[1], 93970[1], 93971[1], 93975[1], 93976[1], 93978[1], 93979[1], 93980[1], 93981[1], 94002[1], 94004[1], 94200[1], 94250[0], 94640[1], 94644[1], 94660[1], 94662[1], 94680[1], 94681[1], 94690[1], 94760[0], 94761[0], 94762[1], 94770[1], 95812[0], 95813[0], 95816[0], 95819[0], 95822[0], 95829[0], 95955[0], 95956[0], 95957[0], 96360[0], 96365[0], 96372[0], 96373[0], 96374[0], 96375[0], 96376[0], 96377[0], 99151[0], 99152[0], 99153[0], 99155[0], 99156[0], 99157[0], 99201[0], 99202[0], 99203[0], 99204[0], 99205[0], 99211[0], 99212[0], 99213[0], 99214[0], 99215[0], 99217[0], 99218[0], 99219[0], 99220[0], 99221[0], 99222[0], 99223[0], 99224[0], 99225[0], 99226[0], 99231[0], 99232[0], 99233[0], 99234[0], 99235[0], 99236[0], 99238[0], 99239[0], 99281[0], 99282[0], 99283[0], 99284[0], 99285[0], 99304[0], 99305[0], 99306[0], 99307[0], 99308[0], 99309[0], 99310[0], 99315[0], 99318[0], 99324[0], 99325[0], 99326[0], 99327[0], 99328[0], 99334[0], 99335[0], 99336[0], 99337[0], 99341[0], 99342[0], 99343[0], 99347[0], 99348[0], 99349[0], 99354[0], 99355[0], 99356[0], 99357[0], 99358[0], 99359[0], 99415[0], 99416[0], 99446[0], 99447[0], 99448[0], 99449[0], 99451[0], 99452[0], 99466[0], 99468[0], 99469[0], 99471[0], 99472[0], 99475[0], 99476[0], 99477[0], 99478[0], 99479[0], 99480[0], 99483[0], 99485[0], 99497[0], C8921[1], C8922[1], C8923[1], C8924[1], C8925[1], C8926[1], C8927[0], C8929[1], C8930[1], G0380[1], G0381[1], G0382[1], G0383[1], G0384[1], G0406[0], G0407[0], G0408[0], G0425[0], G0426[0], G0427[0], G0463[0], G0500[0], G0508[0], G0509[0]
01832	01996[1], 0213T[1], 0216T[1], 0228T[1], 0230T[1], 31505[1], 31515[1], 31527[1], 31622[1], 31634[1], 31645[1], 31647[1], 36000[1], 36010[0], 36011[1], 36012[1], 36013[1], 36014[1], 36015[1], 36400[1], 36405[1], 36406[1], 36410[1], 36420[1], 36425[1], 36430[1], 36440[1], 36591[0], 36592[0], 36600[1], 36640[1], 43752[1], 43753[1], 43754[1], 61026[1], 61055[1], 62280[1], 62281[1], 62282[1], 62284[1], 62320[1], 62321[1], 62322[1], 62323[1], 62324[1], 62325[1], 62326[1], 62327[1], 64400[1], 64402[1], 64405[1], 64408[1], 64410[1], 64413[1], 64415[1], 64416[1], 64417[1], 64418[1], 64420[1], 64421[1], 64425[1], 64430[1], 64435[1], 64445[1], 64446[1], 64447[1], 64448[1], 64449[1], 64450[1], 64461[1], 64463[1], 64479[1], 64483[1], 64486[1], 64487[1], 64488[1], 64489[1], 64490[1], 64493[1], 64505[1], 64510[1], 64517[1], 64520[1], 64530[1], 64553[1], 64555[1], 67500[1], 76000[1], 76970[1], 76998[0], 77002[0], 90865[1], 92511[1], 92512[1], 92516[1], 92520[1], 92537[1], 92538[1], 92950[1], 92953[1], 92960[1], 92961[1], 93000[1], 93005[1], 93010[1], 93040[1], 93041[1], 93042[1], 93050[0], 93303[0], 93304[0], 93306[1], 93307[1], 93308[1], 93312[1], 93313[1], 93314[1], 93315[1], 93316[1], 93317[1], 93318[0], 93351[1], 93355[0], 93451[1], 93456[1], 93457[1], 93561[0], 93562[0], 93701[0], 93922[1], 93923[1], 93924[1], 93925[1], 93926[1], 93930[1], 93931[1], 93970[1], 93971[1], 93975[1], 93976[1], 93978[1], 93979[1], 93980[1], 93981[1], 94002[1], 94004[1], 94200[1], 94250[0], 94640[1], 94644[1], 94660[1], 94662[1], 94680[1], 94681[1], 94690[1], 94760[0], 94761[0], 94762[1], 94770[1], 95812[0], 95813[0], 95816[0], 95819[0], 95822[0], 95829[0], 95955[0], 95956[0], 95957[0], 96360[0], 96365[0], 96372[0], 96373[0], 96374[0], 96375[0], 96376[0], 96377[0], 99151[0], 99152[0], 99153[0], 99155[0], 99156[0], 99157[0], 99201[0], 99202[0], 99203[0], 99204[0], 99205[0], 99211[0], 99212[0], 99213[0], 99214[0], 99215[0], 99217[0], 99218[0], 99219[0], 99220[0], 99221[0], 99222[0], 99223[0], 99224[0], 99225[0], 99226[0], 99231[0], 99232[0], 99233[0], 99234[0], 99235[0], 99236[0], 99238[0], 99239[0], 99281[0], 99282[0], 99283[0], 99284[0], 99285[0], 99304[0], 99305[0], 99306[0], 99307[0], 99308[0], 99309[0], 99310[0], 99315[0], 99318[0], 99324[0], 99325[0], 99326[0], 99327[0], 99328[0], 99334[0], 99335[0], 99336[0], 99337[0], 99341[0], 99342[0], 99343[0], 99347[0], 99348[0], 99349[0], 99354[0],

0 = Modifier usage not allowed or inappropriate 1 = Modifier usage allowed

CPT © 2018 American Medical Association. All Rights Reserved.

Code 1	Code 2
	99355[0], 99356[0], 99357[0], 99358[0], 99359[0], 99415[0], 99416[0], 99446[0], 99447[0], 99448[0], 99449[0], 99451[0], 99452[0], 99466[0], 99468[0], 99469[0], 99471[0], 99472[0], 99475[0], 99476[0], 99477[0], 99478[0], 99479[0], 99480[0], 99483[0], 99485[0], 99497[0], C8921[1], C8922[1], C8923[1], C8924[1], C8925[1], C8926[1], C8927[0], C8929[1], C8930[1], G0380[1], G0381[1], G0382[1], G0383[1], G0384[1], G0406[0], G0407[0], G0408[0], G0425[0], G0426[0], G0427[0], G0463[0], G0500[0], G0508[0], G0509[0]
01840	01996[1], 0213T[1], 0216T[1], 0228T[1], 0230T[1], 31505[1], 31515[1], 31527[1], 31622[1], 31634[1], 31645[1], 31647[1], 36000[1], 36010[0], 36011[1], 36012[1], 36013[1], 36014[1], 36015[1], 36400[1], 36405[1], 36406[1], 36410[1], 36420[1], 36425[1], 36430[1], 36440[1], 36591[0], 36592[0], 36600[1], 36640[1], 43752[1], 43753[1], 43754[1], 61026[1], 61055[1], 62280[1], 62281[1], 62282[1], 62284[1], 62320[1], 62321[1], 62322[1], 62323[1], 62324[1], 62325[1], 62326[1], 62327[1], 64400[1], 64402[1], 64405[1], 64408[1], 64410[1], 64413[1], 64415[1], 64416[1], 64417[1], 64418[1], 64420[1], 64421[1], 64425[1], 64430[1], 64435[1], 64445[1], 64446[1], 64447[1], 64448[1], 64449[1], 64450[1], 64461[1], 64463[1], 64479[1], 64483[1], 64486[1], 64487[1], 64488[1], 64489[1], 64490[1], 64493[1], 64505[1], 64510[1], 64517[1], 64520[1], 64530[1], 64553[1], 64555[1], 67500[1], 76000[1], 76970[1], 76998[0], 77002[0], 90865[1], 92511[1], 92512[1], 92516[1], 92520[1], 92537[1], 92538[1], 92950[1], 92953[1], 92960[1], 92961[1], 93000[1], 93005[1], 93010[1], 93040[1], 93041[1], 93042[1], 93050[0], 93303[0], 93304[0], 93306[1], 93307[1], 93308[1], 93312[1], 93313[1], 93314[1], 93315[1], 93316[1], 93317[1], 93318[0], 93351[1], 93355[0], 93451[1], 93456[1], 93457[1], 93561[0], 93562[0], 93701[0], 93922[1], 93923[1], 93924[1], 93925[1], 93926[1], 93930[1], 93931[1], 93970[1], 93971[1], 93975[1], 93976[1], 93978[1], 93979[1], 93980[1], 93981[1], 94002[1], 94004[1], 94200[1], 94250[0], 94640[1], 94644[1], 94660[1], 94662[1], 94680[1], 94681[1], 94690[1], 94760[0], 94761[0], 94762[1], 94770[1], 95812[0], 95813[0], 95816[0], 95819[0], 95822[0], 95829[0], 95955[0], 95956[0], 95957[0], 96360[0], 96365[0], 96372[0], 96373[0], 96374[0], 96375[0], 96376[0], 96377[0], 99151[0], 99152[0], 99153[0], 99155[0], 99156[0], 99157[0], 99201[0], 99202[0], 99203[0], 99204[0], 99205[0], 99211[0], 99212[0], 99213[0], 99214[0], 99215[0], 99217[0], 99218[0], 99219[0], 99220[0], 99221[0], 99222[0], 99223[0], 99224[0], 99225[0], 99226[0], 99231[0], 99232[0], 99233[0], 99234[0], 99235[0], 99236[0], 99238[0], 99239[0], 99281[0], 99282[0], 99283[0], 99284[0], 99285[0], 99304[0], 99305[0], 99306[0], 99307[0], 99308[0], 99309[0], 99310[0], 99315[0], 99318[0], 99324[0], 99325[0], 99326[0], 99327[0], 99328[0], 99334[0], 99335[0], 99336[0], 99337[0], 99341[0], 99342[0], 99343[0], 99347[0], 99348[0], 99349[0], 99354[0], 99355[0], 99356[0], 99357[0], 99358[0], 99359[0], 99415[0], 99416[0], 99446[0], 99447[0], 99448[0], 99449[0], 99451[0], 99452[0], 99466[0], 99468[0], 99469[0], 99471[0], 99472[0], 99475[0], 99476[0], 99477[0], 99478[0], 99479[0], 99480[0], 99483[0], 99485[0], 99497[0], C8921[1], C8922[1], C8923[1], C8924[1], C8925[1], C8926[1], C8927[0], C8929[1], C8930[1], G0380[1], G0381[1], G0382[1], G0383[1], G0384[1], G0406[0], G0407[0], G0408[0], G0425[0], G0426[0], G0427[0], G0463[0], G0500[0], G0508[0], G0509[0]
01842	01996[1], 0213T[1], 0216T[1], 0228T[1], 0230T[1], 31505[1], 31515[1], 31527[1], 31622[1], 31634[1], 31645[1], 31647[1], 36000[1], 36010[0], 36011[1], 36012[1], 36013[1], 36014[1], 36015[1], 36400[1], 36405[1], 36406[1], 36410[1], 36420[1], 36425[1], 36430[1], 36440[1], 36591[0], 36592[0], 36600[1], 36640[1], 43752[1], 43753[1], 43754[1], 61026[1], 61055[1], 62280[1], 62281[1], 62282[1], 62284[1], 62320[1], 62321[1], 62322[1], 62323[1], 62324[1], 62325[1], 62326[1], 62327[1], 64400[1], 64402[1], 64405[1], 64408[1], 64410[1], 64413[1], 64415[1], 64416[1], 64417[1], 64418[1], 64420[1], 64421[1], 64425[1], 64430[1], 64435[1], 64445[1], 64446[1], 64447[1], 64448[1], 64449[1], 64450[1], 64461[1], 64463[1], 64479[1], 64483[1], 64486[1], 64487[1], 64488[1], 64489[1], 64490[1], 64493[1], 64505[1], 64510[1], 64517[1], 64520[1], 64530[1], 64553[1], 64555[1], 67500[1], 76000[1], 76970[1], 76998[0], 77002[0], 90865[1], 92511[1], 92512[1], 92516[1], 92520[1], 92537[1], 92538[1], 92950[1], 92953[1], 92960[1], 92961[1], 93000[1], 93005[1], 93010[1], 93040[1], 93041[1], 93042[1], 93050[0], 93303[0], 93304[0], 93306[1], 93307[1], 93308[1], 93312[1], 93313[1], 93314[1], 93315[1], 93316[1], 93317[1], 93318[0], 93351[1], 93355[0], 93451[1], 93456[1], 93457[1], 93561[0], 93562[0], 93701[0], 93922[1], 93923[1], 93924[1], 93925[1], 93926[1], 93930[1], 93931[1], 93970[1], 93971[1], 93975[1], 93976[1], 93978[1], 93979[1], 93980[1], 93981[1], 94002[1], 94004[1], 94200[1], 94250[0], 94640[1], 94644[1], 94660[1], 94662[1], 94680[1], 94681[1], 94690[1], 94760[0], 94761[0], 94762[1], 94770[1], 95812[0], 95813[0], 95816[0], 95819[0], 95822[0], 95829[0], 95955[0], 95956[0], 95957[0], 96360[0], 96365[0], 96372[0], 96373[0], 96374[0], 96375[0], 96376[0], 96377[0], 99151[0], 99152[0], 99153[0], 99155[0], 99156[0], 99157[0], 99201[0], 99202[0], 99203[0], 99204[0], 99205[0], 99211[0], 99212[0], 99213[0], 99214[0], 99215[0], 99217[0], 99218[0], 99219[0], 99220[0], 99221[0], 99222[0], 99223[0], 99224[0], 99225[0], 99226[0], 99231[0], 99232[0], 99233[0], 99234[0], 99235[0], 99236[0], 99238[0], 99239[0], 99281[0], 99282[0], 99283[0], 99284[0], 99285[0], 99304[0], 99305[0], 99306[0], 99307[0], 99308[0], 99309[0], 99310[0], 99315[0], 99318[0], 99324[0], 99325[0], 99326[0], 99327[0], 99328[0], 99334[0], 99335[0], 99336[0], 99337[0], 99341[0], 99342[0], 99343[0], 99347[0], 99348[0], 99349[0], 99354[0], 99355[0], 99356[0], 99357[0], 99358[0], 99359[0], 99415[0], 99416[0], 99446[0], 99447[0], 99448[0], 99449[0], 99451[0], 99452[0], 99466[0], 99468[0], 99469[0], 99471[0], 99472[0], 99475[0], 99476[0], 99477[0], 99478[0], 99479[0], 99480[0], 99483[0], 99485[0], 99497[0], C8921[1], C8922[1], C8923[1], C8924[1], C8925[1], C8926[1], C8927[0], C8929[1], C8930[1], G0380[1], G0381[1], G0382[1], G0383[1], G0384[1], G0406[0], G0407[0], G0408[0], G0425[0], G0426[0], G0427[0], G0463[0], G0500[0], G0508[0], G0509[0]
01844	01996[1], 0213T[1], 0216T[1], 0228T[1], 0230T[1], 31505[1], 31515[1], 31527[1], 31622[1], 31634[1], 31645[1], 31647[1], 36000[1], 36010[0], 36011[1], 36012[1], 36013[1], 36014[1], 36015[1], 36400[1], 36405[1], 36406[1], 36410[1], 36420[1], 36425[1], 36430[1], 36440[1], 36591[0], 36592[0], 36600[1], 36640[1], 43752[1], 43753[1], 43754[1], 61026[1], 61055[1], 62280[1], 62281[1], 62282[1], 62284[1], 62320[1], 62321[1], 62322[1], 62323[1], 62324[1], 62325[1], 62326[1], 62327[1], 64400[1], 64402[1], 64405[1], 64408[1], 64410[1], 64413[1], 64415[1], 64416[1], 64417[1], 64418[1], 64420[1], 64421[1], 64425[1], 64430[1], 64435[1], 64445[1], 64446[1], 64447[1], 64448[1], 64449[1], 64450[1], 64461[1], 64463[1], 64479[1], 64483[1], 64486[1], 64487[1], 64488[1], 64489[1], 64490[1], 64493[1], 64505[1], 64510[1], 64517[1], 64520[1], 64530[1], 64553[1], 64555[1], 67500[1], 76000[1], 76970[1], 76998[0], 77002[0], 90865[1], 92511[1], 92512[1], 92516[1], 92520[1], 92537[1], 92538[1], 92950[1], 92953[1], 92960[1], 92961[1], 93000[1], 93005[1], 93010[1], 93040[1], 93041[1], 93042[1], 93050[0], 93303[0], 93304[0], 93306[1], 93307[1], 93308[1], 93312[1], 93313[1], 93314[1], 93315[1], 93316[1], 93317[1], 93318[0], 93351[1], 93355[0], 93451[1], 93456[1], 93457[1], 93561[0], 93562[0], 93701[0], 93922[1], 93923[1], 93924[1], 93925[1], 93926[1], 93930[1], 93931[1], 93970[1], 93971[1], 93975[1], 93976[1], 93978[1], 93979[1], 93980[1], 93981[1], 94002[1], 94004[1], 94200[1], 94250[0], 94640[1], 94644[1], 94660[1], 94662[1], 94680[1], 94681[1], 94690[1], 94760[0], 94761[0], 94762[1], 94770[1], 95812[0], 95813[0], 95816[0], 95819[0], 95822[0], 95829[0], 95955[0], 95956[0], 95957[0], 96360[0], 96365[0], 96372[0], 96373[0], 96374[0], 96375[0], 96376[0], 96377[0], 99151[0], 99152[0], 99153[0], 99155[0], 99156[0], 99157[0], 99201[0], 99202[0], 99203[0], 99204[0], 99205[0], 99211[0], 99212[0], 99213[0], 99214[0], 99215[0], 99217[0], 99218[0], 99219[0], 99220[0], 99221[0], 99222[0], 99223[0], 99224[0], 99225[0], 99226[0], 99231[0], 99232[0], 99233[0], 99234[0], 99235[0], 99236[0], 99238[0], 99239[0], 99281[0], 99282[0], 99283[0], 99284[0], 99285[0], 99304[0], 99305[0], 99306[0], 99307[0], 99308[0], 99309[0], 99310[0], 99315[0], 99318[0], 99324[0], 99325[0], 99326[0], 99327[0], 99328[0], 99334[0], 99335[0], 99336[0], 99337[0], 99341[0], 99342[0], 99343[0], 99347[0], 99348[0], 99349[0], 99354[0], 99355[0], 99356[0], 99357[0], 99358[0], 99359[0], 99415[0], 99416[0], 99446[0], 99447[0], 99448[0], 99449[0], 99451[0], 99452[0], 99466[0], 99468[0], 99469[0], 99471[0], 99472[0], 99475[0], 99476[0], 99477[0], 99478[0], 99479[0], 99480[0], 99483[0], 99485[0], 99497[0], C8921[1], C8922[1], C8923[1], C8924[1], C8925[1], C8926[1], C8927[0], C8929[1], C8930[1], G0380[1], G0381[1], G0382[1], G0383[1], G0384[1], G0406[0], G0407[0], G0408[0], G0425[0], G0426[0], G0427[0], G0463[0], G0500[0], G0508[0], G0509[0]
01850	01996[1], 0213T[1], 0216T[1], 0228T[1], 0230T[1], 31505[1], 31515[1], 31527[1], 31622[1], 31634[1], 31645[1], 31647[1], 36000[1], 36010[0], 36011[1], 36012[1], 36013[1], 36014[1], 36015[1], 36400[1], 36405[1], 36406[1], 36410[1], 36420[1], 36425[1], 36430[1], 36440[1], 36591[0], 36592[0], 36600[1], 36640[1], 43752[1], 43753[1], 43754[1], 61026[1], 61055[1], 62280[1], 62281[1], 62282[1], 62284[1], 62320[1], 62321[1], 62322[1], 62323[1], 62324[1], 62325[1], 62326[1], 62327[1], 64400[1], 64402[1], 64405[1], 64408[1], 64410[1], 64413[1], 64415[1], 64416[1], 64417[1], 64418[1], 64420[1], 64421[1], 64425[1], 64430[1], 64435[1], 64445[1], 64446[1], 64447[1], 64448[1], 64449[1], 64450[1], 64461[1], 64463[1], 64479[1], 64483[1], 64486[1], 64487[1], 64488[1], 64489[1], 64490[1], 64493[1], 64505[1], 64510[1], 64517[1], 64520[1], 64530[1], 64553[1], 64555[1], 67500[1], 76000[1], 76970[1], 76998[0], 77002[0], 90865[1], 92511[1], 92512[1], 92516[1], 92520[1], 92537[1], 92538[1], 92950[1], 92953[1], 92960[1], 92961[1], 93000[1], 93005[1], 93010[1], 93040[1], 93041[1], 93042[1], 93050[0], 93303[0], 93304[0], 93306[1], 93307[1], 93308[1], 93312[1], 93313[1], 93314[1], 93315[1], 93316[1], 93317[1], 93318[0], 93351[1], 93355[0], 93451[1], 93456[1], 93457[1], 93561[0], 93562[0], 93701[0], 93922[1], 93923[1], 93924[1], 93925[1], 93926[1], 93930[1], 93931[1], 93970[1], 93971[1], 93975[1], 93976[1], 93978[1], 93979[1], 93980[1], 93981[1], 94002[1], 94004[1], 94200[1], 94250[0], 94640[1], 94644[1], 94660[1], 94662[1], 94680[1], 94681[1], 94690[1], 94760[0], 94761[0], 94762[1], 94770[1], 95812[0], 95813[0], 95816[0], 95819[0], 95822[0], 95829[0], 95955[0], 95956[0], 95957[0], 96360[0], 96365[0], 96372[0], 96373[0], 96374[0], 96375[0], 96376[0], 96377[0], 99151[0], 99152[0], 99153[0], 99155[0], 99156[0], 99157[0], 99201[0], 99202[0], 99203[0], 99204[0], 99205[0], 99211[0], 99212[0], 99213[0], 99214[0], 99215[0], 99217[0], 99218[0], 99219[0], 99220[0], 99221[0], 99222[0], 99223[0], 99224[0], 99225[0], 99226[0], 99231[0], 99232[0], 99233[0], 99234[0], 99235[0], 99236[0], 99238[0], 99239[0], 99281[0], 99282[0], 99283[0], 99284[0], 99285[0], 99304[0], 99305[0], 99306[0], 99307[0], 99308[0], 99309[0], 99310[0], 99315[0], 99318[0], 99324[0], 99325[0], 99326[0], 99327[0], 99328[0], 99334[0], 99335[0], 99336[0], 99337[0], 99341[0], 99342[0], 99343[0], 99347[0], 99348[0], 99349[0], 99354[0], 99355[0], 99356[0], 99357[0], 99358[0], 99359[0], 99415[0], 99416[0], 99446[0], 99447[0], 99448[0], 99449[0], 99451[0], 99452[0], 99466[0], 99468[0], 99469[0], 99471[0], 99472[0], 99475[0], 99476[0], 99477[0], 99478[0], 99479[0], 99480[0], 99483[0], 99485[0], 99497[0], C8921[1], C8922[1], C8923[1], C8924[1], C8925[1], C8926[1], C8927[0], C8929[1], C8930[1], G0380[1], G0381[1], G0382[1], G0383[1], G0384[1], G0406[0], G0407[0], G0408[0], G0425[0], G0426[0], G0427[0], G0463[0], G0500[0], G0508[0], G0509[0]
01852	01996[1], 0213T[1], 0216T[1], 0228T[1], 0230T[1], 31505[1], 31515[1], 31527[1], 31622[1], 31634[1], 31645[1], 31647[1], 36000[1], 36010[0], 36011[1], 36012[1], 36013[1], 36014[1], 36015[1], 36400[1], 36405[1], 36406[1], 36410[1], 36420[1], 36425[1], 36430[1], 36440[1], 36591[0], 36592[0], 36600[1], 36640[1], 43752[1], 43753[1], 43754[1], 61026[1], 61055[1], 62280[1], 62281[1], 62282[1], 62284[1], 62320[1], 62321[1], 62322[1], 62323[1], 62324[1], 62325[1], 62326[1], 62327[1], 64400[1], 64402[1], 64405[1], 64408[1], 64410[1], 64413[1], 64415[1], 64416[1], 64417[1], 64418[1], 64420[1], 64421[1],

0 = Modifier usage not allowed or inappropriate 1 = Modifier usage allowed

Appendix A: NCCI - CPT Codes

CPT © 2018 American Medical Association. All Rights Reserved.

Code 1	Code 2
	64425[1], 64430[1], 64435[1], 64445[1], 64446[1], 64447[1], 64448[1], 64449[1], 64450[1], 64461[1], 64463[1], 64479[1], 64483[1], 64486[1], 64487[1], 64488[1], 64489[1], 64490[1], 64493[1], 64505[1], 64510[1], 64517[1], 64520[1], 64530[1], 64553[1], 64555[1], 67500[1], 76000[1], 76970[1], 76998[0], 77002[0], 90865[1], 92511[1], 92512[1], 92516[1], 92520[1], 92537[1], 92538[1], 92950[1], 92953[1], 92960[1], 92961[1], 93000[1], 93005[1], 93010[1], 93040[1], 93041[1], 93042[1], 93050[0], 93303[0], 93304[0], 93306[1], 93307[1], 93308[1], 93312[1], 93313[1], 93314[1], 93315[1], 93316[1], 93317[1], 93318[0], 93351[1], 93355[0], 93451[1], 93456[1], 93457[1], 93561[0], 93562[0], 93701[0], 93922[1], 93923[1], 93924[1], 93925[1], 93926[1], 93930[1], 93931[1], 93970[1], 93971[1], 93975[1], 93976[1], 93978[1], 93979[1], 93980[1], 93981[1], 94002[1], 94004[1], 94200[1], 94250[0], 94640[1], 94644[1], 94660[1], 94662[1], 94680[1], 94681[1], 94690[1], 94760[0], 94761[0], 94762[1], 94770[1], 95812[0], 95813[0], 95816[0], 95819[0], 95822[0], 95829[0], 95955[0], 95956[0], 95957[0], 96360[0], 96365[0], 96372[0], 96373[0], 96374[0], 96375[0], 96376[0], 96377[0], 99151[0], 99152[0], 99153[0], 99155[0], 99156[0], 99157[0], 99201[0], 99202[0], 99203[0], 99204[0], 99205[0], 99211[0], 99212[0], 99213[0], 99214[0], 99215[0], 99217[0], 99218[0], 99219[0], 99220[0], 99221[0], 99222[0], 99223[0], 99224[0], 99225[0], 99226[0], 99231[0], 99232[0], 99233[0], 99234[0], 99235[0], 99236[0], 99238[0], 99239[0], 99281[0], 99282[0], 99283[0], 99284[0], 99285[0], 99304[0], 99305[0], 99306[0], 99307[0], 99308[0], 99309[0], 99310[0], 99315[0], 99318[0], 99324[0], 99325[0], 99326[0], 99327[0], 99328[0], 99334[0], 99335[0], 99336[0], 99337[0], 99341[0], 99342[0], 99343[0], 99347[0], 99348[0], 99349[0], 99354[0], 99355[0], 99356[0], 99357[0], 99358[0], 99359[0], 99415[0], 99416[0], 99446[0], 99447[0], 99448[0], 99449[0], 99451[0], 99452[0], 99466[0], 99468[0], 99469[0], 99471[0], 99472[0], 99475[0], 99476[0], 99477[0], 99478[0], 99479[0], 99480[0], 99483[0], 99485[0], 99497[0], C8921[1], C8922[1], C8923[1], C8924[1], C8925[1], C8926[1], C8927[0], C8929[1], C8930[1], G0380[1], G0381[1], G0382[1], G0383[1], G0384[1], G0406[0], G0407[0], G0408[0], G0425[0], G0426[0], G0427[0], G0463[0], G0500[0], G0508[0], G0509[0]
01860	01996[1], 0213T[1], 0216T[1], 0228T[1], 0230T[1], 31505[1], 31515[1], 31527[1], 31622[1], 31634[1], 31645[1], 31647[1], 36000[1], 36010[0], 36011[1], 36012[1], 36013[1], 36014[1], 36015[1], 36400[1], 36405[1], 36406[1], 36410[1], 36420[1], 36425[1], 36430[1], 36440[1], 36591[0], 36592[0], 36600[1], 36640[1], 43752[1], 43753[1], 43754[1], 61026[1], 61055[1], 62280[1], 62281[1], 62282[1], 62284[1], 62320[1], 62321[1], 62322[1], 62323[1], 62324[1], 62325[1], 62326[1], 62327[1], 64400[1], 64402[1], 64405[1], 64408[1], 64410[1], 64413[1], 64415[1], 64416[1], 64417[1], 64418[1], 64420[1], 64421[1], 64425[1], 64430[1], 64435[1], 64445[1], 64446[1], 64447[1], 64448[1], 64449[1], 64450[1], 64461[1], 64463[1], 64479[1], 64483[1], 64486[1], 64487[1], 64488[1], 64489[1], 64490[1], 64493[1], 64505[1], 64510[1], 64517[1], 64520[1], 64530[1], 64553[1], 64555[1], 67500[1], 76000[1], 76970[1], 76998[0], 77002[0], 90865[1], 92511[1], 92512[1], 92516[1], 92520[1], 92537[1], 92538[1], 92950[1], 92953[1], 92960[1], 92961[1], 93000[1], 93005[1], 93010[1], 93040[1], 93041[1], 93042[1], 93050[0], 93303[0], 93304[0], 93306[1], 93307[1], 93308[1], 93312[1], 93313[1], 93314[1], 93315[1], 93316[1], 93317[1], 93318[0], 93351[1], 93355[0], 93451[1], 93456[1], 93457[1], 93561[0], 93562[0], 93701[0], 93922[1], 93923[1], 93924[1], 93925[1], 93926[1], 93930[1], 93931[1], 93970[1], 93971[1], 93975[1], 93976[1], 93978[1], 93979[1], 93980[1], 93981[1], 94002[1], 94004[1], 94200[1], 94250[0], 94640[1], 94644[1], 94660[1], 94662[1], 94680[1], 94681[1], 94690[1], 94760[0], 94761[0], 94762[1], 94770[1], 95812[0], 95813[0], 95816[0], 95819[0], 95822[0], 95829[0], 95955[0], 95956[0], 95957[0], 96360[0], 96365[0], 96372[0], 96373[0], 96374[0], 96375[0], 96376[0], 96377[0], 99151[0], 99152[0], 99153[0], 99155[0], 99156[0], 99157[0], 99201[0], 99202[0], 99203[0], 99204[0], 99205[0], 99211[0], 99212[0], 99213[0], 99214[0], 99215[0], 99217[0], 99218[0], 99219[0], 99220[0], 99221[0], 99222[0], 99223[0], 99224[0], 99225[0], 99226[0], 99231[0], 99232[0], 99233[0], 99234[0], 99235[0], 99236[0], 99238[0], 99239[0], 99281[0], 99282[0], 99283[0], 99284[0], 99285[0], 99304[0], 99305[0], 99306[0], 99307[0], 99308[0], 99309[0], 99310[0], 99315[0], 99318[0], 99324[0], 99325[0], 99326[0], 99327[0], 99328[0], 99334[0], 99335[0], 99336[0], 99337[0], 99341[0], 99342[0], 99343[0], 99347[0], 99348[0], 99349[0], 99354[0], 99355[0], 99356[0], 99357[0], 99358[0], 99359[0], 99415[0], 99416[0], 99446[0], 99447[0], 99448[0], 99449[0], 99451[0], 99452[0], 99466[0], 99468[0], 99469[0], 99471[0], 99472[0], 99475[0], 99476[0], 99477[0], 99478[0], 99479[0], 99480[0], 99483[0], 99485[0], 99497[0], C8921[1], C8922[1], C8923[1], C8924[1], C8925[1], C8926[1], C8927[0], C8929[1], C8930[1], G0380[1], G0381[1], G0382[1], G0383[1], G0384[1], G0406[0], G0407[0], G0408[0], G0425[0], G0426[0], G0427[0], G0463[0], G0500[0], G0508[0], G0509[0]
01916	01996[1], 0213T[1], 0216T[1], 0228T[1], 0230T[1], 31505[1], 31515[1], 31527[1], 31622[1], 31634[1], 31645[1], 31647[1], 36000[1], 36010[0], 36011[1], 36012[1], 36013[1], 36014[1], 36015[1], 36400[1], 36405[1], 36406[1], 36410[1], 36420[1], 36425[1], 36430[1], 36440[1], 36591[0], 36592[0], 36600[1], 36640[1], 43752[1], 43753[1], 43754[1], 61026[1], 61055[1], 62280[1], 62281[1], 62282[1], 62284[1], 62320[1], 62321[1], 62322[1], 62323[1], 62324[1], 62325[1], 62326[1], 62327[1], 64400[1], 64402[1], 64405[1], 64408[1], 64410[1], 64413[1], 64415[1], 64416[1], 64417[1], 64418[1], 64420[1], 64421[1], 64425[1], 64430[1], 64435[1], 64445[1], 64446[1], 64447[1], 64448[1], 64449[1], 64450[1], 64461[1], 64463[1], 64479[1], 64483[1], 64486[1], 64487[1], 64488[1], 64489[1], 64490[1], 64493[1], 64505[1], 64510[1], 64517[1], 64520[1], 64530[1], 64553[1], 64555[1], 67500[0], 76000[1], 76970[1], 76998[0], 77002[0], 90865[1], 92511[1], 92512[1], 92516[1], 92520[1], 92537[1], 92538[1], 92950[1], 92953[1], 92960[1], 92961[1], 93000[1], 93005[1], 93010[1], 93040[1], 93041[1], 93042[1], 93050[0], 93303[0], 93304[0], 93306[1], 93307[1], 93308[1], 93312[1], 93313[1], 93314[1], 93315[1], 93316[1], 93317[1], 93318[0], 93351[1], 93355[0], 93451[1], 93456[1], 93457[1], 93561[0], 93562[0], 93701[0], 93922[1], 93923[1], 93924[1], 93925[1], 93926[1], 93930[1], 93931[1], 93970[1], 93971[1], 93975[1], 93976[1], 93978[1], 93979[1], 93980[1], 93981[1], 94002[1], 94004[1], 94200[1], 94250[0], 94640[1], 94644[1], 94660[1], 94662[1], 94680[1], 94681[1], 94690[1], 94760[0], 94761[0], 94762[1], 94770[1], 95812[0], 95813[0], 95816[0], 95819[0], 95822[0], 95829[0], 95955[0], 95956[0], 95957[0], 96360[0], 96365[0], 96372[0], 96373[0], 96374[0], 96375[0], 96376[0], 96377[0], 99151[0], 99152[0], 99153[0], 99155[0], 99156[0], 99157[0], 99201[0], 99202[0], 99203[0], 99204[0], 99205[0], 99211[0], 99212[0], 99213[0], 99214[0], 99215[0], 99217[0], 99218[0], 99219[0], 99220[0], 99221[0], 99222[0], 99223[0], 99224[0], 99225[0], 99226[0], 99231[0], 99232[0], 99233[0], 99234[0], 99235[0], 99236[0], 99238[0], 99239[0], 99281[0], 99282[0], 99283[0], 99284[0], 99285[0], 99304[0], 99305[0], 99306[0], 99307[0], 99308[0], 99309[0], 99310[0], 99315[0], 99318[0], 99324[0], 99325[0], 99326[0], 99327[0], 99328[0], 99334[0], 99335[0], 99336[0], 99337[0], 99341[0], 99342[0], 99343[0], 99347[0], 99348[0], 99349[0], 99354[0], 99355[0], 99356[0], 99357[0], 99358[0], 99359[0], 99415[0], 99416[0], 99446[0], 99447[0], 99448[0], 99449[0], 99451[0], 99452[0], 99466[0], 99468[0], 99469[0], 99471[0], 99472[0], 99475[0], 99476[0], 99477[0], 99478[0], 99479[0], 99480[0], 99483[0], 99485[0], 99497[0], C8921[1], C8922[1], C8923[1], C8924[1], C8925[1], C8926[1], C8927[0], C8929[1], C8930[1], G0380[1], G0381[1], G0382[1], G0383[1], G0384[1], G0406[0], G0407[0], G0408[0], G0425[0], G0426[0], G0427[0], G0463[0], G0500[0], G0508[0], G0509[0]
01920	01996[1], 0213T[1], 0216T[1], 0228T[1], 0230T[1], 31505[1], 31515[1], 31527[1], 31622[1], 31634[1], 31645[1], 31647[1], 36000[1], 36400[1], 36405[1], 36406[1], 36410[1], 36420[1], 36425[1], 36430[1], 36440[1], 36500[1], 36591[0], 36592[0], 36600[1], 36640[1], 43752[1], 43753[1], 43754[1], 61026[1], 61055[1], 62280[1], 62281[1], 62282[1], 62284[1], 62320[1], 62321[1], 62322[1], 62323[1], 62324[1], 62325[1], 62326[1], 62327[1], 64400[1], 64402[1], 64405[1], 64408[1], 64410[1], 64413[1], 64415[1], 64416[1], 64417[1], 64418[1], 64420[1], 64421[1], 64425[1], 64430[1], 64435[1], 64445[1], 64446[1], 64447[1], 64448[1], 64449[1], 64450[1], 64461[1], 64463[1], 64479[1], 64483[1], 64486[1], 64487[1], 64488[1], 64489[1], 64490[1], 64493[1], 64505[1], 64510[1], 64517[1], 64520[1], 64530[1], 64553[1], 64555[1], 67500[1], 76000[1], 76970[1], 76998[0], 77002[0], 90865[1], 92511[1], 92512[1], 92516[1], 92520[1], 92537[1], 92538[1], 92950[1], 92953[1], 92960[1], 92961[1], 93000[1], 93005[1], 93010[1], 93040[1], 93041[1], 93042[1], 93050[0], 93303[0], 93304[0], 93307[1], 93308[1], 93312[1], 93313[1], 93314[1], 93315[1], 93316[1], 93317[1], 93318[0], 93355[0], 93561[0], 93562[0], 93701[0], 93922[1], 93923[1], 93924[1], 93925[1], 93926[1], 93930[1], 93931[1], 93970[1], 93971[1], 93975[1], 93976[1], 93978[1], 93979[1], 93980[1], 93981[1], 94002[1], 94004[1], 94200[1], 94250[0], 94640[1], 94644[1], 94660[1], 94662[1], 94680[1], 94681[1], 94690[1], 94760[0], 94761[0], 94762[1], 94770[1], 95812[0], 95813[0], 95816[0], 95819[0], 95822[0], 95829[0], 95955[0], 95956[0], 95957[0], 96360[0], 96365[0], 96372[0], 96373[0], 96374[0], 96375[0], 96376[0], 96377[0], 99151[0], 99152[0], 99153[0], 99155[0], 99156[0], 99157[0], 99201[0], 99202[0], 99203[0], 99204[0], 99205[0], 99211[0], 99212[0], 99213[0], 99214[0], 99215[0], 99217[0], 99218[0], 99219[0], 99220[0], 99221[0], 99222[0], 99223[0], 99224[0], 99225[0], 99226[0], 99231[0], 99232[0], 99233[0], 99234[0], 99235[0], 99236[0], 99238[0], 99239[0], 99281[0], 99282[0], 99283[0], 99284[0], 99285[0], 99304[0], 99305[0], 99306[0], 99307[0], 99308[0], 99309[0], 99310[0], 99315[0], 99318[0], 99324[0], 99325[0], 99326[0], 99327[0], 99328[0], 99334[0], 99335[0], 99336[0], 99337[0], 99341[0], 99342[0], 99343[0], 99347[0], 99348[0], 99349[0], 99354[0], 99355[0], 99356[0], 99357[0], 99358[0], 99359[0], 99415[0], 99416[0], 99446[0], 99447[0], 99448[0], 99449[0], 99451[0], 99452[0], 99468[0], 99469[0], 99471[0], 99472[0], 99475[0], 99476[0], 99477[0], 99478[0], 99479[0], 99480[0], 99483[0], 99497[0], C8921[1], C8922[1], C8923[1], C8924[1], C8925[1], C8926[1], C8927[0], C8929[1], G0380[1], G0381[1], G0382[1], G0383[1], G0384[1], G0406[0], G0407[0], G0408[0], G0425[0], G0426[0], G0427[0], G0463[0], G0500[0], G0508[0], G0509[0]
01922	01996[1], 0213T[1], 0216T[1], 0228T[1], 0230T[1], 31505[1], 31515[1], 31527[1], 31622[1], 31634[1], 31645[1], 31647[1], 36000[1], 36010[0], 36011[1], 36012[1], 36013[1], 36014[1], 36015[1], 36400[1], 36405[1], 36406[1], 36410[1], 36420[1], 36425[1], 36430[1], 36440[1], 36591[0], 36592[0], 36600[1], 36640[1], 43752[1], 43753[1], 43754[1], 61026[1], 61055[1], 62280[1], 62281[1], 62282[1], 62284[1], 62320[1], 62321[1], 62322[1], 62323[1], 62324[1], 62325[1], 62326[1], 62327[1], 64400[1], 64402[1], 64405[1], 64408[1], 64410[1], 64413[1], 64415[1], 64416[1], 64417[1], 64418[1], 64420[1], 64421[1], 64425[1], 64430[1], 64435[1], 64445[1], 64446[1], 64447[1], 64448[1], 64449[1], 64450[1], 64461[1], 64463[1], 64479[1], 64483[1], 64486[1], 64487[1], 64488[1], 64489[1], 64490[1], 64493[1], 64505[1], 64510[1], 64517[1], 64520[1], 64530[1], 64553[1], 64555[1], 67500[1], 76000[1], 76970[1], 76998[0], 77002[0], 90865[1], 92511[1], 92512[1], 92516[1], 92520[1], 92537[1], 92538[1], 92950[1], 92953[1], 92960[1], 92961[1], 93000[1], 93005[1], 93010[1], 93040[1], 93041[1], 93042[1], 93050[0], 93303[0], 93304[0], 93307[1], 93308[1], 93312[1], 93313[1], 93314[1], 93315[1], 93316[1], 93317[1], 93318[0], 93355[0], 93451[1], 93456[1], 93457[1], 93561[0], 93562[0], 93701[0], 93922[1], 93923[1], 93924[1], 93925[1], 93926[1], 93930[1], 93931[1], 93970[1], 93971[1], 93975[1], 93976[1], 93978[1], 93979[1], 93980[1], 93981[1], 94002[1], 94004[1], 94200[1], 94250[0], 94640[1], 94644[1], 94660[1], 94662[1], 94680[1], 94681[1], 94690[1], 94760[0], 94761[0], 94762[1], 94770[1], 95812[0], 95813[0], 95816[0], 95819[0], 95822[0], 95829[0], 95955[0], 95956[0], 95957[0], 96360[0], 96365[0], 96372[0], 96373[0], 96374[0], 96375[0], 96376[0], 96377[0], 99151[0], 99152[0], 99153[0], 99155[0], 99156[0], 99157[0], 99201[0], 99202[0], 99203[0], 99204[0], 99205[0], 99211[0], 99212[0], 99213[0], 99214[0], 99215[0], 99217[0], 99218[0], 99219[0], 99220[0], 99221[0], 99222[0], 99223[0], 99224[0], 99225[0], 99226[0],

0 = Modifier usage not allowed or inappropriate 1 = Modifier usage allowed

CPT © 2018 American Medical Association. All Rights Reserved.

Code 1	Code 2
	99231[0], 99232[0], 99233[0], 99234[0], 99235[0], 99236[0], 99238[0], 99239[0], 99281[0], 99282[0], 99283[0], 99284[0], 99285[0], 99304[0], 99305[0], 99306[0], 99307[0], 99308[0], 99309[0], 99310[0], 99315[0], 99318[0], 99324[0], 99325[0], 99326[0], 99327[0], 99328[0], 99334[0], 99335[0], 99336[0], 99337[0], 99341[0], 99342[0], 99343[0], 99347[0], 99348[0], 99349[0], 99354[0], 99355[0], 99356[0], 99357[0], 99358[0], 99359[0], 99415[0], 99416[0], 99446[0], 99447[0], 99448[0], 99449[0], 99451[0], 99452[0], 99468[0], 99469[0], 99471[0], 99472[0], 99475[0], 99476[0], 99477[0], 99478[0], 99479[0], 99480[0], 99483[0], 99497[0], C8921[1], C8922[1], C8923[1], C8924[1], C8925[1], C8926[1], C8927[0], C8929[1], G0380[1], G0381[1], G0382[1], G0383[1], G0384[1], G0406[0], G0407[0], G0408[0], G0425[0], G0426[0], G0427[0], G0463[0], G0500[0], G0508[0], G0509[0]
01924	01916[1], 01996[1], 0213T[1], 0216T[1], 0228T[1], 0230T[1], 0333T[0], 0464T[0], 31505[1], 31515[1], 31527[1], 31622[1], 31634[1], 31645[1], 31647[1], 36000[1], 36010[0], 36011[1], 36012[1], 36013[1], 36014[1], 36015[1], 36400[1], 36405[1], 36406[1], 36410[1], 36420[1], 36425[1], 36430[1], 36440[1], 36591[0], 36592[0], 36600[1], 36640[1], 43752[1], 43753[1], 43754[1], 61026[1], 61055[1], 62280[1], 62281[1], 62282[1], 62284[1], 62320[1], 62321[1], 62322[1], 62323[1], 62324[1], 62325[1], 62326[1], 62327[1], 64400[1], 64402[1], 64405[1], 64408[1], 64410[1], 64413[1], 64415[1], 64416[1], 64417[1], 64418[1], 64420[1], 64421[1], 64425[1], 64430[1], 64435[1], 64445[1], 64446[1], 64447[1], 64448[1], 64449[1], 64450[1], 64461[1], 64463[1], 64479[1], 64483[1], 64486[1], 64487[1], 64488[1], 64489[1], 64490[1], 64493[1], 64505[1], 64510[1], 64517[1], 64520[1], 64530[1], 64553[1], 64555[1], 67500[0], 76000[1], 76970[1], 76998[0], 77002[0], 90865[1], 92511[1], 92512[1], 92516[1], 92520[1], 92537[1], 92538[1], 92585[0], 92950[1], 92953[1], 92960[1], 92961[1], 93000[1], 93005[1], 93010[1], 93040[1], 93041[1], 93042[1], 93050[0], 93303[0], 93304[0], 93306[1], 93307[1], 93308[1], 93312[1], 93313[1], 93314[1], 93315[1], 93316[1], 93317[1], 93318[0], 93351[1], 93355[0], 93451[1], 93561[0], 93562[0], 93701[0], 93922[1], 93923[1], 93924[1], 93925[1], 93926[1], 93930[1], 93931[1], 93970[1], 93971[1], 93975[1], 93976[1], 93978[1], 93979[1], 93980[1], 93981[1], 94002[1], 94004[1], 94200[1], 94250[0], 94640[1], 94644[1], 94660[1], 94662[1], 94680[1], 94681[1], 94690[1], 94760[0], 94761[0], 94762[1], 94770[1], 95812[0], 95813[0], 95816[0], 95819[0], 95822[0], 95829[0], 95860[0], 95861[0], 95863[0], 95864[0], 95865[0], 95866[0], 95867[0], 95868[0], 95869[0], 95870[0], 95907[0], 95908[0], 95909[0], 95910[0], 95911[0], 95912[0], 95913[0], 95925[0], 95926[0], 95927[0], 95928[0], 95929[0], 95930[0], 95933[0], 95937[0], 95938[0], 95939[0], 95940[0], 95955[0], 95956[0], 95957[0], 96360[0], 96365[0], 96372[0], 96373[0], 96374[0], 96375[0], 96376[0], 96377[0], 99151[0], 99152[0], 99153[0], 99155[0], 99156[0], 99157[0], 99201[0], 99202[0], 99203[0], 99204[0], 99205[0], 99211[0], 99212[0], 99213[0], 99214[0], 99215[0], 99217[0], 99218[0], 99219[0], 99220[0], 99221[0], 99222[0], 99223[0], 99224[0], 99225[0], 99226[0], 99231[0], 99232[0], 99233[0], 99234[0], 99235[0], 99236[0], 99238[0], 99239[0], 99281[0], 99282[0], 99283[0], 99284[0], 99285[0], 99304[0], 99305[0], 99306[0], 99307[0], 99308[0], 99309[0], 99310[0], 99315[0], 99318[0], 99324[0], 99325[0], 99326[0], 99327[0], 99328[0], 99334[0], 99335[0], 99336[0], 99337[0], 99341[0], 99342[0], 99343[0], 99347[0], 99348[0], 99349[0], 99354[0], 99355[0], 99356[0], 99357[0], 99358[0], 99359[0], 99415[0], 99416[0], 99446[0], 99447[0], 99448[0], 99449[0], 99451[0], 99452[0], 99466[0], 99468[0], 99469[0], 99471[0], 99472[0], 99475[0], 99476[0], 99477[0], 99478[0], 99479[0], 99480[0], 99483[0], 99485[0], 99497[0], C8921[1], C8922[1], C8923[1], C8924[1], C8925[1], C8926[1], C8927[0], C8929[1], C8930[1], G0380[1], G0381[1], G0382[1], G0383[1], G0384[1], G0406[0], G0407[0], G0408[0], G0425[0], G0426[0], G0427[0], G0453[0], G0463[0], G0500[0], G0508[0], G0509[0]
01925	01916[1], 01996[1], 0213T[1], 0216T[1], 0228T[1], 0230T[1], 0333T[0], 0464T[0], 31505[1], 31515[1], 31527[1], 31622[1], 31634[1], 31645[1], 31647[1], 36000[1], 36010[0], 36011[1], 36012[1], 36013[1], 36014[1], 36015[1], 36400[1], 36405[1], 36406[1], 36410[1], 36420[1], 36425[1], 36430[1], 36440[1], 36591[0], 36592[0], 36600[1], 36640[1], 43752[1], 43753[1], 43754[1], 61026[1], 61055[1], 62280[1], 62281[1], 62282[1], 62284[1], 62320[1], 62321[1], 62322[1], 62323[1], 62324[1], 62325[1], 62326[1], 62327[1], 64400[1], 64402[1], 64405[1], 64408[1], 64410[1], 64413[1], 64415[1], 64416[1], 64417[1], 64418[1], 64420[1], 64421[1], 64425[1], 64430[1], 64435[1], 64445[1], 64446[1], 64447[1], 64448[1], 64449[1], 64450[1], 64461[1], 64463[1], 64479[1], 64483[1], 64486[1], 64487[1], 64488[1], 64489[1], 64490[1], 64493[1], 64505[1], 64510[1], 64517[1], 64520[1], 64530[1], 64553[1], 64555[1], 67500[0], 76000[1], 76970[1], 76998[0], 77002[0], 90865[1], 92511[1], 92512[1], 92516[1], 92520[1], 92537[1], 92538[1], 92585[0], 92950[1], 92953[1], 92960[1], 92961[1], 93000[1], 93005[1], 93010[1], 93040[1], 93041[1], 93042[1], 93050[0], 93303[0], 93304[0], 93306[1], 93307[1], 93308[1], 93312[1], 93313[1], 93314[1], 93315[1], 93316[1], 93317[1], 93318[0], 93351[1], 93355[0], 93451[1], 93561[0], 93562[0], 93701[0], 93922[1], 93923[1], 93924[1], 93925[1], 93926[1], 93930[1], 93931[1], 93970[1], 93971[1], 93975[1], 93976[1], 93978[1], 93979[1], 93980[1], 93981[1], 94002[1], 94004[1], 94200[1], 94250[0], 94640[1], 94644[1], 94660[1], 94662[1], 94680[1], 94681[1], 94690[1], 94760[0], 94761[0], 94762[1], 94770[1], 95812[0], 95813[0], 95816[0], 95819[0], 95822[0], 95829[0], 95860[0], 95861[0], 95863[0], 95864[0], 95865[0], 95866[0], 95867[0], 95868[0], 95869[0], 95870[0], 95907[0], 95908[0], 95909[0], 95910[0], 95911[0], 95912[0], 95913[0], 95925[0], 95926[0], 95927[0], 95928[0], 95929[0], 95930[0], 95933[0], 95937[0], 95938[0], 95939[0], 95940[0], 95955[0], 95956[0], 95957[0], 96360[0], 96365[0], 96372[0], 96373[0], 96374[0], 96375[0], 96376[0], 96377[0], 99151[0], 99152[0], 99153[0], 99155[0], 99156[0], 99157[0], 99201[0], 99202[0], 99203[0], 99204[0], 99205[0], 99211[0], 99212[0], 99213[0], 99214[0], 99215[0], 99217[0], 99218[0], 99219[0], 99220[0], 99221[0], 99222[0], 99223[0], 99224[0], 99225[0], 99226[0], 99231[0], 99232[0], 99233[0], 99234[0], 99235[0], 99236[0], 99238[0], 99239[0], 99281[0], 99282[0], 99283[0], 99284[0], 99285[0], 99304[0], 99305[0], 99306[0], 99307[0], 99308[0], 99309[0], 99310[0], 99315[0], 99318[0], 99324[0], 99325[0], 99326[0], 99327[0], 99328[0], 99334[0], 99335[0], 99336[0], 99337[0], 99341[0], 99342[0], 99343[0], 99347[0], 99348[0], 99349[0], 99354[0], 99355[0], 99356[0], 99357[0], 99358[0], 99359[0], 99415[0], 99416[0], 99446[0], 99447[0], 99448[0], 99449[0], 99451[0], 99452[0], 99466[0], 99468[0], 99469[0], 99471[0], 99472[0], 99475[0], 99476[0], 99477[0], 99478[0], 99479[0], 99480[0], 99483[0], 99485[0], 99497[0], C8921[1], C8922[1], C8923[1], C8924[1], C8925[1], C8926[1], C8927[0], C8929[1], C8930[1], G0380[1], G0381[1], G0382[1], G0383[1], G0384[1], G0406[0], G0407[0], G0408[0], G0425[0], G0426[0], G0427[0], G0453[0], G0463[0], G0500[0], G0508[0], G0509[0]
01926	01916[1], 01996[1], 0213T[1], 0216T[1], 0228T[1], 0230T[1], 0333T[0], 0464T[0], 31505[1], 31515[1], 31527[1], 31622[1], 31634[1], 31645[1], 31647[1], 36000[1], 36010[0], 36011[1], 36012[1], 36013[1], 36014[1], 36015[1], 36400[1], 36405[1], 36406[1], 36410[1], 36420[1], 36425[1], 36430[1], 36440[1], 36591[0], 36592[0], 36600[1], 36640[1], 43752[1], 43753[1], 43754[1], 61026[1], 61055[1], 62280[1], 62281[1], 62282[1], 62284[1], 62320[1], 62321[1], 62322[1], 62323[1], 62324[1], 62325[1], 62326[1], 62327[1], 64400[1], 64402[1], 64405[1], 64408[1], 64410[1], 64413[1], 64415[1], 64416[1], 64417[1], 64418[1], 64420[1], 64421[1], 64425[1], 64430[1], 64435[1], 64445[1], 64446[1], 64447[1], 64448[1], 64449[1], 64450[1], 64461[1], 64463[1], 64479[1], 64483[1], 64486[1], 64487[1], 64488[1], 64489[1], 64490[1], 64493[1], 64505[1], 64510[1], 64517[1], 64520[1], 64530[1], 64553[1], 64555[1], 67500[0], 76000[1], 76970[1], 76998[0], 77002[0], 90865[1], 92511[1], 92512[1], 92516[1], 92520[1], 92537[1], 92538[1], 92585[0], 92950[1], 92953[1], 92960[1], 92961[1], 93000[1], 93005[1], 93010[1], 93040[1], 93041[1], 93042[1], 93050[0], 93303[0], 93304[0], 93306[1], 93307[1], 93308[1], 93312[1], 93313[1], 93314[1], 93315[1], 93316[1], 93317[1], 93318[0], 93351[1], 93355[0], 93451[1], 93561[0], 93562[0], 93701[0], 93922[1], 93923[1], 93924[1], 93925[1], 93926[1], 93930[1], 93931[1], 93970[1], 93971[1], 93975[1], 93976[1], 93978[1], 93979[1], 93980[1], 93981[1], 94002[1], 94004[1], 94200[1], 94250[0], 94640[1], 94644[1], 94660[1], 94662[1], 94680[1], 94681[1], 94690[1], 94760[0], 94761[0], 94762[1], 94770[1], 95812[0], 95813[0], 95816[0], 95819[0], 95822[0], 95829[0], 95860[0], 95861[0], 95863[0], 95864[0], 95865[0], 95866[0], 95867[0], 95868[0], 95869[0], 95870[0], 95907[0], 95908[0], 95909[0], 95910[0], 95911[0], 95912[0], 95913[0], 95925[0], 95926[0], 95927[0], 95928[0], 95929[0], 95930[0], 95933[0], 95937[0], 95938[0], 95939[0], 95940[0], 95955[0], 95956[0], 95957[0], 96360[0], 96365[0], 96372[0], 96373[0], 96374[0], 96375[0], 96376[0], 96377[0], 99151[0], 99152[0], 99153[0], 99155[0], 99156[0], 99157[0], 99201[0], 99202[0], 99203[0], 99204[0], 99205[0], 99211[0], 99212[0], 99213[0], 99214[0], 99215[0], 99217[0], 99218[0], 99219[0], 99220[0], 99221[0], 99222[0], 99223[0], 99224[0], 99225[0], 99226[0], 99231[0], 99232[0], 99233[0], 99234[0], 99235[0], 99236[0], 99238[0], 99239[0], 99281[0], 99282[0], 99283[0], 99284[0], 99285[0], 99304[0], 99305[0], 99306[0], 99307[0], 99308[0], 99309[0], 99310[0], 99315[0], 99318[0], 99324[0], 99325[0], 99326[0], 99327[0], 99328[0], 99334[0], 99335[0], 99336[0], 99337[0], 99341[0], 99342[0], 99343[0], 99347[0], 99348[0], 99349[0], 99354[0], 99355[0], 99356[0], 99357[0], 99358[0], 99359[0], 99415[0], 99416[0], 99446[0], 99447[0], 99448[0], 99449[0], 99451[0], 99452[0], 99466[0], 99468[0], 99469[0], 99471[0], 99472[0], 99475[0], 99476[0], 99477[0], 99478[0], 99479[0], 99480[0], 99483[0], 99485[0], 99497[0], C8921[1], C8922[1], C8923[1], C8924[1], C8925[1], C8926[1], C8927[0], C8929[1], C8930[1], G0380[1], G0381[1], G0382[1], G0383[1], G0384[1], G0406[0], G0407[0], G0408[0], G0425[0], G0426[0], G0427[0], G0453[0], G0463[0], G0500[0], G0508[0], G0509[0]
01930	01916[1], 01996[1], 0213T[1], 0216T[1], 0228T[1], 0230T[1], 0333T[0], 0464T[0], 31505[1], 31515[1], 31527[1], 31622[1], 31634[1], 31645[1], 31647[1], 36000[1], 36010[0], 36011[1], 36012[1], 36013[1], 36014[1], 36015[1], 36400[1], 36405[1], 36406[1], 36410[1], 36420[1], 36425[1], 36430[1], 36440[1], 36591[0], 36592[0], 36600[1], 36640[1], 43752[1], 43753[1], 43754[1], 61026[1], 61055[1], 62280[1], 62281[1], 62282[1], 62284[1], 62320[1], 62321[1], 62322[1], 62323[1], 62324[1], 62325[1], 62326[1], 62327[1], 64400[1], 64402[1], 64405[1], 64408[1], 64410[1], 64413[1], 64415[1], 64416[1], 64417[1], 64418[1], 64420[1], 64421[1], 64425[1], 64430[1], 64435[1], 64445[1], 64446[1], 64447[1], 64448[1], 64449[1], 64450[1], 64461[1], 64463[1], 64479[1], 64483[1], 64486[1], 64487[1], 64488[1], 64489[1], 64490[1], 64493[1], 64505[1], 64510[1], 64517[1], 64520[1], 64530[1], 64553[1], 64555[1], 67500[0], 76000[1], 76970[1], 76998[0], 77002[0], 90865[1], 92511[1], 92512[1], 92516[1], 92520[1], 92537[1], 92538[1], 92585[0], 92950[1], 92953[1], 92960[1], 92961[1], 93000[1], 93005[1], 93010[1], 93040[1], 93041[1], 93042[1], 93050[0], 93303[0], 93304[0], 93306[1], 93307[1], 93308[1], 93312[1], 93313[1], 93314[1], 93315[1], 93316[1], 93317[1], 93318[0], 93351[1], 93355[0], 93451[1], 93456[1], 93457[1], 93561[0], 93562[0], 93701[0], 93922[1], 93923[1], 93924[1], 93925[1], 93926[1], 93930[1], 93931[1], 93970[1], 93971[1], 93975[1], 93976[1], 93978[1], 93979[1], 93980[1], 93981[1], 94002[1], 94004[1], 94200[1], 94250[0], 94640[1], 94644[1], 94660[1], 94662[1], 94680[1], 94681[1], 94690[1], 94760[0], 94761[0], 94762[1], 94770[1], 95812[0], 95813[0], 95816[0], 95819[0], 95822[0], 95829[0], 95860[0], 95861[0], 95863[0], 95864[0], 95865[0], 95866[0], 95867[0], 95868[0], 95869[0], 95870[0], 95907[0], 95908[0], 95909[0], 95910[0], 95911[0], 95912[0], 95913[0], 95925[0], 95926[0], 95927[0], 95928[0], 95929[0], 95930[0], 95933[0], 95937[0], 95938[0], 95939[0], 95940[0], 95955[0], 95956[0], 95957[0], 96360[0], 96365[0], 96372[0], 96373[0], 96374[0], 96375[0], 96376[0], 96377[0], 99151[0], 99152[0], 99153[0], 99155[0], 99156[0], 99157[0], 99201[0], 99202[0], 99203[0], 99204[0], 99205[0], 99211[0], 99212[0], 99213[0], 99214[0], 99215[0], 99217[0], 99218[0], 99219[0], 99220[0], 99221[0], 99222[0], 99223[0], 99224[0], 99225[0], 99226[0], 99231[0], 99232[0], 99233[0], 99234[0], 99235[0], 99236[0],

0 = Modifier usage not allowed or inappropriate   1 = Modifier usage allowed

CPT © 2018 American Medical Association. All Rights Reserved.

Code 1	Code 2
	99238[0], 99239[0], 99281[0], 99282[0], 99283[0], 99284[0], 99285[0], 99304[0], 99305[0], 99306[0], 99307[0], 99308[0], 99309[0], 99310[0], 99315[0], 99318[0], 99324[0], 99325[0], 99326[0], 99327[0], 99328[0], 99334[0], 99335[0], 99336[0], 99337[0], 99341[0], 99342[0], 99343[0], 99347[0], 99348[0], 99349[0], 99354[0], 99355[0], 99356[0], 99357[0], 99358[0], 99359[0], 99415[0], 99416[0], 99446[0], 99447[0], 99448[0], 99449[0], 99451[0], 99452[0], 99466[0], 99468[0], 99469[0], 99471[0], 99472[0], 99475[0], 99476[0], 99477[0], 99478[0], 99479[0], 99480[0], 99483[0], 99485[0], 99497[0], C8921[1], C8922[1], C8923[1], C8924[1], C8925[1], C8926[1], C8927[0], C8929[1], C8930[1], G0380[1], G0381[1], G0382[1], G0383[1], G0384[1], G0406[0], G0407[0], G0408[0], G0425[0], G0426[0], G0427[0], G0453[0], G0463[0], G0500[0], G0508[0], G0509[0]
01931	01916[1], 01996[1], 0213T[1], 0216T[1], 0228T[1], 0230T[1], 31505[1], 31515[1], 31527[1], 31622[1], 31634[1], 31645[1], 31647[1], 36000[1], 36010[0], 36011[1], 36012[1], 36013[1], 36014[1], 36015[1], 36400[1], 36405[1], 36406[1], 36410[1], 36420[1], 36425[1], 36430[1], 36440[1], 36591[0], 36592[0], 36600[1], 36640[1], 43752[1], 43753[1], 43754[1], 61026[1], 61055[1], 62280[1], 62281[1], 62282[1], 62284[1], 62320[1], 62321[1], 62322[1], 62323[1], 62324[1], 62325[1], 62326[1], 62327[1], 64400[1], 64402[1], 64405[1], 64408[1], 64410[1], 64413[1], 64415[1], 64416[1], 64417[1], 64418[1], 64420[1], 64421[1], 64425[1], 64430[1], 64435[1], 64445[1], 64446[1], 64447[1], 64448[1], 64449[1], 64450[1], 64461[1], 64463[1], 64479[1], 64483[1], 64486[1], 64487[1], 64488[1], 64489[1], 64490[1], 64493[1], 64505[1], 64510[1], 64517[1], 64520[1], 64530[1], 64553[1], 64555[1], 67500[0], 76000[1], 76970[1], 76998[0], 77002[0], 90865[1], 92511[1], 92512[1], 92516[1], 92520[1], 92537[1], 92538[1], 92950[1], 92953[1], 92960[1], 92961[1], 93000[1], 93005[1], 93010[1], 93040[1], 93041[1], 93042[1], 93050[0], 93303[0], 93304[0], 93306[1], 93307[1], 93308[1], 93312[1], 93313[1], 93314[1], 93315[1], 93316[1], 93317[1], 93318[0], 93351[1], 93355[0], 93451[1], 93456[1], 93457[1], 93561[0], 93562[0], 93701[0], 93922[1], 93923[1], 93924[1], 93925[1], 93926[1], 93930[1], 93931[1], 93970[1], 93971[1], 93975[1], 93976[1], 93978[1], 93979[1], 93980[1], 93981[1], 94002[1], 94004[1], 94200[1], 94250[0], 94640[1], 94644[1], 94660[1], 94662[1], 94680[1], 94681[1], 94690[1], 94760[0], 94761[0], 94762[1], 94770[1], 95812[0], 95813[0], 95816[0], 95819[0], 95822[0], 95829[0], 95955[0], 95956[0], 95957[0], 96360[0], 96365[0], 96372[0], 96373[0], 96374[0], 96375[0], 96376[0], 96377[0], 99151[0], 99152[0], 99153[0], 99155[0], 99156[0], 99157[0], 99201[0], 99202[0], 99203[0], 99204[0], 99205[0], 99211[0], 99212[0], 99213[0], 99214[0], 99215[0], 99217[0], 99218[0], 99219[0], 99220[0], 99221[0], 99222[0], 99223[0], 99224[0], 99225[0], 99226[0], 99231[0], 99232[0], 99233[0], 99234[0], 99235[0], 99236[0], 99238[0], 99239[0], 99281[0], 99282[0], 99283[0], 99284[0], 99285[0], 99304[0], 99305[0], 99306[0], 99307[0], 99308[0], 99309[0], 99310[0], 99315[0], 99318[0], 99324[0], 99325[0], 99326[0], 99327[0], 99328[0], 99334[0], 99335[0], 99336[0], 99337[0], 99341[0], 99342[0], 99343[0], 99347[0], 99348[0], 99349[0], 99354[0], 99355[0], 99356[0], 99357[0], 99358[0], 99359[0], 99415[0], 99416[0], 99446[0], 99447[0], 99448[0], 99449[0], 99451[0], 99452[0], 99466[0], 99468[0], 99469[0], 99471[0], 99472[0], 99475[0], 99476[0], 99477[0], 99478[0], 99479[0], 99480[0], 99483[0], 99485[0], 99497[0], C8921[1], C8922[1], C8923[1], C8924[1], C8925[1], C8926[1], C8927[0], C8929[1], C8930[1], G0380[1], G0381[1], G0382[1], G0383[1], G0384[1], G0406[0], G0407[0], G0408[0], G0425[0], G0426[0], G0427[0], G0463[0], G0500[0], G0508[0], G0509[0]
01932	01916[1], 01996[1], 0213T[1], 0216T[1], 0228T[1], 0230T[1], 0333T[0], 0464T[0], 31505[1], 31515[1], 31527[1], 31622[1], 31634[1], 31645[1], 31647[1], 36000[1], 36010[0], 36011[1], 36012[1], 36013[1], 36014[1], 36015[1], 36400[1], 36405[1], 36406[1], 36410[1], 36420[1], 36425[1], 36430[1], 36440[1], 36591[0], 36592[0], 36600[1], 36640[1], 43752[1], 43753[1], 43754[1], 61026[1], 61055[1], 62280[1], 62281[1], 62282[1], 62284[1], 62320[1], 62321[1], 62322[1], 62323[1], 62324[1], 62325[1], 62326[1], 62327[1], 64400[1], 64402[1], 64405[1], 64408[1], 64410[1], 64413[1], 64415[1], 64416[1], 64417[1], 64418[1], 64420[1], 64421[1], 64425[1], 64430[1], 64435[1], 64445[1], 64446[1], 64447[1], 64448[1], 64449[1], 64450[1], 64461[1], 64463[1], 64479[1], 64483[1], 64486[1], 64487[1], 64488[1], 64489[1], 64490[1], 64493[1], 64505[1], 64510[1], 64517[1], 64520[1], 64530[1], 64553[1], 64555[1], 67500[0], 76000[1], 76970[1], 76998[0], 77002[0], 90865[1], 92511[1], 92512[1], 92516[1], 92520[1], 92537[1], 92538[1], 92585[0], 92950[1], 92953[1], 92960[1], 92961[1], 93000[1], 93005[1], 93010[1], 93040[1], 93041[1], 93042[1], 93050[0], 93303[0], 93304[0], 93306[1], 93307[1], 93308[1], 93312[1], 93313[1], 93314[1], 93315[1], 93316[1], 93317[1], 93318[0], 93351[1], 93355[0], 93451[1], 93456[1], 93457[1], 93561[0], 93562[0], 93701[0], 93922[1], 93923[1], 93924[1], 93925[1], 93926[1], 93930[1], 93931[1], 93970[1], 93971[1], 93975[1], 93976[1], 93978[1], 93979[1], 93980[1], 93981[1], 94002[1], 94004[1], 94200[1], 94250[0], 94640[1], 94644[1], 94660[1], 94662[1], 94680[1], 94681[1], 94690[1], 94760[0], 94761[0], 94762[1], 94770[1], 95812[0], 95813[0], 95816[0], 95819[0], 95822[0], 95829[0], 95860[0], 95861[0], 95863[0], 95864[0], 95865[0], 95866[0], 95867[0], 95868[0], 95869[0], 95870[0], 95907[0], 95908[0], 95909[0], 95910[0], 95911[0], 95912[0], 95913[0], 95925[0], 95926[0], 95927[0], 95928[0], 95929[0], 95930[0], 95933[0], 95937[0], 95938[0], 95939[0], 95940[0], 95955[0], 95956[0], 95957[0], 96360[0], 96365[0], 96372[0], 96373[0], 96374[0], 96375[0], 96376[0], 96377[0], 99151[0], 99152[0], 99153[0], 99155[0], 99156[0], 99157[0], 99201[0], 99202[0], 99203[0], 99204[0], 99205[0], 99211[0], 99212[0], 99213[0], 99214[0], 99215[0], 99217[0], 99218[0], 99219[0], 99220[0], 99221[0], 99222[0], 99223[0], 99224[0], 99225[0], 99226[0], 99231[0], 99232[0], 99233[0], 99234[0], 99235[0], 99236[0], 99238[0], 99239[0], 99281[0], 99282[0], 99283[0], 99284[0], 99285[0], 99304[0], 99305[0], 99306[0], 99307[0], 99308[0], 99309[0], 99310[0], 99315[0], 99318[0], 99324[0], 99325[0], 99326[0], 99327[0], 99328[0], 99334[0], 99335[0], 99336[0], 99337[0], 99341[0], 99342[0], 99343[0], 99347[0], 99348[0], 99349[0], 99354[0], 99355[0], 99356[0], 99357[0], 99358[0], 99359[0], 99415[0], 99416[0], 99446[0], 99447[0], 99448[0], 99449[0], 99451[0], 99452[0], 99466[0], 99468[0], 99469[0], 99471[0], 99472[0], 99475[0], 99476[0], 99477[0], 99478[0], 99479[0], 99480[0], 99483[0], 99485[0], 99497[0], C8921[1], C8922[1], C8923[1], C8924[1], C8925[1], C8926[1], C8927[0], C8929[1], C8930[1], G0380[1], G0381[1], G0382[1], G0383[1], G0384[1], G0406[0], G0407[0], G0408[0], G0425[0], G0426[0], G0427[0], G0453[0], G0463[0], G0500[0], G0508[0], G0509[0]
01933	01916[1], 01996[1], 0213T[1], 0216T[1], 0228T[1], 0230T[1], 0333T[0], 0464T[0], 31505[1], 31515[1], 31527[1], 31622[1], 31634[1], 31645[1], 31647[1], 36000[1], 36010[0], 36011[1], 36012[1], 36013[1], 36014[1], 36015[1], 36400[1], 36405[1], 36406[1], 36410[1], 36420[1], 36425[1], 36430[1], 36440[1], 36591[0], 36592[0], 36600[1], 36640[1], 43752[1], 43753[1], 43754[1], 61026[1], 61055[1], 62280[1], 62281[1], 62282[1], 62284[1], 62320[1], 62321[1], 62322[1], 62323[1], 62324[1], 62325[1], 62326[1], 62327[1], 64400[1], 64402[1], 64405[1], 64408[1], 64410[1], 64413[1], 64415[1], 64416[1], 64417[1], 64418[1], 64420[1], 64421[1], 64425[1], 64430[1], 64435[1], 64445[1], 64446[1], 64447[1], 64448[1], 64449[1], 64450[1], 64461[1], 64463[1], 64479[1], 64483[1], 64486[1], 64487[1], 64488[1], 64489[1], 64490[1], 64493[1], 64505[1], 64510[1], 64517[1], 64520[1], 64530[1], 64553[1], 64555[1], 67500[0], 76000[1], 76970[1], 76998[0], 77002[0], 90865[1], 92511[1], 92512[1], 92516[1], 92520[1], 92537[1], 92538[1], 92585[0], 92950[1], 92953[1], 92960[1], 92961[1], 93000[1], 93005[1], 93010[1], 93040[1], 93041[1], 93042[1], 93050[0], 93303[0], 93304[0], 93306[1], 93307[1], 93308[1], 93312[1], 93313[1], 93314[1], 93315[1], 93316[1], 93317[1], 93318[0], 93351[1], 93355[0], 93451[1], 93456[1], 93457[1], 93561[0], 93562[0], 93701[0], 93922[1], 93923[1], 93924[1], 93925[1], 93926[1], 93930[1], 93931[1], 93970[1], 93971[1], 93975[1], 93976[1], 93978[1], 93979[1], 93980[1], 93981[1], 94002[1], 94004[1], 94200[1], 94250[0], 94640[1], 94644[1], 94660[1], 94662[1], 94680[1], 94681[1], 94690[1], 94760[0], 94761[0], 94762[1], 94770[1], 95812[0], 95813[0], 95816[0], 95819[0], 95822[0], 95829[0], 95860[0], 95861[0], 95863[0], 95864[0], 95865[0], 95866[0], 95867[0], 95868[0], 95869[0], 95870[0], 95907[0], 95908[0], 95909[0], 95910[0], 95911[0], 95912[0], 95913[0], 95925[0], 95926[0], 95927[0], 95928[0], 95929[0], 95930[0], 95933[0], 95937[0], 95938[0], 95939[0], 95940[0], 95955[0], 95956[0], 95957[0], 96360[0], 96365[0], 96372[0], 96373[0], 96374[0], 96375[0], 96376[0], 96377[0], 99151[0], 99152[0], 99153[0], 99155[0], 99156[0], 99157[0], 99201[0], 99202[0], 99203[0], 99204[0], 99205[0], 99211[0], 99212[0], 99213[0], 99214[0], 99215[0], 99217[0], 99218[0], 99219[0], 99220[0], 99221[0], 99222[0], 99223[0], 99224[0], 99225[0], 99226[0], 99231[0], 99232[0], 99233[0], 99234[0], 99235[0], 99236[0], 99238[0], 99239[0], 99281[0], 99282[0], 99283[0], 99284[0], 99285[0], 99304[0], 99305[0], 99306[0], 99307[0], 99308[0], 99309[0], 99310[0], 99315[0], 99318[0], 99324[0], 99325[0], 99326[0], 99327[0], 99328[0], 99334[0], 99335[0], 99336[0], 99337[0], 99341[0], 99342[0], 99343[0], 99347[0], 99348[0], 99349[0], 99354[0], 99355[0], 99356[0], 99357[0], 99358[0], 99359[0], 99415[0], 99416[0], 99446[0], 99447[0], 99448[0], 99449[0], 99451[0], 99452[0], 99466[0], 99468[0], 99469[0], 99471[0], 99472[0], 99475[0], 99476[0], 99477[0], 99478[0], 99479[0], 99480[0], 99483[0], 99485[0], 99497[0], C8921[1], C8922[1], C8923[1], C8924[1], C8925[1], C8926[1], C8927[0], C8929[1], C8930[1], G0380[1], G0381[1], G0382[1], G0383[1], G0384[1], G0406[0], G0407[0], G0408[0], G0425[0], G0426[0], G0427[0], G0453[0], G0463[0], G0500[0], G0508[0], G0509[0]
01935	01996[1], 0213T[1], 0216T[1], 0228T[1], 0230T[1], 0333T[0], 0464T[0], 31505[1], 31515[1], 31527[1], 31622[1], 31634[1], 31645[1], 31647[1], 36000[1], 36010[0], 36011[1], 36012[1], 36013[1], 36014[1], 36015[1], 36400[1], 36405[1], 36406[1], 36410[1], 36420[1], 36425[1], 36430[1], 36440[1], 36591[0], 36592[0], 36600[1], 36640[1], 43752[1], 43753[1], 43754[1], 61026[1], 62320[1], 62321[1], 62322[1], 62323[1], 62324[1], 62325[1], 62326[1], 62327[1], 64400[1], 64402[1], 64405[1], 64408[1], 64410[1], 64413[1], 64415[1], 64416[1], 64417[1], 64418[1], 64420[1], 64421[1], 64425[1], 64430[1], 64435[1], 64445[1], 64446[1], 64447[1], 64448[1], 64449[1], 64450[1], 64461[1], 64463[1], 64479[1], 64483[1], 64486[1], 64487[1], 64488[1], 64489[1], 64490[1], 64493[1], 64505[1], 64510[1], 64517[1], 64520[1], 64530[1], 64553[1], 64555[1], 67500[1], 76000[1], 76970[1], 76998[0], 77002[0], 90865[1], 92511[1], 92512[1], 92516[1], 92520[1], 92537[1], 92538[1], 92585[0], 92950[1], 92953[1], 92960[1], 92961[1], 93000[1], 93005[1], 93010[1], 93040[1], 93041[1], 93042[1], 93050[0], 93303[0], 93304[0], 93306[1], 93307[1], 93308[1], 93312[1], 93313[1], 93314[1], 93315[1], 93316[1], 93317[1], 93318[0], 93351[1], 93355[0], 93451[1], 93456[1], 93457[1], 93561[0], 93562[0], 93701[0], 93922[1], 93923[1], 93924[1], 93925[1], 93926[1], 93930[1], 93931[1], 93970[1], 93971[1], 93975[1], 93976[1], 93978[1], 93979[1], 93980[1], 93981[1], 94002[1], 94004[1], 94200[1], 94250[0], 94640[1], 94644[1], 94660[1], 94662[1], 94680[1], 94681[1], 94690[1], 94760[0], 94761[0], 94762[1], 94770[1], 95812[0], 95813[0], 95816[0], 95819[0], 95822[0], 95829[0], 95860[0], 95861[0], 95863[0], 95864[0], 95865[0], 95866[0], 95867[0], 95868[0], 95869[0], 95870[0], 95907[0], 95908[0], 95909[0], 95910[0], 95911[0], 95912[0], 95913[0], 95925[0], 95926[0], 95927[0], 95928[0], 95929[0], 95930[0], 95933[0], 95937[0], 95938[0], 95939[0], 95940[0], 95955[0], 95956[0], 95957[0], 96360[0], 96365[0], 96372[0], 96373[0], 96374[0], 96375[0], 96376[0], 96377[0], 99151[0], 99152[0], 99153[0], 99155[0], 99156[0], 99157[0], 99201[0], 99202[0], 99203[0], 99204[0], 99205[0], 99211[0], 99212[0], 99213[0], 99214[0], 99215[0], 99217[0], 99218[0], 99219[0], 99220[0], 99221[0], 99222[0], 99223[0], 99224[0], 99225[0], 99226[0], 99231[0], 99232[0], 99233[0], 99234[0], 99235[0], 99236[0], 99238[0], 99239[0], 99281[0], 99282[0], 99283[0], 99284[0], 99285[0], 99304[0], 99305[0], 99306[0], 99307[0], 99308[0], 99309[0], 99310[0], 99315[0], 99316[0], 99318[0], 99324[0], 99325[0], 99326[0], 99327[0], 99328[0], 99334[0], 99335[0], 99336[0], 99337[0], 99341[0], 99342[0], 99343[0], 99344[0], 99345[0], 99347[0], 99348[0], 99349[0], 99350[0], 99354[0],

0 = Modifier usage not allowed or inappropriate 1 = Modifier usage allowed

CPT © 2018 American Medical Association. All Rights Reserved.

Code 1	Code 2
	99355[0], 99356[0], 99357[0], 99358[0], 99359[0], 99415[0], 99416[0], 99446[0], 99447[0], 99448[0], 99449[0], 99451[0], 99452[0], 99466[0], 99468[0], 99469[0], 99471[0], 99472[0], 99475[0], 99476[0], 99477[0], 99478[0], 99479[0], 99480[0], 99483[0], 99485[0], 99497[0], C8921[1], C8922[1], C8923[1], C8924[1], C8925[1], C8926[1], C8927[0], C8929[1], C8930[1], G0380[1], G0381[1], G0382[1], G0383[1], G0384[1], G0406[0], G0407[0], G0408[0], G0425[0], G0426[0], G0427[0], G0453[0], G0463[0], G0500[0], G0508[0], G0509[0]
01936	01996[1], 0213T[1], 0216T[1], 0228T[1], 0230T[1], 0333T[0], 0464T[0], 31505[1], 31515[1], 31527[1], 31622[1], 31634[1], 31645[1], 31647[1], 36000[1], 36010[0], 36011[1], 36012[1], 36013[1], 36014[1], 36015[1], 36400[1], 36405[1], 36406[1], 36410[1], 36420[1], 36425[1], 36430[1], 36440[1], 36591[0], 36592[0], 36600[1], 36640[1], 43752[1], 43753[1], 43754[1], 61026[1], 62320[1], 62321[1], 62322[1], 62323[1], 62324[1], 62325[1], 62326[1], 62327[1], 64400[1], 64402[1], 64405[1], 64408[1], 64410[1], 64413[1], 64415[1], 64416[1], 64417[1], 64418[1], 64420[1], 64421[1], 64425[1], 64430[1], 64435[1], 64445[1], 64446[1], 64447[1], 64448[1], 64449[1], 64450[1], 64461[1], 64463[1], 64479[1], 64483[1], 64486[1], 64487[1], 64488[1], 64489[1], 64490[1], 64493[1], 64505[1], 64510[1], 64517[1], 64520[1], 64530[1], 64553[1], 64555[1], 67500[1], 76000[1], 76970[1], 76998[0], 77002[0], 90865[1], 92511[1], 92512[1], 92516[1], 92520[1], 92537[1], 92538[1], 92585[0], 92950[1], 92953[1], 92960[1], 92961[1], 93000[1], 93005[1], 93010[1], 93040[1], 93041[1], 93042[1], 93050[0], 93303[0], 93304[0], 93306[1], 93307[1], 93308[1], 93312[1], 93313[1], 93314[1], 93315[1], 93316[1], 93317[1], 93318[0], 93351[1], 93355[0], 93451[1], 93456[1], 93457[1], 93561[0], 93562[0], 93701[0], 93922[1], 93923[1], 93924[1], 93925[1], 93926[1], 93930[1], 93931[1], 93970[1], 93971[1], 93975[1], 93976[1], 93978[1], 93979[1], 93980[1], 93981[1], 94002[1], 94004[1], 94200[1], 94250[0], 94640[1], 94644[1], 94660[1], 94662[1], 94680[1], 94681[1], 94690[1], 94760[0], 94761[0], 94762[1], 94770[1], 95812[0], 95813[0], 95816[0], 95819[0], 95822[0], 95829[0], 95860[0], 95861[0], 95863[0], 95864[0], 95865[0], 95866[0], 95867[0], 95868[0], 95869[0], 95870[0], 95907[0], 95908[0], 95909[0], 95910[0], 95911[0], 95912[0], 95913[0], 95925[0], 95926[0], 95927[0], 95928[0], 95929[0], 95930[0], 95933[0], 95937[0], 95938[0], 95939[0], 95940[0], 95955[0], 95956[0], 95957[0], 96360[0], 96365[0], 96372[0], 96373[0], 96374[0], 96375[0], 96376[0], 96377[0], 99151[0], 99152[0], 99153[0], 99155[0], 99156[0], 99157[0], 99201[0], 99202[0], 99203[0], 99204[0], 99205[0], 99211[0], 99212[0], 99213[0], 99214[0], 99215[0], 99217[0], 99218[0], 99219[0], 99220[0], 99221[0], 99222[0], 99223[0], 99224[0], 99225[0], 99226[0], 99231[0], 99232[0], 99233[0], 99234[0], 99235[0], 99236[0], 99238[0], 99239[0], 99281[0], 99282[0], 99283[0], 99284[0], 99285[0], 99304[0], 99305[0], 99306[0], 99307[0], 99308[0], 99309[0], 99310[0], 99315[0], 99316[0], 99318[0], 99324[0], 99325[0], 99326[0], 99327[0], 99328[0], 99334[0], 99335[0], 99336[0], 99337[0], 99341[0], 99342[0], 99343[0], 99344[0], 99345[0], 99347[0], 99348[0], 99349[0], 99350[0], 99354[0], 99355[0], 99356[0], 99357[0], 99358[0], 99359[0], 99415[0], 99416[0], 99446[0], 99447[0], 99448[0], 99449[0], 99451[0], 99452[0], 99466[0], 99468[0], 99469[0], 99471[0], 99472[0], 99475[0], 99476[0], 99477[0], 99478[0], 99479[0], 99480[0], 99483[0], 99485[0], 99497[0], C8921[1], C8922[1], C8923[1], C8924[1], C8925[1], C8926[1], C8927[0], C8929[1], C8930[1], G0380[1], G0381[1], G0382[1], G0383[1], G0384[1], G0406[0], G0407[0], G0408[0], G0425[0], G0426[0], G0427[0], G0453[0], G0463[0], G0500[0], G0508[0], G0509[0]
01951	01996[1], 0213T[1], 0216T[1], 0228T[1], 0230T[1], 31505[1], 31515[1], 31527[1], 31622[1], 31634[1], 31645[1], 31647[1], 36000[1], 36010[0], 36011[1], 36012[1], 36013[1], 36014[1], 36015[1], 36400[1], 36405[1], 36406[1], 36410[1], 36420[1], 36425[1], 36430[1], 36440[1], 36591[0], 36592[0], 36600[1], 36640[1], 43752[1], 43753[1], 43754[1], 61026[1], 61055[1], 62280[1], 62281[1], 62282[1], 62284[1], 62320[1], 62321[1], 62322[1], 62323[1], 62324[1], 62325[1], 62326[1], 62327[1], 64400[1], 64402[1], 64405[1], 64408[1], 64410[1], 64413[1], 64415[1], 64416[1], 64417[1], 64418[1], 64420[1], 64421[1], 64425[1], 64430[1], 64435[1], 64445[1], 64446[1], 64447[1], 64448[1], 64449[1], 64450[1], 64461[1], 64463[1], 64479[1], 64483[1], 64486[1], 64487[1], 64488[1], 64489[1], 64490[1], 64493[1], 64505[1], 64510[1], 64517[1], 64520[1], 64530[1], 64553[1], 64555[1], 67500[0], 76000[1], 76970[1], 76998[0], 77002[0], 90865[1], 92511[1], 92512[1], 92516[1], 92520[1], 92537[1], 92538[1], 92950[1], 92953[1], 92960[1], 92961[1], 93000[1], 93005[1], 93010[1], 93040[1], 93041[1], 93042[1], 93050[0], 93303[0], 93304[0], 93306[1], 93307[1], 93308[1], 93312[1], 93313[1], 93314[1], 93315[1], 93316[1], 93317[1], 93318[0], 93351[1], 93355[0], 93451[1], 93456[1], 93457[1], 93561[0], 93562[0], 93701[0], 93922[1], 93923[1], 93924[1], 93925[1], 93926[1], 93930[1], 93931[1], 93970[1], 93971[1], 93975[1], 93976[1], 93978[1], 93979[1], 93980[1], 93981[1], 94002[1], 94004[1], 94200[1], 94250[0], 94640[1], 94644[1], 94660[1], 94662[1], 94680[1], 94681[1], 94690[1], 94760[0], 94761[0], 94762[1], 94770[1], 95812[0], 95813[0], 95816[0], 95819[0], 95822[0], 95829[0], 95955[0], 95956[0], 95957[0], 96360[0], 96365[0], 96372[0], 96373[0], 96374[0], 96375[0], 96376[0], 96377[0], 99151[0], 99152[0], 99153[0], 99155[0], 99156[0], 99157[0], 99201[0], 99202[0], 99203[0], 99204[0], 99205[0], 99211[0], 99212[0], 99213[0], 99214[0], 99215[0], 99217[0], 99218[0], 99219[0], 99220[0], 99221[0], 99222[0], 99223[0], 99224[0], 99225[0], 99226[0], 99231[0], 99232[0], 99233[0], 99234[0], 99235[0], 99236[0], 99238[0], 99239[0], 99281[0], 99282[0], 99283[0], 99284[0], 99285[0], 99304[0], 99305[0], 99306[0], 99307[0], 99308[0], 99309[0], 99310[0], 99315[0], 99316[0], 99318[0], 99324[0], 99325[0], 99326[0], 99327[0], 99328[0], 99334[0], 99335[0], 99336[0], 99337[0], 99341[0], 99342[0], 99343[0], 99344[0], 99345[0], 99347[0], 99348[0], 99349[0], 99350[0], 99354[0], 99355[0], 99356[0], 99357[0], 99358[0], 99359[0], 99415[0], 99416[0], 99446[0], 99447[0], 99448[0], 99449[0], 99451[0], 99452[0], 99466[0], 99468[0], 99469[0], 99471[0], 99472[0], 99475[0], 99476[0], 99477[0], 99478[0], 99479[0], 99480[0], 99483[0], 99485[0], 99497[0], C8921[1], C8922[1], C8923[1], C8924[1], C8925[1], C8926[1], C8927[0], C8929[1], C8930[1], G0380[1], G0381[1], G0382[1], G0383[1], G0384[1], G0406[0], G0407[0], G0408[0], G0425[0], G0426[0], G0427[0], G0463[0], G0500[0], G0508[0], G0509[0]
01952	01996[1], 0213T[1], 0216T[1], 0228T[1], 0230T[1], 31505[1], 31515[1], 31527[1], 31622[1], 31634[1], 31645[1], 31647[1], 36000[1], 36010[0], 36011[1], 36012[1], 36013[1], 36014[1], 36015[1], 36400[1], 36405[1], 36406[1], 36410[1], 36420[1], 36425[1], 36430[1], 36440[1], 36591[0], 36592[0], 36600[1], 36640[1], 43752[1], 43753[1], 43754[1], 61026[1], 61055[1], 62280[1], 62281[1], 62282[1], 62284[1], 62320[1], 62321[1], 62322[1], 62323[1], 62324[1], 62325[1], 62326[1], 62327[1], 64400[1], 64402[1], 64405[1], 64408[1], 64410[1], 64413[1], 64415[1], 64416[1], 64417[1], 64418[1], 64420[1], 64421[1], 64425[1], 64430[1], 64435[1], 64445[1], 64446[1], 64447[1], 64448[1], 64449[1], 64450[1], 64461[1], 64463[1], 64479[1], 64483[1], 64486[1], 64487[1], 64488[1], 64489[1], 64490[1], 64493[1], 64505[1], 64510[1], 64517[1], 64520[1], 64530[1], 64553[1], 64555[1], 67500[0], 76000[1], 76970[1], 76998[0], 77002[0], 90865[1], 92511[1], 92512[1], 92516[1], 92520[1], 92537[1], 92538[1], 92950[1], 92953[1], 92960[1], 92961[1], 93000[1], 93005[1], 93010[1], 93040[1], 93041[1], 93042[1], 93050[0], 93303[0], 93304[0], 93306[1], 93307[1], 93308[1], 93312[1], 93313[1], 93314[1], 93315[1], 93316[1], 93317[1], 93318[0], 93351[1], 93355[0], 93451[1], 93456[1], 93457[1], 93561[0], 93562[0], 93701[0], 93922[1], 93923[1], 93924[1], 93925[1], 93926[1], 93930[1], 93931[1], 93970[1], 93971[1], 93975[1], 93976[1], 93978[1], 93979[1], 93980[1], 93981[1], 94002[1], 94004[1], 94200[1], 94250[0], 94640[1], 94644[1], 94660[1], 94662[1], 94680[1], 94681[1], 94690[1], 94760[0], 94761[0], 94762[1], 94770[1], 95812[0], 95813[0], 95816[0], 95819[0], 95822[0], 95829[0], 95955[0], 95956[0], 95957[0], 96360[0], 96365[0], 96372[0], 96373[0], 96374[0], 96375[0], 96376[0], 96377[0], 99151[0], 99152[0], 99153[0], 99155[0], 99156[0], 99157[0], 99201[0], 99202[0], 99203[0], 99204[0], 99205[0], 99211[0], 99212[0], 99213[0], 99214[0], 99215[0], 99217[0], 99218[0], 99219[0], 99220[0], 99221[0], 99222[0], 99223[0], 99224[0], 99225[0], 99226[0], 99231[0], 99232[0], 99233[0], 99234[0], 99235[0], 99236[0], 99238[0], 99239[0], 99281[0], 99282[0], 99283[0], 99284[0], 99285[0], 99304[0], 99305[0], 99306[0], 99307[0], 99308[0], 99309[0], 99310[0], 99315[0], 99316[0], 99318[0], 99324[0], 99325[0], 99326[0], 99327[0], 99328[0], 99334[0], 99335[0], 99336[0], 99337[0], 99341[0], 99342[0], 99343[0], 99344[0], 99345[0], 99347[0], 99348[0], 99349[0], 99350[0], 99354[0], 99355[0], 99356[0], 99357[0], 99358[0], 99359[0], 99415[0], 99416[0], 99446[0], 99447[0], 99448[0], 99449[0], 99451[0], 99452[0], 99466[0], 99468[0], 99469[0], 99471[0], 99472[0], 99475[0], 99476[0], 99477[0], 99478[0], 99479[0], 99480[0], 99483[0], 99485[0], 99497[0], C8921[1], C8922[1], C8923[1], C8924[1], C8925[1], C8926[1], C8927[0], C8929[1], C8930[1], G0380[1], G0381[1], G0382[1], G0383[1], G0384[1], G0406[0], G0407[0], G0408[0], G0425[0], G0426[0], G0427[0], G0463[0], G0500[0], G0508[0], G0509[0]
01953	36000[1], 36591[0], 36592[0], 43752[1], 76970[1], 76998[0], 93050[0], 95812[0], 95813[0], 95816[0], 95819[0], 95822[0], 95829[0], 95956[0], 95957[0], 99151[0], 99152[0], 99153[0], 99155[0], 99156[0], 99157[0], 99358[0], 99359[0], 99446[0], 99447[0], 99448[0], 99449[0], 99451[0], 99452[0], G0500[0]
01958	01996[1], 0213T[1], 0216T[1], 0228T[1], 0229T[1], 0230T[1], 0231T[1], 31505[1], 31515[1], 31527[1], 31622[1], 31634[1], 31645[1], 31647[1], 36000[1], 36010[0], 36011[1], 36012[1], 36013[1], 36014[1], 36015[1], 36400[1], 36405[1], 36406[1], 36410[1], 36420[1], 36425[1], 36430[1], 36440[1], 36591[0], 36592[0], 36600[1], 36640[1], 43752[1], 43753[1], 43754[1], 61026[1], 61055[1], 62280[1], 62281[1], 62282[1], 62284[1], 62320[1], 62321[1], 62322[1], 62323[1], 62324[1], 62325[1], 62326[1], 62327[1], 64400[1], 64402[1], 64405[1], 64408[1], 64410[1], 64413[1], 64415[1], 64416[1], 64417[1], 64418[1], 64420[1], 64421[1], 64425[1], 64430[1], 64435[1], 64445[1], 64446[1], 64447[1], 64448[1], 64449[1], 64450[1], 64461[1], 64463[1], 64479[1], 64480[1], 64483[1], 64484[1], 64486[1], 64487[1], 64488[1], 64489[1], 64490[1], 64493[1], 64505[1], 64510[1], 64517[1], 64520[1], 64530[1], 64553[1], 64555[1], 67500[0], 76000[1], 76970[1], 76998[0], 77002[0], 90865[1], 92511[1], 92512[1], 92516[1], 92520[1], 92537[1], 92538[1], 92950[1], 92953[1], 92960[1], 92961[1], 93000[1], 93005[1], 93010[1], 93040[1], 93041[1], 93042[1], 93050[0], 93303[0], 93304[0], 93306[1], 93307[1], 93308[1], 93312[1], 93313[1], 93314[1], 93315[1], 93316[1], 93317[1], 93318[0], 93351[1], 93355[0], 93451[1], 93456[1], 93457[1], 93561[0], 93562[0], 93701[0], 93922[1], 93923[1], 93924[1], 93925[1], 93926[1], 93930[1], 93931[1], 93970[1], 93971[1], 93975[1], 93976[1], 93978[1], 93979[1], 93980[1], 93981[1], 94002[1], 94004[1], 94200[1], 94250[0], 94640[1], 94644[1], 94660[1], 94662[1], 94680[1], 94681[1], 94690[1], 94760[0], 94761[0], 94762[1], 94770[1], 95812[0], 95813[0], 95816[0], 95819[0], 95822[0], 95829[0], 95955[0], 95956[0], 95957[0], 96360[0], 96365[0], 96372[0], 96373[0], 96374[0], 96375[0], 96376[0], 96377[0], 99151[0], 99152[0], 99153[0], 99155[0], 99156[0], 99157[0], 99201[0], 99202[0], 99203[0], 99204[0], 99205[0], 99211[0], 99212[0], 99213[0], 99214[0], 99215[0], 99217[0], 99218[0], 99219[0], 99220[0], 99221[0], 99222[0], 99223[0], 99224[0], 99225[0], 99226[0], 99231[0], 99232[0], 99233[0], 99234[0], 99235[0], 99236[0], 99238[0], 99239[0], 99281[0], 99282[0], 99283[0], 99284[0], 99285[0], 99304[0], 99305[0], 99306[0], 99307[0], 99308[0], 99309[0], 99310[0], 99315[0], 99316[0], 99318[0], 99324[0], 99325[0], 99326[0], 99327[0], 99328[0], 99334[0], 99335[0], 99336[0], 99337[0], 99341[0], 99342[0], 99343[0], 99344[0], 99345[0], 99347[0], 99348[0], 99349[0], 99350[0], 99354[0], 99355[0], 99356[0], 99357[0], 99358[0], 99359[0], 99415[0], 99416[0], 99446[0], 99447[0], 99448[0], 99449[0], 99451[0], 99452[0], 99466[0], 99468[0], 99469[0], 99471[0], 99472[0], 99475[0], 99476[0], 99477[0], 99478[0], 99479[0], 99480[0], 99483[0], 99485[0], 99497[0], C8921[1], C8922[1], C8923[1], C8924[1], C8925[1],

0 = Modifier usage not allowed or inappropriate 1 = Modifier usage allowed

CPT © 2018 American Medical Association. All Rights Reserved.

Code 1	Code 2
	C8926[1], C8927[0], C8929[1], C8930[1], G0380[1], G0381[1], G0382[1], G0383[1], G0384[1], G0406[0], G0407[0], G0408[0], G0425[0], G0426[0], G0427[0], G0463[0], G0500[0], G0508[0], G0509[0]
01960	01996[1], 0213T[1], 0216T[1], 0228T[1], 0230T[1], 31505[1], 31515[1], 31527[1], 31622[1], 31634[1], 31645[1], 31647[1], 36000[1], 36010[0], 36011[1], 36012[1], 36013[1], 36014[1], 36015[1], 36400[1], 36405[1], 36406[1], 36410[1], 36420[1], 36425[1], 36430[1], 36440[1], 36591[0], 36592[0], 36600[1], 36640[1], 43752[1], 43753[1], 43754[1], 61026[1], 61055[1], 62280[1], 62281[1], 62282[1], 62284[1], 62320[1], 62321[1], 62322[1], 62323[1], 62324[1], 62325[1], 62326[1], 62327[1], 64400[1], 64402[1], 64405[1], 64408[1], 64410[1], 64413[1], 64415[1], 64416[1], 64417[1], 64418[1], 64420[1], 64421[1], 64425[1], 64430[1], 64435[1], 64445[1], 64446[1], 64447[1], 64448[1], 64449[1], 64450[1], 64461[1], 64463[1], 64479[1], 64483[1], 64486[1], 64487[1], 64488[1], 64489[1], 64490[1], 64493[1], 64505[1], 64510[1], 64517[1], 64520[1], 64530[1], 64553[1], 64555[1], 67500[0], 76000[1], 76970[1], 76998[0], 77002[0], 90865[1], 92511[1], 92512[1], 92516[1], 92520[1], 92537[1], 92538[1], 92950[1], 92953[1], 92960[1], 92961[1], 93000[1], 93005[1], 93010[1], 93040[1], 93041[1], 93042[1], 93050[0], 93303[0], 93304[0], 93306[1], 93307[1], 93308[1], 93312[1], 93313[1], 93314[1], 93315[1], 93316[1], 93317[1], 93318[0], 93351[1], 93355[0], 93451[1], 93456[1], 93457[1], 93561[0], 93562[0], 93701[0], 93922[1], 93923[1], 93924[1], 93925[1], 93926[1], 93930[1], 93931[1], 93970[1], 93971[1], 93975[1], 93976[1], 93978[1], 93979[1], 93980[1], 93981[1], 94002[1], 94004[1], 94200[1], 94250[0], 94640[1], 94644[1], 94660[1], 94662[1], 94680[1], 94681[1], 94690[1], 94760[0], 94761[0], 94762[1], 94770[1], 95812[0], 95813[0], 95816[0], 95819[0], 95822[0], 95829[0], 95955[0], 95956[0], 95957[0], 96360[0], 96365[0], 96372[0], 96373[0], 96374[0], 96375[0], 96376[0], 96377[0], 99151[0], 99152[0], 99153[0], 99155[0], 99156[0], 99157[0], 99201[0], 99202[0], 99203[0], 99204[0], 99205[0], 99211[0], 99212[0], 99213[0], 99214[0], 99215[0], 99217[0], 99218[0], 99219[0], 99220[0], 99221[0], 99222[0], 99223[0], 99224[0], 99225[0], 99226[0], 99231[0], 99232[0], 99233[0], 99234[0], 99235[0], 99236[0], 99238[0], 99239[0], 99281[0], 99282[0], 99283[0], 99284[0], 99285[0], 99304[0], 99305[0], 99306[0], 99307[0], 99308[0], 99309[0], 99310[0], 99315[0], 99318[0], 99324[0], 99325[0], 99326[0], 99327[0], 99328[0], 99334[0], 99335[0], 99336[0], 99337[0], 99341[0], 99342[0], 99343[0], 99347[0], 99348[0], 99349[0], 99354[0], 99355[0], 99356[0], 99357[0], 99358[0], 99359[0], 99415[0], 99416[0], 99446[0], 99447[0], 99448[0], 99449[0], 99451[0], 99452[0], 99466[0], 99468[0], 99469[0], 99471[0], 99472[0], 99475[0], 99476[0], 99477[0], 99478[0], 99479[0], 99480[0], 99483[0], 99485[0], 99497[0], C8921[1], C8922[1], C8923[1], C8924[1], C8925[1], C8926[1], C8927[0], C8929[1], C8930[1], G0380[1], G0381[1], G0382[1], G0383[1], G0384[1], G0406[0], G0407[0], G0408[0], G0425[0], G0426[0], G0427[0], G0463[0], G0500[0], G0508[0], G0509[0]
01961	01996[1], 0213T[1], 0216T[1], 0228T[1], 0230T[1], 31505[1], 31515[1], 31527[1], 31622[1], 31634[1], 31645[1], 31647[1], 36000[1], 36010[0], 36011[1], 36012[1], 36013[1], 36014[1], 36015[1], 36400[1], 36405[1], 36406[1], 36410[1], 36420[1], 36425[1], 36430[1], 36440[1], 36591[0], 36592[0], 36600[1], 36640[1], 43752[1], 43753[1], 43754[1], 61026[1], 61055[1], 62280[1], 62281[1], 62282[1], 62284[1], 62320[1], 62321[1], 62322[1], 62323[1], 62324[1], 62325[1], 62326[1], 62327[1], 64400[1], 64402[1], 64405[1], 64408[1], 64410[1], 64413[1], 64415[1], 64416[1], 64417[1], 64418[1], 64420[1], 64421[1], 64425[1], 64430[1], 64435[1], 64445[1], 64446[1], 64447[1], 64448[1], 64449[1], 64450[1], 64461[1], 64463[1], 64479[1], 64483[1], 64486[1], 64487[1], 64488[1], 64489[1], 64490[1], 64493[1], 64505[1], 64510[1], 64517[1], 64520[1], 64530[1], 64553[1], 64555[1], 67500[0], 76000[1], 76970[1], 76998[0], 77002[0], 90865[1], 92511[1], 92512[1], 92516[1], 92520[1], 92537[1], 92538[1], 92950[1], 92953[1], 92960[1], 92961[1], 93000[1], 93005[1], 93010[1], 93040[1], 93041[1], 93042[1], 93050[0], 93303[0], 93304[0], 93306[1], 93307[1], 93308[1], 93312[1], 93313[1], 93314[1], 93315[1], 93316[1], 93317[1], 93318[0], 93351[1], 93355[0], 93451[1], 93456[1], 93457[1], 93561[0], 93562[0], 93701[0], 93922[1], 93923[1], 93924[1], 93925[1], 93926[1], 93930[1], 93931[1], 93970[1], 93971[1], 93975[1], 93976[1], 93978[1], 93979[1], 93980[1], 93981[1], 94002[1], 94004[1], 94200[1], 94250[0], 94640[1], 94644[1], 94660[1], 94662[1], 94680[1], 94681[1], 94690[1], 94760[0], 94761[0], 94762[1], 94770[1], 95812[0], 95813[0], 95816[0], 95819[0], 95822[0], 95829[0], 95955[0], 95956[0], 95957[0], 96360[0], 96365[0], 96372[0], 96373[0], 96374[0], 96375[0], 96376[0], 96377[0], 99151[0], 99152[0], 99153[0], 99155[0], 99156[0], 99157[0], 99201[0], 99202[0], 99203[0], 99204[0], 99205[0], 99211[0], 99212[0], 99213[0], 99214[0], 99215[0], 99217[0], 99218[0], 99219[0], 99220[0], 99221[0], 99222[0], 99223[0], 99224[0], 99225[0], 99226[0], 99231[0], 99232[0], 99233[0], 99234[0], 99235[0], 99236[0], 99238[0], 99239[0], 99281[0], 99282[0], 99283[0], 99284[0], 99285[0], 99304[0], 99305[0], 99306[0], 99307[0], 99308[0], 99309[0], 99310[0], 99315[0], 99318[0], 99324[0], 99325[0], 99326[0], 99327[0], 99328[0], 99334[0], 99335[0], 99336[0], 99337[0], 99341[0], 99342[0], 99343[0], 99347[0], 99348[0], 99349[0], 99354[0], 99355[0], 99356[0], 99357[0], 99358[0], 99359[0], 99415[0], 99416[0], 99446[0], 99447[0], 99448[0], 99449[0], 99451[0], 99452[0], 99466[0], 99468[0], 99469[0], 99471[0], 99472[0], 99475[0], 99476[0], 99477[0], 99478[0], 99479[0], 99480[0], 99483[0], 99485[0], 99497[0], C8921[1], C8922[1], C8923[1], C8924[1], C8925[1], C8926[1], C8927[0], C8929[1], C8930[1], G0380[1], G0381[1], G0382[1], G0383[1], G0384[1], G0406[0], G0407[0], G0408[0], G0425[0], G0426[0], G0427[0], G0463[0], G0500[0], G0508[0], G0509[0]
01962	01996[1], 0213T[1], 0216T[1], 0228T[1], 0230T[1], 31505[1], 31515[1], 31527[1], 31622[1], 31634[1], 31645[1], 31647[1], 36000[1], 36010[0], 36011[1], 36012[1], 36013[1], 36014[1], 36015[1], 36400[1], 36405[1], 36406[1], 36410[1], 36420[1], 36425[1], 36430[1], 36440[1], 36591[0], 36592[0], 36600[1], 36640[1], 43752[1], 43753[1], 43754[1], 61026[1], 61055[1], 62280[1], 62281[1], 62282[1], 62284[1], 62320[1], 62321[1], 62322[1], 62323[1], 62324[1], 62325[1], 62326[1], 62327[1], 64400[1], 64402[1], 64405[1], 64408[1], 64410[1], 64413[1], 64415[1], 64416[1], 64417[1], 64418[1], 64420[1], 64421[1], 64425[1], 64430[1], 64435[1], 64445[1], 64446[1], 64447[1], 64448[1], 64449[1], 64450[1], 64461[1], 64463[1], 64479[1], 64483[1], 64486[1], 64487[1], 64488[1], 64489[1], 64490[1], 64493[1], 64505[1], 64510[1], 64517[1], 64520[1], 64530[1], 64553[1], 64555[1], 67500[0], 76000[1], 76970[1], 76998[0], 77002[0], 90865[1], 92511[1], 92512[1], 92516[1], 92520[1], 92537[1], 92538[1], 92950[1], 92953[1], 92960[1], 92961[1], 93000[1], 93005[1], 93010[1], 93040[1], 93041[1], 93042[1], 93050[0], 93303[0], 93304[0], 93306[1], 93307[1], 93308[1], 93312[1], 93313[1], 93314[1], 93315[1], 93316[1], 93317[1], 93318[0], 93351[1], 93355[0], 93451[1], 93456[1], 93457[1], 93561[0], 93562[0], 93701[0], 93922[1], 93923[1], 93924[1], 93925[1], 93926[1], 93930[1], 93931[1], 93970[1], 93971[1], 93975[1], 93976[1], 93978[1], 93979[1], 93980[1], 93981[1], 94002[1], 94004[1], 94200[1], 94250[0], 94640[1], 94644[1], 94660[1], 94662[1], 94680[1], 94681[1], 94690[1], 94760[0], 94761[0], 94762[1], 94770[1], 95812[0], 95813[0], 95816[0], 95819[0], 95822[0], 95829[0], 95955[0], 95956[0], 95957[0], 96360[0], 96365[0], 96372[0], 96373[0], 96374[0], 96375[0], 96376[0], 96377[0], 99151[0], 99152[0], 99153[0], 99155[0], 99156[0], 99157[0], 99201[0], 99202[0], 99203[0], 99204[0], 99205[0], 99211[0], 99212[0], 99213[0], 99214[0], 99215[0], 99217[0], 99218[0], 99219[0], 99220[0], 99221[0], 99222[0], 99223[0], 99224[0], 99225[0], 99226[0], 99231[0], 99232[0], 99233[0], 99234[0], 99235[0], 99236[0], 99238[0], 99239[0], 99281[0], 99282[0], 99283[0], 99284[0], 99285[0], 99304[0], 99305[0], 99306[0], 99307[0], 99308[0], 99309[0], 99310[0], 99315[0], 99318[0], 99324[0], 99325[0], 99326[0], 99327[0], 99328[0], 99334[0], 99335[0], 99336[0], 99337[0], 99341[0], 99342[0], 99343[0], 99347[0], 99348[0], 99349[0], 99354[0], 99355[0], 99356[0], 99357[0], 99358[0], 99359[0], 99415[0], 99416[0], 99446[0], 99447[0], 99448[0], 99449[0], 99451[0], 99452[0], 99466[0], 99468[0], 99469[0], 99471[0], 99472[0], 99475[0], 99476[0], 99477[0], 99478[0], 99479[0], 99480[0], 99483[0], 99485[0], 99497[0], C8921[1], C8922[1], C8923[1], C8924[1], C8925[1], C8926[1], C8927[0], C8929[1], C8930[1], G0380[1], G0381[1], G0382[1], G0383[1], G0384[1], G0406[0], G0407[0], G0408[0], G0425[0], G0426[0], G0427[0], G0463[0], G0500[0], G0508[0], G0509[0]
01963	01996[1], 0213T[1], 0216T[1], 0228T[1], 0230T[1], 31505[1], 31515[1], 31527[1], 31622[1], 31634[1], 31645[1], 31647[1], 36000[1], 36010[0], 36011[1], 36012[1], 36013[1], 36014[1], 36015[1], 36400[1], 36405[1], 36406[1], 36410[1], 36420[1], 36425[1], 36430[1], 36440[1], 36591[0], 36592[0], 36600[1], 36640[1], 43752[1], 43753[1], 43754[1], 61026[1], 61055[1], 62280[1], 62281[1], 62282[1], 62284[1], 62320[1], 62321[1], 62322[1], 62323[1], 62324[1], 62325[1], 62326[1], 62327[1], 64400[1], 64402[1], 64405[1], 64408[1], 64410[1], 64413[1], 64415[1], 64416[1], 64417[1], 64418[1], 64420[1], 64421[1], 64425[1], 64430[1], 64435[1], 64445[1], 64446[1], 64447[1], 64448[1], 64449[1], 64450[1], 64461[1], 64463[1], 64479[1], 64483[1], 64486[1], 64487[1], 64488[1], 64489[1], 64490[1], 64493[1], 64505[1], 64510[1], 64517[1], 64520[1], 64530[1], 64553[1], 64555[1], 67500[0], 76000[1], 76970[1], 76998[0], 77002[0], 90865[1], 92511[1], 92512[1], 92516[1], 92520[1], 92537[1], 92538[1], 92950[1], 92953[1], 92960[1], 92961[1], 93000[1], 93005[1], 93010[1], 93040[1], 93041[1], 93042[1], 93050[0], 93303[0], 93304[0], 93306[1], 93307[1], 93308[1], 93312[1], 93313[1], 93314[1], 93315[1], 93316[1], 93317[1], 93318[0], 93351[1], 93355[0], 93451[1], 93456[1], 93457[1], 93561[0], 93562[0], 93701[0], 93922[1], 93923[1], 93924[1], 93925[1], 93926[1], 93930[1], 93931[1], 93970[1], 93971[1], 93975[1], 93976[1], 93978[1], 93979[1], 93980[1], 93981[1], 94002[1], 94004[1], 94200[1], 94250[0], 94640[1], 94644[1], 94660[1], 94662[1], 94680[1], 94681[1], 94690[1], 94760[0], 94761[0], 94762[1], 94770[1], 95812[0], 95813[0], 95816[0], 95819[0], 95822[0], 95829[0], 95955[0], 95956[0], 95957[0], 96360[0], 96365[0], 96372[0], 96373[0], 96374[0], 96375[0], 96376[0], 96377[0], 99151[0], 99152[0], 99153[0], 99155[0], 99156[0], 99157[0], 99201[0], 99202[0], 99203[0], 99204[0], 99205[0], 99211[0], 99212[0], 99213[0], 99214[0], 99215[0], 99217[0], 99218[0], 99219[0], 99220[0], 99221[0], 99222[0], 99223[0], 99224[0], 99225[0], 99226[0], 99231[0], 99232[0], 99233[0], 99234[0], 99235[0], 99236[0], 99238[0], 99239[0], 99281[0], 99282[0], 99283[0], 99284[0], 99285[0], 99304[0], 99305[0], 99306[0], 99307[0], 99308[0], 99309[0], 99310[0], 99315[0], 99318[0], 99324[0], 99325[0], 99326[0], 99327[0], 99328[0], 99334[0], 99335[0], 99336[0], 99337[0], 99341[0], 99342[0], 99343[0], 99347[0], 99348[0], 99349[0], 99354[0], 99355[0], 99356[0], 99357[0], 99358[0], 99359[0], 99415[0], 99416[0], 99446[0], 99447[0], 99448[0], 99449[0], 99451[0], 99452[0], 99466[0], 99468[0], 99469[0], 99471[0], 99472[0], 99475[0], 99476[0], 99477[0], 99478[0], 99479[0], 99480[0], 99483[0], 99485[0], 99497[0], C8921[1], C8922[1], C8923[1], C8924[1], C8925[1], C8926[1], C8927[0], C8929[1], C8930[1], G0380[1], G0381[1], G0382[1], G0383[1], G0384[1], G0406[0], G0407[0], G0408[0], G0425[0], G0426[0], G0427[0], G0463[0], G0500[0], G0508[0], G0509[0]
01965	01996[1], 0213T[1], 0216T[1], 0228T[1], 0230T[1], 31505[1], 31515[1], 31527[1], 31622[1], 31634[1], 31645[1], 31647[1], 36000[1], 36010[0], 36011[1], 36012[1], 36013[1], 36014[1], 36015[1], 36400[1], 36405[1], 36406[1], 36410[1], 36420[1], 36425[1], 36430[1], 36440[1], 36591[0], 36592[0], 36600[1], 36640[1], 43752[1], 43753[1], 43754[1], 61026[1], 61055[1], 62280[1], 62281[1], 62282[1], 62284[1], 62320[1], 62321[1], 62322[1], 62323[1], 62324[1], 62325[1], 62326[1], 62327[1], 64400[1], 64402[1], 64405[1], 64408[1], 64410[1], 64413[1], 64415[1], 64416[1], 64417[1], 64418[1], 64420[1], 64421[1], 64425[1], 64430[1], 64435[1], 64445[1], 64446[1], 64447[1], 64448[1], 64449[1], 64450[1], 64461[1], 64463[1], 64479[1], 64483[1], 64486[1], 64487[1], 64488[1], 64489[1], 64490[1], 64493[1], 64505[1], 64510[1], 64517[1], 64520[1], 64530[1], 64553[1], 64555[1], 67500[0], 76000[1], 76970[1], 76998[0],

CPT © 2018 American Medical Association. All Rights Reserved.

Code 1	Code 2
	77002[0], 90865[1], 92511[1], 92512[1], 92516[1], 92520[1], 92537[1], 92538[1], 92950[1], 92953[1], 92960[1], 92961[1], 93000[1], 93005[1], 93010[1], 93040[1], 93041[1], 93042[1], 93050[0], 93303[0], 93304[0], 93306[1], 93307[1], 93308[1], 93312[1], 93313[1], 93314[1], 93315[1], 93316[1], 93317[1], 93318[0], 93351[1], 93355[0], 93451[1], 93456[1], 93457[1], 93561[0], 93562[0], 93701[0], 93922[1], 93923[1], 93924[1], 93925[1], 93926[1], 93930[1], 93931[1], 93970[1], 93971[1], 93975[1], 93976[1], 93978[1], 93979[1], 93980[1], 93981[1], 94002[1], 94004[1], 94200[1], 94250[0], 94640[1], 94644[1], 94660[1], 94662[1], 94680[1], 94681[1], 94690[1], 94760[0], 94761[0], 94762[1], 94770[1], 95812[0], 95813[0], 95816[0], 95819[0], 95822[0], 95829[0], 95955[0], 95956[0], 95957[0], 96360[0], 96365[0], 96372[0], 96373[0], 96374[0], 96375[0], 96376[0], 96377[0], 99151[0], 99152[0], 99153[0], 99155[0], 99156[0], 99157[0], 99201[0], 99202[0], 99203[0], 99204[0], 99205[0], 99211[0], 99212[0], 99213[0], 99214[0], 99215[0], 99217[0], 99218[0], 99219[0], 99220[0], 99221[0], 99222[0], 99223[0], 99224[0], 99225[0], 99226[0], 99231[0], 99232[0], 99233[0], 99234[0], 99235[0], 99236[0], 99238[0], 99239[0], 99281[0], 99282[0], 99283[0], 99284[0], 99285[0], 99304[0], 99305[0], 99306[0], 99307[0], 99308[0], 99309[0], 99310[0], 99315[0], 99318[0], 99324[0], 99325[0], 99326[0], 99327[0], 99328[0], 99334[0], 99335[0], 99336[0], 99337[0], 99341[0], 99342[0], 99343[0], 99347[0], 99348[0], 99349[0], 99354[0], 99355[0], 99356[0], 99357[0], 99358[0], 99359[0], 99415[0], 99416[0], 99446[0], 99447[0], 99448[0], 99449[0], 99451[0], 99452[0], 99466[0], 99468[0], 99469[0], 99471[0], 99472[0], 99475[0], 99476[0], 99477[0], 99478[0], 99479[0], 99480[0], 99483[0], 99485[0], 99497[0], C8921[1], C8922[1], C8923[1], C8924[1], C8925[1], C8926[1], C8927[0], C8929[1], C8930[1], G0380[1], G0381[1], G0382[1], G0383[1], G0384[1], G0406[0], G0407[0], G0408[0], G0425[0], G0426[0], G0427[0], G0463[0], G0500[0], G0508[0], G0509[0]
01966	01965[1], 01996[1], 0213T[1], 0216T[1], 0228T[1], 0230T[1], 31505[1], 31515[1], 31527[1], 31622[1], 31634[1], 31645[1], 31647[1], 36000[1], 36010[0], 36011[1], 36012[1], 36013[1], 36014[1], 36015[1], 36400[1], 36405[1], 36406[1], 36410[1], 36420[1], 36425[1], 36430[1], 36440[1], 36591[0], 36592[0], 36600[1], 36640[1], 43752[1], 43753[1], 43754[1], 61026[1], 61055[1], 62280[1], 62281[1], 62282[1], 62284[1], 62320[1], 62321[1], 62322[1], 62323[1], 62324[1], 62325[1], 62326[1], 62327[1], 64400[1], 64402[1], 64405[1], 64408[1], 64410[1], 64413[1], 64415[1], 64416[1], 64417[1], 64418[1], 64420[1], 64421[1], 64425[1], 64430[1], 64435[1], 64445[1], 64446[1], 64447[1], 64448[1], 64449[1], 64450[1], 64461[1], 64463[1], 64479[1], 64483[1], 64486[1], 64487[1], 64488[1], 64489[1], 64490[1], 64493[1], 64505[1], 64510[1], 64517[1], 64520[1], 64530[1], 64553[1], 64555[1], 67500[0], 76000[1], 76970[1], 76998[0], 77002[0], 90865[1], 92511[1], 92512[1], 92516[1], 92520[1], 92537[1], 92538[1], 92950[1], 92953[1], 92960[1], 92961[1], 93000[1], 93005[1], 93010[1], 93040[1], 93041[1], 93042[1], 93050[0], 93303[0], 93304[0], 93306[1], 93307[1], 93308[1], 93312[1], 93313[1], 93314[1], 93315[1], 93316[1], 93317[1], 93318[0], 93351[1], 93355[0], 93451[1], 93456[1], 93457[1], 93561[0], 93562[0], 93701[0], 93922[1], 93923[1], 93924[1], 93925[1], 93926[1], 93930[1], 93931[1], 93970[1], 93971[1], 93975[1], 93976[1], 93978[1], 93979[1], 93980[1], 93981[1], 94002[1], 94004[1], 94200[1], 94250[0], 94640[1], 94644[1], 94660[1], 94662[1], 94680[1], 94681[1], 94690[1], 94760[0], 94761[0], 94762[1], 94770[1], 95812[0], 95813[0], 95816[0], 95819[0], 95822[0], 95829[0], 95955[0], 95956[0], 95957[0], 96360[0], 96365[0], 96372[0], 96373[0], 96374[0], 96375[0], 96376[0], 96377[0], 99151[0], 99152[0], 99153[0], 99155[0], 99156[0], 99157[0], 99201[0], 99202[0], 99203[0], 99204[0], 99205[0], 99211[0], 99212[0], 99213[0], 99214[0], 99215[0], 99217[0], 99218[0], 99219[0], 99220[0], 99221[0], 99222[0], 99223[0], 99224[0], 99225[0], 99226[0], 99231[0], 99232[0], 99233[0], 99234[0], 99235[0], 99236[0], 99238[0], 99239[0], 99281[0], 99282[0], 99283[0], 99284[0], 99285[0], 99304[0], 99305[0], 99306[0], 99307[0], 99308[0], 99309[0], 99310[0], 99315[0], 99318[0], 99324[0], 99325[0], 99326[0], 99327[0], 99328[0], 99334[0], 99335[0], 99336[0], 99337[0], 99341[0], 99342[0], 99343[0], 99347[0], 99348[0], 99349[0], 99354[0], 99355[0], 99356[0], 99357[0], 99358[0], 99359[0], 99415[0], 99416[0], 99446[0], 99447[0], 99448[0], 99449[0], 99451[0], 99452[0], 99466[0], 99468[0], 99469[0], 99471[0], 99472[0], 99475[0], 99476[0], 99477[0], 99478[0], 99479[0], 99480[0], 99483[0], 99485[0], 99497[0], C8921[1], C8922[1], C8923[1], C8924[1], C8925[1], C8926[1], C8927[0], C8929[1], C8930[1], G0380[1], G0381[1], G0382[1], G0383[1], G0384[1], G0406[0], G0407[0], G0408[0], G0425[0], G0426[0], G0427[0], G0463[0], G0500[0], G0508[0], G0509[0]
01967	01996[1], 0213T[1], 0216T[1], 0228T[1], 0230T[1], 31505[1], 31515[1], 31527[1], 31622[1], 31634[1], 31645[1], 31647[1], 36000[1], 36010[0], 36011[1], 36012[1], 36013[1], 36014[1], 36015[1], 36400[1], 36405[1], 36406[1], 36410[1], 36420[1], 36425[1], 36430[1], 36440[1], 36591[0], 36592[0], 36600[1], 36640[1], 43752[1], 43753[1], 43754[1], 61026[1], 61055[1], 62280[1], 62281[1], 62282[1], 62284[1], 62320[1], 62321[1], 62322[1], 62323[1], 62324[1], 62325[1], 62326[1], 62327[1], 64400[1], 64402[1], 64405[1], 64408[1], 64410[1], 64413[1], 64415[1], 64416[1], 64417[1], 64418[1], 64420[1], 64421[1], 64425[1], 64430[1], 64435[1], 64445[1], 64446[1], 64447[1], 64448[1], 64449[1], 64450[1], 64461[1], 64463[1], 64479[1], 64483[1], 64486[1], 64487[1], 64488[1], 64489[1], 64490[1], 64493[1], 64505[1], 64510[1], 64517[1], 64520[1], 64530[1], 64553[1], 64555[1], 67500[0], 76000[1], 76970[1], 76998[0], 77002[0], 90865[1], 92511[1], 92512[1], 92516[1], 92520[1], 92537[1], 92538[1], 92950[1], 92953[1], 92960[1], 92961[1], 93000[1], 93005[1], 93010[1], 93040[1], 93041[1], 93042[1], 93050[0], 93303[0], 93304[0], 93306[1], 93307[1], 93308[1], 93312[1], 93313[1], 93314[1], 93315[1], 93316[1], 93317[1], 93318[0], 93351[1], 93355[0], 93451[1], 93456[1], 93457[1], 93561[0], 93562[0], 93701[0], 93922[1], 93923[1], 93924[1], 93925[1], 93926[1], 93930[1], 93931[1], 93970[1], 93971[1], 93975[1], 93976[1], 93978[1], 93979[1], 93980[1], 93981[1], 94002[1], 94004[1], 94200[1], 94250[0], 94640[1], 94644[1], 94660[1], 94662[1], 94680[1], 94681[1], 94690[1], 94760[0], 94761[0], 94762[1], 94770[1], 95812[0], 95813[0], 95816[0], 95819[0], 95822[0], 95829[0], 95955[0], 95956[0], 95957[0], 96360[0], 96365[0], 96372[0], 96373[0], 96374[0], 96375[0], 96376[0], 96377[0], 99151[0], 99152[0], 99153[0], 99155[0], 99156[0], 99157[0], 99201[0], 99202[0], 99203[0], 99204[0], 99205[0], 99211[0], 99212[0], 99213[0], 99214[0], 99215[0], 99217[0], 99218[0], 99219[0], 99220[0], 99221[0], 99222[0], 99223[0], 99224[0], 99225[0], 99226[0], 99231[0], 99232[0], 99233[0], 99234[0], 99235[0], 99236[0], 99238[0], 99239[0], 99281[0], 99282[0], 99283[0], 99284[0], 99285[0], 99304[0], 99305[0], 99306[0], 99307[0], 99308[0], 99309[0], 99310[0], 99315[0], 99318[0], 99324[0], 99325[0], 99326[0], 99327[0], 99328[0], 99334[0], 99335[0], 99336[0], 99337[0], 99341[0], 99342[0], 99343[0], 99347[0], 99348[0], 99349[0], 99354[0], 99355[0], 99356[0], 99357[0], 99358[0], 99359[0], 99415[0], 99416[0], 99466[0], 99468[0], 99469[0], 99471[0], 99472[0], 99475[0], 99476[0], 99477[0], 99478[0], 99479[0], 99480[0], 99483[0], 99485[0], 99497[0], C8921[1], C8922[1], C8923[1], C8924[1], C8925[1], C8926[1], C8927[0], C8929[1], C8930[1], G0380[1], G0381[1], G0382[1], G0383[1], G0384[1], G0406[0], G0407[0], G0408[0], G0425[0], G0426[0], G0427[0], G0463[0], G0500[0], G0508[0], G0509[0]
01968	01996[1], 0213T[1], 0216T[1], 0228T[1], 0230T[1], 31505[1], 31515[1], 31527[1], 31622[1], 31634[1], 31645[1], 31647[1], 36000[1], 36010[0], 36011[1], 36012[1], 36013[1], 36014[1], 36015[1], 36400[1], 36405[1], 36406[1], 36410[1], 36420[1], 36425[1], 36430[1], 36440[1], 36591[0], 36592[0], 36600[1], 36640[1], 43752[1], 43753[1], 43754[1], 62280[1], 62281[1], 62282[1], 62284[1], 62320[1], 62321[1], 62322[1], 62323[1], 62324[1], 62325[1], 62326[1], 62327[1], 64400[1], 64402[1], 64405[1], 64408[1], 64410[1], 64413[1], 64415[1], 64416[1], 64417[1], 64418[1], 64420[1], 64421[1], 64425[1], 64430[1], 64435[1], 64445[1], 64446[1], 64447[1], 64448[1], 64449[1], 64450[1], 64461[1], 64463[1], 64479[1], 64483[1], 64486[1], 64487[1], 64488[1], 64489[1], 64490[1], 64493[1], 64505[1], 64510[1], 64517[1], 64520[1], 64530[1], 64553[1], 64555[1], 67500[0], 76000[1], 76970[1], 76998[0], 90865[1], 92511[1], 92512[1], 92516[1], 92520[1], 92537[1], 92538[1], 92950[1], 92953[1], 92960[1], 92961[1], 93000[1], 93005[1], 93010[1], 93040[1], 93041[1], 93042[1], 93050[0], 93303[0], 93304[0], 93306[1], 93307[1], 93308[1], 93312[1], 93313[1], 93314[1], 93315[1], 93316[1], 93317[1], 93318[0], 93351[1], 93355[0], 93451[1], 93456[1], 93457[1], 93701[0], 93922[1], 93923[1], 93924[1], 93925[1], 93926[1], 93930[1], 93931[1], 93970[1], 93971[1], 93975[1], 93976[1], 93978[1], 93979[1], 93980[1], 93981[1], 94002[1], 94004[1], 94200[1], 94250[0], 94640[1], 94660[1], 94662[1], 94680[1], 94681[1], 94690[1], 94760[0], 94761[0], 94762[1], 94770[1], 95812[0], 95813[0], 95816[0], 95819[0], 95822[0], 95829[0], 95955[0], 95956[0], 95957[0], 96373[0], 99151[0], 99152[0], 99153[0], 99155[0], 99156[0], 99157[0], 99201[0], 99202[0], 99203[0], 99204[0], 99205[0], 99211[0], 99212[0], 99213[0], 99214[0], 99215[0], 99217[0], 99218[0], 99219[0], 99220[0], 99221[0], 99222[0], 99223[0], 99224[0], 99225[0], 99226[0], 99231[0], 99232[0], 99233[0], 99238[0], 99281[0], 99282[0], 99283[0], 99284[0], 99285[0], 99304[0], 99305[0], 99306[0], 99307[0], 99308[0], 99309[0], 99310[0], 99318[0], 99324[0], 99325[0], 99326[0], 99327[0], 99328[0], 99334[0], 99335[0], 99336[0], 99337[0], 99341[0], 99342[0], 99343[0], 99347[0], 99348[0], 99349[0], 99354[0], 99355[0], 99356[0], 99357[0], 99358[0], 99359[0], 99415[0], 99416[0], 99446[0], 99447[0], 99448[0], 99449[0], 99451[0], 99452[0], 99468[0], 99469[0], 99471[0], 99472[0], 99475[0], 99476[0], 99477[0], 99478[0], 99479[0], 99480[0], 99483[0], 99497[0], C8929[1], C8930[1], G0463[0], G0500[0]
01969	01996[1], 0213T[1], 0216T[1], 0228T[1], 0230T[1], 31505[1], 31515[1], 31527[1], 31622[1], 31634[1], 31645[1], 31647[1], 36000[1], 36010[0], 36011[1], 36012[1], 36013[1], 36014[1], 36015[1], 36400[1], 36405[1], 36406[1], 36410[1], 36420[1], 36425[1], 36430[1], 36440[1], 36591[0], 36592[0], 36600[1], 36640[1], 43752[1], 43753[1], 43754[1], 62280[1], 62281[1], 62282[1], 62284[1], 62320[1], 62321[1], 62322[1], 62323[1], 62324[1], 62325[1], 62326[1], 62327[1], 64400[1], 64402[1], 64405[1], 64408[1], 64410[1], 64413[1], 64415[1], 64416[1], 64417[1], 64418[1], 64420[1], 64421[1], 64425[1], 64430[1], 64435[1], 64445[1], 64446[1], 64447[1], 64448[1], 64449[1], 64450[1], 64461[1], 64463[1], 64479[1], 64483[1], 64486[1], 64487[1], 64488[1], 64489[1], 64490[1], 64493[1], 64505[1], 64510[1], 64517[1], 64520[1], 64530[1], 64553[1], 64555[1], 67500[0], 76000[1], 76970[1], 76998[0], 90865[1], 92511[1], 92512[1], 92516[1], 92520[1], 92537[1], 92538[1], 92950[1], 92953[1], 92960[1], 92961[1], 93000[1], 93005[1], 93010[1], 93040[1], 93041[1], 93042[1], 93050[0], 93303[0], 93304[0], 93306[1], 93307[1], 93308[1], 93312[1], 93313[1], 93314[1], 93315[1], 93316[1], 93317[1], 93318[0], 93351[1], 93355[0], 93451[1], 93456[1], 93457[1], 93701[0], 93922[1], 93923[1], 93924[1], 93925[1], 93926[1], 93930[1], 93931[1], 93970[1], 93971[1], 93975[1], 93976[1], 93978[1], 93979[1], 93980[1], 93981[1], 94002[1], 94004[1], 94200[1], 94250[0], 94640[1], 94660[1], 94662[1], 94680[1], 94681[1], 94690[1], 94760[0], 94761[0], 94762[1], 94770[1], 95812[0], 95813[0], 95816[0], 95819[0], 95822[0], 95829[0], 95955[0], 95956[0], 95957[0], 96373[0], 99151[0], 99152[0], 99153[0], 99155[0], 99156[0], 99157[0], 99201[0], 99202[0], 99203[0], 99204[0], 99205[0], 99211[0], 99212[0], 99213[0], 99214[0], 99215[0], 99217[0], 99218[0], 99219[0], 99220[0], 99221[0], 99222[0], 99223[0], 99224[0], 99225[0], 99226[0], 99231[0], 99232[0], 99233[0], 99238[0], 99281[0], 99282[0], 99283[0], 99284[0], 99285[0], 99304[0], 99305[0], 99306[0], 99307[0], 99308[0], 99309[0], 99310[0], 99318[0], 99324[0], 99325[0], 99326[0], 99327[0], 99328[0], 99334[0], 99335[0], 99336[0], 99337[0], 99341[0], 99342[0], 99343[0], 99347[0], 99348[0], 99349[0], 99354[0], 99355[0], 99356[0], 99357[0], 99358[0], 99359[0], 99415[0], 99416[0], 99446[0], 99447[0], 99448[0], 99449[0], 99451[0], 99452[0], 99468[0], 99469[0], 99471[0], 99472[0], 99475[0], 99476[0], 99477[0], 99478[0], 99479[0], 99480[0], 99483[0], 99497[0], C8929[1], C8930[1], G0463[0], G0500[0]

0 = Modifier usage not allowed or inappropriate 1 = Modifier usage allowed

Appendix A: NCCI - CPT Codes

CPT © 2018 American Medical Association. All Rights Reserved.

Code 1	Code 2
01990	01996[1], 0213T[1], 0216T[1], 0228T[1], 0230T[1], 31505[1], 31515[1], 31527[1], 31622[1], 31634[1], 31645[1], 31647[1], 36000[1], 36010[0], 36011[1], 36012[1], 36013[1], 36014[1], 36015[1], 36400[1], 36405[1], 36406[1], 36410[1], 36420[1], 36425[1], 36430[1], 36440[1], 36591[0], 36592[0], 36600[1], 36640[1], 43752[1], 43753[1], 43754[1], 61026[1], 61055[1], 62280[1], 62281[1], 62282[1], 62284[1], 62320[1], 62321[1], 62322[1], 62323[1], 62324[1], 62325[1], 62326[1], 62327[1], 64400[1], 64402[1], 64405[1], 64408[1], 64410[1], 64413[1], 64415[1], 64416[1], 64417[1], 64418[1], 64420[1], 64421[1], 64425[1], 64430[1], 64435[1], 64445[1], 64446[1], 64447[1], 64448[1], 64449[1], 64450[1], 64461[1], 64463[1], 64479[1], 64483[1], 64486[1], 64487[1], 64488[1], 64489[1], 64490[1], 64493[1], 64505[1], 64510[1], 64517[1], 64520[1], 64530[1], 64553[1], 64555[1], 67500[1], 76000[1], 76970[1], 76998[0], 77002[0], 90865[1], 92511[1], 92512[1], 92516[1], 92520[1], 92537[1], 92538[1], 92950[1], 92953[1], 92960[1], 92961[1], 93000[1], 93005[1], 93010[1], 93040[1], 93041[1], 93042[1], 93050[0], 93303[0], 93304[0], 93307[1], 93308[1], 93312[1], 93313[1], 93314[1], 93315[1], 93316[1], 93317[1], 93318[0], 93355[0], 93451[1], 93456[1], 93457[1], 93561[0], 93562[0], 93701[0], 93922[1], 93923[1], 93924[1], 93925[1], 93926[1], 93930[1], 93931[1], 93970[1], 93971[1], 93975[1], 93976[1], 93978[1], 93979[1], 93980[1], 93981[1], 94002[1], 94004[1], 94200[1], 94250[1], 94640[1], 94644[1], 94660[1], 94662[1], 94680[1], 94681[1], 94690[1], 94760[0], 94761[0], 94762[1], 94770[1], 95812[0], 95813[0], 95816[0], 95819[0], 95822[0], 95829[0], 95955[0], 95956[0], 95957[0], 96360[0], 96365[0], 96372[0], 96373[0], 96374[0], 96375[0], 96376[0], 96377[0], 99151[0], 99152[0], 99153[0], 99155[0], 99156[0], 99157[0], 99201[0], 99202[0], 99203[0], 99204[0], 99205[0], 99211[0], 99212[0], 99213[0], 99214[0], 99215[0], 99217[0], 99218[0], 99219[0], 99220[0], 99221[0], 99222[0], 99223[0], 99224[0], 99225[0], 99226[0], 99231[0], 99232[0], 99233[0], 99234[0], 99235[0], 99236[0], 99238[0], 99239[0], 99281[0], 99282[0], 99283[0], 99284[0], 99285[0], 99304[0], 99305[0], 99306[0], 99307[0], 99308[0], 99309[0], 99310[0], 99315[0], 99318[0], 99324[0], 99325[0], 99326[0], 99327[0], 99328[0], 99334[0], 99335[0], 99336[0], 99337[0], 99341[0], 99342[0], 99343[0], 99347[0], 99348[0], 99349[0], 99354[0], 99355[0], 99356[0], 99357[0], 99358[0], 99359[0], 99415[0], 99416[0], 99468[0], 99469[0], 99471[0], 99472[0], 99475[0], 99476[0], 99477[0], 99478[0], 99479[0], 99480[0], 99483[0], 99497[0], C8921[1], C8922[1], C8923[1], C8924[1], C8925[1], C8926[1], C8927[0], C8929[1], G0380[1], G0381[1], G0382[1], G0383[1], G0384[1], G0406[0], G0407[0], G0408[0], G0425[0], G0426[0], G0427[0], G0463[0], G0500[0], G0508[0], G0509[0]
01991	01992[1], 01996[1], 0333T[0], 0464T[0], 31505[1], 31515[1], 31527[1], 31622[1], 31634[1], 31645[1], 31647[1], 36000[1], 36010[0], 36011[1], 36012[1], 36013[1], 36014[1], 36015[1], 36400[1], 36405[1], 36406[1], 36410[1], 36420[1], 36425[1], 36430[1], 36440[1], 36591[0], 36592[0], 36600[1], 36640[1], 43752[1], 43753[1], 43754[1], 61026[1], 61055[1], 62280[1], 62281[1], 62282[1], 62284[1], 64553[1], 64555[1], 67500[0], 76000[1], 76970[1], 76998[0], 77002[0], 90865[1], 92511[1], 92512[1], 92516[1], 92520[1], 92537[1], 92538[1], 92585[0], 92950[1], 92953[1], 92960[1], 92961[1], 93000[1], 93005[1], 93010[1], 93040[1], 93041[1], 93042[1], 93050[0], 93303[0], 93304[0], 93306[1], 93307[1], 93308[1], 93312[1], 93313[1], 93314[1], 93315[1], 93316[1], 93317[1], 93318[0], 93351[1], 93355[0], 93451[1], 93456[1], 93457[1], 93561[0], 93562[0], 93701[0], 93922[1], 93923[1], 93924[1], 93925[1], 93926[1], 93930[1], 93931[1], 93970[1], 93971[1], 93975[1], 93976[1], 93978[1], 93979[1], 93980[1], 93981[1], 94002[1], 94004[1], 94200[1], 94250[0], 94640[1], 94644[1], 94660[1], 94662[1], 94680[1], 94681[1], 94690[1], 94760[0], 94761[0], 94762[1], 94770[1], 95812[0], 95813[0], 95816[0], 95819[0], 95822[0], 95829[0], 95860[0], 95861[0], 95863[0], 95864[0], 95865[0], 95866[0], 95867[0], 95868[0], 95869[0], 95870[0], 95907[0], 95908[0], 95909[0], 95910[0], 95911[0], 95912[0], 95913[0], 95925[0], 95926[0], 95927[0], 95928[0], 95929[0], 95930[0], 95933[0], 95937[0], 95938[0], 95939[0], 95940[0], 95955[0], 95956[0], 95957[0], 96360[0], 96365[0], 96372[0], 96373[0], 96374[0], 96375[0], 96376[0], 96377[0], 99151[0], 99152[0], 99153[0], 99155[0], 99156[0], 99157[0], 99201[0], 99202[0], 99203[0], 99204[0], 99205[0], 99211[0], 99212[0], 99213[0], 99214[0], 99215[0], 99217[0], 99218[0], 99219[0], 99220[0], 99221[0], 99222[0], 99223[0], 99224[0], 99225[0], 99226[0], 99231[0], 99232[0], 99233[0], 99234[0], 99235[0], 99236[0], 99238[0], 99239[0], 99281[0], 99282[0], 99283[0], 99284[0], 99285[0], 99304[0], 99305[0], 99306[0], 99307[0], 99308[0], 99309[0], 99310[0], 99315[0], 99318[0], 99324[0], 99325[0], 99326[0], 99327[0], 99328[0], 99334[0], 99335[0], 99336[0], 99337[0], 99341[0], 99342[0], 99343[0], 99347[0], 99348[0], 99349[0], 99354[0], 99355[0], 99356[0], 99357[0], 99358[0], 99359[0], 99415[0], 99416[0], 99446[0], 99447[0], 99448[0], 99449[0], 99451[0], 99452[0], 99468[0], 99469[0], 99471[0], 99472[0], 99475[0], 99476[0], 99477[0], 99478[0], 99479[0], 99480[0], 99483[0], 99497[0], C8921[1], C8922[1], C8923[1], C8924[1], C8925[1], C8926[1], C8927[0], C8929[1], C8930[1], G0380[1], G0381[1], G0382[1], G0383[1], G0384[1], G0406[0], G0407[0], G0408[0], G0425[0], G0426[0], G0427[0], G0453[0], G0463[0], G0500[0], G0508[0], G0509[0]
01992	01996[1], 0333T[0], 0464T[0], 31505[1], 31515[1], 31527[1], 31622[1], 31634[1], 31645[1], 31647[1], 36000[1], 36010[0], 36011[1], 36012[1], 36013[1], 36014[1], 36015[1], 36400[1], 36405[1], 36406[1], 36410[1], 36420[1], 36425[1], 36430[1], 36440[1], 36591[0], 36592[0], 36600[1], 36640[1], 43752[1], 43753[1], 43754[1], 61026[1], 61055[1], 62280[1], 62281[1], 62282[1], 62284[1], 64553[1], 64555[1], 67500[0], 76000[1], 76970[1], 76998[0], 77002[0], 90865[1], 92511[1], 92512[1], 92516[1], 92520[1], 92537[1], 92538[1], 92585[0], 92950[1], 92953[1], 92960[1], 92961[1], 93000[1], 93005[1], 93010[1], 93040[1], 93041[1], 93042[1], 93050[0], 93303[0], 93304[0], 93306[1], 93307[1], 93308[1], 93312[1], 93313[1], 93314[1], 93315[1], 93316[1], 93317[1], 93318[0], 93351[1], 93355[0], 93451[1], 93456[1], 93457[1], 93561[0], 93562[0], 93701[0], 93922[1], 93923[1], 93924[1], 93925[1], 93926[1], 93930[1], 93931[1], 93970[1], 93971[1], 93975[1], 93976[1], 93978[1], 93979[1], 93980[1], 93981[1], 94002[1], 94004[1], 94200[1], 94250[0], 94640[1], 94644[1], 94660[1], 94662[1], 94680[1], 94681[1], 94690[1], 94760[0], 94761[0], 94762[1], 94770[1], 95812[0], 95813[0], 95816[0], 95819[0], 95822[0], 95829[0], 95860[0], 95861[0], 95863[0], 95864[0], 95865[0], 95866[0], 95867[0], 95868[0], 95869[0], 95870[0], 95907[0], 95908[0], 95909[0], 95910[0], 95911[0], 95912[0], 95913[0], 95925[0], 95926[0], 95927[0], 95928[0], 95929[0], 95930[0], 95933[0], 95937[0], 95938[0], 95939[0], 95940[0], 95955[0], 95956[0], 95957[0], 96360[0], 96365[0], 96372[0], 96373[0], 96374[0], 96375[0], 96376[0], 96377[0], 99151[0], 99152[0], 99153[0], 99155[0], 99156[0], 99157[0], 99201[0], 99202[0], 99203[0], 99204[0], 99205[0], 99211[0], 99212[0], 99213[0], 99214[0], 99215[0], 99217[0], 99218[0], 99219[0], 99220[0], 99221[0], 99222[0], 99223[0], 99224[0], 99225[0], 99226[0], 99231[0], 99232[0], 99233[0], 99234[0], 99235[0], 99236[0], 99238[0], 99239[0], 99281[0], 99282[0], 99283[0], 99284[0], 99285[0], 99304[0], 99305[0], 99306[0], 99307[0], 99308[0], 99309[0], 99310[0], 99315[0], 99318[0], 99324[0], 99325[0], 99326[0], 99327[0], 99328[0], 99334[0], 99335[0], 99336[0], 99337[0], 99341[0], 99342[0], 99343[0], 99347[0], 99348[0], 99349[0], 99354[0], 99355[0], 99356[0], 99357[0], 99358[0], 99359[0], 99415[0], 99416[0], 99446[0], 99447[0], 99448[0], 99449[0], 99451[0], 99452[0], 99468[0], 99469[0], 99471[0], 99472[0], 99475[0], 99476[0], 99477[0], 99478[0], 99479[0], 99480[0], 99483[0], 99497[0], C8921[1], C8922[1], C8923[1], C8924[1], C8925[1], C8926[1], C8927[0], C8929[1], C8930[1], G0380[1], G0381[1], G0382[1], G0383[1], G0384[1], G0406[0], G0407[0], G0408[0], G0425[0], G0426[0], G0427[0], G0453[0], G0463[0], G0500[0], G0508[0], G0509[0]
01996	36591[0], 36592[0], 93312[1], 93313[1], 93561[0], 93562[0], 93701[0], 99151[0], 99152[0], 99153[0], 99155[0], 99156[0], 99157[0], C8921[1], C8922[1], C8923[1], C8924[1], C8925[1], C8926[1], C8927[0], G0500[0]
20526	0213T[1], 0216T[1], 0228T[1], 0230T[1], 10030[1], 10160[1], 11900[1], 11901[1], 20500[1], 29075[1], 29105[1], 29125[1], 29260[1], 29584[1], 36000[1], 36400[1], 36405[1], 36406[1], 36410[1], 36420[1], 36425[1], 36430[1], 36440[1], 36591[0], 36592[0], 36600[1], 36640[1], 43752[1], 51701[1], 51702[1], 51703[1], 64400[1], 64402[1], 64405[1], 64408[1], 64410[1], 64413[1], 64415[1], 64416[1], 64417[1], 64418[1], 64420[1], 64421[1], 64425[1], 64430[1], 64435[1], 64445[1], 64446[1], 64447[1], 64448[1], 64449[1], 64461[0], 64462[0], 64463[0], 64479[1], 64480[0], 64483[1], 64484[0], 64486[0], 64487[0], 64488[0], 64489[0], 64490[1], 64491[0], 64492[0], 64493[1], 64494[0], 64495[0], 64505[1], 64510[1], 64517[1], 64520[1], 64530[1], 69990[0], 76000[1], 77001[1], 92012[1], 92014[1], 93000[1], 93005[1], 93010[1], 93040[1], 93041[1], 93042[1], 93318[1], 93355[1], 94002[1], 94200[1], 94250[1], 94680[1], 94681[1], 94690[1], 94770[1], 95812[1], 95813[1], 95816[1], 95819[1], 95822[1], 95829[1], 95955[1], 96360[1], 96361[1], 96365[1], 96366[1], 96367[1], 96368[1], 96372[1], 96374[1], 96375[1], 96376[1], 96377[1], 99155[0], 99156[0], 99157[0], 99211[1], 99212[1], 99213[1], 99214[1], 99215[1], 99217[1], 99218[1], 99219[1], 99220[1], 99221[1], 99222[1], 99223[1], 99231[1], 99232[1], 99233[1], 99234[1], 99235[1], 99236[1], 99238[1], 99239[1], 99241[1], 99242[1], 99243[1], 99244[1], 99245[1], 99251[1], 99252[1], 99253[1], 99254[1], 99255[1], 99291[1], 99292[1], 99304[1], 99305[1], 99306[1], 99307[1], 99308[1], 99309[1], 99310[1], 99315[1], 99316[1], 99334[1], 99335[1], 99336[1], 99337[1], 99347[1], 99348[1], 99349[1], 99350[1], 99374[1], 99375[1], 99377[1], 99378[1], 99446[0], 99447[0], 99448[0], 99449[0], 99451[0], 99452[0], 99495[1], 99496[1], G0463[1], G0471[1], J0670[1], J2001[1]
20550	0232T[1], 0481T[1], 0490T[1], 10030[1], 10160[1], 11010[1], 11900[1], 11901[1], 12032[1], 12042[1], 20500[1], 20526[1], 20551[1], 20552[1], 20553[1], 29075[1], 29105[1], 29125[1], 29130[1], 29260[1], 29405[1], 29425[1], 29450[1], 29515[1], 29530[1], 29540[1], 29550[1], 29580[1], 29581[1], 29584[1], 36000[1], 36400[1], 36405[1], 36406[1], 36410[1], 36420[1], 36425[1], 36430[1], 36440[1], 36591[0], 36592[0], 36600[1], 36640[1], 43752[1], 51701[1], 51702[1], 51703[1], 62320[1], 62321[1], 62322[1], 62323[1], 62324[1], 62325[1], 62326[1], 62327[1], 64408[1], 64410[1], 64435[1], 64455[1], 64461[0], 64463[0], 64480[0], 64484[0], 64486[0], 64487[0], 64488[0], 64489[0], 64494[0], 64495[0], 64505[1], 64510[1], 64517[1], 64520[1], 64530[1], 64714[1], 69990[0], 72240[1], 72265[1], 72295[1], 76000[1], 77001[1], 87076[0], 87077[0], 87102[0], 92012[1], 92014[1], 93000[1], 93005[1], 93010[1], 93040[1], 93041[1], 93042[1], 93318[1], 93355[1], 94002[1], 94200[1], 94250[1], 94680[1], 94681[1], 94690[1], 94770[1], 95812[1], 95813[1], 95816[1], 95819[1], 95822[1], 95829[1], 95907[1], 95908[1], 95909[1], 95910[1], 95911[1], 95912[1], 95913[1], 95955[1], 96360[1], 96361[1], 96365[1], 96366[1], 96367[1], 96368[1], 96372[1], 96374[1], 96375[1], 96376[1], 96377[1], 99155[0], 99156[0], 99157[0], 99211[1], 99212[1], 99213[1], 99214[1], 99215[1], 99217[1], 99218[1], 99219[1], 99220[1], 99221[1], 99222[1], 99223[1], 99231[1], 99232[1], 99233[1], 99234[1], 99235[1], 99236[1], 99238[1], 99239[1], 99241[1], 99242[1], 99243[1], 99244[1], 99245[1], 99251[1], 99252[1], 99253[1], 99254[1], 99255[1], 99291[1], 99292[1], 99304[1], 99305[1], 99306[1], 99307[1], 99308[1], 99309[1], 99310[1], 99315[1], 99316[1], 99334[1], 99335[1], 99336[1], 99337[1], 99347[1], 99348[1], 99349[1], 99350[1], 99374[1], 99375[1], 99377[1], 99378[1], 99446[0], 99447[0], 99448[0], 99449[0], 99451[0], 99452[0], 99495[1], 99496[1], G0463[1], G0471[1], J0670[1], J2001[1]
20551	0232T[1], 0481T[1], 0490T[1], 10030[1], 10160[1], 11000[1], 11001[1], 11004[1], 11005[1], 11006[1], 11042[1], 11043[1], 11044[1], 11045[1], 11046[1], 11047[1], 11900[1], 11901[1], 20500[1], 20526[1], 20552[1], 20553[1], 29075[1], 29105[1], 29125[1], 29130[1], 29260[1], 29405[1], 29425[1], 29450[1], 29515[1], 29530[1], 29540[1], 29550[1], 29580[1], 29581[1], 29584[1], 36000[1], 36400[1], 36405[1], 36406[1], 36410[1], 36420[1], 36425[1], 36430[1], 36440[1], 36591[0], 36592[0], 36600[1], 36640[1], 43752[1], 51701[1], 51702[1], 51703[1], 62320[1], 62321[1], 62322[1], 62323[1], 62324[1], 62325[1],

0 = Modifier usage not allowed or inappropriate   1 = Modifier usage allowed

CPT © 2018 American Medical Association. All Rights Reserved.

Code 1	Code 2
	62326^1, 62327^1, 64408^1, 64410^1, 64435^1, 64455^1, 64461^0, 64463^0, 64480^0, 64484^0, 64486^0, 64487^0, 64488^0, 64489^0, 64494^0, 64495^0, 64505^1, 64510^1, 64517^1, 64520^1, 64530^1, 69990^0, 76000^1, 77001^1, 92012^1, 92014^1, 93000^1, 93005^1, 93010^1, 93040^1, 93041^1, 93042^1, 93318^1, 93355^1, 94002^1, 94200^1, 94250^1, 94680^1, 94681^1, 94690^1, 94770^1, 95812^1, 95813^1, 95816^1, 95819^1, 95822^1, 95829^1, 95955^1, 96360^1, 96361^1, 96365^1, 96366^1, 96367^1, 96368^1, 96372^1, 96374^1, 96375^1, 96376^1, 96377^1, 97597^1, 97598^1, 97602^1, 99155^0, 99156^0, 99157^0, 99211^1, 99212^1, 99213^1, 99214^1, 99215^1, 99217^1, 99218^1, 99219^1, 99220^1, 99221^1, 99222^1, 99223^1, 99231^1, 99232^1, 99233^1, 99234^1, 99235^1, 99236^1, 99238^1, 99239^1, 99241^1, 99242^1, 99243^1, 99244^1, 99245^1, 99251^1, 99252^1, 99253^1, 99254^1, 99255^1, 99291^1, 99292^1, 99304^1, 99305^1, 99306^1, 99307^1, 99308^1, 99309^1, 99310^1, 99315^1, 99316^1, 99334^1, 99335^1, 99336^1, 99337^1, 99347^1, 99348^1, 99349^1, 99350^1, 99374^1, 99375^1, 99377^1, 99378^1, 99446^0, 99447^0, 99448^0, 99449^0, 99451^0, 99452^0, 99495^1, 99496^1, G0463^1, G0471^1, J0670^1, J2001^1
20552	01991^0, 01992^0, 0213T^1, 0216T^1, 0228T^1, 0230T^1, 0490T^1, 10030^1, 10160^1, 11900^1, 11901^1, 20500^1, 20526^1, 29075^1, 29105^1, 29125^1, 29130^1, 29260^1, 29405^1, 29425^1, 29450^1, 29515^1, 29530^1, 29540^1, 29550^1, 29580^1, 29581^1, 29584^1, 36000^1, 36400^1, 36405^1, 36406^1, 36410^1, 36420^1, 36425^1, 36430^1, 36440^1, 36591^0, 36592^0, 36600^1, 36640^1, 43752^1, 51701^1, 51702^1, 51703^1, 64400^1, 64402^1, 64405^1, 64408^1, 64410^1, 64413^1, 64415^1, 64416^1, 64417^1, 64418^1, 64420^1, 64421^1, 64425^1, 64430^1, 64435^1, 64445^1, 64446^1, 64447^1, 64448^1, 64449^1, 64450^1, 64455^1, 64461^1, 64462^1, 64463^1, 64479^1, 64480^1, 64483^1, 64484^1, 64486^0, 64487^0, 64488^0, 64489^0, 64490^1, 64491^1, 64492^1, 64493^1, 64494^1, 64495^1, 64505^1, 64510^1, 64517^1, 64520^1, 64530^1, 69990^0, 76000^1, 76970^1, 76998^1, 77001^1, 77012^1, 92012^1, 92014^1, 93000^1, 93005^1, 93010^1, 93040^1, 93041^1, 93042^1, 93318^1, 93355^1, 94002^1, 94200^1, 94250^1, 94680^1, 94681^1, 94690^1, 94770^1, 95812^1, 95813^1, 95816^1, 95819^1, 95822^1, 95829^1, 95955^1, 96360^1, 96361^1, 96365^1, 96366^1, 96367^1, 96368^1, 96372^1, 96374^1, 96375^1, 96376^1, 96377^1, 99155^0, 99156^0, 99157^0, 99211^1, 99212^1, 99213^1, 99214^1, 99215^1, 99217^1, 99218^1, 99219^1, 99220^1, 99221^1, 99222^1, 99223^1, 99231^1, 99232^1, 99233^1, 99234^1, 99235^1, 99236^1, 99238^1, 99239^1, 99241^1, 99242^1, 99243^1, 99244^1, 99245^1, 99251^1, 99252^1, 99253^1, 99254^1, 99255^1, 99291^1, 99292^1, 99304^1, 99305^1, 99306^1, 99307^1, 99308^1, 99309^1, 99310^1, 99315^1, 99316^1, 99334^1, 99335^1, 99336^1, 99337^1, 99347^1, 99348^1, 99349^1, 99350^1, 99374^1, 99375^1, 99377^1, 99378^1, 99446^0, 99447^0, 99448^0, 99449^0, 99451^0, 99452^0, 99495^1, 99496^1, G0463^1, G0471^1, J0670^1, J2001^1
20553	01991^0, 01992^0, 0213T^1, 0216T^1, 0228T^1, 0230T^1, 0490T^1, 10030^1, 10160^1, 11900^1, 11901^1, 20500^1, 20526^1, 20552^0, 29075^1, 29105^1, 29125^1, 29130^1, 29260^1, 29405^1, 29425^1, 29450^1, 29515^1, 29530^1, 29540^1, 29550^1, 29580^1, 29581^1, 29584^1, 36000^1, 36400^1, 36405^1, 36406^1, 36410^1, 36420^1, 36425^1, 36430^1, 36440^1, 36591^0, 36592^0, 36600^1, 36640^1, 43752^1, 51701^1, 51702^1, 51703^1, 64400^1, 64402^1, 64405^1, 64408^1, 64410^1, 64413^1, 64415^1, 64416^1, 64417^1, 64418^1, 64420^1, 64421^1, 64425^1, 64430^1, 64435^1, 64445^1, 64446^1, 64447^1, 64448^1, 64449^1, 64450^1, 64455^1, 64461^1, 64462^1, 64463^1, 64479^1, 64480^1, 64483^1, 64484^1, 64486^0, 64487^0, 64488^0, 64489^0, 64490^1, 64491^1, 64492^1, 64493^1, 64494^1, 64495^1, 64505^1, 64510^1, 64517^1, 64520^1, 64530^1, 69990^0, 76000^1, 76970^1, 76998^1, 77001^1, 77012^1, 92012^1, 92014^1, 93000^1, 93005^1, 93010^1, 93040^1, 93041^1, 93042^1, 93318^1, 93355^1, 94002^1, 94200^1, 94250^1, 94680^1, 94681^1, 94690^1, 94770^1, 95812^1, 95813^1, 95816^1, 95819^1, 95822^1, 95829^1, 95955^1, 96360^1, 96361^1, 96365^1, 96366^1, 96367^1, 96368^1, 96372^1, 96374^1, 96375^1, 96376^1, 96377^1, 99155^0, 99156^0, 99157^0, 99211^1, 99212^1, 99213^1, 99214^1, 99215^1, 99217^1, 99218^1, 99219^1, 99220^1, 99221^1, 99222^1, 99223^1, 99231^1, 99232^1, 99233^1, 99234^1, 99235^1, 99236^1, 99238^1, 99239^1, 99241^1, 99242^1, 99243^1, 99244^1, 99245^1, 99251^1, 99252^1, 99253^1, 99254^1, 99255^1, 99291^1, 99292^1, 99304^1, 99305^1, 99306^1, 99307^1, 99308^1, 99309^1, 99310^1, 99315^1, 99316^1, 99334^1, 99335^1, 99336^1, 99337^1, 99347^1, 99348^1, 99349^1, 99350^1, 99374^1, 99375^1, 99377^1, 99378^1, 99446^0, 99447^0, 99448^0, 99449^0, 99451^0, 99452^0, 99495^1, 99496^1, G0463^1, G0471^1, J0670^1, J2001^1
20600	00400^0, 01380^0, 0228T^1, 0230T^1, 0232T^1, 0481T^1, 10030^1, 10060^1, 10061^1, 10140^1, 10160^1, 11010^1, 11719^1, 20500^1, 20526^1, 20527^1, 20550^1, 20551^1, 20552^1, 20553^1, 25259^1, 26340^1, 29065^1, 29075^1, 29085^1, 29105^1, 29125^1, 29130^1, 29260^1, 29280^1, 29365^1, 29405^1, 29425^1, 29505^1, 29515^1, 29540^1, 29550^1, 29580^1, 29581^1, 29584^1, 36000^1, 36400^1, 36405^1, 36406^1, 36410^1, 36420^1, 36425^1, 36430^1, 36440^1, 36591^0, 36592^0, 36600^1, 36640^1, 43752^1, 51701^1, 51702^1, 51703^1, 62320^1, 62321^1, 62322^1, 62323^1, 62324^1, 62325^1, 62326^1, 62327^1, 64400^1, 64402^1, 64405^1, 64408^1, 64410^1, 64413^1, 64415^1, 64416^1, 64417^1, 64418^1, 64420^1, 64421^1, 64425^1, 64430^1, 64435^1, 64445^1, 64446^1, 64447^1, 64448^1, 64449^1, 64450^1, 64461^0, 64462^0, 64463^0, 64479^1, 64480^0, 64483^1, 64484^0, 64486^1, 64487^1, 64488^1, 64489^1, 64494^0, 64495^0, 64505^1, 64510^1, 64517^1, 64520^1, 64530^1, 64704^1, 64708^1, 69990^0, 72240^1, 72265^1, 76000^1, 76881^1, 76882^1, 76942^1, 76970^1, 76998^1, 77001^1, 92012^1, 92014^1, 93000^1, 93005^1, 93010^1, 93040^1, 93041^1, 93042^1, 93318^1, 93355^1, 94002^1, 94200^1, 94250^1, 94680^1, 94681^1, 94690^1, 94770^1, 95812^1, 95813^1, 95816^1, 95819^1, 95822^1, 95829^1, 95907^1, 95908^1, 95909^1, 95910^1, 95911^1, 95912^1, 95913^1, 95955^1, 96360^1, 96361^1, 96365^1, 96366^1, 96367^1, 96368^1, 96372^1, 96374^1, 96375^1, 96376^1, 96377^1, 99155^0, 99156^0, 99157^0, 99211^1, 99212^1, 99213^1, 99214^1, 99215^1, 99217^1, 99218^1, 99219^1, 99220^1, 99221^1, 99222^1, 99223^1, 99231^1, 99232^1, 99233^1, 99234^1, 99235^1, 99236^1, 99238^1, 99239^1, 99241^1, 99242^1, 99243^1, 99244^1, 99245^1, 99251^1, 99252^1, 99253^1, 99254^1, 99255^1, 99291^1, 99292^1, 99304^1, 99305^1, 99306^1, 99307^1, 99308^1, 99309^1, 99310^1, 99315^1, 99316^1, 99334^1, 99335^1, 99336^1, 99337^1, 99347^1, 99348^1, 99349^1, 99350^1, 99374^1, 99375^1, 99377^1, 99378^1, 99446^0, 99447^0, 99448^0, 99449^0, 99451^0, 99452^0, 99495^1, 99496^1, G0127^1, G0463^1, G0471^1, J0670^1, J2001^1
20604	00400^0, 01380^0, 0213T^1, 0216T^1, 0228T^1, 0230T^1, 0232T^1, 0481T^1, 10030^1, 10060^1, 10061^1, 10140^1, 10160^1, 11719^1, 12001^1, 12002^1, 12004^1, 12005^1, 12006^1, 12007^1, 12011^1, 12013^1, 12014^1, 12015^1, 12016^1, 12017^1, 12018^1, 12020^1, 12021^1, 12031^1, 12032^1, 12034^1, 12035^1, 12036^1, 12037^1, 12041^1, 12042^1, 12044^1, 12045^1, 12046^1, 12047^1, 12051^1, 12052^1, 12053^1, 12054^1, 12055^1, 12056^1, 12057^1, 13100^1, 13101^1, 13102^1, 13120^1, 13121^1, 13122^1, 13131^1, 13132^1, 13133^1, 13151^1, 13152^1, 13153^1, 20500^1, 20526^1, 20527^1, 20550^1, 20551^1, 20552^1, 20553^1, 20600^1, 25259^1, 26340^1, 29065^1, 29075^1, 29085^1, 29105^1, 29125^1, 29130^1, 29260^1, 29280^1, 29365^1, 29405^1, 29425^1, 29505^1, 29515^1, 29540^1, 29550^1, 29580^1, 29581^1, 29584^1, 36000^1, 36400^1, 36405^1, 36406^1, 36410^1, 36420^1, 36425^1, 36430^1, 36440^1, 36591^0, 36592^0, 36600^1, 36640^1, 43752^1, 51701^1, 51702^1, 51703^1, 62320^1, 62321^1, 62322^1, 62323^1, 62324^1, 62325^1, 62326^1, 62327^1, 64400^1, 64402^1, 64405^1, 64408^1, 64410^1, 64413^1, 64415^1, 64416^1, 64417^1, 64418^1, 64420^1, 64421^1, 64425^1, 64430^1, 64435^1, 64445^1, 64446^1, 64447^1, 64448^1, 64449^1, 64450^1, 64461^0, 64462^0, 64463^0, 64479^1, 64480^0, 64483^1, 64484^0, 64486^1, 64487^1, 64488^1, 64489^1, 64490^1, 64491^0, 64492^0, 64493^1, 64494^0, 64495^0, 64505^1, 64510^1, 64517^1, 64520^1, 64530^1, 64704^1, 64708^1, 69990^0, 72240^1, 72265^1, 76000^1, 76380^1, 76881^1, 76882^1, 76942^1, 76970^1, 76998^1, 77001^1, 77002^1, 77003^1, 77012^1, 77021^1, 92012^1, 92014^1, 93000^1, 93005^1, 93010^1, 93040^1, 93041^1, 93042^1, 93318^1, 93355^1, 94002^1, 94200^1, 94250^1, 94680^1, 94681^1, 94690^1, 94770^1, 95812^1, 95813^1, 95816^1, 95819^1, 95822^1, 95829^1, 95907^1, 95908^1, 95909^1, 95910^1, 95911^1, 95912^1, 95913^1, 95955^1, 96360^1, 96361^1, 96365^1, 96366^1, 96367^1, 96368^1, 96372^1, 96374^1, 96375^1, 96376^1, 96377^1, 99155^0, 99156^0, 99157^0, 99211^1, 99212^1, 99213^1, 99214^1, 99215^1, 99217^1, 99218^1, 99219^1, 99220^1, 99221^1, 99222^1, 99223^1, 99231^1, 99232^1, 99233^1, 99234^1, 99235^1, 99236^1, 99238^1, 99239^1, 99241^1, 99242^1, 99243^1, 99244^1, 99245^1, 99251^1, 99252^1, 99253^1, 99254^1, 99255^1, 99291^1, 99292^1, 99304^1, 99305^1, 99306^1, 99307^1, 99308^1, 99309^1, 99310^1, 99315^1, 99316^1, 99334^1, 99335^1, 99336^1, 99337^1, 99347^1, 99348^1, 99349^1, 99350^1, 99374^1, 99375^1, 99377^1, 99378^1, 99446^0, 99447^0, 99448^0, 99449^0, 99451^0, 99452^0, 99495^1, 99496^1, G0127^1, G0463^1, G0471^1, J0670^1, J2001^1
20605	00400^0, 01380^0, 0232T^1, 0481T^1, 10030^1, 10060^1, 10061^1, 10140^1, 10160^1, 11010^1, 11900^1, 12011^1, 15852^1, 20526^1, 20527^1, 20550^1, 20551^1, 20552^1, 20553^1, 24300^1, 25259^1, 26340^1, 29065^1, 29075^1, 29085^1, 29105^1, 29125^1, 29126^1, 29240^1, 29260^1, 29405^1, 29425^1, 29445^1, 29505^1, 29515^1, 29540^1, 29580^1, 29581^1, 29584^1, 29705^1, 36000^1, 36400^1, 36405^1, 36406^1, 36410^1, 36420^1, 36425^1, 36430^1, 36440^1, 36591^0, 36592^0, 36600^1, 36640^1, 43752^1, 51701^1, 51702^1, 51703^1, 64400^1, 64402^1, 64405^1, 64408^1, 64410^1, 64413^1, 64415^1, 64416^1, 64417^1, 64418^1, 64420^1, 64421^1, 64425^1, 64430^1, 64435^1, 64445^1, 64446^1, 64447^1, 64448^1, 64449^1, 64450^1, 64461^0, 64462^0, 64463^0, 64480^0, 64484^0, 64486^1, 64487^1, 64488^1, 64489^1, 64494^0, 64495^0, 64505^1, 64510^1, 64517^1, 64520^1, 64530^1, 64704^1, 69990^0, 76000^1, 76881^1, 76882^1, 76942^1, 76970^1, 76998^1, 77001^1, 92012^1, 92014^1, 93000^1, 93005^1, 93010^1, 93040^1, 93041^1, 93042^1, 93318^1, 93355^1, 94002^1, 94200^1, 94250^1, 94680^1, 94681^1, 94690^1, 94770^1, 95812^1, 95813^1, 95816^1, 95819^1, 95822^1, 95829^1, 95907^1, 95908^1, 95909^1, 95910^1, 95911^1, 95912^1, 95913^1, 95955^1, 96360^1, 96361^1, 96365^1, 96366^1, 96367^1, 96368^1, 96372^1, 96374^1, 96375^1, 96376^1, 96377^1, 99155^0, 99156^0, 99157^0, 99211^1, 99212^1, 99213^1, 99214^1, 99215^1, 99217^1, 99218^1, 99219^1, 99220^1, 99221^1, 99222^1, 99223^1, 99231^1, 99232^1, 99233^1, 99234^1, 99235^1, 99236^1, 99238^1, 99239^1, 99241^1, 99242^1, 99243^1, 99244^1, 99245^1, 99251^1, 99252^1, 99253^1, 99254^1, 99255^1, 99291^1, 99292^1, 99304^1, 99305^1, 99306^1, 99307^1, 99308^1, 99309^1, 99310^1, 99315^1, 99316^1, 99334^1, 99335^1, 99336^1, 99337^1, 99347^1, 99348^1, 99349^1, 99350^1, 99374^1, 99375^1, 99377^1, 99378^1, 99446^0, 99447^0, 99448^0, 99449^0, 99451^0, 99452^0, 99495^1, 99496^1, G0463^1, G0471^1, J0670^1, J2001^1
20606	00400^0, 01380^0, 0213T^1, 0216T^1, 0228T^1, 0230T^1, 0232T^1, 0481T^1, 10030^1, 10060^1, 10061^1, 10140^1, 10160^1, 11900^1, 12001^1, 12002^1, 12004^1, 12005^1, 12006^1, 12007^1, 12011^1, 12013^1, 12014^1, 12015^1, 12016^1, 12017^1, 12018^1, 12020^1, 12021^1, 12031^1,

0 = Modifier usage not allowed or inappropriate 1 = Modifier usage allowed

CPT © 2018 American Medical Association. All Rights Reserved.

Code 1	Code 2
	12032[1], 12034[1], 12035[1], 12036[1], 12037[1], 12041[1], 12042[1], 12044[1], 12045[1], 12046[1], 12047[1], 12051[1], 12052[1], 12053[1], 12054[1], 12055[1], 12056[1], 12057[1], 13100[1], 13101[1], 13102[1], 13120[1], 13121[1], 13122[1], 13131[1], 13132[1], 13133[1], 13151[1], 13152[1], 13153[1], 15852[1], 20526[1], 20527[1], 20550[1], 20551[1], 20552[1], 20553[1], 20605[1], 24300[1], 25259[1], 26340[1], 29065[1], 29075[1], 29085[1], 29105[1], 29125[1], 29126[1], 29240[1], 29260[1], 29405[1], 29425[1], 29445[1], 29505[1], 29515[1], 29540[1], 29580[1], 29581[1], 29584[1], 29705[1], 36000[1], 36400[1], 36405[1], 36406[1], 36410[1], 36420[1], 36425[1], 36430[1], 36440[1], 36591[0], 36592[0], 36600[1], 36640[1], 43752[1], 51701[1], 51702[1], 51703[1], 62320[1], 62321[1], 62322[1], 62323[1], 62324[1], 62325[1], 62326[1], 62327[1], 64400[1], 64402[1], 64405[1], 64408[1], 64410[1], 64413[1], 64415[1], 64416[1], 64417[1], 64418[1], 64420[1], 64421[1], 64425[1], 64430[1], 64435[1], 64445[1], 64446[1], 64447[1], 64448[1], 64449[1], 64450[1], 64461[0], 64462[0], 64463[0], 64479[1], 64480[0], 64483[1], 64484[0], 64486[1], 64487[1], 64488[1], 64489[1], 64490[1], 64491[0], 64492[0], 64493[1], 64494[0], 64495[0], 64505[1], 64510[1], 64517[1], 64520[1], 64530[1], 64704[1], 69990[0], 76000[1], 76380[1], 76881[1], 76882[1], 76942[1], 76970[1], 76998[1], 77001[1], 77002[1], 77003[1], 77012[1], 77021[1], 92012[1], 92014[1], 93000[1], 93005[1], 93010[1], 93040[1], 93041[1], 93042[1], 93318[1], 93355[1], 94002[1], 94200[1], 94250[1], 94680[1], 94681[1], 94690[1], 94770[1], 95812[1], 95813[1], 95816[1], 95819[1], 95822[1], 95829[1], 95907[1], 95908[1], 95909[1], 95910[1], 95911[1], 95912[1], 95913[1], 95955[1], 96360[1], 96361[1], 96365[1], 96366[1], 96367[1], 96368[1], 96372[1], 96374[1], 96375[1], 96376[1], 96377[1], 99155[0], 99156[0], 99157[0], 99211[1], 99212[1], 99213[1], 99214[1], 99215[1], 99217[1], 99218[1], 99219[1], 99220[1], 99221[1], 99222[1], 99223[1], 99231[1], 99232[1], 99233[1], 99234[1], 99235[1], 99236[1], 99238[1], 99239[1], 99241[1], 99242[1], 99243[1], 99244[1], 99245[1], 99251[1], 99252[1], 99253[1], 99254[1], 99255[1], 99291[1], 99292[1], 99304[1], 99305[1], 99306[1], 99307[1], 99308[1], 99309[1], 99310[1], 99315[1], 99316[1], 99334[1], 99335[1], 99336[1], 99337[1], 99347[1], 99348[1], 99349[1], 99350[1], 99374[1], 99375[1], 99377[1], 99378[1], 99446[0], 99447[0], 99448[0], 99449[0], 99451[0], 99452[0], 99495[1], 99496[1], G0463[1], G0471[1], J0670[1], J2001[1]
20610	00400[0], 01380[0], 0232T[1], 0481T[1], 10030[1], 10060[1], 10061[1], 10140[1], 10160[1], 11010[1], 11900[1], 12001[1], 12002[1], 12020[1], 12031[1], 12044[1], 15851[1], 20500[1], 20501[1], 20527[1], 20550[1], 20551[1], 20552[1], 20553[1], 24300[1], 25259[1], 26340[1], 29065[1], 29075[1], 29085[1], 29105[1], 29125[1], 29130[1], 29240[1], 29260[1], 29345[1], 29355[1], 29365[1], 29405[1], 29425[1], 29505[1], 29515[1], 29530[1], 29540[1], 29580[1], 29581[1], 29584[1], 36000[1], 36400[1], 36405[1], 36406[1], 36410[1], 36420[1], 36425[1], 36430[1], 36440[1], 36591[0], 36592[0], 36600[1], 36640[1], 43752[1], 51701[1], 51702[1], 51703[1], 64400[1], 64402[1], 64405[1], 64408[1], 64410[1], 64413[1], 64415[1], 64416[1], 64417[1], 64418[1], 64420[1], 64421[1], 64425[1], 64430[1], 64435[1], 64445[1], 64446[1], 64447[1], 64448[1], 64449[1], 64450[1], 64461[0], 64462[0], 64463[0], 64480[1], 64484[1], 64486[1], 64487[1], 64488[1], 64489[1], 64494[1], 64495[1], 64505[1], 64510[1], 64517[1], 64520[1], 64530[1], 69990[0], 72255[1], 72265[1], 72295[1], 76000[1], 76080[1], 76881[1], 76882[1], 76942[1], 76970[1], 76998[1], 77001[1], 92012[1], 92014[1], 93000[1], 93005[1], 93010[1], 93040[1], 93041[1], 93042[1], 93318[1], 93355[1], 94002[1], 94200[1], 94250[1], 94680[1], 94681[1], 94690[1], 94770[1], 95812[1], 95813[1], 95816[1], 95819[1], 95822[1], 95829[1], 95907[1], 95908[1], 95909[1], 95910[1], 95911[1], 95912[1], 95913[1], 95955[1], 96360[1], 96361[1], 96365[1], 96366[1], 96367[1], 96368[1], 96372[1], 96374[1], 96375[1], 96376[1], 96377[1], 99155[0], 99156[0], 99157[0], 99211[1], 99212[1], 99213[1], 99214[1], 99215[1], 99217[1], 99218[1], 99219[1], 99220[1], 99221[1], 99222[1], 99223[1], 99231[1], 99232[1], 99233[1], 99234[1], 99235[1], 99236[1], 99238[1], 99239[1], 99241[1], 99242[1], 99243[1], 99244[1], 99245[1], 99251[1], 99252[1], 99253[1], 99254[1], 99255[1], 99291[1], 99292[1], 99304[1], 99305[1], 99306[1], 99307[1], 99308[1], 99309[1], 99310[1], 99315[1], 99316[1], 99334[1], 99335[1], 99336[1], 99337[1], 99347[1], 99348[1], 99349[1], 99350[1], 99374[1], 99375[1], 99377[1], 99378[1], 99446[0], 99447[0], 99448[0], 99449[0], 99451[0], 99452[0], 99495[1], 99496[1], G0168[1], G0463[1], G0471[1], J0670[1], J2001[1]
20611	00400[0], 01380[0], 0213T[1], 0216T[1], 0228T[1], 0230T[1], 0232T[1], 0481T[1], 10030[1], 10060[1], 10061[1], 10140[1], 10160[1], 11900[1], 12001[1], 12002[1], 12004[1], 12005[1], 12006[1], 12007[1], 12011[1], 12013[1], 12014[1], 12015[1], 12016[1], 12017[1], 12018[1], 12020[1], 12021[1], 12031[1], 12032[1], 12034[1], 12035[1], 12036[1], 12037[1], 12041[1], 12042[1], 12044[1], 12045[1], 12046[1], 12047[1], 12051[1], 12052[1], 12053[1], 12054[1], 12055[1], 12056[1], 12057[1], 13100[1], 13101[1], 13102[1], 13120[1], 13121[1], 13122[1], 13131[1], 13132[1], 13133[1], 13151[1], 13152[1], 13153[1], 15851[1], 20500[1], 20501[1], 20527[1], 20550[1], 20551[1], 20552[1], 20553[1], 20610[1], 24300[1], 25259[1], 26340[1], 29065[1], 29075[1], 29085[1], 29105[1], 29125[1], 29130[1], 29240[1], 29260[1], 29345[1], 29355[1], 29365[1], 29405[1], 29425[1], 29505[1], 29515[1], 29530[1], 29540[1], 29580[1], 29581[1], 29584[1], 36000[1], 36400[1], 36405[1], 36406[1], 36410[1], 36420[1], 36425[1], 36430[1], 36440[1], 36591[0], 36592[0], 36600[1], 36640[1], 43752[1], 51701[1], 51702[1], 51703[1], 62320[1], 62321[1], 62322[1], 62323[1], 62324[1], 62325[1], 62326[1], 62327[1], 64400[1], 64402[1], 64405[1], 64408[1], 64410[1], 64413[1], 64415[1], 64416[1], 64417[1], 64418[1], 64420[1], 64421[1], 64425[1], 64430[1], 64435[1], 64445[1], 64446[1], 64447[1], 64448[1], 64449[1], 64450[1], 64461[0], 64462[0], 64463[0], 64479[1], 64480[0], 64483[1], 64484[1], 64486[1], 64487[1], 64488[1], 64489[1], 64490[1], 64491[0], 64492[0], 64493[1], 64494[0], 64495[0], 64505[1], 64510[1], 64517[1], 64520[1], 64530[1], 69990[0], 72255[1], 72265[1], 72295[1], 76000[1], 76080[1], 76380[1], 76881[1], 76882[1], 76942[1], 76970[1], 76998[1], 77001[1], 77002[1], 77003[1], 77012[1], 77021[1], 92012[1], 92014[1], 93000[1], 93005[1], 93010[1], 93040[1], 93041[1], 93042[1], 93318[1], 93355[1], 94002[1], 94200[1], 94250[1], 94680[1], 94681[1], 94690[1], 94770[1], 95812[1], 95813[1], 95816[1], 95819[1], 95822[1], 95829[1], 95907[1], 95908[1], 95909[1], 95910[1], 95911[1], 95912[1], 95913[1], 95955[1], 96360[1], 96361[1], 96365[1], 96366[1], 96367[1], 96368[1], 96372[1], 96374[1], 96375[1], 96376[1], 96377[1], 99155[0], 99156[0], 99157[0], 99211[1], 99212[1], 99213[1], 99214[1], 99215[1], 99217[1], 99218[1], 99219[1], 99220[1], 99221[1], 99222[1], 99223[1], 99231[1], 99232[1], 99233[1], 99234[1], 99235[1], 99236[1], 99238[1], 99239[1], 99241[1], 99242[1], 99243[1], 99244[1], 99245[1], 99251[1], 99252[1], 99253[1], 99254[1], 99255[1], 99291[1], 99292[1], 99304[1], 99305[1], 99306[1], 99307[1], 99308[1], 99309[1], 99310[1], 99315[1], 99316[1], 99334[1], 99335[1], 99336[1], 99337[1], 99347[1], 99348[1], 99349[1], 99350[1], 99374[1], 99375[1], 99377[1], 99378[1], 99446[0], 99447[0], 99448[0], 99449[0], 99451[0], 99452[0], 99495[1], 99496[1], G0168[1], G0463[1], G0471[1], J0670[1], J2001[1]
27096	0216T[0], 0230T[1], 12001[1], 12002[1], 12004[1], 12005[1], 12006[1], 12007[1], 12011[1], 12013[1], 12014[1], 12015[1], 12016[1], 12017[1], 12018[1], 12020[1], 12021[1], 12031[1], 12032[1], 12034[1], 12035[1], 12036[1], 12037[1], 12041[1], 12042[1], 12044[1], 12045[1], 12046[1], 12047[1], 12051[1], 12052[1], 12053[1], 12054[1], 12055[1], 12056[1], 12057[1], 13100[1], 13101[1], 13102[1], 13120[1], 13121[1], 13122[1], 13131[1], 13132[1], 13133[1], 13151[1], 13152[1], 13153[1], 20552[1], 20553[1], 20600[1], 20604[1], 20605[1], 20606[1], 20610[1], 20611[1], 36000[1], 36400[1], 36405[1], 36406[1], 36410[1], 36420[1], 36425[1], 36430[1], 36440[1], 36591[0], 36592[0], 36600[1], 36640[1], 43752[1], 51701[1], 51702[1], 51703[1], 62322[1], 62323[1], 62326[1], 62327[1], 64449[1], 64450[1], 64483[1], 64484[0], 64486[0], 64487[0], 64488[0], 64489[0], 69990[0], 76000[1], 76380[1], 76942[1], 76970[1], 76998[1], 77001[1], 77002[1], 77003[1], 77012[1], 92012[1], 92014[1], 93000[1], 93005[1], 93010[1], 93040[1], 93041[1], 93042[1], 93318[1], 93355[1], 94002[1], 94200[1], 94250[1], 94680[1], 94681[1], 94690[1], 94770[1], 95812[1], 95813[1], 95816[1], 95819[1], 95822[1], 95829[1], 95955[1], 96360[1], 96361[1], 96365[1], 96366[1], 96367[1], 96368[1], 96372[1], 96374[1], 96375[1], 96376[1], 96377[1], 96523[0], 99155[0], 99156[0], 99157[0], 99211[1], 99212[1], 99213[1], 99214[1], 99215[1], 99217[1], 99218[1], 99219[1], 99220[1], 99221[1], 99222[1], 99223[1], 99231[1], 99232[1], 99233[1], 99234[1], 99235[1], 99236[1], 99238[1], 99239[1], 99241[1], 99242[1], 99243[1], 99244[1], 99245[1], 99251[1], 99252[1], 99253[1], 99254[1], 99255[1], 99291[1], 99292[1], 99304[1], 99305[1], 99306[1], 99307[1], 99308[1], 99309[1], 99310[1], 99315[1], 99316[1], 99334[1], 99335[1], 99336[1], 99337[1], 99347[1], 99348[1], 99349[1], 99350[1], 99374[1], 99375[1], 99377[1], 99378[1], 99446[0], 99447[0], 99448[0], 99449[0], 99451[0], 99452[0], 99495[1], 99496[1], G0463[1], G0471[1], J0670[1], J1644[1], J2001[1]
28890	0101T[1], 0102T[1], 01462[0], 01470[0], 0213T[0], 0216T[0], 0228T[0], 0230T[0], 0508T[0], 0512T[1], 0513T[1], 12001[1], 12002[1], 12004[1], 12005[1], 12006[1], 12007[1], 12011[1], 12013[1], 12014[1], 12015[1], 12016[1], 12017[1], 12018[1], 12020[1], 12021[1], 12031[1], 12032[1], 12034[1], 12035[1], 12036[1], 12037[1], 12041[1], 12042[1], 12044[1], 12045[1], 12046[1], 12047[1], 12051[1], 12052[1], 12053[1], 12054[1], 12055[1], 12056[1], 12057[1], 13100[1], 13101[1], 13102[1], 13120[1], 13121[1], 13122[1], 13131[1], 13132[1], 13133[1], 13151[1], 13152[1], 13153[1], 36000[1], 36400[1], 36405[1], 36406[1], 36410[1], 36420[1], 36425[1], 36430[1], 36440[1], 36591[0], 36592[0], 36600[1], 36640[1], 43752[1], 51701[1], 51702[1], 51703[1], 62320[0], 62321[0], 62322[0], 62323[0], 62324[0], 62325[0], 62326[0], 62327[0], 64400[0], 64402[0], 64405[0], 64408[0], 64410[0], 64413[0], 64415[0], 64416[0], 64417[0], 64418[0], 64420[0], 64421[0], 64425[0], 64430[0], 64435[0], 64445[0], 64446[0], 64447[0], 64448[0], 64449[0], 64450[1], 64461[0], 64462[0], 64463[0], 64479[0], 64480[0], 64483[0], 64484[0], 64486[0], 64487[0], 64488[0], 64489[0], 64490[0], 64491[0], 64492[0], 64493[0], 64494[0], 64495[0], 64505[0], 64510[0], 64517[0], 64520[0], 64530[0], 69990[0], 76881[0], 76882[0], 76970[1], 76977[0], 76998[0], 76999[0], 92012[1], 92014[1], 93000[1], 93005[1], 93010[1], 93040[1], 93041[1], 93042[1], 93318[1], 93355[1], 94002[1], 94200[1], 94250[1], 94680[1], 94681[1], 94690[1], 94770[1], 95812[1], 95813[1], 95816[1], 95819[1], 95822[1], 95829[1], 95955[1], 96360[1], 96361[1], 96365[1], 96366[1], 96367[1], 96368[1], 96372[1], 96374[1], 96375[1], 96376[1], 96377[1], 99155[0], 99156[0], 99157[0], 99211[1], 99212[1], 99213[1], 99214[1], 99215[1], 99217[1], 99218[1], 99219[1], 99220[1], 99221[1], 99222[1], 99223[1], 99231[1], 99232[1], 99233[1], 99234[1], 99235[1], 99236[1], 99238[1], 99239[1], 99241[1], 99242[1], 99243[1], 99244[1], 99245[1], 99251[1], 99252[1], 99253[1], 99254[1], 99255[1], 99291[1], 99292[1], 99304[1], 99305[1], 99306[1], 99307[1], 99308[1], 99309[1], 99310[1], 99315[1], 99316[1], 99334[1], 99335[1], 99336[1], 99337[1], 99347[1], 99348[1], 99349[1], 99350[1], 99374[1], 99375[1], 99377[1], 99378[1], 99446[0], 99447[0], 99448[0], 99449[0], 99451[0], 99452[0], 99495[0], 99496[0], G0463[1], G0471[1], J0670[1], J2001[1]
36000	36591[0], 36592[0], 69990[0], 77001[1], 77002[1], 96523[0]
36010	35201[1], 35206[1], 35226[1], 35231[1], 35236[1], 35256[1], 35261[1], 35266[1], 35286[1], 36005[1], 36568[1], 36569[1], 36572[1], 36573[1], 36591[0], 36592[0], 69990[0], 75893[1], 76000[1], 77001[1], 77002[1], 99155[0], 99156[0], 99157[0], J0670[1], J1642[1], J1644[1], J2001[1]
36011	35201[1], 35206[1], 35226[1], 35231[1], 35236[1], 35256[1], 35261[1], 35266[1], 35286[1], 36000[1], 36005[1], 36010[1], 36400[1], 36405[1], 36406[1], 36410[1], 36420[1], 36425[1], 36555[1], 36556[1], 36568[1], 36569[1], 36572[1], 36573[1], 36591[0], 36592[0], 69990[0], 75893[1], 77001[1], 77002[1], J0670[1], J1642[1], J1644[1], J2001[1]

0 = Modifier usage not allowed or inappropriate 1 = Modifier usage allowed

CPT © 2018 American Medical Association. All Rights Reserved.

Code 1	Code 2
36012	35201[1], 35206[1], 35226[1], 35231[1], 35236[1], 35256[1], 35261[1], 35266[1], 35286[1], 36000[1], 36002[1], 36005[1], 36010[1], 36011[1], 36400[1], 36405[1], 36406[1], 36410[1], 36420[1], 36425[1], 36555[1], 36556[1], 36568[1], 36569[1], 36572[1], 36573[1], 36591[0], 36592[0], 69990[0], 75893[1], 76000[1], 77001[1], 77002[1], J0670[1], J1642[1], J1644[1], J2001[1]
36013	35201[1], 35206[1], 35226[1], 35231[1], 35236[1], 35256[1], 35261[1], 35266[1], 35286[1], 35820[1], 36000[1], 36005[1], 36010[1], 36400[1], 36405[1], 36406[1], 36410[1], 36420[1], 36425[1], 36556[1], 36568[1], 36569[1], 36572[1], 36573[1], 36591[0], 36592[0], 69990[0], 75893[1], 76000[1], 77001[1], 77002[1], J0670[1], J1642[1], J1644[1], J2001[1]
36014	35201[1], 35206[1], 35226[1], 35231[1], 35236[1], 35256[1], 35261[1], 35266[1], 35286[1], 36000[1], 36005[1], 36010[1], 36013[1], 36400[1], 36405[1], 36406[1], 36410[1], 36420[1], 36425[1], 36591[0], 36592[0], 69990[0], 75893[1], 76000[1], 77001[1], 77002[1], J0670[1], J1642[1], J1644[1], J2001[1]
36015	35201[1], 35206[1], 35226[1], 35231[1], 35236[1], 35256[1], 35261[1], 35266[1], 35286[1], 36000[1], 36005[1], 36010[1], 36013[1], 36014[1], 36400[1], 36405[1], 36406[1], 36410[1], 36420[1], 36425[1], 36591[0], 36592[0], 69990[0], 75893[1], 76000[1], 77001[1], 77002[1], J0670[1], J1642[1], J1644[1], J2001[1]
36100	01916[0], 01924[0], 01925[0], 01926[0], 35201[1], 35206[1], 35226[1], 35231[1], 35236[1], 35256[1], 35261[1], 35266[1], 35286[1], 36002[1], 36591[0], 36592[0], 69990[1], 76000[1], 77001[1], 77002[1], J0670[1], J1642[1], J1644[1], J2001[1]
36140	01916[0], 01924[0], 01925[0], 01926[0], 35201[1], 35206[1], 35226[1], 35231[1], 35236[1], 35256[1], 35261[1], 35266[1], 35286[1], 35860[1], 36002[1], 36500[1], 36591[0], 36592[0], 69990[1], 75893[1], 76000[1], 77001[1], 77002[1], 99155[0], 99156[0], 99157[0], J0670[1], J2001[1]
36400	36591[0], 36592[0], 69990[0], 99195[1]
36405	36591[0], 36592[0], 69990[0]
36406	36591[0], 36592[0], 69990[0], 99195[1]
36410	36450[0], 36460[0], 36510[0], 36591[0], 36592[0], 69990[0], 96523[0], 99195[1]
36415	36591[0], 36592[0], 99211[1]
36420	36591[0], 36592[0], 69990[0]
36425	36591[0], 36592[0], 69990[0]
36430	36460[1], 36591[0], 36592[0], 69990[0], J1642[1], J1644[1]
36440	36591[0], 36592[0], 69990[0]
36555	11000[1], 11001[1], 11004[1], 11005[1], 11006[1], 11042[1], 11043[1], 11044[1], 11045[1], 11046[1], 11047[1], 12001[1], 12002[1], 12004[1], 12005[1], 12006[1], 12007[1], 12011[1], 12013[1], 12014[1], 12015[1], 12016[1], 12017[1], 12018[1], 12020[1], 12021[1], 12031[1], 12032[1], 12034[1], 12035[1], 12036[1], 12037[1], 12041[1], 12042[1], 12044[1], 12045[1], 12046[1], 12047[1], 12051[1], 12052[1], 12053[1], 12054[1], 12055[1], 12056[1], 12057[1], 13100[1], 13101[1], 13102[1], 13120[1], 13121[1], 13122[1], 13131[1], 13132[1], 13133[1], 13151[1], 13152[1], 13153[1], 35201[1], 35206[1], 35226[1], 35231[1], 35236[1], 35256[1], 35261[1], 35266[1], 35286[1], 35800[1], 35820[1], 35840[1], 35860[1], 36000[1], 36002[1], 36005[1], 36010[1], 36013[1], 36400[1], 36405[1], 36406[1], 36410[1], 36420[1], 36425[1], 36430[1], 36440[1], 36556[1], 36568[1], 36569[1], 36591[0], 36592[0], 36597[1], 36600[1], 36640[1], 43752[1], 51701[1], 51702[1], 51703[1], 64461[0], 64462[0], 64463[0], 64486[0], 64487[0], 64488[0], 64489[0], 64490[0], 64491[0], 64492[0], 64493[0], 64494[0], 64495[0], 69990[0], 71045[1], 71046[1], 71047[1], 76000[1], 76942[1], 76970[1], 76998[1], 77002[1], 92012[1], 92014[1], 93000[1], 93005[1], 93010[1], 93040[1], 93041[1], 93042[1], 93318[1], 93355[1], 94002[1], 94200[1], 94250[1], 94680[1], 94681[1], 94690[1], 94770[1], 95812[1], 95813[1], 95816[1], 95819[1], 95822[1], 95829[1], 95955[1], 96360[1], 96361[1], 96365[1], 96366[1], 96367[1], 96368[1], 96372[1], 96374[1], 96375[1], 96376[1], 96377[1], 97597[1], 97598[1], 97602[1], 99155[1], 99156[1], 99157[1], 99211[1], 99212[1], 99213[1], 99214[1], 99215[1], 99217[1], 99218[1], 99219[1], 99220[1], 99221[1], 99222[1], 99223[1], 99231[1], 99232[1], 99233[1], 99234[1], 99235[1], 99236[1], 99238[1], 99239[1], 99241[1], 99242[1], 99243[1], 99244[1], 99245[1], 99251[1], 99252[1], 99253[1], 99254[1], 99255[1], 99291[1], 99292[1], 99304[1], 99305[1], 99306[1], 99307[1], 99308[1], 99309[1], 99310[1], 99315[1], 99316[1], 99334[1], 99335[1], 99336[1], 99337[1], 99347[1], 99348[1], 99349[1], 99350[1], 99374[1], 99375[1], 99377[1], 99378[1], 99446[0], 99447[0], 99448[0], 99449[0], 99451[0], 99452[0], 99495[1], 99496[1], G0463[1], G0471[1], J0670[1], J1642[1], J1644[1], J2001[1]
36556	11000[1], 11001[1], 11004[1], 11005[1], 11006[1], 11042[1], 11043[1], 11044[1], 11045[1], 11046[1], 11047[1], 12001[1], 12002[1], 12004[1], 12005[1], 12006[1], 12007[1], 12011[1], 12013[1], 12014[1], 12015[1], 12016[1], 12017[1], 12018[1], 12020[1], 12021[1], 12031[1], 12032[1], 12034[1], 12035[1], 12036[1], 12037[1], 12041[1], 12042[1], 12044[1], 12045[1], 12046[1], 12047[1], 12051[1], 12052[1], 12053[1], 12054[1], 12055[1], 12056[1], 12057[1], 13100[1], 13101[1], 13102[1], 13120[1], 13121[1], 13122[1], 13131[1], 13132[1], 13133[1], 13151[1], 13152[1], 13153[1], 35201[1], 35206[1], 35226[1], 35231[1], 35236[1], 35256[1], 35261[1], 35266[1], 35286[1], 35800[1], 35820[1], 35840[1], 35860[1], 36000[1], 36002[1], 36005[1], 36010[1], 36400[1], 36405[1], 36406[1], 36410[1], 36420[1], 36425[1], 36430[1], 36440[1], 36568[1], 36569[1], 36591[0], 36592[0], 36597[1], 36600[1], 36640[1], 43752[1], 51701[1], 51702[1], 51703[1], 69990[0], 71045[1], 71046[1], 71047[1], 76000[1], 76942[1], 76970[1], 76998[1], 77002[1], 92012[1], 92014[1], 93000[1], 93005[1], 93010[1], 93040[1], 93041[1], 93042[1], 93318[1], 93355[1], 94002[1], 94200[1], 94250[1], 94680[1], 94681[1], 94690[1], 94770[1], 95812[1], 95813[1], 95816[1], 95819[1], 95822[1], 95829[1], 95955[1], 96360[1], 96361[1], 96365[1], 96366[1], 96367[1], 96368[1], 96372[1], 96374[1], 96375[1], 96376[1], 96377[1], 97597[1], 97598[1], 97602[1], 99155[1], 99156[1], 99157[1], 99211[1], 99212[1], 99213[1], 99214[1], 99215[1], 99217[1], 99218[1], 99219[1], 99220[1], 99221[1], 99222[1], 99223[1], 99231[1], 99232[1], 99233[1], 99234[1], 99235[1], 99236[1], 99238[1], 99239[1], 99241[1], 99242[1], 99243[1], 99244[1], 99245[1], 99251[1], 99252[1], 99253[1], 99254[1], 99255[1], 99291[1], 99292[1], 99304[1], 99305[1], 99306[1], 99307[1], 99308[1], 99309[1], 99310[1], 99315[1], 99316[1], 99334[1], 99335[1], 99336[1], 99337[1], 99347[1], 99348[1], 99349[1], 99350[1], 99374[1], 99375[1], 99377[1], 99378[1], 99446[0], 99447[0], 99448[0], 99449[0], 99451[0], 99452[0], 99495[1], 99496[1], G0463[1], G0471[1], J0670[1], J1642[1], J1644[1], J2001[1]
36557	0213T[1], 0216T[1], 0228T[1], 0230T[1], 11000[1], 11001[1], 11004[1], 11005[1], 11006[1], 11042[1], 11043[1], 11044[1], 11045[1], 11046[1], 11047[1], 12001[1], 12002[1], 12004[1], 12005[1], 12006[1], 12007[1], 12011[1], 12013[1], 12014[1], 12015[1], 12016[1], 12017[1], 12018[1], 12020[1], 12021[1], 12031[1], 12032[1], 12034[1], 12035[1], 12036[1], 12037[1], 12041[1], 12042[1], 12044[1], 12045[1], 12046[1], 12047[1], 12051[1], 12052[1], 12053[1], 12054[1], 12055[1], 12056[1], 12057[1], 13100[1], 13101[1], 13102[1], 13120[1], 13121[1], 13122[1], 13131[1], 13132[1], 13133[1], 13151[1], 13152[1], 13153[1], 35201[1], 35206[1], 35226[1], 35231[1], 35236[1], 35256[1], 35261[1], 35266[1], 35286[1], 35800[1], 35820[1], 35840[1], 35860[1], 36000[1], 36002[1], 36005[1], 36010[1], 36011[1], 36012[1], 36013[1], 36400[1], 36405[1], 36406[1], 36410[1], 36420[1], 36425[1], 36430[1], 36440[1], 36555[1], 36556[1], 36558[0], 36568[1], 36569[1], 36573[1], 36591[0], 36592[0], 36597[1], 36600[1], 36640[1], 43752[1], 51701[1], 51702[1], 51703[1], 62320[1], 62321[1], 62322[1], 62323[1], 62324[0], 62325[0], 62326[0], 62327[0], 64400[1], 64402[1], 64405[1], 64408[1], 64410[1], 64413[1], 64415[1], 64416[1], 64417[1], 64418[1], 64420[1], 64421[1], 64425[1], 64430[1], 64435[1], 64445[1], 64446[1], 64447[1], 64448[1], 64449[1], 64450[1], 64461[0], 64462[0], 64463[0], 64479[1], 64480[0], 64483[1], 64484[0], 64486[0], 64487[0], 64488[0], 64489[0], 64490[1], 64491[0], 64492[0], 64493[1], 64494[0], 64495[0], 64505[1], 64510[1], 64517[1], 64520[1], 64530[1], 69990[0], 71045[1], 71046[1], 71047[1], 76000[1], 76942[1], 76970[1], 76998[1], 77002[1], 92012[1], 92014[1], 93000[1], 93005[1], 93010[1], 93040[1], 93041[1], 93042[1], 93318[1], 93355[1], 94002[1], 94200[1], 94250[1], 94680[1], 94681[1], 94690[1], 94770[1], 95812[1], 95813[1], 95816[1], 95819[1], 95822[1], 95829[1], 95955[1], 96360[1], 96361[1], 96365[1], 96366[1], 96367[1], 96368[1], 96372[1], 96374[1], 96375[1], 96376[1], 96377[1], 97597[1], 97598[1], 97602[1], 99155[1], 99156[1], 99157[1], 99211[1], 99212[1], 99213[1], 99214[1], 99215[1], 99217[1], 99218[1], 99219[1], 99220[1], 99221[1], 99222[1], 99223[1], 99231[1], 99232[1], 99233[1], 99234[1], 99235[1], 99236[1], 99238[1], 99239[1], 99241[1], 99242[1], 99243[1], 99244[1], 99245[1], 99251[1], 99252[1], 99253[1], 99254[1], 99255[1], 99291[1], 99292[1], 99304[1], 99305[1], 99306[1], 99307[1], 99308[1], 99309[1], 99310[1], 99315[1], 99316[1], 99334[1], 99335[1], 99336[1], 99337[1], 99347[1], 99348[1], 99349[1], 99350[1], 99374[1], 99375[1], 99377[1], 99378[1], 99446[0], 99447[0], 99448[0], 99449[0], 99451[0], 99452[0], 99495[0], 99496[0], G0463[1], G0471[1], J0670[1], J1642[1], J1644[1], J2001[1]
36558	0213T[1], 0216T[1], 0228T[1], 0230T[1], 11000[1], 11001[1], 11004[1], 11005[1], 11006[1], 11042[1], 11043[1], 11044[1], 11045[1], 11046[1], 11047[1], 12001[1], 12002[1], 12004[1], 12005[1], 12006[1], 12007[1], 12011[1], 12013[1], 12014[1], 12015[1], 12016[1], 12017[1], 12018[1], 12020[1], 12021[1], 12031[1], 12032[1], 12034[1], 12035[1], 12036[1], 12037[1], 12041[1], 12042[1], 12044[1], 12045[1], 12046[1], 12047[1], 12051[1], 12052[1], 12053[1], 12054[1], 12055[1], 12056[1], 12057[1], 13100[1], 13101[1], 13102[1], 13120[1], 13121[1], 13122[1], 13131[1], 13132[1], 13133[1], 13151[1], 13152[1], 13153[1], 35201[1], 35206[1], 35226[1], 35231[1], 35236[1], 35256[1], 35261[1], 35266[1], 35286[1], 35800[1], 35820[1], 35840[1], 35860[1], 36000[1], 36002[1], 36005[1], 36010[1], 36011[1], 36012[1], 36013[1], 36400[1], 36405[1], 36406[1], 36410[1], 36420[1], 36425[1], 36430[1], 36440[1], 36555[1], 36556[1], 36568[0], 36569[1], 36572[0], 36573[1], 36591[0], 36592[0], 36597[1], 36600[1], 36640[1], 43752[1], 51701[1], 51702[1], 51703[1], 62320[1], 62321[1], 62322[1], 62323[1], 62324[0], 62325[0], 62326[0], 62327[0], 64400[1], 64402[1], 64405[1], 64408[1], 64410[1], 64413[1], 64415[1], 64416[1], 64417[1], 64418[1], 64420[1], 64421[1], 64425[1], 64430[1], 64435[1], 64445[1], 64446[1], 64447[1], 64448[1], 64449[1], 64450[1], 64461[0], 64462[0], 64463[0], 64479[1], 64480[0], 64483[1], 64484[0], 64486[0], 64487[0], 64488[0], 64489[0], 64490[1], 64491[0], 64492[0], 64493[1], 64494[0], 64495[0], 64505[1], 64510[1], 64517[1], 64520[1], 64530[1], 69990[0], 71045[1], 71046[1], 71047[1], 76000[1], 76942[1], 76970[1], 76998[1], 77002[1], 92012[1], 92014[1], 93000[1], 93005[1], 93010[1], 93040[1], 93041[1], 93042[1], 93318[1], 93355[1], 94002[1], 94200[1], 94250[1], 94680[1], 94681[1], 94690[1], 94770[1], 95812[1], 95813[1], 95816[1], 95819[1], 95822[1], 95829[1], 95955[1], 96360[1], 96361[1], 96365[1], 96366[1], 96367[1], 96368[1], 96372[1], 96374[1], 96375[1], 96376[1], 96377[1], 97597[1], 97598[1], 97602[1], 99155[1], 99156[1], 99157[1], 99211[1], 99212[1], 99213[1], 99214[1], 99215[1], 99217[1], 99218[1], 99219[1], 99220[1], 99221[1], 99222[1], 99223[1], 99231[1], 99232[1], 99233[1], 99234[1], 99235[1], 99236[1], 99238[1], 99239[1], 99241[1], 99242[1], 99243[1], 99244[1], 99245[1], 99251[1], 99252[1], 99253[1], 99254[1], 99255[1], 99291[1], 99292[1], 99304[1], 99305[1], 99306[1], 99307[1], 99308[1], 99309[1], 99310[1], 99315[1], 99316[1], 99334[1], 99335[1], 99336[1], 99337[1], 99347[1], 99348[1], 99349[1], 99350[1], 99374[1], 99375[1], 99377[1], 99378[1], 99446[0], 99447[0],

0 = Modifier usage not allowed or inappropriate 1 = Modifier usage allowed

CPT © 2018 American Medical Association. All Rights Reserved.

Code 1	Code 2
	99448^0, 99449^0, 99451^0, 99452^0, 99495^0, 99496^0, G0463^1, G0471^1, J0670^1, J1642^1, J1644^1, J2001^1
36560	0213T^1, 0216T^1, 0228T^1, 0230T^1, 11000^1, 11001^1, 11004^1, 11005^1, 11006^1, 11042^1, 11043^1, 11044^1, 11045^1, 11046^1, 11047^1, 12001^1, 12002^1, 12004^1, 12005^1, 12006^1, 12007^1, 12011^1, 12013^1, 12014^1, 12015^1, 12016^1, 12017^1, 12018^1, 12020^1, 12021^1, 12031^1, 12032^1, 12034^1, 12035^1, 12036^1, 12037^1, 12041^1, 12042^1, 12044^1, 12045^1, 12046^1, 12047^1, 12051^1, 12052^1, 12053^1, 12054^1, 12055^1, 12056^1, 12057^1, 13100^1, 13101^1, 13102^1, 13120^1, 13121^1, 13122^1, 13131^1, 13132^1, 13133^1, 13151^1, 13152^1, 13153^1, 35201^1, 35206^1, 35226^1, 35231^1, 35236^1, 35256^1, 35261^1, 35266^1, 35286^1, 35800^1, 35820^1, 35840^1, 35860^1, 36000^1, 36005^1, 36010^1, 36011^1, 36012^1, 36013^1, 36400^1, 36405^1, 36406^1, 36410^1, 36420^1, 36425^1, 36430^1, 36440^1, 36555^1, 36556^1, 36557^1, 36558^1, 36561^1, 36563^1, 36565^1, 36568^1, 36569^1, 36570^1, 36571^1, 36572^1, 36573^1, 36591^0, 36592^0, 36600^1, 36640^1, 43752^1, 51701^1, 51702^1, 51703^1, 62320^1, 62321^1, 62322^1, 62323^1, 62324^0, 62325^0, 62326^0, 62327^0, 64400^1, 64402^1, 64405^1, 64408^1, 64410^1, 64413^1, 64415^1, 64416^1, 64417^1, 64418^1, 64420^1, 64421^1, 64425^1, 64430^1, 64435^1, 64445^1, 64446^1, 64447^1, 64448^1, 64449^1, 64450^1, 64461^0, 64462^0, 64463^0, 64479^1, 64480^0, 64483^1, 64484^0, 64486^0, 64487^0, 64488^0, 64489^0, 64490^1, 64491^0, 64492^0, 64493^1, 64494^0, 64495^0, 64505^1, 64510^1, 64517^1, 64520^1, 64530^1, 69990^0, 71045^1, 71046^1, 71047^1, 76000^1, 76942^1, 76970^1, 76998^1, 77002^1, 92012^1, 92014^1, 93000^1, 93005^1, 93010^1, 93040^1, 93041^1, 93042^1, 93318^1, 93355^1, 94002^1, 94200^1, 94250^1, 94680^1, 94681^1, 94690^1, 94770^1, 95812^1, 95813^1, 95816^1, 95819^1, 95822^1, 95829^1, 95955^1, 96360^1, 96361^1, 96365^1, 96366^1, 96367^1, 96368^1, 96372^1, 96374^1, 96375^1, 96376^1, 96377^1, 96522^1, 97597^1, 97598^1, 97602^1, 99155^1, 99156^1, 99157^1, 99211^1, 99212^1, 99213^1, 99214^1, 99215^1, 99217^1, 99218^1, 99219^1, 99220^1, 99221^1, 99222^1, 99223^1, 99231^1, 99232^1, 99233^1, 99234^1, 99235^1, 99236^1, 99238^1, 99239^1, 99241^1, 99242^1, 99243^1, 99244^1, 99245^1, 99251^1, 99252^1, 99253^1, 99254^1, 99255^1, 99291^1, 99292^1, 99304^1, 99305^1, 99306^1, 99307^1, 99308^1, 99309^1, 99310^1, 99315^1, 99316^1, 99334^1, 99335^1, 99336^1, 99337^1, 99347^1, 99348^1, 99349^1, 99350^1, 99374^1, 99375^1, 99377^1, 99378^1, 99446^0, 99447^0, 99448^0, 99449^0, 99451^0, 99452^0, 99495^0, 99496^0, G0463^1, G0471^1, J0670^1, J1642^1, J1644^1, J2001^1
36561	0213T^1, 0216T^1, 0228T^1, 0230T^1, 11000^1, 11001^1, 11004^1, 11005^1, 11006^1, 11042^1, 11043^1, 11044^1, 11045^1, 11046^1, 11047^1, 12001^1, 12002^1, 12004^1, 12005^1, 12006^1, 12007^1, 12011^1, 12013^1, 12014^1, 12015^1, 12016^1, 12017^1, 12018^1, 12020^1, 12021^1, 12031^1, 12032^1, 12034^1, 12035^1, 12036^1, 12037^1, 12041^1, 12042^1, 12044^1, 12045^1, 12046^1, 12047^1, 12051^1, 12052^1, 12053^1, 12054^1, 12055^1, 12056^1, 12057^1, 13100^1, 13101^1, 13102^1, 13120^1, 13121^1, 13122^1, 13131^1, 13132^1, 13133^1, 13151^1, 13152^1, 13153^1, 35201^1, 35206^1, 35226^1, 35231^1, 35236^1, 35256^1, 35261^1, 35266^1, 35286^1, 35800^1, 35820^1, 35840^1, 35860^1, 36000^1, 36005^1, 36010^1, 36011^1, 36012^1, 36013^1, 36400^1, 36405^1, 36406^1, 36410^1, 36420^1, 36425^1, 36430^1, 36440^1, 36555^1, 36556^1, 36557^1, 36558^1, 36565^1, 36568^1, 36569^1, 36570^1, 36571^1, 36572^1, 36573^1, 36591^0, 36592^0, 36600^1, 36640^1, 43752^1, 51701^1, 51702^1, 51703^1, 62320^1, 62321^1, 62322^1, 62323^1, 62324^0, 62325^0, 62326^0, 62327^0, 64400^1, 64402^1, 64405^1, 64408^1, 64410^1, 64413^1, 64415^1, 64416^1, 64417^1, 64418^1, 64420^1, 64421^1, 64425^1, 64430^1, 64435^1, 64445^1, 64446^1, 64447^1, 64448^1, 64449^1, 64450^1, 64461^0, 64462^0, 64463^0, 64479^1, 64480^0, 64483^1, 64484^0, 64486^0, 64487^0, 64488^0, 64489^0, 64490^1, 64491^0, 64492^0, 64493^1, 64494^0, 64495^0, 64505^1, 64510^1, 64517^1, 64520^1, 64530^1, 69990^0, 71045^1, 71046^1, 71047^1, 76000^1, 76942^1, 76970^1, 76998^1, 77002^1, 92012^1, 92014^1, 93000^1, 93005^1, 93010^1, 93040^1, 93041^1, 93042^1, 93318^1, 93355^1, 94002^1, 94200^1, 94250^1, 94680^1, 94681^1, 94690^1, 94770^1, 95812^1, 95813^1, 95816^1, 95819^1, 95822^1, 95829^1, 95955^1, 96360^1, 96361^1, 96365^1, 96366^1, 96367^1, 96368^1, 96372^1, 96374^1, 96375^1, 96376^1, 96377^1, 96522^1, 97597^1, 97598^1, 97602^1, 99155^1, 99156^1, 99157^1, 99211^1, 99212^1, 99213^1, 99214^1, 99215^1, 99217^1, 99218^1, 99219^1, 99220^1, 99221^1, 99222^1, 99223^1, 99231^1, 99232^1, 99233^1, 99234^1, 99235^1, 99236^1, 99238^1, 99239^1, 99241^1, 99242^1, 99243^1, 99244^1, 99245^1, 99251^1, 99252^1, 99253^1, 99254^1, 99255^1, 99291^1, 99292^1, 99304^1, 99305^1, 99306^1, 99307^1, 99308^1, 99309^1, 99310^1, 99315^1, 99316^1, 99334^1, 99335^1, 99336^1, 99337^1, 99347^1, 99348^1, 99349^1, 99350^1, 99374^1, 99375^1, 99377^1, 99378^1, 99446^0, 99447^0, 99448^0, 99449^0, 99451^0, 99452^0, 99495^0, 99496^0, G0463^1, G0471^1, J0670^1, J1642^1, J1644^1, J2001^1
36563	0213T^1, 0216T^1, 0228T^1, 0230T^1, 11000^1, 11001^1, 11004^1, 11005^1, 11006^1, 11042^1, 11043^1, 11044^1, 11045^1, 11046^1, 11047^1, 12001^1, 12002^1, 12004^1, 12005^1, 12006^1, 12007^1, 12011^1, 12013^1, 12014^1, 12015^1, 12016^1, 12017^1, 12018^1, 12020^1, 12021^1, 12031^1, 12032^1, 12034^1, 12035^1, 12036^1, 12037^1, 12041^1, 12042^1, 12044^1, 12045^1, 12046^1, 12047^1, 12051^1, 12052^1, 12053^1, 12054^1, 12055^1, 12056^1, 12057^1, 13100^1, 13101^1, 13102^1, 13120^1, 13121^1, 13122^1, 13131^1, 13132^1, 13133^1, 13151^1, 13152^1, 13153^1, 35201^1, 35206^1, 35226^1, 35231^1, 35236^1, 35256^1, 35261^1, 35266^1, 35286^1, 35800^1, 35820^1, 35840^1, 35860^1, 36000^1, 36005^1, 36010^1, 36011^1, 36012^1, 36013^1, 36400^1, 36405^1, 36406^1, 36410^1, 36420^1, 36425^1, 36430^1, 36440^1, 36555^1, 36556^1, 36557^1, 36558^1, 36561^1, 36565^1, 36568^1, 36569^1, 36570^1, 36571^1, 36572^1, 36573^1, 36591^0, 36592^0, 36600^1, 36640^1, 43752^1, 51701^1, 51702^1, 51703^1, 62320^1, 62321^1, 62322^1, 62323^1, 62324^0, 62325^0, 62326^0, 62327^0, 64400^1, 64402^1, 64405^1, 64408^1, 64410^1, 64413^1, 64415^1, 64416^1, 64417^1, 64418^1, 64420^1, 64421^1, 64425^1, 64430^1, 64435^1, 64445^1, 64446^1, 64447^1, 64448^1, 64449^1, 64450^1, 64461^0, 64462^0, 64463^0, 64479^1, 64480^0, 64483^1, 64484^0, 64486^0, 64487^0, 64488^0, 64489^0, 64490^1, 64491^0, 64492^0, 64493^1, 64494^0, 64495^0, 64505^1, 64510^1, 64517^1, 64520^1, 64530^1, 69990^0, 71045^1, 71046^1, 71047^1, 76000^1, 76942^1, 76970^1, 76998^1, 77002^1, 92012^1, 92014^1, 93000^1, 93005^1, 93010^1, 93040^1, 93041^1, 93042^1, 93318^1, 93355^1, 94002^1, 94200^1, 94250^1, 94680^1, 94681^1, 94690^1, 94770^1, 95812^1, 95813^1, 95816^1, 95819^1, 95822^1, 95829^1, 95955^1, 96360^1, 96361^1, 96365^1, 96366^1, 96367^1, 96368^1, 96372^1, 96374^1, 96375^1, 96376^1, 96377^1, 96522^1, 97597^1, 97598^1, 97602^1, 99155^1, 99156^1, 99157^1, 99211^1, 99212^1, 99213^1, 99214^1, 99215^1, 99217^1, 99218^1, 99219^1, 99220^1, 99221^1, 99222^1, 99223^1, 99231^1, 99232^1, 99233^1, 99234^1, 99235^1, 99236^1, 99238^1, 99239^1, 99241^1, 99242^1, 99243^1, 99244^1, 99245^1, 99251^1, 99252^1, 99253^1, 99254^1, 99255^1, 99291^1, 99292^1, 99304^1, 99305^1, 99306^1, 99307^1, 99308^1, 99309^1, 99310^1, 99315^1, 99316^1, 99334^1, 99335^1, 99336^1, 99337^1, 99347^1, 99348^1, 99349^1, 99350^1, 99374^1, 99375^1, 99377^1, 99378^1, 99446^0, 99447^0, 99448^0, 99449^0, 99451^0, 99452^0, 99495^0, 99496^0, G0463^1, G0471^1, J0670^1, J1642^1, J1644^1, J2001^1
36565	0213T^1, 0216T^1, 0228T^1, 0230T^1, 11000^1, 11001^1, 11004^1, 11005^1, 11006^1, 11042^1, 11043^1, 11044^1, 11045^1, 11046^1, 11047^1, 12001^1, 12002^1, 12004^1, 12005^1, 12006^1, 12007^1, 12011^1, 12013^1, 12014^1, 12015^1, 12016^1, 12017^1, 12018^1, 12020^1, 12021^1, 12031^1, 12032^1, 12034^1, 12035^1, 12036^1, 12037^1, 12041^1, 12042^1, 12044^1, 12045^1, 12046^1, 12047^1, 12051^1, 12052^1, 12053^1, 12054^1, 12055^1, 12056^1, 12057^1, 13100^1, 13101^1, 13102^1, 13120^1, 13121^1, 13122^1, 13131^1, 13132^1, 13133^1, 13151^1, 13152^1, 13153^1, 35201^1, 35206^1, 35226^1, 35231^1, 35236^1, 35256^1, 35261^1, 35266^1, 35286^1, 35820^1, 36000^1, 36005^1, 36011^1, 36012^1, 36013^1, 36400^1, 36405^1, 36406^1, 36410^1, 36420^1, 36425^1, 36430^1, 36440^1, 36555^1, 36556^1, 36557^1, 36558^1, 36568^1, 36569^1, 36570^1, 36571^1, 36572^1, 36573^1, 36591^0, 36592^0, 36600^1, 36640^1, 43752^1, 51701^1, 51702^1, 51703^1, 62320^1, 62321^1, 62322^1, 62323^1, 62324^0, 62325^0, 62326^0, 62327^0, 64400^1, 64402^1, 64405^1, 64408^1, 64410^1, 64413^1, 64415^1, 64416^1, 64417^1, 64418^1, 64420^1, 64421^1, 64425^1, 64430^1, 64435^1, 64445^1, 64446^1, 64447^1, 64448^1, 64449^1, 64450^1, 64461^0, 64462^0, 64463^0, 64479^1, 64480^0, 64483^1, 64484^0, 64486^0, 64487^0, 64488^0, 64489^0, 64490^1, 64491^0, 64492^0, 64493^1, 64494^0, 64495^0, 64505^1, 64510^1, 64517^1, 64520^1, 64530^1, 69990^0, 71045^1, 71046^1, 71047^1, 76000^1, 76942^1, 76970^1, 76998^1, 77002^1, 92012^1, 92014^1, 93000^1, 93005^1, 93010^1, 93040^1, 93041^1, 93042^1, 93318^1, 93355^1, 94002^1, 94200^1, 94250^1, 94680^1, 94681^1, 94690^1, 94770^1, 95812^1, 95813^1, 95816^1, 95819^1, 95822^1, 95829^1, 95955^1, 96360^1, 96361^1, 96365^1, 96366^1, 96367^1, 96368^1, 96372^1, 96374^1, 96375^1, 96376^1, 96377^1, 97597^1, 97598^1, 97602^1, 99155^1, 99156^1, 99157^1, 99211^1, 99212^1, 99213^1, 99214^1, 99215^1, 99217^1, 99218^1, 99219^1, 99220^1, 99221^1, 99222^1, 99223^1, 99231^1, 99232^1, 99233^1, 99234^1, 99235^1, 99236^1, 99238^1, 99239^1, 99241^1, 99242^1, 99243^1, 99244^1, 99245^1, 99251^1, 99252^1, 99253^1, 99254^1, 99255^1, 99291^1, 99292^1, 99304^1, 99305^1, 99306^1, 99307^1, 99308^1, 99309^1, 99310^1, 99315^1, 99316^1, 99334^1, 99335^1, 99336^1, 99337^1, 99347^1, 99348^1, 99349^1, 99350^1, 99374^1, 99375^1, 99377^1, 99378^1, 99446^0, 99447^0, 99448^0, 99449^0, 99451^0, 99452^0, 99495^0, 99496^0, G0463^1, G0471^1, J0670^1, J1642^1, J1644^1, J2001^1
36566	0213T^1, 0216T^1, 0228T^1, 0230T^1, 11000^1, 11001^1, 11004^1, 11005^1, 11006^1, 11042^1, 11043^1, 11044^1, 11045^1, 11046^1, 11047^1, 12001^1, 12002^1, 12004^1, 12005^1, 12006^1, 12007^1, 12011^1, 12013^1, 12014^1, 12015^1, 12016^1, 12017^1, 12018^1, 12020^1, 12021^1, 12031^1, 12032^1, 12034^1, 12035^1, 12036^1, 12037^1, 12041^1, 12042^1, 12044^1, 12045^1, 12046^1, 12047^1, 12051^1, 12052^1, 12053^1, 12054^1, 12055^1, 12056^1, 12057^1, 13100^1, 13101^1, 13102^1, 13120^1, 13121^1, 13122^1, 13131^1, 13132^1, 13133^1, 13151^1, 13152^1, 13153^1, 35201^1, 35206^1, 35226^1, 35231^1, 35236^1, 35256^1, 35261^1, 35266^1, 35286^1, 35800^1, 35820^1, 35840^1, 35860^1, 36000^1, 36005^1, 36010^1, 36011^1, 36012^1, 36013^1, 36400^1, 36405^1, 36406^1, 36410^1, 36420^1, 36425^1, 36430^1, 36440^1, 36555^1, 36556^1, 36557^1, 36558^1, 36560^1, 36561^1, 36563^1, 36565^1, 36568^1, 36569^1, 36570^1, 36571^1, 36572^1, 36573^1, 36591^0, 36592^0, 36600^1, 36640^1, 43752^1, 51701^1, 51702^1, 51703^1, 62320^1, 62321^1, 62322^1, 62323^1, 62324^0, 62325^0, 62326^0, 62327^0, 64400^1, 64402^1, 64405^1, 64408^1, 64410^1, 64413^1, 64415^1, 64416^1, 64417^1, 64418^1, 64420^1, 64421^1, 64425^1, 64430^1, 64435^1, 64445^1, 64446^1, 64447^1, 64448^1, 64449^1, 64450^1, 64461^0, 64462^0, 64463^0, 64479^1, 64480^0, 64483^1, 64484^0, 64486^0, 64487^0, 64488^0, 64489^0, 64490^1, 64491^0, 64492^0, 64493^1, 64494^0, 64495^0, 64505^1, 64510^1, 64517^1, 64520^1, 64530^1, 69990^0, 71045^1, 71046^1, 71047^1, 76000^1, 76942^1, 76970^1, 76998^1, 77002^1, 92012^1, 92014^1, 93000^1, 93005^1, 93010^1, 93040^1, 93041^1, 93042^1, 93318^1, 93355^1,

0 = Modifier usage not allowed or inappropriate 1 = Modifier usage allowed

CPT © 2018 American Medical Association. All Rights Reserved.

Code 1	Code 2
	94002[1], 94200[1], 94250[1], 94680[1], 94681[1], 94690[1], 94770[1], 95812[1], 95813[1], 95816[1], 95819[1], 95822[1], 95829[1], 95955[1], 96360[1], 96361[1], 96365[1], 96366[1], 96367[1], 96368[1], 96372[1], 96374[1], 96375[1], 96376[1], 96377[1], 96522[1], 97597[1], 97598[1], 97602[1], 99155[1], 99156[1], 99157[1], 99211[1], 99212[1], 99213[1], 99214[1], 99215[1], 99217[1], 99218[1], 99219[1], 99220[1], 99221[1], 99222[1], 99223[1], 99231[1], 99232[1], 99233[1], 99234[1], 99235[1], 99236[1], 99238[1], 99239[1], 99241[1], 99242[1], 99243[1], 99244[1], 99245[1], 99251[1], 99252[1], 99253[1], 99254[1], 99255[1], 99291[1], 99292[1], 99304[1], 99305[1], 99306[1], 99307[1], 99308[1], 99309[1], 99310[1], 99315[1], 99316[1], 99334[1], 99335[1], 99336[1], 99337[1], 99347[1], 99348[1], 99349[1], 99350[1], 99374[1], 99375[1], 99377[1], 99378[1], 99446[0], 99447[0], 99448[0], 99449[0], 99451[0], 99452[0], 99495[0], 99496[0], G0463[1], G0471[1], J0670[1], J1642[1], J1644[1], J2001[1]
36568	11000[1], 11001[1], 11004[1], 11005[1], 11006[1], 11042[1], 11043[1], 11044[1], 11045[1], 11046[1], 11047[1], 12001[1], 12002[1], 12004[1], 12005[1], 12006[1], 12007[1], 12011[1], 12013[1], 12014[1], 12015[1], 12016[1], 12017[1], 12018[1], 12020[1], 12021[1], 12031[1], 12032[1], 12034[1], 12035[1], 12036[1], 12037[1], 12041[1], 12042[1], 12044[1], 12045[1], 12046[1], 12047[1], 12051[1], 12052[1], 12053[1], 12054[1], 12055[1], 12056[1], 12057[1], 13100[1], 13101[1], 13102[1], 13120[1], 13121[1], 13122[1], 13131[1], 13132[1], 13133[1], 13151[1], 13152[1], 13153[1], 35201[1], 35206[1], 35226[1], 35231[1], 35236[1], 35256[1], 35261[1], 35266[1], 35286[1], 35800[1], 35820[1], 35840[1], 35860[1], 36000[1], 36002[1], 36005[1], 36400[1], 36405[1], 36406[1], 36410[1], 36420[1], 36425[1], 36430[1], 36440[1], 36569[1], 36572[1], 36573[1], 36591[0], 36592[0], 36597[1], 36600[1], 36640[1], 43752[1], 51701[1], 51702[1], 51703[1], 64461[0], 64462[0], 64463[0], 64486[0], 64487[0], 64488[0], 64489[0], 64490[0], 64491[0], 64492[0], 64493[0], 64494[0], 64495[0], 69990[0], 71045[1], 71046[1], 71047[1], 76000[1], 76380[1], 76937[1], 76942[1], 76970[1], 76998[1], 77001[1], 77002[1], 77012[1], 77021[1], 92012[1], 92014[1], 93000[1], 93005[1], 93010[1], 93040[1], 93041[1], 93042[1], 93318[1], 93355[1], 94002[1], 94200[1], 94250[1], 94680[1], 94681[1], 94690[1], 94770[1], 95812[1], 95813[1], 95816[1], 95819[1], 95822[1], 95829[1], 95955[1], 96360[1], 96361[1], 96365[1], 96366[1], 96367[1], 96368[1], 96372[1], 96374[1], 96375[1], 96376[1], 96377[1], 97597[1], 97598[1], 97602[1], 99155[1], 99156[1], 99157[1], 99211[1], 99212[1], 99213[1], 99214[1], 99215[1], 99217[1], 99218[1], 99219[1], 99220[1], 99221[1], 99222[1], 99223[1], 99231[1], 99232[1], 99233[1], 99234[1], 99235[1], 99236[1], 99238[1], 99239[1], 99241[1], 99242[1], 99243[1], 99244[1], 99245[1], 99251[1], 99252[1], 99253[1], 99254[1], 99255[1], 99291[1], 99292[1], 99304[1], 99305[1], 99306[1], 99307[1], 99308[1], 99309[1], 99310[1], 99315[1], 99316[1], 99334[1], 99335[1], 99336[1], 99337[1], 99347[1], 99348[1], 99349[1], 99350[1], 99374[1], 99375[1], 99377[1], 99378[1], 99446[0], 99447[0], 99448[0], 99449[0], 99451[0], 99452[0], 99495[1], 99496[1], G0463[1], G0471[1], J0670[1], J1642[1], J1644[1], J2001[1]
36569	11000[1], 11001[1], 11004[1], 11005[1], 11006[1], 11042[1], 11043[1], 11044[1], 11045[1], 11046[1], 11047[1], 12001[1], 12002[1], 12004[1], 12005[1], 12006[1], 12007[1], 12011[1], 12013[1], 12014[1], 12015[1], 12016[1], 12017[1], 12018[1], 12020[1], 12021[1], 12031[1], 12032[1], 12034[1], 12035[1], 12036[1], 12037[1], 12041[1], 12042[1], 12044[1], 12045[1], 12046[1], 12047[1], 12051[1], 12052[1], 12053[1], 12054[1], 12055[1], 12056[1], 12057[1], 13100[1], 13101[1], 13102[1], 13120[1], 13121[1], 13122[1], 13131[1], 13132[1], 13133[1], 13151[1], 13152[1], 13153[1], 35201[1], 35206[1], 35226[1], 35231[1], 35236[1], 35256[1], 35261[1], 35266[1], 35286[1], 35800[1], 35820[1], 35840[1], 35860[1], 36000[1], 36002[1], 36005[1], 36400[1], 36405[1], 36406[1], 36410[1], 36420[1], 36425[1], 36430[1], 36440[1], 36572[1], 36573[1], 36591[0], 36592[0], 36597[1], 36600[1], 36640[1], 43752[1], 51701[1], 51702[1], 51703[1], 64461[0], 64462[0], 64463[0], 64486[0], 64487[0], 64488[0], 64489[0], 64490[0], 64491[0], 64492[0], 64493[0], 64494[0], 64495[0], 69990[0], 71045[1], 71046[1], 71047[1], 76000[1], 76380[1], 76937[1], 76942[1], 76970[1], 76998[1], 77001[1], 77002[1], 77012[1], 77021[1], 92012[1], 92014[1], 93000[1], 93005[1], 93010[1], 93040[1], 93041[1], 93042[1], 93318[1], 93355[1], 94002[1], 94200[1], 94250[1], 94680[1], 94681[1], 94690[1], 94770[1], 95812[1], 95813[1], 95816[1], 95819[1], 95822[1], 95829[1], 95955[1], 96360[1], 96361[1], 96365[1], 96366[1], 96367[1], 96368[1], 96372[1], 96374[1], 96375[1], 96376[1], 96377[1], 97597[1], 97598[1], 97602[1], 99155[1], 99156[1], 99157[1], 99211[1], 99212[1], 99213[1], 99214[1], 99215[1], 99217[1], 99218[1], 99219[1], 99220[1], 99221[1], 99222[1], 99223[1], 99231[1], 99232[1], 99233[1], 99234[1], 99235[1], 99236[1], 99238[1], 99239[1], 99241[1], 99242[1], 99243[1], 99244[1], 99245[1], 99251[1], 99252[1], 99253[1], 99254[1], 99255[1], 99291[1], 99292[1], 99304[1], 99305[1], 99306[1], 99307[1], 99308[1], 99309[1], 99310[1], 99315[1], 99316[1], 99334[1], 99335[1], 99336[1], 99337[1], 99347[1], 99348[1], 99349[1], 99350[1], 99374[1], 99375[1], 99377[1], 99378[1], 99446[0], 99447[0], 99448[0], 99449[0], 99451[0], 99452[0], 99495[1], 99496[1], G0463[1], G0471[1], J0670[1], J1642[1], J1644[1], J2001[1]
36570	0213T[1], 0216T[1], 0228T[0], 0230T[0], 11000[1], 11001[1], 11004[1], 11005[1], 11006[1], 11042[1], 11043[1], 11044[1], 11045[1], 11046[1], 11047[1], 12001[1], 12002[1], 12004[1], 12005[1], 12006[1], 12007[1], 12011[1], 12013[1], 12014[1], 12015[1], 12016[1], 12017[1], 12018[1], 12020[1], 12021[1], 12031[1], 12032[1], 12034[1], 12035[1], 12036[1], 12037[1], 12041[1], 12042[1], 12044[1], 12045[1], 12046[1], 12047[1], 12051[1], 12052[1], 12053[1], 12054[1], 12055[1], 12056[1], 12057[1], 13100[1], 13101[1], 13102[1], 13120[1], 13121[1], 13122[1], 13131[1], 13132[1], 13133[1], 13151[1], 13152[1], 13153[1], 35201[1], 35206[1], 35226[1], 35231[1], 35236[1], 35256[1], 35261[1], 35266[1], 35286[1], 35800[1], 35820[1], 35840[1], 35860[1], 36000[1], 36005[1], 36010[1], 36011[1], 36012[1], 36013[1], 36400[1], 36405[1], 36406[1], 36410[1], 36420[1], 36425[1], 36430[1], 36440[1], 36555[1], 36556[1], 36557[1], 36558[1], 36568[1], 36569[1], 36571[1], 36572[1], 36573[1], 36591[0], 36592[0], 36600[1], 36640[1], 43752[1], 51701[1], 51702[1], 51703[1], 62320[0], 62321[0], 62322[0], 62323[0], 62324[1], 62325[1], 62326[1], 62327[1], 64400[0], 64402[0], 64405[0], 64408[0], 64410[0], 64413[0], 64415[1], 64416[1], 64417[1], 64418[0], 64420[0], 64421[0], 64425[0], 64430[0], 64435[0], 64445[0], 64446[0], 64447[0], 64448[0], 64449[0], 64450[1], 64461[0], 64462[0], 64463[0], 64479[0], 64480[0], 64483[0], 64484[0], 64486[0], 64487[0], 64488[0], 64489[0], 64490[1], 64491[0], 64492[0], 64493[1], 64494[0], 64495[0], 64505[0], 64510[0], 64517[0], 64520[0], 64530[0], 69990[0], 71045[1], 71046[1], 71047[1], 76000[1], 76942[1], 76970[1], 76998[1], 77002[1], 92012[1], 92014[1], 93000[1], 93005[1], 93010[1], 93040[1], 93041[1], 93042[1], 93318[1], 93355[1], 94002[1], 94200[1], 94250[1], 94680[1], 94681[1], 94690[1], 94770[1], 95812[1], 95813[1], 95816[1], 95819[1], 95822[1], 95829[1], 95955[1], 96360[1], 96361[1], 96365[1], 96366[1], 96367[1], 96368[1], 96372[1], 96374[1], 96375[1], 96376[1], 96377[1], 96522[1], 97597[1], 97598[1], 97602[1], 99155[0], 99156[0], 99157[0], 99211[1], 99212[1], 99213[1], 99214[1], 99215[1], 99217[1], 99218[1], 99219[1], 99220[1], 99221[1], 99222[1], 99223[1], 99231[1], 99232[1], 99233[1], 99234[1], 99235[1], 99236[1], 99238[1], 99239[1], 99241[1], 99242[1], 99243[1], 99244[1], 99245[1], 99251[1], 99252[1], 99253[1], 99254[1], 99255[1], 99291[1], 99292[1], 99304[1], 99305[1], 99306[1], 99307[1], 99308[1], 99309[1], 99310[1], 99315[1], 99316[1], 99334[1], 99335[1], 99336[1], 99337[1], 99347[1], 99348[1], 99349[1], 99350[1], 99374[1], 99375[1], 99377[1], 99378[1], 99446[0], 99447[0], 99448[0], 99449[0], 99451[0], 99452[0], 99495[0], 99496[0], G0463[1], G0471[1], J0670[1], J1642[1], J1644[1], J2001[1]
36571	0213T[1], 0216T[1], 0228T[0], 0230T[0], 11000[1], 11001[1], 11004[1], 11005[1], 11006[1], 11042[1], 11043[1], 11044[1], 11045[1], 11046[1], 11047[1], 12001[1], 12002[1], 12004[1], 12005[1], 12006[1], 12007[1], 12011[1], 12013[1], 12014[1], 12015[1], 12016[1], 12017[1], 12018[1], 12020[1], 12021[1], 12031[1], 12032[1], 12034[1], 12035[1], 12036[1], 12037[1], 12041[1], 12042[1], 12044[1], 12045[1], 12046[1], 12047[1], 12051[1], 12052[1], 12053[1], 12054[1], 12055[1], 12056[1], 12057[1], 13100[1], 13101[1], 13102[1], 13120[1], 13121[1], 13122[1], 13131[1], 13132[1], 13133[1], 13151[1], 13152[1], 13153[1], 35201[1], 35206[1], 35226[1], 35231[1], 35236[1], 35256[1], 35261[1], 35266[1], 35286[1], 35800[1], 35820[1], 35840[1], 35860[1], 36000[1], 36005[1], 36010[1], 36011[1], 36012[1], 36013[1], 36400[1], 36405[1], 36406[1], 36410[1], 36420[1], 36425[1], 36430[1], 36440[1], 36555[1], 36556[1], 36557[1], 36558[1], 36568[1], 36569[1], 36572[1], 36573[1], 36591[0], 36592[0], 36600[1], 36640[1], 43752[1], 51701[1], 51702[1], 51703[1], 62320[0], 62321[0], 62322[0], 62323[0], 62324[1], 62325[1], 62326[1], 62327[1], 64400[0], 64402[0], 64405[0], 64408[0], 64410[0], 64413[0], 64415[1], 64416[1], 64417[1], 64418[0], 64420[0], 64421[0], 64425[0], 64430[0], 64435[0], 64445[0], 64446[0], 64447[0], 64448[0], 64449[0], 64450[1], 64461[0], 64462[0], 64463[0], 64479[0], 64480[0], 64483[0], 64484[0], 64486[0], 64487[0], 64488[0], 64489[0], 64490[1], 64491[0], 64492[0], 64493[1], 64494[0], 64495[0], 64505[0], 64510[0], 64517[0], 64520[0], 64530[0], 69990[0], 71045[1], 71046[1], 71047[1], 76000[1], 76942[1], 76970[1], 76998[1], 77002[1], 92012[1], 92014[1], 93000[1], 93005[1], 93010[1], 93040[1], 93041[1], 93042[1], 93318[1], 93355[1], 94002[1], 94200[1], 94250[1], 94680[1], 94681[1], 94690[1], 94770[1], 95812[1], 95813[1], 95816[1], 95819[1], 95822[1], 95829[1], 95955[1], 96360[1], 96361[1], 96365[1], 96366[1], 96367[1], 96368[1], 96372[1], 96374[1], 96375[1], 96376[1], 96377[1], 96522[1], 97597[1], 97598[1], 97602[1], 99155[0], 99156[0], 99157[0], 99211[1], 99212[1], 99213[1], 99214[1], 99215[1], 99217[1], 99218[1], 99219[1], 99220[1], 99221[1], 99222[1], 99223[1], 99231[1], 99232[1], 99233[1], 99234[1], 99235[1], 99236[1], 99238[1], 99239[1], 99241[1], 99242[1], 99243[1], 99244[1], 99245[1], 99251[1], 99252[1], 99253[1], 99254[1], 99255[1], 99291[1], 99292[1], 99304[1], 99305[1], 99306[1], 99307[1], 99308[1], 99309[1], 99310[1], 99315[1], 99316[1], 99334[1], 99335[1], 99336[1], 99337[1], 99347[1], 99348[1], 99349[1], 99350[1], 99374[1], 99375[1], 99377[1], 99378[1], 99446[0], 99447[0], 99448[0], 99449[0], 99451[0], 99452[0], 99495[0], 99496[0], G0463[1], G0471[1], J0670[1], J1642[1], J1644[1], J2001[1]
36572	0213T[0], 0216T[0], 0228T[0], 0230T[0], 11000[1], 11001[1], 11004[1], 11005[1], 11006[1], 11042[1], 11043[1], 11044[1], 11045[1], 11046[1], 11047[1], 12001[1], 12002[1], 12004[1], 12005[1], 12006[1], 12007[1], 12011[1], 12013[1], 12014[1], 12015[1], 12016[1], 12017[1], 12018[1], 12020[1], 12021[1], 12031[1], 12032[1], 12034[1], 12035[1], 12036[1], 12037[1], 12041[1], 12042[1], 12044[1], 12045[1], 12046[1], 12047[1], 12051[1], 12052[1], 12053[1], 12054[1], 12055[1], 12056[1], 12057[1], 13100[1], 13101[1], 13102[1], 13120[1], 13121[1], 13122[1], 13131[1], 13132[1], 13133[1], 13151[1], 13152[1], 13153[1], 35201[1], 35206[1], 35207[1], 35211[1], 35216[1], 35221[1], 35226[1], 35231[1], 35236[1], 35241[1], 35246[1], 35251[1], 35256[1], 35261[1], 35266[1], 35271[1], 35276[1], 35281[1], 35286[1], 35800[1], 35820[1], 35840[1], 35860[1], 36000[1], 36002[1], 36005[1], 36400[1], 36405[1], 36406[1], 36410[1], 36420[1], 36425[1], 36430[1], 36440[1], 36555[1], 36556[1], 36557[1], 36591[0], 36592[0], 36597[1], 36600[1], 36640[1], 43752[1], 51701[1], 51702[1], 51703[1], 62320[0], 62321[0], 62322[0], 62323[0], 62324[0], 62325[0], 62326[0], 62327[0], 64400[0], 64402[0], 64405[0], 64408[0], 64410[0], 64413[0], 64415[0], 64416[0], 64417[0], 64418[0], 64420[0], 64421[0], 64425[0], 64430[0], 64435[0], 64445[0], 64446[0], 64447[0], 64448[0], 64449[0], 64450[0], 64461[0], 64462[0], 64463[0], 64479[0], 64480[0], 64483[0], 64484[0], 64486[0], 64487[0], 64488[0], 64489[0], 64490[0], 64491[0], 64492[0], 64493[0], 64494[0], 64495[0], 64505[0], 64510[0], 64517[0], 64520[0], 64530[0], 69990[0], 71045[1], 71046[1], 71047[1], 71048[1], 75810[1], 75820[1], 75822[1], 75825[1], 75827[1], 75831[1], 75833[1], 75840[1], 75842[1], 75860[1], 75870[1], 75872[1], 75880[1], 75889[1], 75891[1], 76000[1], 76380[1], 76937[1], 76942[1], 76970[1], 76998[1], 77001[1], 77002[1], 77012[1], 77021[1], 92012[1], 92014[1],

0 = Modifier usage not allowed or inappropriate 1 = Modifier usage allowed

CPT © 2018 American Medical Association. All Rights Reserved.

Code 1	Code 2
	93000[1], 93005[1], 93010[1], 93040[1], 93041[1], 93042[1], 93318[1], 93355[1], 93503[1], 94002[1], 94200[1], 94250[1], 94680[1], 94681[1], 94690[1], 94770[1], 95812[1], 95813[1], 95816[1], 95819[1], 95822[1], 95829[1], 95955[1], 96360[1], 96361[1], 96365[1], 96366[1], 96367[1], 96368[1], 96372[1], 96374[1], 96375[1], 96376[1], 96377[1], 96523[0], 97597[1], 97598[1], 97602[1], 99155[0], 99156[0], 99157[0], 99211[1], 99212[1], 99213[1], 99214[1], 99215[1], 99217[1], 99218[1], 99219[1], 99220[1], 99221[1], 99222[1], 99223[1], 99231[1], 99232[1], 99233[1], 99234[1], 99235[1], 99236[1], 99238[1], 99239[1], 99241[1], 99242[1], 99243[1], 99244[1], 99245[1], 99251[1], 99252[1], 99253[1], 99254[1], 99255[1], 99291[1], 99292[1], 99304[1], 99305[1], 99306[1], 99307[1], 99308[1], 99309[1], 99310[1], 99315[1], 99316[1], 99334[1], 99335[1], 99336[1], 99337[1], 99347[1], 99348[1], 99349[1], 99350[1], 99374[1], 99375[1], 99377[1], 99378[1], 99446[0], 99447[0], 99448[0], 99449[0], 99495[1], 99496[1], G0463[1], G0471[1], J0670[1], J1642[1], J1644[1], J2001[1]
36573	0213T[0], 0216T[0], 0228T[0], 0230T[0], 11000[1], 11001[1], 11004[1], 11005[1], 11006[1], 11042[1], 11043[1], 11044[1], 11045[1], 11046[1], 11047[1], 12001[1], 12002[1], 12004[1], 12005[1], 12006[1], 12007[1], 12011[1], 12013[1], 12014[1], 12015[1], 12016[1], 12017[1], 12018[1], 12020[1], 12021[1], 12031[1], 12032[1], 12034[1], 12035[1], 12036[1], 12037[1], 12041[1], 12042[1], 12044[1], 12045[1], 12046[1], 12047[1], 12051[1], 12052[1], 12053[1], 12054[1], 12055[1], 12056[1], 12057[1], 13100[1], 13101[1], 13102[1], 13120[1], 13121[1], 13122[1], 13131[1], 13132[1], 13133[1], 13151[1], 13152[1], 13153[1], 35201[1], 35206[1], 35207[1], 35211[1], 35216[1], 35221[1], 35226[1], 35231[1], 35236[1], 35241[1], 35246[1], 35251[1], 35256[1], 35261[1], 35266[1], 35271[1], 35276[1], 35281[1], 35286[1], 35800[1], 35820[1], 35840[1], 35860[1], 36000[1], 36002[1], 36005[1], 36400[1], 36405[1], 36406[1], 36410[1], 36420[1], 36425[1], 36430[1], 36440[1], 36555[1], 36556[1], 36591[0], 36592[0], 36597[1], 36600[1], 36640[1], 43752[1], 51701[1], 51702[1], 51703[1], 62320[0], 62321[0], 62322[0], 62323[0], 62324[0], 62325[0], 62326[0], 62327[0], 64400[0], 64402[0], 64405[0], 64408[0], 64410[0], 64413[0], 64415[0], 64416[0], 64417[0], 64418[0], 64420[0], 64421[0], 64425[0], 64430[0], 64435[0], 64445[0], 64446[0], 64447[0], 64448[0], 64449[0], 64450[0], 64461[0], 64462[0], 64463[0], 64479[0], 64480[0], 64483[0], 64484[0], 64486[0], 64487[0], 64488[0], 64489[0], 64490[0], 64491[0], 64492[0], 64493[0], 64494[0], 64495[0], 64505[0], 64510[0], 64517[0], 64520[0], 64530[0], 69990[0], 71045[1], 71046[1], 71047[1], 71048[1], 75810[1], 75820[1], 75822[1], 75825[1], 75827[1], 75831[1], 75833[1], 75840[1], 75842[1], 75860[1], 75870[1], 75872[1], 75880[1], 75889[1], 75891[1], 76000[1], 76380[1], 76937[1], 76942[1], 76970[1], 76998[1], 77001[1], 77002[1], 77012[1], 77021[1], 92012[1], 92014[1], 93000[1], 93005[1], 93010[1], 93040[1], 93041[1], 93042[1], 93318[1], 93355[1], 94002[1], 94200[1], 94250[1], 94680[1], 94681[1], 94690[1], 94770[1], 95812[1], 95813[1], 95816[1], 95819[1], 95822[1], 95829[1], 95955[1], 96360[1], 96361[1], 96365[1], 96366[1], 96367[1], 96368[1], 96372[1], 96374[1], 96375[1], 96376[1], 96377[1], 96523[0], 97597[1], 97598[1], 97602[1], 99155[0], 99156[0], 99157[0], 99211[1], 99212[1], 99213[1], 99214[1], 99215[1], 99217[1], 99218[1], 99219[1], 99220[1], 99221[1], 99222[1], 99223[1], 99231[1], 99232[1], 99233[1], 99234[1], 99235[1], 99236[1], 99238[1], 99239[1], 99241[1], 99242[1], 99243[1], 99244[1], 99245[1], 99251[1], 99252[1], 99253[1], 99254[1], 99255[1], 99291[1], 99292[1], 99304[1], 99305[1], 99306[1], 99307[1], 99308[1], 99309[1], 99310[1], 99315[1], 99316[1], 99334[1], 99335[1], 99336[1], 99337[1], 99347[1], 99348[1], 99349[1], 99350[1], 99374[1], 99375[1], 99377[1], 99378[1], 99446[0], 99447[0], 99448[0], 99449[0], 99495[1], 99496[1], G0463[1], G0471[1], J0670[1], J1642[1], J1644[1], J2001[1]
36575	0213T[1], 0216T[1], 0228T[0], 0230T[0], 11000[1], 11001[1], 11004[1], 11005[1], 11006[1], 11042[1], 11043[1], 11044[1], 11045[1], 11046[1], 11047[1], 12001[1], 12002[1], 12004[1], 12005[1], 12006[1], 12007[1], 12011[1], 12013[1], 12014[1], 12015[1], 12016[1], 12017[1], 12018[1], 12020[1], 12021[1], 12031[1], 12032[1], 12034[1], 12035[1], 12036[1], 12037[1], 12041[1], 12042[1], 12044[1], 12045[1], 12046[1], 12047[1], 12051[1], 12052[1], 12053[1], 12054[1], 12055[1], 12056[1], 12057[1], 13100[1], 13101[1], 13102[1], 13120[1], 13121[1], 13122[1], 13131[1], 13132[1], 13133[1], 13151[1], 13152[1], 13153[1], 35201[1], 35206[1], 35226[1], 35231[1], 35236[1], 35256[1], 35261[1], 35266[1], 35286[1], 36000[1], 36005[1], 36400[1], 36405[1], 36406[1], 36410[1], 36420[1], 36425[1], 36430[1], 36440[1], 36591[0], 36592[0], 36597[1], 36600[1], 36640[1], 43752[1], 51701[1], 51702[1], 51703[1], 62320[0], 62321[0], 62322[0], 62323[0], 62324[1], 62325[1], 62326[1], 62327[1], 64400[0], 64402[0], 64405[0], 64408[0], 64410[0], 64413[0], 64415[1], 64416[1], 64417[1], 64418[0], 64420[0], 64421[0], 64425[0], 64430[0], 64435[0], 64445[0], 64446[0], 64447[0], 64448[0], 64449[0], 64450[1], 64461[0], 64462[0], 64463[0], 64479[0], 64480[0], 64483[0], 64484[0], 64486[0], 64487[0], 64488[0], 64489[0], 64490[1], 64491[0], 64492[0], 64493[1], 64494[0], 64495[0], 64505[0], 64510[0], 64517[0], 64520[0], 64530[0], 69990[0], 71045[1], 71046[1], 71047[1], 76000[1], 76942[1], 76970[1], 76998[1], 77002[1], 92012[1], 92014[1], 93000[1], 93005[1], 93010[1], 93040[1], 93041[1], 93042[1], 93318[1], 93355[1], 94002[1], 94200[1], 94250[1], 94680[1], 94681[1], 94690[1], 94770[1], 95812[1], 95813[1], 95816[1], 95819[1], 95822[1], 95829[1], 95955[1], 96360[1], 96361[1], 96365[1], 96366[1], 96367[1], 96368[1], 96372[1], 96374[1], 96375[1], 96376[1], 96377[1], 97597[1], 97598[1], 97602[1], 99155[0], 99156[0], 99157[0], 99211[1], 99212[1], 99213[1], 99214[1], 99215[1], 99217[1], 99218[1], 99219[1], 99220[1], 99221[1], 99222[1], 99223[1], 99231[1], 99232[1], 99233[1], 99234[1], 99235[1], 99236[1], 99238[1], 99239[1], 99241[1], 99242[1], 99243[1], 99244[1], 99245[1], 99251[1], 99252[1], 99253[1], 99254[1], 99255[1], 99291[1], 99292[1], 99304[1], 99305[1], 99306[1], 99307[1], 99308[1], 99309[1], 99310[1], 99315[1], 99316[1], 99334[1], 99335[1], 99336[1], 99337[1], 99347[1], 99348[1], 99349[1], 99350[1], 99374[1], 99375[1], 99377[1], 99378[1], 99446[0], 99447[0], 99448[0], 99449[0], 99451[0], 99452[0], 99495[1], 99496[1], G0463[1], G0471[1], J0670[1], J1642[1], J1644[1], J2001[1]
36576	0213T[1], 0216T[1], 0228T[0], 0230T[0], 11000[1], 11001[1], 11004[1], 11005[1], 11006[1], 11042[1], 11043[1], 11044[1], 11045[1], 11046[1], 11047[1], 12001[1], 12002[1], 12004[1], 12005[1], 12006[1], 12007[1], 12011[1], 12013[1], 12014[1], 12015[1], 12016[1], 12017[1], 12018[1], 12020[1], 12021[1], 12031[1], 12032[1], 12034[1], 12035[1], 12036[1], 12037[1], 12041[1], 12042[1], 12044[1], 12045[1], 12046[1], 12047[1], 12051[1], 12052[1], 12053[1], 12054[1], 12055[1], 12056[1], 12057[1], 13100[1], 13101[1], 13102[1], 13120[1], 13121[1], 13122[1], 13131[1], 13132[1], 13133[1], 13151[1], 13152[1], 13153[1], 35201[1], 35206[1], 35226[1], 35231[1], 35236[1], 35256[1], 35261[1], 35266[1], 35286[1], 36000[1], 36005[1], 36400[1], 36405[1], 36406[1], 36410[1], 36420[1], 36425[1], 36430[1], 36440[1], 36591[0], 36592[0], 36597[1], 36600[1], 36640[1], 43752[1], 51701[1], 51702[1], 51703[1], 62320[0], 62321[0], 62322[0], 62323[0], 62324[1], 62325[1], 62326[1], 62327[1], 64400[0], 64402[0], 64405[0], 64408[0], 64410[0], 64413[0], 64415[1], 64416[1], 64417[1], 64418[0], 64420[0], 64421[0], 64425[0], 64430[0], 64435[0], 64445[0], 64446[0], 64447[0], 64448[0], 64449[0], 64450[1], 64461[0], 64462[0], 64463[0], 64479[0], 64480[0], 64483[0], 64484[0], 64486[0], 64487[0], 64488[0], 64489[0], 64490[1], 64491[0], 64492[0], 64493[1], 64494[0], 64495[0], 64505[0], 64510[0], 64517[0], 64520[0], 64530[0], 69990[0], 71045[1], 71046[1], 71047[1], 76000[1], 76942[1], 76970[1], 76998[1], 77002[1], 92012[1], 92014[1], 93000[1], 93005[1], 93010[1], 93040[1], 93041[1], 93042[1], 93318[1], 93355[1], 94002[1], 94200[1], 94250[1], 94680[1], 94681[1], 94690[1], 94770[1], 95812[1], 95813[1], 95816[1], 95819[1], 95822[1], 95829[1], 95955[1], 96360[1], 96361[1], 96365[1], 96366[1], 96367[1], 96368[1], 96372[1], 96374[1], 96375[1], 96376[1], 96377[1], 97597[1], 97598[1], 97602[1], 99155[0], 99156[0], 99157[0], 99211[1], 99212[1], 99213[1], 99214[1], 99215[1], 99217[1], 99218[1], 99219[1], 99220[1], 99221[1], 99222[1], 99223[1], 99231[1], 99232[1], 99233[1], 99234[1], 99235[1], 99236[1], 99238[1], 99239[1], 99241[1], 99242[1], 99243[1], 99244[1], 99245[1], 99251[1], 99252[1], 99253[1], 99254[1], 99255[1], 99291[1], 99292[1], 99304[1], 99305[1], 99306[1], 99307[1], 99308[1], 99309[1], 99310[1], 99315[1], 99316[1], 99334[1], 99335[1], 99336[1], 99337[1], 99347[1], 99348[1], 99349[1], 99350[1], 99374[1], 99375[1], 99377[1], 99378[1], 99446[0], 99447[0], 99448[0], 99449[0], 99451[0], 99452[0], 99495[0], 99496[0], G0463[1], G0471[1], J0670[1], J1642[1], J1644[1], J2001[1]
36578	0213T[0], 0216T[0], 0228T[0], 0230T[0], 11000[1], 11001[1], 11004[1], 11005[1], 11006[1], 11042[1], 11043[1], 11044[1], 11045[1], 11046[1], 11047[1], 12001[1], 12002[1], 12004[1], 12005[1], 12006[1], 12007[1], 12011[1], 12013[1], 12014[1], 12015[1], 12016[1], 12017[1], 12018[1], 12020[1], 12021[1], 12031[1], 12032[1], 12034[1], 12035[1], 12036[1], 12037[1], 12041[1], 12042[1], 12044[1], 12045[1], 12046[1], 12047[1], 12051[1], 12052[1], 12053[1], 12054[1], 12055[1], 12056[1], 12057[1], 13100[1], 13101[1], 13102[1], 13120[1], 13121[1], 13122[1], 13131[1], 13132[1], 13133[1], 13151[1], 13152[1], 13153[1], 35201[1], 35206[1], 35226[1], 35231[1], 35236[1], 35256[1], 35261[1], 35266[1], 35286[1], 36000[1], 36005[1], 36400[1], 36405[1], 36406[1], 36410[1], 36420[1], 36425[1], 36430[1], 36440[1], 36575[1], 36576[1], 36580[1], 36581[1], 36584[1], 36591[0], 36592[0], 36595[1], 36596[1], 36597[1], 36600[1], 36640[1], 43752[1], 51701[1], 51702[1], 51703[1], 62320[0], 62321[0], 62322[0], 62323[0], 62324[0], 62325[0], 62326[0], 62327[0], 64400[0], 64402[0], 64405[0], 64408[0], 64410[0], 64413[0], 64415[0], 64416[0], 64417[0], 64418[0], 64420[0], 64421[0], 64425[0], 64430[0], 64435[0], 64445[0], 64446[0], 64447[0], 64448[0], 64449[0], 64450[0], 64461[0], 64462[0], 64463[0], 64479[0], 64480[0], 64483[0], 64484[0], 64486[0], 64487[0], 64488[0], 64489[0], 64490[0], 64491[0], 64492[0], 64493[0], 64494[0], 64495[0], 64505[0], 64510[0], 64517[0], 64520[0], 64530[0], 69990[0], 71045[1], 71046[1], 71047[1], 76000[1], 76942[1], 76970[1], 76998[1], 77002[1], 92012[1], 92014[1], 93000[1], 93005[1], 93010[1], 93040[1], 93041[1], 93042[1], 93318[1], 93355[1], 94002[1], 94200[1], 94250[1], 94680[1], 94681[1], 94690[1], 94770[1], 95812[1], 95813[1], 95816[1], 95819[1], 95822[1], 95829[1], 95955[1], 96360[1], 96361[1], 96365[1], 96366[1], 96367[1], 96368[1], 96372[1], 96374[1], 96375[1], 96376[1], 96377[1], 97597[1], 97598[1], 97602[1], 99155[0], 99156[0], 99157[0], 99211[1], 99212[1], 99213[1], 99214[1], 99215[1], 99217[1], 99218[1], 99219[1], 99220[1], 99221[1], 99222[1], 99223[1], 99231[1], 99232[1], 99233[1], 99234[1], 99235[1], 99236[1], 99238[1], 99239[1], 99241[1], 99242[1], 99243[1], 99244[1], 99245[1], 99251[1], 99252[1], 99253[1], 99254[1], 99255[1], 99291[1], 99292[1], 99304[1], 99305[1], 99306[1], 99307[1], 99308[1], 99309[1], 99310[1], 99315[1], 99316[1], 99334[1], 99335[1], 99336[1], 99337[1], 99347[1], 99348[1], 99349[1], 99350[1], 99374[1], 99375[1], 99377[1], 99378[1], 99446[0], 99447[0], 99448[0], 99449[0], 99451[0], 99452[0], 99495[0], 99496[0], G0463[1], G0471[1], J0670[1], J1642[1], J1644[1], J2001[1]
36580	0213T[0], 0216T[0], 0228T[0], 0230T[0], 11000[1], 11001[1], 11004[1], 11005[1], 11006[1], 11042[1], 11043[1], 11044[1], 11045[1], 11046[1], 11047[1], 12001[1], 12002[1], 12004[1], 12005[1], 12006[1], 12007[1], 12011[1], 12013[1], 12014[1], 12015[1], 12016[1], 12017[1], 12018[1], 12020[1], 12021[1], 12031[1], 12032[1], 12034[1], 12035[1], 12036[1], 12037[1], 12041[1], 12042[1], 12044[1], 12045[1], 12046[1], 12047[1], 12051[1], 12052[1], 12053[1], 12054[1], 12055[1], 12056[1], 12057[1], 13100[1], 13101[1], 13102[1], 13120[1], 13121[1], 13122[1], 13131[1], 13132[1], 13133[1], 13151[1], 13152[1], 13153[1], 35201[1], 35206[1], 35226[1], 35231[1], 35236[1], 35256[1], 35261[1], 35266[1], 35286[1], 35800[1], 35820[1], 35840[1], 35860[1], 36000[1], 36005[1], 36010[1], 36011[1], 36012[1], 36013[1], 36400[1], 36405[1], 36406[1], 36410[1], 36420[1], 36425[1], 36430[1], 36440[1], 36555[1], 36556[1], 36557[1], 36558[1], 36560[1], 36561[1], 36563[1], 36565[1], 36566[1], 36568[1], 36569[1], 36570[1],

0 = Modifier usage not allowed or inappropriate   1 = Modifier usage allowed

CPT © 2018 American Medical Association. All Rights Reserved.

Code 1	Code 2
	36571[1], 36572[1], 36573[1], 36575[1], 36576[1], 36591[0], 36592[0], 36595[1], 36596[1], 36597[1], 36600[1], 36640[1], 43752[1], 51701[1], 51702[1], 51703[1], 62320[0], 62321[0], 62322[0], 62323[0], 62324[0], 62325[0], 62326[0], 62327[0], 64400[0], 64402[0], 64405[0], 64408[0], 64410[0], 64413[0], 64415[0], 64416[0], 64417[0], 64418[0], 64420[0], 64421[0], 64425[0], 64430[0], 64435[0], 64445[0], 64446[0], 64447[0], 64448[0], 64449[0], 64450[0], 64461[0], 64462[0], 64463[0], 64479[0], 64480[0], 64483[0], 64484[0], 64486[0], 64487[0], 64488[0], 64489[0], 64490[0], 64491[0], 64492[0], 64493[0], 64494[0], 64495[0], 64505[0], 64510[0], 64517[0], 64520[0], 64530[0], 69990[0], 71045[1], 71046[1], 71047[1], 76000[1], 76942[1], 76970[1], 76998[1], 77002[1], 92012[1], 92014[1], 93000[1], 93005[1], 93010[1], 93040[1], 93041[1], 93042[1], 93318[1], 93355[1], 94002[1], 94200[1], 94250[1], 94680[1], 94681[1], 94690[1], 94770[1], 95812[1], 95813[1], 95816[1], 95819[1], 95822[1], 95829[1], 95955[1], 96360[1], 96361[1], 96365[1], 96366[1], 96367[1], 96368[1], 96372[1], 96374[1], 96375[1], 96376[1], 96377[1], 97597[1], 97598[1], 97602[1], 99155[0], 99156[0], 99157[0], 99211[1], 99212[1], 99213[1], 99214[1], 99215[1], 99217[1], 99218[1], 99219[1], 99220[1], 99221[1], 99222[1], 99223[1], 99231[1], 99232[1], 99233[1], 99234[1], 99235[1], 99236[1], 99238[1], 99239[1], 99241[1], 99242[1], 99243[1], 99244[1], 99245[1], 99251[1], 99252[1], 99253[1], 99254[1], 99255[1], 99291[1], 99292[1], 99304[1], 99305[1], 99306[1], 99307[1], 99308[1], 99309[1], 99310[1], 99315[1], 99316[1], 99334[1], 99335[1], 99336[1], 99337[1], 99347[1], 99348[1], 99349[1], 99350[1], 99374[1], 99375[1], 99377[1], 99378[1], 99446[0], 99447[0], 99448[0], 99449[0], 99451[0], 99452[0], 99495[1], 99496[1], G0463[1], G0471[1], J0670[1], J1642[1], J1644[1], J2001[1]
36581	0213T[0], 0216T[0], 0228T[0], 0230T[0], 11000[1], 11001[1], 11004[1], 11005[1], 11006[1], 11042[1], 11043[1], 11044[1], 11045[1], 11046[1], 11047[1], 12001[1], 12002[1], 12004[1], 12005[1], 12006[1], 12007[1], 12011[1], 12013[1], 12014[1], 12015[1], 12016[1], 12017[1], 12018[1], 12020[1], 12021[1], 12031[1], 12032[1], 12034[1], 12035[1], 12036[1], 12037[1], 12041[1], 12042[1], 12044[1], 12045[1], 12046[1], 12047[1], 12051[1], 12052[1], 12053[1], 12054[1], 12055[1], 12056[1], 12057[1], 13100[1], 13101[1], 13102[1], 13120[1], 13121[1], 13122[1], 13131[1], 13132[1], 13133[1], 13151[1], 13152[1], 13153[1], 35201[1], 35206[1], 35226[1], 35231[1], 35236[1], 35256[1], 35261[1], 35266[1], 35286[1], 35800[1], 35820[1], 35840[1], 35860[1], 36000[1], 36005[1], 36010[1], 36011[1], 36012[1], 36013[1], 36400[1], 36405[1], 36406[1], 36410[1], 36420[1], 36425[1], 36430[1], 36440[1], 36555[1], 36556[1], 36557[1], 36558[1], 36560[1], 36561[1], 36563[1], 36565[1], 36566[1], 36568[1], 36569[1], 36570[1], 36571[1], 36572[1], 36573[1], 36575[1], 36576[1], 36591[0], 36592[0], 36595[1], 36596[1], 36597[1], 36600[1], 36640[1], 43752[1], 51701[1], 51702[1], 51703[1], 62320[0], 62321[0], 62322[0], 62323[0], 62324[0], 62325[0], 62326[0], 62327[0], 64400[0], 64402[0], 64405[0], 64408[0], 64410[0], 64413[0], 64415[0], 64416[0], 64417[0], 64418[0], 64420[0], 64421[0], 64425[0], 64430[0], 64435[0], 64445[0], 64446[0], 64447[0], 64448[0], 64449[0], 64450[0], 64461[0], 64462[0], 64463[0], 64479[0], 64480[0], 64483[0], 64484[0], 64486[0], 64487[0], 64488[0], 64489[0], 64490[0], 64491[0], 64492[0], 64493[0], 64494[0], 64495[0], 64505[0], 64510[0], 64517[0], 64520[0], 64530[0], 69990[0], 71045[1], 71046[1], 71047[1], 76000[1], 76942[1], 76970[1], 76998[1], 77002[1], 92012[1], 92014[1], 93000[1], 93005[1], 93010[1], 93040[1], 93041[1], 93042[1], 93318[1], 93355[1], 94002[1], 94200[1], 94250[1], 94680[1], 94681[1], 94690[1], 94770[1], 95812[1], 95813[1], 95816[1], 95819[1], 95822[1], 95829[1], 95955[1], 96360[1], 96361[1], 96365[1], 96366[1], 96367[1], 96368[1], 96372[1], 96374[1], 96375[1], 96376[1], 96377[1], 97597[1], 97598[1], 97602[1], 99155[0], 99156[0], 99157[0], 99211[1], 99212[1], 99213[1], 99214[1], 99215[1], 99217[1], 99218[1], 99219[1], 99220[1], 99221[1], 99222[1], 99223[1], 99231[1], 99232[1], 99233[1], 99234[1], 99235[1], 99236[1], 99238[1], 99239[1], 99241[1], 99242[1], 99243[1], 99244[1], 99245[1], 99251[1], 99252[1], 99253[1], 99254[1], 99255[1], 99291[1], 99292[1], 99304[1], 99305[1], 99306[1], 99307[1], 99308[1], 99309[1], 99310[1], 99315[1], 99316[1], 99334[1], 99335[1], 99336[1], 99337[1], 99347[1], 99348[1], 99349[1], 99350[1], 99374[1], 99375[1], 99377[1], 99378[1], 99446[0], 99447[0], 99448[0], 99449[0], 99451[0], 99452[0], 99495[0], 99496[0], G0463[1], G0471[1], J0670[1], J1642[1], J1644[1], J2001[1]
36582	0213T[0], 0216T[0], 0228T[0], 0230T[0], 11000[1], 11001[1], 11004[1], 11005[1], 11006[1], 11042[1], 11043[1], 11044[1], 11045[1], 11046[1], 11047[1], 12001[1], 12002[1], 12004[1], 12005[1], 12006[1], 12007[1], 12011[1], 12013[1], 12014[1], 12015[1], 12016[1], 12017[1], 12018[1], 12020[1], 12021[1], 12031[1], 12032[1], 12034[1], 12035[1], 12036[1], 12037[1], 12041[1], 12042[1], 12044[1], 12045[1], 12046[1], 12047[1], 12051[1], 12052[1], 12053[1], 12054[1], 12055[1], 12056[1], 12057[1], 13100[1], 13101[1], 13102[1], 13120[1], 13121[1], 13122[1], 13131[1], 13132[1], 13133[1], 13151[1], 13152[1], 13153[1], 35201[1], 35206[1], 35226[1], 35231[1], 35236[1], 35256[1], 35261[1], 35266[1], 35286[1], 35800[1], 35820[1], 35840[1], 35860[1], 36000[1], 36005[1], 36010[1], 36011[1], 36012[1], 36013[1], 36400[1], 36405[1], 36406[1], 36410[1], 36420[1], 36425[1], 36430[1], 36440[1], 36555[1], 36556[1], 36557[1], 36558[1], 36560[1], 36561[1], 36563[1], 36565[1], 36566[1], 36568[1], 36569[1], 36570[1], 36571[1], 36572[1], 36573[1], 36575[1], 36576[1], 36578[1], 36591[0], 36592[0], 36595[1], 36596[1], 36597[1], 36600[1], 36640[1], 43752[1], 51701[1], 51702[1], 51703[1], 62320[0], 62321[0], 62322[0], 62323[0], 62324[0], 62325[0], 62326[0], 62327[0], 64400[0], 64402[0], 64405[0], 64408[0], 64410[0], 64413[0], 64415[0], 64416[0], 64417[0], 64418[0], 64420[0], 64421[0], 64425[0], 64430[0], 64435[0], 64445[0], 64446[0], 64447[0], 64448[0], 64449[0], 64450[0], 64461[0], 64462[0], 64463[0], 64479[0], 64480[0], 64483[0], 64484[0], 64486[0], 64487[0], 64488[0], 64489[0], 64490[0], 64491[0], 64492[0], 64493[0], 64494[0], 64495[0], 64505[0], 64510[0], 64517[0], 64520[0], 64530[0], 69990[0], 71045[1], 71046[1], 71047[1], 76000[1], 76942[1], 76970[1], 76998[1], 77002[1], 92012[1], 92014[1], 93000[1], 93005[1], 93010[1], 93040[1], 93041[1], 93042[1], 93318[1], 93355[1], 94002[1], 94200[1], 94250[1], 94680[1], 94681[1], 94690[1], 94770[1], 95812[1], 95813[1], 95816[1], 95819[1], 95822[1], 95829[1], 95955[1], 96360[1], 96361[1], 96365[1], 96366[1], 96367[1], 96368[1], 96372[1], 96374[1], 96375[1], 96376[1], 96377[1], 97597[1], 97598[1], 97602[1], 99155[0], 99156[0], 99157[0], 99211[1], 99212[1], 99213[1], 99214[1], 99215[1], 99217[1], 99218[1], 99219[1], 99220[1], 99221[1], 99222[1], 99223[1], 99231[1], 99232[1], 99233[1], 99234[1], 99235[1], 99236[1], 99238[1], 99239[1], 99241[1], 99242[1], 99243[1], 99244[1], 99245[1], 99251[1], 99252[1], 99253[1], 99254[1], 99255[1], 99291[1], 99292[1], 99304[1], 99305[1], 99306[1], 99307[1], 99308[1], 99309[1], 99310[1], 99315[1], 99316[1], 99334[1], 99335[1], 99336[1], 99337[1], 99347[1], 99348[1], 99349[1], 99350[1], 99374[1], 99375[1], 99377[1], 99378[1], 99446[0], 99447[0], 99448[0], 99449[0], 99451[0], 99452[0], 99495[0], 99496[0], G0463[1], G0471[1], J0670[1], J1642[1], J1644[1], J2001[1]
36583	0213T[0], 0216T[0], 0228T[0], 0230T[0], 11000[1], 11001[1], 11004[1], 11005[1], 11006[1], 11042[1], 11043[1], 11044[1], 11045[1], 11046[1], 11047[1], 12001[1], 12002[1], 12004[1], 12005[1], 12006[1], 12007[1], 12011[1], 12013[1], 12014[1], 12015[1], 12016[1], 12017[1], 12018[1], 12020[1], 12021[1], 12031[1], 12032[1], 12034[1], 12035[1], 12036[1], 12037[1], 12041[1], 12042[1], 12044[1], 12045[1], 12046[1], 12047[1], 12051[1], 12052[1], 12053[1], 12054[1], 12055[1], 12056[1], 12057[1], 13100[1], 13101[1], 13102[1], 13120[1], 13121[1], 13122[1], 13131[1], 13132[1], 13133[1], 13151[1], 13152[1], 13153[1], 35201[1], 35206[1], 35226[1], 35231[1], 35236[1], 35256[1], 35261[1], 35266[1], 35286[1], 35800[1], 35820[1], 35840[1], 35860[1], 36000[1], 36005[1], 36010[1], 36011[1], 36012[1], 36013[1], 36400[1], 36405[1], 36406[1], 36410[1], 36420[1], 36425[1], 36430[1], 36440[1], 36555[1], 36556[1], 36557[1], 36558[1], 36560[1], 36561[1], 36563[1], 36565[1], 36566[1], 36568[1], 36569[1], 36570[1], 36571[1], 36572[1], 36573[1], 36575[1], 36576[1], 36578[1], 36591[0], 36592[0], 36595[1], 36596[1], 36597[1], 36600[1], 36640[1], 43752[1], 51701[1], 51702[1], 51703[1], 62320[0], 62321[0], 62322[0], 62323[0], 62324[0], 62325[0], 62326[0], 62327[0], 64400[0], 64402[0], 64405[0], 64408[0], 64410[0], 64413[0], 64415[0], 64416[0], 64417[0], 64418[0], 64420[0], 64421[0], 64425[0], 64430[0], 64435[0], 64445[0], 64446[0], 64447[0], 64448[0], 64449[0], 64450[0], 64461[0], 64462[0], 64463[0], 64479[0], 64480[0], 64483[0], 64484[0], 64486[0], 64487[0], 64488[0], 64489[0], 64490[0], 64491[0], 64492[0], 64493[0], 64494[0], 64495[0], 64505[0], 64510[0], 64517[0], 64520[0], 64530[0], 69990[0], 71045[1], 71046[1], 71047[1], 76000[1], 76942[1], 76970[1], 76998[1], 77002[1], 92012[1], 92014[1], 93000[1], 93005[1], 93010[1], 93040[1], 93041[1], 93042[1], 93318[1], 93355[1], 94002[1], 94200[1], 94250[1], 94680[1], 94681[1], 94690[1], 94770[1], 95812[1], 95813[1], 95816[1], 95819[1], 95822[1], 95829[1], 95955[1], 96360[1], 96361[1], 96365[1], 96366[1], 96367[1], 96368[1], 96372[1], 96374[1], 96375[1], 96376[1], 96377[1], 97597[1], 97598[1], 97602[1], 99155[0], 99156[0], 99157[0], 99211[1], 99212[1], 99213[1], 99214[1], 99215[1], 99217[1], 99218[1], 99219[1], 99220[1], 99221[1], 99222[1], 99223[1], 99231[1], 99232[1], 99233[1], 99234[1], 99235[1], 99236[1], 99238[1], 99239[1], 99241[1], 99242[1], 99243[1], 99244[1], 99245[1], 99251[1], 99252[1], 99253[1], 99254[1], 99255[1], 99291[1], 99292[1], 99304[1], 99305[1], 99306[1], 99307[1], 99308[1], 99309[1], 99310[1], 99315[1], 99316[1], 99334[1], 99335[1], 99336[1], 99337[1], 99347[1], 99348[1], 99349[1], 99350[1], 99374[1], 99375[1], 99377[1], 99378[1], 99446[0], 99447[0], 99448[0], 99449[0], 99451[0], 99452[0], 99495[0], 99496[0], G0463[1], G0471[1], J0670[1], J1642[1], J1644[1], J2001[1]
36584	0213T[0], 0216T[0], 0228T[0], 0230T[0], 11000[1], 11001[1], 11004[1], 11005[1], 11006[1], 11042[1], 11043[1], 11044[1], 11045[1], 11046[1], 11047[1], 12001[1], 12002[1], 12004[1], 12005[1], 12006[1], 12007[1], 12011[1], 12013[1], 12014[1], 12015[1], 12016[1], 12017[1], 12018[1], 12020[1], 12021[1], 12031[1], 12032[1], 12034[1], 12035[1], 12036[1], 12037[1], 12041[1], 12042[1], 12044[1], 12045[1], 12046[1], 12047[1], 12051[1], 12052[1], 12053[1], 12054[1], 12055[1], 12056[1], 12057[1], 13100[1], 13101[1], 13102[1], 13120[1], 13121[1], 13122[1], 13131[1], 13132[1], 13133[1], 13151[1], 13152[1], 13153[1], 35201[1], 35206[1], 35226[1], 35231[1], 35236[1], 35256[1], 35261[1], 35266[1], 35286[1], 35800[1], 35820[1], 35840[1], 35860[1], 36000[1], 36005[1], 36010[1], 36011[1], 36012[1], 36013[1], 36400[1], 36405[1], 36406[1], 36410[1], 36420[1], 36425[1], 36430[1], 36440[1], 36555[1], 36556[1], 36557[1], 36558[1], 36560[1], 36561[1], 36563[1], 36565[1], 36566[1], 36568[1], 36569[1], 36570[1], 36571[1], 36572[1], 36573[1], 36575[1], 36576[1], 36591[0], 36592[0], 36595[1], 36596[1], 36597[1], 36600[1], 36640[1], 43752[1], 51701[1], 51702[1], 51703[1], 62320[0], 62321[0], 62322[0], 62323[0], 62324[0], 62325[0], 62326[0], 62327[0], 64400[0], 64402[0], 64405[0], 64408[0], 64410[0], 64413[0], 64415[0], 64416[0], 64417[0], 64418[0], 64420[0], 64421[0], 64425[0], 64430[0], 64435[0], 64445[0], 64446[0], 64447[0], 64448[0], 64449[0], 64450[0], 64461[0], 64462[0], 64463[0], 64479[0], 64480[0], 64483[0], 64484[0], 64486[0], 64487[0], 64488[0], 64489[0], 64490[0], 64491[0], 64492[0], 64493[0], 64494[0], 64495[0], 64505[0], 64510[0], 64517[0], 64520[0], 64530[0], 69990[0], 71045[1], 71046[1], 71047[1], 71048[1], 75810[1], 75820[1], 75822[1], 75825[1], 75827[1], 75831[1], 75833[1], 75840[1], 75842[1], 75860[1], 75870[1], 75872[1], 75880[1], 75889[1], 75891[1], 76000[1], 76380[1], 76937[1], 76942[1], 76970[1], 76998[1], 77001[1], 77002[1], 77012[1], 77021[1], 92012[1], 92014[1], 93000[1], 93005[1], 93010[1], 93040[1], 93041[1], 93042[1], 93318[1], 93355[1], 94002[1], 94200[1], 94250[1], 94680[1], 94681[1], 94690[1], 94770[1], 95812[1], 95813[1], 95816[1], 95819[1], 95822[1], 95829[1], 95955[1], 96360[1], 96361[1], 96365[1], 96366[1], 96367[1], 96368[1], 96372[1], 96374[1], 96375[1], 96376[1], 96377[1], 97597[1], 97598[1], 97602[1], 99155[0], 99156[0], 99157[0], 99211[1], 99212[1], 99213[1], 99214[1], 99215[1], 99217[1], 99218[1], 99219[1], 99220[1], 99221[1], 99222[1], 99223[1], 99231[1], 99232[1], 99233[1], 99234[1], 99235[1], 99236[1], 99238[1], 99239[1], 99241[1], 99242[1],

0 = Modifier usage not allowed or inappropriate   1 = Modifier usage allowed

Appendix A: NCCI - CPT Codes

CPT © 2018 American Medical Association. All Rights Reserved.

Code 1	Code 2
	99243[1], 99244[1], 99245[1], 99251[1], 99252[1], 99253[1], 99254[1], 99255[1], 99291[1], 99292[1], 99304[1], 99305[1], 99306[1], 99307[1], 99308[1], 99309[1], 99310[1], 99315[1], 99316[1], 99334[1], 99335[1], 99336[1], 99337[1], 99347[1], 99348[1], 99349[1], 99350[1], 99374[1], 99375[1], 99377[1], 99378[1], 99446[0], 99447[0], 99448[0], 99449[0], 99451[0], 99452[0], 99495[1], 99496[1], G0463[1], G0471[1], J0670[1], J1642[1], J1644[1], J2001[1]
36585	0213T[0], 0216T[0], 0228T[0], 0230T[0], 11000[1], 11001[1], 11004[1], 11005[1], 11006[1], 11042[1], 11043[1], 11044[1], 11045[1], 11046[1], 11047[1], 12001[1], 12002[1], 12004[1], 12005[1], 12006[1], 12007[1], 12011[1], 12013[1], 12014[1], 12015[1], 12016[1], 12017[1], 12018[1], 12020[1], 12021[1], 12031[1], 12032[1], 12034[1], 12035[1], 12036[1], 12037[1], 12041[1], 12042[1], 12044[1], 12045[1], 12046[1], 12047[1], 12051[1], 12052[1], 12053[1], 12054[1], 12055[1], 12056[1], 12057[1], 13100[1], 13101[1], 13102[1], 13120[1], 13121[1], 13122[1], 13131[1], 13132[1], 13133[1], 13151[1], 13152[1], 13153[1], 35201[1], 35206[1], 35226[1], 35231[1], 35236[1], 35256[1], 35261[1], 35266[1], 35286[1], 35800[1], 35820[1], 35840[1], 35860[1], 36000[1], 36005[1], 36010[1], 36011[1], 36012[1], 36013[1], 36400[1], 36405[1], 36406[1], 36410[1], 36420[1], 36425[1], 36430[1], 36440[1], 36555[1], 36556[1], 36557[1], 36558[1], 36560[1], 36561[1], 36563[1], 36565[1], 36566[1], 36568[1], 36569[1], 36570[1], 36571[1], 36572[1], 36573[1], 36575[1], 36576[1], 36578[1], 36591[0], 36592[0], 36595[1], 36596[1], 36597[1], 36600[1], 36640[1], 43752[1], 51701[1], 51702[1], 51703[1], 62320[0], 62321[0], 62322[0], 62323[0], 62324[0], 62325[0], 62326[0], 62327[0], 64400[0], 64402[0], 64405[0], 64408[0], 64410[0], 64413[0], 64415[0], 64416[0], 64417[0], 64418[0], 64420[0], 64421[0], 64425[0], 64430[0], 64435[0], 64445[0], 64446[0], 64447[0], 64448[0], 64449[0], 64450[0], 64461[0], 64462[0], 64463[0], 64479[0], 64480[0], 64483[0], 64484[0], 64486[0], 64487[0], 64488[0], 64489[0], 64490[0], 64491[0], 64492[0], 64493[0], 64494[0], 64495[0], 64505[0], 64510[0], 64517[0], 64520[0], 64530[0], 69990[0], 71045[1], 71046[1], 71047[1], 76000[1], 76942[1], 76970[1], 76998[1], 77002[1], 92012[1], 92014[1], 93000[1], 93005[1], 93010[1], 93040[1], 93041[1], 93042[1], 93318[1], 93355[1], 94002[1], 94200[1], 94250[1], 94680[1], 94681[1], 94690[1], 94770[1], 95812[1], 95813[1], 95816[1], 95819[1], 95822[1], 95829[1], 95955[1], 96360[1], 96361[1], 96365[1], 96366[1], 96367[1], 96368[1], 96372[1], 96374[1], 96375[1], 96376[1], 96377[1], 97597[1], 97598[1], 97602[1], 99155[0], 99156[0], 99157[0], 99211[1], 99212[1], 99213[1], 99214[1], 99215[1], 99217[1], 99218[1], 99219[1], 99220[1], 99221[1], 99222[1], 99223[1], 99231[1], 99232[1], 99233[1], 99234[1], 99235[1], 99236[1], 99238[1], 99239[1], 99241[1], 99242[1], 99243[1], 99244[1], 99245[1], 99251[1], 99252[1], 99253[1], 99254[1], 99255[1], 99291[1], 99292[1], 99304[1], 99305[1], 99306[1], 99307[1], 99308[1], 99309[1], 99310[1], 99315[1], 99316[1], 99334[1], 99335[1], 99336[1], 99337[1], 99347[1], 99348[1], 99349[1], 99350[1], 99374[1], 99375[1], 99377[1], 99378[1], 99446[0], 99447[0], 99448[0], 99449[0], 99451[0], 99452[0], 99495[0], 99496[0], G0463[1], G0471[1], J0670[1], J1642[1], J1644[1], J2001[1]
36589	0213T[0], 0216T[0], 0228T[0], 0230T[0], 11000[1], 11001[1], 11004[1], 11005[1], 11006[1], 11042[1], 11043[1], 11044[1], 11045[1], 11046[1], 11047[1], 12001[1], 12002[1], 12004[1], 12005[1], 12006[1], 12007[1], 12011[1], 12013[1], 12014[1], 12015[1], 12016[1], 12017[1], 12018[1], 12020[1], 12021[1], 12031[1], 12032[1], 12034[1], 12035[1], 12036[1], 12037[1], 12041[1], 12042[1], 12044[1], 12045[1], 12046[1], 12047[1], 12051[1], 12052[1], 12053[1], 12054[1], 12055[1], 12056[1], 12057[1], 13100[1], 13101[1], 13102[1], 13120[1], 13121[1], 13122[1], 13131[1], 13132[1], 13133[1], 13151[1], 13152[1], 13153[1], 35201[1], 35206[1], 35226[1], 35231[1], 35236[1], 35256[1], 35261[1], 35266[1], 35286[1], 36000[1], 36005[1], 36400[1], 36405[1], 36406[1], 36410[1], 36420[1], 36425[1], 36430[1], 36440[1], 36575[1], 36576[1], 36578[1], 36591[0], 36592[0], 36595[1], 36596[1], 36597[1], 36600[1], 36640[1], 43752[1], 51701[1], 51702[1], 51703[1], 62320[0], 62321[0], 62322[0], 62323[0], 62324[0], 62325[0], 62326[0], 62327[0], 64400[0], 64402[0], 64405[0], 64408[0], 64410[0], 64413[0], 64415[0], 64416[0], 64417[0], 64418[0], 64420[0], 64421[0], 64425[0], 64430[0], 64435[0], 64445[0], 64446[0], 64447[0], 64448[0], 64449[0], 64450[0], 64461[0], 64462[0], 64463[0], 64479[0], 64480[0], 64483[0], 64484[0], 64486[0], 64487[0], 64488[0], 64489[0], 64490[0], 64491[0], 64492[0], 64493[0], 64494[0], 64495[0], 64505[0], 64510[0], 64517[0], 64520[0], 64530[0], 69990[0], 76000[1], 76942[1], 76970[1], 76998[1], 77002[1], 92012[1], 92014[1], 93000[1], 93005[1], 93010[1], 93040[1], 93041[1], 93042[1], 93318[1], 93355[1], 94002[1], 94200[1], 94250[1], 94680[1], 94681[1], 94690[1], 94770[1], 95812[1], 95813[1], 95816[1], 95819[1], 95822[1], 95829[1], 95955[1], 96360[1], 96361[1], 96365[1], 96366[1], 96367[1], 96368[1], 96372[1], 96374[1], 96375[1], 96376[1], 96377[1], 97597[1], 97598[1], 97602[1], 99155[0], 99156[0], 99157[0], 99211[1], 99212[1], 99213[1], 99214[1], 99215[1], 99217[1], 99218[1], 99219[1], 99220[1], 99221[1], 99222[1], 99223[1], 99231[1], 99232[1], 99233[1], 99234[1], 99235[1], 99236[1], 99238[1], 99239[1], 99241[1], 99242[1], 99243[1], 99244[1], 99245[1], 99251[1], 99252[1], 99253[1], 99254[1], 99255[1], 99291[1], 99292[1], 99304[1], 99305[1], 99306[1], 99307[1], 99308[1], 99309[1], 99310[1], 99315[1], 99316[1], 99334[1], 99335[1], 99336[1], 99337[1], 99347[1], 99348[1], 99349[1], 99350[1], 99374[1], 99375[1], 99377[1], 99378[1], 99446[0], 99447[0], 99448[0], 99449[0], 99451[0], 99452[0], 99495[0], 99496[0], G0463[1], G0471[1]
36590	0213T[0], 0216T[0], 0228T[0], 0230T[0], 11000[1], 11001[1], 11004[1], 11005[1], 11006[1], 11042[1], 11043[1], 11044[1], 11045[1], 11046[1], 11047[1], 12001[1], 12002[1], 12004[1], 12005[1], 12006[1], 12007[1], 12011[1], 12013[1], 12014[1], 12015[1], 12016[1], 12017[1], 12018[1], 12020[1], 12021[1], 12031[1], 12032[1], 12034[1], 12035[1], 12036[1], 12037[1], 12041[1], 12042[1], 12044[1], 12045[1], 12046[1], 12047[1], 12051[1], 12052[1], 12053[1], 12054[1], 12055[1], 12056[1], 12057[1], 13100[1], 13101[1], 13102[1], 13120[1], 13121[1], 13122[1], 13131[1], 13132[1], 13133[1], 13151[1], 13152[1], 13153[1], 35201[1], 35206[1], 35226[1], 35231[1], 35236[1], 35256[1], 35261[1], 35266[1], 35286[1], 36000[1], 36005[1], 36400[1], 36405[1], 36406[1], 36410[1], 36420[1], 36425[1], 36430[1], 36440[1], 36575[1], 36576[1], 36578[1], 36589[1], 36591[0], 36592[0], 36595[1], 36596[1], 36597[1], 36600[1], 36640[1], 43752[1], 51701[1], 51702[1], 51703[1], 62320[0], 62321[0], 62322[0], 62323[0], 62324[0], 62325[0], 62326[0], 62327[0], 64400[0], 64402[0], 64405[0], 64408[0], 64410[0], 64413[0], 64415[0], 64416[0], 64417[0], 64418[0], 64420[0], 64421[0], 64425[0], 64430[0], 64435[0], 64445[0], 64446[0], 64447[0], 64448[0], 64449[0], 64450[0], 64461[0], 64462[0], 64463[0], 64479[0], 64480[0], 64483[0], 64484[0], 64486[0], 64487[0], 64488[0], 64489[0], 64490[0], 64491[0], 64492[0], 64493[0], 64494[0], 64495[0], 64505[0], 64510[0], 64517[0], 64520[0], 64530[0], 69990[0], 76000[1], 76942[1], 76970[1], 76998[1], 77002[1], 92012[1], 92014[1], 93000[1], 93005[1], 93010[1], 93040[1], 93041[1], 93042[1], 93318[1], 93355[1], 94002[1], 94200[1], 94250[1], 94680[1], 94681[1], 94690[1], 94770[1], 95812[1], 95813[1], 95816[1], 95819[1], 95822[1], 95829[1], 95955[1], 96360[1], 96361[1], 96365[1], 96366[1], 96367[1], 96368[1], 96372[1], 96374[1], 96375[1], 96376[1], 96377[1], 97597[1], 97598[1], 97602[1], 99155[0], 99156[0], 99157[0], 99211[1], 99212[1], 99213[1], 99214[1], 99215[1], 99217[1], 99218[1], 99219[1], 99220[1], 99221[1], 99222[1], 99223[1], 99231[1], 99232[1], 99233[1], 99234[1], 99235[1], 99236[1], 99238[1], 99239[1], 99241[1], 99242[1], 99243[1], 99244[1], 99245[1], 99251[1], 99252[1], 99253[1], 99254[1], 99255[1], 99291[1], 99292[1], 99304[1], 99305[1], 99306[1], 99307[1], 99308[1], 99309[1], 99310[1], 99315[1], 99316[1], 99334[1], 99335[1], 99336[1], 99337[1], 99347[1], 99348[1], 99349[1], 99350[1], 99374[1], 99375[1], 99377[1], 99378[1], 99446[0], 99447[0], 99448[0], 99449[0], 99451[0], 99452[0], 99495[0], 99496[0], G0463[1], G0471[1], J0670[1], J2001[1]
36591	35201[0], 35206[0], 35226[0], 35231[0], 35236[0], 35256[0], 35261[0], 35266[0], 35286[0]
36592	35201[0], 35206[0], 35226[0], 35231[0], 35236[0], 35256[0], 35261[0], 35266[0], 35286[0], 36591[0], J1642[1], J1644[1]
36593	35201[1], 35206[1], 35226[1], 35231[1], 35236[1], 35256[1], 35261[1], 35266[1], 35286[1], 36005[1], 36591[0], 36592[0], 69990[0], J1642[1], J1644[1]
36595	0213T[0], 0216T[0], 0228T[0], 0230T[0], 11000[1], 11001[1], 11004[1], 11005[1], 11006[1], 11042[1], 11043[1], 11044[1], 11045[1], 11046[1], 11047[1], 12001[1], 12002[1], 12004[1], 12005[1], 12006[1], 12007[1], 12011[1], 12013[1], 12014[1], 12015[1], 12016[1], 12017[1], 12018[1], 12020[1], 12021[1], 12031[1], 12032[1], 12034[1], 12035[1], 12036[1], 12037[1], 12041[1], 12042[1], 12044[1], 12045[1], 12046[1], 12047[1], 12051[1], 12052[1], 12053[1], 12054[1], 12055[1], 12056[1], 12057[1], 13100[1], 13101[1], 13102[1], 13120[1], 13121[1], 13122[1], 13131[1], 13132[1], 13133[1], 13151[1], 13152[1], 13153[1], 35201[1], 35206[1], 35226[1], 35231[1], 35236[1], 35256[1], 35261[1], 35266[1], 35286[1], 36000[1], 36005[1], 36400[1], 36405[1], 36406[1], 36410[1], 36420[1], 36425[1], 36430[1], 36440[1], 36591[0], 36592[0], 36593[1], 36596[1], 36597[1], 36598[0], 36600[1], 36640[1], 37211[1], 37212[1], 37213[1], 37214[1], 43752[1], 51701[1], 51702[1], 51703[1], 61645[1], 62320[0], 62321[0], 62322[0], 62323[0], 62324[0], 62325[0], 62326[0], 62327[0], 64400[0], 64402[0], 64405[0], 64408[0], 64410[0], 64413[0], 64415[0], 64416[0], 64417[0], 64418[0], 64420[0], 64421[0], 64425[0], 64430[0], 64435[0], 64445[0], 64446[0], 64447[0], 64448[0], 64449[0], 64450[0], 64461[0], 64462[0], 64463[0], 64479[0], 64480[0], 64483[0], 64484[0], 64486[0], 64487[0], 64488[0], 64489[0], 64490[0], 64491[0], 64492[0], 64493[0], 64494[0], 64495[0], 64505[0], 64510[0], 64517[0], 64520[0], 64530[0], 69990[0], 71045[1], 71046[1], 71047[1], 76000[1], 76380[1], 76937[1], 76942[1], 76970[1], 76998[1], 77001[1], 77002[1], 77012[1], 77021[1], 92012[1], 92014[1], 93000[1], 93005[1], 93010[1], 93040[1], 93041[1], 93042[1], 93318[1], 93355[1], 94002[1], 94200[1], 94250[1], 94680[1], 94681[1], 94690[1], 94770[1], 95812[1], 95813[1], 95816[1], 95819[1], 95822[1], 95829[1], 95955[1], 96360[1], 96361[1], 96365[1], 96366[1], 96367[1], 96368[1], 96372[1], 96374[1], 96375[1], 96376[1], 96377[1], 97597[1], 97598[1], 97602[1], 99155[0], 99156[0], 99157[0], 99211[1], 99212[1], 99213[1], 99214[1], 99215[1], 99217[1], 99218[1], 99219[1], 99220[1], 99221[1], 99222[1], 99223[1], 99231[1], 99232[1], 99233[1], 99234[1], 99235[1], 99236[1], 99238[1], 99239[1], 99241[1], 99242[1], 99243[1], 99244[1], 99245[1], 99251[1], 99252[1], 99253[1], 99254[1], 99255[1], 99291[1], 99292[1], 99304[1], 99305[1], 99306[1], 99307[1], 99308[1], 99309[1], 99310[1], 99315[1], 99316[1], 99334[1], 99335[1], 99336[1], 99337[1], 99347[1], 99348[1], 99349[1], 99350[1], 99374[1], 99375[1], 99377[1], 99378[1], 99446[0], 99447[0], 99448[0], 99449[0], 99451[0], 99452[0], 99495[1], 99496[1], G0463[1], G0471[1]
36596	0213T[0], 0216T[0], 0228T[0], 0230T[0], 11000[1], 11001[1], 11004[1], 11005[1], 11006[1], 11042[1], 11043[1], 11044[1], 11045[1], 11046[1], 11047[1], 12001[1], 12002[1], 12004[1], 12005[1], 12006[1], 12007[1], 12011[1], 12013[1], 12014[1], 12015[1], 12016[1], 12017[1], 12018[1], 12020[1], 12021[1], 12031[1], 12032[1], 12034[1], 12035[1], 12036[1], 12037[1], 12041[1], 12042[1], 12044[1], 12045[1], 12046[1], 12047[1], 12051[1], 12052[1], 12053[1], 12054[1], 12055[1], 12056[1], 12057[1], 13100[1], 13101[1], 13102[1], 13120[1], 13121[1], 13122[1], 13131[1], 13132[1], 13133[1], 13151[1], 13152[1], 13153[1], 35201[1], 35206[1], 35226[1], 35231[1], 35236[1], 35256[1], 35261[1], 35266[1], 35286[1], 36000[1], 36005[1], 36400[1], 36405[1], 36406[1], 36410[1], 36420[1], 36425[1], 36430[1], 36440[1], 36591[0], 36592[0], 36593[1], 36597[1], 36598[0], 36600[1], 36640[1], 37211[1], 37212[1], 37213[1], 37214[1], 43752[1], 51701[1], 51702[1], 51703[1], 61645[1], 62320[0], 62321[0], 62322[0], 62323[0], 62324[0], 62325[0], 62326[0], 62327[0], 64400[0], 64402[0], 64405[0], 64408[0], 64410[0], 64413[0], 64415[0], 64416[0], 64417[0], 64418[0], 64420[0], 64421[0], 64425[0], 64430[0], 64435[0], 64445[0],

0 = Modifier usage not allowed or inappropriate 1 = Modifier usage allowed

Appendix A: NCCI - CPT Codes

CPT © 2018 American Medical Association. All Rights Reserved.

Code 1	Code 2
	64446[0], 64447[0], 64448[0], 64449[0], 64450[0], 64461[0], 64462[0], 64463[0], 64479[0], 64480[0], 64483[0], 64484[0], 64486[0], 64487[0], 64488[0], 64489[0], 64490[0], 64491[0], 64492[0], 64493[0], 64494[0], 64495[0], 64505[0], 64510[0], 64517[0], 64520[0], 64530[0], 69990[0], 71045[1], 71046[1], 71047[1], 76000[1], 76380[1], 76937[1], 76942[1], 76970[1], 76998[1], 77001[1], 77002[1], 77012[1], 77021[1], 92012[1], 92014[1], 93000[1], 93005[1], 93010[1], 93040[1], 93041[1], 93042[1], 93318[1], 93355[1], 94002[1], 94200[1], 94250[1], 94680[1], 94681[1], 94690[1], 94770[1], 95812[1], 95813[1], 95816[1], 95819[1], 95822[1], 95829[1], 95955[1], 96360[1], 96361[1], 96365[1], 96366[1], 96367[1], 96368[1], 96372[1], 96374[1], 96375[1], 96376[1], 96377[1], 97597[1], 97598[1], 97602[1], 99155[0], 99156[0], 99157[0], 99211[1], 99212[1], 99213[1], 99214[1], 99215[1], 99217[1], 99218[1], 99219[1], 99220[1], 99221[1], 99222[1], 99223[1], 99231[1], 99232[1], 99233[1], 99234[1], 99235[1], 99236[1], 99238[1], 99239[1], 99241[1], 99242[1], 99243[1], 99244[1], 99245[1], 99251[1], 99252[1], 99253[1], 99254[1], 99255[1], 99291[1], 99292[1], 99304[1], 99305[1], 99306[1], 99307[1], 99308[1], 99309[1], 99310[1], 99315[1], 99316[1], 99334[1], 99335[1], 99336[1], 99337[1], 99347[1], 99348[1], 99349[1], 99350[1], 99374[1], 99375[1], 99377[1], 99378[1], 99446[0], 99447[0], 99448[0], 99449[0], 99451[0], 99452[0], 99495[1], 99496[1], G0463[1], G0471[1], J0670[1], J1642[1], J1644[1], J2001[1]
36597	0213T[0], 0216T[0], 0228T[0], 0230T[0], 12001[1], 12002[1], 12004[1], 12005[1], 12006[1], 12007[1], 12011[1], 12013[1], 12014[1], 12015[1], 12016[1], 12017[1], 12018[1], 12020[1], 12021[1], 12031[1], 12032[1], 12034[1], 12035[1], 12036[1], 12037[1], 12041[1], 12042[1], 12044[1], 12045[1], 12046[1], 12047[1], 12051[1], 12052[1], 12053[1], 12054[1], 12055[1], 12056[1], 12057[1], 13100[1], 13101[1], 13102[1], 13120[1], 13121[1], 13122[1], 13131[1], 13132[1], 13133[1], 13151[1], 13152[1], 13153[1], 35201[1], 35206[1], 35226[1], 35231[1], 35236[1], 35256[1], 35261[1], 35266[1], 35286[1], 36000[1], 36002[1], 36005[1], 36400[1], 36405[1], 36406[1], 36410[1], 36420[1], 36425[1], 36430[1], 36440[1], 36591[0], 36592[0], 36600[1], 36640[1], 43752[1], 51701[1], 51702[1], 51703[1], 62320[0], 62321[0], 62322[0], 62323[0], 62324[0], 62325[0], 62326[0], 62327[0], 64400[0], 64402[0], 64405[0], 64408[0], 64410[0], 64413[0], 64415[0], 64416[0], 64417[0], 64418[0], 64420[0], 64421[0], 64425[0], 64430[0], 64435[0], 64445[0], 64446[0], 64447[0], 64448[0], 64449[0], 64450[0], 64461[0], 64462[0], 64463[0], 64479[0], 64480[0], 64483[0], 64484[0], 64486[0], 64487[0], 64488[0], 64489[0], 64490[0], 64491[0], 64492[0], 64493[0], 64494[0], 64495[0], 64505[0], 64510[0], 64517[0], 64520[0], 64530[0], 69990[0], 71045[1], 71046[1], 71047[1], 76942[1], 76970[1], 76998[1], 77001[1], 77002[1], 92012[1], 92014[1], 93000[1], 93005[1], 93010[1], 93040[1], 93041[1], 93042[1], 93318[1], 93355[1], 94002[1], 94200[1], 94250[1], 94680[1], 94681[1], 94690[1], 94770[1], 95812[1], 95813[1], 95816[1], 95819[1], 95822[1], 95829[1], 95955[1], 96360[1], 96361[1], 96365[1], 96366[1], 96367[1], 96368[1], 96372[1], 96374[1], 96375[1], 96376[1], 96377[1], 99155[0], 99156[0], 99157[0], 99211[1], 99212[1], 99213[1], 99214[1], 99215[1], 99217[1], 99218[1], 99219[1], 99220[1], 99221[1], 99222[1], 99223[1], 99231[1], 99232[1], 99233[1], 99234[1], 99235[1], 99236[1], 99238[1], 99239[1], 99241[1], 99242[1], 99243[1], 99244[1], 99245[1], 99251[1], 99252[1], 99253[1], 99254[1], 99255[1], 99291[1], 99292[1], 99304[1], 99305[1], 99306[1], 99307[1], 99308[1], 99309[1], 99310[1], 99315[1], 99316[1], 99334[1], 99335[1], 99336[1], 99337[1], 99347[1], 99348[1], 99349[1], 99350[1], 99374[1], 99375[1], 99377[1], 99378[1], 99446[0], 99447[0], 99448[0], 99449[0], 99451[0], 99452[0], 99495[1], 99496[1], G0463[1], G0471[1], J0670[1], J1642[1], J1644[1], J2001[1]
36598	0213T[0], 0216T[0], 0228T[0], 0230T[0], 12001[1], 12002[1], 12004[1], 12005[1], 12006[1], 12007[1], 12011[1], 12013[1], 12014[1], 12015[1], 12016[1], 12017[1], 12018[1], 12020[1], 12021[1], 12031[1], 12032[1], 12034[1], 12035[1], 12036[1], 12037[1], 12041[1], 12042[1], 12044[1], 12045[1], 12046[1], 12047[1], 12051[1], 12052[1], 12053[1], 12054[1], 12055[1], 12056[1], 12057[1], 13100[1], 13101[1], 13102[1], 13120[1], 13121[1], 13122[1], 13131[1], 13132[1], 13133[1], 13151[1], 13152[1], 13153[1], 35201[1], 35206[1], 35226[1], 35231[1], 35236[1], 35256[1], 35261[1], 35266[1], 35286[1], 36000[1], 36005[1], 36400[1], 36405[1], 36406[1], 36410[1], 36420[1], 36425[1], 36430[1], 36440[1], 36591[0], 36592[0], 36600[1], 36640[1], 43752[1], 51701[1], 51702[1], 51703[1], 62320[0], 62321[0], 62322[0], 62323[0], 62324[0], 62325[0], 62326[0], 62327[0], 64400[0], 64402[0], 64405[0], 64408[0], 64410[0], 64413[0], 64415[0], 64416[0], 64417[0], 64418[0], 64420[0], 64421[0], 64425[0], 64430[0], 64435[0], 64445[0], 64446[0], 64447[0], 64448[0], 64449[0], 64450[0], 64461[0], 64462[0], 64463[0], 64479[0], 64480[0], 64483[0], 64484[0], 64486[0], 64487[0], 64488[0], 64489[0], 64490[0], 64491[0], 64492[0], 64493[0], 64494[0], 64495[0], 64505[0], 64510[0], 64517[0], 64520[0], 64530[0], 76000[1], 77002[1], 92012[1], 92014[1], 93000[1], 93005[1], 93010[1], 93040[1], 93041[1], 93042[1], 93318[1], 93355[1], 94002[1], 94200[1], 94250[1], 94680[1], 94681[1], 94690[1], 94770[1], 95812[1], 95813[1], 95816[1], 95819[1], 95822[1], 95829[1], 95955[1], 96360[1], 96361[1], 96365[1], 96366[1], 96367[1], 96368[1], 96372[1], 96374[1], 96375[1], 96376[1], 96377[1], 99155[0], 99156[0], 99157[0], 99211[1], 99212[1], 99213[1], 99214[1], 99215[1], 99217[1], 99218[1], 99219[1], 99220[1], 99221[1], 99222[1], 99223[1], 99231[1], 99232[1], 99233[1], 99234[1], 99235[1], 99236[1], 99238[1], 99239[1], 99241[1], 99242[1], 99243[1], 99244[1], 99245[1], 99251[1], 99252[1], 99253[1], 99254[1], 99255[1], 99291[1], 99292[1], 99304[1], 99305[1], 99306[1], 99307[1], 99308[1], 99309[1], 99310[1], 99315[1], 99316[1], 99334[1], 99335[1], 99336[1], 99337[1], 99347[1], 99348[1], 99349[1], 99350[1], 99374[1], 99375[1], 99377[1], 99378[1], 99446[0], 99447[0], 99448[0], 99449[0], 99451[0], 99452[0], 99495[1], 99496[1], G0463[1], G0471[1], J1642[1], J1644[1]
36600	36002[1], 36005[1], 36140[1], 36591[0], 36592[0], 36625[1], 69990[0], 76000[1], 77001[1], 77002[1], 93050[0], J0670[1], J2001[1]
36620	12001[1], 12002[1], 12004[1], 12005[1], 12006[1], 12007[1], 12011[1], 12013[1], 12014[1], 12015[1], 12016[1], 12017[1], 12018[1], 12020[1], 12021[1], 12031[1], 12032[1], 12034[1], 12035[1], 12036[1], 12037[1], 12041[1], 12042[1], 12044[1], 12045[1], 12046[1], 12047[1], 12051[1], 12052[1], 12053[1], 12054[1], 12055[1], 12056[1], 12057[1], 13100[1], 13101[1], 13102[1], 13120[1], 13121[1], 13122[1], 13131[1], 13132[1], 13133[1], 13151[1], 13152[1], 13153[1], 35201[1], 35206[1], 35226[1], 35231[1], 35236[1], 35256[1], 35261[1], 35266[1], 35286[1], 35820[1], 36000[1], 36002[1], 36005[1], 36400[1], 36405[1], 36406[1], 36410[1], 36420[1], 36425[1], 36430[1], 36440[1], 36591[0], 36592[0], 36600[1], 43752[1], 51701[1], 51702[1], 51703[1], 69990[0], 76000[1], 77001[1], 77002[1], 92012[1], 92014[1], 93000[1], 93005[1], 93010[1], 93040[1], 93041[1], 93042[1], 93050[0], 93318[1], 93355[1], 94002[1], 94200[1], 94250[1], 94680[1], 94681[1], 94690[1], 94770[1], 95812[1], 95813[1], 95816[1], 95819[1], 95822[1], 95829[1], 95955[1], 96360[1], 96361[1], 96365[1], 96366[1], 96367[1], 96368[1], 96372[1], 96374[1], 96375[1], 96376[1], 96377[1], 99155[1], 99156[1], 99157[1], 99211[1], 99212[1], 99213[1], 99214[1], 99215[1], 99217[1], 99218[1], 99219[1], 99220[1], 99221[1], 99222[1], 99223[1], 99231[1], 99232[1], 99233[1], 99234[1], 99235[1], 99236[1], 99238[1], 99239[1], 99241[1], 99242[1], 99243[1], 99244[1], 99245[1], 99251[1], 99252[1], 99253[1], 99254[1], 99255[1], 99291[1], 99292[1], 99304[1], 99305[1], 99306[1], 99307[1], 99308[1], 99309[1], 99310[1], 99315[1], 99316[1], 99334[1], 99335[1], 99336[1], 99337[1], 99347[1], 99348[1], 99349[1], 99350[1], 99374[1], 99375[1], 99377[1], 99378[1], 99446[0], 99447[0], 99448[0], 99449[0], 99451[0], 99452[0], 99495[1], 99496[1], G0463[1], G0471[1]
36625	12001[1], 12002[1], 12004[1], 12005[1], 12006[1], 12007[1], 12011[1], 12013[1], 12014[1], 12015[1], 12016[1], 12017[1], 12018[1], 12020[1], 12021[1], 12031[1], 12032[1], 12034[1], 12035[1], 12036[1], 12037[1], 12041[1], 12042[1], 12044[1], 12045[1], 12046[1], 12047[1], 12051[1], 12052[1], 12053[1], 12054[1], 12055[1], 12056[1], 12057[1], 13100[1], 13101[1], 13102[1], 13120[1], 13121[1], 13122[1], 13131[1], 13132[1], 13133[1], 13151[1], 13152[1], 13153[1], 35201[1], 35206[1], 35226[1], 35231[1], 35236[1], 35256[1], 35261[1], 35266[1], 35286[1], 35820[1], 36000[1], 36002[1], 36005[1], 36400[1], 36405[1], 36406[1], 36410[1], 36420[1], 36425[1], 36430[1], 36440[1], 36591[0], 36592[0], 36620[1], 43752[1], 51701[1], 51702[1], 51703[1], 64461[0], 64462[0], 64463[0], 64486[0], 64487[0], 64488[0], 64489[0], 64490[0], 64491[0], 64492[0], 64493[0], 64494[0], 64495[0], 69990[0], 92012[1], 92014[1], 93000[1], 93005[1], 93010[1], 93040[1], 93041[1], 93042[1], 93050[0], 93318[1], 93355[1], 94002[1], 94200[1], 94250[1], 94680[1], 94681[1], 94690[1], 94770[1], 95812[1], 95813[1], 95816[1], 95819[1], 95822[1], 95829[1], 95955[1], 96360[1], 96361[1], 96365[1], 96366[1], 96367[1], 96368[1], 96372[1], 96374[1], 96375[1], 96376[1], 96377[1], 99155[1], 99156[1], 99157[1], 99211[1], 99212[1], 99213[1], 99214[1], 99215[1], 99217[1], 99218[1], 99219[1], 99220[1], 99221[1], 99222[1], 99223[1], 99231[1], 99232[1], 99233[1], 99234[1], 99235[1], 99236[1], 99238[1], 99239[1], 99241[1], 99242[1], 99243[1], 99244[1], 99245[1], 99251[1], 99252[1], 99253[1], 99254[1], 99255[1], 99291[1], 99292[1], 99304[1], 99305[1], 99306[1], 99307[1], 99308[1], 99309[1], 99310[1], 99315[1], 99316[1], 99334[1], 99335[1], 99336[1], 99337[1], 99347[1], 99348[1], 99349[1], 99350[1], 99374[1], 99375[1], 99377[1], 99378[1], 99446[0], 99447[0], 99448[0], 99449[0], 99451[0], 99452[0], 99495[1], 99496[1], G0463[1], G0471[1]
61050	0213T[0], 0216T[0], 0228T[0], 0230T[0], 0333T[0], 0464T[0], 12001[1], 12002[1], 12004[1], 12005[1], 12006[1], 12007[1], 12011[1], 12013[1], 12014[1], 12015[1], 12016[1], 12017[1], 12018[1], 12020[1], 12021[1], 12031[1], 12032[1], 12034[1], 12035[1], 12036[1], 12037[1], 12041[1], 12042[1], 12044[1], 12045[1], 12046[1], 12047[1], 12051[1], 12052[1], 12053[1], 12054[1], 12055[1], 12056[1], 12057[1], 13100[1], 13101[1], 13102[1], 13120[1], 13121[1], 13122[1], 13131[1], 13132[1], 13133[1], 13151[1], 13152[1], 13153[1], 36000[1], 36400[1], 36405[1], 36406[1], 36410[1], 36420[1], 36425[1], 36430[1], 36440[1], 36591[0], 36592[0], 36600[1], 36640[1], 43752[1], 51701[1], 51702[1], 51703[1], 62320[0], 62321[0], 62322[0], 62323[0], 62324[0], 62325[0], 62326[0], 62327[0], 64400[0], 64402[0], 64405[0], 64408[0], 64410[0], 64413[0], 64415[0], 64416[0], 64417[0], 64418[0], 64420[0], 64421[0], 64425[0], 64430[0], 64435[0], 64445[0], 64446[0], 64447[0], 64448[0], 64449[0], 64450[0], 64461[0], 64462[0], 64463[0], 64479[0], 64480[0], 64483[0], 64484[0], 64486[0], 64487[0], 64488[0], 64489[0], 64490[0], 64491[0], 64492[0], 64493[0], 64494[0], 64495[0], 64505[0], 64510[0], 64517[0], 64520[0], 64530[0], 69990[0], 92012[1], 92014[1], 92585[0], 93000[1], 93005[1], 93010[1], 93040[1], 93041[1], 93042[1], 93318[1], 93355[1], 94002[1], 94200[1], 94250[1], 94680[1], 94681[1], 94690[1], 94770[1], 95812[1], 95813[1], 95816[1], 95819[1], 95822[0], 95829[1], 95860[0], 95861[0], 95863[0], 95864[0], 95865[0], 95866[0], 95867[0], 95868[0], 95869[0], 95870[0], 95907[0], 95908[0], 95909[0], 95910[0], 95911[0], 95912[0], 95913[0], 95925[0], 95926[0], 95927[0], 95928[0], 95929[0], 95930[0], 95933[0], 95937[0], 95938[0], 95939[0], 95940[0], 95955[1], 96360[1], 96361[1], 96365[1], 96366[1], 96367[1], 96368[1], 96372[1], 96374[1], 96375[1], 96376[1], 96377[1], 99155[0], 99156[0], 99157[0], 99211[1], 99212[1], 99213[1], 99214[1], 99215[1], 99217[1], 99218[1], 99219[1], 99220[1], 99221[1], 99222[1], 99223[1], 99231[1], 99232[1], 99233[1], 99234[1], 99235[1], 99236[1], 99238[1], 99239[1], 99241[1], 99242[1], 99243[1], 99244[1], 99245[1], 99251[1], 99252[1], 99253[1], 99254[1], 99255[1], 99291[1], 99292[1], 99304[1], 99305[1], 99306[1], 99307[1], 99308[1], 99309[1], 99310[1], 99315[1], 99316[1], 99334[1], 99335[1], 99336[1], 99337[1], 99347[1], 99348[1], 99349[1], 99350[1], 99374[1], 99375[1], 99377[1], 99378[1], 99446[0], 99447[0], 99448[0], 99449[0], 99451[0], 99452[0], 99495[1], 99496[1], G0453[0], G0463[1], G0471[1]

0 = Modifier usage not allowed or inappropriate 1 = Modifier usage allowed

CPT © 2018 American Medical Association. All Rights Reserved.

Code 1	Code 2
61055	01935[0], 01936[0], 0213T[0], 0216T[0], 0228T[0], 0230T[0], 0333T[0], 0464T[0], 12001[1], 12002[1], 12004[1], 12005[1], 12006[1], 12007[1], 12011[1], 12013[1], 12014[1], 12015[1], 12016[1], 12017[1], 12018[1], 12020[1], 12021[1], 12031[1], 12032[1], 12034[1], 12035[1], 12036[1], 12037[1], 12041[1], 12042[1], 12044[1], 12045[1], 12046[1], 12047[1], 12051[1], 12052[1], 12053[1], 12054[1], 12055[1], 12056[1], 12057[1], 13100[1], 13101[1], 13102[1], 13120[1], 13121[1], 13122[1], 13131[1], 13132[1], 13133[1], 13151[1], 13152[1], 13153[1], 36000[1], 36400[1], 36405[1], 36406[1], 36410[1], 36420[1], 36425[1], 36430[1], 36440[1], 36591[0], 36592[0], 36600[1], 36640[1], 43752[1], 51701[1], 51702[1], 51703[1], 61050[1], 62320[0], 62321[0], 62322[0], 62323[0], 62324[0], 62325[0], 62326[0], 62327[0], 64400[0], 64402[0], 64405[0], 64408[0], 64410[0], 64413[0], 64415[0], 64416[0], 64417[0], 64418[0], 64420[0], 64421[0], 64425[0], 64430[0], 64435[0], 64445[0], 64446[0], 64447[0], 64448[0], 64449[0], 64450[0], 64461[0], 64462[0], 64463[0], 64479[0], 64480[0], 64483[0], 64484[0], 64486[0], 64487[0], 64488[0], 64489[0], 64490[0], 64491[0], 64492[0], 64493[0], 64494[0], 64495[0], 64505[0], 64510[0], 64517[0], 64520[0], 64530[0], 69990[0], 92012[1], 92014[1], 92585[0], 93000[1], 93005[1], 93010[1], 93040[1], 93041[1], 93042[1], 93318[1], 93355[1], 94002[1], 94200[1], 94250[1], 94680[1], 94681[1], 94690[1], 94770[1], 95812[1], 95813[1], 95816[1], 95819[1], 95822[0], 95829[1], 95860[0], 95861[0], 95863[0], 95864[0], 95865[0], 95866[0], 95867[0], 95868[0], 95869[0], 95870[0], 95907[0], 95908[0], 95909[0], 95910[0], 95911[0], 95912[0], 95913[0], 95925[0], 95926[0], 95927[0], 95928[0], 95929[0], 95930[0], 95933[0], 95937[0], 95938[0], 95939[0], 95940[0], 95955[1], 96360[1], 96361[1], 96365[1], 96366[1], 96367[1], 96368[1], 96372[1], 96374[1], 96375[1], 96376[1], 96377[1], 99155[0], 99156[0], 99157[0], 99211[1], 99212[1], 99213[1], 99214[1], 99215[1], 99217[1], 99218[1], 99219[1], 99220[1], 99221[1], 99222[1], 99223[1], 99231[1], 99232[1], 99233[1], 99234[1], 99235[1], 99236[1], 99238[1], 99239[1], 99241[1], 99242[1], 99243[1], 99244[1], 99245[1], 99251[1], 99252[1], 99253[1], 99254[1], 99255[1], 99291[1], 99292[1], 99304[1], 99305[1], 99306[1], 99307[1], 99308[1], 99309[1], 99310[1], 99315[1], 99316[1], 99334[1], 99335[1], 99336[1], 99337[1], 99347[1], 99348[1], 99349[1], 99350[1], 99374[1], 99375[1], 99377[1], 99378[1], 99446[0], 99447[0], 99448[0], 99449[0], 99451[0], 99452[0], 99495[1], 99496[1], G0453[0], G0463[1], G0471[1]
62270	00635[0], 01935[0], 01936[0], 0213T[0], 0216T[0], 0228T[0], 0230T[0], 12001[1], 12002[1], 12004[1], 12005[1], 12006[1], 12007[1], 12011[1], 12013[1], 12014[1], 12015[1], 12016[1], 12017[1], 12018[1], 12020[1], 12021[1], 12031[1], 12032[1], 12034[1], 12035[1], 12036[1], 12037[1], 12041[1], 12042[1], 12044[1], 12045[1], 12046[1], 12047[1], 12051[1], 12052[1], 12053[1], 12054[1], 12055[1], 12056[1], 12057[1], 13100[1], 13101[1], 13102[1], 13120[1], 13121[1], 13122[1], 13131[1], 13132[1], 13133[1], 13151[1], 13152[1], 13153[1], 36000[1], 36400[1], 36405[1], 36406[1], 36410[1], 36420[1], 36425[1], 36430[1], 36440[1], 36591[0], 36592[0], 36600[1], 36640[1], 43752[1], 51701[1], 51702[1], 51703[1], 62273[1], 62320[1], 62321[1], 62322[0], 62323[0], 64400[0], 64402[0], 64405[0], 64408[0], 64410[0], 64413[0], 64415[0], 64416[0], 64417[0], 64418[0], 64420[0], 64421[0], 64425[0], 64430[0], 64435[0], 64445[0], 64446[0], 64447[0], 64448[0], 64449[0], 64450[0], 64461[0], 64462[0], 64463[0], 64479[0], 64480[0], 64483[0], 64484[0], 64486[0], 64487[0], 64488[0], 64489[0], 64490[0], 64491[0], 64492[0], 64493[0], 64494[0], 64495[0], 64505[0], 64510[0], 64517[0], 64520[0], 64530[0], 69990[0], 76000[1], 77001[1], 77002[1], 92012[1], 92014[1], 93000[1], 93005[1], 93010[1], 93040[1], 93041[1], 93042[1], 93318[1], 93355[1], 94002[1], 94200[1], 94250[1], 94680[1], 94681[1], 94690[1], 94770[1], 95812[1], 95813[1], 95816[1], 95819[1], 95822[0], 95829[1], 95955[1], 96360[1], 96361[1], 96365[1], 96366[1], 96367[1], 96368[1], 96372[1], 96374[1], 96375[1], 96376[1], 96377[1], 99155[0], 99156[0], 99157[0], 99211[1], 99212[1], 99213[1], 99214[1], 99215[1], 99217[1], 99218[1], 99219[1], 99220[1], 99221[1], 99222[1], 99223[1], 99231[1], 99232[1], 99233[1], 99234[1], 99235[1], 99236[1], 99238[1], 99239[1], 99241[1], 99242[1], 99243[1], 99244[1], 99245[1], 99251[1], 99252[1], 99253[1], 99254[1], 99255[1], 99291[1], 99292[1], 99304[1], 99305[1], 99306[1], 99307[1], 99308[1], 99309[1], 99310[1], 99315[1], 99316[1], 99334[1], 99335[1], 99336[1], 99337[1], 99347[1], 99348[1], 99349[1], 99350[1], 99374[1], 99375[1], 99377[1], 99378[1], 99446[0], 99447[0], 99448[0], 99449[0], 99451[0], 99452[0], 99495[1], 99496[1], G0453[0], G0463[1], G0471[1]
62272	00635[0], 01935[0], 01936[0], 0213T[0], 0216T[0], 0228T[0], 0230T[0], 12001[1], 12002[1], 12004[1], 12005[1], 12006[1], 12007[1], 12011[1], 12013[1], 12014[1], 12015[1], 12016[1], 12017[1], 12018[1], 12020[1], 12021[1], 12031[1], 12032[1], 12034[1], 12035[1], 12036[1], 12037[1], 12041[1], 12042[1], 12044[1], 12045[1], 12046[1], 12047[1], 12051[1], 12052[1], 12053[1], 12054[1], 12055[1], 12056[1], 12057[1], 13100[1], 13101[1], 13102[1], 13120[1], 13121[1], 13122[1], 13131[1], 13132[1], 13133[1], 13151[1], 13152[1], 13153[1], 36000[1], 36400[1], 36405[1], 36406[1], 36410[1], 36420[1], 36425[1], 36430[1], 36440[1], 36591[0], 36592[0], 36600[1], 36640[1], 43752[1], 51701[1], 51702[1], 51703[1], 62270[1], 62273[1], 62320[0], 62321[0], 62322[0], 62323[0], 64400[0], 64402[0], 64405[0], 64408[0], 64410[0], 64413[0], 64415[0], 64416[0], 64417[0], 64418[0], 64420[0], 64421[0], 64425[0], 64430[0], 64435[0], 64445[0], 64446[0], 64447[0], 64448[0], 64449[0], 64450[0], 64461[0], 64462[0], 64463[0], 64479[0], 64480[0], 64483[0], 64484[0], 64486[0], 64487[0], 64488[0], 64489[0], 64490[0], 64491[0], 64492[0], 64493[0], 64494[0], 64495[0], 64505[0], 64510[0], 64517[0], 64520[0], 64530[0], 76000[1], 77001[1], 77002[1], 92012[1], 92014[1], 93000[1], 93005[1], 93010[1], 93040[1], 93041[1], 93042[1], 93318[1], 93355[1], 94002[1], 94200[1], 94250[1], 94680[1], 94681[1], 94690[1], 94770[1], 95812[1], 95813[1], 95816[1], 95819[1], 95822[0], 95829[1], 95955[1], 96360[1], 96361[1], 96365[1], 96366[1], 96367[1], 96368[1], 96372[1], 96374[1], 96375[1], 96376[1], 96377[1], 99155[0], 99156[0], 99157[0], 99211[1], 99212[1], 99213[1], 99214[1], 99215[1], 99217[1], 99218[1], 99219[1], 99220[1], 99221[1], 99222[1], 99223[1], 99231[1], 99232[1], 99233[1], 99234[1], 99235[1], 99236[1], 99238[1], 99239[1], 99241[1], 99242[1], 99243[1], 99244[1], 99245[1], 99251[1], 99252[1], 99253[1], 99254[1], 99255[1], 99291[1], 99292[1], 99304[1], 99305[1], 99306[1], 99307[1], 99308[1], 99309[1], 99310[1], 99315[1], 99316[1], 99334[1], 99335[1], 99336[1], 99337[1], 99347[1], 99348[1], 99349[1], 99350[1], 99374[1], 99375[1], 99377[1], 99378[1], 99446[0], 99447[0], 99448[0], 99449[0], 99451[0], 99452[0], 99495[1], 99496[1], G0453[0], G0463[1], G0471[1], J0670[1], J2001[1]
62273	01935[0], 01936[0], 0213T[0], 0216T[0], 0228T[0], 0230T[0], 0333T[0], 0464T[0], 12001[1], 12002[1], 12004[1], 12005[1], 12006[1], 12007[1], 12011[1], 12013[1], 12014[1], 12015[1], 12016[1], 12017[1], 12018[1], 12020[1], 12021[1], 12031[1], 12032[1], 12034[1], 12035[1], 12036[1], 12037[1], 12041[1], 12042[1], 12044[1], 12045[1], 12046[1], 12047[1], 12051[1], 12052[1], 12053[1], 12054[1], 12055[1], 12056[1], 12057[1], 13100[1], 13101[1], 13102[1], 13120[1], 13121[1], 13122[1], 13131[1], 13132[1], 13133[1], 13151[1], 13152[1], 13153[1], 36000[1], 36140[1], 36400[1], 36405[1], 36406[1], 36410[1], 36420[1], 36425[1], 36430[1], 36440[1], 36591[0], 36592[0], 36600[1], 36640[1], 43752[1], 51701[1], 51702[1], 51703[1], 62320[0], 62321[0], 62322[0], 62323[0], 62324[0], 62326[0], 62327[0], 64400[0], 64402[0], 64405[0], 64408[0], 64410[0], 64413[0], 64415[0], 64416[0], 64417[0], 64418[0], 64420[0], 64421[0], 64425[0], 64430[0], 64435[0], 64445[0], 64446[0], 64447[0], 64448[0], 64449[0], 64450[0], 64461[0], 64462[0], 64463[0], 64479[0], 64480[0], 64483[0], 64484[0], 64486[0], 64487[0], 64488[0], 64489[0], 64490[0], 64491[0], 64492[0], 64493[0], 64494[0], 64495[0], 64505[0], 64510[0], 64517[0], 64520[0], 64530[0], 69990[0], 76000[1], 77001[1], 77002[1], 92012[1], 92014[1], 92585[0], 93000[1], 93005[1], 93010[1], 93040[1], 93041[1], 93042[1], 93318[1], 93355[1], 94002[1], 94200[1], 94250[1], 94680[1], 94681[1], 94690[1], 94770[1], 95812[1], 95813[1], 95816[1], 95819[1], 95822[0], 95829[1], 95860[0], 95861[0], 95863[0], 95864[0], 95865[0], 95866[0], 95867[0], 95868[0], 95869[0], 95870[0], 95907[0], 95908[0], 95909[0], 95910[0], 95911[0], 95912[0], 95913[0], 95925[0], 95926[0], 95927[0], 95928[0], 95929[0], 95930[0], 95933[0], 95937[0], 95938[0], 95939[0], 95940[0], 95955[1], 96360[1], 96361[1], 96365[1], 96366[1], 96367[1], 96368[1], 96372[1], 96374[1], 96375[1], 96376[1], 96377[1], 99155[0], 99156[0], 99157[0], 99211[1], 99212[1], 99213[1], 99214[1], 99215[1], 99217[1], 99218[1], 99219[1], 99220[1], 99221[1], 99222[1], 99223[1], 99231[1], 99232[1], 99233[1], 99234[1], 99235[1], 99236[1], 99238[1], 99239[1], 99241[1], 99242[1], 99243[1], 99244[1], 99245[1], 99251[1], 99252[1], 99253[1], 99254[1], 99255[1], 99291[1], 99292[1], 99304[1], 99305[1], 99306[1], 99307[1], 99308[1], 99309[1], 99310[1], 99315[1], 99316[1], 99334[1], 99335[1], 99336[1], 99337[1], 99347[1], 99348[1], 99349[1], 99350[1], 99374[1], 99375[1], 99377[1], 99378[1], 99446[0], 99447[0], 99448[0], 99449[0], 99451[0], 99452[0], 99495[1], 99496[1], G0453[0], G0463[1], G0471[1], J0670[1], J2001[1]
62280	01935[0], 01936[0], 0213T[0], 0216T[0], 0228T[0], 0230T[0], 0333T[0], 0464T[0], 12001[1], 12002[1], 12004[1], 12005[1], 12006[1], 12007[1], 12011[1], 12013[1], 12014[1], 12015[1], 12016[1], 12017[1], 12018[1], 12020[1], 12021[1], 12031[1], 12032[1], 12034[1], 12035[1], 12036[1], 12037[1], 12041[1], 12042[1], 12044[1], 12045[1], 12046[1], 12047[1], 12051[1], 12052[1], 12053[1], 12054[1], 12055[1], 12056[1], 12057[1], 13100[1], 13101[1], 13102[1], 13120[1], 13121[1], 13122[1], 13131[1], 13132[1], 13133[1], 13151[1], 13152[1], 13153[1], 36000[1], 36400[1], 36405[1], 36406[1], 36410[1], 36420[1], 36425[1], 36430[1], 36440[1], 36591[0], 36592[0], 36600[1], 36640[1], 43752[1], 51701[1], 51702[1], 51703[1], 62270[1], 62272[1], 62273[1], 62284[1], 62320[0], 62321[0], 62322[0], 62323[0], 62324[0], 62325[0], 62326[0], 62327[0], 64400[0], 64402[0], 64405[0], 64408[0], 64410[0], 64413[0], 64415[0], 64416[0], 64417[0], 64418[0], 64420[0], 64421[0], 64425[0], 64430[0], 64435[0], 64445[0], 64446[0], 64447[0], 64448[0], 64449[0], 64450[0], 64461[0], 64462[0], 64463[0], 64479[0], 64480[0], 64483[0], 64484[0], 64486[0], 64487[0], 64488[0], 64489[0], 64490[0], 64491[0], 64492[0], 64493[0], 64494[0], 64495[0], 64505[0], 64510[0], 64517[0], 64520[0], 64530[0], 69990[0], 76000[1], 77001[1], 77002[1], 92012[1], 92014[1], 92585[0], 93000[1], 93005[1], 93010[1], 93040[1], 93041[1], 93042[1], 93318[1], 93355[1], 94002[1], 94200[1], 94250[1], 94680[1], 94681[1], 94690[1], 94770[1], 95812[1], 95813[1], 95816[1], 95819[1], 95822[0], 95829[1], 95860[0], 95861[0], 95863[0], 95864[0], 95865[0], 95866[0], 95867[0], 95868[0], 95869[0], 95870[0], 95907[0], 95908[0], 95909[0], 95910[0], 95911[0], 95912[0], 95913[0], 95925[0], 95926[0], 95927[0], 95928[0], 95929[0], 95930[0], 95933[0], 95937[0], 95938[0], 95939[0], 95940[0], 95955[1], 96360[1], 96361[1], 96365[1], 96366[1], 96367[1], 96368[1], 96372[1], 96374[1], 96375[1], 96376[1], 96377[1], 99155[0], 99156[0], 99157[0], 99211[1], 99212[1], 99213[1], 99214[1], 99215[1], 99217[1], 99218[1], 99219[1], 99220[1], 99221[1], 99222[1], 99223[1], 99231[1], 99232[1], 99233[1], 99234[1], 99235[1], 99236[1], 99238[1], 99239[1], 99241[1], 99242[1], 99243[1], 99244[1], 99245[1], 99251[1], 99252[1], 99253[1], 99254[1], 99255[1], 99291[1], 99292[1], 99304[1], 99305[1], 99306[1], 99307[1], 99308[1], 99309[1], 99310[1], 99315[1], 99316[1], 99334[1], 99335[1], 99336[1], 99337[1], 99347[1], 99348[1], 99349[1], 99350[1], 99374[1], 99375[1], 99377[1], 99378[1], 99446[0], 99447[0], 99448[0], 99449[0], 99451[0], 99452[0], 99495[0], 99496[0], G0453[0], G0463[1], G0471[1]
62281	01935[0], 01936[0], 0213T[0], 0228T[0], 0230T[0], 0333T[0], 0464T[0], 12001[1], 12002[1], 12004[1], 12005[1], 12006[1], 12007[1], 12011[1], 12013[1], 12014[1], 12015[1], 12016[1], 12017[1], 12018[1], 12020[1], 12021[1], 12031[1], 12032[1], 12034[1], 12035[1], 12036[1], 12037[1], 12041[1], 12042[1], 12044[1], 12045[1], 12046[1], 12047[1], 12051[1], 12052[1], 12053[1], 12054[1], 12055[1], 12056[1], 12057[1], 13100[1], 13101[1], 13102[1], 13120[1], 13121[1], 13122[1], 13131[1], 13132[1], 13133[1], 13151[1], 13152[1], 13153[1], 36000[1], 36400[1], 36405[1], 36406[1], 36410[1], 36420[1], 36425[1],

0 = Modifier usage not allowed or inappropriate   1 = Modifier usage allowed

CPT © 2018 American Medical Association. All Rights Reserved.

Code 1	Code 2
	36430[1], 36440[1], 36591[0], 36592[0], 36600[1], 36640[1], 43752[1], 51701[1], 51702[1], 51703[1], 62270[1], 62272[1], 62273[1], 62284[1], 62320[0], 62321[0], 62322[0], 62323[0], 62324[0], 62325[0], 64400[0], 64402[0], 64405[0], 64408[0], 64410[0], 64413[0], 64415[0], 64416[0], 64417[0], 64418[0], 64420[0], 64421[0], 64425[0], 64430[0], 64435[0], 64445[0], 64446[0], 64447[0], 64448[0], 64449[0], 64450[0], 64461[0], 64462[0], 64463[0], 64479[0], 64480[0], 64483[0], 64484[0], 64486[0], 64487[0], 64488[0], 64489[0], 64490[0], 64491[0], 64492[0], 64505[0], 64510[0], 64517[0], 64520[0], 64530[0], 69990[0], 72275[1], 76000[1], 77001[1], 77002[1], 92012[1], 92014[1], 92585[0], 93000[1], 93005[1], 93010[1], 93040[1], 93041[1], 93042[1], 93318[1], 93355[1], 94002[1], 94200[1], 94250[1], 94680[1], 94681[1], 94690[1], 94770[1], 95812[1], 95813[1], 95816[1], 95819[1], 95822[0], 95829[1], 95860[0], 95861[0], 95863[0], 95864[0], 95865[0], 95866[0], 95867[0], 95868[0], 95869[0], 95870[0], 95907[0], 95908[0], 95909[0], 95910[0], 95911[0], 95912[0], 95913[0], 95925[0], 95926[0], 95927[0], 95928[0], 95929[0], 95930[0], 95933[0], 95937[0], 95938[0], 95939[0], 95940[0], 95955[1], 96360[1], 96361[1], 96365[1], 96366[1], 96367[1], 96368[1], 96372[1], 96374[1], 96375[1], 96376[1], 96377[1], 99155[0], 99156[0], 99157[0], 99211[1], 99212[1], 99213[1], 99214[1], 99215[1], 99217[1], 99218[1], 99219[1], 99220[1], 99221[1], 99222[1], 99223[1], 99231[1], 99232[1], 99233[1], 99234[1], 99235[1], 99236[1], 99238[1], 99239[1], 99241[1], 99242[1], 99243[1], 99244[1], 99245[1], 99251[1], 99252[1], 99253[1], 99254[1], 99255[1], 99291[1], 99292[1], 99304[1], 99305[1], 99306[1], 99307[1], 99308[1], 99309[1], 99310[1], 99315[1], 99316[1], 99334[1], 99335[1], 99336[1], 99337[1], 99347[1], 99348[1], 99349[1], 99350[1], 99374[1], 99375[1], 99377[1], 99378[1], 99446[0], 99447[0], 99448[0], 99449[0], 99451[0], 99452[0], 99495[0], 99496[0], G0453[0], G0463[1], G0471[1], J2001[1]
62282	01935[0], 01936[0], 0216T[0], 0228T[0], 0230T[0], 0333T[0], 0464T[0], 12001[1], 12002[1], 12004[1], 12005[1], 12006[1], 12007[1], 12011[1], 12013[1], 12014[1], 12015[1], 12016[1], 12017[1], 12018[1], 12020[1], 12021[1], 12031[1], 12032[1], 12034[1], 12035[1], 12036[1], 12037[1], 12041[1], 12042[1], 12044[1], 12045[1], 12046[1], 12047[1], 12051[1], 12052[1], 12053[1], 12054[1], 12055[1], 12056[1], 12057[1], 13100[1], 13101[1], 13102[1], 13120[1], 13121[1], 13122[1], 13131[1], 13132[1], 13133[1], 13151[1], 13152[1], 13153[1], 36000[1], 36400[1], 36405[1], 36406[1], 36410[1], 36420[1], 36425[1], 36430[1], 36440[1], 36591[0], 36592[0], 36600[1], 36640[1], 43752[1], 51701[1], 51702[1], 51703[1], 62270[1], 62272[1], 62273[1], 62320[0], 62321[0], 62322[0], 62323[0], 62326[0], 62327[0], 64400[0], 64402[0], 64405[0], 64408[0], 64410[0], 64413[0], 64415[0], 64416[0], 64417[0], 64418[0], 64420[0], 64421[0], 64425[0], 64430[0], 64435[0], 64445[0], 64446[0], 64447[0], 64448[0], 64449[0], 64450[0], 64461[0], 64462[0], 64463[0], 64479[0], 64480[0], 64483[0], 64484[0], 64486[0], 64487[0], 64488[0], 64489[0], 64493[0], 64494[0], 64495[0], 64505[0], 64510[0], 64517[0], 64520[0], 64530[0], 69990[0], 72275[1], 76000[1], 77001[1], 77002[1], 92012[1], 92014[1], 92585[0], 93000[1], 93005[1], 93010[1], 93040[1], 93041[1], 93042[1], 93318[1], 93355[1], 94002[1], 94200[1], 94250[1], 94680[1], 94681[1], 94690[1], 94770[1], 95812[1], 95813[1], 95816[1], 95819[1], 95822[0], 95829[1], 95860[0], 95861[0], 95863[0], 95864[0], 95865[0], 95866[0], 95867[0], 95868[0], 95869[0], 95870[0], 95907[0], 95908[0], 95909[0], 95910[0], 95911[0], 95912[0], 95913[0], 95925[0], 95926[0], 95927[0], 95928[0], 95929[0], 95930[0], 95933[0], 95937[0], 95938[0], 95939[0], 95940[0], 95955[1], 96360[1], 96361[1], 96365[1], 96366[1], 96367[1], 96368[1], 96372[1], 96374[1], 96375[1], 96376[1], 96377[1], 99155[0], 99156[0], 99157[0], 99211[1], 99212[1], 99213[1], 99214[1], 99215[1], 99217[1], 99218[1], 99219[1], 99220[1], 99221[1], 99222[1], 99223[1], 99231[1], 99232[1], 99233[1], 99234[1], 99235[1], 99236[1], 99238[1], 99239[1], 99241[1], 99242[1], 99243[1], 99244[1], 99245[1], 99251[1], 99252[1], 99253[1], 99254[1], 99255[1], 99291[1], 99292[1], 99304[1], 99305[1], 99306[1], 99307[1], 99308[1], 99309[1], 99310[1], 99315[1], 99316[1], 99334[1], 99335[1], 99336[1], 99337[1], 99347[1], 99348[1], 99349[1], 99350[1], 99374[1], 99375[1], 99377[1], 99378[1], 99446[0], 99447[0], 99448[0], 99449[0], 99451[0], 99452[0], 99495[0], 99496[0], G0453[0], G0463[1], G0471[1], J2001[1]
62284	01935[0], 01936[0], 0213T[0], 0216T[0], 0228T[0], 0230T[0], 0333T[0], 0464T[0], 12001[1], 12002[1], 12004[1], 12005[1], 12006[1], 12007[1], 12011[1], 12013[1], 12014[1], 12015[1], 12016[1], 12017[1], 12018[1], 12020[1], 12021[1], 12031[1], 12032[1], 12034[1], 12035[1], 12036[1], 12037[1], 12041[1], 12042[1], 12044[1], 12045[1], 12046[1], 12047[1], 12051[1], 12052[1], 12053[1], 12054[1], 12055[1], 12056[1], 12057[1], 13100[1], 13101[1], 13102[1], 13120[1], 13121[1], 13122[1], 13131[1], 13132[1], 13133[1], 13151[1], 13152[1], 13153[1], 36000[1], 36400[1], 36405[1], 36406[1], 36410[1], 36420[1], 36425[1], 36430[1], 36440[1], 36591[0], 36592[0], 36600[1], 36640[1], 43752[1], 51701[1], 51702[1], 51703[1], 62270[1], 62272[1], 62273[1], 62282[1], 64400[0], 64402[0], 64405[0], 64408[0], 64410[0], 64413[0], 64415[0], 64416[0], 64417[0], 64418[0], 64420[0], 64421[0], 64425[0], 64430[0], 64435[0], 64445[0], 64446[0], 64447[0], 64448[0], 64449[0], 64450[0], 64461[0], 64462[0], 64463[0], 64479[0], 64480[0], 64483[0], 64484[0], 64486[0], 64487[0], 64488[0], 64489[0], 64490[0], 64491[0], 64492[0], 64493[0], 64494[0], 64495[0], 64505[0], 64510[0], 64517[0], 64520[0], 64530[0], 69990[0], 76000[1], 77001[1], 77002[1], 92012[1], 92014[1], 92585[0], 93000[1], 93005[1], 93010[1], 93040[1], 93041[1], 93042[1], 93318[1], 93355[1], 94002[1], 94200[1], 94250[1], 94680[1], 94681[1], 94690[1], 94770[1], 95812[1], 95813[1], 95816[1], 95819[1], 95822[0], 95829[1], 95860[0], 95861[0], 95863[0], 95864[0], 95865[0], 95866[0], 95867[0], 95868[0], 95869[0], 95870[0], 95907[0], 95908[0], 95909[0], 95910[0], 95911[0], 95912[0], 95913[0], 95925[0], 95926[0], 95927[0], 95928[0], 95929[0], 95930[0], 95933[0], 95937[0], 95938[0], 95939[0], 95940[0], 95955[1], 96360[1], 96361[1], 96365[1], 96366[1], 96367[1], 96368[1], 96372[1], 96374[1], 96375[1], 96376[1], 96377[1], 99155[0], 99156[0], 99157[0], 99211[1], 99212[1], 99213[1], 99214[1], 99215[1], 99217[1], 99218[1], 99219[1], 99220[1], 99221[1], 99222[1], 99223[1], 99231[1], 99232[1], 99233[1], 99234[1], 99235[1], 99236[1], 99238[1], 99239[1], 99241[1], 99242[1], 99243[1], 99244[1], 99245[1], 99251[1], 99252[1], 99253[1], 99254[1], 99255[1], 99291[1], 99292[1], 99304[1], 99305[1], 99306[1], 99307[1], 99308[1], 99309[1], 99310[1], 99315[1], 99316[1], 99334[1], 99335[1], 99336[1], 99337[1], 99347[1], 99348[1], 99349[1], 99350[1], 99374[1], 99375[1], 99377[1], 99378[1], 99446[0], 99447[0], 99448[0], 99449[0], 99451[0], 99452[0], 99495[1], 99496[1], G0453[0], G0463[1], G0471[1]
62290	01935[0], 01936[0], 0228T[0], 0333T[0], 0464T[0], 12001[1], 12002[1], 12004[1], 12005[1], 12006[1], 12007[1], 12011[1], 12013[1], 12014[1], 12015[1], 12016[1], 12017[1], 12018[1], 12020[1], 12021[1], 12031[1], 12032[1], 12034[1], 12035[1], 12036[1], 12037[1], 12041[1], 12042[1], 12044[1], 12045[1], 12046[1], 12047[1], 12051[1], 12052[1], 12053[1], 12054[1], 12055[1], 12056[1], 12057[1], 13100[1], 13101[1], 13102[1], 13120[1], 13121[1], 13122[1], 13131[1], 13132[1], 13133[1], 13151[1], 13152[1], 13153[1], 36000[1], 36400[1], 36405[1], 36406[1], 36410[1], 36420[1], 36425[1], 36430[1], 36440[1], 36591[0], 36592[0], 36600[1], 36640[1], 43752[1], 51701[1], 51702[1], 51703[1], 62267[1], 62322[0], 62323[0], 62326[0], 62327[0], 64415[0], 64416[0], 64417[0], 64425[0], 64430[0], 64435[0], 64445[0], 64446[0], 64447[0], 64448[0], 64449[0], 64450[0], 64461[0], 64462[0], 64463[0], 64479[0], 64480[0], 64483[0], 64484[0], 64486[0], 64487[0], 64488[0], 64489[0], 64493[0], 64494[0], 64495[0], 64505[0], 64510[0], 64517[0], 64520[0], 64530[0], 69990[0], 76000[1], 76800[1], 76942[1], 76970[1], 76998[1], 77001[1], 77002[1], 77003[1], 92012[1], 92014[1], 92585[0], 93000[1], 93005[1], 93010[1], 93040[1], 93041[1], 93042[1], 93318[1], 93355[1], 94002[1], 94200[1], 94250[1], 94680[1], 94681[1], 94690[1], 94770[1], 95812[1], 95813[1], 95816[1], 95819[1], 95822[0], 95829[1], 95860[0], 95861[0], 95863[0], 95864[0], 95865[0], 95866[0], 95867[0], 95868[0], 95869[0], 95870[0], 95907[0], 95908[0], 95909[0], 95910[0], 95911[0], 95912[0], 95913[0], 95925[0], 95926[0], 95927[0], 95928[0], 95929[0], 95930[0], 95933[0], 95937[0], 95938[0], 95939[0], 95940[0], 95955[1], 96360[1], 96361[1], 96365[1], 96366[1], 96367[1], 96368[1], 96372[1], 96374[1], 96375[1], 96376[1], 96377[1], 99155[0], 99156[0], 99157[0], 99211[1], 99212[1], 99213[1], 99214[1], 99215[1], 99217[1], 99218[1], 99219[1], 99220[1], 99221[1], 99222[1], 99223[1], 99231[1], 99232[1], 99233[1], 99234[1], 99235[1], 99236[1], 99238[1], 99239[1], 99241[1], 99242[1], 99243[1], 99244[1], 99245[1], 99251[1], 99252[1], 99253[1], 99254[1], 99255[1], 99291[1], 99292[1], 99304[1], 99305[1], 99306[1], 99307[1], 99308[1], 99309[1], 99310[1], 99315[1], 99316[1], 99334[1], 99335[1], 99336[1], 99337[1], 99347[1], 99348[1], 99349[1], 99350[1], 99374[1], 99375[1], 99377[1], 99378[1], 99446[0], 99447[0], 99448[0], 99449[0], 99451[0], 99452[0], 99495[1], 99496[1], G0453[0], G0463[1], G0471[1]
62291	01935[0], 01936[0], 0213T[0], 0216T[0], 0228T[0], 0230T[0], 0333T[0], 0464T[0], 12001[1], 12002[1], 12004[1], 12005[1], 12006[1], 12007[1], 12011[1], 12013[1], 12014[1], 12015[1], 12016[1], 12017[1], 12018[1], 12020[1], 12021[1], 12031[1], 12032[1], 12034[1], 12035[1], 12036[1], 12037[1], 12041[1], 12042[1], 12044[1], 12045[1], 12046[1], 12047[1], 12051[1], 12052[1], 12053[1], 12054[1], 12055[1], 12056[1], 12057[1], 13100[1], 13101[1], 13102[1], 13120[1], 13121[1], 13122[1], 13131[1], 13132[1], 13133[1], 13151[1], 13152[1], 13153[1], 36000[1], 36400[1], 36405[1], 36406[1], 36410[1], 36420[1], 36425[1], 36430[1], 36440[1], 36591[0], 36592[0], 36600[1], 36640[1], 43752[1], 51701[1], 51702[1], 51703[1], 62320[0], 62321[0], 62324[0], 62325[0], 64400[0], 64402[0], 64405[0], 64408[0], 64410[0], 64413[0], 64415[0], 64416[0], 64417[0], 64418[0], 64420[0], 64421[0], 64425[0], 64430[0], 64435[0], 64445[0], 64446[0], 64447[0], 64448[0], 64450[1], 64461[0], 64462[0], 64463[0], 64479[0], 64480[0], 64486[0], 64487[0], 64488[0], 64489[0], 64490[0], 64491[0], 64492[0], 64505[0], 64510[0], 64517[0], 64520[0], 64530[0], 69990[0], 76000[1], 76800[1], 76942[1], 76970[1], 76998[1], 77001[1], 77002[1], 77003[1], 92012[1], 92014[1], 92585[0], 93000[1], 93005[1], 93010[1], 93040[1], 93041[1], 93042[1], 93318[1], 93355[1], 94002[1], 94200[1], 94250[1], 94680[1], 94681[1], 94690[1], 94770[1], 95812[1], 95813[1], 95816[1], 95819[1], 95822[0], 95829[1], 95860[0], 95861[0], 95863[0], 95864[0], 95865[0], 95866[0], 95867[0], 95868[0], 95869[0], 95870[0], 95907[0], 95908[0], 95909[0], 95910[0], 95911[0], 95912[0], 95913[0], 95925[0], 95926[0], 95927[0], 95928[0], 95929[0], 95930[0], 95933[0], 95937[0], 95938[0], 95939[0], 95940[0], 95955[1], 96360[1], 96361[1], 96365[1], 96366[1], 96367[1], 96368[1], 96372[1], 96374[1], 96375[1], 96376[1], 96377[1], 99155[0], 99156[0], 99157[0], 99211[1], 99212[1], 99213[1], 99214[1], 99215[1], 99217[1], 99218[1], 99219[1], 99220[1], 99221[1], 99222[1], 99223[1], 99231[1], 99232[1], 99233[1], 99234[1], 99235[1], 99236[1], 99238[1], 99239[1], 99241[1], 99242[1], 99243[1], 99244[1], 99245[1], 99251[1], 99252[1], 99253[1], 99254[1], 99255[1], 99291[1], 99292[1], 99304[1], 99305[1], 99306[1], 99307[1], 99308[1], 99309[1], 99310[1], 99315[1], 99316[1], 99334[1], 99335[1], 99336[1], 99337[1], 99347[1], 99348[1], 99349[1], 99350[1], 99374[1], 99375[1], 99377[1], 99378[1], 99446[0], 99447[0], 99448[0], 99449[0], 99451[0], 99452[0], 99495[1], 99496[1], G0453[0], G0463[1], G0471[1]
62302	00600[0], 01935[0], 01936[0], 0213T[0], 0216T[0], 0228T[0], 0230T[0], 12001[1], 12002[1], 12004[1], 12005[1], 12006[1], 12007[1], 12011[1], 12013[1], 12014[1], 12015[1], 12016[1], 12017[1], 12018[1], 12020[1], 12021[1], 12031[1], 12032[1], 12034[1], 12035[1], 12036[1], 12037[1], 12041[1], 12042[1], 12044[1], 12045[1], 12046[1], 12047[1], 12051[1], 12052[1], 12053[1], 12054[1], 12055[1], 12056[1], 12057[1], 13100[1], 13101[1], 13102[1], 13120[1], 13121[1], 13122[1], 13131[1], 13132[1], 13133[1], 13151[1], 13152[1], 13153[1], 36000[1], 36400[1], 36405[1], 36406[1], 36410[1], 36420[1], 36425[1], 36430[1], 36440[1], 36591[0], 36592[0], 36600[1], 36640[1], 43752[1], 51701[1], 51702[1], 51703[1], 61055[1], 62270[1], 62272[1], 62273[1], 62282[1], 62284[1], 62304[0], 62320[0], 62321[0], 62322[0],

0 = Modifier usage not allowed or inappropriate 1 = Modifier usage allowed

Appendix A: NCCI - CPT Codes

CPT © 2018 American Medical Association. All Rights Reserved.

Code 1	Code 2
	62323[0], 62324[0], 62325[0], 62326[0], 62327[0], 64400[0], 64402[0], 64405[0], 64408[0], 64410[0], 64413[0], 64415[0], 64416[0], 64417[0], 64418[0], 64420[0], 64421[0], 64425[0], 64430[0], 64435[0], 64445[0], 64446[0], 64447[0], 64448[0], 64449[0], 64450[0], 64461[0], 64462[0], 64463[0], 64479[0], 64480[0], 64483[0], 64484[0], 64486[0], 64487[0], 64488[0], 64489[0], 64490[0], 64491[0], 64492[0], 64493[0], 64494[0], 64495[0], 64505[0], 64510[0], 64517[0], 64520[0], 64530[0], 69990[0], 72240[1], 72255[1], 72265[1], 72270[1], 76000[1], 77002[1], 77003[1], 92012[1], 92014[1], 92585[0], 93000[1], 93005[1], 93010[1], 93040[1], 93041[1], 93042[1], 93318[1], 93355[1], 94002[1], 94200[1], 94250[1], 94680[1], 94681[1], 94690[1], 94770[1], 95812[1], 95813[1], 95816[1], 95819[1], 95822[0], 95829[1], 95860[0], 95861[0], 95863[0], 95864[0], 95865[0], 95866[0], 95867[0], 95868[0], 95869[0], 95870[0], 95907[0], 95908[0], 95909[0], 95910[0], 95911[0], 95912[0], 95913[0], 95925[0], 95926[0], 95927[0], 95928[0], 95929[0], 95930[0], 95933[0], 95937[0], 95938[0], 95939[0], 95940[0], 95941[0], 95955[1], 96360[1], 96361[1], 96365[1], 96366[1], 96367[1], 96368[1], 96372[1], 96374[1], 96375[1], 96376[1], 96377[1], 99155[0], 99156[0], 99157[0], 99211[1], 99212[1], 99213[1], 99214[1], 99215[1], 99217[1], 99218[1], 99219[1], 99220[1], 99221[1], 99222[1], 99223[1], 99231[1], 99232[1], 99233[1], 99234[1], 99235[1], 99236[1], 99238[1], 99239[1], 99241[1], 99242[1], 99243[1], 99244[1], 99245[1], 99251[1], 99252[1], 99253[1], 99254[1], 99255[1], 99291[1], 99292[1], 99304[1], 99305[1], 99306[1], 99307[1], 99308[1], 99309[1], 99310[1], 99315[1], 99316[1], 99334[1], 99335[1], 99336[1], 99337[1], 99347[1], 99348[1], 99349[1], 99350[1], 99374[1], 99375[1], 99377[1], 99378[1], G0453[0], G0471[1]
62303	00620[0], 01935[0], 01936[0], 0213T[0], 0216T[0], 0228T[0], 0230T[0], 12001[1], 12002[1], 12004[1], 12005[1], 12006[1], 12007[1], 12011[1], 12013[1], 12014[1], 12015[1], 12016[1], 12017[1], 12018[1], 12020[1], 12021[1], 12031[1], 12032[1], 12034[1], 12035[1], 12036[1], 12037[1], 12041[1], 12042[1], 12044[1], 12045[1], 12046[1], 12047[1], 12051[1], 12052[1], 12053[1], 12054[1], 12055[1], 12056[1], 12057[1], 13100[1], 13101[1], 13102[1], 13120[1], 13121[1], 13122[1], 13131[1], 13132[1], 13133[1], 13151[1], 13152[1], 13153[1], 36000[1], 36400[1], 36405[1], 36406[1], 36410[1], 36420[1], 36425[1], 36430[1], 36440[1], 36591[0], 36592[0], 36600[1], 36640[1], 43752[1], 51701[1], 51702[1], 51703[1], 61055[1], 62270[1], 62272[1], 62273[1], 62282[1], 62284[1], 62302[0], 62304[0], 62320[0], 62321[0], 62322[0], 62323[0], 62324[0], 62325[0], 62326[0], 62327[0], 64400[0], 64402[0], 64405[0], 64408[0], 64410[0], 64413[0], 64415[0], 64416[0], 64417[0], 64418[0], 64420[0], 64421[0], 64425[0], 64430[0], 64435[0], 64445[0], 64446[0], 64447[0], 64448[0], 64449[0], 64450[0], 64461[0], 64462[0], 64463[0], 64479[0], 64480[0], 64483[0], 64484[0], 64486[0], 64487[0], 64488[0], 64489[0], 64490[0], 64491[0], 64492[0], 64493[0], 64494[0], 64495[0], 64505[0], 64510[0], 64517[0], 64520[0], 64530[0], 69990[0], 72240[1], 72255[1], 72265[1], 72270[1], 76000[1], 77002[1], 77003[1], 92012[1], 92014[1], 92585[0], 93000[1], 93005[1], 93010[1], 93040[1], 93041[1], 93042[1], 93318[1], 93355[1], 94002[1], 94200[1], 94250[1], 94680[1], 94681[1], 94690[1], 94770[1], 95812[1], 95813[1], 95816[1], 95819[1], 95822[0], 95829[1], 95860[0], 95861[0], 95863[0], 95864[0], 95865[0], 95866[0], 95867[0], 95868[0], 95869[0], 95870[0], 95907[0], 95908[0], 95909[0], 95910[0], 95911[0], 95912[0], 95913[0], 95925[0], 95926[0], 95927[0], 95928[0], 95929[0], 95930[0], 95933[0], 95937[0], 95938[0], 95939[0], 95940[0], 95941[0], 95955[1], 96360[1], 96361[1], 96365[1], 96366[1], 96367[1], 96368[1], 96372[1], 96374[1], 96375[1], 96376[1], 96377[1], 99155[0], 99156[0], 99157[0], 99211[1], 99212[1], 99213[1], 99214[1], 99215[1], 99217[1], 99218[1], 99219[1], 99220[1], 99221[1], 99222[1], 99223[1], 99231[1], 99232[1], 99233[1], 99234[1], 99235[1], 99236[1], 99238[1], 99239[1], 99241[1], 99242[1], 99243[1], 99244[1], 99245[1], 99251[1], 99252[1], 99253[1], 99254[1], 99255[1], 99291[1], 99292[1], 99304[1], 99305[1], 99306[1], 99307[1], 99308[1], 99309[1], 99310[1], 99315[1], 99316[1], 99334[1], 99335[1], 99336[1], 99337[1], 99347[1], 99348[1], 99349[1], 99350[1], 99374[1], 99375[1], 99377[1], 99378[1], G0453[0], G0471[1]
62304	00630[0], 01935[0], 01936[0], 0213T[0], 0216T[0], 0228T[0], 0230T[0], 12001[1], 12002[1], 12004[1], 12005[1], 12006[1], 12007[1], 12011[1], 12013[1], 12014[1], 12015[1], 12016[1], 12017[1], 12018[1], 12020[1], 12021[1], 12031[1], 12032[1], 12034[1], 12035[1], 12036[1], 12037[1], 12041[1], 12042[1], 12044[1], 12045[1], 12046[1], 12047[1], 12051[1], 12052[1], 12053[1], 12054[1], 12055[1], 12056[1], 12057[1], 13100[1], 13101[1], 13102[1], 13120[1], 13121[1], 13122[1], 13131[1], 13132[1], 13133[1], 13151[1], 13152[1], 13153[1], 36000[1], 36400[1], 36405[1], 36406[1], 36410[1], 36420[1], 36425[1], 36430[1], 36440[1], 36591[0], 36592[0], 36600[1], 36640[1], 43752[1], 51701[1], 51702[1], 51703[1], 61055[1], 62270[1], 62272[1], 62273[1], 62282[1], 62284[1], 62320[0], 62321[0], 62322[0], 62323[0], 62324[0], 62325[0], 62326[0], 62327[0], 64400[0], 64402[0], 64405[0], 64408[0], 64410[0], 64413[0], 64415[0], 64416[0], 64417[0], 64418[0], 64420[0], 64421[0], 64425[0], 64430[0], 64435[0], 64445[0], 64446[0], 64447[0], 64448[0], 64449[0], 64450[0], 64461[0], 64462[0], 64463[0], 64479[0], 64480[0], 64483[0], 64484[0], 64486[0], 64487[0], 64488[0], 64489[0], 64490[0], 64491[0], 64492[0], 64493[0], 64494[0], 64495[0], 64505[0], 64510[0], 64517[0], 64520[0], 64530[0], 69990[0], 72240[1], 72255[1], 72265[1], 72270[1], 76000[1], 77002[1], 77003[1], 92012[1], 92014[1], 92585[0], 93000[1], 93005[1], 93010[1], 93040[1], 93041[1], 93042[1], 93318[1], 93355[1], 94002[1], 94200[1], 94250[1], 94680[1], 94681[1], 94690[1], 94770[1], 95812[1], 95813[1], 95816[1], 95819[1], 95822[0], 95829[1], 95860[0], 95861[0], 95863[0], 95864[0], 95865[0], 95866[0], 95867[0], 95868[0], 95869[0], 95870[0], 95907[0], 95908[0], 95909[0], 95910[0], 95911[0], 95912[0], 95913[0], 95925[0], 95926[0], 95927[0], 95928[0], 95929[0], 95930[0], 95933[0], 95937[0], 95938[0], 95939[0], 95940[0], 95941[0], 95955[1], 96360[1], 96361[1], 96365[1], 96366[1], 96367[1], 96368[1], 96372[1], 96374[1], 96375[1], 96376[1], 96377[1], 99155[0], 99156[0], 99157[0], 99211[1], 99212[1], 99213[1], 99214[1], 99215[1], 99217[1], 99218[1], 99219[1], 99220[1], 99221[1], 99222[1], 99223[1], 99231[1], 99232[1], 99233[1], 99234[1], 99235[1], 99236[1], 99238[1], 99239[1], 99241[1], 99242[1], 99243[1], 99244[1], 99245[1], 99251[1], 99252[1], 99253[1], 99254[1], 99255[1], 99291[1], 99292[1], 99304[1], 99305[1], 99306[1], 99307[1], 99308[1], 99309[1], 99310[1], 99315[1], 99316[1], 99334[1], 99335[1], 99336[1], 99337[1], 99347[1], 99348[1], 99349[1], 99350[1], 99374[1], 99375[1], 99377[1], 99378[1], G0453[0], G0471[1]
62305	00600[0], 00620[0], 00630[0], 01935[0], 01936[0], 0213T[0], 0216T[0], 0228T[0], 0230T[0], 12001[1], 12002[1], 12004[1], 12005[1], 12006[1], 12007[1], 12011[1], 12013[1], 12014[1], 12015[1], 12016[1], 12017[1], 12018[1], 12020[1], 12021[1], 12031[1], 12032[1], 12034[1], 12035[1], 12036[1], 12037[1], 12041[1], 12042[1], 12044[1], 12045[1], 12046[1], 12047[1], 12051[1], 12052[1], 12053[1], 12054[1], 12055[1], 12056[1], 12057[1], 13100[1], 13101[1], 13102[1], 13120[1], 13121[1], 13122[1], 13131[1], 13132[1], 13133[1], 13151[1], 13152[1], 13153[1], 36000[1], 36400[1], 36405[1], 36406[1], 36410[1], 36420[1], 36425[1], 36430[1], 36440[1], 36591[0], 36592[0], 36600[1], 36640[1], 43752[1], 51701[1], 51702[1], 51703[1], 61055[1], 62270[1], 62272[1], 62273[1], 62282[1], 62284[1], 62302[0], 62303[0], 62304[0], 62320[0], 62321[0], 62322[0], 62323[0], 62324[0], 62325[0], 62326[0], 62327[0], 64400[0], 64402[0], 64405[0], 64408[0], 64410[0], 64413[0], 64415[0], 64416[0], 64417[0], 64418[0], 64420[0], 64421[0], 64425[0], 64430[0], 64435[0], 64445[0], 64446[0], 64447[0], 64448[0], 64449[0], 64450[0], 64461[0], 64462[0], 64463[0], 64479[0], 64480[0], 64483[0], 64484[0], 64486[0], 64487[0], 64488[0], 64489[0], 64490[0], 64491[0], 64492[0], 64493[0], 64494[0], 64495[0], 64505[0], 64510[0], 64517[0], 64520[0], 64530[0], 69990[0], 72240[1], 72255[1], 72265[1], 72270[1], 76000[1], 77002[1], 77003[1], 92012[1], 92014[1], 92585[0], 93000[1], 93005[1], 93010[1], 93040[1], 93041[1], 93042[1], 93318[1], 93355[1], 94002[1], 94200[1], 94250[1], 94680[1], 94681[1], 94690[1], 94770[1], 95812[1], 95813[1], 95816[1], 95819[1], 95822[0], 95829[1], 95860[0], 95861[0], 95863[0], 95864[0], 95865[0], 95866[0], 95867[0], 95868[0], 95869[0], 95870[0], 95907[0], 95908[0], 95909[0], 95910[0], 95911[0], 95912[0], 95913[0], 95925[0], 95926[0], 95927[0], 95928[0], 95929[0], 95930[0], 95933[0], 95937[0], 95938[0], 95939[0], 95940[0], 95941[0], 95955[1], 96360[1], 96361[1], 96365[1], 96366[1], 96367[1], 96368[1], 96372[1], 96374[1], 96375[1], 96376[1], 96377[1], 99155[0], 99156[0], 99157[0], 99211[1], 99212[1], 99213[1], 99214[1], 99215[1], 99217[1], 99218[1], 99219[1], 99220[1], 99221[1], 99222[1], 99223[1], 99231[1], 99232[1], 99233[1], 99234[1], 99235[1], 99236[1], 99238[1], 99239[1], 99241[1], 99242[1], 99243[1], 99244[1], 99245[1], 99251[1], 99252[1], 99253[1], 99254[1], 99255[1], 99291[1], 99292[1], 99304[1], 99305[1], 99306[1], 99307[1], 99308[1], 99309[1], 99310[1], 99315[1], 99316[1], 99334[1], 99335[1], 99336[1], 99337[1], 99347[1], 99348[1], 99349[1], 99350[1], 99374[1], 99375[1], 99377[1], 99378[1], G0453[0], G0471[1]
62320	01991[0], 01992[0], 0228T[1], 0333T[0], 0464T[0], 12001[1], 12002[1], 12004[1], 12005[1], 12006[1], 12007[1], 12011[1], 12013[1], 12014[1], 12015[1], 12016[1], 12017[1], 12018[1], 12020[1], 12021[1], 12031[1], 12032[1], 12034[1], 12035[1], 12036[1], 12037[1], 12041[1], 12042[1], 12044[1], 12045[1], 12046[1], 12047[1], 12051[1], 12052[1], 12053[1], 12054[1], 12055[1], 12056[1], 12057[1], 13100[1], 13101[1], 13102[1], 13120[1], 13121[1], 13122[1], 13131[1], 13132[1], 13133[1], 13151[1], 13152[1], 13153[1], 20605[1], 20610[1], 36000[1], 36140[1], 36400[1], 36405[1], 36406[1], 36410[1], 36420[1], 36425[1], 36430[1], 36440[1], 36591[0], 36592[0], 36600[1], 36640[1], 43752[1], 51701[0], 51702[0], 51703[0], 62284[0], 64462[0], 64479[1], 64480[0], 69990[0], 72275[1], 76000[1], 76800[1], 76942[1], 76970[1], 76998[1], 77001[1], 77002[1], 77003[1], 77012[1], 92012[1], 92014[1], 92585[0], 93000[1], 93005[1], 93010[1], 93040[1], 93041[1], 93042[1], 93318[1], 93355[1], 94002[1], 94200[1], 94250[1], 94680[1], 94681[1], 94690[1], 94770[1], 95812[1], 95813[1], 95816[1], 95819[1], 95822[0], 95829[1], 95860[0], 95861[0], 95863[0], 95864[0], 95865[0], 95866[0], 95867[0], 95868[0], 95869[0], 95870[0], 95907[0], 95908[0], 95909[0], 95910[0], 95911[0], 95912[0], 95913[0], 95925[0], 95926[0], 95927[0], 95928[0], 95929[0], 95930[0], 95933[0], 95937[0], 95938[0], 95939[0], 95940[0], 95941[0], 95955[1], 96360[1], 96361[1], 96365[1], 96366[1], 96367[1], 96368[1], 96372[1], 96374[1], 96375[1], 96376[1], 96377[1], 96523[0], 99155[0], 99156[0], 99157[0], 99211[1], 99212[1], 99213[1], 99214[1], 99215[1], 99217[1], 99218[1], 99219[1], 99220[1], 99221[1], 99222[1], 99223[1], 99231[1], 99232[1], 99233[1], 99234[1], 99235[1], 99236[1], 99238[1], 99239[1], 99241[1], 99242[1], 99243[1], 99244[1], 99245[1], 99251[1], 99252[1], 99253[1], 99254[1], 99255[1], 99291[1], 99292[1], 99304[1], 99305[1], 99306[1], 99307[1], 99308[1], 99309[1], 99310[1], 99315[1], 99316[1], 99334[1], 99335[1], 99336[1], 99337[1], 99347[1], 99348[1], 99349[1], 99350[1], 99374[1], 99375[1], 99377[1], 99378[1], 99446[0], 99447[0], 99448[0], 99449[0], 99451[0], 99452[0], 99495[1], 99496[1], G0453[0], G0459[1], G0463[1], G0471[0], J2001[1]
62321	01991[0], 01992[0], 0228T[1], 0333T[0], 0464T[0], 12001[1], 12002[1], 12004[1], 12005[1], 12006[1], 12007[1], 12011[1], 12013[1], 12014[1], 12015[1], 12016[1], 12017[1], 12018[1], 12020[1], 12021[1], 12031[1], 12032[1], 12034[1], 12035[1], 12036[1], 12037[1], 12041[1], 12042[1], 12044[1], 12045[1], 12046[1], 12047[1], 12051[1], 12052[1], 12053[1], 12054[1], 12055[1], 12056[1], 12057[1], 13100[1], 13101[1], 13102[1], 13120[1], 13121[1], 13122[1], 13131[1], 13132[1], 13133[1], 13151[1], 13152[1], 13153[1], 20605[1], 20610[1], 36000[1], 36140[1], 36400[1], 36405[1], 36406[1], 36410[1], 36420[1], 36425[1], 36430[1], 36440[1], 36591[0], 36592[0], 36600[1], 36640[1], 43752[1], 51701[0], 51702[0], 51703[0], 62284[0], 62320[0], 64462[0], 64479[1], 64480[0], 69990[0], 72275[1], 76000[1], 76800[1], 76942[1], 76970[1], 76998[1], 77001[1], 77002[1], 77003[1], 77012[1], 92012[1], 92014[1], 92585[0], 93000[1], 93005[1], 93010[1], 93040[1], 93041[1], 93042[1], 93318[1], 93355[1], 94002[1], 94200[1], 94250[1], 94680[1], 94681[1], 94690[1], 94770[1], 95812[1], 95813[1], 95816[1], 95819[1], 95822[0],

0 = Modifier usage not allowed or inappropriate 1 = Modifier usage allowed

CPT © 2018 American Medical Association. All Rights Reserved.

Code 1	Code 2
	95829[1], 95860[0], 95861[0], 95863[0], 95864[0], 95865[0], 95866[0], 95867[0], 95868[0], 95869[0], 95870[0], 95907[0], 95908[0], 95909[0], 95910[0], 95911[0], 95912[0], 95913[0], 95925[0], 95926[0], 95927[0], 95928[0], 95929[0], 95930[0], 95933[0], 95937[0], 95938[0], 95939[0], 95940[0], 95941[0], 95955[1], 96360[1], 96361[1], 96365[1], 96366[1], 96367[1], 96368[1], 96372[1], 96374[1], 96375[1], 96376[1], 96377[1], 96523[0], 99155[0], 99156[0], 99157[0], 99211[1], 99212[1], 99213[1], 99214[1], 99215[1], 99217[1], 99218[1], 99219[1], 99220[1], 99221[1], 99222[1], 99223[1], 99231[1], 99232[1], 99233[1], 99234[1], 99235[1], 99236[1], 99238[1], 99239[1], 99241[1], 99242[1], 99243[1], 99244[1], 99245[1], 99251[1], 99252[1], 99253[1], 99254[1], 99255[1], 99291[1], 99292[1], 99304[1], 99305[1], 99306[1], 99307[1], 99308[1], 99309[1], 99310[1], 99315[1], 99316[1], 99334[1], 99335[1], 99336[1], 99337[1], 99347[1], 99348[1], 99349[1], 99350[1], 99374[1], 99375[1], 99377[1], 99378[1], 99446[0], 99447[0], 99448[0], 99449[0], 99451[0], 99452[0], 99495[1], 99496[1], G0453[0], G0459[1], G0463[1], G0471[0], J2001[1]
62322	01991[0], 01992[0], 0230T[1], 0333T[0], 0464T[0], 12001[1], 12002[1], 12004[1], 12005[1], 12006[1], 12007[1], 12011[1], 12013[1], 12014[1], 12015[1], 12016[1], 12017[1], 12018[1], 12020[1], 12021[1], 12031[1], 12032[1], 12034[1], 12035[1], 12036[1], 12037[1], 12041[1], 12042[1], 12044[1], 12045[1], 12046[1], 12047[1], 12051[1], 12052[1], 12053[1], 12054[1], 12055[1], 12056[1], 12057[1], 13100[1], 13101[1], 13102[1], 13120[1], 13121[1], 13122[1], 13131[1], 13132[1], 13133[1], 13151[1], 13152[1], 13153[1], 20605[1], 20610[1], 36000[1], 36140[1], 36400[1], 36405[1], 36406[1], 36410[1], 36420[1], 36425[1], 36430[1], 36440[1], 36591[0], 36592[0], 36600[1], 36640[1], 43752[1], 51701[0], 51702[0], 51703[0], 62284[0], 64483[1], 64484[0], 69990[0], 72275[1], 76000[1], 76800[1], 76942[1], 76970[1], 76998[1], 77001[1], 77002[1], 77003[1], 77012[1], 92012[1], 92014[1], 92585[0], 93000[1], 93005[1], 93010[1], 93040[1], 93041[1], 93042[1], 93318[1], 93355[1], 94002[1], 94200[1], 94250[1], 94680[1], 94681[1], 94690[1], 94770[1], 95812[1], 95813[1], 95816[1], 95819[1], 95822[0], 95829[1], 95860[0], 95861[0], 95863[0], 95864[0], 95865[0], 95866[0], 95867[0], 95868[0], 95869[0], 95870[0], 95907[0], 95908[0], 95909[0], 95910[0], 95911[0], 95912[0], 95913[0], 95925[0], 95926[0], 95927[0], 95928[0], 95929[0], 95930[0], 95933[0], 95937[0], 95938[0], 95939[0], 95940[0], 95941[0], 95955[1], 96360[1], 96361[1], 96365[1], 96366[1], 96367[1], 96368[1], 96372[1], 96374[1], 96375[1], 96376[1], 96377[1], 96523[0], 99155[0], 99156[0], 99157[0], 99211[1], 99212[1], 99213[1], 99214[1], 99215[1], 99217[1], 99218[1], 99219[1], 99220[1], 99221[1], 99222[1], 99223[1], 99231[1], 99232[1], 99233[1], 99234[1], 99235[1], 99236[1], 99238[1], 99239[1], 99241[1], 99242[1], 99243[1], 99244[1], 99245[1], 99251[1], 99252[1], 99253[1], 99254[1], 99255[1], 99291[1], 99292[1], 99304[1], 99305[1], 99306[1], 99307[1], 99308[1], 99309[1], 99310[1], 99315[1], 99316[1], 99334[1], 99335[1], 99336[1], 99337[1], 99347[1], 99348[1], 99349[1], 99350[1], 99374[1], 99375[1], 99377[1], 99378[1], 99446[0], 99447[0], 99448[0], 99449[0], 99451[0], 99452[0], 99495[1], 99496[1], G0453[0], G0459[1], G0463[1], G0471[0], J2001[1]
62323	01991[0], 01992[0], 0230T[1], 0333T[0], 0464T[0], 12001[1], 12002[1], 12004[1], 12005[1], 12006[1], 12007[1], 12011[1], 12013[1], 12014[1], 12015[1], 12016[1], 12017[1], 12018[1], 12020[1], 12021[1], 12031[1], 12032[1], 12034[1], 12035[1], 12036[1], 12037[1], 12041[1], 12042[1], 12044[1], 12045[1], 12046[1], 12047[1], 12051[1], 12052[1], 12053[1], 12054[1], 12055[1], 12056[1], 12057[1], 13100[1], 13101[1], 13102[1], 13120[1], 13121[1], 13122[1], 13131[1], 13132[1], 13133[1], 13151[1], 13152[1], 13153[1], 20605[1], 20610[1], 36000[1], 36140[1], 36400[1], 36405[1], 36406[1], 36410[1], 36420[1], 36425[1], 36430[1], 36440[1], 36591[0], 36592[0], 36600[1], 36640[1], 43752[1], 51701[0], 51702[0], 51703[0], 62284[0], 62322[0], 64483[1], 64484[1], 69990[0], 72275[1], 76000[1], 76800[1], 76942[1], 76970[1], 76998[1], 77001[1], 77002[1], 77003[1], 77012[1], 92012[1], 92014[1], 92585[0], 93000[1], 93005[1], 93010[1], 93040[1], 93041[1], 93042[1], 93318[1], 93355[1], 94002[1], 94200[1], 94250[1], 94680[1], 94681[1], 94690[1], 94770[1], 95812[1], 95813[1], 95816[1], 95819[1], 95822[0], 95829[1], 95860[0], 95861[0], 95863[0], 95864[0], 95865[0], 95866[0], 95867[0], 95868[0], 95869[0], 95870[0], 95907[0], 95908[0], 95909[0], 95910[0], 95911[0], 95912[0], 95913[0], 95925[0], 95926[0], 95927[0], 95928[0], 95929[0], 95930[0], 95933[0], 95937[0], 95938[0], 95939[0], 95940[0], 95941[0], 95955[1], 96360[1], 96361[1], 96365[1], 96366[1], 96367[1], 96368[1], 96372[1], 96374[1], 96375[1], 96376[1], 96377[1], 96523[0], 99155[0], 99156[0], 99157[0], 99211[1], 99212[1], 99213[1], 99214[1], 99215[1], 99217[1], 99218[1], 99219[1], 99220[1], 99221[1], 99222[1], 99223[1], 99231[1], 99232[1], 99233[1], 99234[1], 99235[1], 99236[1], 99238[1], 99239[1], 99241[1], 99242[1], 99243[1], 99244[1], 99245[1], 99251[1], 99252[1], 99253[1], 99254[1], 99255[1], 99291[1], 99292[1], 99304[1], 99305[1], 99306[1], 99307[1], 99308[1], 99309[1], 99310[1], 99315[1], 99316[1], 99334[1], 99335[1], 99336[1], 99337[1], 99347[1], 99348[1], 99349[1], 99350[1], 99374[1], 99375[1], 99377[1], 99378[1], 99446[0], 99447[0], 99448[0], 99449[0], 99451[0], 99452[0], 99495[1], 99496[1], G0453[0], G0459[1], G0463[1], G0471[0], J2001[1]
62324	01991[0], 01992[0], 01996[0], 0228T[1], 0333T[0], 0464T[0], 12001[1], 12002[1], 12004[1], 12005[1], 12006[1], 12007[1], 12011[1], 12013[1], 12014[1], 12015[1], 12016[1], 12017[1], 12018[1], 12020[1], 12021[1], 12031[1], 12032[1], 12034[1], 12035[1], 12036[1], 12037[1], 12041[1], 12042[1], 12044[1], 12045[1], 12046[1], 12047[1], 12051[1], 12052[1], 12053[1], 12054[1], 12055[1], 12056[1], 12057[1], 13100[1], 13101[1], 13102[1], 13120[1], 13121[1], 13122[1], 13131[1], 13132[1], 13133[1], 13151[1], 13152[1], 13153[1], 20605[1], 20610[1], 36000[1], 36140[1], 36400[1], 36405[1], 36406[1], 36410[1], 36420[1], 36425[1], 36430[1], 36440[1], 36591[0], 36592[0], 36600[1], 36640[1], 43752[1], 51701[0], 51702[0], 51703[1], 62270[0], 62272[0], 62284[0], 62320[1], 62321[1], 64462[0], 64479[1], 64480[0], 69990[0], 72275[1], 76000[1], 76800[1], 76942[1], 76970[1], 76998[1], 77001[1], 77002[1], 77003[1], 77012[1], 92012[1], 92014[1], 92585[0], 93000[1], 93005[1], 93010[1], 93040[1], 93041[1], 93042[1], 93318[1], 93355[1], 94002[1], 94200[1], 94250[1], 94680[1], 94681[1], 94690[1], 94770[1], 95812[1], 95813[1], 95816[1], 95819[1], 95822[0], 95829[1], 95860[0], 95861[0], 95863[0], 95864[0], 95865[0], 95866[0], 95867[0], 95868[0], 95869[0], 95870[0], 95907[0], 95908[0], 95909[0], 95910[0], 95911[0], 95912[0], 95913[0], 95925[0], 95926[0], 95927[0], 95928[0], 95929[0], 95930[0], 95933[0], 95937[0], 95938[0], 95939[0], 95940[0], 95941[0], 95955[1], 96360[1], 96361[1], 96365[1], 96366[1], 96367[1], 96368[1], 96372[1], 96374[1], 96375[1], 96376[1], 96377[1], 96522[1], 96523[0], 99155[0], 99156[0], 99157[0], 99211[1], 99212[1], 99213[1], 99214[1], 99215[1], 99217[1], 99218[1], 99219[1], 99220[1], 99221[1], 99222[1], 99223[1], 99231[1], 99232[1], 99233[1], 99234[1], 99235[1], 99236[1], 99238[1], 99239[1], 99241[1], 99242[1], 99243[1], 99244[1], 99245[1], 99251[1], 99252[1], 99253[1], 99254[1], 99255[1], 99291[1], 99292[1], 99304[1], 99305[1], 99306[1], 99307[1], 99308[1], 99309[1], 99310[1], 99315[1], 99316[1], 99334[1], 99335[1], 99336[1], 99337[1], 99347[1], 99348[1], 99349[1], 99350[1], 99374[1], 99375[1], 99377[1], 99378[1], 99446[0], 99447[0], 99448[0], 99449[0], 99451[0], 99452[0], 99495[1], 99496[1], G0453[0], G0459[1], G0463[1], G0471[0], J2001[1]
62325	01991[0], 01992[0], 01996[0], 0228T[1], 0333T[0], 0464T[0], 12001[1], 12002[1], 12004[1], 12005[1], 12006[1], 12007[1], 12011[1], 12013[1], 12014[1], 12015[1], 12016[1], 12017[1], 12018[1], 12020[1], 12021[1], 12031[1], 12032[1], 12034[1], 12035[1], 12036[1], 12037[1], 12041[1], 12042[1], 12044[1], 12045[1], 12046[1], 12047[1], 12051[1], 12052[1], 12053[1], 12054[1], 12055[1], 12056[1], 12057[1], 13100[1], 13101[1], 13102[1], 13120[1], 13121[1], 13122[1], 13131[1], 13132[1], 13133[1], 13151[1], 13152[1], 13153[1], 20605[1], 20610[1], 36000[1], 36140[1], 36400[1], 36405[1], 36406[1], 36410[1], 36420[1], 36425[1], 36430[1], 36440[1], 36591[0], 36592[0], 36600[1], 36640[1], 43752[1], 51701[0], 51702[0], 51703[1], 62270[0], 62272[0], 62273[0], 62284[0], 62320[1], 62321[1], 62323[0], 64462[0], 64479[1], 64480[0], 69990[0], 72275[1], 76000[1], 76800[1], 76942[1], 76970[1], 76998[1], 77001[1], 77002[1], 77003[1], 77012[1], 92012[1], 92014[1], 92585[0], 93000[1], 93005[1], 93010[1], 93040[1], 93041[1], 93042[1], 93318[1], 93355[1], 94002[1], 94200[1], 94250[1], 94680[1], 94681[1], 94690[1], 94770[1], 95812[1], 95813[1], 95816[1], 95819[1], 95822[0], 95829[1], 95860[0], 95861[0], 95863[0], 95864[0], 95865[0], 95866[0], 95867[0], 95868[0], 95869[0], 95870[0], 95907[0], 95908[0], 95909[0], 95910[0], 95911[0], 95912[0], 95913[0], 95925[0], 95926[0], 95927[0], 95928[0], 95929[0], 95930[0], 95933[0], 95937[0], 95938[0], 95939[0], 95940[0], 95941[0], 95955[1], 96360[1], 96361[1], 96365[1], 96366[1], 96367[1], 96368[1], 96372[1], 96374[1], 96375[1], 96376[1], 96377[1], 96522[1], 96523[0], 99155[0], 99156[0], 99157[0], 99211[1], 99212[1], 99213[1], 99214[1], 99215[1], 99217[1], 99218[1], 99219[1], 99220[1], 99221[1], 99222[1], 99223[1], 99231[1], 99232[1], 99233[1], 99234[1], 99235[1], 99236[1], 99238[1], 99239[1], 99241[1], 99242[1], 99243[1], 99244[1], 99245[1], 99251[1], 99252[1], 99253[1], 99254[1], 99255[1], 99291[1], 99292[1], 99304[1], 99305[1], 99306[1], 99307[1], 99308[1], 99309[1], 99310[1], 99315[1], 99316[1], 99334[1], 99335[1], 99336[1], 99337[1], 99347[1], 99348[1], 99349[1], 99350[1], 99374[1], 99375[1], 99377[1], 99378[1], 99446[0], 99447[0], 99448[0], 99449[0], 99451[0], 99452[0], 99495[1], 99496[1], G0453[0], G0459[1], G0463[1], G0471[0], J2001[1]
62326	01991[0], 01992[0], 01996[0], 0230T[1], 0333T[0], 0464T[0], 12001[1], 12002[1], 12004[1], 12005[1], 12006[1], 12007[1], 12011[1], 12013[1], 12014[1], 12015[1], 12016[1], 12017[1], 12018[1], 12020[1], 12021[1], 12031[1], 12032[1], 12034[1], 12035[1], 12036[1], 12037[1], 12041[1], 12042[1], 12044[1], 12045[1], 12046[1], 12047[1], 12051[1], 12052[1], 12053[1], 12054[1], 12055[1], 12056[1], 12057[1], 13100[1], 13101[1], 13102[1], 13120[1], 13121[1], 13122[1], 13131[1], 13132[1], 13133[1], 13151[1], 13152[1], 13153[1], 20605[1], 20610[1], 36000[1], 36140[1], 36400[1], 36405[1], 36406[1], 36410[1], 36420[1], 36425[1], 36430[1], 36440[1], 36591[0], 36592[0], 36600[1], 36640[1], 43752[1], 51701[0], 51702[0], 51703[1], 62270[0], 62272[0], 62284[0], 62322[1], 62323[1], 64483[1], 64484[0], 69990[0], 72275[1], 76000[1], 76800[1], 76942[1], 76970[1], 76998[1], 77001[1], 77002[1], 77003[1], 77012[1], 92012[1], 92014[1], 92585[0], 93000[1], 93005[1], 93010[1], 93040[1], 93041[1], 93042[1], 93318[1], 93355[1], 94002[1], 94200[1], 94250[1], 94680[1], 94681[1], 94690[1], 94770[1], 95812[1], 95813[1], 95816[1], 95819[1], 95822[0], 95829[1], 95860[0], 95861[0], 95863[0], 95864[0], 95865[0], 95866[0], 95867[0], 95868[0], 95869[0], 95870[0], 95907[0], 95908[0], 95909[0], 95910[0], 95911[0], 95912[0], 95913[0], 95925[0], 95926[0], 95927[0], 95928[0], 95929[0], 95930[0], 95933[0], 95937[0], 95938[0], 95939[0], 95940[0], 95941[0], 95955[1], 96360[1], 96361[1], 96365[1], 96366[1], 96367[1], 96368[1], 96372[1], 96374[1], 96375[1], 96376[1], 96377[1], 96522[1], 96523[0], 99155[0], 99156[0], 99157[0], 99211[1], 99212[1], 99213[1], 99214[1], 99215[1], 99217[1], 99218[1], 99219[1], 99220[1], 99221[1], 99222[1], 99223[1], 99231[1], 99232[1], 99233[1], 99234[1], 99235[1], 99236[1], 99238[1], 99239[1], 99241[1], 99242[1], 99243[1], 99244[1], 99245[1], 99251[1], 99252[1], 99253[1], 99254[1], 99255[1], 99291[1], 99292[1], 99304[1], 99305[1], 99306[1], 99307[1], 99308[1], 99309[1], 99310[1], 99315[1], 99316[1], 99334[1], 99335[1], 99336[1], 99337[1], 99347[1], 99348[1], 99349[1], 99350[1], 99374[1], 99375[1], 99377[1], 99378[1], 99446[0], 99447[0], 99448[0], 99449[0], 99451[0], 99452[0], 99495[1], 99496[1], G0453[0], G0459[1], G0463[1], G0471[0], J2001[1]
62327	01991[0], 01992[0], 01996[0], 0230T[1], 0333T[0], 0464T[0], 12001[1], 12002[1], 12004[1], 12005[1], 12006[1], 12007[1], 12011[1], 12013[1], 12014[1], 12015[1], 12016[1], 12017[1], 12018[1], 12020[1], 12021[1], 12031[1], 12032[1], 12034[1], 12035[1], 12036[1], 12037[1], 12041[1], 12042[1], 12044[1], 12045[1], 12046[1], 12047[1], 12051[1], 12052[1], 12053[1], 12054[1], 12055[1], 12056[1], 12057[1],

0 = Modifier usage not allowed or inappropriate 1 = Modifier usage allowed

Appendix A: NCCI - CPT Codes

CPT © 2018 American Medical Association. All Rights Reserved.

Code 1	Code 2
	13100[1], 13101[1], 13102[1], 13120[1], 13121[1], 13122[1], 13131[1], 13132[1], 13133[1], 13151[1], 13152[1], 13153[1], 20605[1], 20610[1], 36000[1], 36140[1], 36400[1], 36405[1], 36406[1], 36410[1], 36420[1], 36425[1], 36430[1], 36440[1], 36591[0], 36592[0], 36600[1], 36640[1], 43752[1], 51701[0], 51702[0], 51703[1], 62270[0], 62272[0], 62284[0], 62322[1], 62323[1], 62326[0], 64483[1], 64484[0], 69990[0], 72275[1], 76000[1], 76800[1], 76942[1], 76970[1], 76998[1], 77001[1], 77002[1], 77003[1], 77012[1], 92012[1], 92014[1], 92585[0], 93000[1], 93005[1], 93010[1], 93040[1], 93041[1], 93042[1], 93318[1], 93355[1], 94002[1], 94200[1], 94250[1], 94680[1], 94681[1], 94690[1], 94770[1], 95812[1], 95813[1], 95816[1], 95819[1], 95822[0], 95829[1], 95860[0], 95861[0], 95863[0], 95864[0], 95865[0], 95866[0], 95867[0], 95868[0], 95869[0], 95870[0], 95907[0], 95908[0], 95909[0], 95910[0], 95911[0], 95912[0], 95913[0], 95925[0], 95926[0], 95927[0], 95928[0], 95929[0], 95930[0], 95933[0], 95937[0], 95938[0], 95939[0], 95940[0], 95941[0], 95955[1], 96360[1], 96361[1], 96365[1], 96366[1], 96367[1], 96368[1], 96372[1], 96374[1], 96375[1], 96376[1], 96377[1], 96522[1], 96523[0], 99155[0], 99156[0], 99157[0], 99211[1], 99212[1], 99213[1], 99214[1], 99215[1], 99217[1], 99218[1], 99219[1], 99220[1], 99221[1], 99222[1], 99223[1], 99231[1], 99232[1], 99233[1], 99234[1], 99235[1], 99236[1], 99238[1], 99239[1], 99241[1], 99242[1], 99243[1], 99244[1], 99245[1], 99251[1], 99252[1], 99253[1], 99254[1], 99255[1], 99291[1], 99292[1], 99304[1], 99305[1], 99306[1], 99307[1], 99308[1], 99309[1], 99310[1], 99315[1], 99316[1], 99334[1], 99335[1], 99336[1], 99337[1], 99347[1], 99348[1], 99349[1], 99350[1], 99374[1], 99375[1], 99377[1], 99378[1], 99446[0], 99447[0], 99448[0], 99449[0], 99451[0], 99452[0], 99495[1], 99496[1], G0453[0], G0459[1], G0463[1], G0471[0], J2001[1]
62350	0213T[0], 0216T[0], 0228T[0], 0230T[0], 0333T[0], 0464T[0], 11000[1], 11001[1], 11004[1], 11005[1], 11006[1], 11042[1], 11043[1], 11044[1], 11045[1], 11046[1], 11047[1], 12001[1], 12002[1], 12004[1], 12005[1], 12006[1], 12007[1], 12011[1], 12013[1], 12014[1], 12015[1], 12016[1], 12017[1], 12018[1], 12020[1], 12021[1], 12031[1], 12032[1], 12034[1], 12035[1], 12036[1], 12037[1], 12041[1], 12042[1], 12044[1], 12045[1], 12046[1], 12047[1], 12051[1], 12052[1], 12053[1], 12054[1], 12055[1], 12056[1], 12057[1], 13100[1], 13101[1], 13102[1], 13120[1], 13121[1], 13122[1], 13131[1], 13132[1], 13133[1], 13151[1], 13152[1], 13153[1], 36000[1], 36400[1], 36405[1], 36406[1], 36410[1], 36420[1], 36425[1], 36430[1], 36440[1], 36591[0], 36592[0], 36600[1], 36640[1], 43752[1], 51701[1], 51702[1], 51703[1], 62270[1], 62272[1], 62273[1], 62280[1], 62281[1], 62282[1], 62320[0], 62321[0], 62322[0], 62323[0], 62324[0], 62325[0], 62326[0], 62327[0], 64400[0], 64402[0], 64405[0], 64408[0], 64410[0], 64413[0], 64415[0], 64416[0], 64417[0], 64418[0], 64420[0], 64421[0], 64425[0], 64430[0], 64435[0], 64445[0], 64446[0], 64447[0], 64448[0], 64449[0], 64450[0], 64461[0], 64462[0], 64463[0], 64479[0], 64480[0], 64483[0], 64484[0], 64486[0], 64487[0], 64488[0], 64489[0], 64490[0], 64491[0], 64492[0], 64493[0], 64494[0], 64495[0], 64505[0], 64510[0], 64517[0], 64520[0], 64530[0], 69990[0], 76000[1], 77001[1], 77002[1], 77003[1], 92012[1], 92014[1], 92585[0], 93000[1], 93005[1], 93010[1], 93040[1], 93041[1], 93042[1], 93318[1], 93355[1], 94002[1], 94200[1], 94250[1], 94680[1], 94681[1], 94690[1], 94770[1], 95812[1], 95813[1], 95816[1], 95819[1], 95822[0], 95829[1], 95860[0], 95861[0], 95863[0], 95864[0], 95865[0], 95866[0], 95867[0], 95868[0], 95869[0], 95870[0], 95907[0], 95908[0], 95909[0], 95910[0], 95911[0], 95912[0], 95913[0], 95925[0], 95926[0], 95927[0], 95928[0], 95929[0], 95930[0], 95933[0], 95937[0], 95938[0], 95939[0], 95940[0], 95955[1], 95990[1], 95991[1], 96360[1], 96361[1], 96365[1], 96366[1], 96367[1], 96368[1], 96372[1], 96374[1], 96375[1], 96376[1], 96377[1], 96521[1], 96522[1], 97597[1], 97598[1], 97602[1], 99155[0], 99156[0], 99157[0], 99211[1], 99212[1], 99213[1], 99214[1], 99215[1], 99217[1], 99218[1], 99219[1], 99220[1], 99221[1], 99222[1], 99223[1], 99231[1], 99232[1], 99233[1], 99234[1], 99235[1], 99236[1], 99238[1], 99239[1], 99241[1], 99242[1], 99243[1], 99244[1], 99245[1], 99251[1], 99252[1], 99253[1], 99254[1], 99255[1], 99291[1], 99292[1], 99304[1], 99305[1], 99306[1], 99307[1], 99308[1], 99309[1], 99310[1], 99315[1], 99316[1], 99334[1], 99335[1], 99336[1], 99337[1], 99347[1], 99348[1], 99349[1], 99350[1], 99374[1], 99375[1], 99377[1], 99378[1], 99446[0], 99447[0], 99448[0], 99449[0], 99451[0], 99452[0], 99495[0], 99496[0], G0453[0], G0463[1], G0471[1]
62351	0213T[0], 0216T[0], 0228T[0], 0230T[0], 0333T[0], 0464T[0], 11000[1], 11001[1], 11004[1], 11005[1], 11006[1], 11042[1], 11043[1], 11044[1], 11045[1], 11046[1], 11047[1], 12001[1], 12002[1], 12004[1], 12005[1], 12006[1], 12007[1], 12011[1], 12013[1], 12014[1], 12015[1], 12016[1], 12017[1], 12018[1], 12020[1], 12021[1], 12031[1], 12032[1], 12034[1], 12035[1], 12036[1], 12037[1], 12041[1], 12042[1], 12044[1], 12045[1], 12046[1], 12047[1], 12051[1], 12052[1], 12053[1], 12054[1], 12055[1], 12056[1], 12057[1], 13100[1], 13101[1], 13102[1], 13120[1], 13121[1], 13122[1], 13131[1], 13132[1], 13133[1], 13151[1], 13152[1], 13153[1], 36000[1], 36400[1], 36405[1], 36406[1], 36410[1], 36420[1], 36425[1], 36430[1], 36440[1], 36591[0], 36592[0], 36600[1], 36640[1], 43752[1], 51701[1], 51702[1], 51703[1], 62280[1], 62281[1], 62282[1], 62320[0], 62321[0], 62322[0], 62323[0], 62324[0], 62325[0], 62326[0], 62327[0], 62350[1], 63707[1], 63709[1], 64400[0], 64402[0], 64405[0], 64408[0], 64410[0], 64413[0], 64415[0], 64416[0], 64417[0], 64418[0], 64420[0], 64421[0], 64425[0], 64430[0], 64435[0], 64445[0], 64446[0], 64447[0], 64448[0], 64449[0], 64450[0], 64461[0], 64462[0], 64463[0], 64479[0], 64480[0], 64483[0], 64484[0], 64486[0], 64487[0], 64488[0], 64489[0], 64490[0], 64491[0], 64492[0], 64493[0], 64494[0], 64495[0], 64505[0], 64510[0], 64517[0], 64520[0], 64530[0], 69990[0], 76000[1], 77001[1], 77002[1], 77003[1], 92012[1], 92014[1], 92585[0], 93000[1], 93005[1], 93010[1], 93040[1], 93041[1], 93042[1], 93318[1], 93355[1], 94002[1], 94200[1], 94250[1], 94680[1], 94681[1], 94690[1], 94770[1], 95812[1], 95813[1], 95816[1], 95819[1], 95822[0], 95829[1], 95860[0], 95861[0], 95863[0], 95864[0], 95865[0], 95866[0], 95867[0], 95868[0], 95869[0], 95870[0], 95907[0], 95908[0], 95909[0], 95910[0], 95911[0], 95912[0], 95913[0], 95925[0], 95926[0], 95927[0], 95928[0], 95929[0], 95930[0], 95933[0], 95937[0], 95938[0], 95939[0], 95940[0], 95955[1], 95990[1], 95991[1], 96360[1], 96361[1], 96365[1], 96366[1], 96367[1], 96368[1], 96372[1], 96374[1], 96375[1], 96376[1], 96377[1], 96522[1], 97597[1], 97598[1], 97602[1], 99155[0], 99156[0], 99157[0], 99211[1], 99212[1], 99213[1], 99214[1], 99215[1], 99217[1], 99218[1], 99219[1], 99220[1], 99221[1], 99222[1], 99223[1], 99231[1], 99232[1], 99233[1], 99234[1], 99235[1], 99236[1], 99238[1], 99239[1], 99241[1], 99242[1], 99243[1], 99244[1], 99245[1], 99251[1], 99252[1], 99253[1], 99254[1], 99255[1], 99291[1], 99292[1], 99304[1], 99305[1], 99306[1], 99307[1], 99308[1], 99309[1], 99310[1], 99315[1], 99316[1], 99334[1], 99335[1], 99336[1], 99337[1], 99347[1], 99348[1], 99349[1], 99350[1], 99374[1], 99375[1], 99377[1], 99378[1], 99446[0], 99447[0], 99448[0], 99449[0], 99451[0], 99452[0], 99495[0], 99496[0], G0453[0], G0463[1], G0471[1]
62355	0213T[0], 0216T[0], 0228T[0], 0230T[0], 0333T[0], 0464T[0], 11000[1], 11001[1], 11004[1], 11005[1], 11006[1], 11042[1], 11043[1], 11044[1], 11045[1], 11046[1], 11047[1], 12001[1], 12002[1], 12004[1], 12005[1], 12006[1], 12007[1], 12011[1], 12013[1], 12014[1], 12015[1], 12016[1], 12017[1], 12018[1], 12020[1], 12021[1], 12031[1], 12032[1], 12034[1], 12035[1], 12036[1], 12037[1], 12041[1], 12042[1], 12044[1], 12045[1], 12046[1], 12047[1], 12051[1], 12052[1], 12053[1], 12054[1], 12055[1], 12056[1], 12057[1], 13100[1], 13101[1], 13102[1], 13120[1], 13121[1], 13122[1], 13131[1], 13132[1], 13133[1], 13151[1], 13152[1], 13153[1], 36000[1], 36400[1], 36405[1], 36406[1], 36410[1], 36420[1], 36425[1], 36430[1], 36440[1], 36591[0], 36592[0], 36600[1], 36640[1], 43752[1], 51701[1], 51702[1], 51703[1], 62270[1], 62272[1], 62320[0], 62321[0], 62322[0], 62323[0], 62324[0], 62325[0], 62326[0], 62327[0], 62350[1], 62351[1], 64400[0], 64402[0], 64405[0], 64408[0], 64410[0], 64413[0], 64415[0], 64416[0], 64417[0], 64418[0], 64420[0], 64421[0], 64425[0], 64430[0], 64435[0], 64445[0], 64446[0], 64447[0], 64448[0], 64449[0], 64450[0], 64461[0], 64462[0], 64463[0], 64479[0], 64480[0], 64483[0], 64484[0], 64486[0], 64487[0], 64488[0], 64489[0], 64490[0], 64491[0], 64492[0], 64493[0], 64494[0], 64495[0], 64505[0], 64510[0], 64517[0], 64520[0], 64530[0], 69990[0], 76000[1], 77001[1], 77002[1], 77003[1], 92012[1], 92014[1], 92585[0], 93000[1], 93005[1], 93010[1], 93040[1], 93041[1], 93042[1], 93318[1], 93355[1], 94002[1], 94200[1], 94250[1], 94680[1], 94681[1], 94690[1], 94770[1], 95812[1], 95813[1], 95816[1], 95819[1], 95822[0], 95829[1], 95860[0], 95861[0], 95863[0], 95864[0], 95865[0], 95866[0], 95867[0], 95868[0], 95869[0], 95870[0], 95907[0], 95908[0], 95909[0], 95910[0], 95911[0], 95912[0], 95913[0], 95925[0], 95926[0], 95927[0], 95928[0], 95929[0], 95930[0], 95933[0], 95937[0], 95938[0], 95939[0], 95940[0], 95955[1], 96360[1], 96361[1], 96365[1], 96366[1], 96367[1], 96368[1], 96372[1], 96374[1], 96375[1], 96376[1], 96377[1], 97597[1], 97598[1], 97602[1], 99155[0], 99156[0], 99157[0], 99211[1], 99212[1], 99213[1], 99214[1], 99215[1], 99217[1], 99218[1], 99219[1], 99220[1], 99221[1], 99222[1], 99223[1], 99231[1], 99232[1], 99233[1], 99234[1], 99235[1], 99236[1], 99238[1], 99239[1], 99241[1], 99242[1], 99243[1], 99244[1], 99245[1], 99251[1], 99252[1], 99253[1], 99254[1], 99255[1], 99291[1], 99292[1], 99304[1], 99305[1], 99306[1], 99307[1], 99308[1], 99309[1], 99310[1], 99315[1], 99316[1], 99334[1], 99335[1], 99336[1], 99337[1], 99347[1], 99348[1], 99349[1], 99350[1], 99374[1], 99375[1], 99377[1], 99378[1], 99446[0], 99447[0], 99448[0], 99449[0], 99451[0], 99452[0], 99495[0], 99496[0], G0453[0], G0463[1], G0471[1]
62360	0213T[0], 0216T[0], 0228T[0], 0230T[0], 0333T[0], 0464T[0], 11000[1], 11001[1], 11004[1], 11005[1], 11006[1], 11042[1], 11043[1], 11044[1], 11045[1], 11046[1], 11047[1], 12001[1], 12002[1], 12004[1], 12005[1], 12006[1], 12007[1], 12011[1], 12013[1], 12014[1], 12015[1], 12016[1], 12017[1], 12018[1], 12020[1], 12021[1], 12031[1], 12032[1], 12034[1], 12035[1], 12036[1], 12037[1], 12041[1], 12042[1], 12044[1], 12045[1], 12046[1], 12047[1], 12051[1], 12052[1], 12053[1], 12054[1], 12055[1], 12056[1], 12057[1], 13100[1], 13101[1], 13102[1], 13120[1], 13121[1], 13122[1], 13131[1], 13132[1], 13133[1], 13151[1], 13152[1], 13153[1], 36000[1], 36400[1], 36405[1], 36406[1], 36410[1], 36420[1], 36425[1], 36430[1], 36440[1], 36591[0], 36592[0], 36600[1], 36640[1], 43752[1], 51701[1], 51702[1], 51703[1], 62270[1], 62272[1], 62273[1], 62280[1], 62281[1], 62282[1], 62320[0], 62321[0], 62322[0], 62323[0], 62324[0], 62325[0], 62326[0], 62327[0], 62362[1], 62365[0], 62367[1], 62368[1], 62369[1], 62370[1], 64400[0], 64402[0], 64405[0], 64408[0], 64410[0], 64413[0], 64415[0], 64416[0], 64417[0], 64418[0], 64420[0], 64421[0], 64425[0], 64430[0], 64435[0], 64445[0], 64446[0], 64447[0], 64448[0], 64449[0], 64450[0], 64461[0], 64462[0], 64463[0], 64479[0], 64480[0], 64483[0], 64484[0], 64486[0], 64487[0], 64488[0], 64489[0], 64490[0], 64491[0], 64492[0], 64493[0], 64494[0], 64495[0], 64505[0], 64510[0], 64517[0], 64520[0], 64530[0], 69990[0], 76000[1], 77001[1], 77002[1], 92012[1], 92014[1], 92585[0], 93000[1], 93005[1], 93010[1], 93040[1], 93041[1], 93042[1], 93318[1], 93355[1], 94002[1], 94200[1], 94250[1], 94680[1], 94681[1], 94690[1], 94770[1], 95812[1], 95813[1], 95816[1], 95819[1], 95822[0], 95829[1], 95860[0], 95861[0], 95863[0], 95864[0], 95865[0], 95866[0], 95867[0], 95868[0], 95869[0], 95870[0], 95907[0], 95908[0], 95909[0], 95910[0], 95911[0], 95912[0], 95913[0], 95925[0], 95926[0], 95927[0], 95928[0], 95929[0], 95930[0], 95933[0], 95937[0], 95938[0], 95939[0], 95940[0], 95955[1], 95990[1], 95991[1], 96360[1], 96361[1], 96365[1], 96366[1], 96367[1], 96368[1], 96372[1], 96374[1], 96375[1], 96376[1], 96377[1], 96522[1], 97597[1], 97598[1], 97602[1], 99155[0], 99156[0], 99157[0], 99211[1], 99212[1], 99213[1], 99214[1], 99215[1], 99217[1], 99218[1], 99219[1], 99220[1], 99221[1], 99222[1], 99223[1], 99231[1], 99232[1], 99233[1], 99234[1], 99235[1], 99236[1], 99238[1], 99239[1], 99241[1], 99242[1], 99243[1], 99244[1], 99245[1], 99251[1], 99252[1], 99253[1], 99254[1], 99255[1], 99291[1], 99292[1], 99304[1], 99305[1], 99306[1], 99307[1], 99308[1], 99309[1], 99310[1], 99315[1], 99316[1], 99334[1], 99335[1], 99336[1], 99337[1], 99347[1], 99348[1], 99349[1], 99350[1], 99374[1], 99375[1], 99377[1], 99378[1], 99446[0], 99447[0], 99448[0], 99449[0], 99451[0], 99452[0], 99495[0], 99496[0], G0453[0], G0463[1], G0471[1]

0 = Modifier usage not allowed or inappropriate 1 = Modifier usage allowed

CPT © 2018 American Medical Association. All Rights Reserved.

Code 1	Code 2
62361	0213T[0], 0216T[0], 0228T[0], 0230T[0], 0333T[0], 0464T[0], 11000[1], 11001[1], 11004[1], 11005[1], 11006[1], 11042[1], 11043[1], 11044[1], 11045[1], 11046[1], 11047[1], 12001[1], 12002[1], 12004[1], 12005[1], 12006[1], 12007[1], 12011[1], 12013[1], 12014[1], 12015[1], 12016[1], 12017[1], 12018[1], 12020[1], 12021[1], 12031[1], 12032[1], 12034[1], 12035[1], 12036[1], 12037[1], 12041[1], 12042[1], 12044[1], 12045[1], 12046[1], 12047[1], 12051[1], 12052[1], 12053[1], 12054[1], 12055[1], 12056[1], 12057[1], 13100[1], 13101[1], 13102[1], 13120[1], 13121[1], 13122[1], 13131[1], 13132[1], 13133[1], 13151[1], 13152[1], 13153[1], 36000[1], 36400[1], 36405[1], 36406[1], 36410[1], 36420[1], 36425[1], 36430[1], 36440[1], 36591[0], 36592[0], 36600[1], 36640[1], 43752[1], 51701[1], 51702[1], 51703[1], 62270[1], 62272[1], 62273[1], 62280[1], 62281[1], 62282[1], 62320[0], 62321[0], 62322[0], 62323[0], 62324[0], 62325[0], 62326[0], 62327[0], 62360[1], 62365[0], 62367[1], 62368[1], 62369[1], 62370[1], 64400[0], 64402[0], 64405[0], 64408[0], 64410[0], 64413[0], 64415[0], 64416[0], 64417[0], 64418[0], 64420[0], 64421[0], 64425[0], 64430[0], 64435[0], 64445[0], 64446[0], 64447[0], 64448[0], 64449[0], 64450[0], 64461[0], 64462[0], 64463[0], 64479[0], 64480[0], 64483[0], 64484[0], 64486[0], 64487[0], 64488[0], 64489[0], 64490[0], 64491[0], 64492[0], 64493[0], 64494[0], 64495[0], 64505[0], 64510[0], 64517[0], 64520[0], 64530[0], 69990[0], 76000[1], 77001[1], 77002[1], 92012[1], 92014[1], 92585[0], 93000[1], 93005[1], 93010[1], 93040[1], 93041[1], 93042[1], 93318[1], 93355[1], 94002[1], 94200[1], 94250[1], 94680[1], 94681[1], 94690[1], 94770[1], 95812[1], 95813[1], 95816[1], 95819[1], 95822[0], 95829[1], 95860[0], 95861[0], 95863[0], 95864[0], 95865[0], 95866[0], 95867[0], 95868[0], 95869[0], 95870[0], 95907[0], 95908[0], 95909[0], 95910[0], 95911[0], 95912[0], 95913[0], 95925[0], 95926[0], 95927[0], 95928[0], 95929[0], 95930[0], 95933[0], 95937[0], 95938[0], 95939[0], 95940[0], 95955[1], 95990[1], 95991[1], 96360[1], 96361[1], 96365[1], 96366[1], 96367[1], 96368[1], 96372[1], 96374[1], 96375[1], 96376[1], 96377[1], 96522[1], 97597[1], 97598[1], 97602[1], 99155[0], 99156[0], 99157[0], 99211[1], 99212[1], 99213[1], 99214[1], 99215[1], 99217[1], 99218[1], 99219[1], 99220[1], 99221[1], 99222[1], 99223[1], 99231[1], 99232[1], 99233[1], 99234[1], 99235[1], 99236[1], 99238[1], 99239[1], 99241[1], 99242[1], 99243[1], 99244[1], 99245[1], 99251[1], 99252[1], 99253[1], 99254[1], 99255[1], 99291[1], 99292[1], 99304[1], 99305[1], 99306[1], 99307[1], 99308[1], 99309[1], 99310[1], 99315[1], 99316[1], 99334[1], 99335[1], 99336[1], 99337[1], 99347[1], 99348[1], 99349[1], 99350[1], 99374[1], 99375[1], 99377[1], 99378[1], 99446[0], 99447[0], 99448[0], 99449[0], 99451[0], 99452[0], 99495[0], 99496[0], G0453[0], G0463[1], G0471[1]
62362	0213T[0], 0216T[0], 0228T[0], 0230T[0], 0333T[0], 0464T[0], 11000[1], 11001[1], 11004[1], 11005[1], 11006[1], 11042[1], 11043[1], 11044[1], 11045[1], 11046[1], 11047[1], 12001[1], 12002[1], 12004[1], 12005[1], 12006[1], 12007[1], 12011[1], 12013[1], 12014[1], 12015[1], 12016[1], 12017[1], 12018[1], 12020[1], 12021[1], 12031[1], 12032[1], 12034[1], 12035[1], 12036[1], 12037[1], 12041[1], 12042[1], 12044[1], 12045[1], 12046[1], 12047[1], 12051[1], 12052[1], 12053[1], 12054[1], 12055[1], 12056[1], 12057[1], 13100[1], 13101[1], 13102[1], 13120[1], 13121[1], 13122[1], 13131[1], 13132[1], 13133[1], 13151[1], 13152[1], 13153[1], 36000[1], 36400[1], 36405[1], 36406[1], 36410[1], 36420[1], 36425[1], 36430[1], 36440[1], 36591[0], 36592[0], 36600[1], 36640[1], 43752[1], 51701[1], 51702[1], 51703[1], 62270[1], 62272[1], 62273[1], 62280[1], 62281[1], 62282[1], 62320[0], 62321[0], 62322[0], 62323[0], 62324[0], 62325[0], 62326[0], 62327[0], 62361[1], 62365[0], 62367[1], 62368[1], 62369[1], 62370[1], 64400[0], 64402[0], 64405[0], 64408[0], 64410[0], 64413[0], 64415[0], 64416[0], 64417[0], 64418[0], 64420[0], 64421[0], 64425[0], 64430[0], 64435[0], 64445[0], 64446[0], 64447[0], 64448[0], 64449[0], 64450[0], 64461[0], 64462[0], 64463[0], 64479[0], 64480[0], 64483[0], 64484[0], 64486[0], 64487[0], 64488[0], 64489[0], 64490[0], 64491[0], 64492[0], 64493[0], 64494[0], 64495[0], 64505[0], 64510[0], 64517[0], 64520[0], 64530[0], 69990[0], 76000[1], 77001[1], 77002[1], 92012[1], 92014[1], 92585[0], 93000[1], 93005[1], 93010[1], 93040[1], 93041[1], 93042[1], 93318[1], 93355[1], 94002[1], 94200[1], 94250[1], 94680[1], 94681[1], 94690[1], 94770[1], 95812[1], 95813[1], 95816[1], 95819[1], 95822[0], 95829[1], 95860[0], 95861[0], 95863[0], 95864[0], 95865[0], 95866[0], 95867[0], 95868[0], 95869[0], 95870[0], 95907[0], 95908[0], 95909[0], 95910[0], 95911[0], 95912[0], 95913[0], 95925[0], 95926[0], 95927[0], 95928[0], 95929[0], 95930[0], 95933[0], 95937[0], 95938[0], 95939[0], 95940[0], 95955[1], 95990[0], 95991[1], 96360[1], 96361[1], 96365[1], 96366[1], 96367[1], 96368[1], 96372[1], 96374[1], 96375[1], 96376[1], 96377[1], 96522[1], 97597[1], 97598[1], 97602[1], 99155[0], 99156[0], 99157[0], 99211[1], 99212[1], 99213[1], 99214[1], 99215[1], 99217[1], 99218[1], 99219[1], 99220[1], 99221[1], 99222[1], 99223[1], 99231[1], 99232[1], 99233[1], 99234[1], 99235[1], 99236[1], 99238[1], 99239[1], 99241[1], 99242[1], 99243[1], 99244[1], 99245[1], 99251[1], 99252[1], 99253[1], 99254[1], 99255[1], 99291[1], 99292[1], 99304[1], 99305[1], 99306[1], 99307[1], 99308[1], 99309[1], 99310[1], 99315[1], 99316[1], 99334[1], 99335[1], 99336[1], 99337[1], 99347[1], 99348[1], 99349[1], 99350[1], 99374[1], 99375[1], 99377[1], 99378[1], 99446[0], 99447[0], 99448[0], 99449[0], 99451[0], 99452[0], 99495[0], 99496[0], G0453[0], G0463[1], G0471[1]
62367	0213T[1], 0216T[1], 0333T[0], 0464T[0], 36000[1], 36410[1], 36591[0], 36592[0], 61650[1], 62324[1], 62325[1], 62326[1], 62327[1], 64415[1], 64416[1], 64417[1], 64450[1], 64486[1], 64487[1], 64488[1], 64489[1], 64490[1], 69990[0], 92585[0], 95822[0], 95860[0], 95861[0], 95863[0], 95864[0], 95865[0], 95866[0], 95867[0], 95868[0], 95869[0], 95870[0], 95907[0], 95908[0], 95909[0], 95910[0], 95911[0], 95912[0], 95913[0], 95925[0], 95926[0], 95927[0], 95928[0], 95929[0], 95930[0], 95933[0], 95937[0], 95938[0], 95939[0], 95940[0], 96360[1], 96365[1], 96522[1], G0453[0]
62368	0213T[1], 0216T[1], 0333T[0], 0464T[0], 36000[1], 36410[1], 36591[0], 36592[0], 61650[1], 62324[1], 62325[1], 62326[1], 62327[1], 62367[0], 64415[1], 64416[1], 64417[1], 64450[1], 64486[1], 64487[1], 64488[1], 64489[1], 64490[1], 69990[0], 92585[0], 95822[0], 95860[0], 95861[0], 95863[0], 95864[0], 95865[0], 95866[0], 95867[0], 95868[0], 95869[0], 95870[0], 95907[0], 95908[0], 95909[0], 95910[0], 95911[0], 95912[0], 95913[0], 95925[0], 95926[0], 95927[0], 95928[0], 95929[0], 95930[0], 95933[0], 95937[0], 95938[0], 95939[0], 95940[0], 96360[1], 96365[1], 96522[1], G0453[0]
62369	0213T[1], 0216T[1], 0333T[0], 0464T[0], 36000[1], 36410[1], 36591[0], 36592[0], 61650[1], 62324[1], 62325[1], 62326[1], 62327[1], 62367[0], 62368[0], 64415[1], 64416[1], 64417[1], 64450[1], 64486[1], 64487[1], 64488[1], 64489[1], 64490[1], 69990[0], 92585[0], 95822[0], 95860[0], 95861[0], 95863[0], 95864[0], 95865[0], 95866[0], 95867[0], 95868[0], 95869[0], 95870[0], 95907[0], 95908[0], 95909[0], 95910[0], 95911[0], 95912[0], 95913[0], 95925[0], 95926[0], 95927[0], 95928[0], 95929[0], 95930[0], 95933[0], 95937[0], 95938[0], 95939[0], 95940[0], 95990[0], 95991[0], 96360[1], 96365[1], A4220[0], G0453[0]
62370	0213T[1], 0216T[1], 0333T[0], 0464T[0], 36000[1], 36410[1], 36591[0], 36592[0], 61650[1], 62324[1], 62325[1], 62326[1], 62327[1], 62367[0], 62368[0], 62369[0], 64415[1], 64416[1], 64417[1], 64450[1], 64486[1], 64487[1], 64488[1], 64489[1], 64490[1], 69990[0], 92585[0], 95822[0], 95860[0], 95861[0], 95863[0], 95864[0], 95865[0], 95866[0], 95867[0], 95868[0], 95869[0], 95870[0], 95907[0], 95908[0], 95909[0], 95910[0], 95911[0], 95912[0], 95913[0], 95925[0], 95926[0], 95927[0], 95928[0], 95929[0], 95930[0], 95933[0], 95937[0], 95938[0], 95939[0], 95940[0], 95990[0], 95991[0], 96360[1], 96365[1], 96522[1], A4220[0], G0453[0]
62380	0202T[1], 0213T[0], 0216T[0], 0228T[0], 0230T[0], 0275T[1], 0333T[0], 0464T[0], 11000[1], 11001[1], 11004[1], 11005[1], 11006[1], 11042[1], 11043[1], 11044[1], 11045[1], 11046[1], 11047[1], 12001[1], 12002[1], 12004[1], 12005[1], 12006[1], 12007[1], 12011[1], 12013[1], 12014[1], 12015[1], 12016[1], 12017[1], 12018[1], 12020[1], 12021[1], 12031[1], 12032[1], 12034[1], 12035[1], 12036[1], 12037[1], 12041[1], 12042[1], 12044[1], 12045[1], 12046[1], 12047[1], 12051[1], 12052[1], 12053[1], 12054[1], 12055[1], 12056[1], 12057[1], 13100[1], 13101[1], 13102[1], 13120[1], 13121[1], 13122[1], 13131[1], 13132[1], 13133[1], 13151[1], 13152[1], 13153[1], 20251[1], 20926[1], 22102[1], 22208[1], 22505[0], 36000[1], 36400[1], 36405[1], 36406[1], 36410[1], 36420[1], 36425[1], 36430[1], 36440[1], 36591[0], 36592[0], 36600[1], 36640[1], 38220[0], 38222[0], 38230[0], 38232[0], 43752[1], 51701[1], 51702[1], 51703[1], 61783[1], 62284[1], 62290[0], 62320[0], 62321[0], 62322[0], 62323[0], 62324[0], 62325[0], 62326[0], 62327[0], 63707[1], 63709[1], 64400[0], 64402[0], 64405[0], 64408[0], 64410[0], 64413[0], 64415[0], 64416[0], 64417[0], 64418[0], 64420[0], 64421[0], 64425[0], 64430[0], 64435[0], 64445[0], 64446[0], 64447[0], 64448[0], 64449[0], 64450[0], 64461[0], 64462[0], 64463[0], 64479[0], 64480[0], 64483[0], 64484[0], 64486[0], 64487[0], 64488[0], 64489[0], 64490[0], 64491[0], 64492[0], 64493[0], 64494[0], 64495[0], 64505[0], 64510[0], 64517[0], 64520[0], 64530[0], 64722[1], 69990[0], 72295[0], 76000[1], 77001[1], 77002[1], 77003[1], 92012[1], 92014[1], 92585[0], 93000[1], 93005[1], 93010[1], 93040[1], 93041[1], 93042[1], 93318[1], 93355[1], 94002[1], 94200[1], 94250[1], 94680[1], 94681[1], 94690[1], 94770[1], 95812[1], 95813[1], 95816[1], 95819[1], 95822[0], 95829[1], 95860[0], 95861[0], 95863[0], 95864[0], 95865[0], 95866[0], 95867[0], 95868[0], 95869[0], 95870[0], 95907[0], 95908[0], 95909[0], 95910[0], 95911[0], 95912[0], 95913[0], 95925[0], 95926[0], 95927[0], 95928[0], 95929[0], 95930[0], 95933[0], 95937[0], 95938[0], 95939[0], 95940[0], 95941[0], 95955[1], 96360[1], 96361[1], 96365[1], 96366[1], 96367[1], 96368[1], 96372[1], 96374[1], 96375[1], 96376[1], 96377[1], 96523[0], 97597[1], 97598[1], 97602[1], 99155[0], 99156[0], 99157[0], 99211[1], 99212[1], 99213[1], 99214[1], 99215[1], 99217[1], 99218[1], 99219[1], 99220[1], 99221[1], 99222[1], 99223[1], 99231[1], 99232[1], 99233[1], 99234[1], 99235[1], 99236[1], 99238[1], 99239[1], 99241[1], 99242[1], 99243[1], 99244[1], 99245[1], 99251[1], 99252[1], 99253[1], 99254[1], 99255[1], 99291[1], 99292[1], 99304[1], 99305[1], 99306[1], 99307[1], 99308[1], 99309[1], 99310[1], 99315[1], 99316[1], 99334[1], 99335[1], 99336[1], 99337[1], 99347[1], 99348[1], 99349[1], 99350[1], 99374[1], 99375[1], 99377[1], 99378[1], 99446[0], 99447[0], 99448[0], 99449[0], 99451[0], 99452[0], 99495[0], 99496[0], G0276[0], G0453[0], G0463[1], G0471[1]
63650	01935[0], 01936[0], 0213T[0], 0216T[0], 0228T[0], 0230T[0], 0333T[0], 0464T[0], 12001[1], 12002[1], 12004[1], 12005[1], 12006[1], 12007[1], 12011[1], 12013[1], 12014[1], 12015[1], 12016[1], 12017[1], 12018[1], 12020[1], 12021[1], 12031[1], 12032[1], 12034[1], 12035[1], 12036[1], 12037[1], 12041[1], 12042[1], 12044[1], 12045[1], 12046[1], 12047[1], 12051[1], 12052[1], 12053[1], 12054[1], 12055[1], 12056[1], 12057[1], 13100[1], 13101[1], 13102[1], 13120[1], 13121[1], 13122[1], 13131[1], 13132[1], 13133[1], 13151[1], 13152[1], 13153[1], 22505[0], 36000[1], 36400[1], 36405[1], 36406[1], 36410[1], 36420[1], 36425[1], 36430[1], 36440[1], 36591[0], 36592[0], 36600[1], 36640[1], 43752[1], 51701[1], 51702[1], 51703[1], 62320[0], 62321[0], 62322[0], 62323[0], 62324[0], 62325[0], 62326[0], 62327[0], 63610[0], 63655[1], 63661[0], 64400[0], 64402[0], 64405[0], 64408[0], 64410[0], 64413[0], 64415[0], 64416[0], 64417[0], 64418[0], 64420[0], 64421[0], 64425[0], 64430[0], 64435[0], 64445[0], 64446[0], 64447[0], 64448[0], 64449[0], 64450[0], 64461[0], 64462[0], 64463[0], 64479[0], 64480[0], 64483[0], 64484[0], 64486[0], 64487[0], 64488[0], 64489[0], 64490[0], 64491[0], 64492[0], 64493[0], 64494[0], 64495[0], 64505[0], 64510[0], 64517[0], 64520[0], 64530[0], 69990[0], 76000[1], 77001[1], 77002[1], 77003[1], 92012[1], 92014[1], 92585[0], 93000[1], 93005[1], 93010[1], 93040[1], 93041[1], 93042[1], 93318[1], 93355[1], 94002[1], 94200[1], 94250[1], 94680[1], 94681[1], 94690[1], 94770[1], 95812[1],

Appendix A: NCCI - CPT Codes

0 = Modifier usage not allowed or inappropriate 1 = Modifier usage allowed

CPT © 2018 American Medical Association. All Rights Reserved.

Code 1	Code 2
	95813^1, 95816^1, 95819^1, 95822^0, 95829^1, 95860^0, 95861^0, 95863^0, 95864^0, 95865^0, 95866^0, 95867^0, 95868^0, 95869^0, 95870^0, 95907^0, 95908^0, 95909^0, 95910^0, 95911^0, 95912^0, 95913^0, 95925^0, 95926^0, 95927^0, 95928^0, 95929^0, 95930^0, 95933^0, 95937^0, 95938^0, 95939^0, 95940^0, 95955^1, 95970^1, 95971^1, 95972^1, 96360^1, 96361^1, 96365^1, 96366^1, 96367^1, 96368^1, 96372^1, 96374^1, 96375^1, 96376^1, 96377^1, 99155^0, 99156^0, 99157^0, 99211^1, 99212^1, 99213^1, 99214^1, 99215^1, 99217^1, 99218^1, 99219^1, 99220^1, 99221^1, 99222^1, 99223^1, 99231^1, 99232^1, 99233^1, 99234^1, 99235^1, 99236^1, 99238^1, 99239^1, 99241^1, 99242^1, 99243^1, 99244^1, 99245^1, 99251^1, 99252^1, 99253^1, 99254^1, 99255^1, 99291^1, 99292^1, 99304^1, 99305^1, 99306^1, 99307^1, 99308^1, 99309^1, 99310^1, 99315^1, 99316^1, 99334^1, 99335^1, 99336^1, 99337^1, 99347^1, 99348^1, 99349^1, 99350^1, 99374^1, 99375^1, 99377^1, 99378^1, 99446^0, 99447^0, 99448^0, 99449^0, 99451^0, 99452^0, 99495^0, 99496^0, G0453^0, G0463^1, G0471^1
63655	0213T^0, 0216T^0, 0228T^0, 0230T^0, 0333T^0, 0464T^0, 11000^1, 11001^1, 11004^1, 11005^1, 11006^1, 11042^1, 11043^1, 11044^1, 11045^1, 11046^1, 11047^1, 12001^1, 12002^1, 12004^1, 12005^1, 12006^1, 12007^1, 12011^1, 12013^1, 12014^1, 12015^1, 12016^1, 12017^1, 12018^1, 12020^1, 12021^1, 12031^1, 12032^1, 12034^1, 12035^1, 12036^1, 12037^1, 12041^1, 12042^1, 12044^1, 12045^1, 12046^1, 12047^1, 12051^1, 12052^1, 12053^1, 12054^1, 12055^1, 12056^1, 12057^1, 13100^1, 13101^1, 13102^1, 13120^1, 13121^1, 13122^1, 13131^1, 13132^1, 13133^1, 13151^1, 13152^1, 13153^1, 20926^1, 22505^0, 36000^1, 36400^1, 36405^1, 36406^1, 36410^1, 36420^1, 36425^1, 36430^1, 36440^1, 36591^0, 36592^0, 36600^1, 36640^1, 43752^1, 51701^1, 51702^1, 51703^1, 62320^0, 62321^0, 62322^0, 62323^0, 62324^0, 62325^0, 62326^0, 62327^0, 63610^0, 63662^0, 63663^0, 63707^1, 63709^1, 64400^0, 64402^0, 64405^0, 64408^0, 64410^0, 64413^0, 64415^0, 64416^0, 64417^0, 64418^0, 64420^0, 64421^0, 64425^0, 64430^0, 64435^0, 64445^0, 64446^0, 64447^0, 64448^0, 64449^0, 64450^0, 64461^0, 64462^0, 64463^0, 64479^0, 64480^0, 64483^0, 64484^0, 64486^0, 64487^0, 64488^0, 64489^0, 64490^0, 64491^0, 64492^0, 64493^0, 64494^0, 64495^0, 64505^0, 64510^0, 64517^0, 64520^0, 64530^0, 69990^0, 76000^1, 77001^1, 77002^1, 77003^1, 92012^1, 92014^1, 92585^0, 93000^1, 93005^1, 93010^1, 93040^1, 93041^1, 93042^1, 93318^1, 93355^1, 94002^1, 94200^1, 94250^1, 94680^1, 94681^1, 94690^1, 94770^1, 95812^1, 95813^1, 95816^1, 95819^1, 95822^0, 95829^1, 95860^0, 95861^0, 95863^0, 95864^0, 95865^0, 95866^0, 95867^0, 95868^0, 95869^0, 95870^0, 95907^0, 95908^0, 95909^0, 95910^0, 95911^0, 95912^0, 95913^0, 95925^0, 95926^0, 95927^0, 95928^0, 95929^0, 95930^0, 95933^0, 95937^0, 95938^0, 95939^0, 95940^0, 95955^1, 95970^1, 95971^1, 95972^1, 96360^1, 96361^1, 96365^1, 96366^1, 96367^1, 96368^1, 96372^1, 96374^1, 96375^1, 96376^1, 96377^1, 97597^1, 97598^1, 97602^1, 99155^0, 99156^0, 99157^0, 99211^1, 99212^1, 99213^1, 99214^1, 99215^1, 99217^1, 99218^1, 99219^1, 99220^1, 99221^1, 99222^1, 99223^1, 99231^1, 99232^1, 99233^1, 99234^1, 99235^1, 99236^1, 99238^1, 99239^1, 99241^1, 99242^1, 99243^1, 99244^1, 99245^1, 99251^1, 99252^1, 99253^1, 99254^1, 99255^1, 99291^1, 99292^1, 99304^1, 99305^1, 99306^1, 99307^1, 99308^1, 99309^1, 99310^1, 99315^1, 99316^1, 99334^1, 99335^1, 99336^1, 99337^1, 99347^1, 99348^1, 99349^1, 99350^1, 99374^1, 99375^1, 99377^1, 99378^1, 99446^0, 99447^0, 99448^0, 99449^0, 99451^0, 99452^0, 99495^0, 99496^0, G0453^0, G0463^1, G0471^1
63661	01935^0, 01936^0, 0213T^0, 0216T^0, 0228T^0, 0230T^0, 0333T^0, 0464T^0, 11000^1, 11001^1, 11004^1, 11005^1, 11006^1, 11042^1, 11043^1, 11044^1, 11045^1, 11046^1, 11047^1, 12001^1, 12002^1, 12004^1, 12005^1, 12006^1, 12007^1, 12011^1, 12013^1, 12014^1, 12015^1, 12016^1, 12017^1, 12018^1, 12020^1, 12021^1, 12031^1, 12032^1, 12034^1, 12035^1, 12036^1, 12037^1, 12041^1, 12042^1, 12044^1, 12045^1, 12046^1, 12047^1, 12051^1, 12052^1, 12053^1, 12054^1, 12055^1, 12056^1, 12057^1, 13100^1, 13101^1, 13102^1, 13120^1, 13121^1, 13122^1, 13131^1, 13132^1, 13133^1, 13151^1, 13152^1, 13153^1, 22505^0, 36000^1, 36400^1, 36405^1, 36406^1, 36410^1, 36420^1, 36425^1, 36430^1, 36440^1, 36591^0, 36592^0, 36600^1, 36640^1, 43752^1, 51701^1, 51702^1, 51703^1, 62273^1, 62320^0, 62321^0, 62322^0, 62323^0, 62324^0, 62325^0, 62326^0, 62327^0, 63610^0, 64400^0, 64402^0, 64405^0, 64408^0, 64410^0, 64413^0, 64415^0, 64416^0, 64417^0, 64418^0, 64420^0, 64421^0, 64425^0, 64430^0, 64435^0, 64445^0, 64446^0, 64447^0, 64448^0, 64449^0, 64450^0, 64461^0, 64462^0, 64463^0, 64479^0, 64480^0, 64483^0, 64484^0, 64486^0, 64487^0, 64488^0, 64489^0, 64490^0, 64491^0, 64492^0, 64493^0, 64494^0, 64495^0, 64505^0, 64510^0, 64517^0, 64520^0, 64530^0, 69990^0, 76000^1, 77001^1, 77002^1, 77003^1, 92012^1, 92014^1, 92585^0, 93000^1, 93005^1, 93010^1, 93040^1, 93041^1, 93042^1, 93318^1, 93355^1, 94002^1, 94200^1, 94250^1, 94680^1, 94681^1, 94690^1, 94770^1, 95812^1, 95813^1, 95816^1, 95819^1, 95822^0, 95829^1, 95860^0, 95861^0, 95863^0, 95864^0, 95865^0, 95866^0, 95867^0, 95868^0, 95869^0, 95870^0, 95907^0, 95908^0, 95909^0, 95910^0, 95911^0, 95912^0, 95913^0, 95925^0, 95926^0, 95927^0, 95928^0, 95929^0, 95930^0, 95933^0, 95937^0, 95938^0, 95939^0, 95940^0, 95955^1, 95970^1, 95971^1, 95972^1, 96360^1, 96361^1, 96365^1, 96366^1, 96367^1, 96368^1, 96372^1, 96374^1, 96375^1, 96376^1, 96377^1, 97597^1, 97598^1, 97602^1, 99155^0, 99156^0, 99157^0, 99211^1, 99212^1, 99213^1, 99214^1, 99215^1, 99217^1, 99218^1, 99219^1, 99220^1, 99221^1, 99222^1, 99223^1, 99231^1, 99232^1, 99233^1, 99234^1, 99235^1, 99236^1, 99238^1, 99239^1, 99241^1, 99242^1, 99243^1, 99244^1, 99245^1, 99251^1, 99252^1, 99253^1, 99254^1, 99255^1, 99291^1, 99292^1, 99304^1, 99305^1, 99306^1, 99307^1, 99308^1, 99309^1, 99310^1, 99315^1, 99316^1, 99334^1, 99335^1, 99336^1, 99337^1, 99347^1, 99348^1, 99349^1, 99350^1, 99374^1, 99375^1, 99377^1, 99378^1, 99446^0, 99447^0, 99448^0, 99449^0, 99451^0, 99452^0, 99495^0, 99496^0, G0453^0, G0463^1, G0471^1
63662	0213T^0, 0216T^0, 0228T^0, 0230T^0, 0333T^0, 0464T^0, 11000^1, 11001^1, 11004^1, 11005^1, 11006^1, 11042^1, 11043^1, 11044^1, 11045^1, 11046^1, 11047^1, 12001^1, 12002^1, 12004^1, 12005^1, 12006^1, 12007^1, 12011^1, 12013^1, 12014^1, 12015^1, 12016^1, 12017^1, 12018^1, 12020^1, 12021^1, 12031^1, 12032^1, 12034^1, 12035^1, 12036^1, 12037^1, 12041^1, 12042^1, 12044^1, 12045^1, 12046^1, 12047^1, 12051^1, 12052^1, 12053^1, 12054^1, 12055^1, 12056^1, 12057^1, 13100^1, 13101^1, 13102^1, 13120^1, 13121^1, 13122^1, 13131^1, 13132^1, 13133^1, 13151^1, 13152^1, 13153^1, 22505^0, 36000^1, 36400^1, 36405^1, 36406^1, 36410^1, 36420^1, 36425^1, 36430^1, 36440^1, 36591^0, 36592^0, 36600^1, 36640^1, 43752^1, 51701^1, 51702^1, 51703^1, 62263^1, 62273^1, 62320^0, 62321^0, 62322^0, 62323^0, 62324^0, 62325^0, 62326^0, 62327^0, 63610^0, 63650^1, 63661^1, 63663^1, 63707^1, 63709^1, 64400^0, 64402^0, 64405^0, 64408^0, 64410^0, 64413^0, 64415^0, 64416^0, 64417^0, 64418^0, 64420^0, 64421^0, 64425^0, 64430^0, 64435^0, 64445^0, 64446^0, 64447^0, 64448^0, 64449^0, 64450^0, 64461^0, 64462^0, 64463^0, 64479^0, 64480^0, 64483^0, 64484^0, 64486^0, 64487^0, 64488^0, 64489^0, 64490^0, 64491^0, 64492^0, 64493^0, 64494^0, 64495^0, 64505^0, 64510^0, 64517^0, 64520^0, 64530^0, 69990^0, 76000^1, 77001^1, 77002^1, 77003^1, 92012^1, 92014^1, 92585^0, 93000^1, 93005^1, 93010^1, 93040^1, 93041^1, 93042^1, 93318^1, 93355^1, 94002^1, 94200^1, 94250^1, 94680^1, 94681^1, 94690^1, 94770^1, 95812^1, 95813^1, 95816^1, 95819^1, 95822^0, 95829^1, 95860^0, 95861^0, 95863^0, 95864^0, 95865^0, 95866^0, 95867^0, 95868^0, 95869^0, 95870^0, 95907^0, 95908^0, 95909^0, 95910^0, 95911^0, 95912^0, 95913^0, 95925^0, 95926^0, 95927^0, 95928^0, 95929^0, 95930^0, 95933^0, 95937^0, 95938^0, 95939^0, 95940^0, 95955^1, 95970^1, 95971^1, 95972^1, 96360^1, 96361^1, 96365^1, 96366^1, 96367^1, 96368^1, 96372^1, 96374^1, 96375^1, 96376^1, 96377^1, 97597^1, 97598^1, 97602^1, 99155^0, 99156^0, 99157^0, 99211^1, 99212^1, 99213^1, 99214^1, 99215^1, 99217^1, 99218^1, 99219^1, 99220^1, 99221^1, 99222^1, 99223^1, 99231^1, 99232^1, 99233^1, 99234^1, 99235^1, 99236^1, 99238^1, 99239^1, 99241^1, 99242^1, 99243^1, 99244^1, 99245^1, 99251^1, 99252^1, 99253^1, 99254^1, 99255^1, 99291^1, 99292^1, 99304^1, 99305^1, 99306^1, 99307^1, 99308^1, 99309^1, 99310^1, 99315^1, 99316^1, 99334^1, 99335^1, 99336^1, 99337^1, 99347^1, 99348^1, 99349^1, 99350^1, 99374^1, 99375^1, 99377^1, 99378^1, 99446^0, 99447^0, 99448^0, 99449^0, 99451^0, 99452^0, 99495^0, 99496^0, G0453^0, G0463^1, G0471^1
63663	01935^0, 01936^0, 0213T^0, 0216T^0, 0228T^0, 0230T^0, 0333T^0, 0464T^0, 11000^1, 11001^1, 11004^1, 11005^1, 11006^1, 11042^1, 11043^1, 11044^1, 11045^1, 11046^1, 11047^1, 12001^1, 12002^1, 12004^1, 12005^1, 12006^1, 12007^1, 12011^1, 12013^1, 12014^1, 12015^1, 12016^1, 12017^1, 12018^1, 12020^1, 12021^1, 12031^1, 12032^1, 12034^1, 12035^1, 12036^1, 12037^1, 12041^1, 12042^1, 12044^1, 12045^1, 12046^1, 12047^1, 12051^1, 12052^1, 12053^1, 12054^1, 12055^1, 12056^1, 12057^1, 13100^1, 13101^1, 13102^1, 13120^1, 13121^1, 13122^1, 13131^1, 13132^1, 13133^1, 13151^1, 13152^1, 13153^1, 22505^0, 36000^1, 36400^1, 36405^1, 36406^1, 36410^1, 36420^1, 36425^1, 36430^1, 36440^1, 36591^0, 36592^0, 36600^1, 36640^1, 43752^1, 51701^1, 51702^1, 51703^1, 62273^1, 62320^0, 62321^0, 62322^0, 62323^0, 62324^0, 62325^0, 62326^0, 62327^0, 63610^0, 63650^0, 63661^0, 64400^0, 64402^0, 64405^0, 64408^0, 64410^0, 64413^0, 64415^0, 64416^0, 64417^0, 64418^0, 64420^0, 64421^0, 64425^0, 64430^0, 64435^0, 64445^0, 64446^0, 64447^0, 64448^0, 64449^0, 64450^0, 64461^0, 64462^0, 64463^0, 64479^0, 64480^0, 64483^0, 64484^0, 64486^0, 64487^0, 64488^0, 64489^0, 64490^0, 64491^0, 64492^0, 64493^0, 64494^0, 64495^0, 64505^0, 64510^0, 64517^0, 64520^0, 64530^0, 69990^0, 76000^1, 77001^1, 77002^1, 77003^1, 92012^1, 92014^1, 92585^0, 93000^1, 93005^1, 93010^1, 93040^1, 93041^1, 93042^1, 93318^1, 93355^1, 94002^1, 94200^1, 94250^1, 94680^1, 94681^1, 94690^1, 94770^1, 95812^1, 95813^1, 95816^1, 95819^1, 95822^0, 95829^1, 95860^0, 95861^0, 95863^0, 95864^0, 95865^0, 95866^0, 95867^0, 95868^0, 95869^0, 95870^0, 95907^0, 95908^0, 95909^0, 95910^0, 95911^0, 95912^0, 95913^0, 95925^0, 95926^0, 95927^0, 95928^0, 95929^0, 95930^0, 95933^0, 95937^0, 95938^0, 95939^0, 95940^0, 95955^1, 95970^1, 95971^1, 95972^1, 96360^1, 96361^1, 96365^1, 96366^1, 96367^1, 96368^1, 96372^1, 96374^1, 96375^1, 96376^1, 96377^1, 97597^1, 97598^1, 97602^1, 99155^0, 99156^0, 99157^0, 99211^1, 99212^1, 99213^1, 99214^1, 99215^1, 99217^1, 99218^1, 99219^1, 99220^1, 99221^1, 99222^1, 99223^1, 99231^1, 99232^1, 99233^1, 99234^1, 99235^1, 99236^1, 99238^1, 99239^1, 99241^1, 99242^1, 99243^1, 99244^1, 99245^1, 99251^1, 99252^1, 99253^1, 99254^1, 99255^1, 99291^1, 99292^1, 99304^1, 99305^1, 99306^1, 99307^1, 99308^1, 99309^1, 99310^1, 99315^1, 99316^1, 99334^1, 99335^1, 99336^1, 99337^1, 99347^1, 99348^1, 99349^1, 99350^1, 99374^1, 99375^1, 99377^1, 99378^1, 99446^0, 99447^0, 99448^0, 99449^0, 99451^0, 99452^0, 99495^0, 99496^0, G0453^0, G0463^1, G0471^1
63664	0213T^0, 0216T^0, 0228T^0, 0230T^0, 0333T^0, 0464T^0, 11000^1, 11001^1, 11004^1, 11005^1, 11006^1, 11042^1, 11043^1, 11044^1, 11045^1, 11046^1, 11047^1, 12001^1, 12002^1, 12004^1, 12005^1, 12006^1, 12007^1, 12011^1, 12013^1, 12014^1, 12015^1, 12016^1, 12017^1, 12018^1, 12020^1, 12021^1, 12031^1, 12032^1, 12034^1, 12035^1, 12036^1, 12037^1, 12041^1, 12042^1, 12044^1, 12045^1, 12046^1, 12047^1, 12051^1, 12052^1, 12053^1, 12054^1, 12055^1, 12056^1, 12057^1, 13100^1, 13101^1, 13102^1, 13120^1, 13121^1, 13122^1, 13131^1, 13132^1, 13133^1,

0 = Modifier usage not allowed or inappropriate 1 = Modifier usage allowed

CPT © 2018 American Medical Association. All Rights Reserved.

Code 1	Code 2
	13151[1], 13152[1], 13153[1], 22505[0], 36000[1], 36400[1], 36405[1], 36406[1], 36410[1], 36420[1], 36425[1], 36430[1], 36440[1], 36591[0], 36592[0], 36600[1], 36640[1], 43752[1], 51701[1], 51702[1], 51703[1], 62263[1], 62273[1], 62320[0], 62321[0], 62322[0], 62323[0], 62324[0], 62325[0], 62326[0], 62327[0], 63610[0], 63650[0], 63655[0], 63661[0], 63662[1], 63663[0], 63707[1], 63709[1], 64400[0], 64402[0], 64405[0], 64408[0], 64410[0], 64413[0], 64415[0], 64416[0], 64417[0], 64418[0], 64420[0], 64421[0], 64425[0], 64430[0], 64435[0], 64445[0], 64446[0], 64447[0], 64448[0], 64449[0], 64450[0], 64461[0], 64462[0], 64463[0], 64479[0], 64480[0], 64483[0], 64484[0], 64486[0], 64487[0], 64488[0], 64489[0], 64490[0], 64491[0], 64492[0], 64493[0], 64494[0], 64495[0], 64505[0], 64510[0], 64517[0], 64520[0], 64530[0], 69990[0], 76000[1], 77001[1], 77002[1], 77003[1], 92012[1], 92014[1], 92585[0], 93000[1], 93005[1], 93010[1], 93040[1], 93041[1], 93042[1], 93318[1], 93355[1], 94002[1], 94200[1], 94250[1], 94680[1], 94681[1], 94690[1], 94770[1], 95812[1], 95813[1], 95816[1], 95819[1], 95822[0], 95829[1], 95860[0], 95861[0], 95863[0], 95864[0], 95865[0], 95866[0], 95867[0], 95868[0], 95869[0], 95870[0], 95907[0], 95908[0], 95909[0], 95910[0], 95911[0], 95912[0], 95913[0], 95925[0], 95926[0], 95927[0], 95928[0], 95929[0], 95930[0], 95933[0], 95937[0], 95938[0], 95939[0], 95940[0], 95955[1], 95970[1], 95971[1], 95972[1], 96360[1], 96361[1], 96365[1], 96366[1], 96367[1], 96368[1], 96372[1], 96374[1], 96375[1], 96376[1], 96377[1], 97597[1], 97598[1], 97602[1], 99155[0], 99156[0], 99157[0], 99211[1], 99212[1], 99213[1], 99214[1], 99215[1], 99217[1], 99218[1], 99219[1], 99220[1], 99221[1], 99222[1], 99223[1], 99231[1], 99232[1], 99233[1], 99234[1], 99235[1], 99236[1], 99238[1], 99239[1], 99241[1], 99242[1], 99243[1], 99244[1], 99245[1], 99251[1], 99252[1], 99253[1], 99254[1], 99255[1], 99291[1], 99292[1], 99304[1], 99305[1], 99306[1], 99307[1], 99308[1], 99309[1], 99310[1], 99315[1], 99316[1], 99334[1], 99335[1], 99336[1], 99337[1], 99347[1], 99348[1], 99349[1], 99350[1], 99374[1], 99375[1], 99377[1], 99378[1], 99446[0], 99447[0], 99448[0], 99449[0], 99451[0], 99452[0], 99495[0], 99496[0], G0453[0], G0463[1], G0471[1]
63685	01935[0], 01936[0], 0213T[0], 0216T[0], 0228T[0], 0230T[0], 0333T[0], 0424T[1], 0427T[1], 0428T[1], 0431T[1], 0446T[1], 0448T[1], 0464T[0], 11000[1], 11001[1], 11004[1], 11005[1], 11006[1], 11042[1], 11043[1], 11044[1], 11045[1], 11046[1], 11047[1], 12001[1], 12002[1], 12004[1], 12005[1], 12006[1], 12007[1], 12011[1], 12013[1], 12014[1], 12015[1], 12016[1], 12017[1], 12018[1], 12020[1], 12021[1], 12031[1], 12032[1], 12034[1], 12035[1], 12036[1], 12037[1], 12041[1], 12042[1], 12044[1], 12045[1], 12046[1], 12047[1], 12051[1], 12052[1], 12053[1], 12054[1], 12055[1], 12056[1], 12057[1], 13100[1], 13101[1], 13102[1], 13120[1], 13121[1], 13122[1], 13131[1], 13132[1], 13133[1], 13151[1], 13152[1], 13153[1], 36000[1], 36400[1], 36405[1], 36406[1], 36410[1], 36420[1], 36425[1], 36430[1], 36440[1], 36591[0], 36592[0], 36600[1], 36640[1], 43752[1], 51701[1], 51702[1], 51703[1], 62320[0], 62321[0], 62322[0], 62323[0], 62324[0], 62325[0], 62326[0], 62327[0], 63610[0], 63688[1], 64400[0], 64402[0], 64405[0], 64408[0], 64410[0], 64413[0], 64415[0], 64416[0], 64417[0], 64418[0], 64420[0], 64421[0], 64425[0], 64430[0], 64435[0], 64445[0], 64446[0], 64447[0], 64448[0], 64449[0], 64450[0], 64461[0], 64462[0], 64463[0], 64479[0], 64480[0], 64483[0], 64484[0], 64486[0], 64487[0], 64488[0], 64489[0], 64490[0], 64491[0], 64492[0], 64493[0], 64494[0], 64495[0], 64505[0], 64510[0], 64517[0], 64520[0], 64530[0], 69990[0], 76000[1], 77001[1], 77002[1], 77003[1], 92012[1], 92014[1], 92585[0], 93000[1], 93005[1], 93010[1], 93040[1], 93041[1], 93042[1], 93318[1], 93355[1], 94002[1], 94200[1], 94250[1], 94680[1], 94681[1], 94690[1], 94770[1], 95812[1], 95813[1], 95816[1], 95819[1], 95822[0], 95829[1], 95860[0], 95861[0], 95863[0], 95864[0], 95865[0], 95866[0], 95867[0], 95868[0], 95869[0], 95870[0], 95907[0], 95908[0], 95909[0], 95910[0], 95911[0], 95912[0], 95913[0], 95925[0], 95926[0], 95927[0], 95928[0], 95929[0], 95930[0], 95933[0], 95937[0], 95938[0], 95939[0], 95940[0], 95955[1], 95970[1], 95971[1], 95972[1], 95976[1], 95977[1], 96360[1], 96361[1], 96365[1], 96366[1], 96367[1], 96368[1], 96372[1], 96374[1], 96375[1], 96376[1], 96377[1], 97597[1], 97598[1], 97602[1], 99155[0], 99156[0], 99157[0], 99211[1], 99212[1], 99213[1], 99214[1], 99215[1], 99217[1], 99218[1], 99219[1], 99220[1], 99221[1], 99222[1], 99223[1], 99231[1], 99232[1], 99233[1], 99234[1], 99235[1], 99236[1], 99238[1], 99239[1], 99241[1], 99242[1], 99243[1], 99244[1], 99245[1], 99251[1], 99252[1], 99253[1], 99254[1], 99255[1], 99291[1], 99292[1], 99304[1], 99305[1], 99306[1], 99307[1], 99308[1], 99309[1], 99310[1], 99315[1], 99316[1], 99334[1], 99335[1], 99336[1], 99337[1], 99347[1], 99348[1], 99349[1], 99350[1], 99374[1], 99375[1], 99377[1], 99378[1], 99446[0], 99447[0], 99448[0], 99449[0], 99451[0], 99452[0], 99495[0], 99496[0], G0453[0], G0463[1], G0471[1]
63688	01935[0], 01936[0], 0213T[0], 0216T[0], 0228T[0], 0230T[0], 0333T[0], 0447T[1], 0448T[1], 0464T[0], 11000[1], 11001[1], 11004[1], 11005[1], 11006[1], 11042[1], 11043[1], 11044[1], 11045[1], 11046[1], 11047[1], 12001[1], 12002[1], 12004[1], 12005[1], 12006[1], 12007[1], 12011[1], 12013[1], 12014[1], 12015[1], 12016[1], 12017[1], 12018[1], 12020[1], 12021[1], 12031[1], 12032[1], 12034[1], 12035[1], 12036[1], 12037[1], 12041[1], 12042[1], 12044[1], 12045[1], 12046[1], 12047[1], 12051[1], 12052[1], 12053[1], 12054[1], 12055[1], 12056[1], 12057[1], 13100[1], 13101[1], 13102[1], 13120[1], 13121[1], 13122[1], 13131[1], 13132[1], 13133[1], 13151[1], 13152[1], 13153[1], 36000[1], 36400[1], 36405[1], 36406[1], 36410[1], 36420[1], 36425[1], 36430[1], 36440[1], 36591[0], 36592[0], 36600[1], 36640[1], 43752[1], 51701[1], 51702[1], 51703[1], 62320[0], 62321[0], 62322[0], 62323[0], 62324[0], 62325[0], 62326[0], 62327[0], 63610[0], 64400[0], 64402[0], 64405[0], 64408[0], 64410[0], 64413[0], 64415[0], 64416[0], 64417[0], 64418[0], 64420[0], 64421[0], 64425[0], 64430[0], 64435[0], 64445[0], 64446[0], 64447[0], 64448[0], 64449[0], 64450[0], 64461[0], 64462[0], 64463[0], 64479[0], 64480[0], 64483[0], 64484[0], 64486[0], 64487[0], 64488[0], 64489[0], 64490[0], 64491[0], 64492[0], 64493[0], 64494[0], 64495[0], 64505[0], 64510[0], 64517[0], 64520[0], 64530[0], 69990[0], 76000[1], 77001[1], 77002[1], 92012[1], 92014[1], 92585[0], 93000[1], 93005[1], 93010[1], 93040[1], 93041[1], 93042[1], 93318[1], 93355[1], 94002[1], 94200[1], 94250[1], 94680[1], 94681[1], 94690[1], 94770[1], 95812[1], 95813[1], 95816[1], 95819[1], 95822[0], 95829[1], 95860[0], 95861[0], 95863[0], 95864[0], 95865[0], 95866[0], 95867[0], 95868[0], 95869[0], 95870[0], 95907[0], 95908[0], 95909[0], 95910[0], 95911[0], 95912[0], 95913[0], 95925[0], 95926[0], 95927[0], 95928[0], 95929[0], 95930[0], 95933[0], 95937[0], 95938[0], 95939[0], 95940[0], 95955[1], 95970[1], 95971[1], 95972[1], 95976[1], 95977[1], 96360[1], 96361[1], 96365[1], 96366[1], 96367[1], 96368[1], 96372[1], 96374[1], 96375[1], 96376[1], 96377[1], 97597[1], 97598[1], 97602[1], 99155[0], 99156[0], 99157[0], 99211[1], 99212[1], 99213[1], 99214[1], 99215[1], 99217[1], 99218[1], 99219[1], 99220[1], 99221[1], 99222[1], 99223[1], 99231[1], 99232[1], 99233[1], 99234[1], 99235[1], 99236[1], 99238[1], 99239[1], 99241[1], 99242[1], 99243[1], 99244[1], 99245[1], 99251[1], 99252[1], 99253[1], 99254[1], 99255[1], 99291[1], 99292[1], 99304[1], 99305[1], 99306[1], 99307[1], 99308[1], 99309[1], 99310[1], 99315[1], 99316[1], 99334[1], 99335[1], 99336[1], 99337[1], 99347[1], 99348[1], 99349[1], 99350[1], 99374[1], 99375[1], 99377[1], 99378[1], 99446[0], 99447[0], 99448[0], 99449[0], 99451[0], 99452[0], 99495[0], 99496[0], G0453[0], G0463[1], G0471[1]
64400	01991[0], 01992[0], 0333T[0], 0464T[0], 20550[1], 20551[1], 36000[1], 36400[1], 36405[1], 36406[1], 36410[1], 36420[1], 36425[1], 36430[1], 36440[1], 36591[0], 36592[0], 36600[1], 51701[0], 51702[0], 51703[0], 69990[0], 76000[1], 76970[1], 76998[1], 77001[1], 77002[1], 92012[1], 92014[1], 92585[0], 93000[1], 93005[1], 93010[1], 93040[1], 93041[1], 93042[1], 93318[1], 93355[1], 94002[1], 94200[1], 94250[1], 94680[1], 94681[1], 94690[1], 94770[1], 95812[1], 95813[1], 95816[1], 95819[1], 95822[0], 95829[1], 95860[1], 95861[1], 95863[1], 95864[1], 95865[1], 95866[1], 95867[1], 95868[1], 95869[1], 95870[1], 95907[1], 95908[1], 95909[1], 95910[1], 95911[1], 95912[1], 95913[1], 95925[0], 95926[0], 95927[0], 95928[0], 95929[0], 95930[0], 95933[0], 95937[0], 95938[0], 95939[0], 95940[0], 95955[1], 96360[1], 96361[1], 96365[1], 96366[1], 96367[1], 96368[1], 96372[1], 96374[1], 96375[1], 96376[1], 96377[1], 99155[0], 99156[0], 99157[0], 99211[1], 99212[1], 99213[1], 99214[1], 99215[1], 99217[1], 99218[1], 99219[1], 99220[1], 99221[1], 99222[1], 99223[1], 99231[1], 99232[1], 99233[1], 99234[1], 99235[1], 99236[1], 99238[1], 99239[1], 99241[1], 99242[1], 99243[1], 99244[1], 99245[1], 99251[1], 99252[1], 99253[1], 99254[1], 99255[1], 99291[1], 99292[1], 99304[1], 99305[1], 99306[1], 99307[1], 99308[1], 99309[1], 99310[1], 99315[1], 99316[1], 99334[1], 99335[1], 99336[1], 99337[1], 99347[1], 99348[1], 99349[1], 99350[1], 99374[1], 99375[1], 99377[1], 99378[1], 99446[0], 99447[0], 99448[0], 99449[0], 99451[0], 99452[0], 99495[1], 99496[1], G0453[0], G0459[1], G0463[1], G0471[0], J0670[1], J2001[1]
64402	01991[0], 01992[0], 0333T[0], 0464T[0], 20550[1], 20551[1], 36000[1], 36400[1], 36405[1], 36406[1], 36410[1], 36420[1], 36425[1], 36430[1], 36440[1], 36591[0], 36592[0], 36600[1], 51701[0], 51702[0], 51703[0], 69990[0], 76000[1], 76970[1], 76998[1], 77001[1], 77002[1], 92012[1], 92014[1], 92585[0], 93000[1], 93005[1], 93010[1], 93040[1], 93041[1], 93042[1], 93318[1], 93355[1], 94002[1], 94200[1], 94250[1], 94680[1], 94681[1], 94690[1], 94770[1], 95812[1], 95813[1], 95816[1], 95819[1], 95822[0], 95829[1], 95860[1], 95861[1], 95863[1], 95864[1], 95865[1], 95866[1], 95867[1], 95868[1], 95869[1], 95870[1], 95907[1], 95908[1], 95909[1], 95910[1], 95911[1], 95912[1], 95913[1], 95925[0], 95926[0], 95927[0], 95928[0], 95929[0], 95930[0], 95933[0], 95937[0], 95938[0], 95939[0], 95940[0], 95955[1], 96360[1], 96361[1], 96365[1], 96366[1], 96367[1], 96368[1], 96372[1], 96374[1], 96375[1], 96376[1], 96377[1], 99155[0], 99156[0], 99157[0], 99211[1], 99212[1], 99213[1], 99214[1], 99215[1], 99217[1], 99218[1], 99219[1], 99220[1], 99221[1], 99222[1], 99223[1], 99231[1], 99232[1], 99233[1], 99234[1], 99235[1], 99236[1], 99238[1], 99239[1], 99241[1], 99242[1], 99243[1], 99244[1], 99245[1], 99251[1], 99252[1], 99253[1], 99254[1], 99255[1], 99291[1], 99292[1], 99304[1], 99305[1], 99306[1], 99307[1], 99308[1], 99309[1], 99310[1], 99315[1], 99316[1], 99334[1], 99335[1], 99336[1], 99337[1], 99347[1], 99348[1], 99349[1], 99350[1], 99374[1], 99375[1], 99377[1], 99378[1], 99446[0], 99447[0], 99448[0], 99449[0], 99451[0], 99452[0], 99495[1], 99496[1], G0453[0], G0459[1], G0463[1], G0471[0], J0670[1], J2001[1]
64405	01991[0], 01992[0], 0333T[0], 0464T[0], 20550[1], 20551[1], 36000[1], 36400[1], 36405[1], 36406[1], 36410[1], 36420[1], 36425[1], 36430[1], 36440[1], 36591[0], 36592[0], 36600[1], 51701[0], 51702[0], 51703[0], 69990[0], 76000[1], 76970[1], 76998[1], 77001[1], 77002[1], 92012[1], 92014[1], 92585[0], 93000[1], 93005[1], 93010[1], 93040[1], 93041[1], 93042[1], 93318[1], 93355[1], 94002[1], 94200[1], 94250[1], 94680[1], 94681[1], 94690[1], 94770[1], 95812[1], 95813[1], 95816[1], 95819[1], 95822[0], 95829[1], 95860[1], 95861[1], 95863[1], 95864[1], 95865[1], 95866[1], 95867[1], 95868[1], 95869[1], 95870[1], 95907[1], 95908[1], 95909[1], 95910[1], 95911[1], 95912[1], 95913[1], 95925[0], 95926[0], 95927[0], 95928[0], 95929[0], 95930[0], 95933[0], 95937[0], 95938[0], 95939[0], 95940[0], 95955[1], 96360[1], 96361[1], 96365[1], 96366[1], 96367[1], 96368[1], 96372[1], 96374[1], 96375[1], 96376[1], 96377[1], 99155[0], 99156[0], 99157[0], 99211[1], 99212[1], 99213[1], 99214[1], 99215[1], 99217[1], 99218[1], 99219[1], 99220[1], 99221[1], 99222[1], 99223[1], 99231[1], 99232[1], 99233[1], 99234[1], 99235[1], 99236[1], 99238[1], 99239[1], 99241[1], 99242[1], 99243[1], 99244[1], 99245[1], 99251[1], 99252[1], 99253[1], 99254[1], 99255[1], 99291[1], 99292[1], 99304[1], 99305[1], 99306[1], 99307[1], 99308[1], 99309[1], 99310[1], 99315[1], 99316[1], 99334[1], 99335[1], 99336[1], 99337[1], 99347[1], 99348[1], 99349[1], 99350[1], 99374[1], 99375[1], 99377[1], 99378[1], 99446[0], 99447[0], 99448[0], 99449[0], 99451[0], 99452[0], 99495[1], 99496[1], G0453[0], G0459[1], G0463[1], G0471[0], J0670[1], J2001[1]

0 = Modifier usage not allowed or inappropriate 1 = Modifier usage allowed

CPT © 2018 American Medical Association. All Rights Reserved.

Code 1	Code 2
64408	01991[0], 01992[0], 0333T[0], 0464T[0], 36000[1], 36400[1], 36405[1], 36406[1], 36410[1], 36420[1], 36425[1], 36430[1], 36440[1], 36591[0], 36592[0], 36600[1], 51701[0], 51702[0], 51703[0], 69990[0], 76000[1], 76970[1], 76998[1], 77001[1], 77002[1], 92012[1], 92014[1], 92585[0], 93000[1], 93005[1], 93010[1], 93040[1], 93041[1], 93042[1], 93318[1], 93355[1], 94002[1], 94200[1], 94250[1], 94680[1], 94681[1], 94690[1], 94770[1], 95812[1], 95813[1], 95816[1], 95819[1], 95822[0], 95829[1], 95860[1], 95861[1], 95863[1], 95864[1], 95865[1], 95866[1], 95867[1], 95868[1], 95869[1], 95870[1], 95907[1], 95908[1], 95909[1], 95910[1], 95911[1], 95912[1], 95913[1], 95925[0], 95926[0], 95927[0], 95928[0], 95929[0], 95930[0], 95933[0], 95937[0], 95938[0], 95939[0], 95940[0], 95955[1], 96360[1], 96361[1], 96365[1], 96366[1], 96367[1], 96368[1], 96372[1], 96374[1], 96375[1], 96376[1], 96377[1], 99155[0], 99156[0], 99157[0], 99211[1], 99212[1], 99213[1], 99214[1], 99215[1], 99217[1], 99218[1], 99219[1], 99220[1], 99221[1], 99222[1], 99223[1], 99231[1], 99232[1], 99233[1], 99234[1], 99235[1], 99236[1], 99238[1], 99239[1], 99241[1], 99242[1], 99243[1], 99244[1], 99245[1], 99251[1], 99252[1], 99253[1], 99254[1], 99255[1], 99291[1], 99292[1], 99304[1], 99305[1], 99306[1], 99307[1], 99308[1], 99309[1], 99310[1], 99315[1], 99316[1], 99334[1], 99335[1], 99336[1], 99337[1], 99347[1], 99348[1], 99349[1], 99350[1], 99374[1], 99375[1], 99377[1], 99378[1], 99446[0], 99447[0], 99448[0], 99449[0], 99451[0], 99452[0], 99495[1], 99496[1], G0453[0], G0459[1], G0463[1], G0471[0], J0670[1], J2001[1]
64410	01991[0], 01992[0], 0333T[0], 0464T[0], 36000[1], 36400[1], 36405[1], 36406[1], 36410[1], 36420[1], 36425[1], 36430[1], 36440[1], 36591[0], 36592[0], 36600[1], 51701[0], 51702[0], 51703[0], 69990[0], 76000[1], 76970[1], 76998[1], 77001[1], 77002[1], 92012[1], 92014[1], 92585[0], 93000[1], 93005[1], 93010[1], 93040[1], 93041[1], 93042[1], 93318[1], 93355[1], 94002[1], 94200[1], 94250[1], 94680[1], 94681[1], 94690[1], 94770[1], 95812[1], 95813[1], 95816[1], 95819[1], 95822[0], 95829[1], 95860[1], 95861[1], 95863[1], 95864[1], 95865[1], 95866[1], 95867[1], 95868[1], 95869[1], 95870[1], 95907[1], 95908[1], 95909[1], 95910[1], 95911[1], 95912[1], 95913[1], 95925[0], 95926[0], 95927[0], 95928[0], 95929[0], 95930[0], 95933[0], 95937[0], 95938[0], 95939[0], 95940[0], 95955[1], 96360[1], 96361[1], 96365[1], 96366[1], 96367[1], 96368[1], 96372[1], 96374[1], 96375[1], 96376[1], 96377[1], 99155[0], 99156[0], 99157[0], 99211[1], 99212[1], 99213[1], 99214[1], 99215[1], 99217[1], 99218[1], 99219[1], 99220[1], 99221[1], 99222[1], 99223[1], 99231[1], 99232[1], 99233[1], 99234[1], 99235[1], 99236[1], 99238[1], 99239[1], 99241[1], 99242[1], 99243[1], 99244[1], 99245[1], 99251[1], 99252[1], 99253[1], 99254[1], 99255[1], 99291[1], 99292[1], 99304[1], 99305[1], 99306[1], 99307[1], 99308[1], 99309[1], 99310[1], 99315[1], 99316[1], 99334[1], 99335[1], 99336[1], 99337[1], 99347[1], 99348[1], 99349[1], 99350[1], 99374[1], 99375[1], 99377[1], 99378[1], 99446[0], 99447[0], 99448[0], 99449[0], 99451[0], 99452[0], 99495[1], 99496[1], G0453[0], G0459[1], G0463[1], G0471[0], J0670[1], J2001[1]
64413	01991[0], 01992[0], 0333T[0], 0464T[0], 20550[1], 20551[1], 36000[1], 36400[1], 36405[1], 36406[1], 36410[1], 36420[1], 36425[1], 36430[1], 36440[1], 36591[0], 36592[0], 36600[1], 51701[0], 51702[0], 51703[0], 69990[0], 76000[1], 76800[1], 76970[1], 76998[1], 77001[1], 77002[1], 92012[1], 92014[1], 92585[0], 93000[1], 93005[1], 93010[1], 93040[1], 93041[1], 93042[1], 93318[1], 93355[1], 94002[1], 94200[1], 94250[1], 94680[1], 94681[1], 94690[1], 94770[1], 95812[1], 95813[1], 95816[1], 95819[1], 95822[0], 95829[1], 95860[1], 95861[1], 95863[1], 95864[1], 95865[1], 95866[1], 95867[1], 95868[1], 95869[1], 95870[1], 95907[1], 95908[1], 95909[1], 95910[1], 95911[1], 95912[1], 95913[1], 95925[0], 95926[0], 95927[0], 95928[0], 95929[0], 95930[0], 95933[0], 95937[0], 95938[0], 95939[0], 95940[0], 95955[1], 96360[1], 96361[1], 96365[1], 96366[1], 96367[1], 96368[1], 96372[1], 96374[1], 96375[1], 96376[1], 96377[1], 99155[0], 99156[0], 99157[0], 99211[1], 99212[1], 99213[1], 99214[1], 99215[1], 99217[1], 99218[1], 99219[1], 99220[1], 99221[1], 99222[1], 99223[1], 99231[1], 99232[1], 99233[1], 99234[1], 99235[1], 99236[1], 99238[1], 99239[1], 99241[1], 99242[1], 99243[1], 99244[1], 99245[1], 99251[1], 99252[1], 99253[1], 99254[1], 99255[1], 99291[1], 99292[1], 99304[1], 99305[1], 99306[1], 99307[1], 99308[1], 99309[1], 99310[1], 99315[1], 99316[1], 99334[1], 99335[1], 99336[1], 99337[1], 99347[1], 99348[1], 99349[1], 99350[1], 99374[1], 99375[1], 99377[1], 99378[1], 99446[0], 99447[0], 99448[0], 99449[0], 99451[0], 99452[0], 99495[1], 99496[1], G0453[0], G0459[1], G0463[1], G0471[0], J0670[1], J2001[1]
64415	01991[0], 01992[0], 0333T[0], 0464T[0], 20550[1], 20551[1], 36591[0], 36592[0], 51701[0], 51702[0], 69990[0], 76000[1], 76970[1], 76998[1], 77001[1], 77002[1], 92012[1], 92014[1], 92585[0], 93000[1], 93005[1], 93010[1], 93040[1], 93041[1], 93042[1], 93318[1], 93355[1], 94002[1], 94200[1], 94250[1], 94680[1], 94681[1], 94690[1], 94770[1], 95812[1], 95813[1], 95816[1], 95819[1], 95822[0], 95829[1], 95860[1], 95861[1], 95863[1], 95864[1], 95865[1], 95866[1], 95867[1], 95868[1], 95869[1], 95870[1], 95907[1], 95908[1], 95909[1], 95910[1], 95911[1], 95912[1], 95913[1], 95925[0], 95926[0], 95927[0], 95928[0], 95929[0], 95930[0], 95933[0], 95937[0], 95938[0], 95939[0], 95940[0], 95955[1], 96360[1], 96361[1], 96365[1], 96366[1], 96367[1], 96368[1], 96372[1], 96374[1], 96375[1], 96376[1], 96377[1], 99155[0], 99156[0], 99157[0], 99211[1], 99212[1], 99213[1], 99214[1], 99215[1], 99217[1], 99218[1], 99219[1], 99220[1], 99221[1], 99222[1], 99223[1], 99231[1], 99232[1], 99233[1], 99234[1], 99235[1], 99236[1], 99238[1], 99239[1], 99241[1], 99242[1], 99243[1], 99244[1], 99245[1], 99251[1], 99252[1], 99253[1], 99254[1], 99255[1], 99291[1], 99292[1], 99304[1], 99305[1], 99306[1], 99307[1], 99308[1], 99309[1], 99310[1], 99315[1], 99316[1], 99334[1], 99335[1], 99336[1], 99337[1], 99347[1], 99348[1], 99349[1], 99350[1], 99374[1], 99375[1], 99377[1], 99378[1], 99446[0], 99447[0], 99448[0], 99449[0], 99451[0], 99452[0], 99495[1], 99496[1], G0453[0], G0459[1], G0463[1], G0471[0], J0670[1], J2001[1]
64416	01991[0], 01992[0], 01996[0], 0333T[0], 0464T[0], 20550[1], 20551[1], 36000[1], 36410[1], 36591[0], 36592[0], 51701[0], 51702[0], 51703[0], 69990[0], 76000[1], 76970[1], 76998[1], 77001[1], 77002[1], 92012[1], 92014[1], 92585[0], 93000[1], 93005[1], 93010[1], 93040[1], 93041[1], 93042[1], 93318[1], 93355[1], 94002[1], 94200[1], 94250[1], 94680[1], 94681[1], 94690[1], 94770[1], 95812[1], 95813[1], 95816[1], 95819[1], 95822[0], 95829[1], 95860[1], 95861[1], 95863[1], 95864[1], 95865[1], 95866[1], 95867[1], 95868[1], 95869[1], 95870[1], 95907[1], 95908[1], 95909[1], 95910[1], 95911[1], 95912[1], 95913[1], 95925[0], 95926[0], 95927[0], 95928[0], 95929[0], 95930[0], 95933[0], 95937[0], 95938[0], 95939[0], 95940[0], 95955[1], 96360[1], 96361[1], 96365[1], 96366[1], 96367[1], 96368[1], 96372[1], 96374[1], 96375[1], 96376[1], 96377[1], 99155[0], 99156[0], 99157[0], 99211[1], 99212[1], 99213[1], 99214[1], 99215[1], 99217[1], 99218[1], 99219[1], 99220[1], 99221[1], 99222[1], 99223[1], 99231[1], 99232[1], 99233[1], 99234[1], 99235[1], 99236[1], 99238[1], 99239[1], 99241[1], 99242[1], 99243[1], 99244[1], 99245[1], 99251[1], 99252[1], 99253[1], 99254[1], 99255[1], 99291[1], 99292[1], 99304[1], 99305[1], 99306[1], 99307[1], 99308[1], 99309[1], 99310[1], 99315[1], 99316[1], 99334[1], 99335[1], 99336[1], 99337[1], 99347[1], 99348[1], 99349[1], 99350[1], 99374[1], 99375[1], 99377[1], 99378[1], 99446[0], 99447[0], 99448[0], 99449[0], 99451[0], 99452[0], 99495[1], 99496[1], G0453[0], G0459[1], G0463[1], G0471[0], J2001[1]
64417	01991[0], 01992[0], 0333T[0], 0464T[0], 20550[1], 20551[1], 36591[0], 36592[0], 51701[0], 51702[0], 69990[0], 76000[1], 76970[1], 76998[1], 77001[1], 77002[1], 92012[1], 92014[1], 92585[0], 93000[1], 93005[1], 93010[1], 93040[1], 93041[1], 93042[1], 93318[1], 93355[1], 94002[1], 94200[1], 94250[1], 94680[1], 94681[1], 94690[1], 94770[1], 95812[1], 95813[1], 95816[1], 95819[1], 95822[0], 95829[1], 95860[1], 95861[1], 95863[1], 95864[1], 95865[1], 95866[1], 95867[1], 95868[1], 95869[1], 95870[1], 95907[1], 95908[1], 95909[1], 95910[1], 95911[1], 95912[1], 95913[1], 95925[0], 95926[0], 95927[0], 95928[0], 95929[0], 95930[0], 95933[0], 95937[0], 95938[0], 95939[0], 95940[0], 95955[1], 96360[1], 96361[1], 96365[1], 96366[1], 96367[1], 96368[1], 96372[1], 96374[1], 96375[1], 96376[1], 96377[1], 99155[0], 99156[0], 99157[0], 99211[1], 99212[1], 99213[1], 99214[1], 99215[1], 99217[1], 99218[1], 99219[1], 99220[1], 99221[1], 99222[1], 99223[1], 99231[1], 99232[1], 99233[1], 99234[1], 99235[1], 99236[1], 99238[1], 99239[1], 99241[1], 99242[1], 99243[1], 99244[1], 99245[1], 99251[1], 99252[1], 99253[1], 99254[1], 99255[1], 99291[1], 99292[1], 99304[1], 99305[1], 99306[1], 99307[1], 99308[1], 99309[1], 99310[1], 99315[1], 99316[1], 99334[1], 99335[1], 99336[1], 99337[1], 99347[1], 99348[1], 99349[1], 99350[1], 99374[1], 99375[1], 99377[1], 99378[1], 99446[0], 99447[0], 99448[0], 99449[0], 99451[0], 99452[0], 99495[1], 99496[1], G0453[0], G0459[1], G0463[1], G0471[0], J0670[1], J2001[1]
64418	01991[0], 01992[0], 0333T[0], 0464T[0], 20550[1], 20551[1], 36000[1], 36400[1], 36405[1], 36406[1], 36410[1], 36420[1], 36425[1], 36430[1], 36440[1], 36591[0], 36592[0], 36600[1], 51701[0], 51702[0], 51703[0], 69990[0], 76000[1], 76970[1], 76998[1], 77001[1], 77002[1], 92012[1], 92014[1], 92585[0], 93000[1], 93005[1], 93010[1], 93040[1], 93041[1], 93042[1], 93318[1], 93355[1], 94002[1], 94200[1], 94250[1], 94680[1], 94681[1], 94690[1], 94770[1], 95812[1], 95813[1], 95816[1], 95819[1], 95822[0], 95829[1], 95860[1], 95861[1], 95863[1], 95864[1], 95865[1], 95866[1], 95867[1], 95868[1], 95869[1], 95870[1], 95907[1], 95908[1], 95909[1], 95910[1], 95911[1], 95912[1], 95913[1], 95925[0], 95926[0], 95927[0], 95928[0], 95929[0], 95930[0], 95933[0], 95937[0], 95938[0], 95939[0], 95940[0], 95955[1], 96360[1], 96361[1], 96365[1], 96366[1], 96367[1], 96368[1], 96372[1], 96374[1], 96375[1], 96376[1], 96377[1], 99155[0], 99156[0], 99157[0], 99211[1], 99212[1], 99213[1], 99214[1], 99215[1], 99217[1], 99218[1], 99219[1], 99220[1], 99221[1], 99222[1], 99223[1], 99231[1], 99232[1], 99233[1], 99234[1], 99235[1], 99236[1], 99238[1], 99239[1], 99241[1], 99242[1], 99243[1], 99244[1], 99245[1], 99251[1], 99252[1], 99253[1], 99254[1], 99255[1], 99291[1], 99292[1], 99304[1], 99305[1], 99306[1], 99307[1], 99308[1], 99309[1], 99310[1], 99315[1], 99316[1], 99334[1], 99335[1], 99336[1], 99337[1], 99347[1], 99348[1], 99349[1], 99350[1], 99374[1], 99375[1], 99377[1], 99378[1], 99446[0], 99447[0], 99448[0], 99449[0], 99451[0], 99452[0], 99495[1], 99496[1], G0453[0], G0459[1], G0463[1], G0471[0], J0670[1], J2001[1]
64420	01991[0], 01992[0], 0333T[0], 0464T[0], 20550[1], 20551[1], 36000[1], 36400[1], 36405[1], 36406[1], 36410[1], 36420[1], 36425[1], 36430[1], 36440[1], 36591[0], 36592[0], 36600[1], 51701[0], 51702[0], 51703[0], 69990[0], 76000[1], 76970[1], 76998[1], 77001[1], 77002[1], 92012[1], 92014[1], 92585[0], 93000[1], 93005[1], 93010[1], 93040[1], 93041[1], 93042[1], 93318[1], 93355[1], 94002[1], 94200[1], 94250[1], 94680[1], 94681[1], 94690[1], 94770[1], 95812[1], 95813[1], 95816[1], 95819[1], 95822[0], 95829[1], 95860[1], 95861[1], 95863[1], 95864[1], 95865[1], 95866[1], 95867[1], 95868[1], 95869[1], 95870[1], 95907[1], 95908[1], 95909[1], 95910[1], 95911[1], 95912[1], 95913[1], 95925[0], 95926[0], 95927[0], 95928[0], 95929[0], 95930[0], 95933[0], 95937[0], 95938[0], 95939[0], 95940[0], 95955[1], 96360[1], 96361[1], 96365[1], 96366[1], 96367[1], 96368[1], 96372[1], 96374[1], 96375[1], 96376[1], 96377[1], 99155[0], 99156[0], 99157[0], 99211[1], 99212[1], 99213[1], 99214[1], 99215[1], 99217[1], 99218[1], 99219[1], 99220[1], 99221[1], 99222[1], 99223[1], 99231[1], 99232[1], 99233[1], 99234[1], 99235[1], 99236[1], 99238[1], 99239[1], 99241[1], 99242[1], 99243[1], 99244[1], 99245[1], 99251[1], 99252[1], 99253[1], 99254[1], 99255[1], 99291[1], 99292[1], 99304[1], 99305[1], 99306[1], 99307[1], 99308[1], 99309[1], 99310[1], 99315[1], 99316[1], 99334[1], 99335[1], 99336[1], 99337[1], 99347[1], 99348[1], 99349[1], 99350[1], 99374[1], 99375[1], 99377[1], 99378[1], 99446[0], 99447[0], 99448[0], 99449[0], 99451[0], 99452[0], 99495[1], 99496[1], G0453[0], G0459[1], G0463[1], G0471[0], J0670[1], J2001[1]

0 = Modifier usage not allowed or inappropriate 1 = Modifier usage allowed

CPT © 2018 American Medical Association. All Rights Reserved.

Code 1	Code 2
64421	01991[0], 01992[0], 0333T[0], 0464T[0], 20550[1], 20551[1], 36000[1], 36400[1], 36405[1], 36406[1], 36410[1], 36420[1], 36425[1], 36430[1], 36440[1], 36591[0], 36592[0], 36600[1], 51701[0], 51702[0], 51703[0], 64420[1], 69990[0], 76000[1], 76970[1], 76998[1], 77001[1], 77002[1], 92012[1], 92014[1], 92585[0], 93000[1], 93005[1], 93010[1], 93040[1], 93041[1], 93042[1], 93318[1], 93355[1], 94002[1], 94200[1], 94250[1], 94680[1], 94681[1], 94690[1], 94770[1], 95812[1], 95813[1], 95816[1], 95819[1], 95822[0], 95829[1], 95860[1], 95861[1], 95863[1], 95864[1], 95865[1], 95866[1], 95867[1], 95868[1], 95869[1], 95870[1], 95907[1], 95908[1], 95909[1], 95910[1], 95911[1], 95912[1], 95913[1], 95925[0], 95926[0], 95927[0], 95928[0], 95929[0], 95930[0], 95933[0], 95937[0], 95938[0], 95939[0], 95940[0], 95955[1], 96360[1], 96361[1], 96365[1], 96366[1], 96367[1], 96368[1], 96372[1], 96374[1], 96375[1], 96376[1], 96377[1], 99155[0], 99156[0], 99157[0], 99211[1], 99212[1], 99213[1], 99214[1], 99215[1], 99217[1], 99218[1], 99219[1], 99220[1], 99221[1], 99222[1], 99223[1], 99231[1], 99232[1], 99233[1], 99234[1], 99235[1], 99236[1], 99238[1], 99239[1], 99241[1], 99242[1], 99243[1], 99244[1], 99245[1], 99251[1], 99252[1], 99253[1], 99254[1], 99255[1], 99291[1], 99292[1], 99304[1], 99305[1], 99306[1], 99307[1], 99308[1], 99309[1], 99310[1], 99315[1], 99316[1], 99334[1], 99335[1], 99336[1], 99337[1], 99347[1], 99348[1], 99349[1], 99350[1], 99374[1], 99375[1], 99377[1], 99378[1], 99446[0], 99447[0], 99448[0], 99449[0], 99451[0], 99452[0], 99495[1], 99496[1], G0453[0], G0459[1], G0463[1], G0471[0], J0670[1], J2001[1]
64425	01991[0], 01992[0], 0333T[0], 0464T[0], 20550[1], 20551[1], 36000[1], 36400[1], 36405[1], 36406[1], 36410[1], 36420[1], 36425[1], 36430[1], 36440[1], 36591[0], 36592[0], 36600[1], 51701[0], 51702[0], 51703[0], 69990[0], 76000[1], 76970[1], 76998[1], 77001[1], 77002[1], 92012[1], 92014[1], 92585[0], 93000[1], 93005[1], 93010[1], 93040[1], 93041[1], 93042[1], 93318[1], 93355[1], 94002[1], 94200[1], 94250[1], 94680[1], 94681[1], 94690[1], 94770[1], 95812[1], 95813[1], 95816[1], 95819[1], 95822[0], 95829[1], 95860[1], 95861[1], 95863[1], 95864[1], 95865[1], 95866[1], 95867[1], 95868[1], 95869[1], 95870[1], 95907[1], 95908[1], 95909[1], 95910[1], 95911[1], 95912[1], 95913[1], 95925[0], 95926[0], 95927[0], 95928[0], 95929[0], 95930[0], 95933[0], 95937[0], 95938[0], 95939[0], 95940[0], 95955[1], 96360[1], 96361[1], 96365[1], 96366[1], 96367[1], 96368[1], 96372[1], 96374[1], 96375[1], 96376[1], 96377[1], 99155[0], 99156[0], 99157[0], 99211[1], 99212[1], 99213[1], 99214[1], 99215[1], 99217[1], 99218[1], 99219[1], 99220[1], 99221[1], 99222[1], 99223[1], 99231[1], 99232[1], 99233[1], 99234[1], 99235[1], 99236[1], 99238[1], 99239[1], 99241[1], 99242[1], 99243[1], 99244[1], 99245[1], 99251[1], 99252[1], 99253[1], 99254[1], 99255[1], 99291[1], 99292[1], 99304[1], 99305[1], 99306[1], 99307[1], 99308[1], 99309[1], 99310[1], 99315[1], 99316[1], 99334[1], 99335[1], 99336[1], 99337[1], 99347[1], 99348[1], 99349[1], 99350[1], 99374[1], 99375[1], 99377[1], 99378[1], 99446[0], 99447[0], 99448[0], 99449[0], 99451[0], 99452[0], 99495[1], 99496[1], G0453[0], G0459[1], G0463[1], G0471[0], J0670[1], J2001[1]
64430	01991[0], 01992[0], 0333T[0], 0464T[0], 20550[1], 20551[1], 36000[1], 36400[1], 36405[1], 36406[1], 36410[1], 36420[1], 36425[1], 36430[1], 36440[1], 36591[0], 36592[0], 36600[1], 51701[0], 51702[0], 51703[0], 69990[0], 76000[1], 76970[1], 76998[1], 77001[1], 77002[1], 92012[1], 92014[1], 92585[0], 93000[1], 93005[1], 93010[1], 93040[1], 93041[1], 93042[1], 93318[1], 93355[1], 94002[1], 94200[1], 94250[1], 94680[1], 94681[1], 94690[1], 94770[1], 95812[1], 95813[1], 95816[1], 95819[1], 95822[0], 95829[1], 95860[1], 95861[1], 95863[1], 95864[1], 95865[1], 95866[1], 95867[1], 95868[1], 95869[1], 95870[1], 95907[1], 95908[1], 95909[1], 95910[1], 95911[1], 95912[1], 95913[1], 95925[0], 95926[0], 95927[0], 95928[0], 95929[0], 95930[0], 95933[0], 95937[0], 95938[0], 95939[0], 95940[0], 95955[1], 96360[1], 96361[1], 96365[1], 96366[1], 96367[1], 96368[1], 96372[1], 96374[1], 96375[1], 96376[1], 96377[1], 99155[0], 99156[0], 99157[0], 99211[1], 99212[1], 99213[1], 99214[1], 99215[1], 99217[1], 99218[1], 99219[1], 99220[1], 99221[1], 99222[1], 99223[1], 99231[1], 99232[1], 99233[1], 99234[1], 99235[1], 99236[1], 99238[1], 99239[1], 99241[1], 99242[1], 99243[1], 99244[1], 99245[1], 99251[1], 99252[1], 99253[1], 99254[1], 99255[1], 99291[1], 99292[1], 99304[1], 99305[1], 99306[1], 99307[1], 99308[1], 99309[1], 99310[1], 99315[1], 99316[1], 99334[1], 99335[1], 99336[1], 99337[1], 99347[1], 99348[1], 99349[1], 99350[1], 99374[1], 99375[1], 99377[1], 99378[1], 99446[0], 99447[0], 99448[0], 99449[0], 99451[0], 99452[0], 99495[1], 99496[1], G0453[0], G0459[1], G0463[1], G0471[0], J0670[1], J2001[1]
64435	01991[0], 01992[0], 0333T[0], 0464T[0], 36000[1], 36400[1], 36405[1], 36406[1], 36410[1], 36420[1], 36425[1], 36430[1], 36440[1], 36591[0], 36592[0], 36600[1], 51701[0], 51702[0], 51703[0], 69990[0], 76000[1], 76970[1], 76998[1], 77001[1], 77002[1], 92012[1], 92014[1], 92585[0], 93000[1], 93005[1], 93010[1], 93040[1], 93041[1], 93042[1], 93318[1], 93355[1], 94002[1], 94200[1], 94250[1], 94680[1], 94681[1], 94690[1], 94770[1], 95812[1], 95813[1], 95816[1], 95819[1], 95822[0], 95829[1], 95860[1], 95861[1], 95863[1], 95864[1], 95865[1], 95866[1], 95867[1], 95868[1], 95869[1], 95870[1], 95907[1], 95908[1], 95909[1], 95910[1], 95911[1], 95912[1], 95913[1], 95925[0], 95926[0], 95927[0], 95928[0], 95929[0], 95930[0], 95933[0], 95937[0], 95938[0], 95939[0], 95940[0], 95955[1], 96360[1], 96361[1], 96365[1], 96366[1], 96367[1], 96368[1], 96372[1], 96374[1], 96375[1], 96376[1], 96377[1], 99155[0], 99156[0], 99157[0], 99211[1], 99212[1], 99213[1], 99214[1], 99215[1], 99217[1], 99218[1], 99219[1], 99220[1], 99221[1], 99222[1], 99223[1], 99231[1], 99232[1], 99233[1], 99234[1], 99235[1], 99236[1], 99238[1], 99239[1], 99241[1], 99242[1], 99243[1], 99244[1], 99245[1], 99251[1], 99252[1], 99253[1], 99254[1], 99255[1], 99291[1], 99292[1], 99304[1], 99305[1], 99306[1], 99307[1], 99308[1], 99309[1], 99310[1], 99315[1], 99316[1], 99334[1], 99335[1], 99336[1], 99337[1], 99347[1], 99348[1], 99349[1], 99350[1], 99374[1], 99375[1], 99377[1], 99378[1], 99446[0], 99447[0], 99448[0], 99449[0], 99451[0], 99452[0], 99495[1], 99496[1], G0453[0], G0459[1], G0463[1], G0471[0], J0670[1], J2001[1]
64445	01991[0], 01992[0], 0333T[0], 0464T[0], 20550[1], 20551[1], 36000[1], 36400[1], 36405[1], 36406[1], 36410[1], 36420[1], 36425[1], 36430[1], 36440[1], 36591[0], 36592[0], 36600[1], 51701[0], 51702[0], 51703[0], 69990[0], 76000[1], 76800[1], 76970[1], 76998[1], 77001[1], 77002[1], 92012[1], 92014[1], 92585[0], 93000[1], 93005[1], 93010[1], 93040[1], 93041[1], 93042[1], 93318[1], 93355[1], 94002[1], 94200[1], 94250[1], 94680[1], 94681[1], 94690[1], 94770[1], 95812[1], 95813[1], 95816[1], 95819[1], 95822[0], 95829[1], 95860[1], 95861[1], 95863[1], 95864[1], 95865[1], 95866[1], 95867[1], 95868[1], 95869[1], 95870[1], 95907[1], 95908[1], 95909[1], 95910[1], 95911[1], 95912[1], 95913[1], 95925[0], 95926[0], 95927[0], 95928[0], 95929[0], 95930[0], 95933[0], 95937[0], 95938[0], 95939[0], 95940[0], 95955[1], 96360[1], 96361[1], 96365[1], 96366[1], 96367[1], 96368[1], 96372[1], 96374[1], 96375[1], 96376[1], 96377[1], 99155[0], 99156[0], 99157[0], 99211[1], 99212[1], 99213[1], 99214[1], 99215[1], 99217[1], 99218[1], 99219[1], 99220[1], 99221[1], 99222[1], 99223[1], 99231[1], 99232[1], 99233[1], 99234[1], 99235[1], 99236[1], 99238[1], 99239[1], 99241[1], 99242[1], 99243[1], 99244[1], 99245[1], 99251[1], 99252[1], 99253[1], 99254[1], 99255[1], 99291[1], 99292[1], 99304[1], 99305[1], 99306[1], 99307[1], 99308[1], 99309[1], 99310[1], 99315[1], 99316[1], 99334[1], 99335[1], 99336[1], 99337[1], 99347[1], 99348[1], 99349[1], 99350[1], 99374[1], 99375[1], 99377[1], 99378[1], 99446[0], 99447[0], 99448[0], 99449[0], 99451[0], 99452[0], 99495[1], 99496[1], G0453[0], G0459[1], G0463[1], G0471[0], J0670[1], J2001[1]
64446	01991[0], 01992[0], 01996[0], 0333T[0], 0464T[0], 20550[1], 20551[1], 36000[1], 36400[1], 36405[1], 36406[1], 36410[1], 36420[1], 36425[1], 36430[1], 36440[1], 36591[0], 36592[0], 36600[1], 51701[0], 51702[0], 51703[0], 69990[0], 76000[1], 76800[1], 76970[1], 76998[1], 77001[1], 77002[1], 92012[1], 92014[1], 92585[0], 93000[1], 93005[1], 93010[1], 93040[1], 93041[1], 93042[1], 93318[1], 93355[1], 94002[1], 94200[1], 94250[1], 94680[1], 94681[1], 94690[1], 94770[1], 95812[1], 95813[1], 95816[1], 95819[1], 95822[0], 95829[1], 95860[1], 95861[1], 95863[1], 95864[1], 95865[1], 95866[1], 95867[1], 95868[1], 95869[1], 95870[1], 95907[1], 95908[1], 95909[1], 95910[1], 95911[1], 95912[1], 95913[1], 95925[0], 95926[0], 95927[0], 95928[0], 95929[0], 95930[0], 95933[0], 95937[0], 95938[0], 95939[0], 95940[0], 95955[1], 96360[1], 96361[1], 96365[1], 96366[1], 96367[1], 96368[1], 96372[1], 96374[1], 96375[1], 96376[1], 96377[1], 99155[0], 99156[0], 99157[0], 99211[1], 99212[1], 99213[1], 99214[1], 99215[1], 99217[1], 99218[1], 99219[1], 99220[1], 99221[1], 99222[1], 99223[1], 99231[1], 99232[1], 99233[1], 99234[1], 99235[1], 99236[1], 99238[1], 99239[1], 99241[1], 99242[1], 99243[1], 99244[1], 99245[1], 99251[1], 99252[1], 99253[1], 99254[1], 99255[1], 99291[1], 99292[1], 99304[1], 99305[1], 99306[1], 99307[1], 99308[1], 99309[1], 99310[1], 99315[1], 99316[1], 99334[1], 99335[1], 99336[1], 99337[1], 99347[1], 99348[1], 99349[1], 99350[1], 99374[1], 99375[1], 99377[1], 99378[1], 99446[0], 99447[0], 99448[0], 99449[0], 99451[0], 99452[0], 99495[1], 99496[1], G0453[0], G0459[1], G0463[1], G0471[0], J2001[1]
64447	01991[0], 01992[0], 01996[0], 0333T[0], 0464T[0], 20550[1], 20551[1], 36000[1], 36400[1], 36405[1], 36406[1], 36410[1], 36420[1], 36425[1], 36430[1], 36440[1], 36591[0], 36592[0], 36600[1], 51701[0], 51702[0], 51703[0], 69990[0], 76000[1], 76970[1], 76998[1], 77001[1], 77002[1], 92012[1], 92014[1], 92585[0], 93000[1], 93005[1], 93010[1], 93040[1], 93041[1], 93042[1], 93318[1], 93355[1], 94002[1], 94200[1], 94250[1], 94680[1], 94681[1], 94690[1], 94770[1], 95812[1], 95813[1], 95816[1], 95819[1], 95822[0], 95829[1], 95860[1], 95861[1], 95863[1], 95864[1], 95865[1], 95866[1], 95867[1], 95868[1], 95869[1], 95870[1], 95907[1], 95908[1], 95909[1], 95910[1], 95911[1], 95912[1], 95913[1], 95925[0], 95926[0], 95927[0], 95928[0], 95929[0], 95930[0], 95933[0], 95937[0], 95938[0], 95939[0], 95940[0], 95955[1], 96360[1], 96361[1], 96365[1], 96366[1], 96367[1], 96368[1], 96372[1], 96374[1], 96375[1], 96376[1], 96377[1], 99155[0], 99156[0], 99157[0], 99211[1], 99212[1], 99213[1], 99214[1], 99215[1], 99217[1], 99218[1], 99219[1], 99220[1], 99221[1], 99222[1], 99223[1], 99231[1], 99232[1], 99233[1], 99234[1], 99235[1], 99236[1], 99238[1], 99239[1], 99241[1], 99242[1], 99243[1], 99244[1], 99245[1], 99251[1], 99252[1], 99253[1], 99254[1], 99255[1], 99291[1], 99292[1], 99304[1], 99305[1], 99306[1], 99307[1], 99308[1], 99309[1], 99310[1], 99315[1], 99316[1], 99334[1], 99335[1], 99336[1], 99337[1], 99347[1], 99348[1], 99349[1], 99350[1], 99374[1], 99375[1], 99377[1], 99378[1], 99446[0], 99447[0], 99448[0], 99449[0], 99451[0], 99452[0], 99495[1], 99496[1], G0453[0], G0459[1], G0463[1], G0471[0], J0670[1], J2001[1]
64448	01991[0], 01992[0], 01996[0], 0333T[0], 0464T[0], 20550[1], 20551[1], 36000[1], 36400[1], 36405[1], 36406[1], 36410[1], 36420[1], 36425[1], 36430[1], 36440[1], 36591[0], 36592[0], 36600[1], 51701[0], 51702[0], 51703[0], 69990[0], 76000[1], 76970[1], 76998[1], 77001[1], 77002[1], 92012[1], 92014[1], 92585[0], 93000[1], 93005[1], 93010[1], 93040[1], 93041[1], 93042[1], 93318[1], 93355[1], 94002[1], 94200[1], 94250[1], 94680[1], 94681[1], 94690[1], 94770[1], 95812[1], 95813[1], 95816[1], 95819[1], 95822[0], 95829[1], 95860[1], 95861[1], 95863[1], 95864[1], 95865[1], 95866[1], 95867[1], 95868[1], 95869[1], 95870[1], 95907[1], 95908[1], 95909[1], 95910[1], 95911[1], 95912[1], 95913[1], 95925[0], 95926[0], 95927[0], 95928[0], 95929[0], 95930[0], 95933[0], 95937[0], 95938[0], 95939[0], 95940[0], 95955[1], 96360[1], 96361[1], 96365[1], 96366[1], 96367[1], 96368[1], 96372[1], 96374[1], 96375[1], 96376[1], 96377[1], 99155[0], 99156[0], 99157[0], 99211[1], 99212[1], 99213[1], 99214[1], 99215[1], 99217[1], 99218[1], 99219[1], 99220[1], 99221[1], 99222[1], 99223[1], 99231[1], 99232[1], 99233[1], 99234[1], 99235[1], 99236[1], 99238[1], 99239[1], 99241[1], 99242[1], 99243[1], 99244[1], 99245[1],

Appendix A: NCCI - CPT Codes

0 = Modifier usage not allowed or inappropriate 1 = Modifier usage allowed

CPT © 2018 American Medical Association. All Rights Reserved.

Code 1	Code 2
	99251[1], 99252[1], 99253[1], 99254[1], 99255[1], 99291[1], 99292[1], 99304[1], 99305[1], 99306[1], 99307[1], 99308[1], 99309[1], 99310[1], 99315[1], 99316[1], 99334[1], 99335[1], 99336[1], 99337[1], 99347[1], 99348[1], 99349[1], 99350[1], 99374[1], 99375[1], 99377[1], 99378[1], 99446[0], 99447[0], 99448[0], 99449[0], 99451[0], 99452[0], 99495[1], 99496[1], G0453[0], G0459[1], G0463[1], G0471[0], J2001[1]
64449	01991[0], 01992[0], 01996[0], 0333T[0], 0464T[0], 20550[1], 20551[1], 36000[1], 36400[1], 36405[1], 36406[1], 36410[1], 36420[1], 36425[1], 36430[1], 36440[1], 36591[0], 36592[0], 36600[1], 51701[0], 51702[0], 51703[0], 69990[0], 76000[1], 76800[1], 76970[1], 76998[1], 77001[1], 77002[1], 92012[1], 92014[1], 92585[0], 93000[1], 93005[1], 93010[1], 93040[1], 93041[1], 93042[1], 93318[1], 93355[1], 94002[1], 94200[1], 94250[1], 94680[1], 94681[1], 94690[1], 94770[1], 95812[1], 95813[1], 95816[1], 95819[1], 95822[0], 95829[1], 95860[1], 95861[1], 95863[1], 95864[1], 95865[1], 95866[1], 95867[1], 95868[1], 95869[1], 95870[1], 95907[1], 95908[1], 95909[1], 95910[1], 95911[1], 95912[1], 95913[1], 95925[0], 95926[0], 95927[0], 95928[0], 95929[0], 95930[0], 95933[0], 95937[0], 95938[0], 95939[0], 95940[0], 95955[1], 96360[1], 96361[1], 96365[1], 96366[1], 96367[1], 96368[1], 96372[1], 96374[1], 96375[1], 96376[1], 96377[1], 97033[1], 99155[0], 99156[0], 99157[0], 99211[1], 99212[1], 99213[1], 99214[1], 99215[1], 99217[1], 99218[1], 99219[1], 99220[1], 99221[1], 99222[1], 99223[1], 99231[1], 99232[1], 99233[1], 99234[1], 99235[1], 99236[1], 99238[1], 99239[1], 99241[1], 99242[1], 99243[1], 99244[1], 99245[1], 99251[1], 99252[1], 99253[1], 99254[1], 99255[1], 99291[1], 99292[1], 99304[1], 99305[1], 99306[1], 99307[1], 99308[1], 99309[1], 99310[1], 99315[1], 99316[1], 99334[1], 99335[1], 99336[1], 99337[1], 99347[1], 99348[1], 99349[1], 99350[1], 99374[1], 99375[1], 99377[1], 99378[1], 99446[0], 99447[0], 99448[0], 99449[0], 99451[0], 99452[0], 99495[1], 99496[1], G0453[0], G0459[1], G0463[1], G0471[0], J2001[1]
64450	01991[0], 01992[0], 0333T[0], 0464T[0], 20526[1], 20550[1], 20551[1], 29515[0], 29540[0], 29580[0], 36591[0], 36592[0], 51701[0], 51702[0], 64455[1], 69990[0], 76000[1], 76970[1], 76998[1], 77001[1], 77002[1], 92012[1], 92014[1], 92585[0], 93000[1], 93005[1], 93010[1], 93040[1], 93041[1], 93042[1], 93318[1], 93355[1], 94002[1], 94200[1], 94250[1], 94680[1], 94681[1], 94690[1], 94770[1], 95812[1], 95813[1], 95816[1], 95819[1], 95822[0], 95829[1], 95860[1], 95861[1], 95863[1], 95864[1], 95865[1], 95866[1], 95867[1], 95868[1], 95869[1], 95870[1], 95907[1], 95908[1], 95909[1], 95910[1], 95911[1], 95912[1], 95913[1], 95925[0], 95926[0], 95927[0], 95928[0], 95929[0], 95930[0], 95933[0], 95937[0], 95938[0], 95939[0], 95940[0], 95955[1], 96361[1], 96366[1], 96367[1], 96368[1], 96372[1], 96374[1], 96375[1], 96376[1], 96377[1], 99155[0], 99156[0], 99157[0], 99211[1], 99212[1], 99213[1], 99214[1], 99215[1], 99217[1], 99218[1], 99219[1], 99220[1], 99221[1], 99222[1], 99223[1], 99231[1], 99232[1], 99233[1], 99234[1], 99235[1], 99236[1], 99238[1], 99239[1], 99241[1], 99242[1], 99243[1], 99244[1], 99245[1], 99251[1], 99252[1], 99253[1], 99254[1], 99255[1], 99291[1], 99292[1], 99304[1], 99305[1], 99306[1], 99307[1], 99308[1], 99309[1], 99310[1], 99315[1], 99316[1], 99334[1], 99335[1], 99336[1], 99337[1], 99347[1], 99348[1], 99349[1], 99350[1], 99374[1], 99375[1], 99377[1], 99378[1], 99446[0], 99447[0], 99448[0], 99449[0], 99451[0], 99452[0], 99495[1], 99496[1], G0453[0], G0459[1], G0463[1], G0471[0], J0670[1], J2001[1]
64455	01991[0], 01992[1], 0333T[0], 0464T[0], 29515[1], 29540[1], 29550[1], 29580[1], 36000[1], 36400[1], 36405[1], 36406[1], 36410[1], 36420[1], 36425[1], 36430[1], 36440[1], 36591[0], 36592[0], 36600[1], 36640[1], 43752[1], 51701[0], 51702[0], 51703[0], 69990[0], 76000[1], 76970[1], 76998[1], 77001[1], 77002[1], 92012[1], 92014[1], 92585[0], 93000[1], 93005[1], 93010[1], 93040[1], 93041[1], 93042[1], 93318[1], 93355[1], 94002[1], 94200[1], 94250[1], 94680[1], 94681[1], 94690[1], 94770[1], 95812[1], 95813[1], 95816[1], 95819[1], 95822[0], 95829[1], 95860[1], 95861[1], 95863[1], 95864[1], 95865[1], 95866[1], 95867[1], 95868[1], 95869[1], 95870[1], 95907[1], 95908[1], 95909[1], 95910[1], 95911[1], 95912[1], 95913[1], 95925[0], 95926[0], 95927[0], 95928[0], 95929[0], 95930[0], 95933[0], 95937[0], 95938[0], 95939[0], 95940[0], 95955[1], 96360[1], 96361[1], 96365[1], 96366[1], 96367[1], 96368[1], 96372[1], 96374[1], 96375[1], 96376[1], 96377[1], 99155[0], 99156[0], 99157[0], 99211[1], 99212[1], 99213[1], 99214[1], 99215[1], 99217[1], 99218[1], 99219[1], 99220[1], 99221[1], 99222[1], 99223[1], 99231[1], 99232[1], 99233[1], 99234[1], 99235[1], 99236[1], 99238[1], 99239[1], 99241[1], 99242[1], 99243[1], 99244[1], 99245[1], 99251[1], 99252[1], 99253[1], 99254[1], 99255[1], 99291[1], 99292[1], 99304[1], 99305[1], 99306[1], 99307[1], 99308[1], 99309[1], 99310[1], 99315[1], 99316[1], 99334[1], 99335[1], 99336[1], 99337[1], 99347[1], 99348[1], 99349[1], 99350[1], 99374[1], 99375[1], 99377[1], 99378[1], 99446[0], 99447[0], 99448[0], 99449[0], 99451[0], 99452[0], 99495[1], 99496[1], G0453[0], G0463[1], G0471[0], J0670[1], J2001[1]
64461	01991[0], 01992[0], 0333T[0], 0464T[0], 12001[1], 12002[1], 12004[1], 12005[1], 12006[1], 12007[1], 12011[1], 12013[1], 12014[1], 12015[1], 12016[1], 12017[1], 12018[1], 12020[1], 12021[1], 12031[1], 12032[1], 12034[1], 12035[1], 12036[1], 12037[1], 12041[1], 12042[1], 12044[1], 12045[1], 12046[1], 12047[1], 12051[1], 12052[1], 12053[1], 12054[1], 12055[1], 12056[1], 12057[1], 13100[1], 13101[1], 13102[1], 13120[1], 13121[1], 13122[1], 13131[1], 13132[1], 13133[1], 13151[1], 13152[1], 13153[1], 36000[1], 36400[1], 36405[1], 36406[1], 36410[1], 36420[1], 36425[1], 36430[1], 36440[1], 36591[0], 36592[0], 36600[1], 51701[0], 51702[0], 51703[0], 62320[0], 62321[0], 62324[0], 62325[0], 64420[0], 64421[0], 64479[0], 64480[0], 64490[0], 64491[0], 64492[0], 69990[0], 76000[1], 76380[1], 76942[1], 76970[1], 76998[1], 77001[1], 77002[1], 77003[1], 77012[1], 77021[1], 92012[1], 92014[1], 92585[0], 93000[1], 93005[1], 93010[1], 93040[1], 93041[1], 93042[1], 93318[1], 93355[1], 94002[1], 94200[1], 94250[1], 94680[1], 94681[1], 94690[1], 94770[1], 95812[1], 95813[1], 95816[1], 95819[1], 95822[0], 95829[1], 95860[0], 95861[0], 95863[0], 95864[0], 95865[0], 95866[0], 95867[0], 95868[0], 95869[0], 95870[0], 95907[0], 95908[0], 95909[0], 95910[0], 95911[0], 95912[0], 95913[0], 95925[0], 95926[0], 95927[0], 95928[0], 95929[0], 95930[0], 95933[0], 95937[0], 95938[0], 95939[0], 95940[0], 95941[0], 95955[1], 96360[1], 96361[1], 96365[1], 96366[1], 96367[1], 96368[1], 96372[1], 96374[1], 96375[1], 96376[1], 96377[1], 99155[0], 99156[0], 99157[0], 99211[1], 99212[1], 99213[1], 99214[1], 99215[1], 99217[1], 99218[1], 99219[1], 99220[1], 99221[1], 99222[1], 99223[1], 99231[1], 99232[1], 99233[1], 99234[1], 99235[1], 99236[1], 99238[1], 99239[1], 99241[1], 99242[1], 99243[1], 99244[1], 99245[1], 99251[1], 99252[1], 99253[1], 99254[1], 99255[1], 99291[1], 99292[1], 99304[1], 99305[1], 99306[1], 99307[1], 99308[1], 99309[1], 99310[1], 99315[1], 99316[1], 99334[1], 99335[1], 99336[1], 99337[1], 99347[1], 99348[1], 99349[1], 99350[1], 99374[1], 99375[1], 99377[1], 99378[1], 99446[0], 99447[0], 99448[0], 99449[0], 99451[0], 99452[0], 99495[1], 99496[1], G0453[0], G0459[1], G0463[1], G0471[0], J0670[1], J2001[1]
64462	01991[0], 01992[0], 0333T[0], 0464T[0], 12001[0], 12002[1], 12004[1], 12005[1], 12006[1], 12007[1], 12011[1], 12013[1], 12014[1], 12015[1], 12016[1], 12017[1], 12018[1], 12020[1], 12021[1], 12031[1], 12032[1], 12034[1], 12035[1], 12036[1], 12037[1], 12041[1], 12042[1], 12044[1], 12045[1], 12046[1], 12047[1], 12051[1], 12052[1], 12053[1], 12054[1], 12055[1], 12056[1], 12057[1], 13100[1], 13101[1], 13102[1], 13120[1], 13121[1], 13122[1], 13131[1], 13132[1], 13133[1], 13151[1], 13152[1], 13153[1], 20550[1], 20551[1], 36000[1], 36400[1], 36405[1], 36406[1], 36410[1], 36420[1], 36425[1], 36430[1], 36440[1], 36591[0], 36592[0], 36600[1], 36640[1], 43752[1], 51701[0], 51702[0], 51703[0], 64420[0], 64421[0], 64479[0], 64480[0], 64490[0], 64491[0], 64492[0], 69990[0], 76000[1], 76380[1], 76942[1], 76970[1], 76998[1], 77001[1], 77002[1], 77003[1], 77012[1], 77021[1], 92012[1], 92014[1], 92585[0], 93000[1], 93005[1], 93010[1], 93040[1], 93041[1], 93042[1], 93318[1], 93355[1], 94002[1], 94200[1], 94250[1], 94680[1], 94681[1], 94690[1], 94770[1], 95812[1], 95813[1], 95816[1], 95819[1], 95822[0], 95829[1], 95860[0], 95861[0], 95863[0], 95864[0], 95865[0], 95866[0], 95867[0], 95868[0], 95869[0], 95870[0], 95907[0], 95908[0], 95909[0], 95910[0], 95911[0], 95912[0], 95913[0], 95925[0], 95926[0], 95927[0], 95928[0], 95929[0], 95930[0], 95933[0], 95937[0], 95938[0], 95939[0], 95940[0], 95941[0], 95955[1], 96360[1], 96365[1], 96372[1], 96374[1], 96375[1], 96376[1], 96377[1], 99155[0], 99156[0], 99157[0], 99211[1], 99212[1], 99213[1], 99214[1], 99215[1], 99217[1], 99218[1], 99219[1], 99220[1], 99221[1], 99222[1], 99223[1], 99231[1], 99232[1], 99233[1], 99234[1], 99235[1], 99236[1], 99238[1], 99239[1], 99241[1], 99242[1], 99243[1], 99244[1], 99245[1], 99251[1], 99252[1], 99253[1], 99254[1], 99255[1], 99291[1], 99292[1], 99304[1], 99305[1], 99306[1], 99307[1], 99308[1], 99309[1], 99310[1], 99315[1], 99316[1], 99334[1], 99335[1], 99336[1], 99337[1], 99347[1], 99348[1], 99349[1], 99350[1], 99374[1], 99375[1], 99377[1], 99378[1], 99446[0], 99447[0], 99448[0], 99449[0], 99451[0], 99452[0], 99495[1], 99496[1], G0453[0], G0459[1], G0463[1], G0471[0], J0670[1], J2001[1]
64463	01991[0], 01992[0], 0333T[0], 0464T[0], 12001[1], 12002[1], 12004[1], 12005[1], 12006[1], 12007[1], 12011[1], 12013[1], 12014[1], 12015[1], 12016[1], 12017[1], 12018[1], 12020[1], 12021[1], 12031[1], 12032[1], 12034[1], 12035[1], 12036[1], 12037[1], 12041[1], 12042[1], 12044[1], 12045[1], 12046[1], 12047[1], 12051[1], 12052[1], 12053[1], 12054[1], 12055[1], 12056[1], 12057[1], 13100[1], 13101[1], 13102[1], 13120[1], 13121[1], 13122[1], 13131[1], 13132[1], 13133[1], 13151[1], 13152[1], 13153[1], 36000[1], 36400[1], 36405[1], 36406[1], 36410[1], 36420[1], 36425[1], 36430[1], 36440[1], 36591[0], 36592[0], 36600[1], 51701[0], 51702[0], 51703[0], 62320[0], 62321[0], 62324[0], 62325[0], 64420[0], 64421[0], 64479[0], 64480[0], 64490[0], 64491[0], 64492[0], 69990[0], 76000[1], 76380[1], 76942[1], 76970[1], 76998[1], 77001[1], 77002[1], 77003[1], 77012[1], 77021[1], 92012[1], 92014[1], 92585[0], 93000[1], 93005[1], 93010[1], 93040[1], 93041[1], 93042[1], 93318[1], 93355[1], 94002[1], 94200[1], 94250[1], 94680[1], 94681[1], 94690[1], 94770[1], 95812[1], 95813[1], 95816[1], 95819[1], 95822[0], 95829[1], 95860[0], 95861[0], 95863[0], 95864[0], 95865[0], 95866[0], 95867[0], 95868[0], 95869[0], 95870[0], 95907[0], 95908[0], 95909[0], 95910[0], 95911[0], 95912[0], 95913[0], 95925[0], 95926[0], 95927[0], 95928[0], 95929[0], 95930[0], 95933[0], 95937[0], 95938[0], 95939[0], 95940[0], 95941[0], 95955[1], 96360[1], 96361[1], 96365[1], 96366[1], 96367[1], 96368[1], 96372[1], 96374[1], 96375[1], 96376[1], 96377[1], 99155[0], 99156[0], 99157[0], 99211[1], 99212[1], 99213[1], 99214[1], 99215[1], 99217[1], 99218[1], 99219[1], 99220[1], 99221[1], 99222[1], 99223[1], 99231[1], 99232[1], 99233[1], 99234[1], 99235[1], 99236[1], 99238[1], 99239[1], 99241[1], 99242[1], 99243[1], 99244[1], 99245[1], 99251[1], 99252[1], 99253[1], 99254[1], 99255[1], 99291[1], 99292[1], 99304[1], 99305[1], 99306[1], 99307[1], 99308[1], 99309[1], 99310[1], 99315[1], 99316[1], 99334[1], 99335[1], 99336[1], 99337[1], 99347[1], 99348[1], 99349[1], 99350[1], 99374[1], 99375[1], 99377[1], 99378[1], 99446[0], 99447[0], 99448[0], 99449[0], 99451[0], 99452[0], 99495[1], 99496[1], G0453[0], G0459[1], G0463[1], G0471[0], J0670[1], J2001[1]
64479	01991[0], 01992[0], 0228T[0], 0229T[1], 0333T[0], 0464T[0], 20550[1], 20551[1], 20605[1], 20610[1], 36000[1], 36140[1], 36400[1], 36405[1], 36406[1], 36410[1], 36420[1], 36425[1], 36430[1], 36440[1], 36591[0], 36592[0], 36600[1], 51701[0], 51702[0], 51703[0], 69990[0], 72275[1], 76000[1], 76380[1], 76800[1], 76942[1], 76970[1], 76998[1], 77001[1], 77002[1], 77003[1], 77012[1], 92012[1], 92014[1], 92585[0], 93000[1], 93005[1], 93010[1], 93040[1], 93041[1], 93042[1], 93318[1], 93355[1], 94002[1], 94200[1], 94250[1], 94680[1], 94681[1], 94690[1], 94770[1], 95812[1], 95813[1], 95816[1], 95819[1], 95822[0], 95829[1], 95860[1], 95861[1], 95863[1], 95864[1], 95865[1], 95866[1], 95869[1], 95870[1],

Appendix A: NCCI - CPT Codes

0 = Modifier usage not allowed or inappropriate 1 = Modifier usage allowed

CPT © 2018 American Medical Association. All Rights Reserved.

Code 1	Code 2
	95907[1], 95908[1], 95909[1], 95910[1], 95911[1], 95912[1], 95913[1], 95925[0], 95926[0], 95927[0], 95928[0], 95929[0], 95930[0], 95933[0], 95937[0], 95938[0], 95939[0], 95940[0], 95955[1], 96360[1], 96361[1], 96365[1], 96366[1], 96367[1], 96368[1], 96372[1], 96374[1], 96375[1], 96376[1], 96377[1], 99155[0], 99156[0], 99157[0], 99211[1], 99212[1], 99213[1], 99214[1], 99215[1], 99217[1], 99218[1], 99219[1], 99220[1], 99221[1], 99222[1], 99223[1], 99231[1], 99232[1], 99233[1], 99234[1], 99235[1], 99236[1], 99238[1], 99239[1], 99241[1], 99242[1], 99243[1], 99244[1], 99245[1], 99251[1], 99252[1], 99253[1], 99254[1], 99255[1], 99291[1], 99292[1], 99304[1], 99305[1], 99306[1], 99307[1], 99308[1], 99309[1], 99310[1], 99315[1], 99316[1], 99334[1], 99335[1], 99336[1], 99337[1], 99347[1], 99348[1], 99349[1], 99350[1], 99374[1], 99375[1], 99377[1], 99378[1], 99446[0], 99447[0], 99448[0], 99449[0], 99451[0], 99452[0], 99495[1], 99496[1], G0453[0], G0459[1], G0463[1], G0471[0], J2001[1]
64480	01991[0], 01992[0], 0229T[0], 0333T[0], 0464T[0], 36591[0], 36592[0], 69990[0], 76000[1], 76380[1], 76800[1], 76942[1], 76970[1], 76998[1], 77002[1], 77003[1], 77012[1], 92585[0], 93000[1], 93005[1], 93010[1], 93040[1], 93041[1], 93042[1], 95822[0], 95860[1], 95861[1], 95863[1], 95864[1], 95865[1], 95866[1], 95869[1], 95907[1], 95908[1], 95909[1], 95910[1], 95911[1], 95912[1], 95913[1], 95925[0], 95926[0], 95927[0], 95930[0], 95933[0], 95937[0], 95938[0], 95939[0], 95940[0], G0453[0], G0459[1]
64483	01991[0], 01992[0], 0230T[0], 0231T[1], 0333T[0], 0464T[0], 20550[1], 20551[1], 20605[1], 20610[1], 36000[1], 36140[1], 36400[1], 36405[1], 36406[1], 36410[1], 36420[1], 36425[1], 36430[1], 36440[1], 36591[0], 36592[0], 36600[1], 51701[0], 51702[0], 51703[0], 72275[1], 76000[1], 76380[1], 76800[1], 76942[1], 76970[1], 76998[1], 77001[1], 77002[1], 77003[1], 77012[1], 92012[1], 92014[1], 92585[0], 93000[1], 93005[1], 93010[1], 93040[1], 93041[1], 93042[1], 93318[1], 93355[1], 94002[1], 94200[1], 94250[1], 94680[1], 94681[1], 94690[1], 94770[1], 95812[1], 95813[1], 95816[1], 95819[1], 95822[0], 95829[1], 95860[1], 95861[1], 95863[1], 95864[1], 95865[1], 95866[1], 95869[1], 95870[1], 95907[1], 95908[1], 95909[1], 95910[1], 95911[1], 95912[1], 95913[1], 95925[0], 95926[0], 95927[0], 95928[0], 95929[0], 95930[0], 95933[0], 95937[0], 95938[0], 95939[0], 95940[0], 95955[1], 96360[1], 96361[1], 96365[1], 96366[1], 96367[1], 96368[1], 96372[1], 96374[1], 96375[1], 96376[1], 96377[1], 99155[0], 99156[0], 99157[0], 99211[1], 99212[1], 99213[1], 99214[1], 99215[1], 99217[1], 99218[1], 99219[1], 99220[1], 99221[1], 99222[1], 99223[1], 99231[1], 99232[1], 99233[1], 99234[1], 99235[1], 99236[1], 99238[1], 99239[1], 99241[1], 99242[1], 99243[1], 99244[1], 99245[1], 99251[1], 99252[1], 99253[1], 99254[1], 99255[1], 99291[1], 99292[1], 99304[1], 99305[1], 99306[1], 99307[1], 99308[1], 99309[1], 99310[1], 99315[1], 99316[1], 99334[1], 99335[1], 99336[1], 99337[1], 99347[1], 99348[1], 99349[1], 99350[1], 99374[1], 99375[1], 99377[1], 99378[1], 99446[0], 99447[0], 99448[0], 99449[0], 99451[0], 99452[0], 99495[1], 99496[1], G0453[0], G0459[1], G0463[1], G0471[0], J2001[1]
64484	01991[0], 01992[0], 0231T[0], 0333T[0], 0464T[0], 36591[0], 36592[0], 76000[1], 76380[1], 76800[1], 76942[1], 76970[1], 76998[1], 77002[1], 77003[1], 77012[1], 92585[0], 93000[1], 93005[1], 93010[1], 93040[1], 93041[1], 93042[1], 95822[0], 95860[1], 95861[1], 95863[1], 95864[1], 95865[1], 95866[1], 95869[1], 95907[1], 95908[1], 95909[1], 95910[1], 95911[1], 95912[1], 95913[1], 95925[0], 95926[0], 95927[0], 95930[0], 95933[0], 95937[0], 95938[0], 95939[0], 95940[0], G0453[0], G0459[1]
64486	01991[0], 01992[0], 0333T[0], 0464T[0], 12001[1], 12002[1], 12004[1], 12005[1], 12006[1], 12007[1], 12011[1], 12013[1], 12014[1], 12015[1], 12016[1], 12017[1], 12018[1], 12020[1], 12021[1], 12031[1], 12032[1], 12034[1], 12035[1], 12036[1], 12037[1], 12041[1], 12042[1], 12044[1], 12045[1], 12046[1], 12047[1], 12051[1], 12052[1], 12053[1], 12054[1], 12055[1], 12056[1], 12057[1], 13100[1], 13101[1], 13102[1], 13120[1], 13121[1], 13122[1], 13131[1], 13132[1], 13133[1], 13151[1], 13152[1], 13153[1], 36000[1], 36400[1], 36405[1], 36406[1], 36410[1], 36420[1], 36425[1], 36430[1], 36440[1], 36591[0], 36592[0], 36600[1], 51701[1], 51702[1], 69990[0], 76000[1], 76380[1], 76942[1], 76970[1], 76998[1], 77001[1], 77002[1], 77012[1], 77021[1], 92012[1], 92014[1], 92585[0], 93000[1], 93005[1], 93010[1], 93040[1], 93041[1], 93042[1], 93318[1], 93355[1], 94002[1], 94200[1], 94250[1], 94680[1], 94681[1], 94690[1], 94770[1], 95812[1], 95813[1], 95816[1], 95819[1], 95822[0], 95829[1], 95860[0], 95861[0], 95863[0], 95864[0], 95865[0], 95866[0], 95867[0], 95868[0], 95869[0], 95870[0], 95907[0], 95908[0], 95909[0], 95910[0], 95911[0], 95912[0], 95913[0], 95925[0], 95926[0], 95927[0], 95928[0], 95929[0], 95930[0], 95933[0], 95937[0], 95938[0], 95939[0], 95940[0], 95941[0], 95955[1], 96360[1], 96361[1], 96365[1], 96366[1], 96367[1], 96368[1], 96372[1], 96374[1], 96375[1], 96376[1], 96377[1], 99155[0], 99156[0], 99157[0], 99211[1], 99212[1], 99213[1], 99214[1], 99215[1], 99217[1], 99218[1], 99219[1], 99220[1], 99221[1], 99222[1], 99223[1], 99231[1], 99232[1], 99233[1], 99234[1], 99235[1], 99236[1], 99238[1], 99239[1], 99241[1], 99242[1], 99243[1], 99244[1], 99245[1], 99251[1], 99252[1], 99253[1], 99254[1], 99255[1], 99291[1], 99292[1], 99304[1], 99305[1], 99306[1], 99307[1], 99308[1], 99309[1], 99310[1], 99315[1], 99316[1], 99334[1], 99335[1], 99336[1], 99337[1], 99347[1], 99348[1], 99349[1], 99350[1], 99374[1], 99375[1], 99377[1], 99378[1], 99446[0], 99447[0], 99448[0], 99449[0], 99451[0], 99452[0], 99495[1], 99496[1], G0453[0], G0459[1], G0463[1], G0471[1], J0670[1], J2001[1]
64487	01991[0], 01992[0], 0333T[0], 0464T[0], 12001[1], 12002[1], 12004[1], 12005[1], 12006[1], 12007[1], 12011[1], 12013[1], 12014[1], 12015[1], 12016[1], 12017[1], 12018[1], 12020[1], 12021[1], 12031[1], 12032[1], 12034[1], 12035[1], 12036[1], 12037[1], 12041[1], 12042[1], 12044[1], 12045[1], 12046[1], 12047[1], 12051[1], 12052[1], 12053[1], 12054[1], 12055[1], 12056[1], 12057[1], 13100[1], 13101[1], 13102[1], 13120[1], 13121[1], 13122[1], 13131[1], 13132[1], 13133[1], 13151[1], 13152[1], 13153[1], 36000[1], 36400[1], 36405[1], 36406[1], 36410[1], 36420[1], 36425[1], 36430[1], 36440[1], 36591[0], 36592[0], 36600[1], 51701[1], 51702[1], 64486[0], 69990[0], 76000[1], 76380[1], 76942[1], 76970[1], 76998[1], 77001[1], 77002[1], 77012[1], 77021[1], 92012[1], 92014[1], 92585[0], 93000[1], 93005[1], 93010[1], 93040[1], 93041[1], 93042[1], 93318[1], 93355[1], 94002[1], 94200[1], 94250[1], 94680[1], 94681[1], 94690[1], 94770[1], 95812[1], 95813[1], 95816[1], 95819[1], 95822[0], 95829[1], 95860[0], 95861[0], 95863[0], 95864[0], 95865[0], 95866[0], 95867[0], 95868[0], 95869[0], 95870[0], 95907[0], 95908[0], 95909[0], 95910[0], 95911[0], 95912[0], 95913[0], 95925[0], 95926[0], 95927[0], 95928[0], 95929[0], 95930[0], 95933[0], 95937[0], 95938[0], 95939[0], 95940[0], 95941[0], 95955[1], 96360[1], 96361[1], 96365[1], 96366[1], 96367[1], 96368[1], 96372[1], 96374[1], 96375[1], 96376[1], 96377[1], 99155[0], 99156[0], 99157[0], 99211[1], 99212[1], 99213[1], 99214[1], 99215[1], 99217[1], 99218[1], 99219[1], 99220[1], 99221[1], 99222[1], 99223[1], 99231[1], 99232[1], 99233[1], 99234[1], 99235[1], 99236[1], 99238[1], 99239[1], 99241[1], 99242[1], 99243[1], 99244[1], 99245[1], 99251[1], 99252[1], 99253[1], 99254[1], 99255[1], 99291[1], 99292[1], 99304[1], 99305[1], 99306[1], 99307[1], 99308[1], 99309[1], 99310[1], 99315[1], 99316[1], 99334[1], 99335[1], 99336[1], 99337[1], 99347[1], 99348[1], 99349[1], 99350[1], 99374[1], 99375[1], 99377[1], 99378[1], 99446[0], 99447[0], 99448[0], 99449[0], 99451[0], 99452[0], 99495[1], 99496[1], G0453[0], G0459[1], G0463[1], G0471[1], J0670[1], J2001[1]
64488	01991[0], 01992[0], 0333T[0], 0464T[0], 12001[1], 12002[1], 12004[1], 12005[1], 12006[1], 12007[1], 12011[1], 12013[1], 12014[1], 12015[1], 12016[1], 12017[1], 12018[1], 12020[1], 12021[1], 12031[1], 12032[1], 12034[1], 12035[1], 12036[1], 12037[1], 12041[1], 12042[1], 12044[1], 12045[1], 12046[1], 12047[1], 12051[1], 12052[1], 12053[1], 12054[1], 12055[1], 12056[1], 12057[1], 13100[1], 13101[1], 13102[1], 13120[1], 13121[1], 13122[1], 13131[1], 13132[1], 13133[1], 13151[1], 13152[1], 13153[1], 36000[1], 36400[1], 36405[1], 36406[1], 36410[1], 36420[1], 36425[1], 36430[1], 36440[1], 36591[0], 36592[0], 36600[1], 51701[1], 51702[1], 64486[0], 64487[0], 69990[0], 76000[1], 76380[1], 76942[1], 76970[1], 76998[1], 77001[1], 77002[1], 77012[1], 77021[1], 92012[1], 92014[1], 92585[0], 93000[1], 93005[1], 93010[1], 93040[1], 93041[1], 93042[1], 93318[1], 93355[1], 94002[1], 94200[1], 94250[1], 94680[1], 94681[1], 94690[1], 94770[1], 95812[1], 95813[1], 95816[1], 95819[1], 95822[0], 95829[1], 95860[0], 95861[0], 95863[0], 95864[0], 95865[0], 95866[0], 95867[0], 95868[0], 95869[0], 95870[0], 95907[0], 95908[0], 95909[0], 95910[0], 95911[0], 95912[0], 95913[0], 95925[0], 95926[0], 95927[0], 95928[0], 95929[0], 95930[0], 95933[0], 95937[0], 95938[0], 95939[0], 95940[0], 95941[0], 95955[1], 96360[1], 96361[1], 96365[1], 96366[1], 96367[1], 96368[1], 96372[1], 96374[1], 96375[1], 96376[1], 96377[1], 99155[0], 99156[0], 99157[0], 99211[1], 99212[1], 99213[1], 99214[1], 99215[1], 99217[1], 99218[1], 99219[1], 99220[1], 99221[1], 99222[1], 99223[1], 99231[1], 99232[1], 99233[1], 99234[1], 99235[1], 99236[1], 99238[1], 99239[1], 99241[1], 99242[1], 99243[1], 99244[1], 99245[1], 99251[1], 99252[1], 99253[1], 99254[1], 99255[1], 99291[1], 99292[1], 99304[1], 99305[1], 99306[1], 99307[1], 99308[1], 99309[1], 99310[1], 99315[1], 99316[1], 99334[1], 99335[1], 99336[1], 99337[1], 99347[1], 99348[1], 99349[1], 99350[1], 99374[1], 99375[1], 99377[1], 99378[1], 99446[0], 99447[0], 99448[0], 99449[0], 99451[0], 99452[0], 99495[1], 99496[1], G0453[0], G0459[1], G0463[1], G0471[1], J0670[1], J2001[1]
64489	01991[0], 01992[0], 0333T[0], 0464T[0], 12001[1], 12002[1], 12004[1], 12005[1], 12006[1], 12007[1], 12011[1], 12013[1], 12014[1], 12015[1], 12016[1], 12017[1], 12018[1], 12020[1], 12021[1], 12031[1], 12032[1], 12034[1], 12035[1], 12036[1], 12037[1], 12041[1], 12042[1], 12044[1], 12045[1], 12046[1], 12047[1], 12051[1], 12052[1], 12053[1], 12054[1], 12055[1], 12056[1], 12057[1], 13100[1], 13101[1], 13102[1], 13120[1], 13121[1], 13122[1], 13131[1], 13132[1], 13133[1], 13151[1], 13152[1], 13153[1], 36000[1], 36400[1], 36405[1], 36406[1], 36410[1], 36420[1], 36425[1], 36430[1], 36440[1], 36591[0], 36592[0], 36600[1], 51701[1], 51702[1], 64486[0], 64487[0], 64488[0], 69990[0], 76000[1], 76380[1], 76942[1], 76970[1], 76998[1], 77001[1], 77002[1], 77012[1], 77021[1], 92012[1], 92014[1], 92585[0], 93000[1], 93005[1], 93010[1], 93040[1], 93041[1], 93042[1], 93318[1], 93355[1], 94002[1], 94200[1], 94250[1], 94680[1], 94681[1], 94690[1], 94770[1], 95812[1], 95813[1], 95816[1], 95819[1], 95822[0], 95829[1], 95860[0], 95861[0], 95863[0], 95864[0], 95865[0], 95866[0], 95867[0], 95868[0], 95869[0], 95870[0], 95907[0], 95908[0], 95909[0], 95910[0], 95911[0], 95912[0], 95913[0], 95925[0], 95926[0], 95927[0], 95928[0], 95929[0], 95930[0], 95933[0], 95937[0], 95938[0], 95939[0], 95940[0], 95941[0], 95955[1], 96360[1], 96361[1], 96365[1], 96366[1], 96367[1], 96368[1], 96372[1], 96374[1], 96375[1], 96376[1], 96377[1], 99155[0], 99156[0], 99157[0], 99211[1], 99212[1], 99213[1], 99214[1], 99215[1], 99217[1], 99218[1], 99219[1], 99220[1], 99221[1], 99222[1], 99223[1], 99231[1], 99232[1], 99233[1], 99234[1], 99235[1], 99236[1], 99238[1], 99239[1], 99241[1], 99242[1], 99243[1], 99244[1], 99245[1], 99251[1], 99252[1], 99253[1], 99254[1], 99255[1], 99291[1], 99292[1], 99304[1], 99305[1], 99306[1], 99307[1], 99308[1], 99309[1], 99310[1], 99315[1], 99316[1], 99334[1], 99335[1], 99336[1], 99337[1], 99347[1], 99348[1], 99349[1], 99350[1], 99374[1], 99375[1], 99377[1], 99378[1], 99446[0], 99447[0], 99448[0], 99449[0], 99451[0], 99452[0], 99495[1], 99496[1], G0453[0], G0459[1], G0463[1], G0471[1], J0670[1], J2001[1]
64490	01991[0], 01992[0], 0213T[0], 0214T[0], 0215T[0], 0216T[0], 0217T[0], 0218T[0], 0333T[0], 0464T[0], 20550[1], 20551[1], 20600[1], 20605[1], 20610[1], 36140[1], 36410[1], 36591[0], 36592[0], 51701[1], 51702[1], 51703[1], 69990[0], 72275[1], 76000[1], 76380[1], 76800[1], 76942[1], 76970[1], 76998[1], 77001[1], 77002[1], 77003[1], 77012[1], 77021[1], 92012[1], 92014[1], 92585[0], 93000[1], 93005[1], 93010[1], 93040[1], 93041[1], 93042[1], 93318[1], 93355[1], 94002[1], 94200[1], 94250[1], 94680[1], 94681[1], 94690[1], 94770[1], 95812[1], 95813[1], 95816[1], 95819[1], 95822[0], 95829[1], 95860[1], 95861[1], 95863[1], 95864[1], 95865[1], 95866[1], 95867[1], 95868[1], 95869[1], 95870[1], 95907[1],

Appendix A: NCCI - CPT Codes

0 = Modifier usage not allowed or inappropriate   1 = Modifier usage allowed

CPT © 2018 American Medical Association. All Rights Reserved.

Code 1	Code 2
	95908[1], 95909[1], 95910[1], 95911[1], 95912[1], 95913[1], 95925[0], 95926[0], 95927[0], 95928[0], 95929[0], 95930[0], 95933[0], 95937[0], 95938[0], 95939[0], 95940[0], 95955[1], 96360[1], 96361[1], 96365[1], 96366[1], 96367[1], 96368[1], 96372[1], 96374[1], 96375[1], 96376[1], 96377[1], 99155[0], 99156[0], 99157[0], 99211[1], 99212[1], 99213[1], 99214[1], 99215[1], 99217[1], 99218[1], 99219[1], 99220[1], 99221[1], 99222[1], 99223[1], 99231[1], 99232[1], 99233[1], 99234[1], 99235[1], 99236[1], 99238[1], 99239[1], 99241[1], 99242[1], 99243[1], 99244[1], 99245[1], 99251[1], 99252[1], 99253[1], 99254[1], 99255[1], 99291[1], 99292[1], 99304[1], 99305[1], 99306[1], 99307[1], 99308[1], 99309[1], 99310[1], 99315[1], 99316[1], 99334[1], 99335[1], 99336[1], 99337[1], 99347[1], 99348[1], 99349[1], 99350[1], 99374[1], 99375[1], 99377[1], 99378[1], 99446[0], 99447[0], 99448[0], 99449[0], 99451[0], 99452[0], 99495[1], 99496[1], G0453[0], G0459[1], G0463[1], G0471[1], J0670[1], J2001[1]
64491	0213T[0], 0214T[0], 0215T[0], 0216T[0], 0217T[0], 0218T[0], 0333T[0], 0464T[0], 36591[0], 36592[0], 51701[1], 51702[1], 51703[1], 69990[0], 76000[1], 76380[1], 76800[1], 76942[1], 76970[1], 76998[1], 77001[1], 77002[1], 77003[1], 77012[1], 77021[1], 92585[0], 95822[0], 95860[1], 95861[1], 95863[1], 95864[1], 95865[1], 95866[1], 95867[1], 95868[1], 95869[1], 95870[1], 95907[1], 95908[1], 95909[1], 95910[1], 95911[1], 95912[1], 95913[1], 95925[0], 95926[0], 95927[0], 95928[0], 95929[0], 95930[0], 95933[0], 95937[0], 95938[0], 95939[0], 95940[0], G0453[0], G0471[1], J0670[1], J2001[1]
64492	0213T[0], 0214T[0], 0215T[0], 0216T[0], 0217T[0], 0218T[0], 0333T[0], 0464T[0], 36591[0], 36592[0], 51701[1], 51702[1], 51703[1], 69990[0], 76000[1], 76380[1], 76800[1], 76942[1], 76970[1], 76998[1], 77001[1], 77002[1], 77003[1], 77012[1], 77021[1], 92585[0], 95822[0], 95860[1], 95861[1], 95863[1], 95864[1], 95865[1], 95866[1], 95867[1], 95868[1], 95869[1], 95870[1], 95907[1], 95908[1], 95909[1], 95910[1], 95911[1], 95912[1], 95913[1], 95925[0], 95926[0], 95927[0], 95928[0], 95929[0], 95930[0], 95933[0], 95937[0], 95938[0], 95939[0], 95940[0], G0453[0], G0471[1], J0670[1], J2001[1]
64493	01991[0], 01992[0], 0213T[0], 0214T[0], 0215T[0], 0216T[0], 0217T[0], 0218T[0], 0333T[0], 0464T[0], 20550[1], 20551[1], 20600[1], 20605[1], 20610[1], 36140[1], 36591[0], 36592[0], 51701[1], 51702[1], 51703[1], 69990[0], 72275[1], 76000[1], 76380[1], 76800[1], 76942[1], 76970[1], 76998[1], 77001[1], 77002[1], 77003[1], 77012[1], 77021[1], 92012[1], 92014[1], 92585[0], 93000[1], 93005[1], 93010[1], 93040[1], 93041[1], 93042[1], 93318[1], 93355[1], 94002[1], 94200[1], 94250[1], 94680[1], 94681[1], 94690[1], 94770[1], 95812[1], 95813[1], 95816[1], 95819[1], 95822[0], 95829[1], 95860[1], 95861[1], 95863[1], 95864[1], 95865[1], 95866[1], 95867[1], 95868[1], 95869[1], 95870[1], 95907[1], 95908[1], 95909[1], 95910[1], 95911[1], 95912[1], 95913[1], 95925[0], 95926[0], 95927[0], 95928[0], 95929[0], 95930[0], 95933[0], 95937[0], 95938[0], 95939[0], 95940[0], 95955[1], 96360[1], 96361[1], 96365[1], 96366[1], 96367[1], 96368[1], 96372[1], 96374[1], 96375[1], 96376[1], 96377[1], 99155[0], 99156[0], 99157[0], 99211[1], 99212[1], 99213[1], 99214[1], 99215[1], 99217[1], 99218[1], 99219[1], 99220[1], 99221[1], 99222[1], 99223[1], 99231[1], 99232[1], 99233[1], 99234[1], 99235[1], 99236[1], 99238[1], 99239[1], 99241[1], 99242[1], 99243[1], 99244[1], 99245[1], 99251[1], 99252[1], 99253[1], 99254[1], 99255[1], 99291[1], 99292[1], 99304[1], 99305[1], 99306[1], 99307[1], 99308[1], 99309[1], 99310[1], 99315[1], 99316[1], 99334[1], 99335[1], 99336[1], 99337[1], 99347[1], 99348[1], 99349[1], 99350[1], 99374[1], 99375[1], 99377[1], 99378[1], 99446[0], 99447[0], 99448[0], 99449[0], 99451[0], 99452[0], 99495[1], 99496[1], G0453[0], G0459[1], G0463[1], G0471[1], J0670[1], J2001[1]
64494	0213T[0], 0214T[0], 0215T[0], 0216T[0], 0217T[0], 0218T[0], 0333T[0], 0464T[0], 36591[0], 36592[0], 51701[1], 51702[1], 51703[1], 69990[0], 76000[1], 76380[1], 76800[1], 76942[1], 76970[1], 76998[1], 77001[1], 77002[1], 77003[1], 77012[1], 77021[1], 92585[0], 95822[0], 95860[1], 95861[1], 95863[1], 95864[1], 95865[1], 95866[1], 95867[1], 95868[1], 95869[1], 95870[1], 95907[1], 95908[1], 95909[1], 95910[1], 95911[1], 95912[1], 95913[1], 95925[0], 95926[0], 95927[0], 95928[0], 95929[0], 95930[0], 95933[0], 95937[0], 95938[0], 95939[0], 95940[0], G0453[0], G0471[1], J0670[1], J2001[1]
64495	0213T[0], 0214T[0], 0215T[0], 0216T[0], 0217T[0], 0218T[0], 0333T[0], 0464T[0], 36591[0], 36592[0], 51701[1], 51702[1], 51703[1], 69990[0], 76000[1], 76380[1], 76800[1], 76942[1], 76970[1], 76998[1], 77001[1], 77002[1], 77003[1], 77012[1], 77021[1], 92585[0], 95822[0], 95860[1], 95861[1], 95863[1], 95864[1], 95865[1], 95866[1], 95867[1], 95868[1], 95869[1], 95870[1], 95907[1], 95908[1], 95909[1], 95910[1], 95911[1], 95912[1], 95913[1], 95925[0], 95926[0], 95927[0], 95928[0], 95929[0], 95930[0], 95933[0], 95937[0], 95938[0], 95939[0], 95940[0], G0453[0], G0471[1], J0670[1], J2001[1]
64505	01991[0], 01992[0], 0333T[0], 0464T[0], 36000[1], 36400[1], 36405[1], 36406[1], 36410[1], 36420[1], 36425[1], 36430[1], 36440[1], 36591[0], 36592[0], 36600[1], 51701[0], 51702[0], 51703[0], 69990[0], 76000[1], 76970[1], 76998[1], 77001[1], 92012[1], 92014[1], 92585[0], 93000[1], 93005[1], 93010[1], 93040[1], 93041[1], 93042[1], 93318[1], 93355[1], 94002[1], 94200[1], 94250[1], 94680[1], 94681[1], 94690[1], 94770[1], 95812[1], 95813[1], 95816[1], 95819[1], 95822[0], 95829[1], 95860[1], 95861[1], 95863[1], 95864[1], 95865[1], 95866[1], 95867[1], 95868[1], 95869[1], 95870[1], 95907[1], 95908[1], 95909[1], 95910[1], 95911[1], 95912[1], 95913[1], 95925[0], 95926[0], 95927[0], 95928[0], 95929[0], 95930[0], 95933[0], 95937[0], 95938[0], 95939[0], 95940[0], 95955[1], 96360[1], 96361[1], 96365[1], 96366[1], 96367[1], 96368[1], 96372[1], 96374[1], 96375[1], 96376[1], 96377[1], 99155[0], 99156[0], 99157[0], 99211[1], 99212[1], 99213[1], 99214[1], 99215[1], 99217[1], 99218[1], 99219[1], 99220[1], 99221[1], 99222[1], 99223[1], 99231[1], 99232[1], 99233[1], 99234[1], 99235[1], 99236[1], 99238[1], 99239[1], 99241[1], 99242[1], 99243[1], 99244[1], 99245[1], 99251[1], 99252[1], 99253[1], 99254[1], 99255[1], 99291[1], 99292[1], 99304[1], 99305[1], 99306[1], 99307[1], 99308[1], 99309[1], 99310[1], 99315[1], 99316[1], 99334[1], 99335[1], 99336[1], 99337[1], 99347[1], 99348[1], 99349[1], 99350[1], 99374[1], 99375[1], 99377[1], 99378[1], 99446[0], 99447[0], 99448[0], 99449[0], 99451[0], 99452[0], 99495[1], 99496[1], G0453[0], G0459[1], G0463[1], G0471[0], J0670[1], J2001[1]
64510	01991[0], 01992[0], 0333T[0], 0464T[0], 36000[1], 36400[1], 36405[1], 36406[1], 36410[1], 36420[1], 36425[1], 36430[1], 36440[1], 36591[0], 36592[0], 36600[1], 51701[0], 51702[0], 51703[0], 69990[0], 76000[1], 76970[1], 76998[1], 77001[1], 77002[1], 92012[1], 92014[1], 92585[0], 93000[1], 93005[1], 93010[1], 93040[1], 93041[1], 93042[1], 93318[1], 93355[1], 94002[1], 94200[1], 94250[1], 94680[1], 94681[1], 94690[1], 94770[1], 95812[1], 95813[1], 95816[1], 95819[1], 95822[0], 95829[1], 95860[1], 95861[1], 95863[1], 95864[1], 95865[1], 95866[1], 95867[1], 95868[1], 95869[1], 95870[1], 95907[1], 95908[1], 95909[1], 95910[1], 95911[1], 95912[1], 95913[1], 95925[0], 95926[0], 95927[0], 95928[0], 95929[0], 95930[0], 95933[0], 95937[0], 95938[0], 95939[0], 95940[0], 95955[1], 96360[1], 96361[1], 96365[1], 96366[1], 96367[1], 96368[1], 96372[1], 96374[1], 96375[1], 96376[1], 96377[1], 99155[0], 99156[0], 99157[0], 99211[1], 99212[1], 99213[1], 99214[1], 99215[1], 99217[1], 99218[1], 99219[1], 99220[1], 99221[1], 99222[1], 99223[1], 99231[1], 99232[1], 99233[1], 99234[1], 99235[1], 99236[1], 99238[1], 99239[1], 99241[1], 99242[1], 99243[1], 99244[1], 99245[1], 99251[1], 99252[1], 99253[1], 99254[1], 99255[1], 99291[1], 99292[1], 99304[1], 99305[1], 99306[1], 99307[1], 99308[1], 99309[1], 99310[1], 99315[1], 99316[1], 99334[1], 99335[1], 99336[1], 99337[1], 99347[1], 99348[1], 99349[1], 99350[1], 99374[1], 99375[1], 99377[1], 99378[1], 99446[0], 99447[0], 99448[0], 99449[0], 99451[0], 99452[0], 99495[1], 99496[1], G0453[0], G0459[1], G0463[1], G0471[0], J0670[1], J2001[1]
64517	01991[0], 01992[0], 0333T[0], 0464T[0], 36000[1], 36400[1], 36405[1], 36406[1], 36410[1], 36420[1], 36425[1], 36430[1], 36440[1], 36591[0], 36592[0], 36600[1], 51701[0], 51702[0], 51703[0], 69990[0], 76000[1], 76800[1], 76970[1], 76998[1], 77001[1], 92012[1], 92014[1], 92585[0], 93000[1], 93005[1], 93010[1], 93040[1], 93041[1], 93042[1], 93318[1], 93355[1], 94002[1], 94200[1], 94250[1], 94680[1], 94681[1], 94690[1], 94770[1], 95812[1], 95813[1], 95816[1], 95819[1], 95822[0], 95829[1], 95860[1], 95861[1], 95863[1], 95864[1], 95865[1], 95866[1], 95867[1], 95868[1], 95869[1], 95870[1], 95907[1], 95908[1], 95909[1], 95910[1], 95911[1], 95912[1], 95913[1], 95925[0], 95926[0], 95927[0], 95928[0], 95929[0], 95930[0], 95933[0], 95937[0], 95938[0], 95939[0], 95940[0], 95955[1], 96360[1], 96361[1], 96365[1], 96366[1], 96367[1], 96368[1], 96372[1], 96374[1], 96375[1], 96376[1], 96377[1], 99155[0], 99156[0], 99157[0], 99211[1], 99212[1], 99213[1], 99214[1], 99215[1], 99217[1], 99218[1], 99219[1], 99220[1], 99221[1], 99222[1], 99223[1], 99231[1], 99232[1], 99233[1], 99234[1], 99235[1], 99236[1], 99238[1], 99239[1], 99241[1], 99242[1], 99243[1], 99244[1], 99245[1], 99251[1], 99252[1], 99253[1], 99254[1], 99255[1], 99291[1], 99292[1], 99304[1], 99305[1], 99306[1], 99307[1], 99308[1], 99309[1], 99310[1], 99315[1], 99316[1], 99334[1], 99335[1], 99336[1], 99337[1], 99347[1], 99348[1], 99349[1], 99350[1], 99374[1], 99375[1], 99377[1], 99378[1], 99446[0], 99447[0], 99448[0], 99449[0], 99451[0], 99452[0], 99495[1], 99496[1], G0453[0], G0459[1], G0463[1], G0471[0], J0670[1], J2001[1]
64520	01991[0], 01992[0], 0333T[0], 0464T[0], 36000[1], 36400[1], 36405[1], 36406[1], 36410[1], 36420[1], 36425[1], 36430[1], 36440[1], 36591[0], 36592[0], 36600[1], 51701[0], 51702[0], 51703[0], 69990[0], 76000[1], 76800[1], 76970[1], 76998[1], 77001[1], 77002[1], 92012[1], 92014[1], 92585[0], 93000[1], 93005[1], 93010[1], 93040[1], 93041[1], 93042[1], 93318[1], 93355[1], 94002[1], 94200[1], 94250[1], 94680[1], 94681[1], 94690[1], 94770[1], 95812[1], 95813[1], 95816[1], 95819[1], 95822[0], 95829[1], 95860[1], 95861[1], 95863[1], 95864[1], 95865[1], 95866[1], 95867[1], 95868[1], 95869[1], 95870[1], 95907[1], 95908[1], 95909[1], 95910[1], 95911[1], 95912[1], 95913[1], 95925[0], 95926[0], 95927[0], 95928[0], 95929[0], 95930[0], 95933[0], 95937[0], 95938[0], 95939[0], 95940[0], 95955[1], 96360[1], 96361[1], 96365[1], 96366[1], 96367[1], 96368[1], 96372[1], 96374[1], 96375[1], 96376[1], 96377[1], 99155[0], 99156[0], 99157[0], 99211[1], 99212[1], 99213[1], 99214[1], 99215[1], 99217[1], 99218[1], 99219[1], 99220[1], 99221[1], 99222[1], 99223[1], 99231[1], 99232[1], 99233[1], 99234[1], 99235[1], 99236[1], 99238[1], 99239[1], 99241[1], 99242[1], 99243[1], 99244[1], 99245[1], 99251[1], 99252[1], 99253[1], 99254[1], 99255[1], 99291[1], 99292[1], 99304[1], 99305[1], 99306[1], 99307[1], 99308[1], 99309[1], 99310[1], 99315[1], 99316[1], 99334[1], 99335[1], 99336[1], 99337[1], 99347[1], 99348[1], 99349[1], 99350[1], 99374[1], 99375[1], 99377[1], 99378[1], 99446[0], 99447[0], 99448[0], 99449[0], 99451[0], 99452[0], 99495[1], 99496[1], G0453[0], G0459[1], G0463[1], G0471[0], J0670[1], J2001[1]
64530	01991[0], 01992[0], 0333T[0], 0464T[0], 36000[1], 36400[1], 36405[1], 36406[1], 36410[1], 36420[1], 36425[1], 36430[1], 36440[1], 36591[0], 36592[0], 36600[1], 51701[0], 51702[0], 51703[0], 69990[0], 76000[1], 76970[1], 76998[1], 77001[1], 77002[1], 77003[1], 92012[1], 92014[1], 92585[0], 93000[1], 93005[1], 93010[1], 93040[1], 93041[1], 93042[1], 93318[1], 93355[1], 94002[1], 94200[1], 94250[1], 94680[1], 94681[1], 94690[1], 94770[1], 95812[1], 95813[1], 95816[1], 95819[1], 95822[0], 95829[1], 95860[1], 95861[1], 95863[1], 95864[1], 95865[1], 95866[1], 95867[1], 95868[1], 95869[1], 95870[1], 95907[1], 95908[1], 95909[1], 95910[1], 95911[1], 95912[1], 95913[1], 95925[0], 95926[0], 95927[0], 95928[0], 95929[0], 95930[0], 95933[0], 95937[0], 95938[0], 95939[0], 95940[0], 95955[1], 96360[1], 96361[1], 96365[1], 96366[1], 96367[1], 96368[1], 96372[1], 96374[1], 96375[1], 96376[1], 96377[1], 99155[0], 99156[0], 99157[0], 99211[1], 99212[1], 99213[1], 99214[1], 99215[1], 99217[1], 99218[1], 99219[1], 99220[1], 99221[1], 99222[1], 99223[1], 99231[1], 99232[1], 99233[1], 99234[1], 99235[1], 99236[1], 99238[1], 99239[1], 99241[1], 99242[1], 99243[1], 99244[1], 99245[1], 99251[1], 99252[1], 99253[1], 99254[1], 99255[1], 99291[1], 99292[1], 99304[1], 99305[1], 99306[1], 99307[1], 99308[1], 99309[1], 99310[1], 99315[1], 99316[1], 99334[1], 99335[1], 99336[1], 99337[1], 99347[1], 99348[1],

0 = Modifier usage not allowed or inappropriate 1 = Modifier usage allowed

CPT © 2018 American Medical Association. All Rights Reserved.

Code 1	Code 2
	99349[1], 99350[1], 99374[1], 99375[1], 99377[1], 99378[1], 99446[0], 99447[0], 99448[0], 99449[0], 99451[0], 99452[0], 99495[1], 99496[1], G0453[0], G0459[1], G0463[1], G0471[0], J0670[1], J2001[1]
64555	0213T[0], 0216T[0], 0228T[0], 0230T[0], 0333T[0], 0464T[0], 12001[1], 12002[1], 12004[1], 12005[1], 12006[1], 12007[1], 12011[1], 12013[1], 12014[1], 12015[1], 12016[1], 12017[1], 12018[1], 12020[1], 12021[1], 12031[1], 12032[1], 12034[1], 12035[1], 12036[1], 12037[1], 12041[1], 12042[1], 12044[1], 12045[1], 12046[1], 12047[1], 12051[1], 12052[1], 12053[1], 12054[1], 12055[1], 12056[1], 12057[1], 13100[1], 13101[1], 13102[1], 13120[1], 13121[1], 13122[1], 13131[1], 13132[1], 13133[1], 13151[1], 13152[1], 13153[1], 36000[1], 36400[1], 36405[1], 36406[1], 36410[1], 36420[1], 36425[1], 36430[1], 36440[1], 36591[0], 36592[0], 36600[1], 36640[1], 43752[1], 51701[1], 51702[1], 51703[1], 61850[0], 61860[0], 61870[0], 61880[0], 61885[0], 61886[0], 62320[0], 62321[0], 62322[0], 62323[0], 62324[0], 62325[0], 62326[0], 62327[0], 64400[0], 64402[0], 64405[0], 64408[0], 64410[0], 64413[0], 64415[0], 64416[0], 64417[0], 64418[0], 64420[0], 64421[0], 64425[0], 64430[0], 64435[0], 64445[0], 64446[0], 64447[0], 64448[0], 64449[0], 64450[0], 64461[0], 64462[0], 64463[0], 64479[0], 64480[0], 64483[0], 64484[0], 64486[0], 64487[0], 64488[0], 64489[0], 64490[0], 64491[0], 64492[0], 64493[0], 64494[0], 64495[0], 64505[0], 64510[0], 64517[0], 64520[0], 64530[0], 64553[1], 64561[1], 64566[1], 64575[1], 64580[0], 64581[0], 69990[0], 76000[1], 77001[1], 77002[1], 92012[1], 92014[1], 92585[0], 93000[1], 93005[1], 93010[1], 93040[1], 93041[1], 93042[1], 93318[1], 93355[1], 94002[1], 94200[1], 94250[1], 94680[1], 94681[1], 94690[1], 94770[1], 95812[1], 95813[1], 95816[1], 95819[1], 95822[0], 95829[1], 95860[0], 95861[0], 95863[0], 95864[0], 95865[0], 95866[0], 95867[0], 95868[0], 95869[0], 95870[0], 95907[0], 95908[0], 95909[0], 95910[0], 95911[0], 95912[0], 95913[0], 95925[0], 95926[0], 95927[0], 95928[0], 95929[0], 95930[0], 95933[0], 95937[0], 95938[0], 95939[0], 95940[0], 95955[1], 95970[1], 95971[1], 95972[1], 96360[1], 96361[1], 96365[1], 96366[1], 96367[1], 96368[1], 96372[1], 96374[1], 96375[1], 96376[1], 96377[1], 99155[0], 99156[0], 99157[0], 99211[1], 99212[1], 99213[1], 99214[1], 99215[1], 99217[1], 99218[1], 99219[1], 99220[1], 99221[1], 99222[1], 99223[1], 99231[1], 99232[1], 99233[1], 99234[1], 99235[1], 99236[1], 99238[1], 99239[1], 99241[1], 99242[1], 99243[1], 99244[1], 99245[1], 99251[1], 99252[1], 99253[1], 99254[1], 99255[1], 99291[1], 99292[1], 99304[1], 99305[1], 99306[1], 99307[1], 99308[1], 99309[1], 99310[1], 99315[1], 99316[1], 99334[1], 99335[1], 99336[1], 99337[1], 99347[1], 99348[1], 99349[1], 99350[1], 99374[1], 99375[1], 99377[1], 99378[1], 99446[0], 99447[0], 99448[0], 99449[0], 99451[0], 99452[0], 99495[0], 99496[0], G0453[0], G0463[1], G0471[1]
64561	0213T[0], 0216T[0], 0228T[0], 0230T[0], 0333T[0], 0464T[0], 12001[1], 12002[1], 12004[1], 12005[1], 12006[1], 12007[1], 12011[1], 12013[1], 12014[1], 12015[1], 12016[1], 12017[1], 12018[1], 12020[1], 12021[1], 12031[1], 12032[1], 12034[1], 12035[1], 12036[1], 12037[1], 12041[1], 12042[1], 12044[1], 12045[1], 12046[1], 12047[1], 12051[1], 12052[1], 12053[1], 12054[1], 12055[1], 12056[1], 12057[1], 13100[1], 13101[1], 13102[1], 13120[1], 13121[1], 13122[1], 13131[1], 13132[1], 13133[1], 13151[1], 13152[1], 13153[1], 36000[1], 36400[1], 36405[1], 36406[1], 36410[1], 36420[1], 36425[1], 36430[1], 36440[1], 36591[0], 36592[0], 36600[1], 36640[1], 43752[1], 51701[1], 51702[1], 51703[1], 62320[0], 62321[0], 62322[0], 62323[0], 62324[0], 62325[0], 62326[0], 62327[0], 64400[0], 64402[0], 64405[0], 64408[0], 64410[0], 64413[0], 64415[0], 64416[0], 64417[0], 64418[0], 64420[0], 64421[0], 64425[0], 64430[0], 64435[0], 64445[0], 64446[0], 64447[0], 64448[0], 64449[0], 64450[0], 64461[0], 64462[0], 64463[0], 64479[0], 64480[0], 64483[0], 64484[0], 64486[0], 64487[0], 64488[0], 64489[0], 64490[0], 64491[0], 64492[0], 64493[0], 64494[0], 64495[0], 64505[0], 64510[0], 64517[0], 64520[0], 64530[0], 64581[0], 69990[0], 76000[1], 77001[1], 77002[1], 77003[1], 92012[1], 92014[1], 92585[0], 93000[1], 93005[1], 93010[1], 93040[1], 93041[1], 93042[1], 93318[1], 93355[1], 94002[1], 94200[1], 94250[1], 94680[1], 94681[1], 94690[1], 94770[1], 95812[1], 95813[1], 95816[1], 95819[1], 95822[0], 95829[1], 95860[0], 95861[0], 95863[0], 95864[0], 95865[0], 95866[0], 95867[0], 95868[0], 95869[0], 95870[0], 95907[0], 95908[0], 95909[0], 95910[0], 95911[0], 95912[0], 95913[0], 95925[0], 95926[0], 95927[0], 95928[0], 95929[0], 95930[0], 95933[0], 95937[0], 95938[0], 95939[0], 95940[0], 95955[1], 95970[1], 95971[1], 95972[1], 96360[1], 96361[1], 96365[1], 96366[1], 96367[1], 96368[1], 96372[1], 96374[1], 96375[1], 96376[1], 96377[1], 99155[0], 99156[0], 99157[0], 99211[1], 99212[1], 99213[1], 99214[1], 99215[1], 99217[1], 99218[1], 99219[1], 99220[1], 99221[1], 99222[1], 99223[1], 99231[1], 99232[1], 99233[1], 99234[1], 99235[1], 99236[1], 99238[1], 99239[1], 99241[1], 99242[1], 99243[1], 99244[1], 99245[1], 99251[1], 99252[1], 99253[1], 99254[1], 99255[1], 99291[1], 99292[1], 99304[1], 99305[1], 99306[1], 99307[1], 99308[1], 99309[1], 99310[1], 99315[1], 99316[1], 99334[1], 99335[1], 99336[1], 99337[1], 99347[1], 99348[1], 99349[1], 99350[1], 99374[1], 99375[1], 99377[1], 99378[1], 99446[0], 99447[0], 99448[0], 99449[0], 99451[0], 99452[0], 99495[0], 99496[0], A4290[0], G0453[0], G0463[1], G0471[1], J0670[1], J2001[1]
64575	0213T[0], 0216T[0], 0228T[0], 0230T[0], 0333T[0], 0464T[0], 12001[1], 12002[1], 12004[1], 12005[1], 12006[1], 12007[1], 12011[1], 12013[1], 12014[1], 12015[1], 12016[1], 12017[1], 12018[1], 12020[1], 12021[1], 12031[1], 12032[1], 12034[1], 12035[1], 12036[1], 12037[1], 12041[1], 12042[1], 12044[1], 12045[1], 12046[1], 12047[1], 12051[1], 12052[1], 12053[1], 12054[1], 12055[1], 12056[1], 12057[1], 13100[1], 13101[1], 13102[1], 13120[1], 13121[1], 13122[1], 13131[1], 13132[1], 13133[1], 13151[1], 13152[1], 13153[1], 36000[1], 36400[1], 36405[1], 36406[1], 36410[1], 36420[1], 36425[1], 36430[1], 36440[1], 36591[0], 36592[0], 36600[1], 36640[1], 43752[1], 51701[1], 51702[1], 51703[1], 61850[0], 61860[0], 61870[0], 61880[0], 61885[0], 61886[1], 62320[0], 62321[0], 62322[0], 62323[0], 62324[0], 62325[0], 62326[0], 62327[0], 64400[0], 64402[0], 64405[0], 64408[0], 64410[0], 64413[0], 64415[0], 64416[0], 64417[0], 64418[0], 64420[0], 64421[0], 64425[0], 64430[0], 64435[0], 64445[0], 64446[0], 64447[0], 64448[0], 64449[0], 64450[0], 64461[0], 64462[0], 64463[0], 64479[0], 64480[0], 64483[0], 64484[0], 64486[0], 64487[0], 64488[0], 64489[0], 64490[0], 64491[0], 64492[0], 64493[0], 64494[0], 64495[0], 64505[0], 64510[0], 64517[0], 64520[0], 64530[0], 64561[1], 64566[1], 64581[0], 69990[0], 92012[1], 92014[1], 92585[0], 93000[1], 93005[1], 93010[1], 93040[1], 93041[1], 93042[1], 93318[1], 93355[1], 94002[1], 94200[1], 94250[1], 94680[1], 94681[1], 94690[1], 94770[1], 95812[1], 95813[1], 95816[1], 95819[1], 95822[0], 95829[1], 95860[0], 95861[0], 95863[0], 95864[0], 95865[0], 95866[0], 95867[0], 95868[0], 95869[0], 95870[0], 95907[0], 95908[0], 95909[0], 95910[0], 95911[0], 95912[0], 95913[0], 95925[0], 95926[0], 95927[0], 95928[0], 95929[0], 95930[0], 95933[0], 95937[0], 95938[0], 95939[0], 95940[0], 95955[1], 95970[1], 96360[1], 96361[1], 96365[1], 96366[1], 96367[1], 96368[1], 96372[1], 96374[1], 96375[1], 96376[1], 96377[1], 99155[0], 99156[0], 99157[0], 99211[1], 99212[1], 99213[1], 99214[1], 99215[1], 99217[1], 99218[1], 99219[1], 99220[1], 99221[1], 99222[1], 99223[1], 99231[1], 99232[1], 99233[1], 99234[1], 99235[1], 99236[1], 99238[1], 99239[1], 99241[1], 99242[1], 99243[1], 99244[1], 99245[1], 99251[1], 99252[1], 99253[1], 99254[1], 99255[1], 99291[1], 99292[1], 99304[1], 99305[1], 99306[1], 99307[1], 99308[1], 99309[1], 99310[1], 99315[1], 99316[1], 99334[1], 99335[1], 99336[1], 99337[1], 99347[1], 99348[1], 99349[1], 99350[1], 99374[1], 99375[1], 99377[1], 99378[1], 99446[0], 99447[0], 99448[0], 99449[0], 99451[0], 99452[0], 99495[0], 99496[0], G0453[0], G0463[1], G0471[1]
64580	0213T[0], 0216T[0], 0228T[0], 0230T[0], 0333T[0], 0464T[0], 12001[1], 12002[1], 12004[1], 12005[1], 12006[1], 12007[1], 12011[1], 12013[1], 12014[1], 12015[1], 12016[1], 12017[1], 12018[1], 12020[1], 12021[1], 12031[1], 12032[1], 12034[1], 12035[1], 12036[1], 12037[1], 12041[1], 12042[1], 12044[1], 12045[1], 12046[1], 12047[1], 12051[1], 12052[1], 12053[1], 12054[1], 12055[1], 12056[1], 12057[1], 13100[1], 13101[1], 13102[1], 13120[1], 13121[1], 13122[1], 13131[1], 13132[1], 13133[1], 13151[1], 13152[1], 13153[1], 36000[1], 36400[1], 36405[1], 36406[1], 36410[1], 36420[1], 36425[1], 36430[1], 36440[1], 36591[0], 36592[0], 36600[1], 36640[1], 43752[1], 51701[1], 51702[1], 51703[1], 61850[0], 61860[0], 61870[0], 61880[0], 61885[0], 61886[0], 62320[0], 62321[0], 62322[0], 62323[0], 62324[0], 62325[0], 62326[0], 62327[0], 64400[0], 64402[0], 64405[0], 64408[0], 64410[0], 64413[0], 64415[0], 64416[0], 64417[0], 64418[0], 64420[0], 64421[0], 64425[0], 64430[0], 64435[0], 64445[0], 64446[0], 64447[0], 64448[0], 64449[0], 64450[0], 64461[0], 64462[0], 64463[0], 64479[0], 64480[0], 64483[0], 64484[0], 64486[0], 64487[0], 64488[0], 64489[0], 64490[0], 64491[0], 64492[0], 64493[0], 64494[0], 64495[0], 64505[0], 64510[0], 64517[0], 64520[0], 64530[0], 64561[1], 64575[0], 64581[1], 69990[0], 92012[1], 92014[1], 92585[0], 93000[1], 93005[1], 93010[1], 93040[1], 93041[1], 93042[1], 93318[1], 93355[1], 94002[1], 94200[1], 94250[1], 94680[1], 94681[1], 94690[1], 94770[1], 95812[1], 95813[1], 95816[1], 95819[1], 95822[0], 95829[1], 95860[0], 95861[0], 95863[0], 95864[0], 95865[0], 95866[0], 95867[0], 95868[0], 95869[0], 95870[0], 95907[0], 95908[0], 95909[0], 95910[0], 95911[0], 95912[0], 95913[0], 95925[0], 95926[0], 95927[0], 95928[0], 95929[0], 95930[0], 95933[0], 95937[0], 95938[0], 95939[0], 95940[0], 95955[1], 95970[1], 96360[1], 96361[1], 96365[1], 96366[1], 96367[1], 96368[1], 96372[1], 96374[1], 96375[1], 96376[1], 96377[1], 99155[0], 99156[0], 99157[0], 99211[1], 99212[1], 99213[1], 99214[1], 99215[1], 99217[1], 99218[1], 99219[1], 99220[1], 99221[1], 99222[1], 99223[1], 99231[1], 99232[1], 99233[1], 99234[1], 99235[1], 99236[1], 99238[1], 99239[1], 99241[1], 99242[1], 99243[1], 99244[1], 99245[1], 99251[1], 99252[1], 99253[1], 99254[1], 99255[1], 99291[1], 99292[1], 99304[1], 99305[1], 99306[1], 99307[1], 99308[1], 99309[1], 99310[1], 99315[1], 99316[1], 99334[1], 99335[1], 99336[1], 99337[1], 99347[1], 99348[1], 99349[1], 99350[1], 99374[1], 99375[1], 99377[1], 99378[1], 99446[0], 99447[0], 99448[0], 99449[0], 99451[0], 99452[0], 99495[0], 99496[0], G0281[1], G0283[1], G0453[0], G0463[1], G0471[1]
64581	0213T[0], 0216T[0], 0228T[0], 0230T[0], 0333T[0], 0464T[0], 12001[1], 12002[1], 12004[1], 12005[1], 12006[1], 12007[1], 12011[1], 12013[1], 12014[1], 12015[1], 12016[1], 12017[1], 12018[1], 12020[1], 12021[1], 12031[1], 12032[1], 12034[1], 12035[1], 12036[1], 12037[1], 12041[1], 12042[1], 12044[1], 12045[1], 12046[1], 12047[1], 12051[1], 12052[1], 12053[1], 12054[1], 12055[1], 12056[1], 12057[1], 13100[1], 13101[1], 13102[1], 13120[1], 13121[1], 13122[1], 13131[1], 13132[1], 13133[1], 13151[1], 13152[1], 13153[1], 36000[1], 36400[1], 36405[1], 36406[1], 36410[1], 36420[1], 36425[1], 36430[1], 36440[1], 36591[0], 36592[0], 36600[1], 36640[1], 43752[1], 51701[1], 51702[1], 51703[1], 62320[0], 62321[0], 62322[0], 62323[0], 62324[0], 62325[0], 62326[0], 62327[0], 64400[0], 64402[0], 64405[0], 64408[0], 64410[0], 64413[0], 64415[0], 64416[0], 64417[0], 64418[0], 64420[0], 64421[0], 64425[0], 64430[0], 64435[0], 64445[0], 64446[0], 64447[0], 64448[0], 64449[0], 64450[0], 64461[0], 64462[0], 64463[0], 64479[0], 64480[0], 64483[0], 64484[0], 64486[0], 64487[0], 64488[0], 64489[0], 64490[0], 64491[0], 64492[0], 64493[0], 64494[0], 64495[0], 64505[0], 64510[0], 64517[0], 64520[0], 64530[0], 69990[0], 92012[1], 92014[1], 92585[0], 93000[1], 93005[1], 93010[1], 93040[1], 93041[1], 93042[1], 93318[1], 93355[1], 94002[1], 94200[1], 94250[1], 94680[1], 94681[1], 94690[1], 94770[1], 95812[1], 95813[1], 95816[1], 95819[1], 95822[0], 95829[1], 95860[0], 95861[0], 95863[0], 95864[0], 95865[0], 95866[0], 95867[0], 95868[0], 95869[0], 95870[0], 95907[0], 95908[0], 95909[0], 95910[0], 95911[0], 95912[0], 95913[0], 95925[0], 95926[0], 95927[0], 95928[0], 95929[0], 95930[0], 95933[0], 95937[0], 95938[0], 95939[0], 95940[0], 95955[1], 95970[1], 96360[1], 96361[1], 96365[1], 96366[1], 96367[1], 96368[1], 96372[1], 96374[1], 96375[1], 96376[1], 96377[1], 99155[0], 99156[0], 99157[0], 99211[1], 99212[1], 99213[1], 99214[1], 99215[1], 99217[1], 99218[1], 99219[1], 99220[1], 99221[1], 99222[1], 99223[1], 99231[1], 99232[1], 99233[1], 99234[1], 99235[1], 99236[1], 99238[1], 99239[1], 99241[1],

0 = Modifier usage not allowed or inappropriate 1 = Modifier usage allowed

CPT © 2018 American Medical Association. All Rights Reserved.

Code 1	Code 2
	99242[1], 99243[1], 99244[1], 99245[1], 99251[1], 99252[1], 99253[1], 99254[1], 99255[1], 99291[1], 99292[1], 99304[1], 99305[1], 99306[1], 99307[1], 99308[1], 99309[1], 99310[1], 99315[1], 99316[1], 99334[1], 99335[1], 99336[1], 99337[1], 99347[1], 99348[1], 99349[1], 99350[1], 99374[1], 99375[1], 99377[1], 99378[1], 99446[0], 99447[0], 99448[0], 99449[0], 99451[0], 99452[0], 99495[0], 99496[0], G0453[0], G0463[1], G0471[1]
64585	0213T[0], 0216T[0], 0228T[0], 0230T[0], 0333T[0], 0464T[0], 11000[1], 11001[1], 11004[1], 11005[1], 11006[1], 11042[1], 11043[1], 11044[1], 11045[1], 11046[1], 11047[1], 12001[1], 12002[1], 12004[1], 12005[1], 12006[1], 12007[1], 12011[1], 12013[1], 12014[1], 12015[1], 12016[1], 12017[1], 12018[1], 12020[1], 12021[1], 12031[1], 12032[1], 12034[1], 12035[1], 12036[1], 12037[1], 12041[1], 12042[1], 12044[1], 12045[1], 12046[1], 12047[1], 12051[1], 12052[1], 12053[1], 12054[1], 12055[1], 12056[1], 12057[1], 13100[1], 13101[1], 13102[1], 13120[1], 13121[1], 13122[1], 13131[1], 13132[1], 13133[1], 13151[1], 13152[1], 13153[1], 36000[1], 36400[1], 36405[1], 36406[1], 36410[1], 36420[1], 36425[1], 36430[1], 36440[1], 36591[0], 36592[0], 36600[1], 36640[1], 43752[1], 51701[1], 51702[1], 51703[1], 61886[1], 62320[0], 62321[0], 62322[0], 62323[0], 62324[0], 62325[0], 62326[0], 62327[0], 63688[1], 64400[0], 64402[0], 64405[0], 64408[0], 64410[0], 64413[0], 64415[0], 64416[0], 64417[0], 64418[0], 64420[0], 64421[0], 64425[0], 64430[0], 64435[0], 64445[0], 64446[0], 64447[0], 64448[0], 64449[0], 64450[0], 64461[0], 64462[0], 64463[0], 64479[0], 64480[0], 64483[0], 64484[0], 64486[0], 64487[0], 64488[0], 64489[0], 64490[0], 64491[0], 64492[0], 64493[0], 64494[0], 64495[0], 64505[0], 64510[0], 64517[0], 64520[0], 64530[0], 64553[1], 64555[1], 64561[1], 64575[1], 64580[1], 64581[0], 69990[0], 92012[1], 92014[1], 92585[0], 93000[1], 93005[1], 93010[1], 93040[1], 93041[1], 93042[1], 93318[1], 93355[1], 94002[1], 94200[1], 94250[1], 94680[1], 94681[1], 94690[1], 94770[1], 95812[1], 95813[1], 95816[1], 95819[1], 95822[0], 95829[1], 95860[0], 95861[0], 95863[0], 95864[0], 95865[0], 95866[0], 95867[0], 95868[0], 95869[0], 95870[0], 95907[0], 95908[0], 95909[0], 95910[0], 95911[0], 95912[0], 95913[0], 95925[0], 95926[0], 95927[0], 95928[0], 95929[0], 95930[0], 95933[0], 95937[0], 95938[0], 95939[0], 95940[0], 95955[1], 95970[1], 96360[1], 96361[1], 96365[1], 96366[1], 96367[1], 96368[1], 96372[1], 96374[1], 96375[1], 96376[1], 96377[1], 97597[1], 97598[1], 97602[1], 99155[0], 99156[0], 99157[0], 99211[1], 99212[1], 99213[1], 99214[1], 99215[1], 99217[1], 99218[1], 99219[1], 99220[1], 99221[1], 99222[1], 99223[1], 99231[1], 99232[1], 99233[1], 99234[1], 99235[1], 99236[1], 99238[1], 99239[1], 99241[1], 99242[1], 99243[1], 99244[1], 99245[1], 99251[1], 99252[1], 99253[1], 99254[1], 99255[1], 99291[1], 99292[1], 99304[1], 99305[1], 99306[1], 99307[1], 99308[1], 99309[1], 99310[1], 99315[1], 99316[1], 99334[1], 99335[1], 99336[1], 99337[1], 99347[1], 99348[1], 99349[1], 99350[1], 99374[1], 99375[1], 99377[1], 99378[1], 99446[0], 99447[0], 99448[0], 99449[0], 99451[0], 99452[0], 99495[0], 99496[0], G0453[0], G0463[1], G0471[1], J0670[1], J2001[1]
64590	0213T[0], 0216T[0], 0228T[0], 0230T[0], 0333T[0], 0424T[0], 0427T[0], 0428T[0], 0431T[0], 0464T[0], 11000[1], 11001[1], 11004[1], 11005[1], 11006[1], 11042[1], 11043[1], 11044[1], 11045[1], 11046[1], 11047[1], 12001[1], 12002[1], 12004[1], 12005[1], 12006[1], 12007[1], 12011[1], 12013[1], 12014[1], 12015[1], 12016[1], 12017[1], 12018[1], 12020[1], 12021[1], 12031[1], 12032[1], 12034[1], 12035[1], 12036[1], 12037[1], 12041[1], 12042[1], 12044[1], 12045[1], 12046[1], 12047[1], 12051[1], 12052[1], 12053[1], 12054[1], 12055[1], 12056[1], 12057[1], 13100[1], 13101[1], 13102[1], 13120[1], 13121[1], 13122[1], 13131[1], 13132[1], 13133[1], 13151[1], 13152[1], 13153[1], 36000[1], 36400[1], 36405[1], 36406[1], 36410[1], 36420[1], 36425[1], 36430[1], 36440[1], 36591[0], 36592[0], 36600[1], 36640[1], 43752[1], 51701[1], 51702[1], 51703[1], 61885[0], 61886[0], 62320[0], 62321[0], 62322[0], 62323[0], 62324[0], 62325[0], 62326[0], 62327[0], 63685[1], 64400[0], 64402[0], 64405[0], 64408[0], 64410[0], 64413[0], 64415[0], 64416[0], 64417[0], 64418[0], 64420[0], 64421[0], 64425[0], 64430[0], 64435[0], 64445[0], 64446[0], 64447[0], 64448[0], 64449[0], 64450[0], 64461[0], 64462[0], 64463[0], 64479[0], 64480[0], 64483[0], 64484[0], 64486[0], 64487[0], 64488[0], 64489[0], 64490[0], 64491[0], 64492[0], 64493[0], 64494[0], 64495[0], 64505[0], 64510[0], 64517[0], 64520[0], 64530[0], 64595[1], 69990[0], 92012[1], 92014[1], 92585[0], 93000[1], 93005[1], 93010[1], 93040[1], 93041[1], 93042[1], 93318[1], 93355[1], 94002[1], 94200[1], 94250[1], 94680[1], 94681[1], 94690[1], 94770[1], 95812[1], 95813[1], 95816[1], 95819[1], 95822[0], 95829[1], 95860[0], 95861[0], 95863[0], 95864[0], 95865[0], 95866[0], 95867[0], 95868[0], 95869[0], 95870[0], 95907[0], 95908[0], 95909[0], 95910[0], 95911[0], 95912[0], 95913[0], 95925[0], 95926[0], 95927[0], 95928[0], 95929[0], 95930[0], 95933[0], 95937[0], 95938[0], 95939[0], 95940[0], 95955[1], 95970[1], 95976[1], 95977[1], 95981[1], 95982[1], 96360[1], 96361[1], 96365[1], 96366[1], 96367[1], 96368[1], 96372[1], 96374[1], 96375[1], 96376[1], 96377[1], 97597[1], 97598[1], 97602[1], 99155[0], 99156[0], 99157[0], 99211[1], 99212[1], 99213[1], 99214[1], 99215[1], 99217[1], 99218[1], 99219[1], 99220[1], 99221[1], 99222[1], 99223[1], 99231[1], 99232[1], 99233[1], 99234[1], 99235[1], 99236[1], 99238[1], 99239[1], 99241[1], 99242[1], 99243[1], 99244[1], 99245[1], 99251[1], 99252[1], 99253[1], 99254[1], 99255[1], 99291[1], 99292[1], 99304[1], 99305[1], 99306[1], 99307[1], 99308[1], 99309[1], 99310[1], 99315[1], 99316[1], 99334[1], 99335[1], 99336[1], 99337[1], 99347[1], 99348[1], 99349[1], 99350[1], 99374[1], 99375[1], 99377[1], 99378[1], 99446[0], 99447[0], 99448[0], 99449[0], 99451[0], 99452[0], 99495[0], 99496[0], G0453[0], G0463[1], G0471[1], J0670[1], J2001[1]
64595	0213T[0], 0216T[0], 0228T[0], 0230T[0], 0333T[0], 0464T[0], 11000[1], 11001[1], 11004[1], 11005[1], 11006[1], 11042[1], 11043[1], 11044[1], 11045[1], 11046[1], 11047[1], 12001[1], 12002[1], 12004[1], 12005[1], 12006[1], 12007[1], 12011[1], 12013[1], 12014[1], 12015[1], 12016[1], 12017[1], 12018[1], 12020[1], 12021[1], 12031[1], 12032[1], 12034[1], 12035[1], 12036[1], 12037[1], 12041[1], 12042[1], 12044[1], 12045[1], 12046[1], 12047[1], 12051[1], 12052[1], 12053[1], 12054[1], 12055[1], 12056[1], 12057[1], 13100[1], 13101[1], 13102[1], 13120[1], 13121[1], 13122[1], 13131[1], 13132[1], 13133[1], 13151[1], 13152[1], 13153[1], 36000[1], 36400[1], 36405[1], 36406[1], 36410[1], 36420[1], 36425[1], 36430[1], 36440[1], 36591[0], 36592[0], 36600[1], 36640[1], 43752[1], 51701[1], 51702[1], 51703[1], 62320[0], 62321[0], 62322[0], 62323[0], 62324[0], 62325[0], 62326[0], 62327[0], 63688[1], 64400[0], 64402[0], 64405[0], 64408[0], 64410[0], 64413[0], 64415[0], 64416[0], 64417[0], 64418[0], 64420[0], 64421[0], 64425[0], 64430[0], 64435[0], 64445[0], 64446[0], 64447[0], 64448[0], 64449[0], 64450[0], 64461[0], 64462[0], 64463[0], 64479[0], 64480[0], 64483[0], 64484[0], 64486[0], 64487[0], 64488[0], 64489[0], 64490[0], 64491[0], 64492[0], 64493[0], 64494[0], 64495[0], 64505[0], 64510[0], 64517[0], 64520[0], 64530[0], 69990[0], 92012[1], 92014[1], 92585[0], 93000[1], 93005[1], 93010[1], 93040[1], 93041[1], 93042[1], 93318[1], 93355[1], 94002[1], 94200[1], 94250[1], 94680[1], 94681[1], 94690[1], 94770[1], 95812[1], 95813[1], 95816[1], 95819[1], 95822[0], 95829[1], 95860[0], 95861[0], 95863[0], 95864[0], 95865[0], 95866[0], 95867[0], 95868[0], 95869[0], 95870[0], 95907[0], 95908[0], 95909[0], 95910[0], 95911[0], 95912[0], 95913[0], 95925[0], 95926[0], 95927[0], 95928[0], 95929[0], 95930[0], 95933[0], 95937[0], 95938[0], 95939[0], 95940[0], 95955[1], 95970[1], 95976[1], 95977[1], 95981[1], 95982[1], 96360[1], 96361[1], 96365[1], 96366[1], 96367[1], 96368[1], 96372[1], 96374[1], 96375[1], 96376[1], 96377[1], 97597[1], 97598[1], 97602[1], 99155[0], 99156[0], 99157[0], 99211[1], 99212[1], 99213[1], 99214[1], 99215[1], 99217[1], 99218[1], 99219[1], 99220[1], 99221[1], 99222[1], 99223[1], 99231[1], 99232[1], 99233[1], 99234[1], 99235[1], 99236[1], 99238[1], 99239[1], 99241[1], 99242[1], 99243[1], 99244[1], 99245[1], 99251[1], 99252[1], 99253[1], 99254[1], 99255[1], 99291[1], 99292[1], 99304[1], 99305[1], 99306[1], 99307[1], 99308[1], 99309[1], 99310[1], 99315[1], 99316[1], 99334[1], 99335[1], 99336[1], 99337[1], 99347[1], 99348[1], 99349[1], 99350[1], 99374[1], 99375[1], 99377[1], 99378[1], 99446[0], 99447[0], 99448[0], 99449[0], 99451[0], 99452[0], 99495[0], 99496[0], G0453[0], G0463[1], G0471[1], J0670[1], J2001[1]
64600	0213T[0], 0216T[0], 0228T[0], 0230T[0], 0333T[0], 0464T[0], 12001[1], 12002[1], 12004[1], 12005[1], 12006[1], 12007[1], 12011[1], 12013[1], 12014[1], 12015[1], 12016[1], 12017[1], 12018[1], 12020[1], 12021[1], 12031[1], 12032[1], 12034[1], 12035[1], 12036[1], 12037[1], 12041[1], 12042[1], 12044[1], 12045[1], 12046[1], 12047[1], 12051[1], 12052[1], 12053[1], 12054[1], 12055[1], 12056[1], 12057[1], 13100[1], 13101[1], 13102[1], 13120[1], 13121[1], 13122[1], 13131[1], 13132[1], 13133[1], 13151[1], 13152[1], 13153[1], 20550[1], 20551[1], 20552[1], 20553[1], 36000[1], 36400[1], 36405[1], 36406[1], 36410[1], 36420[1], 36425[1], 36430[1], 36440[1], 36591[0], 36592[0], 36600[1], 36640[1], 43752[1], 51701[1], 51702[1], 51703[1], 62320[1], 62321[1], 62322[1], 62323[1], 62324[1], 62325[1], 62326[1], 62327[1], 64400[1], 64402[1], 64405[1], 64408[1], 64410[1], 64413[1], 64415[1], 64416[1], 64417[1], 64418[1], 64420[1], 64421[1], 64425[1], 64430[1], 64435[1], 64445[1], 64446[1], 64447[1], 64448[1], 64449[1], 64450[1], 64461[0], 64462[0], 64463[0], 64479[1], 64480[0], 64483[1], 64484[0], 64486[0], 64487[0], 64488[0], 64489[0], 64490[1], 64491[0], 64492[0], 64493[1], 64494[0], 64495[0], 64505[1], 64510[1], 64517[1], 64520[1], 64530[1], 69990[0], 76000[1], 77001[1], 92012[1], 92014[1], 92585[0], 93000[1], 93005[1], 93010[1], 93040[1], 93041[1], 93042[1], 93318[1], 93355[1], 94002[1], 94200[1], 94250[1], 94680[1], 94681[1], 94690[1], 94770[1], 95812[1], 95813[1], 95816[1], 95819[1], 95822[0], 95829[1], 95860[0], 95861[0], 95863[0], 95864[0], 95865[0], 95866[0], 95867[0], 95868[0], 95869[0], 95870[0], 95907[0], 95908[0], 95909[0], 95910[0], 95911[0], 95912[0], 95913[0], 95925[0], 95926[0], 95927[0], 95928[0], 95929[0], 95930[0], 95933[0], 95937[0], 95938[0], 95939[0], 95940[0], 95955[1], 96360[1], 96361[1], 96365[1], 96366[1], 96367[1], 96368[1], 96372[1], 96374[1], 96375[1], 96376[1], 96377[1], 99155[0], 99156[0], 99157[0], 99211[1], 99212[1], 99213[1], 99214[1], 99215[1], 99217[1], 99218[1], 99219[1], 99220[1], 99221[1], 99222[1], 99223[1], 99231[1], 99232[1], 99233[1], 99234[1], 99235[1], 99236[1], 99238[1], 99239[1], 99241[1], 99242[1], 99243[1], 99244[1], 99245[1], 99251[1], 99252[1], 99253[1], 99254[1], 99255[1], 99291[1], 99292[1], 99304[1], 99305[1], 99306[1], 99307[1], 99308[1], 99309[1], 99310[1], 99315[1], 99316[1], 99334[1], 99335[1], 99336[1], 99337[1], 99347[1], 99348[1], 99349[1], 99350[1], 99374[1], 99375[1], 99377[1], 99378[1], 99446[0], 99447[0], 99448[0], 99449[0], 99451[0], 99452[0], 99495[0], 99496[0], G0453[0], G0463[1], G0471[1], J2001[1]
64605	0213T[0], 0216T[0], 0228T[0], 0230T[0], 0333T[0], 0464T[0], 12001[1], 12002[1], 12004[1], 12005[1], 12006[1], 12007[1], 12011[1], 12013[1], 12014[1], 12015[1], 12016[1], 12017[1], 12018[1], 12020[1], 12021[1], 12031[1], 12032[1], 12034[1], 12035[1], 12036[1], 12037[1], 12041[1], 12042[1], 12044[1], 12045[1], 12046[1], 12047[1], 12051[1], 12052[1], 12053[1], 12054[1], 12055[1], 12056[1], 12057[1], 13100[1], 13101[1], 13102[1], 13120[1], 13121[1], 13122[1], 13131[1], 13132[1], 13133[1], 13151[1], 13152[1], 13153[1], 20550[1], 20551[1], 20552[1], 20553[1], 36000[1], 36400[1], 36405[1], 36406[1], 36410[1], 36420[1], 36425[1], 36430[1], 36440[1], 36591[0], 36592[0], 36600[1], 36640[1], 43752[1], 51701[1], 51702[1], 51703[1], 62320[1], 62321[1], 62322[1], 62323[1], 62324[1], 62325[1], 62326[1], 62327[1], 64400[1], 64402[1], 64405[1], 64408[1], 64410[1], 64413[1], 64415[1], 64416[1], 64417[1], 64418[1], 64420[1], 64421[1], 64425[1], 64430[1], 64435[1], 64445[1], 64446[1], 64447[1], 64448[1], 64449[1], 64450[1], 64461[0], 64462[0], 64463[0], 64479[1], 64480[0], 64483[1], 64484[0], 64486[0], 64487[0], 64488[0], 64489[0], 64490[1], 64491[0], 64492[0], 64493[1], 64494[0], 64495[0], 64505[1], 64510[1], 64517[1], 64520[1], 64530[1], 69990[0], 76000[1], 77001[1], 92012[1], 92014[1], 92585[0], 93000[1], 93005[1], 93010[1], 93040[1], 93041[1], 93042[1], 93318[1], 93355[1], 94002[1], 94200[1], 94250[1], 94680[1], 94681[1], 94690[1], 94770[1], 95812[1], 95813[1], 95816[1], 95819[1], 95822[0],

0 = Modifier usage not allowed or inappropriate   1 = Modifier usage allowed

CPT © 2018 American Medical Association. All Rights Reserved.

Code 1	Code 2
	95829[1], 95860[0], 95861[0], 95863[0], 95864[0], 95865[0], 95866[0], 95867[0], 95868[0], 95869[0], 95870[0], 95907[0], 95908[0], 95909[0], 95910[0], 95911[0], 95912[0], 95913[0], 95925[0], 95926[0], 95927[0], 95928[0], 95929[0], 95930[0], 95933[0], 95937[0], 95938[0], 95939[0], 95940[0], 95955[1], 96360[1], 96361[1], 96365[1], 96366[1], 96367[1], 96368[1], 96372[1], 96374[1], 96375[1], 96376[1], 96377[1], 99155[0], 99156[0], 99157[0], 99211[1], 99212[1], 99213[1], 99214[1], 99215[1], 99217[1], 99218[1], 99219[1], 99220[1], 99221[1], 99222[1], 99223[1], 99231[1], 99232[1], 99233[1], 99234[1], 99235[1], 99236[1], 99238[1], 99239[1], 99241[1], 99242[1], 99243[1], 99244[1], 99245[1], 99251[1], 99252[1], 99253[1], 99254[1], 99255[1], 99291[1], 99292[1], 99304[1], 99305[1], 99306[1], 99307[1], 99308[1], 99309[1], 99310[1], 99315[1], 99316[1], 99334[1], 99335[1], 99336[1], 99337[1], 99347[1], 99348[1], 99349[1], 99350[1], 99374[1], 99375[1], 99377[1], 99378[1], 99446[0], 99447[0], 99448[0], 99449[0], 99451[0], 99452[0], 99495[0], 99496[0], G0453[0], G0463[1], G0471[1], J2001[1]
64610	0213T[0], 0216T[0], 0228T[0], 0230T[0], 0333T[0], 0464T[0], 12001[1], 12002[1], 12004[1], 12005[1], 12006[1], 12007[1], 12011[1], 12013[1], 12014[1], 12015[1], 12016[1], 12017[1], 12018[1], 12020[1], 12021[1], 12031[1], 12032[1], 12034[1], 12035[1], 12036[1], 12037[1], 12041[1], 12042[1], 12044[1], 12045[1], 12046[1], 12047[1], 12051[1], 12052[1], 12053[1], 12054[1], 12055[1], 12056[1], 12057[1], 13100[1], 13101[1], 13102[1], 13120[1], 13121[1], 13122[1], 13131[1], 13132[1], 13133[1], 13151[1], 13152[1], 13153[1], 20550[1], 20551[1], 20552[1], 20553[1], 36000[1], 36400[1], 36405[1], 36406[1], 36410[1], 36420[1], 36425[1], 36430[1], 36440[1], 36591[0], 36592[0], 36600[1], 36640[1], 43752[1], 51701[1], 51702[1], 51703[1], 62320[1], 62321[1], 62322[1], 62323[1], 62324[1], 62325[1], 62326[1], 62327[1], 64400[1], 64402[1], 64405[1], 64408[1], 64410[1], 64413[1], 64415[1], 64416[1], 64417[1], 64418[1], 64420[1], 64421[1], 64425[1], 64430[1], 64435[1], 64445[1], 64446[1], 64447[1], 64448[1], 64449[1], 64450[1], 64461[0], 64462[0], 64463[0], 64479[1], 64480[0], 64483[1], 64484[0], 64486[0], 64487[0], 64488[0], 64489[0], 64490[1], 64491[0], 64492[0], 64493[1], 64494[0], 64495[0], 64505[1], 64510[1], 64517[1], 64520[1], 64530[1], 64605[1], 69990[0], 76000[1], 77001[1], 77002[1], 92012[1], 92014[1], 92585[0], 93000[1], 93005[1], 93010[1], 93040[1], 93041[1], 93042[1], 93318[1], 93355[1], 94002[1], 94200[1], 94250[1], 94680[1], 94681[1], 94690[1], 94770[1], 95812[1], 95813[1], 95816[1], 95819[1], 95822[0], 95829[1], 95860[0], 95861[0], 95863[0], 95864[0], 95865[0], 95866[0], 95867[0], 95868[0], 95869[0], 95870[0], 95907[0], 95908[0], 95909[0], 95910[0], 95911[0], 95912[0], 95913[0], 95925[0], 95926[0], 95927[0], 95928[0], 95929[0], 95930[0], 95933[0], 95937[0], 95938[0], 95939[0], 95940[0], 95955[1], 96360[1], 96361[1], 96365[1], 96366[1], 96367[1], 96368[1], 96372[1], 96374[1], 96375[1], 96376[1], 96377[1], 99155[0], 99156[0], 99157[0], 99211[1], 99212[1], 99213[1], 99214[1], 99215[1], 99217[1], 99218[1], 99219[1], 99220[1], 99221[1], 99222[1], 99223[1], 99231[1], 99232[1], 99233[1], 99234[1], 99235[1], 99236[1], 99238[1], 99239[1], 99241[1], 99242[1], 99243[1], 99244[1], 99245[1], 99251[1], 99252[1], 99253[1], 99254[1], 99255[1], 99291[1], 99292[1], 99304[1], 99305[1], 99306[1], 99307[1], 99308[1], 99309[1], 99310[1], 99315[1], 99316[1], 99334[1], 99335[1], 99336[1], 99337[1], 99347[1], 99348[1], 99349[1], 99350[1], 99374[1], 99375[1], 99377[1], 99378[1], 99446[0], 99447[0], 99448[0], 99449[0], 99451[0], 99452[0], 99495[0], 99496[0], G0453[0], G0463[1], G0471[1]
64612	0213T[0], 0216T[0], 0228T[0], 0230T[0], 0333T[0], 0464T[0], 12001[1], 12002[1], 12004[1], 12005[1], 12006[1], 12007[1], 12011[1], 12013[1], 12014[1], 12015[1], 12016[1], 12017[1], 12018[1], 12020[1], 12021[1], 12031[1], 12032[1], 12034[1], 12035[1], 12036[1], 12037[1], 12041[1], 12042[1], 12044[1], 12045[1], 12046[1], 12047[1], 12051[1], 12052[1], 12053[1], 12054[1], 12055[1], 12056[1], 12057[1], 13100[1], 13101[1], 13102[1], 13120[1], 13121[1], 13122[1], 13131[1], 13132[1], 13133[1], 13151[1], 13152[1], 13153[1], 20550[1], 20551[1], 20552[1], 20553[1], 36000[1], 36400[1], 36405[1], 36406[1], 36410[1], 36420[1], 36425[1], 36430[1], 36440[1], 36591[0], 36592[0], 36600[1], 36640[1], 43752[1], 51701[1], 51702[1], 51703[1], 62320[1], 62321[1], 62322[1], 62323[1], 62324[1], 62325[1], 62326[1], 62327[1], 64400[1], 64402[1], 64405[1], 64408[1], 64410[1], 64413[1], 64415[1], 64416[1], 64417[1], 64418[1], 64420[1], 64421[1], 64425[1], 64430[1], 64435[1], 64445[1], 64446[1], 64447[1], 64448[1], 64449[1], 64450[1], 64461[0], 64462[0], 64463[0], 64479[1], 64480[0], 64483[1], 64484[0], 64486[0], 64487[0], 64488[0], 64489[0], 64490[1], 64491[0], 64492[0], 64493[1], 64494[0], 64495[0], 64505[1], 64510[1], 64517[1], 64520[1], 64530[1], 69990[0], 92012[1], 92014[1], 92585[0], 93000[1], 93005[1], 93010[1], 93040[1], 93041[1], 93042[1], 93318[1], 93355[1], 94002[1], 94200[1], 94250[1], 94680[1], 94681[1], 94690[1], 94770[1], 95812[1], 95813[1], 95816[1], 95819[1], 95822[0], 95829[1], 95860[0], 95861[0], 95863[0], 95864[0], 95865[0], 95866[0], 95867[0], 95868[0], 95870[0], 95907[0], 95908[0], 95909[0], 95910[0], 95911[0], 95912[0], 95913[0], 95925[0], 95926[0], 95927[0], 95928[0], 95929[0], 95930[0], 95933[0], 95937[0], 95938[0], 95939[0], 95940[0], 95955[1], 96360[1], 96361[1], 96365[1], 96366[1], 96367[1], 96368[1], 96372[1], 96374[1], 96375[1], 96376[1], 96377[1], 99155[0], 99156[0], 99157[0], 99211[1], 99212[1], 99213[1], 99214[1], 99215[1], 99217[1], 99218[1], 99219[1], 99220[1], 99221[1], 99222[1], 99223[1], 99231[1], 99232[1], 99233[1], 99234[1], 99235[1], 99236[1], 99238[1], 99239[1], 99241[1], 99242[1], 99243[1], 99244[1], 99245[1], 99251[1], 99252[1], 99253[1], 99254[1], 99255[1], 99291[1], 99292[1], 99304[1], 99305[1], 99306[1], 99307[1], 99308[1], 99309[1], 99310[1], 99315[1], 99316[1], 99334[1], 99335[1], 99336[1], 99337[1], 99347[1], 99348[1], 99349[1], 99350[1], 99374[1], 99375[1], 99377[1], 99378[1], 99446[0], 99447[0], 99448[0], 99449[0], 99451[0], 99452[0], 99495[0], 99496[0], G0453[0], G0463[1], G0471[1], J2001[1]
64615	0213T[0], 0216T[0], 0228T[0], 0230T[0], 0333T[1], 0464T[1], 12001[1], 12002[1], 12004[1], 12005[1], 12006[1], 12007[1], 12011[1], 12013[1], 12014[1], 12015[1], 12016[1], 12017[1], 12018[1], 12020[1], 12021[1], 12031[1], 12032[1], 12034[1], 12035[1], 12036[1], 12037[1], 12041[1], 12042[1], 12044[1], 12045[1], 12046[1], 12047[1], 12051[1], 12052[1], 12053[1], 12054[1], 12055[1], 12056[1], 12057[1], 13100[1], 13101[1], 13102[1], 13120[1], 13121[1], 13122[1], 13131[1], 13132[1], 13133[1], 13151[1], 13152[1], 13153[1], 20550[1], 20551[1], 20552[1], 20553[1], 36000[1], 36400[1], 36405[1], 36406[1], 36410[1], 36420[1], 36425[1], 36430[1], 36440[1], 36591[0], 36592[0], 36600[1], 36640[1], 43752[1], 51701[1], 51702[1], 51703[1], 62320[1], 62321[1], 62322[1], 62323[1], 62324[1], 62325[1], 62326[1], 62327[1], 64400[1], 64402[1], 64405[1], 64408[1], 64410[1], 64413[1], 64415[1], 64416[1], 64417[1], 64418[1], 64420[1], 64421[1], 64425[1], 64430[1], 64435[1], 64445[1], 64446[1], 64447[1], 64448[1], 64449[1], 64450[1], 64461[0], 64462[0], 64463[0], 64479[1], 64480[0], 64483[1], 64484[0], 64486[0], 64487[0], 64488[0], 64489[0], 64490[1], 64491[0], 64492[0], 64493[1], 64494[0], 64495[0], 64505[1], 64510[1], 64517[1], 64520[1], 64530[1], 64612[0], 64616[0], 64642[1], 64643[1], 64644[1], 64645[1], 64646[1], 69990[0], 92012[1], 92014[1], 92585[1], 93000[1], 93005[1], 93010[1], 93040[1], 93041[1], 93042[1], 93318[1], 93355[1], 94002[1], 94200[1], 94250[1], 94680[1], 94681[1], 94690[1], 94770[1], 95812[1], 95813[1], 95816[1], 95819[1], 95822[1], 95829[1], 95860[1], 95861[1], 95863[1], 95864[1], 95865[1], 95866[1], 95867[1], 95868[1], 95870[1], 95907[1], 95908[1], 95909[1], 95910[1], 95911[1], 95912[1], 95913[1], 95925[1], 95926[1], 95927[1], 95928[1], 95929[1], 95930[1], 95933[1], 95937[1], 95938[1], 95939[1], 95940[1], 95955[1], 96360[1], 96361[1], 96365[1], 96366[1], 96367[1], 96368[1], 96372[1], 96374[1], 96375[1], 96376[1], 96377[1], 99155[0], 99156[0], 99157[0], 99211[1], 99212[1], 99213[1], 99214[1], 99215[1], 99217[1], 99218[1], 99219[1], 99220[1], 99221[1], 99222[1], 99223[1], 99231[1], 99232[1], 99233[1], 99234[1], 99235[1], 99236[1], 99238[1], 99239[1], 99241[1], 99242[1], 99243[1], 99244[1], 99245[1], 99251[1], 99252[1], 99253[1], 99254[1], 99255[1], 99291[1], 99292[1], 99304[1], 99305[1], 99306[1], 99307[1], 99308[1], 99309[1], 99310[1], 99315[1], 99316[1], 99334[1], 99335[1], 99336[1], 99337[1], 99347[1], 99348[1], 99349[1], 99350[1], 99374[1], 99375[1], 99377[1], 99378[1], 99446[0], 99447[0], 99448[0], 99449[0], 99451[0], 99452[0], 99495[0], 99496[0], G0453[0], G0463[1], G0471[1], J2001[1]
64616	0213T[1], 0216T[1], 0228T[1], 0230T[1], 0333T[0], 0464T[0], 12001[1], 12002[1], 12004[1], 12005[1], 12006[1], 12007[1], 12011[1], 12013[1], 12014[1], 12015[1], 12016[1], 12017[1], 12018[1], 12020[1], 12021[1], 12031[1], 12032[1], 12034[1], 12035[1], 12036[1], 12037[1], 12041[1], 12042[1], 12044[1], 12045[1], 12046[1], 12047[1], 12051[1], 12052[1], 12053[1], 12054[1], 12055[1], 12056[1], 12057[1], 13100[1], 13101[1], 13102[1], 13120[1], 13121[1], 13122[1], 13131[1], 13132[1], 13133[1], 13151[1], 13152[1], 13153[1], 20550[1], 20551[1], 20552[1], 20553[1], 36000[1], 36400[1], 36405[1], 36406[1], 36410[1], 36420[1], 36425[1], 36430[1], 36440[1], 36591[0], 36592[0], 36600[1], 36640[1], 43752[1], 51701[1], 51702[1], 51703[1], 62320[1], 62321[1], 62322[1], 62323[1], 62324[1], 62325[1], 62326[1], 62327[1], 64400[1], 64402[1], 64405[1], 64408[1], 64410[1], 64413[1], 64415[1], 64416[1], 64417[1], 64418[1], 64420[1], 64421[1], 64425[1], 64430[1], 64435[1], 64445[1], 64446[1], 64447[1], 64448[1], 64449[1], 64450[1], 64461[0], 64462[0], 64463[0], 64479[1], 64480[0], 64483[1], 64484[0], 64486[0], 64487[0], 64488[0], 64489[0], 64490[1], 64491[0], 64492[0], 64493[1], 64494[0], 64495[0], 64505[1], 64510[1], 64517[1], 64520[1], 64530[1], 69990[0], 92012[1], 92014[1], 93000[1], 93005[1], 93010[1], 93040[1], 93041[1], 93042[1], 93318[1], 93355[1], 94002[1], 94200[1], 94250[1], 94680[1], 94681[1], 94690[1], 94770[1], 95812[1], 95813[1], 95816[1], 95819[1], 95829[1], 95860[1], 95861[1], 95863[1], 95864[1], 95865[1], 95866[1], 95867[1], 95868[1], 95869[1], 95870[1], 95930[0], 95933[0], 95937[0], 95940[0], 95941[0], 95955[1], 96360[1], 96361[1], 96365[1], 96366[1], 96367[1], 96368[1], 96372[1], 96374[1], 96375[1], 96376[1], 96377[1], 99155[0], 99156[0], 99157[0], 99211[1], 99212[1], 99213[1], 99214[1], 99215[1], 99217[1], 99218[1], 99219[1], 99220[1], 99221[1], 99222[1], 99223[1], 99231[1], 99232[1], 99233[1], 99234[1], 99235[1], 99236[1], 99238[1], 99239[1], 99241[1], 99242[1], 99243[1], 99244[1], 99245[1], 99251[1], 99252[1], 99253[1], 99254[1], 99255[1], 99291[1], 99292[1], 99304[1], 99305[1], 99306[1], 99307[1], 99308[1], 99309[1], 99310[1], 99315[1], 99316[1], 99334[1], 99335[1], 99336[1], 99337[1], 99347[1], 99348[1], 99349[1], 99350[1], 99374[1], 99375[1], 99377[1], 99378[1], 99446[0], 99447[0], 99448[0], 99449[0], 99451[0], 99452[0], G0453[0], G0463[1], G0471[1], J2001[1]
64620	0213T[0], 0228T[0], 0230T[0], 0333T[0], 0464T[0], 12001[1], 12002[1], 12004[1], 12005[1], 12006[1], 12007[1], 12011[1], 12013[1], 12014[1], 12015[1], 12016[1], 12017[1], 12018[1], 12020[1], 12021[1], 12031[1], 12032[1], 12034[1], 12035[1], 12036[1], 12037[1], 12041[1], 12042[1], 12044[1], 12045[1], 12046[1], 12047[1], 12051[1], 12052[1], 12053[1], 12054[1], 12055[1], 12056[1], 12057[1], 13100[1], 13101[1], 13102[1], 13120[1], 13121[1], 13122[1], 13131[1], 13132[1], 13133[1], 13151[1], 13152[1], 13153[1], 20550[1], 20551[1], 20552[1], 20553[1], 36000[1], 36400[1], 36405[1], 36406[1], 36410[1], 36420[1], 36425[1], 36430[1], 36440[1], 36591[0], 36592[0], 36600[1], 36640[1], 43752[1], 51701[1], 51702[1], 51703[1], 62320[1], 62321[1], 62324[1], 62325[1], 64400[1], 64402[1], 64405[1], 64408[1], 64410[1], 64413[1], 64415[1], 64416[1], 64417[1], 64418[1], 64420[1], 64421[1], 64425[1], 64430[1], 64435[1], 64445[1], 64446[1], 64447[1], 64448[1], 64449[1], 64461[0], 64462[0], 64463[0], 64479[1], 64480[0], 64483[1], 64484[0], 64486[0], 64487[0], 64488[0], 64489[0], 64490[1], 64491[0], 64492[0], 64505[1], 64510[1], 64517[1], 64520[1], 64530[1], 69990[0], 76000[1], 77001[1], 77002[1], 92012[1], 92014[1], 92585[0], 93000[1], 93005[1], 93010[1], 93040[1], 93041[1], 93042[1], 93318[1], 93355[1], 94002[1], 94200[1], 94250[1], 94680[1], 94681[1], 94690[1], 94770[1], 95812[1], 95813[1], 95816[1], 95819[1], 95822[0], 95829[1], 95860[0], 95861[0], 95863[0], 95864[0], 95865[0], 95866[0], 95867[0], 95868[0], 95869[0], 95870[0], 95907[0], 95908[0], 95909[0], 95910[0], 95911[0], 95912[0], 95913[0], 95925[0], 95926[0], 95927[0], 95928[0], 95929[0], 95930[0], 95933[0], 95937[0], 95938[0], 95939[0],

0 = Modifier usage not allowed or inappropriate 1 = Modifier usage allowed

CPT © 2018 American Medical Association. All Rights Reserved.

Code 1	Code 2
	95940[0], 95955[1], 96360[1], 96361[1], 96365[1], 96366[1], 96367[1], 96368[1], 96372[1], 96374[1], 96375[1], 96376[1], 96377[1], 99155[0], 99156[0], 99157[0], 99211[1], 99212[1], 99213[1], 99214[1], 99215[1], 99217[1], 99218[1], 99219[1], 99220[1], 99221[1], 99222[1], 99223[1], 99231[1], 99232[1], 99233[1], 99234[1], 99235[1], 99236[1], 99238[1], 99239[1], 99241[1], 99242[1], 99243[1], 99244[1], 99245[1], 99251[1], 99252[1], 99253[1], 99254[1], 99255[1], 99291[1], 99292[1], 99304[1], 99305[1], 99306[1], 99307[1], 99308[1], 99309[1], 99310[1], 99315[1], 99316[1], 99334[1], 99335[1], 99336[1], 99337[1], 99347[1], 99348[1], 99349[1], 99350[1], 99374[1], 99375[1], 99377[1], 99378[1], 99446[0], 99447[0], 99448[0], 99449[0], 99451[0], 99452[0], 99495[0], 99496[0], G0453[0], G0463[1], G0471[1], J2001[1]
64630	0213T[0], 0216T[0], 0228T[0], 0230T[0], 0333T[0], 0464T[0], 12001[1], 12002[1], 12004[1], 12005[1], 12006[1], 12007[1], 12011[1], 12013[1], 12014[1], 12015[1], 12016[1], 12017[1], 12018[1], 12020[1], 12021[1], 12031[1], 12032[1], 12034[1], 12035[1], 12036[1], 12037[1], 12041[1], 12042[1], 12044[1], 12045[1], 12046[1], 12047[1], 12051[1], 12052[1], 12053[1], 12054[1], 12055[1], 12056[1], 12057[1], 13100[1], 13101[1], 13102[1], 13120[1], 13121[1], 13122[1], 13131[1], 13132[1], 13133[1], 13151[1], 13152[1], 13153[1], 20550[1], 20551[1], 20552[1], 20553[1], 36000[1], 36400[1], 36405[1], 36406[1], 36410[1], 36420[1], 36425[1], 36430[1], 36440[1], 36591[0], 36592[0], 36600[1], 36640[1], 43752[1], 51701[1], 51702[1], 51703[1], 62320[1], 62321[1], 62322[1], 62323[1], 62324[1], 62325[1], 62326[1], 62327[1], 64400[1], 64402[1], 64405[1], 64408[1], 64410[1], 64413[1], 64415[1], 64416[1], 64417[1], 64418[1], 64420[1], 64421[1], 64425[1], 64430[1], 64435[1], 64445[1], 64446[1], 64447[1], 64448[1], 64449[1], 64450[1], 64461[0], 64462[0], 64463[0], 64479[1], 64480[0], 64483[1], 64484[0], 64486[0], 64487[0], 64488[0], 64489[0], 64490[1], 64491[0], 64492[0], 64493[1], 64494[0], 64495[0], 64505[1], 64510[1], 64517[1], 64520[1], 64530[1], 69990[0], 92012[1], 92014[1], 92585[0], 93000[1], 93005[1], 93010[1], 93040[1], 93041[1], 93042[1], 93318[1], 93355[1], 94002[1], 94200[1], 94250[1], 94680[1], 94681[1], 94690[1], 94770[1], 95812[1], 95813[1], 95816[1], 95819[1], 95822[0], 95829[1], 95860[0], 95861[0], 95863[0], 95864[0], 95865[0], 95866[0], 95867[0], 95868[0], 95869[0], 95870[0], 95907[0], 95908[0], 95909[0], 95910[0], 95911[0], 95912[0], 95913[0], 95925[0], 95926[0], 95927[0], 95928[0], 95929[0], 95930[0], 95933[0], 95937[0], 95938[0], 95939[0], 95940[0], 95955[1], 96360[1], 96361[1], 96365[1], 96366[1], 96367[1], 96368[1], 96372[1], 96374[1], 96375[1], 96376[1], 96377[1], 99155[0], 99156[0], 99157[0], 99211[1], 99212[1], 99213[1], 99214[1], 99215[1], 99217[1], 99218[1], 99219[1], 99220[1], 99221[1], 99222[1], 99223[1], 99231[1], 99232[1], 99233[1], 99234[1], 99235[1], 99236[1], 99238[1], 99239[1], 99241[1], 99242[1], 99243[1], 99244[1], 99245[1], 99251[1], 99252[1], 99253[1], 99254[1], 99255[1], 99291[1], 99292[1], 99304[1], 99305[1], 99306[1], 99307[1], 99308[1], 99309[1], 99310[1], 99315[1], 99316[1], 99334[1], 99335[1], 99336[1], 99337[1], 99347[1], 99348[1], 99349[1], 99350[1], 99374[1], 99375[1], 99377[1], 99378[1], 99446[0], 99447[0], 99448[0], 99449[0], 99451[0], 99452[0], 99495[0], 99496[0], G0453[0], G0463[1], G0471[1], J2001[1]
64632	0213T[1], 0216T[1], 0228T[1], 0230T[1], 0333T[0], 0464T[0], 12001[1], 12002[1], 12004[1], 12005[1], 12006[1], 12007[1], 12011[1], 12013[1], 12014[1], 12015[1], 12016[1], 12017[1], 12018[1], 12020[1], 12021[1], 12031[1], 12032[1], 12034[1], 12035[1], 12036[1], 12037[1], 12041[1], 12042[1], 12044[1], 12045[1], 12046[1], 12047[1], 12051[1], 12052[1], 12053[1], 12054[1], 12055[1], 12056[1], 12057[1], 13100[1], 13101[1], 13102[1], 13120[1], 13121[1], 13122[1], 13131[1], 13132[1], 13133[1], 13151[1], 13152[1], 13153[1], 20550[1], 20551[1], 20552[1], 20553[1], 36000[1], 36400[1], 36405[1], 36406[1], 36410[1], 36420[1], 36425[1], 36430[1], 36440[1], 36591[0], 36592[0], 36600[1], 36640[1], 43752[1], 51701[1], 51702[1], 51703[1], 62320[1], 62321[1], 62322[1], 62323[1], 62324[1], 62325[1], 62326[1], 62327[1], 64400[1], 64402[1], 64405[1], 64408[1], 64410[1], 64413[1], 64415[1], 64416[1], 64417[1], 64418[1], 64420[1], 64421[1], 64425[1], 64430[1], 64435[1], 64445[1], 64446[1], 64447[1], 64448[1], 64449[1], 64450[1], 64455[1], 64461[0], 64462[0], 64463[0], 64479[1], 64480[0], 64483[1], 64484[0], 64486[0], 64487[0], 64488[0], 64489[0], 64490[1], 64491[0], 64492[0], 64493[1], 64494[0], 64495[0], 64505[1], 64510[1], 64517[1], 64520[1], 64530[1], 69990[0], 92012[1], 92014[1], 92585[0], 93000[1], 93005[1], 93010[1], 93040[1], 93041[1], 93042[1], 93318[1], 93355[1], 94002[1], 94200[1], 94250[1], 94680[1], 94681[1], 94690[1], 94770[1], 95812[1], 95813[1], 95816[1], 95819[1], 95822[0], 95829[1], 95860[0], 95861[0], 95863[0], 95864[0], 95865[0], 95866[0], 95867[0], 95868[0], 95869[0], 95870[0], 95907[0], 95908[0], 95909[0], 95910[0], 95911[0], 95912[0], 95913[0], 95925[0], 95926[0], 95927[0], 95928[0], 95929[0], 95930[0], 95933[0], 95937[0], 95938[0], 95939[0], 95940[0], 95955[1], 96360[1], 96361[1], 96365[1], 96366[1], 96367[1], 96368[1], 96372[1], 96374[1], 96375[1], 96376[1], 96377[1], 99155[0], 99156[0], 99157[0], 99211[1], 99212[1], 99213[1], 99214[1], 99215[1], 99217[1], 99218[1], 99219[1], 99220[1], 99221[1], 99222[1], 99223[1], 99231[1], 99232[1], 99233[1], 99234[1], 99235[1], 99236[1], 99238[1], 99239[1], 99241[1], 99242[1], 99243[1], 99244[1], 99245[1], 99251[1], 99252[1], 99253[1], 99254[1], 99255[1], 99291[1], 99292[1], 99304[1], 99305[1], 99306[1], 99307[1], 99308[1], 99309[1], 99310[1], 99315[1], 99316[1], 99334[1], 99335[1], 99336[1], 99337[1], 99347[1], 99348[1], 99349[1], 99350[1], 99374[1], 99375[1], 99377[1], 99378[1], 99446[0], 99447[0], 99448[0], 99449[0], 99451[0], 99452[0], 99495[0], 99496[0], G0453[0], G0463[1], G0471[1], J0670[1], J2001[1]
64633	0213T[0], 0216T[0], 0228T[0], 0230T[0], 0333T[0], 0464T[0], 12001[1], 12002[1], 12004[1], 12005[1], 12006[1], 12007[1], 12011[1], 12013[1], 12014[1], 12015[1], 12016[1], 12017[1], 12018[1], 12020[1], 12021[1], 12031[1], 12032[1], 12034[1], 12035[1], 12036[1], 12037[1], 12041[1], 12042[1], 12044[1], 12045[1], 12046[1], 12047[1], 12051[1], 12052[1], 12053[1], 12054[1], 12055[1], 12056[1], 12057[1], 13100[1], 13101[1], 13102[1], 13120[1], 13121[1], 13122[1], 13131[1], 13132[1], 13133[1], 13151[1], 13152[1], 13153[1], 20550[1], 20551[1], 20552[1], 20553[1], 36000[1], 36400[1], 36405[1], 36406[1], 36410[1], 36420[1], 36425[1], 36430[1], 36440[1], 36591[0], 36592[0], 36600[1], 36640[1], 43752[1], 51701[1], 51702[1], 51703[1], 62320[1], 62321[1], 62322[1], 62323[1], 62324[1], 62325[1], 62326[1], 62327[1], 64400[1], 64402[1], 64405[1], 64408[1], 64410[1], 64413[1], 64415[1], 64416[1], 64417[1], 64418[1], 64420[1], 64421[1], 64425[1], 64430[1], 64435[1], 64445[1], 64446[1], 64447[1], 64448[1], 64449[1], 64450[1], 64461[0], 64462[0], 64463[0], 64479[1], 64480[0], 64483[1], 64484[1], 64486[0], 64487[0], 64488[0], 64489[0], 64490[1], 64491[1], 64492[1], 64493[1], 64494[1], 64495[1], 64505[1], 64510[1], 64517[1], 64520[1], 64530[1], 69990[0], 76000[1], 76380[1], 77001[1], 77002[1], 77003[1], 77012[1], 92012[1], 92014[1], 92585[0], 93000[1], 93005[1], 93010[1], 93040[1], 93041[1], 93042[1], 93318[1], 93355[1], 94002[1], 94200[1], 94250[1], 94680[1], 94681[1], 94690[1], 94770[1], 95812[1], 95813[1], 95816[1], 95819[1], 95822[0], 95829[1], 95860[0], 95861[0], 95863[0], 95864[0], 95865[0], 95866[0], 95867[0], 95868[0], 95869[0], 95870[0], 95907[0], 95908[0], 95909[0], 95910[0], 95911[0], 95912[0], 95913[0], 95925[0], 95926[0], 95927[0], 95928[0], 95929[0], 95930[0], 95933[0], 95937[0], 95938[0], 95939[0], 95940[0], 95955[1], 96360[1], 96361[1], 96365[1], 96366[1], 96367[1], 96368[1], 96372[1], 96374[1], 96375[1], 96376[1], 96377[1], 99155[0], 99156[0], 99157[0], 99211[1], 99212[1], 99213[1], 99214[1], 99215[1], 99217[1], 99218[1], 99219[1], 99220[1], 99221[1], 99222[1], 99223[1], 99231[1], 99232[1], 99233[1], 99234[1], 99235[1], 99236[1], 99238[1], 99239[1], 99241[1], 99242[1], 99243[1], 99244[1], 99245[1], 99251[1], 99252[1], 99253[1], 99254[1], 99255[1], 99291[1], 99292[1], 99304[1], 99305[1], 99306[1], 99307[1], 99308[1], 99309[1], 99310[1], 99315[1], 99316[1], 99334[1], 99335[1], 99336[1], 99337[1], 99347[1], 99348[1], 99349[1], 99350[1], 99374[1], 99375[1], 99377[1], 99378[1], 99446[0], 99447[0], 99448[0], 99449[0], 99451[0], 99452[0], 99495[0], 99496[0], G0453[0], G0463[1], G0471[1], J0670[1], J2001[1]
64634	0213T[0], 0216T[0], 0228T[0], 0230T[0], 0333T[0], 0464T[0], 20550[1], 20551[1], 20552[1], 20553[1], 36000[1], 36400[1], 36405[1], 36406[1], 36410[1], 36420[1], 36425[1], 36430[1], 36440[1], 36591[0], 36592[0], 36600[1], 36640[1], 43752[1], 51701[1], 51702[1], 51703[1], 61650[1], 62320[1], 62321[1], 62322[1], 62323[1], 62324[1], 62325[1], 62326[1], 62327[1], 64400[1], 64402[1], 64405[1], 64408[1], 64410[1], 64413[1], 64415[1], 64416[1], 64417[1], 64418[1], 64420[1], 64421[1], 64425[1], 64430[1], 64435[1], 64445[1], 64446[1], 64447[1], 64448[1], 64449[1], 64450[1], 64461[1], 64463[1], 64479[1], 64483[1], 64486[1], 64487[1], 64488[1], 64489[1], 64490[1], 64493[1], 64505[1], 64510[1], 64517[1], 64520[1], 64530[1], 69990[0], 76000[1], 76380[1], 77002[1], 77003[1], 77012[1], 92585[0], 93000[1], 93005[1], 93010[1], 93040[1], 93041[1], 93042[1], 93318[1], 93355[1], 94002[1], 94200[1], 94250[1], 94680[1], 94681[1], 94690[1], 94770[1], 95812[1], 95813[1], 95816[1], 95819[1], 95822[0], 95829[1], 95860[0], 95861[0], 95863[0], 95864[0], 95865[0], 95866[0], 95867[0], 95868[0], 95869[0], 95870[0], 95907[0], 95908[0], 95909[0], 95910[0], 95911[0], 95912[0], 95913[0], 95925[0], 95926[0], 95927[0], 95928[0], 95929[0], 95930[0], 95933[0], 95937[0], 95938[0], 95939[0], 95940[0], 95955[1], 96360[1], 96365[1], 96372[1], 96374[1], 96375[1], 96376[1], 96377[1], 99155[0], 99156[0], 99157[0], G0453[0], G0471[1], J0670[1], J2001[1]
64635	0213T[0], 0216T[0], 0228T[0], 0230T[0], 0333T[0], 0464T[0], 12001[1], 12002[1], 12004[1], 12005[1], 12006[1], 12007[1], 12011[1], 12013[1], 12014[1], 12015[1], 12016[1], 12017[1], 12018[1], 12020[1], 12021[1], 12031[1], 12032[1], 12034[1], 12035[1], 12036[1], 12037[1], 12041[1], 12042[1], 12044[1], 12045[1], 12046[1], 12047[1], 12051[1], 12052[1], 12053[1], 12054[1], 12055[1], 12056[1], 12057[1], 13100[1], 13101[1], 13102[1], 13120[1], 13121[1], 13122[1], 13131[1], 13132[1], 13133[1], 13151[1], 13152[1], 13153[1], 20550[1], 20551[1], 20552[1], 20553[1], 36000[1], 36400[1], 36405[1], 36406[1], 36410[1], 36420[1], 36425[1], 36430[1], 36440[1], 36591[0], 36592[0], 36600[1], 36640[1], 43752[1], 51701[1], 51702[1], 51703[1], 62320[1], 62321[1], 62322[1], 62323[1], 62324[1], 62325[1], 62326[1], 62327[1], 64400[1], 64402[1], 64405[1], 64408[1], 64410[1], 64413[1], 64415[1], 64416[1], 64417[1], 64418[1], 64420[1], 64421[1], 64425[1], 64430[1], 64435[1], 64445[1], 64446[1], 64447[1], 64448[1], 64449[1], 64450[1], 64461[0], 64462[0], 64463[0], 64479[1], 64480[0], 64483[1], 64484[1], 64486[0], 64487[0], 64488[0], 64489[0], 64490[1], 64491[1], 64492[1], 64493[1], 64494[1], 64495[1], 64505[1], 64510[1], 64517[1], 64520[1], 64530[1], 69990[0], 76000[1], 76380[1], 77001[1], 77002[1], 77003[1], 77012[1], 92012[1], 92014[1], 92585[0], 93000[1], 93005[1], 93010[1], 93040[1], 93041[1], 93042[1], 93318[1], 93355[1], 94002[1], 94200[1], 94250[1], 94680[1], 94681[1], 94690[1], 94770[1], 95812[1], 95813[1], 95816[1], 95819[1], 95822[0], 95829[1], 95860[0], 95861[0], 95863[0], 95864[0], 95865[0], 95866[0], 95867[0], 95868[0], 95869[0], 95870[0], 95907[0], 95908[0], 95909[0], 95910[0], 95911[0], 95912[0], 95913[0], 95925[0], 95926[0], 95927[0], 95928[0], 95929[0], 95930[0], 95933[0], 95937[0], 95938[0], 95939[0], 95940[0], 95955[1], 96360[1], 96361[1], 96365[1], 96366[1], 96367[1], 96368[1], 96372[1], 96374[1], 96375[1], 96376[1], 96377[1], 99155[0], 99156[0], 99157[0], 99211[1], 99212[1], 99213[1], 99214[1], 99215[1], 99217[1], 99218[1], 99219[1], 99220[1], 99221[1], 99222[1], 99223[1], 99231[1], 99232[1], 99233[1], 99234[1], 99235[1], 99236[1], 99238[1], 99239[1], 99241[1], 99242[1], 99243[1], 99244[1], 99245[1], 99251[1], 99252[1], 99253[1], 99254[1], 99255[1], 99291[1], 99292[1], 99304[1], 99305[1], 99306[1], 99307[1], 99308[1], 99309[1], 99310[1], 99315[1], 99316[1], 99334[1], 99335[1], 99336[1], 99337[1], 99347[1], 99348[1], 99349[1], 99350[1], 99374[1], 99375[1], 99377[1], 99378[1], 99446[0], 99447[0], 99448[0], 99449[0], 99451[0], 99452[0], 99495[0], 99496[0], G0453[0], G0463[1], G0471[1], J0670[1], J2001[1]

0 = Modifier usage not allowed or inappropriate 1 = Modifier usage allowed

CPT © 2018 American Medical Association. All Rights Reserved.

Code 1	Code 2
64636	0213T[0], 0216T[0], 0228T[0], 0230T[0], 0333T[0], 0464T[0], 20550[1], 20551[1], 20552[1], 20553[1], 36000[1], 36400[1], 36405[1], 36406[1], 36410[1], 36420[1], 36425[1], 36430[1], 36440[1], 36591[0], 36592[0], 36600[1], 36640[1], 43752[1], 51701[1], 51702[1], 51703[1], 61650[1], 62320[1], 62321[1], 62322[1], 62323[1], 62324[1], 62325[1], 62326[1], 62327[1], 64400[1], 64402[1], 64405[1], 64408[1], 64410[1], 64413[1], 64415[1], 64416[1], 64417[1], 64418[1], 64420[1], 64421[1], 64425[1], 64430[1], 64435[1], 64445[1], 64446[1], 64447[1], 64448[1], 64449[1], 64450[1], 64461[1], 64463[1], 64479[1], 64483[1], 64486[1], 64487[1], 64488[1], 64489[1], 64490[1], 64493[1], 64505[1], 64510[1], 64517[1], 64520[1], 64530[1], 69990[0], 76000[1], 76380[1], 77002[1], 77003[1], 77012[1], 92585[0], 93000[1], 93005[1], 93010[1], 93040[1], 93041[1], 93042[1], 93318[1], 93355[1], 94002[1], 94200[1], 94250[1], 94680[1], 94681[1], 94690[1], 94770[1], 95812[1], 95813[1], 95816[1], 95819[1], 95822[0], 95829[1], 95860[0], 95861[0], 95863[0], 95864[0], 95865[0], 95866[0], 95867[0], 95868[0], 95869[0], 95870[0], 95907[0], 95908[0], 95909[0], 95910[0], 95911[0], 95912[0], 95913[0], 95925[0], 95926[0], 95927[0], 95928[0], 95929[0], 95930[0], 95933[0], 95937[0], 95938[0], 95939[0], 95940[0], 95955[1], 96360[1], 96365[1], 96372[1], 96374[1], 96375[1], 96376[1], 96377[1], 99155[0], 99156[0], 99157[0], G0453[0], G0471[1], J0670[1], J2001[1]
64640	0213T[0], 0216T[0], 0228T[0], 0230T[0], 0333T[0], 0464T[0], 12001[1], 12002[1], 12004[1], 12005[1], 12006[1], 12007[1], 12011[1], 12013[1], 12014[1], 12015[1], 12016[1], 12017[1], 12018[1], 12020[1], 12021[1], 12031[1], 12032[1], 12034[1], 12035[1], 12036[1], 12037[1], 12041[1], 12042[1], 12044[1], 12045[1], 12046[1], 12047[1], 12051[1], 12052[1], 12053[1], 12054[1], 12055[1], 12056[1], 12057[1], 13100[1], 13101[1], 13102[1], 13120[1], 13121[1], 13122[1], 13131[1], 13132[1], 13133[1], 13151[1], 13152[1], 13153[1], 20550[1], 20551[1], 20552[1], 20553[1], 36000[1], 36400[1], 36405[1], 36406[1], 36410[1], 36420[1], 36425[1], 36430[1], 36440[1], 36591[0], 36592[0], 36600[1], 36640[1], 43752[1], 51701[1], 51702[1], 51703[1], 62320[1], 62321[1], 62322[1], 62323[1], 62324[1], 62325[1], 62326[1], 62327[1], 64400[1], 64402[1], 64405[1], 64408[1], 64410[1], 64413[1], 64415[1], 64416[1], 64417[1], 64418[1], 64420[1], 64421[1], 64425[1], 64430[1], 64435[1], 64445[1], 64446[1], 64447[1], 64448[1], 64449[1], 64450[1], 64455[1], 64461[0], 64462[0], 64463[0], 64479[1], 64480[0], 64483[1], 64484[0], 64486[0], 64487[0], 64488[0], 64489[0], 64490[1], 64491[0], 64492[0], 64493[1], 64494[0], 64495[0], 64505[1], 64510[1], 64517[1], 64520[1], 64530[1], 64632[1], 69990[0], 92012[1], 92014[1], 92585[0], 93000[1], 93005[1], 93010[1], 93040[1], 93041[1], 93042[1], 93318[1], 93355[1], 94002[1], 94200[1], 94250[1], 94680[1], 94681[1], 94690[1], 94770[1], 95812[1], 95813[1], 95816[1], 95819[1], 95822[0], 95829[1], 95860[0], 95861[0], 95863[0], 95864[0], 95865[0], 95866[0], 95867[0], 95868[0], 95869[0], 95870[0], 95907[0], 95908[0], 95909[0], 95910[0], 95911[0], 95912[0], 95913[0], 95925[0], 95926[0], 95927[0], 95928[0], 95929[0], 95930[0], 95933[0], 95937[0], 95938[0], 95939[0], 95940[0], 95955[1], 96360[1], 96361[1], 96365[1], 96366[1], 96367[1], 96368[1], 96372[1], 96374[1], 96375[1], 96376[1], 96377[1], 99155[0], 99156[0], 99157[0], 99211[1], 99212[1], 99213[1], 99214[1], 99215[1], 99217[1], 99218[1], 99219[1], 99220[1], 99221[1], 99222[1], 99223[1], 99231[1], 99232[1], 99233[1], 99234[1], 99235[1], 99236[1], 99238[1], 99239[1], 99241[1], 99242[1], 99243[1], 99244[1], 99245[1], 99251[1], 99252[1], 99253[1], 99254[1], 99255[1], 99291[1], 99292[1], 99304[1], 99305[1], 99306[1], 99307[1], 99308[1], 99309[1], 99310[1], 99315[1], 99316[1], 99334[1], 99335[1], 99336[1], 99337[1], 99347[1], 99348[1], 99349[1], 99350[1], 99374[1], 99375[1], 99377[1], 99378[1], 99446[0], 99447[0], 99448[0], 99449[0], 99451[0], 99452[0], 99495[0], 99496[0], G0453[0], G0463[1], G0471[1], J0670[1], J2001[1]
64642	0213T[0], 0216T[0], 0228T[0], 0230T[0], 0333T[0], 0440T[1], 0441T[1], 0464T[0], 12001[1], 12002[1], 12004[1], 12005[1], 12006[1], 12007[1], 12011[1], 12013[1], 12014[1], 12015[1], 12016[1], 12017[1], 12018[1], 12020[1], 12021[1], 12031[1], 12032[1], 12034[1], 12035[1], 12036[1], 12037[1], 12041[1], 12042[1], 12044[1], 12045[1], 12046[1], 12047[1], 12051[1], 12052[1], 12053[1], 12054[1], 12055[1], 12056[1], 12057[1], 13100[1], 13101[1], 13102[1], 13120[1], 13121[1], 13122[1], 13131[1], 13132[1], 13133[1], 13151[1], 13152[1], 13153[1], 20550[1], 20551[1], 20552[1], 20553[1], 36000[1], 36400[1], 36405[1], 36406[1], 36410[1], 36420[1], 36425[1], 36430[1], 36440[1], 36591[0], 36592[0], 36600[1], 36640[1], 43752[1], 51701[1], 51702[1], 51703[1], 62320[0], 62321[0], 62322[0], 62323[0], 62324[0], 62325[0], 62326[0], 62327[0], 64400[0], 64402[0], 64405[0], 64408[0], 64410[0], 64413[0], 64415[0], 64416[0], 64417[0], 64418[0], 64420[0], 64421[0], 64425[0], 64430[0], 64435[0], 64445[0], 64446[0], 64447[0], 64448[0], 64449[0], 64450[0], 64461[0], 64462[0], 64463[0], 64479[0], 64480[0], 64483[0], 64484[0], 64486[0], 64487[0], 64488[0], 64489[0], 64490[0], 64491[0], 64492[0], 64493[0], 64494[0], 64495[0], 64505[0], 64510[0], 64517[0], 64520[0], 64530[0], 69990[0], 92012[1], 92014[1], 93000[1], 93005[1], 93010[1], 93040[1], 93041[1], 93042[1], 93318[1], 93355[1], 94002[1], 94200[1], 94250[1], 94680[1], 94681[1], 94690[1], 94770[1], 95812[1], 95813[1], 95816[1], 95819[1], 95829[1], 95930[0], 95933[0], 95937[0], 95940[0], 95941[0], 95955[1], 96360[1], 96361[1], 96365[1], 96366[1], 96367[1], 96368[1], 96372[1], 96374[1], 96375[1], 96376[1], 96377[1], 99155[0], 99156[0], 99157[0], 99211[1], 99212[1], 99213[1], 99214[1], 99215[1], 99217[1], 99218[1], 99219[1], 99220[1], 99221[1], 99222[1], 99223[1], 99231[1], 99232[1], 99233[1], 99234[1], 99235[1], 99236[1], 99238[1], 99239[1], 99241[1], 99242[1], 99243[1], 99244[1], 99245[1], 99251[1], 99252[1], 99253[1], 99254[1], 99255[1], 99291[1], 99292[1], 99304[1], 99305[1], 99306[1], 99307[1], 99308[1], 99309[1], 99310[1], 99315[1], 99316[1], 99334[1], 99335[1], 99336[1], 99337[1], 99347[1], 99348[1], 99349[1], 99350[1], 99374[1], 99375[1], 99377[1], 99378[1], 99446[0], 99447[0], 99448[0], 99449[0], 99451[0], 99452[0], G0453[0], G0463[1], G0471[1]
64643	0213T[0], 0216T[0], 0228T[0], 0230T[0], 0333T[0], 0440T[1], 0441T[1], 0464T[0], 12001[1], 12002[1], 12004[1], 12005[1], 12006[1], 12007[1], 12011[1], 12013[1], 12014[1], 12015[1], 12016[1], 12017[1], 12018[1], 12020[1], 12021[1], 12031[1], 12032[1], 12034[1], 12035[1], 12036[1], 12037[1], 12041[1], 12042[1], 12044[1], 12045[1], 12046[1], 12047[1], 12051[1], 12052[1], 12053[1], 12054[1], 12055[1], 12056[1], 12057[1], 13100[1], 13101[1], 13102[1], 13120[1], 13121[1], 13122[1], 13131[1], 13132[1], 13133[1], 13151[1], 13152[1], 13153[1], 20550[1], 20551[1], 20552[1], 20553[1], 36000[1], 36400[1], 36405[1], 36406[1], 36410[1], 36420[1], 36425[1], 36430[1], 36440[1], 36591[0], 36592[0], 36600[1], 36640[1], 43752[1], 51701[1], 51702[1], 51703[1], 61650[1], 62320[1], 62321[1], 62322[1], 62323[1], 62324[1], 62325[1], 62326[1], 62327[1], 64400[1], 64402[1], 64405[1], 64408[1], 64410[1], 64413[1], 64415[1], 64416[1], 64417[1], 64418[1], 64420[1], 64421[1], 64425[1], 64430[1], 64435[1], 64445[1], 64446[1], 64447[1], 64448[1], 64449[1], 64450[1], 64461[1], 64463[1], 64479[1], 64483[1], 64486[1], 64487[1], 64488[1], 64489[1], 64490[1], 64493[1], 64505[1], 64510[1], 64517[1], 64520[1], 64530[1], 69990[0], 93000[1], 93005[1], 93010[1], 93040[1], 93041[1], 93042[1], 93318[1], 93355[1], 94002[1], 94200[1], 94250[1], 94680[1], 94681[1], 94690[1], 94770[1], 95812[1], 95813[1], 95816[1], 95819[1], 95829[1], 95930[0], 95933[0], 95937[0], 95940[0], 95941[0], 95955[1], 96360[1], 96365[1], 96372[1], 96374[1], 96375[1], 96376[1], 96377[1], 99155[0], 99156[0], 99157[0], 99211[1], 99212[1], 99213[1], 99214[1], 99215[1], 99217[1], 99218[1], 99219[1], 99220[1], 99221[1], 99222[1], 99223[1], 99231[1], 99232[1], 99233[1], 99234[1], 99235[1], 99236[1], 99238[1], 99239[1], 99241[1], 99242[1], 99243[1], 99244[1], 99245[1], 99251[1], 99252[1], 99253[1], 99254[1], 99255[1], 99291[1], 99292[1], 99304[1], 99305[1], 99306[1], 99307[1], 99308[1], 99309[1], 99310[1], 99315[1], 99316[1], 99334[1], 99335[1], 99336[1], 99337[1], 99347[1], 99348[1], 99349[1], 99350[1], 99374[1], 99375[1], 99377[1], 99378[1], 99446[0], 99447[0], 99448[0], 99449[0], 99451[0], 99452[0], G0453[0], G0463[1], G0471[1]
64644	0213T[0], 0216T[0], 0228T[0], 0230T[0], 0333T[0], 0440T[1], 0441T[1], 0464T[0], 12001[1], 12002[1], 12004[1], 12005[1], 12006[1], 12007[1], 12011[1], 12013[1], 12014[1], 12015[1], 12016[1], 12017[1], 12018[1], 12020[1], 12021[1], 12031[1], 12032[1], 12034[1], 12035[1], 12036[1], 12037[1], 12041[1], 12042[1], 12044[1], 12045[1], 12046[1], 12047[1], 12051[1], 12052[1], 12053[1], 12054[1], 12055[1], 12056[1], 12057[1], 13100[1], 13101[1], 13102[1], 13120[1], 13121[1], 13122[1], 13131[1], 13132[1], 13133[1], 13151[1], 13152[1], 13153[1], 20550[1], 20551[1], 20552[1], 20553[1], 36000[1], 36400[1], 36405[1], 36406[1], 36410[1], 36420[1], 36425[1], 36430[1], 36440[1], 36591[0], 36592[0], 36600[1], 36640[1], 43752[1], 51701[1], 51702[1], 51703[1], 62320[0], 62321[0], 62322[0], 62323[0], 62324[0], 62325[0], 62326[0], 62327[0], 64400[0], 64402[0], 64405[0], 64408[0], 64410[0], 64413[0], 64415[0], 64416[0], 64417[0], 64418[0], 64420[0], 64421[0], 64425[0], 64430[0], 64435[0], 64445[0], 64446[0], 64447[0], 64448[0], 64449[0], 64450[0], 64461[0], 64462[0], 64463[0], 64479[0], 64480[0], 64483[0], 64484[0], 64486[0], 64487[0], 64488[0], 64489[0], 64490[0], 64491[0], 64492[0], 64493[0], 64494[0], 64495[0], 64505[0], 64510[0], 64517[0], 64520[0], 64530[0], 64642[0], 69990[0], 92012[1], 92014[1], 93000[1], 93005[1], 93010[1], 93040[1], 93041[1], 93042[1], 93318[1], 93355[1], 94002[1], 94200[1], 94250[1], 94680[1], 94681[1], 94690[1], 94770[1], 95812[1], 95813[1], 95816[1], 95819[1], 95829[1], 95930[0], 95933[0], 95937[0], 95940[0], 95941[0], 95955[1], 96360[1], 96361[1], 96365[1], 96366[1], 96367[1], 96368[1], 96372[1], 96374[1], 96375[1], 96376[1], 96377[1], 99155[0], 99156[0], 99157[0], 99211[1], 99212[1], 99213[1], 99214[1], 99215[1], 99217[1], 99218[1], 99219[1], 99220[1], 99221[1], 99222[1], 99223[1], 99231[1], 99232[1], 99233[1], 99234[1], 99235[1], 99236[1], 99238[1], 99239[1], 99241[1], 99242[1], 99243[1], 99244[1], 99245[1], 99251[1], 99252[1], 99253[1], 99254[1], 99255[1], 99291[1], 99292[1], 99304[1], 99305[1], 99306[1], 99307[1], 99308[1], 99309[1], 99310[1], 99315[1], 99316[1], 99334[1], 99335[1], 99336[1], 99337[1], 99347[1], 99348[1], 99349[1], 99350[1], 99374[1], 99375[1], 99377[1], 99378[1], 99446[0], 99447[0], 99448[0], 99449[0], 99451[0], 99452[0], G0453[0], G0463[1], G0471[1]
64645	0213T[0], 0216T[0], 0228T[0], 0230T[0], 0333T[0], 0440T[1], 0441T[1], 0464T[0], 12001[1], 12002[1], 12004[1], 12005[1], 12006[1], 12007[1], 12011[1], 12013[1], 12014[1], 12015[1], 12016[1], 12017[1], 12018[1], 12020[1], 12021[1], 12031[1], 12032[1], 12034[1], 12035[1], 12036[1], 12037[1], 12041[1], 12042[1], 12044[1], 12045[1], 12046[1], 12047[1], 12051[1], 12052[1], 12053[1], 12054[1], 12055[1], 12056[1], 12057[1], 13100[1], 13101[1], 13102[1], 13120[1], 13121[1], 13122[1], 13131[1], 13132[1], 13133[1], 13151[1], 13152[1], 13153[1], 20550[1], 20551[1], 20552[1], 20553[1], 36000[1], 36400[1], 36405[1], 36406[1], 36410[1], 36420[1], 36425[1], 36430[1], 36440[1], 36591[0], 36592[0], 36600[1], 36640[1], 43752[1], 51701[1], 51702[1], 51703[1], 61650[1], 62320[1], 62321[1], 62322[1], 62323[1], 62324[1], 62325[1], 62326[1], 62327[1], 64400[1], 64402[1], 64405[1], 64408[1], 64410[1], 64413[1], 64415[1], 64416[1], 64417[1], 64418[1], 64420[1], 64421[1], 64425[1], 64430[1], 64435[1], 64445[1], 64446[1], 64447[1], 64448[1], 64449[1], 64450[1], 64461[1], 64463[1], 64479[1], 64483[1], 64486[1], 64487[1], 64488[1], 64489[1], 64490[1], 64493[1], 64505[1], 64510[1], 64517[1], 64520[1], 64530[1], 69990[0], 93000[1], 93005[1], 93010[1], 93040[1], 93041[1], 93042[1], 93318[1], 93355[1], 94002[1], 94200[1], 94250[1], 94680[1], 94681[1], 94690[1], 94770[1], 95812[1], 95813[1], 95816[1], 95819[1], 95829[1], 95930[0], 95933[0], 95937[0], 95940[0], 95941[0], 95955[1], 96360[1], 96365[1], 96372[1], 96374[1], 96375[1], 96376[1], 96377[1], 99155[0], 99156[0], 99157[0], 99211[1], 99212[1], 99213[1], 99214[1], 99215[1], 99217[1], 99218[1], 99219[1], 99220[1], 99221[1], 99222[1], 99223[1], 99231[1], 99232[1], 99233[1], 99234[1], 99235[1], 99236[1], 99238[1], 99239[1], 99241[1], 99242[1], 99243[1], 99244[1], 99245[1], 99251[1], 99252[1], 99253[1], 99254[1], 99255[1], 99291[1], 99292[1], 99304[1], 99305[1], 99306[1], 99307[1], 99308[1], 99309[1], 99310[1], 99315[1], 99316[1], 99334[1], 99335[1],

0 = Modifier usage not allowed or inappropriate 1 = Modifier usage allowed

CPT © 2018 American Medical Association. All Rights Reserved.

Code 1	Code 2
	99336[1], 99337[1], 99347[1], 99348[1], 99349[1], 99350[1], 99374[1], 99375[1], 99377[1], 99378[1], 99446[0], 99447[0], 99448[0], 99449[0], 99451[0], 99452[0], G0453[0], G0463[1], G0471[1]
64646	0213T[0], 0216T[0], 0228T[0], 0230T[0], 0333T[0], 0442T[1], 0464T[0], 12001[1], 12002[1], 12004[1], 12005[1], 12006[1], 12007[1], 12011[1], 12013[1], 12014[1], 12015[1], 12016[1], 12017[1], 12018[1], 12020[1], 12021[1], 12031[1], 12032[1], 12034[1], 12035[1], 12036[1], 12037[1], 12041[1], 12042[1], 12044[1], 12045[1], 12046[1], 12047[1], 12051[1], 12052[1], 12053[1], 12054[1], 12055[1], 12056[1], 12057[1], 13100[1], 13101[1], 13102[1], 13120[1], 13121[1], 13122[1], 13131[1], 13132[1], 13133[1], 13151[1], 13152[1], 13153[1], 20550[1], 20551[1], 20552[1], 20553[1], 36000[1], 36400[1], 36405[1], 36406[1], 36410[1], 36420[1], 36425[1], 36430[1], 36440[1], 36591[0], 36592[0], 36600[1], 36640[1], 43752[1], 51701[1], 51702[1], 51703[1], 62320[0], 62321[0], 62322[0], 62323[0], 62324[0], 62325[0], 62326[0], 62327[0], 64400[0], 64402[0], 64405[0], 64408[0], 64410[0], 64413[0], 64415[0], 64416[0], 64417[0], 64418[0], 64420[0], 64421[0], 64425[0], 64430[0], 64435[0], 64445[0], 64446[0], 64447[0], 64448[0], 64449[0], 64450[0], 64461[0], 64462[0], 64463[0], 64479[0], 64480[0], 64483[0], 64484[0], 64486[0], 64487[0], 64488[0], 64489[0], 64490[0], 64491[0], 64492[0], 64493[0], 64494[0], 64495[0], 64505[0], 64510[0], 64517[0], 64520[0], 64530[0], 69990[0], 92012[1], 92014[1], 93000[1], 93005[1], 93010[1], 93040[1], 93041[1], 93042[1], 93318[1], 93355[1], 94002[1], 94200[1], 94250[1], 94680[1], 94681[1], 94690[1], 94770[1], 95812[1], 95813[1], 95816[1], 95819[1], 95829[1], 95930[0], 95933[0], 95937[0], 95940[0], 95941[0], 95955[1], 96360[1], 96361[1], 96365[1], 96366[1], 96367[1], 96368[1], 96372[1], 96374[1], 96375[1], 96376[1], 96377[1], 99155[0], 99156[0], 99157[0], 99211[1], 99212[1], 99213[1], 99214[1], 99215[1], 99217[1], 99218[1], 99219[1], 99220[1], 99221[1], 99222[1], 99223[1], 99231[1], 99232[1], 99233[1], 99234[1], 99235[1], 99236[1], 99238[1], 99239[1], 99241[1], 99242[1], 99243[1], 99244[1], 99245[1], 99251[1], 99252[1], 99253[1], 99254[1], 99255[1], 99291[1], 99292[1], 99304[1], 99305[1], 99306[1], 99307[1], 99308[1], 99309[1], 99310[1], 99315[1], 99316[1], 99334[1], 99335[1], 99336[1], 99337[1], 99347[1], 99348[1], 99349[1], 99350[1], 99374[1], 99375[1], 99377[1], 99378[1], 99446[0], 99447[0], 99448[0], 99449[0], 99451[0], 99452[0], G0453[0], G0463[1], G0471[1]
64647	0213T[0], 0216T[0], 0228T[0], 0230T[0], 0333T[0], 0442T[1], 0464T[0], 12001[1], 12002[1], 12004[1], 12005[1], 12006[1], 12007[1], 12011[1], 12013[1], 12014[1], 12015[1], 12016[1], 12017[1], 12018[1], 12020[1], 12021[1], 12031[1], 12032[1], 12034[1], 12035[1], 12036[1], 12037[1], 12041[1], 12042[1], 12044[1], 12045[1], 12046[1], 12047[1], 12051[1], 12052[1], 12053[1], 12054[1], 12055[1], 12056[1], 12057[1], 13100[1], 13101[1], 13102[1], 13120[1], 13121[1], 13122[1], 13131[1], 13132[1], 13133[1], 13151[1], 13152[1], 13153[1], 20550[1], 20551[1], 20552[1], 20553[1], 36000[1], 36400[1], 36405[1], 36406[1], 36410[1], 36420[1], 36425[1], 36430[1], 36440[1], 36591[0], 36592[0], 36600[1], 36640[1], 43752[1], 51701[1], 51702[1], 51703[1], 62320[0], 62321[0], 62322[0], 62323[0], 62324[0], 62325[0], 62326[0], 62327[0], 64400[0], 64402[0], 64405[0], 64408[0], 64410[0], 64413[0], 64415[0], 64416[0], 64417[0], 64418[0], 64420[0], 64421[0], 64425[0], 64430[0], 64435[0], 64445[0], 64446[0], 64447[0], 64448[0], 64449[0], 64450[0], 64461[0], 64462[0], 64463[0], 64479[0], 64480[0], 64483[0], 64484[0], 64486[0], 64487[0], 64488[0], 64489[0], 64490[0], 64491[0], 64492[0], 64493[0], 64494[0], 64495[0], 64505[0], 64510[0], 64517[0], 64520[0], 64530[0], 64615[1], 64646[0], 69990[0], 92012[1], 92014[1], 93000[1], 93005[1], 93010[1], 93040[1], 93041[1], 93042[1], 93318[1], 93355[1], 94002[1], 94200[1], 94250[1], 94680[1], 94681[1], 94690[1], 94770[1], 95812[1], 95813[1], 95816[1], 95819[1], 95829[1], 95930[0], 95933[0], 95937[0], 95940[0], 95941[0], 95955[1], 96360[1], 96361[1], 96365[1], 96366[1], 96367[1], 96368[1], 96372[1], 96374[1], 96375[1], 96376[1], 96377[1], 99155[0], 99156[0], 99157[0], 99211[1], 99212[1], 99213[1], 99214[1], 99215[1], 99217[1], 99218[1], 99219[1], 99220[1], 99221[1], 99222[1], 99223[1], 99231[1], 99232[1], 99233[1], 99234[1], 99235[1], 99236[1], 99238[1], 99239[1], 99241[1], 99242[1], 99243[1], 99244[1], 99245[1], 99251[1], 99252[1], 99253[1], 99254[1], 99255[1], 99291[1], 99292[1], 99304[1], 99305[1], 99306[1], 99307[1], 99308[1], 99309[1], 99310[1], 99315[1], 99316[1], 99334[1], 99335[1], 99336[1], 99337[1], 99347[1], 99348[1], 99349[1], 99350[1], 99374[1], 99375[1], 99377[1], 99378[1], 99446[0], 99447[0], 99448[0], 99449[0], 99451[0], 99452[0], G0453[0], G0463[1], G0471[1]
64680	0213T[0], 0228T[0], 0230T[0], 0333T[0], 0464T[0], 12001[1], 12002[1], 12004[1], 12005[1], 12006[1], 12007[1], 12011[1], 12013[1], 12014[1], 12015[1], 12016[1], 12017[1], 12018[1], 12020[1], 12021[1], 12031[1], 12032[1], 12034[1], 12035[1], 12036[1], 12037[1], 12041[1], 12042[1], 12044[1], 12045[1], 12046[1], 12047[1], 12051[1], 12052[1], 12053[1], 12054[1], 12055[1], 12056[1], 12057[1], 13100[1], 13101[1], 13102[1], 13120[1], 13121[1], 13122[1], 13131[1], 13132[1], 13133[1], 13151[1], 13152[1], 13153[1], 20550[1], 20551[1], 20552[1], 20553[1], 36000[1], 36400[1], 36405[1], 36406[1], 36410[1], 36420[1], 36425[1], 36430[1], 36440[1], 36591[0], 36592[0], 36600[1], 36640[1], 43752[1], 51701[1], 51702[1], 51703[1], 62322[1], 62323[1], 62326[1], 62327[1], 64400[1], 64402[1], 64405[1], 64408[1], 64410[1], 64413[1], 64418[1], 64420[1], 64421[1], 64425[1], 64430[1], 64435[1], 64445[1], 64446[1], 64447[1], 64448[1], 64449[1], 64450[1], 64461[0], 64462[0], 64463[0], 64479[1], 64480[0], 64483[1], 64484[0], 64486[0], 64487[0], 64488[0], 64489[0], 64490[1], 64491[0], 64492[0], 64505[1], 64510[1], 64517[1], 64520[1], 64530[1], 69990[0], 76000[1], 77001[1], 77002[1], 77003[1], 92012[1], 92014[1], 92585[0], 93000[1], 93005[1], 93010[1], 93040[1], 93041[1], 93042[1], 93318[1], 93355[1], 94002[1], 94200[1], 94250[1], 94680[1], 94681[1], 94690[1], 94770[1], 95812[1], 95813[1], 95816[1], 95819[1], 95822[0], 95829[1], 95860[0], 95861[0], 95863[0], 95864[0], 95865[0], 95866[0], 95867[0], 95868[0], 95869[0], 95870[0], 95907[0], 95908[0], 95909[0], 95910[0], 95911[0], 95912[0], 95913[0], 95925[0], 95926[0], 95927[0], 95928[0], 95929[0], 95930[0], 95933[0], 95937[0], 95938[0], 95939[0], 95940[0], 95955[1], 96360[1], 96361[1], 96365[1], 96366[1], 96367[1], 96368[1], 96372[1], 96374[1], 96375[1], 96376[1], 96377[1], 99155[0], 99156[0], 99157[0], 99211[1], 99212[1], 99213[1], 99214[1], 99215[1], 99217[1], 99218[1], 99219[1], 99220[1], 99221[1], 99222[1], 99223[1], 99231[1], 99232[1], 99233[1], 99234[1], 99235[1], 99236[1], 99238[1], 99239[1], 99241[1], 99242[1], 99243[1], 99244[1], 99245[1], 99251[1], 99252[1], 99253[1], 99254[1], 99255[1], 99291[1], 99292[1], 99304[1], 99305[1], 99306[1], 99307[1], 99308[1], 99309[1], 99310[1], 99315[1], 99316[1], 99334[1], 99335[1], 99336[1], 99337[1], 99347[1], 99348[1], 99349[1], 99350[1], 99374[1], 99375[1], 99377[1], 99378[1], 99446[0], 99447[0], 99448[0], 99449[0], 99451[0], 99452[0], 99495[0], 99496[0], G0453[0], G0463[1], G0471[1], J2001[1]
64681	0216T[0], 0228T[0], 0230T[0], 0333T[0], 0464T[0], 12001[1], 12002[1], 12004[1], 12005[1], 12006[1], 12007[1], 12011[1], 12013[1], 12014[1], 12015[1], 12016[1], 12017[1], 12018[1], 12020[1], 12021[1], 12031[1], 12032[1], 12034[1], 12035[1], 12036[1], 12037[1], 12041[1], 12042[1], 12044[1], 12045[1], 12046[1], 12047[1], 12051[1], 12052[1], 12053[1], 12054[1], 12055[1], 12056[1], 12057[1], 13100[1], 13101[1], 13102[1], 13120[1], 13121[1], 13122[1], 13131[1], 13132[1], 13133[1], 13151[1], 13152[1], 13153[1], 20550[1], 20551[1], 20552[1], 20553[1], 36000[1], 36400[1], 36405[1], 36406[1], 36410[1], 36420[1], 36425[1], 36430[1], 36440[1], 36591[0], 36592[0], 36600[1], 36640[1], 43752[1], 51701[1], 51702[1], 51703[1], 62320[1], 62321[1], 62322[1], 62323[1], 62324[1], 62325[1], 62326[1], 62327[1], 64400[1], 64402[1], 64405[1], 64408[1], 64410[1], 64413[1], 64415[1], 64416[1], 64417[1], 64418[1], 64420[1], 64421[1], 64425[1], 64430[1], 64435[1], 64445[1], 64446[1], 64447[1], 64448[1], 64449[1], 64450[1], 64461[0], 64462[0], 64463[0], 64479[1], 64480[0], 64483[1], 64484[0], 64486[0], 64487[0], 64488[0], 64489[0], 64493[1], 64494[0], 64495[0], 64505[1], 64510[1], 64517[1], 64520[1], 64530[1], 69990[0], 76000[1], 77001[1], 77002[1], 77003[1], 92012[1], 92014[1], 92585[0], 93000[1], 93005[1], 93010[1], 93040[1], 93041[1], 93042[1], 93318[1], 93355[1], 94002[1], 94200[1], 94250[1], 94680[1], 94681[1], 94690[1], 94770[1], 95812[1], 95813[1], 95816[1], 95819[1], 95822[0], 95829[1], 95860[0], 95861[0], 95863[0], 95864[0], 95865[0], 95866[0], 95867[0], 95868[0], 95869[0], 95870[0], 95907[0], 95908[0], 95909[0], 95910[0], 95911[0], 95912[0], 95913[0], 95925[0], 95926[0], 95927[0], 95928[0], 95929[0], 95930[0], 95933[0], 95937[0], 95938[0], 95939[0], 95940[0], 95955[1], 96360[1], 96361[1], 96365[1], 96366[1], 96367[1], 96368[1], 96372[1], 96374[1], 96375[1], 96376[1], 96377[1], 99155[0], 99156[0], 99157[0], 99211[1], 99212[1], 99213[1], 99214[1], 99215[1], 99217[1], 99218[1], 99219[1], 99220[1], 99221[1], 99222[1], 99223[1], 99231[1], 99232[1], 99233[1], 99234[1], 99235[1], 99236[1], 99238[1], 99239[1], 99241[1], 99242[1], 99243[1], 99244[1], 99245[1], 99251[1], 99252[1], 99253[1], 99254[1], 99255[1], 99291[1], 99292[1], 99304[1], 99305[1], 99306[1], 99307[1], 99308[1], 99309[1], 99310[1], 99315[1], 99316[1], 99334[1], 99335[1], 99336[1], 99337[1], 99347[1], 99348[1], 99349[1], 99350[1], 99374[1], 99375[1], 99377[1], 99378[1], 99446[0], 99447[0], 99448[0], 99449[0], 99451[0], 99452[0], 99495[0], 99496[0], G0453[0], G0463[1], G0471[1]

0 = Modifier usage not allowed or inappropriate   1 = Modifier usage allowed

CPT © 2018 American Medical Association. All Rights Reserved.

Code 1	Code 2
Q9966	Q9951[0], Q9959[0], Q9964[0], Q9965[1]

0 = Modifier usage not allowed or inappropriate 1 = Modifier usage allowed

CPT © 2017 American Medical Association. All Rights Reserved.

APPENDIX B

Clinical Documentation Checklists

Introduction

Appendix B provides checklists for common diagnoses and other conditions which are designed to be used for review of current records to help identify any documentation deficiencies. The checklists begin with the applicable ICD-10-CM categories, subcategories, and/or codes being covered. Definitions and other information pertinent to coding the condition are then provided. This is followed by a checklist that identifies each element needed for assignment of the most specific code. If one or more of the required elements are not documented, this information should be shared with the physician and a corrective action plan initiated to ensure that the necessary information is captured in the future.

Similar documentation and coding checklists for conditions not addressed in this book can be created using the checklists provided as a template. There are a few different formats and styles of checklists so users can determine which style works best for their practice and then create additional checklists using that format and style.

Burns, Corrosions, and Frostbite

ICD-10-CM Categories

Burns and corrosions are classified in the following ICD-10-CM categories:

T20	Burn and corrosion of head, face and neck
T21	Burn and corrosion of trunk
T22	Burn and corrosion of shoulder and upper limb, except wrist and hand
T23	Burn and corrosion of wrist and hand
T24	Burn and corrosion of lower limb, except ankle and foot
T25	Burn and corrosion of ankle and foot
T26	Burn and corrosion confined to eye and adnexa
T27	Burn and corrosion of respiratory tract
T28	Burn and corrosion of internal organ
T30	Burn and corrosion, body region unspecified
T31	Burns classified according to extent of body surface involved
T33	Superficial frostbite

ICD-10-CM Definitions

Burn – A thermal injury due to a heat source such as fire, a hot appliance, friction, hot objects, hot air, hot water, electricity, lightning, and radiation. Burns due to exposure to the sun are not considered burns in ICD-10-CM.

Corrosion – A thermal injury due to chemicals.

Episode of Care – There are three (3) possible 7th character values for burns and corrosions. The 7th character defines the stage of treatment and residual effects related to the initial injury.

A **Initial encounter.** The period when the patient is receiving active treatment for the injury, poisoning, or other consequences of an external cause. An 'A' may be assigned on more than one claim.

D **Subsequent encounter.** Encounter after the active phase of treatment and when the patient is receiving routine care for the injury during the period of healing or recovery.

S **Sequela.** Encounter for complications or conditions that arise as a direct result of an injury.

Extent of body surface – The amount of body surface burned is governed by the rule of nines. These percentages may be modified for infants and children or adults with large buttocks, thighs, and abdomens when those regions are burned.

Head and neck – 9%

Each arm – 9%

Each leg – 18%

Anterior trunk – 18%

Posterior trunk – 18%

Genitalia – 1%

Levels of Burns:

First Degree – Affects only the epidermis causing pain, redness, and swelling.

Second Degree – Affects both the dermis and epidermis causing pain, redness, white or blotchy skin, and swelling. Blistering may occur and pain can be intense. Scarring can develop.

Third Degree – Affects the fat or subcutaneous layer of the skin. The skin will appear white or charred black or may look leathery. Third degree burns can destroy nerves resulting in numbness.

Note: Burns noted as non-healing are coded as acute burns and necrosis of burned skin should be coded as a non-healing burn.

Checklist

1. Identify the type of thermal injury:
   - ☐ Burn
   - ☐ Corrosion
   - ☐ Frostbite (Proceed to #9)
2. Identify the body region:
   - ☐ Eye
   - ☐ Internal organs
   - ☐ Skin (external body surface)
   - ☐ Multiple areas
   - ☐ Unspecified body region

Note: Codes from category T30 Burn and corrosion, body region unspecified, is extremely vague and should rarely be used.

3. Identify the body area
   - ☐ Eye and adnexa
     - ☐ Eyelid and periocular area
     - ☐ Cornea and conjunctival sac
     - ☐ With resulting rupture and destruction of eyeball
     - ☐ Unspecified site – review medical record/query physician
   - ☐ External body surface
     - ☐ Head, face and neck
       - ☐ Scalp
       - ☐ Forehead and cheek
       - ☐ Ear
       - ☐ Nose
       - ☐ Lips
       - ☐ Chin
       - ☐ Neck
       - ☐ Multiple sites of head, face, and neck
       - ☐ Unspecified site – review medical record/query physician
       - ☐ Trunk
         - ☐ Chest wall
         - ☐ Abdominal wall
       - ☐ Upper back
       - ☐ Lower back
       - ☐ Buttocks
       - ☐ Genital region
         - ☐ Female

- ☐ Male
- ☐ Other site
- ☐ Unspecified site – review medical record/query physician

- ☐ Shoulder and upper limb (excluding wrist and hand)
  - ☐ Scapula
  - ☐ Shoulder
  - ☐ Axilla
  - ☐ Upper arm
  - ☐ Elbow
  - ☐ Forearm
  - ☐ Multiple sites shoulder and upper limb (excluding wrist and hand)
  - ☐ Unspecified site – review medical record/query physician
- ☐ Wrist and hand
  - ☐ Wrist
  - ☐ Hand
    - ☐ Back of hand
    - ☐ Palm
    - ☐ Finger
      - ☐ Multiple fingers not including thumb
      - ☐ Multiple fingers including thumb
      - ☐ Single except thumb
      - ☐ Thumb
      - ☐ Unspecified site hand – review medical record/query physician
    - ☐ Multiple sites of wrist and hand
- ☐ Lower limb except ankle and foot
  - ☐ Thigh
  - ☐ Knee
  - ☐ Lower leg
  - ☐ Multiple sites of lower limb
  - ☐ Unspecified site lower limb – review medical record/query physician
- ☐ Ankle and foot
  - ☐ Ankle
  - ☐ Foot
  - ☐ Toe(s)
  - ☐ Multiple sites of ankle and foot
  - ☐ Unspecified site ankle or foot – review medical record/query physician

- ☐ Internal Organs
  - ☐ Ear drum
  - ☐ Esophagus
  - ☐ Genitourinary organs, internal
  - ☐ Mouth and pharynx
  - ☐ Other parts of alimentary tract
  - ☐ Respiratory tract
    - ☐ Larynx and trachea
    - ☐ Larynx and trachea with lung
    - ☐ Other parts of respiratory tract (thoracic cavity)
    - ☐ Unspecified site respiratory tract- review medical record/query physician
  - ☐ Other internal organ
  - ☐ Unspecified internal organ

4. Identify degree of burn:
   - ☐ First degree
   - ☐ Second degree
   - ☐ Third degree
   - ☐ Unspecified degree – review medical record/query physician
5. Identify laterality:
   - ☐ Left
   - ☐ Right
   - ☐ Unspecified – review medical record/query physician

Note: Laterality only applies to burns and corrosions involving the extremities, ears, and eyes.

6. Identify episode of care/stage of healing/complication
   - ☐ A Initial encounter
   - ☐ D Subsequent encounter
   - ☐ S Sequela
7. Identify extent of body surface involved and percent of third degree burns, if over 10% of body surface:
   - ☐ Less than 10% of body surface
   - ☐ 10-19% of body surface
     - ☐ 0% to 9% of third degree burns
     - ☐ 10-19% of third degree burns
   - ☐ 20-29% of body surface
     - ☐ 0% to 9% of third degree burns
     - ☐ 10-19% of third degree burns
     - ☐ 20-29% of third degree burns
   - ☐ 30-39% of body surface
     - ☐ 0% to 9% of third degree burns
     - ☐ 10-19% of third degree burns
     - ☐ 20-29% of third degree burns
     - ☐ 30-39% of third degree burns
   - ☐ 40-49% of body surface
     - ☐ 0% to 9% of third degree burns
     - ☐ 10-19% of third degree burns
     - ☐ 20-29% of third degree burns
     - ☐ 30-39% of third degree burns
     - ☐ 40-49% of third degree burns
   - ☐ 50-59% of body surface
     - ☐ 0% to 9% of third degree burns
     - ☐ 10-19% of third degree burns
     - ☐ 20-29% of third degree burns
     - ☐ 30-39% of third degree burns
     - ☐ 40-49% of third degree burns
     - ☐ 50-59% of third degree burns
   - ☐ 60-69% of body surface
     - ☐ 0% to 9% of third degree burns
     - ☐ 10-19% of third degree burns
     - ☐ 20-29% of third degree burns
     - ☐ 30-39% of third degree burns
     - ☐ 40-49% of third degree burns
     - ☐ 50-59% of third degree burns

- ☐ 6Ø-69% of third degree burns
- ☐ 7Ø-79% of body surface
  - ☐ Ø% to 9% of third degree burns
  - ☐ 1Ø-19% of third degree burns
  - ☐ 2Ø-29% of third degree burns
  - ☐ 3Ø-39% of third degree burns
  - ☐ 4Ø-49% of third degree burns
  - ☐ 5Ø-59% of third degree burns
  - ☐ 6Ø-69% of third degree burns
  - ☐ 7Ø-79% of third degree burns
- ☐ 8Ø-89% of body surface
  - ☐ Ø% to 9% of third degree burns
  - ☐ 1Ø-19% of third degree burns
  - ☐ 2Ø-29% of third degree burns
  - ☐ 3Ø-39% of third degree burns
  - ☐ 4Ø-49% of third degree burns
  - ☐ 5Ø-59% of third degree burns
  - ☐ 6Ø-69% of third degree burns
  - ☐ 7Ø-79% of third degree burns
  - ☐ 8Ø-89% of third degree burns
- ☐ 9Ø% or more of body surface
  - ☐ Ø% to 9% of third degree burns
  - ☐ 1Ø-19% of third degree burns
  - ☐ 2Ø-29% of third degree burns
  - ☐ 3Ø-39% of third degree burns
  - ☐ 4Ø-49% of third degree burns
  - ☐ 5Ø-59% of third degree burns
  - ☐ 6Ø-69% of third degree burns
  - ☐ 7Ø-79% third degree burns
  - ☐ 8Ø-89% third degree burns
  - ☐ 9Ø% or more third degree burns

Note: Extent of body surface is to be coded as a supplementary code for burns of an external body surface when the site is specified. It should only be used as the primary code when the site of the burn is unspecified.

8. Identify the external cause source/chemical agent, intent and place:
   - ☐ If burn, identify the source and intent XØØ-X19, X75-X77, X96-X98
   - ☐ If corrosion, code first the chemical agent and intent (T51-T65)
   - ☐ Place Y92
9. For frostbite, identify extent of tissue involvement:
   - ☐ Superficial
   - ☐ With tissue necrosis
10. For frostbite, identify body area:
    - ☐ Head
      - ☐ Ear
      - ☐ Nose
      - ☐ Other part of head
    - ☐ Neck
    - ☐ Thorax
    - ☐ Abdominal wall, lower back and pelvis
    - ☐ Arm
    - ☐ Wrist, hand, and fingers
      - ☐ Wrist
      - ☐ Hand
      - ☐ Finger(s)
    - ☐ Hip and thigh
    - ☐ Knee and lower leg
    - ☐ Ankle, foot, and toes
      - ☐ Ankle
      - ☐ Foot
      - ☐ Toe(s)
    - ☐ Other sites
    - ☐ Unspecified site
11. Identify laterality (excluding nose, neck, thorax, abdominal wall, lower back and pelvis):
    - ☐ Left
    - ☐ Right
    - ☐ Unspecified – review medical record/query physician
12. For sequencing of multiple burns and/or burns with related conditions:
    - Multiple external burns only. When more than one external burn is present, the first listed diagnosis code is the code that reflects the highest degree burn
    - Internal and external burns. The circumstances of the admission or encounter govern the selection of the principle or first-listed diagnosis
    - Burn injuries and other related conditions such as smoke inhalation or respiratory failure. The circumstances of the admission or encounter govern the selection of the principal or first-listed diagnosis.
    - Assign separate codes for each burn site
    - Classify burns of the same local site (three-digit category level) but of different degrees to the subcategory identifying the highest degree recorded in the diagnosis.

Diabetes Mellitus

ICD-10-CM Categories

E08	Diabetes mellitus due to underlying condition
E09	Drug or chemical induced diabetes mellitus
E10	Type 1 diabetes mellitus
E11	Type 2 diabetes mellitus
E13	Other specified diabetes mellitus

ICD-10-CM Definitions

Codes for diabetes mellitus are combination codes that reflect the type of diabetes, the body system affected, and any specific complications/manifestations affecting that body system.

Other specified diabetes (E13) includes secondary diabetes specified as:

- Due to genetic defects of beta-cell function
- Due to genetic defects in insulin action
- Postpancreatectomy
- Postprocedural
- Secondary diabetes not elsewhere classified

Checklist

1. Identify the type of diabetes mellitus:
   - ☐ Type 1
   - ☐ Type 2 (includes unspecified)
   - ☐ Secondary diabetes
     - ☐ Drug or chemical induced
     - ☐ Due to underlying condition
     - ☐ Other specified diabetes mellitus
2. Identify the body system affected and any manifestations/ complications:
   - ☐ No complications
   - ☐ Arthropathy
     - ☐ Neuropathic
     - ☐ Other arthropathy
   - ☐ Circulatory complications
     - ☐ Peripheral angiopathy
       - ☐ With gangrene
       - ☐ Without gangrene
     - ☐ Other circulatory complication
   - ☐ Hyperglycemia
   - ☐ Hyperosmolarity (except type 1)
     - ☐ With coma
     - ☐ Without coma
   - ☐ Hypoglycemia
     - ☐ With coma
     - ☐ Without coma
   - ☐ Ketoacidosis
     - ☐ With coma
     - ☐ Without coma
   - ☐ Kidney complications
     - ☐ Nephropathy
     - ☐ Chronic kidney disease – Use additional code (N18.1-N18.6) for stage of CKD
     - ☐ Other diabetic kidney complication
   - ☐ Neurological complications
     - ☐ Amyotrophy
     - ☐ Autonomic (poly)neuropathy
     - ☐ Mononeuropathy
     - ☐ Polyneuropathy
     - ☐ Other diabetic neurological complication
     - ☐ Unspecified diabetic neuropathy
   - ☐ Ophthalmic complications
     - ☐ Diabetic retinopathy
       - ☐ Mild nonproliferative
         - ☐ With macular edema
         - ☐ Without macular edema
       - ☐ Moderate nonproliferative
         - ☐ With macular edema
         - ☐ Without macular edema
       - ☐ Severe nonproliferative
         - ☐ With macular edema
         - ☐ Without macular edema
       - ☐ Proliferative
         - ☐ With traction retinal detachment involving the macula
         - ☐ With traction retinal detachment not involving the macula
         - ☐ With combined traction retinal detachment and rhegmatogenous retinal detachment
         - ☐ With macular edema
         - ☐ Without macular edema
       - ☐ Unspecified
         - ☐ With macular edema
         - ☐ Without macular edema
       - ☐ Identify laterality (*except with diabetic cataract, unspecified diabetic retinopathy, and other diabetic ophthalmic complication*)
         - ☐ Right eye
         - ☐ Left eye
         - ☐ Bilateral
         - ☐ Unspecified eye
     - ☐ Diabetic cataract
     - ☐ Diabetic macular edema, resolved following treatment
     - ☐ Other diabetic ophthalmic complication
   - ☐ Oral complications
     - ☐ Periodontal disease
     - ☐ Other oral complications
   - ☐ Skin complications
     - ☐ Dermatitis
     - ☐ Foot ulcer – Use additional code (L97.4-, L97.5-) to identify site of ulcer

- ☐ Other skin ulcer – Use additional code (L97.1-L97.9, L98.41-L98.49) to identify site of ulcer
- ☐ Other skin complication

☐ Other specified complication – Use additional code to identify complication

☐ Unspecified complication

For Type II (E11) and secondary diabetes types (E08, E09, E13), use additional code to identify any long-term insulin use (Z79.4).

For diabetes due to underlying disease (E08), code first the underlying condition.

For diabetes due to drugs or chemicals (E09):

- Code first poisoning due to drug or toxin (T36-T65 with 5th or 6th character 1-4 or 6) – OR-
- Use additional code for adverse effect, if applicable, to identify drug (T36-T5Ø with 5th or 6th character 5)

For other specified diabetes mellitus (E13) documented as due to pancreatectomy:

- Assign first code E89.1 Postprocedural hypoinsulinemia
- Assign the applicable codes from category E13
- Assign a code from Z9Ø.41- Acquired absence of pancreas
- Use additional code (Z79.4, Z79.84) to identify type of control

Fractures

ICD-10-CM Categories

Fractures are classified according to whether the fracture is a result of trauma or due to overuse or an underlying disease process (nontraumatic).

Nontraumatic fractures are classified in the following ICD-10-CM categories:

M48.4	Fatigue fracture of vertebra
M48.5	Collapsed vertebra, not elsewhere classified
M80	Osteoporosis with current pathological fracture
M84.3	Stress fracture
M84.4	Pathological fracture, not elsewhere classified
M84.5	Pathological fracture in neoplastic disease
M84.6	Pathological fracture in other disease
M84.75	Atypical femoral fracture

Traumatic fractures are classified in the following ICD-10-CM categories:

S02	Fracture of skull and facial bones
S12	Fracture of cervical vertebra and other parts of neck
S22	Fracture of ribs, sternum and thoracic spine
S32	Fracture of lumbar spine and pelvis
S42	Fracture of shoulder and upper arm
S49.0	Physeal fracture of upper end of humerus
S49.1	Physeal fracture of lower end of humerus
S52	Fracture of forearm
S59.0	Physeal fracture of lower end of ulna
S59.1	Physeal fracture of upper end of radius
S59.2	Physeal fracture of lower end of radius
S62	Fracture at wrist and hand level
S72	Fracture of femur
S79.0	Fracture of upper end of femur
S79.1	Fracture of lower end of femur
S82	Fracture of lower leg, including ankle
S89.0	Physeal fracture of upper end of tibia
S89.1	Physeal fracture of lower end of tibia
S89.2	Physeal fracture of upper end of fibula
S89.3	Physeal fracture of lower end of fibula
S92	Fracture of foot and toe, except ankle
S99.0	Physeal fracture of calcaneus
S99.1	Physeal fracture of metatarsal
S99.2	Physeal fracture of phalanx of toe

ICD-10-CM Definitions

Closed – A fracture that does not have contact with the outside environment.

Comminuted – A fracture that has more than two pieces.

Displaced – Bone breaks in two or more parts that are not in normal alignment.

Episode of Care – There are sixteen (16) possible 7th character values to select from for fractures depending upon the fracture category. The 7th character defines the stage of treatment, fracture condition for traumatic fractures (open vs. closed), status of healing and residual effects related to the initial fracture.

A. Initial encounter. The period when the patient is receiving active treatment for the injury, poisoning, or other consequences of an external cause. An 'A' may be assigned on more than one claim.

B. Initial encounter for open fracture or (Gustilo) type I or II.

C. Initial encounter for open fracture (Gustilo) type IIIA, IIIB or IIIC.

D. Subsequent encounter for (closed) fracture with routine healing. Encounter after the active phase of treatment and when the patient is receiving routine care for the fracture during the period of healing or recovery.

E. Subsequent encounter for open fracture (Gustilo) type I or II. Encounter after the active phase of treatment and when the patient is receiving routine care for the fracture during the period of healing or recovery.

F. Subsequent encounter for open fracture (Gustilo) type IIIA, IIIB, IIIC with routine healing. Encounter after the active phase of treatment when the patient is receiving routine care for the fracture during the period of healing or recovery.

G. Subsequent encounter for (closed) fracture with delayed healing.

H. Subsequent encounter for open fracture (Gustilo) type I or II with delayed healing.

J. Subsequent encounter for open fracture (Gustilo) type IIIA, IIIB, IIIC with delayed healing.

K. Subsequent encounter for (closed) fracture with nonunion.

M. Subsequent encounter for open fracture (Gustilo) type I or II with nonunion.

N. Subsequent encounter for open fracture (Gustilo) type IIIA, IIIB, IIIC with nonunion.

P. Subsequent encounter for (closed) fracture with malunion.

Q. Subsequent encounter for open fracture (Gustilo) type I or II with malunion.

R. Subsequent encounter for open fracture (Gustilo) type IIIA, IIIB, IIIC with malunion.

S. Sequela. Encounter for complications or conditions that arise as a direct result of a fracture.

Fracture – A disruption or break of the continuity of a bone, epiphyseal plate or cartilaginous surface.

Greenstick – Incomplete fracture in children where one side of the bone breaks, the other side bends. Tends to occur in the shaft of a long bone.

Oblique – A diagonal fracture of a long bone.

Open fracture – An open wound at the site of the fracture resulting in communication with the outside environment. The open may be produced by the bone or the opening can produce the fracture.

> **Gustilo classification** – Classification of open fractures of the forearm (S52), femur (S72) and lower leg (S82) based upon the size of the open wound and the amount of soft tissue injury.

Osteochondral – A break of tear of the articular cartilage along with a fracture of the bone.

Pathologic – Fracture that involves an underlying disease process. It may involve an injury but of the type that would not typically result in a fracture.

Physeal – Fracture in growing children that involves the growth plate.

Spiral – Twisting fracture usually of a long bone resulting in a spiral-shaped fracture line.

Stress – Fracture due to repetitive activity or overexertion without trauma.

Torus – Incomplete fracture of a long bone in children where one side buckles and the other side bulges. Occurs towards the ends of the shaft of the bone.

Transverse – A fracture line that goes across the shaft of a long bone.

Checklist

1. Identify whether the fracture is due to trauma or non-traumatic:
   - ☐ Nontraumatic fracture
     - ☐ Atypical femoral fracture
     - ☐ Pathological fracture
       - ☐ Due to osteoporosis
         - ☐ Age-related
         - ☐ Other
       - ☐ Due to neoplastic disease
         - ☐ Define neoplasm
       - ☐ Due to other disease
         - ☐ Define underlying disease
       - ☐ Not otherwise specified
     - ☐ Stress fracture
   - ☐ Traumatic fracture
2. If non-traumatic, identify nature and anatomic site of fracture:
   - ☐ Due to osteoporosis
     - ☐ Shoulder
     - ☐ Humerus
     - ☐ Forearm
     - ☐ Hand
     - ☐ Femur
     - ☐ Lower leg
     - ☐ Ankle and foot
     - ☐ Vertebra
   - ☐ Pathological, other disease process
     - ☐ Shoulder
     - ☐ Humerus
     - ☐ Radius
     - ☐ Ulna
     - ☐ Hand
     - ☐ Finger(s)
     - ☐ Pelvis
     - ☐ Femur
     - ☐ Hip, unspecified
     - ☐ Tibia
     - ☐ Fibula
     - ☐ Ankle
     - ☐ Foot
     - ☐ Toe(s)
     - ☐ Other site (includes vertebra)
   - ☐ Stress
     - ☐ Shoulder
     - ☐ Humerus
     - ☐ Radius
     - ☐ Ulna
     - ☐ Hand
     - ☐ Finger(s)
     - ☐ Pelvis
     - ☐ Femur
     - ☐ Hip, unspecified
     - ☐ Tibia
     - ☐ Fibula
     - ☐ Ankle
     - ☐ Foot
     - ☐ Toe(s)
     - ☐ Vertebra
       - a. Identify type:
         - ☐ Collapsed/Compression/Wedging
         - ☐ Fatigue
       - b. Identify spinal region:
         - ☐ Occipito-atlanto-axial region
         - ☐ Cervical region
         - ☐ Cervicothoracic region
         - ☐ Thoracic region
         - ☐ Thoracolumbar region
         - ☐ Lumbar region
         - ☐ Lumbosacral region
         - ☐ Sacral/sacrococcygeal region
     - ☐ Other site

3. If traumatic, identify location and specific anatomic site (bone):
   - ☐ Skull
     - ☐ Vault (frontal bone, parietal bone)
     - ☐ Base of skull
     - ☐ Occiput
       - ☐ Occipital condyle
         - ☐ Type I
         - ☐ Type II
         - ☐ Type III
       - ☐ Other bone base of skull
     - ☐ Facial bones
       - ☐ Malar
       - ☐ Mandible
         - ☐ Alveolus of mandible
         - ☐ Angle
         - ☐ Condylar process
         - ☐ Coronoid process
         - ☐ Ramus
         - ☐ Subcondylar process
       - ☐ Maxillary
         - ☐ Maxilla
         - ☐ LeFort
           - ☐ LeFort I
           - ☐ LeFort II
           - ☐ Le Fort III
         - ☐ Alveolus of maxilla
       - ☐ Nasal bones
       - ☐ Orbital floor
       - ☐ Zygomatic
     - ☐ Other skull and facial bones
   - ☐ Vertebra
     - ☐ Cervical
       - ☐ C1
         - ☐ Posterior arch
         - ☐ Lateral mass
         - ☐ Other
         - ☐ Unspecified – review medical record/query physician
       - ☐ C2/Dens
         - ☐ Type II dens
         - ☐ Other dens
         - ☐ Other fracture 2nd cervical
         - ☐ Spondylolisthesis, traumatic
           - ☐ Type III
           - ☐ Other
           - ☐ Unspecified – review medical record/query physician
       - ☐ C3
         - ☐ Other fracture 3rd cervical
         - ☐ Spondylolisthesis, traumatic
           - ☐ Type III
           - ☐ Other
           - ☐ Unspecified – review medical record/query physician
         - ☐ Unspecified – review medical record/query physician
       - ☐ C4
         - ☐ Other fracture 4th cervical
         - ☐ Spondylolisthesis, traumatic
           - ☐ Type III
           - ☐ Other
           - ☐ Unspecified – review medical record/query physician
         - ☐ Unspecified – review medical record/query physician
       - ☐ C5
         - ☐ Other fracture 5th cervical
         - ☐ Spondylolisthesis, traumatic
           - ☐ Type III
           - ☐ Other
           - ☐ Unspecified – review medical record/query physician
         - ☐ Unspecified – review medical record/query physician
       - ☐ C6
         - ☐ Other fracture 6th cervical
         - ☐ Spondylolisthesis, traumatic
           - ☐ Type III
           - ☐ Other
           - ☐ Unspecified – review medical record/query physician
         - ☐ Unspecified – review medical record/query physician
       - ☐ C7
         - ☐ Other fracture 7th cervical
         - ☐ Spondylolisthesis, traumatic
           - ☐ Type III
           - ☐ Other
           - ☐ Unspecified – review medical record/query physician
         - ☐ Unspecified – review medical record/query physician
     - ☐ Thoracic
       - ☐ T1
       - ☐ T2
       - ☐ T3
       - ☐ T4
       - ☐ T5-T6
       - ☐ T7-T8
       - ☐ T9-T1Ø
       - ☐ T11-T12
       - ☐ Unspecified – review medical record/query physician
     - ☐ Lumbar
       - ☐ L1
       - ☐ L2
       - ☐ L3
       - ☐ L4
       - ☐ L5

- ☐ Sacrum
  - ☐ Type 1
  - ☐ Type 2
  - ☐ Type 3
  - ☐ Zone 1
  - ☐ Zone 2
  - ☐ Zone3
  - ☐ Other
  - ☐ Unspecified – review medical record/query physician
- ☐ Coccyx

☐ Clavicle
- ☐ Sternal end
- ☐ Shaft
- ☐ Lateral/acromial end
- ☐ Unspecified – review medical record/query physician

☐ Scapula
- ☐ Acromial end
- ☐ Body
- ☐ Coracoid process
- ☐ Glenoid cavity
- ☐ Neck
- ☐ Other
- ☐ Unspecified – review medical record/query physician

☐ Humerus
- ☐ Upper end
  - ☐ Greater tuberosity
  - ☐ Lesser tuberosity
  - ☐ Physeal
  - ☐ Surgical neck
  - ☐ Other upper/proximal end
  - ☐ Unspecified – review medical record/query physician
- ☐ Shaft
- ☐ Lower end
  - ☐ Condyle
    - ☐ Lateral condyle/capitellum
    - ☐ Medial condyle/trochlea
    - ☐ Supracondylar
    - ☐ Transcondylar
  - ☐ Epicondyle
    - ☐ Lateral
    - ☐ Medial
  - ☐ Physeal
  - ☐ Other lower/distal end
  - ☐ Unspecified – review medical record/query physician
- ☐ Shoulder girdle, part unspecified – review medical record/query physician

☐ Radius
- ☐ Upper end
  - ☐ Head
  - ☐ Neck
  - ☐ Physeal
  - ☐ Other upper/proximal end
  - ☐ Unspecified – review medical record/query physician
- ☐ Shaft
- ☐ Lower end
  - ☐ Physeal
  - ☐ Radial styloid
  - ☐ Other lower/distal end
  - ☐ Unspecified – review medical record/query physician

☐ Ulna
- ☐ Upper end
  - ☐ Coronoid process
  - ☐ Olecranon process
  - ☐ Other upper/proximal end
  - ☐ Unspecified – review medical record/query physician
- ☐ Shaft
- ☐ Lower end
  - ☐ Ulnar styloid
  - ☐ Physeal
  - ☐ Other lower/distal end
  - ☐ Unspecified – review medical record/query physician

☐ Carpal
- ☐ Navicula (scaphoid)
  - ☐ Proximal third (pole)
  - ☐ Middle third (waist)
  - ☐ Distal third (pole)
  - ☐ Unspecified – review medical record/query physician
- ☐ Lunate
- ☐ Triquetrum
- ☐ Pisiform
- ☐ Trapezium
- ☐ Trapezoid
- ☐ Capitate
- ☐ Hamate
  - ☐ Body
  - ☐ Hook

☐ Metacarpal
- ☐ First
  - ☐ Base
  - ☐ Shaft
  - ☐ Neck
  - ☐ Unspecified – review medical record/query physician
- ☐ Second
  - ☐ Base
  - ☐ Shaft
  - ☐ Neck
  - ☐ Other
  - ☐ Unspecified – review medical record/query physician
- ☐ Third

- ☐ Base
- ☐ Shaft
- ☐ Neck
- ☐ Other
- ☐ Unspecified – review medical record/query physician

☐ Fourth
- ☐ Base
- ☐ Shaft
- ☐ Neck
- ☐ Other
- ☐ Unspecified – review medical record/query physician

☐ Fifth
- ☐ Base
- ☐ Shaft
- ☐ Neck
- ☐ Other
- ☐ Unspecified – review medical record/query physician

☐ Phalanx
- ☐ Thumb
  - ☐ Proximal phalanx
  - ☐ Distal phalanx
  - ☐ Unspecified – review medical record/query physician
- ☐ Index finger
  - ☐ Proximal phalanx
  - ☐ Middle phalanx
  - ☐ Distal phalanx
  - ☐ Unspecified – review medical record/query physician
- ☐ Middle finger
  - ☐ Proximal phalanx
  - ☐ Middle phalanx
  - ☐ Distal phalanx
  - ☐ Unspecified – review medical record/query physician
- ☐ Ring finger
  - ☐ Proximal phalanx
  - ☐ Middle phalanx
  - ☐ Distal phalanx
  - ☐ Unspecified – review medical record/query physician
- ☐ Little finger
  - ☐ Proximal phalanx
  - ☐ Middle phalanx
  - ☐ Distal phalanx
  - ☐ Unspecified – review medical record/query physician
- ☐ Other finger
  - ☐ Proximal phalanx
  - ☐ Medial phalanx
  - ☐ Distal phalanx
  - ☐ Unspecified – review medical record/query physician

☐ Unspecified fracture of wrist and hand– review medical record/query physician

☐ Pelvis
- ☐ Ilium
- ☐ Ischium
- ☐ Pubis
  - ☐ Superior rim
  - ☐ Other specified
  - ☐ Unspecified – review medical record/query physician
- ☐ Acetabulum
  - ☐ Anterior column
  - ☐ Anterior wall
  - ☐ Dome
  - ☐ Medial wall
  - ☐ Posterior column
  - ☐ Posterior wall
  - ☐ Transverse
  - ☐ Transverse-posterior
  - ☐ Other specified
  - ☐ Unspecified fracture of acetabulum – review medical record/query physician
- ☐ Multiple fractures of pelvis
- ☐ Other parts of pelvis

☐ Unspecified part of lumbosacral spine and pelvis – review medical record/query physician

☐ Femur
- ☐ Upper end
  - ☐ Apophyseal
  - ☐ Base of neck
  - ☐ Epiphysis (separation)
  - ☐ Greater trochanter
  - ☐ Head (articular)
  - ☐ Intracapsular unspecified/subcapital
  - ☐ Intertrochanteric
  - ☐ Lesser trochanter
  - ☐ Midcervical
  - ☐ Pertrochanteric
  - ☐ Physeal
  - ☐ Subtrochanteric
  - ☐ Other fracture of head and neck
  - ☐ Unspecified fracture head of femur – review medical record/query physician
  - ☐ Unspecified part of neck of femur – review medical record/query physician
  - ☐ Unspecified trochanteric fracture – review medical record/query physician
- ☐ Shaft
- ☐ Lower end
  - ☐ Condyle
    - ☐ Lateral
    - ☐ Medial
    - ☐ Supracondylar

- ☐ with intracondylar extension
- ☐ without intracondylar extension
- ☐ Epiphysis (separation)
- ☐ Physeal
- ☐ Other lower/distal end
- ☐ Other fracture of femur
- ☐ Unspecified fracture of femur – review medical record/query physician
- ☐ Patella
- ☐ Tibia
  - ☐ Upper end
    - ☐ Condyle
      - ☐ Bicondylar
      - ☐ Lateral
      - ☐ Medial
    - ☐ Physeal
    - ☐ Tibial spine
    - ☐ Tibial tuberosity
    - ☐ Other upper/proximal end
    - ☐ Unspecified upper end of tibia – review medical record/query physician
  - ☐ Shaft
  - ☐ Lower end
    - ☐ Physeal
    - ☐ Other lower/distal end
    - ☐ Unspecified lower end of tibia – review medical record/query physician
- ☐ Fibula
  - ☐ Physeal
    - ☐ Upper end
    - ☐ Lower end
  - ☐ Shaft
  - ☐ Upper end
  - ☐ Lower end
  - ☐ Other fracture upper and lower end of fibula
  - ☐ Unspecified fracture of lower leg – review medical record/query physician
- ☐ Ankle
  - ☐ Bimalleolar
  - ☐ Medial malleolus
  - ☐ Lateral malleolus
  - ☐ Pilon/plafond
  - ☐ Trimalleolar
- ☐ Foot
  - ☐ Talus
    - ☐ Body
    - ☐ Dome
    - ☐ Neck
    - ☐ Posterior process
    - ☐ Other fracture of talus
    - ☐ Unspecified fracture of talus – review medical record/query physician
  - ☐ Calcaneus
    - ☐ Anterior process
    - ☐ Body
    - ☐ Extraarticular, other
    - ☐ Intraarticular
    - ☐ Physeal
    - ☐ Tuberosity
    - ☐ Unspecified fracture of calcaneus – review medical record/query physician
  - ☐ Tarsal, other
    - ☐ Navicula
    - ☐ Cuneiform
      - ☐ Medial
      - ☐ Intermediate
      - ☐ Lateral
    - ☐ Cuboid
    - ☐ Unspecified tarsal – review medical record/query physician
  - ☐ Metatarsal
    - ☐ First
    - ☐ Second
    - ☐ Third
    - ☐ Fourth
    - ☐ Fifth
    - ☐ Physeal
    - ☐ Unspecified metatarsal fracture – review medical record/query physician
  - ☐ Toe
    - ☐ Great toe/hallux
      - ☐ Proximal phalanx
      - ☐ Distal phalanx
      - ☐ Other
      - ☐ Unspecified fracture great toe– review medical record/query physician
    - ☐ Lesser toe(s)
      - ☐ Proximal phalanx
      - ☐ Middle phalanx
      - ☐ Distal phalanx
      - ☐ Other
      - ☐ Unspecified fracture lesser toe– review medical record/query physician
    - ☐ Physeal
  - ☐ Other fracture of foot
    - ☐ Sesamoid
  - ☐ Unspecified fracture of foot– review medical record/query physician
  - ☐ Unspecified fracture of toe– review medical record/query physician
- ☐ Other fractures
  - ☐ Neck (includes hyoid, larynx, thyroid cartilage, trachea)
  - ☐ Rib (s)
    - ☐ One
    - ☐ Multiple
    - ☐ Flail chest
  - ☐ Sternum
    - ☐ Body

- ☐ Manubrium
- ☐ Manubrium dissociation
- ☐ Xiphoid process

4. For atypical femoral fractures and traumatic fractures, identify fracture configuration/type, where appropriate:
   - ☐ Atypical femoral fracture
     - ☐ Complete oblique
     - ☐ Complete transverse
     - ☐ Incomplete
   - ☐ Vertebral fractures
     - ☐ C1
       - ☐ Stable burst
       - ☐ Unstable burst
     - ☐ Thoracic and Lumbar
       - ☐ Wedge
       - ☐ Stable burst
       - ☐ Unstable burst
       - ☐ Other
     - ☐ Humerus
       - ☐ Surgical neck
         - ☐ 2-part
         - ☐ 3-part
         - ☐ 4-part
       - ☐ Upper or lower end
         - ☐ Physeal
           - ☐ Salter-Harris Type I
           - ☐ Salter-Harris Type II
           - ☐ Salter-Harris Type III
           - ☐ Salter-Harris Type IV
           - ☐ Other
           - ☐ Unspecified – review medical record/ query physician
         - ☐ Torus
       - ☐ Shaft
         - ☐ Comminuted
         - ☐ Greenstick
         - ☐ Oblique
         - ☐ Segmental
         - ☐ Spiral
         - ☐ Transverse
         - ☐ Other
         - ☐ Unspecified – review medical record/query physician
       - ☐ Supracondylar without intercondylar fracture
         - ☐ Comminuted
         - ☐ Simple
     - ☐ Ulna
       - ☐ Olecranon process
         - ☐ with intercondylar extension
         - ☐ without intercondylar extension
       - ☐ Upper or lower end
         - ☐ Physeal
           - ☐ Salter-Harris Type I
           - ☐ Salter-Harris Type II
           - ☐ Salter-Harris Type III
           - ☐ Salter-Harris Type IV
           - ☐ Other
           - ☐ Unspecified – review medical record/ query physician
         - ☐ Torus
       - ☐ Shaft
         - ☐ Bent bone
         - ☐ Comminuted
         - ☐ Greenstick
         - ☐ Monteggia
         - ☐ Oblique
         - ☐ Segmental
         - ☐ Spiral
         - ☐ Transverse
         - ☐ Other
         - ☐ Unspecified – review medical record/query physician
     - ☐ Radius
       - ☐ Upper or lower end
         - ☐ Physeal
           - ☐ Salter-Harris Type I
           - ☐ Salter-Harris Type II
           - ☐ Salter-Harris Type III
           - ☐ Salter-Harris Type IV
           - ☐ Other
           - ☐ Unspecified – review medical record/ query physician
         - ☐ Torus
       - ☐ Shaft
         - ☐ Bent bone
         - ☐ Comminuted
         - ☐ Galeazzi's
         - ☐ Greenstick
         - ☐ Oblique
         - ☐ Segmental
         - ☐ Spiral
         - ☐ Transverse
         - ☐ Other
         - ☐ Unspecified – review medical record/query physician
       - ☐ Lower end
         - ☐ Extraarticular
           - ☐ Colles'
           - ☐ Smith's
           - ☐ Other
         - ☐ Intraarticular
           - ☐ Barton's
           - ☐ Other
         - ☐ Torus
     - ☐ Pelvis
       - ☐ Ilium
         - ☐ Avulsion
         - ☐ Other
       - ☐ Ischium

    - ☐ Avulsion
    - ☐ Other
  - ☐ Multiple fractures of pelvis
    - ☐ with stable disruption of pelvic ring
    - ☐ with unstable disruption of pelvic ring
    - ☐ without disruption of pelvic ring
- ☐ Femur
  - ☐ Physeal upper end
    - ☐ Salter-Harris Type I
    - ☐ Other
    - ☐ Unspecified
  - ☐ Shaft
    - ☐ Comminuted
    - ☐ Oblique
    - ☐ Segmental
    - ☐ Spiral
    - ☐ Transverse
    - ☐ Other
    - ☐ Unspecified – review medical record/query physician
  - ☐ Lower end
    - ☐ Physeal
      - ☐ Salter-Harris Type I
      - ☐ Salter-Harris Type II
      - ☐ Salter-Harris Type III
      - ☐ Salter-Harris Type IV
      - ☐ Other
      - ☐ Unspecified – review medical record/query physician
    - ☐ Torus
  - ☐ Other
- ☐ Patella
  - ☐ Comminuted
  - ☐ Longitudinal
  - ☐ Osteochondral
  - ☐ Transverse
  - ☐ Other
  - ☐ Unspecified – review medical record/query physician
- ☐ Tibia
  - ☐ Upper or lower end
    - ☐ Physeal
      - ☐ Salter-Harris Type I
      - ☐ Salter-Harris Type II
      - ☐ Salter-Harris Type III
      - ☐ Salter-Harris Type IV
      - ☐ Other
      - ☐ Unspecified – review medical record/query physician
    - ☐ Torus
    - ☐ Other
  - ☐ Shaft
    - ☐ Comminuted
    - ☐ Oblique
    - ☐ Segmental
    - ☐ Spiral
    - ☐ Transverse
    - ☐ Other
    - ☐ Unspecified – review medical record/query physician
- ☐ Fibula
  - ☐ Upper or lower end
    - ☐ Physeal
      - ☐ Salter-Harris Type I
      - ☐ Salter-Harris Type II
      - ☐ Other
      - ☐ Unspecified – review medical record/query physician
    - ☐ Torus
    - ☐ Other
  - ☐ Shaft
    - ☐ Comminuted
    - ☐ Oblique
    - ☐ Segmental
    - ☐ Spiral
    - ☐ Transverse
    - ☐ Other
    - ☐ Unspecified – review medical record/query physician
- ☐ Talus
  - ☐ Avulsion
- ☐ Calcaneus
  - ☐ Avulsion
  - ☐ Physeal
    - ☐ Salter-Harris Type I
    - ☐ Salter-Harris Type II
    - ☐ Salter-Harris Type III
    - ☐ Salter-Harris Type IV
    - ☐ Other
    - ☐ Unspecified – review medical record/query physician
- ☐ Metatarsal
  - ☐ Physeal
    - ☐ Salter-Harris Type I
    - ☐ Salter-Harris Type II
    - ☐ Salter-Harris Type III
    - ☐ Salter-Harris Type IV
    - ☐ Other
    - ☐ Unspecified – review medical record/query physician
- ☐ Phalanx
  - ☐ Physeal
    - ☐ Salter-Harris Type I
    - ☐ Salter-Harris Type II
    - ☐ Salter-Harris Type III
    - ☐ Salter-Harris Type IV
    - ☐ Other
    - ☐ Unspecified – review medical record/query physician

5. For traumatic fractures excluding torus and greenstick, identify displacement unless inherent to fracture configuration:
   - ☐ Displaced
   - ☐ Nondisplaced

Note: Fractures not documented as displaced or nondisplaced, default to displaced.

6. Identify laterality, excluding vertebral fractures:
   - ☐ Left
   - ☐ Right
   - ☐ Unspecified – review medical record/query physician
7. For traumatic fractures, identify status:
   - ☐ Closed
   - ☐ Open
     - ☐ If S52, S72, S82
       - ☐ Gustilo Type I
       - ☐ Gustilo Type II
       - ☐ Gustilo Type IIIA
       - ☐ Gustilo Type IIIB

Note: Fractures not identified as open or closed, default to closed.

8. Identify episode of care/stage of healing/complication:
   - ☐ Pathologic fracture
     - ☐ A Initial encounter
     - ☐ D Subsequent encounter with routine healing
     - ☐ G Subsequent encounter with delayed healing
     - ☐ K Subsequent encounter with nonunion
     - ☐ P Subsequent encounter with malunion
     - ☐ S Sequela
   - ☐ Stress fracture (excluding vertebra)
     - ☐ A Initial encounter
     - ☐ D Subsequent encounter with routine healing
     - ☐ G Subsequent encounter with delayed healing
     - ☐ K Subsequent encounter with nonunion
     - ☐ P Subsequent encounter with malunion
     - ☐ S Sequela
   - ☐ Stress fracture vertebra (fatigue, collapsed vertebra)
     - ☐ A Initial encounter
     - ☐ D Subsequent encounter with routine healing
     - ☐ G Subsequent encounter with delayed healing
     - ☐ S Sequela
   - ☐ Traumatic fracture vertebra
     - ☐ A Initial encounter for closed fracture
     - ☐ B Initial encounter for open fracture
     - ☐ D Subsequent encounter with routine healing
     - ☐ G Subsequent encounter with delayed healing
     - ☐ K Subsequent encounter with nonunion
     - ☐ S Sequela
   - ☐ Traumatic (excluding torus and greenstick and S52, S62, S72, S82)
     - ☐ A Initial encounter for closed fracture

B Initial encounter for open fracture

     - ☐ D Subsequent encounter with routine healing
     - ☐ G Subsequent encounter with delayed healing
     - ☐ K Subsequent encounter with nonunion
     - ☐ P Subsequent encounter with malunion
     - ☐ S Sequela
   - ☐ Traumatic torus and greenstick
     - ☐ A Initial encounter
     - ☐ D Subsequent encounter with routine healing
     - ☐ G Subsequent encounter with delayed healing
     - ☐ K Subsequent encounter with nonunion
     - ☐ P Subsequent encounter with malunion
     - ☐ S Sequela
   - ☐ Traumatic (S52 forearm, S72 femur, S82 lower leg)
     - ☐ A Initial encounter for closed fracture
     - ☐ B Initial encounter for Gustilo type I or II
     - ☐ C Initial encounter for Gustilo type III A or IIIB
     - ☐ D Subsequent encounter closed fracture with routine healing
     - ☐ E Subsequent encounter Gustilo type I or II with routine healing
     - ☐ F Subsequent encounter Gustilo type IIIA or IIIB with routine healing
     - ☐ G Subsequent encounter closed fracture with delayed healing
     - ☐ H Subsequent encounter Gustilo type I or II with delayed healing
     - ☐ J Subsequent encounter Gustilo type IIIA or IIIB with delayed healing
     - ☐ K Subsequent encounter closed fracture with nonunion
     - ☐ M Subsequent encounter Gustilo type I or II with nonunion
     - ☐ N Subsequent encounter Gustilo type IIIA or IIIB with nonunion
     - ☐ P Subsequent encounter closed fracture with malunion
     - ☐ Subsequent encounter Gustilo type I or II with malunion
     - ☐ R Subsequent encounter Gustilo type IIIA or IIIB with malunion
     - ☐ S Sequela
9. Identify any associated injuries:
   - ☐ Fracture of skull and facial bones any associated intracranial injuries SØ6.-
   - ☐ Fracture of cervical vertebra any associated spinal cord injury S14.Ø, S14.1-
   - ☐ Fracture of thoracic vertebra any associated spinal cord injury S24.Ø, S24.1-
   - ☐ Fracture of lumbar vertebra any associated spinal cord/nerve injury S34.Ø-, S34.1-
   - ☐ Fracture of rib(s) and sternum any associated injury intrathoracic organ S27.-
10. Identify the external cause, intent, activity, place, and status where applicable

Gout

ICD-10-CM Categories

Gout is classified in two categories in Chapter 13 as a disease of the musculoskeletal system and connective tissue:

M1A	Chronic gout
M10	Gout

ICD-10-CM Definitions

Chronic gout – Long term gout that develops in cases where uric acid levels remain consistently high over a number of years, resulting in more frequent attacks and pain that may remain constant.

Gout – A complex type of arthritis characterized by the accumulation of uric acid crystals within the joints, causing severe pain, redness, swelling, and stiffness, particularly in the big toe. The needle-like crystal deposits in a joint cause sudden attacks or flares of severe pain and inflammation that intensify before subsiding.

Uric acid – A chemical compound of ions and salts formed by the metabolic breakdown of purines, found in foods such as meats and shellfish, and in cells of the body.

Checklist

1. Identify type of gout:
   - ☐ Acute (attack) (flare)
   - ☐ Chronic
   - ☐ Unspecified
2. Identify cause:
   - ☐ Drug-induced
     - ☐ Use additional code to identify drug and adverse effect, if applicable
   - ☐ Due to renal impairment
     - ☐ Code first causative renal disease
   - ☐ Idiopathic (primary)
   - ☐ Lead-induced
     - ☐ Code first toxic effects of lead and lead compounds
   - ☐ Secondary
     - ☐ Code first associated condition
   - ☐ Unspecified
3. Identify site:
   - ☐ Lower extremity
     - ☐ Ankle/foot
     - ☐ Hip
     - ☐ Knee
   - ☐ Upper extremity
     - ☐ Elbow
     - ☐ Hand
     - ☐ Shoulder
     - ☐ Wrist
   - ☐ Vertebrae
   - ☐ Multiple sites
   - ☐ Unspecified site
4. Identify laterality for extremities:
   - ☐ Left
   - ☐ Right
   - ☐ Unspecified
5. For chronic gout, identify presence/absence of tophi:
   - ☐ With tophi
   - ☐ Without tophi
6. For all types of gout, identify any accompanying conditions with the underlying gout:
   - ☐ Autonomic neuropathy
   - ☐ Cardiomyopathy
   - ☐ Disorders of external ear, iris, or ciliary body
   - ☐ Glomerular disorders
   - ☐ Urinary calculus

Headache Syndromes

ICD-10-CM Subcategories

G44.0	Cluster headaches and other trigeminal autonomic cephalgias (TAC)
G44.1	Vascular headache, not elsewhere classified
G44.2	Tension-type headache
G44.3	Post-traumatic headache
G44.4	Drug-induced headache, not elsewhere classified
G44.5	Complicated headache syndromes
G44.8	Other specified headache syndromes
R51	Headache NOS

ICD-10-CM Definitions

Headache NOS – Headache not further documented as a migraine or other specific headache syndrome is reported with the sign/symptom code R51 in Chapter 18 of ICD-10-CM.

Intractable headache – A headache that is not responding to treatment. Synonymous terms include: pharmacoresistant (pharmacologically resistant) headache, treatment resistant headache, refractory headache, and poorly controlled headache.

Not intractable headache – Headache that is responding to treatment.

Tension headache – Tension headache is synonymous with tension-type headache in ICD-10-CM. Use codes in subcategory G44.2 for headache documented as tension headache.

Checklist

1. Identify the specific type of headache or syndrome:
   - ☐ Cluster headaches and trigeminal autonomic cephalgias
     - ☐ Cluster headache
       - ☐ Chronic
       - ☐ Episodic
       - ☐ Unspecified
     - ☐ Paroxysmal hemicranias
       - ☐ Chronic
       - ☐ Episodic
     - ☐ Short lasting unilateral neuralgiform headache with conjunctival injection and tearing (SUNCT)
     - ☐ Other trigeminal autonomic cephalgias (TAC)
   - ☐ Vascular headache, not elsewhere classified
   - ☐ Tension-type headache
     - ☐ Chronic
     - ☐ Episodic
     - ☐ Unspecified
   - ☐ Post-traumatic headache
     - ☐ Acute
     - ☐ Chronic
     - ☐ Unspecified
   - ☐ Drug-induced headache, not elsewhere classified – Use additional code for adverse effect, if applicable, to identify drug (T36-T5Ø with 5th or 6th character 5)
   - ☐ Complicated headache syndromes
     - ☐ Hemicrania continua
     - ☐ New daily persistent headache (NDPH)
     - ☐ Primary thunderclap headache
     - ☐ Other complicated headache syndrome
   - ☐ Other specified headache syndromes
     - ☐ Hypnic headache
     - ☐ Headache associated with sexual activity
     - ☐ Primary cough headache
     - ☐ Primary exertional headache
     - ☐ Primary stabbing headache
     - ☐ Other specified type headache syndrome – Specify ____________

2. Identify response to treatment for the following types: cluster, paroxysmal hemicranias, SUNCT, other TAC, tension-type, post-traumatic, and drug-induced
   - ☐ Intractable
   - ☐ Not intractable

Migraine

ICD-10-CM Subcategories

G43.0	Migraine without aura
G43.1	Migraine with aura
G43.4	Hemiplegic migraine
G43.5	Persistent migraine aura without cerebral infarction
G43.6	Persistent migraine aura with cerebral infarction
G43.7	Chronic migraine without aura
G43.A	Cyclical vomiting
G43.B	Ophthalmoplegic migraine
G43.C	Periodic headache syndromes in child or adult
G43.D	Abdominal migraine
G43.8	Other migraine
G43.9	Migraine, unspecified

ICD-10-CM Definitions

Migraine – Common neurological disorder that often manifests as a headache. Usually unilateral and pulsating in nature, the headache results from abnormal brain activity along nerve pathways and brain chemical (neurotransmitter) changes. These affect blood flow in the brain and surrounding tissue and may trigger an "aura" or warning sign (visual, sensory, language, motor) before the onset of pain. Migraine headache is frequently accompanied by autonomic nervous system symptoms (nausea, vomiting, sensitivity to light and/or sound).

Intractable headache – A headache that is not responding to treatment. Synonymous terms include: pharmacoresistant (pharmacologically resistant) headache, treatment resistant headache, refractory headache, and poorly controlled headache.

Not intractable headache – Headache that is responding to treatment.

Status migrainosus – Migraine that has lasted more than 72 hours.

Checklist

1. Identify migraine type:
   - ☐ Abdominal
   - ☐ Chronic without aura
   - ☐ Cyclical vomiting
   - ☐ Hemiplegic
   - ☐ Menstrual – Code also associated premenstrual tension syndrome (N94.3)
   - ☐ Ophthalmoplegic
   - ☐ Periodic headache syndromes in child or adult
   - ☐ Persistent aura
     - ☐ With cerebral infarction – Code also type of cerebral infarction (I63.-)
     - ☐ Without cerebral infarction
   - ☐ With aura – Code also any associated seizure (G4Ø.-, R56.9)
   - ☐ Without aura
   - ☐ Other specified migraine
   - ☐ Unspecified migraine
2. Identify presence/absence of intractability:
   - ☐ Intractable
   - ☐ Not intractable
3. Identify presence/absence of status migrainosus (not required for migraines documented as abdominal, cyclical vomiting, ophthalmoplegic, or periodic headache syndromes in child/adult):
   - ☐ With status migrainosus
   - ☐ Without (mention of) status migrainosus
4. Use additional code for adverse effect, if applicable, to identify drug (T36-T50 with 5th or 6th character 5)

Rheumatoid Arthritis

ICD-10-CM Categories

Rheumatoid arthritis may be classified as a combination code according to the type of rheumatoid arthritis, the joint, and organ system involved. Conditions related to rheumatoid arthritis are also included in this category.

Rheumatoid arthritis is classified in the following ICD-10-CM categories/subcategories:

M05	Rheumatoid arthritis with rheumatoid factor
M06	Other rheumatoid arthritis
M08.0	Unspecified juvenile rheumatoid arthritis
M08.1	Juvenile ankylosing spondylitis
M08.2	Juvenile rheumatoid arthritis with systemic onset
M08.3	Juvenile rheumatoid polyarthritis (seronegative)
M08.4	Pauciarticular juvenile rheumatoid arthritis
M45.0	Ankylosing spondylitis

ICD-10-CM Definitions

Ankylosing spondylitis – Also known as Marie-Strumpell disease, rheumatoid spondylitis, and Bechterew's syndrome, ankylosing spondylitis is a chronic, progressive, autoimmune arthropathy that affects the spine and sacroiliac joints, eventually leading to spinal fusion and rigidity. Almost all of the autoimmune spondyloarthropathies share a common genetic marker, HLA-B27, although the cause is still unknown. The disease appears in some predisposed people after exposure to bowel or urinary tract infections. The most common patient is a young male, aged 15-30. It affects men about three times more than women. Swelling occurs in the intervertebral discs and in the joints between the spine and pelvis. Patients have persistent buttock and low back pain and stiffness alleviated with exercise. Over time, the vertebrae may become fused together, progressing up the spine and affecting other organs.

Felty's Syndrome – An atypical form of rheumatoid arthritis that presents with fever, an enlarged spleen, recurring infections, and a decreased white blood count.

Juvenile rheumatoid arthritis with systemic onset – Systemic onset juvenile rheumatoid arthritis (JRA), also known as Still's Disease in children, is an autoimmune inflammatory disease that develops in children up to the age of 16. It is the most uncommon form of JRA. It begins with periods of recurrent high fever spikes up to 103 degrees accompanied by a rash that lasts for at least two weeks. Other symptoms can include enlarged lymph nodes, enlarged liver or spleen, or inflammation of the lining of the heart or lungs (pericarditis or pleuritis). Joint swelling and joint damage may not appear for months or years after the fevers begin. In addition to the joints, other connective tissue organs such as the liver and spleen may also be affected.

Pauciarticular juvenile rheumatoid arthritis – Pauciarticular JRA, also known as oligoarticular JRA, is an autoimmune inflammatory disease that develops in children any time up to 16 years of age that presents with an initial onset affecting 5 or fewer joints. The larger joints, such as the knees, ankles, and elbows are the most commonly affected. Pauciarticular JRA is the most common form of JRA occurring more commonly in girls. Children, particularly boys, who develop the disease after the age of 7 tend to have other joints, including the spine, become affected and will frequently continue with the disease into adulthood. Children who develop the disease at a younger age tend to go into remission and become asymptomatic.

Rheumatoid arthritis – Rheumatoid arthritis (RA) is an autoimmune, systemic, inflammatory disease that normally occurs between the ages of 30 and 50. RA affects the synovial lining of joints resulting in swelling, pain, warmth, and stiffness around the joint, followed by thickening of the synovial lining; bone and cartilage destruction leading to pain; joint deformity and instability; and loss of function. RA commonly begins in the small joints of the hands and wrists and is often symmetrical, affecting the same joints on both sides. RA is accompanied by other physical symptoms including morning pain and stiffness or pain with prolonged sitting; flu-like low grade fever and muscle ache; disease flare-ups followed by remission; and sometimes rheumatoid nodules under the skin, particularly over the elbows. Some people also have an increase in rheumatoid factor antibody that helps direct the production of normal antibodies.

Rheumatoid factor – Rheumatoid factor is an antibody (protein) in the blood that binds with other antibodies and is not present in normal individuals. A value of 14IU/ml or greater is considered positive.

Rheumatoid nodule – Benign lumps or masses that develop under the skin of some patients with rheumatoid arthritis. These masses are firm and generally located near a joint, most commonly occurring on the fingers, elbows, forearm, knees, and backs of the heels.

Still's disease (adult-onset) – Adult-onset Still's disease is a rare inflammatory disease that develops in adults over the age of 45 and affects multiple joints and organ systems. There is no known cause of Still's disease. Common symptoms include fever, joint pain, sore throat, muscle pain, and a rash. This disease may be an isolated episode or reoccur. The knees and wrists are the most common joints destroyed by the disease.

Checklist

1. Identify the type of arthritis:
   - ☐ Ankylosing spondylitis
     - ☐ Ankylosing spondylitis
     - ☐ Juvenile ankylosing spondylitis
   - ☐ Juvenile rheumatoid arthritis
     - ☐ Juvenile rheumatoid arthritis with systemic onset
     - ☐ Juvenile rheumatoid polyarthritis
     - ☐ Pauciarticular juvenile rheumatoid arthritis
     - ☐ With or without rheumatoid factor/unspecified
   - ☐ Rheumatoid arthritis
     - ☐ With rheumatoid factor (seropositive)
       - ☐ Felty's syndrome
       - ☐ Rheumatoid arthritis
       - ☐ Other
     - ☐ Other rheumatoid arthritis

- ☐ Adult-onset Still's disease
- ☐ Rheumatoid bursitis
- ☐ Rheumatoid nodule
- ☐ Other specified
- ☐ Without rheumatoid factor (seronegative)

Note: For Adult-onset Still's disease and juvenile rheumatoid polyarthritis there is no further classification for the code. For Still's disease in children, see juvenile rheumatoid arthritis with systemic onset.

2. For other than ankylosing spondylitis, identify joint:
   - ☐ Shoulder
   - ☐ Elbow
   - ☐ Wrist
   - ☐ Hand
   - ☐ Hip
   - ☐ Knee
   - ☐ Ankle and foot
   - ☐ Vertebrae (excluding Felty's syndrome)
   - ☐ Multiple sites (excluding Felty's syndrome and pauciarticular JRA)
   - ☐ Unspecified site– review medical record/query physician
3. For ankylosing spondylitis (M45), identify vertebral level/region:
   - ☐ Occipito-atlanto-axial spine
   - ☐ Cervical region
   - ☐ Cervicothoracic region
   - ☐ Thoracic region
   - ☐ Thoracolumbar region
   - ☐ Lumbar region
   - ☐ Lumbosacral region
   - ☐ Sacral and sacrococcygeal region
   - ☐ Multiple sites in spine
   - ☐ Unspecified sites in spine– review medical record/query physician

   Note: Juvenile ankylosing spondylitis (M08.1) is not defined by vertebral level/region.
4. For rheumatoid arthritis with rheumatoid factor (excluding other), identify organ system involvement:
   - ☐ Rheumatoid heart disease
   - ☐ Rheumatoid myopathy
   - ☐ Rheumatoid lung disease
   - ☐ Rheumatoid polyneuropathy
   - ☐ Rheumatoid vasculitis
   - ☐ Other organs and systems
   - ☐ Without organ or system involvement
5. Identify laterality excluding vertebrae, multiple sites, and ankylosing spondylitis:
   - ☐ Left
   - ☐ Right
   - ☐ Unspecified – review medical record/query physician

Seizures

ICD-10-CM Categories/Subcategories

Codes for seizures are located across multiple categories in different chapters. Epileptic seizures are the only group classified to Chapter 6 Diseases of the Nervous System. Other types of nonepileptic seizures such as new onset, febrile, or hysterical seizure are classified to other chapters.

F44.5	Conversion disorder with seizures or convulsions
G40	Epilepsy and recurrent seizures
P90	Convulsions of newborn
R56	Convulsions, not elsewhere classified

ICD-10-CM Definitions

Absence seizure – A type of seizure common in children that appears as brief, sudden lapses in attention or vacant staring spells during which the child is unresponsive; often accompanied by other signs such as lip smacking, chewing motions, eyelid fluttering, and small finger or hand movements; formerly called petit mal seizure.

Epilepsy – Disorder of the central nervous system characterized by long-term predisposition to recurring episodes of sudden onset seizures, muscle contractions, sensory disturbance, and loss of consciousness caused by excessive neuronal activity in the brain and resulting in cognitive, psychological, and neurobiological consequences.

Generalized tonic clonic seizure – A type of seizure involving the entire body that usually begins on both sides of the brain and manifests with loss of consciousness, muscle stiffness, and convulsive, jerking movements; also called grand mal seizure.

Juvenile myoclonic epilepsy – A form of generalized epilepsy manifesting in mid or late childhood typically emerging first as absence seizures, then the presence of myoclonic jerks upon awakening from sleep in another 1-9 years as its hallmark feature, followed by generalized tonic clonic seizures some months later in nearly all cases.

Lennox-Gastaut syndrome – Severe form of epilepsy characterized by multiple different seizure types that are hard to control that may be absence, tonic (muscle stiffening), atonic (muscle drop), myoclonic, tonic clonic (grand mal); usually beginning before age 4 and associated with impaired intellectual functioning, developmental delay, and behavioral disturbances.

Localization-related epilepsy – Focal epilepsy generating seizures from one localized area of the brain where excessive or abnormal electrical discharges begin; synonymous with partial epilepsy.

Myoclonic jerks – Irregular, shock-like movements in the arms or legs that occur upon awakening, usually seen affecting both arms but sometimes restricted to the fingers, and may occur unilaterally, typically occurring in clusters and often a warning sign before generalized tonic clonic seizure.

Seizure – A transient occurrence of abnormal or uncontrolled electrical discharges in the brain resulting in an event of physical convulsions, thought and sensory disturbances, other minor physical signs, and possible loss of consciousness.

Checklist

1. Identify type of seizure(s):
   - ☐ Epileptic – Proceed to #2
   - ☐ Other (nonepileptic) type – Proceed to #3
2. Epilepsy and recurrent seizures
   a. Identify type of epilepsy or epileptic syndrome:
      - ☐ Absence epileptic syndrome (G40.A-)
      - ☐ Epileptic spasms (G40.82-)
      - ☐ Generalized
        - ☐ Idiopathic (G40.3-)
        - ☐ Other (G40.4-)
      - ☐ Juvenile myoclonic epilepsy (G40.B-)
      - ☐ Lennox-Gastaut syndrome (G40.81-)
      - ☐ Localization-related (focal) (partial)
        - ☐ Idiopathic (G40.0-)
        - ☐ Symptomatic
          - ☐ With complex partial seizures (G40.2-)
          - ☐ With simple partial seizures (G40.1-)
      - ☐ Other epilepsy (G40.80-)
      - ☐ Other seizures (G40.89)
      - ☐ Related to external causes (G40.5-)
      - ☐ Unspecified epilepsy (G40.9-)

   b. Determine intractability status:
      - ☐ Intractable
      - ☐ Not intractable

   Note: Intractable status does not apply to other seizures or to epileptic seizures related to external causes.

   c. Determine status epilepticus:
      - ☐ With status epilepticus
      - ☐ Without status epilepticus

   Note: Status epilepticus does not apply to other seizures.
3. Other (nonepileptic) type seizures
   a. Identify type of other nonepileptic seizure:
      - ☐ Febrile
        - ☐ Complex (R56.01)
        - ☐ Simple (R56.00)
      - ☐ Hysterical (F44.5)
      - ☐ Newborn (P90)
      - ☐ Post-traumatic (R56.1)
      - ☐ Unspecified (R56.9)

Documentation Guidelines for Evaluation and Management (E/M) Services

I. Introduction

What is documentation and why is it important?

Medical record documentation is required to record pertinent facts, findings, and observations about an individual's health history including past and present illnesses, examinations, tests, treatments, and outcomes. The medical record chronologically documents the care of the patient and is an important element contributing to high-quality care. The medical record facilitates:

An appropriately documented medical record can reduce many of the "hassles" associated with claims processing and may serve as a legal document to verify the care provided, if necessary.

What do payers want and why?

Because payers have a contractual obligation to enrollees, they may require reasonable documentation that services are consistent with the insurance coverage provided. They may request information to validate:

- the site of service;
- the medical necessity and appropriateness of the diagnostic and/or therapeutic services provided; and/or
- that services provided have been accurately reported.

II. General Principles of Medical Record Documentation

The principles of documentation listed below are applicable to all types of medical and surgical services in all settings. For Evaluation and Management (E/M) services, the nature and amount of physician work and documentation varies by type of service, place of service and the patient's status. The general principles listed below may be modified to account for these variable circumstances in providing E/M services.

1. The medical record should be complete and legible.
2. The documentation of each patient encounter should include:
   - reason for the encounter and relevant history, physical examination findings and prior diagnostic test results;
   - assessment, clinical impression or diagnosis;
   - plan for care; and
   - date and legible identity of the observer.
3. If not documented, the rationale for ordering diagnostic and other ancillary services should be easily inferred.
4. Past and present diagnoses should be accessible to the treating and/or consulting physician.
5. Appropriate health risk factors should be identified.
6. The patient's progress, response to and changes in treatment, and revision of diagnosis should be documented.
7. The CPT® and ICD-10-CM codes reported on the health insurance claim form or billing statement should be supported by the documentation in the medical record.

CPT © 2018 American Medical Association. All Rights Reserved.

III. Documentation of E/M Services

This publication provides definitions and documentation guidelines for the three *key* components of E/M services and for visits which consist predominately of counseling or coordination of care. The three key components — history, examination, and medical decision-making — appear in the descriptors for office and other outpatient services, hospital observation services, hospital inpatient services, consultations, emergency department services, nursing facility services, domiciliary care services and home services. While some of the text of CPT® has been repeated in this publication, the reader should refer to CPT® for the complete descriptors for E/M services and instructions for selecting a level of service.

Documentation Guidelines are identified by the symbol • *DG.*

The descriptors for the levels of E/M services recognize seven components which are used in defining the levels of E/M services. These components are:

- history;
- examination;
- medical decision-making;
- counseling;
- coordination of care;
- nature of presenting problem; and
- time.

The first three of these components (i.e., history, examination and medical decision-making) are the key components in selecting the level of E/M services. In the case of visits which consist predominantly of counseling or coordination of care, time is the key or controlling factor to qualify for a particular level of E/M service.

Because the level of E/M service is dependent on two or three *key* components, performance and documentation of one component (e.g., examination) at the highest level does not necessarily mean that the encounter in its entirety qualifies for the highest level of E/M service.

These documentation guidelines for E/M services reflect the needs of the typical adult population. For certain groups of patients, the recorded information may vary slightly from that described here. Specifically, the medical records of infants, children, adolescents and pregnant women may have additional or modified information recorded in each history and examination area.

As an example, newborn records may include under history of the present illness (HPI) the details of mother's pregnancy and the infant's status at birth; social history will focus on family structure; family history will focus on congenital anomalies and hereditary disorders in the family. In addition, the content of a pediatric examination will vary with the age and development of the child. Although not specifically defined in these documentation guidelines, these patient group variations on history and examination are appropriate.

A. Documentation of History

The levels of E/M services are based on four types of history (Problem Focused, Expanded Problem Focused, Detailed and Comprehensive). Each type of history includes some or all of the following elements:

- Chief complaint (CC);
- History of present illness (HPI);
- Review of systems (ROS); and
- Past, family and/or social history (PFSH).

The extent of history of present illness, review of systems and past, family and/or social history that is obtained and documented is dependent upon clinical judgment and the nature of the presenting problem(s).

The chart below shows the progression of the elements required for each type of history. To qualify for a given type of history all three elements in the table must be met. (A chief complaint is indicated at all levels.)

History of Present Illness (HPI)	Review of Systems (ROS)	Past, Family, and/or Social History (PFSH)	Type of History
Brief	N/A	N/A	Problem Focused
Brief	Problem Pertinent	Problem Pertinent	Expanded Problem Focused
Extended	Extended	Pertinent	Detailed
Extended	Complete	Complete	Comprehensive

• *DG: The CC, ROS and PFSH may be listed as separate elements of history, or they may be included in the description of the history of the present illness.*

• *DG: A ROS and/or a PFSH obtained during an earlier encounter does not need to be re-recorded if there is evidence that the physician reviewed and updated the previous information. This may occur when a physician updates his or her own record or in an institutional setting or group practice where many physicians use a common record. The review and update may be documented by:*

- *describing any new ROS and/or PFSH information or noting there has been no change in the information; and*
- *noting the date and location of the earlier ROS and/or PFSH.*

• *DG: The ROS and/or PFSH may be recorded by ancillary staff or on a form completed by the patient. To document that the physician reviewed the information, there must be a notation supplementing or confirming the information recorded by others.*

• *DG: If the physician is unable to obtain a history from the patient or other source, the record should describe the patient's condition or other circumstance which precludes obtaining a history.*

Definitions and specific documentation guidelines for each of the elements of history are listed below.

Chief Complaint (CC)

The CC is a concise statement describing the symptom, problem, condition, diagnosis, physician recommended return, or other factor that is the reason for the encounter, usually stated in the patient's words.

CPT © 2018 American Medical Association. All Rights Reserved.

• *DG: The medical record should clearly reflect the chief complaint.*

History of Present Illness (HPI)

The HPI is a chronological description of the development of the patient's present illness from the first sign and/or symptom or from the previous encounter to the present. It includes the following elements:

- location,
- quality,
- severity,
- duration,
- timing,
- context,
- modifying factors, and
- associated signs and symptoms.

Brief and ***extended*** HPIs are distinguished by the amount of detail needed to accurately characterize the clinical problem(s).

A brief HPI consists of one to three elements of the HPI.

• *DG: The medical record should describe one to three elements of the present illness (HPI).*

An ***extended*** HPI consists of at least four elements of the HPI or the status of at least three chronic or inactive conditions.

• *DG: The medical record should describe at least four elements of the present illness (HPI), or the status of at least three chronic or inactive conditions.*

Review of Systems (ROS)

A ROS is an inventory of body systems obtained through a series of questions seeking to identify signs and/or symptoms which the patient may be experiencing or has experienced.

For purposes of ROS, the following systems are recognized:

- Constitutional symptoms (e.g., fever, weight loss)
- Eyes
- Ears, Nose, Mouth, Throat
- Cardiovascular
- Respiratory
- Gastrointestinal
- Genitourinary
- Musculoskeletal
- Integumentary (skin and/or breast)
- Neurological
- Psychiatric
- Endocrine
- Hematologic/Lymphatic
- Allergic/Immunologic

A ***problem*** pertinent ROS inquires about the system directly related to the problem(s) identified in the HPI.

• *DG: The patient's positive responses and pertinent negatives for the system related to the problem should be documented.*

An ***extended*** ROS inquires about the system directly related to the problem(s) identified in the HPI and a

limited number of additional systems.

• *DG: The patient's positive responses and pertinent negatives for two to nine systems should be documented.*

A ***complete*** ROS inquires about the system(s) directly related to the problem(s) identified in the HPI plus all additional body systems.

• *DG: At least 10 organ systems must be reviewed. Those systems with positive or pertinent negative responses must be individually documented. For the remaining systems, a notation indicating all other systems are negative is permissible. In the absence of such a notation, at least 10 systems must be individually documented.*

Past, Family and/or Social History (PFSH)

The PFSH consists of a review of three areas: past history (the patient's past experiences with illnesses, operations, injuries and treatments); family history (a review of medical events in the patient's family, including diseases which may be hereditary or place the patient at risk); and social history (an age-appropriate review of past and current activities).

For certain categories of E/M services that include only an interval history, it is not necessary to record information about the PFSH. Those categories are subsequent hospital care, follow-up inpatient consultations and subsequent nursing facility care.

A ***pertinent*** PFSH is a review of the history area(s) directly related to the problem(s) identified in the HPI.

• *DG: At least one specific item from any of the three history areas must be documented for a pertinent PFSH.*

A ***complete*** PFSH is of a review of two or all three of the PFSH history areas, depending on the category of the E/M service. A review of all three history areas is required for services that by their nature include a comprehensive assessment or reassessment of the patient. A review of two of the three history areas is sufficient for other services.

• *DG: At least one specific item from two of the three history areas must be documented for a complete PFSH for the following categories of E/M services: office or other outpatient services, established patient; emergency department; domiciliary care, established patient; and home care, established patient.*

• *DG: At least one specific item from each of the three history areas must be documented for a complete PFSH for the following categories of E/M services: office or other outpatient services, new patient; hospital observation services; hospital inpatient services, initial care; consultations; comprehensive nursing facility assessments; domiciliary care, new patient; and home care, new patient.*

B. Documentation of Examination

The levels of E/M services are based on four types of examination:

- ***Problem Focused*** — a limited examination of the affected body area or organ system.
- ***Expanded Problem Focused*** — a limited examination of the affected body area or organ system and any other symptomatic or related body area(s) or organ system(s).

CPT © 2018 American Medical Association. All Rights Reserved.

- ***Detailed*** — an extended examination of the affected body area(s) or organ system(s) and any other symptomatic or related body area(s) or organ system(s).
- ***Comprehensive*** — a general multi-system examination, or complete examination of a single organ system and other symptomatic or related body area(s) or organ system(s).

These types of examinations have been defined for general multi-system and the following single organ systems:

- Cardiovascular
- Ears, Nose, Mouth and Throat
- Eyes
- Genitourinary (Female)
- Genitourinary (Male)
- Hematologic/Lymphatic/Immunologic
- Musculoskeletal
- Neurological
- Psychiatric
- Respiratory
- Skin

A general multi-system examination or a single organ system examination may be performed by any physician regardless of specialty. The type (general multi-system or single organ system) and content of examination are selected by the examining physician and are based upon clinical judgment, the patient's history, and the nature of the presenting problem(s).

The content and documentation requirements for each type and level of examination are summarized below and described in detail in tables. In the tables, organ systems and body areas recognized by CPT® for purposes of describing examinations are shown in the left column. The content, or individual elements, of the examination pertaining to that body area or organ system are identified by bullets (•) in the right column.

Parenthetical examples, "(e.g., …)," have been used for clarification and to provide guidance regarding documentation. Documentation for each element must satisfy any numeric requirements (such as "Measurement of any three of the following seven … ") included in the description of the element. Elements with multiple components but with no specific numeric requirement (such as "Examination of liver and spleen") require documentation of at least one component. It is possible for a given examination to be expanded beyond what is defined here. When that occurs, findings related to the additional systems and/or areas should be documented.

• *DG: Specific abnormal and relevant negative findings of the examination of the affected or symptomatic body area(s) or organ system(s) should be documented. A notation of "abnormal" without elaboration is insufficient.*

• *DG: Abnormal or unexpected findings of the examination of any asymptomatic body area(s) or organ system(s) should be described.*

• *DG: A brief statement or notation indicating "negative" or "normal" is sufficient to document normal findings related to unaffected area(s) or asymptomatic organ system(s).*

General Multi-System Examinations

General multi-system examinations are described in detail below. To qualify for a given level of multi-system examination, the following content and documentation requirements should be met:

- ***Problem Focused Examination*** — should include performance and documentation of one to five elements identified by a bullet (•) in one or more organ system(s) or body area(s).
- ***Expanded Problem Focused Examination*** — should include performance and documentation of at least six elements identified by a bullet (•) in one or more organ system(s) or body area(s).
- ***Detailed Examination*** — should include at least six organ systems or body areas. For each system/area selected, performance and documentation of at least two elements identified by a bullet (•) is expected. Alternatively, a detailed examination may include performance and documentation of at least 12 elements identified by a bullet (•) in two or more organ systems or body areas.
- ***Comprehensive Examination*** — should include at least nine organ systems or body areas. For each system/area selected, all elements of the examination identified by a bullet (•) should be performed, unless specific directions limit the content of the examination. For each area/system, documentation of at least two elements identified by a bullet is expected.

Single Organ System Examinations

The single organ system examinations recognized by CPT® are described in detail previously. Variations among these examinations in the organ systems and body areas identified in the left columns and in the elements of the examinations described in the right columns reflect differing emphases among specialties. To qualify for a given level of single organ system examination, the following content and documentation requirements should be met:

- ***Problem Focused Examination*** — should include performance and documentation of one to five elements identified by a bullet (•), whether in a box with a shaded or unshaded border.
- ***Expanded Problem Focused Examination*** — should include performance and documentation of at least six elements identified by a bullet (•), whether in a box with a shaded or unshaded border.
- ***Detailed Examination*** — examinations other than the eye and psychiatric examinations should include performance and documentation of at least 12 elements identified by a bullet (•), whether in box with a shaded or unshaded border.

CPT © 2018 American Medical Association. All Rights Reserved.

Eye and psychiatric examinations should include the performance and documentation of at least nine elements identified by a bullet (•), whether in a box with a shaded or unshaded border.

- *Comprehensive Examination* — should include performance of all elements identified by a bullet (•), whether in a shaded or unshaded box. Documentation of every element in each box with a shaded border and at least one element in each box with an unshaded border is expected.

General Multi-System Examination

System/Body Area	Elements of Examination
Constitutional	Measurement of **any three of the following seven** vital signs: 1) sitting or standing blood pressure, 2) supine blood pressure, 3) pulse rate and regularity, 4) respiration, 5) temperature, 6) height, 7) weight (May be measured and recorded by ancillary staff) General appearance of patient (e.g., development, nutrition, body habitus, deformities, attention to grooming)
Eyes	Inspection of conjunctivae and lids Examination of pupils and irises (e.g., reaction to light and accommodation, size and symmetry) Ophthalmoscopic examination of optic discs (e.g., size, C/D ratio, appearance) and posterior segments (e.g., vessel changes, exudates, hemorrhages)
Ears, Nose, Mouth, and Throat	External inspection of ears and nose (e.g., overall appearance, scars, lesions, masses) Otoscopic examination of external auditory canals and tympanic membranes Assessment of hearing (e.g., whispered voice, finger rub, tuning fork) Inspection of nasal mucosa, septum and turbinates Inspection of lips, teeth and gums Examination of oropharynx: oral mucosa, salivary glands, hard and soft palates, tongue, tonsils and posterior pharynx
Neck	Examination of neck (e.g., masses, overall appearance, symmetry, tracheal position, crepitus Examination of thyroid (e.g., enlargement, tenderness, mass)
Respiratory	Assessment of respiratory effort (e.g., intercostal retractions, use of accessory muscles, diaphragmatic movement) Percussion of chest (e.g., dullness, flatness, hyperresonance) Palpation of chest (e.g., tactile fremitus) Auscultation of lungs (e.g., breath sounds, adventitious sounds, rubs)
Cardiovascular	Palpation of heart (e.g., location, size, thrills) Auscultation of heart with notation of abnormal sounds and murmurs Examination of: Carotid arteries (e.g., pulse amplitude, bruits) Abdominal aorta (e.g., size, bruits) Femoral arteries (e.g., pulse amplitude, bruits) Pedal pulses (e.g., pulse amplitude) Extremities for edema and/or varicosities
Chest (Breasts)	Inspection of breasts (e.g., symmetry, nipple discharge) Palpation of breasts and axillae (e.g., masses or lumps, tenderness)
Gastrointestinal (Abdomen)	Examination of abdomen with notation of presence of masses or tenderness Examination of liver and spleen Examination for presence or absence of hernia Examination (when indicated) of anus, perineum and rectum, including sphincter tone, presence of hemorrhoids, rectal masses Obtain stool sample for occult blood test when indicated
Genitourinary	Male: Examination of the scrotal contents (e.g., hydrocele, spermatocele, tenderness of cord, testicular mass) Examination of the penis Digital rectal examination of prostate gland (e.g., size, symmetry, nodularity, tenderness) Female: Pelvic examination (with or without specimen collection for smears and cultures), including: Examination of external genitalia (e.g., general appearance, hair distribution, lesions) and vagina (e.g., general appearance, estrogen effect, discharge, lesions, pelvic support, cystocele, rectocele) Examination of urethra (e.g., masses, tenderness, scarring) Examination of bladder (e.g., fullness, masses, tenderness) Cervix (e.g., general appearance, lesions, discharge) Uterus (e.g., size, contour, position, mobility, tenderness, consistency, descent or support) Adnexa/parametria (e.g., masses, tenderness, organomegaly, nodularity)
Lymphatic	Palpation of lymph nodes in **two or more** areas: Neck Axillae Groin Other

CPT © 2018 American Medical Association. All Rights Reserved.

System/Body Area	Elements of Examination
Musculoskeletal	Examination of gait and station Inspection and/or palpation of digits and nails (e.g., clubbing, cyanosis, inflammatory conditions, petechiae, ischemia, infections, nodes) Examination of joints, bones and muscles of **one or more of the following six** areas: 1) head and neck; 2) spine, ribs and pelvis; 3) right upper extremity; 4) left upper extremity; 5) right lower extremity; and 6) left lower extremity. The examination of a given area includes: Inspection and/or palpation with notation of presence of any misalignment, asymmetry, crepitation, defects, tenderness, masses, effusions Assessment of range of motion with notation of any pain, crepitation or contracture Assessment of stability with notation of any dislocation (luxation), subluxation or laxity Assessment of muscle strength and tone (e.g., flaccid, cog wheel, spastic) with notation of any atrophy or abnormal movements
Skin	Inspection of skin and subcutaneous tissue (e.g., rashes, lesions, ulcers) Palpation of skin and subcutaneous tissue (e.g., induration, subcutaneous nodules, tightening)
Neurologic	Test cranial nerves with notation of any deficits Examination of deep tendon reflexes with notation of pathological reflexes (e.g., Babinski) Examination of sensation (e.g., by touch, pin, vibration, proprioception)
Psychiatric	Description of patient's judgment and insight Brief assessment of mental status including: Orientation to time, place and person Recent and remote memory Mood and affect (e.g., depression, anxiety, agitation)

General Multi-System Examination Content and Documentation Requirements

Level of Exam	Perform and Document
Problem Focused	**One to five** elements identified by a bullet
Expanded Problem Focused	**At least six** elements identified by a bullet
Detailed	**At least two** elements identified by a bullet **from each of six areas/systems** OR **at least 12** elements identified by a bullet **in two or more areas/systems.**
Comprehensive	Perform **all elements** identified by a bullet in **at least nine** organ systems or body areas and document **at least two** elements identified by a bullet **from each of nine areas/systems.**

Cardiovascular Examination

System/Body Area	Elements of Examination
Constitutional	Measurement of **any three of the following seven** vital signs: 1) sitting or standing blood pressure, 2) supine blood pressure, 3) pulse rate and regularity, 4) respiration, 5) temperature, 6) height, 7) weight (May be measured and recorded by ancillary staff) General appearance of patient (e.g., development, nutrition, body habitus, deformities, attention to grooming)
Eyes	Inspection of conjunctivae and lids (e.g., xanthelasma)
Ears, Nose, Mouth, and Throat	Inspection of teeth, gums and palate Inspection of oral mucosa with notation of presence of pallor or cyanosis
Neck	Examination of jugular veins (e.g., distension; a, v or cannon a waves) Examination of thyroid (e.g., enlargement, tenderness, mass)
Respiratory	Assessment of respiratory effort (e.g., intercostal retractions, use of accessory muscles, diaphragmatic movement) Auscultation of lungs (e.g., breath sounds, adventitious sounds, rubs)
Cardiovascular	Palpation of heart (e.g., location, size and forcefulness of the point of maximal impact; thrills; lifts; palpable S3 or S4) Auscultation of heart including sounds, abnormal sounds and murmurs Measurement of blood pressure in two or more extremities when indicated (e.g., aortic dissection, coarctation) Examination of: Carotid arteries (e.g., waveform, pulse amplitude, bruits, apical-carotid delay) Abdominal aorta (e.g., size, bruits) Femoral arteries (e.g., pulse amplitude, bruits) Pedal pulses (e.g., pulse amplitude) Extremities for peripheral edema and/or varicosities
Gastrointestinal (Abdomen)	Examination of abdomen with notation of presence of masses or tenderness Examination of liver and spleen Obtain stool sample for occult blood from patients who are being considered for thrombolytic or anticoagulant therapy
Musculoskeletal	Examination of the back with notation of kyphosis or scoliosis Examination of gait with notation of ability to undergo exercise testing and/or participation in exercise programs Assessment of muscle strength and tone (e.g., flaccid, cog wheel, spastic) with notation of any atrophy and abnormal movements
Extremities	Inspection and palpation of digits and nails (e.g., clubbing, cyanosis, inflammation, petechiae, ischemia, infections, Osler's nodes)

CPT © 2018 American Medical Association. All Rights Reserved.

System/Body Area	Elements of Examination
Skin	Inspection and/or palpation of skin and subcutaneous tissue (e.g., stasis dermatitis, ulcers, scars, xanthomas)
Neurological/ Psychiatric	Brief assessment of mental status including: Orientation to time, place and person, Mood and affect (e.g., depression, anxiety, agitation)

Cardiovascular Examination Content and Documentation Requirements

Level of Exam	Perform and Document
Problem Focused	**One to five** elements identified by a bullet
Expanded Problem Focused	**At least six** elements identified by a bullet
Detailed	**At least 12** elements identified by a bullet
Comprehensive	Perform all elements identified by a bullet; document every element in each box with a shaded border and at least one element in each box with an unshaded border.

C. Documentation of the Complexity of Medical Decision-Making

The levels of E/M services recognize four types of medical decision-making (Straightforward, Low Complexity, Moderate Complexity and High Complexity). Medical decision-making refers to the complexity of establishing a diagnosis and/or selecting a management option as measured by:

- the number of possible diagnoses and/or the number of management options that must be considered;
- the amount and/or complexity of medical records, diagnostic tests, and/or other information that must be obtained, reviewed and analyzed; and
- the risk of significant complications, morbidity and/or mortality, as well as comorbidities associated with the patient's presenting problem(s), the diagnostic procedure(s) and/or the possible management options.

The chart below shows the progression of the elements required for each level of medical decision-making. To qualify for a given type of decision-making, two of the three elements in the table must be either met or exceeded.

Number of diagnoses or management options	Amount and/or complexity of data	Risk of complications and/or morbidity or mortality	Type of decision-making
Minimal	Minimal or None	Minimal	**Straightforward**
Limited	Limited	Low	**Low Complexity**
Multiple	Moderate	Moderate	**Moderate Complexity**
Extensive	Extensive	High	**High Complexity**

The following is a description of elements of medical decision-making.

Number of Diagnoses of Management Options

The number of possible diagnoses and/or the number of management options that must be considered is based on the number and types of problems addressed during the encounter, the complexity of establishing a diagnosis and the management decisions that are made by the physician.

Generally, decision-making with respect to a diagnosed problem is easier than that for an identified but undiagnosed problem. The number and type of diagnostic tests employed may be an indicator of the number of possible diagnoses. Problems which are improving or resolving are less complex than those which are worsening or failing to change as expected. The need to seek advice from others is another indicator of complexity of diagnostic or management problems.

- *DG: For each encounter, an assessment, clinical impression, or diagnosis should be documented. It may be explicitly stated or implied in documented decisions regarding management plans and/or further evaluation.*
  - For a presenting problem with an established diagnosis the record should reflect whether the problem is: a) improved, well controlled, resolving or resolved; or, b) inadequately controlled, worsening, or failing to change as expected.
  - For a presenting problem without an established diagnosis, the assessment or clinical impression may be stated in the form of differential diagnoses or as a "possible," "probable," or "rule out" (R/O) diagnosis.
- *DG: The initiation of, or changes in, treatment should be documented. Treatment includes a wide range of management options including patient instructions, nursing instructions, therapies, and medications.*
- *DG: If referrals are made, consultations requested or advice sought, the record should indicate to whom or where the referral or consultation is made or from whom the advice is requested.*

Amount and/or Complexity of Data to be Reviewed

The amount and complexity of data to be reviewed is based on the types of diagnostic testing ordered or reviewed. A decision to obtain and review old medical records and/or obtain history from sources other than the patient increases the amount and complexity of data to be reviewed.

Discussion of contradictory or unexpected test results with the physician who performed or interpreted the test is an indication of the complexity of data being reviewed. On occasion the physician who ordered a test may personally review the image, tracing or specimen to supplement information from the physician who prepared the test report or interpretation; this is another indication of the complexity of data being reviewed.

- *DG: If a diagnostic service (test or procedure) is ordered, planned, scheduled, or performed at the time of the E/M encounter, the type of service, e.g., lab or X-ray, should be documented.*
- *DG: The review of lab, radiology and/or other diagnostic tests should be documented. A simple notation such as "WB elevated" or "chest X-ray unremarkable" is acceptable. Alternatively, the review may be documented by initialing and dating the report containing the test results.*

CPT © 2018 American Medical Association. All Rights Reserved.

• *DG: A decision to obtain old records or decision to obtain additional history from the family, caretaker or other source to supplement that obtained from the patient should be documented.*

• *DG: Relevant findings from the review of old records, and/or the receipt of additional history from the family, caretaker or other source to supplement that obtained from the patient should be documented. If there is no relevant information beyond that already obtained, that fact should be documented. A notation of "old records reviewed" or "additional history obtained from family" without elaboration is insufficient.*

• *DG: The results of discussion of laboratory, radiology or other diagnostic tests with the physician who performed or interpreted the study should be documented.*

• *DG: The direct visualization and independent interpretation of an image, tracing or specimen previously or subsequently interpreted by another physician should be documented.*

Risk of Significant Complications, Morbidity and/or Mortality

The risk of significant complications, morbidity and/or mortality is based on the risks associated with the presenting problem(s), the diagnostic procedure(s) and the possible management options.

• *DG: Comorbidities/underlying diseases or other factors that increase the complexity of medical decision-making by increasing the risk of complications, morbidity, and/or mortality should be documented.*

• *DG: If a surgical or invasive diagnostic procedure is ordered, planned or scheduled at the time of the E/M encounter, the type of procedure, e.g., laparoscopy, should be documented.*

• *DG: If a surgical or invasive diagnostic procedure is performed at the time of the E/M encounter, the specific procedure should be documented.*

• *DG: The referral for or decision to perform a surgical or invasive diagnostic procedure on an urgent basis should be documented or implied.*

The following table may be used to help determine whether the risk of significant complications, morbidity and/or mortality is minimal, low, moderate or high. Because the determination of risk is complex and not readily quantifiable, the table includes common clinical examples rather than absolute measures of risk. The assessment of risk of the presenting problem(s) is based on the risk related to the disease process anticipated between the present encounter and the next one. The assessment of risk of selecting diagnostic procedures and management options is based on the risk during and immediately following any procedures or treatment. **The highest level of risk in any one category (presenting problem(s), diagnostic procedure(s) or management options) determines the overall risk.**

D. Documentation of an Encounter Dominated by Counseling or Coordination of Care

In the case where counseling and/or coordination of care dominates (more than 50%) of the physician/patient and/or family encounter (face-to-face time in the office or other or outpatient setting, floor/unit time in the hospital or nursing facility), time is considered the key or controlling factor to qualify for a particular level of E/M services.

• *DG: If the physician elects to report the level of service based on counseling and/or coordination of care, the total length of time of the encounter (face-to-face or floor time, as appropriate) should be documented and the record should describe the counseling and/or activities to coordinate care.*

CPT © 2018 American Medical Association. All Rights Reserved.

Table of Risk

Level of Risk	Presenting Problem(s)	Diagnostic Procedure(s) Ordered	Management Options Selected
Minimal	One self-limited or minor problem, e.g., cold, insect bite, tinea corporis	Laboratory tests requiring venipuncture Chest X-rays EKG/EEG Urinalysis Ultrasound, e.g., echocardiography KOH prep	Rest Gargles Elastic bandages Superficial dressings
Low	Two or more self-limited or minor problems One stable chronic illness, e.g., well controlled hypertension, non-insulin dependent diabetes, cataract, BPH Acute uncomplicated illness or injury, e.g., cystitis, allergic rhinitis, simple sprain	Physiologic tests not under stress, e.g., pulmonary function test Non-cardiovascular imaging studies with contrast, e.g., barium enema Superficial needle biopsies Clinical laboratory tests requiring arterial puncture Skin biopsies	Over-the-counter drugs Minor surgery with no identified risk factors Physical therapy Occupational therapy IV fluids without additives
Moderate	One or more chronic illnesses with mild exacerbation, progression, or side effects of treatment Two or more stable chronic illnesses Undiagnosed new problem with uncertain prognosis, e.g., lump in breast Acute illness with systemic symptoms, e.g., pyelonephritis, pneumonitis, colitis Acute complicated injury, e.g., head injury with brief loss of consciousness	Physiologic tests under stress, e.g., cardio stress test, fetal contraction stress test Diagnostic endoscopies with no identified risk factors Deep needle or incisional biopsy Cardiovascular imaging studies with contrast and no identified risk factors, e.g., arteriogram, cardiac catheterization Obtain fluid from body cavity, e.g. lumbar puncture, thoracentesis, culdocentesis	Minor surgery with identified risk factors Elective major surgery (open, percutaneous or endoscopic) with no identified risk factors Prescription drug management Therapeutic nuclear medicine IV fluids with additives Closed treatment of fracture or dislocation without manipulation
High	One or more chronic illnesses with severe exacerbation, progression, or side effects of treatment Acute or chronic illnesses or injuries that pose a threat to life or bodily function, e.g., multiple trauma, acute MI, pulmonary embolus, severe respiratory distress, progressive severe rheumatoid arthritis, psychiatric illness with potential threat to self or others, peritonitis, acute renal failure An abrupt change in neurologic status, e.g., seizure, TIA, weakness, sensory loss	Cardiovascular imaging studies with contrast with identified risk factors Cardiac electrophysiological tests Diagnostic endoscopies with identified risk factors Discography	Elective major surgery (open, percutaneous or endoscopic) with identified risk factors Emergency major surgery (open, percutaneous or endoscopic) Parenteral controlled substances Drug therapy requiring intensive monitoring for toxicity Decision not to resuscitate or to deescalate care because of poor prognosis

CPT © 2018 American Medical Association. All Rights Reserved.